Dietary Reference Intakes (DRIs): Recommended Dietary Allowances and Adequate Intakes, Elements

Food and Nutrition Board, Institute of Medicine, National Academies

Life Stage Group	Calcium (mg/d)	Chromium (mcg/d)	Copper (mcg/d)	Fluoride (mg/d)	Iodine (mcg/d)	Iron (mg/d)	Magnesium (mg/d)	Manganese (mg/d)	Molybdenum (mcg/d)	Phosphorus (mg/d)	Selenium (mcg/d)	Zinc (mg/d)	Potassium (g/d)	Sodium (g/d)	Chloride (g/d)
Infants															
Birth to 6 mo	200*	0.2*	200*	0.01*	110*	0.27*	30*	0.003*	2*	100*	15*	2*	0.4*	0.12*	0.18*
6 to 12 mo	260*	5.5*	220*	0.5*	130*	11	75*	0.6*	3*	275*	20*	3	0.7*	0.37*	0.57*
Children															
1-3 yr	700	11*	340	0.7*	90	7	80	1.2*	17	460	20	3	3.0*	1.0*	1.5*
4-8 yr	1000	15*	440	1*	90	10	130	1.5*	22	500	30	5	3.8*	1.2*	1.9*
Males															
9-13 yr	1300	25*	700	2*	120	8	240	1.9*	34	1250	40	8	4.5*	1.5*	2.3*
14-18 yr	1300	35*	890	3*	150	11	410	2.2*	43	1250	55	11	4.7*	1.5*	2.3*
19-30 yr	1000	35*	900	4*	150	8	400	2.3*	45	700	55	11	4.7*	1.5*	2.3*
31-50 yr	1000	35*	900	4*	150	8	420	2.3*	45	700	55	11	4.7*	1.5*	2.3*
51-70 yr	1000	30*	900	4*	150	8	420	2.3*	45	700	55	11	4.7*	1.3*	2.0*
>70 yr	1200	30*	900	4*	150	8	420	2.3*	45	700	55	11	4.7*	1.2*	1.8*
Females															
9-13 yr	1300	21*	700	2*	120	8	240	1.6*	34	1250	40	8	4.5*	1.5*	2.3*
14-18 yr	1300	24*	890	3*	150	15	360	1.6*	43	1250	55	9	4.7*	1.5*	2.3*
19-30 yr	1000	25*	900	3*	150	18	310	1.8*	45	700	55	8	4.7*	1.5*	2.3*
31-50 yr	1000	25*	900	3*	150	18	320	1.8*	45	700	55	8	4.7*	1.5*	2.3*
51-70 yr	1200	20*	900	3*	150	8	320	1.8*	45	700	55	8	4.7*	1.3*	2.0*
>70 yr	1200	20*	900	3*	150	8	320	1.8*	45	700	55	8	4.7*	1.2*	1.8*
Pregnancy															
14-18 yr	1300	29*	1000	3*	220	27	400	2.0*	50	1250	60	12	4.7*	1.5*	2.3*
19-30 yr	1000	30*	1000	3*	220	27	350	2.0*	50	700	60	11	4.7*	1.5*	2.3*
31-50 yr	1000	30*	1000	3*	220	27	360	2.0*	50	700	60	11	4.7*	1.5*	2.3*
Lactation															
14-18 yr	1300	44*	1300	3*	290	10	360	2.6*	50	1250	70	13	5.1*	1.5*	2.3*
19-30 yr	1000	45*	1300	3*	290	9	310	2.6*	50	700	70	12	5.1*	1.5*	2.3*
31-50 yr	1000	45*	1300	3*	290	9	320	2.6*	50	700	70	12	5.1*	1.5*	2.3*

Sources: Dietary Reference Intakes for Calcium, Phosphorus, Magnesium, Vitamin D, and Fluoride (1997); Dietary Reference Intakes for Thiamin, Riboflavin, Niacin, Vitamin B_6, Folate, Vitamin B_{12}, Pantothenic Acid, Biotin, and Choline (1998); Dietary Reference Intakes for Vitamin C, Vitamin E, Selenium, and Carotenoids (2000); and Dietary Reference Intakes for Vitamin A, Vitamin K, Arsenic, Boron, Chromium, Copper, Iodine, Iron, Manganese, Molybdenum, Nickel, Silicon, Vanadium, and Zinc (2001); Dietary Reference Intakes for Water, Potassium, Sodium, Chloride, and Sulfate (2005); and Dietary Reference Intakes for Calcium and Vitamin D (2011). These reports may be accessed via www.nap.edu.

Dietary Reference Intakes of Energy and Protein from Birth to 18 Years of Age Per Day*

	Age	Estimated Energy Requirement	Protein (g)
Infants	0 to 3 months	(89 ×Weight [kg] − 100) + 175 kcal	9.1
	4 to 6 months	(89 × Weight [kg] − 100) + 56 kcal	9.1
	7 to 12 months	(89 × Weight [kg] − 100) + 22 kcal	11
	13 to 36 months	(89 × Weight [kg] − 100) + 20 kcal	13
Boys	3 to 8 years	88.5 − (61.9 × Age [yr] + PA × (26.7 × Weight [kg] + 903 × Height [m]) + 20 kcal	19
	9 to 18 years	88.5 − (61.9 × Age [yr]) + PA × (26.7 × Weight [kg] + 903 × Height [m]) + 25 kcal	34 to 52
Girls	3 to 8 years	135.3 − (30.8 × Age [yr] + PA× (10.0 × Weight [kg] + 934 × Height [m]) + 20 kcal	19
	9 to 18 years	135.3 − (30.8 × Age [yr] + PA × (10.0 × Weight [kg] + 934 × Height [m]) + 25 kcal	34 to 46

*PA, Physical activity level. Data from the Food and Nutrition Board, Institute of Medicine. *Dietary reference intakes for energy, carbohydrate, fiber, fat, fatty acids, cholesterol, protein, and amino acids (macronutrients).* Washington, DC: National Academies Press; 2002.

Dietary Reference Intakes (DRIs): Recommended Dietary Allowances and Adequate Intakes, Total Water and Macronutrients*

Food and Nutrition Board, Institute of Medicine, National Academies

Life Stage Group	Total Water[a] (L/d)	Total Fiber (g/d)	Linoleic Acid (g/d)	α-Linolenic Acid (g/d)	Protein[b] (g/d)
Infants					
Birth to 6 mo	0.7*	ND	4.4*	0.5*	9.1*
6 to 12 mo	0.8*	ND	4.6*	0.5*	11.0
Children					
1-3 yr	1.3*	19*	7*	0.7*	13
4-8 yr	1.7*	25*	10*	0.9*	19
Males					
9-13 yr	2.4*	31*	12*	1.2*	34
14-18 yr	3.3*	38*	16*	1.6*	52
19-30 yr	3.7*	38*	17*	1.6*	56
31-50 yr	3.7*	38*	17*	1.6*	56
51-70 yr	3.7*	30*	14*	1.6*	56
>70 yr	3.7*	30*	14*	1.6*	56
Females					
9-13 yr	2.1*	26*	10*	1.0*	34
14-18 yr	2.3*	26*	11*	1.1*	46
19-30 yr	2.7*	25*	12*	1.1*	46
31-50 yr	2.7*	25*	12*	1.1*	46
51-70 yr	2.7*	21*	11*	1.1*	46
>70 yr	2.7*	21*	11*	1.1*	46
Pregnancy					
14-18 yr	3.0*	28*	13*	1.4*	71
19-30 yr	3.0*	28*	13*	1.4*	71
31-50 yr	3.0*	28*	13*	1.4*	71
Lactation					
14-18 yr	3.8*	29*	13*	1.3*	71
19-30 yr	3.8*	29*	13*	1.3*	71
31-50 yr	3.8*	29*	13*	1.3*	71

Source: *Dietary Reference Intakes for Energy, Carbohydrate, Fiber, Fat, Fatty Acids, Cholesterol, Protein, and Amino Acids* (2002/2005) and *Dietary Reference Intakes for Water, Potassium, Sodium, Chloride, and Sulfate* (2005). The report may be accessed via www.n

***NOTE:** This table (taken from the DRI reports, see www.nap.edu) presents Recommended Dietary Allowances (RDA) in **boldface type** and Adequate Intakes (AIs) in ordinary type followed by an asterisk (*). An RDA is the average daily dietary intake level; sufficient to meet the nutrient requirements of nearly all (97-98%) healthy individuals in a group. It is calculated from an Estimated Average Requirement (EAR)

If sufficient scientific evidence is not available to establish an EAR, and thus calculate an RDA, an AI is usually developed. For healthy breastfed infants, an AI is the mean intake. The AI for other life stage and gender groups is believed to cover the needs of all healthy individuals in the groups, but lack of data or uncertainty in the data prevent being able to specify with confidence the percentage of individuals covered by this intake.

[a]Total water includes all water contained in food, beverages, and drinking water.

[b]Based on grams of protein per kilogram of body weight for the reference body weight (e.g., for adults 0.8 g/kg body weight for the reference body weight).

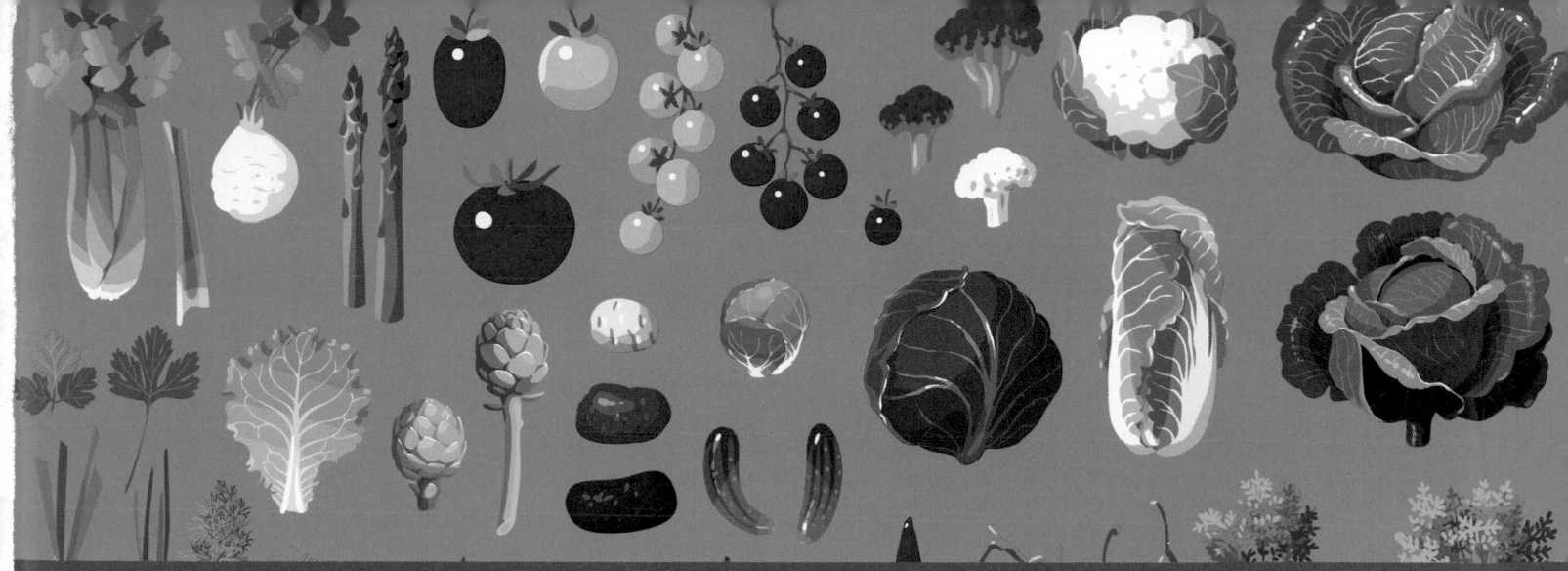

KRAUSE'S

14TH EDITION

FOOD & THE NUTRITION CARE PROCESS

L. KATHLEEN MAHAN, MS, RDN, CD

Functional Nutrition Counselor
Nutrition by Design
Seattle, WA;
Clinical Associate
Department of Pediatrics
School of Medicine
University of Washington
Seattle, WA

JANICE L. RAYMOND, MS, RDN, CD, CSG

Clinical Nutrition Director, Thomas Cuisine Management
Providence Mount St. Vincent
Seattle, WA;
Affiliate Faculty
Bastyr University
Kenmore, WA

ELSEVIER

ELSEVIER

3251 Riverport Lane
St. Louis, Missouri 63043

KRAUSE'S FOOD & THE NUTRITION CARE PROCESS,
FOURTEENTH EDITION

978-0-323-34075-5

Notices

Knowledge and best practice in this field are constantly changing. As new research and experience broaden our understanding, changes in research methods, professional practices, or medical treatment may become necessary.

Practitioners and researchers must always rely on their own experience and knowledge in evaluating and using any information, methods, compounds, or experiments described herein. In using such information or methods they should be mindful of their own safety and the safety of others, including parties for whom they have a professional responsibility.

With respect to any drug or pharmaceutical products identified, readers are advised to check the most current information provided (i) on procedures featured or (ii) by the manufacturer of each product to be administered, to verify the recommended dose or formula, the method and duration of administration, and contraindications. It is the responsibility of practitioners, relying on their own experience and knowledge of their patients, to make diagnoses, to determine dosages and the best treatment for each individual patient, and to take all appropriate safety precautions.

To the fullest extent of the law, neither the Publisher nor the authors, contributors, or editors, assume any liability for any injury and/or damage to persons or property as a matter of products liability, negligence or otherwise, or from any use or operation of any methods, products, instructions, or ideas contained in the material herein.

Previous editions copyrighted 2012, 2008, 2004, 2000, 1996, 1992, 1984, 1979, 1972, 1966, 1961, 1957, 1952.

Library of Congress Cataloging-in-Publication Data

Names: Mahan, L. Kathleen., editor. | Raymond, Janice L., editor.
Title: Krause's food & the nutrition care process / [edited by] L. Kathleen
  Mahan, Janice L. Raymond.
Other titles: Food and the nutrition care process | Krause's food and the
  nutrition care process
Description: Fourteenth edition. | St. Louis, Missouri : Elsevier, [2017] |
  Includes bibliographical references and index.
Identifiers: LCCN 2016004666 | ISBN 9780323340755 (hardcover)
Subjects: | MESH: Diet Therapy | Food | Nutritional Physiological Phenomena
Classification: LCC RM216 | NLM WB 400 | DDC 615.8/54—dc23 LC record available at http://lccn.loc.gov/
2016004666

Director, Traditional Education: Kristin Geen
Content Development Manager: Jean S. Fornango
Content Development Specialist: Danielle M. Frazier
Publishing Services Manager: Jeff Patterson
Project Manager: Lisa A. P. Bushey
Senior Book Designer: Amy Buxton

Printed in Canada

Last digit is the print number: 9   8   7   6   5   4   3   2   1

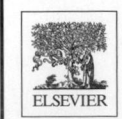 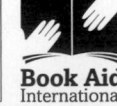

*This 14th edition is dedicated to the students, professors and practitioners
who use this text and consider it their "nutrition bible."
We are most grateful to them for their learning, writing, and insights
and dedication to the field of nutrition and dietetic practice.*

—The Authors, 14th Edition

and
*To Robert who is always there for me with love and a humorous perspective,
to Carly and Justin for their loving energy, to Ana who has known the "book"
her whole life, and to Ailey and Kiera, my grandchildren who bring such joy.*

—Kathleen

*To my parents who are both now deceased. My father, George Raymond, DDS,
sparked my interest in nutrition through his interest in it. And my mother
Betty Raymond, a woman who could whip up delicious foods in minutes and
who was making her own yogurt and sprouting beans when I was a teenager.
Thank you for the inspiration.*

—Janice

CONTRIBUTORS

Diane M. Anderson, PhD, RDN, FADA
Associate Professor of Pediatrics
Baylor College of Medicine
Houston, Texas

Cynthia Taft Bayerl, MS, RDN, LDN, FAND
Nutrition Coordinator
Nutrition Consultant
Taft & Bayerl Associates
Cape Cod, Massachusetts

Geri Brewster, MPH, RDN, CDN
Registered Dietitian—Clinical Nutritionist
Private Practice
Mount Kisco, New York

Virginia H. Carney, MPH, RDN, LDN, IBCLC, RLC, FILCA, FAND
Director, Clinical Nutrition Services
St. Jude Children's Research Hospital
Memphis, Tennessee

Digna I. Cassens, MHA, RDN, CLT
Diversified Nutrition Management Systems
Yucca Valley, California

Karen Chapman-Novakofski, PhD, RDN, LDN
Professor, Nutrition
Department of Food Science and Human Nutrition
Division of Nutritional Sciences
Department of Internal Medicine
University of Illinois Extension
University of Illinois
Champaign-Urbana, Illinois

Pamela Charney, PhD, RD, CHTS-CP
Program Chair
Healthcare Informatics
Bellevue College
Bellevue, Washington

Harriett Cloud, MS, RDN, FAND
Pediatric Nutrition Consultant
Owner, Nutrition Matters
Birmingham, Alabama

Mandy L. Corrigan, MPH, RD, CNSC, FAND
Nutrition Support Dietitian and Consultant
Coram Specialty Pharmacy
St. Louis, Missouri

Sarah C. Couch, PhD, RDN
Professor and Department Chair
Department of Nutritional Sciences
University of Cincinnati Medical Center
Cincinnati, Ohio

Jean T. Cox, MS, RD, LN
Senior Clinical Nutritionist
Department of Obstetrics and Gynecology
University of New Mexico School of Medicine
Albuquerque, New Mexico

Gail Cresci, PhD, RDN, LD, CNSC
Associate Professor
Cleveland Clinic Lerner College of Medicine
Case Western Reserve University School of Medicine
Cleveland, Ohio

Patricia Davidson, DCN, RDN, CDE, LDN, FAND
Assistant Professor
Nutrition Department, College of Health Sciences
West Chester University of Pennsylvania
West Chester, Pennsylvania

Lisa L. Deal, PharmD, BCPS, BSN, RN
Pharmacotherapy Specialist
Beebe Healthcare
Lewes, Delaware

Sheila Dean, DSc, RDN, LD, CCN, CDE
USF Health Morsani College of Medicine
The University of Tampa
Tampa, Florida
Co-Founder, Integrative and Functional Nutrition Academy (IFNA)

Ruth DeBusk, PhD, RDN
Consultant, Clinical Nutrition and Genomics
Family Medicine Residency Program
Tallahassee Memorial Health Care
Tallahassee, Florida

Judith L. Dodd, MS, RDN, LDN, FAND
Community Nutrition Consultant
Assistant Professor
Sports Medicine and Nutrition
Nutrition and Dietetics
University of Pittsburgh
Pittsburgh, Pennsylvania

Kimberly R. Dong, MS, RDN
Project Manager/Research Dietitian
Nutrition and Infection Unit
Department of Public Health and Community Medicine
Tufts University School of Medicine
Boston, Massachusetts

Lisa Dorfman, MS, RDN, CSSD, LMHC, FAND
The Running Nutritionist
CEO/Director Sports Nutrition & Performance
Food Fitness International, Inc
Author – *Legally Lean*
Chair, Miami Culinary Institute Advisory Board
Miami, Florida

Arlene Escuro, MS, RDN, CNSC
Advanced Practice Dietitian
Center for Human Nutrition
Digestive Disease Institute
Cleveland Clinic
Cleveland, Ohio

Alison B. Evert, MS, RDN, CDE
Diabetes Nutrition Specialist
Coordinator Diabetes Education Programs
Endocrine and Diabetes Care Center
University of Washington Medical Center
Seattle, Washington

Sharon A. Feucht, MA, RDN, CD
Nutritionist, LEND Program
Center on Human Development and Disability (CHDD)
Editor, Nutrition Focus Newsletter for Children with Special Health Care Needs
University of Washington
Seattle, Washington

Marion J. Franz, MS, RDN, CDE
Nutrition/Health Consultant
Nutrition Concepts by Franz, Inc
Minneapolis, Minnesota

F. Enrique Gómez, PhD
Head, Laboratory of Nutritional Immunology
Department of Nutritional Physiology
Instituto Nacional de Ciencias Médicas y Nutrición Salvador Zubirán
Ciudad de México, DF México

Barbara L. Grant, MS, RDN, CSO, LD, FAND
Oncology Outpatient Dietitian Nutritionist
Saint Alphonsus Cancer Care Center
Boise, Idaho

Michael Hahn, BA
Scientific Program Analyst
Preferred Solutions Group
National Human Genome Research Institute
National Institutes of Health
Bethesda, Maryland

Kathryn K. Hamilton, MA, RDN, CSO, CDN, FAND
Outpatient Oncology Dietitian Nutritionist
Carol G. Simon Cancer Center
Morristown Medical Center
Morristown, New Jersey

Kathleen A. Hammond, MS, RN, BSN, BSHE, RDN, LD
Consultant, Healthcare Education
Atlanta, Georgia

Jeanette M. Hasse, PhD, RDN, LD, CNSC, FADA
Transplant Nutrition Manager
Annette C. and Harold C. Simmons Transplant Institute
Baylor University Medical Center
Dallas, Texas

Cindy Mari Imai, PhD, MS, RDN
Research Scientist
Unit for Nutrition Research
University of Iceland
Reykjavik, Iceland

Carol S. Ireton-Jones, PhD, RDN, LD, CNSC, FAND, FASPEN
Nutrition Therapy Specialist
Private Practice/Consultant
Good Nutrition for Good Living
Dallas, Texas

Donna A. Israel, PhD, RDN, LPC, FADA, FAND
President, Professional Nutrition Therapists, LLC
Dallas, Texas
Retired, Interim Professor of Nutrition
Baylor University
Waco, Texas

Janice M. Joneja, PhD, RD
Food Allergy Consultant
President, Vickerstaff Health Services, Inc.
British Columbia, Canada

Veena Juneja, MScRD, RDN
Senior Renal Dietitian
St. Joseph's Healthcare
Hamilton, Ontario, Canada

Barbara J. Kamp, MS, RDN
Assistant Professor
College of Culinary Arts
Johnson & Wales University
North Miami, Florida

Ashok M. Karnik, MD, FACP, FCCP, FRCP
Retired Attending Physician
World Trade Center Health Program
Long Island, New York;
Clinical Professor of Medicine
Retired Chief, Division of Pulmonary and Critical Care Medicine
Nassau University Medical Center
East Meadow, New York, and
School of Medicine
Stony Brook University
Stony Brook, New York

Martha Kaufer-Horwitz, DSc, NC
Medical Research Scientist
Obesity and Eating Disorders Clinic
Department of Endocrinology and Metabolism
Instituto Nacional de Ciencias Médicas y Nutrición Salvador Zubirán (Mexican National Institute of Medical Sciences and Nutrition)
Ciudad de México, DF México

Sameera H. Khan, RDN, PA-C, MBA
Bariatric Coordinator
North Shore University Hospital
North Well Health System
Manhasset, New York
Nutrition Adjunct Professor
Nassau Community College
Garden City, New York

Nicole Larson, PhD, MPH, RDN
Senior Research Associate
Division of Epidemiology and Community Health
School of Public Health
University of Minnesota
Minneapolis, Minnesota

Tashara Leak, PhD, RDN
Post Doctoral Scholar
School of Public Health
University of California, Berkeley
Berkeley, California

Ruth Leyse-Wallace, PhD
Retired Adjunct Faculty Member, Mesa Community College
Author – *Nutrition and Mental Health*
Mental Health Resource Professional of Behavioral Health DPG of AND
San Diego, California

Mary Demarest Litchford, PhD, RDN, LDN
President
CASE Software & Books
Greensboro, North Carolina

Betty L. Lucas, MPH
Former LEND Nutritionist
University of Washington
Seattle, Washington

Lucinda K. Lysen, RDN, RN, BSN
Medical Nutrition Therapy Specialist
Consulting and Private Practice
Chicago, Illinois

Ainsley M. Malone, MS, RD, CNSC, FAND, FASPEN
Nutrition Support Team
Mt. Carmel West Hospital
Clinical Practice Specialist
The American Society for Parenteral and Enteral Nutrition
New Albany, Ohio

Gabriela E. Mancera-Chávez, MSc, NC
Escuela de Dietetica y Nutricion-ISSSTE
Ciudad de México, DF México

Laura E. Matarese, PhD, RDN, LDN, CNSC, FADA, FASPEN, FAND
Professor
Division of Gastroenterology, Hepatology and Nutrition
Brody School of Medicine
East Carolina University
Greenville, North Carolina

Lisa Mays, MPH, RDN
Nutrition Services Manager
The Idaho Foodbank
Boise, Idaho

Mari O. Mazon, MS, RDN, CD
Nutritionist
Center on Human Development and Disability (CHDD)
University of Washington
Seattle, Washington

Christine McCullum-Gomez, PhD, RDN
Food and Nutrition Consultant
Cypress, Texas

Kelly N. McKean, MS, RDN, CSP, CD
Clinical Pediatric Dietitian
Seattle Children's Hospital
Seattle, Washington

Kelly Morrow, MS, RDN
Associate Professor, Nutrition Clinic Coordinator
Department of Nutrition and Exercise Science
Bastyr University and the Bastyr Center for Natural Health
Seattle, Washington

Diana Noland, MPH, RD, CCN, LD
Adjunct Faculty
Dietetics and Nutrition
School of Health Professions
University of Kansas Medical Center
Kansas City, Kansas
Clinical Nutrition - Private Practice
Burbank, California

Therese O'Flaherty, MS, RDN
Ketogenic Diet and Interdisciplinary Feeding
    Team
Cincinnati Children's Hospital Medical Center
Cincinnati, Ohio

Beth N. Ogata, MS, RDN, CD, CSP
Lecturer
Department of Pediatrics
Center on Human Development and
    Disability (CHDD)
University of Washington
Seattle, Washington

Mary Purdy, MS, RDN
Arivale Coach and Team Lead
Arivale
Adjunct Professor
Bastyr University
Seattle, Washington

Sudha Raj, PhD, RD, FAND
Director of Graduate Program
Department of Public Health, Food Studies
    and Nutrition
The David B. Falk College of Sport and
    Human Dynamics
Syracuse University
Syracuse, New York

Diane Rigassio Radler, PhD, RDN
Associate Professor
Department of Nutritional Sciences
Director, Institute for Nutrition
    Interventions
School of Health Related Professions
Rutgers University
Newark, New Jersey

Justine Roth, MS, RDN
Director, Nutrition Department
New York State Psychiatric Institute
New York, New York

**Mary Krystofiak Russell, MS, RDN, LDN,
    FAND**
Senior Manager, Global Nutrition Medical Affairs
Baxter Healthcare Corporation
Deerfield, Illinois

Janet E. Schebendach, PhD, RDN
Assistant Professor of Neurobiology
Department of Psychiatry
Columbia University Medical Center
New York, New York

Elizabeth Shanaman, RDN
Renal Dietitian
Nutrition and Fitness Services
Northwest Kidney Centers
Seattle, Washington

Jamie S. Stang, PhD, MPH, RDN
Associate Professor
Division of Epidemiology and Community
    Health
University of Minnesota, School of Public Health
Minneapolis, Minnesota

Erik R. Stegman, MA, JD
Executive Director
Center for Native American Youth
The Aspen Institute
Washington, District of Columbia

Alison Steiber PhD, RDN
Chief Science Officer
Academy of Nutrition and Dietetics
Cleveland, Ohio

Tracy Stopler, MS, RDN
Registered Dietitian/Fitness Trainer;
President, NUTRITION E.T.C. Inc
Plainview, New York; and
Adjunct Professor
Adelphi University
Garden City, New York

**Kathie Madonna Swift, MS, RDN, LDN,
    FAND**
Co-Founder, Integrative and Functional
    Nutrition Academy (IFNA)
Owner, Swift Nutrition
Nutritionist, Canyon Ranch in the Berkshires,
    Kripalu Center for Yoga and Health and
    the Ultrawellness Center
Boston, Massachusetts
Education Director, Center for Mind Body
    Medicine
Washington, District of Columbia

Kelly A. Tappenden, PhD, RDN, FASPEN
Kraft Foods Human Nutrition Endowed
    Professor
University of Illinois at Urbana
Urbana, Illinois

Jacob Teitelbaum, MD
Director, Practitioners Alliance Network
Kona, Hawaii

Cristine M. Trahms, MS, RDN, FADA
Retired Senior Lecturer
Department of Pediatrics
Center on Human Development and
    Disability (CHDD)
University of Washington
Seattle, Washington

**DeeAnna Wales VanReken, MS,
    RDN, CD**
Certified Natural Chef
Clinical Nutrition Specialist
Swedish Medical Center, First Hill
Seattle, Washington

Doris Wales, BA, BS, RPh
Registered Pharmacist
Certified Immunizer
K-Mart Pharmacies
Huntsville, Alabama

Susan Weiner, MS, RDN, CDE
Registered Dietitian-Nutritionist
Certified Diabetes Educator
Owner and President, Susan Weiner
    Nutrition, PLLC
Merrick, New York

Alan Weiss, MD
Director, Annapolis Integrative Medicine
Annapolis, Maryland

Nancy S. Wellman, PhD, RDN, FAND
Adjunct Professor
Friedman School of Nutrition Science
    and Policy
Tufts University
Boston, Massachusetts

Katy G. Wilkens, MS, RDN
Manager
Nutrition and Fitness Services
Northwest Kidney Centers
Seattle, Washington

**Marion F. Winkler, PhD, RD, LDN,
    CNSC, FASPEN**
Department of Surgery and Nutrition
    Support Service
Surgical Nutrition Specialist
Rhode Island Hospital
Associate Professor of Surgery
Alpert Medical School of Brown
    University
Providence, Rhode Island

**Martin M. Yadrick, MBI, MS,
    RDN, FAND**
Director of Nutrition Informatics
Computrition, Inc.
Los Angeles, California

Beth Zupec-Kania, RDN
Consultant Nutritionist
Ketogenic Therapies, LLC
Milwaukee, Wisconsin

Judith Ashley, PhD, RD
Associate Professor
Department of Agriculture, Nutrition and Veterinary Sciences
University of Nevada
Reno, Nevada

Jo Ann S. Carson, PhD, RDN, LD
Professor and Program Director
Department of Clinical Nutrition, University of Texas
    Southwestern Medical Center
Dallas, Texas

Patricia Davidson, DCN, RDN, CDE, LDN, FAND
Assistant Professor
Nutrition Department, College of Health Sciences
West Chester University of Pennsylvania
West Chester, Pennsylvania

Susan Fullmer PhD, RDN, CD
Teaching Professor
Nutrition, Dietetics and Food Science
Brigham Young University
Provo, Utah

Mary Hendrickson-Nelson MSc, RD
Clinical Coordinator/Faculty Lecture
McGill University Dietetics and Human Nutrition Department
Montreal, Quebec, Canada

Janice M. Joneja, PhD, RD
Food Allergy Consultant
President, Vickerstaff Healthy Services, Inc.
British Columbia, Canada

Lydia Kloiber, MS, RDN, LD
Director, Didactic Program in Dietetics & Instructor
Texas Tech University
Lubbock, Texas

Sudha Raj, PhD, RD, FAND
Director of Graduate Program
Department of Public Health, Food Studies and Nutrition
The David B. Falk College of Sport and Human Dynamics
Syracuse University
Syracuse, New York

Louise E. Schneider, DrPH, RD
Associate Professor
Nutrition and Dietetics Department, Loma Linda University
Loma Linda, California

Jessica Setnick, MS, RD, CEDRD
Meadows Senior Fellow
Remuda Ranch Center for the Treatment of Eating
    Disorders
Dallas, Texas

Amandio Vieira, PhD
Associate Professor
Nutrition Research Laboratory, Biomedical Physiology BPK,
    Simon Fraser University
Burnaby, British Columbia, Canada

Ruth Leyse-Wallace, PhD, MS, BS, RD
Retired Adjunct Faculty Member, Mesa Community College
Author – *Nutrition and Mental Health*
Mental Health Resource Professional of Behavioral Health
    DPG of AND
San Diego, California

Mary Width, MS, RD
Senior Lecturer, Coordinated Program in Dietetics
Department of Nutrition and Food Science
Wayne State University
Detroit, Michigan

FOREWORD

"We're not just a textbook; we're your connection to the leaders in nutrition." This statement has been true since the first edition of *Krause's Food and the Nutrition Care Process* was published in 1952. The reason this nutrition and diet therapy textbook became and has remained the go-to book for teaching about food and the nutrition care process is the editors have been in the forefront of dietetics practice. In addition, the editors have selected authors who not only have expertise on the topic of their chapter, but also are engaged in cutting-edge practice in the specific area that is being addressed.

With each edition, one thinks it cannot get better, but it does. The well-known and highly respected editors of this 14th edition, Kathleen Mahan and Janice Raymond, as well as the authors, read like a who's who of dietetics practice. Both editors have been and are authors of chapters in this and prior editions, Kathleen for more than 35 years. Early on one author could cover one or more topics. With the ever-increasing explosion of information, it often takes two or three authors to cover a topic. The editors have done an excellent job selecting authors who are clinical specialists with the specific expertise to address each of the topics – writers, researchers, and practitioners who have provided in-depth coverage with many practical and evidence-based recommendations. The authors, at the request of the editors, have taken an integrative approach to nutrition care.

The comprehensiveness of the book continues in this edition with a new chapter on "Inflammation and the Physiology of Chronic Disease," which underlies so much of the therapy, including nutrition, of chronic disease. This edition also includes the 2015 Dietary Guidelines for Americans, more visuals, and high-lighted *Focus On* boxes, *Clinical Insights*, and *Clinical Case Studies* that help translate scientific knowledge into practical patient care.

The editors and authors are also leaders in the dietetics profession. They are often selected to make presentations at national meetings. It is exciting for students and young professionals, who have been exposed to the latest information in the Krause textbook, to attend national meetings and hear presentations by the authors who provide even newer and more exciting information on their topic for which they have extensive expertise. It is even more exciting to be able to meet and talk with them.

This remarkable food and nutrition textbook has been in existence throughout my almost 50 years in the dietetics profession. I fully expect it to be a leading textbook for the next 50 years!

Sonja L. Connor, MS, RD, LD, FAND
Research Associate Professor
Oregon Health & Science University
Portland, Oregon
President, Academy of Nutrition and Dietetics 2014–2015

Over its 14 editions this classic text has continued to change in response to the ever-dynamic field of nutrition. And because it remains the most comprehensive nutrition text book available it is the reference students take into their internships and careers.

AUDIENCE

Scientific knowledge and clinical information is presented in a form that is useful to students in dietetics, nursing, and other allied health professions in an interdisciplinary setting. It is valuable as a reference for other disciplines such as medicine, dentistry, child development, physical and occupational therapy, health education, and lifestyle counseling. Nutrient and assessment appendices, tables, illustrations, and clinical insight boxes provide practical hands-on procedures and clinical tools for students and practitioners alike.

This textbook accompanies the graduating student into clinical practice as a treasured shelf reference. The popular features remain: having basic information on nutrition in the life cycle all the way through to protocols for clinical nutrition practice in one place, clinical management algorithms, focus boxes that give "nice-to- know" detailed insight, sample nutrition diagnoses for clinical scenarios, useful websites, and extensive appendices for patient education. All material reflects current evidence-based practice as contributed by authors, experts in their fields. This text is the first choice in the field of dietetics for students, interns, educators, and clinicians.

ORGANIZATION

This edition follows the Conceptual Framework for Steps of the Nutrition Care Process (see inside of back cover). All nutritional care process components are addressed to enhance or improve the nutritional well-being of individuals, their families, or populations. The chapters flow according to the steps of assessment, nutrition diagnosis, intervention, monitoring, and evaluation with the separation of the pediatric medical nutrition therapy (MNT) chapters into their own section to assist with that specialty practice.

Part 1, Nutrition Assessment, organizes content for an effective assessment. Chapters here provide an overview of the digestive system, as well as calculation of energy requirements and expenditure, macronutrient and micronutrient needs, nutritional genomics, and food intake. A thorough review of biochemical tests, acid-base balance issues, and medications promote the necessary insight for provision of excellent care. A new approach for this edition is a chapter titled "Inflammation and the Pathophysiology of Chronic Disease," which addresses the latest knowledge about inflammation as a cause of chronic disease and the necessity of assessing for it. The final chapter in this section addresses the behavioral aspects of an individual's food choices within the community, a safe food supply, and available resources for sufficient food access.

Part 2, Nutrition Diagnosis and Intervention, describes the critical thinking process from assessment to selection of relevant, timely, and measurable nutrition diagnoses. These nutrition diagnoses can be resolved by the dietitian nutritionist (RDN) or trained health professional. The process is generally used for individuals but can be applied when helping families, teaching groups, or evaluating the nutritional needs of a community or a population. A nutrition diagnosis requires an intervention, and interventions relate to food and nutrient delivery (including nutrition support), use of bioactive substances and integrative medical nutrition, education, counseling, and referral when needed.

Part 3, Nutrition in the Life Cycle, presents in-depth information on the nutrition for life stages from conception and nutrition in the womb and pregnancy and through lactation and infancy. There is a chapter on nutrition in adolescence and another that deals with the nutrition issues and chronic disease that usually start appearing in adulthood. Finally, nutrition and the aging adult is discussed in detail because much of the employment of nutrition professionals in the future is going to be in providing nutrition services to this rapidly expanding percentage of the population.

Part 4, Nutrition for Health and Fitness, provides nutrition concepts for the achievement and maintenance of health and fitness, as well as the prevention of many disease states. Weight management, problems with eating disorders, dental health, bone health, and sports nutrition focus on the role of nutrition in promoting long-term health.

Part 5, Medical Nutrition Therapy, reflects evidence-based knowledge and current trends in nutrition therapies. All of the chapters are written and reviewed by experts in their fields who present nutritional aspects of conditions such as cardiovascular disorders; diabetes; liver disease; renal disease; pulmonary disease; HIV; endocrine disorders, especially thyroid disease; and rheumatologic, neurologic, and psychiatric disorders.

Part 6, Pediatric Specialties, describes the role of nutrition therapies in childhood. Chapters provide details for low-birth-weight, neonatal intensive-care conditions, genetic metabolic disorders, and developmental disabilities.

NEW TO THIS EDITION

- Provides the most current content throughout, including the 2015 Dietary Guidelines for Americans, due to be finalized in 2016.
- Includes a new chapter titled "Inflammation and the Pathophysiology of Chronic Disease."
- Worksheets on calculating parenteral and enteral nutrition needs are included in Chapter 12: "Food and Nutrient Delivery: Nutrition Support Methods."
- Standards of Care recommendations have been incorporated throughout the book as appropriate.
- The latest recommendations from the National Institutes of Health are discussed in Chapter 33: "Medical Nutrition Therapy for Cardiovascular Disease."
- Now includes detailed Clinical Case Studies and Clinical Applications boxes designed to help translate academic knowledge into practical patient care.
- New Appendix on The Anti-inflammatory Diet.
- Many new content highlight boxes such as "Nutrition and the Affordable Care Act" and "Human Milk Banking and Vending Machine Labeling Law."

PEDAGOGY

- UNIQUE! Pathophysiology algorithms present the cause, pathophysiology, and the medical nutrition management for a variety of disorders and conditions. They equip the reader with an understanding of the illness as background for providing optimal nutritional care.
- *Clinical Insight* boxes expand on clinical information in the text and highlight areas that may go unnoticed. These boxes contain information on studies and clinical resources for the student and practitioner.
- *New Directions* boxes suggest areas for further research by spotlighting emerging areas of interest within the field
- *Focus On* boxes provide thought-provoking information on key concepts for well-rounded study and the promotion of further discussion within the classroom.
- Useful Websites direct the reader to online resources that relate to the chapter topics.
- Sample Nutrition Diagnosis boxes present a problem, its etiology, and its signs and symptoms, before concluding with a sample nutrition diagnosis, providing both students and practitioners with "real-life" scenarios they may encounter in practice.
- Key Terms are defined at the beginning of each chapter and bolded within the text where they are discussed in more detail.
- Chapter References: References are current and extensive, with the purpose of giving the student and instructor lots of opportunity for further reading and understanding.

ANCILLARIES

Accompanying this edition is the Evolve website, which includes updated and invaluable resources for instructors and students. These materials can be accessed by going to http://evolve.elsevier.com/Mahan/nutrition/.

INSTRUCTOR RESOURCES

- PowerPoint presentations: More than 900 slides to help guide classroom lectures.
- Image Collection: Approximately 200 images from the text are included in the PowerPoint presentations, as well as more illustrations that can be downloaded and used to develop other teaching resources.
- Audience Response System Questions (for use with iClicker and other systems): Three to five questions per chapter help aid incorporation of this new technology into the classroom.
- Test Bank: Each chapter includes NCLEX-formatted questions with page references specific to that chapter's content to bring you more than 900 multiple-choice questions.
- Animations: Animations have been developed to visually complement the text and the processes described.
- Nutrition Care Process Tools: Consisting of assessment and monitoring tools and intervention tools, this information can be used by the new student and practitioner in teaching and guiding the client in his or her specific nutritional care.

STUDENT RESOURCES

- Study Exercises with Answers: With more than 600 questions, these exercises give instant feedback on questions related to the chapter's content.

We strive to create a text that is current, relevant and interesting to read.

L. Kathleen Mahan, MS, RDN, CD
Janice L. Raymond, MS, RDN, CD, CSG

ACKNOWLEDGMENTS

We sincerely thank the reviewers and especially contributors for this edition who have devoted hours and hours of time and commitment to researching the book's content for accuracy, reliability, and practicality. We are greatly in debt to them and realize that we could not continue to produce this book without them. Thank you!

We also wish to acknowledge the hard work of Kristin Geen, Director of Traditional Education, who keeps the vision, and Danielle Frazier, Senior Developmental Editor, who can get the "hot off the press" items we'd like included, and Alex Kluesner, Project Manager at Graphic World, who amazingly keeps the manuscript moving forward as he juggles between us and all others. Thank you!

CONTENTS

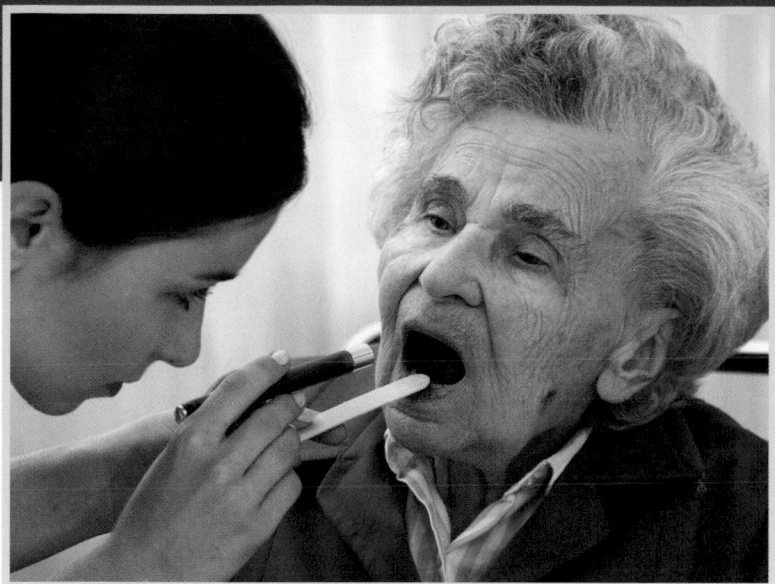

PART I

Nutrition Assessment

Food provides energy and building materials for countless substances that are essential for the growth and survival of every human being. This section opens with a brief overview of the digestion, absorption, transportation, and excretion of nutrients. These remarkable processes convert myriads of complex foodstuffs into individual nutrients ready to be used in metabolism. Macronutrients (proteins, fats, and carbohydrates) each contribute to the total energy pool, but ultimately the energy they yield is available for the work of the muscles and organs of the body. The way nutrients become integral parts of the body and contribute to proper functioning depends heavily on the physiologic and biochemical processes that govern their actions. It is now known that these metabolic processes are altered in the presence of acute and chronic inflammation. Understanding the biomarkers and other indicators of inflammation are a critical component of nutrition assessment.

For the health provider, nutrition assessment is the first step in the nutrition care process. To implement a successful nutrition plan, the assessment must include key elements of the patient's clinical or medical history, current situation, anthropometric measurements, biochemical and laboratory values, information on medication and herbal supplement use for potential food-drug interactions, plus a thorough food and nutrition intake history. Genetic research is rapidly clarifying how genes and nutrition are interrelated. Nutrigenomics is the study of the effects of foods and nutrients on gene expression and thus nutritional requirements. Thus, the chapters in Part 1 provide an organized way to develop the skills needed to make an assessment in the nutrition care process.

Intake: Digestion, Absorption, Transport, and Excretion of Nutrients

Kelly A. Tappenden, PhD, RDN, FASPEN

KEY TERMS

amylase, pancreatic
amylase, salivary
brush border membrane
chelation
cholecystokinin (CCK)
chyme
colonic salvage
diffusion, facilitated
diffusion, passive
dysbiosis
enterohepatic circulation
enterokinase
gastrin
ghrelin
glucagon-like peptide 2 (GLP-2)

gut-brain axis
isomaltase
lactase
lipase, gastric
lipase, pancreatic
lipase, salivary
maltase
micelle
microbiota
microbiome
microvilli
motilin
parietal cells
pepsin

peristalsis
prebiotic
probiotic
proteolytic enzymes
secretin
somatostatin
sucrase
synbiotic
transport, active
transport, passive
trypsinogen
trypsin
unstirred water layer (UWL)
villi

One of the primary considerations for a complete nutrition assessment is to consider the three-step model of "ingestion, digestion, and utilization." In this model, consideration is given to each step to identify all areas of inadequacy or excess. If there is any reason why a step is altered from physical, biochemical, or behavioral-environmental causes, the astute nutrition provider must select an appropriate nutrition diagnosis for which intervention is required. Intake and assimilation of nutrients should lead to a desirable level of nutritional health.

THE GASTROINTESTINAL TRACT

Assessment of the function of the gastrointestinal tract (GIT) is essential to the nutrition care process. For the nutrition care process, several nutrition diagnoses can be identified when assessing GIT function. Common or possible nutrition diagnoses related to digestion or metabolism include:

Altered gastrointestinal function
Imbalance of nutrient intake
Altered nutrient utilization
Altered nutrition biomarkers
Inadequate or excessive fluid intake
Food-drug interaction

The GIT is designed to (1) digest the macronutrients protein, carbohydrates, and lipids from ingested foods and beverages; (2) absorb fluids, micronutrients, and trace elements; (3) provide a physical and immunologic barrier to pathogens,

Sections of the chapter were written by Peter L. Beyer, MS, RD, for previous editions of this text.

foreign material, and potential antigens consumed with food or formed during the passage of food through the GIT; and (4) provide regulatory and biochemical signaling to the nervous system, often involving the intestinal microbiota, via a pathway known as the gut-brain axis.

The human GIT is well suited for digesting and absorbing nutrients from a tremendous variety of foods, including meats, dairy products, fruits, vegetables, grains, complex starches, sugars, fats, and oils. Depending on the nature of the diet consumed, 90% to 97% of food is digested and absorbed; most of the unabsorbed material is of plant origin. Compared with ruminants and animals with a very large cecum, humans are considerably less efficient at extracting energy from grasses, stems, seeds, and other coarse fibrous materials. Humans lack the enzymes to hydrolyze the chemical bonds that link the molecules of sugars that make up plant fibers. However, fibrous foods and any undigested carbohydrates are fermented to varying degrees by bacteria in the human colon; this process can contribute 5% to 10% of the energy needed by humans.

The GIT is one of the largest organs in the body, has the greatest surface area, has the largest number of immune cells, and is one of the most metabolically active tissues in the body (Figure 1-1). The unique structure of the GIT enables ample processing capacity in healthy humans. The human GIT is about 9 m long, extending from the mouth to the anus and including the oropharyngeal structures, esophagus, stomach, liver and gallbladder, pancreas, and small and large intestine. The lining of this hollow tube, called the mucosa, is configured in a pattern of folds, pits, and fingerlike projections called villi. The villi are lined with epithelial cells and even smaller, cylindrical

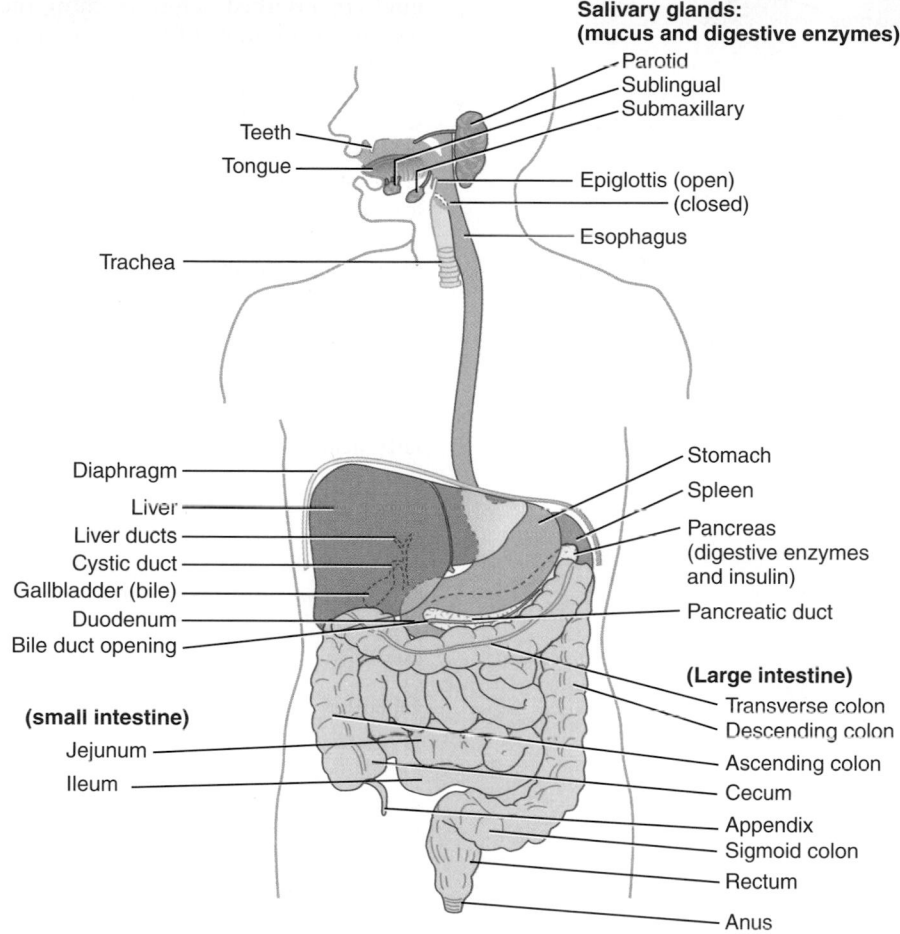

FIGURE 1-1 The digestive system.

extensions called microvilli. The result is a tremendous increase in surface area compared with that expected from a smooth, hollow cylinder. The cells lining the intestinal tract have a life span of approximately 3 to 5 days, and then they are sloughed into the lumen and "recycled," adding to the pool of available nutrients. The cells are fully functional only for the last 2 to 3 days as they migrate from the crypts to the distal third of the villi.

The health of the body depends on a healthy, functional GIT. Because of the unusually high turnover rate and metabolic requirements of the GIT, the cells lining it are more susceptible than most tissues to micronutrient deficiencies, protein-energy malnutrition, and damage resulting from toxins, drugs, irradiation, food allergy reactions, or interruption of its blood supply. Approximately 45% of the energy requirement of the small intestine and 70% of the energy requirement of cells lining the colon are supplied by nutrients passing through its lumen. After only a few days of starvation or intravenous feeding (parenteral nutrition), the GIT atrophies (i.e., the surface area decreases and secretions, synthetic functions, blood flow, and absorptive capacity are all reduced). Resumption of food intake, even with less-than-adequate calories, results in cellular proliferation and return of normal GI function after only a few days. Optimum function of the human GIT seems to depend on a constant supply of foods rather than on consumption of large amounts of foods interrupted by prolonged fasts. This knowledge justifies the clinical practice of feeding an individual orally and/or

enterally (via tube), as opposed to intravenously (or parenterally) when adequate GIT function is present (see Chapter 13).

BRIEF OVERVIEW OF DIGESTIVE AND ABSORPTIVE PROCESSES

The sight, smell, taste, and even thought of food starts the secretions and movements of the GIT. In the mouth, chewing reduces the size of food particles, which are mixed with salivary secretions that prepare them for swallowing. A small amount of starch is degraded by salivary amylase, but digestion in the mouth is minimal. The esophagus transports food and liquid from the oral cavity and pharynx to the stomach. In the stomach, food is mixed with acidic fluid and proteolytic and lipolytic enzymes. Small amounts of lipid digestion take place, and some proteins are changed in structure or partially digested to large peptides. When food reaches the appropriate consistency and concentration, it is now called chyme and passes from the stomach into the small intestine, where most digestion takes place.

In the first 100 cm of small intestine, a flurry of activity occurs, resulting in the digestion and absorption of most ingested food (Figure 1-2). Here the presence of food stimulates the release of hormones which stimulate the production and release of powerful enzymes from the pancreas as well as bile from the gallbladder. Starches and proteins are reduced to smaller-molecular-weight carbohydrates and small to medium-size peptides. Dietary fats are reduced from visible globules of fat to microscopic droplets of

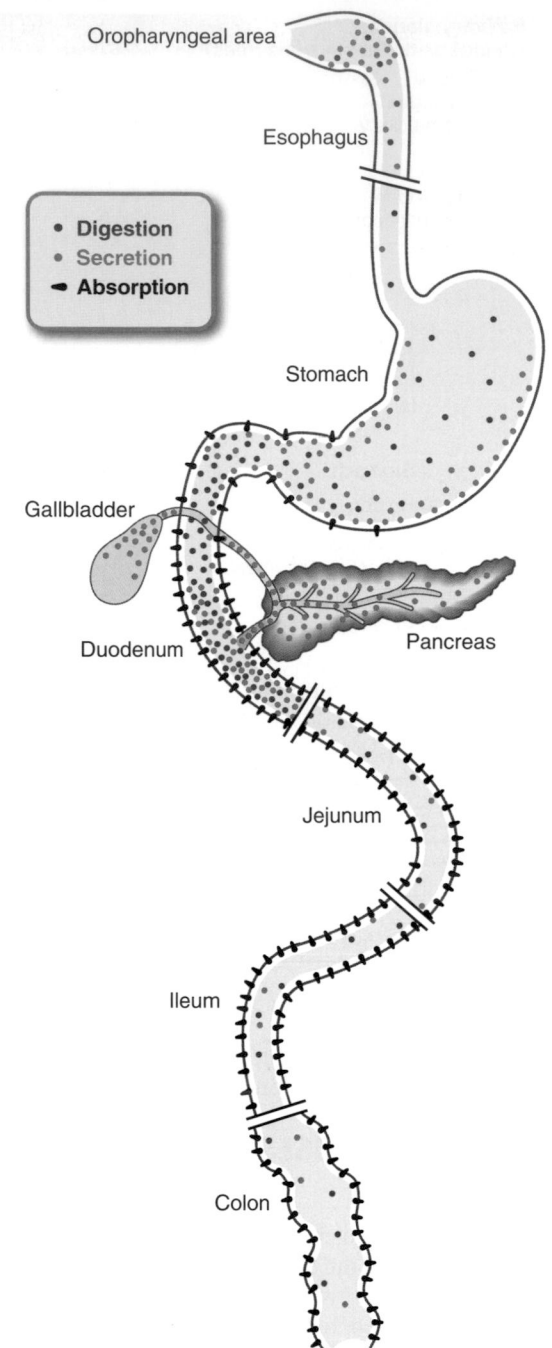

FIGURE 1-2 Sites of secretion, digestion, and absorption.

fluid are absorbed before reaching the colon. The colon and rectum absorb most of the remaining fluid delivered from the small intestine. The colon absorbs electrolytes and only a small amount of remaining nutrients. The movement of ingested and secreted material in the GIT is regulated primarily by hormones, nerves, and enteric muscles.

Most nutrients absorbed from the GIT enter the portal vein for transport to the liver where they may be stored, transformed into other substances, or released into circulation. End products of most dietary fats are transported into the bloodstream via the lymphatic circulation.

Nutrients reaching the distal small intestine and large intestine, most notably dietary fiber and resistant starches, are fermented by the microbiota located within the lumen of the ileum and large intestine. Fermentation produces short-chain fatty acids (SCFAs) and gas. SCFAs provide a preferred fuel source for cells of the intestine, stimulate intestinal cell renewal and function, enhance immune function, and regulate gene expression. In addition, some carbohydrates have "prebiotic" functions that induce the growth and activity of beneficial microbes within the intestinal microbiota. The large intestine also provides temporary storage for waste products. The distal colon, rectum, and anus control defecation.

Enzymes in Digestion

Digestion of food is accomplished by enzymatic hydrolysis. Cofactors such as hydrochloric acid, bile, and sodium bicarbonate facilitate the digestive and absorptive processes. Digestive enzymes synthesized in specialized cells of the mouth, stomach, and pancreas are released into the GIT lumen, whereas digestive enzymes synthesized in enterocytes of the small intestine remain embedded within the brush border membrane. Except for fiber and resistant carbohydrates, digestion and absorption of intake is completed essentially in the small intestine. Table 1-1 summarizes digestive enzymes and their functions within the GIT.

Regulators of Gastrointestinal Activity: Neural and Hormonal Mechanisms

GIT movement, including contraction, mixing, and propulsion of luminal contents, is the result of the coordinated movement of smooth muscle and the activity of the enteric nervous system, enteroendocrine hormones, and smooth muscle. The enteric nervous system is integrated throughout the lining of the GIT. Mucosal receptors sense the composition of chyme and distention of the lumen (i.e., fullness) and send impulses that coordinate the processes of digestion, secretion, absorption, and immunity.

Neurotransmitters and neuropeptides with small molecular weights signal nerves to contract or relax muscles, increase or decrease fluid secretions, or change blood flow. The GIT then largely regulates its own motility and secretory activity. However, signals from the central nervous system can override the enteric system and affect GIT function. Hormones, neuropeptides, and neurotransmitters in the GIT not only affect intestinal function but also have an effect on other nerves and tissues in many parts of the body. Some examples of neurotransmitters released from enteric nerve endings are listed in Table 1-2. In people with gastrointestinal disease (e.g., infections, inflammatory bowel disease, irritable bowel syndrome), the enteric nervous system may be overstimulated, resulting in abnormal secretion, altered blood flow, increased permeability, and altered immune function.

triglycerides, then to free fatty acids and monoglycerides. Enzymes from the brush border of the small intestine further reduce the remaining carbohydrates to monosaccharides and the remaining peptides to single amino acids, dipeptides, and tripeptides. Large volumes of fluid are used to digest and absorb nutrients. Together with salivary and gastric secretions, secretions from the pancreas, small intestine, and gallbladder secrete 7 L of fluid into the GIT lumen each day—far more than the 2 L ingested through dietary intake each day. All but 100 mL of the total fluid entering the lumen is reabsorbed: about 7 L in the small intestine and about 2 L in the large intestine.

Along the remaining length of the small intestine, almost all the macronutrients, minerals, vitamins, trace elements, and

TABLE 1-1   Summary of Enzymatic Digestion and Absorption

Secretion and Source	Enzymes	Substrate	Action and Resulting Products	Final Products Absorbed
Saliva from salivary glands in mouth	α-amylase	Starch (α-linked polysaccharides)	Hydrolysis to form dextrins and maltose	—
	Lingual lipase	Triglyceride	Hydrolysis to form diglyceride and free fatty acids	—
Gastric secretion from gastric glands in stomach mucosa	Pepsin (activated from pepsinogen in the presence of hydrochloric acid)	Protein	Hydrolysis of peptide bonds to form peptides and amino acids	—
	Gastric lipase	Triglyceride	Hydrolysis to form diglyceride and free fatty acids	—
Exocrine secretions from pancreatic acinar cells, acting in duodenum	Lipase	Fat (in the presence of bile salts)	Hydrolysis to form monoglycerides and fatty acids; incorporated into micelles	Fatty acids into mucosal cells; reesterified as triglycerides
	Cholesterol esterase	Sterols (such as cholesterol)	Hydrolysis to form esters of cholesterol and fatty acids; incorporated into micelles	Cholesterol into mucosal cells; transferred to chylomicrons
	α-Amylase	Starch and dextrins	Hydrolysis to form dextrins and maltose	—
	Trypsin (activated trypsinogen)	Proteins and polypeptides	Hydrolysis of interior peptide bonds to form polypeptides	—
	Chymotrypsin (activated chymotrypsinogen)	Proteins and peptides	Hydrolysis of interior peptide bonds to form polypeptides	—
	Carboxypeptidase (activated pro-carboxypeptidase)	Polypeptides	Hydrolysis of terminal peptide bonds (carboxyl end) to form amino acids	Amino acids
	Ribonuclease and deoxyribonuclease	Ribonucleic acids (RNA) and deoxyribonucleic acids (DNA)	Hydrolysis to form mononucleotides	Mononucleotides
	Elastase	Fibrous protein (elastin)	Hydrolysis to form peptides and amino acids	—
Small intestine enzymes (embedded in the brush border membrane)	Enterokinase	Trypsinogen	Activates trypsin	Dipeptides and tripeptides
	Aminopeptidase and dipeptidase (also located within the enterocyte cytosol)	Polypeptides	Cleavage of amino acids from the amino terminus of protein (N-terminus) or peptide substrates	Amino acids
	Sucrase	Sucrose	Hydrolysis to form glucose and fructose	Glucose and fructose
	α-Dextrinase (isomaltase)	Dextrin (isomaltose)	Hydrolysis to form glucose	Glucose
	Maltase	Maltose	Hydrolysis to form glucose	Glucose
	Lactase	Lactose	Hydrolysis to form glucose and galactose	Glucose and galactose
	Nucleotidases	Nucleic acids	Hydrolysis to form nucleotides and phosphates	Nucleotides
	Nucleosidase and phosphorylase	Nucleosides	Hydrolysis to form purines, pyrimidines, and pentose phosphate	Purine and pyrimidine bases

Autonomic innervation is supplied by the sympathetic fibers that run along blood vessels and by the parasympathetic fibers in the vagal and pelvic nerves. In general, sympathetic neurons, which are activated by fear, anger, and stress, tend to slow transit of intestinal contents by inhibiting neurons affecting muscle contraction and inhibiting secretions. The parasympathetic nerves innervate specific areas of the alimentary tract and contribute to certain functions. For example, the sight or smell of food stimulates vagal activity and subsequent secretion of acid from parietal cells within the stomach. The enteric nervous system also sends signals to the central nervous system that are perceived as pain, nausea, urgency or gastric fullness, or gastric emptiness by way of the vagal and spinal nerves. Inflammation, dysmotility, and various types of intestinal damage may intensify these perceptions.

Gastrointestinal Hormones

Regulation of the GIT involves numerous hormones that are secreted by enteroendocrine cells located within the epithelium lining of the GIT. These regulators can regulate function of the cell from which they were secreted (autocrine), on neighboring cells (paracrine), or distant cells by traveling through the blood to their target organs (endocrine). More than 100 peptide hormones and hormone-like growth factors have been identified. Their actions are often complex and extend well beyond the

TABLE 1-2 Examples of Neurotransmitters and their Actions

Neurotransmitter	Site of Release	Primary Action
GABA	Central nervous system	Relaxes lower esophageal sphincter
Norepinephrine	Central nervous system, spinal cord, sympathetic nerves	Decreases motility, increases contraction of sphincters, inhibits secretions
Acetylcholine	Central nervous system, autonomic system, other tissues	Increases motility, relaxes sphincters, stimulates secretion
Neurotensin	GI tract, central nervous system	Inhibits release of gastric emptying and acid secretion
Serotonin (5-HT)	GI tract, spinal cord	Facilitates secretion and peristalsis
Nitric oxide	Central nervous system, GI tract	Regulates blood flow, maintains muscle tone, maintains gastric motor activity
Substance P	Gut, central nervous system, skin	Increases sensory awareness (mainly pain), and peristalsis

5-HT, 5-hydroxytryptamine; *GABA*, α-aminobutyric acid; *GI*, gastrointestinal.

GIT. Some of the hormones (e.g., of the cholecystokinin [CCK] and somatostatin family) also serve as neurotransmitters between neurons.

The GIT secretes more than 30 hormone families, making it the largest hormone-producing organ in the body (Rehfeld, 2014). Gastrointestinal hormones are involved in initiating and terminating feeding, signaling hunger and satiety, pacing movements of the GIT, governing gastric emptying, regulating blood flow and permeability, priming immune functions, and stimulating the growth of cells (within and beyond the GIT). Ghrelin, a neuropeptide secreted from the stomach, and motilin, a related hormone secreted from the duodenum, send a "hungry" message to the brain. Once food has been ingested, hormones PYY 3-36, CCK, glucagon-like peptide-1 (GLP-1), oxyntomodulin, pancreatic polypeptide, and gastrin-releasing polypeptide (bombesin) send signals to decrease hunger and increase satiety (Rui, 2013). Some of the GI hormones, including some of those that affect satiety, also tend to slow gastric emptying and decrease secretions (e.g., somatostatin). Other GI hormones (e.g., motilin) increase motility.

The signaling agents of the GIT also are involved in several metabolic functions. Glucose-dependent insulinotropic polypeptide (GIP) and GLP-1 are called incretin hormones because they help lower blood sugar by facilitating insulin secretion, decreasing gastric emptying, and increasing satiety. Several of these hormones and analogs are used in management of obesity, inflammatory bowel disease, diarrhea, diabetes, GI malignancies, and other conditions. This area of research is critically important.

Some functions of the hormones that affect gastrointestinal cell growth, deoxyribonucleic acid (DNA) synthesis, inflammation, proliferation, secretion, movement, or metabolism have not been fully identified. Knowledge of major hormone functions becomes especially important when the sites of their secretion or action are diseased or removed in surgical procedures, or when hormones and their analogs are used to suppress or enhance some aspect of gastrointestinal function. Glucagon-like peptide-2 (GLP-2) is an example of a hormone secreted from the distal GIT that increases intestinal surface area and enhances nutrient processing capacity. An analog of GLP-2, named teduglutide, recently has become available for treatment of patients with short bowel syndrome who are dependent on parenteral nutrition to meet their nutrient and fluid requirements (Seidner et al, 2013; see the Clinical Insight box in Chapter 28). The key GIT hormones are summarized in Table 1-3.

Gastrin, a hormone that stimulates gastric secretions and motility, is secreted primarily from endocrine "G" cells in the antral mucosa of the stomach. Secretion is initiated by (1) impulses from the vagus nerve, such as those triggered by the smell or sight of food; (2) distention of the antrum after a meal; and (3) the presence of secretagogues in the antrum, such as partially digested proteins, fermented alcoholic beverages, caffeine, or food extracts (e.g., bouillon). When the lumen gets more acidic, feedback involving other hormones inhibits gastrin release (Chu and Schubert, 2013). Gastrin binds to receptors on parietal cells and histamine-releasing cells to stimulate gastric acid, to receptors on chief cells to release pepsinogen, and to receptors on smooth muscle to increase gastric motility.

Secretin, the first hormone to be named, is released from "S" cells in the wall of the proximal small intestine into the bloodstream. It is secreted in response to gastric acid and digestive end products in the duodenum, wherein it stimulates the secretion of pancreatic juice and inhibits gastric acid secretion and emptying (the opposite of gastrin). Neutralized acidity protects the duodenal mucosa from prolonged exposure to acid and provides the appropriate environment for intestinal and pancreatic enzyme activity. The human receptor is found in the stomach and ductal and acinar cells of the pancreas. In different species, other organs may express secretin, including the liver, colon, heart, kidney, and brain (Chey and Chang, 2014).

Small bowel mucosal "I" cells secrete CCK, an important multifunctional hormone released in response to the presence of protein and fat. Receptors for CCK are in pancreatic acinar cells, pancreatic islet cells, gastric somatostatin-releasing D cells, smooth muscle cells of the GIT, and the central nervous system. Major functions of CCK are to (1) stimulate the pancreas to secrete enzymes, bicarbonate, and water; (2) stimulate gallbladder contraction; (3) increase colonic and rectal motility; (4) slow gastric emptying; and (5) increase satiety. CCK is also widely distributed in the brain and plays a role in neuronal functioning (Dockray, 2012).

Motilin is released by endocrine cells in the duodenal mucosa during fasting to stimulate gastric emptying and intestinal migrating contractions. Erythromycin, an antibiotic, has been shown to bind to motilin receptors; thus analogs of erythromycin and motilin have been used as therapeutic agents to treat delayed gastric emptying (De Smet et al, 2009).

Somatostatin, released by "D" cells in the antrum and pylorus, is a hormone with far-reaching actions. Its primary roles are inhibitory and antisecretory. It decreases motility of the stomach and intestine and inhibits or regulates the release of several gastrointestinal hormones. Somatostatin and its analog, octreotide, are being used to treat certain malignant diseases, as well as numerous gastrointestinal disorders such as diarrhea,

TABLE 1-3   Functions of Major Gastrointestinal Hormones

Hormone	Site of Release	Stimulants for Release	Organ Affected	Effect on Target Organ
Gastrin	G cells of gastric mucosa and duodenum	Peptides, amino acids, caffeine Distention of the antrum Some alcoholic beverages, vagus nerve	Stomach, esophagus, GIT in general	Stimulates secretion of HCl and pepsinogen Increases gastric antral motility Increases lower esophageal sphincter tone
			Gallbladder	Weakly stimulates contraction of gallbladder
			Pancreas	Weakly stimulates pancreatic secretion of bicarbonate
Secretin	S cells of duodenum	Acid in small intestine	Pancreas	Increases output of H_2O and bicarbonate; increases enzyme secretion from the pancreas and insulin release
			Duodenum	Decreases motility Increases mucus output
CCK	I cells of duodenum	Peptides, amino acids, fats, HCl	Pancreas	Stimulates secretion of pancreatic enzymes
			Gallbladder	Causes contraction of gallbladder
			Stomach	Slows gastric emptying
			Colon	Increases motility May mediate feeding behavior
GIP	K cells of duodenum and jejunum	Glucose, fat	Stomach	Reduced intestinal motility
Motilin	M cells of duodenum and jejunum	Interdigestive periods, alkaline pH in duodenum	Stomach, small bowel, colon	Promotes gastric emptying and GI motility
GLP-1	L cells of small intestine and colon (density increases in distal GIT)	Glucose, fat, short–chain fatty acids	Stomach	Prolongs gastric emptying
			Pancreas	Inhibits glucagon release; Stimulates insulin release
GLP-2	L cells of small intestine and colon (density increases in distal GIT)	Glucose, fat, short-chain fatty acids	Small intestine, colon	Stimulates intestinal growth and nutrient digestion and absorption

CCK, Cholecystokinin; *GI,* gastrointestinal; *GIP,* glucose-dependent insulinotropic polypeptide; *GIT,* gastrointestinal tract; *GLP-1,* glucagon-like peptide-1; *GLP-2,* glucagon-like peptide-2; *H_2O,* water; *HCl,* hydrochloric acid.

short bowel syndrome, pancreatitis, dumping syndrome, and gastric hypersecretion (Van Op den Bosch et al, 2009; see Chapters 27 and 28).

Digestion in the Mouth

In the mouth, the teeth grind and crush food into small particles. The food mass is simultaneously moistened and lubricated by saliva. Three pairs of salivary glands – the parotid, submaxillary, and sublingual glands – produce approximately 1.5 L of saliva daily. Enzymatic digestion of starch and lipid is initiated in the mouth due to the presence of amylase and salivary lipase, respectively, in saliva. This digestion is minimal, and the salivary amylase becomes inactive when it reaches the acidic contents of the stomach. Saliva also contains mucus, a protein that causes particles of food to stick together and lubricates the mass for swallowing.

The masticated food mass, or bolus, is passed back to the pharynx under voluntary control, but throughout the esophagus, the process of swallowing (deglutition) is involuntary. Peristalsis then moves the food rapidly into the stomach (see Chapter 40 for detailed discussion of swallowing).

Digestion in the Stomach

Food particles are propelled forward and mixed with gastric secretions by wavelike contractions that progress forward from the upper portion of the stomach (fundus), to the midportion (corpus), and then to the antrum and pylorus. In the stomach, gastric secretions are mixed with food and beverages. An average of 2000 to 2500 ml of fluid is secreted daily in the stomach. These gastric secretions contain hydrochloric acid (secreted by the parietal cells), pepsinogen, gastric lipase, mucus, intrinsic factor (a glycoprotein that facilitates vitamin B_{12} absorption in the ileum), and gastrin. The protease, pepsin, is secreted in an inactive form, pepsinogen, which is converted by hydrochloric acid to its active form. Pepsin is active only in the acidic environment of the stomach and primarily changes the shape and size of some of the proteins found in a normal meal.

An acid-stable lipase is secreted into the stomach by chief cells. Although this lipase is considerably less active than pancreatic lipase, it contributes to the overall processing of dietary triglycerides. Gastric lipase is more specific for triglycerides composed of medium- and short-chain fatty acids, but the usual diet contains few of these fats. Lipases secreted in the upper portions of the GIT may have a relatively important role in the liquid diet of infants; however, when pancreatic insufficiency occurs, it becomes apparent that lingual and gastric lipases are not sufficient to prevent lipid malabsorption. In the process of gastric digestion, most of the food becomes semiliquid chyme, which is 50% water. When food is consumed, significant numbers of microorganisms are also consumed. The stomach pH is low, ranging from about 1 to 4. The combined actions of hydrochloric acid and proteolytic enzymes result in a significant reduction in the concentration of viable microorganisms. Some microbes may escape and enter the intestine if consumed in sufficient concentrations or if achlorhydria, gastrectomy, gastrointestinal dysfunction or disease, poor nutrition, or drugs that suppress acid secretions are present. This may increase the risk of pathogenic infection in the intestine.

The lower esophageal sphincter (LES), which lies above the entrance to the stomach, prevents reflux of gastric contents into the esophagus. The pyloric sphincter in the distal portion of the stomach helps regulate the exit of gastric contents, preventing backflow of chyme from the duodenum into the stomach. Obesity, certain food, gastrointestinal regulators, and irritation from nearby ulcers may alter the performance of sphincters. Certain foods and beverages may alter LES pressure, permitting reflux of stomach contents back into the esophagus (see Chapter 27).

The stomach continuously mixes and churns food and normally releases the mixture in small quantities into the small intestine through the pyloric sphincter. The amount emptied with each contraction of the antrum and pylorus varies with the volume and type of food consumed, but only a few milliliters are released at a time. The presence of acid and nutrients in the duodenum stimulate the regulatory hormone, GIP, to slow gastric emptying.

Most of a liquid meal empties within 1 to 2 hours, and most of a solid meal empties within 2 to 3 hours. When eaten alone, carbohydrates leave the stomach the most rapidly, followed by protein, fat, and fibrous food. In a meal with mixed types of foods, emptying of the stomach depends on the overall volume and characteristics of the foods. Liquids empty more rapidly than solids, large particles empty more slowly than small particles, and energy-dense foods empty more slowly than those containing less energy. These factors are important considerations for practitioners who counsel patients with nausea, vomiting, diabetic gastroparesis, or weight management concerns (see Chapters 27, 30, and 21).

Digestion in the Small Intestine

The small intestine is the primary site for digestion of foods and nutrients. The small intestine is divided into the duodenum, the jejunum, and the ileum (Figure 1-2). The duodenum is approximately 0.5 m long, the jejunum is 2 to 3 m, and the ileum is 3 to 4 m. Most of the digestive process is completed in the duodenum and upper jejunum, and the absorption of most nutrients is largely complete by the time the material reaches the middle of the jejunum. The acidic chyme from the stomach enters the duodenum, where it is mixed with secretions from the pancreas, gallbladder, and duodenal epithelium. The sodium bicarbonate contained within these secretions neutralizes the acidic chyme and allows the digestive enzymes to work more effectively at this location.

The entry of partially digested foods, primarily fats and protein, stimulates the release of CCK, secretin, and GIP, which, in turn, stimulate the secretion of enzymes and fluids and affect gastrointestinal motility and satiety. Bile, which is predominantly a mixture of water, bile salts, and small amounts of pigments and cholesterol, is secreted from the liver and gallbladder. Through their surfactant properties, the bile salts facilitate the digestion and absorption of lipids, cholesterol, and fat-soluble vitamins. Bile acids are also regulatory molecules; they activate the vitamin D receptor and cell-signaling pathways in the liver and GIT that alter gene expression of enzymes involved in the regulation of energy metabolism (Hylemon et al, 2009). Furthermore, bile acids play an important role in hunger and satiety.

The pancreas secretes potent enzymes capable of digesting all of the major nutrients, and enzymes from the small intestine help complete the process. The primary lipid-digesting enzymes secreted by the pancreas are **pancreatic lipase** and colipase. **Proteolytic enzymes** include trypsin and chymotrypsin, carboxypeptidase, aminopeptidase, ribonuclease, and deoxyribonuclease. Trypsin and chymotrypsin are secreted in their inactive forms and are activated by enterokinase (also known as enteropeptidase), which is bound within the brush border membrane of enterocytes within the small intestine. **Pancreatic amylase** eventually hydrolyzes large starch molecules into units of approximately two to six sugars. Disaccharidase enzymes bound in the enterocyte brush border membrane further break down the carbohydrate molecules into monosaccharides before absorption. Varying amounts of resistant starches and most ingested dietary fiber escape digestion in the small intestine and may add to fibrous material available for fermentation by colonic microbes.

Intestinal contents move along the small intestine at a rate of approximately 1 cm per minute, taking from 3 to 8 hours to travel through the entire intestine to the ileocecal valve; along the way, remaining substrates continue to be digested and absorbed. The ileocecal valve, like the pyloric sphincter, paces the entry of chyme into the colon and limits the amount of material passed back and forth between the small intestine and the colon. A damaged or nonfunctional ileocecal valve results in the entry of significant amounts of fluid and substrate into the colon and increases the chance for microbial overgrowth in the small intestine (see Chapter 28).

THE SMALL INTESTINE: PRIMARY SITE OF NUTRIENT ABSORPTION

The primary organ of nutrient and water absorption is the small intestine, which has an expansive absorptive area. The surface area is attributable to its extensive length, as well as to the organization of the mucosal lining. The small intestine has characteristic folds in its surface called *valvulae conniventes*. These convolutions are covered with fingerlike projections called *villi* (Figure 1-3), which in turn are covered by enterocytes that contain microvilli, or the **brush border membrane**. The combination of folds, villous projections, and microvillous border creates an enormous absorptive surface of approximately 200 to 300 m² - a surface area equivalent to a tennis court. The villi rest on a supporting structure called the *lamina propria*. Within the lamina propria, which is composed of connective tissue, the blood and lymph vessels receive the products of digestion.

Each day, on average, the small intestine absorbs 150 to 300 g of monosaccharides, 60 to 100 g of fatty acids, 60 to 120 g of amino acids and peptides, and 50 to 100 g of ions. The capacity for absorption in the healthy individual far exceeds the normal macronutrient and energy requirements. Approximately 95% of the bile salts secreted from the liver and gallbladder are reabsorbed as bile acids in the distal ileum. Without recycling bile acids from the GIT (enterohepatic circulation), synthesis of new bile acids in the liver would not keep pace with needs for adequate digestion. Bile salt insufficiency becomes clinically important in patients who have resections of the distal small bowel and diseases affecting the small intestine, such as Crohn's disease, radiation enteritis, and cystic fibrosis. The distal ileum is also the site for vitamin B_{12} (with intrinsic factor) absorption.

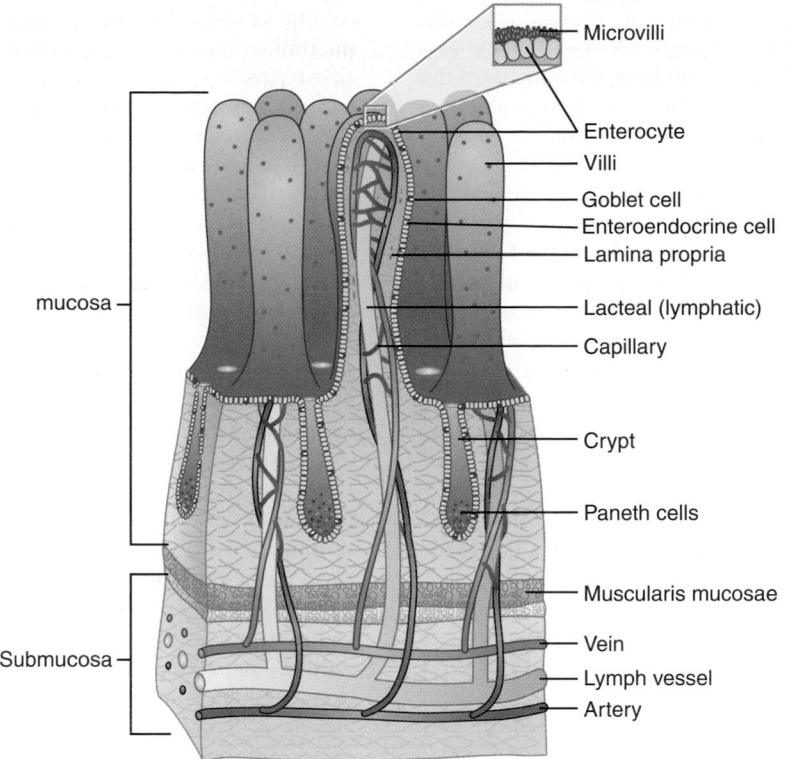

FIGURE 1-3 Structure of the human intestine showing crypt-villus architecture and blood and lymph vessels.

Absorptive and Transport Mechanisms

Absorption is a complex process involving many distinct pathways for specific nutrients and/or ions. However, the two basic transport mechanisms used are active and passive transport. The primary differences between the two are whether (1) energy in the form of ATP is required and (2) the nutrient being transported is moving with or against a concentration gradient.

Passive transport does not require energy, and nutrients move from a location of high concentration to low concentration. With passive transport a transport protein may or may not be involved. If the nutrient moves through the brush border membrane without a transport protein, this is termed passive diffusion, or simple passive transport. However, in cases in which a transport protein assists the passage of the nutrient across the brush border membrane, this process is termed facilitated diffusion (Figure 1-4).

Active transport is the movement of molecules across cell membranes in the direction *against* their concentration gradient and therefore requires a transporter protein and energy in the form of ATP. Some nutrients may share the same transporter and thus compete for absorption. Transport or carrier systems also can become saturated, slowing the absorption of the nutrient. A notable example of such a carrier is intrinsic factor, which is responsible for the absorption of vitamin B_{12} (see Chapter 27).

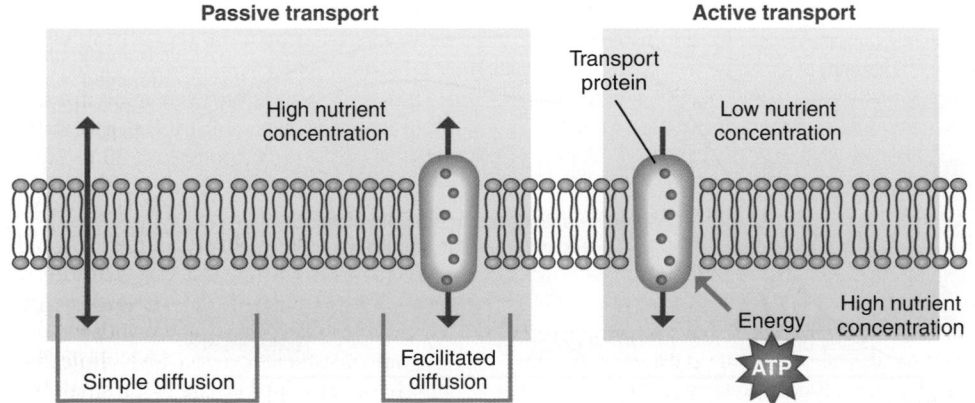

FIGURE 1-4 Transport pathways through the cell membrane, as well as basic transport mechanisms. *ATP,* Adenosine triphosphate.

THE LARGE INTESTINE

The large intestine is approximately 1.5 m long and consists of the cecum, colon, rectum, and anal tract. Mucus secreted by the mucosa of the large intestine protects the intestinal wall from excoriation and bacterial activity and provides the medium for binding the feces together. Bicarbonate ions secreted in exchange for absorbed chloride ions help to neutralize the acidic end products produced from bacterial action. Approximately 2 L of fluids are taken from food and beverages during the day, and 7 L of fluid is secreted along the GIT. Under normal circumstances, most of that fluid is absorbed in the small intestine, and approximately 2 L of fluid enters the large intestine. All but 100 to 150 ml of this fluid is absorbed; the remainder is excreted in the feces.

The large intestine is also the site of bacterial fermentation of remaining carbohydrates and amino acids, synthesis of a small amount of vitamins (particularly vitamin K), storage, and excretion of fecal residues. Colonic contents move forward slowly at a rate of 5 cm/h, and some remaining nutrients may be absorbed.

Defecation, or expulsion of feces through the rectum and anus, occurs with varying frequency, ranging from three times daily to once every 3 or more days. Average stool weight ranges from 100 to 200 g, and mouth-to-anus transit time may vary from 18 to 72 hours. The feces generally consist of 75% water and 25% solids, but the proportions vary greatly. Approximately two thirds of the contents of the wet weight of the stool is bacteria, with the remainder coming from gastrointestinal secretions, mucus, sloughed cells, microbiota, and undigested foods. A diet that includes abundant fruits, vegetables, legumes, and whole grains typically results in a shorter overall GIT transit time, more frequent defecation, and larger and softer stools.

Intestinal Microbiota: The Microbiome

The intestinal microbiota, also called the microbiome, is a dynamic mixture of essential microbes that develops under key influences of genetics, environment, diet, and disease. Bacterial population profiles differ along the gastrointestinal tract, from the lumen to the mucosa, and among individuals. The total microbiota population outnumbers the cells in the human body by a factor of 10 and accounts for 35% to 50% of the volume of the colonic content. Key physiologic functions of the commensal microbiota include (1) protective effects exerted directly by specific bacterial species, (2) control of epithelial cell proliferation and differentiation, (3) production of essential mucosal nutrients, such as short-chain fatty acids and amino acids, (4) prevention of overgrowth of pathogenic organisms, (5) stimulation of intestinal immunity, and (6) development of the gut-brain axis (Kostic et al, 2014; see Chapter 41). Reduced abundance or changes in the relative proportions of these beneficial bacteria, a state called dysbiosis, is associated with various diseases in both children and adults (Buccigrossi et al, 2013; Figure 1-5).

Normally, relatively few bacteria remain in the stomach or small intestine after meals because bile, hydrochloric acid, and pepsin work as germicides. However, decreased gastric secretions can increase the risk of inflammation of the gastric mucosa (*gastritis*), increase the risk of bacterial overgrowth in the small intestine, or increase the numbers of microbes reaching the colon. An acid-tolerant bacterium is known to infect the stomach (*Helicobacter pylori*) and may cause gastritis and ulceration in the host (see Chapter 27).

Bacterial action is most intense in the distal small intestine and the large intestine. After a meal, dietary fiber, resistant starches, remaining bits of amino acids, and mucus sloughed from the intestine are fermented by the microbes present. This process of fermentation produces gases (e.g., hydrogen, carbon dioxide, nitrogen, and, in some individuals, methane) and SCFAs (e.g., acetic, propionic, butyric, and some lactic acids). During the process, several nutrients are formed by bacterial synthesis, such as vitamin K, vitamin B_{12}, thiamin, and riboflavin.

Strategies to stabilize and fortify the beneficial microbes within the microbiota in an attempt to maintain or improve health include the consumption of prebiotics, probiotics, and synbiotics.

Probiotics are live microorganisms, which, when administered in adequate amounts, provide a health benefit to the host. Probiotics can be found within fermented food products (such as miso or sauerkraut) or as a nutritional supplement (Hill et al, 2014). Knowledge of their role in preventing and treating a host of gastrointestinal and systemic disorders has expanded tremendously (Tappenden and Deutsch, 2007; Floch, 2014) in recent years. However, when recommending a probiotic,

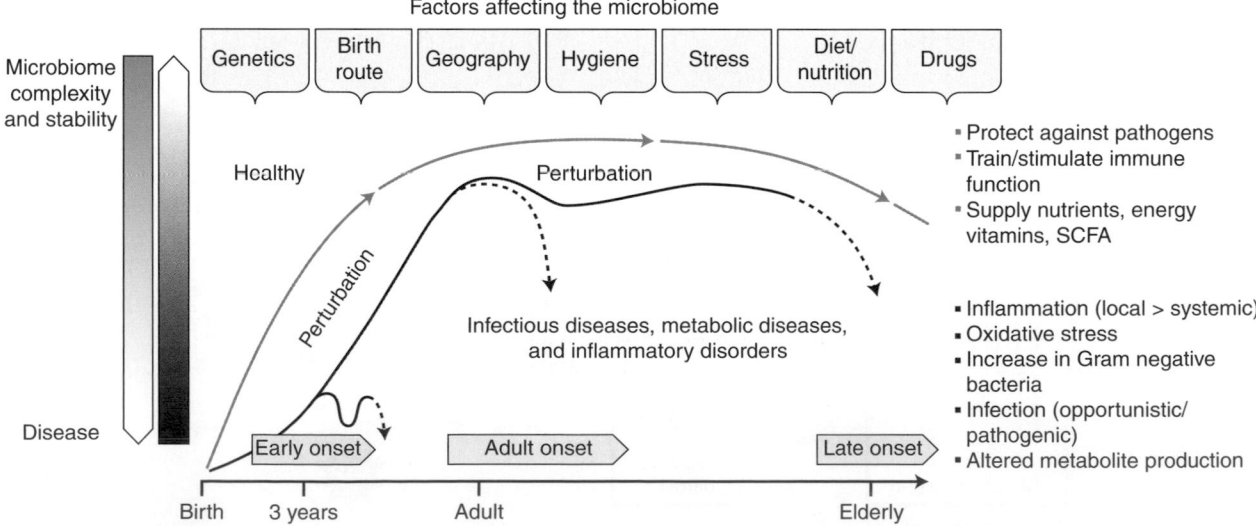

FIGURE 1-5 Factors affecting stability and complexity of intestinal microbiota in health and disease. (Redrawn from Kostic AD et al: The microbiome in inflammatory bowel disease: current status and the future ahead, *Gastroenterology* 146:1489, 2014.)

practitioners must ensure that the specific microbial species has been shown in properly controlled studies to provide benefits to health (see Chapter 12).

Prebiotics are nondigestible food ingredients that have a specific stimulatory effect upon selected populations of GIT bacteria. Prebiotics typically require the following three attributes to benefit "beneficial" microbes such as *Lactobacilli* and *Bifidobacteria* spp.: (1) be able to escape digestion in the upper GIT, (2) be able to be fermented by the microbiota to SCFA(s), and (3) be able to increase the abundance and/or relative proportion of bacteria known to contribute to human health. Good dietary sources of prebiotic carbohydrates are vegetables, grains, and legumes, chicory, Jerusalem artichokes, soybeans, and wheat bran. Strong evidence exists for the use of specific prebiotics in reducing the extent of diarrhea and immune stimulation, and improving mineral bioavailability (Rastall and Gibson, 2014). **Synbiotics** are a synergistic combination of probiotics and prebiotics in the same food or supplement.

Colonic Salvage of Malabsorbed Energy Sources and Short-Chain Fatty Acids

Normally, varying amounts of some small-molecular-weight carbohydrates and amino acids remain in the chyme after leaving the small intestine. Accumulation of these small molecules could become osmotically important were it not for the action of bacteria in the colon. The disposal of residual substrates through production of SCFAs is called colonic salvage. SCFAs produced in fermentation are rapidly absorbed and take water with them. They also serve as fuel for the colonocytes and the microbiota, stimulate colonocyte proliferation and differentiation, enhance the absorption of electrolytes and water, and reduce the osmotic load of malabsorbed sugars. SCFAs also may help slow the movement of GI contents and participate in several other regulatory functions.

The ability to salvage carbohydrates is limited in humans. Colonic fermentation normally disposes of 20 to 25 g of carbohydrate over 24 hours. Excess amounts of carbohydrate and fermentable fiber in the colon can cause increased gas production, abdominal distention, bloating, pain, flatulence, decreased colonic pH, and diarrhea. Over time, adaptation occurs in individuals consuming diets high in fiber. Current recommendations are for the consumption of approximately 14 g of dietary fiber per 1000 kcal consumed each day. This recommendation can be met by consuming ample fruits, vegetables, legumes, seeds, and whole grains and is aimed to (1) maintain the health of the colonic epithelium, (2) prevent constipation, and (3) support stable, health-promoting microbiota.

Digestion and Absorption of Specific Types of Nutrients
Carbohydrates and Fiber

Most dietary carbohydrates are consumed in the form of starches, disaccharides, and monosaccharides. Starches, or polysaccharides, usually make up the greatest proportion of carbohydrates. Starches are large molecules composed of straight or branched chains of sugar molecules that are joined together, primarily in alpha 1-4 or 1-6 linkages. Most of the dietary starches are *amylopectins,* the branching polysaccharides, and *amylose,* the straight chain–type polymers.

Dietary fiber also is made largely of chains and branches of sugar molecules, but in this case the hydrogens are positioned on the beta (opposite) side of the oxygen in the link instead of the alpha side. Humans have significant ability to digest starch but not most fiber; this exemplifies the "stereospecificity" of enzymes.

In the mouth, the enzyme salivary amylase operates at a neutral or slightly alkaline pH and starts the digestive action by hydrolyzing a small amount of the starch molecules into smaller fragments (Figure 1-6). Amylase deactivates after contact with hydrochloric acid. If digestible carbohydrates remained in the stomach long enough, acid hydrolysis could eventually reduce most of them into monosaccharides. However, the stomach usually empties before significant digestion can take place. By far, most carbohydrate digestion occurs in the proximal small intestine.

Pancreatic amylase breaks the large starch molecules at the 1-4 linkages to create maltose, maltotriose, and "alpha-limit" dextrins remaining from the amylopectin branches. Enzymes from the brush border of the enterocytes further break the disaccharides and oligosaccharides into monosaccharides. For example, maltase located at the enterocyte brush border membrane breaks down the disaccharide maltose into two molecules

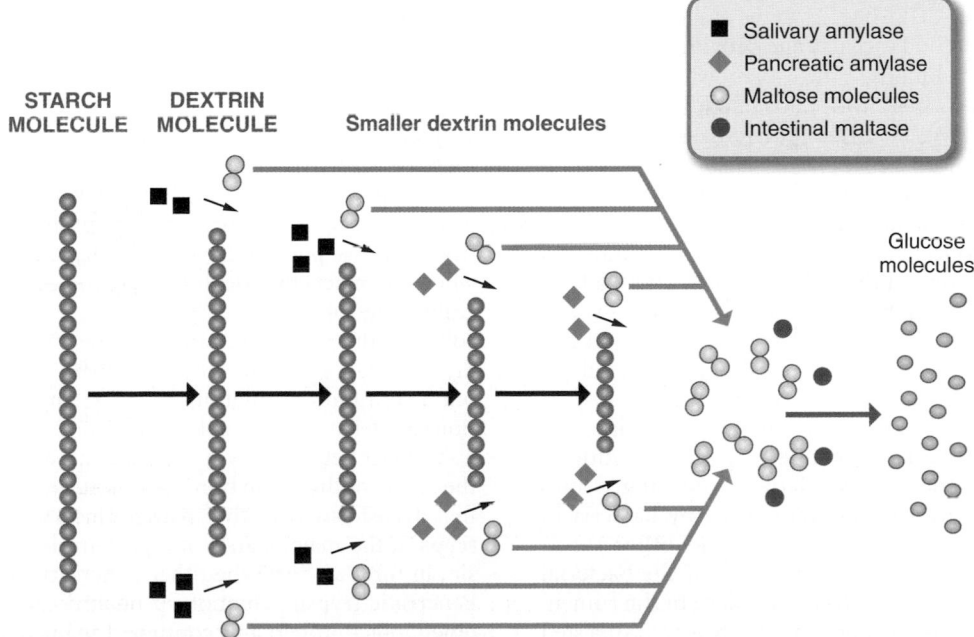

FIGURE 1-6 The gradual breakdown of large starch molecules into glucose by digestion enzymes.

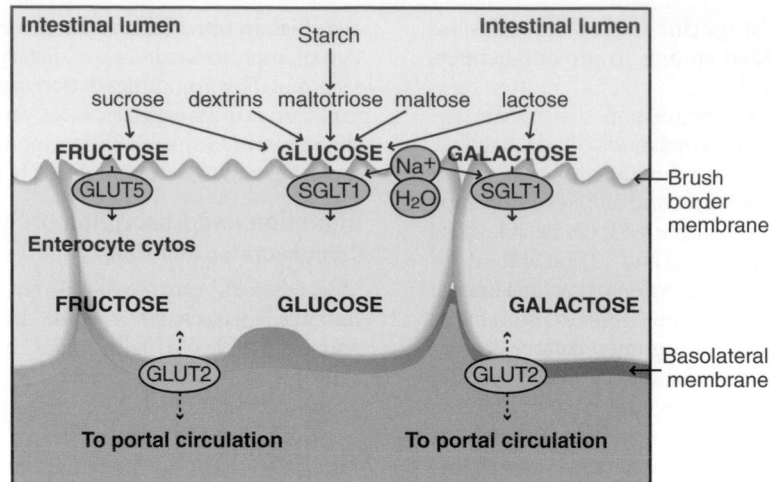

FIGURE 1-7 Starch, sucrose, maltotriose, and galactose are digested to their constituent sugars. Glucose and galactose are transported through the apical brush border membrane of the enterocyte by a sodium-dependent transporter, glucose (galactose) cotransporter; fructose is transported by glucose transporter 5 (GLUT5). Glucose, fructose, and galactose are transported across the serosal membrane by the sodium-independent transporter, GLUT2.

of glucose. The brush border membrane also contains the enzymes **sucrase**, **lactase**, and isomaltase, which act on sucrose, lactose, and isomaltose, respectively (Figure 1-7).

The resultant monosaccharides (i.e., glucose, galactose, and fructose) pass through the enterocytes and into the bloodstream via the capillaries of the villi, where they are carried by the portal vein to the liver. At low concentrations, glucose and galactose are absorbed by active transport, primarily by a sodium-dependent active transporter called the sodium-glucose cotransporter (SGLT1). At higher luminal concentrations of glucose, the facilitative transporter GLUT2 becomes a primary route for transport of glucose from the lumen into the enterocyte. Fructose is absorbed from the intestinal lumen across the brush border membrane using the facilitative transporter, GLUT5. All three monosaccharides—glucose, galactose, and fructose—exit the basolateral membrane of the enterocyte into portal circulation using the facilitative transporter, GLUT2.

The active transporter, SGLT1, is key to the ability of the small intestine to absorb 7 L of fluid each day and provides the basis for why oral rehydration solutions, rather than water or sugary drinks, should be used to treat hydration. In addition to transporting sodium and glucose, SGLT1 functions as a molecular water pump. For each molecule of glucose absorbed by SGLT1, two molecules of sodium and 210 molecules of water also are absorbed. Given that this is a major pathway for water absorption in the small intestine, to facilitate water absorption, sodium and glucose also must be present in the right amounts. This explains why the most effective oral rehydration solutions often include both sugar and salt, in addition to water (see Chapters 6 and 23).

Some forms of carbohydrates (i.e., cellulose, hemicellulose, pectin, gum, and other forms of fiber) cannot be digested by humans because neither salivary nor pancreatic amylase has the ability to split the linkages connecting the constituent sugars. These carbohydrates pass relatively unchanged into the colon, where they are partially fermented by bacteria in the colon. However, unlike humans, cows and other ruminants can subsist on high-fiber food because of the bacterial digestion of these carbohydrates that takes place in the rumen. Other resistant starches and sugars are also less well digested or absorbed by humans; thus their consumption may result in

significant amounts of starch and sugar in the colon. These resistant starches and some types of dietary fiber are fermented into SCFAs and gases. Starches resistant to digestion tend to include plant foods with a high protein and fiber content such as those from legumes and whole grains. One form of dietary fiber, lignin, is made of cyclopentane units and is neither readily soluble nor fermentable.

Proteins

Protein intake in the Western world ranges from approximately 50 to 100 g daily, and a good deal of the protein consumed is from animal sources. Additional protein is added all along the GIT from gastrointestinal secretions and sloughed epithelial cells. The GIT is one of the most active synthetic tissues in the body, and the life span of enterocytes migrating from the crypts of the villi until they are shed is only 3 to 4 days. The number of cells shed daily is in the range of 10 to 20 billion. The latter accounts for an additional 50 to 60 g of protein that is digested and "recycled" and contributes to the daily supply. In general, animal proteins are more efficiently digested than plant proteins, but human physiology allows for very effective digestion and absorption of large amounts of ingested protein sources.

Protein digestion begins in the stomach, where some of the proteins are split into proteoses, peptones, and large polypeptides. Inactive pepsinogen is converted into the enzyme pepsin when it contacts hydrochloric acid and other pepsin molecules. Unlike any of the other proteolytic enzymes, pepsin digests collagen, the major protein of connective tissue. Most protein digestion takes place in the upper portion of the small intestine, but it continues throughout the GIT. Any residual protein fractions are fermented by colonic microbes.

Contact between chyme and the intestinal mucosa allows for the action of the brush border–bound **enterokinase**, an enzyme that transforms inactive pancreatic **trypsinogen** into active **trypsin**, the major pancreatic protein-digesting enzyme. Trypsin, in turn, activates the other pancreatic proteolytic enzymes. Pancreatic trypsin, chymotrypsin, and carboxypeptidase break down intact protein and continue the breakdown started in the stomach until small polypeptides and amino acids are formed.

Proteolytic peptidases located on the brush border also act on polypeptides, breaking them down into amino acids, dipeptides, and tripeptides. The final phase of protein digestion takes place in the brush border, where some of the dipeptides and tripeptides are hydrolyzed into their constituent amino acids by peptide hydrolases.

End products of protein digestion are absorbed as both amino acids and small peptides. Several transport molecules are required for the different amino acids, probably because of the wide differences in the size, polarity, and configuration of the different amino acids. Some of the transporters are sodium or chloride dependent, and some are not. Considerable amounts of dipeptides and tripeptides also are absorbed into intestinal cells using a peptide transporter, a form of active transport (Wuensch et al, 2013). Absorbed peptides and amino acids are transported to the liver via the portal vein for metabolism by the liver and are released into the general circulation.

The presence of antibodies to many food proteins in the circulation of healthy individuals indicates that immunologically significant amounts of large intact peptides escape hydrolysis and can enter the portal circulation. The exact mechanisms that cause a food to become an allergen are not entirely clear, but these foods tend to be high in protein, to be relatively resistant to complete digestion, and to produce an immunoglobulin response (see Chapter 26). With new technology, it is possible to map and characterize allergenic peptides; this eventually will lead to better diagnosis and development of safe immunotherapy treatments (Melioli et al, 2014).

Almost all protein is absorbed by the time it reaches the end of the jejunum, and only 1% of ingested protein is found in the feces. Small amounts of amino acids may remain in the epithelial cells and are used for synthesis of new proteins, including intestinal enzymes and new cells.

Lipids

Approximately 97% of dietary lipids are in the form of triglycerides, and the rest are found as phospholipids and cholesterol. Only small amounts of fat are digested in the mouth by lingual lipase and in the stomach from the action of gastric lipase. Gastric lipase hydrolyzes some triglycerides, especially short-chain triglycerides (such as those found in butter), into fatty acids and glycerol. However, most fat digestion takes place in the small intestine as a result of the emulsifying action of bile salts and hydrolysis by pancreatic lipase. As in the case of carbohydrates and protein, the capacity for digestion and absorption of dietary fat is in excess of ordinary needs.

Entrance of fat and protein into the small intestine stimulates the release of CCK, secretin, and GIP, which inhibit gastric secretions and motility, thus slowing the delivery of lipids. As a result, a portion of a large, fatty meal may remain in the stomach for 4 hours or longer. In addition to its many other functions, CCK stimulates biliary and pancreatic secretions. The combination of the peristaltic action of the small intestine and the surfactant and emulsification action of bile reduces the fat globules into tiny droplets, thus making them more accessible to digestion by the most potent lipid-digesting enzyme, pancreatic lipase.

Bile is a liver secretion composed of bile acids (primarily conjugates of cholic and chenodeoxycholic acids with glycine or taurine), bile pigments (which color the feces), inorganic salts, some protein, cholesterol, lecithin, and many compounds such as detoxified drugs that are metabolized and secreted by the liver. From its storage organ, the gallbladder, approximately 1 L

of bile is secreted daily in response to the stimulus of food in the duodenum and stomach.

Emulsification of fats in the small intestine is followed by their digestion, primarily by pancreatic lipase, into free fatty acids and monoglycerides. Pancreatic lipase typically cleaves the first and third fatty acids, leaving a single fatty acid esterified to the middle glycerol carbon. When the concentration of bile salts reaches a certain level, they form micelles (small aggregates of fatty acids, monoglycerides, cholesterol, bile salts, and other lipids), which are organized with the polar ends of the molecules oriented toward the watery lumen of the intestine. The products of lipid digestion are solubilized rapidly in the central portion of the micelles and carried to the intestinal brush border (Figure 1-8).

At the surface of the unstirred water layer (UWL), the slightly acidic and watery plate that forms a boundary between the intestinal lumen and the brush border membranes, the lipids detach from the micelles. Remnants of the micelles return to the lumen for further transport. The monoglycerides and fatty acids thus are left to make their way across the lipophobic UWL to the more lipid-friendly membrane cells of the brush border. Upon release of the lipid components, luminal bile salts are reabsorbed actively in the terminal ileum and returned to the liver to reenter the gut in bile secretions. This efficient recycling process is known as the enterohepatic circulation. The pool of bile acids may circulate from 3 to 15 times per day, depending on the amount of food ingested.

The cellular mechanism(s) whereby fatty acids traverse the brush-border membrane include both passive diffusion (a form of transport that does not require energy), and active transport processes. Traditionally, the absorption of lipid was thought to be passive, wherein lipid molecules would solubilize through the brush border membrane in a manner driven by diffusion down the concentration gradient into the enterocyte. The inwardly directed concentration gradient was thought to be maintained in the fed state by the high concentration of fatty acids within the intestinal lumen and the rapid scavenging of free fatty acids for triglyceride reformation once inside the enterocyte. Current theories indicate that passive diffusion and carrier-mediated mechanisms contribute to lipid absorption. At low fatty acid concentrations, carrier-mediated mechanisms take precedence with little passive diffusion occurring. However, when free fatty acid concentration in the intestinal lumen is high, absorption of fatty acids via passive diffusion becomes quantitatively important.

In the enterocyte, the fatty acids and monoglycerides are reassembled into new triglycerides. Others are further digested into free fatty acids and glycerol and then reassembled to form triglycerides. These triglycerides, along with cholesterol, fat-soluble vitamins, and phospholipids, are surrounded by a lipoprotein coat, forming chylomicrons (see Figure 1-8). The lipoprotein globules pass into the lymphatic system instead of entering portal blood and are transported to the thoracic duct and emptied into the systemic circulation at the junction of the left internal jugular and left subclavian veins. The chylomicrons then are carried through the bloodstream to several tissues, including liver, adipose tissue, and muscle. In the liver, triglycerides from the chylomicrons are repackaged into very low–density lipoproteins and transported primarily to the adipose tissue for metabolism and storage.

Under normal conditions approximately 95% to 97% of ingested fat is absorbed into lymph vessels. Because of their shorter length and thus increased solubility, fatty acids of 8 to 12 carbons (i.e., medium-chain fatty acids) can be absorbed directly into colonic mucosal cells without the presence of bile and micelle formation. After entering mucosal cells, they are

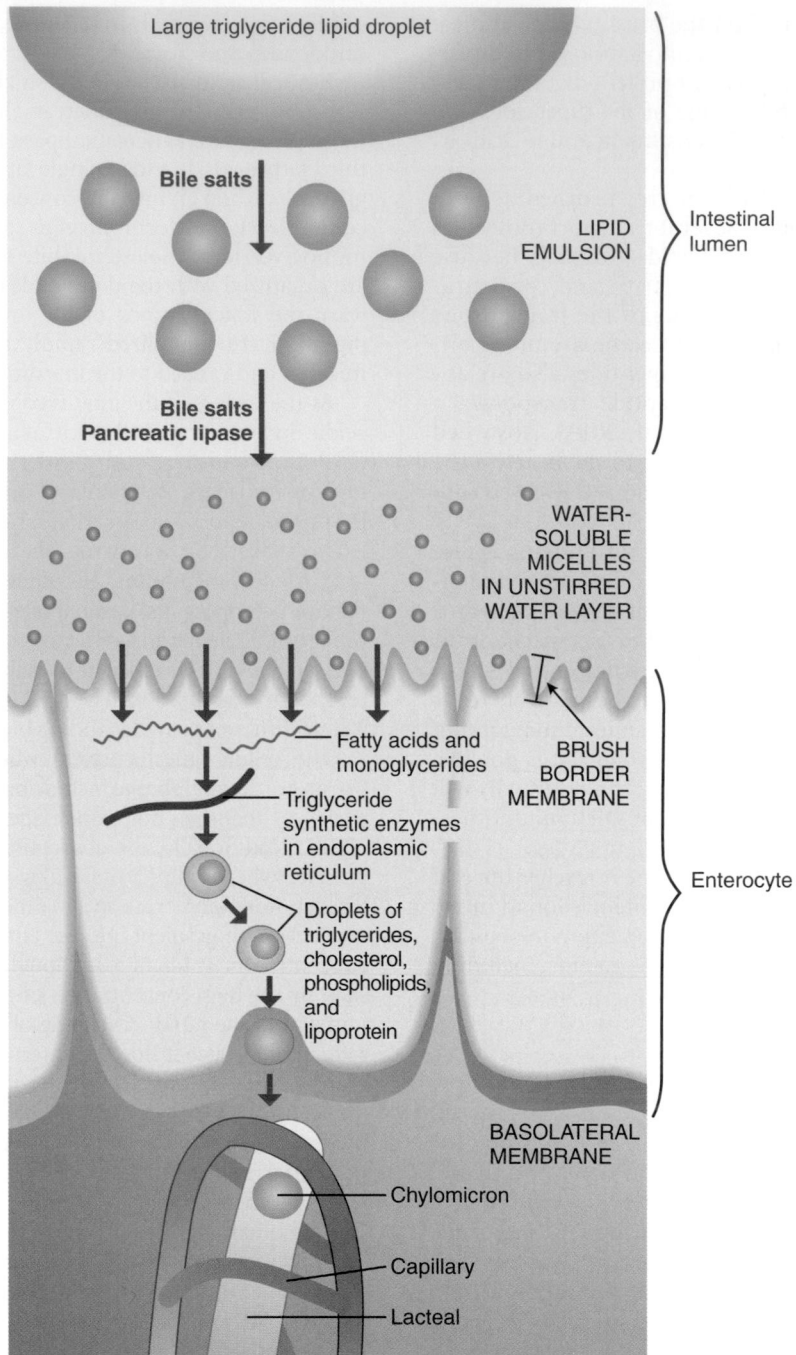

FIGURE 1-8 Summary of fat absorption.

able to go directly without esterification into the portal vein, which carries them to the liver.

Increased motility, intestinal mucosal changes, pancreatic insufficiency, or the absence of bile can decrease the absorption of fat. When undigested fat appears in the feces, the condition is known as steatorrhea (see Chapter 28). Medium-chain triglycerides (MCTs) have fatty acids 8 to 12 carbons long; MCTs are clinically valuable for individuals who lack necessary bile salts for long-chain fatty acid metabolism and transport. Supplements for clinical use normally are provided in the form of oil or a dietary beverage with other macronutrients and micronutrients.

Vitamins and Minerals

Vitamins and minerals from foods are made available as macronutrients and are digested and absorbed across the mucosal layer, primarily in the small intestine (Figure 1-9). Besides adequate passive and transporter mechanisms, various factors affect the bioavailability of vitamins and minerals, including the presence or absence of other specific nutrients, acid or alkali, phytates, and oxalates. The liters of fluid that are secreted each day from the GIT serve as a solvent, a vehicle for chemical reactions, and a medium for transfer of several nutrients.

At least some vitamins and water pass unchanged from the small intestine into the blood by passive diffusion, but several

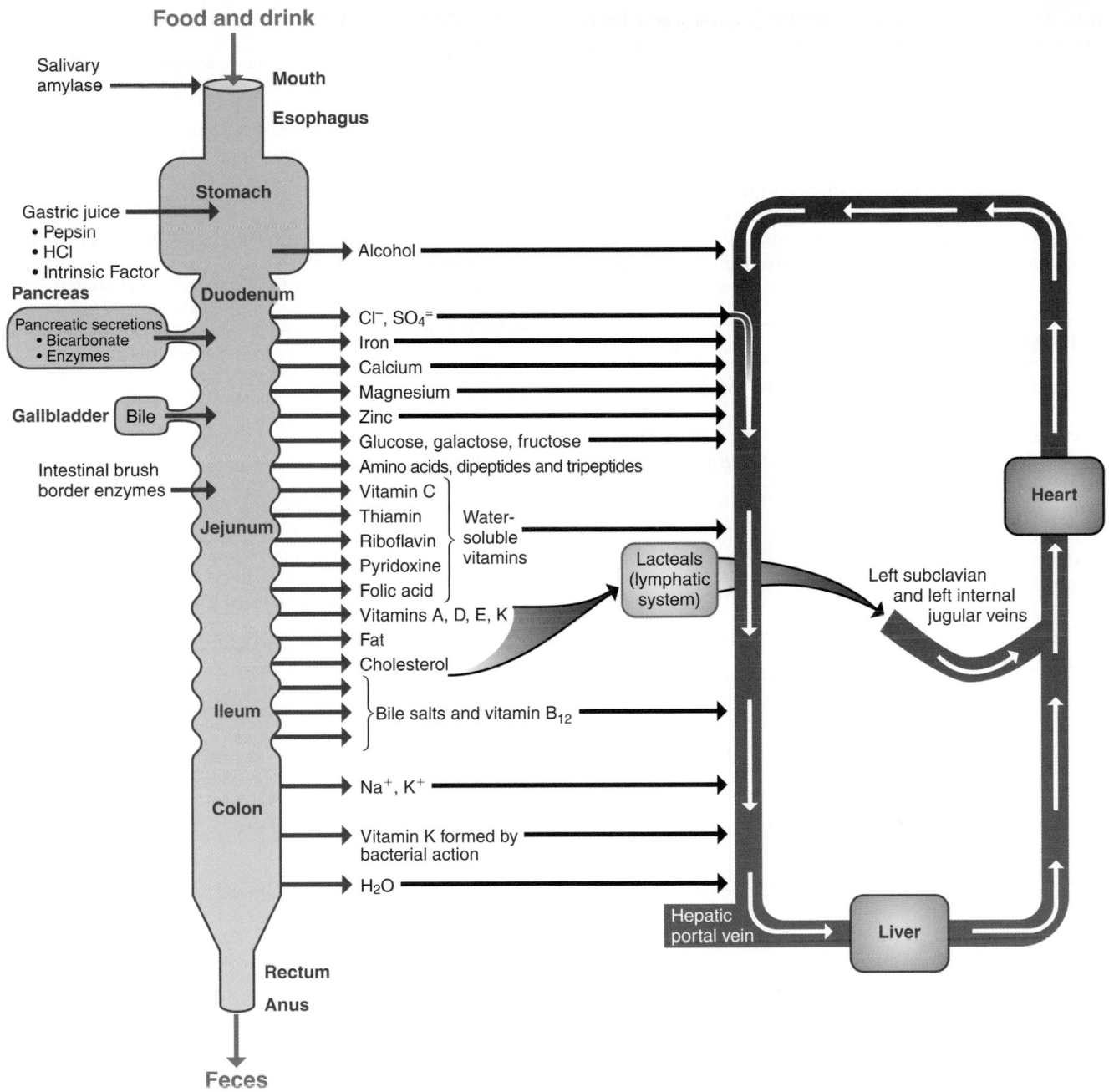

FIGURE 1-9 Sites of secretion and absorption in the gastrointestinal tract.

different mechanisms may be used to transport individual vitamins across the mucosa. Drugs are absorbed by a number of mechanisms but often by passive diffusion. Thus drugs may share or compete with mechanisms for the absorption nutrients into intestinal cells (see Chapter 8).

Mineral absorption is more complex, especially the absorption of the cation minerals. These cations, such as selenium, are made available for absorption by the process of **chelation**, in which a mineral is bound to a ligand—usually an acid, an organic acid, or an amino acid—so that it is in a form absorbable by intestinal cells.

Iron and zinc absorption share several characteristics in that the efficiency of absorption partly depends on the needs of the host. They also use at least one transport protein, and each has mechanisms to increase absorption when stores are inadequate. Because

phytates and oxalates from plants impair the absorption of iron and zinc, absorption is better when animal sources are consumed. The absorption of zinc is impaired with disproportionately increased amounts of magnesium, calcium, and iron. Calcium absorption into the enterocyte occurs through channels in the brush border membrane, where it is bound to a specific protein carrier for transportation across the basolateral membrane. The process is regulated by the presence of vitamin D. Phosphorus is absorbed by a sodium phosphorus cotransporter, which also is regulated by vitamin D or low phosphate intake.

The GIT is the site of important interactions among minerals. Supplementation with large amounts of iron or zinc may decrease the absorption of copper. In turn, the presence of copper may lower iron and molybdenum absorption. Cobalt absorption is increased in patients with iron deficiency, but cobalt and iron compete and inhibit one another's absorption. These interactions are probably the result of an overlap of mineral absorption mechanisms.

Minerals are transported in blood bound to protein carriers. The protein binding is either specific (e.g., transferrin, which binds with iron, or ceruloplasmin, which binds with copper) or general (e.g., albumin, which binds with a variety of minerals). A fraction of each mineral also is carried in the serum as amino acid or peptide complexes. Specific protein carriers are usually not completely saturated; the reserve capacity may serve as a buffer against excessive exposure. Toxicity from minerals usually results only after this buffering capacity is exceeded.

USEFUL WEBSITES

American Gastroenterological Association (AGA)
http://www.gastro.org/
AGA Center for Gut Microbiome Research and Education
http://www.gastro.org/research/aga-center-for-gut-microbiome-research-and-education
NIH Digestive Diseases
http://digestive.niddk.nih.gov/
NIH Human Microbiome Project
http://commonfund.nih.gov/hmp/index

REFERENCES

Buccigrossi V, et al: Functions of intestinal microflora in children, *Curr Opin Gastroenterol* 29:31, 2013.

Chey WY, Chang TM: Secretin: historical perspective and current status, *Pancreas* 43:162, 2014.

Chu S, Schubert ML: Gastric secretion, *Curr Opin Gastroenterol* 29:636, 2013.

De Smet B, et al: Motilin and ghrelin as prokinetic drug targets, *Pharmacol Ther* 123:207, 2009.

Dockray GJ: Cholecystokinin, *Curr Opin Endocrinol Diabetes Obes* 19:8, 2012.

Floch MH: Recommendations for probiotic use in humans—a 2014 update, *Pharmaceuticals (Basel)* 7:999, 2014.

Hill C, et al: Expert consensus document. The International Scientific Association for Probiotics and Prebiotics statement on the scope and appropriate use of the term probiotic, *Nat Rev Gastroenterol Hepatol* 11:506, 2014.

Hylemon PB, et al: Bile acids as regulatory molecules, *J Lipid Res* 50:1509, 2009.

Kellett G, Brot-Laroche E: Apical GLUT2: a major pathway of intestinal sugar absorption, *Diabetes* 54:3056, 2005.

Kostic AD, et al: The microbiome in inflammatory bowel disease: current status and the future ahead, *Gastroenterology* 146:1489, 2014.

Melioli G, et al: Novel in silico technology in combination with microarrays: a state-of-the-art technology for allergy diagnosis and management? *Expert Rev Clin Immunol* 10:1559, 2014.

Rastall RA, Gibson GR: Recent developments in prebiotics to selectively impact beneficial microbes and promote intestinal health, *Curr Opin Biotechnol* 32C:42, 2014.

Rehfeld JF: Gastrointestinal hormones and their targets, *Adv Exp Med Biol* 817:157, 2014.

Rui L: Brain regulation of energy balance and body weight, *Rev Endocr Metab Disord* 14:387, 2013.

Seidner DL, et al: Increased intestinal absorption in the era of teduglutide and its impact on management strategies in patients with short bowel syndrome-associated intestinal failure, *JPEN J Parenter Enteral Nutr* 37:201, 2013.

Tappenden KA, Deutsch AS: The physiological relevance of the intestinal microbiota-contributions to human health, *J Am Coll Nutr* 26:679S, 2007.

Van Op den Bosch J, et al: The role(s) of somatostatin, structurally related peptides and somatostatin receptors in the gastrointestinal tract: a review, *Regul Pept* 156:1, 2009.

Wuensch T, et al: The peptide transporter PEPT1 is expressed in distal colon in rodents and humans and contributes to water absorption, *Am J Physiol Gastrointest Liver Physiol* 305:G66, 2013.

Intake: Energy

Carol S. Ireton-Jones, PhD, RDN, LD, CNSC, FAND, FASPEN

KEY TERMS

activity thermogenesis (AT)
basal energy expenditure (BEE)
basal metabolic rate (BMR)
calorie
direct calorimetry
estimated energy requirement (EER)
excess postexercise oxygen consumption (EPOC)
facultative thermogenesis

fat-free mass (FFM)
high-metabolic-rate organ (HMRO)
indirect calorimetry (IC)
kilocalorie (kcal)
lean body mass (LBM)
metabolic equivalents (METs)
nonexercise activity thermogenesis (NEAT)

obligatory thermogenesis
physical activity level (PAL)
resting energy expenditure (REE)
resting metabolic rate (RMR)
respiratory quotient (RQ)
thermic effect of food (TEF)
total energy expenditure (TEE)

Energy may be defined as "the capacity to do work." The ultimate source of all energy in living organisms is the sun. Through the process of photosynthesis, green plants intercept a portion of the sunlight reaching their leaves and capture it within the chemical bonds of glucose. Proteins, fats, and other carbohydrates are synthesized from this basic carbohydrate to meet the needs of the plant. Animals and humans obtain these nutrients and the energy they contain by consuming plants and the flesh of other animals.

The body makes use of the energy from dietary carbohydrates, proteins, fats, and alcohol; this energy is locked in chemical bonds within food and is released through metabolism. Energy must be supplied regularly to meet needs for the body's survival. Although all energy eventually takes the form of heat, which dissipates into the atmosphere, unique cellular processes first make possible its use for all of the tasks required for life. These processes involve chemical reactions that maintain body tissues, electrical conduction of the nerves, mechanical work of the muscles, and heat production to maintain body temperature.

ENERGY REQUIREMENTS

Energy requirements are defined as the dietary energy intake that is required for growth or maintenance in a person of a defined age, gender, weight, height, and level of physical activity. In children and pregnant or lactating women, energy requirements include the needs associated with the deposition of tissues or the secretion of milk at rates consistent with good health. In ill or injured people, the stressors have an effect by increasing or decreasing energy expenditure.

Body weight is one indicator of energy adequacy or inadequacy. The body has the unique ability to shift the fuel mixture of carbohydrates, proteins, and fats to accommodate energy needs. However, consuming too much or too little energy over time results in body weight changes. Thus body weight reflects adequacy of energy intake, but it is not a reliable indicator of macronutrient or micronutrient adequacy.

In addition, because body weight is affected by body composition, a person with a higher lean mass to body fat mass or body fat mass to lean mass may require differing energy intakes compared with the norm or "average" person. Obese individuals have higher energy needs as a result of an increase in body fat mass and lean body mass (Kee et al, 2012).

COMPONENTS OF ENERGY EXPENDITURE

Energy is expended by the human body in the form of basal energy expenditure (BEE), thermic effect of food (TEF), and activity thermogenesis (AT). These three components make up a person's daily total energy expenditure (TEE).

Basal and Resting Energy Expenditure

BEE, or basal metabolic rate (BMR), is the minimum amount of energy expended that is compatible with life. An individual's BEE reflects the amount of energy used during 24 hours while physically and mentally at rest in a thermoneutral environment that prevents the activation of heat-generating processes, such as shivering. Measurements of BEE should be done before an individual has engaged in any physical activity (preferably on awakening from sleep) and 10 to 12 hours after the ingestion of any food, drink, or nicotine. The BEE remains remarkably constant on a daily basis.

Resting energy expenditure (REE), or resting metabolic rate (RMR), is the energy expended in the activities necessary to sustain normal body functions and homeostasis. These activities include respiration and circulation, the synthesis of organic compounds, and the pumping of ions across membranes. REE, or RMR, includes the energy required by the central nervous system and for the maintenance of body temperature. It does not include thermogenesis, activity, or other energy expenditure and is higher than the BEE by 10% to 20% (Ireton-Jones, 2010). The terms *REE* and *RMR* and *BEE* and *BMR* can be used interchangeably, but *REE* and *BEE* are used in this chapter.

Factors Affecting Resting Energy Expenditure

Numerous factors cause the REE to vary among individuals, but body size and composition have the greatest effect. See Chapter 7 for discussion of methods used to determine body composition.

Age. Because REE is highly affected by the proportion of lean body mass (LBM), it is highest during periods of rapid growth, especially the first and second years of life. Growing infants may store as much as 12% to 15% of the energy value of their food in the form of new tissue. As a child becomes older, the energy requirement for growth is reduced to approximately 1% of TEE. After early adulthood there is a decline in REE of 1% to 2% per kilogram of fat-free mass (FFM) per decade (Keys et al, 1973). Fortunately, exercise can help maintain a higher LBM and a higher REE. Decreases in REE with increasing age may be partly related to age-associated changes in the relative size of LBM components (Cooper et al, 2013).

Body composition. FFM, or LBM, makes up the majority of metabolically active tissue in the body and is the primary predictor of REE. FFM contributes to approximately 80% of the variations in REE (Bosy-Westphal et al, 2004). Because of their greater FFM, athletes with greater muscular development have an approximately 5% higher resting metabolism than nonathletic individuals. Organs in the body contribute to heat production (Figure 2-1). Approximately 60% of REE can be accounted for by the heat produced by high-metabolic-rate organs (HMROs): the liver, brain, heart, spleen, intestines, and kidneys (McClave and Snider, 2001). Indeed, differences in FFM between ethnic groups may be related to the total mass of these as well as musculature (Gallagher et al, 2006). Relatively small individual variation in the mass of the liver, brain, heart, spleen, and kidneys, collectively or individually, can significantly affect REE (Javed et al, 2010). As a result, estimating the percentage of energy expenditure that appendages (arms and legs) account for in overall daily energy expenditure is difficult, although it is presumably a small amount.

Body size. Larger people generally have higher metabolic rates than smaller people, but tall, thin people have higher metabolic rates than short, stocky people. For example, if two people weigh the same but one person is taller, the taller person has a larger body surface area and a higher metabolic rate. The amount of LBM is highly correlated with total body size. For example, obese children have higher REEs than nonobese children, but, when REE is adjusted for body composition, FFM, and fat mass, no REE differences are found (Byrne et al, 2003). This provides a conundrum for the practitioner when using the BMI to assess health (see Chapter 7).

Climate. The REE is affected by extremes in environmental temperature. People living in tropical climates usually have REEs that are 5% to 20% higher than those living in temperate areas. Exercise in temperatures greater than 86°F imposes a small additional metabolic load of approximately 5% from increased sweat gland activity. The extent to which energy metabolism increases in extremely cold environments depends on the insulation available from body fat and protective clothing (Dobratz et al, 2007).

Gender. Gender differences in metabolic rates are attributable primarily to differences in body size and composition. Women, who generally have more fat in proportion to muscle than men, have metabolic rates that are approximately 5% to 10% lower than men of the same weight and height. However, with aging, this difference becomes less pronounced (Cooper et al, 2013).

Hormonal status. Hormones affect metabolic rate. Endocrine disorders, such as hyperthyroidism and hypothyroidism, increase or decrease energy expenditure, respectively (see Chapter 31). Stimulation of the sympathetic nervous system during periods of emotional excitement or stress causes the release of epinephrine, which promotes glycogenolysis and increased cellular activity. Ghrelin and peptide YY are gut hormones involved in appetite regulation and energy homeostasis (Larson-Meyer et al, 2010). The metabolic rate of women fluctuates with the menstrual cycle. During the luteal phase (i.e., the time between ovulation and the onset of menstruation), metabolic rate increases slightly (Ferraro et al, 1992). During pregnancy, growth in uterine, placental, and fetal tissues, along with the mother's increased cardiac workload, contributes to gradual increases in BEE (Butte et al, 2004).

Temperature. Fevers increase REE by approximately 7% for each degree of increase in body temperature above 98.6° F or 13% for each degree more than 37° C, as noted by classic studies (Hardy and DuBois, 1937).

Other factors. Caffeine, nicotine, and alcohol stimulate metabolic rate. Caffeine intakes of 200 to 350 mg in men or 240 mg in women may increase mean REE by 7% to 11% and 8% to 15%, respectively (Compher et al, 2006). Nicotine use increases REE by approximately 3% to 4% in men and by 6% in women; alcohol consumption increases REE in women by 9% (Compher et al, 2006). Under conditions of stress and disease, energy expenditure may increase or decrease, based on the clinical situation. Energy expenditure may be higher in people who are obese (Dobratz et al, 2007) but depressed during starvation or chronic dieting and in people with bulimia (Sedlet and Ireton-Jones, 1989).

Thermic Effect of Food

The thermic effect of food (TEF) is the increase in energy expenditure associated with the consumption, digestion, and absorption of food. The TEF accounts for approximately 10% of TEE (Ireton-Jones, 2010). The TEF may also be called diet-induced thermogenesis, specific dynamic action, or the specific effect of food. TEF can be separated into obligatory and facultative

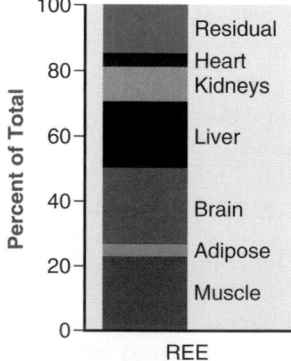

FIGURE 2-1 Proportional contribution of organs and tissues to calculated resting energy expenditure. (Modified and used with permission from Gallagher D et al: Organ-tissue mass measurement allows modeling of REE and metabolically active tissue mass, *Am J Physiol Endocrinol Metab* 275:E249, 1998. Copyright American Physiological Society.)

(or adaptive) subcomponents. **Obligatory thermogenesis** is the energy required to digest, absorb, and metabolize nutrients, including the synthesis and storage of protein, fat, and carbohydrate. Adaptive or **facultative thermogenesis** is the "excess" energy expended in addition to the obligatory thermogenesis and is thought to be attributable to the metabolic inefficiency of the system stimulated by sympathetic nervous activity.

The TEF varies with the composition of the diet, with energy expenditure increasing directly after food intake, particularly after consumption of a meal higher in protein compared with a meal higher in fat (Tentolouris et al, 2008). Fat is metabolized efficiently, with only 4% waste, compared with 25% waste when carbohydrate is converted to fat for storage. The macronutrient oxidation rate is not different in lean and obese individuals (Tentolouris et al, 2008). Although the extent of TEF depends on the size and macronutrient content of the meal, TEF decreases after ingestion over 30 to 90 minutes, so effects on TEE are small. For practical purposes, TEF is calculated as no more than an additional 10% of the REE. Spicy foods enhance and prolong the effect of the TEF. Caffeine, capsaicin, and different teas such as green, white, and oolong tea also may increase energy expenditure and fat oxidation and suppress hunger (Hursel and Westerterp-Plantenga, 2010; Reinbach et al, 2009). The role of TEF in weight management is discussed in Chapter 21.

Enteral nutrition (tube feeding) as well as parenteral nutrition exert a thermic effect on energy expenditure, which should be considered in patients receiving nutrition support. Leuck and colleagues found that energy expenditure of patients receiving enteral nutrition intermittently vs. continuously was increased at night and increased in association with each intermittent feeding (Leuck et al, 2013). A case study of a long-term home parenteral nutrition patient showed an increase in energy expenditure when the intravenous nutrition was being infused (Ireton-Jones, 2010). These are important considerations when predicting overall energy needs for patients receiving enteral or parenteral nutrition (see Chapter 13).

Activity Thermogenesis

Beyond REE and TEF, energy is expended in physical activity, either exercise-related or as part of daily work and movement. This is referred to as **activity thermogenesis**. Activity thermogenesis (AT) includes nonexercise activity thermogenesis (NEAT), the energy expended during activities of daily living, and the energy expended during sports or fitness exercise. T(Levine and Kotz, 2005).

The contribution of physical activity is the most variable component of TEE, which may be as low as 100 kcal/day in sedentary people or as high as 3000 kcal/day in athletes. **NEAT** represents the energy expended during the workday and during leisure-type activities (e.g., shopping, fidgeting, even gum chewing), which may account for vast differences in energy costs among people (Levine and Kotz, 2005; see Appendix 20). TEE reflects REE, TEF, and energy expended for exercise, as depicted in Figure 2-2.

Individual AT varies considerably, depending on body size and the efficiency of individual habits of motion. The level of fitness also affects the energy expenditure of voluntary activity because of variations in muscle mass. AT tends to decrease with age, a trend that is associated with a decline in FFM and an increase in fat mass. In general, men have greater skeletal muscle

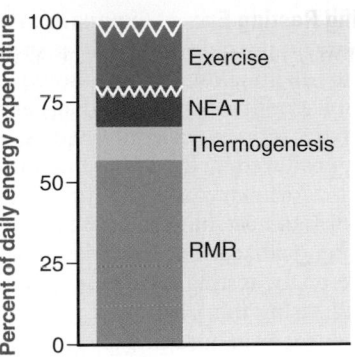

FIGURE 2-2 The components of total energy expenditure: activity, thermic effect of food (TEF), and basal or resting metabolic rate.

than women, which may account for their higher AT. The measurement of physical activity is very difficult whether related to children, adolescents, or adults (Mindell et al, 2014). However, this remains an important component of the overall energy intake recommendation suggesting that low-cost quantitative assessment methods are needed (e.g., heart rate monitoring) along with the typical questionnaire and estimate.

Additional Considerations in Energy Expenditure

Excess postexercise oxygen consumption (EPOC) is influenced by the duration and magnitude of physical activity. In a study of high-intensity intermittent exercise, there was an increase in energy expenditure during activity, although the effect on metabolic rate post-activity was minor (Kelly et al, 2013). Habitual exercise does not cause a significantly prolonged increase in metabolic rate unless FM is decreased and FFM is increased, and then this increase in energy expenditure is mostly during the activity itself.

Amputations resulting from trauma, wounds, or disease processes affect body size; presumably then, they would affect activity energy expenditure. However, a study of energy expenditure related to level of amputation (partial foot to transfemoral) at various speeds of walking was done in unilateral amputees, and no differences in energy expenditure were found between levels of amputation or speed when walking (Göktepe et al, 2010).

Measurement of Energy Expenditure

The standard unit for measuring energy is the **calorie**, which is the amount of heat energy required to raise the temperature of 1 ml of water at 15°C by 1°C. Because the amount of energy involved in the metabolism of food is fairly large, the kilocalorie (kcal), 1000 calories, is used to measure it. A popular convention is to designate kilocalorie by Calorie (with a capital C). In this text, however, kilocalorie is abbreviated kcal. The *joule* (J) measures energy in terms of mechanical work and is the amount of energy required to accelerate with a force of 1 Newton (N) for a distance of 1 m; this measurement is widely used in countries other than the United States. One kcal is equivalent to 4.184 kilojoules (kJ).

Because various methods are available to measure human energy expenditure, it is important to gain an understanding of the differences in these methods and how they can be applied in practical and research settings.

Direct Calorimetry

Direct calorimetry is possible only with specialized and expensive equipment. An individual is monitored in a room-type structure (a whole-room calorimeter) that permits a moderate amount of activity. It includes equipment that monitors the amount of heat produced by the individual inside the chamber or room. Direct calorimetry provides a measure of energy expended in the form of heat, but provides no information on the kind of fuel being oxidized. The method also is limited by the confined nature of the testing conditions. Therefore the measurement of TEE using this method is not representative of a free-living (i.e., engaged in normal daily activities) individual in a normal environment, because physical activity within the chamber is limited. High cost, complex engineering, and scarcity of appropriate facilities around the world also limit the use of this method.

Indirect Calorimetry

Indirect calorimetry (IC) is a more commonly used method for measuring energy expenditure. An individual's oxygen consumption and carbon dioxide production are quantified over a given period. The Weir equation (1949) and a constant respiratory quotient value of 0.85 are used to convert oxygen consumption to REE. The equipment varies but usually involves an individual breathing into a mouthpiece (with nose clips), a mask that covers the nose and mouth, or a ventilated hood that captures all expired carbon dioxide (Figure 2-3). Ventilated hoods are useful for short- and long-term measurements.

IC measurements are achieved using equipment called a metabolic measurement cart or an indirect calorimeter. There are various types of metabolic measurement carts, varying from larger equipment that measures oxygen consumption and carbon dioxide production only, to equipment that also has the capability of providing pulmonary function and exercise testing parameters. These larger carts are more expensive because of the expanded capabilities, including measurement interface for IC measurements of hospitalized patients who are ventilator dependent. Metabolic carts often are used at hospitals to assess energy requirements and are found most typically in the intensive care unit (Ireton-Jones, 2010). Individuals and patients who are breathing spontaneously may have their energy expenditure measured with smaller "handheld" indirect calorimeters designed specifically for measuring oxygen consumption while using a static value for carbon dioxide production. These have easy mobility and are relatively low cost (Hipskind et al, 2011).

A strict protocol should be followed before performing IC measurement. For healthy people, a minimum of a 5-hour fast after meals and snacks is recommended. Caffeine should be avoided for at least 4 hours, and alcohol and smoking for at least 2 hours. Testing should occur no sooner than 2 hours after moderate exercise; after vigorous resistance exercise, a 14-hour period is advised (Compher et al, 2006). To achieve a steady-state measurement, there should be a rest period of 10 to 20 minutes before the measurement is taken. An IC measurement duration of 10 minutes, with the first 5 minutes deleted and the remaining 5 minutes having a coefficient of variation less than 10%, indicates a steady-state measurement (Compher et al, 2006). When the measurement conditions listed here are met and a steady state is achieved, energy expenditure can be measured at any time during the day.

Energy expenditure can be measured for ill or injured individuals as well (Cooney and Frankenfield, 2012). Equipment used for the patient who is ventilator dependent may be different from that used for the ambulatory individual; however, a protocol specifying the conditions of measurement should be used for these patients as well (Ireton-Jones, 2010). When these conditions are met, IC can be applied for measuring the energy expenditure of acute or critically ill inpatients, outpatients, or healthy individuals.

Respiratory Quotient

When oxygen consumption and carbon dioxide production are measured, the respiratory quotient (RQ) may be calculated as noted in the following equation. The RQ indicates the fuel mixture being metabolized. The RQ for carbohydrate is 1 because the number of carbon dioxide molecules produced is equal to the number of oxygen molecules consumed.

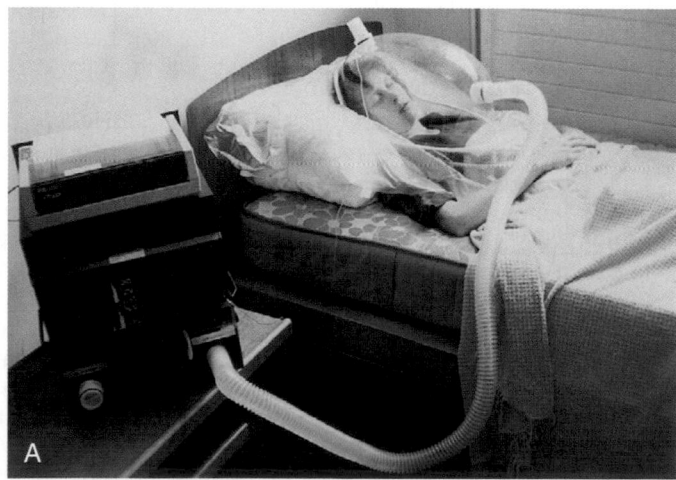
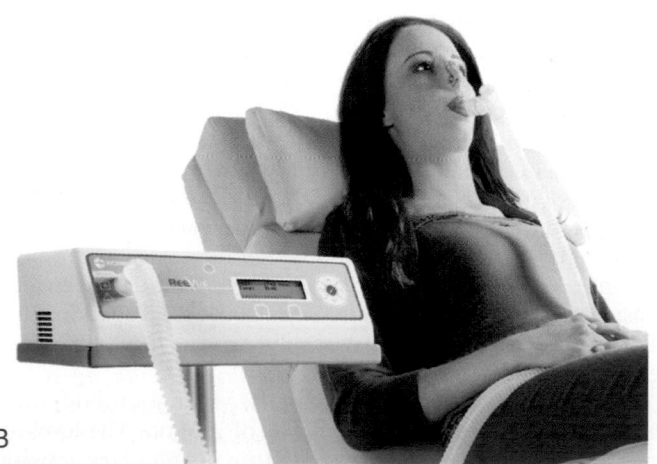

FIGURE 2-3 A: Measuring resting energy expenditure using a ventilated hood system. (Courtesy MRC Mitochondrial Biology Unit, Cambridge, England.). **B:** Measuring resting energy expenditure using a handheld system. (Courtesy Korr.)

$$RQ = \text{volume of CO expired/volume of O}_2 \text{ consumed (VO}_2/\text{VCO}_2)$$

RQ values:
1 = carbohydrate
0.85 = mixed diet
0.82 = protein
0.7 = fat
≤0.65 = ketone production

RQs greater than 1 are associated with net fat synthesis, carbohydrate (glucose) intake, or total caloric intake that is excessive, whereas a very low RQ may be seen under conditions of inadequate nutrient intake (McClave et al, 2003). Although RQ has been used to determine the efficacy of nutrition support regimens for hospitalized patients, McClave found that changes in RQ failed to correlate to percent calories provided or required, indicating low sensitivity and specificity that limits the efficacy of RQ as an indicator of overfeeding or underfeeding. However, use of RQ is appropriate as a marker of test validity (to confirm measured RQ values are in physiologic range) and a marker for respiratory tolerance of the nutrition support regimen.

Other Methods of Measuring Energy Expenditure

Alternative methods of measuring energy expenditure remain in the research setting because of the need for specialized equipment and expertise.

Doubly labeled water. The doubly labeled water (DLW) technique for measuring TEE is considered the gold standard for determining energy requirements and energy balance in humans. The DLW method is based on the principle that carbon dioxide production can be estimated from the difference in the elimination rates of body hydrogen and oxygen. After an oral loading dose of water labeled with deuterium oxide (^2H_2O) and oxygen-18 ($H_2^{18}O$)—hence the term doubly labeled water—is administered, the ^2H_2O is eliminated from the body as water, and the $H_2^{18}O$ is eliminated as water and carbon dioxide. The elimination rates of the two isotopes are measured for 10 to 14 days by periodic sampling of body water from urine, saliva, or plasma. The difference between the two elimination rates is a measure of carbon dioxide production. Carbon dioxide production then can be equated to TEE using standard IC techniques for the calculation of energy expenditure.

The caloric value of AT can be estimated by using the DLW method in conjunction with IC and also can be used to determine adherence to recommended intake and body composition longitudinally (Wong et al, 2014). The DLW technique is most applicable as a research tool; the stable isotopes are expensive, and expertise is required to operate the highly sophisticated and costly mass spectrometer for the analysis of the isotope enrichments. These disadvantages make the DLW technique impractical for daily use by clinicians.

Measuring Activity-Related Energy Expenditure

Triaxial monitors. A triaxial monitor has also been used to measure energy related to activity. It more efficiently measures multidirectional movement by employing three uniaxial monitors. In a review of numerous articles, Plasqui and Westerterp (2007) found that a triaxial monitor correlated with energy expenditure measured using DLW technique. Application of an easily accessible and useable monitor allows determination of real activity levels, thereby reducing errors related to overreporting or underreporting of actual energy expenditure for weight management.

Physical Activity Questionnaire

Physical activity questionnaires (PAQs) are the simplest and least expensive tools for gaining information about an individual's activity level (Winters-Hart et al, 2004). Reporting errors are common among PAQs, which can lead to discrepancies between calculated energy expenditure and that determined by DLW (Neilson et al, 2008). For healthy individuals, this may account for slowed weight loss or gain and, as such, a need to modify caloric intake.

ESTIMATING ENERGY REQUIREMENTS

Equations for Estimating Resting Energy Expenditure

Over the years several equations have been developed to estimate the REE. Equations are available that allow the estimation of REE as derived from measurement using IC in adults. Until recently, the Harris-Benedict equations were some of the most widely used equations to estimate REE in normal and ill or injured individuals (Harris and Benedict, 1919). The Harris-Benedict formulas have been found to overestimate REE in normal weight and obese individuals by 7% to 27% (Frankenfield et al, 2003). A study comparing measured REE with estimated REE using the Mifflin-St. Jeor equations, Owen equations, and Harris-Benedict equations for males and females found that the Mifflin-St. Jeor equations were most accurate in estimating REE in both normal weight and obese people (Frankenfield et al, 2003). The Mifflin-St Jeor equations were developed from measured REE using IC in 251 males and 247 females; 47% of these individuals had a body mass index (BMI) between 30 and 42 kg/m^2 (Mifflin et al, 1990). Mifflin-St. Jeor equations are used today to estimate energy expenditure of healthy individuals and in some patients and are as follows:

$$\text{Males: kcal/day} = 10\,(\text{wt}) + 6.25\,(\text{ht}) - 5\,(\text{age}) + 5$$
$$\text{Females: kcal/day} = 10\,(\text{wt}) + 6.25\,(\text{ht}) - 5\,(\text{age}) - 161$$
$$\text{Weight} = \text{actual body weight in kilograms}$$
$$\text{Height} = \text{centimeters; age} = \text{years}$$

Although the Harris-Benedict equations have been applied to ill and injured people, these equations, as well as those of Mifflin, were developed for use in healthy individuals, and their application to any other population is questionable. In addition, the database from which the Harris-Benedict equations were developed no longer reflects the population, and therefore use of these equations is not recommended.

Energy expenditure of ill or injured patients also can be estimated or measured using IC. For energy requirements for critically ill patients, see Chapter 38.

Determining TEE

The equations for estimating or measuring energy expenditure begin with resting energy expenditure or REE. Additional factors for TEF and activity must be added. As stated previously, the TEF may be considered as an overall additive factor within activity thermogenesis in calculations of TEE. A simplified way of predicting physical activity additions to REE is through the use of estimates of the level of physical activity, which are then multiplied by the measured or predicted REE. To estimate TEE for minimal activity, increase REE by 10% to 20%; for moderate activity, increase REE by 25% to 40%; for strenuous activity, increase REE by 45% to 60%. These levels are ranges used in practice and can be considered "expert opinion" rather than evidence based at this time.

Estimating Energy Requirements from Energy Intake

Traditionally, recommendations for energy requirements were based on self-recorded estimates (e.g., diet records) or self-reported estimates (e.g., 24-hour recalls) of food intake. However, these methods do not provide accurate or unbiased estimates of an individual's energy intake. The percentage of people who underestimate or underreport their food intake ranges from 10% to 45%, depending on the person's age, gender, and body composition. This occurs in the compromised patient population as well (Ribeiro et al, 2014). See Chapter 4.

Many online programs are available in which an individual can enter the food and quantity consumed into a program that estimates the macronutrient and micronutrient content. These programs allow users to enter data and receive a summary report, often with a detailed report provided to the health professional as well. Widely available programs include Food Prodigy and the MyPlate Tracker from the United States Department of Agriculture (see Chapter 4).

Other Prediction Equations

The National Academy of Sciences, Institute of Medicine (IOM), and Food and Nutrition Board, in partnership with Health Canada, developed the estimated energy requirements for men, women, children, and infants and for pregnant and lactating women (IOM, 2005). The **estimated energy requirement (EER)** is the average dietary energy intake predicted to maintain energy balance in a healthy adult of a defined age, gender, weight, height, and level of physical activity consistent with good health. In children and pregnant and lactating women, the EER is taken to include the energy needs associated with the deposition of tissues or the secretion of milk at rates consistent with good health. Table 2-1 lists average dietary reference intake (DRI) values for energy in healthy, active people of reference height, weight, and age for each life-stage group (IOM, 2002; 2005).

Supported by DLW studies, prediction equations have been developed to estimate energy requirements for people according to their life-stage group. Box 2-1 lists the EER prediction equations for people of normal weight. TEE prediction equations also are listed for various overweight and obese groups, as well as for weight maintenance in obese girls and boys. All equations have been developed to maintain current body weight (and promote growth when appropriate) and current levels of physical activity for all subsets of the population; they are not intended to promote weight loss (IOM, 2002; 2005).

The EER incorporates age, weight, height, gender, and level of physical activity for people ages 3 years and older. Although variables such as age, gender, and feeding type (i.e., breast milk, formula) can affect TEE among infants and young children, weight has been determined as the sole predictor of TEE needs (IOM, 2002; 2005). Beyond TEE requirements, additional calories are required for infants, young children, and children ages 3 through 18 to support the deposition of tissues needed for growth, and for pregnant and lactating women. Thus the EER among these subsets of the population is the sum of TEE plus the caloric requirements for energy deposition.

TABLE 2-1   Dietary Reference Intake Values for Energy for Active Individuals

Life-Stage Group	Criterion	ACTIVE PAL EER (kcal/day)	
		Male	**Female**
Infants			
0-6 mo	Energy expenditure + Energy deposition	570	520 (3 mo)
7-12 mo	Energy expenditure + Energy deposition	743	676 (9 mo)
Children			
1-2 yr	Energy expenditure + Energy deposition	1046	992 (24 mo)
3-8 yr	Energy expenditure + Energy deposition	1742	1642 (6 yr)
9-13 yr	Energy expenditure + Energy deposition	2279	2071 (11 yr)
14-18 yr	Energy expenditure + Energy deposition	3152	2368 (16 yr)
Adults			
>18 yr	Energy expenditure	3067[†]	2403[†] (19 yr)
Pregnant Women			
14-18 yr	Adolescent female EER + Change in TEE + Pregnancy energy deposition		
First trimester			2368 (16 yr)
Second trimester			2708 (16 yr)
Third trimester			2820 (16 yr)
19-50 yr	Adult female EER + Change in TEE + Pregnancy energy deposition		
First trimester			2403[†] (19 yr)
Second trimester			2743[†] (19 yr)
Third trimester			2855[†] (19 yr)
Lactating Women			
14-18 yr	Adolescent female EER + Milk energy output − Weight loss		
First 6 mo			2698 (16 yr)
Second 6 mo			2768 (16 yr)
19-50 yr	Adult female EER + Milk energy output − Weight loss		
First 6 mo			2733[†] (19 yr)
Second 6 mo			2803[†] (19 yr)

From Institute of Medicine of The National Academies: *Dietary reference intakes for energy, carbohydrate, fiber, fat, fatty acids, cholesterol, protein, and amino acids.* Washington, DC, 2002/2005, The National Academies Press.
EER, Estimated energy requirement; *PAL,* physical activity level; *TEE,* total energy expenditure.
*For healthy active Americans and Canadians at the reference height and weight.
[†]Subtract 10 kcal/day for men and 7 kcal/day for women for each year of age above 19 years.

The prediction equations include a physical activity (PA) coefficient for all groups except infants and young children (see Box 2-1). PA coefficients correspond to four **physical activity level (PAL)** lifestyle categories: sedentary, low active, active, and very active. Because PAL is the ratio of TEE to BEE, the energy spent during activities of daily living, the sedentary lifestyle category has a PAL range of 1 to 1.39. PAL categories beyond sedentary are determined according to the energy spent by an adult walking at a set pace (Table 2-2). The walking equivalents that correspond to each PAL category for an average-weight adult walking at 3 to 4 mph are 2, 7, and 17 miles per day, for low active, active and very active (IOM, 2002; 2005). All equations

---

BOX 2-1 Estimated Energy Expenditure* Prediction Equations at Four Physical Activity Levels†

EER for Infants and Young Children 0 to 2 Years (Within the 3rd to 97th Percentile for Weight-for-Height)

EER = TEE‡ Energy deposition

0-3 months (89 × Weight of infant [kg] − 100) + 175 (kcal for energy deposition)

4-6 months (89 × Weight of infant [kg] − 100) + 56 (kcal for energy deposition)

7-12 months (89 × Weight of infant [kg] −100) + 22 (kcal for energy deposition)

13-35 months (89 × Weight of child [kg] − 100) + 20 (kcal for energy deposition)

EER for Boys 3 to 8 Years (Within the 5th to 85th Percentile for BMI)§

EER = TEE‡ Energy deposition

EER = 88.5 − 61.9 × Age (yr) + PA × (26.7 × Weight [kg] + 903 × Height [m]) + 20 (kcal for energy deposition)

EER for Boys 9 to 18 Years (Within the 5th to 85th Percentile for BMI)

EER = TEE Energy deposition

EER = 88.5 − 61.9 × Age (yr) + PA × (26.7 × Weight [kg] + 903 × Height [m]) + 25 (kcal for energy deposition)

in which

PA = Physical activity coefficient for boys 3-18 years:

PA = 1 if PAL is estimated to be ≥ 1 < 1.4 (Sedentary)

PA = 1.13 if PAL is estimated to be ≥ 1.4 < 1.6 (Low active)

PA = 1.26 if PAL is estimated to be ≥ 1.6 < 1.9 (Active)

PA = 1.42 if PAL is estimated to be ≥ 1.9 < 2.5 (Very active)

EER for Girls 3 to 8 Years (Within the 5th to 85th Percentile for BMI)

EER = TEE Energy deposition

EER = 135.3 − 30.8 × Age (yr) + PA × (10 × Weight [kg] + 934 × Height [m]) + 20 (kcal for energy deposition)

EER for Girls 9 to 18 Years (Within the 5th to 85th Percentile for BMI)

EER = TEE + Energy deposition

EER = 135.3 − 30.8 × Age (yr) + PA × (10 × Weight [kg] + 934 × Height [m]) + 25 (kcal for energy deposition)

in which

PA = Physical activity coefficient for girls 3-18 years:

PA = 1 (Sedentary)

PA = 1.16 (Low active)

PA = 1.31 (Active)

PA = 1.56 (Very active)

EER for Men 19 Years and Older (BMI 18.5 to 25 kg/m²)

EER = TEE

EER = 662 − 9.53 × Age (yr) + PA × (15.91 × Weight [kg] + 539.6 × Height [m])

in which

PA = Physical activity coefficient:

PA = 1 (Sedentary)

PA = 1.11 (Low active)

PA = 1.25 (Active)

PA = 1.48 (Very active)

EER for Women 19 Years and Older (BMI 18.5 to 25 kg/m²)

EER = TEE

EER = 354 − 6.91 × Age (yr) + PA × (9.36 × Weight [kg] + 726 × Height [m])

in which

PA = Physical activity coefficient:

PA = 1 (Sedentary)

PA = 1.12 (Low active)

PA = 1.27 (Active)

PA = 1.45 (Very active)

EER for Pregnant Women

14-18 years: EER = Adolescent EER + Pregnancy energy deposition

First trimester = Adolescent EER + 0 (Pregnancy energy deposition)

Second trimester = Adolescent EER + 160 kcal (8 kcal/wk 1 × 20 wk) + 180 kcal

Third trimester = Adolescent EER + 272 kcal (8 kcal/wk × 34 wk) + 180 kcal

19-50 years: = Adult EER + Pregnancy energy deposition

First trimester = Adult EER + 0 (Pregnancy energy deposition)

Second trimester = Adult EER + 160 kcal (8 kcal/wk × 20 wk) + 180 kcal

Third trimester = Adult EER + 272 kcal (8 kcal/wk × 34 wk) + 180 kcal

EER for Lactating Women

14-18 years: EER = Adolescent EER + Milk energy output − Weight loss

First 6 months = Adolescent EER + 500 − 170 (Milk energy output − Weight loss)

Second 6 months = Adolescent EER + 400 − 0 (Milk energy output − Weight loss)

19-50 years: EAR = Adult EER + Milk energy output − Weight loss

First 6 months = Adult EER + 500 − 70 (Milk energy output − Weight loss)

Second 6 months = Adult EER + 400 − 0 (Milk energy output − Weight loss)

Weight Maintenance TEE for Overweight and At-Risk for Overweight Boys 3 to 18 Years (BMI >85th Percentile for Overweight)

TEE = 114 − 50.9 × Age (yr) + PA × (19.5 × Weight [kg] + 1161.4 × Height [m])

in which

PA = Physical activity coefficient:

PA = 1 if PAL is estimated to be ≥ 1.0 < 1.4 (Sedentary)

PA = 1.12 if PAL is estimated to be ≥ 1.4 < 1.6 (Low active)

PA = 1.24 if PAL is estimated to be ≥ 1.6 < 1.9 (Active)

PA = 1.45 if PAL is estimated to be ≥ 1.9 < 2.5 (Very active)

Weight Maintenance TEE for Overweight and At-Risk for Overweight Girls 3-18 Years (BMI >85th Percentile for Overweight)

TEE = 389 − 41.2 × Age (yr) + PA × (15 × Weight [kg] + 701.6 × Height [m])

in which

PA = Physical activity coefficient:

PA = 1 if PAL is estimated to be ≥ 1 < 1.4 (Sedentary)

PA = 1.18 if PAL is estimated to be ≥ 1.4 < 1.6 (Low active)

PA = 1.35 if PAL is estimated to be ≥ 1.6 < 1.9 (Active)

PA = 1.60 if PAL is estimated to be ≥ 1.9 < 2.5 (Very active)

Continued

BOX 2-1   **Estimated Energy Expenditure Prediction Equations at Four Physical Activity Levels—cont'd**

Overweight and Obese Men 19 Years and Older (BMI ≥25 kg/m²)

TEE = 1086 − 10.1 × Age (yr) + PA × (13.7 × Weight [kg] + 416 × Height [m])

in which

  PA = Physical activity coefficient:

  PA = 1 if PAL is estimated to be ≥ 1 < 1.4 (Sedentary)

  PA = 1.12 if PAL is estimated to be ≥ 1.4 < 1.6 (Low active)

  PA = 1.29 if PAL is estimated to be ≥ 1.6 < 1.9 (Active)

  PA = 1.59 if PAL is estimated to be ≥ 1.9 < 2.5 (Very active)

Overweight and Obese Women 19 Years and Older (BMI ≥25 kg/m²)

TEE = 448 − 7.95 × Age (yr) + PA × (11.4 × Weight [kg] + 619 × Height [m])

where

  PA = Physical activity coefficient:

  PA = 1 if PAL is estimated to be ≥ 1 < 1.4 (Sedentary)

  PA = 1.16 if PAL is estimated to be ≥ 1.4 < 1.6 (Low active)

  PA = 1.27 if PAL is estimated to be ≥ 1.6 < 1.9 (Active)

  PA = 1.44 if PAL is estimated to be ≥ 1.9 < 2.5 (Very active)

Normal and Overweight or Obese Men 19 Years and Older (BMI ≥18.5 kg/m²)

TEE = 864 − 9.72 × Age (yr) + PA × (14.2 × Weight [kg] + 503 × Height [m])

in which

  PA = Physical activity coefficient:

  PA = 1 if PAL is estimated to be ≥ 1 < 1.4 (Sedentary)

  PA = 1.12 if PAL is estimated to be ≥ 1.4 < 1.6 (Low active)

  PA = 1.27 if PAL is estimated to be ≥ 1.6 < 1.9 (Active)

  PA = 1.54 if PAL is estimated to be ≥ 1.9 < 2.5 (Very active)

Normal and Overweight or Obese Women 19 Years and Older (BMI ≥18.5 kg/m²)

TEE = 387 − 7.31 × Age (yr) + PA × (10.9 × Weight [kg] + 660.7 × Height [m])

in which

  PA = Physical activity coefficient:

  PA = 1 if PAL is estimated to be ≥ 1 < 1.4 (Sedentary)

  PA = 1.14 if PAL is estimated to be ≥ 1.4 < 1.6 (Low active)

  PA = 1.27 if PAL is estimated to be ≥ 1.6 < 1.9 (Active)

  PA = 1.45 if PAL is estimated to be ≥ 1.9 < 2.5 (Very active)

From Institute of Medicine, Food and Nutrition Board: *Dietary reference intakes for energy, carbohydrate, fiber, fat, fatty acids, cholesterol, protein, and amino acids,* Washington, DC, 2002, The National Academies Press, www.nap.edu.

BMI, Body mass index; *EER,* estimated energy requirement; *PA,* physical activity; *PAL,* physical activity level; *TEE,* total energy expenditure.

EER is the average dietary energy intake that is predicted to maintain energy balance in a healthy adult of a defined age, gender, weight, height, and level of physical activity consistent with good health. In children and pregnant and lactating women, the EER includes the needs associated with the deposition of tissues or the secretion of milk at rates consistent with good health.

†PAL is the physical activity level that is the ratio of the total energy expenditure to the basal energy expenditure.

‡TEE is the sum of the resting energy expenditure, energy expended in physical activity, and the thermic effect of food.

§BMI is determined by dividing the weight (in kilograms) by the square of the height (in meters).

TABLE 2-2   Physical Activity Level Categories and Walking Equivalence*

PAL Category	PAL Values	Walking Equivalence (Miles/Day at 3-4 mph)
Sedentary	1-1.39	
Low active	1.4-1.59	1.5, 2.2, 2.9 for PAL = 1.5
Active	1.6-1.89	3, 4.4, 5.8 for PAL = 1.6
		5.3, 7.3, 9.9 for PAL = 1.75
Very active	1.9-2.5	7.5, 10.3, 14 for PAL = 1.9
		12.3, 16.7, 22.5 for PAL = 2.2
		17, 23, 31 for PAL = 2.5

From Institute of Medicine, The National Academies: Dietary reference intakes for energy, carbohydrate, fiber, fat, fatty acids, cholesterol, protein, and amino acids, Washington, DC, 2002/2005, The National Academies Press.

PAL, Physical activity level.

*In addition to energy spent for the generally unscheduled activities that are part of a normal daily life. The low, middle, and high miles/day values apply to relatively heavy-weight (120-kg), midweight (70-kg), and lightweight (44-kg) individuals, respectively.

are only estimates and individual variations may be wide and unexpected (O'Riordan et al, 2010).

Estimated Energy Expended in Physical Activity

Energy expenditure in physical activity can be estimated using either the method shown in Appendix 20, which represents energy spent during common activities and incorporates body weight and the duration of time for each activity as variables, or using information in Figure 2-3, which represents energy spent by adults during various intensities of physical activity—energy

that is expressed as metabolic equivalents (METs) (IOM, 2002; 2005).

Estimating Energy Expenditure of Selected Activities Using Metabolic Equivalents

METs are units of measure that correspond with a person's metabolic rate during selected physical activities of varying intensities and are expressed as multiples of REE. A MET value of 1 is the oxygen metabolized at rest (3.5 ml of oxygen per kilogram of body weight per minute in adults) and can be expressed as 1 kcal/kg of body weight per hour. Thus the energy expenditure of adults can be estimated using MET values (1 MET = 1 kcal/kg/hr). For example, an adult who weighs 65 kg and is walking moderately at a pace of 4 mph (which is a MET value of 4.5) would expend 293 calories in 1 hour (4.5 kcal × 65 kg × 1 = 293) (Table 2-3).

Estimating a person's energy requirements using the Institute of Medicine's EER equations requires identifying a PAL value for that person. A person's PAL value can be affected by various activities performed throughout the day and is referred to as the change in physical activity level (Δ PAL). To determine Δ PAL, take the sum of the Δ PALs for each activity performed for 1 day from the DRI tables (IOM, 2002; 2005). To calculate the PAL value for 1 day, take the sum of activities and add the BEE (1) plus 10% to account for the TEF (1 + 0.1 = 1.1). For example, to calculate an adult woman's PAL value, take the sum of the Δ PAL values for activities of daily living, such as walking the dog (0.11) and vacuuming (0.14) for 1 hour each, sitting for 4 hours doing light activity (0.12), and then performing moderate to vigorous activities such as

TABLE 2-3   Intensity and Effect of Various Activities on Physical Activity Level in Adults*

Physical Activity	METs*	Δ PAL/10 min[†]	Δ PAL/hr[‡]
Daily Activities			
Lying quietly	1	0	0
Riding in a car	1	0	0
Light activity while sitting	1.5	0.005	0.03
Watering plants	2.5	0.014	0.09
Walking the dog	3	0.019	0.11
Vacuuming	3.5	0.024	0.14
Doing household tasks (moderate effort)	3.5	0.024	0.14
Gardening (no lifting)	4.4	0.032	0.19
Mowing lawn (power mower)	4.5	0.033	0.20
Leisure Activities: Mild			
Walking (2 mph)	2.5	0.014	0.09
Canoeing (leisurely)	2.5	0.014	0.09
Golfing (with cart)	2.5	0.014	0.09
Dancing (ballroom)	2.9	0.018	0.11
Leisure Activities: Moderate			
Walking (3 mph)	3.3	0.022	0.13
Cycling (leisurely)	3.5	0.024	0.14
Performing calisthenics (no weight)	4	0.029	0.17
Walking (4 mph)	4.5	0.033	0.20
Leisure Activities: Vigorous			
Chopping wood	4.9	0.037	0.22
Playing tennis (doubles)	5	0.038	0.23
Ice skating	5.5	0.043	0.26
Cycling (moderate)	5.7	0.045	0.27
Skiing (downhill or water)	6.8	0.055	0.33
Swimming	7	0.057	0.34
Climbing hills (5-kg load)	7.4	0.061	0.37
Walking (5 mph)	8	0.067	0.40
Jogging (10-min mile)	10.2	0.088	0.53
Skipping rope	12	0.105	0.63

Modified from Institute of Medicine of The National Academies: *Dietary reference intakes for energy, carbohydrate, fiber, fat, fatty acids, protein, and amino acids,* Washington, DC, 2002, The National Academies Press.
MET, Metabolic equivalent; *PAL,* physical activity level.
*PAL is the physical activity level that is the ratio of the total energy expenditure to the basal energy expenditure.
[†]METs are multiples of an individual's resting oxygen uptakes, defined as the rate of oxygen (O_2) consumption of 3.5 ml of O_2/min/kg body weight in adults.
[‡]The Δ PAL is the allowance made to include the delayed effect of physical activity in causing excess postexercise oxygen consumption and the dissipation of some of the food energy consumed through the thermic effect of food.

walking for 1 hour at 4 mph (0.20) and ice skating for 30 minutes (0.13) for a total of 0.7. To that value add the BEE adjusted for the 10% TEF (1.1) for the final calculation:

$$0.7 + 1.1 = 1.8$$

For this woman, the PAL value (1.8) falls within an active range. The PA coefficient that correlates with an active lifestyle for this woman is 1.27.

To calculate the EER for this adult woman, age 30, use the EER equation for women 19 years and older (BMI 18.5-25 kg/m^2); see Box 2-1. The following calculation estimates the EER for a 30-year-old active woman who weighs 65 kg, is 1.77 m tall, with a PA coefficient (1.27):

$$EER = 354 - 6.91 \times Age\ (yr) + PA \times (9.36 \times Weight\ [kg] + 726 \times Height\ [m])$$

$$EER = 354 - (6.91 \times 30) + 1.27 \times ([9.36 \times 65] + [726 \times 1.77])$$

$$EER = 2551\ kcal$$

Energy spent during various activities and the intensity and impact of selected activities also can be determined for children and teens (see Box 2-1).

Physical Activity in Children

CALCULATING FOOD ENERGY

The total energy available from a food is measured with a bomb calorimeter. This device consists of a closed container in which a weighed food sample, ignited with an electric spark, is burned in an oxygenated atmosphere. The container is immersed in a known volume of water, and the rise in the temperature of the water after igniting the food is used to calculate the heat energy generated.

Not all of the energy in foods and alcohol is available to the body's cells, because the processes of digestion and absorption are not completely efficient. In addition, the nitrogenous portion of amino acids is not oxidized but is excreted in the form of urea. Therefore, the biologically available energy from foods and alcohol is expressed in values rounded off slightly below those obtained using the calorimeter. These values for protein, fat, carbohydrate, and alcohol (Figure 2-4) are 4, 9, 4, and 7 kcal/g, respectively. Fiber is an "unavailable carbohydrate" that resists digestion and absorption; its energy contribution is minimal.

Although the energy value of each nutrient is known precisely, only a few foods, such as oils and sugars, are made up of a single nutrient. More commonly, foods contain a mixture of protein, fat, and carbohydrate. For example, the energy value of one medium (50 g) egg calculated in terms of weight is derived from protein (13%), fat (12%), and carbohydrate (1%) as follows:

Protein: 13% × 50 g = 6.5 g × 4 kcal/g = 26 kcal

Fat: 12% × 50 g = 6 g × 9 kcal/g = 54 kcal

Carbohydrate: 1% × 50 g = 0.05g × 4 kcal/g = 2 kcal

Total = 82 kcal

The energy value of alcoholic beverages can be determined using the following equation:

Alcohol kcal = amount of beverage (oz) x proof x .8 kcal/proof/oz.

Proof is the proportion of alcohol to water or other liquids in an alcoholic beverage. The standard in the United States defines 100-proof as equal to 50% of ethyl alcohol by volume. To determine the percentage of ethyl alcohol in a beverage, divide the proof value by 2. For example, 86-proof whiskey contains 43% ethyl alcohol. The latter part of the equation—0.8 kcal/proof/1 oz—is the factor that accounts

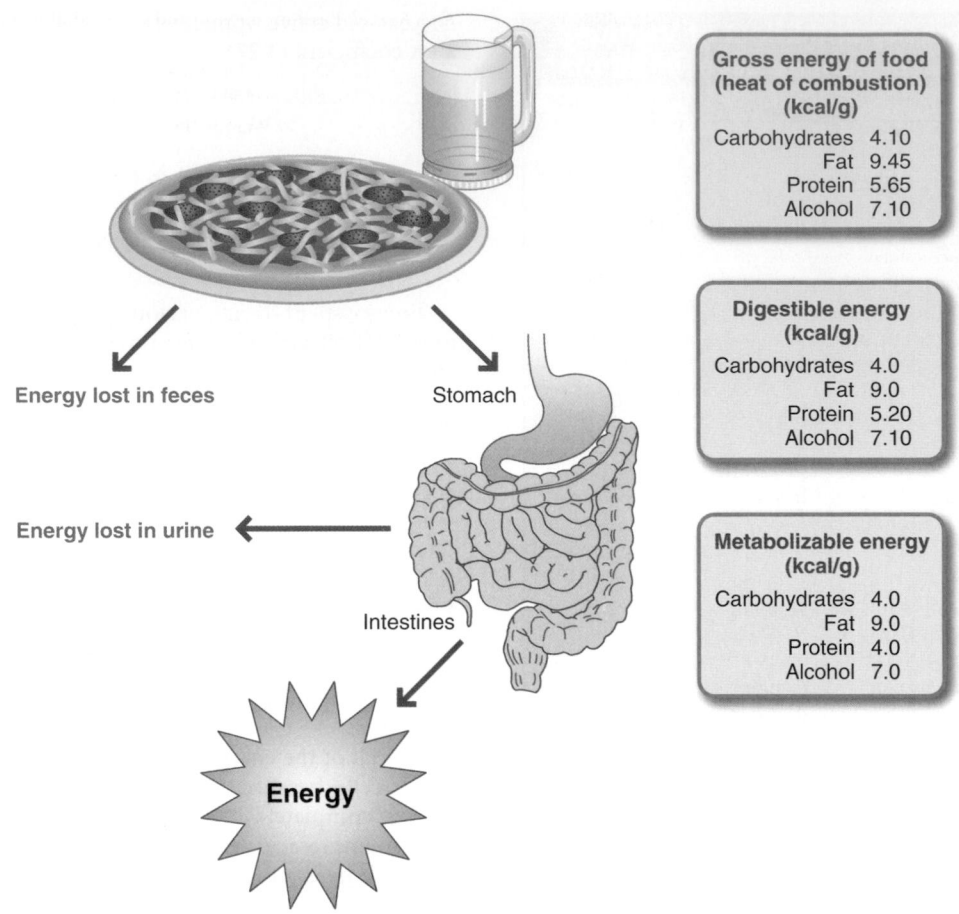

Gross energy of food (heat of combustion) (kcal/g)	
Carbohydrates	4.10
Fat	9.45
Protein	5.65
Alcohol	7.10

Digestible energy (kcal/g)	
Carbohydrates	4.0
Fat	9.0
Protein	5.20
Alcohol	7.10

Metabolizable energy (kcal/g)	
Carbohydrates	4.0
Fat	9.0
Protein	4.0
Alcohol	7.0

FIGURE 2-4 Energy value of food.

for the caloric density of alcohol (7 kcal/g) and the fact that not all of the alcohol in liquor is available for energy. For example, the number of kilocalories in 1½ oz of 86-proof whiskey would be determined as follows:

$$1\frac{1}{2}\text{ oz} \times 86\% \text{ proof} \times 0.8 \text{ kcal/proof/1 oz} = 103 \text{ kcal}$$

See Appendix 32 for the caloric content of alcoholic beverages.

Energy values of foods based on chemical analyses may be obtained from the U.S. Department of Agriculture (USDA) Nutrient Data Laboratory website or from *Bowes and Church's Food Values of Portions Commonly Used* (Pennington and Spungen, 2009).

Many computer software programs that use the USDA nutrient database as the standard reference are also available and many online websites can be used. See Chapter 4.

Recommendations for macronutrient percentages vary based on the goal of the client and any underlying or overriding disease process. This is discussed in other chapters.

USEFUL WEBSITES/APPS

The Academy of Nutrition and Dietetics: Evidence Analysis Library
www.andevidencelibrary.com
American Society for Parenteral and Enteral Nutrition
www.nutritioncare.org/

Food Prodigy
www.esha.com/foodprodigy
National Academy Press—Publisher of Institute of Medicine DRIs for Energy
www.fnic.nal.usda.gov/dietary-guidance/dietary-reference-intakes/dri-reports
My Fitness Pal
www.myfitnesspal.com/
MyPlate Tracker
www.chooseMyPlate.gov/tracker
U.S. Department of Agriculture Food Composition Tables
www.ars.usda.gov/main/site_main.htm?modecode=12-35-45-00

REFERENCES

Bosy-Westphal A, et al: Effect of organ and tissue masses on resting energy expenditure in underweight, normal weight and obese adults, *Int J Obes Relat Metab Disord* 28:72, 2004.

Butte NF, et al: Energy requirements during pregnancy based on total energy expenditure and energy deposition, *Am J Clin Nutr* 79:1078, 2004.

Byrne NM, et al: Influence of distribution of lean body mass on resting metabolic rate after weight loss and weight regain: comparison of responses in white and black women, *Am J Clin Nutr* 77:1368, 2003.

Compher C, et al: Best practice methods to apply to measurement of resting metabolic rate in adults: a systematic review, *J Am Diet Assoc* 106:881, 2006.

Cooney RN, Frankenfield DC: Determining energy needs in critically ill patients: equations or indirect calorimeters, *Curr Opin Crit Care* 18:174, 2012.

Cooper JA, et al: Longitudinal change in energy expenditure and effects on energy requirements of the elderly, *Nutr J* 12(1):73, 2013.

Dobratz JR, et al: Prediction of energy expenditure in extremely obese women, *J Parenter Enteral Nutr* 31:217, 2007.

Ferraro R, et al: Lower sedentary metabolic rate in women compared with men, *J Clin Invest* 90:780, 1992.

Frankenfield DC, et al: Validation of several established equations for resting metabolic rate in obese and nonobese people, *J Am Diet Assoc* 103:1152, 2003.

Gallagher D, et al: Small organs with a high metabolic rate explain lower resting energy expenditure in African American than in white adults, *Am J Clin Nutr* 83:1062, 2006.

Göktepe AS, et al: Energy expenditure of walking with prostheses: comparison of three amputation levels, *Prosthet Orthot Int* 34(1):31, 2010.

Hardy JD, DuBois EF: Regulation of heat loss from the human body, *Proc Natl Acad Sci U S A* 23:624, 1937.

Harris JA, Benedict FG: *A biometric study of basal metabolism in man, Pub no. 279*, Washington, DC, 1919, Carnegie Institute of Washington.

Hipskind P, et al: Do handheld calorimeters have a role in assessment of nutrition needs in hospitalized patients? A systematic review of literature, *Nutr Clin Pract* 26:426, 2011.

Hursel R, Westerterp-Plantenga MS: Thermogenic ingredients and body weight regulation, *Int J Obes (Lond)* 34:659, 2010.

Institute of Medicine, Food and Nutrition Board: *Dietary reference intakes for energy, carbohydrate, fiber, fat, fatty acids, cholesterol, protein, and amino acids*, Washington, DC, 2002, The National Academies Press.

Institute of Medicine of the National Academies, Food and Nutrition Board: *Dietary reference intakes for energy, carbohydrate, fiber, fat, fatty acids, cholesterol, protein, and amino acids*, Washington, DC, 2005, The National Academies Press.

Ireton-Jones C: Indirect calorimetry. In Skipper A, editor: *The dietitian's handbook of enteral and parenteral nutrition*, ed 3, Sudbury, Mass, 2010, Jones and Bartlett.

Javed F, et al: Brain and high metabolic rate organ mass: contributions to resting energy expenditure beyond fat-free mass, *Am J Clin Nutr* 91:907, 2010.

Kee AL, et al: Resting energy expenditure of morbidly obese patients using indirect calorimetry: a systematic review, *Obes Rev* 13:753, 2012.

Kelly B, et al: The impact of high-intensity intermittent exercise on resting metabolic rate in healthy males, *Eur J Appl Physiol* 113:3039, 2013.

Keys A, et al: Basal metabolism and age of adult man, *Metabolism* 22:579, 1973.

Larson-Meyer DE, et al: Ghrelin and peptide YY in postpartum lactating and nonlactating women, *Am J Clin Nutr* 91:366, 2010.

Leuck M, et al: Circadian rhythm of energy expenditure and oxygen consumption, *J Parenter Enteral Nutr* 38:263, 2013.

Levine JA, Kotz CM: NEAT—non-exercise activity thermogenesis—egocentric & geocentric environmental factors vs. biological regulation, *Acta Physiol Scand* 184:309, 2005.

McClave SA, Snider HL: Dissecting the energy needs of the body, *Curr Opin Clin Nutr Metab Care* 4:143, 2001.

McClave SA, et al: Clinical use of the respiratory quotient obtained from indirect calorimetry, *J Parenter Enteral Nutr* 27:21, 2003.

Mifflin MD, St. Jeor ST, et al: A new predictive equation for resting energy expenditure in healthy individuals, *Am J Clin Nutr* 51:241, 1990.

Mindell JS, et al: Measuring physical activity in children and adolescents for dietary surveys: practicalities, problems and pitfalls, *Proc Nutr Soc* 15:1, 2014.

Neilson HK, et al: Estimating activity energy expenditure: how valid are physical activity questionnaires? *Am J Clin Nutr* 87:279, 2008.

O'Riordan CF, et al: Reliability of energy expenditure prediction equations in the weight management clinic, *J Hum Nutr Diet* 23:169, 2010.

Pennington JA, Spungen JS: *Bowes and Church's food values of portions commonly used*, ed 19, Philadelphia, 2009, Lippincott Williams & Wilkins.

Plasqui G, Westerterp KR: Physical activity assessment with accelerometers: an evaluation against doubly labeled water, *Obesity* 15:2371, 2007.

Reinbach HC, et al: Effects of capsaicin, green tea and CH-19 sweet pepper on appetite and energy intake in humans in negative and positive energy balance, *Clin Nutr* 28:260, 2009.

Ribeiro HS, et al: Energy expenditure and balance among long-term liver recipients, *Clin Nutr* 33:1147–1152, Jan 3, 2014, [Epub ahead of print].

Sedlet KL, Ireton-Jones CS: Energy expenditure and the abnormal eating pattern of a bulimic: a case study, *J Am Diet Assoc* 89:74, 1989.

Tentolouris N, et al: Diet induced thermogenesis and substrate oxidation are not different between lean and obese women after two different isocaloric meals, one rich in protein and one rich in fat, *Metabolism* 57:313, 2008.

Winters-Hart CS, et al: Validity of a questionnaire to assess historical physical activity in older women, *Med Sci Sports Exerc* 36:2082, 2004.

Wong WW, et al: The doubly labeled water method produces highly reproducible longitudinal results in nutrition studies, *J Nutr* 144:777, 2014.

Inflammation and the Pathophysiology of Chronic Disease

Diana Noland, MPH, RD, CCN, LD

KEY TERMS

allostasis
adipokines
antecedents
autophagy
biochemical individuality
body fluid viscosity
C-reactive protein- hs
coenzyme Q-10
conditionally essential
curcumin
cyclooxygenases (COX)
cytochrome P450 enzymes
cytokines
delta-6-desaturase
eicosanoid cascade
enteroimmunology

genesis of disease
glutathione
health continuum
hyperinsulinemia
inflammation
interleukin-6 (IL-6)
leukotrienes
lipoic acid
lipoxygenases (LOX)
long-latency nutrient insufficiencies
mediators
metabolic syndrome
"new-to-nature" molecules
nutrient-partner principle
nutrition transition
prolonged inflammation

prostaglandins
reactive oxygen species (ROS)
resolvins
quercitin
sarcopenia
sedimentation rate
smoldering disease
specialized pro-resolving mediators (SPM)
systems biology
TNF-alpha
total inflammatory load
triage theory
triggers
visceral adipose tissue (VAT)
xenobiotics

EPIDEMIC OF CHRONIC DISEASE

Now that the biochemical and lifestyle components of chronic disease have become more evident, the question of how to change the lifelong diet and lifestyle habits of people, as well as a food industry, an agricultural industry, the political climate, and a culture became the challenge we face today.

Sydney Baker, MD, 2009

Chronic disease in the twenty-first century is a recent phenomenon in the history of the human race (Murray et al, 2012; UN, 2011; World Health Organization [WHO], 2011; Yach, 2004). Its recognition began after World War II at the same time the very significant nutrition transition began to occur, first in industrialized countries, then globally. The nutrition transition includes technology that enables synthesis of "new-to-nature" molecules (Bland, 1998, 2007), rapid increases in environmental toxin exposure, and decreased physical activity. New behavior patterns have promoted a decrease in home cooking along with increases in convenience food consumption and eating out. All of these changes are accompanied by the increased use of processed, less nutrient-dense food, decreased intake of whole fruits and vegetables, and increased consumption of sugar and high-sugar–containing foods. These components of the nutrition transition do not appear to have been beneficial

to the human race, because the effects are rapidly and globally increasing the risk of being overweight and obese, along with producing epidemic levels of chronic diseases at earlier ages (Hruby and Hu, 2014; Olshansky, 2005). (see *New Directions:* Is Chronic Disease an Epidemic?).

Despite the fact that the United States spends more money on health care than any other country, according to a report by

✺ NEW DIRECTIONS

Is Chronic Disease an Epidemic?

- If the current trend continues, 1 out of 3 U.S. adults will have diabetes by 2050 (CDC, 2011).
- 70% of U.S. deaths are from chronic disease (CDC, 2015).
- Global cancer rates could increase by 70% 2015 to 2035 (WHO, 2015).
- Two of three U.S. adults are overweight or obese.
- One third of cancer deaths are due to the five leading behavioral and dietary risks (WHO, 2015).
- Younger Americans will likely face a greater risk of mortality throughout life than previous generations (related to obesity) (Olshansky, 2005).
- The three most preventable risk factors are unhealthy diet, smoking, and physical inactivity (CDC, 2014).

the Centers for Disease Control and Prevention (CDC), 86% of the health care dollars in the United States are spent on chronic disease management (CDC, 2015). As people are living longer, the number of years spent living with disability has increased. The fact of the growing incidence of chronic disease has driven the global civilian and governmental health care systems to seek new answers to this nearly universal challenge.

The global effort to improve understanding of this chronic disease phenomenon is bringing the realization that these chronic diseases have long incubation periods (years to decades), thus they may not be observable during their early stages and may be present in an otherwise healthy-looking person. Focus on preventive care with earlier detection of signs, symptoms, and biomarkers that were previously thought insignificant allows for a chance of reversing the disease process before it becomes a serious affliction. The new phenotype of "fat, fatigued, and painful" in combination with associated conditions is descriptive of many chronic disease states considered to be preventable "lifestyle" diseases. The genotype, or genetic makeup, of a person may increase the propensity toward a chronic disease, but lifestyle—what one eats and thinks and where one lives—may be the most powerful cause of these "lifestyle" chronic diseases (CDC, 2015; Elwood et al, 2013).

CONCEPTS OF CHRONIC DISEASE PATHOPHYSIOLOGY

An understanding of the following basic concepts is essential when addressing the newly identified characteristics of chronic disease pathophysiology: systems biology, allostasis, autophagy, the health continuum, genesis of disease, long-latency nutrient insufficiencies, and nutrient-partner principle.

Systems Biology

The emerging new paradigm of systems biology (Aderem et al, 2011; Potthast, 2009) is the basis for a broader understanding of chronic disease. Systems biology encompasses viewing the whole person, the whole organism, and all systems working together interdependently. It provides a working model for assessing and monitoring the whole person. Chronic disease is complex and never involves just one organ or organ system. It involves underlying physiologic systems affecting the whole organism. With use of a systematic examination of an individual's physiologic imbalances that include mind, body, and spirit, a more robust identification of metabolic priorities can be achieved by members of the health care team.

The global movement in health care toward systems biology and personalized medicine is expanding. The registered dietitian nutritionist (RDN), as a member of the health care team, has a larger role to improve the nutritional status of each individual with dietary and lifestyle modifications as a foundational component of addressing chronic disease.

Allostasis

This is a condition of metabolic stability with adjustments for environmental influences and stresses through physiologic changes. Allostasis will be established even under inflammatory conditions but not always for optimal function. The maintenance of allostatic changes over a long period of time can lead to wear and tear of the system and body. Inflammation may be initiated for tissue adaptation and yet may involve collateral damage. Inflammation is particularly relevant to obesity and its associated adverse health conditions, such as type 2 diabetes, cardiovascular disease, and cancer. The ensuing systemic low-grade inflammation promotes a multitude of pathologic and self-perpetuating events, such as insulin resistance, endothelial dysfunction, and activation of oncogenic pathways (Baffy and Loscalzo, 2014).

For the nutritionist in clinical practice, the challenge is assessing metabolism and levels of inflammation at the cellular-molecular level available indirectly by using improved laboratory testing technology and scientific discovery of biochemical markers. For example, the biomarker C-reactive protein-high sensitivity (CRP-hs) has been shown to be the strongest univariate predictor of the risk of cardiovascular events (Ridker, 2000). It is a systemic marker of inflammation related most often to bacterial infection, trauma, and neoplastic activity with acute and chronic expression. Strong evidence indicates that the omega-3 fat EPA from fish oil has a powerful antiinflammatory effect and suppresses CRP-hs. Its measurement shows if the nutrients are balanced and working to create an allostatic microenvironment of wellness, or if there are imbalances that must be identified and restored (Baffy and Loscalzo, 2014).

Autophagy

Autophagy, or "self-eating," results in the lysosomal degradation of organelles, unfolded proteins, or foreign extracellular material. It is a survival mechanism required for maintaining cellular homeostasis after infection, mitochondrial damage, or endothelial reticulum stress. Defects in autophagy have been shown to result in pathologic inflammation (Abraham and Medzhitov, 2011; Prado et al, 2014).

Health Continuum

Health is a continuum from birth to death. "Health is the perfect, continuing adjustment of an organism to its environment" (Wyle, 1970). Chronic disease management for an individual must include considering the entire health continuum history to determine which factors along the way relate to one's current health condition. When collecting the patient's history during the assessment, clinicians should think of a life timeline to put the health continuum in perspective (see Figure 7-9).

Genesis of Disease

Triggers, antecedents, and mediators are critical terms that are part of the genesis of disease that underlies the patient's signs and symptoms, illness behaviors, and demonstrable pathology. Triggers are the distinct entities or events that provoke disease or its symptoms. They are usually insufficient for disease formation; host response is an essential component (Jones, 2005). Antecedents are congenital or developmental aspects of the individual that can include gender, family history, and genomics. These act to set the stage for the body's response to the trigger. Mediators are intermediates that are the primary drivers of disease; these are biochemical (Di Gennaro, 2012) but can be influenced by psychosocial factors such as smoking or stress (Avitsur et al, 2015; see Figure 7-9).

Long-Latency Nutrient Insufficiencies

Long-latency nutrient insufficiencies (i.e., subclinical [below-optimum] or deficient nutrient pools resulting from chronic poor intake and genotype) contribute over time to development of chronic disease. New tools have to be included in nutrition practice to expand beyond just detection of overt clinical deficiencies (Heaney, 2012). There must be further identification of biomarkers, usually biochemical and phenotypic, which are indicative of early chronic disease and are evidence based.

The nutrient deficiencies defined in the early 1900s are the end-stage and the result of specific index diseases. An example of this is the discovery that vitamin C deficiency caused scurvy in British sailors. Scurvy produces obvious clinical symptoms and death within months of the absence of vitamin C intake. In contrast, a more recent discovery is that years of subclinical vitamin C deficiency (without classic scurvy symptoms) can cause a less recognizable form of scorbutic progression in the form of periodontal gum disease (periodontitis) (Alagl and Bhat, 2015; Japatti et al, 2013; Popovich et al, 2009). Many other functions of vitamin C are compromised because of this "subclinical" deficiency (see Figure 7-2).

Nutrient-Partner Principle

Nutrient balance is the foundation of nutrition science, and this concept is expanding to appreciate the principle that, besides all macronutrients requiring balance, there are known partner nutrients involved in an individual's nutrition and inflammatory status. An example of application of the **nutrient partner principle** is the common recommendation for adults to take calcium supplements along with vitamin D. Another example is calcium and magnesium. For years, no attempt was made to routinely assess an individual's intake of magnesium, even though the NHANES studies showed that 70% to 80% of the U.S. population had magnesium intakes below the RDA for magnesium. With recent recognition of this calcium-magnesium partnership, many calcium supplements now contain magnesium in a 2:1 or 1:1 Ca:Mg ratio, and nutrition guidelines include the consumption of more vegetables and greens containing magnesium and calcium. The principle of nutrients as well as metabolic systems having synergistic relationships are seen in Box 3-1.

Triage Theory

The concept of nutrient **triage theory** states that "during poor dietary supply, nutrients are preferentially utilized for functions that are important for survival." This infers that some tissues may be lacking during times of insufficiency. This may be chronic in the person with an inadequate diet week after week, month after month, year after year, and often for decades (Ames 2010; McCann and Ames, 2011). To summarize (Heaney, 2014; Maggio, 2014):

- Most tissues need most nutrients.
- Inadequate intakes of most nutrients impair the function of most systems.
- The classical deficiency diseases occur at only the extremes of "inadequacy" (see Figure 7-2).
- The role of nutritional status as a key factor of successful aging is very well recognized (McCann and Ames, 2011).
- "Adequate" adult nutrition can be best conceptualized as preventive maintenance.

INFLAMMATION: COMMON DENOMINATOR OF CHRONIC DISEASE

Inflammation is the natural healthy reaction of the immune system as it responds to injury or infection, or flight or fright scenarios. See Box 3-2 for a classic description of inflammation.

The immune system's response to physiologic and metabolic stress is to produce pro-inflammatory molecules such as **adipokines** and **cytokines** - cell-signaling molecules that aid cell-to-cell communication and stimulate the movement of cells toward sites of inflammation in conditions of infection and injury. Thus immune system responses and the resulting inflammation are intimately connected.

Inflammation is the complex biological response of vascular tissue to harmful stimuli such as pathogens, damaged cells or irritants that consists of both vascular and cellular responses. Inflammation is a protective attempt by the organism to remove the injurious stimuli and initiate the healing process and to restore both structure and function. Inflammation may be local or systemic. It may be acute or chronic.

Undurti N. Das, MD
Molecular Basis of Health and Disease (2011)

Optimally, the immune system's function is to keep the body healthy, responding appropriately with an inflammatory response to environmental influences, such as short-lived infection and injury, and then returning the body to an alert system of defense. This function depends on the body's ability to recognize "self" and "non-self." When the immune response is successful, the tissue returns to a state of wellness, or metabolic stability described as **allostasis**. If many areas of the body's defense system, such as the gastrointestinal barrier, stomach acidity, skin, or various orifices (e.g., eye, ear, nose, lung, vagina, uterus), are compromised, there is diminishing recognition of "self" and

---

BOX 3-1   Nutrient and System Partner Principles

Nutrient Partners
- Calcium – Zinc – Copper
- Omega 6 GLA/DGLA - Arachidonic Acid – Omega 3 EPA/DHA
- Sodium chloride – potassium - calcium
- B Complex (B1-B2-B3-B5-B6-B9 (folate)-B12-Biotin-Choline)
- Antioxidants – reactive oxygen species (ROS)
- Albumin – globulin

System Partners and Rhythm Cycles:
- Autonomic Nervous System: sympathetic – parasympathetic
- Circadian Rhythm: 24 hour balanced rhythm
- Acid-Base Balance
- Microbiome: oral, nasal, skin, lung, vaginal, gastrointestinal
- Hormones-biochemistry
  - Cortisol - insulin - glucose
  - Estrogen – progesterone -testosterone
  - T4-T3 (total and free forms)
  - HPTA axis – Hippocampus – Pituitary – Thyroid - Adrenal

BOX 3-2   The five classic signs of inflammation, first described and documented by Aulus Cornelius Celsus (ca 25 BC-ca 50), a Roman physician and encyclopaedist

- **Dolor** - "pain"
- **Calor** - "heat"
- **Rubor** - "redness"
- **Tumor** - "swelling"
- **Functio laesa** - "injured function" or "loss of function".

"non-self" until the body is repaired. The longer the physiologic injury continues, the greater the loss of the ability to recognize "self" and "non-self" (Fasano, 2012; Wu et al, 2014).

If the underlying cause is not resolved, the immune response can get "stuck" in a state of prolonged inflammation. Locked into this state for a while, the immune system loses its ability to recognize "self" and "non-self," a critical survival skill and the core of immunology (Paul, 2010; Queen, 1998).

Prolonged Inflammation

Prolonged inflammation, known as chronic inflammation, sustained inflammation, or non-resolving inflammation, leads to a progressive shift in the type of cells present at the site of inflammation and is characterized by simultaneous destruction and healing of the tissue from the inflammatory process. Multiple studies have suggested that prolonged inflammation plays a primary role in the pathogenesis of chronic diseases (e.g., arthritis), when the immune response is to increase the ratio of proinflammatory to antiinflammatory cytokines (Bauer et al, 2014; Franceschi and Campisi, 2014).

One of the most fundamental characteristics of all chronic diseases is the initiation and continuation of a prolonged inflammation over all or part of the lifespan, leading to clinical chronic disease (Bauer et al, 2014). In the chronology of chronic disease progression, inflammation is at first subclinical, often referred to as "silent inflammation." This insidious inflammation remains below the threshold of clinical diagnosis. Cellular and tissue damage occurs in the body for years before being noticed. It is like a "smoldering" fire with a small whiff of smoke and heat being evident before it finally bursts into a flame. Some refer to early chronic disease as a "smoldering disease" (Noland, 2013). Chronic disease inflammation is described as:

Low-grade, chronic, systemic inflammation may be defined as a 2- to 3-fold elevation of circulating inflammatory mediators, usually associated with the innate arm of the immune system. It is a state that develops slowly (in contrast to pathological acute inflammatory responses, to sepsis for example), and its origin cannot be easily identified (in contrast to chronic inflammatory diseases such as rheumatoid arthritis and inflammatory bowel disease, where additional symptoms identify local dysregulated inflammation). This makes it difficult to develop appropriate therapeutic strategies that target both cause and symptom (inflammation) in a concerted fashion (Calcada et al, 2014).

Of grave concern is the initiation of prolonged inflammation in utero from the maternal inflammatory environment, thereby programming the fetus for a lifetime of chronic disease (Barker, 1998; Delisle, 2002; European Foundation for the Care of Newborn Infants [EFCNI], 2015; Fisher et al, 2012; Fleisch et al, 2012; see Chapter 15).

Clinical elevations of inflammatory biomarkers, such as high-sensitivity C-reactive protein (CRP-hs) (plasma), sedimentation rate, interleukin-6 (IL-6), and TNF-alpha, represent systemic markers of inflammation that are exacerbated by insulin resistance (IR) and hyperinsulinemia (Das, 2012, 2014; see Table 3-1). Diseases well characterized by these markers include heart disease, diabetes, autoimmune diseases, and possibly cancer and Alzheimer's disease (Birch et al, 2014; Wu, 2013).

There are other common physiologies shared by these inflammatory conditions that include changes in nutrient tissue pools, plasma, and RBC membrane composition of polyunsaturated fatty acids and antioxidants. This multifactorial syndrome (often referred to as metabolic syndrome) is related to obesity, and more importantly, insulin resistance and central adiposity evidenced by the presence of visceral adipose tissue (VAT). (See Chapters 7 and 30 for discussion of the metabolic syndrome). However, the expression of the prolonged inflammation is individual, and all individuals need not necessarily have all the characteristics described above.

TABLE 3-1 Biomarkers of Prolonged Inflammation

Test	Reference	Association
Blood Speciman		
8-hydroxy-2-deoxyquanosine	< 7.6 ng/ml	DNA increased ROS and cell proliferation*
Asymmetric dimethylarginine (ADMA)	<18 years: not established ≥18 years: 63-137 ng/mL	Inhibitor of L-arginine (Arg)-derived nitric oxide (NO)
C-reactive protein hi sensitivity	≤3.0 mg/l	Systemic inflammation related to bacterial infection, trauma, VAT, neoplastic activity
CA-125	0-35 U/mL	Inflammation in abdomen Ovarian cancer Uterine fibroids
CA 15-3/CA 27-29	<32 U/mL	Breast Cancer, advanced
CA-19-9	<55 U/mL	Pancreatic cancer
Carbohydrate Ag 19-9 (screening test)	Up to 20% of individuals do not express CA 19-9.	Infections in your liver, gallbladder, and pancreas.
CEA (other specimens also)	12-100 years: 0-5.0 ng/mL	Cancer
CD4 Lymphocyte CD4 percent		HIV infections, autoimmune
CD8 Count		Infections Lymphoma
Ceruloplasmin (bound copper/ acute phase reactant)	18-46 mg/dL	Acute Phase Reactant Cancer (elevated) Wilson's Disease (low) Menkes syndrome (low)

Continued

TABLE 3-1 Biomarkers of Prolonged Inflammation—cont'd

Test	Reference	Association
Eosinophils	1-4%	Elevated inflammatory marker of Allergies/ sensitivities, helminthic, parasites, autoimmune, neoplasms
Ferritin (storage iron)	Males ≥5 years: 24-150 ng/mL Females ≥5 years: 12-150 ng/mL	Acute Phase Reactant Hemochromatosis (genetic) Iron Toxicity
Fibrinogen / Platelets	150-450 mg/dL / 150-450 billion/L	Disseminated intravascular coagulation (DC) Liver disease
Homocysteine (Hcy)	0-15 umol/L	Block in homocysteine metabolism to cystothionine relate to B_6, B_{12}, folate, betaine co-factors
IgA Total or IgA specific	50-350 mg/dl	Elevated in lymphoproliferative disorders; chronic infections; autoimmune; celiac disease.
IgE Total or IgE specific	800-1500 mg/dl	Elevated immediate-response inflammatory allergic disorders; parasitic infections;
IgG Total or IgG specific	800-1500 mg/dl	Elevated inflammation marker of delayed sensitivities; chronic infections.
Interleukin-1 (IL-1)	<3.9 pg/mL	Bone formation, insulin secretion, appetite regulation, fever reduction, neuronal development
Interleukin 8 (IL-8)	<17.4 pg/mL < or = 5 pg/mL (2014)	Neoplasms /promotes angiogenesis Obesity Oxidative Stress
Insulin (Korkmaz 2014)	2.0-12.0 ulU/ml	Elevated inflammatory insulin resistance.
Lipid Peroxides	<2.60 nmol/ml	Inflammatory elevation when risk of oxidative stress/ elevated triglycerides.
Liver enzyme: ALT	0-35/U/L	Inflammatory elevation in liver disease
Liver enzyme: AST	0-35 U/L	Inflammatory elevation with liver, kidney, muscle infection or injury.
Liver enzymes: Alk Phos	30-120 U/L	Inflammatory elevation related to liver, bone, placenta
Liver enzyme: GGT	0-30 U/L	Elevated inflammatory marker of liver disease, neoplasms, toxicity
Liver enzyme: LDH	50-150 U/L	
Prostate Specific Antigen (PSA)	Total PSA ≤4.0 ng/mL % Free PSA >25 % (calc)	Prostate inflammation Prostate cancer
Rheumatoid factor (RF)	Less than 40-60 u/mL Less than 1:80 (1 to 80) titer	Rheumatoid Arthritis Sjorgrens Autoimmune disease
Sedimentation Rate/ ESR Westergren	Male <50 years old:<15 mm/hr Male>50 years old:<20 mm/hr Female<50years old:<20 mm/hr Female >50 years old:<30 mm/hr	Systemic inflammation marker related to autoimmune; viral infections; rouleaux; carcinoid influence.
Total Protein	60-80g/L. 6.0-8.0g/dl),	Total Protein in serum
Albumin	35 - 50 g/L (3.5 - 5.0 g/dL) (half-life ~ 20 days)	Acute Phase Reactant
Globulin	2.6-4.6 g/dL.	Chronic inflammation, low albumin levels and other disorders
TH17 Interlukin 17 (IL-17)	0.0 – 1.9 pg.ml	Fungal, bacterial, viral infections, autoimmune conditions
TNF-a	1.2-15.3 pg/mL	Systemic inflammation Acute Phase Reactant Alzheimer's, infection, depression, IBD, cancer
Uric Acid	2-7 mg/dl	Antioxidant, elevated in abnormal urate cycle exacerbated by protein in diet, gout, other.
VEGF	31-86 pg/mL	Cancer, angiogensis
White blood cell count	4.5- 11 x10E3/uL	(elevated) Leukocytosis , bacterial infections, anemia, cigarette smoking (Low) Cancer, radiation, severe infection
Stool Specimen		
Calprotectin	2–9 years 166 µg/g of feces 10–59 years 51 µg/g of feces ≥ 60 years 112 µg/g of feces	Inflammatory Bowel Disease Intestinal inflammation Neoplasms
Lactoferrin	Negative	Intestinal inflammation
Pancreatic elastase I	> 200 mcg/g	Exocrine pancreatic function
Urine		
5-hydroxyindoleacetate (5-HIAA)	1.6-10.9 mcg/ml creatinine	Elevated with inflammatory breakdown of serotonin.
p-hydroxyphenyllactate (HPLA)	<1.45 mcg/ml creatinine	Inverse relationship to depletion of ascorbic acid

*Normal value ranges may vary slightly among different labs

For the nutritionist to incorporate the related factors of prolonged inflammation into the nutrition assessment, it is useful to conceptualize an overview of a person's **total inflammatory load** (see Figure 3-1). It is a compilation of every factor in the patient's history or story that contributes to the inflammation that a person carries.

As various factors are identified within diet, lifestyle, environment, and genetics, the pattern of where the most inflammatory risk is being generated becomes clear and gives a basis of how to intervene with a plan for medical nutrition therapy (MNT).

Antigens

Antigens are a source of inflammation that become chronic with chronic exposure (see Chapter 26). During assessment of the total inflammatory load of an individual, the "antigenic load" is important. Antigens usually are thought to come from foods to which one is either allergic or sensitive, but also can be derived from cosmetics, clothing, inhalants, furniture, household building materials, and other substances in the environment. Antigens from food are much more likely to be significant when a person has lost gut barrier integrity and a situation of intestinal permeability, sometimes referred to as "leaky gut" exists (Fasano, 2012). This condition provides access of larger molecules into the internal microenvironment, setting off a cascade of immunologic responses (see Chapters 26 and 28).

Genomics

Predictive genomic testing, family history, and personal history are gathered as the practitioner hears the patient's story during an assessment. This information helps to paint a picture of biochemical individuality (Williams, 1956), which influences the response to inflammation. Since the completion of the Human Genome Project (2003), the rapid development of genomic testing for clinical application has greatly enhanced the toolbox of the nutrition practitioner. Nutrigenomics, nutrigenetics, and epigenetics are new fields of study about the way the individual metabolically interacts with their environment (Dick, 2015; see Chapter 5).

Body Composition

Chronic diseases are related directly to increased body fat exacerbated by physical inactivity, poor diet, lack of restorative sleep, and immune stress, all of which drive increased inflammation. Of equal importance with increased body fat percentage is the fat distribution. Central adiposity at all ages is the most serious health concern. **Visceral adipose tissue (VAT)** has been discovered to have endocrine functions with the secretion of several known inflammatory adipokines, such as resistin, leptin, and adiponectin, and tumor necrosis-factor-alpha (TNF-alpha)—all contributing to the systemic total inflammatory load (Hughes-Austin et al, 2014). **Sarcopenia** results from a wasting of lean body mass from the ongoing inflammatory burden and is exacerbated by decreased physical activity. Most often the sarcopenia is accompanied by increased body fat percentage, especially the deposit of VAT with increasing waist circumference.

Body composition can be assessed (see Chapter 7), and if found to be abnormal based an individual's lean body mass (LBM) and fat mass (FM), it should be considered a primary marker for monitoring prolonged inflammation (Biolo et al, 2015; Juby, 2014; Stenholm et al, 2008).

Obesity today stands at the intersection between inflammation and metabolic disorders causing an aberration of immune activity, and resulting in increased risk for diabetes, atherosclerosis, fatty liver, and pulmonary inflammation to name a few.

Khan et al, 2014a

In addition to assessing those who are overweight, obese, and have VAT, it is important to assess those with normal or low BMIs. However, body composition phenotypes cannot be determined based solely on BMI (Roubenoff, 2004). See Chapter 7 for assessment of body composition (see *Clinical Insight:* Sarcopenic Obesity).

Energy Dysregulation

Another underlying physiologic system involved in inflammation is compromised mitochondrial production of adenosine triphosphate (ATP) (Cherry and Piantadosi, 2015). Assessment of mitochondrial function focuses on structure and function by considering co-nutrients such as coenzyme Q10 and alpha-lipoic acid (already produced by the body) and their protective effects against oxidative stress. Quelling systemic prolonged inflammation promotes a healthier microenvironment for improved mitochondrial function and energy production.

Mitochondrial disease or dysfunction is an energy production problem. Almost all cells in the body have mitochondria, which are tiny "power plants" that produce a body's essential energy. Mitochondrial disease means the power plants in cells do not function properly. When that happens, some functions in the body do not work normally. It is as if the body has a power failure: there is a gradation of effects, like a "brown out" or a "black out."

The ratios of carbohydrate, fat, and protein affect mitochondrial function, primarily affecting glucose-insulin regulation. During each assessment, determination of the most favorable macronutrient ratios and individual nutrient requirements provides the foundation for the most effective interventions for restoring mitochondrial health and general wellness. The complaint of "fatigue" is the most common phenotypic expression of mitochondrial dysfunction (http://mitochondrialdiseases.org/mitochondrial-disease/, 2013. Accessed 02.07.15.) (see *New Directions:* Inflammaging).

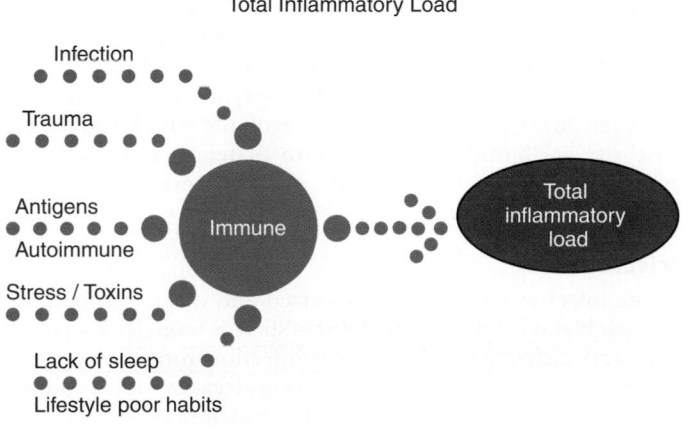

Total Inflammatory Load

Infection
Trauma
Antigens
Autoimmune
Stress / Toxins
Lack of sleep
Lifestyle poor habits

Immune

Total inflammatory load

FIGURE 3-1 Total Inflammatory Load

CLINICAL INSIGHT
Sarcopenic Obesity

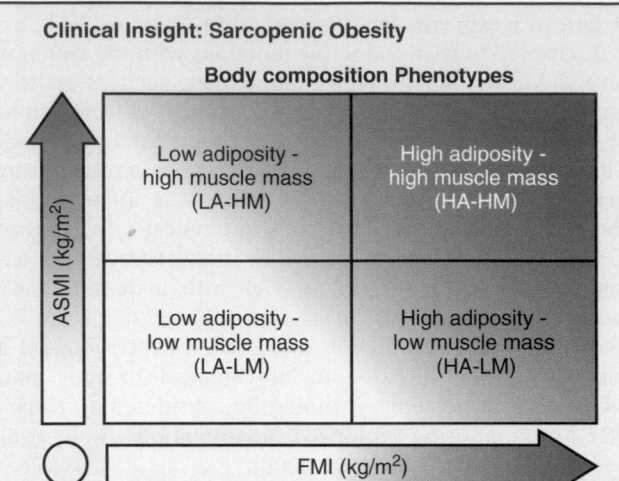

Clinical Insight: Sarcopenic Obesity

Body composition Phenotypes

	Low adiposity - high muscle mass (LA-HM)	High adiposity - high muscle mass (HA-HM)
ASMI (kg/m²) ↑	Low adiposity - low muscle mass (LA-LM)	High adiposity - low muscle mass (HA-LM)

○ → **FMI (kg/m²)**

In this figure, body composition is depicted by a spectrum of ASMI and FMI (low to high). On the basis of the Baumgartner model (Waters and Baumgartner, 2011), these phenotypes can be depicted as follows:

LA-HM = low adiposity with high muscle mass (individuals with low FMI and high ASMI)

HA-HM= high adiposity with high muscle mass (individuals with high FMI and ASMI)

LA-LM = low adiposity with low muscle mass (individuals with low ASMI and FMI)

HA- LM = high adiposity with low muscle mass (individuals with high FMI and low ASMI).

Those with **LA-HM would be the least healthiest.**

Cutoffs were defined according to the following deciles:

LA-HM (ASMI: 50–100; FMI: 0–49.99)
HA-HM (ASMI: 50–100; FMI: 50–100)
LA-LM (ASMI: 0–49.99; FMI: 0–49.99)
HA-LM (ASMI: 0–49.99; FMI: 50–100).

ASMI, appendicular skeletal muscle mass index; **FMI**, fat mass index
A population-based approach to define body-composition phenotypes
Carla MM Prado et. al: Am J Clin Nutr, 99:1369, 2014.

✳ NEW DIRECTIONS
Inflammaging

Aging is a ubiquitous complex phenomenon that results from environmental, stochastic, genetic, and epigenetic events in different cell types and tissues and their interactions throughout life. A pervasive feature of aging tissues and most if not all age-related diseases is chronic inflammation. "Inflammaging" describes the low-grade, chronic, systemic inflammation in aging, in the absence of overt infection ("sterile" inflammation) and is a highly significant risk factor for morbidity and mortality in the elderly (Franceschi and Campisi, 2014).

Microbiome

After the Human Genome Project, the National Institutes of Health (NIH) launched studies for genomic identification and characterization of the microorganisms associated with healthy and diseased humans. The exciting findings focus on five body sites (mouth, skin, vagina, gastrointestinal (GI)

tract, and nose/lung) and reveal data that exceed expectations. The total number of genes in the human microbiome exceeds the human genome tenfold. When the delicate microbiome community in and on the body is disturbed and altered from healthy baseline, it becomes a factor in promoting prolonged inflammation and affects the way food is used. The loss of microbiome diversity and the presence of specific undesirable or virulent bacteria appears to be a common finding related to various diseases (Fasano, 2012; Viladomiu, 2013).

The cause of these changes in the patterns of microbiota from "healthy" to dysfunctional appears to be influenced by genetics, diet, exposure to environmental toxins, and antibiotic use (National Institutes of Health [NIH], 2014). After pathology has been determined, the systems biology-based practitioner often uses the functional Comprehensive Digestive Stool Analysis (CDSA) testing to provide more quantitative and specific information regarding the condition of the gut environment and microbiology. The CDSA tests for inflammatory markers such as calprotectin, lactoferrin, and pancreatic elastase 1 in the gut, much like sedimentation rate or C-reactive protein-ultra sensitive (CRPus) and IgA are markers of inflammation in the blood (Gommerman, 2014). Because the GI tract contains about 70% of the immune system, it is important to assess the condition of the GI tract—from the mouth to the anus—as part of the total inflammatory load of an individual (Underwood, 2014). A new field of study regarding diseases that are related to disturbances in the gut environment and the immune system is called **enteroimmunology** (Lewis, 2014; see Figure 3–2).

Hypercoagulation

With inflammation comes an increasingly unhealthy degree of coagulation within body fluids. At some point, the microenvironment becomes too sluggish and congested, facilitating the development of chronic diseases such as cancer, cardiovascular disease, and infectious diseases (Karabudak et al, 2008). This increase in **body fluid viscosity** promotes secretion of more pro-inflammatory immune cytokines and chemokines that can set the stage for any of the chronic disease conditions. Autophagy is the normal response to raise the level of proteolytic enzymes to "clean up" the cell debris and prepare it for recycling or elimination (Gottleib and Mentzer, 2010; Gurkar et al, 2013; Wallace et al, 2014).

Dietary factors helping to maintain healthy fluid viscosity are hydration, vitamin E with significant gamma-tocopherol, polyunsaturated fatty acids (PUFAs), monounsaturated fats (MUFAs), and avoidance of any chronic subclinical infections and foods or substances that may act as antigens (see Chapter 26). Common biomarkers of increased body fluid viscosity are blood fibrinogen with platelets, and urinalysis measurements of specific gravity and the presence of "cloudiness" or mucus.

Infection

Acute infections are easily recognized and diagnosed because of their blatant signs and symptoms such as fever, leukocytosis, pus, and tachycardia. Subclinical infection processes, on the contrary, may go unnoticed for years or decades while promoting a "smoldering," under-the-radar, inflammatory condition

ENTEROIMMUNOLOGY

Enteroimmunology includes underlying pathophysiologies of many, if not all, autoimmune diseases. About 50% of the body's immune cells are housed in the intestine. The intestine secretes the largest amount of inflammatory cytokines in the body. What happens in an inflamed GUT has the potential to exacerbate inflammation throughout the body.

Common nonspecific symptoms
in enteroimmune disease

Area Affected	Symptoms
Cognitive	Mental fog, poor concentration, learning difficulties, poor memory, lethargy, apathy, rage, restlessness, hyperactivity
Sensory	Vertigo, lightheadedness, tinnitus
Emotional	Anxiety, moodiness, depression, aggressiveness, irritability
Somatic	Headaches, insomnia, fatigue, joint pain, muscle pain, stiffness, weakness, weight gain, fluid retention, non-ischemic chest pain
Gastrointestinal	Dyspepsia, bloating, belching, constipation, abdominal cramping, nausea, excessive flatulence
Respiratory	Congestion, excessive phlegm and mucous, dyspnea, chronic cough, gagging
Adapted from Lewis (2013)	

Some neurologic diseases
associated with enteroimmunopathies

- Autism
- Alzheimer's disease
- Parkinson's disease
- Multiple sclerosis
- Depression
- Bipolar disorder
- Schizophrenia
- Migraine headaches
- Cerebellar ataxia
- Certain seizure disorders

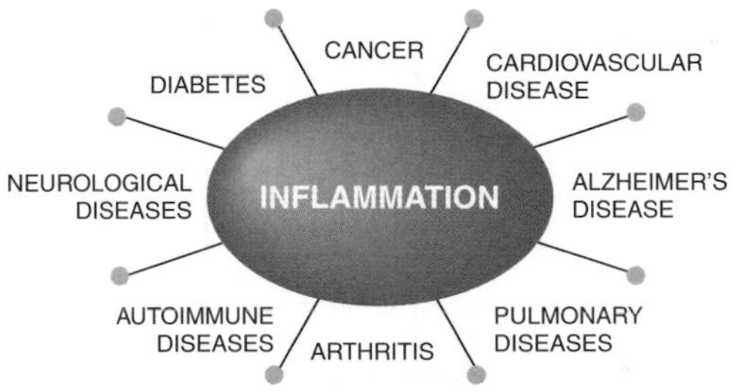

Copyright 2013 Diana Noland, MPH RD CCN

FIGURE 3-2 Enteroimmunology

that wears away at the integrity of the body cells and tissues. Good examples are hepatitis C virus (HCV), which begins as an acute infection but persists as a chronic infection in the liver (Vescovo et al, 2014), and human papilloma virus (HPV), which becomes chronic in cervical tissue and may lead to cervical cancer.

All chronic infections raise the level of immune response to produce inflammatory mediators and are exacerbated by nutrient insufficiencies and deficiencies and imbalances between prooxidant and antioxidant conditions (Cokluk et al, 2015). Other nutrients, when insufficient for optimum function, are involved in permitting chronic infections to persist over decades include vitamin D, vitamin C, and methylation nutrients such as folate, B_{12}, B_6, and B_2, which act as co-nutrients in inflammation and immune-control mechanisms (Ames, 2010). In addition, the health of the microbiome in the gastrointestinal tract, the skin, and other body orifices plays a critical role in inflammation and immune strength or weakness.

Stress

Stress is inflammatory. The sources of metabolic stress may include injury, infection, musculoskeletal misalignment, lack of sleep, emotions, unhealthy diet, smoking, quality of life challenges, or lack or excess of physical activity. Whatever the source, stress can increase nutrient requirements contributing to depletion and the level of oxidative stress risks of damage to body cells and tissues.

NUTRIENT MODULATORS OF INFLAMMATION

For the prostaglandins formed from the eicosanoid cascade, there are vitamin, mineral, and antioxidant nutrients that act as rate-limiting cofactors for the shared delta-5 and delta-6 desaturase and the elongase enzymes required for conversion of the essential fatty acids (EFA) and polyunsaturated fatty acids (PUFAs) to prostaglandins. These co-nutrients, listed in Figure 3-3, have the important ability to modulate the fatty acids and their antiinflammatory products

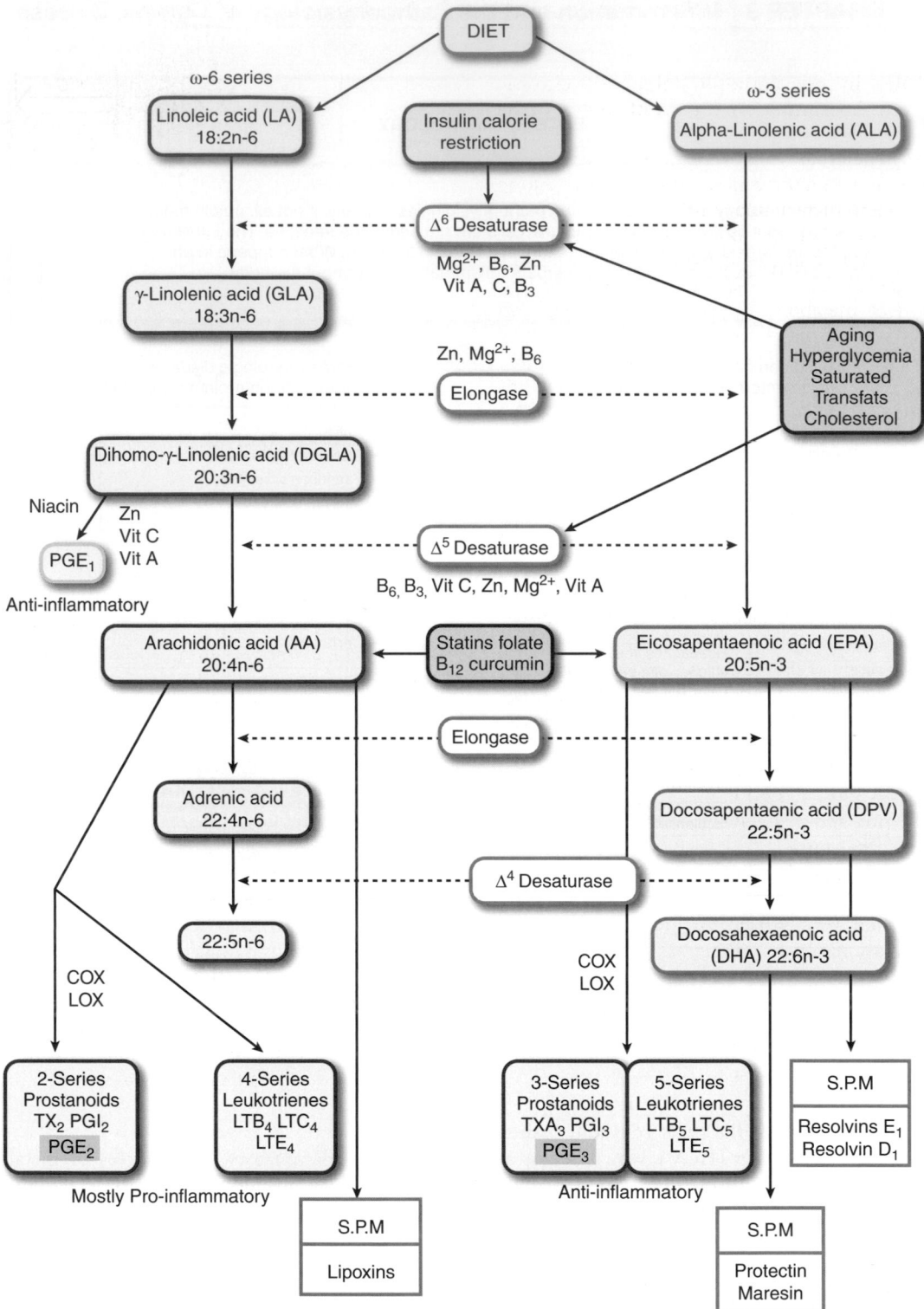

FIGURE 3-3 Mechanisms of essential fatty acids and Eicosanoid metabolites in modulating inflammation Inflammatory biological responses are driven by a balance between feedback loops, much like a "toggle" switch, influenced by messages from hormones, lifestyle and nutrient co-factors (see primary enzyme nutrient-co-factors listed in diagram). The Eicosanoid biological cascade responses receive environmental messages from diet, lifestyle, infection and trauma. From the essential fatty acids (LA, ALA), downstream metabolites are produced dependent on hormonal messages, genotype and adequate nutrient co-factors of enzymatic conversion activity. Acute inflammatory triggers to initiate a healing response from infection or trauma are then resolved to homeostasis by specialized proresolving mediators (SPM) in healthy subjects. This complex dance of biochemical activity is handicapped by interferring conditions (see (circle with X in it) noted in the diagram above). Nutrition status from regular intake over the lifespan of essential fatty acids and nutrient dense whole foods build the foundation for healthy Eicosanoid management of acute and prolonged inflammation.

that have key roles in the pathophysiology of chronic disease and systemic inflammation that contributes to its progression.

Nutrient insufficiencies and imbalances that accompany prolonged inflammation initially can go unrecognized. Along with possible insufficient dietary intake of nutrients, there can potentially be imbalances of the body nutrient reservoirs. Various stressors or genomic single nucleotide polymorphisms (SNPs) (see Chapter 5) can also cause increased nutrient requirements to meet metabolic needs, and those depleted nutrients become "conditionally essential" for an individual. Dr. Robert P. Heaney has provided a simplified conceptual diagram called the sigmoid curve to illustrate the concepts of dynamic varied nutrient needs of the physiologic "nutrient needs spectrum." (see Figure 3-4).

Nutriture is the state of nutrition. This skill of assessing the *nutriture* condition of body tissues relies on evidence-based research, physiologic science–based, individual nutrient therapy skills, and the awareness that no nutrient functions in isolation but has extensive interaction with other molecular compounds (e.g., hormones, nutrients, ROS). Manipulating biologic function with nutrition always must include consideration of the "rate limiting" restrictions on a biochemical system. Like a food recipe, if any "ingredient" in the "biology of life recipe" is depleted or missing, the final product is flawed (see http://blogs.creighton.edu/heaney/2013/06/25/some-rules-for-studies-evaluating-nutrient-effects/).

Examples of some critical nutrient-partner balances are omega-6 and omega-3 fatty acids, vitamin D and vitamin A, magnesium and calcium, and folate, B_6, B_2, and B_{12}. In whole or unprocessed foods, these nutrients naturally exist in balance, such as vitamin A and D in cod liver oil, in liver, and in eggs (see Box 3-1).

The nutrient partners most strongly associated with influencing prolonged inflammation are discussed below.

Omega-6 Linoleic Acid and Omega-3 Alpha-Linolenic Acid (Essential Fatty Acids)

Fish ingestion several times a week has been associated with reduced risk of chronic disease, especially cardiac disease. It is a characteristic of the Mediterranean Diet (Pallauf et al, 2013), the Asian Diet (Kruk, 2014), and the more recently studied Nordic or Viking Diet described in the Systems Biology in Controlled Dietary Interventions and Cohort Studies (SYSDIET) (Kolehmainem, 2015; Uusitupa et al, 2013). The human metabolism of oils in fish and their bioactive mediators provide important factors in inflammatory processes. The relationship of diet to inflammatory biochemistry supports a strong position for the nutritionist to develop individualized interventions to ensure adequate balance of the eicosanoid-producing foods that decrease inflammation.

Three main groups of prostaglandin metabolites are formed from the two initial essential fatty acids in the eicosanoid cascade (linoleic acid [LA] and alpha-linolenic acid [ALA]): prostaglandin 1 (PGE1) (omega 6 di-homo gamma-linoleic acid [DGLA]-derived antiinflammatory), prostaglandin 2 (PGE2) (omega 6-arachidonic-derived pro-inflammatory), and prostaglandin 3 (PGE3) (omega 3-derived antiinflammatory). These metabolites are precursors for a wide range of bioactive lipid mediators influencing inflammation within the body. Again, like making a recipe in the kitchen, the nutritionist

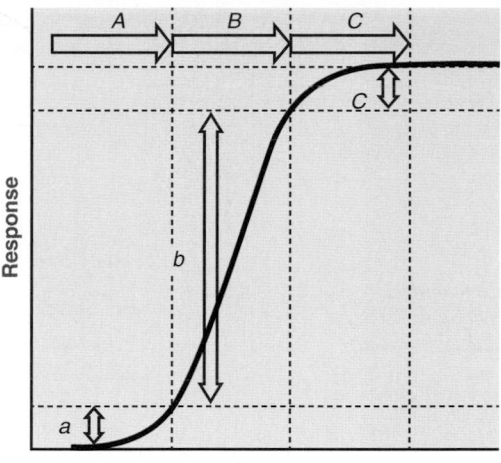

Typical sigmoid curve showing physiological response as a function of nutrient intake. Depicted are the expected responses from *equal* increments in intake, starting from a low basal intake, and moving to progressively higher starting levels. Intake increments *A*, *B*, and *C* produce responses, *a*, *b*, and *c*, respectively. Only intakes in the *B* region produce responses large enough adequately to test the hypothesis that the nutrient concerned elicits the response in question. (Copyright Robert P. Heaney, MD., 2010. All rights reserved. Used with permission.)

FIGURE 3-4 Sigmoid Curve (Heaney 2010) PERMISSION BY ROBERT HEANEY Heaney RP: The Nutrient Problem, *Nutr Rev* 70:165, 2012.

can assess and then develop an individualized intervention "recipe" to return the individual's metabolic balance in these three groups of metabolites of the eicosanoid series toward wellness for the individual. The most accurate way to assess fatty acid status is to evaluate dietary fat intake (see Table 3-2), absorptive capacity (bile adequacy, pancreatic function), and red blood cell (RBC) fatty acids (Kelley, 2009). Collecting this nutrition data for an individual during assessment can reveal important underlying physiologic imbalances. (See Chapters 4 and 7.)

The balance between the two eicosanoid pathways, omega-3 and omega-6, exert inflammatory control in response to the metabolic environment (Gil et al, 2015). Prostaglandins contribute to the regulation of vascular tone, platelet function, and fertility (Ricciotti and FitzGerald, 2011; Stipanuk and Caudill, 2013). They also play key roles as inflammatory mediators and modulators of tumor biology and are major regulators of growth and transport in epithelial cells (Varga et al, 2014). Although technically hormonal in function (autocrine/paracrine), because they do not have a specific organ of secretion, they are not often referred to as such.

The prostaglandins formed as downstream metabolites are the primary metabolic control for acute and chronic inflammation. The seminal observation that omega-3 EPA could modulate eicosanoid biosynthesis to suppress arachidonic acid biosynthesis, an omega-6 fatty acid, was first made in 1962 (Machlin) and 1963 (Mohrhauer and Holman) and initiated the plethora of research on the use of fish oil supplements to calm inflammation.

TABLE 3-2   Fat-Oil Dietary Intake Survey

Fats and Oils

Please indicate how many times PER WEEK you eat the following fats/oils.

OMEGA 9 (stabilizer) ~50% of daily fat calories Oleic Fatty Acid	__ Almond Oil __ Almonds/Cashews __ Almond butter __ Avocados __ Peanuts __ Peanut butter (natural/soft)	__ Olives __ Olive Oil __ Sesame Seeds/Tahini __ Hummus (tahini oil) __ Macadamia Nuts __ Pine Nuts
OMEGA 6 (controllers) *Essential Fatty Acid Family* ~30% of daily fat calories LA→GLA→DGLA→AA	__ Eggs (whole), organic (AA) __ Meats (commercial) (AA) __ Meats (grass-fed, org) (AA) __ Brazil nuts (raw) __ Pecan (raw) __ Hazelnuts/Filberts (raw) __ Hemp Seeds	__ Evening Primrose (GLA) __ Black Currant Oil (GLA) __ Borage Oil (GLA) __ Hemp Oil __ Grapeseed Oil __ Sunflower Seeds (raw) __ Pumpkin seeds (raw)
OMEGA 3 (fluidity/communicators) *Essential Fatty Acid Family* ~10% of daily fat calories ALA→EPA→DHA	__ Fish Oil capsule:↑DHA __ Fish Oil capsule: ↑TEPA __ Fish (salmon/fin-fish) __ Fish (shellfish) __ Flax seeds/meal	__ Flax Oil __ UDO's DHA Oil __ Algae __ Greens Powder w/algae __ Chia seeds
BENEFICIAL SATURATED (structure) ~10% of daily fat calories Short Chain/Medium-chain Triglycerides	__ Coconut Oil __ Butter, organic __ Ghee (clarified butter) __ Dairy, raw & organic	__ Meats, grass-fed __ Wild game __ Poultry, organic __ Eggs, whole organic
DAMAGED FATS/OILS (promoting stress to cells & tissues) Should be <5% (try to avoid) Trans Fats Acrylamides Odd-Chain Fatty Acids VLCFA/damaged	__ Margarine __ Reg. vegetable oils (corn, sunflower, canola) __ Mayonnaise (Commercial) __ Hydrogenated Oil (as an ingredient) __ "Imitation" cheeses __ Tempura	__ Doughnuts (fried) __ Deep-fried foods __ Chips fried in oil __ Regular salad dressing __ Peanut Butter (JIF, etc) __ Roasted nuts/seeds __ Products with hydrogenated fats

An interesting molecule is formed from the eicosanoid cascade, omega-3 DHA, a C22 with antiinflammatory effects (Shichiri et al, 2014), collaborating with the omega-3 EPA. EPA and DHA are found in fish oil, and they are biochemically reversible, meaning they can be metabolized from one molecule to the other. DHA is a critical component of many body tissues such as the eye and brain, and it contributes to modulation of metabolic inflammation. It illustrates the enormous capacity of the body to have redundant and multiple systems to provide essential molecules for metabolism.

The key eicosanoid metabolic intersections in the eicosanoid cascade are omega-6 gamma-linolenic acid (GLA), di-homo-gamma linolenic acid (DGLA), and arachidonic acid (AA) co-existing with omega-3 eicosapentaenoic acid (EPA) and docosahexaenoic acid (DHA). As the knowledge of the functions of these eicosanoid metabolites has matured over the past 50 years, their synergistic relationships and the need to keep them in homeostatic balance is now appreciated (Das, 2011). The omega-6 and omega-3 eicosanoids share the same desaturase and elongase enzymes, so there is a competition between the two, ready to move in response to the environment and availability of cofactor nutrients (Reed, 2014).

Today, knowledge that fatty acid intake can change physiologic responses by modification of eicosanoid metabolism to favor synthesis of antiinflammatory prostaglandins and leukotrienes (produced by the oxidation of arachidonic acid) can help manage chronic inflammation (Arm et al, 2013). As more RCT studies are available, it is hoped this will result in an improved model for study of nutrient synergistic influences on metabolism. Wergeland and colleagues designed a multivariable study of a combination of fatty acid therapies that showed a suppression of inflammation in multiple sclerosis described as "beneficial disease-modifying effect of increased intake of polyunsaturated fatty acids (PUFAs)" (Wergeland et al, 2012). Even as far back as 1993, Berth-Jones hypothesized that "since both ω6 and ω3 essential fatty acids may possess this property [anti-inflammatory], it is possible that giving both together will have a synergistic effect" (1993).

Metabolically the five primary eicosanoids (GLA, DGLA, AA, EPA, DHA) collaborate and compete for shared enzymes in forming the prostaglandin groups: prostaglandin 1 (PGE1), prostaglandin 2 (PGE2), and prostaglandin 3 (PGE3) series (see Figure 3-3). Each plays a critical role in the control of inflammatory conditions. Until the research interest in the 1990s of the dynamic influence omega-3 EPA has on elevated omega-6 AA, dietary intake of the essential fatty acids was the main determinant of the levels of these fatty acids in tissue composition.

However, as awareness of omega-3 and its function increased, a large portion of the U.S. population is now adding omega-3 fatty acids to their regular nutraceutical intake. This has resulted in some individuals who take more than 500 mg EPA and/or DHA daily with the result that arachidonic acid and gamma-linolenic acid (GLA) biosynthesis is suppressed with the potential to unbalance the levels of these two molecules (Horribin, 2000). Nutrient partners require balance for optimum metabolic function. A nutrition assessment should consider the fatty acid supplements a client is taking and for how long, in addition to the amount in the diet to assess the potential for imbalance. If laboratory testing of fatty acid parameters is available, it can add a quantitative evaluation to the assessment (Djousse et al, 2012; Guo et al, 2010; Mouglos et al, 1995) (see Chapter 7).

Prostaglandin 1 Series (PGE1): Antiinflammatory

PGE1 metabolites are part of the balancing act between prostaglandin groups to manage inflammation, with a primary antiinflammatory effect on the tissue microenvironment. PGE1 is particularly important for the effects of GLA and its conversion to DGLA in managing inflammation. GLA not only attenuates intracellular inflammation by converting to DGLA (Arm et al, 2013) but also reduces inflammation in the extracellular matrix present in diabetic nephropathy (Kim et al, 2012). Evidence suggests skin integrity and other inflammatory conditions have a "conditionally essential" (Kendler, 2006) need for GLA (Harbige, 2003; Muggli, 2005).

Another physiologic function of the fatty acids is that GLA, DGLA, EPA, and DHA, if kept in balance, can function as inhibitors of tumor cell proliferation and migration in in-vitro and in-vivo conditions (Rahman et al, 2013; Wang et al, 2012; Yao et al, 2014).

Prostaglandin 2 Series (PGE2): Pro-inflammatory When in Excess

PGE2's ability to increase tissue inflammation is part of the cause of inflammation with pain, swelling, fever, redness, and constriction of blood vessels that lead to loss of function. Arachidonic acid (AA) increases with acute injury to bring inflammation and increased healing blood flow, but with chronic disease's prolonged character, AA can get "stuck" in an elevated state and continue to damage tissue and encourage degeneration. The neoplastic disease overproduction of PGE2 in the tumor environment has been found to simulate the growth and formation of a substantial number of carcinomas (Goodwin, 2010).

AA can become dangerously elevated, especially when dietary intake has deficient levels of omega-3 ALA, EPA, and DHA to act as an AA counterbalance. The United States and most industrialized countries' populations live with high AA levels because of low intake of omega-3 oils and large intakes of highly processed PUFAs and trans fats.

With all the reporting over the past 20 years of elevated AA being the generator of the fire of chronic disease, AA function in a healthy human must be acknowledged for its positive contribution to stable cell membranes and inflammation control. AA has essential functions in platelet aggregation and vasoconstriction, for example. Targeted nutrition therapy must have a goal of healthy homeostasis requiring monitoring to ensure omega-3 supplementation does not cause AA levels to fall too low (Khan et al, 2014).

Prostaglandin 3 Series (PGE3): Antiinflammatory

Another aspect of antiinflammatory action lies in the PGE3 group and their metabolites, leukotriene-5 series and others, which promote suppression of AA, GLA, and DGLA. They are most studied in relation to cardiovascular pathologies such as vascular and coagulation health, but often the suppression of GLA goes unnoticed and unappreciated.

Lipoxygenases (LOX)

Lipoxygenases (LOX) are intermediates that produce inflammatory leukotrienes-4 (PGE2) or antiinflammatory leukotrienes-5 (PGE3). LOX-4 and LOX-5 molecules can modulate inflammation, mostly as mediators of cell signaling and as modifiers of cell membrane structures. Practical examples of structural changes are in red blood cell maturation, modification of lung barrier function to improve bronchial function in asthma conditions, and others. The LOX molecules also act as a substrate in the mobilization of fatty acids in membranes involving beta-oxidation metabolism of fatty acids. The LOX are expressed more intensely under physiologic stress (Brash, 1999; Allaj, 2013).

Cyclooxygenases (COX)

Another group of eicosanoid metabolites, the cyclooxygenase (COX) products, have an important role in reproduction and in the inflammatory response with inflammatory COX (PGE2) molecules and antiinflammatory COX (PGE1 and PGE3).

Specialized Pro-resolving Mediators (SPM)

More recent recognition of further downstream metabolites of a different class are called SPM derived from both w3 and w6 PUFA. These SPM lipid molecules are capable of initiating a resolution phase of inflammation to return metabolism to homeostasis. These SPMs are lipoxins, resolvins, protectins and maresins (See Fig 3-3). These mediators appear to explain some of the anti-inflammatory effects of PGE1, PGE2 and PGE3 metabolites (Calder, 2009).

REDUCING INFLAMMATION IN THE BODY

Modern research of essential fatty acids (EFA) and their metabolites has been concerned mainly with the therapeutic impact on the inflammatory process. However, as with all systems in the body, there are opposing mediators in the body's regulation of these systems to achieve homeostasis or allostasis to promote survival. Among the primary mediators of inflammation are biogenic amines, such as histamine and serotonin, cytokines, prostaglandins, thromboxanes, and leukotrienes. The PGE1 and PGE3 antiinflammatory action oppose and balance the PGE2 inflammatory systems. Both are required for healthy metabolism. For instance, derivatives of the omega-6 GLA and DGLA acids regulate the inflammatory process through their opposed activity and synergism with EPA, by directing formation at the crossroads to the antiinflammatory PGE1, or the inflammatory PGE2 molecules. In parallel metabolism the derivatives of the omega-3 ALA, EPA, DHA, and others form the antiinflammatory PGE3 metabolites, while at the same time inhibiting the transformation of AA to leukotrienes and conversion of DGLA to the PGE1 molecules. This antiinflammatory action of the omega-3 eicosanoids is most researched because of their powerful suppression of AA associated with cardiovascular disease (Tousoulis et al, 2014).

It is important to understand the enzymes responsible for healthy metabolic conversions from the essential fatty acids, LA and ALA, and how to target them with foods and nutrients. These enzymes are illustrated on the eicosanoid cascade (see Figure 3-3). The desaturase enzymes (delta-5 and delta-6) and the elongase enzymes are shared and are in competition between the omega-6 and omega-3 pathways. Delta-6-desaturase transforms LA into GLA and ALA to EPA by making additional double bonds. Of all the endogenous conversion steps in the eicosanoid cascade, the one driven by delta-6-desaturase is the least efficient and not biochemically equipped to handle the conversion of high dietary intake of LA found in the standard American diet (Kurotani et al, 2012). In the competition for the enzyme between the omega-6 and omega-3 metabolites, a preference has been shown toward the omega-3s. However, these enzyme systems are affected by the adequacy of nutrient cofactors such as zinc, vitamin B_6, and magnesium and other physiologic and pathologic factors, such as hyperglycemia, that can lead to GLA deficiency.

This is seen often in type 2 diabetes related to the hyperglycemia in the early stages of that disease. GLA supplementation has been shown to bypass the inefficient rate-limiting delta-6-desaturase system in the formation of LA to GLA and then DGLA, and which pathway it will follow—either antiinflammatory PG1 or inflammatory AA-PG2 and their derivatives. EPA has been shown in the omega-3 pathway to bypass the delta-6-desaturase conversion of ALA to EPA (Innis, 2014; see Figure 3–3). The biology of essential fatty acids and particularly the role of GLA is important as part of the quelling of excessive prolonged inflammation (Dobryniewski, 2007; Miyake, 2009).

A targeted approach using dietary, nutraceutical, or enteral and parenteral lipids directs PUFAs to shift the metabolism of eicosanoids toward homeostasis, thereby attributing potent antiinflammatory effects (Triana et al, 2014; Waitzberg, 2014; see Chapter 13). There are promising data out of Europe, where olive oil–based intravenous lipids have been used for a decade, which indicate that by using different intravenous fat sources, inflammation can be reduced.

Short-term and long-term inflammatory stimulation influence COX pathways in shifting them to the "less inflammatory" COX (PGE3 and thromboxane [TX]-3), and the resolvins derived from EPA and DHA polyunsaturated fatty acids (LC PUFAs) through Cox-2 enzymatic epoxidation (5-lipoxygenase), thereby offering protection against inflammation (Kahn SA, 2014; Uddin 2011).

Dietary therapies to improve balance and promote adequate GLA to DGLA conversion that directs DGLA toward conversion to the PGE1 prostanoids include weight management, improving insulin sensitivity, and adequate nutrient stores of vitamin D, EFA, zinc, magnesium, B_6, and others. Nutraceuticals studied include GLA-rich plant oils from evening primrose, black currant, and borage (Pickens et al, 2014).

The nutritionist who is skilled in assessing an individual's fatty acid balance, by first performing a dietary intake survey (see Table 3-2), and more specifically by obtaining an RBC fatty acid analysis, can more accurately target interventions to see improved outcomes in managing inflammation. With the information from a RBC fatty acid test, one can calculate an Omega-3 Index, a prognostic indicator of cardiovascular disease (CVD) (Harris et al, 2004; von Schacky, 2014; see Figure 3–5).

These assessment parameters provide a roadmap that is able to guide individualized lipid interventions. With this information, the levels of lipids in the body can be manipulated toward a healthy composition, restoring a degree of optimum inflammation-immune response in all systems of the body. Targeted

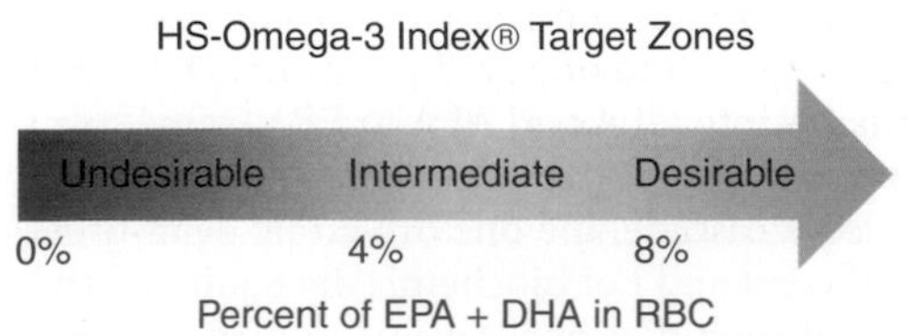

HS-Omega-3 Index® Target Zones

FIGURE 3-5 HS-Omega-3 Index® Target Zones

nutrient therapy using dietary supplements, functional foods, or therapeutic herbal compounds can be mediators of these metabolic enzyme systems and help take advantage of the membrane and tissue malleability affected by dietary and lifestyle changes. These therapies usually require 2 to 12 months of nutrient therapy to achieve successful outcomes.

Cytochrome P450 Enzymes

Cytochrome P450 (CYP450) enzymes are essential for the production of cholesterol, steroids, prostacyclins, and thromboxane A_2. They are also involved in the first pass hydroxylation of endogenous and exogenous toxic molecules in the detoxification transport of toxins for elimination via the feces and bile, urine, and sweat. If the enzyme function is suppressed by poor integrity of the enzyme structure, abnormal pH microenvironment, hepatic inflammation, altered availability of nutrient cofactors, or CYP450 genotype, then there is a backup of toxins and an increase in an individual's toxic load. These CYP450 enzymes are expressed primarily in the liver, but they also occur in the small intestine, kidneys, lungs, and placenta.

More tools for assessment of all the systems of the body's metabolism are becoming available. Testing for the CYP450 single nucleotide polymorphisms (SNP), for instance, allows recognition of a person's metabolic strengths and weaknesses that can influence nutritional interventions (see Chapter 5). The increased availability of nutrigenomic testing is supporting clinical application of a person's genome to provide more detail in understanding the patient's story and the foods and nutrients that enable these biochemical and genomic systems to function.

Vitamin D

Vitamin D (cholecalciferol) actually functions as a prohormone with multiple roles, including hormone and immune modulation, antiinflammatory and antitumor effects, and apoptosis support (Alele and Kamen, 2010; Maruotti and Cantatore, 2010). This suggests that vitamin D is able to physiologically contribute to the regulation of all immune responses, by means of the vitamin D receptor (VDR) expressed in the nucleus of these cells. Epidemiologic, genetic, and basic studies indicate a potential role of vitamin D in the pathogenesis of certain systemic and organ-specific autoimmune diseases (Agmon-Levin et al, 2013).

Vitamin D is made in the skin upon exposure to UV sunlight or artificial rays (therapeutically used in northern and southern extreme latitudes), as well as obtained by dietary sources (fatty fish, fish eggs or caviar, organ meats, egg yolk, and mushrooms; see Appendix 51). The past decade has spotlighted attention on an apparent global epidemic of low vitamin D status without a known cause. Many chronic diseases are associated with increased prevalence of lowered vitamin D levels as vitamin D 25-OH vit D levels fall below 30 ng/ml (75 nmol/L) (see Chapter 7). Recommendations to test for 25-OH vit D and supplement vitamin D are becoming more common to increase blood levels to a goal of 40 to 50 ng/ml (90 to 100 nmol/L). A serum 25(OH) vit D level of approximately 52 ng/ml has been shown to be associated with a reduction by 50% in the incidence of breast cancer (Krishnan et al, 2012). An estimate is that for each additional 1000 IU/day of vitamin D intake, the serum 25(OH) vit D may increase by 4 to 5 ng/ml (10 to 20 nmol/L) (Stipanuk and Caudill, 2013).

Vitamin D is well evidenced to exhibit antiinflammatory effects (Khan, 2014; Krishnan et al, 2012; Krishnan et al, 2013).

Also, as a nutrient partner, the vitamin A (retinol/retinyl palmitate) relationship with vitamin D lies in the sharing of the RXR nuclear receptor with the vitamin D receptor (VDR), establishing a synergistic effect between the two. In nature vitamins A and D are always found together (e.g., liver, egg yolk; see Appendix 41). Because of the close proximity to this RXR nuclear receptor in all cells, there is a synergistic relationship. If one is too high or too low, it can affect the function of the other. Vitamin A (retinol) has been shown to relate to vitamin D function, so prudent testing of vitamin A retinol and 25(OH) vit D when investigating a person's vitamin D status is recommended before supplementation (Schmutz et al, 2015).

Minerals
Magnesium

Magnesium is involved with more than 300 identified enzyme systems in metabolism. It is a key partner as the counterpart of calcium: magnesium being the "relaxing" parasympathetic promoting partner with the "contracting" and sympathetic promoting calcium. They function in balance in a healthy metabolism. Magnesium is inversely related to the systemic inflammatory C-reactive protein blood values (Dibaba et al, 2015). The potential beneficial effect of magnesium intake on chronic disease may be, at least in part, explained by its inhibition of inflammation (Dibaba et al, 2015).

The NHANES 1999-2000 study revealed that 60% of the U.S. population consumed inadequate dietary magnesium from low vegetable and whole grain intake. Low dietary magnesium intake has been related to several health outcomes, including those related to metabolic and inflammatory processes such as hypertension, metabolic syndrome (He et al, 2006; Rayssiguier et al, 2006; Song et al, 2005), type 2 diabetes (Song et al, 2004), cardiovascular diseases (Liu and Chacko, 2013; Stevanovic et al, 2011), osteoporosis, and some cancers (e.g., colon, breast) (Nielsen, 2010).

Magnesium requires the microenvironment of other essential nutrients, especially its nutrient-partners, calcium and zinc. Dietary intake of chlorophyll-rich vegetables, nuts, and seeds and whole grains provides adequate magnesium if digestion and absorption are functioning well (see Appendix 50). Recently, López-Alarcón and colleagues, in their study linking low-grade inflammation with obesity in children, looked at several inflammation-related biomarkers and concluded that the most significant determinants of inflammation were a magnesium-deficient diet and central obesity (López-Alarcón et al, 2014).

Zinc

Zinc is a primary cofactor for more than 300 enzymes, many of which are involved in inflammatory processes. See Appendix 53 for food sources of zinc. Intracellular zinc is required for cell signaling within the intestinal tissue triggered by the inflammatory cytokine TNF-alpha (Ranaldi et al, 2013). Zinc deficiency leads to thymic atrophy and decreased function. The thymus gland is responsible for the production of T-lymphocytes, a critical part of immunity.

Zinc is the nutrient partner to copper, so when assessing zinc status, copper also should be considered. Gibson (2008) has described loss of taste (especially in the elderly) with zinc deficiency, and this should be noted when taking a history from an individual. Also, as a metabolic "hint," because alkaline phosphatase (Alk Phos) is a zinc-dependent/zinc sensitive enzyme, its measurement may suggest further investigation for zinc insufficiency.

Currently, zinc status assessment includes only dietary intake data because there are no reliable functional zinc status tests. However, useful indicators are copper status, the erythrocyte zinc/copper ratio, and hair mineral testing (Stipanuk and Caudill, 2013). In a nutrition-focused physical exam, white spots under the nails (if injury has been ruled out), loss of appetite, anorexia nervosa, loss of normal taste sensation, alopecia, hyperkeratinization of skin, dermatitis, and reproductive abnormalities can indicate possible zinc deficiencies. (Stipanuk and Caudill, 2013; see Appendices 21 and 22).

Methylation

Methylation is universal throughout metabolism, and methyl factor nutrients are one of the primary promoters of healthy methylation. The B complex vitamins work synergistically and are critical to the methylation process. Folate, B_6, B_2 and B_{12} have been shown to be the most rate-limiting when insufficient. More recent research has identified various advantages of vitamin forms when used as dietary supplement therapy to manage inflammation of chronic disease. This is true, for example, with the SNPs MTHFR 677C or MTHFR 1298C when the 5-MTHF form of folate rather than the synthetic folic acid is used (Bailey, 2010; Manshadi, 2014; Miller, 2010; Vollset, 2014) (see *Clinical Insight*: Synthetic and Bioactive B-Complex Vitamins).

CLINICAL INSIGHT

Synthetic and Bioactive B-Complex Vitamins

B-Complex Vitamins	Synthetic form/ common name	Bioactive Natural Form in Foods
B1	Thiamin mononitrate Thiamin hydrochloride	Thiamin (benfotiamine)
B2	Riboflavin	Riboflavin-5-phosphate
B3	Nicotinic acid	Nicotinamide adenine dinucleotide (NAD)
	Niacin (generic term)	NAD phosphate (NADP) Niacinamide
B5	Pantothenic acid D pantothenate Panthenol	Pantothenate
B6	Pyridoxine-HCl	Pyridoxine-5-phosphate (P5P)
B12	Cyanocobalamin	Methylcobalamin Hydroxycobalamin Adenoylcobalamin
B9	Folic Acid	Folinic Acid 5-Methyltetrahydrofolate 5-Formyltetrahydrofolate
B7	Biotin	Biotin (Biocytin)

To date, the methylation system most associated with inflammation of chronic disease is the methylation of DNA, which is especially sensitive. Chronic diseases related to methylation from epigenetic influences from the environment relate to potential development and promotion of cancer (Ehrlich, 2002), inflammatory bowel disease such as Crohn's disease (Karatzas et al, 2014), cognitive function, mood disorders (Hing et al, 2014), and cardiovascular disease (Delbridge, 2015).

The mechanisms supporting this methylation have important implications in inflammation and immune responses

(Kominsky et al, 2010). These mechanisms rely on B vitamin cofactors and the role they play in the methylation metabolism involving folate and homocysteine (Nazki et al, 2014), as well as the eicosanoid cascade producing the inflammation-controlling prostaglandins. These methyl factors are involved in upregulating gene expression concerned with neurotransmitters, nitric oxide (eNO), and methionine metabolism, precursors to antiinflammatory compounds that protect from oxidative stress damage, and other mechanisms (Das, 2007).

CLINICAL INSIGHT

Understanding the Eicosanoid Cascade

A primary nutrient group involved in the control of inflammation is the essential fatty acids, omega-3 alpha-linolenic acid (ALA) and omega-6 linoleic acid (LA), and their downstream metabolites described as the eicosanoid cascade (see Figure 3-3). A nutrition assessment skill for managing prolonged inflammation of chronic disease is a thorough working knowledge of the eicosanoid cascade pathway and the enzymes and nutrient cofactors involved. The polyunsaturated fatty acid (PUFA) metabolites of the essential fatty acids and their hormone-like prostaglandins respond like on/off switches that react to the internal and external environment stimulating anti- or pro-inflammatory signals. In chronic diseases, the switches become dominated by the pro-inflammatory signals. Imbalances in the metabolism of eicosanoid prostaglandin metabolites produced by the essential fatty acids linoleic and alpha-linolenic acids hold particular significance in determining the onset of prolonged inflammation and are influenced by dietary intake.

The methylation genes are currently the most studied of the single nucleotide polymorphisms (SNPs) and able to provide data for clinical application. Most national laboratories provide testing for these genes MTHFR C667T, MTHFR 1298C, and COMT. Others are available at specialty labs (see Chapter 5 and Figure 3-6).

Flavonoids and Antioxidant Nutrients

Flavonoids or bioflavonoids are phytonutrients associated with the varied colors found in fruits and vegetables. These phytonutrients provide antiinflammatory antioxidant functions beneficially messaging the immune system (Grimble, 1994; Jeena et al, 2013). They provide protection against free radical and reactive oxygen species (ROS) activity that cause inflammation, and they modulate epigenetic effects by collaborating with the fatty acid and prostaglandin status of a person.

When the antioxidant and flavonoid status is inadequate to protect cells and tissues, accelerated damage occurs, promoting degeneration, and depleting the health of the individual. The most studied flavonoid compound researched to date is **curcumin**, a component of the spice turmeric (Agrawal, 2015; Tuorkey, 2014). Another example is **quercitin**, a component of citrus pulp, apples, and onions, which is a yellow flavonoid with antiinflammatory action towards mast cells. Quercitin-rich foods are helpful in quelling allergic or sensitivity reactions (Kim et al, 2014; Lee, 2013). Both of these flavonoid compounds, as well as others, are also available in supplemental form for targeted nutritional therapy when indicated (see Box 3-3).

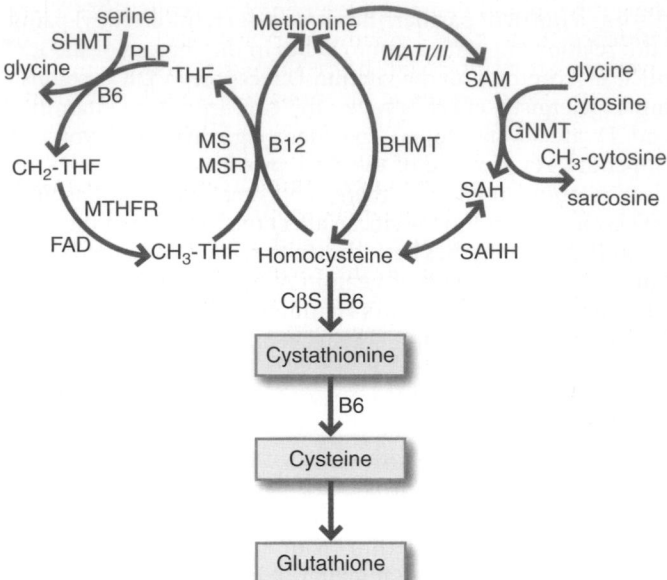

FIGURE 3-6 Methylation Mechanism

BOX 3-3	**Selected Flavonoid Antioxidants**
Alpha Lipoic Acid	Glutathione
Astaxanthin	Lutein
Citrus Bioflavonoids	Lycopene
CoQ10	Quercetin
Curcumin	Reseveratrol
Epigallocatechin 3 Gallate (EGCG)	Zeaxanthin

Several antioxidant systems are involved in protection against these ROS—especially within the electron transport system in the mitochondria. Among the 80 or more known antioxidants, ascorbate (vitamin C) has been shown to react with other biologic antioxidants referred to as the "antioxidant network." Ascorbate acts as a central reducing agent regenerating other biologic antioxidants (Stipanuk and Caudill, 2013). Ascorbate interacts with the vitamin E complex to provide protection to water- and lipid-soluble surfaces in membranes. Other key members of the antioxidant network are **glutathione**, another water-soluble antioxidant that is synthesized in all cells and which supports the central role of ascorbate and vitamin E; **lipoic acid** with its water and lipid molecular components and sometimes considered the "universal antioxidant"; and **coenzyme Q-10** that functions in protecting lipid structures, especially in cardiac muscle and mitochondrial membranes. Antioxidants work synergistically to quell ROS activity. These nutrients are natural metabolites in healthy individuals and can be used as supplements for health-compromised individuals if indicated.

Gut Ecology and the Microbiome

The gastrointestinal tract has many functions in the health of an individual, and one of them is in immune integrity. This is because the largest immune organ is located within the gastrointestinal tract as gut-associated lymphoid tissue (GALT) and mucosa-associated lymphoid tissue (MALT) containing innate and acquired immune systems as well as about 3 pounds of symbiotic microbial organisms. The condition of the gut lymphoid tissue and the microbial ecology has a large influence on the body's inflammatory state (Lewis, 2014). The inverse relationship of gut barrier integrity and ecology with organ specific or systemic inflammation is well documented (Goldman and Schafer, 2012; Hold et al, 2014; Kinnebrew and Pamer, 2012; Pastorelli, 2013; Ruth, 2013).

Medical nutrition therapy recommendations for increasing fermented foods, lowering intake of processed foods, avoiding gastrointestinal irritating foods and any known antigens for an individual, are basic to improving the microbial ecology. Therapeutic use of functional foods (Abuajah, 2015), pre- and probiotics (Isolauri and Salminen, 2015), and supplements can sometimes be indicated to restore optimum gut function and reduce inflammation (Luoto et al, 2013; see chapters 26 and 28).

Lifestyle

Chronic diseases are known as "lifestyle diseases," and total inflammation management requires lifestyle factors be addressed for improved outcomes. Modifications of lifestyle factors such as sleep, physical activity, and smoking cessation have been widely disseminated from public health agencies. More recently, recommendations for environmental toxin exposure protection, stress management, and community relationships have been identified as significantly influencing factors in chronic disease and inflammation (Tay, 2013; Umberson, 2010).

Sleep: Circadian Rhythm

The CDC targets sleep insufficiency as an important public health challenge with 50 to 70 million U.S. adults diagnosed with sleep disorders (CDC, 2014a). Sleep quality and duration, "feeling refreshed" and vital upon awaking, and having good energy throughout the day until bedtime are the signs of adequate sleep. Sleep specialists report that sleep is one of the "most anti-inflammatory" activities (Lombardo, 2005). That is a profound statement. Common habits of TV watching right before bed, and sometimes in bed, produce penetrating light that reduces the body's production of melatonin (the natural sleep hormone responding to darkness). Sleep apnea, snoring disturbing spousal sleep, and stimulant drinks during the day and evening contribute to poor sleep quality. Without quality sleep, the body does not get quality parasympathetic healing time (Ayurveda and Chinese Medicine philosophies) that calms the inflammation of the day.

The cumulative effects of poor sleep affect metabolic activities that lead to weight gain, mood disorders, stressful emotions, and increased nutrient requirements (Heancy, 2012). Sleep problems can contribute to diseases such as hypertension, heart disease, depression, and diabetes, and they add stress and inflammation to already hectic lives. Sleep affects the balance of the 24-hour circadian rhythm involving hormone, mood, immune, organ, and digestive balance. Poor sleep can affect all of those systems and affect the degree of prolonged inflammation and nutrient status (Lopresti et al, 2013).

Physical Activity

Exercise physiology research is revealing new guidelines on the effect physical activity has on inflammation in the body. Too much exercise for too long can produce high levels of reactive oxygen species (ROS), a normal byproduct of metabolism of oxygen. When ROS levels rise too high, they cause oxidative stress damage to cell structures. Current recommendations are for intermittent activity throughout the day, with mild to moderate activity. Strenuous exercise should be for only those who have trained to avoid the damaging effects of the free radicals generated (Lopresti et al, 2013). Nutrition assessment of antioxidant status can provide identification of metabolic excess activity of ROS and guidance for dietary antioxidant protection as part of the investigation into the total inflammatory load of a person (Akil et al, 2015; Mankowski et al, 2015; see Chapter 7).

Stress of Life

Some health professionals and researchers in human body stress state that prolonged unresolved stress on the body is one of the worst promoters of early aging and chronic disease. The unresolved state of stress, whether emotional, physical, or perceived, or from infection or injury, triggers the immune system to respond with more inflammatory cytokines. The analogy used to describe unrelenting stress is getting ready for the "fright or flight" response, with nowhere to run. If animals or humans are frightened they run away and work out the metabolic inflammatory chemicals. When safe, they come to a rest to restore balance (Sapolisky, 1998). That cannot happen with unrelenting chronic stress.

Toxin Load

Toxins are endogenous and exogenous xenobiotics, toxic substances within a biologic organism, that damage the metabolism.

In the modern world, since WWII, there have been 80,000 or more synthetic chemicals and many toxic metals released into the environment, increasing the exposure of plant and animal life to an unprecedented level (NRDC 2010, 2015). Although many historical compounds such as smoking are toxic (Adams, 2015; Jin, 2008), many toxic compounds are "new-to-nature" molecules not before present in the environment (Aris and Leblanc, 2011; Bland, 1998). An example is trans fatty acids (Ganguly and Pierce, 2015).

The metabolisms of plants and animals usually have difficulty providing the systems to process and eliminate these toxins when incorporated into the organism. Industrial and food industry pressures have challenged attempts at governmental regulation of these toxic compounds. The result has been increasing tissue levels of some of these toxins when tissue testing is performed. Examples of these increased levels are shown in the Environmental Working Group (EWG) (http://www.ewg.org) studies of newborn cord blood, which have found more than 260 known-toxic substances present in 100% of U.S. newborns (EWG, 2005).

Another example is studies of toxic cadmium and lead metals in Korean populations residing near abandoned metal mines. A study of more than 5000 Koreans found notably higher toxic metal levels in those residing within a 2-km radius of the mines than in the general population in Korea and other countries (Park et al, 2014). Cadmium and lead are known carcinogens and are related to CNS disturbances and cardiovascular and renal diseases with accompanying prolonged inflammation.

A study on hermetic (low-level) exposure to cadmium and arsenic related to clinical symptoms found that low dietary protein intake affected enzyme activity such that depressed biologic systems and long-term adaptations were inadequate. (Dudka et al, 2014). Lack of dietary vegetable micronutrient and phytonutrient intake has repeatedly been shown to be a potentially significant marker of inflammatory effects of toxins such as toxic metals, chemicals, and pesticides (Bakırcı et al, 2014, Jeena et al, 2013). In summary, there is beneficial protection against toxic damage when there is adequate macro- and micronutrient intake and nutrient bioavailability provided to the human organism, from a high intake of vegetables and adequate protein.

Assessment and Reducing Prolonged Inflammation in Chronic Diseases

The Patient's Story

Nutrition assessment includes gathering information about the whole person and begins by hearing the patient's story and forming the therapeutic relationship that is foundational for the most effective outcomes. It is a type of detective work partnering with the client to uncover root causes of underlying physiological imbalances that frame the intervention.

The patient's story is a term inclusive of the whole of the patient's history and the current state of their health; it is a collection of all data that potentially can contribute to the individual's metabolic health. In the therapeutic encounter the data is collected from the personal interview, study of medical records, family history, clinical observation and current laboratory records. Collection of family history is gathered best by requesting an intake form for health histories of the two previous generations to be completed before an assessment session. Most often a pattern suggesting metabolic genotypes can be recognized. Examples like cardiovascular, autoimmune or neurological events repeated in family members, especially at young ages or in multiple relatives, should prompt the nutritionist to investigate possible metabolic mechanisms and single nucleotide polymorphisms (SNPs). Quantitative laboratory or clinical confirmation of an altered metabolism may be appropriate before planning an intervention.

Personal health history starting with an individual's gestational history and place of birth, and developing a timeline can give insight into recognizing patterns that lead to a better understanding of the individual's current metabolic nutritional health. For example, infants not breastfed are found to have more difficulty in maintaining healthy gut microbiota, and increased incidence of allergies and asthma. These infants may benefit from probiotic supplementation (Prescott 2011, Ip 2007).

Medical History and Data

The common denominator of prolonged inflammation is identifiable in every chronic disease. Most evidence of this phenotype among humans, centers around various aspects of the metabolic syndrome described as presenting with a cluster of risk factors including insulin resistance (IR)/hyperinsulinemia, increased VAT (increased body fat percentage, waist circumference), elevated blood triglycerides (TG)/lowered high-density cholesterol (HDL-chol), hypertension, and raised fasting glucose (dysglycemia) (Watson, 2014). An additional biomarker is seen commonly as elevated CRP-hs blood values greater than

1.0. Increased understanding of dysregulation of glucose metabolism and its various causes helps define the complex condition of prolonged inflammation (Alberti et al, 2009; Grundy et al, 2005).

Biochemical markers also can be important factors in personalizing an individual's "total inflammatory load." In 2004 it became clear that slow increases in inflammatory markers such as sedimentation rate (blood) were significant in the progression of chronic disease degenerative processes (see Table 3-1).

Predictive genomic testing has provided new tools for personalizing assessment of individual metabolism. The use of SNP testing is currently in a preliminary stage as far as clinical application, but growing at a rapid pace. Integrative and functional medicine practitioners currently are adding SNP testing to their assessment as part of the patient's story to guide effective interventions. It is important to appreciate the SNP as a "predictive" value and not as a "diagnostic" tool. An example of use of an SNP with breast cancer is the vitamin D receptor (VDR genes such as CDX2 and BGL) that currently suggest an association (Khan MI, 2014). The VDR gene may influence risks of some cancers and their prognosis. This encourages closer monitoring of vitamin D status in cancer patients (Mun, 2015). Current consensus for cancer prevention recommends maintaining 25(OH)vit D in the range of 30 to 80 ng/ml (90 to 110 nmol/L) (Mohr, 2014).

Vitamin D is involved in enhancing the management of metabolic inflammation because of its almost "pro-hormone" immune and hormone modulating effects. This comprehensive candidate-gene analysis demonstrates that the risk of multiple VDR polymorphisms results in lower VDR mRNA levels. Polymorphisms of the vitamin D receptor gene (VDR) have been shown to be associated with several complex diseases, including osteoporosis. This could affect the vitamin D signaling efficiency and may contribute to the increased fracture risk observed for these risk haplotype alleles (Fang et al, 2005).

Gathering the patient's story and combining it with other data like anthropometrics, medical history, and the nutrition focused physical exam (see Appendix 21) allows a pattern to emerge of nutritional and metabolic priorities. This provides the clinician with important information to develop a nutrition intervention to promote optimal health and wellness.

PROLONGED INFLAMMATION EXPRESSION SPECIFIC TO MAJOR CHRONIC DISEASES

Heart Disease/Cardiometabolic Syndrome

Atherosclerosis is a chronic inflammatory disease. The term most used to describe the multi-factored physiologic condition including all chronic diseases in some form is metabolic syndrome (MetS). Cardiovascular disease (CVD) and diabetes are associated most closely, but increasing connections with the other major chronic diseases are occurring (see Chapters 30 and 33). MetS involves the cardiovascular system and the immune response of building atherosclerotic plaque on the vascular walls. In the 1970s, it was recognized that the atherosclerotic plaque was the result of a highly inflammatory process involving sometimes infection, but always macrophages and

---

BOX 3-4   Cardiometabolic Specific Inflammatory Markers

- Increased body fat%, most often with elevated BMI and VAT.
  - BMI,
  - Waist Circumference
  - Waist/Height Ratio
  - Waist/Hip Ratio
  - Body fat % (bioelectric impedance, Air or water displacement plethysmograph, DEXA, calipers)
- Blood Biomarkers of prolonged inflammation in CVD/cardiometabolic syndrome with Diabetes
  - Hyperlipidemia/Hypertriglyceridemia
  - Total Cholesterol/HDL Ratio
  - Fasting Glucose/Fasting Insulin
  - HgbA1C
  - C-Reactive Protein-hi sensitivity (CRPhs or CRP-cardio)
  - Homocysteine
- Imaging: Coronary calcium scan
- Myeloperoxidase (blood)
- Other associations for CVD/cardiometabolic syndrome /diabetes:
  - Sympathetic dominant metabolism (metabolic stress)
  - Stress (biochemical, glandular, emotional, environmental, smoking)
  - Poor sleep
  - Apnea

BOX 3-5   Cancer Specific Inflammatory Markers

- Various metabolic markers measuring inflammatory hallmarks of cancer
  - Adhesion: Fibrinogen and platelets (blood)
  - Metastasis promoters:
  - Copper (Cu): Zinc Ratio 1.0 or less (rate limiting to metastatic enzymes)
  - Ceruloplasmin (contributes to the total Cu load)
  - Angiogenesis promotors (Bingling, 2014): VEGF, adhesion factors.
- Tumor-promoting inflammation: Specific type of cancer markers (examples: ovarian cancer CA 125, breast cancer CA 15-3), prostate cancer PSA). Various proinflammatory cytokines and chemokines: TNF-a, IL-8, IL-6, etc.
  - Glycolysis (Warburg Effect: (sugar is primary fuel of cancer cells))
  - Growth factors
  - Genome instability/mitochondrial DNA
  - Loss of apoptosis / cell immortality

---

foam cells cementing with free calcium and cholesterol. Other factors of MetS are hypertension, strokes, infections, and stress. The most common biomarkers of inflammation related to metabolic syndrome and CVD are lipids, homocysteine, CRP-hs, myeloperoxidase, and ferritin—all acute phase reactants synonymous with inflammation (Smith, 2010; see Box 3-4 and Table 7-6).

Cancer

Cancer can be considered a cousin of cardiometabolic syndrome sharing many of the same characteristics of prolonged inflammation. Cancer deaths occur because of metastatic growth of a tumor and malnutrition. Metastases of solid tumors require new increased blood supply with neovascularization (angiogenesis) to thrive (Albini, 2011; see Chapter 36). Angiogenesis is essential to adult tissue remodeling and regeneration, solid tumor growth, and coronary artery disease (Bingling et al, 2014). This awareness has brought a research focus to food, herbs and medications that can inhibit angiogenesis (Bodai, 2015; Kunnumakkara et al, 2008).

When assessing the metabolic and nutritional status of a cancer patient, the clinician should use the same factors listed for metabolic syndrome and add cancer-specific markers (see Box 3-5).

Autoimmune Conditions

Autoimmune conditions share the fundamental processes of cardiometabolic disease with a stronger genetic component. Conditions such as rheumatoid arthritis, celiac disease, inflammatory bowel disease, lupus, Sjögren syndrome, and others have identified genetic susceptibilities. All have specific inflammatory markers particular to the disease process. They are exacerbated by obesity, chronic infections, antigenic exposures, and stress (Table 3-3).

Neurologic Conditions

Neurologic conditions range from mitochondrial dysfunction diseases such as Parkinson's disease and Alzheimer's disease (AD) (Hroudová et al, 2014) to mood disorders associated with altered methylation pathways from variations in the MTHFR and COMT genes to nutrient insufficiencies. Inflammation and the cardiometabolic parameters are present with naming of AD as type 3 diabetes (de la Monte and Wands, 2008). The neurologic system appears to be more vulnerable to toxic exposures because of the fact that 90% of toxins are lipophilic, fat-loving, and neurons and the central nervous system (CNS) are high-fat cells and tissues (see Table 3-4).

Endocrine Abnormalities

Endocrine (non-cancer) abnormalities seem to be increasing in the population. For example, infertility has increased globally with 10% of women facing this challenge (CDC, 2015; Inhorn and Patrizio, 2015). Inflammatory conditions of endometriosis, PCOS, and unexplained infertility are the most common related diseases worldwide (Gupta, 2014). Oxidative stress and its accompanying inflammation are postulated as the most important pathways in female infertility. All of the cardiometabolic markers suffice in assessing endocrine risks of chronic disease along with markers specific to the condition. Other conditions such as "estrogen dominance" carry inflammatory problems as in uterine fibroids, fibrocystic breasts, hypothyroid or autoimmune thyroiditis, diabetes type 1 and type 2, and adrenal stress (see Table 3-5).

Developmental Inflammatory-Related Conditions

Developmental inflammatory-related conditions bring a focus to the uterine environment, where there is recognition of the importance of preprogramming the fetus for a lifetime phenotype. The epigenetic messages to the fetal genotype are powerful modulators of the life expression. In the infant and toddler years brain development and behavioral wellness, including self-esteem and forming of relationships are vulnerable. If the fetus and young child do not grow in a healthy environment, the inflammatory processes of chronic disease take root and will challenge the individual lifelong.

TABLE 3-3   Autoimmune Specific Inflammatory Markers

Biomarker Test	Reference Range	Speciman	Association
Sedimentation Rate (ESR)	men: 0-15 mm/h women: 0-20 mm/h	Blood serum	Collagen diseases Inflammatory diseases Infections Toxicity, heavy metals
C-Reactive Protein-hs (CRP-hs)	<1.0 mg/dl	blood	Systemic inflammation Metabolic Syndrome
Rheumatoid Factor (RF)	0-39 IU/ml non-reactive 40-79 IU/ml weakly reactive >80 reactive	blood	Rheumatoid arthritis Sjogren's syndrome Joint pain Rheumatoid conditions
Anti-gliadin Antibody Deamidated Gliadin Antibody, IgA, IgG	0-19 Negative 20-30 Weak Positive >30 Moderate to Strong positive	Blood serum	Celiac disease Dermatitis herpatiforme Non-Celiac gluten sensitivity
Endomysial antibody test (IgA-EMA)	Negative normal individuals Negative Gluten-free diet		Dermatitis herpetiforme, celiac disease
Tissue Transglutaminase IgA/IgG (tTG-IgA)	<4.0 U/mL (negative) 4.0-10.0 U/mL (weak positive) >10.0 U/mL (positive) Reference values apply to all ages.	Blood serum	Celiac disease (indicates Rx biopsy, gene HLA_DQ2/DQ8)) Dermatitis herpetiforme Villi Atrophy
SS-A Sjorgrens/Ro IgG	<1.0 U (negative) > or =1.0 U (positive) Reference values apply to all ages.	blood	Connective tissue disease (Systemic lupus erythematosus, Sjorgrens, Rheumatoid arthritis)
SS-B Sjorgrens	<1.0 U (negative) > or =1.0 U (positive) Reference values apply to all ages.	blood	Connective tissue disease, including Sjogren syndrome, systemic lupus erythematosus (SLE).
ANA antibody titer	<1:40 normal (or < 1/0 IU) is negative.	Blood serum	Multiple autoimmune conditions, systemic lupus erythematosus (SLE).
Anti-dsDNA Test IgG	<30.0 IU/mL (negative) 30.0-75.0 IU/mL (borderline) >75.0 IU/mL (positive) Negative is considered normal. Reference values apply to all ages.	blood	
Cyclic Citrullinated Peptide Antibody (Anti-CCP)	<20.0 U (negative) 20.0-39.9 U (weak positive) 40.0-59.9 U (positive) > or =60.0 U (strong positive) Reference values apply to all ages.	blood	Rheumatoid arthritis Arthritis
Anti-Desmoglein 1/3 IgG antibody Blister biopsy	negative	Blood Skin tissue	Pemphigus vulgaris Pemphigus foliaceus Epidermolysis bullosa acquisita

TABLE 3-4   Neurological Specific Inflammatory Markers

Biomarker Test	Reference	Specimen	Association
RBC Fatty Acid Analysis	Mean +/− SD	Blood	Membrane integrity
Lipid Panel			
Triglycerides	170-200 mg/dL	Blood	
Total Cholesterol	50-80 mg/dL		
HDL	Men: 37-40 mg/dL Women: 40-85 mg/dL	Blood	CHD risk
LDL	Adult <130 mg/dL or <3.4 mmol/L Child <110 mg/dL or <2.8 mmol/L	Blood	Adult: CHD risk Child: abnormal cholesterol metabolism
Creatine Kinase			
Creatinine	0.76-1.27 mg/dL	Blood	Kidney Function
BUN	8-27 mg/dL		
GFR	>60 mL/min/BSA		
Glucose, fasting	65-99 mg/dL	Blood, urine	Glucose status
Insulin, fasting	2.0-19.6 μIU/mL	Blood	Insulin status
HgbA1C	4.8%-6.4%	Blood	Average BS over 120 days
25OH vit D	30-150 ng/ml	Blood, saliva	Vitamin D status

TABLE 3-5   Endocrine (non-cancer) Specific Inflammatory Markers

Biomarker Test (Mother)	Reference	Specimen	Association
RBC Fatty Acid Analysis	Mean +/− SD	Blood	Membrane integrity
Lipid Panel		Blood	CHD
Total Cholesterol	170-200 mg/dL		Cholesterol/lipid metabolism
HDL-chol	Men: 37-40 mg/dL		Liver stress
	Women: 40-85 mg/dL		CHD risk
LDL-chol	Adult <130 mg/dL or <3.4 mmol/L		CHD risk
	Child <110 mg/dL or <2.8 mmol/L		Abnormal cholesterol
Triglycerides	<150 mg/dL		Metabolic syndrome
			Carnitine insufficiency
			High simple sugar/alcohol diet
			CHD risk
Celiac Panel			
tTG IgG/IgA	<4 U/mL no antibody detected		Small intestine villi atrophy
Anti-Gliadin antibody	<20 Units antibody not detected		Gluten sensitivity
			Gluten-free diet
tissueTransglutaminase IgG/IgA			
Antigen (Food IgG/IgE)	Per lab		
Insulin, fasting	2.0-19.6 μIU/mL	Blood	Insulin status
HgbA1C	4.8%-6.4%	Blood	Average BS over 120 days
TSH	Adult 0.2-5.4 mU/L blood	Blood	Thyroid function
Vitamin D25-OH	30-150 ng/ml	Blood, saliva	Vitamin D status

SUMMARY

Chronic disease is an epidemic that is affected by diet and lifestyle, and chronic disease pathophysiology is the result of genetics and epigenetic influences. Sustained inflammation is the common denominator of all chronic disease. Nutrition and lifestyle are modulators of sustained inflammation (see Box 3-6).

The nutritionist has an important role in the interdisciplinary management of chronic disease. The skills to recognize the early signs and symptoms of smoldering inflammation enable the nutritionist to identify nutritional priorities and individual strategies to reduce inflammation and restore health and well-being.

Whole foods, "functional foods," targeted dietary supplements when indicated, and lifestyle changes can be foundational in achieving wellness. The nutritionist, with an understanding of the inflammation and immune response of chronic disease pathophysiology, possesses the capability for more effective nutrition assessment and intervention.

USEFUL WEBSITES

Agroecology in Action
http://nature.berkeley.edu/~miguel-alt/modern_agriculture.html
American Academy of Sleep Medicine
http://www.aasmnet.org/
Angiogenesis Foundation
http://www.angio.org
https://www.ted.com/talks/william_li
Dietitians in Integrative and Functional Medicine
www.integrativeRD.org
Genetic testing for dietitian practitioners
Nutrigenomix.com
KU Integrative Medicine Program
http://www.kumc.edu/school-of-medicine/integrative-medicine.html

BOX 3-6   Food, Nutraceuticals and Lifestyle as Medicine to Manage Inflammation

Food
Whole Foods Diet
Mediterranean Diet
Med-Asian Diet
Nordic Diet
Fruits and vegetables
Beneficial Fats
Pure Water
Targeted nutrients
Low Antigen Foods for the Individual
Low toxin containing foods
Foods and Cookware toxin-free (aluminum, BPA, perfluorooctanoic acid (PFOA)-free)

Nutraceuticals
Quercitin
Rutin
Curcumin
Proteolytic enzymes
Enzyme therapy
Rx Nutrition Therapy
Guidance for dietary supplements

Lifestyle
Sleep
Physical Activity
Beliefs
Community

National Geographic Documentary: Sleepless in America.
https://www.youtube.com/watch?v=1qlxKFEE7Ec
Arizona Center for Integrative Medicine
http://integrativemedicine.arizona.edu/

REFERENCES

Abraham C, Medzhitov R: Interactions between the host innate immune system and microbes in inflammatory bowel disease, *Gastroenterology* 140:1729, 2011.

Abuajah CI: Functional components and medicinal properties of food: a review, *J Food Sci Technol* 52:2522, 2015.

Adams T, Wan E, Wei Y, et al: Secondhand smoking is associated with vascular inflammation, *Chest* 148(1):112, 2015.

Aderem A, Adkins JN, Ansong C, et al: A systems biology approach to infectious disease research: innovating the pathogen-host research paradigm, *MBio* 2:e00325, 2011.

Agmon-Levin N, Theodor E, Segal RM, et al: Vitamin D in systemic and organ-specific autoimmune diseases, *Clin Rev Allergy Immunol* 45:256, 2013.

Agrawal R, Sandhu SK, Sharma I, et al: Development and evaluation of curcumin-loaded elastic vesicles as an effective topical anti-inflammatory formulation, *AAPS PharmSciTech* 16:364, 2015.

Akil M, Gurbuz U, Bicer M, et al: Selenium prevents lipid peroxidation in liver and lung tissues of rats in acute swimming exercise, *Bratisl Lek Listy* 116:233, 2015.

Alagl AS, Bhat SG: Ascorbic acid: new role of an age-old micronutrient in the management of periodontal disease in older adults, *Geriatr Gerontol Int* 15:241, 2015.

Alberti KG, Eckel RH, Grundy SM, et al: Harmonizing the metabolic syndrome –a joint interim statement of the International Diabetes Federation Task Force on Epidemiology and Prevention; National Heart, Lung, and Blood Institute; American Heart Association; World Heart Federation; International Atherosclerosis Society; and International Association for the Study of Obesity, *Circulation* 120:1640, 2009.

Alele JD, Kamen DL: The importance of inflammation and vitamin D status in SLE-associated osteoporosis, *Autoimmun Rev* 9:137, 2010.

Allaj V, Guo C, Nie D: Non-steroid anti-inflammatory drugs, prostaglandins, and cancer, *Cell Biosci* 3:8, 2013.

Ames BN: Prevention of mutation, cancer, and other age-associated diseases by optimizing micronutrient intake, *J Nucleic Acids* 2010. doi:10.4061/2010/725071.

Aris A, Leblanc S: Maternal and fetal exposure to pesticides associated to genetically modified foods in Eastern Townships of Quebec, Canada, *Reprod Toxicol* 31:528, 2011.

Arm JP, Boyce JA, Wang L, et al: Impact of botanical oils on polyunsaturated fatty acid metabolism and leukotriene generation in mild asthmatics, *Lipids Health Dis* 12:141, 2013.

Avitsur R, Levy S, Goren N, et al: Early adversity, immunity and infectious disease, *Stress* 18(3):289, February 2015 [Epub ahead of print].

Baffy G, Loscalzo J: Complexity and network dynamics in physiological adaptation: an integrated view, *Physiol Behav* 131:49, 2014.

Bailey RL, Mills JL, Yetley EA, et al: Unmetabolized serum folic acid and its relation to folic acid intake from diet and supplements in a nationally representative sample of adults aged ≥60 y in the United States, *Am J Clin Nutr* 92:383, 2010.

Bakırcı GT, Yaman Acay DB, Bakırcı F, et al: Pesticide residues in fruits and vegetables from the Aegean region, Turkey, *Food Chem* 160:379, 2014.

Barker DJ: In utero programming of chronic disease, *Clin Sci (Lond)* 95:115, 1998.

Bauer UE, Briss PA, Goodman RA, et al: Prevention of chronic disease in the 21st century: elimination of the leading preventable causes of premature death and disability in the USA, *Lancet* 384:45, 2014.

Berth-Jones J, Graham-Brown RA: Placebo-controlled trial of essential fatty acid supplementation in atopic dermatitis, *Lancet* 341:1557, 1993.

Bingling D, et al: A novel tissue model for angiogenesis: evaluation of inhibitors or promoters in tissue level, *Scientific Reports* 4:3693, 2014.

Biolo G, Di Girolamo FG, Breglia A, et al: Inverse relationship between "a body shape index" (ABSI) and fat-free mass in women and men: insights into mechanisms of sarcopenic obesity, *Clin Nutr* 34:323, 2015.

Birch AM, Katsouri L, Sastre M: Modulation of inflammation in transgenic models of Alzheimer's disease, *J Neuroinflammation* 11:25, 2014.

Bland J: *Nutritional management of inflammatory disorders*, Gig Harbor, Wash, 1998, The Institute for Functional Medicine Inc.

Bland J: The correct therapy for diagnosis: new-to-nature molecules vs natural, *Integrative Med* 6:20, 2007.

Bodai BI, Tuso P: Breast cancer survivorship: a comprehensive review of long-term medical issues and lifestyle recommendations, *Perm J* 19:48, 2015.

Bourlier V, Bouloumie A: Role of macrophage tissue infiltration in obesity and insulin resistance, *Diabetes Metab* 35:251, 2009.

Brash AR: Lipoxygenases: occurrence, functions, catalysis, and acquisition of substrate, *J Biol Chem* 274:23679, 1999.

Calçada D, Vianello D, Giampieri E, et al: The role of low-grade inflammation and metabolic flexibility in aging and nutritional modulation thereof: a systems biology approach, *Mech Ageing Dev* 136:136, 2014.

Calder, PC. Polyunsaturated fatty acids and inflammatory processes: New twists in an old tale. Biochimie 91(6):791, 2009.

Centers for Disease Control and Prevention (CDC): *Chronic Disease Prevention and Health Promotion*, 2015. http://www.cdc.gov/nccdphp/overview.html. Accessed April 4, 2015.

Centers for Disease Control and Prevention (CDC): *Insufficient Sleep Is a Public Health Epidemic*, 2014a. http://www.cdc.gov/features/dssleep/. Accessed April 4, 2015.

Centers for Disease Control and Prevention (CDC): *R2-p: Research to Practice at NIOSH*, 2011. http://www.cdc.gov/niosh/r2p/. Accessed April 4, 2015.

Cherry AD, Piantadosi CA: Regulation of mitochondrial biogenesis and its intersection with inflammatory responses, *Antioxid Redox Signal* 22(12):965, 2015. [Epub ahead of print].

Cokluk E, Sekeroglu MR, Aslan M, et al: Determining oxidant and antioxidant status in patients with genital warts, *Redox Rep* 20(5):210, Jan 13, 2015. [Epub ahead of print].

Das UN: A defect in the activity of Delta6 and Delta5 desaturases may be a factor in the initiation and progression of atherosclerosis, *Prostaglandins Leukot Essent Fatty Acids* 76:251, 2007.

Das UN: *Metabolic syndrome pathophysiology: the role of essential fatty acids*, 2010, Wiley-Blackwell.

Das UN: *Molecular basis of health and disease*, Netherlands, 2011, Springer.

de la Monte SM, Wands R: Alzheimer's disease is type 3 diabetes–evidence reviewed, *J Diabetes Sci Technol* 2:1101, 2008.

Delbridge LM, Mellor KM, Wold LE: Epigenetics and cardiovascular disease, *Life Sci* 129:1, 2015.

Delisle H: *Programming of Chronic Disease by Impaired Fetal Nutrition*, 2002. http://www.who.int/nutrition/publications/programming_chronicdisease.pdf/. Accessed April 4, 2015.

Dibaba DT, Xun P, He K: Dietary magnesium intake is inversely associated with serum C-reactive protein levels: meta-analysis and systematic review, *Eur J Clin Nutr* 69:409, 2015.

Dick DM, Agrawal A, Keller MC, et al: Candidate gene-environment interaction research: reflections and recommendations, *Perspect Psychol Sci* 10:37, 2015.

Di Gennaro A, Haeggström JZ: The leukotrienes: immune-modulating lipid mediators of disease, *Adv Immunol* 116:51, 2012.

Djoussé L, Matthan NR, Lichtenstein AH, et al: Red blood cell membrane concentration of cis-palmitoleic and cis-vaccenic acids and risk of coronary heart disease, *Am J Cardiol* 110:539, 2012.

Dobryniewski J, Szajda SD, Waszkiewicz N, et al: Biology of essential fatty acids (EFA), *Przegl Lek* 64:91, 2007. (in Polish).

Dudka I, Kossowska B, Senhadri H, et al: Metabonomic analysis of serum of workers occupationally exposed to arsenic, cadmium and lead for biomarker research: a preliminary study, *Environ Int* 68:71, 2014.

Ehrlich M: DNA methylation in cancer: too much, but also too little, *Oncogene* 21:5400, 2002.

Elwood P, Galante J, Pickering J, et al: Healthy lifestyles reduce the incidence of chronic diseases and dementia: evidence from the caerphilly cohort study, *PLoS One* 8:e81877, 2013.

Environmental Working Group (EWG): *The Pollution of Newborns: A Benchmark Investigation of Industrial Chemicals*, Pollutants and Pesticides in Umbilical Cord Blood, 2005. http://www.ewg.org/research/body-burden-pollution-newborns. Accessed April 4, 2015.

European Foundation for the Care of Newborn Infants (EFCNI): *Healthy Pregnancy: Fetal Programming and Chronic Diseases in Later Life*, 2015. http://www.efcni.org/fileadmin/Daten/Web/Brochures_Reports_Factsheets_

Position_Papers/Factsheet_Healthy_pregnancy__Fetal_programming.pdf. Accessed April 4, 2015.

Fang Y, van Meurs JB, d'Alesio A, et al: Promoter and 3'-untranslated-region haplotypes in the vitamin D receptor gene predispose to osteoporotic fracture: the Rotterdam Study, *Am J Hum Genet* 77:807, 2005.

Fasano A: Leaky gut and autoimmune diseases, *Clin Rev Allergy Immunol* 42:71, 2012.

Feldman D, et al: *Vitamin D*, ed 3, San Diego, Calif, 2011, Academic Press.

Fisher RE, Steele M, Karrow NA: Fetal programming of the neuroendocrine-immune system and metabolic disease, *J Pregnancy* 2012:792, 2012.

Fleisch AF, Wright RO, Baccarelli AA: Environmental epigenetics: a role in endocrine disease. *J Mol Endocrinol* 49:R61, 2012.

Franceschi C, Campisi J: Chronic inflammation (inflammaging) and its potential contribution to age-associated diseases, *J Gerontol A Biol Sci Med Sci* 69(Suppl 1):S4, 2014.

Ganguly R, Pierce GN: The toxicity of dietary trans fats, *Food Chem Toxicol* 78:170, 2015.

Gibson RS, Hess SY, Hotz C, et al: Indicators of zinc status at the population level: a review of the evidence, *Br J Nutr* 99(Suppl 3):S14, 2008.

Gil Á, Martinez de Victoria E, Olza J: Indicators for the evaluation of diet quality, *Nutr Hosp* 31:128, 2015.

Goldman L, Schafer A: *Goldman's Cecil medicine*, ed 24, Philadelphia, 2012, Elsevier.

Gommerman JL, Rojas OL, Fritz JH: Re-thinking the functions of IgA(+) plasma cells, *Gut Microbes* 5:652, 2014.

Goodwin GM: *Prostaglandins: biochemistry*, functions, types and roles (cell biology research progress), ed 1, 2010, Nova Science Publishers, Inc.

Gottlieb RA, Mentzer RM: Autophagy during cardiac stress: joys and frustrations of autophagy, *Annu Rev Physiol* 72:45, 2010.

Grimble RF: Nutritional antioxidants and the modulation of inflammation: theory and practice, *New Horiz* 2:175, 1994.

Grundy SM, Cleeman JI, Daniels SR, et al: Diagnosis and management of the metabolic syndrome: an American Heart Association/National Heart, Lung, and Blood Institute scientific statement, *Circulation* 112:2735, 2005.

Guo Z, Miura K, Turin TC, et al: Relationship of the polyunsaturated to saturated fatty acid ratio to cardiovascular risk factors and metabolic syndrome in Japanese: the INTERLIPID study, *J Atheroscler Thromb* 17:777, 2010.

Gupta S, Ghulmiyyah J, Sharma R, et al: Power of proteomics in linking oxidative stress and female infertility, *Biomed Res Int* 2014:916212, 2014.

Gurkar AU, Chu K, Raj L, et al: Identification of ROCK1 kinase as a critical regulator of Beclin1-mediated autophagy during metabolic stress, *Nat Commun* 4:2189, 2013.

Harbige LS: Fatty acids, the immune response, and autoimmunity: a question of n-6 essentiality and the balance between n-6 and n-3, *Lipids* 38:323, 2003.

Harris WS, Pottala JV, Lacey SM, et al: Clinical correlates and heritability of erythrocyte eicosapentaenoic and docosahexaenoic acid content in the Framingham Heart Study, *Atherosclerosis* 225:425, 2012.

He K, Liu K, Daviglus ML, et al: Magnesium intake and incidence of metabolic syndrome among young adults, *Circulation* 113:1675, 2006.

Heaney RP: *Albion Webinar: Multi-Target Supplementation for Bone Health*. Accessed on April 2, 2014.

Heaney RP: The nutrient problem, *Nutr Rev* 70:165, 2012.

Hing B, Gardner C, Potash JB, et al: Effects of negative stressors on DNA methylation in the brain: implications for mood and anxiety disorders, *Am J Med Genet B Neuropsychiatr Genet* 165B:541, 2014.

Hold GL, Smith M, Grange C, et al: Role of the gut microbiota in inflammatory bowel disease pathogenesis: what have we learnt in the past 10 years. *World J Gastroenterol* 20:1192, 2014.

Hroudová J, Singh N, Fišar Z, et al: Mitochondrial dysfunctions in neurodegenerative diseases: relevance to Alzheimer's Disease, *Biomed Res Int* 2014:175062, 2014. [Epub ahead of print].

Hruby A, Hu FB: The epidemiology of obesity: a big picture, *Pharmacoeconomics* Dec 4, 2014. [Epub ahead of print].

Hughes-Austin JM, Wassel CL, Jiménez J, et al: The relationship between adiposity associated inflammation and coronary artery and abdominal aortic calcium differs by strata of central adiposity: the Multi-Ethnic Study of Atherosclerosis (MESA), *Vasc Med* 19:264, 2014.

ICD10data.com: *Inflammation Syndrome*. ICD10data.com, 2014. Accessed April 5, 2015.

Inhorn MC, Patrizio P: Infertility around the globe: new thinking on gender, reproductive technologies and global movements in the 21st century, *Hum Reprod Update* 21(4):411. Mar 22, 2015. [Epub ahead of print].

Innis SM: Omega-3 fatty acid biochemistry: perspectives from human nutrition, *Mil Med* 179(Suppl 11):82, 2014.

Ip S, et al: *Breastfeeding and Maternal and Infant Health Outcomes in Developed Countries*, 2007. http://archive.ahrq.gov/downloads/pub/evidence/pdf/brfout/brfout.pdf. Accessed May 27, 2015.

Isolauri E, Salminen S: The impact of early gut microbiota modulation on the risk of child disease: alert to accuracy in probiotic studies, *Benef Microbes* 6(2):167, 2015. [Epub ahead of print].

Japatti SR, Bhatsange A, Reddy M, et al: Scurvy-scorbutic siderosis of gingiva: a diagnostic challenge - a rare case report, *Dent Res J (Isfahan)* 10:394, 2013.

Jeena K, Liju VB, Kuttan R, et al: Antioxidant, anti-inflammatory and antinociceptive activities of essential oil from ginger, *Indian J Physiol Pharmacol* 57:51, 2013.

Jin L: An update on periodontal aetiopathogenesis and clinical implications, *Ann R Australas Coll Dent Surg* 19:96, 2008.

Jones D, editor: *The textbook of functional medicine*, 2005, Institute for Functional Medicine.

Juby AG: A healthy body habitus is more than just a normal BMI: implications of sarcopenia and sarcopenic obesity, *Maturitas* 78:243, 2014.

Karabudak O, Ulusoy RE, Erikci AA, et al: Inflammation and hypercoagulable state in adult psoriatic men, *Acta Derm Venereol* 88:337, 2008.

Karatzas PS, et al: DNA methylation profile of genes involved in inflammation and autoimmunity in inflammatory bowel disease, *Medicine (Baltimore)* 93:e309, 2014.

Kelley DS, Siegel D, Fedor DM, et al: DHA supplementation decreases serum C-reactive protein and other markers of inflammation in hypertriglyceridemic men, *J Nutr* 139:495, 2009.

Kendler BS: Supplemental conditionally essential nutrients in cardiovascular disease therapy, *J Cardiovasc Nurs* 21:9, 2006.

Khan MI, Bielecka ZF, Najm MZ, et al: Vitamin D receptor gene polymorphisms in breast and renal cancer: current state and future approaches (review), *Int J Oncol* 44:349, 2014.

Khan SA, Ali A, Khan SA, et al: Unraveling the complex relationship triad between lipids, obesity, and inflammation, *Mediators Inflamm* 2014:502749, 2014a.

Kim B, Choi YE, Kim HS, et al: Eruca sativa and its flavonoid components, quercetin and isorhamnetin, improve skin barrier function by activation of peroxisome proliferator-activated receptor (PPAR)-α and suppression of inflammatory cytokines, *Phytother Res* 28:1359, 2014.

Kim DH, Yoo TH, Lee SH, et al: Gamma linolenic acid exerts anti-inflammatory and anti-fibrotic effects in diabetic nephropathy, *Yonsei Med J* 53:1165, 2012.

Kinnebrew MA, Pamer EG: Innate immune signaling in defense against intestinal microbes, *Immunol Rev* 245:113, 2012.

Kolehmainen M, Ulven SM, Paananen J, et al: Healthy Nordic diet downregulates the expression of genes involved in inflammation in subcutaneous adipose tissue in individuals with features of the metabolic syndrome, *Am J Clin Nutr* 101:228, 2015.

Kominsky DJ, Campbell EL, Colgan SP: Metabolic shifts in immunity and inflammation, *J Immunol* 184:4062, 2010.

Krishnan AV, Swami S, Feldman D: Equivalent anticancer activities of dietary vitamin D and calcitriol in an animal model of breast cancer: importance of mammary CYP27B1 for treatment and prevention, *J Steroid Biochem Mol Biol* 136:289, 2013.

Krishnan AV, Swami S, Feldman D: The potential therapeutic benefits of vitamin D in the treatment of estrogen receptor positive breast cancer, *Steroids* 77:1107, 2012.

Kruk J: Lifestyle components and primary breast cancer prevention, *Asian Pac J Cancer Prev* 15:10543, 2014.

Kunnumakkara AB, Anand P, Aggarwal BB: Curcumin inhibits proliferation, invasion, angiogenesis and metastasis of different cancers through interaction with multiple cell signaling proteins, *Cancer Lett* 269:199, 2008.

Kurotani K, Sato M, Ejima Y, et al: High levels of stearic acid, palmitoleic acid, and dihomo-γ-linolenic acid and low levels of linoleic acid in serum cholesterol ester are associated with high insulin resistance, *Nutr Res* 32:669, 2012.

Lee CC, Shen SR, Lai YJ, et al: Rutin and quercetin, bioactive compounds from tartary buckwheat, prevent liver inflammatory injury, *Food Funct* 4:794, 2013.

Lewis CA: *Enteroimmunology: a guide to the prevention and treatment of chronic inflammatory disease*, ed 3, Carrabelle, Fla, 2014, Psy Press.

Liu S, Chacko S: Dietary Mg intake and biomarkers of inflammation and endothelial dysfunction. In Watson RR, et al, editors: *Magnesium in human health and disease*, New York, 2013, Humana Press.

Lombardo GT: *Sleep to save your life: the complete guide to living longer and healthier through restorative sleep*, New York, 2005, HarperCollins.

López-Alarcón M, Perichart-Perera O, Flores-Huerta S, et al: Excessive refined carbohydrates and scarce micronutrients intakes increase inflammatory mediators and insulin resistance in prepubertal and pubertal obese children independently of obesity, *Mediators Inflamm* 2014:849031, 2014.

Lopresti AL, Hood SD, Drummond PD, et al: A review of lifestyle factors that contribute to important pathways associated with major depression: diet, sleep and exercise, *J Affect Disord* 148:12, 2013.

Luoto R, Collado MC, Salminen S, et al: Reshaping the gut microbiota at an early age: functional impact on obesity risk. *Ann Nutr Metab* 63(Suppl 2): 17, 2013.

Machlin LJ: Effect of dietary linolenate on the proportion of linoleate and arachidonate in liver fat, *Nature* 194:868, 1962.

Maggio R, Viscomi C, Andreozzi P, et al: Normocaloric low cholesterol diet modulates Th17/Treg balance in patients with chronic hepatitis C virus infection, *PLoS One* 9(12):e112346, 2014.

Mankowski RT, Anton SD, Buford TW, et al: Dietary antioxidants as modifiers of physiologic adaptations to exercise, *Med Sci Sports Exerc* 47(9): 1857, 2015.

Manshadi D, Ishiguro L, Sohn KJ, et al: Folic acid supplementation promotes mammary tumor progression in a rat model, *PLoS ONE* 9:e84635, 2014.

Maruotti N, Cantatore FP: Vitamin D and the immune system, *J Rheumatol* 37:491, 2010.

McCann JC, Ames BN: Adaptive dysfunction of selenoproteins from the perspective of the triage theory: why modest selenium deficiency may increase risk of diseases of aging, *FASEB J* 25:1793, 2011.

Miller ER, Juraschek S, Pastor-Barriuso R, et al: Meta-analysis of folic acid supplementation trials on risk of cardiovascular disease and risk interaction with baseline homocysteine levels, *Am J Cardiol* 106:517, 2010.

Miyake JA, Benadiba M, Colquhoun A: Gamma-linolenic acid inhibits both tumour cell cycle progression and angiogenesis in the orthotopic C6 glioma model through changes in VEGF, Flt1, ERK1/2, MMP2, cyclin D1, pRb, p53 and p27 protein expression, *Lipids Health Dis* 8:8, 2009.

Mohrhauer H, Holman RT: The effect of dose level of essential fatty acids upon fatty acid composition of the rat liver, *J Lipid Res* 4:151, 1963.

Mougios V, Kotzamanidis C, Koutsari C, et al: Exercise-induced changes in the concentration of individual fatty acids and triacylglycerols of human plasma, *Metabolism* 44:681, 1995.

Muggli R: Systemic evening primrose oil improves the biophysical skin parameters of healthy adults, *Int J Cosmet Sci* 27:243, 2005.

Murray CJ, Vos T, Lozano R, et al: Disability-adjusted life-years (DALYs) for 291 diseases and injuries in 21 regions, 1990–2010: a systematic analysis for the Global Burden of Disease Study 2010, *Lancet* 380:2197, 2012.

National Institutes of Health (NIH), National Human Genome Research Institute: *Skin Microbiome*, 2014. http://www.genome.gov/dmd/img.cfm?node=Photos/Graphics&id=85320. Accessed April 5, 2015.

National Resources Defense Council (NRDC): *Take Out Toxics*. http://www.nrdc.org/health/toxics.asp. Accessed April 5, 2015.

National Resources Defense Council (NRDC): *The President's Cancer Panel Report: Implications for Reforming Our Nation's Policies on Toxic Chemicals*, 2010. http://docs.nrdc.org/health/files/hea_11020101a.pdf. Accessed April 5, 2015.

Nazki FH, Sameer AS, Ganaie BA: Folate: metabolism, genes, polymorphisms and the associated diseases, *Gene* 533:11, 2014.

Nielsen FH: Magnesium, inflammation, and obesity in chronic disease, *Nutr Rev* 68:333, 2010.

Noland D: *DN 881 Introduction to Dietetics and Integrative Medicine*, 2013, University of Kansas Medical Center, Kansas City, MO.

Olshansky SJ, Passaro DJ, Hershow RC, et al: A potential decline in life expectancy in the United States in the 21st century, *N Engl J Med* 352:1138, 2005.

Pallauf K, Giller K, Huebbe P, et al: Nutrition and healthy ageing: calorie restriction or polyphenol-rich "MediterrAsian" diet. *Oxid Med Cell Longev* 2013:707421, 2013.

Park DU, Kim DS, Yu SD, et al: Blood levels of cadmium and lead in residents near abandoned metal mine areas in Korea, *Environ Monit Assess* 186:5209, 2014.

Pastorelli L, De Salvo C, Mercado JR, et al: Central role of the gut epithelial barrier in the pathogenesis of chronic intestinal inflammation: lessons learned from animal models and human genetics, *Front Immunol* 4:280, 2013.

Paul WE: Self/nonself—immune recognition and signaling: a new journal tackles a problem at the center of immunological science, *Self Nonself* 1:2, 2010.

Pickens CA, Sordillo LM, Comstock SS, et al: Plasma phospholipids, non-esterified plasma polyunsaturated fatty acids and oxylipids are associated with BMI, *Prostaglandins Leukot Essent Fatty Acids* 95:31, 2015.

Popovich D, McAlhany A, Adewumi AO, et al: Scurvy: forgotten but definitely not gone, *J Pediatr Health Care* 23:405, 2009.

Potthast T: Paradigm shifts versus fashion shifts. Systems and synthetic biology as new epistemic entities in understanding and making "life," *EMBO Rep* 10(Suppl 1):S42, 2009.

Prado CM, Siervo M, Mire E, et al: A population-based approach to define body-composition phenotypes, *Am J Clin Nutr* 99:1369, 2014.

Prescott S, Mowak-Wegrzyn A: Strategies to prevent or reduce allergic disease, *Ann Nutr Metab* 59(Suppl 1):28, 2011.

Queen HL: *Rebuilding your patients' health through free radical therapy and a mouthful of evidence*, 1998, Institute for Health Realities.

Rahman MM, Veigas JM, Williams PJ, et al: DHA is a more potent inhibitor of breast cancer metastasis to bone and related osteolysis than EPA, *Breast Cancer Res Treat* 141:341, 2013.

Ranaldi G, Ferruzza S, Canali R, et al: Intracellular zinc is required for intestinal cell survival signals triggered by the inflammatory cytokine TNFα, *J Nutr Biochem* 24:967, 2013.

Rayssiguier Y, Gueux E, Nowacki W, et al: High fructose consumption combined with low dietary magnesium intake may increase the incidence of the metabolic syndrome by inducing inflammation, *Magnes Res* 19:237, 2006.

Reed S, Qin X, Ran-Ressler R, et al: Dietary zinc deficiency affects blood linoleic acid: dihomo-γ-linolenic acid (LA:DGLA) ratio; a sensitive physiological marker of zinc status in vivo (Gallus gallus), *Nutrients* 6:1164, 2014.

Ricciotti E, FitzGerald GA: Prostaglandins and inflammation, *Arterioscler Thromb Vasc Biol* 31:986, 2011.

Roubenoff R: Sarcopenic obesity: the confluence of two epidemics, *Obes Res* 12:887, 2004.

Ruth MR, Field CJ: The immune modifying effects of amino acids on gut-associated lymphoid tissue, *J Anim Sci Biotechnol* 4:27, 2013.

Sapolsky RM: *Why zebras don't get ulcers: an updated guide to stress, stress-related diseases and coping*, 1998, WH Freeman and Company.

Schmutz EA, Zimmermann MB, Rohrmann S: The inverse association between serum 25-hydroxyvitamin D and mortality may be modified by vitamin A status and use of vitamin A supplements, *Eur J Nutr* Feb 21, 2015. [Epub ahead of print].

Shichiri M, Adkins Y, Ishida N, et al: DHA concentration of red blood cells is inversely associated with markers of lipid peroxidation in men taking DHA supplement, *J Clin Biochem Nutr* 55:196, 2014.

Smith JD: Myeloperoxidase, Inflammation, and Dysfunctional HDL, *J Clin Lipidol* 4(5):382–388, Sep–Oct 2010.

Song Y, Manson JE, Buring JE, et al: Dietary magnesium intake in relation to plasma insulin levels and risk of type 2 diabetes in women, *Diabetes Care* 27:59, 2004.

Song Y, Ridker PM, Manson JE, et al: Magnesium intake, C-reactive protein, and the prevalence of metabolic syndrome in middle-aged and older U.S. women, *Diabetes Care* 28:1438, 2005.

Stenholm S, Harris TB, Rantanen T, et al: Sarcopenic obesity - definition, cause and consequences, *Curr Opin Clin Nutr Metab Care* 11:693, 2008.

Stevanovic S, Nikolic M, Stankovic A, et al: Dietary magnesium intake and coronary heart disease risk: a study from Serbia, *Med Glas* 8:203, 2011.

Stipanuk MH, Caudill MA, editors: *Biochemical, physiological, and molecular aspects of human nutrition*, ed 3, St Louis, MO, 2013, Elsevier.

Tay L, Tan K, Diener E, et al: Social relations, health behaviors, and health outcomes: a survey and synthesis, *Appl Psychol Health Well Being* 5:28, 2013.

Tousoulis D, Plastiras A, Siasos G, et al: Omega-3 PUFAs improved endothelial function and arterial stiffness with a parallel antiinflammatory effect in adults with metabolic syndrome, *Atherosclerosis* 232:10, 2014.

Triana Junco M, García Vázquez N, Zozaya C, et al: An exclusively based parenteral fish-oil emulsion reverses cholestasis, *Nutr Hosp* 31:514, 2014.

Tuorkey MJ: Curcumin a potent cancer preventive agent: mechanisms of cancer cell killing, *Interv Med Appl Sci* 6:139, 2014.

Uddin M, Levy BD: Resolvins: Natural Agonists for Resolution of Pulmonary Inflammation, *Prog Lipid Res* 50(1):75. Jan 2011. Published online Sep 29, 2010.

Umberson D, Montez JK: Social relationships and health: a flashpoint for health policy, *J Health Soc Behav* 51:S54, 2010.

Underwood MA: Intestinal dysbiosis: novel mechanisms by which gut microbes trigger and prevent disease, *Prev Med* 65:133, 2014.

United Nations General Assembly: *Political declaration of the high-level meeting of the general assembly on the prevention and control of non-communicable diseases*, 2011. http://www.who.int/entity/nmh/events/un_ncd_summit2011/en/. Accessed April 5, 2015.

Uusitupa M, Hermansen K, Savolainen MJ, et al: Effects of an isocaloric healthy Nordic diet on insulin sensitivity, lipid profile and inflammation markers in metabolic syndrome— a randomized study (SYSDIET), *J Intern Med* 274:52, 2013.

Varga J, De Oliveira T, Greten FR: The architect who never sleeps: tumor-induced plasticity, *FEBS Lett* 588:2422, 2014.

Vescovo T, Refolo G, Romagnoli A, et al: Autophagy in HCV infection: keeping fat and inflammation at bay, *Biomed Res Int* 2014:265353, 2014.

Viladomiu M, Hontecillas R, Yuan L, et al: Nutritional protective mechanisms against gut inflammation, *J Nutr Biochem* 24:929, 2013.

Vollset SE, Clarke R, Lewington S, et al: Effects of folic acid supplementation on overall and site-specific cancer incidence during the randomised trials: meta-analyses of data on 50,000 individuals, *Lancet* 381:1029, 2013.

von Schacky C: Omega-3 index and cardiovascular health, *Nutrients* 6:799, 2014.

Waitzberg DL: The complexity of prescribing intravenous lipid emulsions, *World Rev Nutr Diet* 112:150, 2015.

Wallace KL, Zheng LB, Kanazawa Y, et al: Immunopathology of inflammatory bowel disease, *World J Gastroenterol* 20:6, 2014.

Wang X, Lin H, Gu Y: Multiple roles of dihomo-g-linolenic acid against proliferation diseases, *Lipids Health Dis* 11:25, 2012.

Watson RR, editor: *Nutrition in the prevention and treatment of abdominal obesity*, Waltham, Mass, 2014, Elsevier.

Wergeland S, Torkildsen Ø, Bø L, et al: Polyunsaturated fatty acids in multiple sclerosis therapy, *Acta Neurol Scand Suppl* 195:70, 2012.

Williams RJ: *Biochemical individuality*, Austin and London, 1956, John Wiley & Sons.

World Health Organization (WHO): *Cancer*, 2015. http://www.who.int/mediacentre/factsheets/fs297/en/. Accessed April 8, 2015.

World Health Organization (WHO): *High-Level Meeting on Prevention and Control of Non-Communicable Diseases*, 2011. http://www.un.org/en/ga/ncdmeeting2011/. Accessed April 6, 2015.

Wu C, Li F, Niu G, et al: PET imaging of inflammation biomarkers, *Theranostics* 3:448, 2013.

Wu Y, Lach B, Provias JP, et al: Statin-associated autoimmune myopathies: a pathophysiologic spectrum, *Can J Neurol Sci* 41:638, 2014.

Wyle CM: The definition and measurement of health and disease, *Public Health Rep* 85:100, 1970.

Yach D, Hawkes C, Gould CL, et al: The global burden of chronic diseases: overcoming impediments to prevention and control, *JAMA* 291:2616, 2004.

Yao QH, Zhang XC, Fu T, et al: ω-3 polyunsaturated fatty acids inhibit the proliferation of the lung adenocarcinoma cell line A549 in vitro, *Mol Med Rep* 9:401, 2014.

4

Intake: Analysis of the Diet

Kathleen A. Hammond, MS, RN, BSN, BSHE, RDN, LD,
L. Kathleen Mahan, RDN, MS, CD

KEY TERMS

24-hour recall
ageusia
anosmia
diet history
dietary intake data
Dietary Supplements Database
dysgeusia
FDA Total Diet Study Database
Food and Nutrient Database for
    Dietary Studies (FNDDS)

food diary
food frequency questionnaire
Mini Nutritional Assessment (MNA)
    Short Form
Mini Nutritional Assessment (MNA),
    Long Form
Malnutrition Screening Tool (MST)
Malnutrition Universal Screening Tool
    (MUST)
nutrient intake analysis (NIA)

nutrition assessment
nutrition risk screening
nutrition status
Subjective Global Assessment (SGA)
USDA National Nutrient Database
    for Standard Reference (SR)

Nutrition status reveals the degree to which physiologic nutrient needs are met for an individual. Assessment of nutrition status is the foundation of nutritional care; it is the important base for personalizing an individual's nutritional care in the context of the cause, prevention, or management of disease or promotion of health. Chronic diseases, including heart disease, stroke, diabetes, and osteoporosis, as well as many gastrointestinal disorders and most cancers, are influenced by the underlying nutritional status. In addition, an individual's nutritional status affects gene expression and vice versa, with implications for many disorders (see Chapter 5). In promotion of health, regular assessment can detect a nutritional insufficiency in the early stages, allowing dietary intake and lifestyle to be improved through nutrition support and counseling before a more severe deficiency and functional change develops.

Nutrition assessment often begins with collection of dietary intake data, the information on the food, drink, and supplements consumed. This personal dietary intake is influenced by factors such as economic situation, availability of food, eating behavior, emotional climate, cultural background, effects of disease, and the ability to acquire and absorb nutrients. Once the dietary intake data are collected, they are analyzed for nutrient and phytonutrient content. This is compared with dietary recommendations and requirements particular to that individual (Figure 4-1). These requirements depend on age, gender, periods of growth such as pregnancy or adolescence, presence of chronic disease or inflammation, coexistence of stressors such as injury or psychologic trauma, and medical treatments or medications.

Nutritional well-being and the continuum of nutritional health are essential concepts to understand. Figure 4-2 illustrates the general sequence of steps leading to nutritional decline and the development of a nutritional deficiency, as well as areas in which an assessment can identify problems.

Screening and assessment are integral parts of the nutrition care process (NCP), which has four steps: (1) assessment of nutrition status; (2) identification of nutritional diagnoses; (3) interventions such as food and nutrient delivery, education, counseling, coordination of care; and (4) monitoring and evaluation of the effectiveness of the interventions (Academy of Nutrition and Dietetics [AND], 2013; see Chapter 10).

NUTRITION SCREENING

Nutrition risk is determined through a nutrition screening process. Factors to consider in determining whether an individual is at nutritional risk are listed in Table 4-1. They include food, nutrient, and botanicals intake patterns; psychosocial and economic factors; physical conditions; abnormal laboratory findings; and medication and treatment regimens.

Ideally, everyone should undergo periodic nutrition screening throughout life. Just as a health care provider conducts an annual health examination, a trained nutrition provider can conduct regular nutritional evaluations. To provide cost-effective nutrition services in today's health care environment, it is important first to screen patients to find those who are at nutritional risk. The purpose of a nutrition screen is to quickly identify individuals who are malnourished or at nutritional risk and determine whether a more detailed assessment is warranted. Nutrition screening is defined as "the process of identifying patients, clients, or groups who may have a nutrition diagnosis and benefit from nutrition assessment and intervention by a

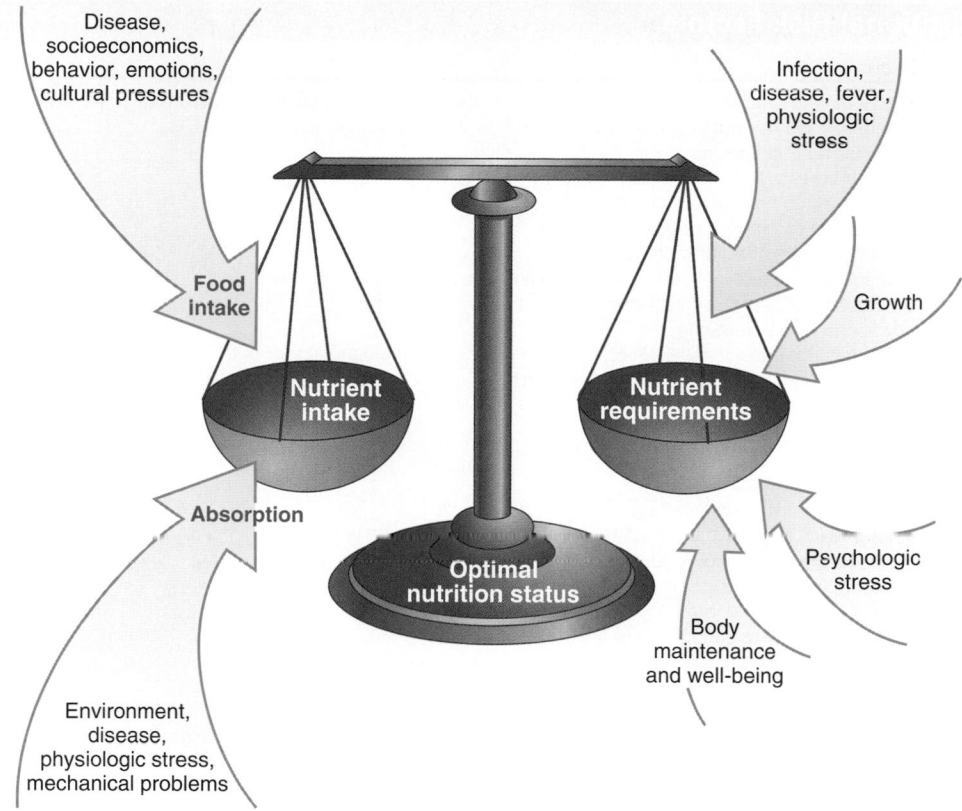

FIGURE 4-1 Optimal nutrition status: a balance between nutrient intake and nutrient requirements.

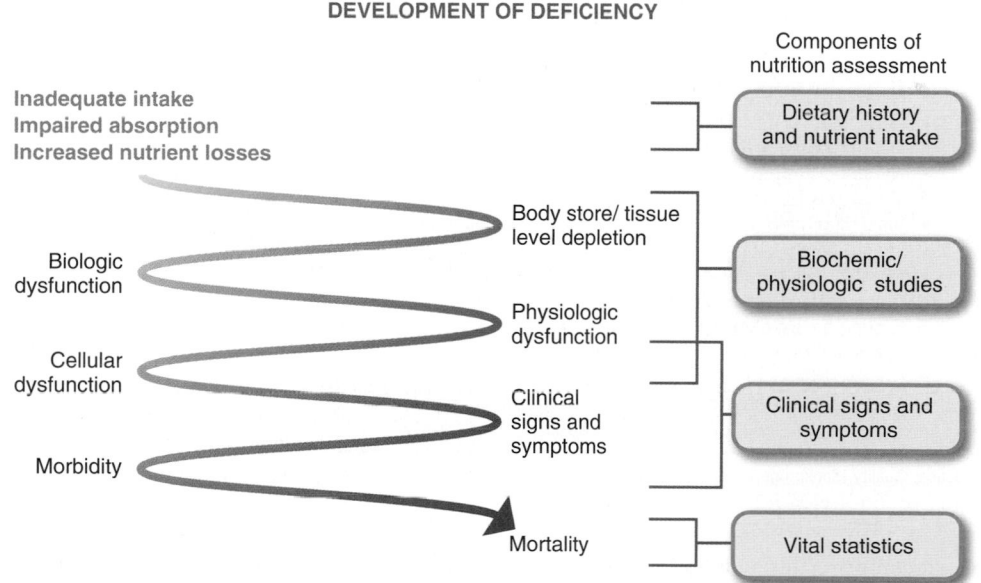

FIGURE 4-2 Development of clinical nutritional deficiency with corresponding dietary, biochemical, and clinical evaluations.

registered dietitian nutritionist (RDN)." Key considerations for nutrition screening include:

1. Tools should be quick, easy to use, and able to be conducted in any practice setting.
2. Tools should be valid and reliable for the patient population or setting.
3. Tools and parameters are established by RDNs, but the screening process may be performed by dietetic technicians, registered, or other trained personnel.
4. Screening and rescreening should occur within an appropriate time frame for the setting (AND, 2013a; Skipper et al, 2012).

TABLE 4-1 Nutritional Risk Factors

Category	Factors
Food and nutrient intake patterns	• Calorie and protein intake greater or less than that required for age and activity level • Vitamin and mineral intake greater or less than that required for age • Swallowing difficulties • Gastrointestinal disturbances • Unusual food habits (e.g., pica) • Impaired cognitive function or depression • Nothing by mouth for more than 3 days • Inability or unwillingness to consume food • Increase or decrease in activities of daily living • Misuse of supplements • Inadequate transitional feeding, tube feeding or parenteral nutrition, or both • Bowel irregularity (e.g., constipation, diarrhea) • Restricted diet • Feeding limitations
Psychologic and social factors	• Low literacy • Language barriers • Cultural or religious factors • Emotional disturbances associated with feeding difficulties (e.g., depression) • Limited resources for food preparation or obtaining food and supplies • Alcohol or drug addiction • Limited or low income • Lack of ability to communicate needs • Limited use or understanding of community resources
Physical conditions	• Extreme age: adults older than 80 years, premature infants, very young children • Pregnancy: adolescent, closely spaced, or three or more pregnancies • Alterations in anthropometric measurements: marked overweight or underweight for height, age, or both; head circumference less than normal; depressed somatic fat and muscle stores; amputation • Fat or muscle wasting • Obesity or overweight • Chronic renal or cardiac disease and related complications • Diabetes and related complications • Pressure ulcers or altered skin integrity • Cancer and related treatments • Acquired immune deficiency syndrome • Gastrointestinal complications (e.g., malabsorption, diarrhea, digestive or bowel changes) • Catabolic or hypermetabolic stress (e.g., trauma, sepsis, burns, stress) • Immobility • Osteoporosis, osteomalacia • Neurologic impairments, including impairment in sensory function • Visual impairments
Abnormal laboratory values	• Visceral proteins (e.g., albumin, transferrin, prealbumin) • Lipid profile (cholesterol, high-density lipoproteins, low-density lipoproteins, triglycerides) • Hemoglobin, hematocrit, and other hematologic tests • Blood urea nitrogen, creatinine, and electrolyte levels • Fasting serum blood glucose level • Other laboratory indexes as indicated
Medications	• Chronic use • Multiple and concurrent administration (polypharmacy) • Drug-nutrient interactions and side effects

Adapted from the Council on Practice, Quality Management Committee: Identifying patients at risk: ADA's definitions for nutrition screening and nutrition assessment, *J Am Diet Assoc* 94:838, 1994.

The most common screening criteria include history of weight loss, current need for nutrition support, presence of skin breakdown, poor dietary intake, and chronic use of modified or unusual diets. Further information collected during a nutrition screen depends on (1) the setting in which the information is obtained (e.g., home, clinic, hospital, long-term care facility), (2) the life stage or disease type, (3) the available data, and (4) a definition of risk priorities. Regardless of the information gathered, the goal of screening is to identify individuals who are at nutritional risk, those likely to become at nutritional risk, and those who need further assessment. For example, being 85 years or older, having low nutrient intake, losing the ability to eat independently, having swallowing and chewing difficulties, becoming bedridden, having pressure ulcers or a hip fracture or dementia, and suffering from two or more chronic illnesses are factors of concern in a nutritional screen.

Nutrition Screening Tools

Commonly used nutrition screening tools were evaluated by the AND. The results can be found in the Evidence Analysis Library (EAL) (AND, 2013b; AND, 2015). A screen that is simple to use is the Malnutrition Screening Tool (MST) by Ferguson (1999). The parameters include recent weight loss and recent poor dietary intake. The tool is useful for the acute hospitalized adult population and was the only one of the 11 evaluated by the EAL shown to be *valid* and *reliable* for identifying problems in acute care and hospital-based ambulatory care settings (AND, 2013b; Box 4-1).

BOX 4-1 Malnutrition Screening Tool (MST)

Question	Score
Have you lost weight recently without trying?	
No	0
Unsure	2
If yes, how much weight (kilograms) have you lost?	
1-5	1
6-10	2
11-15	3
>15	4
Unsure	2
Have you been eating poorly because of a decreased appetite?	
No	0
Yes	1
Total score:	

Score of 2 or more = patient at risk of malnutrition.
From Ferguson M et al: Development of a valid and reliable malnutrition screening tool from adult acute hospital patients, *Nutrition* 15:458, 1999, p 461.

Another screening tool is the **Malnutrition Universal Screening Tool (MUST)** developed by Stratton and colleagues (2004) to assess for malnutrition rapidly and completely; it is designed to be used by professionals of different disciplines (AND, 2015; Figure 4-3). Three independent criteria are used: (1) current weight and height with determination of body mass index (BMI), (2) unintentional weight loss using specific cutoff points, and (3) the effect of acute disease on dietary and nutrition intake for more than 5 days.

These three components work better together to predict outcome rather than the individual components separately. Once the scores are added, the overall risk of malnutrition can be determined using three categories: 0 = low risk, 1 = medium risk, and 2 and above = high risk. Nutritional management guidelines can then be put into place (Stratton et al, 2004).

The **Nutrition Risk Screening** (NRS 2002) is a screening tool that is useful for medical-surgical hospitalized patients (AND, 2015). This tool contains the nutritional components of the MUST and a grading of disease severity as reflected by increased nutritional requirements. Screening parameters for this tool include recent weight loss percentage, body mass index (BMI), severity of disease, consideration of >70 years of age, and food intake/eating problems and skipping of meals (AND, 2013b; Table 4-2).

The **Mini Nutritional Assessment (MNA) Short Form** is a rapid and reliable screening method for the subacute and ambulatory elderly populations. Nutrition screening parameters include recent dietary intake, recent weight loss, mobility, recent acute disease or psychologic stress, neuropsychologic problems, and body mass index (ANDb, 2013; Figure 4-4).

NUTRITION ASSESSMENT

Nutrition assessment is a comprehensive evaluation carried out by an RDN using medical and health, social, dietary and nutritional, medication, and supplement and herbal use histories; physical examination; anthropometric measurements; and laboratory data. Nutrition assessment interprets data from the

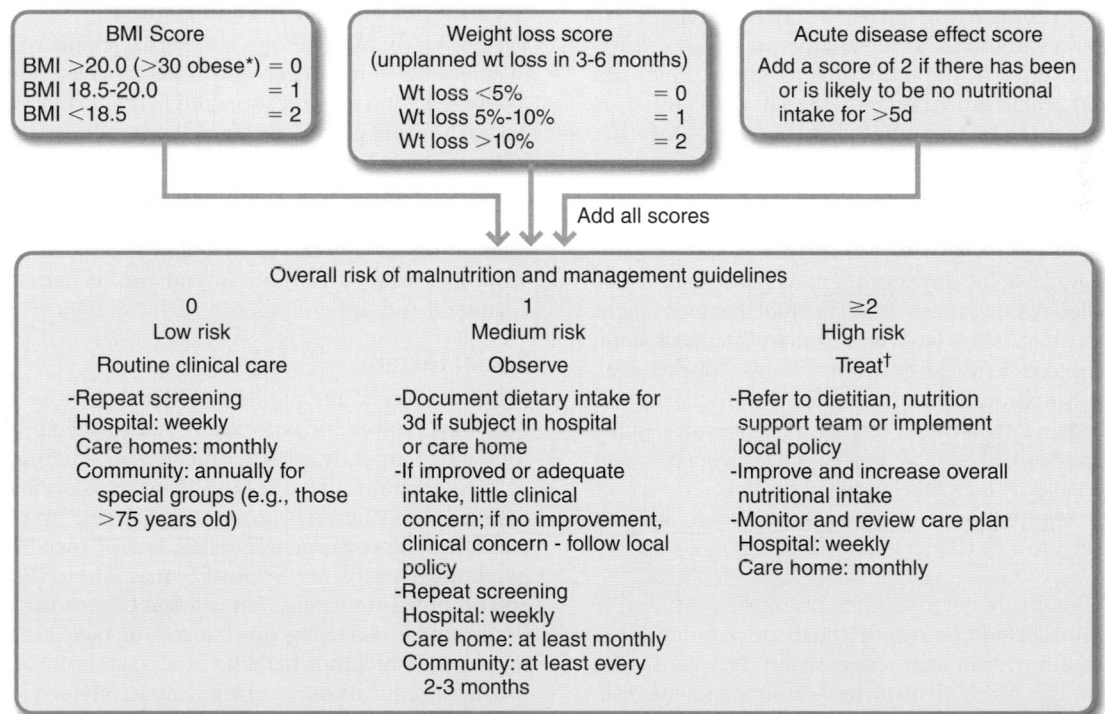

FIGURE 4-3 The Malnutrition Universal Screening Tool (MUST) for adults. Record malnutrition risk category, presence of obesity and/or need for special diets and follow local policy for those identified at risk. If unable to obtain height and weight, alternative measurements and subjective criteria are provided (Elia, 2003).
*In the obese, underlying acute conditions are generally controlled before treatment of obesity.
†Unless detrimental or no benefit is expected from nutritional support (e.g., imminent death).
(Courtesy Professor Marinos Elia, Editor: BAPEN, 2003 ISBN 1 899467 70X. Copies of the full report are available from the BAPEN Office, Secure Hold Business Centre, Studley Road, Redditch, Worcs BN98 7LG Tel: 01527 457850.)

TABLE 4-2 Nutritional Risk Screening 2002 (ESPEN Guidelines)

Impaired Nutritional Status		Severity of Disease (= Requirement/Stress-Metabolism)	
Mild	Wt loss >5% in 3 mo	Mild	Hip fracture
	or	Score 1	Chronic patients, in particular with acute complication:
Score 1	Food intake <50% to 75% of normal requirement in preceding week		cirrhosis, COPD
			Chronic hemodialysis, diabetes, malignant oncology
Moderate	Wt loss >5% in 2 mo	Moderate	Major abdominal surgery
	or		Stroke
Score 2	BMI 18.5 – 20.5 + impaired general condition	Score 2	*Severe pneumonia, malignant hematology*
	or		
	Food intake 25% to 50% of normal requirement in preceding week		
Severe	Wt loss ≥ 5% in 1 mo (= 15% in 3 mo)	Severe	Head injury
	or		Bone marrow transplantation
Score 3	BMI <18.5 + impaired general condition	Score 3	*Intensive care patients (APACHE> 10)*
	or		
	Food intake 0 to 25% of normal requirement in preceding week		
Score:	+	Score: = TOTAL SCORE	

ESPEN, European Society for Parenteral and Enteral Nutrition.

Modified from Kondrup J et al: ESPEN guidelines for nutrition screening 2002, *Clin Nutr* 22:415, 2003.

nutrition screen and incorporates additional information. It is the first step in the nutrition care process (see Chapter 7).

The purpose of assessment is to gather adequate information in which to make a professional judgment about nutrition status. The nutrition assessment is defined as a systematic approach to collect, record, and interpret relevant data from patients, clients, family members, caregivers, and other individuals and groups. It is an ongoing, dynamic process that involves initial data collection and continued reassessment and analysis of nutritional status in comparison to specific criteria (Table 4-3).

The information gathered depends on the particular setting, the present health status of the individual or group, how data are related to particular outcomes, whether it is an initial or follow-up assessment, and recommended practices. Once the nutrition assessment process is complete and a nutrition diagnosis made, the plan of care can be developed (see Chapter 10).

Tools for Assessment of Nutritional Status

Several tools are available for the assessment of nutritional status. The Subjective Global Assessment (SGA) is a tool that uses weight history, diet history data, stress level, and primary diagnosis along with physical symptoms to assess nutritional status (Mueller et al, 2011). The **Mini Nutrition Assessment (MNA) Long Form** tool evaluates independence, medication therapy, pressure sores, number of full meals consumed per day, protein intake, consumption of fruits and vegetables, fluid intake, mode of feeding, self-view of nutritional status, comparison with peers, and mid-arm and calf circumferences (Figure 4-5) (Bauer et al, 2008; Guigoz, 2006).

Histories

The information collected about individuals or populations is used as part of the nutrition status assessment. Frequently the information is in the form of histories—health and medical, social, medication and herbal use, and dietary and nutritional.

Medical or Health History

The medical or health history usually includes the following information: chief complaint, present and past illness, current health, allergies, past or recent surgeries, family history of disease, psychosocial data, and a review of problems—by body system—from the patient's perspective (Hammond, 2006). These histories usually provide much insight into nutrition-related problems. Alcohol and drug use, increased metabolic

needs, increased nutritional losses, chronic disease, recent major surgery or illness, disease or surgery of the gastrointestinal tract, and recent significant weight loss may contribute to malnutrition. In older patients, additional review is recommended to detect mental deterioration, constipation or incontinence, poor eyesight, hearing or taste sensation, slowed reactions, major organ diseases, effects of prescription and over-the-counter drugs, and physical disabilities.

Medication and Herbal Use History

Various foods, medications, and herbal supplements can interact in many ways that affect nutrition status and drug therapy effectiveness; thus a medication and herbal history is an important part of any nutrition assessment. Those who are older, are chronically ill, have a history of marginal or inadequate nutritional intake, or are receiving multiple drugs for a long time are susceptible to drug-induced nutritional deficiencies. The effects of medication therapy can be altered by specific foods, the timing of food and meal consumption, and use of herbal products (see Chapter 8 and Appendix 23).

Social History

Social aspects of the medical or health history also may affect nutrition intake. Socioeconomic status, the ability to purchase food independently, whether the person is living alone, physical or mental handicaps, smoking, drug or alcohol addiction, confusion caused by environmental changes, unsuitable housing conditions, environmental toxins, lack of socialization at meals, psychologic problems, or poverty may add to the risks for inadequate nutrition intake. Knowledge of various cultures is also important in assessing diverse groups of clients. Cultural factors include religious beliefs, rituals, symbols, language, dietary practices, education, communication style, views on health, wellness, and illness, and racial identity. See Chapter 11 for more guidance on nutrition and cultural competency.

Nutrition or Diet History

Inadequate dietary intake and nutritional inadequacy can result from anorexia, ageusia (loss of the sense of taste), dysgeusia (diminished or distorted taste), anosmia (loss of smell), excessive alcohol intake, fad dieting, chewing or swallowing problems, frequent eating of highly processed foods, adverse food and drug interactions, cultural or religious restrictions of diet, an inability

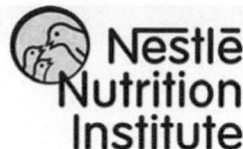

Mini Nutritional Assessment
MNA®

Last name: _____ First name: _____

Sex: _____ Age: _____ Weight, kg: _____ Height, cm: _____ Date: _____

Complete the screen by filling in the boxes with the appropriate numbers. Total the numbers for the final screening score.

Screening

A Has food intake declined over the past 3 months due to loss of appetite, digestive problems, chewing or swallowing difficulties?
0 = severe decrease in food intake
1 = moderate decrease in food intake
2 = no decrease in food intake ☐

B Weight loss during the last 3 months
0 = weight loss greater than 3 kg (6.6 lbs)
1 = does not know
2 = weight loss between 1 and 3 kg (2.2 and 6.6 lbs)
3 = no weight loss ☐

C Mobility
0 = bed or chair bound
1 = able to get out of bed / chair but does not go out
2 = goes out ☐

D Has suffered psychological stress or acute disease in the past 3 months?
0 = yes   2 = no ☐

E Neuropsychological problems
0 = severe dementia or depression
1 = mild dementia
2 = no psychological problems ☐

F1 Body Mass Index (BMI) (weight in kg) / (height in m^2)
0 = BMI less than 19
1 = BMI 19 to less than 21
2 = BMI 21 to less than 23
3 = BMI 23 or greater ☐

IF BMI IS NOT AVAILABLE, REPLACE QUESTION F1 WITH QUESTION F2.
DO NOT ANSWER QUESTION F2 IF QUESTION F1 IS ALREADY COMPLETED.

F2 Calf circumference (CC) in cm
0 = CC less than 31
3 = CC 31 or greater ☐

Screening score ☐☐
(max. 14 points)

12-14 points: Normal nutritional status
8-11 points: At risk of malnutrition
0-7 points: Malnourished

For a more in-depth assessment, complete the full MNA® which is available at **www.mna-elderly.com**

Ref.   Vellas B, Villars H, Abellan G, et al. *Overview of the MNA® - Its History and Challenges.* J Nutr Health Aging 2006;10:456-465.
Rubenstein LZ, Harker JO, Salva A, Guigoz Y, Vellas B. *Screening for Undernutrition in Geriatric Practice: Developing the Short-Form Mini Nutritional Assessment (MNA-SF).* J. Geront 2001;56A: M366-377.
Guigoz Y. *The Mini-Nutritional Assessment (MNA®) Review of the Literature - What does it tell us?* J Nutr Health Aging 2006; 10:466-487.
® Société des Produits Nestlé, S.A., Vevey, Switzerland, Trademark Owners
© Nestlé, 1994, Revision 2009. N67200 12/99 10M
For more information: www.mna-elderly.com

FIGURE 4-4 Mini Nutritional Assessment Short Form. (Permission by Nestlé Healthcare Nutrition.)

TABLE 4-3   Nutrition Care Process: Step 1: Nutrition Assessment

Data sources/tools for assessment	Screening or referral form. Patient/client interview. Medical or health records. Consultation with other caregivers, including family members. Community-based surveys and focus groups. Statistical reports, administrative data, and epidemiologic studies.
Types of data collected	Food- and nutrition-related history. Anthropometric measurements. Biochemical data, medical tests, and procedures. Nutrition-focused physical examination findings. Client history.
Nutrition assessment components	Review data collected for factors that affect nutrition and health status. Cluster individual data elements to identify a nutrition diagnosis as described in diagnosis reference sheets. Identify standards by which data will be compared.
Critical thinking	Determine appropriate data to collect. Determine the need for additional information. Select assessment tools and procedures that match the situation. Apply assessment tools in valid and reliable ways. Distinguish relevant from irrelevant data. Distinguish important from unimportant data. Validate data.
Determination for continuation of care	If on completion of an initial or reassessment it is determined that the problem cannot be modified by further nutrition care, discharge or discontinuation from this episode of nutrition care may be appropriate.

From Writing Group of the Nutrition Care Process/Standardized Language Committee: Nutrition care process and model part 1: the 2008 update, *J Am Diet Assoc* 108:1113, 2008.

to eat for more than 7 to 10 days, intravenous fluid therapy alone for more than 5 days, or the need for assistance with eating. Problems faced by older adults include ill-fitting dentures and poor dentition, changes in taste and smell, long-established poor food habits, poverty and food insecurity, and inadequate knowledge of nutrition (see Chapter 20). Self-prescribed therapies, including use of megadoses of vitamins and minerals, use of various herbs, macrobiotic diets, probiotics, and fatty acid or amino acid supplements, also must be addressed because they affect a person's nutritional and overall health.

A **diet history** is perhaps the best means of obtaining dietary intake information and refers to a review of an individual's usual patterns of food intake and the food selection variables that dictate the food intake. See Box 4-2 for the kind of information collected from a dietary history. **Dietary intake data** may be assessed either by collecting retrospective intake data (e.g., a 24-hour recall or food frequency questionnaire) or by summarizing prospective intake data (e.g., a food record kept for a number of days by an individual or the caretaker). Each method has specific purposes, strengths, and weaknesses. Any self-reported method of obtaining data can be challenging because it is difficult for people to remember what they ate, the content, and the amounts (Thompson et al, 2010). The choice of data collection depends on the purpose and setting, but the goal is to determine the food and nutrient intake that is typical for that individual.

A daily food record, or **food diary**, involves documenting dietary intake as it occurs and is often used in outpatient clinic settings. The food diary is usually completed by the individual client (Figure 4-6). A food diary or record is usually most accurate if the food and amounts eaten are recorded at the time of consumption, minimizing error from incomplete memory or attention. The individual's nutrient intake is then calculated and averaged at the end of the desired period, usually 3 to 7 days, and compared with dietary reference intakes (DRIs) (see inside front cover), government dietary guidelines as in the MyPlate guide (Chapter 11), or personalized dietary recommendations for disease management or prevention.

With the current emphasis on self-management, electronic food diaries and records are gaining in popularity, including mobile applications (apps) that store food intake data along with allowing the sharing of reports with friends or health professionals. (see Focus On: Does Your App Know What You are Eating?).

◎ FOCUS ON

Does Your App Know What You are Eating?

In addition, a variety of nutrition apps can be downloaded to smartphones to further assist in assessing nutrient intake. Using an app, an individual can self-monitor their nutrition and exercise lifestyle. They can record calorie and nutrient intake as well as energy expenditure in exercise. Electronic diaries can be more accurate and useful compared with handwritten entries. With some apps it is also possible for the client to share this information with a dietitian or other health professional and receive feedback on changes or improvements that can be made. Many of these apps support access from a personal computer, a mobile phone, or other hand-held device as well as search in a food database and create graphs from food intake data (Rusin, 2013). Recording electronic devices can link a kitchen scale used to weigh food eaten directly to a computer, making recording of portion sizes more accurate.

Mobile devices can be used to photograph meals and document portion sizes. This process can either be active (i.e., the user takes an image before and after a meal) or passive (i.e., a wearable camera takes images during daily activities, including mealtime). These options can assist with more accurate reporting of intake, which previously relied completely on recall. However, if images are not of satisfactory quality, or if they do not provide a reference point to judge portion size, they may underestimate intake (Gemming et al, 2015). Other apps use a bar code reader to transmit data from food labels to a food record (Six et al, 2011; Thompson et al, 2010; Some of the popular apps are:

Lose It!
MyFitnessPal
Meal Snap
Fooducate

LaGesse D: Lose weight with your phone. <http://www.aarp.org/health/fitness/info-04-2011/lose-weight-with-your-phone.1.html>, 2011. Accessed February 10, 2015.

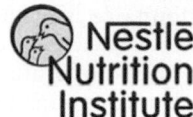

Mini Nutritional Assessment
MNA®

Last name:	First name:

Sex:	Age:	Weight, kg:	Height, cm:	Date:

Complete the screen by filling in the boxes with the appropriate numbers. Add the numbers for the screen. If score is 11 or less, continue with the assessment to gain a Malnutrition Indicator Score.

Screening

A Has food intake declined over the past 3 months due to loss of appetite, digestive problems, chewing or swallowing difficulties?
0 = severe decrease in food intake
1 = moderate decrease in food intake
2 = no decrease in food intake ☐

B Weight loss during the last 3 months
0 = weight loss greater than 3kg (6.6lbs)
1 = does not know
2 = weight loss between 1 and 3kg (2.2 and 6.6 lbs)
3 = no weight loss ☐

C Mobility
0 = bed or chair bound
1 = able to get out of bed / chair but does not go out
2 = goes out ☐

D Has suffered psychological stress or acute disease in the past 3 months?
0 = yes   2 = no ☐

E Neuropsychological problems
0 = severe dementia or depression
1 = mild dementia
2 = no psychological problems ☐

F Body Mass Index (BMI) (weight in kg) / (height in m²)
0 = BMI less than 19
1 = BMI 19 to less than 21
2 = BMI 21 to less than 23
3 = BMI 23 or greater ☐

Screening score ☐☐
(subtotal max. 14 points)

12-14 points: Normal nutritional status
8-11 points: At risk of malnutrition
0-7 points: Malnourished

For a more in-depth assessment, continue with questions G-R

Assessment

G Lives independently (not in nursing home or hospital)
1 = yes   0 = no ☐

H Takes more than 3 prescription drugs per day
0 = yes   1 = no ☐

I Pressure sores or skin ulcers
0 = yes   1 = no ☐

J How many full meals does the patient eat daily?
0 = 1 meal
1 = 2 meals
2 = 3 meals ☐

K Selected consumption markers for protein intake
- At least one serving of dairy products (milk, cheese, yoghurt) per day   yes ☐   no ☐
- Two or more servings of legumes or eggs per week   yes ☐   no ☐
- Meat, fish or poultry every day   yes ☐   no ☐
0.0 = if 0 or 1 yes
0.5 = if 2 yes
1.0 = if 3 yes ☐.☐

L Consumes two or more servings of fruit or vegetables per day?
0 = no   1 = yes ☐

M How much fluid (water, juice, coffee, tea, milk...) is consumed per day?
0.0 = less than 3 cups
0.5 = 3 to 5 cups
1.0 = more than 5 cups ☐.☐

N Mode of feeding
0 = unable to eat without assistance
1 = self-fed with some difficulty
2 = self-fed without any problem ☐

O Self view of nutritional status
0 = views self as being malnourished
1 = Is uncertain of nutritional state
2 = views self as having no nutritional problem ☐

P In comparison with other people of the same age, how does the patient consider his / her health status?
0.0 = not as good
0.5 = does not know
1.0 = as good
2.0 = better ☐.☐

Q Mid-arm circumference (MAC) in cm
0.0 = MAC less than 21
0.5 = MAC 21 to 22
1.0 = MAC 22 or greater ☐.☐

R Calf circumference (CC) in cm
0 = CC less than 31
1 = CC 31 or greater ☐

Assessment (max. 16 points) ☐☐.☐

Screening score ☐☐.☐

Total Assessment (max. 30 points) ☐☐.☐

Ref. Vellas B, Villars H, Abellan G, et al. *Overview of MNA® - Its History and Challenges.* J Nut Health Aging 2006; 10: 456-465.
Rubenstein LZ, Harker JO, Salva A, Guigoz Y, Vellas B. Screening for Undernutrition in Geriatric Practice: *Developing the Short-Form Mini Nutritional Assessment (MNA-SF).* J. Geront 2001; 56A: M366-377.
Guigoz Y. The Mini-Nutritional Assessment (MNA®) *Review of the Literature – What does it tell us?* J Nutr Health Aging 2006; 10: 466-487.
® Société des Produits Nestlé, S.A., Vevey, Switzerland, Trademark Owners
© Nestlé, 1994, Revision 2006. N67200 12/99 10M
For more information: www.mna-elderly.com

Malnutrition Indicator Score

24 to 30 points	☐	normal nutritional status
17 to 23.5 points	☐	at risk of malnutrition
Less than 17 points	☐	malnourished

FIGURE 4-5 Mini Nutritional Assessment Long Form. (Permission by Nestlé Healthcare Nutrition.)

BOX 4-2 Diet History Information

Category

Allergies, intolerances, or food avoidances	Foods avoided and reason for avoidance
	Length of avoidance
	Description of problems caused by foods
Appetite	Good, poor, any changes
	Factors that affect individual's appetite
	Changes in taste or smell perception
Attitude toward food and eating	Disinterest in food
	Irrational ideas about food, eating, or body weight
	Parental interest in child's eating
Chronic disease, treatments, and medications	Treatments or medications
	Length of treatment time
	Length of medication use
	Dietary modification: self-imposed or physician prescribed, date of modification
	Past nutrition and diet education, compliance with diet
Culture and background	Influence of culture on eating habits
	Religious practices, holiday rituals
	Educational background
	Health beliefs
Dental and oral health	Problems with chewing
	Foods that cannot be eaten
	Problems with swallowing, salivation, choking, food sticking
Economics	Income: frequency and steadiness of employment
	Amount of money for food each week or month
	Individual's perception of food security
	Eligibility for SNAP
	Public aid assistance status
Gastrointestinal factors	Problems with heartburn, bloating, gas
	Problems with diarrhea, vomiting, constipation, distention
	Frequency of problems
	Use of OTC medications
	Use of herbal or home remedies
	Antacid, laxative, or other drug use
Home life and meal patterns	Number in household (eat together?)
	Who does shopping
	Who does cooking
	Food storage and cooking facilities (e.g., stove, refrigerator)
	Type of housing (e.g., home, apartment, room)
	Ability to shop and prepare foods, disabilities
Supplements, herbal remedies	Vitamin and mineral supplements: frequency of use, type, amount
	Other nutraceuticals (e.g., coenzyme CoQ10, omega-3 fats): frequency of use, type, and amount
	Medications: type, amount, frequency of administration, length of time on medication
	Herbal remedies: type, amount, purpose
Nutritional problems	Concerns as perceived by patient and family
	Referrals from physician, nurse, other therapist, agency
Physical activity, stress, leisure time	Occupation: type, hours/week, shift, energy expenditure
	Exercise: type, amount, frequency (seasonal?)
	Sleep: hours/day (uninterrupted?)
	Stress: amount, frequency, chronic?
	Relaxation and leisure activities: type, amount, frequency
	Handicaps
Weight pattern and history	Loss or gain: how many pounds and over what length of time?
	Intentional or nonvolitional
	% Usual weight; healthy weight; desirable weight
Environment and toxin exposure	Exposure to known toxins: when, amount, length of time
	Possible exposure to toxins: when
	Sequelae

The **food frequency questionnaire** is a retrospective review of intake based on frequency (i.e., food consumed per day, per week, or per month). For ease of evaluation, the food frequency chart organizes foods into groups that have common nutrients. Because the focus of the food frequency questionnaire is the frequency of consumption of food groups without portion sizes, the information obtained is general, not specific, and cannot be applied to certain nutrients. During illness, food consumption patterns can change, depending on the stage of illness. Therefore it is helpful to complete food frequency questionnaires for the period immediately before hospitalization or before illness to obtain a complete and accurate history. Box 4-3 shows a food frequency questionnaire. Another more specific, quantified questionnaire is online at http://sharedresources.fhcrc.org/content/ffq-sample-booklets.

The **24-hour recall** method of data collection requires individuals to remember the specific foods and amounts of foods they consumed in the past 24 hours. The nutrition professional asks the person to recall his or her intake using a specific set of questions to gain as much detailed information as possible. For example, when told that the person had cereal for breakfast, the nutritionist may ask, "What kind of cereal?" The next question may be, "How much did you have?" at the same time that the person is being shown a bowl or measuring cup to jog the memory on portion size.

Problems commonly associated with this method of data collection include (1) an inability to recall accurately the kinds and amounts of food eaten, (2) difficulty in determining whether the day being recalled represents an individual's typical intake or was exceptional, and (3) the tendency for persons to exaggerate low intakes and underreport high intakes of foods. Concurrent use of food frequency questionnaires with 24-hour recalls or food diaries (i.e., doing a cross-check) improves the accuracy of dietary intake data.

Reliability and validity of dietary recall methods are important issues. When attention is directed toward the diet, people may consciously or unconsciously alter their intake either to simplify recording or impress the interviewer, thus decreasing the information's validity. The validity of dietary recall information from obese individuals is often questionable, because they tend to underreport their intakes. The same can be true for patients with eating disorders, those who are critically ill, those who abuse drugs or alcohol, individuals who are confused, and those whose intake is unpredictable. Table 4-4 describes the advantages and disadvantages of the various methods used to obtain accurate dietary intake data.

Nutrient Intake Analysis

A **nutrient intake analysis (NIA)** also may be referred to as a nutrient intake record analysis or calorie count, depending on the information collected and the analysis done. The NIA is a tool used in various inpatient settings to identify nutritional inadequacies by monitoring intakes before deficiencies develop. Information about actual intake is collected through direct observation or an inventory of foods eaten based on observation of what remains on the individual's tray or plate after a meal. In many cases, photographs taken by smartphones are useful in documenting amount of food consumed (LaGesse, 2011). Intake from enteral and parenteral tube feedings is also recorded.

Food Diary: DAY _____

MEAL Foods (list)	AMOUNT EATEN	HOW PREPARED	WHERE EATEN (home, work, etc.)
Breakfast:			
Snack:			
Lunch:			
Dinner:			
Snack:			

Food Supplements   Cans/Day: _____   Name: _____
Vitamins/Mineral Supplement:_____

FIGURE 4-6 Food diary format.

BOX 4-3   General Food Frequency Questionnaire*

To determine the frequency of food consumption, the following pattern of questions may be useful. However, questions may have to be modified based on information from the 24-hour recall. For instance, if a woman states that she drank a glass of milk the day before, do not ask, "Do you drink milk?" Rather, ask, "How much milk do you drink?" Record answers with the appropriate time frame designated (e.g., 1/day, 1/wk, 3/mo) or as accurately as possible. The frequency may have to be recorded as "occasionally" or "rarely" if the patient cannot be more specific.

1. Do you drink milk? If so, how much? What kind?   Whole   Skim   Low-fat
2. Do you use fat? If so, what kind? How much?   Butter   Oil   Other
3. How often do you eat meat?   Eggs?   Cheese?   Beans?
4. Do you eat snack foods? If so, which ones?   How often?   How much?
5. Which vegetables (in each group) do you eat?   How often?
   a. Broccoli   Cauliflower   Brussels sprouts   Kale
   b. Tomatoes or tomato juice   Raw cabbage   Green peppers
   c. Asparagus   Beets   Green peppers   Corn   Cooked cabbage   Celery   Peas   Lettuce
   d. Cooked greens   Sweet potatoes   Yams   Carrots
6. Which fruits do you eat?   How often?
   a. Apples or applesauce   Apricots   Bananas   Berries   Cherries   Grapes or grape juice   Peaches   Pears   Pineapple   Plums   Prunes   Raisins
   b. Oranges, orange juice   Grapefruit, grapefruit juice   Lemons, lemon juice

7. Bread and cereal products
   Do you eat bread? What kind? Whole wheat? High fiber? White? Gluten-free? How much per day?
   Do you eat cereal? (daily? weekly?) What type?   Cooked   Dry
   How often do you eat foods such as macaroni, spaghetti, and noodles?
   Do you eat crackers or chips? How often? What kind?
8. Do you use salt? Do you salt your food before tasting it? Do you cook with salt? Do you crave salt or salty foods?
9. How many teaspoons of sugar do you use daily? Include sugar on cereal, fruit, toast, and in beverages such as coffee and tea.
10. Do you eat desserts? How often?
11. Do you drink sugar-containing beverages such as soda pop or sweetened juice drinks? How often? How much?
12. How often do you eat candy or cookies?
13. Do you drink water? How often during the day? How much each time? How much water do you drink each day?
14. Do you use sugar substitutes in packet form or in drinks? What type do you use? How often?
15. Do you drink alcohol? Which type: beer, wine, liquor? How often? How much?
16. Do you drink caffeinated beverages such as coffee, tea, or energy drinks? How often? How much per day?

A NIA should be recorded for at least 72 hours to reflect daily variations in intake. Complete records for this period usually accurately reflect an average intake for most individuals. If the record is incomplete, it may be necessary to extend the duration of the recorded intake. Eating habits or meals consumed during the weekend and during the week may differ, so ideally a weekend day is included.

ANALYSIS OF DIETARY INTAKE DATA

Once all data has been collected, the record of total intake can be analyzed for its nutrient content using one of several available computerized methods. Several database choices for estimation of intake vary by the nutrients analyzed, other data factored in, and how the data are presented. For example,

TABLE 4-4 Methods for Obtaining Dietary Intake Data

Method	Advantages	Disadvantages
Inpatient nutrient intake analysis (NIA)	Allows actual observation of food intake in clinical setting for good reliability Weight of foods measured before and after meals allows for most accurate analysis of intake	Does not reflect intake of free-living individual
Daily food record or diary	Provides daily record of food consumption Can provide information on quantity of food, how food is prepared, and timing of meals and snacks Inclusion of weekend days and weekdays results in more accurate analysis of intake More days recorded results in more accurate analysis of intake	Depends on variable literacy skills of participants Requires ability to measure or judge portion size Actual food intake possibly influenced by the recording process Reliability of records is questionable
Food frequency questionnaire	Easily standardized Can be beneficial when considered in combination with usual daily intake Provides overall picture of intake	Requires literacy skills Does not provide meal pattern data
24-hour recall	Quick and easy	Relies on patient's memory Requires knowledge of portion sizes May not represent usual intake Requires nutrition professional to have interviewing skills

besides the amounts of various nutrients, are the data presented for each day in addition to an average for the week? Is information on the individual's gender, height, weight, and age factored in so that the data can be compared with the DRI (see inside cover) for that individual? Or are the food intake data general (as from a completed food frequency questionnaire) and can be compared only with MyPlate.com or other general guidelines?

Nutrient Databases

The USDA National Nutrient Database for Standard Reference (SR), which is maintained by the Agricultural Research Service (ARS) of the U.S. Department of Agriculture, is updated annually. The SR is the major source of food composition data in the United States, and, as of this writing, is at version SR27 (USDA ARS, 2014; Pennington, 2007).

The Food and Nutrient Database for Dietary Studies (FNDDS), also maintained by the ARS, is a database of foods, their nutrient values, and weights for typical food portions. It includes 10 data files, plus comprehensive documentation and a user's guide for ease of use. The FNDDS is used to analyze data from the survey "*What We Eat in America,*" the dietary intake component of the National Health and Nutrition Examination Survey (NHANES).

The FDA Total Diet Study Database includes 280 core foods. It provides analytical data for dietary minerals, folic acid, heavy metals, radionuclides, pesticide residues, industrial chemicals, and chemical contaminants.

The Dietary Supplements Database from the NIH Office of Dietary Supplements offers information on dietary supplements via its website and its My Dietary Supplements (MYDS) mobile application. The **Nutrient Data System for Research** from the University of Minnesota provides ongoing updates for generic and branded products, as well as a dietary supplement assessment module. The **ProNutra** database, from VioCare, Inc., is designed for research diets controlled in many nutrients. It includes customizable calculation algorithms, with research kitchen outputs (Viocare, 2009).

Food and nutrition management software systems such as Computrition or CBORD are designed for institutional

use and typically include extensive nutrient databases. These systems may regularly import data from the SR. Other food database software programs designed and priced for individual use are available; however, their cost and their comprehensiveness vary. Only certain software programs are approved for use in the USDA School Meals program (Stein, 2011).

USEFUL WEBSITES

Automated Self-administered 24-hour Dietary Recall
http://riskfactor.cancer.gov/tools/instruments/asa24/
Food Frequency Questionnaires
http://sharedresources.fhcrc.org/content/ffq-sample-booklets
International Food Information Council
http://www.foodinsight.org/
Malnutrition Universal Screening Tool
http://www.bapen.org.uk/must_tool.html
National Cancer Institute (NCI) Diet History
http://riskfactor.cancer.gov/DHQ/
National Health and Nutrition Examination Survey Food Frequency Questionnaire
http://riskfactor.cancer.gov/diet/usualintakes/ffq.html
National Heart, Lung, and Blood Institute
http://www.nhlbi.nih.gov/index.htm
Nutrition Analysis Tool
http://nat.illinois.edu/
Personal Mobile Dietary Assessment Apps
www.fooducate.com
www.loseit.com/
www.myfitnesspal.com/
http://mealsnap.com/
U.S. Department of Agriculture
http://fnic.nal.usda.gov/food-composition
U.S. Department of Agriculture Healthy Eating Index
http://www.cnpp.usda.gov/HealthyEatingIndex.htm
U.S. Department of Agriculture Nutrient Content of the Food Supply
http://www.cnpp.usda.gov/USFoodSupply.htm

CASE STUDY

Laverne, a 66 year-old woman, has contacted you to set up an outpatient nutrition screening appointment. She works full time and lives by herself. She has type 2 diabetes, hypertension, and a history of colon cancer. She is 5 ft, 8 in tall and weighs 203 lb. Her current medications are glyburide and a diuretic. (She does not know its name.) She tells you that she eats throughout the day and sometimes gets up during the night for a snack. She finds eating fast-food a convenience with her busy schedule and tends to frequent these type of restaurants three to four times per week. She does not have an exercise routine and is usually too tired to exercise after her long day at work and commute.

Nutrition Diagnostic Statement

Overweight/obesity related to poor food choices as evidenced by a BMI of 31.

Nutrition Care Questions

1. What would you include in a nutrition screening for Laverne?
2. What would you include in a nutrition assessment for Laverne?
3. How could you identify her medications?
4. What additional information is needed for assessment of her dietary and nutrient intake?
5. If you need more details, what questions would you ask her physician?

BMI, Body mass index.

REFERENCES

Academy of Nutrition and Dietetics (AND): *Evidence Analysis Library (EAL)*, 2015. http://andevidencelibrary.com/search.cfm?keywords=nutrition+screening. (Accessed November 02, 2015).

Academy of Nutrition and Dietetics (AND): *International dietetics & nutrition terminology (IDNT) reference manual*, ed 4, Chicago, 2013, Academy of Nutrition and Dietetics.

Academy of Nutrition and Dietetics (AND): Nutrition assessment. In *Nutrition Care Manual On-line*, Chicago, 2013a, Academy of Nutrition and Dietetics.

Academy of Nutrition and Dietetics (AND): Nutrition screening. In *Nutrition Care Manual On-line*, Chicago, 2013b, Academy of Nutrition and Dietetics.

Barker LA, Gout BS, Crowe TC: Hospital malnutrition: prevalence, identification and impact on patients and the healthcare system, *Int J Environ Res Public Health* 8:514, 2011.

Bauer JM, Kaiser MJ, Anthony P, et al: The Mini Nutritional Assessment—its history, today's practice, and future perspectives, *Nutr Clin Pract* 23:388, 2008.

Ferguson M, Capra S, Bauer J, et al: Development of a valid and reliable malnutrition screening tool for adult acute hospital patients, *Nutrition* 15:458, 1999.

Gemming L, Utter J, Ni Mhurchu C: Image-assisted dietary assessment: a systematic review of the evidence, *J Acad Nutr Diet* 115:64, 2015.

Guigoz Y: The mini nutrition assessment (MNA®) review of the literature—what does it tell us? *J Nutr Health Aging* 10:466, 2006.

Hammond KA: Physical assessment. In Lysen LK, editor: *Quick reference to clinical dietetics*, ed 2, Boston, 2006, Jones and Bartlett.

LaGesse D: *Lose weight with your phone*, 2011. http://www.aarp.org/health/fitness/info-04-2011/lose-weight-with-your-phone.1.html. Accessed February 10, 2015.

Mueller C, Compher C, Ellen DM, et al: A.S.P.E.N. clinical guidelines: nutrition screening, assessment, and interventions in adults, *JPEN J Parenter Enteral Nutr* 35:16, 2011.

Pennington JA, Stumbo PJ, Murphy SP, et al: Food composition data: the foundation of dietetic practice and research, *J Am Diet Assoc* 107:2105, 2007.

Rusin M, Arsand E, Hartvigsen G: Functionalities and input methods for recording food intake: a systematic review, *Int J Med Inform* 82:653, 2013.

Six BL, Schap TE, Kerr DA, et al: Evaluation of the food and nutrient database for dietary studies for use with a mobile telephone food record, *J Food Compost Anal* 24:1160, 2011.

Skipper A, Ferguson M, Thompson K, et al: Nutrition screening tools: an analysis of the evidence, *JPEN J Parenter Enteral Nutr* 36:292, 2012.

Stein K: It all adds up: nutrition analysis software can open the door to professional opportunities, *J Am Diet Assoc* 111:214, 2011.

Stratton RJ, Hackston A, Longmore D, http://www.ncbi.nlm.nih.gov/pubmed/?term=Dixon R%5BAuthor%5D&cauthor=true&cauthor_uid=15533269 et al: Malnutrition in hospital outpatients and inpatients: prevalence, concurrent validity and ease of use of the "malnutrition universal screening tool" ("MUST") for adults, *Br J Nutr* 92:799, 2004.

Thompson FE, Subar AF, Loria CM, et al: Need for technological innovation in dietary assessment, *J Am Diet Assoc* 110:48, 2010.

U.S. Department of Agriculture, Agricultural Research Service, Nutrient Data Laboratory: *USDA National Nutrient Database for Standard Reference, Release 27*, 2014. http://www.ars.usda.gov/ba/bhnrc/ndl. Accessed February 10, 2015.

Viocare: *Pronutra*, 2009. http://www.viocare.com/pronutra.aspx. Accessed February 10, 2015.

5

Clinical: Nutritional Genomics

Ruth DeBusk, PhD, RDN

KEY TERMS

allele
autosomal dominant
autosomal recessive
autosome
bioactive food components
bioinformatics
chromosome
coding region
codon
copy number variant
CpG island
deletion
deoxyribonucleic acid (DNA)
DNA code
DNA methylation
DNA sequencing
dominant
Encyclopedia of DNA Elements (ENCODE)
environmental factors
epigenetics
epigenetic code
epigenetic gene silencing
epigenetic inheritance
epigenetic marks
epigenome
epigenomics
exon
gene
gene X environment (GxE)
genetic code
genetics
Genetic Information Nondiscrimination Act (GINA)
genetic variation/gene variant
genome
genome-wide association studies (GWAS)

genomic imprinting
genomics
genotype
haplotype
heterozygous
histone
homozygous
Human Genome Project
inborn errors of metabolism (IEM)
insertions
inversions
International HapMap Project
intervening sequences
intron
karyotype
junk DNA
ligand
meiosis
mendelian inheritance
messenger RNA (mRNA)
metabolomics
methylome
microarray technology (DNA "chips")
microbiomics
microRNAs (miRNA)
mitochondrial DNA (mtDNA)
mitochondrial (maternal) inheritance
mitosis
model system
mutation
National Human Genome Research Institute
nucleosome
nucleotide
nutritional epigenetics
nutrigenetics

nutrigenomics
nutritional genomics
pedigree
penetrance, reduced penetrance
peroxisome proliferator-activated receptor (PPAR)
pharmacogenomics
phenotype
polymerase chain reaction (PCR)
polymorphism
posttranscriptional processing
promoter region
proteomics
recessive
recombinant DNA
regulatory region
response element
restriction endonuclease (restriction enzyme)
RNA interference (RNAi)
sex chromosome
sex linked
signal transduction
silent mutation
single nucleotide polymorphism (SNP)
small interfering RNA (siRNA)
transcription
transcription factor
transgenerational epigenetic inheritance
translation
translocation
xenobiotics
X-linked dominant
X-linked recessive
Y-linked inheritance

Imagine being able to factor into the medical nutrition therapeutic intervention a client's genetic susceptibilities and environmental influences so that therapy could be targeted to optimizing health and minimizing disease. Does such an approach sound a bit like science fiction? For the immediate future, perhaps, but not for the long term. The prevalence of chronic disorders, such as heart disease, cancer, diabetes, and obesity, has been rising steadily throughout the world, accompanied by a decreasing quality of life for individuals and a soaring economic burden for the countries in which they live. Chronic disease is lifestyle disease, the result of lifelong inappropriate daily choices, particularly nutrition, interacting with each individual's genetic makeup, their deoxyribonucleic acid (DNA). These disease-promoting habits typically begin in early childhood and, for many, prenatally. Delivering effective lifestyle therapy will be a major focus of clinical nutrition in the decades ahead and will involve knowledge, skills, and tools that target the molecular, biochemical, physiologic, and social aspects of health and disease.

The success of the Human Genome Project in identifying the nucleotide building blocks of human DNA has elevated substantially our knowledge of the importance of understanding how chronic disease occurs at the molecular level. At this level common variations in DNA interact with a multitude of environmental factors, such as the foods consumed, to influence physiologic outcomes (i.e., a tendency toward wellness or illness). Health care for individuals with chronic conditions has focused on managing disease, primarily through the use of medications. Insight into the root causes of these disorders and identification of the underlying mechanisms responsible for the development and perpetuation of chronic disorders is providing new approaches that bring the promise of restoring health to those with chronic disease and, ultimately, preventing its development.

Nutrition research is focused increasingly on the mechanisms that underlie these interactions and on projecting how this understanding can be translated into clinical interventions for more effective chronic disease management and prevention. Health is a continuum that spans wellness at one end and illness at the other. Genes are an important component in determining at which end of this continuum we find ourselves; they determine our unique signature of susceptibility to being well or ill. However, research into chronic disease is teaching us that environmental factors such as diet and other lifestyle choices made on a daily basis strongly influence who among the susceptible will actually develop dysfunction and disease. Food choices, physical activity habits, sleep patterns, thoughts and emotions, and systems of meaning—relationships with self and others and one's sense of purpose in life—affect cellular function at the molecular, biochemical, and physiologic levels. The influence of these environmental factors is modifiable through daily choices and, when appropriate to the genetic makeup, has the potential for changing the health trajectory from a poor quality of life filled with disease and disability to one of thriving and flourishing.

This understanding of the key role of choices regarding these modifiable lifestyle factors is enabling clinicians to drill down to the root cause of chronic disease, to identify the molecular and biochemical mechanisms that underlie symptoms, and to tailor therapy to the individual's uniqueness. As a result, the promise of the molecular era is not only to manage chronic disease more effectively but also to restore health and, ultimately, to prevent chronic disease from developing. The interactions among genes, diet and other lifestyle factors, and their influence on health and disease are the focus of nutritional genomics. This emerging subdiscipline of clinical nutrition provides the tools for identifying genetic variations that portend increased susceptibility to developing chronic disease and the knowledge for modifying lifestyle choices to promote health rather than disease.

Considerable research is needed to realize the full potential of nutrition to prevent disease and promote health, from building a deep foundation of scientific knowledge to developing new technologies and tools, to applying targeted interventions in the clinic. Nutritional genomics is an important assessment tool that provides the ability to (1) identify the genetic signature of each individual, (2) assess the health and disease susceptibilities of that individual, and (3) project, for each modifiable lifestyle factor that influences health, which choices are most likely to promote health and prevent disease throughout the lifespan.

THE HUMAN GENOME PROJECT AND THE "OMIC" DISCIPLINES

Nutritional genomics has been an active research area within the genetics community for decades. However, this discipline has come to the forefront only recently as a result of the success of the Human Genome Project and the resultant widespread understanding that genetic makeup directly relates to state of health and disease. Fifty years after the elucidation of the structure of DNA, the genetic material, and its clues as to how information is encoded and translated into proteins, the Human Genome Project identified the sequence of nucleotide building blocks in the DNA and projected an estimate of approximately 19,000 genes, the sequences of nucleotides that encode each protein's structural information.

The "Omics"

The Human Genome Project was completed in 2003 but was just the beginning of the move to integrate genetic principles into health care. From this multinational effort has come numerous new disciplines (often called the "omics"), technologies, and tools applicable to health care. The sum of an organism's genetic material is its genome. Within the genome are the individual genes, stretches of DNA that contain the information for synthesizing a protein and the regulatory sequences that control expression of this information and thus the synthesis of these proteins.

Genomics is the study of genomes, their composition, organization, and function. Interest in the human genome and how this knowledge can improve health care is paramount at this time, but the genomes of numerous animals and plants also are being sequenced. This work has provided the opportunity to compare the size, nucleotide sequence, and organizational complexity of the human genome with other organisms, from bacteria to plants to mammals. Many aspects of the genome have been conserved across species, which provides useful information as to which regions of the genome are critical to life. Because of this genetic homogeneity, it has been possible to develop a variety of model systems whose genes can be manipulated experimentally and the influence on function determined. In this way model systems, such as the laboratory mouse, whose genome is similar to that of humans, have served as valuable sources of information about human health and disease at the molecular and biochemical levels.

The Human Genome Project has ended, but it has spawned a host of new projects, disciplines, and technologies, which are discussed briefly in this chapter. The Encyclopedia of DNA Elements (ENCODE) is a follow-up to the Human Genome Project. Whereas the Human Genome Project focused on defining genes within the total genome, the ENCODE project's goal is to investigate the nongene sequences, which make up approximately 99% of the human genome. Originally thought to be "junk DNA" because a substantial proportion of this DNA does not code for proteins, these nongene sequences appear to be critical to regulating the expression of genes and their encoded proteins. For additional information see http://ghr.nlm.nih.gov/handbook/genomicresearch/encode.

Among the disciplines spawned by the Human Genome Project are proteomics, metabolomics, microbiomics, and **bioinformatics**. This latter is an important tool for managing the vast amount of data generated by the various "omic" disciplines. **Proteomics** focuses on identifying the protein encoded within each gene in an organism's genome and on determining its function. **Metabolomics** is concerned with identifying metabolites that are produced in all aspects of metabolism, typically as a result of the action of proteins. **Microbiomics** is a relatively new discipline that recognizes the importance of the microbial ecology (the microbiome) of the digestive tract and other body cavities, such as the mouth and vagina. Beneficial and pathogenic microbes colonize these cavities. The contributions of these microbes and their metabolites to human health and disease are currently under investigation.

DNA sequencing analysis is used to identify pathogenic organisms and is replacing rapidly the time-consuming growth assays used in the clinical laboratory to identify which microbial strains are present in a patient's digestive tract, for example, along with the relative concentrations of each strain. In this way antimicrobial therapy can be initiated quickly. For the beneficial microbes, researchers are investigating which strains help to promote human health and how diet and lifestyle choices can support their vitality and successful colonization within the body.

The vast amount of data generated by these disciplines has led to rapid growth in the field of **bioinformatics**, a field that sits at the crossroads of computer science, information science, biology, and medicine. The development of sophisticated computers that can organize, store, and retrieve massive amounts of data has been integral to the rapid advances of the genomics era. Researchers around the world are able to share data and compare various "omic" profiles across a variety of microbes, plants, and animals.

For a more complete explanation of these fields and their nomenclature and associated technologies, see current genetics and molecular biology texts as well as the online resources available through the **National Human Genome Research Institute** (www.genome.gov).

Clinical Applications

These "omic" disciplines that have arisen from the Human Genome Project increasingly are being integrated into clinical applications. The earliest application has been in **pharmacogenomics**, which involves using genomics to analyze the genetic variations in the genes that direct the synthesis of the drug-metabolizing enzymes and using this information to predict a patient's response to a drug. Genetic variability can lead to differing function in these enzymes, which explains why a drug may have the intended effects for one person, be ineffective for another, and be harmful to a third. Examples of drugs for which genetic testing is being incorporated before initiation of therapy include warfarin (the *CYP2C9* and *VKORC1* genes) (Johnson, 2014) and clopidogrel (the *CYP2C19* gene) (Goswami, 2012; Mega, 2009).

Additional clinical applications in current use involve assisting with diagnosis and selection of therapeutic interventions. Knowing the gene associated with a particular disease and the gene's DNA sequence, its protein product, and the function of the protein in promoting health or disease provides the basis for diagnostic assays and effective interventions. Oncologists routinely use genetic profiling for screening and therapy. Tumors that appear pathologically identical can be distinguished by their genetic profiles. This distinction is important for effective therapy because different types of tumors respond to different therapeutic approaches. Oncologists also have been using genomic analysis to monitor therapeutic response and to project which individuals are most likely to experience treatment failure early in the therapy so that they can be switched to another therapy as quickly as possible.

Beyond diagnosis, intervention, and monitoring, genomic analysis can be used to detect dysfunction in those without symptoms. This aspect is particularly important to health promotion because it allows for assessment of genetic susceptibilities and early intervention before disease symptoms become apparent.

Metabolomics, coupled to genomics, is expected to enhance treatment efficacy. Genomic analysis can provide information about an individual's genetic susceptibilities but does not provide insight as to where on the spectrum between illness and wellness the individual currently falls nor the efficacy of the therapeutic intervention being followed. **Metabolomics** is useful in filling in these gaps by measuring which metabolites are present and at what concentrations. This information reflects how functional the gene variant's protein product is, which in turn can be helpful in projecting how well an individual will function in a particular environment. **Epigenomics** enhances genomics further through its focus on the interactions between the genome and the information coming in from the environment. Each of these disciplines is part of the larger picture of increasing focus of nutrition therapy at the molecular and biochemical levels.

For these technologies to be helpful in the clinic, clients must be comfortable with their use. Of particular concern to clients has been whether their information would be used for their benefit and not lead to discrimination in obtaining employment and insurance. These concerns thus far have not been realized. From the beginning of the Human Genome Project attention has been given to addressing the ethical, legal, and social implications of genetic research and technology to protect against just such concerns. The passage of the **Genetic Information Nondiscrimination Act (GINA)** in 2008 is seen as an important milestone in ensuring that Americans will not be discriminated against with respect to employment and health insurance.

Nutritional Genomics

Among the "omic" disciplines of particular importance to nutrition professionals are nutritional genomics and epigenetics. Nutritional genomics is the field itself, and includes nutrigenetics, nutrigenomics, and epigenetics. **Nutritional genomics** focuses on diet- and lifestyle-related disorders that result from the interaction between the genome and environmental factors, such as nutrients and other bioactives in food, toxins and other xenobiotics (new-to-nature molecules), physical activity, sleep, and stress.

Nutritional genomics is conceptually similar to pharmacogenomics in that, like drugs, food requires enzymatic processing into nutrients before absorption and circulation in the body's tissues and cells. Changes in the genes that encode the proteins involved can lead to changes in nutrient availability at the cellular level. This emerging field incorporates the various "omic" disciplines in multiple ways, such as identifying an individual's genetic susceptibilities by virtue of the gene variants in his or her genome (genomics), analyzing the influence of these variants on the expression of the proteins encoded by the gene variants and the functioning of the expressed proteins (proteomics), and detecting the metabolites produced and their concentration (metabolomics).

Nutrigenetics is concerned with how an individual's set of genetic variations affects function. For example, an often-cited illustration of nutrigenetics involves the 5,10-methylenetetrahydrofolate reductase (*MTHFR*) gene. Human beings have two copies of this gene. **Mutations** (changes to the DNA) in this gene can result in a substantial decrease in enzymatic activity, which is responsible for converting dietary folate or folic acid into 5-methyl folate, the active form. Individuals with such a mutation in both copies of the *MTHFR* gene require the active form of folate for optimal health. **Nutrigenomics**, in contrast, is the study of the interaction of genes and environmental factors that result in a change in gene expression. In the *MTHFR* example, mutation in even a single nucleotide within the region of the gene that controls gene expression could result in insufficient reductase enzyme production, which essentially mimics the outcome of having two copies of an altered *MTHFR* gene. This individual also would need the activated form of folate for optimal health. In addition, the frequency of particular genetic variations differs among populations. For example, the frequency of occurrence of the most common *MTHFR* gene variant is low in African Americans, moderate in Caucasians, and relatively high in Hispanics. Clinicians alert to this type of information are particularly diligent about assessing folate status of preconception Hispanic females to forestall complications such as miscarriages and neural tube defects (see Chapter 15).

Epigenetics provides an additional influence on functional outcomes beyond those at the genomic level by controlling whether genes can be expressed, which in turn determines whether nutrigenetic or nutrigenomic influences can occur. The *epi-* prefix is from the Greek meaning "above," in this case meaning "above the genome." By attaching chemical groups to the DNA or its associated proteins, epigenetic processes allow or disallow gene expression in a heritable fashion but without changing the nucleotide sequence of the DNA. Each different cell type, whether a liver, heart, or brain cell, has the complete set of genetic information, yet only a portion of the total genome is expressed once the cell has differentiated. The control of gene expression is the result of the **epigenetic marks** on the genetic material of that cell, the "epigenetic signature" of that cell type. The genome has not changed; the DNA is the same from cell type to cell type. What is different, and what results in the differential gene expression, is the unique set of epigenetic "marks" or "tags" of each cell type (the total of all the epigenetic markings in that cell type is the **epigenome**). In this way cells become specialized and perform roles unique to the needs of a specific type of tissue. A bone cell does not need to produce insulin but the beta-cells of the pancreas do. Epigenetic markings control which regions of a cell's genome are translated into the needed proteins. Further, the timing of gene expression is critical during fetal development and is orchestrated exquisitely.

Epigenetics research is of increasing importance with respect to chronic disease management and prevention, because the composition of the epigenome in various cell types is influenced by our lifelong diet-and-lifestyle choices (i.e., "environmental factors"). Thus the potential exists for these choices to be modified by the individual in ways that will promote health rather than disease. The main emphasis of research to date has centered around epigenetics and cancer, and the role of diet and lifestyle modification (Supic et al, 2013). The main categories of environmental factors in this regard are nutrition, physical activity, sleep and recovery, thoughts and emotions and the stress they induce, and relationships and sense of life purpose. Technically each of the modifiable lifestyle factors has its own subdiscipline of epigenetics that describes how a specific type of environmental factor "talks" to the DNA through chemical modification, such as **nutritional epigenetics**, behavioral epigenetics, and so on. However, in practice epigenetics embraces this whole study of how the environment communicates with an organism's DNA to modulate gene expression and what this interaction portends for one's health status. Ultimately, diet and other lifestyle choices are expected to be geared toward the particular variants of each individual to provide the most appropriate support for that individual's unique genome. (See Waterland, 2014 for an overview of the emerging field of epigenetics.)

Epigenetics is a significant enhancement to our understanding of the role of genes in living organisms. Traditional theory was that genes contain information that, when translated into proteins, determines an organism's functional ability, and that this situation was permanent for life. Instead, genes can be thought of as the organism's hardware; the environmental factors washing over the genes throughout a lifetime supply the software that provides the functional outcomes. That is, it is not just our genes; it is the interaction of our genes with lifestyle choices throughout life that determines function. Identical twins, who have the same DNA nucleotide sequence, provide an excellent descriptive example of the influence of epigenetics. These siblings appear to be identical in looks and function when they are young but, as they age, distinctions gradually begin to emerge in a variety of characteristics, from physical appearance to disease conditions. It is not unusual for one identical twin to develop a disease and for the other twin to remain healthy. Studies of identical twins have been a mainstay of genetic research and will continue to help us understand the physiologic consequences of changes at the molecular level, particularly how environmental factors change gene expression and therefore health outcomes.

GENOTYPE AND NUTRITION ASSESSMENT

The application expected to have the most dramatic effect on clinical nutrition professionals is the ability to associate a unique genotype with that person's susceptibility to particular diseases. This advance is an important enhancement in the nutrition assessment, diagnosis, and intervention phases of the nutrition care process. As understanding of how genotype influences the ability to function within a particular environment and how environmental factors influence gene expression progresses, nutrition protocols will be developed. Specific counseling and nutrient recommendations will be guided increasingly by the client's genetic profile.

Nutrition professionals must be able to translate client genotypes to develop appropriate interventions. If nutrition professionals are going to be prepared for the era of genomic-directed health care, they must develop a foundation in genetics, biochemistry, molecular biology, metabolism, and other fundamental sciences of twenty-first–century nutrition.

GENETIC FUNDAMENTALS

Genetics is the science of inheritance and forms the foundation of the disciplines of genomics, epigenomics, pharmacogenomics, and nutritional genomics. Historically genetic research focused on identifying the mechanisms by which traits were passed from parent to child, such as physical traits or certain rare diseases that appeared within extended families. Genetic diseases were considered to be a separate category of disease that were limited to those rare heritable disorders that resulted either from changes to a single gene that produced a detectable change in function or alterations at the chromosomal level, which affected multiple genes and often had a devastating effect on the functional ability of the individual. Today it is recognized that, directly or indirectly, all disease is connected to the information in the genes and how that information is translated into functional ability. Furthermore, depending on the role of the protein encoded by a gene; where within a gene a change occurs; and the extent of its impact on the ability of the protein to fulfill its role, there is a continuum in terms of the extent of dysfunction that occurs. Whereas particular changes in some genes have a devastating effect on function and that dysfunction is identified readily as a disease, changes in other genes may be silent or have a much less drastic functional impact. Even within the cystic fibrosis transmembrane conductance regulator gene (*CFTR*) associated with the development of cystic fibrosis, more than 1000 different changes (mutations) have been detected in that one gene (http://ghr.nlm.nih.gov/gene/CFTR). Some changes are associated with severe cystic fibrosis and others with much milder disease (see Chapter 34). For additional exploration, the National Coalition for Health Professional Education in Genetics website provides a good overview of characteristics of this gene and the physiologic effects of different mutations within this gene (http://www.nchpeg.org/nutrition/index.php).

Again, what is observed (the **phenotype**) is a continuum of physiologic outcomes reflecting which mutation is involved. This realization has contributed to the shift away from the concept of "genetic disease" being distinct and rare and to an understanding that each different change within a gene's nucleotide structure has the potential to affect physiologic outcomes differently. Some are so devastating that dysfunction (disease) is readily detectable whenever that change is present, whereas others are mild or even silent unless triggered by an environmental factor. The latter is particularly important with respect to chronic disease in which an individual may have the genetic susceptibility but not manifest disease unless exposed to an inappropriate environment. A well-established example is celiac disease, in which a genetic change results in the inability to fully digest to single amino acids a protein common to wheat, barley, and rye. When exposed to these foods, the individual with celiac disease develops an immune reaction to the incompletely digested protein, an inflammatory response within the digestive tract, erosion of the lining of the gut, and resultant disruption of essential digestive and absorptive processes. However, if the environment is changed—in this case eliminating exposure to the offending protein—the pathology characteristic of celiac disease can be avoided, even though the individual still has the genetic potential to react to this type of protein and trigger celiac symptoms.

These examples highlight the value of knowing the client's genetic makeup, the underlying mechanisms involved, and the appropriate nutritional therapy that can prevent disease from occurring and potentially can restore health in those who already have developed disease. For nutrition professionals to maximize the potential of nutrition genomics,

however, it is helpful to have a solid command of genetics and genomics, from the fundamentals to current research into chronic disease and its underlying **gene X environment interaction (GxE)**. This chapter briefly reviews the basic principles of genetics at the molecular and chromosomal levels, modes of inheritance, mechanisms of disease, and then addresses the newer discipline of epigenetics and epigenomics, which is of particular importance to chronic disease, and a summary of how nutritional genomics is being used in various diseases. For a more in-depth exploration of these topics, there are numerous resources for learning foundational genetics and genomics, from current textbooks to online resources, such as the Genetics Home Reference site (http://ghr.nlm.nih.gov/handbook) and the National Human Genome Research Institute (www.genome.gov), as well as various resources from the Online Genetics Education Resources (http://www.genome.gov/10000464). Please see the Useful Websites list at the end of this chapter for additional recommended resources.

Genetic Basics

Genetics as a discipline historically developed from the observation that physical traits could be inherited among generations, first in plants and later in humans and other mammals. In time the inheritance patterns for human traits were explained by the distribution of chromosomes during egg and sperm formation and the reconstitution of the diploid state at fertilization. The later discovery that DNA was the essential chromosomal component responsible for inheritance led to the molecular era in which genes, mutations, proteins, function, and dysfunction came to be understood. Extensive research over the past six decades has revealed many of the details of these processes and their relationship to each other, such as the chemical makeup of the genetic material DNA, how it stores information and how that information is retrieved and translated into proteins that do the work of the cells, and how those proteins contribute to the individual's functional ability.

Deoxyribonucleic acid (DNA) is the genetic material of all living organisms. In higher organisms the DNA is housed within the nucleus of cells. The molecule is a double helix consisting of two strands of **nucleotide** subunits held together by hydrogen bonds. The human genome contains approximately 3 billion nucleotides. Each nucleotide contains the sugar deoxyribose, the mineral phosphorus, and one of four nitrogenous bases: adenine (A), thymine (T), guanine (G), or cytosine (C). The nucleotides are arranged side by side, and this linear arrangement determines the particular information encoded in a stretch of DNA that results in the synthesis of a protein.

The large amount of genetic material in the nucleus is distributed among multiple **chromosomes**, which are a combination of DNA and specific proteins called **histones**. Human beings have 23 pairs of chromosomes, 22 autosomes, and 2 sex chromosomes. One copy of each member of a pair comes from the mother and the other copy from the father. Females have two X chromosomes; males have one X and one Y chromosome. The nucleus of each human cell contains all 46 chromosomes, which are typically in a highly condensed state to fit all the genetic material into the nucleus. Condensation is achieved by the DNA winding around core structures of eight histone proteins. The combination of DNA wrapped around histone structures forms the **nucleosome**.

To be useful to the cells, information in the DNA first must be decoded and translated into proteins, which perform the work of the organism at the cellular level. A sequence of DNA nucleotides that encodes the information for synthesizing a protein is called a **gene**. There are approximately 19,000 genes. Each gene has a location or "address" at a specific site on a particular chromosome. Long stretches of nucleotides often are found between one gene and the next along the chromosome. Such sequences are called **intervening sequences** and compose the majority of the DNA in humans. These sequences do not code for proteins, but they are not "junk DNA." Instead, they perform structural and regulatory functions, such as controlling when, where, and how much of a protein is produced.

To initiate the process of decoding the DNA, the condensed chromosomes housing the genes first must open (decondense) to allow access to the information in the DNA nucleotide sequence. A common mechanism employed is the covalent attachment of acetyl groups to the histone proteins associated with the chromosomes. This action relaxes the DNA and makes it accessible to the transcription (decoding) process. Information decoding involves **transcription** by RNA polymerase into **messenger RNA** (mRNA) and subsequent **translation** of mRNA into the amino acid sequence of the protein according to a universal **genetic code**. The architecture of a gene typically includes a **promoter region**, where the RNA polymerase attaches and a **coding region** (also called a "structural region") that contains the encoded information for the structure of a protein. Within the coding region are sequences of nucleotides (**exons**) that correspond to the order of the amino acids in the gene's protein product. The coding region also contains **introns** (sequences that are interspersed between exons and do not code for amino acids needed for synthesizing proteins).

Upstream from the promoter region is the **regulatory region** that controls the ability of the polymerase to attach to the promoter, thereby influencing whether transcription occurs. Within this region are **response elements**, DNA sequences that serve as binding sites for regulatory proteins such as **transcription factors** and their bound **ligands**. The binding of transcription factors triggers the recruitment of additional proteins to form a protein complex that in turn changes the expression of that gene by changing the conformation of the promoter region, increasing or decreasing the ability of RNA polymerase to attach and transcribe (express) the gene. The array of response elements within the promoter region can be complex, allowing for the binding of multiple transcription factors that in turn fine-tune the control of gene expression. It is through the binding of transcription factors to response elements that environmental factors such as the bioactive components in food essentially "talk" to a gene, conveying information that more or less of its protein product is needed.

Once transcribed, the mRNA must be processed (**posttranscriptional processing**) so that the introns are removed before the protein is synthesized. At this point, each set of three nucleotides in the transcribed and processed exon makes up a **codon**, which in turn specifies a particular amino acid and its position within the protein. Some proteins need further posttranslational processing before they are active, such as occurs with glycoproteins, proenzymes, and prohormones that must be enzymatically processed before becoming active.

The regulation of transcription (i.e., gene expression) is complex. The need to first decondense the chromosomes that contain the genes is one step in the control of gene expression.

A second level of control of gene expression is epigenetic control, which occurs at the level of the DNA. A common control mechanism involves the attachment of methyl groups to the DNA within the regulatory region of a gene. When methyl groups are attached, transcription is impeded and gene expression is silenced. Alternatively, removal of the methyl groups permits gene expression to take place.

In addition to the information in the nucleotide sequence of DNA (the "**DNA code**"), there are two other sources of information: the **epigenetic code** and the environmental factors to which cells are exposed. Epigenetics is nature's "pen-and-pencil set" (Gosden and Feinberg, 2007). Acetyl or methyl groups, covalently attached to histone proteins associated with DNA or to the DNA itself, respectively, affect whether DNA is accessible for decoding. These groups can be added and removed as needed and are influenced by exposure to various environmental factors such as traditional nutrients, phytochemicals, cytokines, toxins, hormones, and drugs. These environmental factors communicate information as to the state of the environment and ultimately influence when and whether particular genes are expressed. The majority of these environmental factors are lifestyle factors and modifiable based on the individual's choices. The science of **nutritional genomics** is concerned particularly with the interactions between dietary factors and DNA, their influence on health outcomes, and how nutrition therapy can be used to optimize health and minimize disease. Figures 5-1 through 5-6 review these fundamental genetic principles.

The proteins coded for by the genes provide the metabolic machinery for the cells, such as enzymes, receptors, transporters, antibodies, hormones, and communicators. Changes within a gene can alter the amino acid sequence of the protein. Such changes are called **mutations**, which historically have been associated with the concept of severely impairing the function of that protein and creating dysfunction within the cells and, ultimately, the organism. A single nucleotide change may be all that is needed to cause a debilitating disease. For example, in those with sickle cell disease, a single nucleotide change causes a

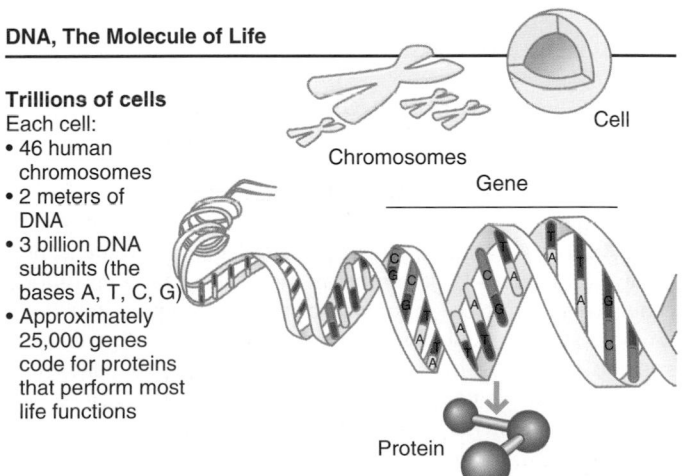

DNA, The Molecule of Life

Trillions of cells
Each cell:
- 46 human chromosomes
- 2 meters of DNA
- 3 billion DNA subunits (the bases A, T, C, G)
- Approximately 25,000 genes code for proteins that perform most life functions

Cell

Chromosomes

Gene

Protein

FIGURE 5-1 Cells are the fundamental working units of every living system. All the instructions needed to direct their activities are contained within the chemical deoxyribonucleic acid. (From U.S. Department of Energy, Human Genome Program: www.ornl.gov/hgmis.)

DNA Replication Prior to Cell Division

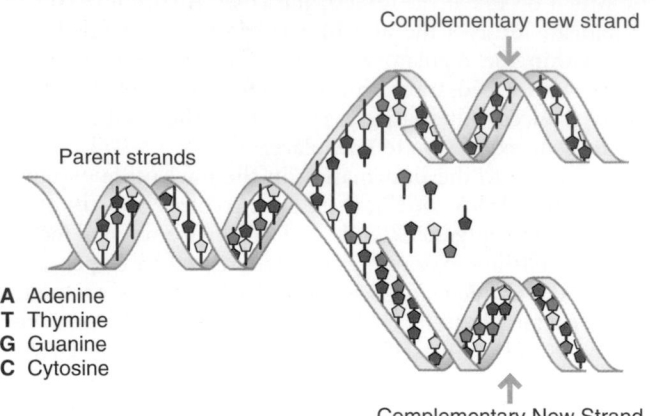

- **A** Adenine
- **T** Thymine
- **G** Guanine
- **C** Cytosine

FIGURE 5-2 Each time a cell divides into two daughter cells, its full genome is duplicated; for humans and other complex organisms, this duplication occurs in the nucleus. During cell division the deoxyribonucleic acid (DNA) molecule unwinds, and the weak bonds between the base pairs break, allowing the strands to separate. Each strand directs the synthesis of a complementary new strand, with free nucleotides matching up with their complementary bases on each of the separated strands. Strict base-pairing rules are adhered to (i.e., adenine pairs only with thymine [an A-T pair] and cytosine with guanine [a C-G pair]). Each daughter cell receives one old and one new DNA strand. The cells' adherence to these base-pairing rules ensures that the new strand is an exact copy of the old one. This minimizes the incidence of errors (mutations) that may greatly affect the resulting organism or its offspring. (From U.S. Department of Energy, Human Genome Program: www.ornl.gov/hgmis.)

DNA Genetic Code Dictates Amino Acid Identity and Order

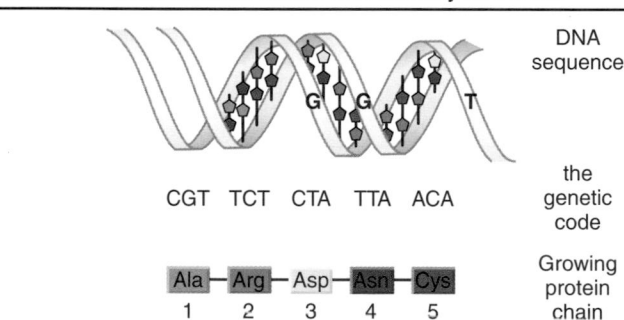

FIGURE 5-3 All living organisms are composed largely of proteins. Proteins are large, complex molecules made up of long chains of subunits called *amino acids.* Twenty different kinds of amino acids are usually found in proteins. Within the gene, each specific sequence of three deoxyribonucleic acid bases (codons) directs the cells protein-synthesizing machinery to add specific amino acids. For example, the base sequence ATG codes for the amino acid methionine. Because three bases code for one amino acid, the protein coded by an average-sized gene (3000 bp) contains 1000 amino acids. The genetic code is thus a series of codons that specify which amino acids are required to make up specific proteins. *A,* adenine; *bp,* base pairs; *C,* cytosine; *G,* guanine; *T,* thymine. (From U.S. Department of Energy, Human Genome Program: www.ornl.gov/hgmis.)

DNA Sequence Variation in a Gene Can Change the Protein Produced by the Genetic Code

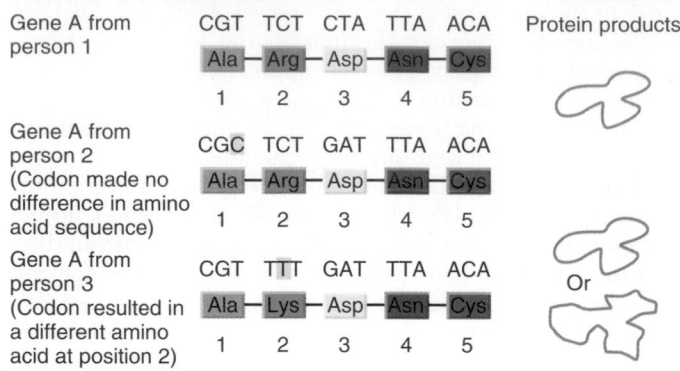

FIGURE 5-4 Some variations in a person's genetic code will have no effect on the protein that is produced; others can lead to disease or an increased susceptibility to a disease. (From U.S. Department of Energy, Human Genome Program: www.ornl.gov/hgmis.)

Health or Disease?

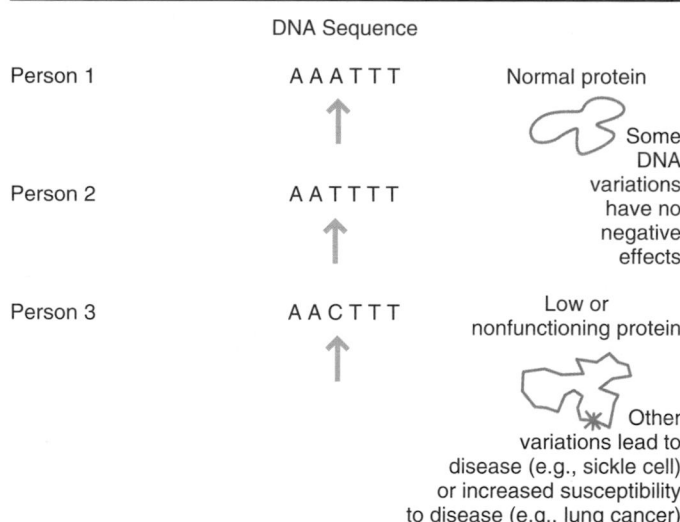

FIGURE 5-5 Human beings differ from each other in only an estimated 0.1% of the total sequence of nucleotides that compose deoxyribonucleic acid. These variations in genetic information are thought to be the basis for the physical and functional differences between individuals. (From U.S. Department of Energy, Human Genome Program: www.ornl.gov/hgmis.)

single amino acid change in the hemoglobin molecule, resulting in severe anemia (see Chapter 32).

Changes in the DNA are the basis for evolution; thus clearly not all mutations are harmful. Some changes actually improve function, and many **silent mutations** have no effect. The effect of the mutation on the functioning of the encoded protein is what determines the outcome, from debilitating disease to no effect at all. All changes to the DNA are technically mutations. However, at this point in the development of genomics and its lexicon, the term **mutation** tends to be applied to those changes that sufficiently influence function such that a measurable outcome results. In contrast, the term **genetic variation** (or **gene**

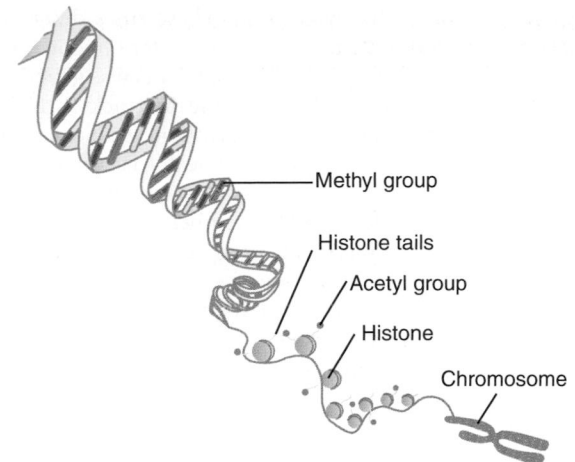

FIGURE 5-6 Epigenetic regulation of gene expression through histone modification and DNA methylation.

variant) is reserved for those mutations with an effect on function that is not strong enough to lead to a disease or other measurable outcome by itself. Nutritional genomics is concerned primarily with those variations that interact with dietary and other environmental factors.

Thus a gene can exist in slightly different forms as a result of a seemingly minor change, such as a substitution of a single nucleotide with another (e.g., guanine can replace cytosine). The term for the different forms of a gene is an **allele** or **polymorphism**. As a result, genes have protein products with differing amino acid sequences (isoforms) and often different functions. Polymorphism (allelism) is an important concept because it explains why human beings, although 99.9% alike genetically, are distinctly different. The 0.1% difference is sufficient to explain the obvious physical variations among humans. It is also the basis for more subtle differences that may not be readily observable, such as in the functional ability of a key metabolic enzyme to catalyze its reaction. Such variations likely underlie many of the inconsistencies observed in therapeutic outcomes and in nutritional intervention research.

The **single nucleotide polymorphism (SNP)** is the structural variant best studied and by far the most common change in DNA. As the name for this genetic variation suggests, the change involves a single nucleotide within DNA. Depending on where in the gene the change occurs and the effect on the encoded protein's function, the nucleotide alteration may result in no change in function, improved change in function, or dysfunction and disease susceptibility. A major ongoing research effort is to identify the SNPs that exist within the human genome and to associate each with their effect on function, particularly with respect to health and disease.

The rate of progress of nutritional genomics in terms of clinical applications is associated strongly with progress in identifying SNPs associated with disease so that diagnostic tests and appropriate diet and lifestyle interventions can be developed and tested for efficacy. The **International HapMap Project** is a multicountry collaboration designed to catalog in the DNA of human beings common patterns of genetic variants that are associated with health and disease. The HapMap Project figures prominently in the efforts to develop a deep scientific foundation upon which to base nutritional genomics-related diagnosis and therapy. "HapMap" is short for haplotype.

A **haplotype** occurs when several SNPs are clustered together in the same region of a chromosome, which typically results in their being inherited as a group. Because the human genome contains approximately 10 million SNPs, studying each one is not practical at this time, but studying haplotypes allows for large-scale studies of SNPs (called **genome-wide association studies**, or **GWAS**) and their association to human disease across multiple populations. Remember that each gene pool (i.e., population) has its own signature set of SNPs, slightly different from any other population. This feature is important to keep in mind in reference to the application of nutrition therapy because what is appropriate for one human population is not necessarily appropriate for all other populations because of the differences in gene pools. For additional information on the HapMap Project, see the Project's website at http://hapmap.ncbi.nlm.nih.gov/abouthapmap.html.

Ongoing analysis of the human genome suggests that, in addition to SNPs, other structural variations also may play an important role in the genotypic and phenotypic variation among humans. Loss or gain of one or more nucleotides (**deletions** and **insertions**, respectively), duplication of nucleotide sequences, **copy number variants**, and restructuring of regions within a chromosome (**inversions** and **translocations**) also have important consequences to function. A chromosome may contain thousands of genes and the order of the nucleotides must remain intact to produce the proteins encoded in each gene's original nucleotide sequence. Whereas a single nucleotide may result in no effect or even an improved effect on function, changes in multiple genes tend to be lethal.

Understanding the prevalence and significance of genetic variation is a primary focus of twenty-first century nutrition, which represents a major departure from nutrition research and therapy to date. Each person is susceptible to a different set of diseases, handles environmental toxins differently, metabolizes molecules somewhat differently, and has slightly unique nutritional requirements. These exciting discoveries are revolutionizing the way clinicians think about the clinical aspects of medicine, pharmacology, and nutrition. Personalized therapy using individualized dietary requirements will become increasingly common in nutrition therapy.

Control of Gene Expression

The control of gene expression occurs at two levels: genomic and epigenomic. Genomic control takes place within the regulatory region of genes, upstream from the promoters. Transcription factors, specialized proteins that have one site for binding DNA and one for binding a small molecular weight ligand, bind to the DNA and regulate whether the RNA polymerase can attach to the promoter and initiate transcription. Factors that influence binding are mutations within the nucleotides that make up the DNA binding site and ligands. Mutations and ligands can promote or inhibit transcription, depending on the gene involved. Among the numerous ligands identified are bioactive food components such as the omega-3 and omega-6 fatty acids, derivatives of vitamin A, vitamin D, and numerous phytonutrients. These molecules bind to transcription factors to form an active complex that directs the conformation of the DNA, which in turn influences the facility with which the RNA polymerase can bind to the promoter and initiate transcription.

From a nutrition therapy perspective, a fruitful research approach has been to investigate whether changing the nature of the ligand can potentially influence transcription and therefore physiologic outcomes. A variety of bioactive components in food (**bioactive food components**) have been tested, particularly for the ability to attenuate inflammation as an important underlying mechanism in the development of cancer (see Chapter 36). The majority of the work to date is either laboratory or animal based. Numerous food bioactives can alter gene expression and interfere with the expression of proinflammatory genes, a central underlying mechanism in cancer and other chronic diseases. In addition to omega-3 and omega-6 fatty acids, vitamin D, and conjugated linoleic acid from dairy products, the phytonutrients curcumin from the spice turmeric, sulforaphane from cruciferous vegetables, resveratrol from purple grapes, genistein from soybeans, quercetin from onion and garlic, (-)-epigallocatechin-3-gallate (EGCG) from green tea, luteolin from celery, broccoli, and numerous other plants have been shown to inhibit proinflammatory transcription factors such as tumor necrosis factor alpha, interleukin-1 beta, interleukin-6, and nuclear factor kappa B, which in turn decreases the expression of proinflammatory genes (Gupta and Prakash, 2014; Ong et al, 2012; see Chapter 3).

Epigenetic control can occur at the level of histone modification or DNA modification and is discussed in the section titled Epigenetic Inheritance. **Epigenetic marks** control the availability of DNA for transcription and translation. Because gene expression changes are critical in normal development and disease progression, epigenetics is widely applicable to many aspects of biological research. The influences of nutrients and bioactive food components on epigenetic phenomena, such as DNA methylation and various types of histone modifications, have been investigated extensively. An individual's epigenetic patterns are established during early pregnancy and are personalized further through the interaction with various environmental factors over his or her lifetime. Epigenetics is, understandably, critically important during development. Alterations of genome-wide DNA methylation have been observed during adulthood, which has led to the hypothesis that epigenetics is also relevant to the aging process as well as the emergence of diseases such as cancer, obesity, diabetes, and cardiovascular disease (Brunet and Berger, 2014; Chaturvedi and Tyagi, 2014; Choi et al, 2013). Of importance to nutrition professionals is the understanding that diet and lifestyle exposure throughout the lifespan are key modifiers of the epigenetic patterns that, in turn, influence long-term health (Jiménez-Chillarón JC et al, 2012; Lillycrop and Burdge, 2012; Milagro et al, 2013).

Modes of Inheritance

Traits are transmitted from one generation to the next in three ways: mendelian inheritance, mitochondrial inheritance, and epigenetic inheritance.

Mendelian Inheritance

Each cell's nucleus contains a complete set of genetic material (**genome**), divided among 22 pairs of chromosomes (called **autosomes**) and 2 **sex chromosomes** for a total of 46 chromosomes. During cell division (**mitosis**) all 46 chromosomes are duplicated and distributed to each new cell. During **meiosis**, one member of each of the autosome and sex chromosome pairs is distributed to each egg or sperm; the full set of 46 chromosomes then is restored to the diploid state upon fertilization.

Because genes are carried on chromosomes, the rules governing the distribution of chromosomes during mitosis and meiosis govern the distribution of genes and any changes

(mutations, variations) they contain. These rules describe the **mendelian inheritance** of a gene, named after Gregor Mendel, who first deduced that the inheritance of traits was governed by a predictable set of rules. It is possible to track a mutation through multiple generations by knowing these rules of inheritance. This transmission is depicted typically as a **pedigree** and can be used to predict the probability of a genetic change being inherited by a particular family member. When the change causes a disease, a pedigree can be helpful in predicting the probability that another family member will inherit the disease. The Family History Initiative, implemented by the U.S. Surgeon General, helps people construct their family pedigree (www.cdc.gov/genomics/famhistory).

Mendelian transmission can be autosomal or **sex linked**, dominant or recessive. There are five classic modes of mendelian inheritance: autosomal dominant, autosomal recessive, X-linked dominant, X-linked recessive, and Y-linked. An individual's **genotype** obeys the laws of inheritance, but the **phenotype** (the observable/measurable expression of the genotype) may not. Each gene in an individual is present in two copies (alleles), one on each chromosome. When the alleles are the same (either both are the common or usual version or both are the mutant or variant form), the individual is said to be **homozygous**. If the alleles are different, the individual is **heterozygous** (also called a *carrier*).

Dominance and recessiveness refer to whether a trait is expressed (can be measured, observed) in a heterozygous individual who has one common allele and one variant allele. If a trait is expressed when only a single copy of a variant allele is present, the allele is said to be **dominant** (i.e., the phenotype of the variant allele is the predominant one). Alleles that do not dominate the genotype when only a single copy is present are called **recessive**. The variant allele is present in the genome, but the trait is not expressed unless two copies of the variant allele are present.

Further confounding the nomenclature is the concept of **penetrance**. Even when a pedigree suggests that a gene is present that should lead to the individual displaying a certain phenotype, the disease may not be evident. Such a gene is said to have reduced penetrance, meaning that not everyone who has the gene expresses it in a measurable form. "Measurable form" very much depends on what is able to be measured. Many alleles thought to be recessive 50 years ago can be detected today as the result of new and more sensitive technologies. Penetrance is of interest to nutrition professionals because it reflects the inability of a genetic variation to impair function and cause disease unless the individual is exposed to specific environmental triggers, such as diet and lifestyle factors. Modifying these factors potentially can improve outcomes for those with such variants. Expect the terminology to continue to be updated as understanding advances.

Mitochondrial Inheritance

In addition to genetic material in the nucleus, the mitochondria in each cell also contain DNA that codes for a limited number of proteins. The majority of these genes are involved in maintenance of the mitochondrion and its energy-producing activities. As with nuclear DNA, changes in **mitochondrial DNA (mtDNA)** can lead to disease. Traits resulting from mitochondrial genes have a characteristic inheritance pattern; they are non-mendelian because mitochondria and their genetic material typically pass from mother to child, called **mitochondrial** or **maternal inheritance**. This biologic principle has become the basis for anthropological studies that trace lineage and population migration patterns through the centuries. It also has provided a way to trace familial diseases caused by changes in mtDNA. However, as with other biologic processes, occasional mistakes occur; reports exist of some mtDNA being passed from father to child.

Epigenetic Inheritance, Genomic Imprinting

Epigenetic inheritance illustrates another mechanism by which genetic information is passed between generations. Epigenetics provides an additional set of instructions beyond that contained in the DNA nucleotide sequence. It affects gene expression but does not change the nucleotide sequence (Villagra et al, 2009). At least three mechanisms are involved: histone modification, DNA modification, and RNA interference (RNAi). Like DNA nucleotide inheritance, the epigenetic "marks" ("tags") also can be passed down through the generations. Just how far the reach extends is not yet known but there is a clear pattern at least from grandparents to children to grandchildren. The importance here to nutrition professionals is that what grandparents ate has the potential to influence the functioning of their grandchildren.

Histones are proteins associated with DNA that assist the chromosome to condense. Units of histone proteins form a scaffolding around which DNA is wrapped, which creates the nucleosome, similar to thread wrapped around a spool. Similar in concept to condensing data on a hard drive, this mechanism helps to fit the large amount of DNA into the small space of the nucleus. When DNA is condensed, it is not available for transcribing into mRNA. The attachment and removal of acetyl groups is an important mechanism for controlling whether DNA is relaxed and available for transcription to proceed or condensed and closed to transcription, respectively.

Similarly, DNA itself can be modified by the covalent attachment and removal of functional groups, such as methyl groups. In somatic (body) cells, **DNA methylation** takes place at cytosine residues that occur within CpG islands found near a gene's promoter region. **CpG islands** (the *p* refers to the phosphodiester bond between [C]cytosine and [G] guanine nucleotides) are DNA sequences enriched in cytosine and guanine that, when methylated, interfere with transcription and therefore gene expression. In general, methylation silences gene expression and demethylation promotes gene expression.

DNA methylation and histone modification can contribute to genomic imprinting and affect gene expression. **Genomic imprinting** is an unusual phenomenon in which only one of the two alleles (version) of a gene is expressed, either the allele contributed by the mother or by the father. If each allele contains a different mutation that leads to a measurable phenotype, the individual's phenotype differs depending on whether the mother's or the father's allele is the one expressed. Prader-Willi syndrome and Angelman syndrome involve DNA on chromosome 15 and provide examples of genomic imprinting. When the father's allele is expressed, the child develops Prader-Willi syndrome. When the mother's allele is expressed, the child develops Angelman syndrome. Both syndromes are characterized by intellectual disabilities, but individuals with Prader-Willi also experience a lack of perception of satiety, which leads to overeating and morbid obesity. The suspected underlying basis for the phenotypic differences is the different pattern of epigenetic markings (either histone acetylation or DNA methylation)

between the two parents rather than differences in the DNA sequence itself. Genomic imprinting represents epigenetic erasure and reestablishment of the epigenetic marks in the germline and has important implications for health and disease, with documented metabolic, neurologic, and behavioral effects (Adalsteinsson and Ferguson-Smith, 2014; Giradot et al, 2012; Peters, 2014).

The third mechanism, **RNA interference (RNAi)**, is the subject of considerable research. Two types of small (21 to 23 nucleotides) RNA molecules, **microRNAs** (miRNA) and **small interfering RNAs** (siRNA), are transcribed from noncoding DNA that formerly was thought to be "junk DNA." If the RNA is complementary to the DNA of a gene's promoter region, increased transcription can occur, but more commonly these RNAs attach to the transcribed messenger RNA and interfere with gene expression by preventing translation of the gene into its encoded protein. Alternatively, attaching to DNA leads to silencing of whole regions of chromosomes, a phenomenon called **epigenetic gene silencing**, which is the basis for X-inactivation in mammalian females in which one of the two X chromosomes is silenced. In this way the amount of information contributed by the X chromosome is equalized between females and males, the latter having only a single X chromosome. The details of these processes are beyond the scope of this chapter, but readers should be aware that diet and other environmental factors are suspected of being primary influencers of epigenetic mechanisms. Therefore expect that in time, understanding epigenetic mechanisms will be essential for the development of effective nutrition therapy in the clinic.

In a landmark study using the mouse as a mammalian model system for dissecting this complex process, Waterland and Jirtle (2003) selected a strain of mice with a mutation in the *agouti* gene. The wild-type (usual, "normal") *agouti* allele causes the mouse's coat color to be brown. The A^{vy} mutation (*agouti viable yellow* allele) causes the coat color to be yellow and, because this allele is dominant, all mice with at least one copy of A^{vy} have the potential to develop the yellow coat color. The researchers bred genetically identical female mice with brown coats (two copies of the usual *agouti* allele) with genetically identical males that had two copies of the A^{vy} mutation and had yellow coats. On a standard mouse chow diet, the coat color of the mothers would be brown, that of the fathers would be yellow, and the coat color of the offspring, who have one *agouti* allele and one A^{vy} allele, would be yellow because the A^{vy} allele is dominant. Waterland and Jirtle asked whether diet could make a difference in coat color by feeding half of the females the usual mouse chow diet and half a methyl-rich diet in which methyl donors such as folate, vitamin B$_{12}$, choline, and betaine were added to the chow. Most of the unsupplemented mothers had offspring with yellow coats. Most of the offspring from the mothers on the methyl-rich diet, however, had a mottled coat with a mix of brown and yellow (called *pseudoagouti*). Remember that ALL the offspring had one copy of the normal allele and one copy of the A^{vy} allele. Clearly, the mother's diet affected the coat color of the offspring and this effect persisted into adulthood. An investigation into what may be causing the difference in phenotype among genotypically identical siblings detected a correlation between mottled coat and degree of methylation of the *agouti* gene, which suggested that the methyl-rich diet led to epigenetic silencing of the A^{vy} allele.

Furthermore, this effect of diet could be inherited. In subsequent experiments (Cropley et al, 2006) found that feeding the females of the "grandmother" generation a methyl-rich diet but not enriching the daughter offspring's diet with methyl donors still produced a number of second generation ("grandchildren") offspring with mottled brown coats, suggesting that the effect the diet had on coat color could be transmitted between generations. Diet and possibly other environmental factors may have a transgenerational effect through their influence on epigenetic markings that affect gene expression without altering the DNA sequence (Jiménez-Chillarón et al, 2012). To transpose the significance of these results to humans, this type of gene-diet epigenetic mechanism could explain why identical twins, although having the exact same genotype, typically do not have identical phenotypes and that the extent of the differences appear to increase as the twins age. This observation in human identical twins has baffled researchers for a long time and now is believed to be due to epigenetics and the influence of diet and other environmental factors. In a series of studies focused on overfeeding-induced phenotypes, studies with rodents suggest that epigenetic inheritance can be sustained for at least two to three generations. In male rats, overfeeding led to impaired glucose and insulin metabolism and altered gene expression in the female offspring over the next two generations (Ng et al, 2014). In mice, feeding males a high-fat diet and then mating them to females fed the usual diet was correlated with heritable impairment of insulin secretion and blood glucose disposition in the daughters as a result of changes in pancreatic beta-cell gene expression (Pentinat et al, 2010). In female mice fed a high-fat diet, the effect was detected into the third generation and was passed from the male line, which suggests that genomic imprinting is involved (Dunn and Bale, 2009; Dunn and Bale, 2011).

A retrospective cohort study in humans also supports the possibility of transgenerational epigenetic inheritance. The Dutch Hunger Winter Families Study investigated the offspring of mothers who were pregnant during the Dutch Hunger Winter famine that followed World War II (Bygren, 2013). Female but not male offspring of these mothers had dyslipidemia compared with unexposed same-sex females from mothers not exposed to the famine. The children subsequently born to these females with dyslipidemia had greater neonatal adiposity and a higher prevalence of metabolic disease compared with controls born to unaffected females. Other environmental factors beyond nutrition also have been shown to be associated with heritable epigenetic markings. These studies, however, have been conducted in animal models and have yet to be substantiated for humans. The molecular mechanisms underlying transgenerational epigenetic inheritance are not yet known but may include mechanisms beyond DNA methylation and histone modification. Heard and Martienssen (2014) provide a current understanding of transgenerational epigenetic inheritance.

Inheritance and Disease

Changes to the genetic material, whether to the chromosomal DNA, mtDNA, or even a single nucleotide, have the potential to alter one or more proteins that may be critical to the operation of the cells, tissues, and organs of the body. There are important consequences from changes to the genetic material at each of these levels.

Disease at the Chromosomal Level

Change in the number of chromosomes, or the arrangement of the DNA within a chromosome, is almost always detrimental and often fatal to the individual. Chromosomal disorders are detected by means of a karyotype, a visualization of all the chromosomes in picture form. An example of a nonfatal chromosomal abnormality is trisomy 21 (Down syndrome), which results from an addition of genetic material to chromosome 21.

Some syndromes are caused by the loss of a portion of a chromosome (a partial deletion). In Beckwith-Wiedemann syndrome (a chromosome 11 deletion), changes are characterized by organ overgrowth, including an oversized tongue, which leads to feeding difficulties and hypoglycemia. Nutrition professionals play an important role in the therapy of those with chromosomal disorders, because these individuals often have oral-motor problems that affect their nutritional status and cause growth problems in early life. Later in development, obesity may become an issue, and nutrition therapy is helpful in controlling weight, diabetes, and cardiovascular complications. In people with such chromosomal abnormalities, varying degrees of mental retardation often complicate therapy. A knowledgeable nutrition professional can mitigate the detrimental effects of these disorders on nutritional status (see Chapter 43).

Disease at the Mitochondrial Level

Mitochondria are subcellular organelles that are thought to have originated from bacteria and function primarily to produce adenosine triphosphate (ATP). Human mtDNA codes for 13 proteins, 2 ribosomal RNAs, and 22 transfer RNAs to synthesize these proteins; the remainder of the proteins are coded for by nuclear DNA. In contrast to nuclear DNA, mtDNA is small (16,569 base pairs), circular, and exists in hundreds to thousands of copies in each mitochondrion. As noted earlier, mtDNA typically is passed from the mother to her offspring.

Not surprisingly, alterations in mtDNA are frequently degenerative and affect tissues primarily with a high demand for oxidative phosphorylation. They also have varied clinical manifestations because of the multiple copies of mtDNA, not all of which may contain the genetic change. Mutations in mtDNA can manifest at any age and include neurologic diseases, cardiomyopathies, and skeletal myopathies. For example, Wolfram syndrome, a form of diabetes with associated deafness, was one of the earliest disorders to be traced to mtDNA. More than 60 diseases that result from changes in mtDNA have been identified thus far. See MITOMAP, a human mitochondrial genome database, for specifics on human mitochondrial DNA variants (www.mitomap.org).

Disease at the Molecular Level

The majority of disease conditions associated with nutritional genomics involve changes at the molecular level. Changes to the DNA typically involve a single nucleotide change or several nucleotides within a single gene through substitutions, additions, or deletions. Further, larger-scale changes involving the deletion or addition of multiple nucleotides also can occur in the regulatory or protein coding regions of a gene. Alterations in the regulatory region may increase or decrease the quantity of protein produced or alter the ability of the gene to respond to environmental signals. Alterations in the coding region may affect the amino acid sequence of the protein, which in turn can affect the conformation and function of the protein and thereby the functioning of the organism. Because the majority of human genes reside on nuclear chromosomes, gene variations are transmitted according to mendelian inheritance and are subject to modification from epigenetic markings.

Autosomal dominant single-gene disorders that have nutritional implications include several that may result in oral-motor problems, growth problems, susceptibility to weight gain, and difficulties with constipation. Examples include Albright hereditary osteodystrophy, which commonly results in dental problems, obesity, hypocalcemia, and hyperphosphatemia; chondrodysplasias, which often result in oral-motor problems and obesity; and Marfan syndrome, which involves cardiac disease, excessive growth, and increased nutritional needs. Familial hypercholesterolemia results in a defective low-density lipoprotein (LDL) receptor, elevated levels of cholesterol, and susceptibility to atherosclerosis.

Autosomal recessive disorders are much more common and include metabolic disorders of amino acid, carbohydrate, and lipid metabolism. Traditionally these disorders were detected because the mutation had a detrimental effect on the newborn infant that led to serious developmental consequences or death. These disorders were heritable, ultimately associated with a particular mutation, and designated **inborn errors of metabolism (IEM)**.

IEM disorders are the earliest known examples of nutritional genomics, and dietary modification is the primary treatment modality (see Chapter 43). A brief overview of IEM from a genetic perspective is included here to emphasize the important role of the nutrition professional in restoring health to these individuals and to contrast IEM with chronic disorders, which result from the same type of genetic change but affect function less severely.

Currently the United States has no uniform guidelines for newborn screening; some states test for a handful of conditions and other states test for 30 or more conditions. With the belief that the early detection of IEM allows earlier initiation of therapy, which results in better health prospects of the child, and at the request of the Health Services and Research Administration (HRSA), in 2011 the American College of Medical Genetics submitted a proposed set of uniform guidelines for consideration.

A classic example of an IEM of amino acid metabolism is phenylketonuria (PKU). PKU results from a mutation in the gene coding for the enzyme phenylalanine hydroxylase, leading to an inability to convert phenylalanine to tyrosine. Lifelong dietary restriction of phenylalanine enables individuals with PKU to live into adulthood and enjoy a quality life (see Chapter 43). In maple syrup urine disease (MSUD), the metabolic defect is branched-chain alpha-keto acid decarboxylase, an enzyme complex encoded by six genes. A mutation in any one of these genes can result in accumulation of alpha-keto acids in the urine, which produces an odor somewhat similar to maple syrup. Failure to limit branched-chain amino acid intake can lead to mental retardation, seizures, and death in individuals with MSUD (see Chapter 43).

Hereditary fructose intolerance (HFI) is an example of an autosomal recessive IEM of carbohydrate metabolism (see Table 43-1). A mutation in the *ALDOB* gene encoding aldolase B (fructose-1,6-biphosphate aldolase) impairs the catalytic activity of the enzyme and prevents fructose from being converted to glucose. Breast-fed infants are typically asymptomatic until fruit is added to the diet. Nutrition therapy involves the elimination of fructose and the fructose-containing disaccharide sucrose as well as sorbitol. In the absence of understanding the presence of this genetic lesion and the need to eliminate these sweeteners from the diet, the individual typically proceeds to develop hypoglycemia, vomiting, and ultimately kidney failure, leading to death.

This disease is a good example of the power of understanding the underlying genetic lesion when developing nutrition therapeutic approaches (see Chapter 43). First, the family history may give a hint that HFI is present. Second, although the genetic lesion (genotype) is permanent, the phenotype is not. In spite of an individual having the ALDOB mutation, eliminating the exposure to these sweeteners essentially keeps the disease susceptibility silent, and the infant will enjoy normal development. Often it is the nutrition professional that detects the problem and recommends the appropriate therapy sufficiently early to prevent disease symptoms from manifesting.

An example of an autosomal recessive disorder of lipid metabolism is the deficiency of medium-chain acyl-coenzyme A (acyl-CoA) dehydrogenase, which prevents medium-chain fatty acids from being oxidized to provide energy during periods of fasting. Nutrition therapy focuses on preventing the accumulation of toxic fatty acid intermediates that, when not controlled, can lead to death (see Chapter 43).

The **X-linked dominant** fragile X syndrome also affects nutritional status. Fragile X syndrome is characterized by developmental delays, mental impairment, and behavioral problems. The lesion occurs within the *FMR1* gene on the X chromosome in which a CGG segment is repeated more times than the usual number for human beings. The multiple repeats of this trinucleotide make the X chromosome susceptible to breakage. Another X-linked dominant disorder is a form of hypophosphatemic rickets. This disorder is found in males and females, is resistant to vitamin D therapy, and is characterized by bone anomalies, which include dental malformations and resultant feeding challenges.

X-linked recessive conditions include nephrogenic diabetes insipidus, adrenoleukodystrophy, and Duchenne muscular dystrophy (DMD) disorders. Individuals with X-linked recessive nephrogenic diabetes insipidus are unable to concentrate urine and exhibit polyuria and polydipsia. This disorder usually is detected in infancy and can manifest as dehydration, poor feeding, vomiting, and failure to thrive. X-linked recessive adrenoleukodystrophy results from a defect in the enzyme that degrades long-chain fatty acids. These fats accumulate and lead to brain and adrenal dysfunction and ultimately motor dysfunction. X-linked recessive DMD is characterized by fatty infiltration of muscles and extreme muscle wasting. Children typically are confined to a wheelchair by the time they reach their teens and need assistance with feeding.

Y-linked inheritance disorders involve male sex determination and physiologic "housekeeping functions." No nutrition-related disorders have been assigned conclusively to the Y chromosome.

In summary, any gene potentially can undergo mutation, which can affect the function of its protein and the health of the individual. Its location within the nuclear or mtDNA determines its mode of inheritance.

Genetic Technologies

Progressing beyond knowing the chromosomal location of a disease trait to associating the disease with a particular mutation and understanding its functional consequences has required the development of sophisticated molecular genetic technologies. One of the most critical technologic advances occurred in the early 1970s with the introduction of **recombinant DNA** technology, which allowed major progress in terms of studying genes, their functions, and the regulation of their expression. Using bacteria-derived restriction endonucleases (restriction enzymes), researchers could cut the DNA in precise, reproducible locations along the nucleotide chain, isolate the fragments and, using polymerase chain reaction (PCR) technology, make unlimited copies of the DNA for various applications. This basic approach has been the cornerstone of many routine techniques, such as genetic engineering and the production of therapeutic proteins such as insulin and growth hormone as well as new genetic strains of crops and food for animal consumption. See Focus On: *GMO or Genetically Engineered (GE) Foods* in chapter 26.

Recombinant DNA technology is the basis for detecting variations in DNA sequences that can be used to identify individuals for forensic and paternity purposes and to predict disease susceptibilities. This technology also paved the way for DNA sequencing, which is used to identify the sequence of nucleotides within a gene, pinpoint the exact location of any change, and identify each of the nucleotides in an individual's genome. DNA sequencing technology has evolved rapidly, from a labor- and time-intensive process to one of high-throughput sequencing techniques that have lowered significantly the cost of sequencing whole genomes. The benefit for health care is the expectation that it will soon be inexpensive to sequence the human genome to detect large numbers of genetic susceptibilities in one analysis, which can provide individuals with their genetic signature.

One of the outgrowths of these earlier technologies is DNA microarray technology. Microarrays, also called DNA "chips," are used to determine which genes are expressed at a particular time under particular conditions, such as during the different stages of fetal development. They also can be used to determine which genes are turned on in response to environmental factors, such as nutrients. A useful clinical application is the comparison of gene expression between normal and diseased cells, with important implications for cancer therapeutics.

Another type of genetic technology involves interfering with a gene's expression to determine the function of that gene and its encoded protein. The concept originally was exploited in model systems involving transgenic animals, particularly the laboratory mouse ("knockout mouse"). In the knockout mouse, a gene is altered ("knocked out") so that the normal protein is no longer made. Alternatively, a gene can be altered so that it expresses too much or too little of its product. Regulatory sequences can be altered so that a gene no longer responds appropriately to environmental signals. In these ways the normal function of a gene can be determined, the effects of overexpressing or underexpressing a gene can be studied, and details of the communication process between signals outside the organism and the genetic material inside the organism can be determined. Transgenic mice are particularly valuable for studying gene-diet interactions. A recent application of this concept involves RNAi. Short sequences of RNA bind to mRNA and interfere with translation of the mRNA into protein ("knock down"). By measuring the outcome of a decrease in a particular protein, researchers can gain insight into the role of the protein and its contribution to the organism's function.

The combination of the data available from the Human Genome Project and the HapMap Project coupled with the new technologies that have been developed as a result of these projects made it possible to conduct GWAS. Such studies allow more rapid analysis of whole-genome sequences for the presence of genetic variations and their association with various traits and disease states. Two groups of subjects are studied, those with the disease of interest and those without. A set of SNPs is analyzed in both groups and if certain ones are found more frequently in those with the disease, these SNPs are proposed to be associated with the disease, which helps to pinpoint the region of the human genome where the culprit genes are located.

The SNPs themselves may be a causative factor or they simply may be located near the causal variants. Typically researchers sequence the regions where the associated SNPs are located to identify the specific genetic changes associated with the disease. Until a genetic region detected in a GWAS study has been mapped to a definitive locus (location on a chromosome) and the gene identified, its location is referred to as a Quantitative Trait Locus (QTL). One of the more notable nutrition-related GWAS successes has been the detection of the *FTO* (fat mass and obesity–associated) gene, which is the most common gene variant to be associated definitively with obesity and across multiple populations (Frayling et al, 2007; Harbron et al, 2014).

The final key technology that has become essential is DNA methylation profiling to detect the epigenetic state of the individual, often referred to as the methylome. Various techniques are currently in use. The methyl group is attached covalently to the cytosine residues of CpG islands, which makes it possible to distinguish between methylated and unmethylated cytosines. The total methylation load can be determined and compared between samples, or specific regions of the genome can be analyzed and compared.

GENETICS AND NUTRITION THERAPY

Chromosomal or single-gene mutations can alter nutritional status and are helpful in illustrating the importance of nutrition therapy for health. The rapid development of molecular nutrition and nutritional genomics expands the role of the nutrition professional beyond rare disorders and into more prevalent chronic diseases such as cardiovascular disease (CVD), cancer, diabetes, inflammatory disorders, osteoporosis, and obesity. Typically these disorders are managed at best, yet diet-and-lifestyle therapy potentially can restore the individual's health.

Nutritional genomics is unique in its focus on how the interactions between genetic variations and environmental factors influence the genetic potential of individuals and populations, the GxE premise. Nutrition professionals play a critical role in this transition to health promotion and disease prevention.

Nutrigenetic Influences on Health and Disease

The interplay between nutrition and genetics varies from being straightforward to being highly complex. The most straightforward is the direct correlation between a faulty gene, a defective protein, a deficient level of a metabolite, and a resultant disease state passed on through mendelian inheritance and is responsive to nutrition therapy. The IEM already discussed are good examples of such interactions. IEM are characterized as rare mutations that result in protein dysfunction, which leads to metabolic disorders. In actuality they are on the far end of the personal health continuum, on the dysfunction/illness end of this spectrum. Far more common are the mutations that occur frequently, have less severe consequences on function, and thus fall on the function/wellness end. The effect of these mutations is far more subtle, which makes detection more challenging for the health care professional, yet no less important if the individual is to make appropriate lifelong choices in terms of the environmental factors that promote health and prevent disease.

All humans have mutations that result in protein dysfunction that leads to metabolic disease. The human species requires certain amino acids, fatty acids, vitamins, and minerals, and mutations limit the ability to synthesize these important nutrients. The diet must supply them to prevent dysfunction and disease. For example, humans lack the gene for the enzyme gulonolactone oxidase and cannot synthesize vitamin C. If dietary vitamin C intake is below needed levels, individuals are at risk for developing scurvy, which can be fatal.

New is the understanding of the genetic basis for nutrient requirements, the realization that nutrition therapy can circumvent genetic limitations by supplying the missing nutrients, and that each individual may require a different level of nutrient because of his or her particular set of genetic variations. In a seminal paper in 2002, Ames and colleagues called attention to this fact by detailing more than 50 metabolic reactions that involve enzymes with decreased affinities for their cofactors and that require high levels of a nutrient to restore function (Ames et al, 2002). Many of the supplementation levels are well in excess of the usual recommended nutrient levels, which highlights the importance of remembering that each individual is genetically unique and has distinct metabolic needs.

Although generalized guidelines for recommended nutrient levels are helpful, individuals may have genetic variations that require them to consume significantly more or less of certain nutrients than the general recommendation. Nutritional genomics has changed the thinking about global dietary recommended intakes, from an age- and sex-related orientation to incorporating nutrigenetic makeup and its influence on protein function. Nutrition assessment, then, is a critical tool for compensating for changes in the DNA that can lead to increased risk of disease (see Chapter 7).

The inborn error of amino acid metabolism classic homocystinuria is of particular interest because it led to the realization that an elevated blood level of homocysteine may be an independent risk factor for CVD. A defect in the vitamin B_6–requiring enzyme cystathionine beta-synthase prevents the conversion of homocysteine to cystathionine. Homocysteine accumulates, appears to promote atherogenesis, and forms the dipeptide homocystine, which leads to abnormal collagen crosslinking and osteoporosis. Nutrition therapy is multipronged, depending on the specific genetic defect. Some individuals have an enzyme defect that requires a high concentration of the vitamin B_6 cofactor for activity. Others are not responsive to B_6 and need a combination of folate, vitamin B_{12}, choline, and betaine to convert homocysteine to methionine. Others must limit their methionine intake. At least three forms of homocystinuria exist, each requiring a different nutritional approach. The ability to use genetic analysis to distinguish these similar disorders has been a useful technological advance (see Chapters 7, 32, and 33).

The consequences of genetic variation in the *MTHFR* gene were discussed earlier and provide an excellent example of nutrigenetics as well as how genetic variation can influence nutrient requirements. Specific variants of this gene can influence the body's ability to supply the active form of the B vitamin folate. Enzymatic impairment also results in insufficient conversion of homocysteine to *S*-adenosylmethionine, a critical methyl donor to numerous metabolic reactions, including

those involved in synthesizing and repairing nucleic acids (see Chapters 32 and 33). A common variation in the *MTHFR* gene is the 677C>T gene variant, which involves substitution of thymine (T) for cytosine (C) at nucleotide position 677 within the coding region of the *MTHFR* gene. The resultant enzyme has reduced activity, which leads to decreased production of active folate and accumulation of homocysteine. Elevated homocysteine levels often can be lowered through supplementation with one or more of the B vitamins, folate, B_2, B_6, and B_{12}, and key mineral cofactors. However, the genotype of the individual is an important factor in exactly which concentration of nutrients at which level is needed to elicit this response, which supports the need for tailoring nutrient recommendations.

In addition to the increased risk of CVD, elevated serum homocysteine increases the risk of neural tube defects in developing fetuses. As a result of these risks, in the United States cereal grains now are fortified with folic acid to ensure adequate levels in women of childbearing age (see Chapter 15). This public policy response brings to our attention the importance of having nutrition professionals knowledgeable about nutritional genomics in positions of influence at the policy-making level. If folate/folic acid is the primary supplier of methyl groups for epigenetic regulation of gene expression via DNA methylation, and excessive methylation of DNA leads to the silencing of gene expression, how do we determine a safe level sufficient to ensure folate levels are high enough to prevent neural tube defects, but low enough not to silence inappropriately genes that are critical to development, the effects of which may not show up until adulthood?

Disease-causing changes also can occur in genes coding for other types of proteins, such as transport proteins, structural proteins, membrane receptors, hormones, and transcription factors. Mutations that increase the transport of iron (hereditary hemochromatosis) or copper (Wilson's disease) to higher-than-normal levels have nutritional implications (see Chapter 32). Mutations in vitamin D receptors are associated with deleterious effects on bone health and throughout the body, because vitamin D is a hormone involved in hundreds of metabolic and regulatory processes. Changes in the gene coding for insulin can result in structural changes in the insulin hormone and lead to dysglycemia, as can mutations in the insulin receptor. Many proteins such as kinases, cytokines, and transcription factors that are involved in critical signaling cascades are subject to mutational changes, altered activities, and health consequences.

Nutrigenomic Influences on Health and Disease

In addition to compensating for metabolic limitations, nutrients and other bioactive components in food can influence gene expression, as seen in studies with lower organisms, such as is seen with the *lac* and *trp* operons of bacteria. In these situations the organism "senses" the presence of a nutrient in its external environment and alters its gene expression accordingly. In the case of lactose, the proteins required to use lactose as an energy source are induced by transcriptional regulation of the genes that code for the lactose transport system and for the enzyme that cleaves lactose into its monosaccharides. The opposite occurs when tryptophan is present in the environment: the organism inhibits the endogenous biosynthesis of tryptophan by inhibiting transcription of the genes that encode tryptophan biosynthetic proteins. Gene X environment interactions, such as monitoring and responding to environmental signals by changing gene expression, are fundamental processes of living systems, allowing them to use resources efficiently.

Higher organisms such as humans have similar mechanisms by which they monitor the environment that bathes their cells and alter cellular or molecular activities as needed. An example is the response of cells to the presence of glucose. Insulin is secreted and binds to its receptor on the surface of skeletal muscle cells and initiates a stepwise biochemical signaling cascade (**signal transduction**). Signaling results in the translocation of glucose transporter type 4 (GLUT4), a receptor involved in glucose entry into cells, from the interior of the cell to the cell surface. Exercise also promotes the translocation of GLUT4, which helps in controlling blood sugar levels. A drop in blood sugar triggers the release of epinephrine and glucagon that, in turn, bind to cell surface receptors in the liver and skeletal muscle and, through signal transduction, stimulate glycogen breakdown to glucose to restore blood sugar levels.

Nutrients and other bioactive food components also can serve as ligands, molecules that bind to specific nucleotide sequences (response elements) within a gene's regulatory region. Binding results in a change in gene expression through the regulation of transcription. Examples of such food components are the polyunsaturated omega-3 fatty acids. These fats decrease inflammation by serving as precursors for the synthesis of anti-inflammatory eicosanoids and by decreasing the expression of genes that lead to the production of inflammatory cytokines, such as the tumor necrosis factor–alpha and the interleukin-1 genes (Calder, 2015; see Chapter 3).

The omega-3 and omega-6 fatty acids also have been found to serve as ligands for the **peroxisome proliferator-activated receptor (PPAR)** family of transcription factors. The PPARs function as lipid sensors and regulate lipid and lipoprotein metabolism, glucose homeostasis, adipocyte proliferation and differentiation, and the formation of foam cells from monocytes during atherogenic plaque formation. They are important components in the sequence of events by which a high-fat diet promotes insulin resistance and obesity (Christodoulides and Vidal-Puig, 2010).

To influence the expression of the genes under its control, a PPAR transcription factor must complex with a second transcription factor, the retinoic X receptor (RXR). Each has its ligand attached—polyunsaturated fatty acid and a derivative of vitamin A—respectively. The PPAR-RXR complex then can bind to the appropriate response element within the regulatory region of a gene under its control. Binding results in a conformational change in the structure of the DNA molecule that allows RNA polymerase to bind and transcribe the PPAR-regulated genes, leading to a host of lipogenic and pro-inflammatory activities. A large number of transcription factors have been identified and the mechanisms of action are under investigation.

The bioactive components that serve as ligands for these transcription factors are either provided by the diet or made endogenously. Examples are omega-3 and omega-6 fatty acids, cholesterol, steroid hormones, bile acids, **xenobiotics** (foreign chemicals, or "new-to-nature" molecules), the active form of vitamin D, and numerous phytonutrients, to name just a few. In all cases these bioactives must communicate their presence to the DNA sequestered within the nucleus. Depending on their size and lipid solubility, some bioactives can penetrate the various membrane barriers and interact directly with the DNA, as in the fatty acid example discussed previously. Others,

including phytochemicals found in the cruciferous vegetables, may not be able to cross the cell membrane and instead interact with a receptor on the cell surface and set into motion the cascade of signal transduction events that results in a transcription factor being translocated to the nucleus.

Identification of the genetic and biochemical mechanisms underlying health and disease provides the basis for developing individualized intervention and prevention strategies. In the case of the omega-3 fatty acids, researchers are actively seeking conditions under which dietary omega-3s can be used to decrease inflammation and increase insulin sensitivity. An understanding of the mechanisms by which gene expression is controlled is also helpful in developing drugs that can target various aspects, including gene expression. For example, the thiazolidinedione class of antidiabetes drugs targets the PPAR mechanism described previously to improve insulin sensitivity.

Identifying bioactive components in fruits, vegetables, and whole grains that are responsible for positive health effects and the mechanisms by which they influence gene expression is of considerable interest. Small-molecular-weight lipophilic molecules can penetrate the cellular and nuclear membranes and serve as ligands for transcription factors that control gene expression. Depending on the gene and the particular bioactive, expression may be turned on or off or increased or decreased in magnitude in keeping with the information received. Examples include resveratrol from purple grape skins; along with a large number of flavonoids such as the catechins found in tea, dark chocolate, and onions and the isoflavones genistein and daidzein from soy. The potential therapeutic use of phytonutrients is being investigated for a variety of chronic disorders (Grabacka et al, 2014; Gupta and Prakash, 2014; Lee et al, 2014; Ong et al., 2011; see *Focus On*: Epigenetics and Colorful Eating).

For bioactive phytochemicals that are too large or too hydrophilic to penetrate the cell's membrane barriers, communication occurs by means of signal transduction. The bioactive interacts with a receptor protein at the cell surface and initiates a cascade of biochemical reactions that ultimately results in one or more transcription factors interacting with DNA and modulating gene expression. Examples of this type of indirect communication are seen with the organosulfur compounds such as sulforaphane and other glucosinolates from the cabbage family vegetables. As a result of the signaling pathway, transcription factors (e.g., *nrf*) are activated and increase transcription of the glutathione-S-transferases needed for phase II detoxification,

---

◉ FOCUS ON

Epigenetics and Colorful Eating

It can be challenging to communicate the specifics of phytonutrients to consumers because they do not think in terms of the food they eat containing bioactive substances. Attempts have been made to simplify the message, such as focusing on thinking of food in terms of its dominant color and understanding that each color contributes different valuable phytonutrients. For example, eating one to two servings from a wide variety of fruits, vegetables, legumes, grains, nuts, and seeds within the red, orange, yellow, green, purple, and white color categories daily supplies a variety of health-promoting phytonutrients. Individuals with particular disease susceptibilities or environmental challenges should increase the number of servings within a particular category to meet their specific health needs. Practitioners can provide a valuable service by translating these research findings into practical food solutions for consumers (Gupta and Prakash, 2014; see Table 36-1).

which helps to protect against cancer. Flavonoids such as naringenin, found in citrus fruits, and quercetin from onions and apples activate signaling pathways, leading to increased apoptosis of cancer cells (see Chapter 36).

Nutritional Genomics and Chronic Disease

Chronic disorders (e.g., CVD, cancer, diabetes, osteoporosis, inflammatory disorders) are typically more complex than single-gene disorders, in which the change in the DNA is known, the abnormal protein can be identified and analyzed, and the resulting phenotype is defined clearly. Either the influence on function of a particular genetic variation is subtle or even silent and/or multiple genes and their genetic variations contribute in small ways to the overall chronic condition rather than a single variant having a dramatic effect. The genes involved with chronic disease are influenced by environmental factors in addition to the genetic variation. An individual may have gene variants that predispose to a particular chronic disorder, but the disorder may or may not develop. Obviously this situation is challenging because of its complexity but nonetheless must be factored into the nutrition assessment and diagnosis if therapeutic interventions are to be successful.

Genetic Variability

Given the genetic variability among individuals in a population, the high degree of variability in client response to nutrition therapy should not be surprising. Although a change in a gene—including diet- and lifestyle-related genes—can affect function severely enough to cause disease outright, the majority of these genetic variations appear to affect the magnitude of response and do not pose a life-threatening situation. They confer an increased susceptibility to dysfunction and disease but not a sure bet. Many are responsive to diet and lifestyle changes, providing the opportunity to minimize their effect through informed lifestyle choices.

The major focus of nutritional genomics research is on identifying (1) gene-disease associations, (2) the dietary components that influence these associations, (3) the mechanisms by which dietary components exert their effects, and (4) the genotypes that benefit most from particular diet and lifestyle choices. The practical applications of this research include a new set of tools that nutrition professionals can use. The growing body of knowledge supports strategies for disease prevention and intervention that are targeted specifically to the underlying mechanisms.

The following section takes a brief look at some of the key diet-related genes, their known variants, and how these variants affect a person's response to diet. Chronic disease involves complex interactions among genes and bioactive food components. Unraveling the details requires population and intervention studies large enough to have the statistical power needed to draw meaningful conclusions.

Cardiovascular Disease

Cardiovascular disease (CVD) remains the number one disease plaguing developed countries. Not surprisingly, a major focus of nutritional genomics has been to identify gene-diet associations for CVD and to study the influence of diet and exercise parameters in managing and preventing this chronic disease. Nutrition professionals who work with clients with dyslipidemia know firsthand the high degree of individual variability of responses to standard dietary interventions. These therapies are used primarily to lower elevated blood levels of LDL cholesterol (LDL-C), raise high-density lipoprotein cholesterol (HDL-C), and lower triglycerides (TGs). Until recently the standard approach is a diet low in saturated fat, with increased content of polyunsaturated fats (PUFAs). Response across a population varies, ranging from reduced LDL-C levels and TGs in some to decreased HDL-C levels or elevated TGs in others. Furthermore, some have had their LDL-C levels respond dramatically to dietary oat bran and other soluble fibers, whereas others have had more modest responses. In some a low-fat diet has caused a shift to a lipid pattern that is more atherogenic than the original. Genotype is an important factor; dietary interventions must be matched to genotypes to accomplish the intended lipid-lowering response (see Chapter 33).

A number of contributing genes already have been identified and include those involved with postprandial lipoprotein and triglyceride response, homocysteine metabolism, hypertension, blood-clotting, and inflammation. Gene-diet interactions have been reported for those that code for apolipoprotein E (*APOE*), apolipoprotein A-1 (*APOA1*), cholesterol esteryl transport protein (*CETP*), hepatic lipase (*LIPC*), lipoxygenase-5 (*ALOX5*), *MTHFR*, angiotensinogen (*AGT*), angiotensin-converting enzyme (*ACE*), the interleukin-1 family (*IL1*), interleukin-6 (*IL6*), and tumor necrosis factor-alpha (*TNF*). Among the more recently discovered interactions are those involving the monoglyceride lipase (*MGLL*) gene, omega-3 fatty acids, and LDL cholesterol levels and LDL particle size (Ouellette et al, 2014). Work with the omega-6 fatty acids and gene-diet-cardiovascular disease associations have involved variants in the fatty acid synthase (FADS) gene and their effect on heart health (Li et al, 2013) as well as gene variants that lead to increased arachidonic acid metabolism to proinflammatory, vasoconstrictive, and platelet-aggregating family of eicosanoids (Chilton et al, 2014). Examining haplotypes of the sterol regulatory element binding protein-1 (SREBP1) gene in postmenopausal women, consumption of omega-6 PUFAs but not omega-3 PUFAs was associated with the progression of atherosclerosis, as measured by decreased arterial diameter (Kalantarian et al, 2014).

An additional link of carbohydrate metabolism to heart health has been reported (Ortega-Azorín et al, 2014). The MLXIPL (Max-like protein X interacting protein-like) gene encodes the carbohydrate response element binding protein. These researchers found that those with one or more copies of the rs3812316 variant had lower blood levels of triglyceride and decreased incidence of myocardial infarcts when consuming a Mediterranean-style diet compared with a control diet and compared with subjects who had no copies of the variant.

The possibilities for nutritional intervention are numerous, with the Mediterranean-style diet being of particular interest in terms of heart health (Gotsis et al, 2015). However, this type of diet is beneficial for some individuals but not for others. Researchers continue to probe potential mechanisms that explain the heart-healthy outcomes of this type of diet and why there are interindividual differences in response to the diet. They also recommend developing sound guidelines for dietary intervention for dyslipidemic conditions (Corella and Ordovás, 2014).

CVD is, at its basis, an inflammatory disorder (Rocha and Libby, 2009), and variants of *TNF*, *IL1*, and *IL6* are being investigated for their effect on CVD susceptibility. Further, cardiovascular disease and other chronic disorders tend to involve multiple comorbidities, which makes it increasingly critical that practitioners become aware of the underlying, intersecting mechanisms and the need for effective interventions for management and prevention. Knowing the genotype of clients provides additional important information as to how they are likely to respond to particular dietary interventions.

In summary of the current state of knowledge of nutritional genomics with respect to cardiovascular disease, considerable research is being conducted globally. The identification of numerous gene variants with associations to different aspects of cardiovascular health suggests that progress is being made in identifying susceptibility variants that can be modulated through judicious diet and lifestyle choices (Merched and Chan, 2013).

Inflammatory Disorders

Inflammation now is recognized as an underlying factor in chronic disorders, from heart disease to cancer to diabetes to obesity to more traditional inflammatory disorders such as arthritis and the inflammatory bowel disorders. Inflammation is a normal and desirable response to insult by the body. Typically inflammation is an acute phase response; once the threat has passed, inflammation subsides and healing ensues. Certain genetic variations predispose individuals to be in a chronic inflammatory state, making them more reactive to proinflammatory triggers and extending the inflammation phase so that inflammation becomes a chronic state. The regular assault of proinflammatory mediators such as the cytokines and eicosanoids on tissues leads to oxidative stress and cellular degeneration rather than the healing that is characteristic of the acute phase (see Chapter 3).

Among the genes known to be of particular importance to the inflammatory response are the proinflammatory cytokine genes *IL1*, which encodes the interleukin-1β cytokine (also known as IL-1F2), *IL6* (encoding the interleukin-6 cytokine), and *TNF* (produces the tumor necrosis factor cytokine). Variants in each of these genes have been discovered that increase the susceptibility of humans to be in a proinflammatory state, which in turn increases the risk of developing one or more chronic disorders. Certain diet and lifestyle approaches can minimize susceptibility and dampen existing inflammation. Examples include the inclusion of fish and foods that contain omega-3 fatty acids and plant foods rich in various polyphenols. Currently the role of the microbiome in chronic inflammation and immunity is receiving increased attention (Belkaid and Hand, 2014). The hypothesis is that current diets and lifestyles may be decreasing the benefits of the symbiotic relationship between humans and the microbes that colonize the digestive tract and may be at least in part responsible for the increase in inflammatory and autoimmune disorders seen in developed countries (see Chapters 3 and 26).

Immune Health and Cancer

The relationship of gene variants and gene-diet interactions to immune health and cancer is of considerable interest to researchers around the world (Trottier et al, 2010; Villagra et al, 2009). One of the key mechanisms by which the body protects against cancer is detoxification, the process of neutralizing potentially harmful molecules (see *Focus On:* Eating to Detoxify in Chapter 19). Among the better characterized genes involved in various aspects of detoxification are the cytochrome P450 isozymes (*CYPs*), glutathione *S*-transferases (*GSTs*), and superoxide dismutases (*SOD1, SOD2, SOD3*). The *CYP* and *GST* genes

are part of the phase I and phase II detoxification system, respectively, found in the liver and the gut. The *SOD* genes code for proteins that dismantle the reactive oxygen species superoxide. Each of these genes has nutritional implications, and variants have been identified that result in decreased detoxification. Nutritional genomics provides the basis for directing nutrition therapy to protect against cancer by augmenting endogenous detoxification activity and by identifying genetic variants that can decrease phase I or phase II activity and including foods that can help compensate for the decreased activity.

Epidemiologic studies have suggested that consuming plant foods is cancer protective. Numerous dietary factors play a role in protecting against cancer (see Chapter 36). Examples include curcumin from the spice turmeric, resveratrol from purple grape skins, glucosinolates in cruciferous vegetables, epigallocatechin gallate catechins from green tea, isoflavones from soybeans, folic acid, and vitamin D. Numerous labs are investigating the underlying mechanisms by which these phytochemicals exert their protective effects (see reviews by Gupta and Prakash [2014], Howes and Simmonds [2014], Lee et al [2011], Martin et al [2013], Ong et al [2011]). See Table 36-1.

Blood Sugar Regulation

Glucose is the preferred source of energy for the body's cells. Accordingly, blood glucose levels are controlled carefully through an intricate system of checks and balances. When glucose levels are higher than normal (hyperglycemia), the hormone insulin is secreted from the beta-cells of the pancreas, glucose is taken up by the cells, and a normal blood sugar level (euglycemia) is restored. When blood glucose levels fall (hypoglycemia), the hormone glucagon is secreted by the liver, glycogen is hydrolyzed to glucose, and euglycemia is again restored. When this process goes awry, the stage is set for the chronic conditions of insulin resistance, metabolic syndrome, and, ultimately, T2DM (see Chapter 30).

Identification of gene variants that lead to T2DM would allow individuals with this susceptibility to be identified early in the lifespan so that intervention could be initiated. A few rare mutations have been associated with the development of T2DM, but they do not explain the high prevalence of the disease. It is likely that multiple gene variants contribute to the development of this condition. One promising variant is the transcription factor 7-like 2 (*TCF7L2*) identified by Grant and colleagues (2006). The variant occurs frequently within multiple populations. Evidence suggests the gene is involved in insulin secretion from pancreatic beta-cells (Villareal et al, 2010).

Bone Mineralization and Maintenance

Healthy bone tissue depends on a balance between the action of the osteoblasts that synthesize new bone tissue and resorption by osteoclasts. Important components in this dynamic balance are vitamin D, calcium, other nutrients, and hormones such as parathyroid hormone and estrogen. When resorption predominates, bones become fragile, are subject to fracture, and osteoporosis results. Osteoporosis can occur in men and women as they age; it is prevalent among older postmenopausal women (see Chapter 24).

Numerous genes and their protein products are involved in the overall process. In fact, more than 60 loci are being investigated for their association with bone health and disease (Mitchell and Streeten, 2013). The gene VDR, which codes for the vitamin D receptor present on the surface of many cell types, is an obvious candidate. Vitamin D has multiple roles in metabolism, but its control of the absorption of dietary calcium from the digestive tract truly affects bone health. Four *VDR* variants have been studied over several years (*ApaI, BsmI, FokI,* and *TaqI*), but no clear association has emerged (Horst-Sikorska et al, 2013). Further research regarding gene variants and risk of osteoporosis is imperative given the aging of the global population and the growing prevalence of osteoporosis.

Weight Management

The ability to maintain a healthy weight is another challenge for modern society. As with the other chronic disorders, the regulation of body weight is a complex process and offers multiple points at which a gene variant can give rise to an impaired protein that, when combined with the appropriate environmental trigger, promotes body fat storage. Similar to T2DM, variations in single genes have been associated with excess weight, but these genetic changes are not likely the basis for the rapid rise in prevalence of excess body weight during the past several generations (Hetherington and Cecil, 2010).

A variant in the *FTO* gene has been identified and found to occur frequently among multiple populations (Chu et al, 2008; Dina et al, 2007). An SNP in the *FTO* gene is associated with increased risk of obesity, and the effect was correlated directly with the number of copies of the SNP. That is, those with one copy of the risk allele weighed more than those with no copies, and those with two copies weighed the most of the three groups (Frayling et al, 2007). In 2009 two large genome-wide association studies found the *FTO* variant to be associated with BMI (Thorleifsson et al, 2009; Willer et al, 2009). Harbron and colleagues (2014) provide a useful overview of the current status of *FTO* and its variants in terms of association with several environmental factors that contribute to susceptibility to overweight and obesity. A number of other gene variants have been implicated in weight management, including ADRB3, FABP2, POMC, and PPARG, but none so dramatically as *FTO*. The *FTO* variant also may increase risk for T2DM and CVD through its effect on susceptibility to increased body fat.

Adipose tissue is dynamic tissue that is highly vascularized and produces hormones, inflammatory peptides (cytokines), and new adipocytes in addition to storing excess calories as triglycerides and hydrolyzing them as energy is needed. The multistep process of transporting free fatty acids into the adipocyte, esterifying them into triglycerides, and mobilizing the triglycerides potentially provides many proteins that could be affected by genetic variation such that fat is stored more readily or mobilized more slowly than normal. Adipocytes have cell surface receptors that respond to various environmental factors, such as catecholamines produced during exercise, to mobilize stored fat. An example is the receptor encoded by the *ADRB2* gene, which has a greater propensity to store dietary fat as body fat. Individuals with either of these variants will find it more challenging to maintain a healthy weight and may need to restrict their dietary fat intake or engage in regular, vigorous exercise to achieve and maintain a healthy weight.

Ethnicity is an additional confounder in maintaining a healthy weight. Joffe and colleagues extensively investigated novel dietary fat-inflammatory gene interactions in black and in white South African women and detected complex interrelationships linking obesity, inflammation, serum lipids, dietary fat intake and ethnicity (Joffe et al, 2010, 2011, 2012, 2013). This extensive work points up the influence of genetic variation on dietary response and could suggest that nutrition professionals proceed with caution in extrapolating findings from one population to another. Obesity is a state of low-grade inflammation, which likely contributes to some populations being more susceptible to becoming obese but also to developing other chronic conditions in addition to obesity. The interconnectedness of obesity, inflammation, insulin resistance, dyslipidemia, and nonalcoholic fatty liver disease and suggest potential common mechanisms (Jung and Choi, 2014).

Other Chronic Diseases

Candidate genes, gene variants, and diet-gene interactions are being investigated for many chronic disorders. Populations differ in the types and frequencies of the gene variants; dietary approaches that are most appropriate vary accordingly. As gene variants and their health implications are identified, attention also is being paid to examining the frequency of particular variants among populations so that guidelines can be developed that take into account the most frequently occurring genetic susceptibilities within specific populations.

ETHICAL, LEGAL, AND SOCIAL IMPLICATIONS

If nutritional genomics is to realize its potential as a valuable tool, genetic testing is an essential component of identifying the variations in each individual. Such testing is not, however, without controversy. Consumers worry that genetic testing for any purpose could be used against them, primarily to deny insurance coverage or employment; they are particularly uncomfortable with insurers and employers having access to their personal genetic information (Genetics & Public Policy Center, 2010).

Although theoretically possible, according to existing case law such discrimination rarely has occurred. Furthermore, identifying gene variants that increase susceptibility to diet- and lifestyle-related diseases that can be addressed through readily available diet and lifestyle measures may also lead to legal debate. Many legislators and legal experts believe the Americans with Disabilities Act sufficiently protects against discrimination, but, as an added measure of protection, GINA was passed by Congress and went into effect on November 21, 2009. GINA defines genetic testing and genetic information, bans discrimination based on genetic information, and penalizes those who violate the provisions of this law. Consumers and health care professionals can feel comfortable in adopting this new service.

Consumers and health care professionals should ask critical questions before consent for genetic testing. The laboratory itself should have the appropriate credentials and state licensing, if required (at a minimum, Clinical Laboratory Improvement Amendment (CLIA) certification according to the CLIA of 1988) and should have an appropriately credentialed health professional available for assistance in interpreting the test results. The laboratory should have written, readily available policies concerning how it will protect the privacy of the individual being tested and whether the DNA sample will be retained by the laboratory or destroyed after testing. Transparency in each of these areas increases consumer comfort.

A second concern on the part of consumers and health care professionals is that nutritional genomics is elitist by nature, in that only the wealthy will be able to benefit. At this early stage in its development, the cost of nutritional genomics testing precludes its use as a public health measure and effectively

BOX 5-1   Discussion Points Related to Genetic Testing

Which laboratory will analyze the deoxyribonucleic acid?

What measures are in place in that laboratory to protect privacy?

What is the total cost of the test?

Which gene variants are tested?

Is there a lifestyle action that can be taken for each variant?

Has the test been scientifically validated for accuracy and reliability?

When will the test results be received?

How and to whom will the test results be presented?

Who should be tested?

Should individuals be tested for a disease for which there is no cure?

Do parents have the right to have their minor children tested for a genetic susceptibility?

Do parents have the right to withhold the results from the children?

Should gene therapy be allowed on reproductive cells so that any corrected genes can be inherited by subsequent generations?

Should human cloning be allowed?

What is the best way to educate those who are already in practice as health care professionals?

What changes are needed so that future health care practitioners can be educated properly?

restricts access to those with sufficient disposable income. However, like any other new technology, as the sales volume increases, the cost will decrease.

Numerous additional issues must be discussed thoroughly in the course of integrating genetic technologies into health care. Box 5-1 lists key questions to be answered in the development of nutritional genomics practices. These and other ethical, legal, and social issues relating to nutritional genomics in particular have been explored. One particular question is whether nutritional genomics may be used for "nutrition-based doping" in athletic competition, and it is recommended that international sports organizations begin to consider such a situation (Bragazzi, 2013).

SUMMARY

The steady rise in chronic disease globally is fueling the need for health care to shift from a focus on acute care to one of managing and, ultimately, preventing chronic disorders. The decreasing quality of life and soaring economic burden of escalating chronic disease is untenable and unsustainable. Chronic disease is diet-and-lifestyle disease, the result of inappropriate daily choices over a lifetime interacting with each individual's DNA.

Nutrition therapy increasingly will have to address chronic disease management and prevention from a new perspective. Among the key drivers of chronic disease are such environmental factors as food choices, whether an individual chooses to exercise, the quality and quantity of sleep and relaxation, how effectively a person manages stress and thoughts and emotions in general, the extent of toxicity of the environment, and the relationships with one's self and others along with a sense of purpose in life. These key drivers contribute to each person's unique health spectrum that spans wellness to illness. Where someone falls on that spectrum is the result of interactions among genes and the environment that bathes the genes throughout a lifetime. When these factors are inappropriate for meeting needs, over time the foundation for health erodes. Normal function (health) cannot be maintained and dysfunction (disease) emerges at some point along the lifespan. Fortunately each of these key factors is modifiable through behavioral change. As health care professionals are well aware, behavioral

change is a slow, steady process requiring excellent counseling skills coupled with the specific guidance needed for each modifiable lifestyle factor.

Increasingly the field of nutrition is recognizing the need to take a whole systems approach to the use of food as a therapeutic intervention. Nutritional genomics is expected to provide a greater understanding of how to use nutrition therapy to promote health and prevent disease. This subdiscipline of nutrition focuses on how genetic makeup influences the ability to digest, absorb, and use the nutrients in food and on how food and other environmental factors influence the expression of genes. As the understanding grows that it is not just genes that contribute to our disease potential but the interaction between genes and environmental factors, it has become important to identify the changes in genes that provide the increased potential for being susceptible to chronic disease. Changes in genes can lead to changes in the information encoded with the genes, which in turn can lead to changes in functional ability. These changes can be inherited from one generation to the next but may lie dormant in their influence on function unless triggered by the interaction with particular environmental factors, such as food. Being able to identify changes within genes that result in altered proteins and function or in the control of the expression of a gene and its encoded protein gives the practitioner insight into potential disease susceptibility and thereby an idea of how to correct the metabolic imbalances that ensue.

Aspects of nutritional genomics have been applied to clinical nutrition for decades. Changes to single genes that cause sufficient dysfunction as to manifest as disease in the individual have been known for a long time. This situation describes the molecular, biochemical, and physiologic basis for the inborn errors of metabolism, which result from errors in single genes and occur rarely. Nutrition professionals have long used food and particular nutrients to address the nutrient imbalances that result. Today nutritional genomics has a far greater reach by being able to detect changes within genes that result in increased susceptibility to chronic disease and provide insight into effective management and preventive interventions.

It is not enough to simply manage chronic disease. Nutrition professionals can and must take the lead in preventing chronic disease and in restoring health to those in whom chronic disease already exists. To do so will entail making use of the extensive scientific training of nutrition professionals to understand the molecular, biochemical, physiologic, and psychosocial mechanisms that underlie chronic disease and provide the targets against which nutrition therapy can be directed effectively. This comprehensive, whole systems biology approach to the functioning of the human organism will form the basis for more effective clinical interventions.

Studies over the past decade have suggested that most nutrition professionals are in the early stage of preparedness regarding nutritional genomics. Most recently registered dietitians in Quebec were surveyed (Cormier et al, 2014), and the majority were not yet comfortable in their knowledge of nutritional genomics and had questions about the clinical validity and utility of nutrigenetic testing. The Academy of Nutrition and Dietetics has provided recommendations in its position paper on nutritional genomics (Camp and Trujillo, 2014). Although cautionary regarding nutrigenetic testing not being ready for clinical application as yet, the Academy supports preparing appropriately for the new opportunities that nutritional genomics affords nutrition professionals.

The nutrition profession will be pivotal in this new era of health promotion and disease prevention. The role includes assessing disease susceptibilities and then recommending preventive therapy and lifestyle approaches. Increasingly, genotyping must be incorporated into the nutrition assessment and recommendations customized to the genetic uniqueness of individuals. Such a pivotal role requires that the nutrition professional be well versed in the molecular and biochemical bases for health. Appropriately trained individuals will be able to converse with physicians in their language, which increasingly will involve therapies targeted to underlying molecular, biochemical, and physiologic mechanisms involved in the disease process (see Chapters 3 and 7). Remember that the nutrients and other bioactive components in food are critical players in these underlying mechanisms. The nutrition professional will be able to recommend therapeutic interventions in which food can be used to target the specific underlying mechanisms of complex disease processes and to ensure that negative interactions with other therapies, such as drugs and medical procedures, are minimized. Further, the translation of the medical therapies into practical applications for the patients and the coaching of patients as they modify their lifestyle choices is a primary role of the nutrition professional that will become increasingly important for the success of patient outcomes.

CLINICAL CASE STUDY

Jared and Matthew are identical twins who grew up together but have lived apart since college. Jared lives in New York City and is a certified public accountant in a high-profile accounting firm, working long hours in a stressful environment. Matthew attended college in California, where he studied nutrition and exercise physiology and now manages the wellness program at a large fitness center. At age 30 the two brothers are noticeably different in weight and body shape. Jared has a body mass index of 29 compared with Matthew's 23. Jared has developed central obesity, hypertension, and problems with blood sugar regulation, all signs of a tendency toward developing type 2 diabetes. In contrast, Matthew is lean and has normal blood pressure and normal blood sugar levels.

Nutrition Diagnostic Statement

Overweight related to possible genetic susceptibility, limited physical activity, overeating with snacks and consumption of large meals as evidenced by diet history, central obesity, and body mass index

Nutrition Care Questions

1. Because they are identical twins, would you have expected the two brothers to have similar health profiles?
2. How would you expect their diets to be different?
3. What is going on? Does Matthew not have the same genetic susceptibilities that Jared has? If not, why not? If so, why doesn't Matthew exhibit the same phenotype as Jared? This question is complex: think about the twins' deoxyribonucleic acid but also their environmental influences and their epigenetic markings.
4. How could you confirm your suspicion that Jared is genetically predisposed to type 2 diabetes?
5. What would you advise Jared to do to decrease his genetic susceptibility to diabetes?
6. As part of the nutrition assessment, Jared is found to be homozygous for IL1 -511C>T and heterozygous for IL6 -174G>C. These genes code for the proinflammatory cytokines interleukin-1 and interleukin-6 and these particular single nucleotide polymorphisms have been strongly associated with chronic inflammation. What would you discuss with Jared about the implications of these genotype findings and his susceptibility to chronic disease?

USEFUL WEBSITES

American College of Medical Genetics and Genomics
www.acmg.net
CDC Genomics
www.cdc.gov/genomics
Epigenetics/Epigenomics, from the National Human Genome Research Institute at the National Institutes of Health
http://www.genome.gov/27532724
Epigenetics NOVA: *Ghost in Your Genes* video
http://www.youtube.com/watch?v=D44cu7v9x1w
Ethical, Legal, and Social Issues, from the Human Genome Project Archive
http://www.ornl.gov/sci/techresources/Human_Genome/elsi/elsi.shtml
Fact Sheets About Genetics and Genomics
http://www.genome.gov/10000202
Family History Initiative, from the U.S. Department of Health and Human Services
http://www.hhs.gov/familyhistory
Genetic and Rare Diseases Information Center (GARD)
http://rarediseases.info.nih.gov/gard
Genetics Core Competencies
http://www.nchpeg.org/index.php?option=com_content&view=article&id=26&Itemid=64
Genetics and Genomics
http://www.genome.gov/Education/
Genetics and Nutrition
http://www.nchpeg.org/nutrition/index.php?option=com_content&view=article&id=398
Genetics Home Reference Handbook: Help Me Understand Genetics
http://ghr.nlm.nih.gov/handbook/basics/dna
Genetic Information and Nondiscrimination Act of 2008
https://www.genome.gov/24519851
Human Genome Project
www.ornl.gov/hgmis/project/info.html
Nutrigenomics—New Zealand
www.nutrigenomics.org.nz
Your Genome
www.yourgenome.org

REFERENCES

Adalsteinsson BT, Ferguson-Smith AC: Epigenetic control of the genome-lessons from genomic imprinting, *Genes* 5:635, 2014.
Ames BN, et al: High-dose vitamin therapy stimulates variant enzymes with decreased coenzyme binding affinity (increased K[m]): relevance to genetic disease and polymorphisms, *Am J Clin Nutr* 75:616, 2002.
Belkaid Y, Hand TW: Role of the microbiota in immunity and inflammation, *Cell* 157:121, 2014.
Bragazzi NL: Situating nutri-ethics at the junction of nutrigenomics and nutriproteomics in postgenomics medicine, *Curr Pharmacogenomics Person Med* 11:162, 2013.
Brunet A, Berger SL: Epigenetics of aging and aging-related disease, *J Gerontol A Biol Sci Med Sci* 69(Suppl 1):S17, 2014.
Bygren LO: Intergenerational health responses to adverse and enriched environments, *Annu Rev Public Health* 34:49, 2013.
Calder PC: Marine omega-3 fatty acids and inflammatory processes: effects, mechanisms and clinical relevance, *Biochim Biophy Acta* 1851:469, 2015.
Camp KM, Trujillo E: Position of the Academy of Nutrition and Dietetics: nutritional genomics, *J Acad Nutr Diet* 14:299, 2014.
Chaturvedi P, Tyagi SC: Epigenetic mechanisms underlying cardiac degeneration and regeneration, *Int J Cardiol* 173:1, 2014.

Chilton FH, et al: Diet-gene interactions and PUFA metabolism: a potential contributor to health disparities and human diseases, *Nutrients* 6:1993, 2014.

Christodoulides C, Vidal-Puig A: PPARS and adipocyte function, *Mol Cell Endocrinol* 318:61, 2010.

Choi SW, et al: Nutritional epigenomics: a portal to disease prevention, *Adv Nutr* 4:530, 2013.

Chu X, et al: Association of morbid obesity with FTO and INSIG2 allelic variants, *Arch Surg* 143:235, 2008.

Corella D, Ordovás JM: How does the Mediterranean diet promote cardiovascular health? Current progress toward molecular mechanisms: gene-diet interactions at the genomic, transcriptomic, and epigenomic levels provide novel insights into new mechanisms, *Bioessays* 36:526, 2014.

Cormier H, et al: Nutrigenomics—perspectives from registered dietitians: a report from the Quebec-wide e-consultation on nutrigenomics among registered dietitians, *J Hum Nutr Diet* 27:391, 2014.

Cropley JE, et al: Germ-line epigenetic modification of the murine A^{vy} allele by nutritional supplementation, *Proc Natl Acad Sci USA* 103:17308, 2006.

Dina C, et al: Variation in FTO contributes to childhood obesity and severe adult obesity, *Nat Genet* 39:724, 2007.

Dunn GA, Bale TL: Maternal high-fat diet effects on third-generation female body size via the paternal lineage, *Endocrinology* 152:2228, 2011.

Dunn GA, Bale TL: Maternal high-fat diet promotes body length increases and insulin insensitivity in second-generation mice, *Endocrinology* 150:4999, 2009.

Frayling TM, et al: A common variant in the FTO gene is associated with body mass index and predisposes to childhood and adult obesity, *Science* 316:889, 2007.

Genetics Home Reference: *CFTR*. http://ghr.nlm.nih.gov/gene/CFTR. Accessed May, 28 2015.

Genetics & Public Policy Center: *Johns Hopkins University*, 2007. http://www.dnapolicy.org/images/reportpdfs/GINAPublic_Opinion_Genetic_Information_Discrimination.pdf. Accessed November 10, 2014.

Girardot M, et al: Small regulatory RNAs controlled by genomic imprinting and their contribution to human disease, *Epigenetics* 7:1341, 2012.

Gosden RG, Feinberg AP: Genetics and epigenetics—nature's pen-and-pencil set, *N Engl J Med* 356:731, 2007.

Goswami S, et al: Clopidogrel and genetic testing: is it necessary for everyone? *Cardiol Rev* 20:96, 2012.

Gotsis E, et al: Health benefits of the Mediterranean diet: an update of research over the last 5 years, *Angiology* 66:304, 2015.

Grabacka MM, et al: Phytochemical modulators of mitochondria: the search for chemopreventive agents and supportive therapeutics, *Pharmaceuticals (Basel)* 7:913, 2014.

Grant SF, et al: Variation of transcription factor 7-like 2 (TCF7L2)—a novel gene confers risk of type 2 diabetes, *Nat Genet* 38:320, 2006.

Gupta C, Prakash D: Phytonutrients as therapeutic agents, *J Complement Integr Med* 11:151, 2014.

Harbron J, et al: Fat mass and obesity-associated (FTO) gene polymorphisms are associated with physical activity, food intake, eating behaviors, psychological health, and modeled change in body mass index in overweight/obese Caucasian adults, *Nutrients* 6:3130, 2014.

Heard E, Martienssen RA: Transgenerational epigenetic inheritance: myths and mechanisms, *Cell* 157:95, 2014.

Hetherington MM, Cecil JE: Gene-environment interactions in obesity, *Forum Nutr* 63:195, 2010.

Horst-Sikorska W, et al: Vitamin D receptor gene polymorphisms, bone mineral density and fractures in postmenopausal women with osteoporosis, *Mol Biol Rep* 40:383, 2013.

Howes MJ, Simmonds MS: The role of phytochemicals as micronutrients in health and disease, *Curr Opin Clin Nutr Metab Care* 17:558, 2014.

Jiménez-Chillarón JC, et al: The role of nutrition on epigenetic modifications and their implications on health, *Biochimie* 94:2242, 2012.

Joffe YT, et al: The relationship between dietary fatty acids and inflammatory genes on the obese phenotype and serum lipids, *Nutrients* 5:1672, 2013.

Joffe YT, et al: Tumor necrosis factor-alpha gene-308 G/A polymorphism modulates the relationship between dietary fat intake, serum lipids, and obesity risk in black South African women, *J Nutr* 140:901, 2010.

Joffe YT, et al: The -308 G/A polymorphism of the tumour necrosis factor-α gene modifies the association between saturated fat intake and serum total cholesterol levels in white South African women, *Genes Nutr* 6:353, 2011.

Joffe YT, et al: The tumor necrosis factor-α gene -238G>A polymorphism, dietary fat intake, obesity risk and serum lipid concentrations in black and white South African women, *Eur J Clin Nutr* 66:1295, 2012.

Johnson M, et al: Warfarin dosing in a patient with CYP2C9(*)3(*)3 and VKORC1-1639 AA Genotypes, *Case Rep Genet* 2014:413743, 2014.

Jung UJ, Choi MS: Obesity and its metabolic complications: the role of adipokines and the relationship between obesity, inflammation, insulin resistance, dyslipidemia and nonalcoholic fatty liver disease, *Int J Mol Sci* 15:6184, 2014.

Kalantarian S, et al: Dietary macronutrients, genetic variation, and progression of coronary atherosclerosis among women, *Am Heart J* 167:627, 2014.

Lee J, et al: Adaptive cellular stress pathways as therapeutic targets of dietary phytochemicals: focus on the nervous system, *Pharmacol Rev* 66:815, 2014.

Lee KW, et al: Molecular targets of phytochemicals for cancer prevention, *Nat Rev Cancer* 11:211, 2011.

Lillycrop KA, Burdge GC: Epigenetic mechanisms linking early nutrition to long term health, *Best Pract Res Clin Endocrinol Metab* 26:667, 2012.

Li SW, et al: FADS gene polymorphisms confer the risk of coronary artery disease in a Chinese Han population through the altered desaturase activities: based on high-resolution melting analysis, *PLoS One* 8:e55869, 2013.

Martin C, et al: Plants, diet, and health, *Annu Rev Plant Biol* 64:19, 2013.

Mega JL, et al: Cytochrome p-450 polymorphisms and response to clopidogrel, *N Engl J Med* 360:354, 2009.

Merched AJ, Chan L: Nutrigenetics and nutrigenomics of atherosclerosis, *Curr Atheroscler Rep* 15:328, 2013.

Milagro FI, et al: Dietary factors, epigenetic modifications and obesity outcomes: progresses and perspectives, *Mol Aspects Med* 34:782, 2013.

Mitchell BD, Streeten EA: Clinical impact of recent genetic discoveries in osteoporosis, *Appl Clin Genet* 6:75, 2013.

NCHPEG site: *Cystic fibrosis and the CFTR gene*. http://www.nchpeg.org/nutrition/index.php?option=com_content&view=article&id=462&Itemid=564&limitstart=4. Accessed May 28, 2015.

Ng SF, et al: Paternal high-fat diet consumption induces common changes in the transcriptomes of retroperitoneal adipose and pancreatic islet tissues in female rat offspring, *FASEB J* 28:1830, 2014.

Ong PT, et al: Targeting the epigenome with bioactive food components for cancer prevention, *J Nutrigenet Nutrigenomic* 4:275, 2011.

Ortega-Azorín C, et al: Amino acid change in the carbohydrate response element binding protein is associated with lower triglycerides and myocardial infarction incidence depending on level of adherence to the Mediterranean diet in the PREDIMED trial, *Circ Cardiovasc Genet* 7:49, 2014.

Ouellette C, et al: Gene-diet interactions with polymorphisms of the MGLL gene on plasma low-density lipoprotein cholesterol and size following an omega-3 polyunsaturated fatty acid supplementation: a clinical trial, *Lipids Health Dis* 13:86, 2014.

Pentinat T, et al: Transgenerational inheritance of glucose intolerance in a mouse model of neonatal overnutrition, *Endocrinology* 151:5617, 2010.

Peters J: The role of genomic imprinting in biology and disease: an expanding view, *Nat Rev Genet* 15:517, 2014.

Rocha VZ, Libby P: Obesity, inflammation and atherosclerosis, *Nat Rev Cardiol* 6:399, 2009.

Supic G, et al: Epigenetics: a new link between nutrition and cancer, *Nutr Cancer* 65:781, 2013.

Thorleifsson G, et al: Genome-wide association yields new sequence variants at seven loci associated with measures of obesity, *Nat Genet* 41:18, 2009.

Trottier G, et al: Nutraceuticals and prostate cancer prevention: a current review, *Nat Rev Urol* 7:21, 2010.

Villagra A, et al: The histone deacetylase HDAC11 regulates the expression of interleukin 10 and immune tolerance, *Nat Immunol* 10:92, 2009.

Villareal DT, et al: TCF7L2 variant rs7903146 affects the risk of type 2 diabetes by modulating incretin action, *Diabetes* 59:479, 2010.

Waterland RA: Epigenetic mechanisms affecting regulation of energy balance: many questions, few answers, *Annu Rev Nutr* 34:337, 2014.

Waterland RA, Jirtle RL: Transposable elements: targets for early nutritional effects on epigenetic gene regulation, *Mol Cell Biol* 23:5293, 2003.

Willer, et al: Six new loci associated with body mass index highlight a neuronal influence on body weight regulation, *Nat Genet* 41:25, 2009.

6

Clinical: Water, Electrolytes, and Acid-Base Balance

Mandy L. Corrigan, MPH, RD, CNSC, FAND

KEY TERMS

acid-base balance
acidemia
alkalemia
anion gap
buffer
contraction alkalosis
corrected calcium
edema
electrolytes
extracellular fluid (ECF)

extracellular water
insensible water loss
intracellular fluid (ICF)
metabolic acidosis
metabolic alkalosis
metabolic water
Na/K-ATPase pump
oncotic pressure (colloidal osmotic
  pressure)
osmolality

osmolarity
osmotic pressure
renin-angiotensin system
respiratory acidosis
respiratory alkalosis
sensible water loss
"third space" fluid
vasopressin
water intoxication

Fluid, electrolyte, and acid-base management is complex and requires an understanding of the functions and homeostatic mechanisms the body uses to maintain an optimal environment for cell function. Alterations in fluid, electrolyte, and acid-base balance are commonly seen in hospitalized patients and can affect homeostasis both acutely and chronically. If untreated these imbalances have consequences with varying degrees of severity including death. Understanding the function and regulation of fluid and electrolytes lends the ability to prevent and treat these imbalances in patients across any disease state.

The volume, composition, and distribution of body fluids have profound effects on cell function. A stable internal environment is maintained through a sophisticated network of homeostatic mechanisms, which are focused on ensuring that water intake and water loss are balanced. Protein-energy malnutrition, disease, trauma, and surgery can disrupt fluid, electrolyte, and acid-base balance and alter the composition, distribution, or amount of body fluids. Even small changes in pH, electrolyte concentrations, and fluid status can adversely affect cell function. If these derangements are not corrected, severe consequences or death can ensue.

BODY WATER

Water is the largest single component of the body. At birth, water accounts for approximately 75% to 85% of total body weight; this proportion decreases with age and adiposity. Water accounts for 60% to 70% of total body weight in the lean adult but only 45% to 55% in the obese adult. Metabolically active cells of the muscle and viscera have the highest concentration of water; calcified tissue cells have the lowest. Total body water

Portions of this chapter were written by Pamela Charney, PhD, RD

is higher in athletes than in nonathletes and decreases with age and diminished muscle mass (Figure 6-1). Although the proportion of body weight accounted for by water varies with gender, age, and body fat, there is little day-to-day variation in an individual (Cheuvront et al, 2010).

Functions

Water makes solutes available for cellular reactions, regulates body temperature, maintains blood volume, transports nutrients, and is involved with digestion, absorption, and excretion (Armstrong 2005, Whitmire 2010). Loss of 20% of body water (**dehydration**) may cause death; loss of only 10% may lead to damage to essential body systems (Figure 6-2). Even mild dehydration (loss of 1% to 2%) can lead to loss of cognitive function and alertness, an increase in heart rate, and a decrease in exercise performance (Armstrong, 2005; Maughan et al, 2007). Healthy adults can live up to 10 days without water, and children can live up to 5 days, whereas a person can survive for several weeks without food.

Distribution

Total body water (TBW) is mainly distributed in the intracellular fluid (ICF) and extracellular fluid (ECF). The transcellular fluid is comprised of 3% of TBW and is the small amount of fluid making up cerebral spinal, pericardial, and pleural fluids as well as fluid surrounding the eye (Whitmire 2008, Rhoda 2011). **ICF** is contained within cells and accounts for two thirds of total body water. ECF accounts for the remaining one third of total body water. ECF is the water and dissolved substances in the plasma, lymph, and also includes interstitial fluid (the fluid around the cells in tissues) (Kingley 2005, Lanley 2012, Whitmire 2008). While the distribution of body water varies under different circumstances, the total amount in the body remains relatively constant. Water intake of foods and beverages is balanced by water lost through urination, perspiration, feces,

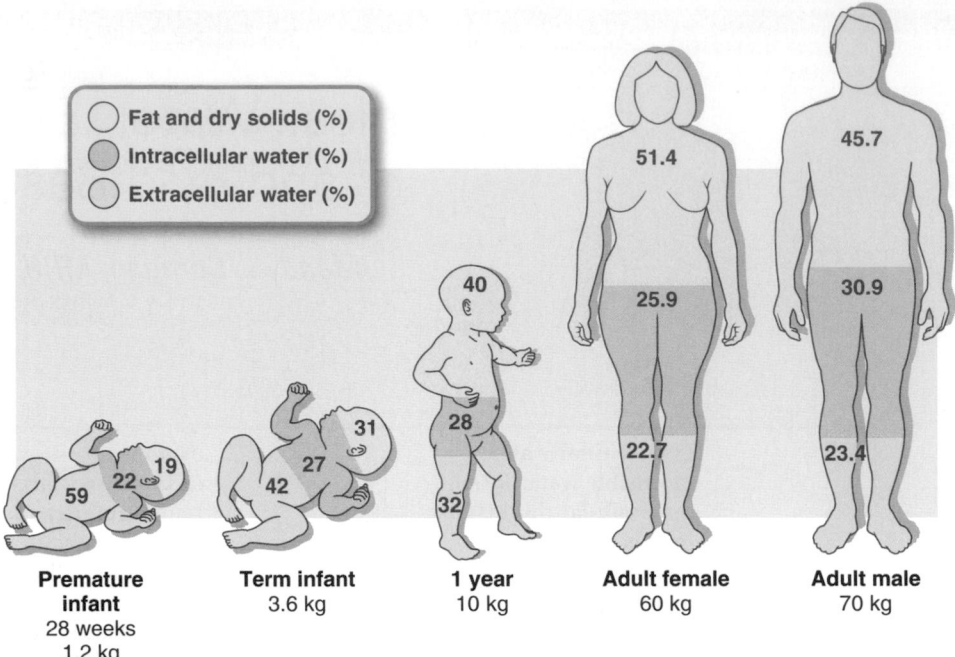

FIGURE 6-1 Distribution of body water as a percentage of body weight.

PERCENTAGE OF BODY WEIGHT LOST

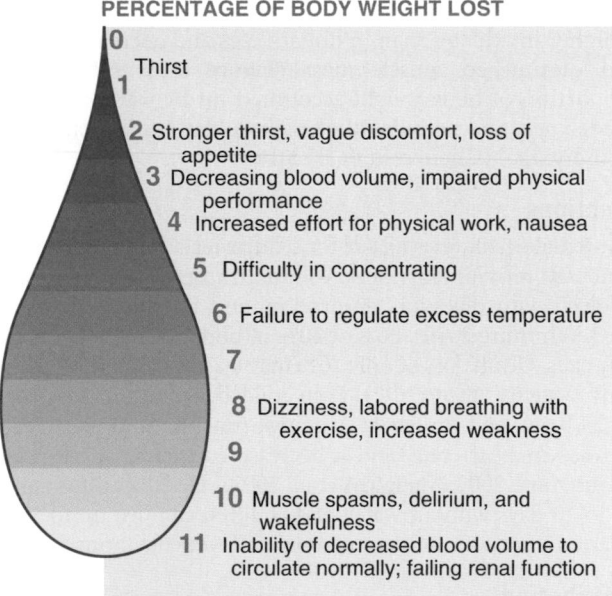

FIGURE 6-2 Adverse effects of dehydration.

CLINICAL INSIGHT

Edema

Edema is the abnormal accumulation of fluid in the "third space," including intercellular tissue spaces or body cavities. Fluid in the "third space" is isolated and therefore does not contribute to the functional duties of body water within the body. Edema is graded based on severity (grades 1, 2, 3, 4+) and can be classified as pitting or nonpitting. If pressure is applied by a finger or thumb to an area with edema, it is classified as pitting edema when an impression or "pit" remains after the finger is removed.

The causes of edema can be multifactorial and have four main causes. Circulating plasma proteins decrease as part of the acute phase response to injury or inflammation. Circulating proteins normally draw water into the vascular space, but with less circulating proteins there is a decrease in oncotic pressure (the pressure at the capillary membrane). To compound the issue, there is an increase in the permeability of the capillaries, which allows protein leaks into the interstitial space, thereby attracting more water out of the vascular space.

Edema also can occur when there is an increase in hydrostatic pressure as seen in disease states such as cirrhosis, congestive heart failure, and pulmonary edema. The force from the increased pressure pushes fluid into the interstitial space. Lymph edema is the final type and usually is localized to specific areas of the body when there is an obstruction of the lymphatic vessels. It occurs when fluid and protein cannot return to circulation, and the trapped protein-rich lymph fluid attracts water. Lymph edema can be seen in cancer patients who have had surgery for lymph node dissection.

and respiration. Edema is the abnormal accumulation of fluid in the "third space," including intercellular tissue spaces or body cavities. Fluid in the "third space" is isolated and therefore does not contribute to the functional duties of body water within the body.

Water Balance

Water movement is dictated by hydrostatic pressure, diffusion, osmosis, and active transport. Water moves in and out of the ICF and ECF based the osmolarity (ability for osmotic pressure to move fluid between compartments) to obtain equilibrium. Osmotic pressure is directly proportional to the number of particles in the solution and usually refers to the pressure at the cell membrane. The sodium-potassium adenosine triphosphatase pump (Na/K-ATPase pump) plays a key role in regulating water balance. In simple terms, osmotic pressure of the ICF is a function of its potassium content because potassium is the predominant intracellular cation. The osmotic pressure of ECF is relative to the sodium content because sodium is the major

TABLE 6-1 Content of Common Intravenous Fluids

Fluid	Dextrose (g/L)	Sodium (mEq/L)	Chloride (mEq/L)	Additional Components (mEq/L)
0.45%NaCl (half normal saline)	0	77	77	n/a
0.9%NaCl (normal saline)	0	154	154	n/a
3% Saline	0	513	513	n/a
5% Dextrose in water (D₅W)	50	0	0	n/a
D₅0.45% NaCl	50	77	77	n/a
D₅0.9% NaCl	50	154	154	n/a
10% Dextrose	100	0	0	n/a
Lactated Ringer's (LR)	0	130	109	Potassium 4 Calcium 3 Lactate 28
D₅LR	50	130	109	Potassium 4 Calcium 3 Lactate 28

extracellular cation. Although variations in the distribution of sodium and potassium ions are the principal causes of water shifts between the various fluid compartments, chloride and phosphate also are involved with water balance.

Osmolality is a measure of the osmotically active particles per kilogram of the solvent in which the particles are dispersed (Langley 2012, Whitmire 2008, Rhoda 2011). The average sum of the concentration of all the cations in serum is approximately 150 mEq/L. The cation concentration is balanced by 150 mEq/L of anions, yielding a total serum osmolality of approximately 300 mOsm/L. Osmolality or tonicity are words used interchangeably in clinical practice. Normal osmolality or tonicity is 280-300 mOsms and values above or below this range are termed hypotonic (typically a sign of water excess) or hypertonic (often a sign of water deficit).

Shifts in water balance can have adverse consequences. Homeostatic regulation by the gastrointestinal (GI) tract, kidneys, and brain keeps body water content fairly constant. In general, the amount of water intake is approximately equivalent to output each day.

Mechanisms to maintain water equilibrium come from a number of hormones including antidiuretic hormone (aka vasopressin), aldosterone, angiotensin II, cortisone, norepinephrine, and epinephrine (Kingley 2005, Rhoda 11, Whitmire 08, Whitmire 03). Increased serum osmolality or decreased blood volume lead to the release of antidiuretic hormone which signals the kidneys to conserve water. In the presence of low ECF volume, the kidneys release renin to produce angiotensin II (the renin-angiotensin system). Angiotensin II has several functions, including stimulation of vasoconstriction and the thirst centers (whitmire 2008, Langley 2012, Harrisons).

Water Intake

Thirst is regulated by the hypothalamus and controls water intake in healthy individuals. Sensitivity to thirst is decreased in older individuals, chronically or acutely ill patients, infants, and athletes leading to a higher potential for water deficits. Sources of water include fluids (oral, enteral tube feeding, parenteral fluids), food, and oxidative metabolism (Tables 6-1 and 6-2). The oxidation of foods in the body produces metabolic water as an end product. The oxidation of 100 g of fat, carbohydrate,

TABLE 6-2 Percentage of Water in Common Foods

Food	Percentage
Lettuce, iceberg	96
Celery	95
Cucumbers	95
Cabbage, raw	92
Watermelon	92
Broccoli, boiled	91
Milk, nonfat	91
Spinach	91
Green beans, boiled	89
Carrots, raw	88
Oranges	87
Cereals, cooked	85
Apples, raw, without skin	84
Grapes	81
Potatoes, boiled	77
Eggs	75
Bananas	74
Fish, haddock, baked	74
Chicken, roasted, white meat	70
Corn, boiled	65
Beef, sirloin	59
Cheese, Swiss	38
Bread, white	37
Cake, angel food	34
Butter	16
Almonds, blanched	5
Saltines	3
Sugar, white	1
Oils	0

From U.S. Department of Agriculture (USDA), Agricultural Research Service (ARS): Nutrient database for standard reference. <http://ndb.nal.usda.gov>, 2011. Accessed February 20, 2015.

or protein yields 107, 55, or 41 g of water, respectively, for a total of approximately 200 to 300 ml/day (Whitmire, 2008).

Tonicity of body fluids can be measured (serum osmolality) or estimated from the following formula:

$$\text{Osmolality (mOsms)} = (2 \times \text{Serum sodium mEq/L}) + (\text{BUN mg/dL}) + (\text{Blood glucose mg/dL})$$

CLINICAL INSIGHT

Osmotic Forces

Osmotic pressure is directly proportional to the number of particles in solution and usually refers to the pressure at the cell membrane. It is convenient (although not entirely accurate) to consider the osmotic pressure of intracellular fluid as a function of its potassium content because potassium is the predominant cation there. In contrast, the osmotic pressure of extracellular fluid may be considered relative to its sodium content because sodium is the major cation present in extracellular fluid. Although variations in the distribution of sodium and potassium ions are the principal causes of water shifts between the various fluid compartments, chloride and phosphate also influence water balance. Proteins cannot diffuse because of their size and thus also play a key role in maintaining osmotic equilibrium. **Oncotic pressure**, or **colloidal osmotic pressure**, is the pressure at the capillary membrane. It is maintained by dissolved proteins in the plasma and interstitial fluids. Oncotic pressure helps to retain water within blood vessels, preventing its leakage from plasma into the interstitial spaces. In patients with an exceptionally low plasma protein content, such as those who are under physiologic stress or have certain diseases, water leaks into the interstitial spaces, causing edema or third spacing, thus the fluid is called "third space" fluid.

Osmoles and Milliosmoles

Concentrations of individual ionic constituents of extracellular or intracellular fluids are expressed in terms of milliosmoles per liter (mOsm/L). One mole equals the gram molecular weight of a substance; when dissolved in 1 L of water, it becomes 1 osmole (osm). One milliosmole (mOsm) equals 1/1000th of an osmole. The number of milliosmoles per liter equals the number of millimoles per liter times the number of particles into which the dissolved substance dissociates. Thus 1 mmol of a nonelectrolyte (e.g., glucose) equals 1 mOsm; similarly, 1 mmol of an electrolyte containing only monovalent ions (e.g., sodium chloride [NaCl]) equals 2 mOsm. One mOsm dissolved in 1 L of water has an osmotic pressure of 17 mm Hg.

Osmolality is a measure of the osmotically active particles per kilogram of the solvent in which the particles are dispersed. It is expressed as milliosmoles of solute per kilogram of solvent (mOsm/kg). **Osmolarity** is the term formerly used to describe concentration—milliosmoles per liter of the entire solution; but osmolality is now the measurement for most clinical work. However, in reference to certain conditions such as hyperlipidemia, it makes a difference whether osmolality is stated as milliosmoles per kilogram of solvent or per liter of solution.

The average sum of the concentration of all the cations in serum is about 150 mEq/L. The cation concentration is balanced by 150 mEq/L of anions, yielding a total serum osmolality of about 300 mOsm/L. An osmolar imbalance is caused by a gain or loss of water relative to a solute. *An osmolality of less than 285 mOsm/L generally indicates a water excess; an osmolality of greater than 300 mOsm/L indicates a water deficit.*

Water Intoxication

Water intoxication occurs as a result of water intake in excess of the body's ability to excrete water. The increased **intracellular fluid** volume is accompanied by osmolar dilution. The increased volume of intracellular fluid causes the cells, particularly the brain cells, to swell, leading to headache, nausea, vomiting, muscle twitching, blindness, and convulsions with impending stupor. If left untreated, water intoxication can be fatal. Water intoxication is not commonly seen in normal, healthy individuals. It may be seen in endurance athletes who consume large amounts of electrolyte-free beverages during events, individuals with psychiatric illness, or as a result of water drinking contests (Goldman, 2009; Rogers and Hew-Butler, 2009; Adetoki 2013.)

Water Elimination

Water loss normally occurs through the kidneys as urine and through the GI tract in the feces (measurable, sensible water loss), as well as through air expired from the lungs and water vapor lost through the skin (nonmeasurable, insensible water loss). The kidney is the primary regulator of sensible water loss. Under normal conditions the kidneys have the ability to adjust to changes in body water composition by either decreasing or increasing water loss in the urine. Natural diuretics are substances in the diet that increase urinary excretion, such as alcohol and caffeine.

Insensible water loss is continuous and usually unconscious. High altitude, low humidity, and high temperatures can increase insensible fluid loss through the lungs and through sweat. Athletes can lose 3 to 4 lb from fluid loss when exercising in a temperature of 80° F and low humidity or even more at higher temperatures.

The GI tract can be a major source of water loss. Under normal conditions the water contained in the 7 to 9 L of digestive juices and other extracellular fluids secreted daily into the GI tract is reabsorbed almost entirely in the ileum and colon, except for about 100 ml that is excreted in the feces. Because this volume of reabsorbed fluid is about twice that of the blood plasma, excessive GI fluid losses through diarrhea may have serious consequences, particularly for very young and very old individuals.

Choleric diarrhea is responsible for the loss of many lives in developing countries and can be successfully corrected without intravenous fluids. Oral rehydration solution, an isotonic fluid, is a simple mixture of water, sugar, and salt is highly effective in improving hydration status (Kelly 2004). Other abnormal fluid losses may occur as a result of emesis, hemorrhage, fistula drainage, burn and wound exudates, gastric and surgical tube drainage, and the use of diuretics.

When water intake is insufficient or water loss is excessive, healthy kidneys compensate by conserving water and excreting more concentrated urine. The renal tubules increase water reabsorption in response to the hormonal action of vasopressin. However, the concentration of the urine made by the kidneys has a limit: approximately 1400 mOsm/L. Once this limit has been reached, the body loses its ability to excrete solutes. The ability of the kidneys to concentrate urine may be compromised in older individuals or in young infants, resulting in increased risk of developing dehydration or hypernatremia, especially during illness.

Signs of dehydration include headache, fatigue, decreased appetite, lightheadedness, poor skin turgor (although this may be present in well-hydrated older persons), skin tenting on the forehead, concentrated urine, decreased urine output, sunken eyes, dry mucous membranes of the mouth and nose, orthostatic blood pressure changes, and tachycardia (Armstrong, 2005). In a dehydrated person the specific gravity, a measure of the dissolved solutes in urine, increases above the normal levels of 1.008 to 1.030, and the urine becomes remarkably darker (Shirreffs, 2003).

High ambient temperature and dehydration adversely affect exercise performance; changes may be mediated by serotonergic and dopaminergic alterations in the central nervous system (Maughan et al, 2007). Fluids of appropriate composition in appropriate amounts are essential (see *Clinical Insight:* Water Requirements: When Eight Is Not Enough).

Clinical Assessment of Fluid Status

A variety of methods to estimate fluid requirements are based on age, caloric intake, and weight. Obesity has lead to challenges with using weight-based calculations for fluid requirements as water accounts for only 45% to 55% of body weight for patients with lower proportions of lean body mass. In clinical practice fluid estimations should be individualized to each patient, especially those with cardiac, liver, or renal failure, and in the presence of ongoing high-volume GI losses.

Unfortunately there is no gold standard to assess hydration status. Clinicians must carefully assess data from a variety of sources, including physical examination by the medical team, nutrition-focused physical examinations, imaging reports (e.g., identifying abnormal fluid collections within the lungs, ascites), laboratory studies, subjective report of symptoms from patients, sudden weight changes, medications, and vital signs. In clinical settings it is important to acknowledge all sources of fluid delivery (oral, enteral feeding tube, intravenous fluids, parenteral nutrition, and intravenous fluids given with medications) and all sources of fluid losses urine, diuretic medications, and GI secretions (e.g., emesis, gastric secretions, surgical drains, stool, fistulas) (Popkin et al, 2010).

CLINICAL INSIGHT

Water Requirements: When Eight is Not Enough

The body has no provision for water storage; therefore the amount of water lost every 24 hours must be replaced to maintain health and equilibrium. Under ordinary circumstances, a reasonable allowance based on recommended caloric intake is 1 ml/kcal for adults and 1.5 ml/kcal for infants. This translates into approximately 35 ml/kg of usual body weight in adults, 50 to 60 ml/kg in children, and 150 ml/kg in infants.

In most cases a suitable daily allowance for water from all sources, including foods, is approximately 3.7 L (15.5 cups) for adult males and 2.7 L (11+ cups) for adult females, depending on body size (Institute of Medicine [IOM] Food and Nutrition Board, 2004). Because solid food provides 19% of total daily fluid intake, this equals 750 ml of water or approximately 3 cups daily. When this is added to the 200 to 300 ml (about 1 cup) of water contributed by oxidative metabolism, men should consume about 11.5 cups and women need 7 cups of fluids daily. Although the annual consumption of bottled water in the United States equals about 1 cup (8 fl oz) of water daily, this volume alone is not sufficient (Campbell, 2007). Total fluid intake comes from drinking water, other liquids, and food; the AIs for water are for total daily water intake and include all dietary water sources.

Infants need more water because of the limited capacity of their kidneys to handle a large renal solute load, their higher percentage of body water, and their large surface area per unit of body weight. A lactating woman's need for water also increases, approximately 600 to 700 mL (2.5 to 3 cups) per day, for milk production.

Thirst is a less effective signal to consume water in infants, heavily exercising athletes, sick individuals, and older adults who may have a diminished thirst sensation. Anyone sick enough to be hospitalized, regardless of the diagnosis, is at risk for water and electrolyte imbalance. Older adults are particularly susceptible because of factors such as impaired renal concentrating ability, fever, diarrhea, vomiting, and a decreased ability to care for themselves. In situations involving extreme heat or excessive sweating, thirst may not keep pace with the actual water requirements of the body.

ELECTROLYTES

Electrolytes are minerals with electric charges that dissociate in a solution into positive or negatively charged ions. Electrolytes can be simple inorganic salts of sodium, potassium, or magnesium, or complex organic molecules; they play a key role in a host of normal metabolic functions (see Table 6-3). One milliequivalent (mEq) of any substance has the capacity to combine chemically with 1 mEq of a substance with an opposite charge. For univalent ions (e.g., Na^+) 1 millimole (mmol) equals 1 mEq; for divalent ions (e.g., Ca^{++}) 1 mmol equals 2 mEq (see Appendix 2 for conversion guidelines).

The major **extracellular** electrolytes are sodium, calcium, chloride, and bicarbonate. Potassium, magnesium, and phosphate are the major **intracellular** electrolytes. These elements, which exist as ions in body fluids, are distributed throughout all body fluids. Electrolytes are responsible for maintenance of physiologic body functions, cellular metabolism, neuromuscular function, and osmotic equilibrium. Although oral intake varies, the homeostatic mechanisms regulate the concentrations of electrolytes throughout the body.

Changes in either intracellular or extracellular electrolyte concentrations can have a major impact on bodily functions. The Na/K-ATPase pump closely regulates cellular electrolyte contents by actively pumping sodium out of cells in exchange for potassium. Other electrolytes follow ion gradients.

Calcium

Although approximately 99% of the body's calcium (Ca^{++}) is stored in the skeleton (bones and teeth) the remaining 1% has important physiologic functions. Ionized calcium within the vascular compartment is a cation, with a positive charge. Approximately half of the calcium found in the intravascular compartment is bound to the serum protein albumin. Thus, when serum albumin levels are low, total calcium levels decrease because of hypoalbuminemia. The corrected calcium formula, often used in renal disease, is:

$$\text{Serum calcium} + 0.8 (4 - \text{Serum albumin})$$

The binding ability of calcium and its ionized content in blood have implications for normal homeostatic mechanisms.

TABLE 6-3 Normal Electrolyte Concentration of Serum

Electrolyte	Normal Range	Location
Cations		
Sodium	136-145 mEq/L	Extracellular cation
Potassium	3.5-5 mEq/L	Intracellular cation
Calcium	4.5-5.5 mEq/L (9-11 mg/dl)	Extracellular cation
Magnesium	1.5-2.5 mEq/L (1.8-3 mg/dl)	Intracellular cation
Anions		
Chloride	96-106 mEq/L	Extracellular Anion
CO_2	24-28.8 mEq/L	Extracellular Anion
Phosphorus (inorganic)	3-4.5 mg/dl (1.9-2.85 mEq/L as HPO_4^{2-})	Intracellular Anion

Blood tests for calcium levels often measure total and ionized calcium levels. This is because ionized (or free, unbound calcium) is the active form of calcium and is not affected by hypoalbuminemia. In healthy adults, normal levels for serum total calcium are about 8.5 to 10.5 mg/dl, whereas normal levels for ionized calcium are 4.5 to 5.5 mEq/L.

Functions

Calcium serves as an extracellular cation that regulates nerve transmission, muscle contraction, bone metabolism, and blood pressure regulation and is necessary for blood clotting. Calcium is regulated by parathyroid hormone (PTH), calcitonin, vitamin D, and phosphorus. Through a complex system of regulation among multiple organs, including the kidney, GI tract, and bone, calcium absorption can be enhanced to increase calcium reabsorption to maintain homeostasis. When serum calcium levels are low, PTH causes release of calcium from the bones and stimulates increased absorption from the GI tract. Calcitonin works in the opposite direction, shutting off the release of calcium from the bone and decreasing GI absorption. Vitamin D stimulates while phosphorus inhibits calcium absorption in the GI tract.

In the setting of hypoalbuminemia, serum calcium levels are not accurate because nearly 50% of calcium is protein bound. An ionized calcium level is the most accurate assay for calcium because it is the active form and is not affected by protein levels. In healthy adults, normal levels for serum total calcium are approximately 8.5 to 10.5 mg/dl, whereas normal levels for ionized calcium are 4.5 to 5.5 mEq/L. When ionized calcium levels are not available, a simple formula may be used. The corrected calcium formula accounts for a 0.8 mg/dl decrease in calcium for each 1 g/dl decrease in serum albumin below 4 g/dl. The corrected calcium formula is

$$([4 - \text{Serum albumin (g/dL)}] \times 0.8) + \text{Measured calcium (mg/dL)}$$

Ionized calcium levels are altered inversely by changes in acid-base balance; as serum pH rises, calcium binds with protein, leading to decreased ionized calcium levels. As pH is lowered, the opposite occurs. Because calcium has an important role in cardiac, nervous system, and skeletal muscle function, hypocalcemia and hypercalcemia can become life threatening.

Common causes of hypercalcemia are cancer with the presence of bone metastases or hyperparathyroidism, when there is a large amount of calcium moved into the ECF. Symptoms of hypercalcemia include lethargy, nausea, vomiting, muscle weakness, and depression. Treatment usually is directed at treating the underlying cause of the problem, discontinuation of calcium containing medications, and increasing the excretion of calcium though the kidneys (by delivery of intravenous fluids followed by diuretic medications).

Hypocalcemia often is marked with numbness or tingling, hyperactive reflexes, tetany, lethargy, muscle weakness, confusion, and seizures. Causes of hypocalcemia include low serum phosphorus or magnesium levels, medications that cause calcium losses, hypoalbuminemia, vitamin D deficiency, or hypoparathyroidism. Oral calcium supplements are most often the first-line therapy in the absence of symptoms. Because other hormones, electrolytes, and vitamins are involved in calcium regulation, these are assessed in the setting of true hypocalcemia. Low phosphorus and magnesium levels must be repleted before calcium levels can be corrected (Rhoda, 2011).

Absorption and Excretion

Approximately 20% to 60% of dietary calcium is absorbed and is tightly regulated because of the need to maintain steady serum calcium levels in the face of fluctuating intake. The ileum is the most important site of calcium absorption. Calcium is absorbed via passive transport and through a vitamin D–regulated transport system.

The kidney is the main site of calcium excretion. The majority of serum calcium is bound to proteins and not filtered by the kidneys; only about 100 to 200 mg is excreted in the urine in normal adults.

Sources

Dairy products are the main source of calcium in the American diet, with some green vegetables, nuts, canned fish including bones, and calcium-enriched tofu having moderate amounts of calcium. Food manufacturers fortify many foods with additional calcium that may have some bioavailability.

Recommended Intakes

Recommended intakes of calcium range from 1000 to 1300 mg/day, depending on age and gender. An upper limit for calcium intake has been estimated to be approximately 2500 to 3000 mg/day (see inside cover).

Sodium

Sodium (Na^+) is the major cation of extracellular fluid with a normal range of 135 to 145 mEq/L. Secretions such as bile and pancreatic juice contain substantial amounts of sodium. Gastric secretions and diarrhea also contain sodium, but contrary to common belief sweat is hypotonic and contains a relatively small amount of sodium. Approximately 35% to 40% of the total body sodium is in the skeleton and the remainder is in body fluids.

Functions

As the predominant ion of the extracellular fluid, sodium thus regulates extracellular and plasma volume. Sodium is also important in neuromuscular function and maintenance of acid-base balance. Maintenance of serum sodium levels is vital, because severe hyponatremia can lead to seizures, coma, and death.

Extracellular sodium concentrations are much higher than intracellular levels (normal serum sodium is around 135 mEq/L, whereas intracellular levels are around 10 mEq/L). The sodium-potassium ATP pump is an active transport system that works to keep sodium outside the cell through exchange with potassium. The sodium-potassium ATP pump requires carriers for sodium and potassium along with energy for proper function. Exportation of sodium from the cell is the driving force for facilitated transporters, which import glucose, amino acids, and other nutrients into the cells.

Hyponatremia. Assessing hyponatremia or hypernatremia takes into consideration sodium's role in regulating fluid balance and requires evaluation of overall hydration status. Hyponatremia is one of the most common electrolyte disorders among hospitalized patients and occurs in 25% of inpatients. When hyponatremia is below 125 mEq/L, symptoms generally become apparent. Patients may display signs of headache, lethargy, restlessness, decreased reflexes, seizures, or coma in extreme cases. There are three basic causes for hyponatremia. Hypertonic hyponatremia is due to excess delivery of mannitol or hyperglycemia, which causes serum sodium to increase by

1.6 mEq for every 100 mg/dl rise in serum glucose. Isotonic hyponatremia occurs in the presence of hyperlipidemia or hyperprotenemia, because the aqueous component that sodium is dissolved in results in a falsely low value (this is mainly a laboratory artifact and is not often seen in clinical practice). The final type is hypotonic hyponatremia. Evaluation depends on fluid status to evaluate the three subtypes.

Isovolemic hyponatremia can be caused by malignancies, adrenal insufficiency, or the syndrome of inappropriate antidiuretic hormone secretion (SIADH). SIADH can result from central nervous system disorders, pulmonary disorders, tumors, and certain medications. The treatment is usually water restriction. Hypervolemic hypotonic hyponatremia is characterized by excess TBW and sodium (overall higher excess water than sodium) because of reduced excretion of water or excess free water administration. Cardiac, renal, or hepatic failure is often a contributing factor, and patients have edema or ascites on physical examination. The treatment is fluid restriction or diuretics to aid in decreasing TBW, and oral sodium restriction also may be beneficial. The final type is hypovolemic hypotonic hyponatremia, characterized by a deficit in TBW and sodium that requires treatment with fluid replacement. Often fluid losses leading to hypovolemia hyponatremia include excessive vomiting, excessive sweating (marathon athletes), diarrhea, wound drainage/burns, high-volume gastrointestinal secretions, or excessive diuretic use. Equations to calculate fluid deficits can be used to replace half of the fluid deficit in the first 24 hours. Correcting sodium levels must be done slowly (max of 8 to 12 mEq in 24 hours) to prevent osmotic demyelinating syndrome that is seen with rapid correction (Rhoda et al, 2011).

Hypernatremia. A serum sodium level greater than 145 mEq/L is classified as hypernatremia, and there are various types. Hypovolemic hypernatremia is caused by a loss of sodium and TBW when water losses exceed sodium losses. It is important to identify the cause of the fluid losses so that they can be corrected and prevented in the future. The treatment is to slowly replace fluid volume with a hypotonic fluid solution. Hypervolemic hypernatremia is caused by excessive intake of sodium resulting in higher sodium gain than water gains. The treatment is to restrict sodium (especially in intravenous fluids) and possibly the use of diuretics. Isovolemic hypernatremia is seen with disease states such as diabetes insipidus. Signs of hypernatremia include lethargy, thirst, hyperreflexia, seizures, coma, or death. Formulas for calculating a water deficit are helpful to guide fluid replacement. Free water deficit is calculated as follows (Kingley, 2005):

$$[0.6 \times \text{Weight (kg)}] \times 1 - [140 / \text{Na mEq/L}]$$

Absorption and Excretion

Sodium is absorbed readily from the intestine and carried to the kidneys, where it is filtered and returned to the blood to maintain appropriate levels. The amount absorbed is proportional to the intake in healthy adults.

About 90% to 95% of normal body sodium loss is through the urine; the rest is lost in feces and sweat. Normally the quantity of sodium excreted daily is equal to the amount ingested. Sodium excretion is maintained by a mechanism involving the glomerular filtration rate, the cells of the juxtaglomerular apparatus of the kidneys, the renin-angiotensin-aldosterone system, the sympathetic nervous system, circulating catecholamines, and blood pressure.

Sodium balance is regulated in part by aldosterone, a mineralocorticoid secreted by the adrenal cortex. When blood sodium levels rise, the thirst receptors in the hypothalamus stimulate the thirst sensation. Ingestion of fluids returns sodium levels to normal. Under certain circumstances sodium and fluid regulation can be disrupted, resulting in abnormal blood sodium levels. The syndrome of inappropriate antidiuretic hormone secretion (SIADH) is characterized by concentrated, low-volume urine and dilutional hyponatremia as water is retained. SIADH can result from central nervous system disorders, pulmonary disorders, tumors, and certain medications.

Estrogen, which is slightly similar to aldosterone, also causes sodium and water retention. Changes in water and sodium balance during the menstrual cycle, during pregnancy, and while taking oral contraceptives are attributable partially to changes in progesterone and estrogen levels.

Dietary Reference Intake

The dietary reference intakes (DRI) give an upper limit of 2.3 g of sodium per day (or 5.8 g sodium chloride per day). The mean daily salt intake in Western societies is approximately 10 to 12 g (4 to 5 g of sodium), which is in excess of the adequate intake for sodium of 1.2 to 1.5 g per day, depending on age, with lower amounts recommended for the elderly (see Table 6-4).

Healthy kidneys are usually able to excrete excess sodium intake; however, persistent excessive sodium intake has been implicated in development of hypertension. In addition to its role in hypertension, excessive salt intake has been associated with increased urinary calcium excretion, kidney stones, and some cases of osteoporosis (Teucher 2003; He 2010, Caudarella et al, 2009). Higher sodium consumption has been associated with higher weight status, and a positive relationship has been observed between sodium intake and obesity independent of energy intake (Song et al, 2013; Yoon 2013; Zhu 2014). In addition, a positive association has been identified between sodium intake and increased circulation of leptin (secreted by fat cells and influences inflammatory response and sodium excretion) and tumor necrosis factor alpha (plays a role in inflammation) (Zhu et al, 2014).

Sources

The major source of sodium is sodium chloride, or common table salt, of which sodium constitutes 40% by weight. Protein foods generally contain more naturally existing sodium than do

TABLE 6-4	**Dietary Reference Intakes for Sodium, Potassium, and Chloride Daily Intake**			
Age	Sodium	Potassium	Chloride	Salt (Sodium Chloride)
Adult 19-49	1.5 g (65 mmol)	4.7 g (120 mmol)	2.3 g (65 mmol)	3.8 g (65 mmol)
Adult 50-70	1.3 g (55 mmol)	4.7 g (120 mmol)	2.0 g (55 mmol)	3.2 g (55 mmol)
Adult 71	1.2 g (50 mmol)	4.7 g (120 mmol)	1.8 g (50 mmol)	2.9 g (50 mmol)
UL	2.3 g (100 mmol)	n/a	3.6 g (100 mmol)	na

Institute of Medicine, Food and Nutrition Board: *Dietary reference intakes for water, potassium, sodium, chloride, and sulfate,* Washington, DC, 2004, National Academies Press.
UL, Tolerable upper intake level.

vegetables and grains, whereas fruits contain little or none. The addition of table salt, flavored salts, flavor enhancers, and preservatives during food processing accounts for the high sodium content of most convenience and fast-food products. For instance ½ cup of frozen vegetables prepared without salt contains 10 mg of sodium, whereas ½ cup of canned vegetables contains approximately 260 mg of sodium. Similarly, 1 ounce of plain meat contains 30 mg of sodium, whereas 1 ounce of luncheon meat contains approximately 400 mg of sodium. The larger portion sizes offered by dining establishments to consumers are increasing the sodium intake even more.

Magnesium

Magnesium is the second most prevalent intracellular cation. Approximately half of the body's magnesium is located in bone, whereas another 45% resides in soft tissue; only 1% of the body's magnesium content is in the extracellular fluids. Normal serum magnesium levels are about 1.6 to 2.5 mEq/L; however, about 70% of serum magnesium is free or ionized. The remainder is bound to proteins and is not active.

Function

Magnesium (Mg^{2+}) is an important cofactor in many enzymatic reactions in the body and is also important in bone metabolism as well as central nervous system and cardiovascular function. Many of the enzyme systems regulated by magnesium are involved in nutrient metabolism and nucleic acid synthesis, leading to the body's need to carefully regulate magnesium status.

As with calcium, severe hypo- or hypermagnesemia can have life-threatening sequelae. Physical symptoms of magnesium abnormalities are similar to those observed with other electrolyte deficiencies, and the challenges with serum measurements discussed earlier make assessment of magnesium status difficult. Symptoms of hypomagnesemia include muscle weakness, tetany, ataxia, nystagmus, and in severe cases ventricular arrhythmia. Frequent causes of hypomagnesemia include excessive stool losses (as seen in short bowel syndrome or malabsorption), inadequate magnesium in the diet (oral, enteral, or parenteral nutrition), intracellular shifts during refeeding syndrome, acute pancreatitis, burns, alcoholism, diabetic ketoacidosis, and medications causing increased magnesium losses via the urine. Longterm use of proton pump inhibitors also may be a rare cause.

Often hypomagnesemia is treated with oral supplementation if no physical symptoms are noted. However, dietitians should monitor cautiously for diarrhea with oral magnesium supplements if they are not given in divided doses (such as magnesium oxide), which often can increase magnesium losses through the stool. Increased losses through the stool is avoided with supplementation from salts such as magnesium gluconate or magnesium lactate. Intravenous repletion with magnesium is required with symptomatic signs of deficiency or if serum levels are below 1 mg/dl.

Hypermagnesemia, a serum value greater than 2.5 mg/dl, can be due to excess supplementation or magnesium containing-medications, severe acidosis, or dehydration. Treatment options include omission of magnesium-containing medications and correction of the fluid imbalance.

Absorption/Excretion

Approximately 30-50% of magnesium ingested from the diet is absorbed (within the jejunum and ileum though passive and active transport mechanisms). Magnesium is regulated by the intestine, kidney, and bone. Magnesium absorption is regulated to maintain serum levels; if levels drop, more is absorbed and if levels increase, less is absorbed. The kidney is the major regulator of magnesium excretion, but some magnesium is also lost via the stool. As magnesium is a cofactor for the Na-K ATPase pump, low magnesium levels should be evaluated and corrected especially when hypokalemia is refractory to repletion. Additionally, the kidneys increase potassium excretion in light of hypomagnesemia (Kraft, Langley 2012, Rhoda 2011).

Sources

Magnesium is found in a variety of foods, making an isolated magnesium deficiency unlikely in otherwise healthy individuals. Highly processed foods tend to have lower magnesium content, whereas green leafy vegetables, legumes, and whole grains are thought to be good sources. The high magnesium content of vegetables helps to alleviate some concerns about the potential for phytate binding. Intakes of magnesium, potassium, fruits, and vegetables have been associated with higher alkaline status and a subsequent beneficial effect on bone health; enhanced mineral-water consumption may be an easy, inexpensive way to reduce the onset of osteoporosis (Wynn et al, 2010).

Dietary Reference Intakes

The recommended intake of magnesium ranges from 310 to 420 mg/day, depending on age and gender (see inside cover).

Phosphorus

Phosphorus is the primary intracellular anion and its role in adenosine triphosphate (ATP) is vital in energy metabolism. In addition, phosphorus is important in bone metabolism. About 80% of the body's phosphorus is found in bones. Normal levels for serum phosphorus are between 2.4 and 4.6 mg/dl.

Functions

Large amounts of free energy are released when the phosphate bonds in ATP are split. In addition to this role, phosphorus is vital for cellular function in phosphorylation and dephosphorylation reactions, as a buffer in acid-base balance, and in cellular structure as part of the phospholipid membrane. Because of the vital role that phosphorus plays in energy production, severe hypophosphatemia can be a life-threatening event. This is seen most often clinically in refeeding syndrome and occurs with the increased use of phosphorus for the phosphorylation of glucose (Skipper, 2012; Rhoda 2011; Kraft 2005). In addition to intracellular shifts, hypophosphatemia can be medication related (insulin, epinephrine, dopamine, erythropoietin, phosphorus-binding medications). Severe and symptomatic hypophosphatemia (<1 mg/dl) can be critical and includes impaired cardiac function, reduced contractions of the diaphragm leading to a weakened respiratory state, confusion, reduced oxygen delivery to tissues, coma, and even death.

Absorption and Excretion

Phosphorus absorption is dependent on serum levels and vitamin D status. Around 80% of phosphorus intake is absorbed in the small bowel when hypophosphatemia is present. The kidney is the major site of phosphorus excretion and regulates phosphorus absorption based on parathyroid hormone and acid base status. Phosphorus absorption decreases when vitamin D deficiency occurs or with certain medications that bind phosphorus (certain antacids or phosphate binders used in patients with chronic kidney disease).

Sources

Phosphorus is found mainly in animal products, including meats and milk; some dried beans are also good sources.

Dietary Reference Intakes

The recommended intake of phosphorus is approximately 700 mg per day, depending on age and gender, with an upper limit of 3500 to 4000 mg (see inside cover).

Potassium

With approximately 98% of Potassium (K^+) in the intracellular space, K^+ is the major cation of intracellular fluid. The normal serum potassium concentration is 3.5 to 5 mEq/L.

Functions

With sodium, potassium is involved in maintaining a normal water balance, osmotic equilibrium, and acid-base balance. In addition to calcium, K^+ is important in the regulation of neuromuscular activity. Concentrations of sodium and potassium determine membrane potentials in nerves and muscle. Potassium also promotes cellular growth. The potassium content of muscle is related to muscle mass and glycogen storage; therefore, if muscle is being formed, an adequate supply of potassium is essential. Potassium has an integral role in the Na/K-ATPase pump.

Hypokalemia and hyperkalemia can have devastating cardiac implications. When hypokalemia is less than 3 mEq/L, symptoms are more apparent and critical. Symptoms of hypokalemia include muscle weakness, cramping in the extremities, vomiting, and weakness. Clinically, hypokalemia occurs with large volume losses of gastrointestinal fluids that contain potassium, insulin delivery, excessive losses through the urine caused by certain medications (diuretics), and diabetic ketoacidosis. Guidelines exist for the treatment of hypokalemia (oral or intravenous medications) and are adjusted in renal impairment because potassium is excreted by the kidneys.

Hyperkalemia can be critical, especially when levels exceed 6.5 mEq/L and are accompanied by symptoms of muscle weakness, paralysis, respiratory failure, and arrhythmias/ECG changes. Causes of hyperkalemia in a clinical setting include hemolysis causing falsely elevated laboratory results, kidney disease impairing K^+ excretion, medications such as potassium-sparing diuretics, gastrointestinal hemorrhage, rhabdomyolysis, catabolism, metabolic acidosis, or overzealous K^+ supplementation.

Absorption and Excretion

Potassium is absorbed readily from the small intestine. Approximately 80% to 90% of ingested potassium is excreted in the urine; the remainder is lost in the feces. The kidneys maintain normal serum levels through their ability to filter, reabsorb, and excrete potassium under the influence of aldosterone. In the setting of hypokalemia, aldosterone secretions are lower and the kidneys shifts to reabsorb potassium and excrete sodium.

Sources

Potassium-rich food sources include fruits, vegetables, fresh meat, and dairy products. Salt substitutes commonly contain potassium. Box 6-1 categorizes select foods according to their potassium content. When evaluating potassium sources and losses, clinicians must consider other nonfood sources of potassium, such as intravenous fluids with added potassium, certain medications containing potassium, and medications that may cause the body to excrete potassium.

Dietary Reference Intakes

The adequate intake level for potassium for adults is 4700 mg per day. No upper limit has been set. Potassium intake is inadequate in a large number of Americans, as many as 50% of adults. The reason for the poor potassium intakes is simply inadequate consumption of fruits and vegetables. Insufficient potassium intakes have been linked to hypertension and cardiac arrhythmia.

ACID-BASE BALANCE

An acid is any substance that tends to release hydrogen ions in solution, whereas a base is any substance that tends to accept hydrogen ions in solution. The hydrogen ion concentration [H^+] determines acidity. Because the magnitude of hydrogen ion concentration is small compared with that of other serum electrolytes, acidity is expressed more readily in terms of pH units. A low blood pH indicates a higher hydrogen ion concentration and greater acidity, whereas a high pH value indicates a lower hydrogen ion concentration and greater alkalinity.

Acid-base balance is the dynamic equilibrium state of hydrogen ion concentration. Maintaining the arterial blood pH level within the normal range of 7.35 to 7.45 is crucial for many physiologic functions and biochemical reactions. Regulatory mechanisms of the kidneys, lungs, and buffering systems enable the body to maintain the blood pH level despite the enormous acid load from food consumption and tissue metabolism. A disruption of the acid-base balance occurs when acid or base losses or gains exceed the body's regulatory capabilities or when normal regulatory mechanisms become ineffective. These regulatory disturbances may develop in association with certain diseases, toxin ingestion, shifts in fluid status, and certain medical and surgical treatments (Table 6-5). If a disrupted acid-base balance is left untreated, multiple detrimental effects ranging from electrolyte abnormalities to death can ensue.

Acid Generation

The body produces a large amount of acids daily though routine processes such as metabolism and oxidation of food, endogenous production of acid from tissue metabolism, and ingestion of acid precursors. The main acid is carbon dioxide (CO_2), termed a volatile acid, which is produced from the oxidation of carbohydrates, amino acids, and fat. Nonvolatile or fixed acids, including phosphoric and sulfuric acids, are produced from the metabolism of phosphate-containing compounds to form phosphates and phosphoric acid and sulfur-containing amino acids (such as the metabolism of methionine and cystine). Organic acids, such as lactic, uric, and keto acids, come from the incomplete metabolism of carbohydrates and fats. These organic acids typically accumulate only during exercise, acute illness, or fasting. Under normal conditions, the body is able to maintain normal acid-base status through a wide range of acid intake from foods.

Regulation

Various regulatory mechanisms maintain the pH level within very narrow physiologic limits. At the cellular level, **buffer**

BOX 6-1   Classification of Select Foods by Potassium Content

Low (0-100 mg/serving)*	Medium (100-200 mg/serving)*	High (200-300 mg/serving)*	Very High (>300 mg/serving)*
Fruits	Fruits	Fruits	Fruits
Applesauce	Apple, 1 small	Apricots, canned	Avocados, ¼ small
Blueberries	Apple juice	Grapefruit juice	Banana, 1 small
Cranberries	Apricot nectar	Kiwi, ½ medium	Cantaloupe, ¼ small
Lemon, ½ medium	Blackberries	Nectarine, 1 small	Dried fruit, ¼ cup
Lime, ½ medium	Cherries, 12 small	Orange, 1 small	Honeydew melon, ⅛ small
Pears, canned	Fruit cocktail	Orange juice	Mango, 1 medium
Pear nectar	Grape juice	Peach, fresh, 1 medium	Papaya, ½ medium
Peach nectar	Grapefruit, ½ small	Pear, fresh, 1 medium	Prune juice
Vegetables	Grapes, 12 small	Vegetables	Vegetables
Cabbage, raw	Mandarin oranges	Asparagus, fresh, cooked, 4	Artichoke, 1 medium
Cucumber slices	Peaches, canned	spears	Bamboo shoots, fresh
Green beans, frozen	Pineapple, canned	Beets, fresh, cooked	Beet greens, ¼ cup
Leeks	Plum, 1 small	Brussels sprouts	Corn on the cob, 1 ear
Lettuce, iceberg, 1 cup	Raspberries	Kohlrabi	Chinese cabbage, cooked
Water chestnuts, canned	Rhubarb	Mushrooms, cooked	Dried beans
Bamboo shoots canned	Strawberries	Okra	Potatoes, baked, ½ medium
	Tangerine, 1 small	Parsnips	Potatoes, French fries, 1 oz
	Watermelon, 1 cup	Potatoes, boiled or mashed	Spinach
	Vegetables	Pumpkin	Sweet potatoes, yams
	Asparagus, frozen	Rutabagas	Swiss chard, ¼ cup
	Beets, canned	Miscellaneous	Tomato, fresh, sauce, or juice; tomato
	Broccoli, frozen	Granola	paste, 2 tbsp
	Cabbage, cooked	Nuts and seeds, 1 oz	Winter squash
	Carrots	Peanut butter, 2 tbsp	Miscellaneous
	Cauliflower, frozen	Chocolate, 1.5-oz bar	Bouillon, low sodium, 1 cup
	Celery, 1 stalk		Cappuccino, 1 cup
	Corn, frozen		Chili, 4 oz
	Eggplant		Coconut, 1 cup
	Green beans, fresh, raw		Lasagna, 8 oz
	Mushrooms, fresh, raw		Milk, chocolate milk, 1 cup
	Onions		Milkshakes, 1 cup
	Peas		Molasses, 1 tbsp
	Radishes		Pizza, 2 slices
	Turnips		Salt substitutes, ¼ tsp
	Zucchini, summer squash		Soy milk, 1 cup
			Spaghetti, 1 cup
			Yogurt, 6 oz

*One serving equals ½ cup unless otherwise specified.

TABLE 6-5   Four Major Acid-Base Imbalances

Acid-base Imbalance	pH	Primary Disturbance	Compensation	Possible Causes
Respiratory				
Respiratory acidosis	Low	Increased pCO_2	Increased renal net acid excretion with resulting increase in serum bicarbonate	Emphysema; COPD; neuromuscular disease where respiratory function is impaired; excessive retention of CO_2
Respiratory alkalosis	High	Decreased pCO_2	Decreased renal net acid excretion with resulting decrease in serum bicarbonate	Heart failure, pregnancy, sepsis, meningitis, anxiety, pain, excessive expiration of CO_2
Metabolic				
Metabolic acidosis	Low	Decreased HCO_3^-	Hyperventilation with resulting low pCO_2	Diarrhea; uremia; ketoacidosis from uncontrolled diabetes mellitus; starvation; high-fat, low-carbohydrate diet; drugs, alcoholism, kidney disease
Metabolic alkalosis	High	Increased HCO_3^-	Hypoventilation with resulting increase in pCO_2	Diuretics use; increased ingestion of alkali; loss of chloride; vomiting/nasogastric tube suction

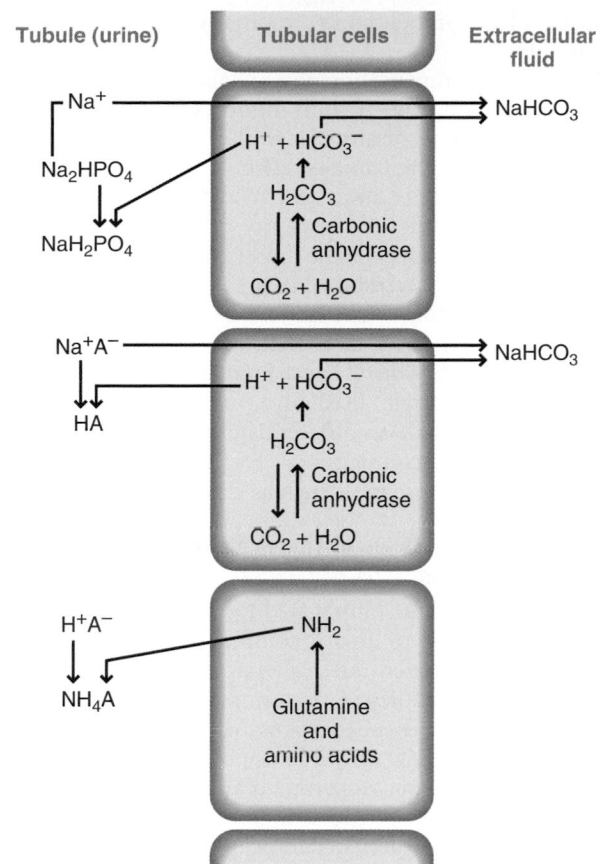

Tubule (urine)   Tubular cells   Extracellular fluid

FIGURE 6-3 Generation of NaHCO$_3$ and clearance of H$^+$ by the three buffer systems that function in the kidney. *HA,* Any acid in the body.

TABLE 6-6 Normal Arterial Blood Gas Values	
Clinical Test	**ABG Value**
pH	7.35-7.45
pCO$_2$	35-45 mm Hg
pO$_2$	80-100 mm Hg
HCO$_3$– (bicarbonate)	22-26 mEq/L
O$_2$ saturation	>95%

ABG, Arterial blood gas.

systems composed of weak acids or bases and their corresponding salts minimize the effect on pH of the addition of a strong acid or base. The buffering effect involves formation of a weaker acid or base in an amount equivalent to the strong acid or base that has been added to the system (Figure 6-3).

Proteins and phosphates are the primary intracellular buffers, whereas the bicarbonate and carbonic acid system is the primary extracellular buffer. The acid-base balance also is maintained by the kidneys and lungs. The kidneys regulate hydrogen ion (H$^+$) secretion and bicarbonate resorption. The kidneys regulate the pH of the urine by excreting H$^+$ or HCO$_3^-$ and can make bicarbonate. The kidneys are the slowest responding mechanism to maintain acid-base balance. The lungs control H$^+$ through the amount of CO$_2$ that is exhaled. When more CO$_2$ is exhaled, it reduces the H$^+$ concentration in the body. The respiratory system responds quickly to alter either the depth or rate of air movement in the lungs.

ACID-BASE DISORDERS

Acid-base disorders can be differentiated based on whether they have metabolic or respiratory causes. The evaluation of acid-base status requires analysis of serum electrolytes and arterial blood gas (ABG) values (Table 6-6). There are four main acid-base abnormalities: metabolic acidosis, metabolic alkalosis, respiratory acidosis and respiratory alkalosis. It is important to

characterize the type of acid-base disorder because this will dictate the treatment and response or "compensation" mechanism enacted by the body. Metabolic acid-base imbalances result in changes in bicarbonate (i.e., base) levels, which are reflected in the total carbon dioxide (TCO$_2$) portion of the electrolyte profile. TCO$_2$ includes bicarbonate (HCO$_3^-$), carbonic acid (H$_2$CO$_3$) and dissolved carbon dioxide; however, all but 1 to 3 mEq/L is in the form of bicarbonate. Thus, for ease of interpretation, TCO$_2$ should be equated with bicarbonate. Respiratory acid-base imbalances result in changes in the partial pressure of dissolved carbon dioxide (pCO$_2$). This is reported in the arterial blood gas values in addition to the pH, which reflects the overall acid-base status.

Metabolic Acidosis

Metabolic acidosis results from increased production or accumulation of acids or loss of base (i.e., bicarbonate) in the extracellular fluids. Simple, acute metabolic acidosis results in a low blood pH (or acidemia), low HCO$_3^-$ and normal pCO$_2$. Examples of metabolic acidosis include diabetic ketoacidosis, lactic acidosis, toxin ingestion, uremia, and excessive bicarbonate loss via the kidneys or intestinal tract. Multiple deaths previously have been attributed to lactic acidosis caused by administration of parenteral nutrition devoid of thiamin. In patients with metabolic acidosis, the anion gap is calculated to help determine cause and appropriate treatment. An anion gap is the measurement of the interval between the sum of "routinely measured" cations minus the sum of the "routinely measured" anions in the blood. The anion gap is

$$(Na^+ + K^+) - (Cl^- + HCO_3–)$$

where Na$^+$is sodium, K$^+$ is potassium, Cl$^-$ is chloride, and HCO$_3$– is bicarbonate. Normal is 12 to 14 mEq/L.

Anion gap metabolic acidosis occurs when a decrease in bicarbonate concentration is balanced by increased acid anions other than chloride. This causes the calculated anion gap to exceed the normal range of 12 to 14 mEq/L. This normochloremic metabolic acidosis may develop in association with the following conditions, represented by the acronym *MUD PILES* (Wilson, 2003):

Methanol ingestion	Paraldehyde ingestion
Uremia	Iatrogenic
Diabetic ketoacidosis	Lactic acidosis
	Ethylene glycol or ethanol ingestion
	Salicylate intoxication

Nongap metabolic acidosis occurs when a decrease in bicarbonate concentration is balanced by an increase in chloride concentration, resulting in a normal anion gap. This hyperchloremic metabolic acidosis may develop in association with the following, represented by the acronym *USED CARP* (Wilson, 2003):

Ureterosigmoidostomy *Carbonic anhydrase inhibitor*
Small bowel fistula *Adrenal insufficiency*
Extra chloride ingestion *Renal tubular acidosis*
Diarrhea *Pancreatic fistula*

Metabolic Alkalosis

Metabolic alkalosis results from the administration or accumulation of bicarbonate (i.e., base) or its precursors, excessive loss of acid (e.g., during gastric suctioning), or loss of extracellular fluid containing more chloride than bicarbonate (e.g., from villous adenoma or diuretic use). Simple, acute metabolic alkalosis results in a high blood pH, or alkalemia. Metabolic alkalosis also may result from volume depletion; decreased blood flow to the kidneys stimulates reabsorption of sodium and water, increasing bicarbonate reabsorption. This condition is known as contraction alkalosis. Alkalosis also can result from severe hypokalemia (serum potassium concentration <2 mEq/L). As potassium moves from the intracellular to the extracellular fluid, hydrogen ions move from the extracellular to the intracellular fluid to maintain electroneutrality. This process produces intracellular acidosis, which increases hydrogen ion excretion and bicarbonate reabsorption by the kidneys.

Respiratory Acidosis

Respiratory acidosis is caused by decreased ventilation and consequent carbon dioxide retention. Simple, acute respiratory acidosis results in a low pH, normal HCO_3^- and elevated pCO_2. Acute respiratory acidosis can occur as a result of sleep apnea, asthma, aspiration of a foreign object, or acute respiratory distress syndrome (ARDS). Chronic respiratory acidosis is associated with obesity hypoventilation syndrome, chronic obstructive pulmonary disease (COPD) or emphysema, certain neuromuscular diseases, and starvation cachexia. Prevention of overfeeding is prudent as it can worsen acidosis (Ayers 2012).

Respiratory Alkalosis

Respiratory alkalosis results from increased ventilation and elimination of carbon dioxide. The condition may be mediated centrally (e.g., from head injury, pain, anxiety, cerebrovascular accident, or tumors) or by peripheral stimulation (e.g., from pneumonia, hypoxemia, high altitudes, pulmonary embolism, congestive heart failure, or interstitial lung disease). Simple, acute respiratory alkalosis results in a high pH, (or alkalemia), normal HCO^{3-}, and decreased pCO_2.

Compensation

When an acid-base imbalance occurs, the body attempts to restore the normal pH by developing an opposite acid-base imbalance to offset the effects of the primary disorder, a response known as compensation. For example, the kidneys of a patient with a primary respiratory acidosis (decreased pH) compensate by increasing bicarbonate reabsorption, thereby creating a metabolic alkalosis. This response helps to increase the pH. Similarly, in response to a primary metabolic acidosis (decreased pH), the lungs compensate by increasing ventilation and carbon dioxide elimination, thereby creating a respiratory alkalosis. This compensatory respiratory alkalosis helps to increase pH.

Respiratory compensation for metabolic acid-base disturbances occurs quickly—within minutes. In contrast, renal compensation for respiratory acid-base imbalances may take 3 to 5 days to be maximally effective (Ayers et al, 2015). Compensation does not always occur; and when it does, it is not completely successful (i.e., does not result in a pH of 7.4). The pH level still reflects the underlying primary disorder. Clinicians must distinguish between primary disturbances and compensatory responses because treatment always is directed toward the primary acid-base disturbance and its underlying cause. As the primary disturbance is treated, the compensatory response corrects itself. Predictive values for compensatory responses are available to differentiate between primary acid-base imbalances and compensatory responses (Whitmire 2002). Clinicians also may use tools such as clinical algorithms.

Acid Base Balance: Rules of Thumb and Applications to Dietetics Practice

Acid-base balance is a complicated topic that requires a high-level understanding of many complex processes. Table 6-5 displays the anticipated ABG alterations and compensation mechanisms. A few rules of thumb may be helpful to understanding this topic. In uncompensated and simple acid base disorders, pH and pCO_2 move in opposite directions in respiratory disorders. In uncompensated and simple acid base disorders, pH and HCO_3^- move in the same direction. When mixed acid base disorders occur, pCO_2 and HCO_3^- generally move in opposite directions. Regardless of the disorder, the medical team directs the treatment at the underlying cause and uses supporting information from the medical history, current clinical condition, medications, laboratory values, intake and output records, and physical examination to determine the cause. Dietetics professionals play an important role in understanding the physiologic process and how it relates to regulation of electrolyte and fluid balance. Adjustments to the nutrition care plan related to acid-base balance can include shifting chloride and acetate salts in Parenteral Nutrition, manipulation of macronutrients to prevent overfeeding, or adjustments in fluid and electrolytes.

USEFUL WEBSITES, TOOLS/CALCULATORS, AND APPS

Interactive DRI (Healthcare Professional site)
http://fnic.nal.usda.gov/fnic/interactiveDRI/
Tools and Calculators
www.medcalc.com
http://www.medcalc.com/acidbase.html
iTunes Apps
KalcuLytes
Electrolytes Calc
Lytes
Dysnatremia
MedCalcPro
Acid Base Calculator
ABG Stat
Merck Manual, Professional Edition ($)

REFERENCES

Adetoki A, Evans R, Cassidy G: Polydipsia with water intoxication in treatment resistant schizophrenia, *Progress in Neurology & Psychiatry* 3:20, 2013.

Adrogu HJ, Madias NE: Hyponatremia, *New Engl J Med* 342:1581, 2000.

Armstrong LE: Hydration assessment techniques, *Nutr Rev* 63:S40, 2005.

Ayers P, Dixon C, Mays A: Acid-base disorders: learning the basics, *Nutr Clin Pract* 30:14, 2015.

Ayers P, Dixon C: Simple acid-base tutorial, *JPEN J Parenter Enteral Nutr* 36(1):18, 2012.

Campbell SM: Hydration needs throughout the lifespan, *J Am Coll Nutr* 26(Suppl 5):S585, 2007.

Caudarella R, Vescini F, Rizzoli E, et al: Salt intake, hypertension, and osteoporosis, *J Endocrinol Invest* 32(Suppl 4):15, 2009.

Cheuvront SN, Ely BR, Kenefick RW, et al: Biological variation and diagnostic accuracy of dehydration assessment markers, *Am J Clin Nutr* 92:565, 2010.

Goldman MB: The mechanism of life-threatening water imbalance in schizophrenia and its relationship to the underlying psychiatric illness, *Brain Res Rev* 61:210, 2009.

Hawkins RC: Age and gender as risk factors for hyponatremia and hypernatremia, *Clinica Chimica Acta* 337:169, 2003.

He FJ, MacGregor GA: Reducing population salt intake worldwide: from evidence to implementation, *Prog Cardiovasc Dis* 52:363, 2010.

Hoffmann IS, Cubeddu LX: Salt and the metabolic syndrome, *Nutr Metab Cardiovasc Dis* 19(2):123, 2009.

Institute of Medicine, Food and Nutrition Board: *Dietary Reference Intakes for water, potassium, sodium, chloride, and sulfate*, Washington, DC, 2004, National Academies Press.

Kelly DG, Nadeau J: Oral rehydration solution, *Pract Gastroenterol* 21:51, 2004.

Kingley J: Fluid and electrolyte management in parenteral nutrition, *Support Line* 27:13, 2005.

Kraft MD, Btaiche IF, Sacks GS: Review of the refeeding syndrome, *Nutr Clin Pract* 20:625, 2005.

Langley G, Tajchmans S: Fluid, electrolytes and acid-base disorders. In Mueller CM, Kovacevich DS, McClave SA, et al, editors: *The ASPEN adult nutrition support core curriculum*, ed 2, Silver Spring, MD, 2012, American Society for Parenteral and Enteral Nutrition, 98.

Maughan RJ, Shirreffs SM, Watson P: Exercise, heat, hydration and the brain, *J Am Coll Nutr* 26(Suppl 5):S604, 2007.

Popkin BM, D'Anci KE, Rosenberg IH: Water hydration, and health, *Nutr Rev* 68:439, 2010.

Rhoda KM, Porter MJ, Quintini C: Fluid and electrolyte management: putting a plan in motion, *JPEN J Parenter Enteral Nutr* 35:675, 2011.

Rogers IR, Hew-Butler T: Exercise-associated hyponatremia: overzealous fluid consumption, *Wilderness Environ Med* 20:139, 2009.

Shirreffs SM: Markers of hydration status, *Eur J Clin Nutr* 57(Suppl 2):S6, 2003.

Skipper A: Refeeding syndrome or refeeding hypophosphatemia: a systematic review of cases, *Nutr Clin Pract* 27:34, 2012.

Song HJ, Cho YG, Lee HJ: Dietary sodium intake and prevalence of overweight in adults, *Metabolism* 62:703, 2013.

Teucher B, Fairweather-Tait S: Dietary sodium as a risk factor for osteoporosis: where is the evidence? *Proc Nutr Soc* 62:859, 2003.

Whitmire SJ: Nutrition focused evaluation and management of dysnatremias, *Nutr Clin Pract* 23:108, 2008.

Whitmire SJ: Fluid, electrolytes and acid-base balance. In Matarese LE, Gottschlich MM, editors: *Contemporary Nutrition Support Practice, A clinical guide*, St Louis, MO, 2003, Saunders. 122.

Wilson RF: Acid-base problems. In Tintinalli JE, et al, editors: *Emergency medicine: a comprehensive study guide*, ed 6, New York, 2003, McGraw-Hill.

Wynn E, Krieg MA, Lanham-New SA, et al: Postgraduate symposium: positive influence of nutritional alkalinity on bone health, *Proc Nutr Soc* 69:166, 2010.

Yoon YS, Oh SW: Sodium density and obesity; the Korea national health and nutrition examination survey 2007–2010, *Eur J Clin Nutr* 67(2):141, 2013.

Zhu H, Pollock NK, Kotak I, et al: Dietary sodium, adiposity, and inflammation in healthy adolescents, *Pediatrics* 133:e635, 2014.

7

Clinical: Biochemical, Physical, and Functional Assessment

Mary Demarest Litchford PhD, RDN, LDN

KEY TERMS

25-hydroxy vitamin D 25-[OH]D
air displacement plethysmogram (ADP)
albumin
analyte
anemia of chronic and inflammatory disease (ACD)
anthropometry
basic metabolic panel (BMP)
bioelectrical impedance analysis (BIA)
body composition
body mass index (BMI)
complete blood count (CBC)
comprehensive metabolic panel (CMP)
C-reactive protein (CRP)
Creatinine
dehydration
differential count
dual-energy x-ray absorptiometry (DXA)

edema
ferritin
folate
functional medicine
Functional Nutrition Assessment (FNA)
head circumference
height-for-age curve
hematocrit (Hct)
hemoglobin (Hgb)
hemoglobin A1C (Hgb A1C)
high-sensitivity CRP (hs-CRP)
homocysteine
ideal body weight (IBW)
inflammation
length-for-age curve
macrocytic anemia
methylmalonic acid (MMA)
microcytic anemia
midarm circumference (MAC)

negative acute-phase reactants
osteocalcin
positive acute-phase reactants
prealbumin (PAB)
retinol
retinol-binding protein (RBP)
serum iron
statiometer
total iron-binding capacity (TIBC)
transferrin
transthyretin (TTHY)
urinalysis
usual body weight (UBW)
waist circumference
waist-to-height ratio (WHtR)
waist-to-hip ratio (WHR)
weight-for-age curve
weight-for-length curve

Nutrition assessment may be completed within the context of a traditional medical model or a functional integrative medical model. Clinicians must demonstrate critical thinking skills to observe, interpret, analyze, and infer data to detect new nutrition diagnoses or determine that nutrition-related issues have resolved (Charney et al, 2013). The three sources of information—biochemical data, physical attributes, and functional changes—are viewed in the context of each other, and the trends of data over time are useful to identify patterns consistent with nutrition and medical diagnoses (Figure 7-1).

Health care reforms are changing the practice of dietetics specific to nutrition assessment in several ways. First, the practice of ordering diets is changing to allow RDNs the privilege of writing diet orders within the parameters set by the governing body of the health care organization. Second, the practice of ordering routine laboratory tests is changing and health care providers must justify the need for each laboratory test ordered. Third, the use of evidence-based medical guidelines is reshaping the types and frequency of biochemical testing, physical assessments, and functional tests ordered. These changes augment the value of physical and functional assessment as pivotal components of nutrition assessment.

Practitioners should assess patients from a global perspective, requesting necessary tests, and not be limited by the history of reimbursement for testing. Also, many consumers are seeking health care services that are not covered currently by traditional insurance and government-funded health care programs. The nutrition professional can determine the validity and usefulness of these requests for testing. Before recommending a biochemical test to be performed, the dietitian should consider, "How will the test results change my intervention?"

BIOCHEMICAL ASSESSMENT OF NUTRITION STATUS

Laboratory tests are ordered to diagnose diseases, support nutrition diagnoses, monitor effectiveness of nutrition preventions, evaluate medication effectiveness, and evaluate NCP interventions or medical nutrition therapy (MNT). Acute illness, surgery, or injury can trigger dramatic changes in laboratory test results, including rapidly deteriorating nutrition status. However, chronic diseases that develop slowly over time also influence these results, making them useful in preventive care.

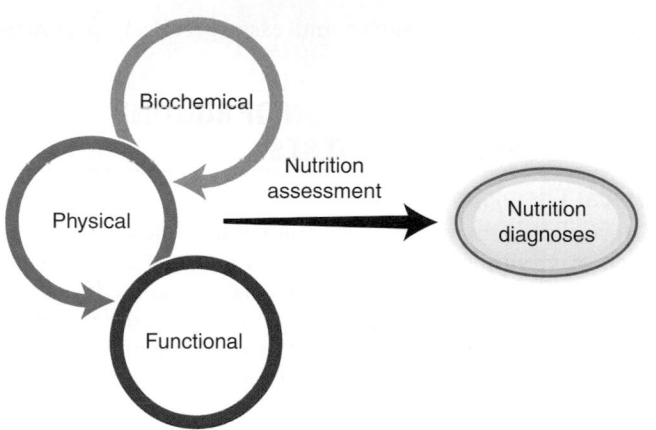

FIGURE 7-1 Interrelationship of biochemical data, physical attributes, and functional status.

Definitions and Applications of Laboratory Test Results

Laboratory assessment is a stringently controlled process. It involves comparing control samples with predetermined substance or chemical constituent (**analyte**) concentrations with every patient specimen. The results obtained must compare favorably with predetermined acceptable values before the patient data can be considered valid. Laboratory data are the only *objective data* used in nutrition assessment that are "controlled"—that is, the validity of the method of its measurement is checked each time a specimen is assayed by also assaying a sample with a known value.

Laboratory-based nutrition testing, used to estimate nutrient concentration in biologic fluids and tissues, is critical for assessment of clinical and subclinical nutrient deficiencies. As shown in Figure 7-2, the size of a nutrient pool can vary continuously from a frank deficit to insufficiency to adequate to toxic. Most of these states can be assessed in the laboratory so that nutritional intervention can occur before a clinical or anthropometric change or a frank deficiency occurs (Litchford, 2015). Single test results must be evaluated in light of the patient's current medical condition, nutrition-focused physical assessment data, medications, lifestyle choices, age, hydration status, fasting status at the time of specimen collection, and reference standards used by the clinical laboratory. Single test results may be useful for screening or to confirm an assessment based on changing clinical, anthropometric, and dietary status. Comparison of current test results to historic baseline test results from the same laboratory is desirable when available. It is vital to monitor trends in test results and patterns of results in the context of genetic and environmental factors. Changes in laboratory test results that occur over time are often an objective measure of nutrition or pharmacologic interventions and modified lifestyle choices.

Specimen Types

Ideally, the specimen to be tested reflects the total body content of the nutrient to be assessed. However, the best specimen may not be readily available. The most common specimens for analysis of nutrients and nutrient-related substances include the following:

- Whole blood: Collected with an anticoagulant if entire content of the blood is to be evaluated; none of the elements are removed; contains red blood cells (RBCs), white blood cells (WBCs), and platelets suspended in plasma
- Serum: The fluid obtained from blood after the blood has been clotted and then centrifuged to remove the clot and blood cells
- Plasma: The transparent (slightly straw-colored) liquid component of blood, composed of water, blood proteins, inorganic electrolytes, and clotting factors
- Blood cells: Separated from anticoagulated whole blood for measurement of cellular analyte content
- Erythrocytes: RBCs
- Leukocytes: WBCs and leukocyte fractions
- Blood spots: Dried whole blood from finger or heel prick that is placed on paper and can be used for selected hormone tests and other tests such as infant phenylketonuria screening
- Other tissues: Obtained from scrapings or biopsy samples
- Urine (from random samples or timed collections): Contains a concentrate of excreted metabolites

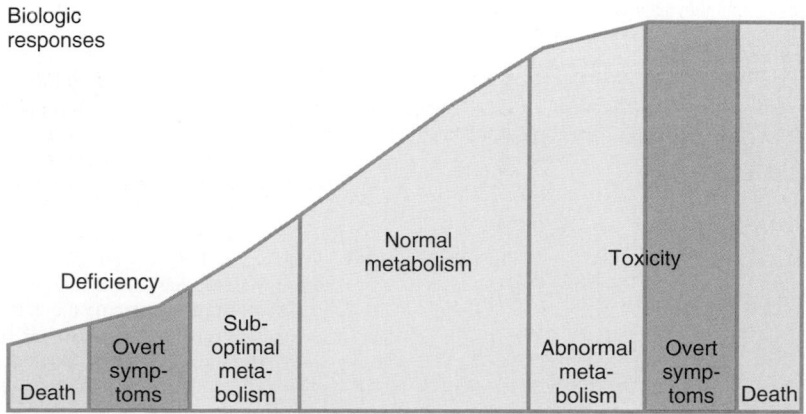

FIGURE 7-2 The size of a nutrient pool can vary continuously from frankly deficient, to adequate, to toxic.

- Feces (from random samples or timed collections): Important in nutritional analyses when nutrients are not absorbed and therefore are present in fecal material or to determine composition of gut flora or microbiota

Less commonly used specimens include the following:

- Breath tests: Noninvasive tool to evaluate nutrient metabolism and malabsorption, particularly of sugars
- Hair and nails: Easy-to-collect tissue for determining exposure to selected toxic metals
- Saliva: Noninvasive medium with a fast turnover; currently is used to evaluate functional adrenal and other hormone levels
- Sweat: Electrolyte test used to detect sweat chloride levels to determine presence of cystic fibrosis
- Hair and nails specimens have significant drawbacks, including lack of standardized procedures for processing, assay, and quality control and there is potential environmental contamination. Nutrient levels or indices may be less than the amounts that can be measured accurately. Hair can be used for deoxyribonucleic acid (DNA) testing and may be useful in the future as a noninvasive methodology to predict genetic predisposition to disease and effectiveness of medical nutrition therapy (see Chapter 5). Considerable research is being done to improve the usefulness of noninvasive and easy-to-collect specimens that are not routinely ordered.

NUTRITION INTERPRETATION OF ROUTINE MEDICAL LABORATORY TESTS

Clinical Chemistry Panels

Historically the majority of laboratory tests were ordered as panels or groupings; however, the current practice is that the professional ordering the test must justify the medical need for each test ordered. The bundling or grouping of laboratory tests is changing as health care reforms reshape medical practices to be more cost effective. The most commonly ordered groups of tests are the basic metabolic panel (BMP) and the comprehensive metabolic panel (CMP) that include groups of laboratory tests defined by the Centers for Medicare and Medicaid Services for reimbursement purposes. The BMP and CMP require the patient to fast for 10 to 12 hours before testing. The BMP includes eight tests used for screening blood glucose level, electrolyte and fluid balance, and kidney function. The CMP includes all the tests in the BMP and six additional tests to evaluate liver function. Table 7-1 explains these tests (see Appendix 22).

TABLE 7-1	Constituents of the Basic Metabolic Panel and Comprehensive Metabolic Panel		
Analytes	**Reference Range***	**Purpose**	**Significance**
Basic Metabolic Panel (BMP) (All Tests Reflect Fasting State)			
Glucose	70-99 mg/dl; 3.9-5.5 mmol/L(fasting)	Used to screen for diabetes and to monitor patients with diabetes. Individuals experiencing severe stress from injuries or surgery have hyperglycemia related to catecholamine release	Fasting glucose >125 mg/dl indicates DM (oral glucose tolerance tests are not needed for diagnosis); fasting glucose >100 mg/dl is indicator of insulin resistance. Monitor levels along with triglycerides in those receiving total parenteral nutrition for glucose intolerance
Total calcium	8.5-10.5 mg/dl; 2.15-2.57 mmol/L Normal dependent on albumin level	Reflects the calcium levels in the body that are not stored in bones. Used to evaluate parathyroid hormone function, calcium metabolism and monitor patients with renal failure, renal transplant, and some cancers	Hypercalcemia associated with endocrine disorders, malignancy, and hypervitaminosis D. Hypocalcemia associated with vitamin D deficiency and inadequate hepatic or renal activation of vitamin D, hypoparathyroidism, magnesium deficiency, renal failure, and nephrotic syndrome. When serum albumin is low, ionized calcium is measured
Na^+	135-145 mEq/L†	Reflects the relationship between total body sodium and extracellular fluid volume as well as the balance between dietary intake and renal excretory function	Used in monitoring various patients, such as those receiving total parenteral nutrition or who have renal conditions, uncontrolled DM, various endocrine disorders, ascitic and edematous symptoms, or acidotic or alkalotic conditions; water dysregulation, and diuretics. Increased with dehydration and decreased with overhydration
K^+	3.6-5 mEq/L†	Levels often change with sodium levels. As sodium increases, potassium decreases and vice versa. Reflects kidney function, changes in blood pH, and adrenal gland function	Used in monitoring various patients, such as those receiving total parenteral nutrition or who have renal conditions, uncontrolled DM, various endocrine disorders, ascitic and edematous symptoms, or acidotic or alkalotic conditions; decreased K^+ associated with diarrhea, vomiting, or nasogastric aspiration, water dysregulation, some drugs, licorice ingestion, and diuretics; increased K^+ associated with renal diseases, crush injuries, infection, and hemolyzed blood specimens
Cl^-	101-111 mEq/L†	Reflects acid-base balance, water balance, and osmolality	Used in monitoring various patients, such as those receiving total parenteral nutrition or who have renal conditions, chronic obstructive pulmonary disease, diabetes insipidus, acidotic or alkalotic conditions; increased with dehydration and decreased with overhydration
HCO_3^- (or total CO_2)	21-31 mEq/L†	Used to assess acid-base balance and electrolyte status	Used in monitoring various patients, such as those receiving total parenteral nutrition or who have renal conditions, chronic obstructive pulmonary disease, uncontrolled DM, various endocrine disorders, ascitic and edematous symptoms, or acidotic or alkalotic conditions

TABLE 7-1   Constituents of the Basic Metabolic Panel and Comprehensive Metabolic Panel—cont'd

Analytes	Reference Range*	Purpose	Significance
Basic Metabolic Panel (BMP) (All Tests Reflect Fasting State)			
BUN or urea	5-20 mg urea nitrogen/dl 1.8-7 mmol/L	Used to assess excretory function of kidney and metabolic function of liver	Increased in those with renal disease and excessive protein catabolism and overhydration; decreased in those with liver failure and negative nitrogen balance and in females who are pregnant
Creatinine	0.6-1.2 mg/dl; 53-106 μmol/L (males) 0.5-1.1 mg/dl; 44-97 μmol/L (females)	Used to assess excretory function of kidney	Increased in those with renal disease and after trauma or surgery; and decreased in those with malnutrition (i.e., BUN/creatinine ratio >15:1)
Comprehensive Metabolic Panel (CMP) (All Tests Reflect Fasting State and Includes All of the Tests in the BMP and Six Additional Tests)			
Albumin	3.5-5 mg/dl; 30-50 g/L	Reflects severity of illness, inflammatory stress and serves as marker for mortality	Decreased in those with liver disease or acute inflammatory disease and overhydration. Increases with dehydration. It is not a biomarker of protein status
Total protein	6.4-8.3 g/dl;64-83 g/L	Reflects albumin and globulin in blood	Not a useful measure of nutrition or protein status
ALP	30-120 units/L; 0.5-2 μKat/L	Reflects function of liver; may be used to screen for bone abnormalities	Increased in those with any of a variety of malignant, muscle, bone, intestinal, and liver diseases or injuries
ALT	4-36 units/L at 37° C; 4-36 units/L	Reflects function of liver	Used in monitoring liver function in those receiving parenteral nutrition
AST	0-35 IU/L; 0-0.58 μKat/L	Reflects function of liver; may be used to screen for cardiac abnormalities	Used in monitoring liver function in those receiving parenteral nutrition
Bilirubin	Total bilirubin 0.3-1 mg/dl; 5.1-17 μmol/L Indirect bilirubin 0.2-0.8 mg/dl; 3.4-12 μmol/L Direct bilirubin 0.1-0.3 mg/dl; 1.7-5.1 μmol/L	Reflects function of liver; also used to evaluate blood disorders, and biliary tract blockage	Increased in association with drugs, gallstones, and other biliary duct diseases; intravascular hemolysis and hepatic immaturity; decreased with some anemias
Phosphorous (phosphate)	3-4.5 mg/dl; 0.97-1.45 mmol/L		Hyperphosphatemia associated with hypoparathyroidism and hypocalcemia; hypophosphatemia associated with hyperparathyroidism, chronic antacid ingestion, and renal failure
Total cholesterol	<200 mg/dl; 5.20 mmol/L		Decreased in those with malnutrition, malabsorption, liver diseases, and hyperthyroidism
Triglycerides	<100 mg/dl; <1.13 mmol/L (age and gender dependent)		Increased in those with glucose intolerance (e.g., in those receiving parenteral nutrition who have combined hyperlipidemia) or in those who are not fasting

*Reference ranges may vary slightly among laboratories.
†mEq/L = 1 mmol/L.

ALP, Alkaline phosphate; *ALT*, alanine aminotransferase; *AST*, aspartate aminotransferase; *BUN*, blood urea nitrogen; *Cl⁻*, chlorine; *CO₂*, carbon dioxide; *DM*, diabetes mellitus; *HCO₃⁻*, bicarbonate; *K⁺*, potassium; *Na⁺*, sodium; *PEM*, protein-energy malnutrition.

Complete Blood Count

The **complete blood count** (CBC) provides a count of the cells in the blood and description of the RBCs. A hemogram is a CBC with a white blood cell **differential count** (often called a *differential* or *diff*). Table 7-2 provides a list of the basic elements of the CBC and differential, with reference ranges and explanatory comments.

Stool Testing

Mucosal changes in the gastrointestinal (GI) tract are indicated by problems such as diarrhea and bloody or black stool. Tests may be done on a stool sample and can reveal excessive amounts of fat (an indication of malabsorption), the status of the GI flora, and the amounts and types of bacteria present in the gut. Fecal samples may be tested for the presence of blood, pathogens, and gut flora. The fecal occult blood test is ordered routinely for adults older than age 50 and younger adults with unexplained anemia. Stool culture testing may be ordered in patients with prolonged diarrhea, especially if foodborne illness is suspected. If pathogenic bacteria are isolated in stool culture,

appropriate pharmacologic interventions are initiated. Patients with chronic GI symptoms such as maldigestion or unexplained weight loss or gain may benefit from gut flora testing to identify pathologic flora or an imbalance of physiologic flora. In addition, stool tests may be helpful to evaluate the gut microbiota and the effectiveness of probiotic, prebiotic, and synbiotic use.

Urinalysis

The **urinalysis** test is used as a screening or diagnostic tool to detect substances or cellular material in the urine associated with different metabolic and kidney disorders. Some urinalysis data have broader medical and nutritional significance (e.g., glycosuria suggests abnormal carbohydrate metabolism and possibly diabetes). The full urinalysis includes a record of (1) the appearance of the urine, (2) the results of basic tests done with chemically impregnated reagent strips (often called dipsticks) that can be read visually or by an automated reader, and (3) the microscopic examination of urine sediment. Table 7-3 provides a list of the chemical tests performed in a urinalysis and their significance.

TABLE 7-2 Constituents of the Hemogram: Complete Blood Count and Differential

Analytes	Reference Range*	Significance
Red blood cells	$4.7\text{-}6.1 \times 10^6/\mu l$ (males); $4.7\text{-}6.1\ 10^{12}/L$ $4.2\text{-}5.4 \times 10^6/\mu l$ (females); $4.2\text{-}5.4\ 10^{12}/L$	In addition to nutritional deficits, may be decreased in those with hemorrhage, hemolysis, genetic aberrations, marrow failure, or renal disease or who are taking certain drugs; not sensitive for iron, vitamin B_{12}, or folate deficiencies
Hemoglobin concentration	14-18 g/dl; 8.7-11.2 mmol/L (males) 12-16 g/dl; 7.4-9.9 mmol/L (females) >11 g/dl; >6.8 mmol/L (pregnant females) 14-24 g/dl; 8.7-14.9 mmol/L (newborns)	In addition to nutritional deficits, may be decreased in those with hemorrhage, hemolysis, genetic aberrations, marrow failure, or renal disease or who are taking certain drugs
Hematocrit	42%-52% (males) 35%-47% (females) 33% (pregnant females) 44%-64% (newborns)	In addition to nutritional deficits, may be decreased in those with hemorrhage, hemolysis, genetic aberrations, marrow failure, or renal disease or who are taking certain drugs Somewhat affected by hydration status
MCV	80-99 fl 96-108 fl (newborns)	Decreased (microcytic) in presence of iron deficiency, thalassemia trait and chronic renal failure; normal or decreased in anemia of chronic disease; increased (macrocytic) in presence of vitamin B_{12} or folate deficiency and genetic defects in DNA synthesis; neither microcytosis nor macrocytosis sensitive to marginal nutrient deficiencies
MCH	27-31 pg/cell 23-34 pg (newborns)	Causes of abnormal values similar to those for MCV
MCHC	32-36 g/dl; 32-36% 32-33 g/dl; 32-33% (newborns)	Decreased in those with iron deficiency and thalassemia trait; not sensitive to marginal nutrient deficiencies
WBC	$5\text{-}10 \times 10^9/L$; 5,000-10,000/mm3 (2 yr-adult) $6\text{-}17 \times 10^9/L$; 6,000-17,000/mm3 (<2 yr) $9\text{-}30 \times 10^9$; 9,000-30,000/mm3 (newborns)	Increased (leukocytosis) in those with infection, neoplasia; stress decreased (leucopenia) in those with malnutrition, autoimmune diseases, or overwhelming infections or who are receiving chemotherapy or radiation therapy
Differential	55%-70% neutrophils 20-40% lymphocytes 2-8% monocytes 1%-4% eosinophils 0.5%-1% basophils	*Neutrophilia:* Ketoacidosis, trauma, stress, pus-forming infections, leukemia *Neutropenia:* malnutrition, aplastic anemia, chemotherapy, overwhelming infection *Lymphocytosis:* Infection, leukemia, myeloma, mononucleosis *Lymphocytopenia:* Leukemia, chemotherapy, sepsis, AIDS *Eosinophilia:* Parasitic infestation, allergy, eczema, leukemia, autoimmune disease *Eosinopenia:* Increased steroid production *Basophilia:* Leukemia *Basopenia:* Allergy

AIDS, Acquired immune deficiency syndrome; *DNA,* deoxyribonucleic acid; *MCH,* mean corpuscular hemoglobin; *MCHC,* mean corpuscular hemoglobin concentration; *MCV,* mean corpuscular volume.

*Reference ranges may vary slightly among laboratories.

TABLE 7-3 Chemical Tests in a Urinalysis

Analyte	Expected Value	Significance
Specific gravity	1.010-1.025	Can be used to test and monitor the concentrating and diluting abilities of the kidney and hydration status; low in those with diabetes insipidus, glomerulonephritis, or pyelonephritis; high in those with vomiting, diarrhea, sweating, fever, adrenal insufficiency, hepatic diseases, or heart failure
pH	4.6-8 (normal diet)	Acidic in those with a high-protein diet or acidosis (e.g., uncontrolled DM or starvation), during administration of some drugs, and in association with uric acid, cystine, and calcium oxalate kidney stones; alkaline in individuals consuming diets rich in vegetables or dairy products and in those with a urinary tract infection, immediately after meals, with some drugs, and in those with phosphate and calcium carbonate kidney stones
Protein	2-8 mg/dl	Marked proteinuria in those with nephrotic syndrome, severe glomerulonephritis, or congestive heart failure; moderate in those with most renal diseases, preeclampsia, or urinary tract inflammation; minimal in those with certain renal diseases or lower urinary tract disorders
Glucose	Not detected (2-10 g/dl in DM)	Positive in those with DM; rarely in benign conditions
Ketones	Negative	Positive in those with uncontrolled DM (usually type 1); also positive in those with a fever, anorexia, certain GI disturbances, persistent vomiting, or cachexia or who are fasting or starving
Blood	Negative	Indicates urinary tract infection, neoplasm, or trauma; also positive in those with traumatic muscle injuries or hemolytic anemia
Bilirubin	Not detected	Index of unconjugated bilirubin; increase in those with certain liver diseases (e.g., gallstones)
Urobilinogen	0.1-1 units/dl	Index of conjugated bilirubin; increased in those with hemolytic conditions; used to distinguish among hepatic diseases
Nitrite	Negative	Index of bacteriuria
Leukocyte esterase	Negative	Indirect test of bacteriuria; detects leukocytes

DM, Diabetes mellitus; *GI,* gastrointestinal.

ASSESSMENT OF HYDRATION STATUS

Assessment of hydration status is vital because water dysregulation can be associated with other imbalances such as electrolyte imbalance. Types of water dysregulation include volume depletion or extracellular fluid contraction, dehydration or sodium intoxication, and overhydration or excessive fluid shift into interstitial-lymph fluid compartment. Dehydration often is due to excessive loss of water and electrolytes from vomiting, diarrhea, excessive laxative abuse, diuretics, fistulas, GI suction, polyuria, fever, excessive sweating, decreased intake caused by anorexia, nausea, depression, or limited access to fluids. Characteristics include rapid weight loss, decreased skin turgor, dry mucous membranes, dry and furrowed tongue, postural hypotension, a weak and rapid pulse, slow capillary refill, a decrease in body temperature (95° to 98° F), decreased urine output, cold extremities, or disorientation. See Figure 6-2 in Chapter 6.

Volume depletion is a state of vascular instability resulting from blood loss, GI bleeding, burns, vomiting, and diarrhea. Volume depletion may occur with hyponatremia, hypernatremia, or normal serum sodium levels.

Edema (overhydration), occurs when there is an increase in the extracellular fluid volume. The fluid shifts from the extracellular compartment to the interstitial fluid compartment (see Chapter 6). Overhydration is caused by an increase in capillary hydrostatic pressure or capillary permeability, or a decrease in colloid osmotic pressure. It often is associated with renal failure, congestive heart failure, cirrhosis of the liver, Cushing syndrome, excess use of sodium-containing intravenous fluids, and excessive intake of sodium-containing food or medications. Characteristics include rapid weight gain, peripheral edema, distended neck veins, slow emptying of peripheral veins, a bounding and full pulse, rales in the lungs, polyuria, ascites, and pleural effusion. Pulmonary edema may occur in severe cases.

Laboratory measures of hydration status include serum sodium, blood urea nitrogen (elevated out of proportion to serum creatinine), serum osmolality, and urine specific gravity. Although the laboratory tests are important, decisions regarding hydration should only be made only in conjunction with other information from physical examination, nutrition-focused physical assessment, and the clinical condition of the patient. In addition, many other labs may be affected by overhydration or dehydration, and accurate interpretation of laboratory results is critical in assessing patients (see Table 7-1).

Inflammation and Biochemical Assessment

Inflammation is a protective response by the immune system to infection, acute illness, trauma, toxins, many chronic diseases, and physical stress. Biochemical indices are affected by inflammation primarily by redirection to synthesis of acute phase reactants. Inflammatory conditions trigger the immune response to release eicosanoids and cytokines, which mobilize nutrients required to synthesize positive acute-phase reactants (which increase in response to inflammation) and leukocytes. Cytokines (interleukin-1beta [IL-1β], tumor necrosis factor-alpha [TNF-α], interleukin-6 [IL-6]) and eicosanoids (prostaglandin E2 [PGE2]) influence whole-body metabolism, body composition, and nutritional status. Cytokines reorient hepatic synthesis of plasma proteins and increase the breakdown of muscle protein to meet the demand for protein and energy during the inflammatory response. Moreover, there is a redistribution of albumin to the interstitial compartment, resulting in

edema. Declining values of the negative acute-phase reactants (i.e., serum albumin, prealbumin, and transferrin) also reflect the inflammatory processes and severity of tissue injury. In the acute inflammatory state, negative acute phase reactant values do not reflect current dietary intake or protein status (Friedman and Fadem, 2010).

Cytokines impair the production of erythrocytes and reorient iron stores from hemoglobin and serum iron to ferritin. During infection IL-1β inhibits the production and release of transferrin while stimulating the synthesis of ferritin. Therefore laboratory test results used to predict the risk of nutritional anemias (see Chapter 32) are not useful in assessing the patient with an inflammatory response. Refer to Chapter 3 for more information on the effects of cytokines on organ systems.

As the body responds to acute inflammation, TNF-α, IL-1β, IL-6, and PGE2 increase to a set threshold, then IL-6 and PGE2 inhibit TNF-α synthesis and IL-1β secretion, creating a negative feedback cycle. Hepatic synthesis of positive acute-phase reactants diminishes, and synthesis of negative acute-phase reactants increases. Albumin shifts from the interstitial compartment to the extravascular space. Iron stores shift from ferritin to transferrin and hemoglobin.

Markers of Inflammation

Biochemical markers of inflammation include positive acute phase reactants and negative acute phase reactants. In the presence of inflammation, the hepatic synthesis of positive acute phase reactants is *increased* while the synthesis of the negative acute phase reactants is *depressed*. See Table 7-4 for acute phase reactants.

Positive Acute Phase Reactants
C-Reactive Protein

C-reactive protein (CRP) is a nonspecific marker of inflammation that may help to estimate and monitor the severity of illness. High-sensitivity CRP (hs-CRP) is a more sensitive measure of chronic inflammation seen in patients with atherosclerosis and other chronic diseases (Bajpai et al, 2010). Although the exact function of CRP is unclear, it increases in the initial stages of acute stress—usually within 4 to 6 hours of surgery or other trauma. Furthermore, its level can increase as much as 1000-fold, depending on the intensity of the stress response. When the CRP level begins to decrease, the patient has entered the anabolic period of the inflammatory response and the beginning of recovery when more intensive nutrition

TABLE 7-4 Acute Phase Reactants	
Positive Acute-Phase Reactants	**Negative Acute-Phase Proteins**
C-reactive protein	Albumin
a-1 antichymotrypsin	Transferrin
a₁-antitrypsin	Prealbumin (transthyretin)
Haptoglobins	Retinol-binding protein
Ceruloplasmin	
Serum amyloid A	
Fibrinogen	
Ferritin	
Complement and components C3 and C4	
Orosomucoid	

therapy may be beneficial. Ongoing assessment and follow-up are required to address changes in nutrition status.

Ferritin

Ferritin is a positive acute-phase protein, meaning that synthesis of ferritin increases in the presence of inflammation. Ferritin is not a reliable indicator of iron stores in patients with acute inflammation, uremia, metastatic cancer, or alcoholic-related liver diseases. Cytokines and other inflammatory mediators can increase ferritin synthesis, ferritin leakage from cells, or both. Elevations in ferritin occur 1 to 2 days after the onset of the acute illness and peak at 3 to 5 days. If iron deficiency also exists, it may not be diagnosed because the level of ferritin would be falsely elevated.

Negative Acute Phase Reactants
Albumin

Albumin is responsible for the transport of major blood constituents, hormones, enzymes, medications, minerals, ions, fatty acids, amino acids, and metabolites. Its major purpose is to maintain colloidal osmotic pressure, providing approximately 80% of colloidal osmotic pressure of the plasma. When serum albumin levels decrease, the water in the plasma moves into the interstitial compartment and edema results. This loss of plasma fluid results in hypovolemia, which triggers renal retention of water and sodium.

Albumin has a half-life of 18 to 21 days. Levels of albumin remain nearly normal during uncomplicated starvation as redistribution from the interstitium to the plasma occurs. Levels of albumin fall precipitously in inflammatory stress and often do not improve with aggressive nutrition support. Serum levels reflect the severity of illness but do not reflect current protein status or the effects of nutrient-dense supplemental nutrition. For these reasons, a well-nourished but stressed patient may have low levels of albumin and the hepatic transport proteins, whereas a patient who has had significant weight loss and undernutrition may have normal or close to normal levels. Albumin is very sensitive to hydration status, and the practitioner must be aware and document the true cause of an elevated or depressed albumin level.

Albumin is synthesized in the liver and is a measure of liver function. When disease affects the liver, the synthesis of albumin, by the hepatocytes, is impaired. Because of the half-life of albumin, significant changes in liver function are not immediately apparent.

Prealbumin (Transthyretin)

Prealbumin (PAB), officially transthyretin (TTHY), is a hepatic protein transported in the serum as a complex of retinol-binding protein and vitamin A. It transports the thyroid hormones triiodothyronine and thyroxine (T_4), along with T_4-binding globulin. It has a short half-life ($t\frac{1}{2} = 2$ days), and currently it is considered a marker of inflammation. Levels of PAB plummet in inflammatory stress and often do not improve with aggressive nutrition support. Moreover, serum levels decrease with malignancy and protein-wasting diseases of the intestines or kidneys. Serum levels do not reflect protein status or the effects of refeeding in the individual with depleted protein reserves. Serum levels also decrease in the presence of a zinc deficiency because zinc is required for hepatic synthesis and secretion of PAB. Consider zinc status from dietary intake and medical history,

in addition to inflammation, when interpreting low plasma PAB levels.

PAB levels are often normal in starvation-related malnutrition but decreased in well-nourished individuals who have undergone recent stress or trauma. During pregnancy, the changed estrogen levels stimulate PAB synthesis and serum levels may increase. In nephrotic syndrome, PAB levels also may be increased. Proteinuria and hypoproteinemia are common in nephrotic syndrome, and because PAB is synthesized rapidly, a disproportionate percentage of PAB can exist in the blood, whereas other proteins take longer to produce (Litchford, 2015).

Retinol-Binding Protein

The hepatic protein with the shortest half-life ($t\frac{1}{2} = 12$ hr) is retinol-binding protein (RBP), a small plasma protein that does not pass through the renal glomerulus because it circulates in a complex with PAB. As implied by its name, RBP binds retinol, and transport of this vitamin A metabolite seems to be its exclusive function. RBP is synthesized in the liver and released with retinol. After RBP releases retinol in peripheral tissue, its affinity for PAB decreases, leading to dissociation of the PAB-RBP complex and filtration of apoprotein (apo)-RBP by the glomerulus.

The plasma RBP concentration has been shown to decrease in starvation-related malnutrition. However, RBP levels also fall in the presence of inflammatory stress and may not improve with refeeding. RBP may not reflect protein status in acutely stressed patients. It may even be elevated with renal failure because the RBP is not being catabolized by the renal tubule.

RBP4 is an adipocyte-derived peptide of RBP that influences glucose homeostasis and may play a role in lipoprotein metabolism. Human clinical trials have demonstrated increased RBP4 levels in obesity, insulin resistance, gestational diabetes, proliferative diabetic retinopathy, and nondiabetic stage 5 chronic kidney disease, suggesting a possible relationship between these conditions. Larger clinical trials are needed to define this relationship (Klein et al, 2010; Li et al, 2010).

Transferrin

Transferrin is a globulin protein that transports iron to the bone marrow for production of hemoglobin (Hgb). The plasma transferrin level is controlled by the size of the iron storage pool. When iron stores are depleted, transferrin synthesis increases. It has a shorter half-life ($t\frac{1}{2} = 8$ days) than albumin. Levels diminish with acute inflammatory reactions, malignancies, collagen vascular diseases, and liver diseases. Transferrin levels reflect inflammation and are not useful as a measure of protein status.

Immunocompetence

Inflammation-related malnutrition is associated with impaired immunocompetence, including depressed cell-mediated immunity, phagocyte dysfunction, decreased levels of complement components, reduced mucosal secretory antibody responses, and lower antibody affinity. Assessing immunocompetence is also useful in the patient who is being treated for allergies (see Chapter 26).

There is no single marker for immunocompetence except for the clinical outcome of infection or allergic response. Laboratory markers with a high degree of sensitivity include vaccine-specific serum antibody production, delayed-type hypersensitivity response, vaccine-specific or total secretory immunoglobulin A in saliva, and the response to attenuated pathogens. Less sensitive markers include natural killer cell cytotoxicity, oxidative burst of phagocytes, lymphocyte proliferation, and the cytokine pattern produced by activated immune cells. Using a combination of markers is currently the best approach to measuring immunocompetence.

ASSESSMENT FOR NUTRITIONAL ANEMIAS

Anemia is a condition characterized by a reduction in the number of erythrocytes per unit of blood volume or a decrease in the Hgb of the blood to below the level of usual physiologic need. By convention, anemia is defined as Hgb concentration below the 95th percentile for healthy reference populations of men, women, or age-grouped children. Anemia is not a disease but a symptom of various conditions, including extensive blood loss, excessive blood cell destruction, or decreased blood cell formation. It is observed in many hospitalized patients and is often a symptom of a disease process; its cause should be investigated. Clinical nutritionists must distinguish between anemia caused by nutritional inadequacies and that caused by other factors (i.e., dehydration masking falsely low blood values). See Chapter 32 for discussion of the management of anemias.

Classification of Anemia

Nutritional deficits are a major cause of decreased Hgb and erythrocyte production. The initial descriptive classification of anemia is derived from the hematocrit (Hct) value or CBC as explained in Table 7-2. Anemias associated with a mean RBC volume of less than 80 fl (femtoliters) are microcytic; those with values of 80 to 99 fl are normocytic; those associated with values of 100 fl or more are macrocytic. (See Chapter 32.) Data from the CBC are helpful in identifying nutritional causes of anemia. Microcytic anemia is associated most often with iron deficiency, whereas macrocytic anemia generally is caused by either folate- or vitamin B_{12}–deficient erythropoiesis. However, because of the low specificity of these indexes, additional data are needed to distinguish between the various nutritional causes and nonnutritional causes, such as thalassemia trait and chronic renal insufficiency. Normocytic anemia is associated with the anemia of chronic and inflammatory disease (ACD). This type of anemia is associated with autoimmune diseases, rheumatic diseases, chronic heart failure, chronic infection, Hodgkin disease and other types of cancer, inflammatory bowel disease and other chronic inflammatory conditions, severe tissue injury, and multiple fractures. ACD does not respond to iron supplementation.

Other information from the CBC that helps to differentiate the nonnutritional causes of anemia includes leukocyte, reticulocyte, and platelet counts. When these levels are low, marrow failure is indicated and elevated counts are associated with anemia caused by leukemia or infection. Erythrocyte sedimentation rate testing is ordered when symptoms are nonspecific and if inflammatory autoimmune diseases are suspected. Reticulocytes are large, nucleated, immature RBCs that are released in small numbers with mature cells. When RBC production rates increase, reticulocyte counts also increase. Any time anemia is accompanied by a high reticulocyte count, elevated erythropoietic activity in response to bleeding should be considered. In such cases, stool specimens can be tested for occult blood to rule out chronic GI blood loss. Other causes of a high reticulocyte count include intravascular hemolysis syndromes and an erythropoietic response to therapy for iron, vitamin B_{12}, or folic acid deficiencies.

Normocytic or microcytic anemia may be caused by chronic or acute blood loss, such as from recent surgery, injury, or from the GI tract as indicated by a positive occult stool test. Note that in those with hemolytic anemias and early iron deficiency anemia, the RBC size may still be normal. Macrocytic anemias include folate deficiency and vitamin B_{12} deficiency. The presence of macrocytic RBCs requires evaluation of folate and vitamin B_{12} status. DNA synthesis is affected negatively by deficiencies of folic acid and vitamin B_{12}, resulting in impaired RBC synthesis and maturation of RBCs. These changes cause large, nucleated cells to be released into the circulation. Although vitamin B_{12}–related anemia is categorized as a macrocytic normochromic anemia, approximately 40% of the cases are normocytic.

Markers of Iron Deficiency Anemias
Hematocrit or Packed Cell Volume and Hemoglobin

Hct and Hgb are part of a routine CBC and are used together to evaluate iron status. Hct is the measure of the percentage of RBCs in total blood volume. Usually the Hct percentage is three times the Hgb concentration in grams per deciliter. The Hct value is affected by an extremely high WBC count and hydration status. Individuals living in high altitudes often have increased values. It is common for individuals older than age 50 to have slightly lower levels than younger adults.

The Hgb concentration is a measure of the total amount of Hgb in the peripheral blood. It is a more direct measure of iron deficiency than Hct because it quantifies total Hgb in RBCs rather than a percentage of total blood volume. Hgb and Hct are below normal in the four types of nutritional anemias and always should be evaluated in light of other laboratory values and recent medical history (see Chapter 32).

Serum Ferritin

Ferritin is the storage protein that sequesters the iron normally gathered in the liver (reticuloendothelial system), spleen, and marrow. As the iron supply increases, the intracellular level of ferritin increases to accommodate iron storage. A small amount of this ferritin leaks into the circulation. This ferritin can be measured by assays that are available in most clinical laboratories. In individuals with normal iron storage, 1 ng/ml of serum ferritin equals approximately 8 mg of stored iron. In healthy adults, the measurement of ferritin that has leaked into the serum is an excellent indicator of the size of the body's iron storage pool.

ACD is the primary condition in which ferritin fails to correlate with iron stores. ACD, a common form of anemia in hospitalized patients, occurs in those with cancer or inflammatory or infectious disorders. It occurs during inflammation because red cell production decreases as the result of inadequate mobilization of iron from its storage sites. In those with arthritis, depletion of stored iron develops partly because of reduced absorption of iron from the gut. Also the regular use of nonsteroidal antiinflammatory drugs can cause occult GI blood loss. ACD has many forms and must be distinguished from iron deficiency anemia so that inappropriate iron supplementation is not initiated.

Serum Iron

Serum iron measures the amount of circulating iron that is bound to transferrin. However, it is a relatively poor index of iron status because of large day-to-day changes, even in healthy individuals. Diurnal variations also occur, with the highest concentrations occurring midmorning (from 6 AM to 10 AM), and a nadir, averaging 30% less than the morning level, occurring mid afternoon. Serum iron should be evaluated in light of other laboratory values and recent medical history to assess iron status.

Total Iron-Binding Capacity and Transferrin Saturation

Total iron-binding capacity (TIBC) is a direct measure of all proteins available to bind mobile iron and depends on the number of free binding sites on the plasma iron-transport protein transferrin. Intracellular iron availability regulates the synthesis and secretion of transferrin (i.e., transferrin concentration increases in those with iron deficiency).

Transferrin saturation reflects iron availability to tissues (bone marrow erythropoiesis). It is determined by the following equation:

$$\% \text{ Transferrin saturation} = (\text{Serum Fe} / \text{TIBC}) \times 100$$

In addition, when the amount of stored iron available for release to transferrin decreases and dietary iron intake is low, saturation of transferrin decreases.

There are exceptions to the general rule that transferrin saturation decreases and TIBC increases in patients with iron deficiency. For example, TIBC increases in those with hepatitis. It also increases in people with hypoxia, women who are pregnant, or those taking oral contraceptives or receiving estrogen replacement therapy. On the other hand, TIBC decreases in those with malignant disease, nephritis, and hemolytic anemias. Furthermore, the plasma level of transferrin may be decreased in those with protein energy malnutrition (PEM), fluid overload, and liver disease. Thus, although TIBC and transferrin saturation are more specific than Hct or Hgb values, they are not perfect indicators of iron status.

An additional concern about the use of serum iron, TIBC, and transferrin saturation values is that normal values persist until frank deficiency actually develops. Thus these tests cannot detect decreasing iron stores and iron insufficiencies.

Tests for Macrocytic Anemias from B Vitamin Deficiencies

Macrocytic anemias include folate deficiency and vitamin B_{12} deficiency. The nutritional causes of macrocytic anemia are related to the availability of folate and vitamin B_{12} in the bone marrow and require evaluation of both nutrient levels. Both nutrients decrease DNA synthesis by preventing the formation of thymidine monophosphate. Folate and vitamin B_{12} are used at different steps of the synthetic pathway. Impaired RBC synthesis occurs and large, nucleated RBCs then are released into the circulation (see Chapter 32).

Assessing Folate and Vitamin B_{12} Status

Evaluation for macrocytic anemia includes static measurement of folate and vitamin B_{12} deficiency in blood. They can be assayed using tests of the ability of the patient's blood specimen to support the growth of microbes that require either folate or vitamin B_{12}, or radiobinding assays, or immunoassays.

Serum Homocysteine. Folate and vitamin B_{12} are required for the synthesis of S-adenosylmethionine (SAM), the biochemical precursor involved in the transfer of one-carbon (methyl) groups during many biochemical syntheses. SAM is synthesized from the amino acid methionine by a reaction that includes the addition of a methyl group and the purine base adenine (from adenosine triphosphate, or ATP). For example, when SAM donates a methyl group for the synthesis of thymidine, choline, creatine, epinephrine, and protein and DNA methylation, it is converted to S-adenosylhomocysteine. After losing the adenosyl group, the remaining homocysteine can be converted either to cysteine by the vitamin B6–dependent transsulfuration pathway or back to methionine in a reaction that depends on adequate folate and vitamin B_{12}.

When either folate or vitamin B_{12} is lacking, the homocysteine-to-methionine reaction is blocked, causing homocysteine to build up in the affected tissue and spill into the circulation. The vitamin B6–dependent transsulfuration pathway can metabolize excess homocysteine. Homocysteine has been shown to be sensitive to folate and vitamin B_{12} deficiency.

Therefore an elevated homocysteine level indicates either genetic defects involved in the enzymes that catalyze these reactions, or a deficiency in folate, vitamin B_{12}, or vitamin B_6. Research indicates that several folate gene polymorphisms affecting the methylation of folate and B_{12} contribute risk for several chronic cardiovascular and neurologic disorders (Fan et al, 2010; see Chapters 5 and 41).

Folate Assessment. Folate most often is measured simultaneously in whole blood with its combined amount from plasma and blood cells, and in the serum alone. The difference between whole-blood folate and serum folate levels then is used to calculate total RBC folate concentration. RBC folate concentration is a better indicator of folate status than serum folate, because folate is much more concentrated in RBCs than in the serum. RBC folate measurement more closely reflects tissue stores and is considered the most reliable indicator of folate status. Folate is absorbed in the jejunum, and its malabsorption has several causes, but a specific test for folate absorption is not available. The presence and extent of deficiency should be assessed in patients with celiac disease, those who have had bariatric surgery, those with a history of long-term use of medications such as anticonvulsants and sulfasalazine, those with chronic alcohol consumption, those with methyltetrahydrofolate reductase (MTHFR) genetic polymorphisms, and those with rheumatoid arthritis taking methotrexate (see Chapters 5 and 8).

Vitamin B_{12} Assessment. Vitamin B_{12} is measured in the serum, and all indications are that the serum level gives as much information about vitamin B_{12} status as does the RBC level. If vitamin B_{12} status is compromised, intrinsic factor antibodies (IFAB) and parietal cell antibodies are measured; the presence of antibodies suggests the main cause of macrocytic anemia. Historically the Schilling test was used to detect defects in vitamin B_{12} absorption; it rarely is used today because the test requires that the patient be given radioactive vitamin B_{12} (see Chapter 32). **Methylmalonic acid (MMA)** levels in serum or urine are more useful to assess B_{12} status.

Vitamin B_{12} and Methylmalonic Acid. Once a genetic or autoimmune cause is ruled out, the most straightforward biochemical method for differentiating between folate and vitamin B_{12} deficiencies is by measuring the serum or urinary MMA level. MMA is formed during the degradation of the amino acid valine and odd-chain fatty acids. MMA is the side product in this metabolic pathway that increases when the conversion of methylmalonic coenzyme A (CoA) to succinyl CoA is blocked by lack of vitamin B$_{12}$, a coenzyme for this reaction. Therefore deficiency leads to an increase in the MMA pool, which is reflected by the serum or urinary MMA level. The urinary MMA test is more sensitive than the serum B$_{12}$ test because it indicates true tissue B$_{12}$ deficiency. The serum MMA test may give falsely high values in renal insufficiency and intravascular volume depletion. The urinary MMA test is the only B$_{12}$ deficiency assay that has been validated as a screening tool. Homocysteine and MMA tend to detect impending vitamin deficiencies better than the static assays. This is especially important when assessing the status of certain patients such as vegans or older adults, who could have vitamin B$_{12}$ deficiency associated with central nervous system impairment.

FAT-SOLUBLE VITAMINS

Fat malabsorption often results in impaired absorption of vitamins A, E, D, and K. Factors including low luminal pH, bile salts below the critical micellar concentration, and inadequate triglyceride hydrolysis can interfere with normal bile salt micelle formation, causing impaired absorption of fat-soluble vitamins. Individuals with fat malabsorptive disorders, including those who have had bariatric surgery, are at greatest risk of deficiencies of fat-soluble vitamins. See Appendix 22 for further discussion of tests for assessing specific vitamin adequacy.

Vitamin A

Vitamin A status can be estimated using serum retinol, and the normal level in adults is 30 to 80 mcg/dl. A primary deficiency of vitamin A can result from inadequate intake, fat malabsorption, or liver disorders. A secondary deficiency of vitamin A may be due to decreased bioavailability of provitamin A carotenoids or interference with vitamin A absorption, storage, or transport (e.g., celiac disease, cystic fibrosis, pancreatic insufficiency, malabsorptive weight loss surgery, or bile duct obstruction). Vitamin A deficiency is common in prolonged malnutrition and reported a year or longer after gastric bypass surgery and biliopancreatic weight loss surgery (Ledoux et al, 2006; Maden et al, 2006; Zalesin et al, 2011). The oxidative stress associated with major surgeries, including gastric bypass surgery, also may interfere with vitamin A absorption and use. Because of shared absorptive mechanisms with vitamin D, serum retinol always should be assessed in the presence of vitamin D supplementation.

Acute or chronic vitamin A toxicity is defined as retinol levels greater than 100 mcg/dl. Hypervitaminosis A has been reported in almost 50% of patients taking 150% of the RDA for vitamin A, in the form of retinol, between 6 to 12 months after laparoscopic sleeve gastrectomy (Aarts, 2011). Chronic vitamin A toxicities are associated with loss of hair; dry mucous membranes; dry, rough skin; and even cortical bone loss and fractures. See Appendix 22.

Vitamin D

Individual vitamin D status can be estimated by measuring plasma **25-hydroxy vitamin D (25-[OH]D$_3$)** levels. Current clinical practice reference ranges have been updated by the IOM (IOM, 2011). Traditional levels defining vitamin D sufficiency have been based on the lowest threshold value for plasma 25-(OH)D$_3$ (approximately 80 nmol/L or 32 ng/ml) that

prevents secondary hyperparathyroidism, increased bone turnover, bone mineral loss, or seasonal variations in plasma parathyroid hormone. The IOM review concluded that individuals are at risk of deficiency at serum 25(OH)D$_3$ levels below 30 nmol or 12 ng/ml and that practically all persons have sufficient serum levels at 50 nmol or 20 ng/ml. The American Geriatric Society (AGS) published a new consensus statement on vitamin D and calcium supplementation for reduction of falls and fractures in adults 65 years and older and for high-risk populations with malabsorption syndromes, those using medications that accelerate vitamin D metabolism, the obese, and those with minimal sun exposure (AGS, 2014).

Vitamin D sufficiency is defined as 25(OH)D$_3$ at 75 nmol/L, or 30 ng/mL (AGS, 2014). Serum levels even higher at 90 to 100 nmol/L (36 to 40 ng/ml) are recommended by some (Bischoff-Ferrari, 2014). Optimal levels of 25(OH)D$_3$ have not been defined, and the measurement of serum levels lacks standardization and calibration.

A vitamin D deficiency may be due to inadequate dietary intake, inadequate exposure to sunlight, or malabsorption. Deficiency of vitamin D also can lead to secondary malabsorption of calcium. Calcium malabsorption occurs in chronic renal failure because renal hydroxylation is required to activate vitamin D, which promotes synthesis of a calcium-binding protein in intestinal absorptive cells (see Chapter 35). Vitamin D toxicity is rare, but it has been reported in a few patients taking megadoses of vitamin D. Reported adverse effects include hypercalcemia, hyperphosphatemia, suppressed parathyroid-hormone levels, and hypercalciuria (Klontz and Acheson, 2007).

Vitamin E

Vitamin E status can be estimated by measuring serum alpha-tocopherol or the ratio of serum alpha-tocopherol to total serum lipids. A low ratio suggests vitamin E deficiency. Deficiencies are uncommon in the developed world except in individuals with fat malabsorption syndromes. The main symptoms of a vitamin E deficiency include mild hemolytic anemia and nonspecific neurologic effects. In adults, alpha-tocopherol levels is less than 5 μg/ml (<11.6 μmol/L) are associated with a deficiency. In adults with hyperlipidemia, a low ratio of serum alpha-tocopherol to lipids (<0.8 mg/g total lipid) is the most accurate indicator.

Vitamin E toxicity is uncommon, but intakes of vitamin E greater than 1000 mg/d may result in a significant bleeding risk, especially if the individual is taking anticoagulation medications. Although adverse effects are rarely observed even in individuals taking very high dosages of vitamin E, a meta-analysis showed a possible increase in mortality at dosages of 400 IU/d and higher (alpha-tocopherol only) (Miller et al, 2005).

Vitamin K

Vitamin K status can be estimated using prothrombin time (PT). PT is used to evaluate the common pathway of blood clotting. The synthesis of clotting factors II, VII, IX, and X are vitamin K dependent. **Osteocalcin** or bone G1a protein (BGP), a bone turnover marker, may also be used to assess vitamin K status. The production of BGP is stimulated by 1,25 dihydroxy vitamin D (1,25[OH]2D3) and depends on vitamin K. Vitamin K increases the carboxylation of osteocalcin or BGP, but it does not increase its overall rate of synthesis. A reduced vitamin K status is associated with reduced BGP or serum osteocalcin levels. This relationship may explain the pathophysiologic findings of vitamin K–deficiency osteoporosis. The function of osteocalcin is unclear; however, it may exist as a deposition site for hydroxyapatite crystals or it also may affect energy metabolism via the production and action of insulin (Hammami, 2014).

WATER-SOLUBLE VITAMINS AND TRACE MINERALS

Ascorbic Acid

Ascorbic acid or vitamin C is a water-soluble vitamin and also an antioxidant. Vitamin C status can be determined by measuring blood ascorbic acid levels. Values less than 6 mg/dl (<34 micromol/L) suggest insufficiency and values less than 2 mg/dl (<11 micromol/L) suggest a deficiency. Deficiencies are rare in developed countries unless self-imposed dietary intake is highly restrictive. Symptoms of a deficiency include bleeding gums, loose teeth, poor wound healing, and perifollicular hemorrhages. Toxicities have been reported in individuals taking more than 2 g/d for an extended period of time.

Vitamin B$_{12}$ and folate are the most common water-soluble vitamin deficiencies reported in adults. Frank deficiencies of other water-soluble vitamins and trace minerals are uncommon in populations that consume a variety of whole foods and fortified foods. Thiamin deficiency has been reported in individuals who chronically consume high levels of alcohol with inadequate thiamin intake, in those with persistent vomiting, when someone is on high doses of diruetics and has poor intake, in those with impaired absorption because of disease or surgery as well as individuals on long-term PN without adequate vitamin added. To assess thiamin status, thiamin diphosphate in whole blood is measured because plasma and serum levels reflect recent dietary changes and may be misleading. Subclinical deficiencies of water-soluble vitamins and other trace minerals may be present in some individuals. However, the current methodologies for evaluating nutritional status of these components are expensive and controversial. See Appendix 22 for further discussion of tests for assessing specific vitamin and trace mineral adequacy.

Markers of Body Composition

Creatinine

Creatinine is formed from creatine, found almost exclusively in muscle tissue. Serum creatinine is used along with BUN to assess kidney function (see Chapter 35). Urinary creatinine has been used to assess somatic (muscle) protein status. Creatine is synthesized from the amino acids glycine and arginine with addition of a methyl group from the folate- and cobalamin-dependent methionine–SAM–homocysteine cycle. Creatine phosphate is a high-energy phosphate buffer that provides a constant supply of ATP for muscle contraction. When creatine is dephosphorylated, some of it is converted spontaneously to creatinine by an irreversible, nonenzymatic reaction. Creatinine has no specific biologic function; it is released continuously from the muscle cells and excreted by the kidneys with little reabsorption.

The use of urinary creatinine to assess somatic protein status is confounded by omnivorous diets. Because creatine is stored in muscle, muscle meats are rich sources. The creatinine formed from dietary creatine cannot be distinguished from endogenously produced creatinine. When a person follows a meat-restricted diet, the size of the somatic (muscle) protein pool is directly proportional to the amount of creatinine excreted.

Therefore men generally have higher serum levels and excrete larger amounts of creatinine than women, and individuals with greater muscular development have higher serum levels and excrete larger amounts than those who are less muscular. Total body weight is not proportional to creatinine excretion, but muscle mass is. Creatinine excretion rate is related to muscle mass and is expressed as a percentage of a standard value as shown by the following equation for creatinine-height index (CHI):

$$CHI = 24\text{-hr urine creatinine (mg)} \times 100 \div \text{Expected 24-hr urine creatinine/cm height}$$

Calculated CHI greater than 80% is normal, 60% to 80% suggests mild skeletal muscle depletion, 40% to 60% suggests moderate depletion, and less than 40% suggests severe depletion (Blackburn et al, 1977).

Daily creatinine excretion varies significantly within individuals, probably because of losses in sweat. In addition, the test is based on 24-hour urine collections, which are difficult to obtain. Because of these limitations, urinary creatinine concentration as a marker of muscle mass has limited use in health care settings and is used typically only in research (Table 7-5).

Nitrogen Balance

Nitrogen balance studies are used primarily in research studies to estimate the balance between exogenous nitrogen intake (orally, enterally, or parenterally) and removal of nitrogen-containing compounds (urinary, fecal, wound), and other nitrogen sources. These studies are not a measure of protein anabolism and catabolism because true protein turnover studies require consumption of labeled (stable isotope) protein to track protein use. Even if useful, nitrogen balance studies are difficult because valid 24-hour urine collections are tedious unless the patient has a catheter. In addition, changes in renal function are common in patients with inflammatory metabolism, making standard nitrogen balance calculations inaccurate without calculation of nitrogen retention (Gottschlich et al, 2001). Clinicians using nitrogen balance to estimate protein

TABLE 7-5 Expected Urinary Creatinine Excretions for Adults Based on Height			
ADULT MALES*		**ADULT FEMALES†**	
Height (cm)	Creatinine (mg)	Height (cm)	Creatinine (mg)
157.5	1288	147.3	830
160.0	1325	149.9	851
162.6	1359	152.9	875
165.1	1386	154.9	900
167.6	1426	157.5	925
170.2	1467	160.0	949
172.7	1513	162.6	977
175.3	1555	165.1	1006
177.8	1596	167.6	1044
180.3	1642	170.2	1076
182.9	1691	172.7	1109
185.4	1739	175.3	1141
188.0	1785	177.8	1174
190.5	1831	180.3	1206
193.0	1891	182.9	1240

*Creatinine coefficient males 23 mg/kg "ideal" body weight.
†Creatinine coefficient females 18 mg/kg "ideal" body weight.

flux in critically ill patients must remember the limitations of these studies and that positive nitrogen balance may not mean that protein catabolism has decreased, particularly in inflammatory (disease and trauma) conditions.

CHRONIC DISEASE RISK ASSESSMENT

Lipid Indices of Cardiovascular Risk

The American College of Cardiology (ACC) and American Heart Association (AHA) released new practice guidelines for the assessment of cardiovascular risk (Stone et al, 2014). These guidelines are referred to as the Adult Treatment Panel 4 (ATP 4) and replace the Adult Treatment Panel 3 (ATP 3). Four high-risk groups are identified:

- Adults with atherosclerotic cardiovascular disease
- Adults with diabetes, aged 40 to 75 years, with low-density lipoprotein (LDL) levels 70 to 189 mg/dl
- Adults with LDL cholesterol levels of at least 190 mg/dl
- Adults aged 40 to 75 years who have LDL levels 70 to 189 mg/dl and at least 7.5% 10-year risk of atherosclerotic cardiovascular disease

Ten-year risk of atherosclerotic cardiovascular disease is determined using the Framingham 10-year general cardiovascular disease risk equations. Risk factors include age, gender, total cholesterol, HDL cholesterol, smoking status, systolic blood pressure, and current treatment for high blood pressure (Box 7-1). The new ACC/AHA Guidelines deemphasize use of

---

BOX 7-1 **Lipid and Lipoprotein Atherosclerotic Cardiovascular Risk Factors**

Laboratory test cutpoints used to calculate 10-year risk of ACVD
Total cholesterol: >200 mg/dl
HDL: <40 mg/dl
LDL: >131 mg/dl
In selected high-risk individuals, these laboratory test cutpoints may be considered:
hs-CRP cutpoints used to assign risk
- <1.0 mg/L = low risk
- 1.1-3.0 mg/L = average risk
- 3.1-9.9 mg/L = high risk
- ≥10 mg/L = very high risk
- If initial value is >3.0 but <10 mg/L, repeat in 2 weeks

Lipoprotein-associated phospholipase A₂ (Lp-PLA₂): used in conjunction with hs-CRP with intermediate or high risk
Apolipoprotein A-1: May be used in addition to LDL-C monitoring as a non-HDL-C marker in patients with serum triglycerides >200 mg/dl; decreased level is atherogenic
Apolipoprotein B/A ratio: May be used in addition to LDL-C monitoring as a non-HDL-C marker in patients with serum triglycerides ≥200 mg/dl
Other laboratory test results associated with cardiovascular risk, but not recommended in ATP 4
VLDL density: Remnants are atherogenic
Lp(a): Elevated levels are atherogenic
Serum homocysteine: Increased = greater risk
RBP4: Elevated levels may identify early insulin resistance and associated cardiovascular risk factors

Adapted from Stone NJ et al: 2013 ACC/AHA guideline on the treatment of blood cholesterol to reduce atherosclerotic cardiovascular risk in adults: a report of the American College of Cardiology/American Heart Association Task Force on practice guidelines, *Circulation* 129 (25 Suppl 2):S1, 2014.
HDL, High-density lipoprotein; *hs-CRP,* high-sensitivity C-reactive protein; *IDL,* intermediate-density lipoprotein; *LDL,* low-density lipoprotein; *Lp(a),* lipoprotein little a; *RBP4,* retinol-binding protein 4; *VLDL,* very low density lipoprotein.

---

any markers other than LDL cholesterol and HDL cholesterol. Emerging risk markers for atherosclerotic cardiovascular disease (ACVD) that are not recommended in ATP 4 include differentiating subparticles of LDL by size and grouping by pattern, apolipoprotein B (apoB), and apolipoprotein E (apoE) phenotype. The Cholesterol Expert Panel determined that these markers are not independent markers for risk and do not add to prediction equations. Other researchers propose mathematical models that predict the risk of plaque formation for combined levels of LDL and HDL (Hao and Friedman, 2014). See Chapter 33 for further discussion of the lipid profile and cardiovascular risk.

The National Lipid Association (NLA) Expert Panel presents somewhat different treatment goals from the ATP 4. The NLA includes treatment goals for non–HDL cholesterol, LDL cholesterol, and apolipoprotein B (Jacobson et al, 2014; see Chapter 33).

Patients undergoing lipid assessments should be fasting for 12 hours at the time of blood sampling. Fasting is necessary primarily because triglyceride levels rise and fall dramatically in the postprandial state, and LDL cholesterol values are calculated from measured total serum cholesterol and high-density lipoprotein cholesterol concentrations. This calculation, based on the Friedewald equation, is most accurate when triglyceride concentrations are less than 400 mg/dl. The Friedewald equation gives an estimate of fasting LDL cholesterol levels that is generally within 4 mg/dl of the true value when triglyceride concentrations are less than 400 mg/dl.

Hemoglobin A1C and Diabetes

In adults with normal glucose control, approximately 4% to 6% of the total Hgb is glycosylated. The percent of this glycohemoglobin or hemoglobin A1C (Hgb A1C) in the blood is related directly to the average blood glucose levels for the preceding 2 to 3 months and does not reflect more recent changes in glucose levels. It is useful in differentiating between short-term hyperglycemia in individuals under stress or who have had an acute myocardial infarction and those with diabetes. It has been added as a diagnostic criteria for diagnosis of diabetes mellitus once the initial value is confirmed by a repeat Hgb A1C above 6.5%, or plasma glucose above 200 mg/dl (11 mmol/L). Hgb A1C is not used as a diagnostic criterion for gestational diabetes because of changes in red cell turnover (American Diabetes Association [ADA], 2011).

Hgb A1C can be correlated with daily mean plasma glucose. Each 1% change in Hgb A1C represents approximately 35 mg/dl change in mean plasma glucose. Test results are useful to provide feedback to patients about changes they have made in their nutritional intakes (ADA, 2011). See Chapter 30 for further discussion of Hgb A1C and diabetes management.

Markers of Oxidative Stress and Inflammation

Biomarkers of oxidative stress status and inflammation have been associated with many chronic conditions and risk factors (see Chapter 3). Aging and many diseases, including rheumatoid arthritis, Parkinson disease, Alzheimer disease, cardiovascular disease, and cancer, are initiated, in part, by oxidative stress as evidenced by free radical oxidation of lipids, nucleic acids, or proteins. An indirect way of assessing the level of oxidative stress is to measure the levels of antioxidant compounds present in body fluids. Oxidative stress is related to levels of the following:

- Antioxidant vitamins (tocopherols and ascorbic acid)
- Dietary phytochemicals with antioxidant properties (e.g., carotenoids)

- Minerals with antioxidant roles (e.g., selenium)
- Endogenous antioxidant compounds and enzymes (e.g., superoxide dismutase, glutathione)

More precisely, the concentration of these compounds correlates with the balance between their intake and production, and their use during the inhibition of free radical compounds produced by oxidative stress.

Measurement of intracellular antioxidant thiols such as glutathione can be estimated using the free oxygen radical test via spectrophotometric techniques on specimens obtained from finger sticks. However, further standardization of protocols for assays and methods of combining and integrating multiple panels of biomarkers of oxidative stress and inflammation are needed to facilitate evaluation of biomarkers for risk factor prediction. Although some intervention studies examining the effects of dietary supplements, diet, and exercise on biomarkers of oxidative stress and inflammation have been done, the data have been inconclusive, and more studies are needed to understand the underlying mechanisms.

The most commonly used chemical markers of oxidative stress are presented in Table 7-6. Some tests measure the presence of one class of free radical products, and others measure the global antioxidant capacity of plasma or a plasma fraction. For example, one noninvasive test measures antioxidant capacity by using Raman spectroscopy with a laser scanner to measure the amount of carotenoids at the cellular level. (See New Directions: *Raman Spectroscopy Used to Measure Antioxidant Capacity.*) These tests have been promoted on the assumption that knowledge of the total antioxidant capacity of the plasma or plasma fraction may be more useful than knowledge of the individual concentrations of free radical markers or antioxidants. This total antioxidant activity is determined by a test that assesses the combined antioxidant capacities of the constituents. Unfortunately, the results of these tests include the antioxidant capacities of compounds such as uric acid and albumin, which are not compounds of interest. In other words, no one type of assay is likely to provide a global picture of the oxidative stress to which an individual is exposed.

TABLE 7-6 Advantages and Disadvantages of Various Biomarkers of Oxidative Stress

Biomarker	Advantages	Disadvantages	Comments
IsoPs (isoprostanes)	Can be detected in various samples (serum, urine) and has been shown to be elevated in the presence of a range of CV risk factors	Current methods of quantification are impractical for large-scale screening.	No evidence linking this biomarker to clinical outcomes yet. F_2-IsoPs show most potential.
MDA (malondialdehyde)	Technically easy to quantify spectrophotometrically using the TBARS assay ELISA kits to detect MDA also have good performance. Studies show MDA can predict progression of CAD and carotid atherosclerosis at 3 years	TBARS assay is nonspecific (can detect aldehydes other than MDA) and sample preparation can influence results.	Shows promise as a clinical biomarker; however does not have a functional impact on the pathophysiology of CVD
Nitrotyrosine (3-NO2-tyr)	Human studies have demonstrated association with CAD independent of traditional risk factors	Circulating levels are not equivalent to tissue levels. Current detection methods are expensive and impractical.	Nitrotyrosine formation on particular cardiovascular proteins has direct effect on function
S-glutathionylation	S-glutathionylation of SERCA, eNOS and Na$^+$–K$^+$ pump demonstrated as biomarkers as well as role in pathogenesis	Detection of S-glutationylation prone to methodological artifact. Access to tissue (myocardium, vasculature), where modification occurs presents a clinical obstacle	Modified hemoglobin currently being investigated as biomarker
Myeloperoxidase (MPO)	Commercial assays available. An enzyme abundant in granules in inflammatory cells. Strong evidence that MPO correlates with CVD risk	Influenced by sample storage and time to analysis	MPO is a promising biomarker for CVD risk prediction.
Oxidized LDL cholesterol (OxLDL)	Forms and occurs in vascular walls as foam cells and stimulates production of proinflammatory cytokines by endothelial cells. Elevated in CAD, increasing OxLDL correlates with increasing clinical severity. Also is predictive of future CAD in healthy population. Good reproducibility from frozen samples	Reduction in OxLDL by antioxidant pharmacotherapy has not been matched by reduction in CVD severity.	ELISAs for OxLDL detection readily available
ROS-induced changes to gene expression	The expression of several genes involved in regulating oxidative stress may be measured simultaneously using microarray technology, potentially increasing the power of this biomarker	Microarray technology can be manually and computationally expensive	It is unclear if expression profiles of cells in biologic samples reflect that in cardiovascular tissues
Serum antioxidant capacity	Activity of antioxidant enzymes such as glutathione peroxidase 1 (GPX-1) and superoxide dismutase (SOD) are demonstrated to be inversely proportional to CAD. Commercial kits available to measure antioxidant capacity. Reproducibly quantified despite frozen sample storage	Antioxidant activity in serum may not reflect that of the cells that are important to the pathogenesis of CVD	Clinical relevance of antioxidant quantification to CVD risk needs further investigation

CAD, Coronary artery disease; *CV*, cardiovascular, ; *CVD*, cardiovascular disease; *ELISA*, enzyme-linked immunosorbent assay; *TBARS*, thiobarbituric acid (TBA) reacting substances; *eNOS*, endothelial nitric oxide synthase; *GPX-1*, glutathione peroxidase-1, *ROS*, reactive oxygen species; *SERCA*, sarcoplasmic reticulum Ca^{2+}-ATPase , *SOD*, superoxide dismutase.
Adapted from Ho E et al: Biological markers of oxidative stress: applications to cardiovascular research and practice, *Redox Biology* 1:483, 2013.

Raman Spectroscopy Used to Measure Antioxidant Capacity

Noninvasive measurements of clinical parameters are always preferable to those requiring blood, urine, or tissue. Raman spectroscopy, or resonance Raman spectroscopy (RRS) is just such a measurement technique, and is being used to measure the antioxidant capacity of an individual. It measures the antioxidant capacity by measuring the amount of skin carotenoids. Carotenoids are powerful antioxidants, and because they are part of the "antioxidant network," a measure of their presence can give a good assessment of the antioxidant capacity of the cell and thus the individual.

A laser light is pointed toward the skin (usually the fat pad of the palm). As the laser light penetrates the skin, the amount of skin carotenoids (all-trans-beta-carotene, lycopene, alpha-carotene, gamma-carotene, phytoene, phytofluene, sepapreno-beta-carotene, dihydro-beta-carotene, astaxanthin, canthaxanthin, zeaxanthin, lutein, violaxanthins, and rhodoxanthin) is measured because carotenoids have a carbon backbone with alternating carbon double and single bonds, and the vibration of these bonds can be detected with RRS.

Serum carotenoids as measured by high performance liquid chromatography (HPLC) significantly correlate with skin carotenoids, as measured using RSS. (Ermakov and Gellerman, 2015, Aguilar et al, 2014, Nguyen et al, 2015). The measurement of skin carotenoids, or the RRS score, also correlates with reported fruit and vegetable and dietary carotenoid intake; the greater the intake of fruits and vegetables, the higher the score. (Jahns et al, 2014). This was found in both adults and children. (Nguyen et al, 2015). The use of skin carotenoid status can be used as an objective biomarker of change in fruit and vegetable based intervention studies or clinical dietary protocols (Mayne et al, 2013, Jahns et al, 2014).

This score, or the numeric result from this scan, can also be used to determine how well a person is processing the consumed carotenoid antioxidants, and whether the antioxidants are reaching the cell where they exert their protective functions. The RRS score is higher in those with optimal health, and besides increasing with greater consumption of fruits and vegetables, it also increases with consumption of carotenoid-containing nutritional supplements, smoking cessation, and loss of excess body fat (Carlson et al., 2006). It has also been found to be lower in those with an ongoing oxidative stress such as with metabolic syndrome (Holt et al, 2014). RRS has also been used to assess carotenoids in precancerous skin lesions, and to assess early stages of macular degeneration in the retina (Carlson et al., 2006).

With the development of portable scanners, RRS measurement is quick, easy, and inexpensive, making it a possible nutritional assessment tool for professionals in the future.

Aguilar SS et al: Skin carotenoids: A biomarker of fruit and vegetable intake in children *J Acad Nutr Diet* 114:1174, 2014.

Carlson JJ et al: Associations of antioxidant status, oxidative stress with skin carotenoids assessed by Raman spectroscopy (RS), *FASEB J* 20:1318, 2006.

Ermakov, IV and Gellerman, W: Optical detection methods for carotenoids in human skin, *Arch Biochem Biophys* 572:101, 2015.

Holt EW et al: Low skin carotenoid concentration measured by resonance Raman spectroscopy is associated with metabolic syndrome in adults, *Nutr Res* 34:821, 2014.

Jahns L et al: Skin and plasma carotenoid response to a provided intervention diet high in vegetables and fruit: uptake and depletion kinetics, *Am J Clin Nutr* 100: 930, 2014.

Mayne ST et al: Resonance raman spectroscopic evaluation of skin carotenoids as a biomarker of carotenoid status for human studies, *Arch Biochem Biophys* 539:163, 2013.

Nguyen LM et al: Evaluating the relationship between plasma and skin carotenoids and reported dietary intake in elementary school children to assess fruit and vegetable intake, *Arch Biochem Biophys* 572: 73, 2015.

Despite this lack of correlation or specificity of assays of oxidative stress, three assays seem promising. One is the immunoassay myeloperoxidase used in conjunction with CRP to predict CVD mortality risk (Heslop et al, 2010). The second assay is the measurement of the compounds F_2 isoprostanes either in plasma or urine (Harrison and Nieto, 2011). This test measures the presence of a continuously formed free radical compound that is produced by free radical oxidation of specific polyunsaturated fatty acids. Isoprostanes are prostaglandin-like compounds that are produced by free radical mediated peroxidation of lipoproteins. Elevated isoprostane levels are associated with oxidative stress, and clinical situations of oxidative stress such as hepatorenal syndrome, rheumatoid arthritis, atherosclerosis, and carcinogenesis (Roberts and Fessel, 2004). The third test is urinary 8-hydroxy-2′ deoxyguanosine (8-OH-d-g), in which elevated levels are associated with inadequate intake of carotenoids and antioxidant-rich foods (see Table 7-6).

PHYSICAL ASSESSMENTS

Anthropometry

Anthropometry involves obtaining physical measurements of an individual, comparing them to standards that reflect the growth and development of that individual, and using them for evaluating overnutrition, undernutrition, or the effects of nutrition preventions over a period of time. Accurate and consistent measurements require training in the proper techniques using calibrated instruments. Measurements of accuracy can be established by several clinicians taking the same measurement and comparing results. Valuable anthropometric measurements include height, weight, and girth measurements. Skinfold thicknesses and circumference measurements are used in some settings but are associated with a higher rate of inconsistency. Head circumference and length are used in pediatric populations. Birth weight and ethnic, familial, and environmental factors affect these parameters and should be considered when anthropometric measures are evaluated.

Interpretation of Height and Weight in Children and Teens

Currently, reference standards are based on a statistical sample of the U.S. population. The WHO international growth standards are based on data from multiple countries and ethnic populations and have been adopted for use in numerous countries. In the United States, the expert review panel of WHO and CDC growth charts recommend the WHO growth standards for children aged less than 24 months and the CDC growth charts for children aged 24 months to 18 years.

Height and weight measurements of children are recorded as percentiles, which reflect the percentage of the total population of children of the same sex who are at or below the same height or weight at a certain age. Children's growth at every age can be monitored by mapping data on growth curves, known as **height-for-age**, **length-for-age**, **weight-for-age**, and **weight-for-length curves**. Appendices 4 through 11 provide pediatric growth charts and percentile interpretations.

Length and Height

The methodology used for determining the length or height of children is determined by the age of the child. Recumbent length measurements are used for infants and children younger

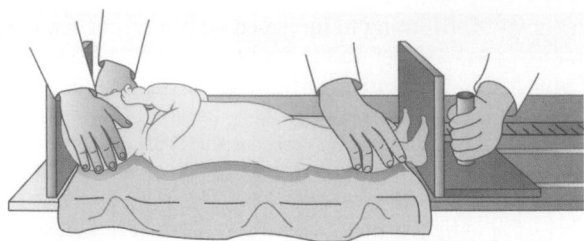

FIGURE 7-3 Measurement of the length of an infant.

than 2 or 3 years of age. Ideally these young children should be measured using a length board as shown in Figure 7-3. Recumbent lengths in children ages 2 and younger should be recorded on the birth to 24-month growth grids. Standing height is determined in children using a measuring rod, or *statiometer*, and should be recorded on the 2- to 20-year growth grids, as in Appendices 6, 7, 10, and 11. Sitting heights may be measured in children who cannot stand (see Figure 44-1). Recording on the proper growth grids provides a record of a child's gain in height over time and compares the child's height with that of other children of the same age. The rate of length or height gain reflects long-term nutritional adequacy.

Weight

Weight in children and teens is a more sensitive measure of nutritional adequacy than height, because it reflects more recent nutritional intake and provides a rough estimate of overall fat and muscle reserves. For children who are obese or have edema, weight alone makes it difficult to assess overall nutritional status. Weight should be recorded on the age- and gender-appropriate growth grid.

Body weight is interpreted using various methods, including **body mass index (BMI)**, usual weight, and actual weight. BMI is used as a screening tool to identify overweight and obese children and teens. Although the calculation of BMI is the same for adults and children, the interpretation of BMI is different in children and teens. BMI is plotted on the CDC BMI-for-age growth charts from which a percentile ranking can be determined. These percentiles are the most commonly used indicator to assess the size and growth patterns of children and teens aged 2 to 20 years in the United States (see Appendices 7 and 11). BMI-for-age weight status categories are noted in Box 7-2.

Interpretation of Height and Weight in Adults

In adults, height and weight measurements are also useful for evaluating nutrition status. Both should be measured because the tendency is to overestimate height and underestimate weight, resulting in an underestimation of the relative weight or BMI. In addition, many adults are losing height as a result of osteoporosis, joint deterioration, and poor posture, and this should be documented (Box 7-3).

BOX 7-2	**Interpretation of BMI-for-Age Percentiles in Children and Teens**	
Percentile Range	**Interpretation**
Less than 5th percentile	Underweight
5th percentile to less than 85th percentile	Healthy weight
85th percentile to less than the 95th percentile	Overweight
Equal to or greater than the 95th percentile	Obese

BOX 7-3 Using Height and Weight to Assess a Hospitalized Patient's Nutritional Status

- Measure. Do not just ask a person's height.
- Measure weight (at admission, current, and usual).
- Determine percentage of weight change over time (weight pattern).
- Determine percentage above or below usual or ideal body weight.

Measurements of height can be obtained using a direct or an indirect approach. The direct method involves a statiometer, and the adult must be able to stand or recline flat. Indirect methods, including knee-height measurements, arm span, or recumbent length using a tape measure, may be options for those who cannot stand or stand straight, such as individuals with scoliosis, kyphosis (curvature of the spine), cerebral palsy, muscular dystrophy, contractures, paralysis, or who are bedridden (see Appendix 15). Recumbent height measurements made with a tape measure while the person is in bed may be appropriate for individuals in institutions who are comatose, critically ill, or unable to be moved. However, this method can be used only with patients who do not have musculoskeletal deformities or contractures.

Ideal weight for height reference standards such as the Metropolitan Life Insurance Tables from 1959 and 1983 or the National Health and Nutrition Examination Survey percentiles are no longer used. A commonly used method of determining ideal body weight is the Hamwi Equation (Hamwi, 1964). It does not adjust for age, race, or frame size and its validity is questionable. Nonetheless, it is in widespread use by clinicians as a quick method for estimation of ideal weight:

Men: 106 lb for first 5 feet of height and 6 lb per inch over 5 feet; or 6 lb subtracted for each inch under 5 feet

Women: 100 lb for first 5 feet of height and 5 lb per inch over 5 feet; or 5 lb subtracted for each inch under 5 feet

Using the Hamwi method a female who is 5 feet 5 inches tall would have an ideal weight of 125 pounds.

Actual body weight is the weight measurement obtained at the time of examination. This measurement may be influenced by changes in the individual's fluid status. Weight loss can reflect dehydration but also can reflect a pattern of suboptimal food intake. The percentage of weight loss is highly indicative of the extent and severity of an individual's illness. The Characteristics of Malnutrition defined by the Academy of Nutrition and Dietetics (AND) and ASPEN serve as a benchmark for evaluating weight loss (White et al, 2012):

- Significant weight loss: 5% loss in a month, 7.5% loss in 3 months, 10% loss in 6 months
- Severe weight loss: >5% weight loss in a month, >7.5% weight loss in 3 months, >10% weight loss in 6 months

$$\text{Percentage weight loss} = \text{Usual wt} - \text{Actual wt/ Usual wt} \times 100$$

- For example if a person's usual weight is 200 lb and he now weighs 180 lb, that is a weight loss of 20 lb.

$$200 \text{ to } 180 = 20\text{lb}/200\text{lb} = 0.10 \text{ or } 10\%$$

- If this person has lost this 10% in 2 months, that would be more than 7.5% in 3 months and considered SEVERE weight loss.

Another method for evaluating the percentage of weight loss is to calculate an individual's current weight as a percentage of usual weight. **Usual body weight (UBW)** is a more useful parameter than **ideal body weight (IBW)** for those who are experiencing involuntary weight loss. However, one problem with using UBW is that it may depend on the patient's memory.

Body Mass Index

The Quetelet index (W/H^2) or the BMI is used to determine whether an adult's weight is appropriate for height and can indicate overnutrition or undernutrition. BMI accounts for differences in body composition by defining the level of adiposity and relating it to height, thus eliminating dependence on frame size (Stensland and Margolis, 1990). The BMI has the least correlation with body height and the highest correlation with independent measures of body fat for adults. The BMI is an indirect measure of body fat and correlates with the direct body fat measures such as underwater weighing and dual x-ray absorptiometry (Keys et al, 1972; Mei et al, 2002). BMI is calculated as follows:

Metric : BMI = Weight (kg) ÷ Height (m)2
English: BMI = Weight (lb) ÷ Height (in)2 × 703

Nomograms are also available to calculate BMI, as are various charts (see Appendix 18). The Clinical Insight box: *Calculating BMI and Determining Appropriate Body Weight* gives an example of the BMI calculation.

Standards classify a BMI of less than 18.5 for an adult as underweight, a BMI between 25 and 29 as overweight, and a BMI greater than 30 as obese. A healthy BMI for adults is considered between 18.5 and 24.9 (CDC, 2014). Although a strong correlation exists between total body fat and BMI, individual variations must be recognized before making conclusions regarding appropriate body fatness (Mueller, 2012).

Differences in race, sex, and age must be considered when evaluating the BMI. BMI values tend to increase with age, yet the relationship between BMI and mortality appears to be 0U-shaped in adults aged 65 and older. The risk of mortality increased in older adults with a BMI of less than 23 (Winter, 2014; see Chapter 20).

Body Composition

Body composition is a critical component of nutrition assessment and medical status. It is used concurrently with other assessment factors to differentiate the estimated proportions of fat mass, soft tissue body mass, and bone mass. For example, muscular athletes may be classified as overweight because of excess muscle mass contributing to increased weight rather than excessive adipose tissue. Older adults tend to have lower bone density and reduced lean body mass and therefore may weigh less than younger adults of the same height and yet have greater adiposity. Variation in body composition exists among different population groups as well as within the same group. The majority of body composition studies that were performed on whites may not be valid for other ethnic groups. There are differences and similarities between blacks and whites relative to fat-free body mass, fat patterning, and body dimensions and proportions; blacks have greater bone mineral density and body protein compared with whites (Wagner and Heyward, 2000). In addition, optimal BMIs for Asian populations must be in the lower ranges of "normal" for optimal health to reflect their higher cardiovascular risks (Zheng et al, 2009). These factors must be considered to avoid inaccurate estimation of body fat and interpretation of risk.

Imaging techniques such as dual-energy x-ray absorptiometry (DXA) and magnetic resonance imaging (MRI) are used in research and clinical settings to assess body composition. The focus of the research on different imaging methodologies is to quantify characteristics of lean soft tissue (LST) that predicts clinical risk and nutrition status. Areas of greatest research are to assess for sarcopenia, sarcopenic obesity, and osteosarcopenic obesity (Prado, 2014).

Subcutaneous Fat in Skinfold Thickness

In research studies and selected health care settings, fat-fold or skinfold thickness measurements may be used to estimate body fat in an individual. Skinfold measurement assumes that 50% of body fat is subcutaneous. Because of limitations with accuracy and reproducibility, these measurements are not used routinely in clinical settings.

Circumference Measurements

Circumference measurements may be useful in health care settings in which these measurements are recorded periodically (e.g., monthly or quarterly) and tracked over time to identify trends and potential risk factors for chronic conditions. However, in acutely ill individuals with daily fluid shifts measures of arm circumference and TSF measurements usually are not performed. (See New Directions: Measuring the Neck: What Can it Mean?)

Circumference Measurements in Children

Head circumference measurements are useful in children younger than 3 years of age, primarily as an indicator of nonnutritional abnormalities. Undernutrition must be very severe to affect head circumference; see Box 7-4.

Measuring Head Circumference

Midarm circumference (MAC) is measured in centimeters halfway between the acromion process of the scapula and the olecranon process at the tip of the elbow. MAC should be measured when assessing for nutritional status of children and compared with the standards developed by WHO for children aged 6 to 59 months of age (de Onis et al, 1997). It is an independent anthropometric assessment tool in determining malnutrition in children.

Circumference Measurements in Adults

MAC is measured the same way in adults as in children. Combining MAC with TSF measurements allows indirect determination of the arm muscle area (AMA) and arm fat area. Because of

---

CLINICAL INSIGHT

Calculating BMI and Determining Appropriate Body Weight

Example: Woman who is 5'8" (68 in) tall and weighs 185 pounds (lb)
Step 1: Calculate current BMI:
Formula: (Metric)   Weight (kg) 84 kg ÷ Height (m2) (1.72 m) ×
                     (1.72 m) = 84 ÷ 2.96 m2 = BMI = 28.4 =
                     overweight
Step 2: Appropriate weight range to have a BMI that falls between
     18.5 and 24.9
18.5   (18.5) × (2.96) = 54.8 kg = 121 pounds
24.9   (24.9) × (2.96) = 73.8 kg = 162 pounds
Appropriate weight range = 121 − 162 lb or 54.8 − 73.8 kg

Formula (English) Weight (lb) ÷ (Height [in] × Height [in]) × 703 = BMI
BMI, Body mass index.

✳ NEW DIRECTIONS

"Measuring the Neck: What Can it Mean?"

Neck circumference (NC) is an emerging marker of overweight, obesity, and associated disease risk in children and adults. Its measurement is a novel, noninvasive screening tool that is easy to do without the privacy concerns associated with waist and hip circumference measurements. Neck circumference is measured on bare skin between the midcervical spine and midanterior neck just below the laryngeal prominence (the Adam's apple) with the head in the Frankfurt plane (looking straight ahead). The tape should be as close to horizontal as anatomically feasible (i.e., the tape line in the front of the neck will be at the same height as the tape line in the back of the neck) (Arnold, 2014).

Studies of adults report that neck circumference is associated highly with waist circumference, weight, BMI, and percent body fat. Findings from study of a predominantly African American cohort include significant correlations between serum insulin, triglycerides, and LDL cholesterol levels, and neck circumference (Arnold, 2014).

Neck circumference can be used as a reliable tool to identify adolescents with high body mass indexes (Androutsos, 2010). The Canadian Health Measures Survey has published reference data for interpretation of neck circumference measurements in Canadian children (Katz, 2014). More research is needed to determine cutoff points for identifying children at risk of central obesity-associated conditions associated with disease risk. In children and adults study is needed to establish possible neck circumference predictors for obesity-related chronic disease.

Androutsos O et al: Neck circumference: a useful screening tool of cardiovascular risk in children. *Pediatric Obesity* Jun;7(3):187, 2010.
Arnold TJ et al: Neck and waist circumference biomarkers of cardiovascular risk in a cohort of predominantly African-American college students: a preliminary study, *J Acad Nutr Dietetics* 114(1):107, 2014.
Katz S et al: Creation of a reference dataset of neck sizes in children: standardizing a potential new tool for prediction of obesity-associated diseases? *BMC Pediatr* 21;14:159, 2014.

---

limitations with accuracy and reproducibility, these measurements are rarely used to assess adult nutrition status.

Waist and Hip Circumference, Waist-to-Hip Ratio, and Waist-to-Height Ratio

Selected circumference measurements may be useful in determining estimated risk for chronic diseases and assessing changes in body composition. Waist circumference (WC) is obtained by measuring the distance around the narrowest area of the waist between the lowest rib and iliac crest and above the umbilicus using a nonstretchable tape measure. Hip circumference is measured at the widest area of the hips at the greatest protuberance of the buttocks. Because fat distribution is an indicator of risk, circumferential or girth measurements may be used. The presence of excess body fat around the abdomen out of proportion to total body fat is a risk factor for chronic diseases associated with obesity and the metabolic syndrome. A WC of greater than 40 inches (102 cm) for men and greater than 35 inches (88 cm) for women is an independent risk factor for disease (CDC, 2014; Stone, 2013). These measurements may not be as useful for those less than 60 inches tall or with a BMI of 35 or greater (CDC, 2014). WC is used as a risk indicator supplementary to BMI.

To determine the waist-to-hip ratio (WHR), divide the waist measurement by the hip measurement. The WHO defines the ratios of greater than 9.0 in men and greater than 8.5 in women as one of the decisive benchmarks for metabolic syndrome and is consistent with findings of research predicting all cause and cardiovascular disease mortality (Srikanthan et al, 2009; Welborn and Dhaliwal, 2007).

Figure 7-4 shows the proper location to measure waist (abdominal) circumference.

The waist-to-height ratio (WHtR) is defined as the waist circumference divided by the measured height. WHtR is a measure of the distribution of adipose tissue. Generally speaking, the higher the values of WHtR , the greater the risk of metabolic syndrome and obesity-related atherosclerotic cardiovascular diseases (Schneider et al, 2010). Desirable ratios are less than 0.5 in adults 40 years and younger, between 0.5 and 0.6 in adults aged 40 to 50 years, and 0.6 or less in adults over 50. These targets apply to both males and females and a variety of ethnic groups. For example, a BMI of 25 is equivalent to a WHtR of 0.51. Table 7-7 provides a guide to interpreting WHtR by gender.

Some experts have concluded that WHtR is a superior measure of cardiovascular disease than BMI (Ashwell et al, 2012). However WHtR is not identified as a risk marker in the ACC/AHA ATP 4.

Researchers have proposed A Body Shape Index (ABSI) based on WC, height, and weight as a complementary health risk indicator to be used in conjunction with BMI. More research is needed to validate this methodology (Krakauer and Krakauer, 2012).

BOX 7-4   Measuring Head Circumference

Indications
- Head circumference is a standard measurement for serial assessment of growth in children from birth to 36 months and in any child whose head size is in question.

Equipment
- Paper or metal tape measure (cloth can stretch) marked in tenths of a centimeter because growth charts are listed in 0.5-cm increments

Technique
- The head is measured at its greatest circumference.
- The greatest circumference is usually above the eyebrows and pinna of the ears and around the occipital prominence at the back of the skull.
- More than one measurement may be necessary because the shape of the head can affect the location of the maximum circumference.
- Compare the measurement with the National Center for Health Statistics standard curves for head circumference (see Appendices 5 and 9).

Data from Hockenberry MJ, Wilson D: *Wong's nursing care of infants and children*, ed 9, St Louis, 2015, Mosby.

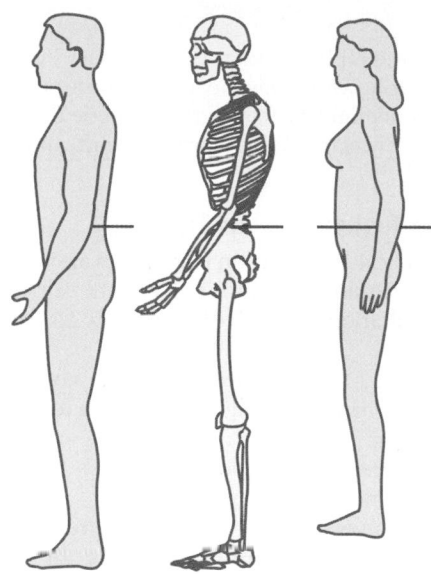

FIGURE 7-4 Measuring tape position for waist circumference.

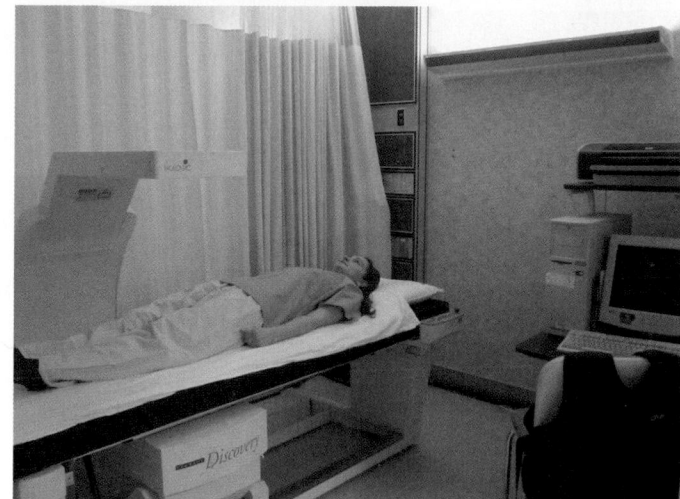

FIGURE 7-5 A patient undergoing a dual-energy x-ray absorptiometry scan. (Courtesy the Division of Nutrition, University of Utah.)

TABLE 7-7	Interpretation of Waist-to-Height Ratio by Gender	
Females	**Males**	
WHtR	WHtR	Interpretation
< 0.35	< 0.35	Underweight
0.35-0.42	0.35-0.43	Slim
0.42-0.49	0.43-0.53	Healthy
0.49-0.54	0.53-0.58	Overweight
0.54-0.58	0.58-0.63	Obese
> 0.58	> 0.63	Very obese

WHtR, Weight-to-height ratio.

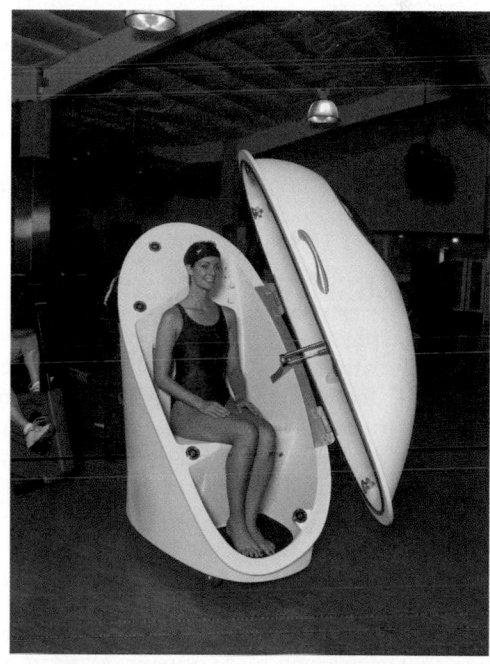

FIGURE 7-6 The BOD-POD measures body fat and fat-free mass. (Courtesy COSMED USA, Inc., Concord, CA.)

Other Methods of Measuring Body Composition

Dual-Energy X-Ray Absorptiometry

Dual-energy x-ray absorptiometry (DXA) measures fat, bone mineral, and fat-free soft tissue. The energy source in DXA is an x-ray tube that contains an energy beam. The amount of energy loss depends on the type of tissue through which the beam passes; the result can be used to measure mineral, fat, and lean tissue compartments (Russell, 2007). DXA is easy to use, emits low levels of radiation, and is available in the hospital setting, making it a useful tool. Generally, it is found to be a reliable measurement of percentage body fat; however, the patient must remain still for more than a few minutes, which may be difficult for older adults and those in chronic pain. Measurements are influenced by the thickness of tissues and hydration status (Prado and Heymsfield, 2014). Figure 7-5 illustrates a DXA scan.

Air Displacement Plethysmogram

Air displacement plethysmogram (ADP) relies on measurements of body density to estimate body fat and fat-free masses. Performing an ADP with the BOD-POD device is a densitometry technique found to be an accurate method to measure body composition. ADP appears to be a reliable instrument in body composition assessment; it is of particular interest with obese individuals. ADP does not rely on body water content to determine body density and body composition, which makes it potentially useful in those adults with end-stage renal disease (Flakoll et al, 2004; Figure 7-6).

Bioelectrical Impedance Analysis

Bioelectrical impedance analysis (BIA) is a body composition analysis technique based on the principle that, relative

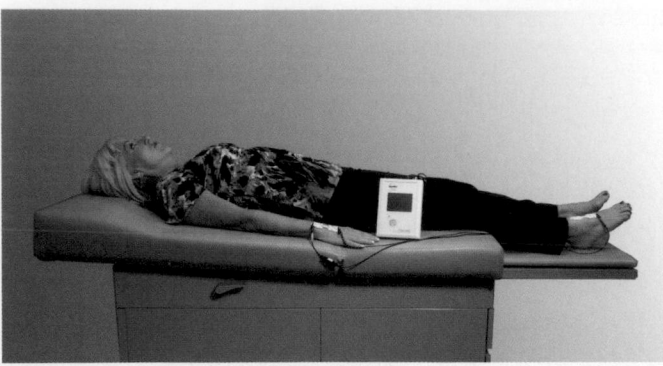

FIGURE 7-7 Image reproduced with permission of ImpediMed Limited.

to water, lean tissue has a higher electrical conductivity and lower impedance than fatty tissue because of its electrolyte content. BIA has been found to be a reliable measurement of body composition (fat-free mass and fat mass) compared with BMI or skinfold measurements or even height and weight measurements. The BIA method is safe, noninvasive, portable, and rapid (Figure 7-7). For accurate results the patient should be well hydrated; have not exercised in the previous 4 to 6 hours; and have not consumed alcohol, caffeine, or diuretics in the previous 24 hours (see Appendix 22). If the person is dehydrated, a higher percentage of body fat than really exists is measured. Fever, electrolyte imbalance, and extreme obesity also may affect the reliability of measurements.

NUTRITION-FOCUSED PHYSICAL ASSESSMENT

Nutrition-focused physical assessment (NFPA) is one of the components of nutrition assessment in the nutrition care process model. Data gathered in the NFPA are used in conjunction with food and nutrition history, laboratory and diagnostic test results, physical measurements, and client history to accurately make one or more nutrition diagnoses. The *International Dietetics & Nutrition Terminology Reference Manual* (IDNT) (AND, 2013) defines nutrition-focused physical examination as "findings from an evaluation of body systems, muscle and subcutaneous fat wasting, oral health, suck, swallow/breathe ability, appetite and affect." Unlike a comprehensive clinical examination that reviews all body systems, NFPA is a focused assessment that addresses specific signs and symptoms by reviewing selected body systems.

Approach

A systems approach is used when performing the NFPA, which should be conducted in an organized, logical way to ensure efficiency and thoroughness (Litchford, 2013). Body systems include the following:

- Overall appearance
- Vital signs
- Skin
- HEENT (head, ears, eyes, nose, and throat)
- Cardiopulmonary system
- Extremities, muscles, and bones
- Digestive system
- Nerves and cognition

Equipment

The extent of the NFPA dictates the necessary equipment. Any or all of the following may be used: examination gloves, a stethoscope, a penlight or flashlight, a tongue depressor, scales, calipers, a tape measure, a blood pressure cuff, and a watch with a second hand.

Examination Techniques and Findings

Four basic physical examination techniques are used during the NFPA. These techniques include inspection, palpation, percussion, and auscultation (Table 7-8). Appendix 21 discusses NFPA in more detail.

Interpretation of data collected in each component of an NFPA requires critical thinking skills and the following steps in clinical reasoning:

- Identify abnormal findings or symptoms.
- Localize the findings anatomically.
- Interpret findings in terms of probable process.
- Make a hypothesis about the nature of the patient's problem.
- Test the hypothesis by collaborating with other medical professionals and establish a working nutrition diagnosis.
- Develop a plan agreeable to the patient following all the steps of the NCP model (Bickley, 2009). See Chapter 10.

Guidelines for Assessing Malnutrition in Children

Definitions and guidelines to identify malnutrition in children are evolving. Pediatric malnutrition is defined as an imbalance between nutrient requirements and dietary intake that results in deficits of energy, protein, and micronutrients stores, resulting in impaired growth and development. Pediatric malnutrition is either related to an illness or injury or caused by an environmental circumstance or behavioral factor (Mehta et al, 2014). Specific parameters for determining pediatric undernutrition and malnutrition are being standardized (Becker et al, 2014).

Guidelines for Assessing Malnutrition in Adults

The Academy and the ASPEN Consensus Statement: Characteristics Recommended for the Identification and Documentation of Adult Malnutrition provides a standardized and measureable set of criteria for all health professionals to use to

TABLE 7-8	**Physical Examination Techniques**
Technique	**Description**
Inspection	General observation that progresses to a more focused observation using the senses of sight, smell, and hearing; note appearance, mood, behavior, movement, facial expressions, most frequently used technique
Palpation	Gentle tactile examination to feel pulsations and vibrations; assessment of body structures, including texture, size, temperature, tenderness, and mobility
Percussion	Assessment of sounds to determine body organ borders, shape, and position; not always used in a nutrition-focused physical examination
Auscultation	Use of the naked ear or bell or diaphragm of stethoscope to listen to body sounds (e.g., heart and lung sounds, bowel sounds, blood vessels)

Adapted from Litchford MD: *Nutrition focused physical assessment: making clinical connections,* Greensboro, NC, 2013, CASE Software & Books.

identify malnutrition (White et al, 2012). It uses a cause-based nomenclature that reflects the current understanding of the role of inflammatory response on the incidence, progression, and resolution of adult malnutrition. Moreover, malnutrition syndromes are defined by patient settings, including acute illness or surgery, chronic disease, and environmental or social circumstances. In addition, the presence and degree of inflammation further differentiates types of malnutrition as nonsevere and severe. Nonsevere does not mean not urgent; it means mild to moderate malnutrition or undernutrition (Figure 7-8).

No single parameter defines malnutrition. The Consensus guidelines identify six characteristics of malnutrition. From these, the clinician must identify a minimum of two characteristics that relate to the context of the concurrent medical condition for a nutrition diagnosis of malnutrition. The characteristics of nonsevere and severe malnutrition are noted in Table 7-9.

Measures of Functionality

Loss of functionality and mobility has a ripple effect on achieving activities of daily living (ADLs) and nutrition-related ADLs. An emerging component of nutrition-focused assessment is assessment for muscle strength and functionality. Clinicians may work collaboratively with rehabilitation therapists to assess this and identify strategies to improve physical strength and mobility using diet and exercise.

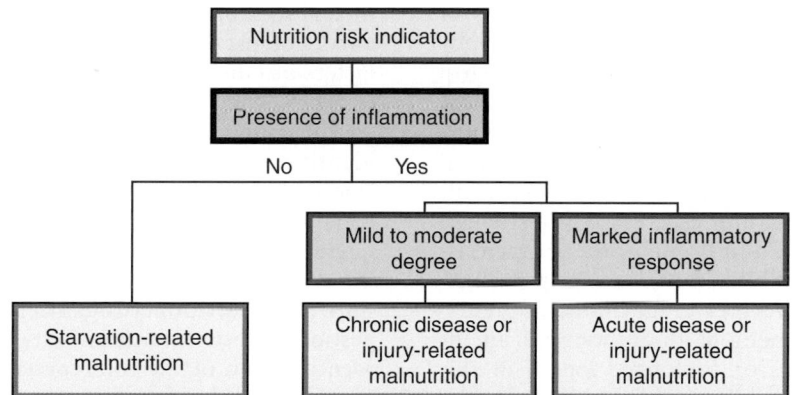

FIGURE 7-8 Cause-based malnutrition. (Adapted from White JV et al: Consensus statement of the Academy of Nutrition and Dietetics/American Society for Parenteral and Enteral Nutrition: characteristics recommended for the identification and documentation of adult malnutrition (undernutrition), *J Acad Nutr Diet* 112(5):730, 2012.)

TABLE 7-9   Characteristics of Adult Malnutrition

ACUTE ILLNESS OR INJURY		CHRONIC ILLNESS		SOCIAL OR ENVIRONMENTAL CIRCUMSTANCES	
Nonsevere	**Severe**	**Nonsevere**	**Severe**	**Nonsevere**	**Severe**
Interpretation of Weight Loss for Malnutrition by Cause					
1-2% in 1 wk	>2% in 1 wk	5% in 1 wk	>5% in 1 wk	>5% in 1 wk	>5% in 1 wk
5% in 1 mo	>5% in 1 mo	7.5% in 3 mo	>7.5% in 3 mo	>7.5% in 3 mo	>7.5% in 3 mo
7.5% in 3 mo	>7.5% in 3 mo	10% in 6 mo	>10% in 6 mo	>10% in 6 mo	>10% in 6 mo
		20% in 1 yr	>20% in 1 yr	>20% in 1 yr	>20% in 1 yr
Interpretation of Reduced Energy Intake for Malnutrition by Cause					
For >7 days < 75% of estimated energy needs	For > or = to 5 days < or = to 50% of estimated energy needs	For > or = to 1 mo <75% of estimated energy needs	For > or = to 1 mo < or = to 75% of estimated energy needs	For > or = to 3 mo <75% of estimated energy needs	For > or − to 1 mo < or − to 50% of estimated energy needs
Loss of Body Fat					
Mild	Moderate	Mild	Severe	Mild	Severe
Loss of Muscle					
Mild	Moderate	Mild	Severe	Mild	Severe
Fluid Accumulation					
Mild	Moderate to severe	Mild	Severe	Mild	Severe
Reduced Grip Strength					
N/A	Measurably reduced	N/A	Measurably reduced	N/A	Measurably reduced

(Adapted from White JV et al: Consensus statement of the Academy of Nutrition and Dietetics/American Society for Parenteral and Enteral Nutrition: characteristics recommended for the identification and documentation of adult malnutrition (undernutrition), J Acad Nutr Diet 112(5):730, 2012.)

Physical Activity Assessment

Inclusion of a physical activity assessment is part of a comprehensive nutrition assessment because lifestyle and behavioral factors play a role in the cause and prevention of chronic diseases. Electronic tracking of physical activity through smartphones and other wearable fitness and health tracking devices are useful in collecting, compiling and preparing summary reports useful to clinicians and patients. Box 7-5 provides a series of questions that can be asked to identify the current levels and interest in future activity levels for ambulatory patients and clients.

Measures of Strength

With aging, the balanced cycle of muscle synthesis and degradation shifts toward more breakdown than synthesis of muscle tissue (See Chapter 20). The consequence is atrophy of muscle mass and loss of strength and power. Handgrip dynamometry can provide a baseline nutritional assessment of muscle function by measuring grip strength and endurance and is useful in serial measurements. Measurements of handgrip dynamometry are compared with reference standards provided by the manufacturer. Decreased grip strength is an important sign of frailty and is one of the characteristics of severe malnutrition (White, 2012). Low grip strength is associated consistently with a greater likelihood of premature mortality, the development of disability, and an increased risk of complications or prolonged length of stay after hospitalization or surgery in middle-aged and older adults (McLean, 2014).

Rehabilitation therapists use a number of evidence-based measures of upper and lower extremity physical function and performance that include muscle resistance testing, walking tests, stair climbing, rising from a chair, and balance. A score is determined for each test and summed for interpretation (Ha, 2010). Working collaboratively with rehabilitation therapists allows for a better understanding of functional measures of performance and how they relate to nutritional status.

Functional Medicine

Functional medicine is an evolving, evidence-based discipline that sees the body with its mutually interactive systems as a whole, rather than as a set of isolated signs and symptoms. The Institute of Functional Medicine (IFM) promotes an evaluation process that recognizes the biochemical, genetic, and environmental individuality of each person. The focus is patient centered, not just disease centered. Lifestyle and health-promoting factors include nutrition, exercise, adequate sleep, healthy relationships, and a positive mind-body-belief system.

The **Functional Nutrition Assessment (FNA)** approach identifies root causes of chronic disease by integrating traditional dietetic practice with nutritional genomics (see Chapter 3, the restoration of gastrointestinal function, the quelling of chronic inflammation (see Chapter 3), and the interpretation of nutritional biomarkers. The functional nutrition practitioner organizes the data collected from ingestion, digestion, and utilization (IDU) factors, leading to identification of the root causes for each individual within the framework of the nutrition care process (NCP). See Table 7-10 and Figure 7-9.

BOX 7-5 Physical Activity Assessment Questionnaire

To be considered physically active, you must get at least:
- 30 minutes of moderate physical activity on 5 or more days a week, OR
- 20 minutes of vigorous physical activity on 3 or more days a week

How physically active do you plan to be over the next 6 months? *(Choose the best answer.)*

____ I am not currently active and do not plan to become physically active in the next 6 months.

____ I am thinking about becoming more physically active.

____ I intend to become more physically active in the next 6 months.

____ I have been trying to get more physical activity.

____ I am currently physically active and have been for the last 1 to 5 months.

____ I have been regularly physically active for the past 6 months or more.

Compared with how physically active you have been over the last 3 months, how would you describe the last 7 days: *(Check one)*

_____ More active_____ Less active_____ About the same

Recall your participation in activities or in sedentary behaviors, over the past 24 hours:
- Reading, watching TV, or computer time _____ minutes/day
- Fast walking ____ minutes/day
- Physical activity (swimming, tennis, racquetball, similar) _____ minutes/day
- Other physical activity (describe _____) _____ minutes/day

What are the 3 most important reasons why you would consider increasing your physical activity?

☐ Improve my health ☐ Control my weight ☐ Lower my stress

TABLE 7-10 Selected Components of Functional Nutrition Assessment

Ingestion	Digestion	Utilization—Cellular and Molecular Functional Relationships
Food, fiber, water, supplements, medication	Adequate microflora	Antioxidants: water-soluble vitamin C, phytonutrients
Intake patterns affected by emotional or disordered eating	Allergies	Methylation and acetylation: dependence on adequate B complex vitamins and minerals
Toxins entering the body via food, skin, inhalants, water, environment (including pesticides and chemicals)	Genetic enzyme deficits	Oils and fatty acids: prostaglandin balance, cell membrane function, vitamin E function
	Hydration	Protein metabolism: connective tissue, enzymes, immune function, etc.
	Infection/inflammatory response	Vitamin D in concert with functional metabolic partner nutrients vitamins A and K
	Lifestyle: sleep, exercise, stressors	

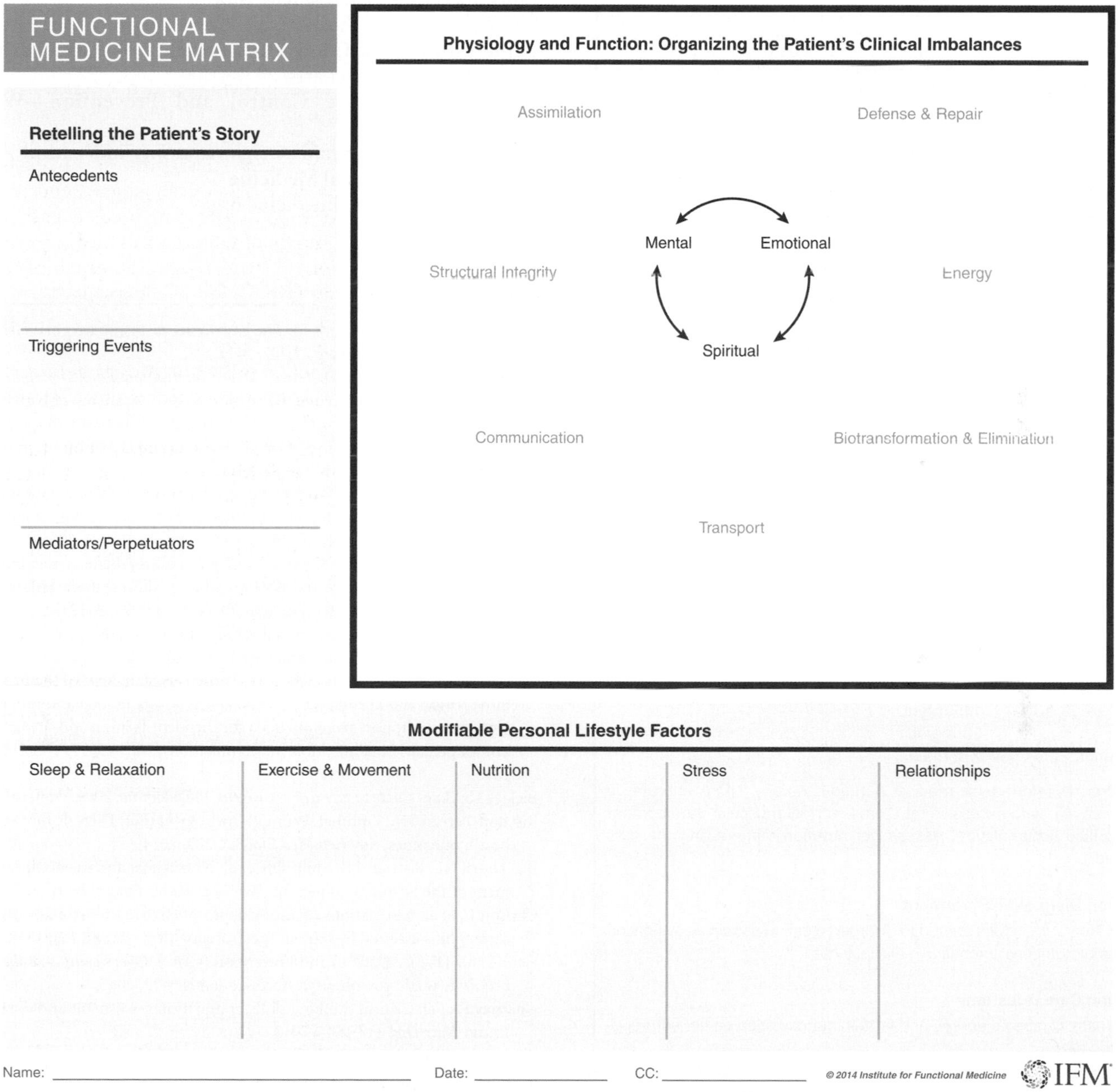

FUNCTIONAL MEDICINE MATRIX

Physiology and Function: Organizing the Patient's Clinical Imbalances

Retelling the Patient's Story

Antecedents

Triggering Events

Mediators/Perpetuators

Assimilation

Defense & Repair

Structural Integrity

Mental ⟷ Emotional

Spiritual

Energy

Communication

Biotransformation & Elimination

Transport

Modifiable Personal Lifestyle Factors

Sleep & Relaxation	Exercise & Movement	Nutrition	Stress	Relationships

Name: _____ Date: _____ CC: _____ © 2014 Institute for Functional Medicine ⚙IFM

FIGURE 7-9 Functional Medicine Matrix Model.

CLINICAL CASE STUDY

Winifred, a 38 year old F, is seen at City Hospital emergency department (ED). She has a history of hypertension, obesity and unsuccessful weight loss attempts. She loves fried foods, soft drinks, beer and pretzels. She has a history of binge eating. Winifred is required to have a yearly physical by her employer, but has put off scheduling the appointment until she can lose some weight. She fell down some stairs in a work-related accident and was sent to the ED for observation. The emergency department doctor determined that Winifred has no broken bones, but is concerned about her elevated blood pressure, 185/98. The doctor orders laboratory tests and Winifred is admitted to the hospital. Her medical profile today is:

Age	38 years old	Normal
Height	5'1"	
Weight	285 lb	
Glucose	142 mg/dL; 7.8 mmol/L	
Calcium	9.1 mg/dL; 2.27 mmol/L	
Sodium	140 mEq/L; 140 mmol/L	
Potassium	3.6 mEq/L; 3.6mmol/L	
CO_2	25 mEq/L/ 25 mmol/L	
Chloride	96 mEq/L; 96 mmol/L	
BUN	30 mg/dL; 10.7 mmol/L	
Creatinine	0.9 mg/dL; 79.6 µmol/L	
Albumin	3.8 g/dL; 38 g/L	
Total protein	8.0 g/dL; 80 g/L	
ALP	35 U/L; 0.5 µkat/L	
ALT	28 units/L; 28 units/L	
AST	23 units/L; 0.38 µkat/L	
Bilirubin, total	1.5 mg/dL; 25.65 µmol/L	
RBC	5.1×10^6 mL; 5.1×10^{12} L	
Hgb	11 g/dL; 7 mmol/L	
Hct	30%; 0.30	
MCV	78 mm³; 78 fL	
MCH	23 pg	
MCHC	40 g/dL; 40%	
WBC	$8 \times 10 \, 9$	
Total cholesterol	245 mg/dL	
LDL	145 mg/dL	
HDL	30 mg/dL	
Triglycerides	210 mg/dL	

Winifred is referred for medical nutrition therapy. NFPA indicates a robust female, with excessive fat stores, normal muscular development and no fluid accumulation. Assess her nutrition status using the data provided.

Nutrition Diagnostic Statement

Altered laboratory values related to disordered eating pattern as evidenced by signs of nutritional anemia and dyslipidemia.

Nutrition Care Questions

1. Estimate Winifred's energy and protein needs based on her anthropometric data.
2. Considering Winifred's medical history, what does her laboratory report for hemoglobin, hematocrit, mean corpuscular volume, mean corpuscular hemoglobin, and mean corpuscular hemoglobin concentration suggest?
3. What does her laboratory report for total cholesterol, LDL, HDL and triglycerides values suggest?
4. What does her laboratory report for sodium, blood urea nitrogen and glucose suggest?
5. What additional laboratory tests would be helpful for a comprehensive nutrition assessment?

ALP, Alkaline phosphate; *ALT,* alanine aminotransferase; *AST,* aspartate aminotransferase; *BUN,* blood urea nitrogen; *CO₂,* carbon dioxide; *Hct,* hematocrit; *Hgb,* hemoglobin; *MCH,* mean corpuscular hemoglobin; *MCHC,* mean corpuscular hemoglobin concentration; *MCV,* mean corpuscular volume; *RBC,* red blood cell; *WBC,* white blood cell.

USEFUL WEBSITES

Academy of Nutrition and Dietetics, Evidence Analysis Library
http://www.adaevidencelibrary.com/topic.cfm?cat=1225
Assessment Tools for Weight-Related Health Risks
http://www.columbia.edu/itc/hs/medical/nutrition/dat/dat.html
Body Mass Index Assessment Tool
http://www.cdc.gov/healthyweight/assessing/bmi/index.html
Centers for Disease Control and Prevention—Growth Charts
www.cdc.gov/growthcharts/
Centers for Disease Control and Prevention—Weight Assessment
http://www.cdc.gov/healthyweight/assessing/index.html
Institute of Functional Medicine
http://www.functionalmedicine.org/

REFERENCES

Aarts EO, Janssen IM, Berends FJ: The gastric sleeve: losing weight as fast as micronutrients? *Obes Surg* 21:207, 2011.

Academy of Nutrition and Dietetics (AND): *International dietetics and nutrition terminology reference manual*, Chicago, 2013, Academy of Nutrition and Dietetics.

American Diabetes Association (ADA): Diagnosis and classification of diabetes mellitus, *Diabetes Care* 343:62, 2011.

American Geriatric Society Workgroup on vitamin D supplementation for older adults: Consensus Statement: Vitamin D for prevention of falls and the consequences in older adults, *J Am Geriatr Soc* 62:147, 2014.

Ashwell M, Gunn P, Gibson S: Waist-to-height ratio is a better screening tool than waist circumference and BMI for adult cardiometabolic risk factors: systematic review and meta-analysis, *Obes Rev* 13:275, 2012.

Bajpai A, Goyal A, Sperling L: Should we measure C-reactive protein on earth or just on JUPITER? *Clin Cardiol* 33:190, 2010.

Becker P, Carney LN, Corkins MR, et al: Consensus Statement of the Academy of Nutrition and Dietetics/American Society for Parenteral and Enteral Nutrition: indicators recommended for the identification and documentation of pediatric malnutrition (undernutrition), *Nutr Clin Prac* 30:147, 2015.

Bickley LS: *Bates Guide to physical assessment*, Philadelphia, 2009, Wolters Kluwer.

Bischoff-Ferrari HA: Optimal serum 25-hydroxyvitamin D levels for multiple health outcomes, *Adv Exp Med Biol* 810:500, 2014.

Blackburn GL, Bistrian BR, Maini BS, et al: Nutritional and metabolic assessment of the hospitalized patient, *JPEN J Parenter Enteral Nutr* 1:11, 1977.

Carlson JJ, et al: Associations of antioxidant status, oxidative stress with skin carotenoids assessed by Raman spectroscopy (RS), *FASEB J* 20:1318, 2006.

Centers for Disease Control and Prevention (CDC): *Overweight and obesity.* http://www.cdc.gov/obesity/. Accessed January 22, 2015.

Charney P, et al: Critical thinking skills in nutrition assessment and diagnosis, *J Acad Nutr Diet* 113:1545, 2013.

de Onis M, Yip R, Mei Z, et al: The development of MUAC-for-age reference data recommended by a WHO expert committee, *Bull World Health Organ* 75:11, 1997.

Fan AZ, Yesupriya A, Chang MH, et al: Gene polymorphisms in association with emerging cardiovascular risk markers in adult women, *BMC Med Genet* 11:6, 2010.

Flakoll PJ, Kent P, Neyra R, et al: Bioelectrical impedance vs air displacement plethysmography and dual-energy X-ray absorptiometry to determine body composition in patients with end-stage renal disease, *J Parenter Enteral Nutr* 28:13, 2004.

Friedman AN, Fadem SZ: Reassessment of albumin as a nutritional marker in kidney disease, *J Am Soc Nephrol* 21:223, 2010.

Gottschlich MM, et al, editors: *The science and practice of nutrition support: a case-based core curriculum*, Dubuque, Iowa, 2001, Kendall/Hunt Publishing.

Ha L, Hauge T, Spenning AB, et al: Individual, nutritional support prevents undernutrition, increases muscle strength and improves QoL among elderly at nutritional risk hospitalized for acute stroke: a randomized controlled trial, *Clin Nutr* 29:567, 2010.

Hammami MB: *Serum osteocalcin*. http://emedicine.medscape.com/article/2093955-overview. Accessed January 20, 2015.

Hamwi GJ: *Diabetes mellitus, diagnosis and treatment*, New York, 1964, American Diabetes Association.

Hao W, Friedman A: The LDL-HDL profile determines the risk of atherosclerosis: a mathematical model, *PLoS One* 9:e90497, 2014.

Harrison DG, Nieto FJ: *Oxidative stress, inflammation and heart, lung, blood, and sleep disorders meeting summary*. http://www.nhlbi.nih.gov/meetings/workshops/oxidative-stress.htm. Accessed January 22, 2015.

Heslop CL, Frohlich JJ, Hill JS: Myeloperoxidase and C-reactive protein have combined utility for long-term prediction of cardiovascular mortality after coronary angiography, *J Am Coll Cardiol* 55:1102, 2010.

Jacobson TA, Ito MK, Maki KC, et al: National Lipid Association recommendations for patient-center management of dyslipidemia, *J Clin Lipidol* 8:473, 2014.

Keys A, Fidanza F, Karvonen MJ, et al: Indices of relative weight and obesity, *J Chronic Dis* 25:329, 1972.

Klein K, Bancher-Todesca D, Leipold H, et al: Retinol-binding protein 4 in patients with gestational diabetes mellitus, *J Womens Health* 19:517, 2010.

Klontz KC, Acheson DW: Dietary supplement-induced vitamin D intoxication, *N Engl J Med* 357:308, 2007.

Krakauer NY, Krakauer JC: A new shape index predicts mortality hazard independently of body mass index, *PLoS One* 7:e39504, 2012.

Ledoux S, Msika S, Moussa F, et al: Comparison of nutritional consequences of conventional therapy of obesity, adjustable gastric banding, and gastric bypass, *Obes Surg* 16:1041, 2006.

Litchford MD: *Laboratory assessment of nutritional status: bridging theory & practice*, Greensboro, NC, 2015, CASE Software & Books.

Litchford MD: *Nutriton-focused physical assessment: making clinical connections*, Greensboro, NC, 2013, Case Software and Books.

Li ZZ, Lu XZ, Liu JB, et al: Serum retinol-binding protein 4 levels in patients with diabetic retinopathy, *J Int Med Res* 38:95, 2010.

Madan AK, Orth WS, Tichansky DS, et al: Vitamin and trace mineral levels after laparoscopic gastric bypass, *Obes Surg* 16:603, 2006.

McLean RR, Shardell MD, Alley DE, et al: Criteria for clinically relevant weakness and low lean mass and their longitudinal association with incident mobility impairment and mortality: the foundation for the National Institutes of Health (FNIH) sarcopenia project, *J Gerontol A Biol Sci Med Sci* 69:576, 2014.

Mehta NM, Corkins MR, Lyman B, et al: Defining pediatric malnutrition: a paradigm shift toward etiology-related definitions, *J Parenter Enteral Nutr* 37:460, 2013.

Mei Z, Grummer-Strawn LM, Pietrobelli A, et al: Validity of body mass index compared with other body-composition screening indexes for the assessment of body fatness in children and adolescents, *Am J Clin Nutr* 75:978, 2002.

Miller ER 3rd, Pastor-Barriuso R, Dalal D, et al: Meta-analysis: high-dosage vitamin E supplementation may increase all-cause mortality, *Ann Intern Med* 142:37, 2005.

Mueller C: *ASPEN Adult nutrition support core curriculum*, Silver Springs, Md, 2012, ASPEN.

Prado CM, Heymsfield SB: Lean tissue imaging: a new era for nutritional assessment and intervention, *J Parenter Enteral Nutr* 38:940, 2014.

Roberts LJ, Fessel JP: The biochemistry of the isoprostane, neuroprostane and isofuran pathways of lipid peroxidation, *Chem Phys Lipids* 128:173, 2004.

Schneider HJ, Friedrich N, Klotsche J, et al: The predictive value of different measures of obesity for incident cardiovascular events and mortality, *J Clin Endocrinol Metab* 95:1777, 2010.

Srikanthan P, Seeman TE, Karlamangla AS, et al: Waist-hip-ratio as a predictor of all-cause mortality in high-functioning older adults, *Ann Epidemiol* 19:724, 2009.

Stensland SH, Margolis S: Simplifying the calculation of body mass index for quick reference, *J Am Diet Assoc* 90:856, 1990.

Stone NJ, Robinson JG, Lichtenstein AH, et al: 2013 ACC/AHA guideline on the treatment of blood cholesterol to reduce atherosclerotic cardiovascular risk in adults: a report of the American College of Cardiology/American Heart Association Task Force on Practice Guidelines, *J Am Coll Cardiol* 63(25 Pt B):2889, 2014.

Wagner DR, Heyward VH: Measures of body composition in blacks and whites: a comparative review, *Am J Clin Nutr* 71:1392, 2000.

Welborn TA, Dhaliwal SS: Preferred clinical measures of central obesity for predicting mortality, *Eur J Clin Nutr* 61:1373, 2007.

White JV, Guenter P, Jensen G, et al: Consensus Statement of the Academy of Nutrition and Dietetics/American Society for Parenteral and Enteral Nutrition: characteristics recommended for the identification and documentation of adult malnutrition (undernutrition), *J Acad Nutr Diet* 112:730, 2012.

Winter JE, MacInnis RJ, Wattanapenpaiboon N, et al: BMI and all-cause mortality in older adults: a meta-analysis, *Am J Clin Nutr* 99:875, 2014.

Zalesin KC, Miller WM, Franklin B, et al: Vitamin A deficiency after gastric bypass surgery: an underreported postoperative complication, *J Obes* 2011;2011, doi:10.1155/2011/760695.

Zheng Y, Stein R, Kwan T, et al: Evolving cardiovascular disease prevalence, mortality, risk factors, and the metabolic syndrome in China, *Clin Cardiol* 32:491, 2009.

8

Clinical: Food-Drug Interactions

Lisa L. Deal, PharmD, BCPS, BSN, RN,
DeeAnna Wales VanReken, MS, RDN, CD

KEY TERMS

absorption
acetylation
bioavailability
biotransformation
black box warning
cytochrome P-450 enzyme system
distribution
drug-nutrient interaction

excipient
excretion
first-pass
food-drug interaction
gastrointestinal pH
half-life
pharmacodynamics
pharmacogenomics

pharmacokinetics
physical incompatibility
polypharmacy
side effect
tubular reabsorption
unbound fraction
vasopressor agents

Progression in the fields of medicine and pharmacology have led to the development of a wide variety of medications for various disease states and conditions. Drugs, by definition, are any chemicals that can affect living processes. Interactions between drugs and food can range from inconsequential to life-threatening. Toxicity can be related to alterations in drug levels within the body, leading to either increased or decreased efficacy.

The terms *drug-nutrient interaction* and *food-drug interaction* often are used interchangeably. In actuality, drug-nutrient interactions are a subsection of the many possible food-drug interactions. **Drug-nutrient interactions** include specific changes to the activity of a drug caused by a nutrient or nutrients, or changes to the kinetics of a nutrient caused by a drug. **Food-drug interaction** is a broader term that also includes the effects of a medication on nutritional status. For example, nutritional status may be affected by the side effects of a medication such as gastrointestinal effects (eg. dry mouth, stomatitis), appetite changes, metabolic effects (blood glucose or lipid abnormalities), or renal or urinary effects (retention, frequency, or acute renal failure).

For clinical, economic, and legal reasons, it is important to recognize and anticipate food-drug interactions. Food-drug interactions that reduce the efficacy of a drug can result in longer or repeated stays in health care facilities, disease progression and increased morbidity and mortality. **Polypharmacy**, or the use of four or more medications during a single time period, can potentiate the risks for food-drug interactions. See Box 8-1 for other situations that put individuals as risk.

Medical team members should be aware of the positive and negative food-drug interactions, and being diligent to review medications and nutrients during every hospital admission,

outpatient office visit, and encounter with the patient. See Box 8-2 for some potential benefits of minimizing drug interactions over time.

PHARMACOLOGIC ASPECTS OF FOOD-DRUG INTERACTIONS

Pharmacology is the study of drugs and their interactions with systems. Drugs are administered to produce a pharmacologic effect in a target organ or tissue. To achieve this goal, the drug must move from the site of administration into the bloodstream and eventually to the site of drug action. In due course, the drug may be changed to active or inactive metabolites, and ultimately is eliminated from the body. An interaction between the drug and food, a food component, or a nutrient can alter this process at any point.

Food-drug interactions are divided into two broad types: (1) pharmacodynamic interactions, which affect the activity at the site of action in the body; and (2) pharmacokinetic interactions, which affect the absorption, distribution, metabolism, and excretion of the drug.

Pharmacodynamics is the study of the biochemical and physiologic effects of a drug. The mechanism of action of a drug may include the binding of the drug molecule to a receptor, enzyme, or ion channel, resulting in the observable physiologic response. This response may be enhanced or attenuated by the addition of other substances with similar or opposing actions.

Pharmacokinetics is the study of the time course of a drug in the body involving the absorption, distribution, metabolism (biotransformation), and excretion of the drug, otherwise known as drug disposition, or "ADME" (Figure 8-1).

Absorption is the process of the movement of the drug from the site of administration to the bloodstream. This process depends on (1) the route of administration, (2) the

---

Sections of this chapter were written by Zaneta M. Pronsky, MS, RD, LDN, FADA and Sr. Jeanne P. Crowe, PharmD, RPh, RPI for previous editions of this text.

BOX 8-1   Individuals at Risk for Drug-Nutrient Interactions

Persons considered at higher risk for drug-nutrient interactions include:
- Those who have a poor diet
- Those who have serious health problems
- Growing children
- Pregnant women
- Older adults
- Patients taking two or more medications at the same time
- Those using prescription and over-the-counter medications together at the same time
- Patients not following medication directions
- Patients taking medications for long periods of time
- Those who drink alcohol or smoke excessively

From Hermann J: *Drug-nutrient interactions,* Oklahoma Cooperative Extension Service (website): http://pods.dasnr.okstate.edu/docushare/dsweb/Get/Document-2458/T-3120web.pdf. Accessed January 14, 2015.

BOX 8-2   Benefits of Minimizing Drug Interactions

- Medications achieve their intended effects.
- Patients do not discontinue their drug.
- The need for additional medication is minimized.
- Fewer caloric or nutrient supplements are required.
- Adverse side effects are avoided.
- Optimal nutritional status is preserved.
- Accidents and injuries are avoided.
- Disease complications are minimized.
- The cost of health care services is reduced.
- There is less professional liability.
- Licensing agency requirements are met.
- Prevention of nutrient deficiencies with long term use.

From Pronsky ZM et al: *Food-medication interactions,* ed 18, Birchrunville, PA, 2015, Food-Medication Interactions.

chemistry of the drug and its ability to cross biologic membranes, and (3) the rate of gastric emptying (for orally administered drugs) and gastrointestinal (GI) motility. Food, food components, and nutrition supplements can interfere with the absorption process, especially when the drug is administered orally.

Distribution occurs when the drug leaves the systemic circulation and travels to various regions of the body. Distribution varies based on the chemistry of the drug molecule. The rate and extent of blood flow to an organ or tissue strongly affect the amount of drug that reaches the sites. Many drugs are bound to plasma proteins such as albumin. The bound fraction of drug does not leave the vasculature and therefore does not produce a pharmacologic effect. Only the **unbound fraction**, medication that is not bound to plasma proteins, is able to produce an effect at a target organ (Figure 8-2).

A drug is eliminated from the body as either an unchanged drug or a metabolite of the original compound. The major organ of metabolism, or **biotransformation**, in the body is the liver, although other sites, such as the intestinal membrane, kidneys, and lungs, contribute to variable degrees of metabolism. One of the more important enzyme systems that facilitates drug metabolism is the **cytochrome P-450 enzyme system**. This is a multi-enzyme system in the smooth endoplasmic reticulum of numerous tissues that is involved in phase I of liver detoxification (see Focus On Box on Detoxification Chapter 19). Food or dietary supplements may either induce or inhibit the activity of this enzyme system, which can significantly alter the rate or extent of drug metabolism. The general tendency of the process of metabolism is to transform a drug from a lipid-soluble to a more water-soluble compound that can be handled more easily by the kidneys and excreted in the urine.

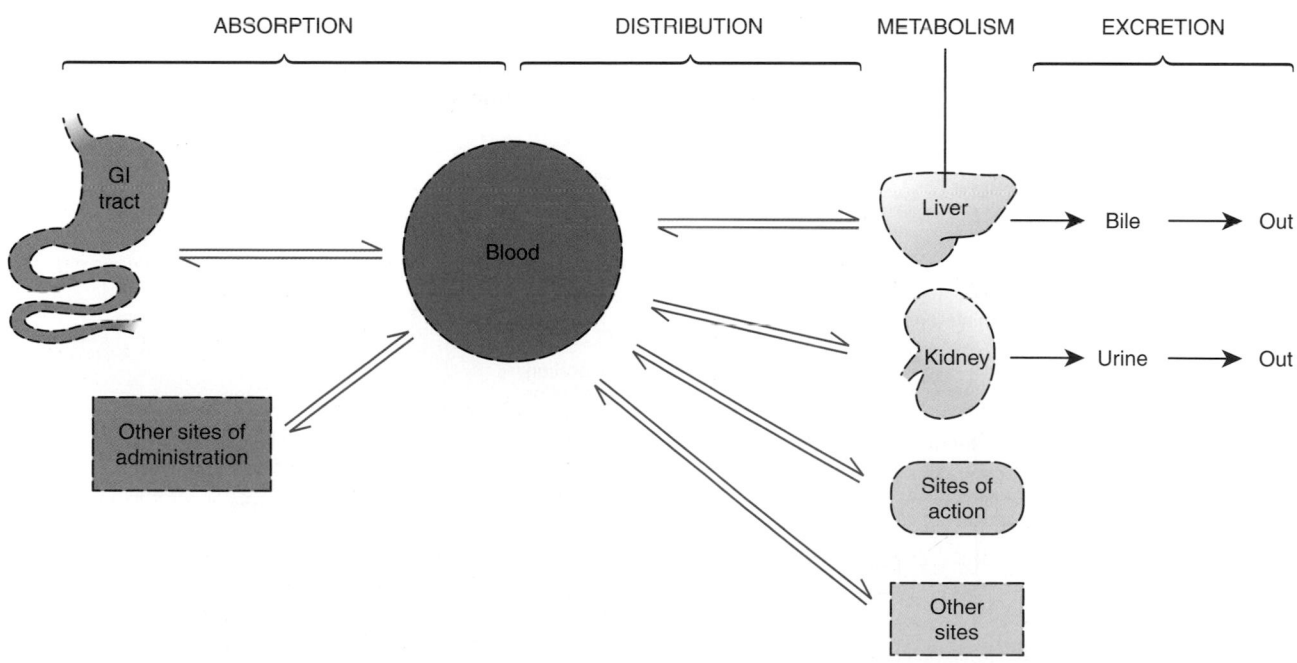

FIGURE 8-1 The four basic pharmacokinetic processes. Dotted lines represent membranes that must be crossed as drugs move throughout the body. (From Lehne et al: *Pharmacology of nursing care,* ed 8, St Louis, Missouri, 2012, Elsevier.)

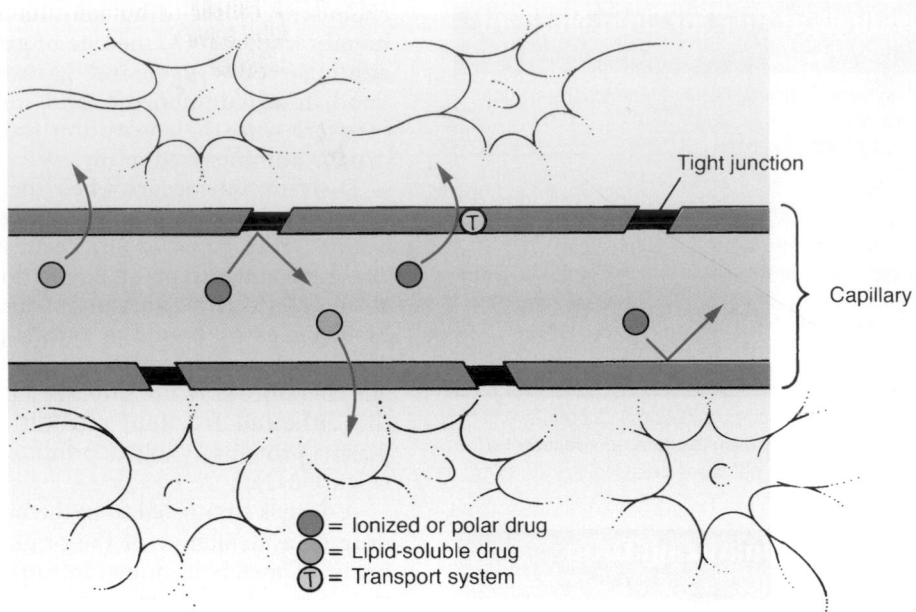

FIGURE 8-2 Drug movement across the blood-brain barrier. Tight junctions between cells that compose the walls of capillaries in the CNS prevent drugs from passing between cells to exit the vascular system. Consequently, to reach sites of action within the brain, a drug must pass directly through cells of the capillary wall. To do this, the drug must be lipid soluble or be able to use an existing transport system. (From Lehne et al: *Pharmacology of nursing care,* ed 8, St Louis, 2012, Elsevier.)

Renal **excretion** is the major route of elimination for drugs and drug metabolites either by glomerular filtration or tubular secretion. To a lesser extent drugs may be eliminated in feces, bile, tears, breast milk, and other body fluids. Under certain circumstances, such as a change in urinary pH, drugs that have reached the renal tubule may pass back into the bloodstream. This process is known as **tubular reabsorption**. The recommended dose of a drug generally assumes normal liver and kidney function, although drug references have sections dedicated to medications that require dosage adjustments based on alterations in kidney function. The dose and dosing interval of an excreted drug or

active metabolite must be adjusted to meet the degree of renal and hepatic dysfunction in patients with kidney disease or hepatic disease (see Chapters 29 and 35; Figure 8-3).

RISK FACTORS FOR FOOD-DRUG INTERACTIONS

Patients must be assessed individually for the effect of food on drug action and nutrition status. Interactions can be caused or complicated by a multitude of patient specific variables, including polypharmacy, nutrition status, genetics, underlying illness, diet, nutrition supplements, herbal or phytonutrient products,

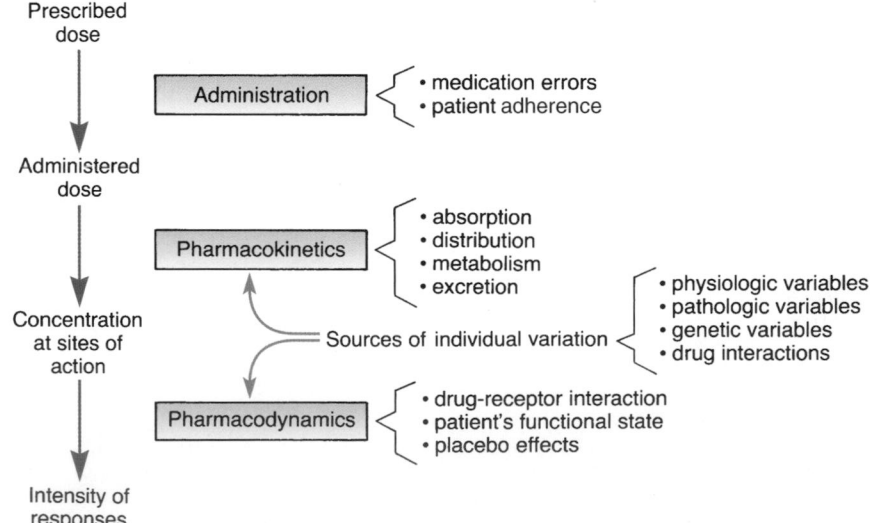

FIGURE 8-3 Factors that determine the intensity of drug responses. (From Lehne et al: *Pharmacology of nursing care,* ed 8, St Louis, 2012, Elsevier.)

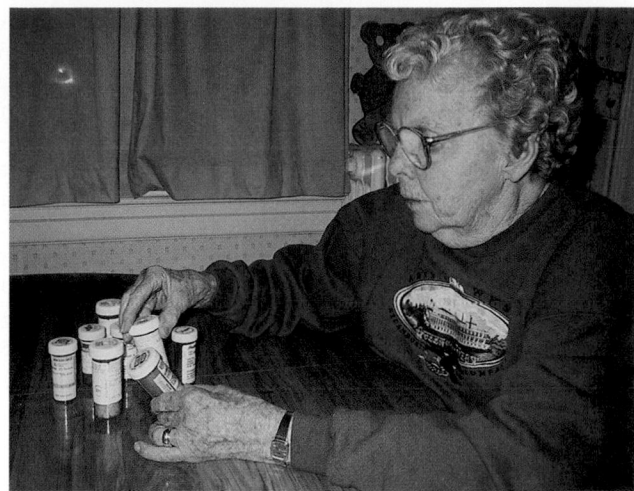

FIGURE 8-4 As a result of the increased potential for illness with aging, older adults often take multiple drugs, both prescription and over-the-counter preparations. This places them at increased risk for drug-drug and food-drug interactions.

alcohol intake, drugs of abuse, gut microbiome, excipients in drugs or food, allergies, and intolerances. Poor patient compliance and physicians' prescribing patterns further complicate the risk. Drug-induced malnutrition occurs most commonly during long-term treatment for chronic disease (see Focus On: Polypharmacy in Older Adults; Figure 8-4).

Existing malnutrition places patients at greater risk for drug-nutrient interactions. Protein alterations and changes in body composition secondary to malnutrition can affect drug disposition by altering protein binding and drug distribution. Patients

◎ FOCUS ON

Polypharmacy in Older Adults

Older patients are more likely to take multiple drugs, prescription and over-the-counter, than are younger patients. They have a higher risk of food-drug interactions because of physical changes related to aging, such as the increase in the ratio of fat tissue to lean body mass, a decrease in liver mass and blood flow, and impairment of kidney function. Illness, cognitive or endocrine dysfunction, and ingestion of restricted diets also increase this risk. Malnutrition and dehydration affect drug kinetics. The use of herbal or phytonutrient products has increased significantly in all developed countries, including use by older adults. Drugs of abuse or excessive alcohol intake often are missed in the older patient.

Central nervous system side effects of drugs can interfere with the ability or desire to eat. Drugs that cause drowsiness, dizziness, ataxia, confusion, headache, weakness, tremor, or peripheral neuropathy can lead to nutritional compromise, particularly in older patients. Recognition of these problems as a drug side effect rather than a consequence of disease or aging can be overlooked.

Care must be taken to evaluate intake of interacting nutrients (in the oral diet, supplements, or tube feedings) when specific drugs are used. Examples are vitamin K with warfarin (Coumadin); calcium and vitamin D with tetracycline; and potassium, sodium, and magnesium with loop diuretics such as furosemide (Lasix). Patients with Parkinson disease may be concerned with the amount and timing of protein intake because of interaction with levodopa (Sinemet, Dopar). The interdisciplinary team, which includes the physician, pharmacist, nurse, and dietitian, must work together to plan and coordinate the medication regimen and diet and nutritional supplements to preserve optimal nutrition status and minimize food-drug interactions.

with active cancer or human immunodeficiency virus (HIV) infection who have significant anorexia and wasting are at special risk because of the high prevalence of malnutrition and reduced dietary intake. Treatment modalities such as chemotherapy and radiation also may exacerbate nutritional disturbances. For example, cisplatin (Platinol-AQ) and other cytotoxic agents commonly cause mouth sores, nausea, vomiting, diarrhea, anorexia, and thus reduced food intake. Many drugs have loss of appetite as a side effect. Drug disposition can be affected by alterations in the GI tract, such as vomiting, diarrhea, hypochlorhydria, mucosal atrophy, and motility changes. Malabsorption caused by intestinal damage from cancer, celiac disease, inflammatory bowel disease, or surgical removal of intestinal tissue for various reasons, creates greater potential for food-drug interactions. Body composition is another important consideration in determining drug response. In obese or older patients, the proportion of adipose tissue to lean body mass is increased. In theory, accumulation of fat-soluble drugs such as the long-acting benzodiazepines (e.g., diazepam [Valium]) is more likely to occur. Accumulation of a drug and its metabolites in adipose tissue may result in prolonged clearance and increased toxicity. In older patients this interaction may also be complicated by decreased hepatic and or renal clearance of the drug.

The developing fetus, infant, and pregnant woman are also at high risk for drug-nutrient interactions. Many drugs have not been tested on these populations, making it difficult to assess the risks of negative drug effects, including food-drug interactions. Medications should be assessed for risk versus benefit with regard to the developing fetus.

Pharmacogenomics

Gene-nutrient interactions reflect the genetic heterogeneity of humans with diverse physiologies, in combination with unique environmental factors and dietary chemicals. Because the efficacy and safety disparity of drugs varies according to race and genetic variants, pharmacogenetic knowledge is important for the interpretation and prediction of drug interaction-induced adverse events.

Pharmacogenomics involves genetically determined variations that are revealed solely by the effects of drugs and can be a driver for nutrigenomics, as discussed in Chapter 5. Food-drug interaction ramifications are seen in glucose-6-phosphate dehydrogenase (G6PD) enzyme deficiency, slow inactivation of isoniazid (Nydrazid) or phenelzine (Nardil), and warfarin (Coumadin) resistance. Warfarin resistance affects individual requirements for and response to warfarin.

Slow inactivation of isoniazid, used in tuberculosis (TB), represents the effect of slow **acetylation**, a conjugation reaction that metabolizes and inactivates amines, hydrazines, and sulfonamides. "Slow acetylators" are persons who metabolize these drugs more slowly than average because of inherited lower levels of the hepatic enzyme acetyl transferase. Therefore unacetylated drug levels remain higher for longer periods in these persons than in those who are "rapid acetylators." For example, the **half-life** (the period of time required for the concentration or amount of drug in the body to be reduced to one-half of a given concentration or amount) of isoniazid for fast acetylators is approximately 70 minutes, compared to more than 3 hours for slow acetylators. A dose of drug prescribed normally for fast acetylators can be toxic for slow acetylators. Elevated blood levels of affected drugs in slow acetylators increase the potential for food-drug interactions. Slow inactivation of isoniazid increases the risk of pyridoxine deficiency and peripheral neuropathy. Slow inactivation of phenelzine, a monoamine oxidase inhibitor (MAOI), increases the risk for hypertensive crisis if foods high in tyramine are consumed. See Chapter 26.

Deficiency of G6PD is an X-chromosome–linked deficiency of G6PD enzyme in red blood cells that can lead to neonatal jaundice, hemolytic anemia, or acute hemolysis. Most common in African, Middle Eastern, and Southeast Asian populations, it is also called *favism*. Intake of fava beans (broad beans), aspirin, sulfonamides, and antimalarial drugs can cause hemolysis and acute anemia in G6PD-deficient persons. The potential exists for food-drug interactions in G6PD deficiency resulting from the ingestion of fava beans, as well as vitamin C or vitamin K.

Another factor that affects drug metabolism is genetic variation of activity of the cytochrome P450 (CYP) enzymes. These enzymes are a group of 12 enzyme families that function in the metabolism of drugs. Therapeutic proteins affect the disposition of drugs that are metabolized by these enzymes (Lee et al, 2010). "Slow metabolizers" may have less of a specific enzyme or their enzymes may be less active. Such individuals have a higher risk of adverse drug effects, as there is an increase in the amount of unbound or active drug. Slow CYP2D6 metabolizers make up approximately 5% to 10% of whites, whereas approximately 20% of Asians are CYP2C19 poor metabolizers (Fohner et al, 2013). The nomenclature of CYP-Number-Letter-Number represents the various enzyme families. Tests are now available to analyze the client's DNA to determine variations in the activity of these two enzymes. The CYP2D6 and CYP2C19 enzyme systems are responsible for metabolizing approximately 25% of all drugs, including many antipsychotics, antidepressants, and narcotics. Slow metabolizers achieve a higher drug blood level with usual doses of such drugs, whereas fast metabolizers may have an unpredictable response as a result of rapid metabolism of the drug (Medical Letter, 2005).

Drug response genotyping helps to determine which drugs will be effective, depending on an individual's genetic makeup (see Chapter 5). The ability to predict response to specific drugs determines more effective treatments for cancer, mental illness, and even pain management. Genotyping helps reduce adverse drug reactions, including food-medication interactions. This is a rapidly growing field, which will change the way medicine is practiced in the future, leading to the development of patient specific medications based on genotypes.

EFFECTS OF FOOD ON DRUG THERAPY

Drug Absorption

The presence of food and nutrients in the stomach or intestinal lumen may alter the absorption of a drug. **Bioavailability** describes the fraction of an administered drug that reaches the systemic circulation (Figure 8-5). If a medication is administered intravenously, its bioavailability is 100%, whereas bioavailability decreases with oral administration as absorption

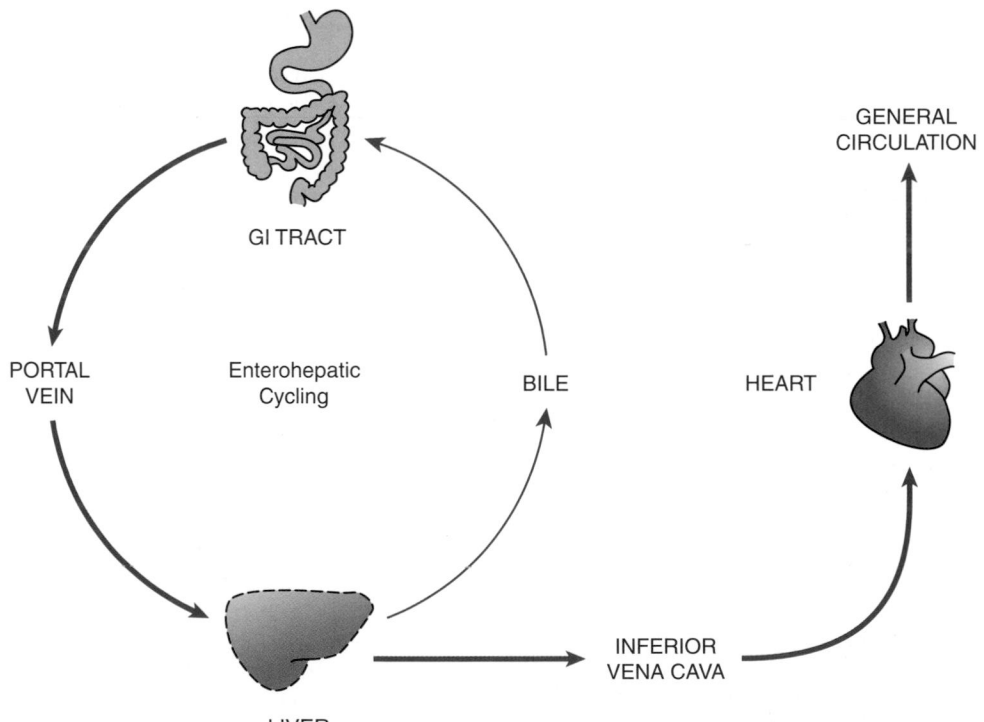

FIGURE 8-5 Movement of drugs after GI absorption. All drugs absorbed from sites along the GI tract—stomach, small intestine, and large intestine (but not the oral mucosa or distal rectum)—must go through the liver, via the portal vein, on their way to the heart and then the general circulation. For some drugs, passage is uneventful. Others undergo extensive hepatic metabolism. Still others undergo *enterohepatic recirculation,* a repeating cycle in which a drug moves from the liver into the duodenum (via the bile duct) and then back to the liver (via the portal blood). As discussed in the text under Enterohepatic Recirculation, the process is limited to drugs that have first undergone hepatic glucuronidation. (From Lehne et al: *Pharmacology of nursing care,* ed 8, St Louis, 2012, Elsevier.)

and metabolism are incomplete. Examples of a critically significant reduction in drug absorption are the bisphosphonate drugs alendronate (Fosamax), risedronate (Actonel), or ibandronate (Boniva) used in the treatment of osteoporosis. Absorption is negligible if these drugs are given with food and reduced by 60% if taken with coffee or orange juice. The manufacturer's instructions for alendronate or risedronate are to take the drug on an empty stomach with plain water at least 30 minutes before any other food, drink, or other medication. Ibandronate must be taken at least 60 minutes before any other food, drink, or medication.

The absorption of the iron from supplements can be decreased by 50% if taken with food. Iron is better absorbed when taken with 8 oz of water on an empty stomach, although orange juice, because of its vitamin C content, actually can increase absorption by 85% when taken concurrently. If iron must be taken with food to avoid GI distress, it should not be taken with bran, eggs, high-phytate foods, fiber supplements, tea, coffee, dairy products, or calcium supplements, because each of these can decrease iron absorption.

Various mechanisms may contribute to the reduction in the rate or extent of drug absorption in the presence of food or nutrients. The presence and type of meal or food ingested influence the rate of gastric emptying. Gastric emptying may be delayed by the consumption of high-fiber or high-fat meals. In general, a delay in drug absorption is not clinically significant as long as the extent of absorption is not affected. However, delayed absorption of antibiotics or analgesics may be clinically significant.

Chelation reactions occur between certain medications and divalent or trivalent cations, such as iron, calcium, magnesium, zinc, or aluminum, where the absorption of drugs may be reduced. Chelation reactions are seen most commonly with tetracycline and fluoroquinolone antibiotics.

The Parkinson disease drug entacapone (Comtan) chelates with iron; therefore the iron must be taken 1 hour before or 2 hours after taking the drug. The fluoroquinolone antibiotics and tetracycline form insoluble complexes with calcium in dairy products or calcium-fortified foods and beverages, or supplements, or aluminum in antacids, thus preventing or reducing the absorption of drugs and nutrients (Pronsky and Crowe, 2012). The optimal approach to avoid this interaction is to stop noncritical supplements for the duration of the antibiotic prescription. If this is not possible, particularly with magnesium, or with long-term antibiotic use, the drug should be administered at least 2 hours before or 6 hours after the mineral.

Gastrointestinal pH is another important factor in the absorption of drugs. Any situations resulting in changes in gastric acid pH, such as achlorhydria or hypochlorhydria, may reduce drug absorption. An example of such an interaction is the failure of antifungal medication, ketoconazole (Nizoral), to clear a *Candida* infection in patients with HIV or in persons taking potent acid-reducing agents for gastroesophageal reflux disease (GERD). Ketoconazole achieves optimal absorption in an acid medium. Because of the high prevalence of achlorhydria in patients infected with HIV, dissolution of ketoconazole tablets in the stomach is reduced, leading to impaired drug absorption. This is also a concern with hypochlorhydria in persons receiving chronic acid suppression therapy, such as antacids, histamine-2 (H2) receptor antagonists (e.g., famotidine [Pepcid]), or proton-pump inhibitors (e.g., omeprazole [Prilosec]). Ingestion of ketoconazole with an acidic liquid such as cola, cranberry juice, orange juice, or a dilute hydrochloric acid (HCl) solution may improve bioavailability in these patients (Pronsky and Crowe, 2012).

The presence of food in the stomach enhances the absorption of some medications, such as the antibiotic cefuroxime axetil (Ceftin) or the antiretroviral drug saquinavir (Invirase). These drugs are prescribed to be taken after a meal to reduce the dose that must be taken to reach an effective level. The bioavailability of cefuroxime axetil is substantially greater when taken with food, compared with taking it in the fasting state.

MEDICATION AND ENTERAL NUTRITION INTERACTIONS

Continuous enteral feeding is an effective method of providing nutrients to patients who are unable to swallow or eat adequately. However, use of the feeding tube to administer medication can be problematic. When liquid medications are mixed with enteral formulas, incompatibilities may occur. Types of physical incompatibility include granulation, gel formation, and separation of the enteral product. This leads to clogged feeding tubes and interruption of delivery of nutrition to the patient. Examples of drugs that can cause granulation and gel formation are ciprofloxacin suspension (Cipro), chlorpromazine (Thorazine) concentrate, ferrous sulfate elixir, guaifenesin (Robitussin expectorant), and metoclopramide (Reglan) syrup (Wohlt et al, 2009).

Most compatibility studies of medication and enteral products have looked at the effect of the drug on the integrity of the enteral product, which in turn changes the bioavailability. This area requires much more research because feeding tube placement is now a common practice. Bioavailability problems are common with phenytoin (Dilantin) suspension and tube feeding. Because blood levels of phenytoin are performed routinely to monitor the drug, much information exists about the reduction of phenytoin bioavailability when given with enteral feedings. Stopping the tube feeding before and after the phenytoin dose generally is suggested; a 1-2-hour feeding-free interval before and after the dose of phenytoin is administered can be recommended safely and can vary based on hospital system policies.

Information may not be readily available concerning a drug and enteral product interactions, even though the manufacturer may have unpublished information about the drug's interaction with enteral products. Checking with the manufacturer's medical information department may yield more information.

Drug Distribution

Albumin is the most important drug-binding protein in the blood. Low serum albumin levels are often the result of acute and chronic inflammatory conditions, and the low albumin leads to fewer binding sites for highly protein-bound drugs. Fewer binding sites mean that a larger free fraction of drug is present in the serum. Only the free fraction (unbound fraction) of a drug is able to leave the vasculature and exert a pharmacologic effect at the target organ. Patients with albumin levels below 3 g/dl are at increased risk for adverse effects. Usual adult doses of highly protein-bound drugs in such persons may produce more pronounced pharmacologic effects than the same dose in persons with normal serum albumin levels. A lower dose of such drugs often is recommended for patients with low albumin levels. In addition, the risk for displacement of one drug from albumin-binding sites by another drug is greater when albumin levels are less than 3 g/dl.

The anticoagulant warfarin, which is 99.9% serum protein bound, and the anticonvulsant phenytoin, which is greater than 90% protein bound, are used commonly in older patients. Low albumin levels tend to be more common in older patients and in critically ill patients. In the case of warfarin, higher levels of free drug lead to risk of excessive anticoagulation and bleeding. Phenytoin toxicity can result from too high or low serum levels of free phenytoin, resulting in seizures.

Drug Metabolism

Enzyme systems in the intestinal tract and the liver, although not the only sites of drug metabolism, account for a large portion of the drug metabolizing activity in the body. Food can inhibit and enhance the metabolism of medication by altering the activity of these enzyme systems. A diet high in protein and low in carbohydrates can increase the hepatic metabolism of the asthma management drug theophylline (Theo-24), which leads to toxicity because theophylline has a narrow therapeutic window.

Conversely, components found in grapefruit (juice, segments, extract) and related citrus fruits (Seville oranges, tangelos, minneolas, pummelos, and certain exotic oranges) called *furanocoumarins* inhibit the cytochrome P-450 3A4 enzyme system responsible for the oxidative metabolism of many orally administered drugs (Pronsky and Crowe, 2012). The intestinal metabolism of drugs such as calcium channel blockers that are dihydropyridine derivatives (felodipine [Plendil]) and some 3-hydroxy-3-methylglutaryl (HMG)–coenzyme A (CoA) reductase inhibitors such as simvastatin (Zocor) are affected (Sica, 2006). This interaction appears to be clinically significant for drugs with low oral bioavailability, which are substantially metabolized and inactivated in the intestinal tract by the cytochrome P-450 3A4 enzyme in the intestinal wall. When grapefruit or grapefruit juice is ingested, the metabolizing enzyme is inhibited irreversibly, which reduces the normal metabolism of the drug. This reduction in metabolism allows more of the drug to reach the systemic circulation; the increase in blood levels of unmetabolized drug results in a greater pharmacologic effect and possible toxicity. Unfortunately, the effects of grapefruit on intestinal cytochrome P-450 3A4 last up to 72 hours. Therefore separating the ingestion of the grapefruit and the daily dose of drug does not appear to alleviate this interaction.

Competition between food and drugs such as propranolol (Inderal) and metoprolol (Lopressor) for metabolizing enzymes in the liver may alter the first-pass metabolism of these medications. The term **first-pass** refers to the hepatic inactivation of oral medications when they are given initially. Drugs absorbed from the intestinal tract by the portal circulation first are transported to the liver before they reach the systemic circulation. Because many drugs are metabolized during this first pass through the liver, only a small percentage of the original dose is actually available to the systemic circulation and the target organ. In some cases, however, this percentage can be increased by concurrent ingestion of food with the drug. When food and drug compete for the same metabolizing enzymes in the liver, more of the drug is likely to reach the systemic circulation, which can lead to a toxic effect if the dose titration occurs in a fasting state.

Drug Excretion

Food and nutrients can alter the reabsorption of drugs from the renal tubule. Reabsorption of the bipolar medication lithium (Lithobid) is associated closely with the reabsorption of sodium. Patients who are concurrently hyponatremic and taking lithium are at risk for toxicity, as the body reabsorbs lithium instead of excreting it due to the similar molecular structure of sodium and lithium. Likewise, when excess sodium is ingested, the kidneys eliminate more sodium in the urine and more lithium. This produces lower lithium levels and possible therapeutic failure.

Drugs that are weak acids or bases are resorbed from the renal tubule into the systemic circulation only in the nonionic state, meaning that they are not carrying a charge. An acidic drug is largely in the nonionic state in urine with an acidic pH, whereas a basic drug is largely in a nonionic state in urine with an alkaline pH. A change in urinary pH by food may change the amount of drug existing in the nonionic state, thus increasing or decreasing the amount of drug available for tubular reabsorption. Foods such as milk, fruits (including citrus fruits), and vegetables are urinary alkalinizers (see the Clinical Insight box: Urinary pH—How Does Diet Affect It? in Chapter 35). This change can affect the ionic state of a basic drug such as the antiarrhythmic agent quinidine. In alkaline urine, quinidine is predominantly in the nonionic state and available for reabsorption from the urine into the systemic circulation, which may lead to higher blood levels. The excretion of memantine (Namenda), a drug used to treat neurodegenerative disorders, also is decreased by alkaline pH, thus raising the drug blood levels. Elevated drug levels may increase the risk of toxicity. This interaction is most likely to be clinically significant when the diet is composed exclusively of a single food or food group. Patients should be cautioned against initiating major diet changes without consulting their physician, dietitian nutritionist, or pharmacist.

Licorice, or glycyrrhizic acid, is an extract of glycyrrhiza root used in "natural" licorice candy. Approximately 100 g of licorice (the amount in two or more twists of natural licorice) can increase cortisol concentration, resulting in pseudohyperaldosteronism, which can lead to hypernatremia, water retention, increased blood pressure, and greater excretion of potassium, which can lead to hypokalemia and electrocardiographic changes. The action of diuretics and antihypertensive drugs may be antagonized. The resultant hypokalemia may alter the action of some drugs (Pronsky et al, 2015).

EFFECTS OF DRUGS ON FOOD AND NUTRITION

Many of the interactions discussed in this section are the opposite of those discussed previously in the Effects of Food on Drug Therapy. For instance, the chelation of a mineral with a medication not only decreases the absorption and therefore the action of the drug but also decreases the absorption and availability of the nutrient.

Nutrient Absorption

Medication can decrease or prevent nutrient absorption. Chelation reactions between medications and minerals (metal ions) reduce the amount of mineral available for absorption. An example is tetracycline and ciprofloxacin, which chelate calcium found in supplements or in dairy products such as milk or yogurt. This is also true for other divalent or trivalent cations such as iron, magnesium, and zinc found in individual mineral supplements or multivitamin-mineral supplements. Standard advice is to take the minerals at least 2 to 6 hours apart from the drug.

Drugs can reduce nutrient absorption by influencing the transit time of food and nutrients in the gut. Cathartic agents and laxatives reduce transit time and may cause diarrhea, leading to losses of calcium and potassium. Diarrhea may be induced by drugs containing sorbitol, such as syrup or solution forms of furosemide (Lasix), valproic acid (Depakene), carbamazepine (Tegretol), trimethoprim/sulfamethoxazole (Bactrim). Drugs that increase peristalsis such as the gastric mucosa protectant misoprostol (Cytotec) or the hyperosmotic, lactulose (Enulose) can also lead to this unpleasant side effect.

Drugs can also prevent nutrient absorption by changing the GI environment. H_2-receptor antagonists, such as famotidine (Pepcid) or ranitidine (Zantac), and proton pump inhibitors (PPIs), such as omeprazole (Prilosec) or esomeprazole (Nexium), are antisecretory drugs used to treat ulcer disease and GERD. They inhibit gastric acid secretion and raise gastric pH. These effects may impair absorption of vitamin B_{12} by reducing cleavage from its dietary sources. Cimetidine (Tagamet) is a H_2-receptor antagonist that also reduces intrinsic factor secretion, which can be problematic for vitamin B_{12} absorption, resulting in vitamin B_{12} deficiency with long-term use. The effect on calcium absorption of proton pump inhibitors may raise the risk of osteoporosis in at risk individuals, and the effect appears to be stronger with PPIs than with H_2-receptor antagonists.(Corley et al, 2010 and Kwok et al, 2011). Aside from these well-known concerns, a number of recent studies have also shown correlations between PPI therapy, Small Intestine Bacterial Overgrowth (SIBO), and IBS (Chey and Spiegel, 2010). Further studies of this type are needed to determine the long-term effects of chronic disruption in the gastric environment and its impact on gut health.

Drugs with the greatest effect on nutrient absorption are those that damage the intestinal mucosa. Damage to the structure of the villi and microvilli can inhibit the brush-border enzymes and intestinal transport systems involved in nutrient absorption. The result is varying degrees of specific malabsorption, which can alter the ability of the GI tract to absorb minerals, specifically iron and calcium. Damage to the gut mucosa commonly results from chemotherapeutic agents, nonsteroidal antiinflammatory drugs (NSAIDs), and long-term antibiotic therapy. NSAIDs may adversely affect the colon by causing a nonspecific colitis or by exacerbating a preexisting colonic disease (Tonolini, 2013). Patients with NSAID-induced colitis present with bloody diarrhea, weight loss, and iron deficiency anemia; the pathogenesis of this colitis is still controversial.

Drugs that affect intestinal transport mechanisms include (1) colchicine (Colcrys), an antiinflammatory agent used to treat gout; (2) sulfasalazine (Azulfidine), used to treat ulcerative colitis; (3) trimethoprim (antibiotic in sulfamethoxazole-trimethoprim [Bactrim]) and (4) antiprotozoal agent pyrimethamine (Daraprim). The colchicine impairs absorption of vitamin B_{12}, while the others are competitive inhibitors of folate transport mechanisms.

Nutrient Metabolism

Drugs may increase the metabolism of a nutrient, potentiating excretion and resulting in higher nutrient requirements. Drugs may cause vitamin antagonism by blocking conversion of a vitamin to the active form. Anticonvulsants phenobarbital and phenytoin induce hepatic enzymes and increase the metabolism of vitamins D, K, and folic acid. Supplementation of these vitamins often is prescribed with phenobarbital and phenytoin. Carbamazepine (Tegretol) has been reported to affect the metabolism of biotin, vitamin D, and folic acid, leading to possible depletion. Regular measurement of vitamin D levels and supplementation are recommended with carbamazepine.

The anti-tuberculosis drug, isoniazid, blocks the conversion of pyridoxine (vitamin B_6) to its active form, pyridoxal

5-phosphate. Patients with low pyridoxine intake who are taking isoniazid may develop pyridoxine deficiency and peripheral neuropathy. Pyridoxal 5-phosphate supplementation (25 to 50 mg/day) generally is recommended with the prescription of isoniazid. Some other drugs that function as pyridoxine antagonists are hydralazine (Apresoline), penicillamine, levodopa (Dopar), and cycloserine (Seromycin).

Methotrexate (Rheumatrex) is a folic acid antagonist used in the treatment of ectopic pregnancies, cancer, and rheumatoid arthritis. Without folic acid, DNA synthesis is inhibited and cell replication stops, resulting in cell death. Pyrimethamine is used to treat HIV, malaria, and toxoplasmosis and is also a folic acid antagonist. Both methotrexate and pyrimethamine bind to and inhibit the enzyme dihydrofolate reductase, preventing conversion of folate to its active form, which can lead to megaloblastic anemia from folate deficiency (see Chapter 32). Leucovorin (folinic acid, the reduced form of folic acid) is used with folic acid antagonists to prevent anemia and GI damage, most commonly with high-dose methotrexate. Leucovorin does not require reduction by dihydrofolate reductase; thus, unlike folic acid, it is not affected by folic acid antagonists. Therefore leucovorin may "rescue" normal cells from methotrexate damage by competing for the same transport mechanisms into the cells. Administration of daily folic acid supplements or folinic acid can lower toxicity without affecting efficacy of the drug. Patients receiving methotrexate should be assessed for their folic acid status (see Chapter 7).

Statin drugs (HMG-CoA reductase inhibitors) such as atorvastatin (Lipitor) affect the formation of coenzyme Q_{10} (CoQ$_{10}$; ubiquinone); See Box 8-3 on the mechanism of this effect. When HMG-CoA reductase is inhibited by statins, the production of cholesterol is decreased; a reasonable conclusion is that the production of CoQ$_{10}$ is also decreased. Studies have shown that circulatory, platelet, and lymphocyte levels of CoQ$_{10}$ are diminished. While initial small studies suggested that the muscle pain and weakness side effect of statins could be relieved by CoQ$_{10}$ supplementation, newer meta-analyses fail to show the same results, and conclude that more large-scale studies are needed (Banach et al, 2015). Overall, it is still considered prudent to advise CoQ$_{10}$ supplementation with 100 mg CoQ$_{10}$ daily for the purposes of repletion in patients taking HMG-CoA reductase inhibitors (Littarru and Langsjoen, 2007).

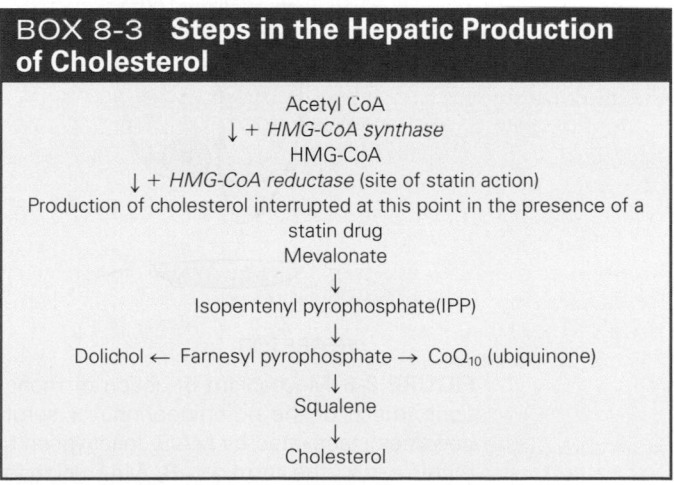

BOX 8-3 Steps in the Hepatic Production of Cholesterol

Acetyl CoA
↓ + *HMG-CoA synthase*
HMG-CoA
↓ + *HMG-CoA reductase* (site of statin action)
Production of cholesterol interrupted at this point in the presence of a statin drug
↓
Mevalonate
↓
Isopentenyl pyrophosphate(IPP)
↓
Dolichol ← Farnesyl pyrophosphate → CoQ$_{10}$ (ubiquinone)
↓
Squalene
↓
Cholesterol

CoA, Coenzyme A; *CoQ$_{10}$*, coenzyme Q$_{10}$; *HMG*, 3-hydroxy-3-methylglutaryl.

Nutrient Excretion

Some drugs either increase or decrease the urinary excretion of nutrients. Drugs can increase the excretion of a nutrient by interfering with nutrient reabsorption by the kidneys. For instance, loop diuretics including furosemide (Lasix) and bumetanide (Bumex) can increase the excretion of potassium while also increasing the excretion of magnesium, sodium, chloride, and calcium. Potassium supplements routinely are prescribed with loop diuretics, as hypokalemia can lead to serious cardiovascular toxicities. In addition, clinicians have to consider supplementation of magnesium and calcium, specifically with long-term or high doses of diuretics, or poor dietary intake. Electrolyte levels should be monitored for alterations.

Prolonged use of high-dose diuretics, particularly by older patients on low-sodium diets, can cause sodium depletion. Hyponatremia may be overlooked in older patients because the mental confusion that is symptomatic of sodium depletion may be misdiagnosed as organic brain syndrome or dementia. Thiazide diuretics such as hydrochlorothiazide (HCTZ) increase the excretion of potassium and magnesium, but reduce the excretion of calcium by enhancing renal reabsorption of calcium, although this is much less significant than with the loop diuretics.

Potassium-sparing diuretics such as spironolactone (Aldactone) or triamterene (Dyrenium) increase excretion of sodium, chloride, and calcium. Blood levels of potassium can rise to dangerous levels if patients also take potassium supplements or suffer from renal insufficiency. Antihypertensive angiotensin-converting enzyme (ACE) inhibitors such as enalapril (Vasotec) decrease potassium excretion, leading to increased serum potassium levels. The combination of a potassium-sparing diuretic and an ACE inhibitor increases the danger of hyperkalemia.

Corticosteroids such as prednisone decrease sodium excretion, resulting in sodium and water retention. Conversely, enhanced excretion of potassium and calcium is caused by these drugs; so a low-sodium, high-potassium diet is recommended.

Calcium and vitamin D supplements generally are recommended with long-term corticosteroid use to prevent osteoporosis. With corticosteroid use this risk is important because not only is calcium lost in the urine, but corticosteroids may also impair intestinal calcium absorption.

Phenothiazine-class antipsychotic drugs such as chlorpromazine (Thorazine) increase excretion of riboflavin and can lead to riboflavin deficiency in those with poor dietary intake. A complication associated with the use of anti-neoplastic drug, cisplatin, is the development of acute hypomagnesemia resulting from nephrotoxicity; hypocalcemia, hypokalemia, and hypophosphatemia are also common. Hypomagnesemia can result from cisplatin use even with high-dose magnesium replacement therapy. Magnesium level monitoring and repletion are essential for cardiovascular stability. Hypomagnesemia can persist for months or even years after the final course of cisplatin (See Appendix 23). Magnesium repletion is determined based on nutritional and cardiovascular status. If the patient is experiencing cardiovascular compromise then intravenous repletion is necessary, while patients with stable cardiac status may be repleted via oral methods.

MODIFICATION OF DRUG ACTION BY FOOD AND NUTRIENTS

Food or nutrients can alter the intended pharmacologic action of a medication by enhancing the medication effects or by opposing them. The classic example of an enhanced drug effect is the interaction between monoamine oxidase inhibitors (MAOIs) drugs such as phenelzine (Nardil) or tranylcypromine (Parnate) and vasopressor agents, such as dopamine, tyramine, (Figure 8-6). Other classes of medications including decongestants and antidepressants may also have similar properties. These biologically active amines are normally present in many foods (Box 8-4), but they rarely constitute a hazard because they are deaminated rapidly by monoamine oxidase (MAO) and diamine oxidase (DAO). Inhibition of MAO by medication prevents the

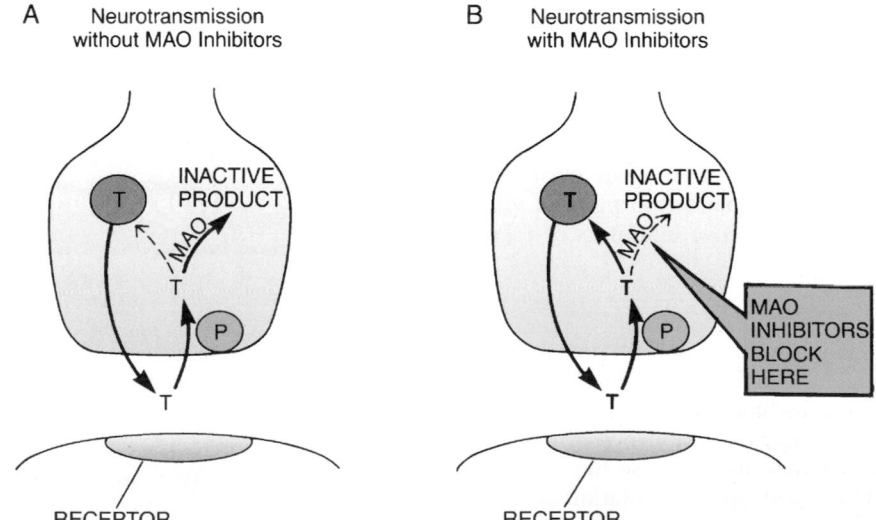

FIGURE 8-6 Mechanism of action of monoamine oxidase inhibitors. **A,** Under drug-free conditions, much of the norepinephrine or serotonin that undergoes reuptake into nerve terminals becomes inactivated by MAO. Inactivation helps maintain an appropriate concentration of transmitter within the terminal. **B,** MAO inhibitors prevent inactivation of norepinephrine and serotonin, thereby increasing the amount of transmitter available for release. Release of supranormal amounts of transmitter intensifies transmission. (From Lehne et al: *Pharmacology of nursing care,* ed 8, St Louis, 2012, Elsevier.)

BOX 8-4 Pressor Agents in Foods and Beverages (Tyramine, Dopamine, Histamine and Phenylethylamine)

Avoid with MAOI medications: phenelzine (Nardil), tranylcypromine (Parnate), isocarboxazid (Marplan), selegiline (Eldepryl) in doses >10 mg/day, and the antibiotic linezolid (Zyvox)

Foods That Must Be Avoided

Aged cheeses (e.g., cheddar, blue, Gorgonzola, Stilton)
Aged meats (e.g., dry sausage such as salami, mortadella, Chinese dried duck)
Soy sauce
Fermented soya beans, soya bean paste, teriyaki sauce
Tofu/fermented bean curd, tempeh
Miso
Fava (broad) beans or pods, snow pea pods (contain dopamine)
Sauerkraut, kim chee
Tap beer, Korean beer
Concentrated yeast extracts (Marmite, Vegemite)
Banana peel
Meats, fish, or poultry stored longer than 3-4 days in the refrigerator

Foods That May Be Used with Caution

Red or white wine 2-4 oz per day
Coffee, cola*
Pizza (homemade or gourmet pizzas may have higher content)
Bottled beer, two 12-oz bottles, maximum

Alcohol-free beer, two 12-oz bottles, maximum
Liquors or distilled spirits (two 1½-oz servings per day)

Foods Not Limited (Based on Current Analyses)

Unfermented cheeses (cream, cottage, ricotta, mozzarella, processed American if refrigerated less than 2-3 weeks)
Smoked white fish, salmon, carp, or anchovies
Pickled herring
Fresh meat poultry or fish
Canned figs, raisins
Fresh pineapple
Beetroot, cucumber
Sweet corn, mushrooms
Salad dressings, tomato sauce
Worcestershire sauce
Baked raised/yeast products, English cookies
Boiled egg, yogurt, junket, ice cream
Avocado, figs, banana, raspberries
Brewer's yeast (vitamin supplements)
Curry powder
Peanuts, chocolate
Packaged or processed meats (e.g., hot dogs, bologna, liverwurst), although they should be stored in refrigerator immediately and eaten as soon as possible; histamine content is highest in improperly stored or spoiled fish, tuna

MAOI, Monoamine oxidase inhibitor.
From Pronsky ZM et al: *Food medication-interactions,* ed 18, Birchrunville, Penn, 2015, Food-Medication Interactions.
*Contains caffeine, a weak pressor agent; in quantities >500 mg/day may exacerbate reactions

---

breakdown of tyramine and other vasopressor agents. Tyramine is a vasoconstrictor that raises blood pressure. Significant ingestion of high-tyramine foods such as aged cheeses and cured meats while being treated with an MAOI antidepressant can cause a hypertensive crisis and may lead to increased heart rate, flushing, headache, stroke, and even death. This reaction may be avoided with use of a transdermal administration method that bypasses the GI tract and omits contact with the indicated foods.

Caffeine in foods or beverages (see Appendix 33) increases the adverse effects of stimulant drugs such as amphetamines, methylphenidate (Ritalin), or theophylline, resulting in nervousness, tremor, and insomnia. Conversely, the central nervous system (CNS) stimulatory properties of caffeine can oppose or counteract the antianxiety effect of benzodiazapines such as lorazepam (Ativan).

Warfarin is an oral anticoagulant that reduces the hepatic production of four vitamin K–dependent clotting factors, II, VII, IX, and X, by inhibiting the conversion of vitamin K to a usable form. Because this is a competitive interaction, the ingestion of vitamin K in the usable form opposes the action of warfarin and allows the production of more clotting factors. To achieve an optimal level of anticoagulation, a balance must be maintained between the dose of the drug and the ingestion of vitamin K. Counseling of a person taking oral anticoagulation therapy should include nutrition therapy to maintain a *consistent* dietary vitamin K intake rather than prohibiting all high–vitamin K foods, such as dark green leafy vegetables (Pronsky and Crowe, 2012). CoQ10, St. John's wort, green tea, and avocado also may counteract the effect of warfarin. Ingestion of other substances may enhance the anticoagulant effect of warfarin, including: onions, garlic, ginger, quinine, papaya, mango, or vitamin E supplements in doses greater than 400 IU. Certain herbal products, such as dong quai, which contain coumarin-like substances, or ginseng, which is a platelet inhibitor, also enhance the effect of the

warfarin. Enhancement of the anticoagulation effects of warfarin may lead to serious bleeding events.

Alcohol

Ethanol combined with certain medications can produce additive toxicities. Ethanol combined with CNS-depressant medications such as a benzodiazepine (e.g., diazepam) or a barbiturate (e.g., phenobarbital) may produce excessive drowsiness, incoordination, and other signs of CNS depression, including death.

In the GI tract ethanol acts as a stomach mucosal irritant. Combining ethanol with other mucosal irritants such as aspirin or other NSAIDs (ibuprofen [Advil or Motrin]) may increase the risk of GI ulceration and bleeding. Because of the hepatotoxic potential of ethanol, it should not be combined with other hepatotoxic medications such as acetaminophen (Tylenol), amiodarone (Cordarone), or methotrexate.

Ethanol can inhibit gluconeogenesis, particularly when consumed in a fasting state. Inhibition of gluconeogenesis prolongs a hypoglycemic episode caused by insulin or an oral hypoglycemic agent such as glyburide (Diabeta).

The combination of disulfiram (Antabuse) and ethanol produces a potentially life-threatening reaction characterized by flushing, rapid heartbeat, palpitations, and elevation of blood pressure. Disulfiram inhibits aldehyde dehydrogenase, an enzyme necessary for the normal catabolism of ethanol by the liver. As a result of this enzyme inhibition, high levels of acetaldehyde accumulate in the blood. Symptoms such as flushing, headache, and nausea appear within 15 minutes of alcohol ingestion. Because these symptoms are unpleasant, the drug is sometimes used as an aid to prevent alcoholics from returning to drinking. However, because these symptoms also may be life threatening, candidates for this drug must be chosen carefully. Other medications, when ingested concurrently with ethanol, may produce disulfiram-like reactions, including: the antibiotic metronidazole

(Flagyl), the oral hypoglycemic agent chlorpropamide (Diabinese), and the antineoplastic agent procarbazine (Matulane).

Ethanol also can affect the physical characteristics of a medication. The FDA required a change in the labeling of the extended-release capsules of morphine sulfate (Avinza) which now includes a black box warning that patients must not consume alcoholic beverages or take morphine sulfate with medications containing alcohol. Black box warnings are given to medications (and are required on their labels or package inserts to be "boxed") with increased risks of adverse events and mortality. In the presence of alcohol, morphine can dissolve rapidly, delivering a potentially fatal dose, instead of the timed release mechanism of the medication.

EFFECTS OF DRUGS ON NUTRITION STATUS

The desired effects of medications often are accompanied by effects that are considered undesirable, or side effects. Side effects are often an extension of the desired effect. An example is the bacterial overgrowth that can occur from the use of an antibiotic that then results in pseudomembranous colitis (*Clostridium Difficile or "C.Diff."*). Suppression of natural oral bacteria may lead to oral yeast overgrowth, or candidiasis (see Chapters 27 and 28).

Taste and Smell

Many drugs affect the ability to taste or smell foods (Box 8-5). Drugs can cause an alteration in taste sensation (dysgeusia), reduced acuity of taste sensation (hypogeusia), or an unpleasant aftertaste, any of which may affect food intake. The mechanisms by which drugs alter the chemical senses are not well understood. They may alter the turnover of taste cells, interfere with transduction mechanisms inside taste cells; or alter neurotransmitters that process chemosensory information. Common drugs that cause dysgeusia include the antihypertensive drug captopril (Capoten), the antineoplastic cisplatin, and the anticonvulsant phenytoin. When exploring taste changes related to medication use it is important to consider changes in zinc absorption related to the medication, as underlying zinc deficiency may affect the sense of taste.

BOX 8-5 **Selected Examples of Drugs that Cause Altered Taste, or Dysgeusia**

Antineoplastic Drugs
carboplatin (Paraplatin)
cisplatin (Platinol-AQ)
dactinomycin (Actinomycin-D)
fluorouracil (5-FU)
interferon α-2a (Roferon-A)
interferon α-2b (Intron-A)
methotrexate (Rheumatrex)
oxaliplatin (Eloxatin)

Antiinfective Drugs
cefuroxime (Ceftin)
clarithromycin (Biaxin)
clotrimazole (Mycelex)
metronidazole (Flagyl)

Cardiovascular/ Antihyperlipidemic Drugs
captopril (Capoten)

amiodarone (Pacerone)
gemfibrozil (Lopid)

Central Nervous System Drugs
clomipramine (Anafranil)
eszopiclone (Lunesta)
levodopa (Dopar)
phenytoin (Dilantin)
phentermine (Adipex-P)
sumatriptan (Imitrex)

Miscellaneous
disulfiram (Antabuse)
docusate (Colace)

From Pronsky ZM et al: Food-medication interactions, ed 18, Birchrunville, Penn, 2015, Food-Medication Interactions.
Box edits reviewed by Doris Dudley Wales, BA, BS, RPh.

Captopril may cause a metallic or salty taste and the loss of taste perception. The antibiotic clarithromycin (Biaxin) enters the saliva and has a bitter taste that stays in the mouth as long as the drug is present in the body. An unpleasant or metallic taste has been reported by up to 34% of patients taking the sleep aid eszopiclone (Lunesta).

Antineoplastic drugs, chemotherapy for cancer, affect cells that reproduce rapidly, including the mucous membranes. Inflammation of the mucous membranes, or mucositis, occurs and is manifest as stomatitis (mouth inflammation), glossitis (tongue inflammation), or cheilitis (lip inflammation and cracking). Mucositis can be extremely painful to the point that patients are not able to eat or even drink (see Chapter 36). Aldesleukin, also called interleukin-2 (Proleukin), paclitaxel (Taxol), and carboplatin are examples of antineoplastic agents that commonly cause severe mucositis.

Anticholinergic drugs compete with the neurotransmitter acetylcholine for its receptor sites, thereby inhibiting transmission of parasympathetic nerve impulses. This results in decreased secretions, including salivary secretions, causing dry mouth (xerostomia). Tricyclic antidepressants such as amitriptyline (Elavil), antihistamines such as diphenhydramine (Benadryl), and antispasmodic bladder control agents such as oxybutynin (Ditropan) are particularly problematic. Dry mouth immediately causes loss of taste sensation. Long-term dry mouth can cause dental caries and loss of teeth, gum disease, stomatitis, and glossitis, as well as nutritional imbalance and undesired weight loss (see Chapter 25).

Gastrointestinal Effects

GI irritation and ulceration are serious problems with many drugs. The osteoporosis medication, alendronate, is contraindicated in patients who are unable to sit upright for at least 30 minutes after taking it because of the danger of esophagitis. NSAIDs such as ibuprofen or aspirin can cause stomach irritation, dyspepsia, gastritis, ulceration, and sudden serious gastric bleeding, sometimes leading to fatalities. Fluoxetine (Prozac) and other selective serotonin reuptake inhibitors (SSRIs) also can cause serious gastric irritation, leading to hemorrhage, especially when aspirin or NSAIDs also are used (Box 8-6).

Antineoplastic drugs often cause severe nausea and vomiting. Severe, prolonged nausea and vomiting, lasting as long as a week and requiring hospitalization, have been reported with cisplatin and other chemotherapeutic medications. Dehydration and electrolyte imbalances are of immediate concern with nausea and vomiting. Weight loss and malnutrition are common long-term effects of these drugs, although it is often difficult to distinguish these effects from the complications of the disease itself (see Chapter 36). Serotonin antagonists such as ondansetron (Zofran) help to reduce these GI side effects, which decrease activity of the chemoreceptor trigger zone in the brain, thus reducing nausea and vomiting.

Drugs can cause changes in bowel function that can lead to constipation or diarrhea. Narcotic agents such as codeine and morphine cause a nonproductive increase in smooth muscle tone of the intestinal muscle wall, thereby decreasing peristalsis and causing constipation. Methylnaltrexone (Relistor) is a laxative, administered subcutaneously, and specifically indicated for severe opioid-induced constipation.

Drugs with anticholinergic effects can also cause GI distress by decreasing intestinal secretions, slowing peristalsis, and causing constipation. The atypical antipsychotics, tricyclic antidepressants, and antihistamines can cause constipation and

---

BOX 8-6 Selected Examples of Drugs that Cause Gastrointestinal Bleeding and Ulceration

Antiinfective Drugs
amphotericin B (Fungizone)
ganciclovir (Cytovene)

Antineoplastic Drugs
erlotinib (Tarceva)
fluorouracil (5-FU)
leuprolide (Lupron)
imatinib (Gleevec)
mitoxantrone (Novantrone)
methotrexate (Rheumatrex)
vinblastine (Velban)

Bisphosphonates
alendronate (Fosamax)
ibandronate (Boniva)
risedronate (Actonel)

Immunosuppressants
prednisone (Deltasone)
myophenolate (CellCept)

Central Nervous System Drugs
bromocriptine (Parlodel)
donepezil (Aricept)
fluoxetine (Prozac)
levodopa (Dopar)
paroxetine (Paxil)
sertraline (Zoloft)
trazodone (Desyrel)

NSAIDs, Analgesic, Antiarthritic Drugs
aspirin/salicylate (Bayer)
celecoxib (Celebrex)
diclofenac (Voltaren)
etodolac (Lodine)
ibuprofen (Motrin)
indomethacin (Indocin)
meloxicam (Mobic)
nabumetone (Relafen)
naproxen (Naprosyn)

From Pronsky ZM et al: Food-medication interactions, ed 18, Birchrunville, Penn, 2015, Food-Medication Interactions.
Box edits reviewed by Doris Dudley Wales, BA, BS, RPh.

BOX 8-7 Selected Examples of Drugs that Cause Diarrhea

Antiinfective Drugs
amoxicillin (Amoxil)
amoxicillin/clavulanic acid (Augmentin)
amphotericin B (Fungizone)
ampicillin (Principen)
azithromycin (Zithromax)
cefdinir (Omnicef)
cefixime (Suprax)
cefuroxime (Ceftin)
cephalexin (Keflex)
clindamycin (Cleocin)
levofloxacin (Levaquin)
linezolid (Zyvox)
metronidazole (Flagyl)
rifampin (Rifadin)
tetracycline (Sumycin)

Antigout Drug
colchicine (Colcrys)

Antineoplastics
capecitabine (Xeloda)
carboplatin (Paraplatin)
fluorouracil (5-FU)
imatinib (Gleevec)

irinotecan (Camptosar)
methotrexate (Rheumatrex)
mitoxantrone (Novantrone)
paclitaxel (Taxol)

Antiviral Drugs
didanosine (Videx)
lopinavir (Kaletra)
nelfinavir (Viracept)
ritonavir (Norvir)
stavudine (Zerit)

Gastrointestinal Drugs
lactulose (Chronulac)
magnesium hydroxide (Milk of Magnesia)
magnesium gluconate (Magonate)
metoclopramide (Reglan)
misoprostol (Cytotec)
docusate (Colace)
orlitstat (Alli)

Antihyperglycemic Drugs
acarbose (Precose)
metformin (Glucophage)
miglitol (Glyset)

From Pronsky ZM et al: Food-medication interactions, ed 18, Birchrunville, Penn, 2015, Food-Medication Interactions.
Box edits reviewed by Doris Dudley Wales, BA, BS, RPh.

BOX 8-8 Selected Examples of Drugs that Cause Anorexia

Antiinfective Drugs
amphotericin B (Fungizone)
didanosine (Videx)
hydroxychloroquine (Plaquenil)
metronidazole (Flagyl)

Antineoplastic Drugs
bleomycin (Blenoxane)
capecitabine (Xeloda)
carboplatin (Paraplatin)
cytarabine (Cytosar-U)
dacarbazine (DTIC-Dome)
fluorouracil (5-FU)
hydroxyurea (Hydrea)
imatinib (Gleevec)
irinotecan (Camptosar)
methotrexate (Rheumatrex)
vinblastine (Velban)
vinorelbine (Navelbine)

Bronchodilators
albuterol (Proventil)
theophylline (Theo-24)

Cardiovascular Drugs
amiodarone (Pacerone)
hydralazine (Apresoline)

Stimulant Drugs
amphetamines (Adderall)
methylphenidate (Ritalin)
phentermine (Adipex-P)

Miscellaneous
fluoxetine (Prozac)
galantamine (Reminyl)
naltrexone (ReVia)
oxycodone (OxyContin)
rivastigmine (Exelon)
topiramate (Topamax)

From Pronsky ZM et al: Food-medication interactions, ed 18, Birchrunville, Penn, 2015, Food-Medication Interactions.
Box edits reviewed by Doris Dudley Wales, BA, BS, RPh.

---

possibly impaction. Patients on any of these drugs should be monitored closely and kept adequately hydrated.

Some drugs are used to inhibit intestinal enzymes, such as the diabetic drugs acarbose (Precose) and miglitol (Glyset), which are α-glucosidase inhibitors. These medications lead to a delayed and reduced rise in postprandial blood glucose levels and plasma insulin responses. The major adverse effect is GI intolerance, specifically diarrhea, flatulence, and cramping secondary to the osmotic effect and bacterial fermentation of undigested carbohydrates in the distal bowel.

The use of antibiotics and particularly broad-spectrum antibiotics, when taken for long periods of time, destroy all sensitive bacteria of the gut flora and often lead to diarrhea (Box 8-7). Opportunistic intestinal flora that are not sensitive to the antibiotic continue to grow because they are no longer inhibited by the bacteria that have been destroyed. An example of this situation is the overgrowth of *Clostridium difficile,* causing pseudomembranous colitis, which is associated with very strong-smelling yellow diarrhea and can lead to death or serious morbidity (see Chapter 28). Administration of a probiotic containing healthy bacteria for the gastrointestinal tract, such as lactobacillus and bifidus, should be considered with antibiotic therapy. Recent meta-analyses have shown that using probiotics concurrently with antibiotics can reduce the risk of antibiotic associated diarrhea and *C.Diff* infections (Pattani et al, 2013) (see Chapter 28).

Appetite Changes

Drugs can suppress appetite (Box 8-8), leading to undesired weight changes, nutritional imbalances, and impaired growth in children. In the past the stimulant drug dextroamphetamine (Dexedrine) was used as an appetite suppressant.

In general, most CNS stimulants, including the amphetamine mixture (Adderall) and methylphenidate (Ritalin), suppress appetite or cause anorexia. These drugs are used extensively to treat ADHD and may cause weight loss and inhibit growth (see Chapter 44).

Side effects of CNS stimulant drugs such as these include: hypertension, chest pain, and lowering of the seizure threshold, Use is contraindicated in hypertensive patients or those who have seizures or cardiac disease.

CNS side effects can interfere with the ability or desire to eat. Drugs that cause drowsiness, dizziness, ataxia, confusion, headache, weakness, tremor, or peripheral neuropathy can lead to nutritional compromise, particularly in older or chronically ill patients. Recognition of these problems as a drug side effect rather than a consequence of disease or aging is often overlooked, particularly in the elderly, who may instead be misdiagnosed with dementia (see Chapter 41).

Many medications stimulate appetite and cause weight gain (Box 8-9). Antipsychotic drugs such as clozapine and olanzapine (Zyprexa), tricyclic antidepressant drugs such as amitriptyline, and the anticonvulsant divalproex (Depakote) often lead to weight gain. Patients complain of a ravenous appetite and the inability to "feel full." Weight gains of 40 to 60 lb in a few months are not uncommon. Corticosteroid use is also associated with dose-dependent weight gain in many patients. Sodium and water retention, as well as appetite stimulation, cause weight increases with corticosteroids. Medical nutrition therapy (MNT) is essential, as is routine exercise while taking these medications (see Chapter 21).

Appetite stimulation is desirable for patients suffering from wasting (cachexia) resulting from disease states such as cancer, HIV, or the acquired immunodeficiency (AIDS) virus. Drugs indicated as appetite stimulants include the hormone megestrol acetate (Megace), antidepressant mirtazapine (Remeron), human growth hormone somatropin (Serostim), the anabolic steroid oxandrolone (Oxandrin), and the marijuana derivative dronabinol (Marinol).

With the successful advent of highly active antiretroviral therapy (HAART) for HIV infections, lipodystrophy is a common side effect from the therapy. Redistribution of body fat, fat wasting, glucose intolerance, hypertension, and hyperlipidemia are common side effects from antiviral medications. Antidiabetic drugs such as metformin (Glucophage) and rosiglitazone (Avandia) are used to normalize glucose and insulin levels in patients receiving HAART. Antihyperlipidemic drugs such as atorvastatin (Lipitor), pravastatin (Pravachol), and fenofibrate (Tricor) are used to control elevated triglycerides and cholesterol and may assist in the treatment of HAART associated adverse drug reactions (see Chapter 37).

Organ System Toxicity

Drugs can cause specific organ system toxicity. MNT may be indicated as part of the treatment of these toxicities. Although all toxicities are of concern, hepatotoxicity and nephrotoxicity are addressed here as the liver and kidneys are common elimination pathways for most medications.

Examples of drugs that cause hepatotoxicity (liver damage) including hepatitis, jaundice, hepatomegaly, or even liver failure include amiodarone, amitriptyline, antihyperlipidemic drugs, divalproex, carbamazepine (Tegretol), and methotrexate. Monitoring of hepatic function through routine blood work for liver enzyme levels generally is prescribed with use of these drugs (see Appendix 22 and Chapter 7). Toxicity related to liver failure can increase the amount of free drug and lead to toxicity from the medication as well.

Nephrotoxicity (kidney damage) may change the excretion of specific nutrients or cause acute or chronic renal insufficiency, which may not resolve with cessation of drug use. Examples of drugs that cause nephrotoxicity are antiinfectives amphotericin B (intravenous desoxycholate form [Fungizone]) and cidofovir (Vistide), antineoplastics cisplatin, gentamicin (Garamycin), ifosfamide (Ifex), methotrexate, and pentamidine. Hydration before drug infusion via intravenous administration can prevent renal toxicity. For example, with cidofovir, 1 L of intravenous normal saline (0.9% sodium chloride [NaCl]) is infused 1 to 2 hours before infusion of the drug. If tolerated, up to an additional liter may be infused after the drug infusion. Oral probenecid also is prescribed with cidofovir to reduce nephrotoxicity; this allows a dose reduction via increased contact with the gastrointestinal mucosa.

Glucose Levels

Many drugs affect glucose metabolism, causing hypoglycemia or hyperglycemia and in some cases diabetes (Box 8-10). The mechanisms of these effects vary. Drugs may stimulate glucose production or impair glucose uptake. They may inhibit insulin secretion, decrease insulin sensitivity, or increase insulin clearance.

Glucose levels may be altered related to medication use such as hypokalemia induced by thiazide diuretics or weight gain induced by antipsychotic medications (Izzedine et al, 2005). Corticosteroids, particularly prednisone, prednisolone, and hydrocortisone, may increase blood glucose because of increased gluconeogenesis, but they also cause insulin resistance and therefore inhibit glucose uptake. Second-generation antipsychotics, particularly clozapine or olanzapine, have been reported to cause hyperglycemia. Recently the FDA added a labeling requirement on all second-generation antipsychotics to warn of the possibility of developing hyperglycemia and diabetes.

EXCIPIENTS AND FOOD-DRUG INTERACTIONS

An **excipient** is added to drug formulations for its action as a buffer, binder, filler, diluent, disintegrant, glidant, flavoring,

---

BOX 8-9 Selected Examples of Drugs that Increase Appetite

Psychotropics
alprazolam (Xanax)
chlordiazepoxide (Librium)

Antipsychotics, Typical
haloperidol (Haldol)
perphenazine (Trilafon)

Antipsychotics, Atypical
olanzapine (Zyprexa)
quetiapine (Seroquel)
risperidone (Risperdal)

Antidepressants, Tricyclic
amitriptyline (Elavil)
clomipramine (Anafranil)
doxepin (Sinequan)
imipramine (Tofranil)
selegiline (Eldepryl) with doses >10 mg/day

Antidepressants, MAOI
isocarboxazid (Marplan)
phenelzine (Nardil)
tranylcypromine (Parnate)

Antidepressants, Other
mirtazapine (Remeron)
paroxetine (Paxil)

Anticonvulsants
divalproex (Depakote)
gabapentin (Neurontin)

Hormones
methylprednisolone (Medrol)
prednisone (Deltasone)
medroxyprogesterone (Depo-Provera)
megestrol acetate (Megace)
oxandrolone (Oxandrin)
testosterone (Androderm)

Miscellaneous
cyproheptadine (Periactin)
dronabinol (Marinol)

From Pronsky ZM et al: Food-medication interactions, ed 18, Birchrunville, Penn, 2015, Food-Medication Interactions.
Box edits reviewed by Doris Dudley Wales, BA, BS, RPh.

BOX 8-10 Selected Examples of Drugs that Affect Glucose Levels

Drugs That Lower or Normalize Glucose Levels

acarbose (Precose)
exenatide (Byetta)
glimepiride (Amaryl)
glipizide (Glucotrol)
glyburide (DiaBeta)
insulin (Humulin)
metformin (Glucophage)
miglitol (Glyset)
nateglinide (Starlix)
pioglitazone (Actos)
pramlintide (Symlin)
repaglinide (Prandin)
rosiglitazone (Avandia)

Drugs That Can Cause Hypoglycemia

ethanol (EtOH)
glipizide (Glucotrol)
glyburide (Diabeta)
glimepiride (Amaryl)

Drugs That Can Cause Hyperglycemia

Antiretroviral agents, protease inhibitors
  nelfinavir mesylate (Viracept)
  ritonavir (Norvir)
  saquinavir (Invirase)
Diuretics, Antihypertensives
  furosemide (Lasix)
  hydrochlorothiazide (HCTZ)
  indapamide (Lozol)

Hormones

prednisone (Deltasone)
medroxyprogesterone (Depo-Provera)
megestrol (Megace)
oral contraceptives

Miscellaneous

niacin (nicotinic acid)
baclofen (Lioresal)
caffeine (No-Doz)
olanzapine (Zyprexa)
cyclosporine (Sandimmune)
interferon α-2a (Roferon-A)
interferon α-2b (Intron-A)

From Pronsky ZM et al: Food-medication interactions, ed 18, Birchrunville, Penn, 2015, Food-Medication Interactions.
Box edits reviewed by Doris Dudley Wales, BA, BS, RPh.

BOX 8-11 Examples of Potential Interactive Drug Excipients

Albumin (egg or human): May cause allergic reaction. Human albumin is a blood product.

Alcohol (ethanol): CNS depressant used as a solvent. All alcohol and alcohol-containing products and drugs must be avoided with medications such as disulfiram (Antabuse) or limited with other drugs to prevent additive CNS or hepatic toxicity. Most elixirs contain 4% to 20% alcohol. Some solution, syrup, liquid, or parenteral forms contain alcohol.

Aspartame: A nonnutritive sweetener composed of the amino acids aspartic acid and phenylalanine. Patients with PKU lack the enzyme phenylalanine hydroxylase. If patients with PKU ingest aspartame in significant quantities, accumulation of phenylalanine causes toxicity to brain tissue.

Benzyl alcohol: A bacteriostatic agent used in parenteral solutions that can cause allergic reactions in some people. It has been associated with a fatal "Gasping Syndrome" in premature infants.

Caffeine: A member of the methylxanthine family of drugs which are CNS and heart muscle stimulants, cerebral vasoconstrictors and diuretics. Coffee, green and black teas, guarana, mate and cola nut are sources of caffeine and may affect medication action.

Lactose: Lactose is used as a filler. The natural sugar in milk, lactose is hydrolyzed in the small intestine by the enzyme lactase to glucose and galactose. Lactose intolerance (caused by lactase deficiency) results in gastrointestinal distress when lactose is ingested. Lactose in medications may cause this reaction.

Licorice (glycyrrhizic acid): Natural extract of glycyrrhiza root used in "natural" black licorice candy. Two or more twists per day (about 100 gm) of natural (usually imported), can increase cortisol concentration resulting in pseudohyperaldosteronism and increased sodium reabsorption, water retention, and K excretion and increased blood blood pressure. It antagonizes the action of diuretics and antihypertensives. The resultant hypokalemia may alter the action of some drugs.

Maltodextrin: In the US it is considered to be gluten-free since it can only be manufactured from corn.

Mannitol: The alcohol form of the sugar mannose, used as a filler. Mannitol is absorbed more slowly, yielding half as many calories per gram as glucose. Because of slow absorption, mannitol can cause soft stools and diarrhea.

Oxalate: A salt or ester of oxalic acid. Oxalate-containing foods must be avoided with some minerals due to formation of nonabsorbable complexes or oxalate kidney stones.

Phytate (phytic acid): Phosphorus-containing compound found in the outer husks of cereal grains. Amount of phosphate increases with maturity of the seed or grain. Phytate containing foods need to be avoided with some minerals (Ca, Fe, Mg, Zn) due to formation of nonabsorbable complexes.

Saccharin: Nonnutritive sweetener. Extensive human research has found no evidence of carcinogenicity.

Sorbitol: The alcohol form of sucrose. Absorbed more slowly than sucrose, sorbitol inhibits the rise in blood glucose. Because of slow absorption, sorbitol can cause soft stools or diarrhea.

Starch: Starch from wheat, corn, or potato is added to medication as a filler, binder, or diluent. Celiac disease patients have a permanent intolerance to gluten, a protein in wheat, barley, rye, and a contaminant of oat. In celiac disease, gluten causes damage to the lining of the small intestine.

Sulfites: Sulfiting agents are used as antioxidants. Sulfites may cause severe hypersensitivity reactions in some people, particularly asthmatics. They include sulfur dioxide, sodium sulfite, and sodium and potassium metabisulfite. The FDA requires the listing of sulfites when present in foods or drugs.

Tartrazine: Tartrazine is a yellow dye No. 5 color additive, which causes severe allergic reactions in some people (1 in 10,000). The FDA requires the listing of tartrazine on labels when present in foods or drugs.

Tyramine and other pressor agents (dopamine, phenethylamine, histamine): Tyramine is the decarboxylated product of the amino acid tyrosine. It is a vasoconstrictor which, in combination with some drugs such as monoamine oxidase inhibitors (MAOI), may cause a hypertensive crisis evidenced by dangerous increases in blood pressure, increased heart rate, flushing, headache, stroke and death. It is highest in aged, fermented or spoiled foods. See Chapter 26.

Vegetable oil: Soy, sesame, cottonseed, corn, or peanut oil is used in some drugs as a solvent or vehicle. Hydrogenated vegetable oil is a tablet or capsule lubricant. May cause allergic reactions in sensitive people.

Modified from Pronsky ZM et al: *Food-medication interactions*, ed 18, Birchrunville, Penn, 2015, Food-Medication Interactions.
CNS, Central nervous system; *FDA,* Food and Drug Administration; *PKU,* phenylketonuria.

dye, preservative, suspending agent, or coating. Excipients are also called *inactive ingredients* (Box 8-11). Hundreds of excipients are approved by the FDA for use in pharmaceuticals. Several common excipients have potential for interactions in persons with an allergy or enzyme deficiency. Often just one brand of a drug or one formulation or strength of a particular brand may contain the excipient of concern. For example, tartrazine, listed as yellow dye no. 5, is used in a brand of clindamycin (Cleocin) capsules in the 75- and 150-mg strengths but not in the 300-mg strength. Certain formulations of the same medication in different dosage strengths may have different excipients, including lactose, peanuts, and lecithin. Micronized progesterone (Prometrium) capsules contain peanut oil and lecithin, whereas other progesterone forms do not. Micronized progesterone labeling includes a warning that anyone allergic to peanuts should not use the drug.

Lactose is used commonly as a filler in many pills and capsules. The amount of lactose may be significant enough to cause GI problems for lactase-deficient patients, particularly those on multiple drugs throughout the day (see Chapter 28). Product information on prescription drugs and labeling on OTC drugs contain information on excipients, usually called "inactive ingredients," including lactose.

Patients with celiac disease have gluten sensitivity and must practice lifelong abstinence from wheat, barley, rye, and oats (which may be contaminated with gluten; see Chapter 28). They are concerned particularly with the composition and source of excipients such as wheat starch or flour, which may contain gluten. Only a few pharmaceutical companies guarantee their products to be gluten free. Excipients such as dextrin and sodium starch glycolate usually are made from corn and potato, respectively, but can be made from wheat or barley. For example, the excipient dextrimaltose, a mixture of maltose and dextrin, is produced by the enzymatic action of barley malt on corn flour (Pronsky and Crowe, 2012). The source of each drug ingredient, if not specified, should be checked with the manufacturer.

Finally, some drug brands may contain enough excipient to be nutritionally significant (see Table 8-1), magnesium in quinapril (Accupril), calcium in calcium polycarbophil (Fibercon), and soybean oil lipid emulsion in propofol (Diprivan). Propofol is used commonly for sedation of patients in the intensive care unit. Its formulation includes 10% emulsion, which contributes 1.1 kcal/mL. When infused at doses up to 9 mg/kg/hr in a patient weighing 70 kg, for instance, it may contribute an additional 1663 kcal/day from the emulsion and enteral and/or parenteral goals must be adjusted accordingly. For a patient receiving total parenteral nutrition, limiting the use of long-chain fatty acids and using medium-chain

triglyceride (MCT) oil may also be recommended while taking propofol and triglyceride levels must be monitored closely. Specific brands or formulations of a specific brand provide significant amounts of sodium and therefore may be contraindicated for patients who need to limit sodium.

MEDICAL NUTRITION THERAPY

Medical nutrition therapy (MNT) can be divided into prospective and retrospective care.

Prospective Medical Nutrition Therapy

Prospective MNT occurs when the patient first starts a drug. A diet history must be obtained, including information about the use of OTC (nonprescription) drugs, alcohol, vitamin and mineral supplements, and herbal or phytonutrient supplements. The patient should be evaluated for genetic characteristics, weight and appetite changes, altered taste, and GI problems (see Chapter 4).

Prospective drug MNT provides basic information about the drug: the name, purpose, and duration of prescription of the drug including when and how to take the drug. This information includes whether to take the drug with or without food. Specific foods and beverages to avoid while taking the drug, and potential interactions between drug and vitamin or mineral supplements must be emphasized. For instance, the patient taking tetracycline or ciprofloxacin should be warned not to combine the drug with milk, yogurt, or supplements containing divalent cations, calcium, iron, magnesium, zinc, or vitamin-minerals containing any of these cations.

Potential significant side effects must be delineated, and possible dietary suggestions to relieve the side effects should be described. For instance, information about a high-fiber diet with adequate fluids should be part of MNT about an anticholinergic drug such as oxybutynin, which often causes constipation. Conversely, diarrhea can be controlled by the use of psyllium (Metamucil) or probiotics, such as *Lactobacillus acidophilus*, particularly for antibiotic-associated diarrhea, even in children. However, probiotics are contraindicated for some individuals such as those with pancreatitis and should be

TABLE 8-1	Examples of Drugs That Contain Nutritionally Significant Ingredients		
Trade Name	**Generic Name**	**Ingredient**	**Nutritional Significance**
Accupril	Quinapril	Magnesium carbonate Magnesium stearate	Provides 50-200 mg magnesium daily
Accutane	Isotretinoin	Drug is related to vitamin A; contains soybean oil	Avoid vitamin A or β-carotene May cause allergic reaction
Atrovent (inhaler)	Ipratropium bromide	Soya lecithin	May cause allergic reaction
Fibercon/ Fiber-Lax	Calcium polycarbophil	Calcium polycarbophil	100 mg Ca/tablet; up to 6 tablets/day = 600 mg calcium total
Marinol	Dronabinol	Sesame oil	May cause allergic reaction
Phazyme	Simethicone	Soybean oil in capsule	May cause allergic reaction
Prometrium	Micronized progesterone	Peanut oil	May cause allergic reaction
Diprivan	Propofol	10% soybean oil emulsion Egg yolk phospholipids	Oil is significant caloric source, providing 1.1 kcals/mL of drug May cause allergic reaction
Videx	Didanosine	Sodium buffer in powder	≥2760 mg Na/adult daily dose
Zantac	Ranitidine	Sodium in *prescription* granules and tablets; Zantac 75 (nonprescription) is sodium free	350-730 mg Na/adult daily dose

Data from Pronsky ZM & Crowe JP: *Food-medication interactions*, ed 16, Birchrunville, Penn, 2010, Food-Medication Interactions.

prescribed and monitored by the physician. A commonly prescribed probiotic contains the yeast *Saccharomyces boulardii*. It should not be used in any patient with a central line for intravenous therapy, including those on dialysis.

Patients should be warned about potential nutritional problems, particularly when dietary intake is inadequate, such as hypokalemia with a potassium-depleting diuretic. Dietary changes that may alter drug action should be included, such as the effect of an increase in foods high in vitamin K on warfarin action. Special diet information, such as an anti-inflammatory, limited-sugar diet that includes healthy fats with atorvastatin (Lipitor) or other antihyperlipidemic drugs, is essential information. Written information should list medication ingredients such as nonnutrient excipients in the medication. Examples include lactose, starch, tartrazine, aspartame, and alcohol. Patients with lactose intolerance, celiac disease, allergies, phenylketonuria, or alcoholism need to avoid or limit one or more of these ingredients.

Prospective MNT also should cover potential concerns with OTC drugs and herbal and natural products. The pharmacokinetic and pharmacodynamic interactions explained in this chapter occur with all medications, whether obtained by prescription, OTC, or as natural or herbal products.

Retrospective MNT evaluates symptoms to determine whether medical problems or nutritional deficiencies may be the result of food-drug interactions. To determine whether a patient's symptoms are the result of a food-drug interaction, a complete medical and nutrition history is essential, including prescription and nonprescription drugs, vitamin-mineral supplements, and herbal or phytonutrient products (see Chapter 4). The date of beginning to take the drugs versus the date of symptom onset is significant information. It is important to identify the use of nutrition supplements or significant dietary changes such as fad diets during the course of drug prescription. Finally, the reported incidence of side effects (by percentage compared with a placebo) must be investigated. For example, vomiting occurs in 1.5% of those taking omeprazole (Prilosec) compared with 4.7% of those taking a placebo. Therefore in a patient treated with omeprazole, it would be appropriate to consider other causes for vomiting. A rare drug effect is less likely to be the reason for a negative symptom than an effect that is common.

In summary, although food provides energy for sustenance and physiologic benefits for good health, and drugs prevent or treat many diseases, together the synergistic effects can be very positive. The medical nutrition therapist must assess, intervene, and evaluate the mixtures with care. As always, working in collaboration with each patient's medical team, including physicians and pharmacists, ensures provision of the highest quality care.

CLINICAL SCENARIO

Charles is a 29-year-old man who began to suffer seizures after a head trauma injury from a motorcycle accident at the age of 18. For the first 2 years after the accident, he was prescribed various anticonvulsant regimens. The combination of phenytoin (Dilantin), 300 mg daily, and phenobarbital, 120 mg daily, has proven to be the most effective therapy to control his seizures. Charles has been stabilized on this regimen for the last 11 years.

Charles is a senior computer programmer for a large corporation. He is 6 feet 2 inches tall and weighs 187 lb. He admits to having an aversion for exercise and athletics. In his free time, he enjoys reading, playing computer games, and watching television. During the past year, Charles has broken his left femur and tibia on two separate occasions. He broke his femur when he missed the bottom step on the stairway in his office building. Several months later he broke his tibia when he tripped over a broken branch in his yard. Charles recently complained to his orthopedic surgeon about hip and pelvic pain of several weeks' duration. An orthopedic examination with x-ray examination, bone scan, and DXA scan revealed that Charles is suffering from osteomalacia. A review of Charles

typical diet reveals a nutritionally marginal diet that commonly includes fast foods and frozen dinners. His diet is generally deficient in fresh fruits, vegetables, and dairy products.

Nutrition Diagnostic Statement

Food-medication interaction related to inadequate calcium and vitamin D intake while taking anticonvulsant medications as evidenced by osteomalacia.

Nutrition Care Questions

1. Is osteomalacia common in young men?
2. How does Charles' lifestyle contribute to the development of osteomalacia?
3. What vitamin or mineral deficiency may have contributed to the current state of Charles' bones?
4. Describe the food-drug interaction that has contributed to Charles' osteomalacia.
5. What medical nutritional therapy would you recommend for Charles?

USEFUL WEBSITES

Access to MedLine
www.pubmed.com
Food and Drug Administration Center for Drug Evaluation and Research
www.fda.gov/cder/
Food and Nutrition Information Center
www.nal.usda.gov/fnic/
Food Medication Interactions
www.foodmedinteractions.com
Grapefruit-Drug Interactions
http://www.medicinenet.com/grapefruit_juice_and_medication_interactions/views.htm
National Institutes of Health Patient Handouts
www.cc.nih.gov/ccc/patient_education/

REFERENCES

Banach M, Serban C, Sahebkar A, et al: Effects of coenzyme Q10 on statin-induced myopathy: a meta-analysis of randomized controlled trials, *Mayo Clin Proc* 90(1):24, 2015.

Chey WD, Spiegel B: Proton Pump Inhibitors, Irritable Bowel Syndrome, and Small Intestinal Bacterial Overgrowth: Coincidence or Newton's third law revisited? *Clin Gastroenterol Hepatol* 8(6):480, 2010.

Corley DA, Kubo A, Zhao W, et al: Proton pump inhibitors and histamine-2 receptor antagonists are associated with hip fractures among at-risk patients, *Gastroenterol* 139:93, 2010.

Fohner A, Muzquiz LI, Austin MA, et al: Pharmacogenetics in American Indian populations: analysis of CYP2D6, CYP3A4, CYP3A5, and CYP2C9 in the Confederated Salish and Kootenai Tribes, *Pharmacogenet Genomics* 23:403, 2013.

Izzedine H, Launay-Vacher V, Deybach C, et al: Drug-induced diabetes mellitus, *Expert Opin Surg Saf* 4:1097, 2005.

Lee JI, Zhang L, Men AY, et al: CYP-mediated therapeutic protein-drug interactions: clinical findings, proposed mechanisms and regulatory implications, *Clin Pharmacokinet* 49:295, 2010.

Kwok CS, Yeong JK, Loke YK: Meta-analysis: risk of fractures with acid-suppressing medication, *Bone* 48:768, 2011.

Littarru GP, Langsjoen P: Coenzyme Q10 and statins: biochemical and clinical implications, *Mitochondrion* 7:S168, 2007.

Medical Letter: AmpliChip CYP450 test, *Med Lett Drugs Ther* 47:71, 2005.

Pattani R, Palda VA, Hwang SW, et al: Probiotics for the prevention of antibiotic-associated diarrhea and *Clostridium difficile* among hospitalized patients: systemic review and meta-analysis, *Open Med* 7(2):e56, 2013.

Pronsky ZM, Crowe JP: *Food medication interactions*, ed 17, Birchrunville, Penn, 2012, Food-Medication Interactions.

Pronsky ZM, Elbe D, Ayoob K: *Food medication interactions*, ed 18, Birchrunville, PA, 2015, Food-Medication Interactions.

Sica DA: Interaction of grapefruit juice and calcium channel blockers, *Am J Hypertens* 19:768, 2006.

Targownik LE, Lix LM, Leung S, et al: Proton-pump inhibitor use is not associated with osteoporosis of accelerated bone mineral density loss, *Gastroenterology* 138:896, 2010.

Tonolini M: Acute nonsteroidal anti-inflammatory drug-induced colitis, *J Emerg Trauma Shock* 6:301, 2013.

Truven Health Analytics, Inc.: *Lunesta. DrugPoints Summary. Micromedex 2.0.* Greenwood Village, CO.

Wohlt PD, Zheng L, Gunderson S, et al: Recommendations for use of medications with continuous enteral nutrition, *Am J Health-Syst Pharm* 66: 1458, 2009.

Behavioral-Environmental: The Individual in the Community

Judith L. Dodd, MS, RDN, LDN, FAND
Cynthia Taft Bayerl, MS, RDN, LDN, FAND, Lisa Mays, MPH, RDN

KEY TERMS

biosecurity
bioterrorism
community needs assessment
Department of Homeland Security (DHS)
Federal Emergency Management Agency (FEMA)
food desert
Food Safety and Inspection Service (FSIS)
foodborne illness
food security
genetically modified organisms (GMOs)

Hazard Analysis Critical Control Points (HACCP)
National Food and Nutrition Survey (NFNS)
National Health and Nutrition Examination Survey (NHANES)
National Nutrient Databank (NND)
National Nutrition Monitoring and Related Research (NNMRR) Act
nutrition policy
pandemic
policy development
primary prevention
public health assurance

risk assessment
risk management
secondary prevention
social determinants of health
Special Supplemental Nutrition Program for Women, Infants, and Children (WIC)
Supplemental Nutrition Assistance Program (SNAP; formerly the food stamp program)
tertiary prevention
U.S. Department of Health and Human Services (USDHHS)
What We Eat in America

Community nutrition is a constantly evolving and growing area of practice with the broad focus of serving the general population. Although this practice area encompasses the goals of public health, in the United States the current model has been shaped and expanded by prevention and wellness initiatives that evolved in the 1960s. Because the thrust of community nutrition is to be proactive and responsive to the needs of the community, current emphasis areas include access to a nutritionally adequate and safe food supply along with disaster and pandemic control, food and water safety, and controlling environmental risk factors related to obesity and other health risks. Food safety has entered the public health picture in new ways. Although traditional safety concerns continue to exist, potential safety issues such as genetic modification of the food supply is a new and growing concern and must be recognized as a part of community nutrition. (See *Focus On:* GMO or Genetically Engineered (GE) Foods in Chapter 26.)

Historically public health was defined as "the science and art of preventing disease, prolonging life, and promoting health and efficiency through organized community effort". The public health approach, also known as a *population-based* or *epidemiologic* approach, differs from the clinical or patient care model generally seen in hospitals and other clinical settings. In the public health model the client is the community, a geopolitical entity. The focus of the traditional public health approach is primary prevention with health promotion, as opposed to secondary prevention with the goal of risk reduction, or tertiary prevention with rehabilitation efforts. Changes in the health care system, technology, and attitudes of the nutrition consumer have influenced the expanding responsibilities of community

nutrition providers. Growing involvement in and access to technology, especially social media, has framed new opportunities and challenges in public health and community nutrition.

In 1988 the Institute of Medicine published a landmark report that promoted the concept that the scope of community nutrition is a work in progress. This report defined a mission and delineated roles and responsibilities that remain the basis for community nutrition practice. The scope of community-based nutrition encompasses efforts to prevent disease and promote positive health and nutritional status for individuals and groups in settings where they live and work. The focus is on well-being and quality of life. "Well-being" goes beyond the usual constraints of physical and mental health and includes other factors that affect the quality of life within the community. Community members need a safe environment and access to housing, food, income, employment, and education. The mission of community nutrition is to promote standards and conditions in which people can be healthy.

SOCIAL DETERMINANTS OF HEALTH

The social determinants of health are the conditions in which people are born, grow, live, work, and age. These circumstances are shaped by the distribution of money, power, and other resources at global, national, and local levels. A summary report of conditions throughout the world, including the United States, by the World Health Organization (WHO) describes how stress, social exclusion, working conditions, unemployment, social support, addiction, quality of the food, and transport affect opportunities (WHO, 2011). The report describes how people with fewer economic resources suffer from more acute and chronic disease and ultimately have shorter lives than their wealthier counterparts. This disparity has drawn attention to the remarkable sensitivity of health to the social environment, including psychological and social influences, and how these factors affect physical health and longevity. The report proposes that public policy can shape a social environment, making it more conducive to better health for all. Although it is a challenging task, if policy makers and advocates focus on policy and action for health needs to address the social determinants of health, the stage can be set for attacking the causes of ill health before they lead to problems (WHO, 2011; Wilkinson and Marmot, 2011).

Programming and services can be for any segment of the population. The program or service should reflect the diversity of the designated community, such as the politics, geography, culture, ethnicity, ages, genders, socioeconomic issues, and overall health status. Along with primary prevention, community nutrition provides links to programs and services with goals of disease risk reduction and rehabilitation.

In the traditional model, funding sources for public health efforts were monies allocated from official sources (government) at the local, state, or federal level. Currently nutrition programs and services are funded alone or from partnership between a broad range of sources, including public (government), private, and voluntary health sectors. As public source funding has declined, the need for private funding has become more crucial. The potential size and diversity of a designated "community" makes collaboration and partnerships critical, because a single agency may be unable to fund or deliver the full range of services. In addition, it is likely that the funding will be for services or product (in-kind) rather than cash. Creative funding and management skills are crucial for a community nutrition practitioner.

NUTRITION PRACTICE IN THE COMMUNITY

Nutrition professionals recognize that successful delivery of food and nutrition services involves actively engaging people in their own community. The pool of nutrition professionals delivering medical nutrition therapy (MNT) and nutrition education in community-based or public health settings continues to expand. An example of community growth is the presence of registered dietitians (RD), registered dietitian nutritionists (RDN), and other health professionals in for-profit or retail settings such as supermarkets, big-box stores, or pharmacies as well as in gyms and fitness-oriented clubs.

The objectives of *Healthy People 2020* offer a framework of measurable public health outcomes that can be used to assess the overall health of a community. Although the settings may vary, there are three core functions in community nutrition practice: (1) community needs assessment, (2) policy development, and (3) public health assurance. These areas are also the components of community nutrition practice, especially community needs assessment as it relates to nutrition. The findings of these needs assessments shape policy development and protect the nutritional health of the public.

Although there is shared responsibility for completion of the core functions of public health, official state health agencies have primary responsibility for this task. Under this model, state public health agencies, community organizations, and leaders have responsibility for assessing the capacity of their state to perform the essential functions and to attain or monitor the goals and objectives of *Healthy People 2020*.

A Framework for Public Health Action: Friedan's Pyramid

Local health agencies are charged with protecting the health of their population groups by ensuring that effective service delivery systems are in place. In 2010 Dr. Thomas Frieden, MD, at the Centers for Disease Control published an article that described a new way of thinking about community-based health services (Frieden, 2010). In his article "A Framework for Public Health Action: The Health Impact Pyramid," Frieden describes a five-tier pyramid derived from evidence-based research (Figure 9-1). The Pyramid describes the potential impact of various types of public health interventions and provides a framework to

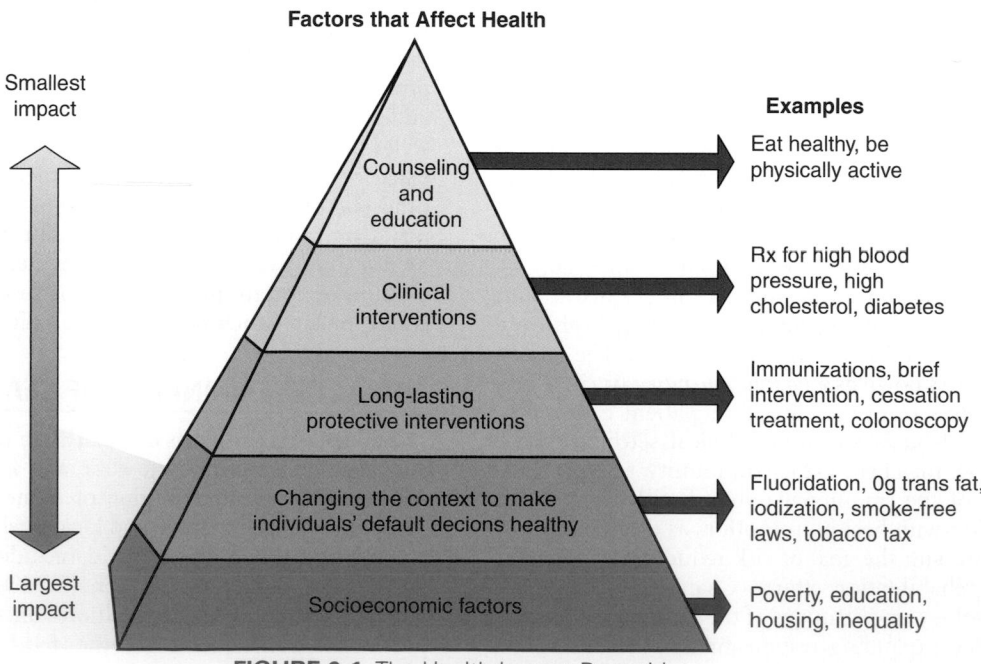

FIGURE 9-1 The Health Impact Pyramid.

improve health. Each layer describes the spheres that influence the involvement of the community in health services including nutrition. The foundation of this Pyramid (graph X) depicts the largest and broadest involvement of partners and communities, which Frieden describes as more powerful in influencing positive health outcome than the more traditional model of one-to-one intervention (depicted at the top of the figure).

Friedan's Pyramid illustrates, in ascending order, the interventions that could change the context to make an individual's default decisions healthy (Frieden, 2010). In addition, the Pyramid includes clinical interventions that require limited contact but confer long-term protection, ongoing direct clinical care, health education, and counseling. Friedan's point is that interventions focusing on lower levels of the Pyramid tend to be more effective because they reach broader segments of society and require less individual effort. Implementing interventions at each of the levels can achieve the maximum possible sustained public health.

Government's Role in Public Health

The federal government can support the development and dissemination of public health knowledge and provide funding. Box 9-1 provides a list of government agencies related to food and nutrition. Typical settings for community nutrition include public health agencies (state and local), including the Special Supplemental Nutrition Program for Women, Infants, and

---

BOX 9-1 Government Agencies Related to Food and Nutrition

Centers for Disease Control and Prevention (Department of Health and Human Services)
http://www.cdc.gov/
Central website for access to all U.S. government information on nutrition
http://www.nutrition.gov
Environmental Protection Agency
http://www.epa.gov/
Federal Trade Commission
http://www.ftc.gov
Food and Agriculture Organization of the United Nations
http://www.fao.org
Food and Drug Administration
http://www.fda.gov
Food and Drug Administration Center for Food Safety and Applied Nutrition
http://www.vm.cfsan.fda.gov
Food and Nutrition Service—Assistance Programs
http://www.fns.usda.gov/programs-and-services
National Cancer Institute (Department of Health and Human Services)
http://www.nci.nih.gov
National Health Information Center
http://www.health.gov/nhic
National Institutes of Health (Department of Health and Human Services)
http://www.nih.gov
National Institutes of Health—Office of Dietary Supplements
http://ods.od.nih.gov
National Marine Fisheries Service
http://www.nmfs.noaa.gov/
USDA Center for Nutrition Policy and Promotion
http://www.usda.gov/cnpp
USDA Food and Nutrition Service
http://www.fns.usda.gov/fns
USDA Food Safety and Inspection Service
http://www.fsis.usda.gov
USDA National Agriculture Library
http://www.nal.usda.gov/fnic

Children (WIC). WIC is a federal program that allocates funds to states and territories for specific foods, health care referrals, and nutrition education for low-income, nutritionally at-risk pregnant, breastfeeding, and non-breastfeeding postpartum women; infants; and children up to age 5 years. This program is a specific, nutrition-based food package that has evolved over the years to provide for the individual needs of the client and has adapted to changes in society. It is an illustration of a nutrition-based program tailored to current needs.

The expansion of community-based practice beyond the scope of traditional public health has opened new employment and outreach opportunities for nutrition professionals. Nutrition professionals often serve as consultants or may establish community-based practices. Nutrition services are often available in programs for senior adults, in community health centers, in early intervention programs, within health maintenance organizations, at food banks and shelters, in schools (including Head Start), and in physicians' offices or clinics.

Effective practice in the community requires a nutrition professional who understands the effect of economic, social, and political issues on health. Many community-based efforts are funded or guided by legislation resulting in regulations and policies. Community practice requires an understanding of the legislative process and an ability to translate policies into action. In addition, the community-based professional needs a working knowledge of funding sources and resources at the federal, state, regional, and local level in the official, nonprofit, and private sectors.

NEEDS ASSESSMENT FOR COMMUNITY-BASED NUTRITION SERVICES

Nutrition services should be organized to meet the needs of a "community." Once that community has been defined, a **community needs assessment** is developed to shape the planning, implementation, and evaluation of nutrition services. Evidence-based, assessment tools are available to aid in this process. One such tool is the Centers for Disease Control and Prevention's (CDC) *The Guide to Community Preventive Services*. This provides evidence-based recommendations for interventions and policies that can improve health and prevent disease in communities. It contains information on various topics related to health risk factors, such as nutrition, obesity, physical activity, tobacco use, and diabetes. Information on policies, programs or services, funding, research, and education are included in this guide (CDC, 2014).

Other sources are organizations and centers such as ChangeLabSolutions, the American Public Health Association, and the Rudd Policy Center at Yale University. Resources are available to communities for use in health and **nutrition policy** (course of action adopted by government or business) that include technical assistance to support communities in the process of developing policies and conducting assessments. Such tools and assistance can result in meaningful strategies and programming.

Community Needs Assessment

A *community needs assessment* is a current snapshot of a defined community with a goal of identifying the health risks or areas of greatest concern to the community's well-being. To be effective, the needs assessment must be a dynamic document responsive to changes in the community. A plan is only as good as the research used to shape the decisions, so a mechanism for ongoing review and revision should be built into the planning.

A needs assessment is based on objective data, including demographic information and health statistics. Information should represent the community's diversity and be segmented by such factors as age, gender, socioeconomic status, disability, and ethnicity. Examples of information to be gathered include current morbidity and mortality statistics, number of low-birth-weight infants, deaths attributed to chronic diseases with a link to nutrition, and health-risk indicators such as incidence of smoking or obesity. *Healthy People 2020* outlines the leading health indicators that can be used to create target objectives. Ongoing evaluation of progress on these indicators builds on objectives and adds new direction. Subjective information such as input from community members, leaders, and health and nutrition professionals can be useful in supporting the objective data or in emphasizing questions or concerns. The process mirrors what the business world knows as *market research.*

Another step should be cataloging accessible community resources and services. As an example, consider how environmental, policy, and societal changes have contributed to the rapid rise in obesity over the past few decades. Resources to consider are affordable access to walkable neighborhoods, recreation facilities, and health-promoting foods (CDC, 2014).

In nutrition planning the goal is to determine who and what resources are available to community members when they need food or nutrition-related products or services. For example, what services are available for medical nutrition therapy (MNT), nutrition and food education, homecare, child care, or homemaker skills training? Are there safe areas for exercise or recreation? Is there access to transportation? Is there compliance with disability legislation? Are mechanisms in place for emergencies that may affect access to adequate and safe food and water?

At first glance some of the data gathered in this process may not appear to relate directly to nutrition, but an experienced community nutritionist or a community-based advisory group with public health professionals can help connect this information to nutrition- and diet-related issues. Often the nutritional problems identified in a review of nutrition indicators are associated with dietary inadequacies, excesses, or imbalances that can be triggers for disease risk (Box 9-2). Careful attention should be paid to the special needs of adults and children with disabilities or other lifestyle-limiting conditions. Once evaluated, the information is used to propose needed services, including MNT as discussed in other chapters, as part of the strategy for improving the overall health of the community.

Sources for Assessment Information

Community practitioners must know how to locate relevant resources and evaluate the information for validity and reliability. Knowing the background and intent of any data source and

---

BOX 9-2 Possible Nutrition Trigger Areas in a Community Needs Assessment

- Presence of risk factors for cardiovascular disease; diabetes and stroke
  - Elevated blood cholesterol and lipid levels
  - Inactivity
  - Smoking
  - Elevated blood glucose levels
  - High body mass index (BMI)
  - Elevated blood pressure
- Presence of risk factors for osteoporosis
- Evidence of eating disorders
- High incidence of teenage pregnancy
- Evidence of hunger and food insecurity

BOX 9-3 Community Nutrition Assessment Sources

NHANES, National Health and Nutrition Examination Survey
NFNS, National Food and Nutrition Survey
CSFII, Continuing Survey of Food Intake of Individuals

---

identifying the limitations and the dates when the information was collected are critical points to consider when selecting and using such sources. Census information is a starting point for beginning a needs assessment. Morbidity and mortality and other health data collected by state and local public health agencies, the CDC, and the National Center for Health Statistics (NCHS) are useful. Federal agencies and their state program administration counterparts are data sources; these agencies include the **U.S. Department of Health and Human Services (USDHHS)**, U.S. Department of Agriculture (USDA), and the Administration on Aging. Local providers such as community hospitals, WIC, child care agencies, health centers, and universities with a public health or nutrition department are additional sources of information. Nonprofit organizations such as the March of Dimes, the American Heart Association (AHA), the American Diabetes Association, and the American Cancer Society (ACS) also maintain population statistics. Health insurers are a source for information related to health care consumers and geographic area. Food banks and related agencies also may be able to provide insights into food access and security (Box 9-3).

NATIONAL NUTRITION SURVEYS

Nutrition and health surveys at the federal and state level provide information on the dietary status of a population, the nutritional adequacy of the food supply, the economics of food consumption, and the effects of food assistance and regulatory programs. Public guidelines for food selection usually are based on survey data. The data are also used in policy setting; program development; and funding at the national, state, and local levels. Until the late 1960s, the USDA was the primary source of food and nutrient consumption data. Although much of the data collection is still at the federal level, other agencies and states are now generating information that provides comprehensive information on the health and nutrition of the public.

National Health and Nutrition Examination Survey

The **National Health and Nutrition Examination Survey (NHANES)** provides a framework for describing the health status of the nation. Sampling the noninstitutionalized population, the initial study began in the early 1960s, with subsequent studies on a periodic basis from 1971 to 1994. NHANES has been collected on a continuous basis since 1999. The process includes interviewing approximately 6000 individuals each year in their homes and following approximately 5000 individuals with a complete health examination. Since its inception, each successive NHANES has included changes or additions that make the survey more responsive as a measurement of the health status of the population. NHANES I to III included medical history, physical measurements, biochemical evaluation, physical signs and symptoms, and diet information using food frequency questionnaires and a 24-hour recall. Design changes added special population studies to increase information on underrepresented groups. NHANES III (1988 to 1994) included a large proportion of persons age 65 years and older.

This information enhanced understanding of the growing and changing population of senior adults. Currently, reports are released in 2-year cycles. Sampling methodology is planned to oversample high-risk groups not previously covered adequately (low income, those older than the age of 60, blacks, and Hispanic Americans). Information on NHANES is available in a pdf document at http://www.cdc.gov/nchs/data/nhanes/survey_content_99_14.pdf. This report catalogs NHANES findings from its inception until 2014 (CDC, 2014).

The most current additions to NHANES include a sampling of the population from 3 to 15 years of age. The 2012 NHANES National Youth Fitness Survey (NNYFS) was a 1-year survey that set up the next phase of NHANES. The design of this part of NHANES was described in a report released November of 2013 (http://www.cdc.gov/nchs/data/nnyfs/NNYFS_Plan_Ops.pdf).

Continuing Survey of Food Intake of Individuals: Diet and Health Knowledge Survey

The Continuing Survey of Food Intake of Individuals (CSFII) was a nationwide dietary survey instituted in 1985 by the USDA. In 1990 CSFII became part of the USDA National Nutrition Monitoring System. Information from previous surveys is available from the 1980s and 1990s. The Diet and Health Knowledge Survey (DHKS), a telephone follow-up to CFSII, began in 1989. The DHKS was designed as a personal interview questionnaire that allowed individual attitudes and knowledge about healthy eating to be linked with reported food choices and nutrient intakes. Early studies focused on dietary history and a 24-hour recall of dietary intake from adult men and women ages 19 to 50. The 1989 and 1994 surveys questioned men, women, and children of all ages and included a 24-hour recall (personal interview) and a 2-day food diary. Household data for these studies were determined by calculating the nutrient content of foods reported to be used in the home during the survey. These results were compared with nutrition recommendations for persons matching in age and gender. The information derived from the CSFII and DHKS is still useful for decision makers and researchers in monitoring the nutritional adequacy of American diets, measuring the effect of food fortification on nutrient intakes, tracking trends, and developing dietary guidance and related programs. In 2002 both surveys merged with NHANES to become the National Food and Nutrition Survey (NFNS), or What We Eat in America.

National Food and Nutrition Survey: What We Eat in America

The integrated survey What We Eat in America is collected as part of NHANES. Food-intake data are linked to health status from other NHANES components, allowing for exploration of relationships between dietary indicators and health status. The USDHHS is responsible for sample design and data, whereas the USDA is responsible for the survey's collection and maintenance of the dietary data. Data are released at 2-year intervals and are accessible from the NHANES website (USDA, Agricultural Research Service, 2014).

National Nutrition Monitoring and Related Research Act

In 1990 Congress passed Public Law 101-445, the National Nutrition Monitoring and Related Research (NNMRR) Act. The purpose of this law is to provide organization, consistency, and unification to the survey methods that monitor the food habits and nutrition of the U.S. population and to coordinate the efforts of the 22 federal agencies that implement or review

nutrition services or surveys. Data obtained through NNMRR are used to direct research activities, develop programs and services, and make policy decisions regarding nutrition programs such as food labeling, food and nutrition assistance, food safety, and nutrition education. Reports of the various activities are issued approximately every 5 years and provide information on trends, knowledge, attitudes and behavior, food composition, and food supply determinants. They are available from the National Agricultural Library database.

National Nutrient Databank

The National Nutrient Databank (NND), maintained by the USDA, is the United States' primary resource of information from private industry, academic institutions, and government laboratories on the nutrient content of foods. Historically the information was published as the series *Agriculture Handbook 8*. Currently, the databases are available to the public on tapes and on the Internet. The bank is updated frequently and includes supplemental sources, international databases, and links to other sites. This databank is a standard and updated source of nutrient information for commercial references and data systems. When using sources other than the USDA site, clinicians should check the sources and the dates of the updates for evidence that these sources are reliable and current.

The Centers for Disease Control and Prevention

The CDC is a component of the USDHHS. It monitors the nation's health, detects and investigates health problems, and conducts research to enhance prevention. The CDC is also a source of information on health for international travel. Housed at CDC is the NCHS, the lead agency for NHANES, morbidity and mortality, BMI, and other health-related measures. Public health threats, such as the H1N1 virus, also are monitored by CDC.

NATIONAL NUTRITION GUIDELINES AND GOALS

Policy development describes the process by which society makes decisions about problems, chooses goals, and prepares the means to reach them. Such policies may include health priorities and dietary guidance.

Early dietary guidance had a specific disease approach. The 1982 National Cancer Institute (NCI) landmark report, *Diet, Nutrition and Cancer*, evolved into *Dietary Guidelines for Cancer Prevention*. These were updated and broadened in 2004, combining recommendations on energy balance, nutrition, and physical activity. The ACS and the American Institute for Cancer Research (AICR) are excellent resources along with materials from the NCI. Another federal agency, the National Heart, Lung, and Blood Institute, provided three sets of landmark guidelines for identifying and treating lipid disorders between 1987 and 2010.

The most recent AHA guidelines continue to focus on reducing risks for hypertension and coronary artery disease with reduction of obesity, incorporation safe and regular exercise, control of individuals' sodium intake and cholesterol levels, and moderation of the type of dietary fat eaten. Additionally they focus on increasing the intake of fruits and vegetables, legumes and nuts. (See Chapter 33). In 2014 the issue of smoking was again updated.

Building on another consumer-friendly, single health guideline (5-a-Day for Better Health), the NCI, the NIH, and the Produce for Better Health Foundation put the focus on fruits and vegetables. This guidance was built around the message that fruits and vegetables are naturally low in fat and good sources of fiber, several vitamins and minerals, and phytonutrients. In keeping with evidence-based messages, five to nine servings of fruits and vegetables a day are recommended to promote good health under the name of "Fruits and Veggies: More Matters". The *More Matters* banner continues as the branding for health guidelines and is an ongoing message for My Plate and the Dietary Guidelines for Americans. (Produce for Better Health, 2015).

The release of My Plate after the update on The Dietary Guidelines for Americans in 2010 made this a source of a strong and ongoing public health message with materials focusing across the life cycle, professional and consumer updates, and a robust social media presence (http://fnic.nal.usda.gov/dietary-guidance/fruits-veggies-more-matters-resources/fruits-veggies-more-matters). See Chapter 11.

Dietary Guidelines for Americans

Senator George McGovern and the Senate Select Committee on Nutrition and Human Needs presented the first *Dietary Goals for the United States* in 1977. In 1980 the goals were modified and issued jointly by the USDHHS and the USDA as the *Dietary Guidelines for Americans (DGA)*. The original guidelines were a response to an increasing national concern for the rise in overweight, obesity, and chronic diseases such as diabetes, coronary artery disease, hypertension, and certain cancers. The approach continues to be one of health promotion and disease prevention, with special attention paid to specific population groups (see Chapter 11).

The release of the DGA led the way for a synchronized message to the community. The common theme has been a focus on a diet lower in sodium and saturated fat, with emphasis on foods that are sources of fiber, complex carbohydrates, and lean or plant-based proteins. The message is based on food choices for optimal health using appropriate portion sizes and calorie choices related to a person's physiologic needs. Exercise, activity, and food safety guidance are standard parts of this dietary guidance. The current DGA are evidence-based rather than just "good advice." The expert committee report provides scientific documentation that is used widely in health practice. The DGA have become a central theme in community nutrition assessment, program planning, and evaluation; they are incorporated into programs such as School Lunch and Congregate Meals. Updated every 5 years, the DGA recently have undergone revision in 2010 and are currently undergoing revision (see Chapter 11). The 2010 DGA set the path for our current food guide, My Plate, and set the stage for programs such as More Matters to evolve. The 2015 DGA are scheduled to be released at the time of this updated chapter. Emphasis continues to be on the 2010 DGA with emerging evidence on plant-based choices, total fat, types of fat, saturated fat, added sugars and sodium (Dietary Guidelines 2015).

Food Guides

In 1916 the USDA initiated the idea of food grouping in the pamphlet *Food for Young Children.* Food grouping systems have changed in shape (wheels, boxes, pyramids, and plates) and numbers of groupings (four, five, and seven groups), but the intent remains consistent: to present an easy guide for healthful eating. In 2005 an Internet-based tool called *MyPyramid.gov: Steps to a Healthier You* was released. In 2011 MyPyramid.gov was replaced with My Plate (chooseMyPlate.gov.) along with a version for children called *chooseMyPlate.gov/kids*. These food guidance systems focus on health promotion and disease prevention and are updated whenever DGA guidance

changes. This program has become a leading public education resource with My Tracker (a way to set and evaluate one's own diet), downloadable tip sheets, and a list of well-done social media efforts that brings application to the food guide (see Chapter 11).

Healthy People and the Surgeon General's Report on Nutrition and Health

The 1979 report of the Surgeon General, *Promoting Health/Preventing Disease: Objectives for the Nation,* outlined the prevention agenda for the nation with a series of health objectives to be accomplished by 1990. In 1988 *The Surgeon General's Report on Nutrition and Health* further stimulated health promotion and disease prevention by highlighting information on dietary practices and health status. Along with specific health recommendations, documentation of the scientific basis was provided. Because the focus included implications for the individual as well as for future public health policy decisions, this report remains a useful reference and tool. *Healthy People 2000: National Health Promotion and Disease Prevention Objectives* and *Healthy People 2010* were the next generations of these landmark public health efforts. Both reports outlined the progress made on previous objectives and set new objectives for the next decade.

During the evaluation phase for setting the 2010 objectives, it was determined that the United States made progress in reducing the number of deaths from cardiovascular disease, stroke, and certain cancers. Dietary evaluation indicated a slight decrease in total dietary fat intake. However, during the previous decade there has been an increase in the number of persons who are overweight or obese, a risk factor for cardiovascular disease, stroke, and other leading chronic diseases and causes of death.

Objectives for *Healthy People 2020* have specific goals that address nutrition and weight, heart disease and stroke, diabetes, oral health, cancer, and health for seniors. These goals are important for consumers and health care providers. The website for *Healthy People 2020* offers an opportunity to monitor the progress on past objectives as well as on the shaping of future health initiatives (https://www.healthypeople.gov/).

National School Lunch Program

The National School Lunch Program (NSLP) is a federal assistance program that provides free or reduced-cost meals for low-income students in public schools and in nonprofit private residential institutions. It is administered at a state level through the education agencies that generally employ dietitians. In 1998 the program was expanded to include after-school snacks in schools with after-hours care. Currently the guidelines for calories, percent of calories from fat, percent of saturated fat, and the amount of protein and key vitamins and minerals must meet the DGA, but there is ongoing evaluation and interpretation. Efforts have been made to meet My Plate guidelines for whole grains, more fruits and vegetables, and skim or 1% milk. In addition, the issues of education of recipients to accept these foods and use of local foods and community gardens are evolving processes that are happening in communities.

A requirement for wellness policies in schools that participate in the NSLP is in place (Edelstein et al, 2010). However, the School Nutrition Dietary Assessment Study, a nationally representative study fielded during school year 2004 to 2005 to evaluate nutritional quality of children's diets, identified that

80% of children had excessive intakes of saturated fat and 92% had excessive intakes of sodium (Clark and Fox, 2009). An increase in whole grains, fresh fruits, and a greater variety of vegetables is needed (Condon et al, 2009). The state of Texas made changes to their school lunches by restricting portion sizes of high-fat and high-sugar snacks and sweetened beverages, fat content of foods, and high-fat vegetables such as French fries; this led to a desired reduction in energy density (Mendoza et al, 2010). Other states and local programs have followed suit, partially because of new guidelines issued by the USDA.

On December 14, 2010, the Hunger-Free Kids Act was signed into law. It expanded the after-school meal program, created a process for a universal meal program that allows schools with a high percentage of low-income children to receive meals at no charge, allowed states to increase WIC coverage from 6 months to 1 year, mandated WIC use electronic benefits by 2020, and improved the nutritional quality of foods served in school-based and preschool settings by developing new nutrition standards.

The Recommended Dietary Allowances and Dietary Reference Intakes

The recommended dietary allowances (RDAs) were developed in 1943 by the Food and Nutrition Board of the National Research Council of the National Academy of Sciences. The first tables were developed at a time when the U.S. population was recovering from a major economic depression and World War II; nutrient deficiencies were a concern. The intent was to develop intake guidelines that would promote optimal health and lower the risk of nutrient deficiencies. As the food supply and the nutrition needs of the population changed, the intent of the RDAs was adapted to prevention of nutrition-related disease. Until 1989 the RDAs were revised approximately every 10 years.

The RDAs always have reflected gender, age, and life-phase differences: there have been additions of nutrients and revisions of the age groups. However, recent revisions are a major departure from the single list some professionals still view as the RDAs. Beginning in 1998 an umbrella of nutrient guidelines known as the *dietary reference intakes (DRIs)* was introduced. Included in the DRIs are RDAs, as well as new designations, including guidance on safe upper limits (ULs) of certain nutrients. As a group the DRIs are evaluated and revised at intervals, making these tools reflective of current research and population base needs (see Chapter 11).

FOOD ASSISTANCE AND NUTRITION PROGRAMS

Public health assurance addresses the implementation of legislative mandates, maintenance of statutory responsibilities, support of crucial services, regulation of services and products provided in the public and private sector, and maintenance of accountability. This includes providing for food security, which translates into having access to an adequate amount of healthful and safe foods.

In the area of food security, or access by individuals to a readily available supply of nutritionally adequate and safe foods programs have continued to evolve. The Supplemental Nutrition Assistance Program (SNAP), formerly known as food stamps, along with food pantries, home-delivered meals, child nutrition programs, supermarkets, and other food sources have been highlighted to focus on the issues of quality, access, and

use. For example, research on neighborhood food access indicates that low availability of healthy food in area stores is associated with low quality diets of area residents (Rose et al, 2010). See Table 9-1 for a list of food and nutrition assistance programs. *Clinical Insight:* The History of the Supplemental Nutrition Assistance Program (SNAP) provides additional information on this program.

There is an ongoing movement to encourage goals emphasized in My Plate, to add more vegetables and fruits and increase minimally processed foods, and to increase education for SNAP recipients as well as other food and nutrition assistance programs. The presence of food deserts is a concept that has become a focus of research and community planning. Food deserts are described by the Agricultural Marking Service of USDA as urban neighborhoods and rural areas with limited access to fresh, healthy, affordable food (http://apps.ams.usda.gov/fooddeserts/foodDeserts.aspx). The Economic Research Service (ERS) of the USDA estimated in 2013 that 23.5 million people live in food deserts and more than half of those are low income. Although the definition of a food desert is controversial, the USDA defines it as a neighborhood where the nearest supermarket or grocery store is located 1 to 3 miles away for urban residents and 10 miles from home for those in rural settings.

FOODBORNE ILLNESS

CDC estimates that each year one in six Americans (or 48 million people) get sick, 128,000 are hospitalized, and 3000 die of foodborne diseases. The majority of foodborne illness outbreaks reported to the CDC result from bacteria, followed by viral outbreaks, chemical causes, and parasitic causes. Segments of the population are particularly susceptible to foodborne illnesses; vulnerable individuals are more likely to become ill and experience complications. Some of the nutritional complications associated with foodborne illness include reduced appetite and reduced nutrient absorption from the gut.

The 2000 edition of the DGA was the first to include food safety, important for linking the safety of the food and water supply with health promotion and disease prevention. This acknowledges the potential for foodborne illness to cause acute illness and long-term chronic complications. Since 2000 all revisions of the DGA have made food safety a priority. Persons at increased risk for foodborne illnesses include young children; pregnant women; older adults; persons who are immunocompromised because of human immunodeficiency virus or acquired immunodeficiency syndrome, steroid use, chemotherapy, diabetes mellitus, or cancer; alcoholics; persons with liver disease, decreased stomach acidity, autoimmune disorders, or malnutrition; persons who take antibiotics; and persons living in institutionalized settings. Costs associated with foodborne illness include those related to investigation of foodborne outbreaks and treatment of victims, employer costs related to lost productivity, and food industry losses related to lower sales and lower stock prices (American Dietetic Association, 2009). Table 9-2 describes common foodborne illnesses and their signs and symptoms, timing of onset, duration, causes, and prevention.

All food groups have ingredients associated with food safety concerns. There are concerns about microbial contamination of fruits and vegetables, especially those imported from other countries. An increased incidence of foodborne illness occurs with new methods of food production or distribution and with

Text continued on page 150

TABLE 9-1 U.S. Food Assistance and Nutrition Programs

Program Name	Goal/Purpose	Services Provided	Target Audience	Eligibility	Funding	Level of Prevention*
After-School Snack Program	Provides reimbursement for snacks served to students after school	Provides cash reimbursement to schools for snacks served to students. Snacks must contain two of four components: fluid milk, meat/meat alternate, vegetable or fruit or full-strength juice, whole-grain or enriched bread.	Children younger than 18 whose school sponsor a structured, supervised after-school enrichment program and provide lunch through the NSLP	School programs located within the boundaries of eligible low-income areas may be reimbursed for snacks served at no charge to students.	USDA	Primary, secondary
Child and Adult Care Food Program	Provides nutritious meals and snacks to infants, young children, and adults receiving day care services, as well as infants and children living in emergency shelters	Provides commodities or cash to help centers serve nutritious meals that meet federal guidelines	Infants, children, and adults receiving day care at childcare centers, family day care homes, and homeless shelters		USDA FNS	Primary, secondary
Commodity Supplemental Food Program	Provides no-cost monthly supplemental food packages composed of commodity foods to populations perceived to be at nutritional risk	Provides food packages; nutrition education services are available often through extension service programs; program referrals provided	Generally children ages 5-6, postpartum non-breastfeeding mothers from 6-12 months' postpartum, seniors	Between 130% and 185% of the poverty guideline	USDA FNS	Primary, secondary
Disaster Feeding Program	Makes commodities available for distribution to disaster relief agencies	Commodities are provided to disaster victims through congregate dining settings and direct distribution to households.	Those experiencing a natural disaster	Those experiencing a natural disaster	USDA FNS	Primary
TEFAP	Commodities are made available to local emergency food providers for preparing meals for the needy or for distribution of food packages.	Surplus commodity foods are provided for distribution.	Low-income households	Low-income households at 150% of the federal poverty income guideline	USDA FNS	Primary
EFSP	Funds are used to purchase food and shelter to supplement and extend local services.	EFSP provides funding for the purchase of food products, operation costs associated with mass feeding and shelter, limited rent or mortgage assistance, providing assistance for first month's rent, limited off-site emergency lodging, and limited utility assistance.	Those in need of emergency services	Primary	FEMA	Primary
Head Start	Provides agencies and schools with support and guidance for half- and full-day child development programs for low-income children	Programs receive reimbursement for nutritious meals and snacks and USDA-donated commodities, support for curriculum, social services, and health screenings.	Low-income children ages 3-5; parents are encouraged to volunteer and be involved	Same as NSLP	USDA (food) USDHHS (health)	Primary Secondary
National School Breakfast Program	Provides nutritionally balanced, low-cost or free breakfasts to children enrolled in participating schools	Participating schools receiving cash subsidies and USDA-donated commodities in return for offering breakfasts that meet same criteria as school lunch and offering free and reduced-price meals to eligible children	Children preschool age through grade 12 in schools; children and teens 20 years of age in residential childcare and juvenile correctional institutions	Same as NSLP	USDA FNS	Primary, secondary

Program	Description	Details	Target audience	Eligibility	Administering agency	Level of prevention
NSLP	Provides nutritionally balanced, low-cost or free lunches to children enrolled in participating schools	Participating schools receive cash subsidies and USDA-donated commodities in return for offering lunches that meet dietary guidelines and 1/3 of RDA for protein, iron, calcium, vitamins A and C, and calories and for offering free and reduced-price meals to eligible children	Children preschool age through grade 12 in schools; children and teenagers 20 years of age and younger in residential childcare and juvenile correctional institutions	185% of federal poverty income guideline for reduced-price lunches; 130% for free lunches	USDA FNS	Primary, secondary
Nutrition Program for the Elderly/Area Agencies on Aging	Provides commodity and cash assistance to programs providing meal services to older adults	Provides nutritious meals for older adults through congregate dining or home-delivered meals	Older adults	No income standard applied	USDHHS administers through state and local agencies; USDA cash and commodity assistance	Primary
Seniors' Farmers Market Nutrition Program	Provides fresh, nutritious, unprepared, locally grown fruits, vegetables, and herbs from farmers' markets, roadside stands, and community-supported agriculture programs to low-income seniors	Coupons for use at authorized farmers' markets, roadside stands, and community-supported agriculture programs (Foods that are not eligible for purchase with coupons by seniors are dried fruits or vegetables, potted plants and herbs, wild rice, nuts, honey, maple syrup, cider, and molasses.)	Low-income adults older than age 60	Low-income seniors with household incomes not exceeding 195% of the federal poverty income guideline	USDA FNS	Primary
SNAP	Provides benefits to low-income people that they can use to buy food to improve their diets	Provides assistance such as food stamps	Any age	For households in the 48 contiguous states and the District of Columbia. To get SNAP benefits, households must meet certain tests, including resource and income tests.	USDA FNS	Primary Secondary
Special Milk Program	Provides milk to children in participating schools who do not have access to other meal programs	Provides cash reimbursement for milk with vitamins A and D at RDA levels served at low or no cost to children; milk programs must be run on nonprofit basis	Same target audience as school lunch and school breakfast programs	Eligible children do *not* have access to other supplemental foods programs.	USDA FNS	Primary, secondary
Summer Food Service Program	Provides healthy meals (per federal guidelines) and snacks to eligible children when school is out, using agriculture commodity foods	Reimburses for up to two or three meals and snacks served daily free to eligible children when school is not in session; cash based on income level of local geographic area or of enrolled children	Infants and children 18 years of age and younger served at variety of feeding sites		USDA FNS	Primary, secondary
WIC	Provides supplemental foods to improve health status of participants	Nutrition education, free nutritious foods (protein, iron, calcium, vitamins A and C), referrals, breastfeeding promotion	Pregnant, breastfeeding and postpartum women up to 1 year; Infants, children up to 5 yrs.	185% of federal poverty income guideline nutritional risk	UDSA FNS, home state support	Primary, secondary, tertiary
WIC FMNP	Provides fresh, unprepared, locally grown fruits and vegetables to WIC recipients, and to expand the awareness, use of and sales at farmers' markets	FMNP food coupons for use at participating farmers' markets stands; nutrition education through arrangements with state agency	Same as WIC recipients	Same as WIC recipients	USDA FNS	Primary

EFSP, Emergency Food and Shelter Program; *FEMA,* Federal Emergency Management Agency; *FMNP,* Farmers Market Nutrition Program; *FNS,* Food and Nutrition Service; *NSLP,* National School Lunch Program; *RDA,* recommended daily allowance; *SNAP,* Special Nutrition Assistance Program; *USDA,* U.S. Department of Agriculture; *USDHHS,* U.S. Department of Health and Human Services; *WIC,* Special Supplemental Nutrition Program for Women, Infants, and Children.

*Level of prevention rationale: Programs that provide food only are regarded as primary; programs that provide food, nutrients at a mandated level of recommended dietary allowances, or an educational component are regarded as secondary; and programs that used health screening measures on enrollment were regarded as tertiary.

CLINICAL INSIGHT

The History of the Supplemental Nutrition Assistance Program (SNAP)

Erik R. Stegman, MA, JD

In the years after World War II, hunger and extreme malnutrition was a serious and pervasive problem in the United States. By the mid-1960s, one fifth of American households had poor diets. Among low-income households, this rate nearly doubled to 36% (United States Department of Agriculture [USDA], Agricultural Research Service [ARS], 1969). According to studies at the time, these rates of hunger, especially in low-income areas of the South, had a serious effect on the public at the time because of malnutrition and vitamin deficiency (Wheeler, 1967). Many Americans learned how serious the problem was in their living rooms when CBS News aired a landmark documentary, *Hunger in America, in* 1968 (Dole Institute of Politics, 2011). The documentary featured malnourished children with distended bellies and stories from everyday people about how hunger affected their lives—something that other Americans couldn't believe was happening in their backyard.

A public outcry resulted in the federal government's modern nutrition assistance system that began in the early 1960s as the Food Stamp program. Originally created as a small program during World War II to help bridge the gap between plentiful farm surpluses and urban hunger, it was discontinued in the 1950s because of the prosperous economy. President John F. Kennedy reintroduced it through an executive order in 1961 as a broader pilot program. As part of President Lyndon B. Johnson's War on Poverty initiative, Congress finally made it permanent. It has since been reauthorized and strengthened several times and is today known as the Supplemental Nutrition Assistance Program (SNAP) (USDA, Food and Nutrition Service [FNS], 2010). Another important supplemental food program is for Women, Infants and Children (WIC) and was developed in the 1970s to provide specialized nutrition assistance and support to low-income pregnant women, infants, and children up to age 5 (USDA, Economic Research Service [ERS], 2009).

In 2013 SNAP helped more than 47 million Americans afford a nutritionally adequate diet in a typical month. It also kept about 4.9 million people out of poverty in 2012, including 1.3 million children (Center on Budget and Policy Priorities, 2015). A recent study has shown that after these expansions in the 1960s and 1970s, disadvantaged children with access to nutrition assistance in early childhood and who had mothers that received assistance during pregnancy, had improved health and education outcomes, better growth curves, and fewer diagnoses of heart disease and obesity (Hoynes et al, 2012). Today, state agencies administering SNAP have the option of providing nutrition education to SNAP participants through federal grants and matching fund programs (USDA, 2015).

TABLE 9-2 Common Foodborne Illnesses

Illness	Signs and Symptoms	Onset and Duration	Causes and Prevention	Comments
Bacillus cereus	Watery diarrhea, abdominal cramping, vomiting	6-15 hours after consumption of contaminated food; duration 24 hours in most instances	Meats, milk, vegetables, and fish have been associated with the diarrheal type; vomiting-type outbreaks have generally been associated with rice products; potato, pasta, and cheese products; food mixtures such as sauces, puddings, soups, casseroles, pastries, and salads may also be a source.	*B. cereus* is a gram-positive, aerobic spore former.
Campylobacter jejuni	Diarrhea (often bloody), fever, and abdominal cramping	2-5 days after exposure; duration 2-10 days	Drinking raw milk or eating raw or undercooked meat, shellfish, or poultry; to prevent exposure, avoid raw milk and cook all meats and poultry thoroughly; it is safest to drink only pasteurized milk; the bacteria also may be found in tofu or raw vegetables. Hand-washing is important for prevention; wash hands with soap before handling raw foods of animal origin, after handling raw foods of animal origin, and before touching anything else; prevent cross-contamination in the kitchen; proper refrigeration and sanitation are also essential.	Top source of foodborne illness; some people develop antibodies to it, but others do not. In persons with compromised immune systems, it may spread to the bloodstream and cause sepsis; may lead to arthritis or to GBS; 40% of GBS in the United States is caused by campylobacteriosis and affects the nerves of the body, beginning several weeks after the diarrheal illness; can lead to paralysis that lasts several weeks and usually requires intensive care.
Clostridium botulinum	Muscle paralysis caused by the bacterial toxin: double or blurred vision, drooping eyelids, slurred speech, difficulty swallowing, dry mouth, and muscle weakness; infants with botulism appear lethargic, feed poorly, are constipated, and have a weak cry and poor muscle tone	In foodborne botulism symptoms generally begin 18-36 hours after eating contaminated food; can occur as early as 6 hours or as late as 10 days; duration days or months	Home-canned foods with low acid content such as asparagus, green beans, beets, and corn; outbreaks have occurred from more unusual sources such as chopped garlic in oil, hot peppers, tomatoes, improperly handled baked potatoes wrapped in aluminum foil, and home-canned or fermented fish. Persons who home-can should follow strict hygienic procedures to reduce contamination of foods; oils infused with garlic or herbs should be refrigerated; potatoes that have been baked while wrapped in aluminum foil should be kept hot until served or refrigerated; because high temperatures destroy the botulism toxin, persons who eat home-canned foods should boil the food for 10 minutes before eating.	If untreated, these symptoms may progress to cause paralysis of the arms, legs, trunk, and respiratory muscles; long-term ventilator support may be needed. Throw out bulging, leaking, or dented cans and jars that are leaking; safe home-canning instructions can be obtained from county extension services or from the U.S. Department of Agriculture; honey can contain spores of *C. botulinum* and has been a source of infection for infants; children younger than 12 months old should not be fed honey.

TABLE 9-2 Common Foodborne Illnesses—cont'd

Illness	Signs and Symptoms	Onset and Duration	Causes and Prevention	Comments
Clostridium perfringens	Nausea with vomiting, diarrhea, and signs of acute gastroenteritis lasting 1 day	Within 6-24 hours from the ingestion	Ingestion of canned meats or contaminated dried mixes, gravy, stews, refried beans, meat products, and unwashed vegetables. Cook foods thoroughly; leftovers must be reheated properly or discarded.	
Cryptosporidium parvum	Watery stools, diarrhea, nausea, vomiting, slight fever, and stomach cramps	2-10 days after being infected	Contaminated food from poor handling. Hand washing is important.	Protozoa causes diarrhea among immuno-compromised patients.
Enterotoxigenic *Escherichia coli* (ETEC)	Watery diarrhea, abdominal cramps, low-grade fever, nausea and malaise	With high infective dose, diarrhea can be induced within 24 hours	Contamination of water with human sewage may lead to contamination of foods; infected food handlers may also contaminate foods; dairy products such as semisoft cheeses may cause problems, but this is rare.	More common with travel to other countries; in infants or debilitated elderly persons, electrolyte replacement therapy may be necessary.
Escherichia coli O157:H7 Enterohemorrhagic *E. coli* (EHEC)	Hemorrhagic colitis (painful, bloody diarrhea)	Onset is slow, usually approximately 3-8 days after ingestion. Duration 5-10 days	Undercooked ground beef and meats, from unprocessed apple cider, or from unwashed fruits and vegetables; sometimes water sources; alfalfa sprouts, unpasteurized fruit juices, dry-cured salami, lettuce, spinach, game meat, and cheese curds. Cook meats thoroughly, use only pasteurized milk, and wash all produce well.	Antibiotics are not used because they spread the toxin further; the condition may progress to hemolytic anemia, thrombocytopenia, and acute renal failure, requiring dialysis and transfusions; HUS can be fatal, especially in young children; there are several outbreaks each year, particularly from catering operations, church events, and family picnics; *E. coli* O157:H7 can survive in refrigerated acid foods for weeks
Listeria monocytogenes (LM)	Mild fever, headache, vomiting, and severe illness in pregnancy; sepsis in the immunocompromised patient; meningoencephalitis in infants; and febrile gastroenteritis in adults	Onset 2-30 days. Duration variable	Processed, ready-to-eat products such as undercooked hot dogs, deli or lunchmeats, and unpasteurized dairy products; post pasteurization contamination of soft cheeses such as feta or Brie, milk, and commercial coleslaw; cross-contamination between food surfaces has also been a problem. Use pasteurized milk and cheeses; wash produce before use; reheat foods to proper temperatures; wash hands with hot, soapy water after handling these ready-to-eat foods; discard foods by their expiration dates.	May be fatal. Caution must be used by pregnant women, who may pass the infection on to their unborn child.
Norovirus	Gastroenteritis with nausea, vomiting, and/or diarrhea accompanied by abdominal cramps; headache, fever/chills, and muscle aches also may be present.	24-48 hours after ingestion of the virus, but can appear as early as 12 hours after exposure	Foods can be contaminated either by direct contact with contaminated hands or work surfaces that are contaminated with stool or vomit or by tiny droplets from nearby vomit that can travel through air to land on food; although the virus cannot multiply outside of human bodies, once on food or in water, it can cause illness; most cases occur on cruise ships.	Symptoms are usually brief and last only 1 or 2 days; however, during that brief period, people can feel very ill and vomit, often violently and without warning, many times a day; drink liquids to prevent dehydration.
Salmonella	Diarrhea, fever, and abdominal cramps	12-72 hours after infection. Duration usually 4-7 days	Ingestion of raw or undercooked meat, poultry, fish, eggs, unpasteurized dairy products; unwashed fruits and raw vegetables (melons and sprouts). Prevent by thorough cooking, proper sanitation, and hygiene.	There are many different kinds of *Salmonella* bacteria; *S. typhimurium* and *S. enteritidis* are the most common in the United States. Most people recover without treatment, but some have diarrhea that is so severe that the patient needs to be hospitalized; this patient must be treated promptly with antibiotics; the elderly, infants, and those with impaired immune systems are more likely to have a severe illness.
Shigellosis	Bloody diarrhea, fever, and stomach cramps	24-48 hours after exposure. Duration 4-7 days	Milk and dairy products; cold mixed salads such as egg, tuna, chicken, potato, and meat salads. Proper cooking, reheating, and maintenance of holding temperatures should aid in prevention; careful hand washing is essential.	This is caused by a group of bacteria called *Shigella*; it may be severe in young children and the elderly; severe infection with high fever may be associated with seizures in children younger than 2 years old.

Continued

TABLE 9-2   Common Foodborne Illnesses—cont'd

Illness	Signs and Symptoms	Onset and Duration	Causes and Prevention	Comments
Staphylococcus aureus	Nausea, vomiting, retching, abdominal cramping, and prostration	Within 1-6 hours; rarely fatal Duration 1-2 days	Meat, pork, eggs, poultry, tuna salad, prepared salads, gravy, stuffing, cream-filled pastries Cooking does not destroy the toxin; proper handling and hygiene are crucial for prevention.	Refrigerate foods promptly during preparation and after meal service.
Streptococcus pyogenes	Sore and red throat, pain on swallowing; tonsillitis, high fever, headache, nausea, vomiting, malaise, rhinorrhea; occasionally a rash occurs	Onset 1-3 days	Milk, ice cream, eggs, steamed lobster, ground ham, potato salad, egg salad, custard, rice pudding, and shrimp salad; in almost all cases, the foodstuffs were allowed to stand at room temperature for several hours between preparation and consumption.	Entrance into the food is the result of poor hygiene, ill food handlers, or the use of unpasteurized milk. Complications are rare; treated with antibiotics.
Vibrio vulnificus	Vomiting, diarrhea, or both; illness is mild	Gastroenteritis occurs about 16 hours after eating contaminated food. Duration about 48 hours	Seafood, especially raw clams and oysters, that has been contaminated with human pathogens; although oysters can only be harvested legally from waters free from fecal contamination, even these can be contaminated with *V. vulnificus* because the bacterium is naturally present.	This is a bacterium in the same family as those that cause cholera; it yields a Norovirus; it may be fatal in immunocompromised individuals.
Yersinia enterocolitica	Common symptoms in children are fever, abdominal pain, and diarrhea, which is often bloody; in older children and adults, right-sided abdominal pain and fever may be predominant symptom and may be confused with appendicitis.	1-2 days after exposure Duration 1-3 weeks or longer	Contaminated food, especially raw or undercooked pork products; postpasteurization contamination of chocolate milk, reconstituted dry milk, pasteurized milk, and tofu are also high-risk foods; cold storage does not kill the bacteria. Cook meats thoroughly; use only pasteurized milk; proper hand washing is also important.	Infectious disease caused by the bacterium *Yersinia*; in the United States most human illness is caused by *Y. enterocolitica*; it most often occurs in young children. In a small proportion of cases, complications such as skin rash, joint pains, or spread of bacteria to the bloodstream can occur.

Adapted with permission from Escott-Stump S: *Nutrition and diagnosis-related care,* ed 7, Baltimore, 2011, Lippincott Williams & Wilkins. Other sources: http://www.cdc.gov/health/diseases;, accessed December 26, 2013.
GBS, Guillian-Barré Syndrome; *HUS,* hemolytic uremic syndrome.

increased reliance on commercial food sources (AND, 2014). Improperly cooked meats can harbor organisms that trigger a foodborne illness. Even properly cooked meats have the potential to cause foodborne illness if the food handler allows raw meat juices to contaminate other foods during preparation. Sources of a foodborne illness outbreak vary, depending on such factors as the type of organism involved, the point of contamination, and the duration and temperature of food during holding.

Targeted food safety public education campaigns are important. However, the model for food safety has expanded beyond the individual consumer and now includes the government, the food industry, food growers, and the general public. Several government agencies provide information through websites with links to the CDC, the USDA Food Safety and Inspection Service (FSIS), the Environmental Protection Agency (EPA), the National Institute of Allergy and Infectious Diseases (NIAID), and the Food and Drug Administration (FDA). A leading industry program, ServSafe, provides food safety and training certification and was developed and administered by the National Restaurant Association. Because the U.S. food supply comes from a global market, food safety concerns are worldwide. The 2009 Country of Origin Labeling (COOL) legislation requires that retailers provide customers with the source of foods such as meats, fish, shellfish, fresh and frozen fruits and vegetables, and certain nuts and herbs (USDA, 2013). The USDA Agricultural Marketing Service has responsibility

for COOL implementation. Future practice must include awareness of global food safety issues (see *Focus On: Global Food Safety*).

Hazard Analysis Critical Control Points

An integral strategy to reduce foodborne illness is risk assessment and management. Risk assessment entails hazard identification, characterization, and exposure. Risk management covers risk evaluation, option assessment and implementation,

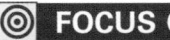 **FOCUS ON**

Global Food Safety

The United States imports produce, meat, and seafood from other countries to meet the consumer demands for foods that are not readily available in the country. Global importation creates potential danger to the public. Our current food supply is becoming much harder to trace to a single source. Because of this, safety concerns must be addressed globally, as well as in the United States. Leadership from food growers, producers, distributors, and those involved in food preparation is essential to ensure a safe food supply. Protecting the food supply chain requires several safety management systems such as hazard analysis, critical control points, good manufacturing practice, and good hygiene practice (Aruoma, 2006). Food safety also includes attention to issues such as the use of toxins and pesticides in countries where standards and enforcement may be variable, as well as the importance of clean water. Finally, the effect of global warming on food production is an increasing concern.

and monitoring and review of progress. One formal program, organized in 1996, is the Hazard Analysis Critical Control Points (HACCP), a systematic approach to the identification, evaluation, and control of food safety hazards. HACCP involves identifying any biologic, chemical, or physical agent that is likely to cause illness or injury in the absence of its control. It also involves identifying points at which control can be applied, thus preventing or eliminating the food safety hazard or reducing it to an acceptable level. Restaurants and health care facilities are obligated to use HACCP procedures in their food handling practices.

Those who serve populations at the greatest risk for foodborne illness have a special need to be involved in the network of food safety education and to communicate this information to their clients (Figure 9-2). Adoption of the HACCP regulations, food quality assurance programs, handling of fresh produce guidelines, technologic advances designed to reduce contamination, increased food supply regulations, and a greater emphasis on food safety education have contributed to a substantial decline in foodborne illness.

FOOD AND WATER SAFETY

Although individual educational efforts are effective in raising awareness of food safety issues, food and water safety must be examined on a national, systems-based level (AND, 2014). Several federal health initiatives include objectives relating to food and water safety, pesticide and allergen exposure, food-handling practices, reducing disease incidence associated with water, and reducing food- and water-related exposure to environmental pollutants. Related agencies can be found in Table 9-3.

Contamination

Controls and precautions in the area of limiting potential contaminants in the water supply are of continuing importance. Water contamination with arsenic, lead, copper, pesticides and herbicides, mercury, dioxin, polychlorinated biphenyls (PCBs), chlorine, and *Escherichia coli* continues to be highlighted by the media. It was estimated that many public water systems, built using early twentieth-century technology, will need to invest more than $138 billion during the next 20 years to ensure

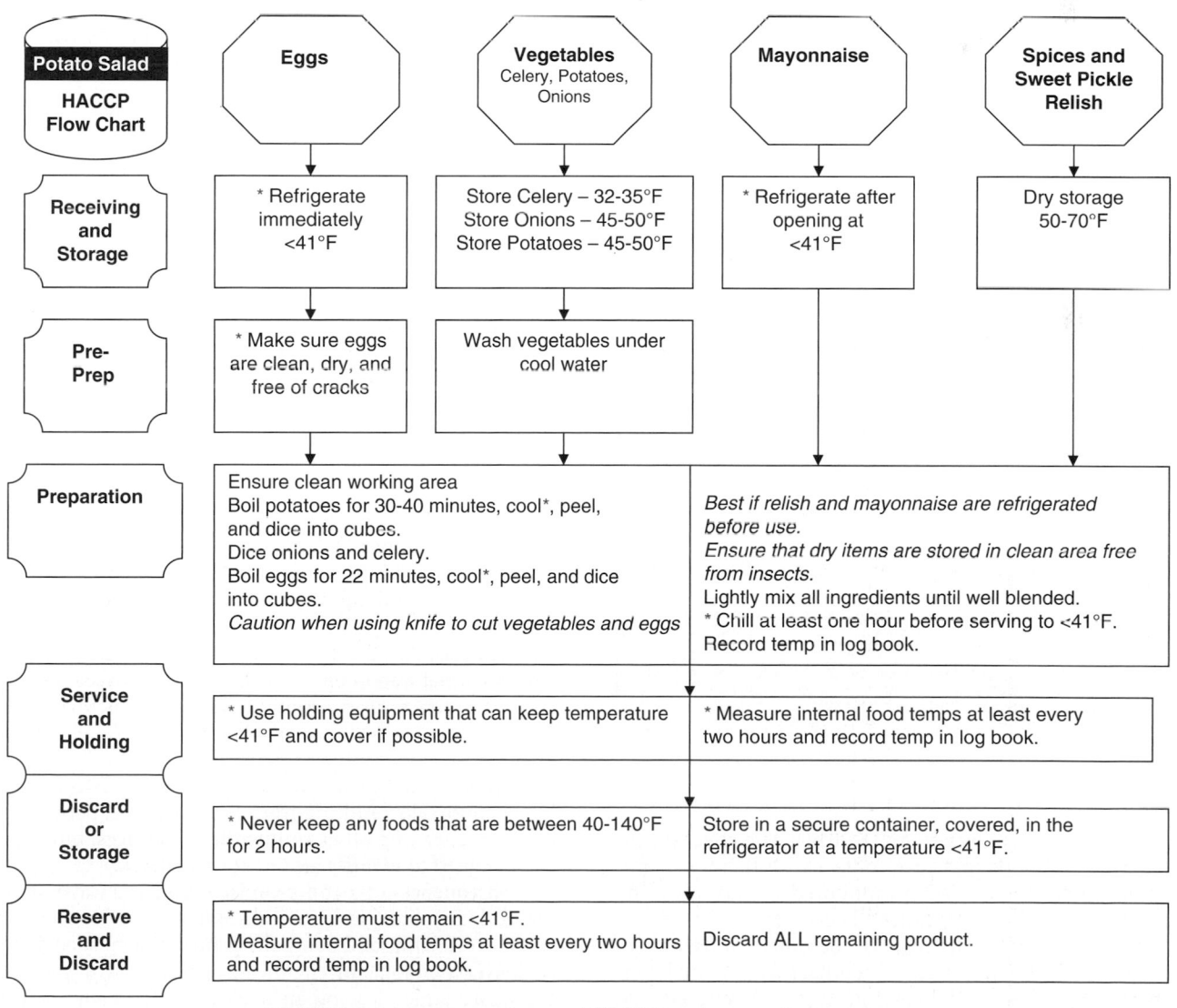

FIGURE 9-2 The Seven Steps of HACCP and a sample flow chart.

TABLE 9-3 Food and Water Safety Resources

Academy of Nutrition and Dietetics	http://www.eatright.org/
Agricultural Marketing Services, USDA	http://www.ams.usda.gov/AMSv1.0/
American Egg Board	http://www.aeb.org
The Academy of Nutrition and Dietetics Duplicate	http://www.eatright.org/
American Meat Institute	http://www.meatami.com
CFSAN	http://www.fda.gov/Food/
CFSCAN—Food and Water Safety—Recalls, Outbreaks & Emergencies	http://www.fda.gov/Food/RecallsOutbreaksEmergencies/default.htm
CDC	http://www.cdc.gov
CDC Disaster	http://www.bt.cdc.gov/disasters/
FEMA	http://www.fema.gov
Food Chemical News	http://www.foodchemicalnews.com
Food Marketing Institute	http://www.fmi.org
Food Marketing Institute—Food Safety	http://www.fmi.org/docs/facts-figures/foodsafety.pdf?sfvrsn=2
FoodNet	http://www.cdc.gov/foodnet/
Food Safety, Iowa State University	http://www.extension.iastate.edu/foodsafety/
Foundation for Food Irradiation Education	http://www.food-irradiation.com
Grocery Manufacturers of America	http://www.gmabrands.org
International Food Information Council	http://www.foodinsight.org/
Fruits and Veggies: More Matters	http://www.fruitsandveggiesmorematters.org/
National Broiler Council	http://www.eatchicken.com
National Cattleman's Beef Association	http://www.beef.org/
National Institutes of Health	http://www.nih.gov
National Food Safety Database	http://www.foodsafety.gov
National Restaurant Association Educational Foundation	http://www.nraef.org/
The Partnership for Food Safety Education	http://www.fightbac.org
Produce Marketing Association	http://www.pma.com
PulseNet	http://www.cdc.gov/pulsenet/
U.S. Department of Agriculture	http://www.usda.gov
U.S. Department of Agriculture Food Safety and Inspection Service	http://www.fsis.usda.gov
U.S. Department of Education	http://www.ed.gov
U.S. Department of Health and Human Services	http://www.hhs.gov/
U.S. EPA—Office of Ground and Drinking Water	http://www.epa.gov/safewater
U.S. EPA Seafood Safety	http://www.epa.gov/ost/fish
U.S. Food and Drug Administration	http://www.fda.gov
U.S. Poultry and Egg Association	http://www.uspoultry.org/

NOTE: Websites are updated frequently. Go to the home website and use a search to find the desired resources.

continued safe drinking water (AND, 2014). The effect on the potential safety of foods that have contact with these contaminants is an ongoing issue being monitored by advocacy and professional groups and governmental agencies.

Of interest to many is the issue of the potential hazards of ingestion of seafood that has been in contact with methyl mercury present naturally in the environment and released into the air from industrial pollution. Mercury has accumulated in bodies of water (i.e., streams, rivers, lakes, and oceans) and in the flesh of seafood in these waters (USDA and EPA, 2013). The body of knowledge on issues such as this is being updated constantly, and current recommendations are to restrict the consumption of certain fish such as shark, mackerel, tilefish, tuna, and swordfish by pregnant women (FDA 2013 and Centers for Food Safety and Applied Nutrition 2013). (See Chapter 15 for further discussion.) Other contaminants in fish, such as PCBs, and dioxin are also of concern (California Office of Environmental Health Hazard Assessment [OEHHA], 2014).

Precautions are in place at the federal, state, and local levels that must be addressed by dietetics professionals whose roles include advocacy, communication, and education. Members of the public and local health officials must understand the risks and the importance of carrying out measures for food and water safety and protection. The EPA and the Center for Food Safety and Applied Nutrition (CFSAN) provide ongoing monitoring and guidance. In addition, food and water safety and foodborne illness issues are monitored by state and local health departments.

Organic Foods and Pesticide Use

The use of pesticides and contaminants from the water supply affect produce quality. The debate continues about whether organic foods are worth the extra cost. However, the beneficial effects of organic farming also must be considered (see *Focus On: Is It Really Organic, and Is It Healthier?*).

Genetic Modification/Genetic Engineering

An emerging safety issue is that of genetically modified organisms (GMOs). A GMO is a plant or animal in which the genetic material has been altered in a way that does not occur naturally. The process of making GMOs is called *genetic engineering*. More than 20 countries have banned the use of GMO crops, but it remains controversial in the United States. Currently labeling of GMO/GE foods is voluntary, but there has been considerable public outcry to require it be labeled. FDA is studying the issue (see *Focus On:* GMO or Genetically Engineered (GE) Foods in Chapter 26).

Bioterrorism and Food-Water Safety

Bioterrorism is the deliberate use of microorganisms or toxins from living organisms to induce death or disease. Threats to the nation's food and water supplies have made food biosecurity, or precautions to minimize risk, an issue when addressing preparedness planning. The CDC has identified seven foodborne pathogens as having the potential to be used by bioterrorists to attack the food supply: tularemia, brucellosis, *Clostridium botulinum* toxin, epsilon toxin of *Clostridium perfringens, Salmonella, Escherichia coli,* and *Shigella*. These pathogens, along with potential water contaminants, such as mycobacteria, *Legionella, Giardia,* viruses, arsenic, lead, copper, methyl butyl ether, uranium, and radon, are the targets of federal systems put in place to monitor the safety of the food and water supply. Current surveillance systems are designed to detect foodborne illness outbreaks resulting from food spoilage, poor food handling practices, or other unintentional sources, but they were not designed to identify an intentional attack.

Consequences of a compromised food and water supply are physical, psychologic, political, and economic. Compromise could occur with food being the primary agent such as a vector to deliver a biologic or chemical weapon or with food being a secondary target, leaving an inadequate food supply to feed a region or the nation. Intentional use of a foodborne pathogen

◎ FOCUS ON

Is It Really Organic, and Is It Healthier?

Christine McCullum-Gomez, PhD, RD

There are a variety of reasons why organic foods can be considered to facilitate the creation of a healthful, sustainable food system (Scialabba, 2013; McCullum-Gómez and Scott, 2009). First, some organic fruits, vegetables, and juices may contain more antioxidants and polyphenols compared with their conventionally grown counterparts (Baranski et al, 2014), although there is an ongoing debate regarding the potential nutritional advantages of consuming organic versus conventional fruits and vegetables and other plant products (Baranski et al, 2014; Smith-Spangler et al, 2012). Second, organically raised meat may reduce the development of human antibiotic resistance and lessen air and water pollution (American Medical Association, 2009). Researchers have found a lower prevalence of antibiotic-resistant *Salmonella* spp. (Sapkota et al, 2014) and antibiotic-resistant *Enterococci* (Sapkota et al, 2011) on U.S. conventional poultry farms that transitioned to organic practices. Third, a published meta-analysis (Palupi et al, 2012) found that organic dairy products contained significantly higher protein, total omega-3 fatty acids, and conjugated linoleic acid than those of conventional types. Another study reported that individual omega-3 fatty acid concentrations and the concentration of conjugated linoleic acid were higher in organic milk (Benbrook et al, 2013). In an ongoing cohort study, consumption of organic dairy products was associated with a lower risk of eczema during the first 2 years of life. These authors hypothesize that "a high intake of omega-3 fatty acids and/or conjugated linoleic acids from organic dairy products by the child is protective against eczema (independent of atopy) and that…the mother's intake of these fatty acids during pregnancy and lactation contributes to this protection" (Kummeling et al, 2008).

Fortunately, the presence of organic foods is increasing in the marketplace. Organic sales account for more than 4% of total U.S. food sales, although organic products account for a much larger share in some food product categories. Certified organic acreage and livestock have been expanding in the United States, particularly for fruits, vegetables, dairy, and poultry (Greene, 2014). These foods are produced following practices described in the USDA National Organic Program (NOP), a marketing program with a certification process throughout the production and manufacturing chain, which describes the practices that are required for labeling a product "organic" (USDA, 2011). Organic foods that are certified through the USDA NOP also must meet the same state and federal food safety requirements as nonorganic foods (Riddle and Markhart, 2010).

In organic farming, raw animal manure must be composted (§205.203), "unless it is: i) applied to land used for a crop not intended for human consumption; ii) incorporated into the soil not less than 120 days prior to the harvest of a product whose edible portion has direct contact with the soil surface or soil particles; or iii) incorporated into the soil not less than 90 days prior to the harvest of a product whose edible portion does not have direct contact with the soil surface or soil particles" (Electronic Code of Federal Regulations, 2014).

Organic agriculture offers numerous opportunities to reduce exposure to agricultural pesticides through the community food and water supply, which may be detrimental to human health, particularly for high-risk groups, including pregnant women, infants, young children, and farmers (American College of Obstetricians and Gynecologists Committee, 2013; Costa et al, 2014). Studies with children reveal that there are dramatic reductions in organophosphate (OP) pesticide exposure with the consumption of organic food (Lu et al, 2008). Research with adults found that the consumption of an organic diet for 1 week significantly reduced OP pesticide exposure. These authors recommend consumption of organic food as a precautionary approach to reducing pesticide exposure (Oates et al, 2014).

Organically grown foods also can cultivate a more sustainable food system by reducing energy requirements for production, reducing soil erosion, rehabilitating poor soils, and sequestering carbon in soil, which may reduce carbon levels in the atmosphere (Gattinger et al, 2012; Scialabba, 2013). In addition, biodiversity is enhanced in organic agricultural systems (Tuck et al, 2014), which makes these farms more resilient to unpredictable weather patterns and pest outbreaks, as is predicted with climate change. Public investment in organic agriculture facilitates wider access to organic food for consumers, helps farmers capture high-value markets, and conserves natural resources, including soil and water.

---

as the primary agent may be mistaken as a routine outbreak of foodborne illness. Distinguishing normal illness fluctuation from an intentional attack depends on having in place a system for preparedness planning, rapid communication, and central analysis.

Experience with the series of hurricanes in 2005 emphasizes the need to provide access to a safe food and water supply after emergencies and disasters. Access to food and water may be limited, which results in social disruption and self-imposed quarantine. These situations require a response different from the traditional approach to disaster relief, during which it is assumed that hungry people will seek assistance and have confidence in the safety of the food that is offered (FDA, 2014). In the event of a disaster, dietetics professionals can play a key role by being aware of their environment, knowing available community and state food and nutrition resources, and participating in coordination and delivery of relief to victims of the disaster.

DISASTER PLANNING

Dietetics and health professionals working in food service are expected to plan for the distribution of safe food and water in any emergency situation. This may include choosing food preparation and distribution sites, establishing temporary kitchens, preparing foods with limited resources, and keeping prepared food safe to eat through HACCP procedures. The Academy of Nutrition and Dietetics (AND) published two papers: *Emergency Preparedness: Infant Feeding During Disasters* and *Special Needs and Vulnerable Groups* (http://www.eatright.org/search.aspx?search=disaster%20planning).

Planning, surveillance, detection, response, and recovery are the key components of public health disaster preparedness. The key agencies are the USDA, the Department of Homeland Security (DHS), the Federal Emergency Management Agency (FEMA), the CDC, and the FDA. In conjunction with DHS, USDA operates Protection of the Food Supply and Agricultural Production (PFSAP). PFSAP handles issues related to food production, processing, storage, and distribution. It addresses threats against the agricultural sector and border surveillance. PFSAP conducts food safety activities concerning meat, poultry, and egg inspection and provides laboratory support, research, and education on outbreaks of foodborne illness.

Ready.gov (www.ready.gov) is an education tool informing the public on how to prepare for a national emergency, including possible terrorist attacks. In addition, the USDA Food Safety and Inspection Service (FSIS) operates the Food Threat Preparedness Network (PrepNet) and the Food Biosecurity Action Team (F-Bat). PrepNet ensures effective coordination of food security efforts, focusing on preventive activities to protect the food supply. F-Bat assesses potential vulnerabilities along the farm-to-table continuum, provides guidelines to industry on food security and increased plant security, strengthens FSIS's coordination and cooperation with law enforcement agencies, and enhances security features of FSIS laboratories (Bruemmer, 2003).

CDC has three operations relating to food security and disaster planning: PulseNet, FoodNet, and the Centers for Public Health Preparedness. PulseNet is a national network of public health laboratories that performs deoxyribonucleic acid fingerprinting on foodborne bacteria, assists in detecting foodborne illness outbreaks and tracing them back to their source, and provides linkages among sporadic cases. FoodNet is the Foodborne Diseases Active Surveillance Network, which functions as the principle foodborne disease component of the CDC's Emerging Infections Program, providing active laboratory-based surveillance. The Centers for Public Health Preparedness fund academic centers linking schools of public health with state, local, and regional bioterrorism preparedness and public health infrastructure needs.

CFSAN in the FDA is concerned with regulatory issues such as seafood HACCP, safety of food and color additives, safety of foods developed through biotechnology, food labeling, dietary supplements, food industry compliance, and regulatory programs to address health risks associated with foodborne chemical and biologic contaminants. CFSAN also runs cooperative programs with state and local governments.

The FEMA, under the DHS, provides emergency support functions after a disaster or emergency. FEMA identifies food and water needs, arranges delivery, and provides assistance with temporary housing and other emergency services. Agencies that assist FEMA include the USDA, the Department of Defense, the USDHHS, the EPA, and the General Services Administration. Major players include nonprofit volunteer agencies such as the American Red Cross, the Salvation Army, and community-based agencies and organizations. Disaster management is evolving as it is tested by manufactured and natural disasters.

HEALTHY FOOD AND WATER SYSTEMS AND SUSTAINABILITY

This chapter began with a note that community nutrition is a constantly evolving and growing area of practice with the broad focus of serving the population at large with a thrust to be proactive and responsive to the needs of the community. Today's community and the community needs differ, but regardless of environmental, social, and geographic variations, a goal of all nutrition and dietetics professionals is to promote and sustain access to a safe, affordable, and health-promoting food sources.

In 2014 The Academy of Nutrition and Dietetics issued Standards of Professional Performance that addressed building and supporting sustainable, resilient, and healthy food and water systems (AND, 2014). These standards are meant to provide guidance to every RDN beyond the usual safety standards. This paper identifies sustainability as the ability to maintain the system for the long term. Resilience means a system can withstand interruptions that occur. From a community nutrition aspect, a practical example of resilience is that standards are in place for access to health-supporting and safe food and water even after a flood, natural disaster, or funding interruption. The sustainability is rooted in how the system is built, guided, and nourished. Public and private programs and resources are critical components and must meet the tests of resiliency to be sustainable to meet funding requirements.

The safety, adequacy, and quality of the food and water supply along with energy sources are components that build sustainability and resiliency. The nutrition and dietetics professional can be a major player but must have the expertise and competency as well as the initiative to build as well as promote standards and conditions in which people can reach the goal of being healthy. Additional resources are available at http://www.andjrnl.org/content/sop#2012 http://www.hendpg.org/page/professional-development.

SUMMARY: A WORK IN PROGRESS

This chapter is indeed a work in progress, a snapshot of the evolving world of community nutrition. Changes are inherent in food, health, food access and safety, and our global environment. The Dietetics Professional is an important player but needs to be current and engaged. Box 9-7 notes some useful websites, many with access to regular updates on problems, issues and solutions.

USEFUL WEBSITES

The Academy of Nutrition and Dietetics
http://www.eatright.org/
American Heart Association
http://www.americanheart.org
Centers for Disease Control
http://www.cdc.gov/
Centers for Science in the Public Interest (CSPI)
http://www.cspinet.org/
ChangeLabSolutions
http://www.linkedin.com/company/changelab-solutions
Dietary Guidance and Dietary Guidelines for Americans
http://www.health.gov/dietaryguidelines/
http://www.cnpp.usda.gov/
Environmental Protection Agency (Fish)
http://www.epa.gov/ost/fish
Federal Emergency Management Agency
http://www.fema.gov/
Feeding America
http://feedingamerica.org/
Homeland Security
http://www.dhs.gov/dhspublic
Food Safety
http://www.foodsafety.gov/
http://www.billmarler.com
Hazard Analysis Critical Control Points
http://www.fda.gov/food/guidanceregulation/haccp/ucm2006801.htm
Fruits and Vegetables: More Matters
http://www.fruitsandveggiesmorematters.org/
Head Start
http://www.acf.hhs.gov/programs/ohs
Healthy People 2010 and 2020
http://www.healthypeople.gov/
MyPlate
http://www.chooseMyPlate.gov
National Academy Press—Dietary Reference Intakes
http://www.nap.edu/topics.php?topic=380
National Center for Health Statistics
http://www.cdc.gov/nchs/

National Health and Nutrition Examination Study
http://www.cdc.gov/nchs/nhanes.htm
Robert Wood Johnson Foundation
http://www.rwjf.org/
Yale Rudd Center for Food Policy & Obesity
www.yaleruddcenter.org
U.S. Department of Agriculture Farm to School Initiative
http://www.fns.usda.gov/cnd/F2S/Default.htm
U.S. Department of Agriculture Nutrition Assistance Programs
http://www.fns.usda.gov/fns/

REFERENCES

Academy of Nutrition and Dietetics (AND), Cody MM, Stretch T: Position of the Academy of Nutrition and Dietetics: food and water safety, *J Acad Nutr Diet* 114:1819, 2014.

Adelson SF, Peterkin, B: *Dietary levels of households in the United States spring 1965*, Washington, DC, 1969, US Agricultural Research Service.

American College of Obstetricians and Gynecologists (ACOG), Committee on Health Care for Underserved Women, American Society for Reproductive Medicine Practice Committee, et al: Exposure to toxic environmental agents, *Fertil Steril* 100:931, 2013.

American Medical Association: *Report of the Council on Science and Public Health. (CSAPH). Sustainable Food, Resolution 405: A-08.2008*. http://www.ama-assn.org/ama1/pub/upload/mm/443/csaph-rep8-a09.pdf. CSAPH Report 8-A-09. Accessed 19 December 2013.

Aruoma OI: The impact of food regulation on the food supply chain, *Toxicology* 221:119, 2006.

Baranski M, Srednicka-Tober D, Volakakis N, et al: Higher antioxidant concentrations, and less cadmium and pesticide residues in organically grown crops: a systematic literature review and meta-analyses, *Br J Nutr* 112:794, 2014.

Benbrook CM, Butler G, Latif MA, et al: Organic production enhances milk nutritional quality by shifting fatty composition: a United States-wide, 18-month study, *PLoS ONE* 8:e82429, 2013, doi:10.1371/journal.pone.0082429.

Bruemmer B: Food biosecurity, *J Am Diet Assoc* 103:687, 2003.

California Office of Environmental Health Hazard Assessment (OEHHA): *Chemicals in fish*. http://oehha.ca.gov/fish/chems/. Accessed November 6, 2014.

Center on Budget and Policy Priorities: *Introduction to the Supplemental Nutrition Assistance Program (SNAP)*. http://www.cbpp.org/cms/index.cfm?fa=view&id=2226. Accessed January 18, 2015.

Centers for Disease Control: *National Health and Examination Survey 1999–2014*. http://www.cdc.gov/nchs/data/nhanes/survey_content_99_14.pdf. Accessed January 2014.

Center for Food Safety and Applied Nutrition (CFSAN), U.S. Department of Health and Human Services, Food and Drug Administration: *Food*. http://www.fda.gov/food/default.htm. Accessed 19 December 2013.

The Community Guide: *What is the community guide*. http://www.thecommunityguide.org/. Accessed November 3, 2014.

Clark MA, Fox MK: Nutritional quality of the diets of US public school children and the role of the school meal programs, *J Am Diet Assoc* 109 (Suppl 2):S44, 2009.

Condon EM, Crepinsek MK, Fox MK: School meals: types of foods offered to and consumed by children at lunch and breakfast, *J Am Diet Assoc* 109(Suppl 2):S67, 2009.

Costa C, García-Lestón J, Costa S, et al: Is organic farming safer to farmers' health? A comparison between organic and traditional farming, *Toxicol Lett* 230:166, 2014. http://dx.doi.org/10.1016/j.toxlet.2014.02.011.

Dietary Guidelines For Americans 2015: http://health.gov/dietaryguidelines/2015-scientific-report/. Accessed June 16, 2015.

Dole Institute of Politics: *History of food stamp program* (video file). https://www.youtube.com/watch?v=-0_OWueb_8Y&feature=youtu.be&t=3m6s/. Accessed January 18, 2015.

Edelstein S: Reaching out to those at highest nutritional risk. In *Nutrition in public health*, ed 2, Sudbury, Mass, 2010, Jones and Bartlett, 122.

Electronic Code of Federal Regulations (e-CFR): *Title 7: Agriculture. Part 205—National Organic Program*. http://www.ecfr.gov/cgi-bin/retrieveECFR?gp=1&SID=2583b0f2fc78f95e7763297d55d36441&ty=HTML&h=L&n=7y3.1.1.9.32&r=PART. Accessed May 13, 2014.

Food and Drug Administration (FDA): *Building a stronger defense against bioterrorism*. http://www.fda.gov/ForConsumers/ConsumerUpdates/ucm048251.htm. Accessed November 11, 2014.

Food and Drug Administration (FDA), Environmental Protection Agency (EPA): *Mercury and fish*. http://www.epa.gov/ost/fish. Accessed December 26, 2013.

Frieden TR: A framework for public health action: the health impact pyramid, *Am J Public Health* 100:590, 2010.

Fruits and Veggies More Matters: *About fruits and veggies more matters*. http://www.fruitsandveggiesmorematters.org/. Accessed December 26, 2014.

Gattinger A, Muller A, Haeni M, et al: Enhanced top soil carbon stocks under organic farming, *Proc Natl Acad Sci* 109:18226, 2012.

Greene C: *Overview – Organic agriculture*. http://www.ers.usda.gov/topics/natural-resources-environment/organic-agriculture.aspx. Washington DC, April 7, 2014, United States Department of Agriculture, Economic Research Service. Accessed May 12, 2014.

Healthy People 2010: *National health promotion and disease prevention objectives*, Washington, DC, 2000, U.S. Department of Health and Human Services.

Healthy People 2020: *Leading Health Indicators*. http://www.healthypeople.gov/2020/topicsobjectives2020/overview.aspx?topicid=29.

Healthy People 2020: *National health promotion and disease prevention objectives*. http://www.healthypeople.gov/2020/default.aspx. Washington, DC, 2010, U.S. Department of Health and Human Services. Accessed December 2013.

Hoynes H, Schanzenbach DW, Almond D: *Long run impacts of childhood access to safety net [White paper]*. http://www.nber.org/papers/w18535. Accessed January 18, 2015.

Kummeling I, Thijs C, Huber M, et al: Consumption of organic food and risk of atopic disease during the first 2 years of life in the Netherlands, *Br J Nutr* 99:598, 2008.

Lu C, Barr DB, Pearson MA, et al: Dietary intake and its contribution to longitudinal pesticide exposure in urban/suburban children, *Environ Health Perspect* 116:537, 2008.

Mayerhauser CM: Survival of enterhemorrhagic Escherichia coli 0157: H7 in retail mustard, *J Food Prot* 64:783, 2001.

McCullum-G001. C, Scott AM: *Hot topic: perspective on the benefit of organic foods* (website). http://www.hendpg.org/docs/Resources%20-%20public/Hot-Topic-Perspective-Benefits-Organic-Foods-2009.pdf. Accessed May 8, 2014.

Mendoza JA, Watson K, Cullen KW: Change in dietary energy density after implementation of the Texas Public School Nutrition Policy, *J Am Diet Assoc* 110:434, 2010.

Oates L, Cohen M, Braun L, et al: Reduction in urinary organophosphate pesticide metabolites in adults after a week-long organic diet, *Environ Res* 132:105, 2014.

Palupi E, Jayanegara A, Ploeger A, et al: Comparison of nutritional quality between conventional and organic dairy products: a meta-analysis, *J Sci Food Agric* 92:2774, 2012.

Produce for Better Health Foundation Brand: *Guidelines*. http://www.pbhfoundation.org/pdfs/licensing/gra/fvmm/2012_Brand_Guidelines.pdf. Accessed June 16, 2015.

Riddle J, Markhart B, University of Minnesota, et al: *What is organic food and why should I care?*. http://swroc.cfans.umn.edu/prod/groups/cfans/

Rose D, Bodor JN, Hutchinson PL, et al: The importance of a multi-dimensional approach for studying the links between food access and consumption, *J Nutr* 140:1170, 2010.

Sapkota A, Kinney EL, George A, et al: Lower prevalence of antibiotic-resistant Salmonella on large-scale U.S. conventional poultry farms that transitioned to organic practices, *Sci Total Environ* 476:387, 2014.

Sapkota A, Hulet RM, Zhang G, et al: Lower prevalence of antibiotic-resistant Enterococci on U.S. conventional poultry farms that transitioned to organic practices, *Environ Health Perspect* 119:1622, 2011.

Scialabba N: Organic agriculture's contribution to sustainability, *Crop Management* 12:2013, doi:10.1094/CM-2013-0429-09-PS.

Smith-Spangler C, Brandeau ML, Hunter GE, et al: Are organic foods safer or healthier than conventional alternatives?: a systematic review, *Ann Intern Med* 157:348, 2012.

Tuck S, Winqvist C, Mota F, et al: Land-use intensity and the effects of organic farming on biodiversity: a hierarchical meta-analysis, *J Appl Ecol* 51: 746, 2014, doi: 10.1111/1365-2664.12219.

United States Department of Agriculture: *Emergency preparedness and response*. http://www.usda.gov/wps/portal/usda/usdahome?contentidonly= true&contentid=Emergency_Preparedness_and_Response.html. Accessed November 11, 2014.

United States Department of Agriculture (USDA): *State SNAP-Ed contacts*. http://snap.nal.usda.gov/state-contacts. Accessed January 18, 2015.

U.S. Department of Agriculture (USDA), Agricultural Marketing Service: *Country of origin labeling*. http://www.ams.usda.gov/AMSv1.0/cool. Accessed December 26, 2013.

U.S. Department of Agriculture (USDA), Agricultural Marketing Service: *Food deserts*. http://apps.ams.usda.gov/fooddeserts/foodDeserts.aspx. Accessed January 2014.

U.S. Department of Agriculture, Agricultural Marketing Service, National Organic Program (NOP): *Organic production and handling standards*. http://www.ams.usda.gov/AMSv1.0/getfile?dDocName=STELDEV300444 5&acct=nopgeninfo. Accessed May 12, 2014.

U.S. Department of Agriculture (USDA), Agricultural Research Service (ARS): *Dietary levels of households in the United States, Spring 1965*, 1969. http://www.ars.usda.gov/SP2UserFiles/Place/80400530/pdf/6566/hfcs6566_rep_6.pdf. Accessed January 18, 2015.

U.S. Department of Agriculture (USDA), Agricultural Research Service (ARS): *What we eat in America (WWEIA), NHANES*. http://www.ars.usda.gov/Services/docs.htm?docid=13793. Accessed December 26, 2014.

U.S. Department of Agriculture (USDA), Economic Research Service (ERS): *The WIC program: background, trends, and economic issues* (website). http://www.ers.usda.gov/media/159295/err73.pdf. Accessed January 18, 2015.

U.S. Department of Agriculture (USDA), Food and Nutrition Service (FNS): *From food stamps to the supplemental nutrition assistance program: legislative timeline*. http://www.fns.usda.gov/sites/default/files/timeline.pdf. Accessed January 18, 2015.

U.S. Department of Health and Human Services (USDHHA): *Dietary guidelines*. 2015. http://www.health.gov/dietaryguidelines/. Accessed June 16, 2015.

Wheeler R: Hungry children: special report, *The Journal of the Southern Regional Council* 6:15, 1967.

Wilkinson RG, Marmot MG, editors: *Social determinants of health: the solid facts*, ed 2, Denmark, 2011, World Health Organization.

Winslow CEA: The untilled field of public health, *Mod Med* 2:183, 1920.

World Health Organization (WHO): *Closing the gap: policy to practice on social determinants of health*, 2011.

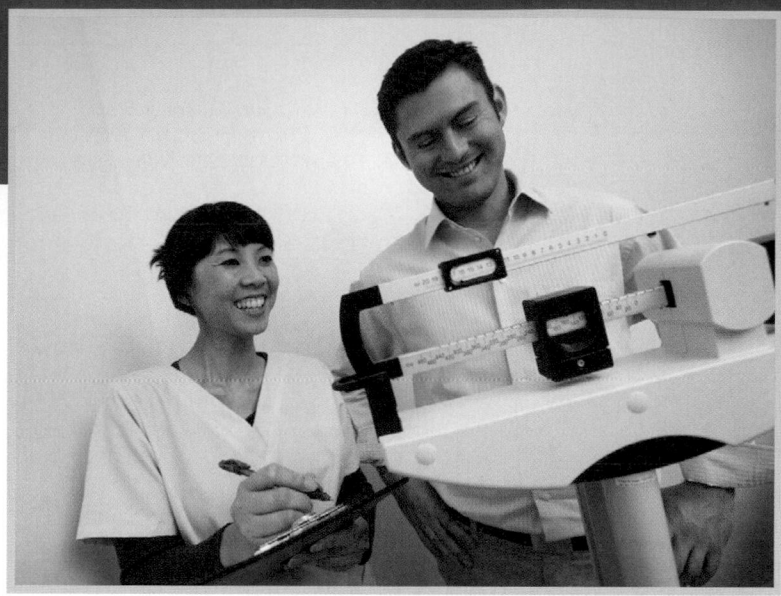

PART II

Nutrition Diagnosis and Intervention

The type of nutrition care provided for an individual varies depending on the findings of the assessment process. The environment, surgery or trauma, food allergies, inadequate access to safe or sufficient food, stage of growth and development, harmful beliefs, lack of knowledge, and socioeconomic issues can all affect whether the individual has an adequate diet. In the healthy individual, omission of a specific food group or intake of high-energy, nutrient-poor foods does not lead to failed nutritional status overnight. It is the prolonged imbalanced intake that leads to chronic disease. Dramatic and acute insufficiency combined with acute disease also leads to undesirable nutritional consequences. Indeed, inadequacy of the types or amounts of macro- or micronutrients, fluid, or even physical activity may cause a decline in health status or immunity and dysfunction and disease.

The establishment of nutrition diagnoses helps to define and promote effective care according to specific nutrition problems. Such problems may be found in an individual, a group (such as persons who have diabetes or celiac disease), or even a community (such as sites where local produce is grown in mineral-depleted soil.)

Step two of the nutrition care process involves an analysis of the factors affecting adequacy of the current nutritional intake and overall nutritional status. In most cases, institutions use standards of care or national practice guidelines that describe recommended actions in the nutrition care process. These standards serve as the basis for assessing the quality of care provided.

Step three of the nutrition care process requires planning and goal-setting, followed by the selection of interventions that deal with the cause of the problem. For example, nutrition education is an appropriate intervention for the person who has little knowledge of how to manage his or her gluten-free diet. And, this requires a counseling approach, keeping the person's level of readiness to change in mind. It may be helpful to refer the individual to available cookbooks, health services, and support groups. Manipulation of dietary components, provision of enteral or parenteral nutrition, or in-depth nutrition counseling may also be needed. Coordination of care between hospital and home and community is important for life long management of nutrition and chronic disease.

The final step of the nutrition care process is specific to the individual patient or client, and is related to the signs and symptoms identified in the assessment. A separate chapter is not written here because this fourth step (monitoring and evaluation) would be developed according to the nutrition diagnoses, assessment factors, and outcomes for the individual being served.

10

Overview of Nutrition Diagnosis and Intervention

Pamela Charney, PhD, RD, CHTS-CP,
Alison Steiber, PhD, RDN

Nutrition care is an organized group of activities allowing identification of nutritional needs and provision of care to meet these needs. Nutrition care can occur in a variety of settings and populations, involving members of the multidisciplinary team, as appropriate. For example, nutrition care occurs in schools with children and in collaboration with a school nurse and the education staff as well as in public health departments with low socioeconomic populations and in collaboration with public health officials. Conversely, nutrition care also occurs in clinical settings (e.g., skilled nursing facilities, dialysis clinics, and hospital settings) in populations who are acutely or chronically ill and in collaboration with the medical team (e.g., nurses, physicians, pharmacists, physical therapists). Comprehensive care may involve different health care providers (e.g., the physician, registered dietitian nutritionist [RDN], nurse, pharmacist, physical or occupational therapist, social worker, speech therapist, and case manager) who are integral in achieving desired outcomes, regardless of the care setting. The patient or client and family are core members of the team and must be included in all major decisions throughout the care process.

A collaborative approach helps to ensure that care is coordinated and that team members and the patient are aware of all goals and priorities. Team conferences, formal or informal, are useful in all settings: a clinic, a hospital, the home, the community,

a long-term care facility, or any other site where nutrition problems may be identified. Coordinating the activities of health care professionals also requires documentation of the process and regular discussions to offer complete nutritional care. Standardization of the care process (the Nutrition Care Process, NCP) improves consistency and quality of care as well as enables collection and assessment of nutrition related outcome measures.

THE NUTRITION CARE PROCESS

The Nutrition Care Process (NCP) is a standardized process for the provision of nutrition care established by the Academy of Nutrition and Dietetics (AND, known as the Academy, formerly the American Dietetic Association [ADA]). Per the Academy the NCP is a process for identifying, planning for, and meeting nutritional needs. The nutritional needs referred to in this definition may be of an individual, specific group, or population. Furthermore, the NCP gives the profession a framework for critical thinking and decision making, which may assist in defining the roles and responsibilities of registered dietitian nutritionists (RDN) and registered nutrition and dietetic technicians (NDTR) in all practice settings (AND, 2014).

The patient or client is the central focus of the NCP (Figure 10-1). The NCP includes four steps that are the responsibility of the RD: (1) nutrition assessment, (2) nutrition diagnosis, (3) nutrition intervention, and (4) monitoring and evaluation (AND, 2010a). Nutrition screening and outcomes management are also vital to safe, high-quality nutrition care; however, they are not included as

---

Sections of this chapter were written by Sylvia Escott-Stump, MA,RDN, LDN for previous editions of this text.

THE NUTRITION CARE PROCESS MODEL

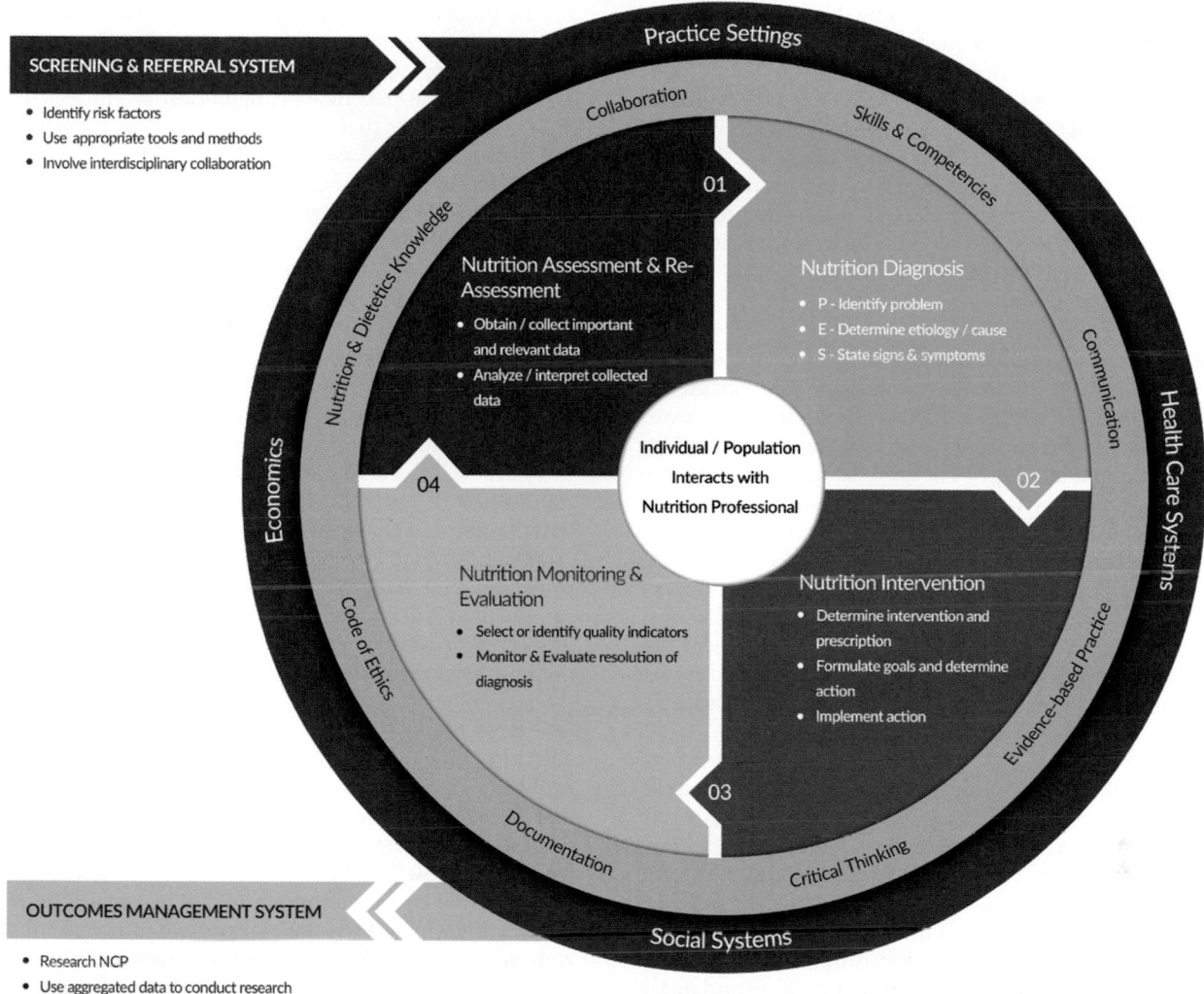

FIGURE 10-1 The nutrition care process. (Copyright 2011 American Dietetic Association. Reprinted with permission.)

separate steps in the NCP because they are not specific to dietetics practice.

Each step of the NCP has corresponding terminology that allows for standardized documentation. This terminology is called the nutrition care process terminology (previously the international dietetics and nutrition terminology [IDNT]). It was previously available as a book published by the Academy but is now available only in a web-based format (http://ncpt.webauthor.com/) for a nominal cost. Using standardized terminology within the documentation process is critical. Systematic and accurate collection of outcomes data allows caregivers a process to determine whether interventions are effective in improving or resolving the nutrition diagnosis. For example, if an RDN were working in a public health department and implemented a program for reducing obesity in an inner city population, he or she would have to be able to collect standardized parameters pre- (assessment) and post (monitoring) intervention and compare

them for change (evaluation) to determine whether the intervention was effective. Without standardized language and corresponding definitions, different terms are used for the same condition and thus reduce the ability to show effectiveness of interventions.

Nutrition Screening

Nutrition screening helps to identify patients or clients who are at nutrition risk and thus should be referred to the RDN for assessment of nutritional status. Nutrition screening can be done in all settings: hospitals, long-term care facilities, schools, food banks, clinics, and hospital settings. When available, population-specific, validated tools should be used for screening (see Chapter 4). Regulatory agencies, including The Joint Commission (TJC), include nutrition screening in their standards. Most health care facilities have developed a multidisciplinary admission screening process that is completed by nursing staff during admission to the facility. Nutrition screening can be incorporated into this admission assessment. Facilities that use an electronic health record (EHR) should build an automatic referral to the RDN when screening criteria are met. The nutrition risk screen should be quick, easy to administer, and cost effective. Table 10-1 lists information that is included frequently in a nutrition screen.

When the Academy's Evidence Analysis Library (EAL) team conducted a systematic review of acute care screening tools, they determined that the Malnutrition Screening Tool (MST), the Mini-Nutrition Assessment-short form (MNA), and the Nutrition Risk Screen-2002 (NRS) had acceptable reliability and validity in various hospital settings (AND, 2010b). See Chapter 4 for a description of these screening tools. When used in a hospital setting, rescreening should occur at regular intervals during the admission. Policies for nutrition rescreening should take into account the average length of time a patient will stay at the facility.

Nutrition Assessment

Nutrition assessment is needed when the screening tool identifies the patient or client to be at nutritional risk (see Chapters 4 through Chapter 7 for detailed discussion of nutrition assessment). The radial in Figure 10-2 presents a summary of all the aspects of the patient and his or her lifestyle that go into a complete assessment as designated in the center with ADIME and Personalized Nutrition Care. Nutrition assessment parameters have specific corresponding terms, which should be used during documentation. These terms are classified into five domains (food/nutrition related history, anthropometrics, biochemical, nutrition-focused physical examination findings, and client history) and can be found online (http://ncpt.webauthor.com/pubs/idnt-en/category-1). See Chapter 7 and Appendices 21 and 22.

Nutrition Diagnosis

RDNs evaluate all of the information from the nutrition assessment to determine a nutrition diagnosis. Accurate diagnosis of nutrition problems is guided by critical evaluation of each component of the assessment combined with critical judgment and decision-making skills. The purpose of identifying the presence of a nutrition diagnosis is "to identify and describe a specific nutrition problem that can be improved or resolved through nutrition treatment/nutrition intervention by a food and nutrition professional" (AND, 2014a). Patients with nutrition diagnoses may be at higher risk for nutrition-related complications,

such as increased morbidity, increased length of hospital stay, and infection with or without complications. Nutrition-related complications can lead to a significant increase in costs associated with hospitalization, lending support to the early diagnosis of nutrition problems followed by prompt intervention (AND, 2009).

The process of aggregating assessment data and using critical thinking to determine appropriate nutrition diagnoses can also allow for identification of the "cause" of the problem. For example, while assessing a patient with significant recent weight loss, the RDN may discover that the person is food insecure because of a lack of money or food assistance. Although the RDN can diagnose "unintended weight loss" and begin providing a high calorie diet to the patient within a hospital stay, this treatment will not resolve the root cause of the diagnosis (lack of food in the home). Conversely, by provision of nutrition education to the patient while in the hospital *and* enrolling the patient into a food assistance program such as Meals on Wheels after he gets home, the RDN may prevent the diagnosis from reoccurring. Identification of the cause (or etiology) is not always possible; however, when it is, it allows for greater understanding of the conditions in which the diagnosis came about and increased individualization of the intervention.

Many facilities use standardized formats to facilitate communication of nutrition diagnoses. It has been recommended that the nutrition diagnosis be documented using the problem, etiology, signs and symptoms (PES) format in a simple, clear statement. However, methods used for documenting nutrition care in the medical record are determined at the facility level. RDNs in private practice should also develop a systematic method for documenting care provided.

Nutrition Intervention

Nutrition interventions are the actions taken to treat nutrition problems. Nutrition intervention involves two steps: planning and implementation. Whenever possible, the nutrition intervention should target the etiology identified during the assessment step of NCP. Thus, if the nutrition diagnosis is *Excessive Carbohydrate* and the etiology is *lack of knowledge about high carbohydrate foods,* then the appropriate intervention would be *education on which foods are high in carbohydrate.*

As previously stated, intervention directed at the etiology is not always possible. When the RDN cannot treat the etiology of the nutrition diagnosis directly, the treatment should focus on ameliorating the signs and symptoms of the diagnosis. For example, a frequent etiology of malnutrition in hospitalized adult patients is inflammation. The RDN may not be able to intervene directly in the inflammatory process; however, inflammation can increase the patient's nutritional needs. Therefore, although the RDN may not be able to reduce the inflammation, the RDN can increase the amount of nutrients provided to the patient through high-calorie foods, nutritional supplements, or other nutrition support therapies.

During the planning phase of the nutrition intervention, the RDN, patient or client, and others as needed, collaborate to identify goals and objectives that will signify success of the intervention. Whether in an inpatient or outpatient clinical setting, a significant component of the plan is the patient prescription. A patient's prescription is a detailed description of the nutrient needs of that particular person. Typically, this should include estimated needs for calories, protein, and fluid but also may include nutrients pertinent to the patient's condition such as carbohydrate needs for patients with diabetes, calcium needs for patients with renal disease, or sodium needs for patients with hypertension.

TABLE 10-1	**Nutrition Risk Screening**	
Responsible Party	**Action**	**Documentation**
Admitting health care professional	Assess weight status— Has the patient lost weight without trying before admission?	Check yes or no on admission screen.
Admitting health care professional	Assess GI symptoms— Has the patient had GI symptoms preventing usual intake over the past 2 weeks?	Check yes or no on admission screen.
Admitting health care professional	Determine need to consult RD.	If either screening criterion is "yes," consult RD for nutrition assessment.

GI, Gastrointestinal; *RD,* registered dietitian.

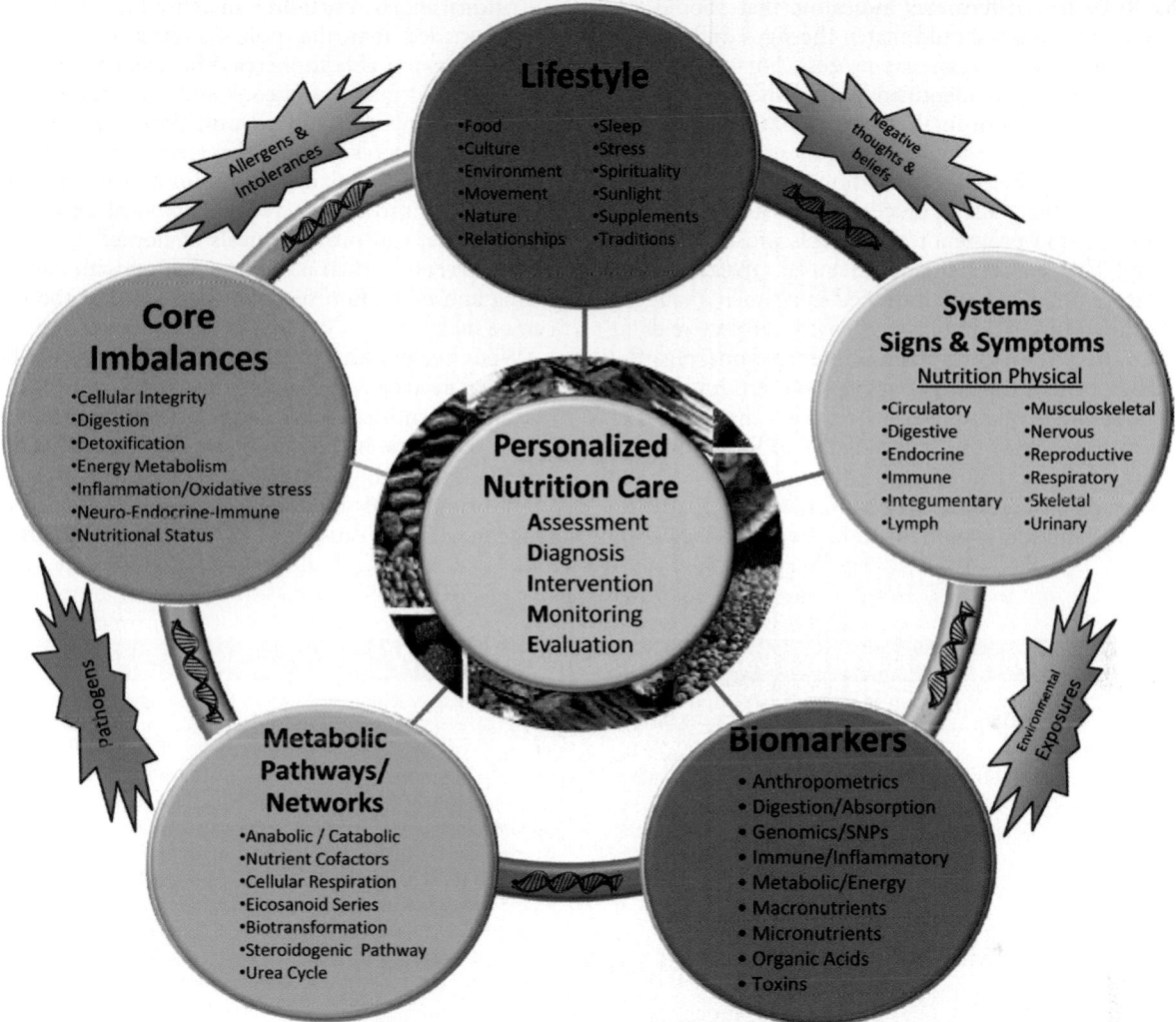

FIGURE 10-2 The radial. (From Ford D et al: American Dietetic Association: Standards of Practice and Standards of Professional Performance for Registered Dietitians (Competent, Proficient, and Expert) in Integrative and Functional Medicine, *J Acad Nutr Diet* 111:902, 2011. Copyright Kathie Madonna Swift, MS, RD, LDN; Diana Noland, MPH, RD; and Elizabeth Redmond, PhD, MMSc, RD, LD. http://www.andjrnl.org/cms/attachment/2002774838/2010029064/gr5_lrg.jpg)

Patient-centered goals and objectives are set, and then implementation begins. Interventions may include food and nutrition therapies, nutrition education, counseling, or coordination of care such as providing referral for financial or food resources. Because the care process is continuous, the initial plan may change as the condition of the patient changes, as new needs are identified, or if the interventions prove to be unsuccessful.

Interventions should be specific; they are the "what, where, when, and how" of the care plan. For example, in a patient with "inadequate oral food or beverage intake," an objective may be to increase portion sizes at two meals per day. This could be implemented through provision of portions that are initially 5% larger with a gradual increase to 25% larger portion sizes. Plans should be communicated to the health care team and the patient to ensure understanding of the plan and its rationale. Thorough communication by the RDN increases the likelihood of adherence to the plan. Box 10-1 presents the NCP applied to a sample patient, JW.

Four categories of interventions are within the Nutrition Care Process Terminology (eNCPT): (1) food and nutrient delivery, (2) nutrition education, (3) nutrition counseling, and (4) coordination of nutrition care by a nutrition professional. Interventions can occur in all settings. For example, a woman with little knowledge of heart-healthy foods may need a group class on cooking or an educational session on lowering saturated fat in her diet (nutrition education). An RDN working for the Women Infant and Children (WIC) clinic may counsel a pregnant woman on initiating breastfeeding as an intervention (nutrition counseling). A clinical RDN may write orders for initiation and progression of enteral feeding for a child with cystic fibrosis (delivery of nutrients). Finally, the RDN may communicate to the social worker the nutrition needs for a patient post discharge to ensure that the patient continues to improve (coordination of care). All of these are types of interventions that RDNs may recommend and implement.

Monitoring and Evaluation of Nutrition Care

The fourth step in the NCP involves monitoring and evaluation of the effect of nutrition interventions. This clarifies the effect that the RDN has in the specific setting, whether health care, education, consulting, food services, or research. During this step, the RDN first determines indicators that should be monitored. These indicators should match the signs and symptoms identified during the assessment process. For example, if excessive sodium intake was identified during the assessment, then an evaluation of sodium intake is needed at a designated time for follow-up.

In the clinical setting the goal of nutrition care is to meet the nutritional needs of the patient or client; thus interventions must be monitored and progress toward goals must be evaluated frequently. This ensures that unmet objectives are addressed and care is evaluated and modified in a timely manner. Evaluation of the monitored indicators provides objective data to demonstrate effectiveness of nutrition interventions, regardless of the setting or focus. If objectives are written in measurable terms, evaluation is relatively easy because a change in the indicator is compared with the status of the indicator before implementation of the nutrition intervention.

An example in clinical practice is the sample case in Box 10-1. Here, monitoring and evaluation include weekly reviews of nutritional intake, including an estimation of energy intake. If intake was less than the goal of 1800 kcal, the evaluation may be: "JW was not able to increase his calorie intake to 1800 kcal because of his inability to cook and prepare meals for himself." This also points to a missed nutrition diagnosis: JW does not have access to tools and supplies needed to cook for himself. A revision in the care plan at this point may include the following: "JW will be provided a referral to local agencies (Meals on Wheels) that can provide meals at home." The new diagnosis and intervention then are implemented with continued monitoring and evaluation to determine whether the new objective can be met.

When evaluation reveals that objectives are not being met or that new needs have arisen, the process begins again with reassessment, identification of new nutrition diagnoses, and formulation of a new NCP. For example, in JW's case, during his hospitalization, high-calorie snacks were provided. However, monitoring reveals that JW's usual eating pattern does not include snacks, and thus he was not consuming them when in the

---

BOX 10-1 Applying the Nutrition Care Process for Patient JW

JW is a 70-year-old male who was admitted to the hospital for mitral valve replacement surgery. JW lives alone in his own home. JW is a widower and states that he hasn't been able to prepare meals for the past 6 months. The nutrition risk screen reveals that he has lost weight without trying and has been eating poorly for several weeks before admission, leading to referral to the RD for nutrition assessment (Step 1 of the nutrition care process).

Assessment: Chart review, patient interview, and nutrition-focused physical examination reveal the following:

Laboratory Data and Medications
Glucose and electrolytes: WNL
Albumin: 3.8 g/dl
Cholesterol/triglycerides: WNL
Medications: Inderal, Lipitor, and and levothyroxine

Anthropometric Data
Height: 70"
Weight: 130 lb (15 lb weight loss over 3 months)

Nutrition Interview Findings
Caloric intake: 1200 kcal/day (less than energy requirements as stated in the recommended dietary allowances)
Meals: irregular throughout the day; drinks 4-6 cups of coffee throughout the day

Medical History
History of hypertension, thyroid dysfunction, asthma, prostate surgery

Psychosocial Data
• New widower; indicates depression and loneliness without his wife
• Has some social support from neighbors and community center but doesn't like to ask for help

Nutrition Diagnosis: JW has been consuming fewer calories than he requires and has little interest in eating. There is support available in the community but JW doesn't like to "impose" on others.
RDN diagnoses nutrition problems and establishes objectives for his care.

Nutrition Diagnostic (PES) Statements:
• Unintended weight loss related to poor oral food and beverage intake as evidenced by 15-lb loss in 3 months.

• Inadequate oral intake related to lack of interest in eating as evidenced by reported intake less than 75% of estimated requirements
• Limited access to food related to inability to prepare meals as evidenced by patient report.

Identification of the nutrition diagnoses allows the RDN to focus the nutrition intervention on treatment of the cause of the problem (in this case the missing meals). Goal setting is the first step, and short-term and long-term plans are established. In the education process the client and the RDN must jointly establish achievable goals. Objectives should be expressed in behavioral terms and stated in terms of what the patient will do or achieve when the objectives are met. Objectives should reflect the educational level and the economic and social resources available to the patient and the family.

Short-Term Objectives
During the hospitalization, JW will maintain his current weight; after discharge he will begin to slowly gain weight up to a target weight of 145 lb.
Interventions:
While in the hospital, JW will include nutrient-dense foods in his diet, especially if his appetite is limited.

Long-Term Objectives
JW will modify his diet to include adequate calories and protein through the use of nutrient-dense foods to prevent further weight loss and eventually promote weight gain.
After discharge, JW will attend a local senior center for lunch on a daily basis to help improve his socialization and caloric intake.
Interventions:
Provide diet to meet JW's needs during hospitalization
Monitor weight
Refer to social services following discharge
Monitoring and Evaluation: Choosing the means for monitoring if the interventions, and nutritional care activities have met the objectives or goals is important. Evaluation of the monitoring criteria will provide the RDN with information on outcomes, and this should occur over time. Finally, documentation is important for each step of the process to ensure communication between all parties.
For JW, weekly weight measurements and nutrient intake analyses are required while he is in the hospital and biweekly weight measurements are taken at the senior center or clinic when he is back at home. If nutrition status is not improving, which in this case would be evidenced by JW's weight records, and the goals are not being met, it is important to reassess JW and perhaps develop new goals and definitely create plans for new interventions.

PES, Problem, etiology, and signs and symptoms; *RDN,* registered dietitian nutritionist; *WNL,* within normal limits.

hospital. The evaluation showed these snacks to be an ineffective intervention. JW agrees to a new intervention: the addition of one more food to his meals. Further monitoring and evaluation will be needed to ascertain if this new intervention improves his intake.

Evidence-Based Guidelines

In health care, providers must use the best available evidence in caring for patients. The Center for Evidence Based Medicine defines evidence-based practice as "the conscientious, explicit and judicious use of current best evidence in making decisions about the care of individual patients." Best evidence includes properly designed and executed prospective, randomized controlled trials (PRCT), systematic reviews of the literature, and meta-analysis to support decisions made in practice (CEBM, 2014; Sackett et al, 1996). Evidence-based guidelines (EBGs) are developed by first conducting a systematic review and then using the conclusion of the systematic review to develop practice-based guidelines. A work group of subject matter experts and specially trained analysts work together to evaluate the research and to develop recommendations for patient care. These guidelines give providers a summary of the best available evidence by which to conduct their practice.

Appropriate use of EBGs may lead to improved quality of care. RDNs must be able to evaluate the EBG and determine whether a given guideline is appropriate in a given situation for a given patient. Many health care professional organizations and practice specialties have developed EBGs, leading to a "glut of guidelines." The National Guideline Clearinghouse, sponsored by the Agency for Healthcare Research and Quality (AHRQ), contains thousands of guidelines for a variety of health conditions (AHRQ, 2014). Because of potential significant differences in quality and applicability, RDNs must be able to evaluate these guidelines.

In the 1990s, the Academy began developing nutrition practice guidelines and evaluating how guideline use affected clinical outcomes; diabetes management was among the first clinical situations examined. These evidence-based nutrition practice guidelines (EBNPG) are disease- and condition-specific recommendations with corresponding toolkits. The EBNPG include major recommendations, background information, and a reference list. To assist the RDN in implementing the EBNPG into their routine care, the guidelines are organized by the NCP steps as appropriate, and NCPT is used throughout the guidelines and within the toolkits.

Medical nutrition therapy (MNT) evidence-based guides are available to assist dietetic practitioners in providing nutrition care, especially for patients with diabetes and early stages of chronic kidney disease (CKD). MNT provided by a Medicare Part B licensed provider can be reimbursed when the EBNPG are used and all procedural forms are documented properly and coded (White et al, 2008). Benefits of nutrition therapy can be communicated to physicians, insurance companies, administrators, or other health care providers using evidence provided from these guidelines.

To define professional practice by the RDN, the Academy published a Scope of Dietetics Practice Framework, a Code of Ethics, and the Standards of Professional Performance (SOPPs) (AND Quality Management Committee, 2013). Specialized standards for knowledge, skills, and competencies required to provide care at the generalist, specialist, and advanced practice level for a variety of populations are now complete for many areas of practice.

The Academy's Evidence Analysis Library (EAL) is a good starting point to answer questions that arise during provision of nutrition care. Use of the EAL may protect the practitioner and the public from the consequences of ineffective care. These guidelines are extremely valuable for staff orientation, competence verification, and training of RDNs.

Accreditation and Surveys

Accreditation by The Joint Commission (TJC) and other accrediting agencies involves review of the systems and processes used to deliver health care along with evaluation of actual care processes. TJC survey teams evaluate health care institutions to determine the level of compliance with established minimum standards. For example, TJC requires that nutrition screening be completed within 24 hours of admission to acute care but does not mandate a method to accomplish screening. However, policies must be applied consistently and must reflect commitment to provision of high-quality, timely nutrition services to all patients.

The "Care of the Patient" section of the *TJC Accreditation Manual for Hospitals* contains standards that apply specifically to medication use, rehabilitation, anesthesia, operative and other invasive procedures, and special treatments, as well as nutrition care standards. The focus of the nutrition care standards is provision of appropriate nutrition care in a timely and effective manner using an interdisciplinary approach. Appropriate care requires screening of patients for nutrition needs, assessing and reassessing patient needs, developing a nutrition care plan, ordering and communicating the diet order, preparing and distributing the diet order, monitoring the process, and continually reassessing and improving the nutrition care plan. A facility can define who, when, where, and how the process is accomplished; but TJC specifies that a qualified dietitian must be involved in establishing this process. A plan for the delivery of nutrition care may be as simple as providing a regular diet for a patient who is not at nutritional risk or as complex as managing enteral feedings in a ventilator-dependent patient, which involves the collaboration of multiple disciplines.

RDNs are involved actively in the survey process. Standards set by TJC play a large role in influencing the standards of care delivered to patients in all health care disciplines. For more information, see the TJC website at www.jointcommission.org.

Dietitians also are involved with surveys from other regulatory bodies, such as a state or local health department, a department of social services, or licensing organizations. Introduction of diagnostic-related groups (DRG) in the mid-1980s led to decreasing acute care length of stay (LOS). However, some patients who no longer need acute hospital care but are not ready to care for themselves at home are admitted to "subacute" care units that are regulated by Center for Medicare-Medicaid Services (CMS). Subacute units also undergo an annual review by CMS. (See Chapter 20 for more information.)

Sentinel events are unanticipated events that involve death, serious physical or psychologic injury, or the risk thereof (TJC, 2014). When there is a sentinel event, the outcomes must be documented in the medical record and there must be clinical and administrative follow-up to document steps taken to prevent recurrence of the event. Regardless of the source of the survey, clinicians must follow all regulations and guidelines at all times and not just when a survey is due.

DOCUMENTATION IN THE NUTRITION CARE RECORD

MNT and other nutrition care provided must be documented in the health or medical record. The medical record is a legal document; if interventions are not recorded, it is assumed that they have not occurred. Documentation affords the following advantages:

- It ensures that nutrition care will be relevant, thorough, and effective by providing a record that identifies the problems and sets criteria for evaluating the care.
- It allows the entire health care team to understand the rationale for nutrition care, the means by which it will be provided, and the role each team member must play to reinforce the plan and ensure its success.

The medical record serves as a tool for communication among members of the health care team. Most health care facilities are using or in the process of implementing EHRs to document patient care, store and manage laboratory and test results, communicate with other entities, and maintain information related to an individual's health. During the transition to EHRs, those using paper documentation maintain paper charts that typically include sections for physician orders, medical history and physical examinations, laboratory test results, consults, and progress notes. Although the format of the medical record varies depending on facility policies and procedures, in most settings all professionals document care in the medical record. The RDN must ensure that all aspects of nutrition care are summarized succinctly in the medical record.

Medical Record Charting

Problem-oriented medical records (POMR) are used in many facilities. The POMR is organized according to the patient's primary problems. Entries into the medical record can be done in many styles. One of the most common forms is the subjective, objective, assessment, plan (SOAP) note format (Table 10-2).

The assessment, diagnosis, interventions, monitoring, evaluation (ADIME) format reflects the steps of the NCP (Box 10-2; Table 10-3). See Table 10-4 for examples of nutrition diagnostic (PES) statements. However, each patient and situation is different, and the NCP should be individualized appropriately.

Documentation must be accurate, clear, and concise and must be able to convey important information to the physician and other health care team members. All entries made by the RDN should address the issues of nutrition status and needs. Those using EHRs must use great caution when using "copy and paste" functions to document care.

Electronic Health Records and Nutrition Informatics

Beginning in the 1990s costs for computer memory decreased, hardware became more portable, and computer science advanced to make computers and technology a permanent fixture in health care. Additional impetus to change standard practice came with publication of several Institute of Medicine (IOM) reports that brought to light a high rate of preventable medical errors along with the recommendation to use technology as a tool to improve health care quality and safety. (See: http://www.iom.edu/Reports/1999/To-Err-is-Human-Building-A-Safer-Health-System.aspx.)

Clinical information systems used in health care are known by different names; although some use electronic medical record (EMR), EHR, and personal health record (PHR) interchangeably, there are important differences. An EHR describes information systems that contain all the health information for an individual over time regardless of

---

TABLE 10-2 Evaluation of a Note in SOAP Format

	Outstanding 2 Points	Above Expectations 1 Point	Below Expectations 0 Points	Score
DATE & TIME		Present	Not present	
S (SUBJECTIVE)	Pertinent components documented	Accurately summarizes most of the pertinent information	One or more pertinent elements missing	
Tolerance of current diet				
Reports of wt loss or appetite decrease	Captures essence of pt's perception of medical problem			
Chewing or swallowing difficulties				
Previously unreported food allergies				
Pertinent diet hx information				
O (OBJECTIVE)	All necessary elements documented accurately	Necessary elements documented	One or more pertinent elements omitted and irrelevant data documented	
Diet order √ Pt dx				
Ht, wt, DBW, %DBW √ UBW, % UBW		No more than one item missing or irrelevant data documented		
Pertinent laboratory values √ Diet-related meds				
Estimated nutrient needs (EER & protein)				
A (ASSESSMENT)	Sophisticated assessment drawn from items documented in S & O	Appropriate, effective assessment, but not based on documentation in S & O	Unacceptable assessment or no assessment	
S + O = A				
Nutritional status assessed			Disease pathophysiologic findings documented as assessment of nutritional status	
Appropriateness of current diet order noted	Appropriate conclusions drawn			
Interpretation of abnormal laboratory values (to assess nutritional status)				
Comments on diet hx (if appropriate)				
Comments on tolerance of diet (if appropriate)				
Rationale for suggested changes (if appropriate)				
SIGNATURE & CREDENTIALS		Present	Not present	

Courtesy Sara Long, PhD, RD.

DBW, Desired body weight; *Dx,* diagnosis; *EER,* estimated energy requirements; *F/U,* follow up; *ht,* height; *hx,* history; *PO,* by mouth; *PRN,* as necessary; *pt,* patient; *Rx,* prescription; *SOAP,* subjective, objective, assessment, plan; *TF,* tube feeding; *TPN,* total parenteral nutrition; *UBW,* usual body weight; *wt,* weight.

BOX 10-2 Chart Note Using ADIME

Nutrition Assessment

- Pt is 66-year-old woman admitted with heart failure: Ht: 62 cm; Wt: 56 kg; IBW: 52-58 kg
- Laboratory values within normal limits
- Estimated energy requirement: 1570-1680 calories (28-30 cal/kg)
- Estimated protein requirement: 56-73 g protein (1-1.3 g/kg)
- Current diet order is "no added salt" with pt consuming 95% of meals recorded
- Consult for education received

Nutrition Diagnosis

- Food- and nutrition-related knowledge deficit related to no previous education on low sodium diet as evidenced by client report.

Nutrition Intervention

- Education: Provided pt with written and verbal instruction on a no added salt diet (3 gm) diet.
- Goals: Develop 1-day menu using dietary restrictions.

Monitoring and Evaluation

- Follow up with pt regarding questions about diet indicated no further questions; good comprehension.
- Evaluation: anticipate no problems following diet at home. Provided contact information for outpatient clinic.

J Wilson, MS, RDN 1/2/15 15 AM

ht, height; *IBW,* ideal body weight; *pt,* patient; *wt,* weight.

TABLE 10-3 Evaluation of a Note in ADIME Format

	Outstanding 2 Points	Above Expectations 1 Point	Below Expectations 0 Points	Score
DATE & TIME		Present	Not present	
A (ASSESSMENT) Reports of wt loss or appetite decrease Chewing or swallowing difficulties Previously unreported food allergies Pertinent diet hx information Estimated nutrient needs (EER & protein) Diet order √ Pt dx Ht, wt, DBW, %DBW √ UBW, % UBW if appropriate Pertinent laboratory values √ Diet-related meds	Pertinent components documented Captures essence of pt's perception of medical problem	Accurately summarizes most of the pertinent information	One or more pertinent elements missing or irrelevant data documented	
D (NUTRITION DIAGNOSIS) Written in PES statement(s) using standardized language for the nutrition care process	Necessary PES statement(s) stated accurately & prioritized	No more than one item missing	Not written in PES statement format or standardized language not used Medical dx listed as nutrition dx	
I (INTERVENTION) Aimed at cause of nutr dx; can be directed at reducing effects of signs & symptoms Planning: prioritize nutr dx, jointly establish goals w/ pt, define nutrition Rx, identify specific nutr interventions Implementation: action phase, includes carrying out & communicating plan of care, continuing data collection & revising nutr intervention as warranted based on pt's response	Appropriate & specific plan(s) AND implementation to remedy nutr dx documented	Plans or implementation missing Vague plans or intervention documented	MD's orders documented as intervention, or inappropriate plan or intervention documented.	
M (MONITORING) & E (EVALUATION) Determines progress made by pt & if goals are being met Tracks pt outcomes relevant to nutr dx Can be organized into one or more of following: Nutr-Related Behavioral & Environmental Outcomes Food & Nutrient Intake Outcomes Nutr-Related Physical Sign & Symptom Outcome Nutr-Related Pt-Centered Outcome	Appropriate nutr care outcomes relevant to nutr dx & intervention plans & goals documented. Nutr care outcomes defined, specific indicators (can be measured & compared with established criteria) identified	No more than one item missing	Nutr care outcome not relevant to nutr dx, intervention, or plans/ goals. Nutr care outcomes cannot be measured or compared with established criteria.	
SIGNATURE & CREDENTIALS		Present	Not present	

Courtesy Sara Long, PhD, RD.

ADIME, Assessment, diagnosis, intervention, monitoring, evaluation; *DBW,* desirable body weight; *dx,* diagnosis; *EER,* estimated energy requirement; *ht,* height; *hx,* history; *MD,* medical doctor; *meds,* medications; *nutr,* nutrition; *PES,* problem, etiology, signs and symptoms; *pt,* patient; *Rx,* prescription; *UBW,* usual body weight; *w/,* with; *wt,* weight.

TABLE 10-4 Sample PES Statements Based on Medical Diagnosis*

Medical Diagnosis	Nutrition Diagnosis** (Problem)	Etiology (E)	Signs/Symptoms (S)
Obesity	Obesity	Energy intake >> estimated requirements and physical inactivity	Current weight 175% desired body weight
	Excessive energy intake	Intake greater than estimated requirements	Diet history; intake approximately 150% estimated requirements
	Lack of physical activity	Lack of time to exercise	Patient report
Unintentional weight loss	Unintended weight loss	Nausea after chemotherapy	Loss of 10% usual body weight in past month
	Inadequate oral intake	Inability to consume more than 25% of most meals	Intake approximately 25% of most meals
Newly diagnosed type 2 diabetes	Food/nutrition-related knowledge deficit	No previous instruction on nutrition management of type 2 diabetes	Patient report
Major trauma	Inadequate oral food/beverage intake	Intubation after surgery	NPO × 48 hours.
GI surgery with complications			
Anorexia nervosa	Inadequate energy intake	Parents report skipping most meals	Intake <25% estimated requirements at least 7 days before admission
Congestive heart failure	Excessive fluid intake	Patient reports excessive thirst	Estimated fluid intake 150% of physician-ordered restriction
	Inability to self-manage daily activities	Patient reports being "thirsty all the time"	Three admissions for fluid overload in past 2 months
Dysphagia	Inadequate oral food/beverage intake	Swallowing difficulty	Inability to consume most foods served
	Swallowing difficulty	Cerebrovascular accident	Requires thickened liquids and does better with thickened liquids
Referral for social services	Limited access to food	Financial constraints	Patient/SWS reports disqualified from SNAP program

*These are only examples. Each patient is different; each nutrition problem diagnosed by the RDN has an etiology and signs/symptoms that are unique to that patient.
**Each patient can have more than one nutrition diagnosis.

the care setting. An EMR is a clinical information system used by a health care organization to document patient care during one episode of care or admission. EHRs and EMRs are maintained by health care providers or organizations. In contrast, the PHR is a system used by individuals to maintain health information. A PHR can be web or paper based or integrated into a facility's EMR. Information in the PHR is controlled by the person, not the provider or healthcare organization.

EHRs include all of the information typically found in a paper-based documentation system along with tools such as clinical decision support (CDS), electronic medication records, computerized provider order entry (CPOE), and alert systems that support clinicians in making decisions regarding patient care. Current government regulations include requirements to implement and "meaningfully use" EHRs to enter, store, retrieve, and manage information related to patient care. Dietitians must have at least a basic understanding of technology and health information management to ensure a smooth transition from paper to EHR and to use effectively the powerful tools provided by a well-designed EHR. Such transitions include development of nutrition screens for patient admission, documentation, information sharing, decision support tools, and order entry protocols. Customization capabilities vary depending on vendor contracts and facility requirements. Because it can take several years to implement an EHR, RDNs managing nutrition services must be involved in EHR system decisions from the very beginning.

In paper and electronic formats, medical records and the information contained are vital conduits for communicating patient care to others, providing information for quality evaluation and improvement and as a legal document. RDN documentation includes information related to NCPs. Documentation must follow the facility policy and be brief and concise while accurately describing actions taken to those authorized to view the record. Figure 10-3 shows how a computerized medical record may look when using the ADIME method.

Current efforts are focused on ensuring that health information stored in clinical information systems can be exchanged safely and securely between providers and facilities. Systems that are able to share information seamlessly are said to be "interoperable." Although this concept seems simple on the surface, problems with interoperability will be very difficult and expensive to overcome. RDNs in private practice and ambulatory care must ensure that systems they are using have the capability to share health information.

The transition from paper medical records to EHRs is facilitated by thorough planning, training, and support. Many health care professionals do not have sufficient experience with health care technology to understand the practice improvement that can be realized with proper implementation and use of technology. Others may resist any change in the workplace that interrupts their current workflow. These clinicians are not resisting change because they are afraid of technology; instead, resistance is based on real or imagined fears that technology will impede their workflow or hinder patient care. Change is never easy but

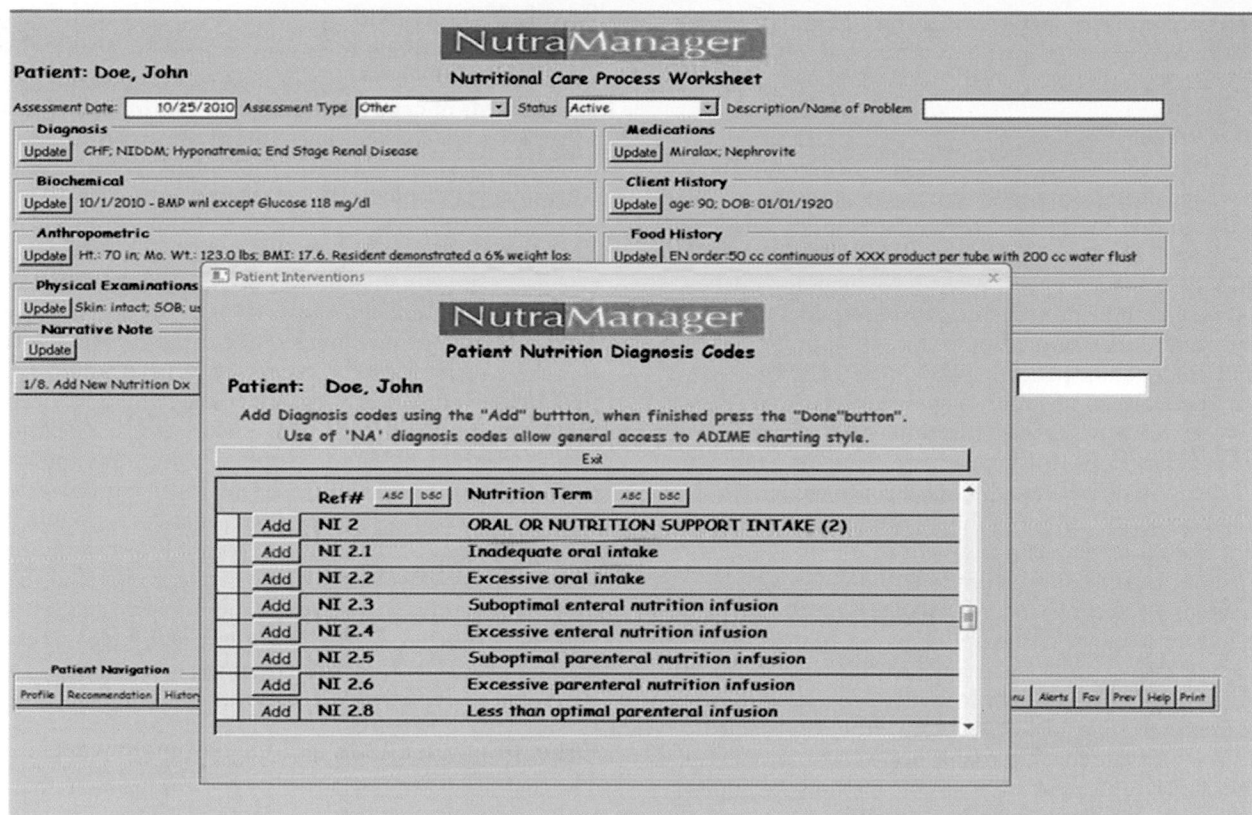

FIGURE 10-3 Example of electronic chart note using drop-down boxes on computer. (Courtesy Maggie Gilligan, RD, owner of NUTRA-MANAGER, 2010.)

proper attention to all of the implications of change can lessen its impact (Schifalacqua, 2009).

INFLUENCES ON NUTRITION AND HEALTH CARE

The health care environment has undergone considerable change related to the provision of care and reimbursement in the last decade. Governmental influences, cost containment issues, changing demographics, and the changing role of the patient as a "consumer" have influenced the health care arena. The United States currently spends more on health care than any other nation, yet health care outcomes lag far behind those seen in other developed nations. Exponential increases in health care costs in the United States have been a major impetus for drives to reform how health care is provided and paid for in the United States (Ross, 2009).

Affordable Health Care for America: Reconciliation Bill

The intent of the Affordable Care Act (ACA), passed by the U.S. Senate in 2009, is to ensure that Americans have access to quality, affordable health care. Other aims are to protect Americans from predatory insurance industry practices, offer the uninsured and small businesses the opportunity to obtain affordable health care plans, cover 32 million uninsured Americans, and reduce the deficit by $143 billion over the next decade.

Final regulations require group health plans and health insurance issuers to provide coverage of dependent children younger than age 26 (see *Clinical Insight:* The ACA: How Does Nutrition Fit?).

Confidentiality and the Health Insurance Portability and Accountability Act

Privacy and security of personal information are a concern in all health care settings. In 1996 Congress passed the Health Insurance Portability and Accountability Act (HIPAA) (Centers for Medicare and Medicaid Services, 2013). The initial intent of HIPAA was to ensure that health insurance eligibility is maintained when people change or lose jobs. The Administrative Simplification provisions of HIPAA require development of national standards that maintain privacy of electronically transmitted protected health information (PHI). In 2013 the HIPAA Omnibus Rule expanded patient rights to their own health information, strengthened rules surrounding privacy and confidentiality of PHI, and increased penalties for unauthorized sharing or loss of PHI (U.S. Department of Health and Human Services, 2015).

HIPAA requires that health care facilities and providers (covered entities) take steps to safeguard PHI. Although HIPAA does not prevent sharing of patient data required for care, patients must be notified if their medical information is to be shared outside of the care process, or if protected information (e.g., address, e-mail, income) is to be shared. Violations of HIPAA rules have resulted in large fines, loss of jobs, and criminal prosecution. In an effort to avoid the serious repercussions of HIPAA violations, health care institutions have implemented mandatory annual education on HIPAA for each employee.

Payment Systems

One of the largest influences on health care delivery in the last decade has been changes in health care payment methods. There are several common methods of reimbursement: private insurance, cost-based reimbursement, negotiated bids, and DRGs. Under the DRG system, a facility receives payment for a patient's admission based on the principal diagnosis, secondary diagnosis (comorbid conditions), surgical procedure (if appropriate), and the age and gender of the patient. Approximately 500 DRGs cover the entire spectrum of medical diagnoses and surgical treatments. Preferred-provider organizations (PPOs) and managed-care organizations (MCOs) also are changing health care. MCOs finance and deliver care through a contracted network of providers in exchange for a monthly premium, changing reimbursement from a fee-for-service system to one in which fiscal risk is borne by health care organizations and physicians.

The Patient Protection and Affordable Care Act (PPACA) was signed into law by President Obama on March 23, 2010. PPACA is the most significant change to the U.S. health care system since the 1965 passage of legislation that created Medicare and Medicaid. The goal of PPACA or the Affordable Care Act (ACA) is to ensure that affordable health insurance is available to all Americans. ACA uses several methods to improve access to health insurance including an individual mandate, subsidies, state insurance exchanges, and assurance of coverage for preexisting conditions (U.S. Government Publishing Office, 2010) (see *Clinical Insight: The ACA: How Does Nutrition Fit?*)

Quality Management

To contain health care costs while providing efficient and effective care that is consistently of high quality, practice guidelines, or standards of care, are used. These sets of recommendations serve as a guide for defining appropriate care for a patient with a specific diagnosis or medical problem. They help to ensure consistency and quality for providers and clients in a health care system and, as such, are specific to an institution or health care organization. Critical pathways, or care maps, identify essential elements that should occur in the patient's care and define a timeframe in which each activity should occur to maximize patient outcomes. They often use an algorithm or flowchart to indicate the necessary steps required to achieve the desired outcomes. Disease management is designed to prevent a specific disease progression or exacerbation and to reduce the frequency and severity of symptoms and complications. Education and other strategies maximize compliance with disease treatment. Educating a patient with type 1 diabetes regarding control of blood glucose levels would be an example of a disease management strategy aimed at decreasing the complications (nephropathy, neuropathy, and retinopathy) and the frequency with which the client needs to access the care provider. Decreasing the number of emergency room visits related to hypoglycemic episodes is a sample goal.

Patient-Centered Care and Case Management

The case management process strives to promote the achievement of patient care goals in a cost-effective, efficient manner. It is an essential component in delivering care that provides a positive experience for the patient, ensures achievement of clinical outcomes, and uses resources wisely. Case management

---

CLINICAL INSIGHT

The ACA: How Does Nutrition Fit?

Patricia Davidson DCN, MS, RD, CDE

To get paid for their services of nutritional counseling under the new Affordable Care Act (ACA), registered dietitian nutritionists (RDNs) must gain an understanding of the language and steps involved in reimbursement as well as how to become a provider. According to Medicare standards, an MNT provider must have completed the educational and clinical experience required of an RDN (AND, 2014; ADA, 2011). Next, he or she has to obtain the 10-digit National Provider Identifier (NPI), required for billing and credentialing (a term used by insurance companies, the payers, for enrolling service providers). Credentialing is a binding contract of services, conditions, and diseases for which nutritional counseling will be paid, codes to use, and the fee schedule. The diagnosis code (ICD-10) and Common Procedure Terminology (CPT) are required for billing purposes. The ICD-10 describes the person's medical condition, obtained from the physician, and the CPT documents the procedure performed by the RDN. Since 2002, MNT has been designated as 97802 (initial visit) and 97803 (follow-up) procedural codes that are applicable for nutritional counseling for the ACA.

By researching insurance companies, RDNs can find out if MNT is covered, if RDNs are accepted into network, the covered diagnosis and procedure codes, the limits to MNT, and the fee schedules. The fee schedule is the payment per billing unit (blocks of 15 minutes, or per visit). Plans differ, even if they are offered by the same insurance company.

From changes stimulated by the passage of the ACA, it is evident that the chronic care model is replacing the acute care model. A chronic care model (CCM) is a multidisciplinary and multifaceted approach for chronic disease management and prevention, whose premise is the development of self-management skills while enhancing the patients' relationships to their care and the team providing that care (Coleman et al, 2009). With this CCM comes development of the Patient-Centered Medical Home (PCMH), Accountable Care Organizations (ACOs) and Comprehensive Primary Care Initiative Projects (CPCI), which combine PCMH and ACOs. A PCMH's focus is on the patient-provider relationship incorporating the team approach (Boyce, 2012).

After the passage of the ACA, ACOs were formed to provide a team approach for coordinating the care provided by doctors, hospitals, and other allied health providers for Medicare patients. Seven states and regions participate in the CPCI, but it is expected to grow, requiring the dietitian-nutritionist to think beyond the traditional MNT model of fee for service, to comprehensive care and new areas of practice, such as primary care settings rather than hospitals (AND, 2013). A survey conducted in 2009 demonstrated that RDNs have a poor awareness of and participation in the PCMH, which adds to the urgency for RDNs to become educated about the ACA and their activity in its implementation (AND, 2013).

Academy of Nutrition and Dietetics: *Coding, Coverage and Compliance* (website): http://www.eatright.org/Members/content.aspx?id=7184. Accessed April 27, 2014. Academy of Nutrition and Dietetics: *Integrating the Registered Dietitian (RD) into Primary Care: Comprehensive Primary Care Initiative (CPCI) Tool Kit* (website): https://www.eatright.org/shop/product.aspx?id=6442476253, 2013. Accessed January 25, 2015. American Dietetic Association: *MNT Provider* (website): http://www.eatright.org/publications/mntprovider/june2011/index.html, 2011. Accessed April 27, 2014. Boyce B: Paradigm shift in health care reimbursement: a look at ACOs and bundled service payments, *J Acad Nutr Diet* 112:974, 2012. Coleman K et al: Evidence on the Chronic Care Model in the new millennium, *Health Aff* 28:75, 2009.

involves assessing, evaluating, planning, implementing, coordinating, and monitoring care, especially in patients with chronic disease or those who are at high risk. In some areas, dietitians have added skill sets that enable them to serve as case managers. Patient-centered care has become a movement in the United States that puts more decision making in the hands of the consumer. It places more emphasis on outcomes, sometimes at the expense of physician autonomy (Bardes, 2012). In long-term care the goal is focused on ensuring dignity as well as choice (see Chapter 20).

Utilization management is a system that strives for cost efficiency by eliminating or reducing unnecessary tests, procedures, and services. Here, a manager usually is assigned to a group of patients and is responsible for ensuring adherence to pre-established criteria.

The patient-centered medical home (PCMH) is a new development that focuses on the relationship between the patient and his or her personal physician. The personal physician takes responsibility for coordinating health care for the patient and coordinates and communicates with other providers as needed. Other providers such as nurses, dietitian nutritionists, health educators, and allied health professionals may be called on by the patient or personal physician for preventive and treatment services. When specialty care is needed, the personal physician becomes responsible for ensuring that care is seamless and that transitions between care sites go smoothly. The RDN should be considered part of the medical home treatment plan.

Regardless of model, the facility must manage patient care prudently. Nutrition screening can be important in identifying patients who are at nutrition risk. Early identification of these factors allows for timely intervention and helps prevent the comorbidities often seen with malnutrition, which may cause the length of stay and costs to increase. The Centers for Medicare and Medicaid Services (CMS) has identified conditions such as heart failure, heart attack, and pneumonia, to name a few, for which no additional reimbursement will be received if a patient is readmitted to acute care within 30 days of a prior admission. Although many view this rule as punitive, it does provide an opportunity for RDNs to demonstrate how nutrition services, including patient education, can save money through decreased readmissions.

Other recent developments include "never events." Never events are those occurrences that should never happen in a facility that provides high-quality, safe, person-focused care. CMS will not reimburse facilities for additional costs of care related to "never events." RDNs must pay attention to new or worsening pressure ulcers and central line infections as potential "never events."

Staffing

Staffing also affects the success of nutrition care. Clinical RDNs may be centralized (all are part of a core nutrition department) or decentralized (individual dietitians are part of a unit or service that provides care to patients), depending on the model adopted by a specific institution. Certain departments such as food service, accounting, and human resources remain centralized in most models because some of the functions for which these departments are responsible are not related directly to patient care. Dietitians should be involved in the planning for any redesign of patient care (see *Focus On:* Nutrition Standardized Language and Coding Practices).

◎ FOCUS ON

Nutrition Standardized Language and Coding Practices

The history of the International Classification of Diseases (ICD) can be traced to the mid-1600s and the London Bills of Mortality. It was not until the late 1800s that ICD codes were introduced in health care. The ICD coding system has been revised and updated several times and is used by most countries. Because ICD initially was developed as a system to track causes of death, its use for coding medical diagnoses has been criticized. The United States has been using ICD-9-CM (version 9, clinical modifications) for several years, whereas most other developed nations have been using ICD-10. It currently is mandated that the United States move to ICD-10 in October 2015, but there is ongoing discussion about the difficulties associated with the move.

Medical records departments review medical records and assign codes to the medical diagnoses based on specific findings documented by health care providers as well as complicating factors ("comorbidities") to determine reimbursement rates. Commonly, pulmonary, gastrointestinal, endocrine, mental disorders, and cancer can lead to malnutrition as a comorbid factor. Thus coordinated nutrition care and coding for malnutrition are important elements in patient services.

A study by White et al (2008) found that self-employed RDNs are more likely to be reimbursed by private or commercial payers, and RDNs working in clinic settings are more likely to be reimbursed by Medicare. RDNs must know and be accountable for the business and clinical side of their nutrition practices (White et al, 2008).

In private practice, use of correct codes and following payers' claims processing policies and procedures are essential. For example, an NPI is a 10-digit number that is required on claims. To apply for an NPI, registered dietitians can complete the online application at the NPPES website at https://nppes.cms.hhs.gov/NPPES/Welcome.do.

ADA, American Dietetic Association; *ICD*, International Classification of Disease; *NPI*, National Provider Identifier; *NPPES*, National Plan and Provider Enumeration System; *RD*, registered dietitian.

NUTRITION INTERVENTIONS

The RDN is responsible for provision of food and nutrition services that are reliable and highly individualized. RDNs are responsible for using evidence-based practice that is not compromised by market forces.

The evaluation of general and modified diets requires in-depth knowledge of the nutrients contained in different foods. In particular, it is essential to be aware of the nutrient-dense foods that contribute to dietary adequacy and how foods can be fortified to increase their nutrition value (see *Focus On:* Food First in Chapter 20.) Balance and judgment are needed. Sometimes a vitamin-mineral supplement is necessary to meet the patient's needs when the intake is limited.

Interventions: Food and Nutrient Delivery

The nutrition prescription, written by the RDN, designates the type, amount, and frequency of nutrition based on the individual's disease process and disease management goals. The prescription may specify a caloric level or other restriction to be implemented. It also may limit or increase various components of the diet, such as carbohydrate, protein, fat, alcohol, fiber, water, specific vitamins or minerals, bioactive substances such as phytonutrients, or probiotics. RDNs write the nutrition prescription after the diagnosis of nutrition problems.

A diet order differs from a nutrition prescription. In most states, only a licensed independent health care provider can enter diet orders into a patient's medical record. Typically, physicians, physician assistants, and advanced practice nurses are considered to be licensed independent providers. In some facilities, RDNs have been granted order-writing privileges, usually under the supervision of a licensed independent provider. The ability to enter orders does not absolve the RDN of the need to communicate and coordinate care with the provider who is ultimately responsible for all aspects of patient care.

Therapeutic or modified diets are based on a general, adequate diet that has been altered to provide for individual requirements, such as digestive and absorptive capacity, alleviation or arrest of a disease process, and psychosocial factors. In general, the therapeutic diet should vary as little as possible from the individual's normal diet. Personal eating patterns and food preferences should be recognized, along with socioeconomic conditions, religious practices, and any environmental factors that influence food intake, such as where the meals are eaten and who prepares them (see "Cultural Aspects of Dietary Planning" in Chapter 11).

A nutritious and adequate diet can be planned in many ways. One foundation of such a diet is the MyPlate Food Guidance System (see Figure 11-1). This is a basic plan; additional foods or more of the foods listed are included to provide additional energy and increase the intake of required nutrients for the individual. The Dietary Guidelines for Americans also are used in meal planning and to promote wellness. The dietary reference intakes (DRIs) and specific nutrient recommended dietary allowances are formulated for healthy persons, but they also are used as a basis for evaluating the adequacy of therapeutic diets. Nutrient requirements specific to a particular person's genetic makeup, disease state, or disorder always must be kept in mind during diet planning.

Modifications of the Normal Diet

Normal nutrition is the foundation on which therapeutic diet modifications are based. Regardless of the type of diet prescribed, the purpose of the diet is to supply needed nutrients to the body in a form that it can handle. Adjustment of the diet may take any of the following forms:

- Change in consistency of foods (liquid diet, pureed diet, low-fiber diet, high-fiber diet)
- Increase or decrease in energy value of diet (weight-reduction diet, high-calorie diet)
- Increase or decrease in the type of food or nutrient consumed (sodium-restricted diet, lactose-restricted diet, fiber-enhanced diet, high-potassium diet)
- Elimination of specific foods (allergy diet, gluten-free diet)
- Adjustment in the level, ratio, or balance of protein, fat, and carbohydrate (diet for diabetes, ketogenic diet, renal diet, cholesterol-lowering diet)
- Rearrangement of the number and frequency of meals (diet for diabetes, postgastrectomy diet)
- Change in route of delivery of nutrients (enteral or parenteral nutrition)

Diet Modifications in Hospitalized Patients

Food is an important part of nutrition care. Attempts must be made to honor patient preferences during illness and recovery from surgery. This means that the patient must be involved in the decision to follow a therapeutic diet. Imagination and ingenuity in menu planning are essential when planning meals acceptable to a varied patient population. Attention to color, texture, composition, and temperature of the foods, coupled with a sound knowledge of therapeutic diets, are required for

menu planning. However, to the patient, good taste and attractive presentation are most important. When possible, patient choices of food are most likely to be consumed. The ability to make food selections gives the patient an option in an otherwise limiting environment.

Hospitals and long-term care facilities are required to adopt a diet manual that serves as the reference for the diets served in the facility. The Academy has an online manual that can be purchased for several users per facility. All hospitals or health care institutions have basic, routine diets designed for uniformity and convenience of service. These standard diets are based on the foundation of an adequate diet pattern with nutrient levels as derived from the DRIs. Types of standard diets vary but generally can be classified as general or regular or modified in consistency. The diets should be realistic and meet the nutritional requirements of the patients. The most important consideration of the type of diet offered is providing foods that the patient is willing and able to eat and that accommodate any required dietary modifications. Shortened lengths of stay in many health care settings result in the need to optimize intake of calories and protein, and this often translates into a liberal approach to therapeutic diets. This is especially true when the therapeutic restrictions may compromise intake and subsequent recovery from surgery, stress, or illness.

Regular or General Diet

"Regular" or "general" diets are used routinely and serve as a foundation for more diversified therapeutic diets. In some institutions a diet that has no restrictions is referred to as the *regular* or *house* diet. It is used when the patient's medical condition does not warrant any limitations. This is a basic, adequate, general diet of approximately 1600 to 2200 kcal; it usually contains 60 to 80 g of protein, 80 to 100 g of fat, and 180 to 300 g of carbohydrate. Although there are no particular food restrictions, some facilities have instituted regular diets that are low in saturated fat, sugar, and salt to follow the dietary recommendations for the general population. In other facilities the diet focuses on providing foods the patient is willing and able to eat, with less focus on restriction of nutrients. Many institutions have a selective menu that allows the patient certain choices; the adequacy of the diet varies based on the patient's selections. More recent developments in healthcare food service include use of "room service" similar to the hotel room service model; patients have complete freedom to choose what and when they will eat.

Consistency Modifications

Modifications in consistency may be needed for patients who have limited chewing or swallowing ability. Chopping, mashing, pureeing, or grinding food modifies its texture. See Chapter 40 and Appendix 28 for more information on consistency modifications and patients with neurologic changes that require these diets.

Clear liquid diets include some electrolytes and small amounts of energy from tea, broth, carbonated beverages, clear fruit juices, and gelatin. Milk and liquids prepared with milk are omitted, as are fruit juices that contain pulp. Fluids and electrolytes often are replaced intravenously until the diet can be advanced to a more nutritionally adequate one.

Little scientific evidence supports the use of clear liquid diets as transition diets after surgery (Jeffery et al, 1996). The average clear liquid diet contains only 500 to 600 kcal, 5 to 10 g of protein, minimum fat, 120 to 130 g of carbohydrate, and small amounts of sodium and potassium. It is inadequate in calories, fiber, and all other essential nutrients and should be used only for short periods. In addition, full liquid diets also are not recommended for a prolonged time. If needed, oral supplements may be used to provide more protein and calories and could be offered as liquids with which to take medications if appropriate.

Food Intake

Food served does not necessarily represent the actual intake of the patient. Prevention of malnutrition in the health care setting requires observation and monitoring of the adequacy of patient intake. This nutrient intake analysis (NIA) is described in Chapter 4. If food intake is inadequate, measures should be taken to provide foods or supplements that may be better accepted or tolerated. Regardless of the type of diet prescribed, the food served and the amount actually eaten must be considered to obtain an accurate determination of the patient's energy and nutrient intake. Nourishments and calorie-containing beverages consumed between meals also are considered in the overall intake. The RDN must maintain communication with nursing and food service personnel to determine adequacy of intake.

Acceptance and Psychologic Factors

Meals and between-meal nourishments are often highlights of the day and are anticipated with pleasure by the patient. Mealtime should be as positive an experience as possible. Whatever setting the patient is eating in should be comfortable for the patient. Food intake is encouraged in a pleasant room with the patient in a comfortable eating position in bed or sitting in a chair located away from unpleasant sights or odors. Eating with others often promotes better intake.

Arrangement of the tray should reflect consideration of the patient's needs. Dishes and utensils should be in a convenient location. Independence should be encouraged in those who require assistance in eating. The caregiver can accomplish this by asking patients to specify the sequence of foods to be eaten and having them participate in eating, if only by holding their bread. Even visually impaired persons can eat unassisted if they are told where to find foods on the tray. Patients who require eating assistance should be fed when the foods are still at an optimal temperature. The assisted eating process requires about 20 minutes as a general rule.

Poor acceptance of foods and meals may be caused by unfamiliar foods, a change in eating schedule, improper food temperatures, the patient's medical condition, or the effects of medical therapy. Food acceptance is improved when personal selection of menus is encouraged.

Patients should be given the opportunity to share concerns regarding meals, which may improve acceptance and intake. The attitude of the caregiver is important for encouraging acceptance of a therapeutic diet. The nurse who understands that the diet contributes to the restoration of the patient's health communicates this conviction by actions, facial expressions, and conversation. Patients who understand that the diet is important to the success of their recovery usually accept it more willingly. When the patient must adhere to a therapeutic dietary program indefinitely, a counseling approach helps him or her achieve nutritional goals (see Chapter 14). Because they have frequent contact with patients, nurses play an important role in a patient's acceptance of nutrition care. Ensuring that the nursing staff is aware of the patient's nutrition care plan can greatly improve the probability of success.

Interventions: Nutrition Education and Counseling

Nutrition education is an important part of the MNT provided to many patients. The goal of nutrition education is to help the patient acquire the knowledge and skills needed to make changes, including modifying behavior to facilitate sustained change. Nutrition education and dietary changes can result in many benefits, including control of the disease or symptoms, improved health status, enhanced quality of life, and decreased health care costs.

As the average length of hospital stays has decreased, the role of the inpatient dietitian in educating inpatients has changed to providing brief education or "survival skills." This education includes the types of foods to limit, timing of meals, and portion sizes. Many patients now transfer to a rehabilitation facility to complete their recovery because of the lower cost of care. RDNs are able to follow them for longer periods of time and are able to continue the diet counseling started in the hospital. Follow-up outpatient counseling should be encouraged at discharge. See Chapter 13 for managing nutrition support and Chapter 14 for counseling.

Intervention: Coordination of Care

Nutrition care is part of **discharge planning**. Education, counseling, and mobilization of resources to provide home care and nutrition support are included in discharge procedures. Completing a discharge nutritional summary for the next caregiver is imperative for optimal care. Appropriate discharge documentation includes a summary of nutrition therapies and outcomes; pertinent information such as weights, laboratory values, and dietary intake; potential drug-nutrient interactions; expected progress or prognosis; and recommendations for follow-up services. Types of therapy attempted and failed can be very useful information. The amount and type of instruction given, the patient's comprehension, and the expected degree of adherence to the prescribed diet are included. An effective discharge plan increases the likelihood of a positive outcome for the patient.

Regardless of the setting to which the patient is discharged, effective coordination of care begins on day 1 of a hospital or nursing home stay and continues throughout the institutionalization. The patient should be included in every step of the planning process whenever possible to ensure that decisions made by the health care team reflect the desires of the patient.

When needed, the RDN refers the patient or client to other caregivers, agencies, or programs for follow-up care or services. For example, use of the home-delivered meal program of the Older Americans Act Nutrition Program traditionally has served frail, homebound, older adults, yet studies show that older adults who have been discharged recently from the hospital may be at high nutritional risk but not referred to this service (Sahyoun et al, 2010; see Chapter 20). Thus the RD plays an essential role in making the referral and coordinating the necessary follow-up.

NUTRITION FOR THE TERMINALLY ILL OR HOSPICE PATIENT

Maintenance of comfort and quality of life are most typically the goals of nutrition care for the terminally ill patient. Dietary restrictions are rarely appropriate. Nutrition care should be mindful of strategies that facilitate symptom and pain control. Recognition of the various phases of dying—denial, anger, bargaining, depression, and acceptance—will help the health care practitioner understand the patient's response to food and nutrition support.

The decision as to when life support should be terminated often involves the issue of whether to continue enteral or parenteral nutrition. With advance directives, the patient can advise family and health care team members of his or her individual preferences with regard to end-of-life issues. Food and hydration issues may be discussed, such as whether tube feeding should be initiated or discontinued, and under what circumstances. Nutrition support should be continued as long as the patient is competent to make this choice (or as specified in the patient's advance directives).

In advanced dementia, the inability to eat orally can lead to weight loss (see Chapter 20). One clear goal-oriented alternative to tube feeding may be the order for "comfort feeding only" to ensure an individualized eating plan (Palecek et al, 2010). Palliative care encourages the alleviation of physical symptoms, anxiety, and fear while attempting to maintain the patient's ability to function independently.

Hospice home care programs allow terminally ill patients to stay at home and delay or avoid hospital admission. Quality of life is the critical component. Indeed, individuals have the right to request or refuse nutrition and hydration as medical treatment. RDN intervention may benefit the patient and family as they adjust to issues related to the approaching death. Families who may be accustomed to a modified diet should be reassured if they are uncomfortable about easing dietary restrictions. Ongoing communication and explanations to the family are important and helpful. RDNs should work collaboratively to make recommendations on providing, withdrawing, or withholding nutrition and hydration in individual cases and serve as active members of institutional ethics committees. The RDN, as a member of the health care team, has a responsibility to promote use of advanced directives of the individual patient and to identify their nutritional and hydration needs.

CLINICAL CASE STUDY

Mr. B, a 47-year-old man, 6 ft 2 in tall and weighing 200 lb, is admitted to the hospital with chest pain. Three days after admission, at patient care rounds, it is discovered that Mr. B has gained 30 pounds over the last 2 years. Review of the medical record reveals the following laboratory data: LDL: 240 (desirable 130), HDL 30 (desirable >50), triglyceride 350 (desirable <200). Blood pressure is 120/85. Current medications: multivitamin/mineral daily. Cardiac catheterization is scheduled for tomorrow. Diet history reveals frequent consumption of high fat foods.

Nutrition Diagnostic Statements

Altered nutrition-related laboratory values related to undesirable food choices as evidenced by elevated LDL and low HDL.

Excessive fat and energy intake related to consumption of high fat foods at all meals as evidenced by patient report.

Nutrition Care Questions

1. What other information do you need to develop a nutrition care plan?
2. Was nutrition screening completed in a timely manner? Discuss the implications of timing of screening versus implementing care.
3. Develop a chart note, using ADIME format, based on this information and the interview you conduct with the patient.
4. What nutrition care goals would you develop for this patient during his hospital stay?
5. What goals would you develop for this patient after discharge? Discuss how the type of health care insurance coverage the patient has might influence this plan.

HDL, High-density lipoprotein; *LDL,* low-density lipoprotein.

USEFUL WEBSITES

Academy of Nutrition and Dietetics
www.eatright.org
Centers for Medicare and Medicaid Services
www.cms.hhs.gov
The Joint Commission
www.jointcommission.org
Nutrition Care Process Terminology (eNCPT)
http://ncpt.webauthor.com

REFERENCES

Academy of Nutrition and Dietetics (AND): *About eNCPT* (website), 2014a. http://ncpt.webauthor.com/. Accessed January 25, 2015.

Academy of Nutrition and Dietetics (AND): *International nutrition and diagnostic terminology,* ed 3, Chicago, 2010a, American Dietetic Association.

Academy of Nutrition and Dietetics (AND): *The nutrition care process model—FAQs* (website), 2014b. http://ncpt.webauthor.com/faqs-1#2. Accessed January 25, 2015.

Academy of Nutrition and Dietetics (AND), Evidence Analysis Library (EAL): *NSCR: adult nutrition screening tool comparison (2009)* (website), 2010b. http://www.andeal.org/topic.cfm?menu=3584&cat=4079. Accessed January 25, 2015.

Academy of Nutrition and Dietetics (AND), Evidence Analysis Library (EAL): *MNT: comparative effectiveness of MNT services (2009)* (website), 2009. http://www.andeal.org/topic.cfm?menu=3949&cat=3676. Accessed January 25, 2015.

Academy of Nutrition and Dietetics Quality Management Committee: Academy of Nutrition and Dietetics: revised 2012 standards of practice in nutrition care and standards of professional performance for registered dietitians, *J Acad Nutr Diet* 113(Suppl 1):S29, 2013.

Agency for Healthcare Research and Quality (AHRQ), National guideline clearinghouse: *About* (website), 2014. http://www.guideline.gov/about/index.aspx. Accessed January 25, 2015.

Bardes CL: Defining patient-centered medicine, *N Engl J Med* 366:782, 2012.

Centers for Medicare and Medicaid Services: *HIPAA general information* (website), 2013. https://www.cms.gov/hipaageninfo/. Accessed January 25, 2015.

Centre for Evidence-Based Medicine: *What is evidence based medicine* (website), 2014. http://www.cebm.net/. Accessed January 25, 2015.

Jeffery KM, Harkins B, Cresci GA, et al: The clear liquid diet is no longer necessary in the routine postoperative management of surgical patients, *Am J Surg* 62:167, 1996.

Joint Commission: *Sentinel event policy and procedures* (website), 2014. http://www.jointcommission.org/Sentinel_Event_Policy_and_Procedures/. Accessed January 25, 2015.

Palecek EJ, Teno JM, Casarett DJ, et al: Comfort feeding only: a proposal to bring clarity to decision-making regarding difficulty with eating for persons with advanced dementia, *J Am Geriatr Soc* 58:580, 2010.

Ross JS: Health reform redux: learning from experience and politics, *Am J Public Health* 99:779, 2009.

Sackctt DL, Rosenberg WM, Gray JA, et al: Evidence based medicine: what it is and what it isn't, *BMJ* 312:71, 1996.

Sahyoun NR, Anyanwu UO, Sharkey JR, et al: Recently hospital-discharged older adults are vulnerable and may be underserved by the Older Americans Act nutrition program, *J Nutr Elder* 29:227, 2010.

Schifalacqua M, Costello C, Denman W: Roadmap for planned change, part I: change leadership and project management, *Nurse Leader* 7:26, 2009.

U.S. Department of Health and Human Services: *Omnibus HIPAA rulemaking* (website). http://www.hhs.gov/ocr/privacy/hipaa/administrative/omnibus/index.html. Accessed January 25, 2015.

U.S. Government Publishing Office: *Public law 111 – 148 - patient protection and affordable care act* (website), 2010. http://www.gpo.gov/fdsys/granule/PLAW-111publ148/PLAW-111publ148/content-detail.html. Accessed January 25, 2015.

White JV, Ayoob KT, Benedict MA, et al: Registered dietitians' coding practices and patterns of code use, *J Am Diet Assoc* 108:1242, 2008.

11

Food and Nutrient Delivery: Diet Guidelines, Nutrient Standards, and Cultural Competence

Martin M. Yadrick, MBI, MS, RDN, FAND

KEY TERMS

adequate intake (AI)
daily reference value (DRV)
daily value (DV)
Dietary Guidelines for Americans (DGA)
dietary reference intake (DRI)
estimated average requirement (EAR)
flexitarian
food insecurity

functional food
health claim
Healthy Eating Index (HEI)
lactovegetarian
lactoovovegetarian
locavore
MyPlate Food Guidance System
nutrition facts label

phytochemicals
recommended dietary allowance (RDA)
reference daily intake (RDI)
semivegetarian
tolerable upper intake level (UL)
vegan
vegetarian

An appropriate diet is adequate and balanced and considers the individual's characteristics, such as age and stage of development, taste preferences, and food habits. It also reflects the availability of food, storage and preparation facilities, socioeconomic conditions, cultural practices and family traditions, and cooking skills. An adequate and balanced diet meets all the nutritional needs of an individual for maintenance, repair, living processes, growth, and development. It includes energy and all nutrients in proper amounts and in proportion to each other. The presence or absence of one essential nutrient may affect the availability, absorption, metabolism, or dietary need for others. The recognition of nutrient interrelationships provides further support for the principle of maintaining food variety to provide the most complete diet.

Dietitians translate food, nutrition, and health information into food choices and diet patterns for groups and individuals. With increasing knowledge of the relationship of diet to incidence of chronic disease among Americans, the importance of an appropriate diet cannot be overemphasized. In this era of vastly expanding scientific knowledge, food intake messages for health promotion and disease prevention change frequently.

DETERMINING NUTRIENT NEEDS

According to the Food and Nutrition Board (FNB) of the Institute of Medicine (IOM), choosing a variety of foods should provide adequate amounts of nutrients. A varied diet also may ensure that a person is consuming sufficient amounts

of functional food constituents that, although not defined as nutrients, have biologic effects and may influence health and susceptibility to disease. Examples include foods containing dietary fiber and carotenoids, as well as lesser known phytochemicals (components of plants that have protective or disease-preventive properties) such as isothiocyanates in Brussels sprouts or other cruciferous vegetables and lycopene in tomato products (see Chapter 19).

WORLDWIDE GUIDELINES

Numerous standards serve as guides for planning and evaluating diets and food supplies for individuals and population groups. The Food and Agriculture Organization (FAO) and the World Health Organization (WHO) of the United Nations have established international standards in many areas of food quality and safety, as well as dietary and nutrient recommendations. In the United States the FNB has led the development of nutrient recommendations since the 1940s. Since the mid-1990s, nutrient recommendations developed by the FNB have been used by the United States and Canada.

The U.S. Departments of Agriculture (USDA) and Health and Human Services (DHHS) have a shared responsibility for issuing dietary recommendations, collecting and analyzing food composition data, and formulating regulations for nutrition information on food products. Health Canada is the agency responsible for Canadian dietary recommendations. In Australia, the guidelines are available through the National Health and Medical Research Council of the Department of Health. In 1996 the WHO and FAO published guidelines for the development and use of food-based dietary guidelines (FAO/WHO, 1996). On the African continent, dietary guidelines have been developed in Namibia, Nigeria, and South

Portions of this chapter were written by Deborah H. Murray, David H. Holben and Janice L. Raymond.

Africa. In South America, several countries such as Argentina, Brazil, Chile, Uruguay, and Venezuela released dietary guidelines in the late 1990s or early 2000s. The same is true for Asian countries, including Bangladesh, India, Indonesia, Malaysia, Nepal, Philippines, Singapore, and Thailand.

Several countries have developed food-based dietary guidelines that are illustrated using images including a pyramid, a house, a staircase, or a palm tree. In the United States the MyPlate Food Guidance System, shown in Figure 11-1, replaced the previous MyPyramid diagram. For comparison, see Eating Well with Canada's Food Guide as shown in *Clinical Insight:* Nutrition Recommendations for Canadians and Figure 11-2. Mexico's *El Plato del Bien Comer,* with its five plate sections including one for legumes, is shown in Figure 11-3. The Australian Guide for Healthy Eating uses a pie-shaped image with the five food groups represented proportionally in terms of recommended intakes (Figure 11-4). In Japan, the Ministry of Health, Labour and Welfare and the Ministry of Agriculture, Forestry and Fisheries jointly develop and update their Dietary Guidelines, and in 2005 created the "Japanese Food Guide Spinning Top" to encourage a well-balanced diet (Figure 11-5). The Chinese Nutrition Society released its latest update to its dietary Pagoda in 2008 (Figure 11-6). Several other countries use images to illustrate their food-based dietary guidelines, including the Netherlands (Figure 11-7), France (Figure 11-8), Greece (Figure 11-9),

Hungary (Figure 11-10), Ireland (Figure 11-11), Saudi Arabia (Figure 11-12), Slovenia (Figure 11-13), South Korea (Figure 11-14), and the United Kingdom (Figure 11-15). The latest dietary guidelines from Brazil include mention of the environment in which one eats, the time spent consuming a meal, and the importance of developing cooking skills (Guia alimentar para a população Brasileira, 2014). The Brazilian guidelines also offer advice on choosing fresh or freshly made foods at the grocery store and at restaurants, and suggest that the consumer look objectively at food product advertisements.

Dietary Reference Intakes

American standards for nutrient requirements have been the recommended dietary allowances (RDAs) established by the FNB of the IOM. They were first published in 1941 and most recently revised in 2010. Each revision incorporates the most recent research findings. In 1993 the FNB developed a framework for the development of nutrient recommendations, called dietary reference intakes (DRIs). Nutrition and health professionals always should use updated food composition databases and tables and inquire whether data used in computerized nutrient analysis programs have been revised to include the most up-to-date information. An interactive DRI calculator is available at http://fnic.nal.usda.gov/interactiveDRI/. This can be used to determine an individual's daily nutrient recommendations based on the DRI, including energy, macronutrients, vitamins, and minerals, as well as calculating BMI.

DRI Components

The DRI model expands the previous RDA and RNI (Canada's Recommended Nutrient Intakes), which focused only on levels of nutrients for healthy populations to prevent deficiency diseases. To respond to scientific advances in diet and health throughout the life cycle, the DRI model now includes four reference points: adequate intake (AI), estimated average requirement (EAR), recommended dietary allowance (RDA), and tolerable upper intake level (UL), as well as Acceptable Macronutrient Distribution Ranges (AMDR).

The adequate intake (AI) is an average daily intake level that is based on observed or experimentally determined approximations of nutrient intake by a group (or groups) of healthy people when sufficient scientific evidence is not available to calculate an RDA. Some key nutrients are expressed as an AI, including potassium (see Chapter 6). The estimated average requirement (EAR) is the average daily requirement of a nutrient for healthy individuals based on gender and stage of life. It is the amount of a nutrient with which approximately one half of individuals would have their needs met and one half would not. The EAR should be used for assessing the nutrient adequacy of populations, but not for individuals.

The recommended dietary allowance (RDA) presents the amount of a nutrient needed to meet the requirements of almost all (97% to 98%) of the healthy population of individuals for whom it was developed. An RDA for a nutrient should serve as a goal for intake for individuals, not as a benchmark for adequacy of diets of populations. Finally the tolerable upper intake level (UL) was established for many nutrients to reduce the risk of adverse or toxic effects from consumption of nutrients in concentrated forms—either alone or combined with others (not in

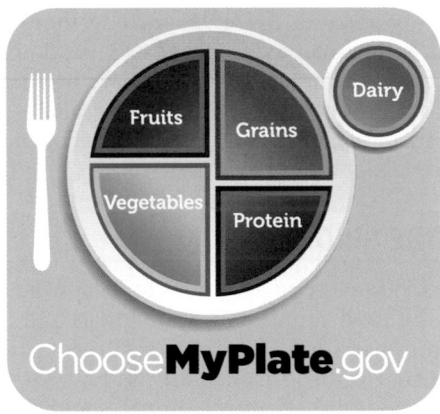

Balancing Calories
- Enjoy your food, but eat less.
- Avoid oversized portions.

Foods to Increase
- Make half your plate fruits and vegetables.
- Make at least half your grains whole grains.
- Switch to fat-free or low-fat (1%) milk.

Foods to Reduce
- Compare sodium in foods like soup, bread, and frozen meals – and choose the foods with lower numbers.
- Drink water instead of sugary drinks.

FIGURE 11-1 MyPlate showing the five essential food groups. (Courtesy from the United States Department of Agriculture. Accessed October 2014 from http://www.choosemyplate.gov/)

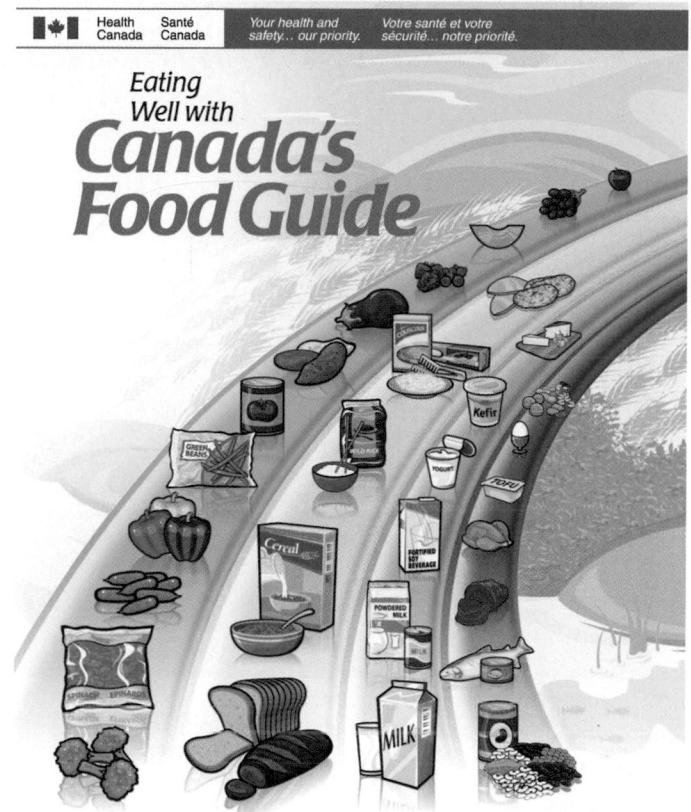

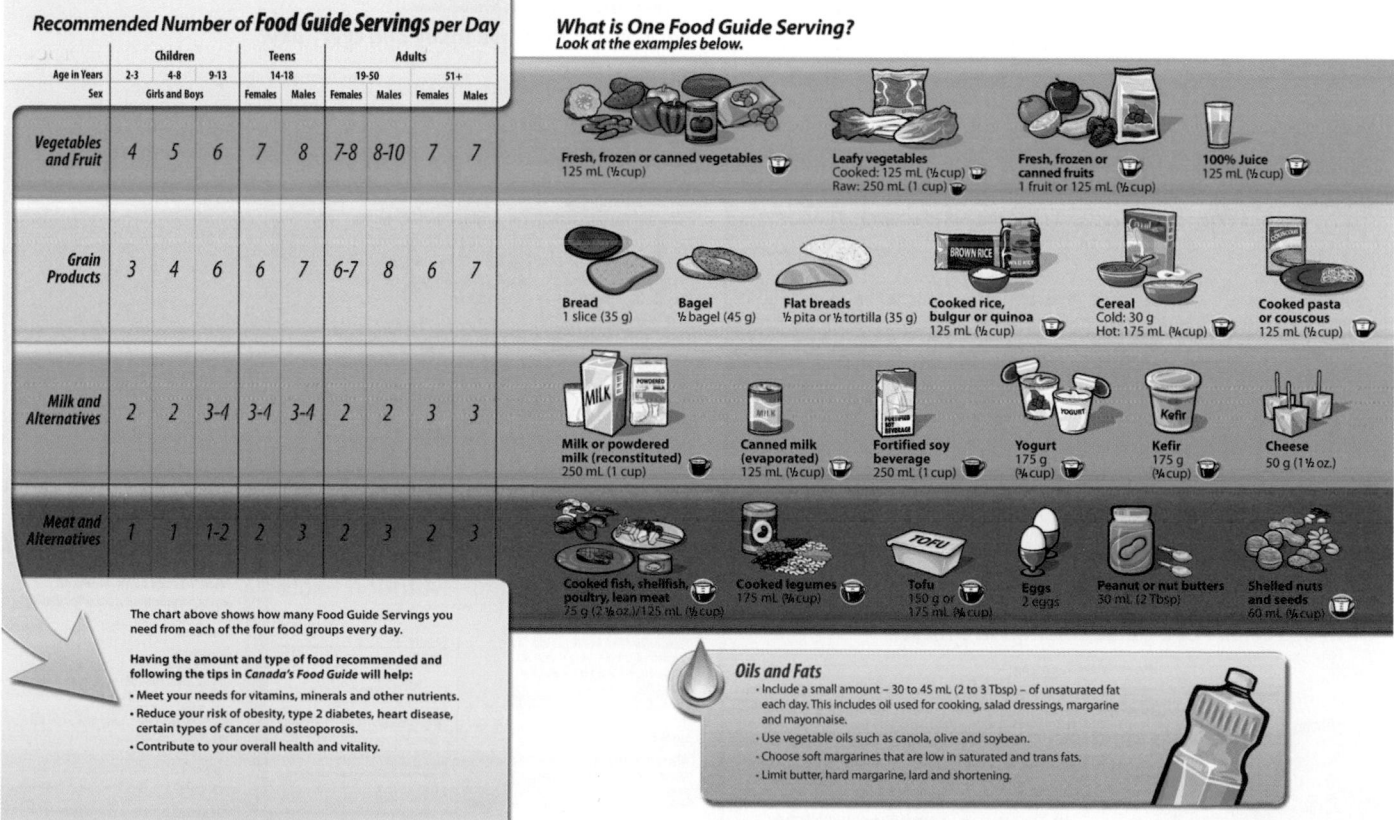

FIGURE 11-2 Eating Well with Canada's Food Guide. (Courtesy from Health Canada. Data from Health Canada: Eating well with Canada's food guide, Her Majesty the Queen in Right of Canada, represented by the Minister of Health Canada, 2011. Accessed October 2014 from http://www. hc-sc.gc.ca/fn-an/food-guide-aliment/index-eng.php.)

Continued

Make each Food Guide Serving count...
wherever you are – at home, at school, at work or when eating out!

▸ **Eat at least one dark green and one orange vegetable each day.**
 · Go for dark green vegetables such as broccoli, romaine lettuce and spinach.
 · Go for orange vegetables such as carrots, sweet potatoes and winter squash.

▸ **Choose vegetables and fruit prepared with little or no added fat, sugar or salt.**
 · Enjoy vegetables steamed, baked or stir-fried instead of deep-fried.

▸ **Have vegetables and fruit more often than juice.**

▸ **Make at least half of your grain products whole grain each day.**
 · Eat a variety of whole grains such as barley, brown rice, oats, quinoa and wild rice.
 · Enjoy whole grain breads, oatmeal or whole wheat pasta.

▸ **Choose grain products that are lower in fat, sugar or salt.**
 · Compare the Nutrition Facts table on labels to make wise choices.
 · Enjoy the true taste of grain products. When adding sauces or spreads, use small amounts.

▸ **Drink skim, 1%, or 2% milk each day.**
 · Have 500 mL (2 cups) of milk every day for adequate vitamin D.
 · Drink fortified soy beverages if you do not drink milk.

▸ **Select lower fat milk alternatives.**
 · Compare the Nutrition Facts table on yogurts or cheeses to make wise choices.

▸ **Have meat alternatives such as beans, lentils and tofu often.**

▸ **Eat at least two Food Guide Servings of fish each week.***
 · Choose fish such as char, herring, mackerel, salmon, sardines and trout.

▸ **Select lean meat and alternatives prepared with little or no added fat or salt.**
 · Trim the visible fat from meats. Remove the skin on poultry.
 · Use cooking methods such as roasting, baking or poaching that require little or no added fat.
 · If you eat luncheon meats, sausages or prepackaged meats, choose those lower in salt (sodium) and fat.

Enjoy a variety of foods from the four food groups.

Satisfy your thirst with water!
Drink water regularly. It's a calorie-free way to quench your thirst. Drink more water in hot weather or when you are very active.

* Health Canada provides advice for limiting exposure to mercury from certain types of fish. Refer to www.healthcanada.gc.ca for the latest information.

Advice for different ages and stages...

Children
Following *Canada's Food Guide* helps children grow and thrive.

Young children have small appetites and need calories for growth and development.

· Serve small nutritious meals and snacks each day.
· Do not restrict nutritious foods because of their fat content. Offer a variety of foods from the four food groups.
· Most of all... be a good role model.

Women of childbearing age
All women who could become pregnant and those who are pregnant or breastfeeding need a multivitamin containing **folic acid** every day. Pregnant women need to ensure that their multivitamin also contains **iron**. A health care professional can help you find the multivitamin that's right for you.

Pregnant and breastfeeding women need more calories. Include an extra 2 to 3 Food Guide Servings each day.

Here are two examples:
· Have fruit and yogurt for a snack, or
· Have an extra slice of toast at breakfast and an extra glass of milk at supper.

Men and women over 50
The need for **vitamin D** increases after the age of 50.

In addition to following *Canada's Food Guide*, everyone over the age of 50 should take a daily vitamin D supplement of 10 µg (400 IU).

Eat well and be active today and every day!

The benefits of eating well and being active include:
· Better overall health.
· Lower risk of disease.
· A healthy body weight.
· Feeling and looking better.
· More energy.
· Stronger muscles and bones.

Be active
To be active every day is a step towards better health and a healthy body weight.

Canada's Physical Activity Guide recommends building 30 to 60 minutes of moderate physical activity into daily life for adults and at least 90 minutes a day for children and youth. You don't have to do it all at once. Add it up in periods of at least 10 minutes at a time for adults and five minutes at a time for children and youth.

Start slowly and build up.

Eat well
Another important step towards better health and a healthy body weight is to follow *Canada's Food Guide* by:
· Eating the recommended amount and type of food each day.
· Limiting foods and beverages high in calories, fat, sugar or salt (sodium) such as cakes and pastries, chocolate and candies, cookies and granola bars, doughnuts and muffins, ice cream and frozen desserts, french fries, potato chips, nachos and other salty snacks, alcohol, fruit flavoured drinks, soft drinks, sports and energy drinks, and sweetened hot or cold drinks.

Read the label
· Compare the Nutrition Facts table on food labels to choose products that contain less fat, saturated fat, trans fat, sugar and sodium.
· Keep in mind that the calories and nutrients listed are for the amount of food found at the top of the Nutrition Facts table.

Limit trans fat
When a Nutrition Facts table is not available, ask for nutrition information to choose foods lower in trans and saturated fats.

Take a step today...
✓ Have breakfast every day. It may help control your hunger later in the day.
✓ Walk wherever you can – get off the bus early, use the stairs.
✓ Benefit from eating vegetables and fruit at all meals and as snacks.
✓ Spend less time being inactive such as watching TV or playing computer games.
✓ Request nutrition information about menu items when eating out to help you make healthier choices.
✓ Enjoy eating with family and friends!
✓ Take time to eat and savour every bite!

For more information, interactive tools, or additional copies visit Canada's Food Guide on-line at:
www.healthcanada.gc.ca/foodguide

or contact:
Publications
Health Canada
Ottawa, Ontario K1A 0K9
E-Mail: publications@hc-sc.gc.ca
Tel.: 1-866-225-0709
Fax: (613) 941-5366
TTY: 1-800-267-1245

Également disponible en français sous le titre :
Bien manger avec le Guide alimentaire canadien

This publication can be made available on request on diskette, large print, audio-cassette and braille.

How do I count Food Guide Servings in a meal?

Here is an example:

Vegetable and beef stir-fry with rice, a glass of milk and an apple for dessert		
250 mL (1 cup) mixed broccoli, carrot and sweet red pepper	=	**2 Vegetables and Fruit** Food Guide Servings
75 g (2½ oz.) lean beef	=	**1 Meat and Alternatives** Food Guide Serving
250 mL (1 cup) brown rice	=	**2 Grain Products** Food Guide Servings
5 mL (1 tsp) canola oil	=	part of your **Oils and Fats** intake for the day
250 mL (1 cup) 1% milk	=	**1 Milk and Alternatives** Food Guide Serving
1 apple	=	**1 Vegetables and Fruit** Food Guide Serving

Nutrition Facts
Per 0 mL (0 g)

Amount		% Daily Value
Calories 0		
Fat 0 g		0 %
Saturates 0 g		0 %
+ Trans 0 g		
Cholesterol 0 mg		
Sodium 0 mg		0 %
Carbohydrate 0 g		0 %
Fibre 0 g		0 %
Sugars 0 g		
Protein 0 g		
Vitamin A 0 %	Vitamin C	0 %
Calcium 0 %	Iron	0 %

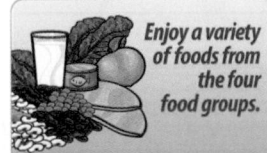
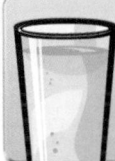
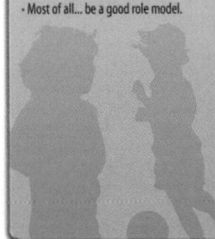

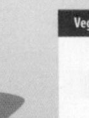

FIGURE 11-2, cont'd

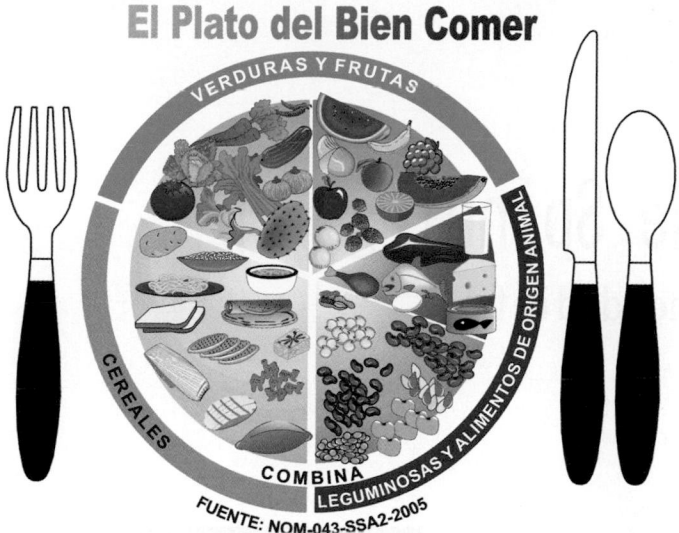

FIGURE 11-3 El Plato del Bien Comer (The Plate of Good Eating). (Courtesy of Mexico Ministry of Health. Accessed January 2014 from http://www.promocion.salud.gob.mx/dgps/descargas1/programas/6_1_plato_bien_comer.pdf.)

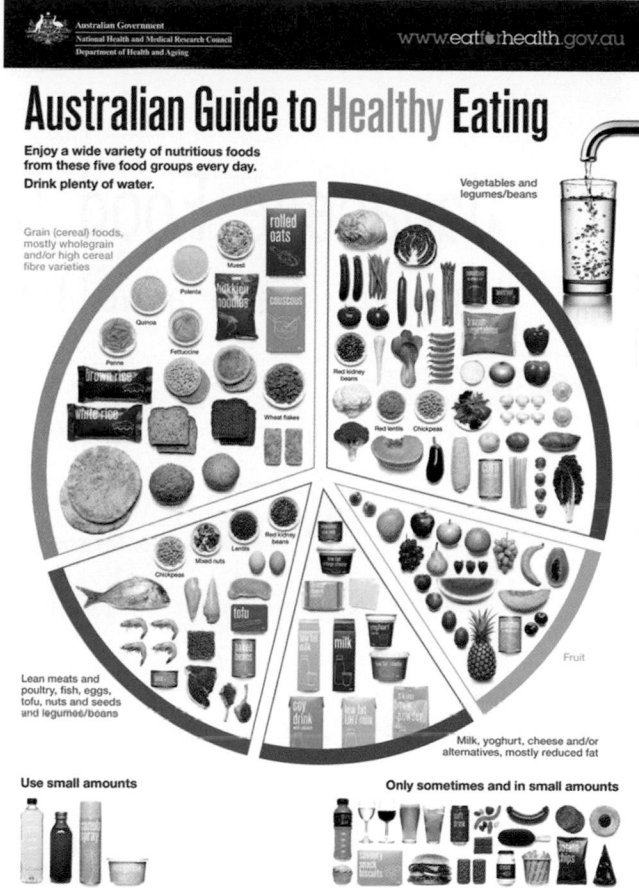

FIGURE 11-4 Australian Guide to Healthy Eating (*Courtesy from the Australian Government, National Health and Medical Research Council, Department of Health and Ageing. Accessed June 2015 from* http://eatforhealth.gov.au/guidelines.)

food)—or from enrichment and fortification. A UL is the highest level of daily nutrient intake that is unlikely to have any adverse health effects on almost all individuals in the general population. The DRIs for the macronutrients, vitamins, and minerals, including the ULs, are presented on the inside front and back covers and opening page of this text. The AMDRs are ranges of intakes of macronutrients associated with reduced risk of chronic disease. The AMDRs for fat, carbohydrate, and protein are based on energy intake by age group. See Table 11-1 and the DRI tables on the inside front and back covers of this text.

Target Population

Each of the nutrient recommendation categories in the DRI system is used for specific purposes among individuals or populations. As noted previously, the EAR is used for evaluating the nutrient intake of populations. The AI and RDA can be used for individuals. Nutrient intakes between the RDA and the UL may further define intakes that may promote health or prevent disease in the individual.

Age and Gender Groups

Because nutrient needs are highly individualized depending on age, gender, and the reproductive status of females, the DRI framework has 10 age groupings, including age group categories for children, adolescents, men and women 51 to 70 years of age, and those older than 70 years of age. It separates three age group categories each for pregnancy and lactation—14 to 18 years, 19 to 30 years, and 31 to 50 years of age.

Reference Men and Women

The requirement for many nutrients is based on body weight, according to reference heights and weights that are specific to gender and stage of life. Reference height and weight information used in determining the DRIs was obtained from the Centers for Disease Control and Prevention (CDC)/National Center for Health Statistics (NCHS) growth charts. Although this does not necessarily imply that these weight-for-height values are ideal, at least they make it possible to define recommended allowances appropriate for the greatest number of people.

NUTRITIONAL STATUS OF AMERICANS

Food and Nutrient Intake Data

Information about the diet and nutritional status of Americans and the relationship between diet and health is collected primarily by the CDC via its NCHS and National Health and Nutrition Examination Survey (NHANES).

Unfortunately, gaps still exist between actual consumption and government recommendations in certain population subgroups. Nutrition-related health measurements indicate that overweight and obesity are increasing from lack of physical activity. Data from the combined NHANES and NHANES National Youth Fitness Survey showed that only about 25% of youth ages 12 to 15 engage in moderate to vigorous physical

Text continued on page 181

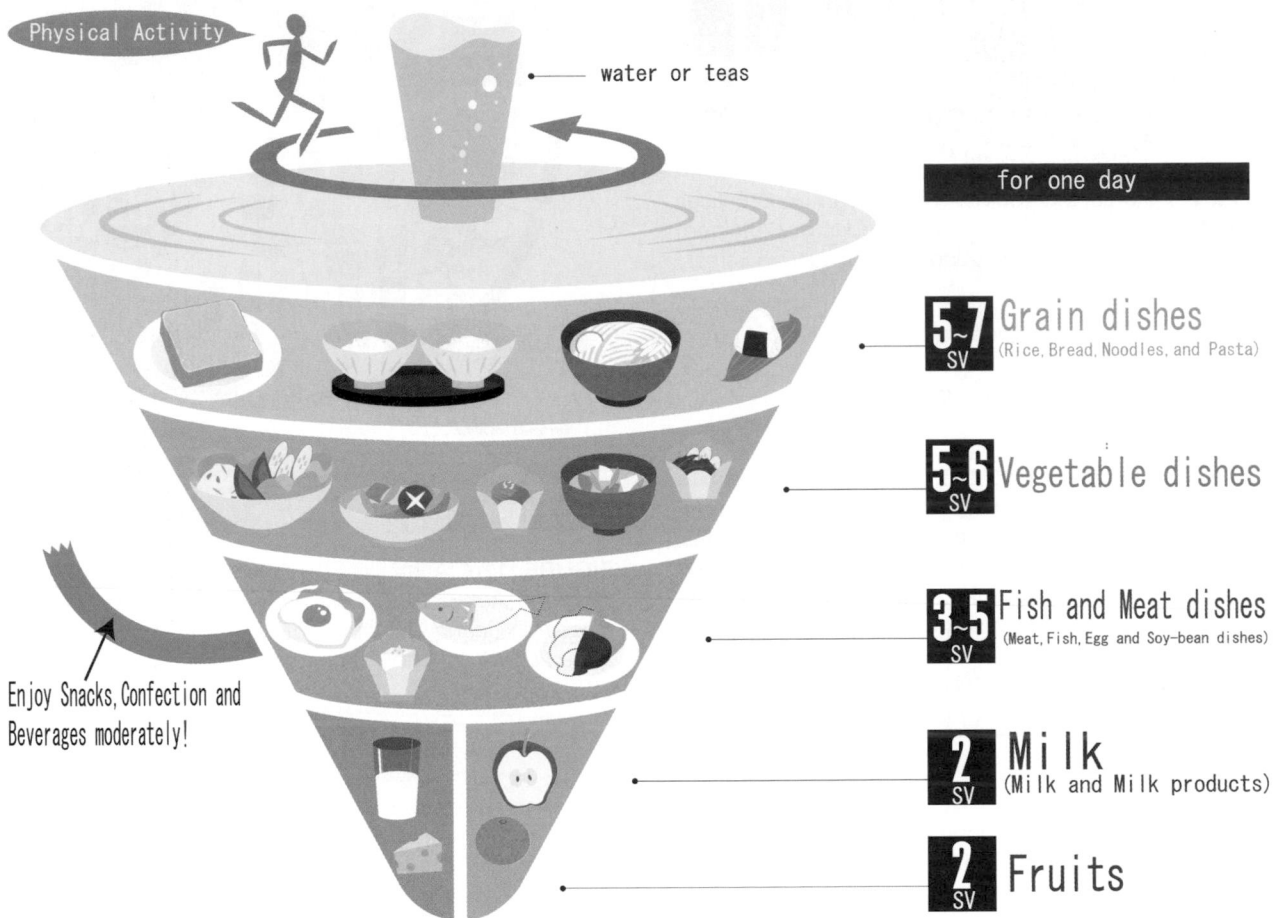

Japanese Food Guide Spinning Top

Do you have a well-balanced diet?

Physical Activity

water or teas

for one day

5~7 SV Grain dishes (Rice, Bread, Noodles, and Pasta)

5~6 SV Vegetable dishes

3~5 SV Fish and Meat dishes (Meat, Fish, Egg and Soy-bean dishes)

2 SV Milk (Milk and Milk products)

2 SV Fruits

Enjoy Snacks, Confection and Beverages moderately!

※ SV is an abbreviation of "Serving", which is a simply countable number describing the approximated amount of each dish or food served to one person

Decided by Ministry of Health, Labour and Welfare and Ministry of Agriculture, Forestry and Fisheries.

FIGURE 11-5 Japanese Food Guide Spinning Top (Courtesy from the Ministry of Health, Labour and Welfare and the Ministry of Agriculture, Forestry and Fisheries. Accessed June 2015 from http://www.mhlw.go.jp/bunya/kenkou/pdf/eiyou-syokuji5.pdf.)

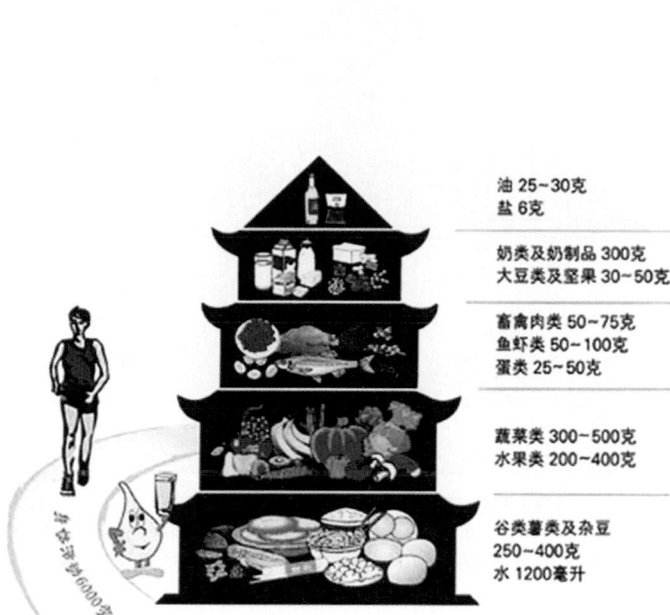

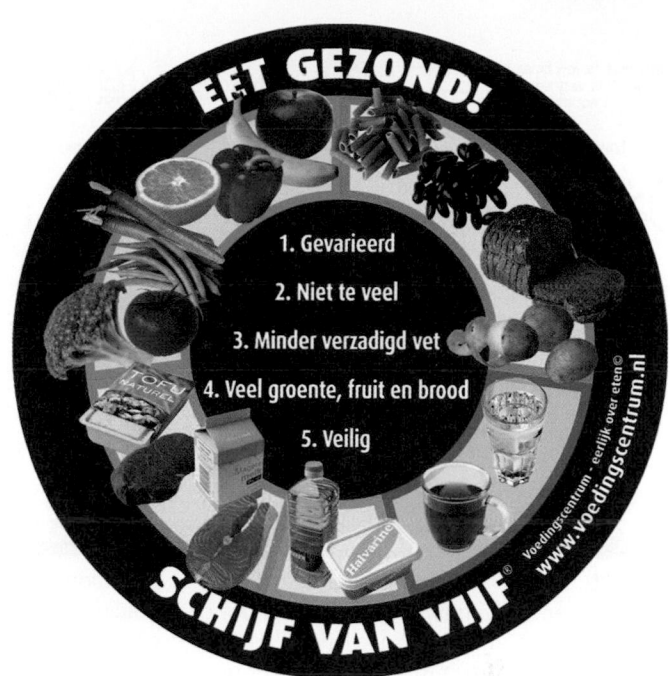

FIGURE 11-6 The Food Guide Pagoda for Chinese People Courtesy from the Chinese Nutrition Society. (Accessed October 2014 from http://www.fao.org/nutrition/education/food-dietary-guidelines/regions/countries/china/en/.)

FIGURE 11-7 The Wheel of Five (Netherlands) (Courtesy from the Netherlands Nutrition Center. Accessed June 2015 from http://www.afvallenkanwel.nl/wp-content/uploads/2010/12/schijfvanvijf.jpg.)

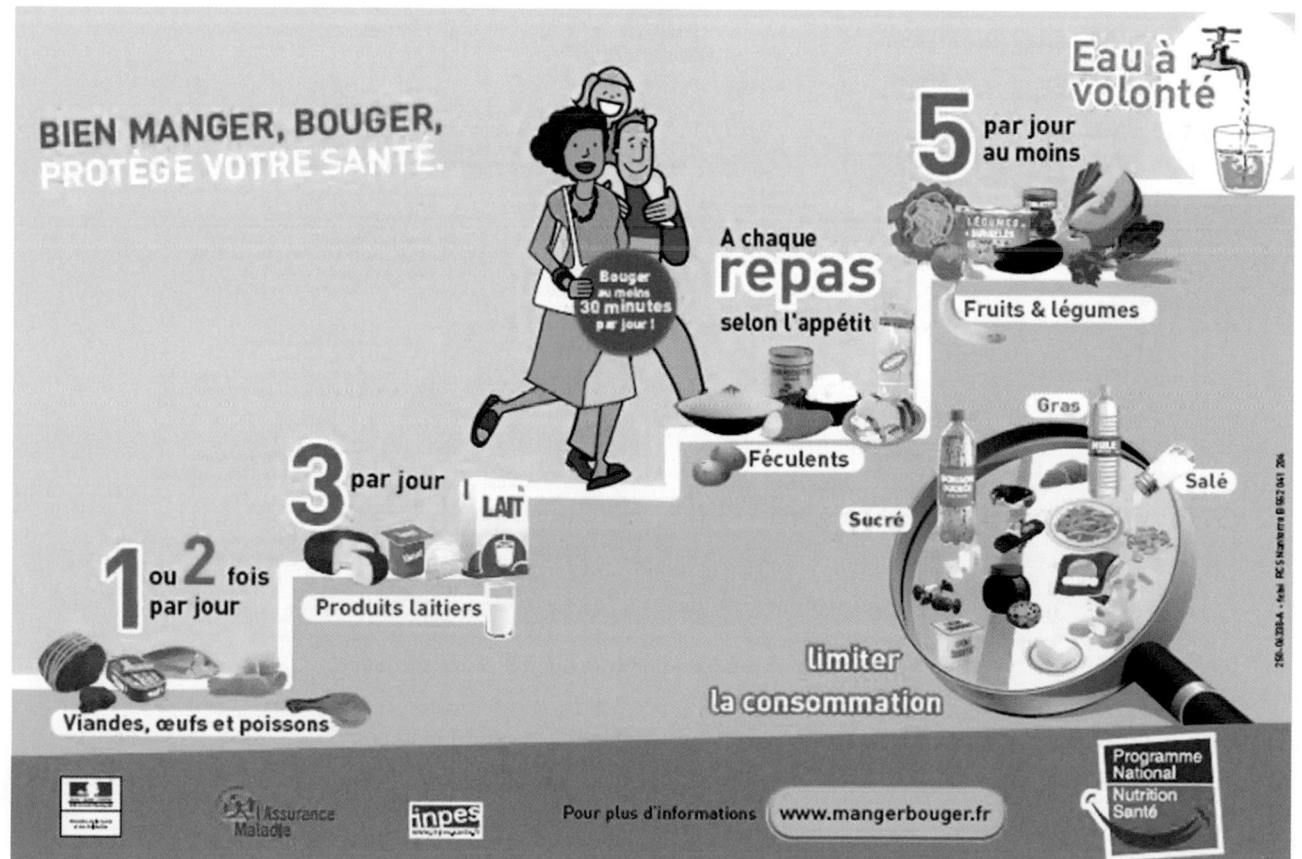

FIGURE 11-8 French Stairs. (Courtesy of Institut national de prévention et d'éducation pour la santé. Accessed June 2015 from http://www.eufic.org/article/en/expid/food-based-dietary-guidelines-in-europe/)

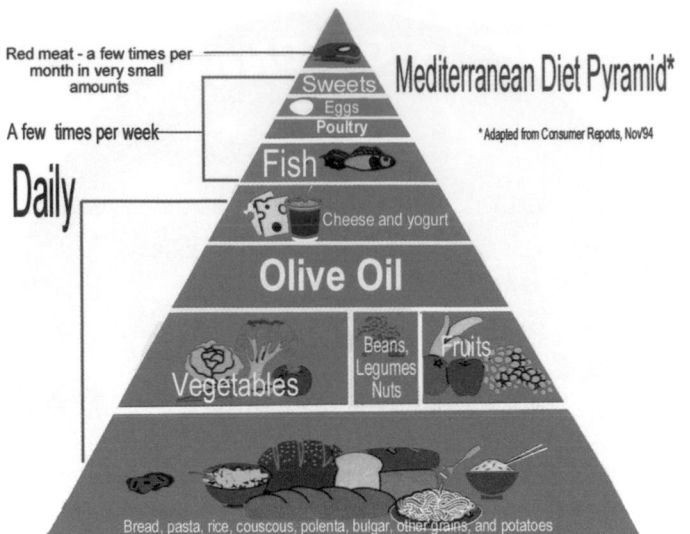

FIGURE 11-9 Greek Food Pyramid. (Courtesy of National and Kapodistrian University of Athens, School of Medicine - WHO Collaborating Center for Food and Nutrition Policies. Accessed October 2014 from http://www.mednet.gr/archives/1999-5/pdf/516.pdf.)

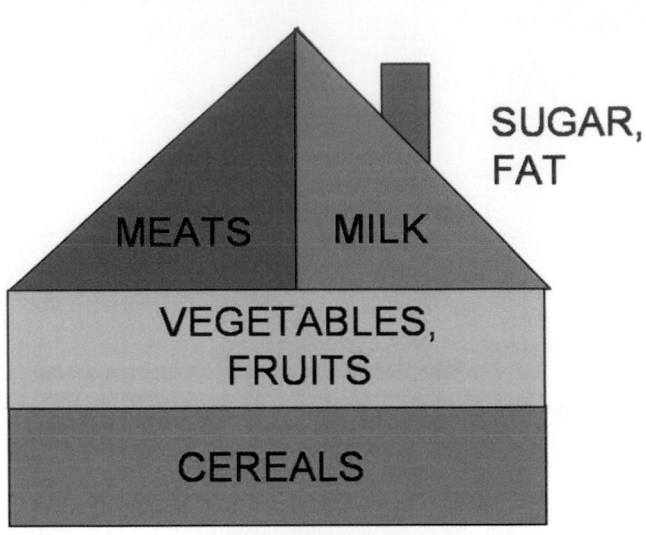

FIGURE 11-10 House of Healthy Nutrition - Hungary (Courtesy of National Institute for Food and Nutrition Science. Accessed June 2015 from ftp://ftp.fao.org/es/esn/nutrition/dietary_guidelines/hun.pdf.)

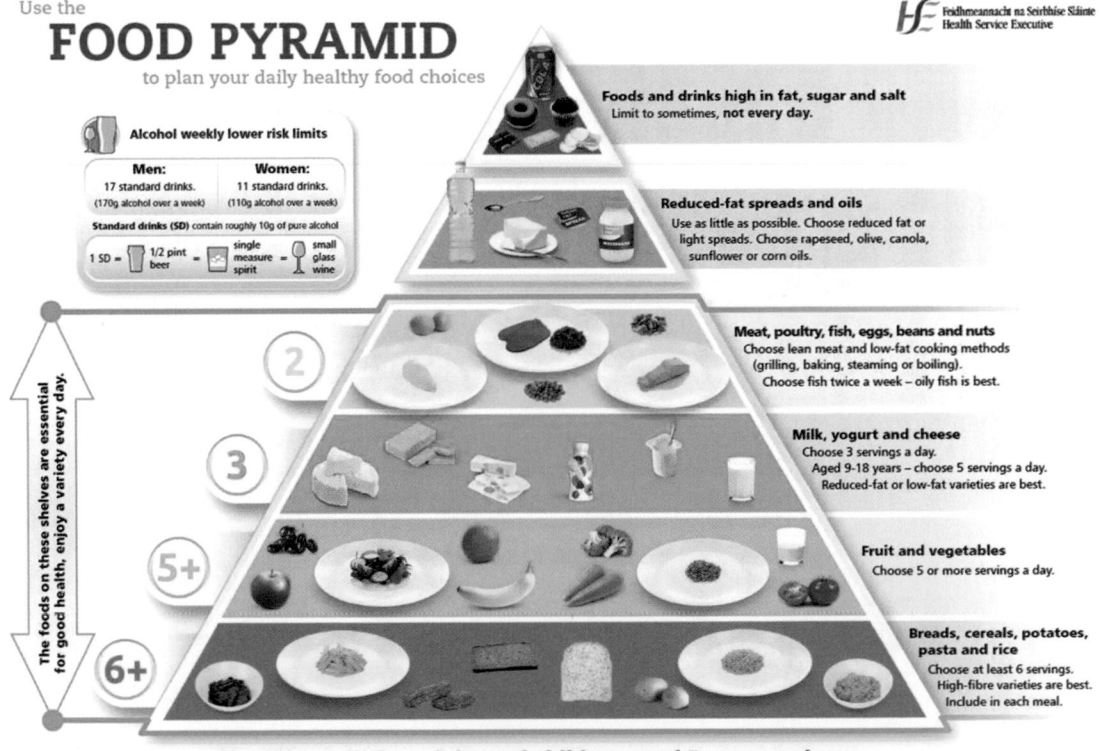

FIGURE 11-11 Food Pyramid – Ireland (Courtesy of Ireland Department of Health. Accessed June 2015 from https://www.healthpromotion.ie/hp-files/docs/HPM00833.pdf.)

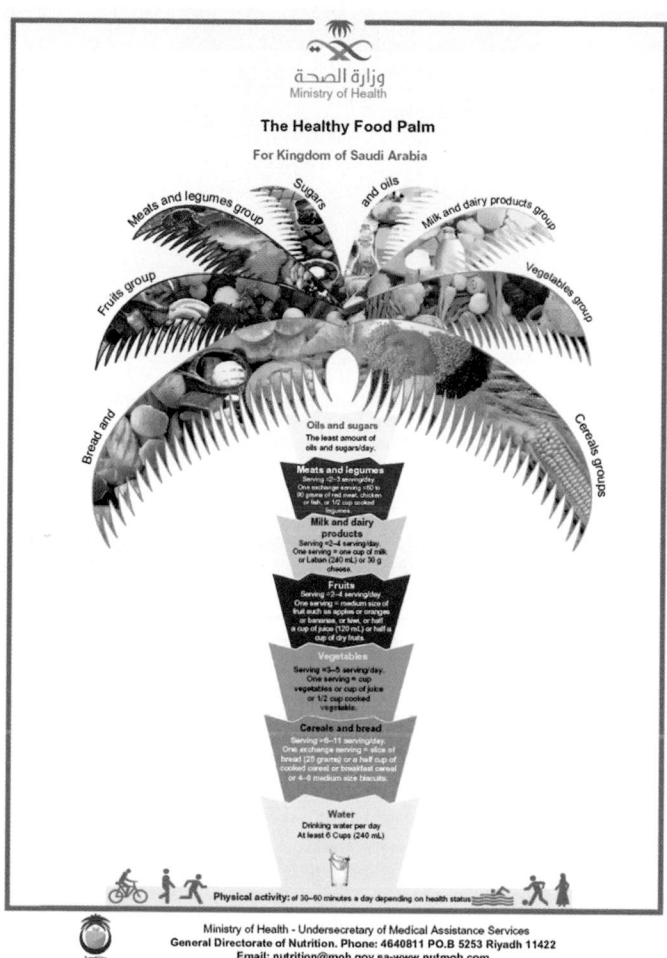

FIGURE 11-12 The Health Food Palm – For Kingdom of Saudi Arabia (Courtesy Ministry of Health. Accessed June 2015 from http://www.moh.gov.sa/en/Ministry/MediaCenter/Publications/Documents/2013-01-16-003.jpg.)

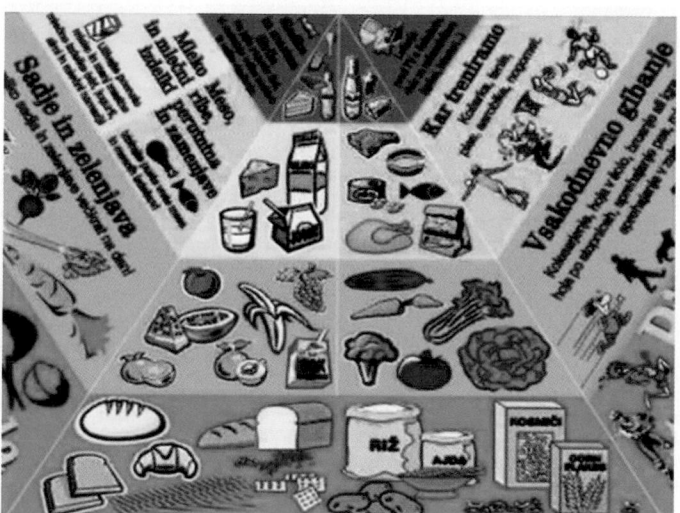

FIGURE 11-13 Food Pyramid – Slovenia (Courtesy National Institute of Public Health. Food Pyramid – Slovenia (Accessed June 2015 from http://www.eufic.org/article/en/expid/food-based-dietaryguidelines-in-europe/.)

Food Balance Wheels

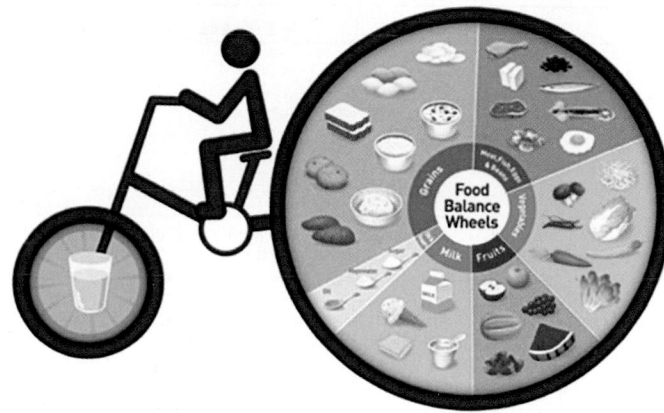

Copyright © 2010 The Korean Nutrition Society.

FIGURE 11-14 The Food Balance Wheels – Republic of Korea (Courtesy of Ministry of Health and Welfare, Republic of Korea and the Korean Nutrition Society Accessed October 2014 from http://www.inpes.sante.fr/CFESBases/catalogue/pdf/581.pdf.)

FIGURE 11-15 The eatwell plate – United Kingdom (Courtesy from Crown copyright. Public Health England in association with the Welsh government, the Scottish government and the Food Standards Agency in Northern Ireland. Accessed June 2015 from http://www.nhs.uk/Livewell/Goodfood/Pages/eatwell-plate.aspx.)

activity for more than 60 minutes daily. In males, this number decreased as weight increased (NHANES, 2012). Hypertension remains a major public health problem in middle-age and older adults and in non-Hispanic blacks in whom it increases the risk of stroke and coronary heart disease (see Chapter 33). Osteoporosis develops more often among non-Hispanic whites than non-Hispanic blacks (see Chapter 24). Concern about preventable conditions, along with an increased emphasis on sustainability, has led to many hospitals taking on the challenge for healthier food intake (see *Focus On:* The "Healthy Food in Health Care" Pledge).

TABLE 11-1 **Acceptable Macronutrient Distribution Ranges**

NUTRIENT	AMDR (PERCENTAGE OF DAILY ENERGY INTAKE)			AMDR SAMPLE DIET ADULT, 2000-KCAL/DAY DIET	
	1-3 Years	4-18 Years	>19 Years	%Reference*	g/Day
Protein[†]	5-20	10-30	10-35	10	50
Carbohydrate	45-65	45-65	45-65	60	300
Fat	30-40	25-35	20-35	30	67
α-Linolenic acid (*omega-3)[‡]	0.6-1.2	0.6-1.2	0.6-1.2	0.8	1.8
Linoleic acid (omega-6)	5-10	5-10	5-10	7	16
Added sugars[§]	≤25% of total calories			500	125

Modified from Food and Nutrition Board, Institute of Medicine: *Dietary reference intakes for energy, carbohydrate, fiber, fat, fatty acids, cholesterol, protein, and amino acids,* Washington, DC, 2002/2005: National Academies Press.
AMDR, Acceptable macronutrient distribution range; *DHA,* docosahexaenoic acid; *DRI,* dietary reference intakes; *EPA,* eicosapentaenoic acid.
*Suggested maximum.
[†]Higher number in protein AMDR is set to complement AMDRs for carbohydrate and fat, not because it is a recommended upper limit in the range of calories from protein.
[‡]Up to 10% of the AMDR for α-linolenic acid can be consumed as EPA, DHA, or both (0.06%-0.12% of calories).
[§]Reference percentages chosen based on average DRI for protein for adult men and women, then calculated back to percentage of calories. Carbohydrate and fat percentages chosen based on difference from protein and balanced with other federal dietary recommendations.

◎ FOCUS ON

The "Healthy Food in Health Care" Pledge

Health care facilities across the nation have recognized that their systems of purchasing, producing, and distributing food may be misaligned with the U.S. dietary guidelines and have joined a movement to change their practices. One organization promoting this plan is called "Health Care Without Harm." In 2009, The American Medical Association (AMA) approved a new policy resolution in support of practices and policies within health care systems that promote and model a healthy and ecologically sustainable food system. The resolution also calls on the AMA to work with health care and public health organizations to educate the health care community and the public about the importance of healthy and ecologically sustainable food systems. Hospitals are using the online pledge form to commit to these eight steps:

1. Increase offerings of nutritionally dense foods, including fruits and vegetables.
2. Communicate to Group Purchasing Organizations an interest in identifying the source and production practices of procured foods.
3. Develop a program to source from producers that uphold the dignity of family, farmers, workers, and their communities and support sustainable systems.
4. Work with farmers, organizations, and suppliers to increase the availability of locally produced food.
5. Educate patients and the community about nutritious, socially just, and ecologically sustainable food practices and procedures.
6. Minimize or beneficially reuse food waste and support the use of food packaging that is ecologically protective.
7. Encourage vendors and food management companies to supply food that is produced in systems that support farm and farm worker health and welfare and use ecologically protective and restorative agriculture.
8. Report annually on implementation.

Modified from *Health Care without Harm* (website): https://noharm-uscanada.org/civicrm/petition/sign?sid=2. Accessed October 2014.

CLINICAL INSIGHT

Nutrition Recommendations for Canadians

The revision to Canada's Food Guide to Healthy Eating, released in 2007, developed age- and gender-specific food intake patterns. These suggested patterns include 4 to 7 servings of vegetables and fruits, 3 to 7 servings of grain products, 2 to 3 servings of milk or milk alternatives, and 1 to 3 servings of meat or meat alternatives. Canada's Eating Well with Canada's Food Guide contains four main food groupings presented in a rainbow shape.

Tips include the following:
- Eat at least one dark green and one orange vegetable each day.
- Make at least half of your grain products whole grain each day.
- Compare the Nutrition Facts table on food labels to choose products that contain less fat, saturated fat, trans fat, sugar, and sodium.
- Drink skim, 1% or 2% milk, or fortified soy beverages each day.
- Include a small amount — 30-45 ml (2-3 Tbsp) — of unsaturated fat each day.
- Eat at least two Food Guide Servings of fish each week.

It is recommended that adults accumulate at least 2½ hours of moderate to vigorous physical activity each week and that children and youth accumulate at least 60 minutes per day. The Canadian Food Guide recognizes the cultural, spiritual, and physical importance of traditional Aboriginal foods as well as the role of nontraditional foods in contemporary diets, with a First Nations, Inuit, and Métis guide available. The guide is available in 12 languages.

Data from Health Canada: *Eating Well with Canada's Food Guide, Her Majesty the Queen in Right of Canada, represented by the Minister of Health Canada, 2011* (website): from http://www.hc-sc.gc.ca/fn-an/food-guide-aliment/index-eng.php. Eating Well with Canada's Food Guide – First Nations, Inuit, and Métis accessed October 2014 from http://hc-sc.gc.ca/fn-an/pubs/fnim-pnim/index-eng.php. Accessed October 2014.

Finally, in spite of available choices, many Americans experience **food insecurity**, meaning that they lack access to adequate and safe food for an active, healthy life. Table 11-2 provides a list of food components and public health concerns related to those components.

Healthy Eating Index

The Center for Nutrition Policy and Promotion of the USDA releases the **Healthy Eating Index (HEI)** to measure how well people's diets conform to recommended healthy eating patterns. The index provides a picture of foods people are

TABLE 11-2 Food Components and Public Health Concerns

Food Component	Relevance to Public Health
Energy	The high prevalence of overweight indicates that an energy imbalance exists among Americans because of physical inactivity and underreporting of energy intake or food consumption in national surveys.
Total fat, saturated fat, and cholesterol	Intakes of fat, saturated fatty acids, and cholesterol among all age groups older than 2 years of age are above recommended levels. Cholesterol intakes are generally within the recommended range of 300 mg/dl or less.
Alcohol	Intake of alcohol is a public health concern because it displaces food sources of nutrients and has potential health consequences.
Iron and calcium	Low intakes of iron and calcium continue to be a public health concern, particularly among infants and females of childbearing age. Prevalence of iron deficiency anemia is higher among these groups than among other age and sex groups. Low calcium intake is a particular concern among adolescent girls and adult women in most racial and ethnic groups.
Sodium*	Sodium intake exceeds government recommendations of 2300 mg/day in most age and sex groups. Strategies to lower intake can be found at the Institute of Medicine website at http://www.iom.edu/Reports/2010/Strategies-to-Reduce-Sodium-Intake-in-the-United-States.aspx.
Other nutrients at potential risk	Some population or age groups may consume insufficient amounts of total carbohydrate and carbohydrate constituents such as dietary fiber; protein; vitamin A; carotenoids; antioxidant vitamins C and E; folate, vitamins B_6 and B_{12}; magnesium, potassium, zinc, copper, selenium, phosphorus, and fluoride. Studies also suggest that vitamin D deficiency is very common.
Imbalanced Nutrients	Intakes of polyunsaturated and monounsaturated fatty acids, trans-fatty acids, and fat substitutes are often excessive.

*Recommended intake of 1500 mg or less in at-risk populations defined as African Americans, people with hypertension, diabetes, or chronic kidney disease, and anyone 51 years or older (Dietary Guidelines for Americans, 2010).

eating, the amount of variety in their diets, and compliance with specific recommendations in the Dietary Guidelines for Americans (DGA). The HEI is designed to assess and monitor the dietary status of Americans by evaluating 12 components, each representing different aspects of a healthy diet. The HEI was last updated after the release of the 2010 DGA. The dietary components used in HEI-2010 include nine related to adequacy: whole fruit, total fruit, whole grains, dairy, total protein foods, seafood and plant proteins, greens and beans, total vegetables, fatty acids, and three for which moderation is recommended: refined grains, sodium, and empty calories (Guenther et al, 2013). The reports from HEI-2010 noted the suboptimal quality of the American diet, for adults as well as children and adolescents, revealing an inadequate intake of beans and dark green vegetables, and the need to substitute whole grains for refined grains more frequently. Americans also need to decrease sodium intake and reduce consumption of empty calories from added sugars and solid fats.

NATIONAL GUIDELINES FOR DIET PLANNING

Eating can be one of life's greatest pleasures. People eat for enjoyment and to obtain energy and nutrients. Although many genetic, environmental, behavioral, and cultural factors affect health, diet is equally important for promoting health and preventing disease. Over the past several decades, attention has been focused increasingly on the relationship of nutrition to chronic diseases and conditions. Although this interest derives somewhat from the increasing percentage of older adults in the population as well as their longevity, it also is prompted by the desire to prevent premature deaths from diseases such as coronary heart disease, diabetes mellitus, and cancer. Approximately two thirds of deaths in the United States are caused by chronic disease.

Current Dietary Guidance

In 1969 President Nixon convened the White House Conference on Nutrition and Health (White House conference on food, nutrition and health, 1969). Increased attention was being given to prevention of hunger and disease. The development of dietary guidelines in the United States is discussed in Chapter 9. Guidelines directed toward prevention of a

particular disease, such as those from the National Cancer Institute; the American Diabetes Association; the American Heart Association; and the National Heart, Lung, and Blood Institute's cholesterol education guidelines, contain recommendations unique to particular conditions. The Academy of Nutrition and Dietetics supports a total diet approach, in which the overall pattern of food eaten, consumed in moderation with appropriate portion sizes and combined with regular physical activity, is key (Academy of Nutrition and Dietetics, 2013). Various guidelines that can be used by health counselors throughout the developed world are summarized in Box 11-1.

Implementing the Guidelines

The task of planning nutritious meals centers on including the essential nutrients in sufficient amounts as outlined in the most recent DRIs, in addition to appropriate amounts of energy, protein, carbohydrate (including fiber and sugars), fat (especially saturated and trans fats), cholesterol, and sodium. Suggestions are included to help people meet the specifics of the recommendations. When specific numeric recommendations differ, they are presented as ranges.

BOX 11-1 Universal Prescription for Health and Nutritional Fitness

- Adjust energy intake and exercise level to achieve and maintain appropriate body weight.
- Eat a wide variety of foods to ensure nutrient adequacy.
- Increase total carbohydrate intake, especially complex carbohydrates.
- Eat less total fat and less saturated fat.
- Eat more fiber-rich foods, including whole grains, fruits, and vegetables.
- Limit or omit high-sodium foods.
- Reduce intake of concentrated sugars.
- Drink alcohol in moderation or not at all.
- Meet the recommendations for calcium, especially important for adolescents and women.
- Meet the recommendation for iron, especially for children, adolescents, and women of childbearing age.
- Limit protein to no more than twice the recommended dietary allowance.
- If using a daily multivitamin, choose dietary supplements that do not exceed the recommended dietary allowance.
- Drink fluoridated water.

BOX 11-2 The 2015 Dietary Guidelines for Americans

1. Follow a healthy eating pattern across the lifespan.
2. Focus on variety, nutrient density, and amount.
3. Limit calories from added sugars and saturated fats and reduce sodium intake.
4. Shift to healthier food and beverage choices.
5. Support healthy eating patterns for all.

Accessed January 2016 from http://www.health.gov/dietaryguidelines/2015/guidelines/.

To help people select an eating pattern that achieves specific health promotion or disease prevention objectives, nutritionists should assist individuals in making food choices (e.g., to reduce saturated fat, to increase fiber). Although numerous federal agencies are involved in the issuance of dietary guidance, the USDA and DHHS lead the effort. The DGA first were published in 1980 and are revised every 5 years; the 2015 guidelines are included (Box 11-2). The DGA are designed to help nutrition and health professionals assist the public (> age 2) in consuming a healthy diet. The information in the DGA is used by the Federal government to create educational materials for consumers and helps guide development of Federal health policies and programs. initiatives (U.S. Department of Health and Human Services, 2015).

FOOD AND NUTRIENT LABELING

To help consumers make choices between similar types of food products that can be incorporated into a healthy diet, the FDA established a voluntary system of providing selected nutrient information on food labels. The regulatory framework for nutrition information on food labels was revised and updated by the USDA (which regulates meat, poultry products and eggs) and the FDA (which regulates all other foods) with enactment of the Nutrition Labeling and Education Act (NLEA) in 1990. The labels became mandatory in 1994. In 2014 changes to the layout of information on the food label were proposed, to help consumers make better informed decisions, placing greater emphasis on calorie content and serving size, as well as replacing nutrients abundant in the food supply (e.g., vitamin A) with those that are underconsumed by certain population groups (e.g., potassium). The new labels also include a separate line for added sugars, because many health experts recommend decreasing intake of sugars in favor of more nutrient-dense foods, as well as to help decrease overall caloric intake (Figure 11-15).

Mandatory Nutrition Labeling

As a result of the NLEA, nutrition labels must appear on most foods, except products that provide few nutrients (such as coffee and spices), restaurant foods, and ready-to-eat foods prepared on site, such as supermarket bakery and deli items. Providing nutrition information on many raw foods is voluntary. However, the FDA and USDA have called for a voluntary point-of-purchase program in which nutrition information is available in most supermarkets. Nutrition information is provided through brochures or point-of-purchase posters for the 20 most popular fruits, vegetables, and fresh fish and the 45 major cuts of fresh meat and poultry. In addition, many food processors in the United States and elsewhere are using front-of-package labeling that employs a score, symbols, or color coding to reflect a product's overall nutrient content. Examples of front-of-package labeling include Smart Choices, NuVal, Guiding Stars, or the "traffic light" color-coding system used in the United Kingdom.

Nutrition information for foods purchased in restaurants is widely available at the point of purchase or from websites. New FDA regulations require restaurant chains, retail food establishments, and vending machines with 20 or more locations to disclose calorie information on their menus or menu board (or on a sign or sticker on or adjacent to the vending machine). Additional nutrient information that must be made available upon request include total calories, calories from fat, total fat, saturated fat, trans fat, cholesterol, sodium, total carbohydrates, fiber, sugars, and protein.

The new regulations also cover ready-to-eat unpackaged foods in delicatessens or supermarkets that meet requirements above. If a food makes the claim of being organic, it also must meet certain criteria and labeling requirements.

Standardized Serving Sizes on Food Labels

Serving sizes of products are set by the United States government based on reference amounts commonly consumed by Americans. For example, a serving of milk is 8 oz, and a serving of salad dressing is 2 tbsp. Standardized serving sizes make it easier for consumers to compare the nutrient contents of similar products (Figure 11-16).

Nutrition Facts Label

The **nutrition facts label** on a food product provides information on its per-serving calories and calories from fat. The label must list the amount (in grams) of total fat, saturated fat, trans fat, cholesterol, sodium, total carbohydrate, dietary fiber, sugar, and protein. For most of these nutrients the label also shows the

Nutrition Facts

Serving Size:About (20g)
Servings Per Container:16

	Amount Per Serving	%Daily Value*
Total Calories	60	
Calories From Fat	15	
Total Fat	2 g	3%
Saturated Fat	1 g	4%
Trans Fat	0 g	
Cholesterol	0 mg	0%
Sodium	45 mg	2%
Total Carbohydrates	15 g	5%
Dietary Fiber	4 g	17%
Sugars	4 g	
Sugar Alcohols (Polyols)	3 g	
Protein	2 g	
Vitamin A		0%
Vitamin C		0%
Calcium		2%
Iron		2%

*Percent Daily Values are based on a 2,000 calorie diet.

Ingredients: Wheat flour,unsweetened chocolate, erythritol, inulin, oat flour, cocoa power, evaporated cane juice, whey protein concencrate, corn starch (low glycemic), natural flavors, salt, baking soda, wheat gluten, guar gurn

FIGURE 11-16 Standard food label showing serving size.

percentage of the **daily value (DV)** supplied by a serving, showing how a product fits into an overall diet by comparing its nutrient content with recommended intakes of those nutrients (Table 11-3). DVs are not recommended intakes for individuals; they are simply reference points to provide some perspective on daily nutrient needs and are based on a 2000-kcal diet. For example, individuals who consume diets supplying more or fewer calories can still use the DVs as a rough guide to ensure that they are getting adequate amounts of vitamin C, for example, but not too much saturated fat.

The DVs are listed for nutrients for which RDAs already exist (in which case they are known as **reference daily intakes [RDIs]**) (Table 11-4) and for which no RDAs exist (in which case they are known as **daily reference values [DRVs]** [Table 11-5]). However, food labels use only the term *daily value*. RDIs provide a large margin of safety; in general, the RDI for a nutrient is greater than the RDA for a specific age group. As new DRIs are developed in various categories, labeling laws are updated. Box 11-3 provides tips for reading and understanding food labels.

Nutrient Content Claims

Nutrient content terms such as *reduced sodium, fat free, low-calorie,* and *healthy* must meet government definitions that apply to all foods (Box 11-4). For example, *lean* refers to a serving of meat, poultry, seafood, or game meat with less than 10 g of fat, less than 4 g of saturated fat, and less than 95 mg of

TABLE 11-3 Daily Value (Based on 2000 kcal Diet)

Nutrient	Amount
Total Fat	65 grams (g)
Saturated Fat	20 g
Cholesterol	300 milligrams (mg)
Sodium	2,400 mg
Potassium	3,500 mg
Total Carbohydrate	300 g
Dietary Fiber	25 g
Protein	50 g
Vitamin A	5,000 International Units (IU)
Vitamin C	60 mg
Calcium	1,000 mg
Iron	18 mg
Vitamin D	400 IU
Vitamin E	30 IU
Vitamin K	80 micrograms μg
Thiamin	1.5 mg
Riboflavin	1.7 mg
Niacin	20 mg
Vitamin B$_6$	2 mg
Folate	400 μg
Vitamin B$_{12}$	6 μg
Biotin	300 μg
Pantothenic acid	10 mg
Phosphorus	1,000 mg
Iodine	150 μg
Magnesium	400 mg
Zinc	15 mg
Selenium	70 μg
Copper	2 mg
Manganese	2 mg
Chromium	120 μg
Molybdenum	75 μg
Chloride	3,400 mg

From Guidance for Industry: A Food Labeling Guide (14. Appendix F: Calculate the Percent Daily Value for the Appropriate Nutrients)

TABLE 11-4 Reference Daily Intakes

Nutrient	Amount
Vitamin A	5000 IU
Vitamin C	60 mg
Thiamin	1.5 mg
Riboflavin	1.7 mg
Niacin	20 mg
Calcium	1000 mg
Iron	18 mg
Vitamin D	400 IU
Vitamin E	30 IU
Vitamin B$_6$	2 mg
Folic acid	400 μg
Vitamin B$_{12}$	6 μg
Phosphorus	1000 mg
Iodine	150 μg
Magnesium	400 mg
Zinc	15 mg
Copper	2 mg
Biotin	300 μg
Pantothenic acid	10 mg
Selenium	70 μg

From Center for Food Safety & Applied Nutrition: *A food labeling guide*, College Park, Md, 1994, US Department of Agriculture, revised 2013.

TABLE 11-5 Daily Reference Values

Food Component	DRV	Calculation
Fat	65 g	30% of kcal
Saturated fat	20 g	10% of kcal
Cholesterol	300 mg	Same regardless of kcal
Carbohydrates (total)	300 g	60% of calories
Fiber	25 g	11.5 g per 1000 kcal
Protein	50 g	10% of kcal
Sodium	2400 mg	Same regardless of kcal
Potassium	3500 mg	Same regardless of kcal

DRV, Daily reference value.
NOTE: The DRVs were established for adults and children over 4 years old. The values for energy yielding nutrients below are based on 2000 calories per day.

BOX 11-3 Tips for Reading and Understanding Food Labels

Interpret the Percent Daily Value.

- Nutrients with %DV of 5 or less are considered low or poor sources
- Nutrients with %DV of 10-19 or less are considered moderate or "good sources."
- Nutrients with %DV of 20 or more are considered high or "rich sources."

Prioritize nutrient needs and compare %DV levels accordingly. For example, if a consumer wishes to lower osteoporosis risk versus limiting sodium, a packaged food containing 25%DV calcium and 15%DV sodium may be considered a sensible food selection.

Note the calories per serving and the servings per container. Consider how the energy value of a specific food fits into the total energy intake "equation." Be conscious of the portion size that is consumed and "do the math" as to how many servings per container that portion would be.

Be aware of specific nutrient content claims. As shown in Box 11-4, there are many nutrient content claims, but only specific ones may relate to personal health priorities. For example, if there is a positive family history for heart disease, the "low fat" nutrient claim of 3 grams or less per serving may serve as a useful guide during food selection.

Review the ingredient list. Ingredients are listed in order of prominence. Pay particular attention to the top five items listed. Ingredients that contain sugar often end in *-ose*. The term *hydrogenated* signals that trans fats may be present. Sodium-containing additives also may be present in multiple forms.

BOX 11-4 Nutrient Content Claims

Free: *Free* means that a product contains no amount of, or only trivial or "physiologically inconsequential" amounts of, one or more of these components: fat, saturated fat, cholesterol, sodium, sugar, or calories. For example, *calorie-free* means the product contains fewer than 5 calories per serving, and *sugar-free* and *fat-free* both mean the product contains less than 0.5 g per serving. Synonyms for *free* include *without, no,* and *zero.* A synonym for fat-free milk is *skim.*

Low: *Low* can be used on foods that can be eaten frequently without exceeding dietary guidelines for one or more of these components: fat, saturated fat, cholesterol, sodium, and calories. Synonyms for low include *little, few, low source of,* and *contains a small amount of.*
- **Low fat:** 3 g or less per serving
- **Low saturated fat:** 1 g or less per serving
- **Low sodium:** 140 mg or less per serving
- **Very low sodium:** 35 mg or less per serving
- **Low cholesterol:** 20 mg or less and 2 g or less of saturated fat per serving
- **Low calorie:** 40 calories or less per serving

Lean and extra lean: *Lean* and *extra lean* can be used to describe the fat content of meat, poultry, seafood, and game meats.
- **Lean:** less than 10 g fat, 4.5 g or less saturated fat, and less than 95 mg cholesterol per serving and per 100 g
- **Extra lean:** less than 5 g fat, less than 2 g saturated fat, and less than 95 mg cholesterol per serving and per 100 g

Reduced: *Reduced* means that a nutritionally altered product contains at least 25% less of a nutrient or of calories than the regular, or reference, product. However, a *reduced* claim cannot be made on a product if its reference food already meets the requirement for a "low" claim.

Less: *Less* means that a food, whether altered or not, contains 25% less of a nutrient or of calories than the reference food. For example, pretzels that have 25% less fat than potato chips could carry a *less* claim. *Fewer* is an acceptable synonym.

Light: *Light* can mean two things:
- First, that a nutritionally altered product contains one-third fewer calories or half the fat of the reference food. If the food derives 50% or more of its calories from fat, the reduction must be 50% of the fat.
- Second that the sodium content of a low-calorie, low-fat food has been reduced by 50%. In addition, *light in sodium* may be used on food in which the sodium content has been reduced by at least 50%.
- The term *light* still can be used to describe such properties as texture and color, as long as the label explains the intent (e.g., *light brown sugar* and *light and fluffy*).

High: *High* can be used if the food contains 20% or more of the daily value for a particular nutrient in a serving.

Good source: *Good source* means that one serving of a food contains 10% to 19% of the daily value for a particular nutrient.

More: *More* means that a serving of food, whether altered or not, contains a nutrient that is at least 10% of the daily value more than the reference food. The 10% of daily value also applies to *fortified, enriched, added, extra,* and *plus* claims, but in these cases the food must be altered.

Data adapted from Food and Drug Administration. Accessed October 2014 from http://www.fda.gov/food/guidanceregulation/guidancedocumentsregulatoryinformation/labelingnutrition/ucm064911.htm and http://www.fda.gov/Food/GuidanceRegulation/GuidanceDocumentsRegulatoryInformation/LabelingNutrition/ucm064916.htm.

cholesterol per serving or per 100 g. Extra lean meat or poultry contains less than 5 g of fat, less than 2 g of saturated fat, and the same cholesterol content as lean, per serving, or per 100 g of product.

Health Claims

A health claim is allowed only on appropriate food products that meet specified standards. The government requires that health claims be worded in ways that are not misleading (e.g., the claim cannot imply that the food product itself helps prevent disease). Health claims cannot appear on foods that supply more than 20% of the DV for fat, saturated fat, cholesterol, and sodium. The following is an example of a health claim for dietary fiber and cancer: "Low-fat diets rich in fiber-containing grain products, fruits, and vegetables may reduce the risk of some types of cancer, a disease associated with many factors." Box 11-5 lists health claims that manufacturers can use to describe food-disease relationships. In 2013 the FDA added a regulation that defines "gluten-free," to clarify its voluntary use in food labeling and to help consumers with celiac disease to avoid foods containing gluten (see Chapters 26 and 28).

BOX 11-5 Health Claims for Diet-Disease Relationships

Calcium and Osteoporosis
- "Adequate calcium throughout life, as part of a well-balanced diet, may reduce the risk of osteoporosis."

Calcium, Vitamin D, and Osteoporosis
- "Adequate calcium and vitamin D, as part of a well-balanced diet, along with physical activity, may reduce the risk of osteoporosis."

Sodium and Hypertension
- "Diets low in sodium may reduce the risk of high blood pressure, a disease associated with many factors."

Dietary Fat and Cancer
- "Development of cancer depends on many factors. A diet low in total fat may reduce the risk of some cancers."

Dietary Saturated Fat and Cholesterol and Risk of Coronary Heart Disease
- "While many factors affect heart disease, diets low in saturated fat and cholesterol may reduce the risk of this disease."

Fiber-Containing Grain Products, Fruits, and Vegetables and Cancer
- "Low-fat diets rich in fiber-containing grain products, fruits, and vegetables may reduce the risk of some types of cancer, a disease associated with many factors."

Fruits, Vegetables and Grain Products That Contain Fiber, Particularly Soluble Fiber, and Risk of Coronary Heart Disease
- "Diets low in saturated fat and cholesterol and rich in fruits, vegetables, and grain products that contain some types of dietary fiber, particularly soluble fiber, may reduce the risk of heart disease, a disease associated with many factors."

Fruits and Vegetables and Cancer
- "Low-fat diets rich in fruits and vegetables [*foods that are low in fat and may contain dietary fiber, vitamin A, or vitamin C*] may reduce the risk of some types of cancer, a disease associated with many factors. Broccoli is high in vitamin A and C, and it is a good source of dietary fiber."

BOX 11-5   Health Claims for Diet-Disease Relationships—cont'd

Folate and Neural Tube Defects

- "Healthful diets with adequate folate may reduce a woman's risk of having a child with a brain or spinal cord defect."

Dietary Noncariogenic Carbohydrate Sweeteners and Dental Caries

- Full claim: "Frequent between-meal consumption of foods high in sugars and starches promotes tooth decay. The sugar alcohols in [name of food] do not promote tooth decay"; Shortened claim on small packages only: "Does not promote tooth decay."

Soluble Fiber from Certain Foods and Risk of Coronary Heart Disease

- "Soluble fiber from foods such as [name of soluble fiber source, and, if desired, name of food product], as part of a diet low in saturated fat and cholesterol, may reduce the risk of heart disease. A serving of [name of food product] supplies __ grams of the [necessary daily dietary intake for the benefit] soluble fiber from [name of soluble fiber source] necessary per day to have this effect."

Soy Protein and Risk of Coronary Heart Disease

- "25 grams of soy protein a day, as part of a diet low in saturated fat and cholesterol, may reduce the risk of heart disease. A serving of [name of food] supplies __ grams of soy protein."
- "Diets low in saturated fat and cholesterol that include 25 grams of soy protein a day may reduce the risk of heart disease. One serving of [name of food] provides __ grams of soy protein."

Plant Sterol/Stanol Esters and Risk of Coronary Heart Disease

"Foods containing at least 0.65 gram per of vegetable oil sterol esters, eaten twice a day with meals for a daily total intake of least 1.3 grams, as part of a diet low in saturated fat and cholesterol, may reduce the risk of heart disease. A serving of [name of food] supplies __ grams of vegetable oil sterol esters."

"Diets low in saturated fat and cholesterol that include two servings of foods that provide a daily total of at least 3.4 grams of plant stanol esters in two meals may reduce the risk of heart disease. A serving of [name of food] supplies __ grams of plant stanol esters."

FDA Modernization Act Health Claims

Whole Grain Foods and Risk of Heart Disease and Certain Cancers

- "Diets rich in whole grain foods and other plant foods and low in total fat, saturated fat, and cholesterol may reduce the risk of heart disease and some cancers."

Potassium and the Risk of High Blood Pressure and Stroke

- "Diets containing foods that are a good source of potassium and that are low in sodium may reduce the risk of high blood pressure and stroke."

Fluoridated Water and Reduced Risk of Dental Carries

- "Drinking fluoridated water may reduce the risk of [dental caries or tooth decay]."

Saturated Fat, Cholesterol, and Trans Fat, and Reduced Risk of Heart Disease

- "Diets low in saturated fat and cholesterol, and as low as possible in trans fat, may reduce the risk of heart disease."

Substitution of Saturated Fat in the Diet with Unsaturated Fatty Acids and Reduced Risk of Heart Disease

- "Replacing saturated fat with similar amounts of unsaturated fats may reduce the risk of heart disease. To achieve this benefit, total daily calories should not increase."

Data from Food and Drug Administration (website): http://www.fda.gov/Food/GuidanceRegulation/GuidanceDocumentsRegulatoryInformation/LabelingNutrition/ucm2006828.htm. Accessed October 2014.

DIETARY PATTERNS AND COUNSELING TIPS

Vegetarian Diet Patterns

Vegetarian diets are popular. Those who choose them may be motivated by philosophic, religious, or ecologic concerns, or by a desire to have a healthier lifestyle. Considerable evidence attests to the health benefits of a vegetarian diet. For example, studies of Seventh-Day Adventists indicate that the diet helps lower rates of metabolic syndrome (Rizzo et al, 2011).

Of the millions of Americans who call themselves **vegetarians**, many eliminate "red" meats but eat fish, poultry, and dairy products. A **lactovegetarian** does not eat meat, fish, poultry, or eggs but does consume milk, cheese, and other dairy products. A **lactoovovegetarian** also consumes eggs. A **vegan** does not eat any food of animal origin. The vegan diet is the only vegetarian diet that has any real risk of providing inadequate nutrition, but this risk can be avoided by careful planning (American Dietetic Association, 2009). A type of **semivegetarian** is known as a **flexitarian**. Flexitarians generally adhere to a vegetarian diet for the purpose of good health and do not follow a specific ideology. They view an occasional meat meal as acceptable. A public health awareness campaign called Meatless Monday advocates that Americans have a vegetarian meal at least one day per week to help reduce the incidence of preventable chronic health conditions such as diabetes, obesity, and cardiovascular disease.

Vegetarian diets tend to be lower in iron than omnivorous diets, although the nonheme iron in fruits, vegetables, and unrefined cereals usually is accompanied either in the food or in the meal by large amounts of ascorbic acid that aids in iron assimilation. Vegetarians do not have a greater risk of iron deficiency than those who are not vegetarians (American Dietetic Association, 2009). Vegetarians who consume no dairy products may have low calcium intakes, and vitamin D intakes may be inadequate among those in northern latitudes where there is less exposure to sunshine. The calcium in some vegetables is made unavailable for absorption by the presence of oxalates. Although phytates in unrefined cereals also can make calcium unavailable, this is not a problem for Western vegetarians, whose diets tend to be based more on fruits and vegetables than on the unrefined cereals of Middle Eastern cultures.

Long-term vegans may develop megaloblastic anemia because of a deficiency of vitamin B_{12}, found only in foods of animal origin. The high levels of folate in vegan diets may mask the neurologic damage of a vitamin B_{12} deficiency. Vegans should have a reliable source of vitamin B_{12} such as fortified breakfast cereals, soy beverages, or a supplement. Although most vegetarians meet or exceed the requirements for protein, their diets tend to be lower in protein than those of omnivores. Lower protein intake usually results in lower saturated fat intake because many high-protein animal products are also rich in saturated fat (American Dietetic Association, 2009).

Well-planned vegetarian diets are safe for infants, children, and adolescents and can meet all of their nutritional requirements for growth. They are also adequate for pregnant and lactating females. The key is that the diets be well planned. Vegetarians should pay special attention to ensure that they get adequate calcium, iron, zinc, and vitamins B_{12} and D. Calculated combinations of complementary protein sources is not necessary, especially if protein sources are reasonably varied. Useful information on vegetarian meal planning is available at http://www. eatright.org/Public/list.aspx?TaxID=6442452074&page=1 through the Academy of Nutrition and Dietetics.

CULTURAL ASPECTS OF DIETARY PLANNING

To plan diets for individuals or groups that are appropriate from a health and nutrition perspective, registered dietitian nutritionists and health providers must use resources that are targeted to the specific client or group. Numerous population subgroups in the United States and throughout the world have specific cultural, ethnic, or religious beliefs and practices to consider. These groups have their own set of dietary practices, which are important when considering dietary planning (Diabetes Care and Education Dietetic Practice Group, 2010). The IOM report entitled *Unequal Treatment* recommended that all health care professionals receive training in cross-cultural communication to help reduce ethnic and racial disparities in health care. Cultural competence training improves the skills and attitudes of the clinician and can facilitate a dialogue that encourages the client to share more information during a session (Betancourt and Green, 2010).

Attitudes, rituals, and practices surrounding food are part of every culture in the world, and there are so many cultures that it defies enumeration. Many world cultures have influenced American cultures as a result of immigration and intermarriage. This makes planning a menu that embraces cultural diversity and is sensitive to the needs of a specific group of people a major challenge. It is tempting to simplify the role of culture by attempting to categorize dietary patterns by race, ethnicity, or religion. However, this type of generalizing can lead to inappropriate labeling and misunderstanding.

To illustrate this point, consider the case of Native Americans. There are more than 550 different federally recognized tribes in 35 states. The food and customs of the tribes in the Southwest are different from those of the Northwest. With traditional foods among Native Americans, the situation is complicated further by the fact that many tribes were removed from their traditional lands in the nineteenth century by the government. Another example of the complexity of diet and culture in the United States is that of African Americans. "Soul food" is commonly identified with African Americans from the South. Traditional food choices, likely borne out of hard times, limited choices, and creativity, may include greens such as collards, mustard, kale, prepared with pork; beans, field peas, yams, fried meats, grits, and cornbread. However, this by no means represents the diet of all African Americans. Similarly, the diet of Mexican Americans does not necessarily equal that of immigrants from Central America.

When faced with planning a diet to meet the needs of an unfamiliar culture, it is important to avoid forming opinions that are based on inaccurate information or stereotyping (see Chapter 14). Some cultural food guides have even been developed for specific populations to help manage disease conditions.

Religion and Food

Dietary practices have been a component of religious practice for all of recorded history. Some religions forbid the eating of certain foods and beverages; others restrict foods and drinks during holy days. Specific dietary rituals may be assigned to members with designated authority or with special spiritual power (e.g., a *shohet,* certified to slaughter animals in accordance with Jewish law). Sometimes dietary rituals or restrictions are observed based on gender. Dietary and food preparation practices (e.g., halal and kosher meat preparation) can be associated with rituals of faith.

Fasting is practiced by many religions. It has been identified as a mechanism that allows one to improve one's body, to earn approval or to understand and appreciate the sufferings of others. Attention to specific eating behaviors such as overeating, use of alcoholic or stimulant-containing beverages, and vegetarianism also are considered by some religions. Before planning menus for members of any religious group, clinicians must gain an understanding of the traditions or dietary practices (Table 11-6). In all

TABLE 11-6   Some Religious Dietary Practices

	Buddhist	Hindu	Jewish (Orthodox)	Muslim	Christian Roman Catholic	Christian Eastern Orthodox	Christian Mormon	Christian Seventh Day Adventist
Beef	A	X						A
Pork	A	A	X	X				X
Meats, all	A	A	R	R	R	R		A
Eggs/dairy	O	O	R			R		O
Fish	A	R	R			R		A
Shellfish	A	R	X			O		X
Alcohol		A		X			X	X
Coffee/tea				A			X	X
Meat/dairy at same meal			X					
Leavened foods			R					
Ritual slaughter of meats			+	+				
Moderation	+			+				+
Fasting*	+	+	+	+	+	+	+	+

Modified from Kittler PG et al: *Food and culture,* ed 6, Belmont, Calif, 2011, Wadsworth/Cengage Learning; Escott-Stump S: *Nutrition and diagnosis-related care,* ed 7, Baltimore, Md, 2011, Lippincott Williams & Wilkins.

+, Practiced; *A,* avoided by the most devout; *O,* permitted, but may be avoided at some observances; *R,* some restrictions regarding types of foods or when a food may be eaten; *X,* prohibited or strongly discouraged.

*Fasting varies from partial (abstention from certain foods or meals) to complete (no food or drink).

cases, discussing the personal dietary preferences of an individual is imperative (Kittler et al, 2011).

Health Literacy

A critical yet often overlooked aspect of communication with individuals or groups about an optimal diet is the audience's level of health literacy. The average American reads at an eighth grade level and 20% read at or below a fifth grade level. A systematic review of nutrition and health literacy found that several gaps exist, including lack of training in health literacy and unfamiliarity with readability assessments and other health literacy screening tools (Carbone and Zoellner, 2012). Several readability tests exist that use criteria such as sentence length and number of multisyllabic words to produce a score and then either translate that score to a U.S. grade level, or compare it to a desired value. For example, the Flesch Reading Ease algorithm uses the average number of words in a sentence and average number of syllables per word, producing a score that ideally should be 60 or higher. Nutrition professionals should be familiar with these indices, especially if they write for the media or contribute to or manage a website.

◎ FOCUS ON

What Is a Locavore?

There is a growing movement in the United States fueled by books like *Animal, Vegetable, Miracle: A Year of Food Life* (Kingsolver, 2007) and *The Omnivore's Dilemma* (Pollan, 2008) to build a more locally based, self-reliant food economy. The movement is one in which sustainable food production, processing, distribution, and consumption are integrated to enhance the economic, environmental, and social health of a particular area. A *locavore,* a term whose creation is attributed to Jessica Prentice in conjunction with World Environment Day in 2005 (Oxford University Press blog, 2007), is one who eats food grown or produced locally or within a certain limited radius. The locavore movement encourages consumers to buy from farmers' markets or even to produce their own food. They argue that locally produced food is fresher and more nutritious and uses less fossil fuel to grow and transport. Another component of this movement is the condemnation of the factory farming method of grain feeding animals, known as concentrated animal feeding operations. There is a growing demand for meat that is grass or range fed and not transported long distances.

The locavore movement is not without its critics, however. In his essay, *"Green" Eggs and Ham? The Myth of Sustainable Meat and the Danger of the Local,* Vasile Stănescu challenges the "food miles" concept that long-distance distribution of food creates greater greenhouse gas emissions, noting that the production phase actually produces significantly more emissions than the distribution phase (Stănescu, 2010). As an example, he cites a study showing that fewer emissions were produced when consumers in the United Kingdom bought certain food items from New Zealand compared with the same items produced in Britain (Saunders et al, 2006). Some authors have suggested that a shift from a meat-based to a plant-based diet would have the greatest impact on greenhouse gas emissions (Weber and Matthews, 2008). In any case, concern about the environment among nutrition professionals, particularly as it relates to food production and distribution, has moved from the fringe to the mainstream.

◎ FOCUS ON

Nutrition Transition

Sudha Raj PhD, RDN, FAND

The term *nutrition transition,* coined in the early 1990s, describes alterations in diet, body composition, and physical activity patterns in people in developing countries undergoing rapid urbanization, and demographic, socioeconomic and acculturative changes (Popkin, 2001; Shetty, 2013). The shifts in traditional ways, value systems and behaviors experienced in emerging economies such as India, China, the Middle East, North Africa, and Latin America are associated with notable increases in nutrition related chronic diseases, while infectious and nutrition related deficiency diseases persist. Consequently, these populations face a double burden of disease—the struggles of undernutrition coexist with the maladies of overnutrition within the same individual, family, or community (Schmidhuber and Shetty, 2005).

Rapid advancements in medicine, food production, and agricultural technologies, along with the liberalization of markets leading to changes in food distribution and retail, have proven to be a double-edged sword in these countries. On the one hand, enormous economic developments and health benefits have accrued; on the other, a myriad of challenges marked by nutritional imbalances and chronic disease trajectories have risen (WHO/FAO, 2013). Inequalities in income and access to quality food and health care exist. Inactive lifestyles and increased toxic burden exposure and processed food consumption at the expense of indigenous foods are important nutrition transition determinants. In addition, there is increased vulnerability of individuals because of epigenetic fetal programming changes (Barker, 2006).

Several holistic, sustainable nutrition intervention approaches using a food-based and community involvement focus are currently underway to address nutrition transition worldwide (Sunguya et al, 2014; Vorster et al, 2011). These initiatives are directed at achieving optimal and balanced nutrition for all using evidence-based interventions and timely policies (Garmendia et al, 2013).

CLINICAL CASE STUDY

Jacob is a 45-year-old Jewish male who emigrated from Israel to the United States 3 years ago. He follows a strict kosher diet. In addition, he does not drink milk but does consume other dairy products. He has a body mass index of 32 and a family history of heart disease. He has come to you for advice on increasing his calcium intake.

Nutrition Diagnostic Statement

Knowledge deficit related to calcium as evidenced by request for nutrient and dietary information

Nutrition Care Questions

1. What type of dietary guidance would you offer Jacob?
2. What type of dietary plan following strict kosher protocols would meet his daily dietary needs and promote weight loss?
3. What suggestions would you offer him about dietary choices for a healthy heart?
4. Which special steps should Jacob take to meet calcium requirements without using supplements?
5. How can food labeling information be used to help Jacob meet his weight loss and nutrient goals and incorporate his religious dietary concerns?

USEFUL WEBSITES

Academy of Nutrition and Dietetics
http://www.eatright.org

Center for Nutrition Policy and Promotion, U.S. Department of Agriculture
http://www.usda.gov/cnpp/

Centers for Disease Control—Health Literacy
http://www.cdc.gov/healthliteracy/gettraining.html

Cost of Food at Home
http://www.cnpp.usda.gov/USDAFoodCost-Home.htm

Dietary Guidelines for Americans
http://www.health.gov/DietaryGuidelines

Ethnic Food Guides
http://fnic.nal.usda.gov/professional-and-career-resources/ethnic-and-cultural-resources

European Food and Information Council
http://www.eufic.org

Food and Drug Administration, Center for Food Safety and Applied Nutrition
http://www.fda.gov/AboutFDA/CentersOffices/OfficeofFoods/CFSAN/default.htm

Food and Nutrition Information Center, National Agricultural Library, U.S. Department of Agriculture
http://www.nal.usda.gov/fnic/

Health Canada
http://www.hc-sc.gc.ca/fn-an/index_e.html

Healthy Eating Index
http://www.cnpp.usda.gov/HealthyEatingIndex.htm

Institute of Medicine, National Academy of Sciences
http://www.iom.edu/

International Food Information Council Foundation
http://www.foodinsight.org

MyPlate Food Guidance System
http://www.chooseMyPlate.gov/

National Center for Health Statistics—National Health and Nutrition Examination Survey
http://www.cdc.gov/nchs/nhanes.htm

Nutrition.gov (U.S. government nutrition site)
http://www.nutrition.gov

U.S. Department of Agriculture
http://www.usda.gov

REFERENCES

Academy of Nutrition and Dietetics: Position of the Academy of Nutrition and Dietetics: Total diet approach to healthy eating, *J Acad Nutr Diet* 113:307, 2013.

American Dietetic Association (ADA): Position of the American Dietetic Association: Vegetarian diets, *J Am Diet Assoc* 109:1266, 2009.

Barker D: Commentary: birthweight and coronary heart disease in a historical cohort, *Int J Epidemiol* 35:886, 2006.

Betancourt JR, Green AR: Commentary: linking cultural competence training to improved health outcomes: perspectives from the field, *Acad Med* 85:583, 2010.

Carbone E, Zoellner J: Nutrition and health literacy: a systematic review to inform nutrition research and practice, *J Acad Nutr Diet* 112:254, 2012.

Diabetes Care and Education Dietetic Practice Group, Goody CM, Drago L, editors: Cultural food practices, Chicago, 2010, American Dietetic Association, 2010.

FAO/WHO: Preparation and use of Food-Based Dietary Guidelines. Report of a joint FAO/WHO consultation. Nicosia, Cyprus: WHO, 1996. Accessed October 2014 from www.fao.org/docrep/X0243E/x0243e00.htm.

Garmendia ML et al: Addressing malnutrition while avoiding obesity: minding the balance, *Eur J Clin Nutr* 67:513, 2013.

Guenther PM et al: Update of the Healthy eating index: HEI-2010, *J Acad Nutr Diet* 113:569, 2013.

Guia alimentar para a população Brasileira (Dietary guidelines for Brazilians). Accessed October 2014 from http://www.incaper.es.gov.br/por_dentro_incaper/uploads/files/7abd8-brazils-dietary-guidelines_2014.pdf.

Kingsolver B: *Animal, vegetable, mineral: a year of food life,* New York, 2007, HarperCollins.

Kittler PG et al: *Food and culture*, ed 6, Belmont, Calif, 2011, Wadsworth/Cengage Learning.

NHANES National Youth Fitness Survey, Centers for Disease Control and Prevention, 2012. Accessed February 2014 from http://www.cdc.gov/nchs/nnyfs.htm.

The birth of locavore, Oxford University Press blog, November 20, 2007, available at http://blog.oup.com/2007/11/prentice/.

Pollan M: *The omnivore's dilemma: a natural history of four meals,* New York, 2008, Penguin Press.

Popkin BM: The nutrition transition and obesity in the developing world, *J Nutr* 131:871S, 2001.

Rizzo NS et al: Vegetarian dietary patterns are associated with a lower risk of metabolic syndrome: The Adventist Health Study 2, *Diabetes Care* 34:1225, 2013.

Saunders C et al: Food miles—comparative energy/emissions performance of New Zealand's agriculture industry, Research Report No. 285, Lincoln University, New Zealand, 2006.

Schmidhuber J, Shetty P: The nutrition transition to 2030. Why developing countries are likely to bear the major burden, *Acta Agr Scand* 2:150, 2005.

Shetty P: Nutrition transition and its health outcomes, *Indian J Pediatr* 80(Suppl 1): S21, 2013.

Stănescu V: "Green" eggs and ham? The myth of sustainable meat and the danger of the local, *J Crit Animal Studies* 8:32, 2010.

Sunguya BF et al: Strong nutrition governance is a key to addressing nutrition transition in low and middle –income countries: review of countries' nutrition policies, *Nutr J* 13:65, 2014.

U.S. Department of Health and Human Services and U.S. Department of Agriculture. 2015 – 2020 Dietary Guidelines for Americans. 8th Edition. December 2015. Available at http://health.gov/dietaryguidelines/2015/guidelines/.

Vorster HH et al: The nutrition transition in Africa: Can it be steered into a more positive direction? *Nutrients* 3:429, 2011.

Weber CL, Matthews HS: Food-miles and the relative climate impacts of food choices in the United States, *Environ Sci Technol* 42:3508, 2008.

White House conference on food, nutrition and health, *Am J Clin Nutr* 11:1543, 1969.

WHO/FAO: Diet, nutrition and the prevention of chronic diseases, Report of Joint WHO/FAO

Expert Consultation, Geneva, 2013, World Health Organization.

12

Food and Nutrient Delivery: Complementary and Integrative Medicine and Dietary Supplementation

Kelly Morrow, MS, RDN

KEY TERMS

Adverse events (AEs)
Acupuncture
Alternative medicine
Ayurveda
Bioactive compound
Botanical medicine
Chi (Qi)
Chiropractic
Codex Alimentarius Commission (Codex)
Commission E Monographs
Complementary medicine
Complementary and alternative medicine (CAM)

Dietary supplement
Dietary Supplement Health and Education Act (DSHEA)
Dietary Supplement Label Database
Drug Nutrient Interaction (DNI)
East Asian Medicine
Excipients
Functional medicine
Generally Recognized As Safe (GRAS)
Health claim
Holistic medicine
Homeopathy

Integrative medicine
Megadose
Meridians
Moxibustion
Naturopathy
New Dietary Ingredient (NDI)
Pharmacognosy
Phytochemical
Phytotherapy
Structure-function claim
Subluxation
Third party certification
Vis Medicatrix Naturae

COMPLEMENTARY AND INTEGRATIVE MEDICINE

Some people may be confused by the multiple names used to describe natural medicine approaches. **Holistic medicine**, from the Greek word *holos* means "whole." Holistic therapies are based on the theory that health is a vital dynamic state and is more than just the absence of disease. **Vis medicatrix naturae**, the healing force of nature, is the underlying precept of holistic medicine. The philosophy states that when a person lives according to the laws of nature, the body has the ability to self-heal. **Alternative medicine** refers to holistic therapies used *in place* of conventional medicine. **Integrative medicine** and **complementary medicine** refer to holistic therapies used *in addition* to conventional medicine (National Center for Complementary and Integrative Health [NCCIH], 2015. (see Tables 12-1 and 12-2).

Functional medicine is another iteration of holistic medicine that has gained esteem in recent years. It shifts the disease-centered focus of traditional medical practice to a more patient-centered approach (IFM, 2015). The goal is to evaluate the whole person rather than individual symptoms and to consider care in relation to prevention and treatment of chronic disease. Functional medicine practitioners acknowledge a web-like interconnectedness of internal physiologic factors within the body and use nutrition therapy, dietary supplements, and physical manipulations as the foundation of medical care. They assess for core imbalances, including dietary intake, hormones and neurotransmitters, markers of oxidative stress, detoxification, immune function, and psychologic and spiritual health.

The Academy of Nutrition and Dietetics (AND) practice group, Dietitians in Integrative and Functional Medicine (DIFM), has developed a nutrition-oriented functional medicine radial for dietetics practitioners to assess clients using Integrative and Functional Medical Nutrition Therapy (IFMNT) (Ford et al, 2011). A functional nutrition assessment can overlap with the nutrition care process (NCP) and includes expanded categories in the clinical, biochemical, and physical domains. (See Chapter 10 and Fig 10-1).

USE OF COMPLEMENTARY AND INTEGRATIVE THERAPIES

According to the National Center for Complementary and Integrative health (NCCIH), almost 40% of adults and 12% of children in the United States use health care approaches that are outside of the mainstream. Worldwide, the prevalence is 12% of

---

Portions of this chapter were written by Cynthia A. Thomson, PhD, RD. for the previous edition of this text.

TABLE 12-1 Common Holistic Therapies According to the National Center for Complementary and Integrative Health (NCCIH)

Complementary and Integrative Medical systems	**Naturopathy,** Traditional Chinese Medicine (also known as **East Asian Medicine**), **Ayurveda,** and **Homeopathy**
Mind /Body therapies	Meditation, prayer, art or music therapy, and cognitive behavior therapy
Biologically based therapies	Herbs, whole-foods diets, and nutrient supplementation
Manipulative therapies	Massage, chiropractic medicine, osteopathy, and yoga
Energy therapies	Qi gong, magnetic therapy, or reiki

National Center for Complementary and Integrative Health (NCCIH). Complementary, Alternative or Integrative Health: What's In a Name? http://nccam.nih.gov/health/whatiscam. Accessed June 19, 2015.

TABLE 12-2 Description of Commonly Used Complementary and Integrative Therapies

	Description
Naturopathy (naturopathic medicine)	Is a primary care medicine that uses the healing power of nature, *Vis Medicatrix Naturae,* to restore and maintain optimum health. Guiding principles include the following: *Primum Non Nocere*—First do no harm *Tolle Causam*—Treat the root cause of illness *Docere*—Doctor as teacher Therapeutic methods and substances are used that work in harmony with a person's self-healing process, including diet and nutrient therapy, **botanical medicine**, psychotherapy, physical and manipulative therapy, minor surgery, prescription medicines, naturopathic obstetrics (natural childbirth), homeopathy, and acupuncture. Licensed in the United States to practice in 17 states and 2 territories. Training includes pathology, microbiology, histology, and physical and clinical diagnosis; **pharmacognosy** (clinical training in botanical medicine), hydrotherapy, physiotherapy, therapeutic nutrition, and homeopathy.
Chiropractic	Embraces many of the same principles as naturopathy, particularly the belief that the body has the ability to heal itself and that the practitioner's role is to assist the body in doing so. Like naturopathy, chiropractic focuses on wellness and prevention and favors noninvasive treatments. Chiropractors do not prescribe drugs or perform surgery. Focus on locating and removing interferences to the body's natural ability to maintain health, called **subluxations** (specifically musculoskeletal problems that lead to interference with the proper function of the nervous and musculoskeletal systems) Therapeutic approach is the manual manipulation of the body, such as spinal adjustment and massage and lifestyle recommendations, including physical exercises and stretching. Two fundamental precepts: (1) the structure and condition of the body influence how well the body functions, and (2) the mind-body relationship is important in maintaining health and in promoting healing Licensed and regulated in all 50 states and in some 30 countries. Must complete a 4-year program from a federally accredited college of chiropractic and, like other licensed practitioners, successfully pass an examination administered by a national certifying body
Homeopathy	The root words of *homeopathy* are derived from the Greek *homios,* meaning *like* and *pathos,* meaning *suffering.* Homeopathy is a medical theory and practice advanced to counter the conventional medical practices of 200 years ago. It endeavors to help the body heal itself by treating like with like, commonly known as the "law of similars." The law of similars is based on the theory that, if a large amount of a substance causes symptoms in a healthy person, a smaller amount of the same substance can be used to treat an ill person Samuel Hahnemann, an eighteenth-century German physician, is credited with founding homeopathy. The amounts of the remedies used in homeopathic medicines are extremely diluted. According to homeopathic principles, remedies are potentized and become more powerful through a shaking process called succussion. Homeopathic tinctures are made from a variety of source materials including botanicals, minerals, and animal tissues. Dosages are based on the following dilutions. A remedy becomes stronger the more it is diluted. X: 1 drop tincture in 10 drops water C: 1 drop tincture in 100 drops water M: 1 drop tincture in 1000 drops water The minimum-dose principle means that many homeopathic remedies are so dilute that no actual molecules of the healing substance can be detected by chemical tests. The goal of homeopathy is to select a remedy that will bring about a sense of well-being on all levels—physical, mental, and emotional—and that will alleviate physical symptoms and restore the patient to a state of wellness and creative energy. Although this form of medicine has a long history of use, clinical evidence on the efficacy of homeopathy is highly contradictory.
East Asian Medicine	Based on the concept that energy, also termed **chi (Qi)** or life-force energy, is central to the functioning of the body. Chi is the intangible force that animates life and enlivens all activity. Wellness is a function of the balanced and harmonious flow of chi, whereas illness or disease results from disturbances in its flow. Wellness also requires preserving equilibrium between the contrasting states of yin and yang (the dual nature of all things). The underlying principle is preventive in nature, and the body is viewed as a reflection of the natural world. Four substances—blood, jing (essence, substance of all life), shen (spirit), and fluids (body fluids other than blood)—constitute the fundamentals. The nutritional modality has several components: food as a means of obtaining nutrition, food as a tonic or medicine, and the abstention from food (fasting). Foods are classified according to taste (sour, bitter, sweet, spicy, and salty) and property (cool, cold, warm, hot, and plain) to regulate yin, yang, chi, and blood. The **meridians** are channels that carry chi and blood throughout the body. These are not channels per se, but rather they are invisible vertical networks that act as energy circuits, unifying all parts of the body and connecting the inner and the outer body; organs are not viewed as anatomic concepts but as energetic fields.

TABLE 12-2	**Description of Commonly Used Complementary and Integrative Therapies—cont'd**
	Description
Acupuncture	Acupuncture is the use of thin needles, inserted into points on the meridians, to stimulate the body's chi, or vital energy. **Moxibustion,** the application of heat using moxa, dried leaves from mugwart, along meridian acupuncture points for the purpose of affecting chi and blood so as to balance substances and organs, is related to acupuncture. This therapy is used to treat disharmony in the body, which leads to disease. Disharmony, or loss of balance, is caused by a weakening of the yin force in the body, which preserves and nurtures life, or a weakening of the yang force, which generates and activates life. The concept of yin and yang expresses the dual nature of all things, the opposing but complementary forces that are interdependent on each other and must exist in equilibrium. Acupuncturists are licensed to practice in 44 states and the District of Columbia.
Ayurveda	Is a 5,000-year-old system of natural healing that originated in India *Ayur* means life and *Veda* means science of knowledge. Assessment and treatment is based on three fundamental forces that govern the internal and external environments and determine an individuals constitution and overall health: Vata (wind): energetic, creative, and adaptable. If out of balance can be anxious, dry, thin, and have poor concentration Pitta (fire): intense, driven, and strong. If out of balance can be compulsive, irritable, inflamed, and have poor digestion Kapha (earth): nurturing, methodical, and stable. When out of balance can be sluggish, phlegmatic, and gain weight easily. Mental and physical health are achieved when these forces are in balance. Therapeutic modalities include diet, herbal, and lifestyle recommendations, massage and aromatherapy.
Massage therapy/ body work	The philosophy behind massage therapy and body work is that there is a healing that occurs through the action of touching. Massage therapy became a profession in the United States in the 1940s and has grown in use over the last several decades. The key principles of body work are the importance of increasing blood circulation, moving lymphatic tissue to remove waste and release toxins, calming of the spirit, enhancing physiologic functions of body systems, and improving musculoskeletal function. This therapy also has been widely used to reduce stress and increase energy.

the adult population in Canada, 26% in the United Kingdom, 56% in Malaysia, and 76% in Japan (Harris et al, 2012). Preferences in medical care are influenced by economic and sociocultural factors. In poor countries where access to modern medicine is limited, there is a heavy reliance on herbalists and traditional healers. In affluent countries, the decision to use natural therapies usually aligns with personal beliefs and preferences and is used commonly in addition to western medicine (Harris et al, 2012).

The use of integrative therapies has been evaluated three times in the National Health Interview Survey (NHIS)—in 2002, 2007, and most recently in 2012. In U.S. adults, the most popular integrative modalities include the use of nonvitamin, nonmineral supplements such as herbs, phytochemicals, fiber, and glucosamine (17.9%), chiropractic or osteopathic manipulation (8.5%), yoga (8.4%), and massage (6.8%). The report also highlighted regional differences in the United States: the Pacific, Mountain, and West North Central regions have the

highest use and the Middle and South Atlantic regions have the lowest use (Peregoy et al, 2014).

Figure 12-1 highlights the most common forms of integrative medicine used by adults in the United States.

A significant number of Americans use some form of integrative therapy more frequently than the services of a primary care physician. Use has been shown to be greatest among women, people ages 30 to 69, people with higher education, those residing in the western United States, and people who were hospitalized in the previous 12 months (Barnes et al, 2008). Factors associated with greater use among children include having college-educated parents, concurrent prescription medication use, reported anxiety or stress, as well as sinusitis, dermatologic, or musculoskeletal conditions (Birdee et al, 2010). By race or ethnicity, Native Americans (50.3%) and Hawaiians and Pacific Islanders (43.2%) report the highest use, followed by non-Hispanic whites (43.1%) (Barnes et al, 2008).

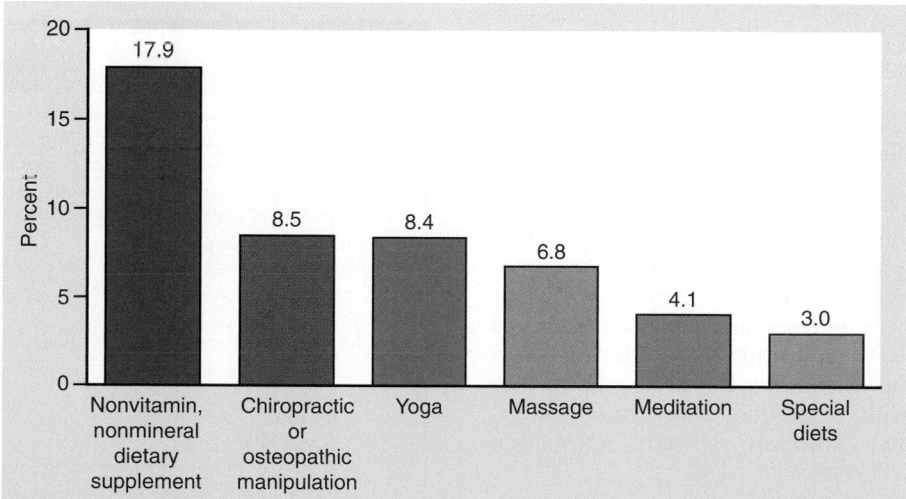

FIGURE 12-1 Percentage of adults who used complementary health approaches in the past 12 months, by type of approach: United States, 2012. (Retrieved from http://www.cdc.gov/nchs/data/databriefs/db146.pdf.)

Integrative therapies are often considered when conventional medicine is not perceived as effective by the patient (as often found in insomnia, pain, and anxiety), when integrative approaches are shown to be effective (chiropractic medicine for back pain, acupuncture for pain relief, select dietary supplementation for conditions such as macular degeneration, depression, and diarrhea), and when integrative approaches are supported by significant historical evidence of efficacy. The NHIS survey also suggested that integrative medicine use increased when conventional treatments were too costly.

As a result of the increased interest in these therapies, the Office of Alternative Medicine of the National Institutes of Health (NIH) was created in 1992 to evaluate their effectiveness. This office became the twenty-seventh institute or center within the NIH in 1998, when it was renamed the National Center for Complementary and Alternative Medicine (NCCAM). In 2015, the name was changed again to the National Center for Complementary and Integrative Health (NCCIH) because the use of holistic medicine in the US is so common, it no longer warrants the term "alternative". Complementary and alternative medicine (CAM) had been the most common term used to describe the use of holistic medicine, although this term may be falling out of favor. The NCCIH explores complementary and integrative healing practices scientifically using research, training, outreach, and integration (National Center for Complementary and Integrative Health [NCCIH], 2015). In recent years, there has been an expansion of training opportunities and medical reimbursement for integrative therapies in the conventional medical system. Increasingly, nursing and medical curricula include integrative training.

In 2011 the Bravewell Collaborative, a philanthropic organization that works to improve health care, published results from a national survey on the use of integrative medicine among 29 major integrative medical centers and programs across the United States. Top conditions for which the centers reported the most success in treatment included chronic pain, gastrointestinal disorders, depression, anxiety, and stress. The most common interventions included nutrition, dietary supplements, yoga, meditation, acupuncture, massage, and pharmaceuticals (Horrigan et al, 2012).

DIETARY SUPPLEMENTATION

More than half of all Americans are taking some form of dietary supplement, and many of them may not be well informed (ADA, 2009; Gahche et al, 2014). Historically, dietetics professionals focused their assessment, care plan, and counseling on diet or food-related recommendations. The demand for information about dietary supplements from dietetics professionals is high. In fact, the 2009 Position Paper of the Academy of Nutrition (formerly the American Dietetic Association) on nutrient supplementation calls on registered dietitian nutritionists (RDN) to be the "first source" of information on nutrient supplementation by keeping up to date on issues associated with regulation, safety, and efficacy of dietary supplements (American Dietetic Association [ADA], 2009).

Defining Dietary Supplements

According to the Food and Drug Administration (FDA), a dietary supplement is a substance that is taken orally and is intended to add nutritional value to the diet. Dietary supplements can come in many forms, including tablets, capsules, powders, and liquid. A complete description can be found in Box 12-1.

Herbal Medicine

Herbal medicine has been used since the beginning of time and has a written history of more than 5000 years. In many parts of the world it is the primary source of medicine (AHG, 2015). Herbs and plants provide a large array of phytochemicals and bioactive compounds (plant based chemicals and compounds) that have biologic activity within the human body. Although some of the phytochemicals have been identified and characterized, many of them have unknown actions and may interact with pharmaceutical drugs (Gurley, 2012). When herbs are used in combination with each other or in concentrated forms, the likelihood for a drug nutrient interaction (DNI) or side effect increases.

Botanical Medicines are made up of a variety of plant parts including leaves, flowers, stems, bark, rhizomes, and roots. They are produced in a variety of forms and are used orally and topically, including teas, infusions, decoctions, extracts, and pills as shown in Box 12-2. Topical application of botanicals or nutrients such as salves and aroma therapy are not classified as dietary supplements under the current regulatory definition because they are not ingested. The Commission E Monographs on phytomedicines were developed in Germany by an expert commission of scientists and health care professionals as references for practice of phytotherapy, the science of using plant-based medicines to prevent or treat illness. Other useful herbal references are listed at the end of the chapter.

Trends in Dietary Supplement Use

According to the National Health and Nutrition Examination Survey (NHANES) 1999-2010, about 50% of U.S. adults and 30% of children regularly take dietary supplements (CDC, 2012; Gahche, 2014). The most common reasons to supplement are to improve or maintain health, supplement the diet, support bone health (in women), lower cholesterol, and improve immunity (Bailey et al, 2013).

BOX 12-1 FDA Definition of a Dietary Supplement

Intended to be a supplement to the diet
Intended to be taken by mouth; this excludes other routes of administration, such as intranasal, transdermal, and suppository
Contains one or more dietary ingredients, including the following:
  Macronutrients (protein, carbohydrates, fats)
  Vitamins and minerals
  Herbs and botanicals
  "Other" dietary substances that are either grandfathered in or are approved as:
    New Dietary Ingredients (NDIs), such as
      Phytochemicals
      Bee pollen
      Probiotics
      Glandulars
      Some hormones, including melatonin and DHEA
Does not contain any unapproved ingredients, such as:
  Thyroid hormone, cortisol, estrogen, progesterone, or testosterone
  Pathogenic bacteria
  Human tissue

BOX 12-2 Botanical Formulations

Type	Form
Bulk Herbs	
	Sold loose to be used as teas, in cooking, and to prepare capsules; rapidly lose potency; should be stored in opaque containers, away from heat and light
Beverages	
Teas	Beverage weak in concentration; steep fresh or dried herbs in a cup of hot water for a few minutes, strain, and drink
Infusions	More concentrated than teas; steep fresh or dried herbs for approximately 15 min to allow more of the active ingredients to be extracted than for teas. A cold infusion is made by steeping an herb over time in a cold liquid.
Decoctions	Most concentrated of the beverages, made by simmering the root, rhizome, bark or berries for 30-60 min to extract the active ingredients
Extracts	
	Herbs are extracted with an organic solvent to dissolve the active components; forms a concentrated form of the active ingredients. *Standardized extracts* concentrate a specific constituent(s) of an herb. Removal of the solvent creates a *solid extract.*
Tinctures	Extract in which the solvent is alcohol, glycerine, honey or occasionally vinegar. Rations are listed herb:quantity of solvent. A 1:1 tincture is equal parts herb and solvent.
Glycerites	Extract in which the solvent is glycerol or a mixture of glycerol and water; more appropriate for children than a tincture
Salve	An infusion of herbs in oil and beeswax that is used topically. This preparation is not considered to be a dietary supplement under DSHEA.
Pill Forms	
	Pills should be taken with at least 4-8 oz of water to avoid leaving residue in the esophagus.
Capsules	Herbal material is enclosed in a hard shell made from animal-derived gelatin or plant-derived cellulose (vegetarian caps).
Tablets	Herbal material is mixed with filler material to form the hard tablet; may be uncoated or coated with starches and polymers
Lozenges	Also called *troches;* method of preparation allows the active components to be readily released in the mouth when chewed or sucked
Soft gels	Soft capsule used to encase liquid extracts such as fatty acids or vitamin E
Essential oils	Fragrant, volatile plant oils; used for aromatherapy, bathing; concentrated form and not to be used internally unless specifically directed (such as enteric-coated peppermint oil)

The industry has grown steadily for the past 30 years. Industry sales were more than $32 billion in 2012 and sales are expected to continue to increase (National Institutes of Health/ Office of Dietary Supplements, [NIH/ODS], 2015). The most common supplements taken are multivitamin-minerals (MVM), calcium, vitamin C, herbals, fish oil, probiotics, vitamin D, glucosamine, and products for weight management and athletic enhancement (Bailey et al, 2013). Sales of herbal dietary supplements rose 7.9% in 2013. The most popular were turmeric (*Curcuma longa*), wheat and barley grass (*Triticum aestivum* and *Hordeum vulgare*), aloe (Aloe vera) and spirulina (*Arthrospira* spp.) (Lindstrom et al, 2013).

Use of dietary supplements has been shown to increase with advancing age, higher education and socioeconomic status, white race, and female gender. Reports find that use of dietary supplements is highest among those who: are in the best state of health, have a body mass index less than 25 kg/m², are nonsmokers, are physically active, report good health, adhere to a healthy diet, and use food labels in making food choices (NIH, 2015).

Multivitamin Efficacy

Many people take an MVM to increase nutrient levels in the diet. Dietary surveillance data from the National Center for Health Statistics (NCHS) and NHANES reveal that most adults and children in the United States are not meeting dietary guidelines and are under-consuming dark greens, orange vegetables, legumes, and whole grains (Krebs-Smith et al, 2010). Total nutrient intakes for vitamin D, vitamin E, calcium, vitamin A, vitamin C, and magnesium have been found to be significantly below the estimated average requirement (EAR), and less than 3% of the population is meeting the adequate intake (AI) for potassium (Fulgoni et al, 2011).

Use of multivitamins and minerals has been shown to improve micronutrient status among adults and children (Bailey et al, 2012; Murphy et al, 2007; NIH, 2006). Unfortunately, increased nutrient intake has not translated into reduced risk of chronic disease in people without overt nutrient deficiencies. Research reviews by the National Institutes of Health State of Science Panel and the U.S. Preventive Services Task Force have evaluated observational and randomized controlled trials (RCTs) of more than 400,000 people using single or paired vitamins or MVM and have not found evidence that they reduce chronic disease or prevent early death (Fortman et al, 2013; Neuhouser et al, 2009; NIH, 2006). Two trials, the Supplementation in Vitamins and Mineral Antioxidants Study (SU.VI.MAX) and the Physicians Health Study II (PHS-II), found a small reduction in cancer incidence for men only after 12½ years (SU.VI.MAX) and 8 years (PHS-II) of supplementation (Fortman et al, 2013). Trials looking at cardiovascular disease, cognitive decline, and all-cause mortality have not shown statistically significant incidence of either harm or benefit (Fortman et al, 2013). Chronic diseases are complex and usually have multifactorial causes. Studying the effect of an MVM on nutrient intake and overall health is a difficult undertaking. Almost all Americans are taking in supplemental forms of nutrients via fortified foods, which complicates efforts to quantify the impact of taking a MVM supplement. In observational trials, people take a variety of MVMs with differing compositions and potencies. People who self-select to take a MVM are usually healthier and have better diets, suggesting that MVMs are probably not helpful for most well nourished people. A few long-term RCTs evaluated the merits of MVMs, and the results have been population or gender specific and not generalizable to the entire U.S. population (Fortman et al, 2013). MVMs may have efficacy based on assessment of individual needs but are not useful for all people.

Antioxidant Supplements

Oxidative stress is implicated in a variety of disease states, and many Americans take antioxidant supplements. A recent Cochrane review of 78 RCTs with 296,707 participants found that all-cause mortality was increased slightly with regular antioxidant use. The effect was strongest with beta carotene in smokers, and high-dose vitamin E and vitamin A. Vitamin C and selenium were not found to increase mortality but also did not improve longevity (Bjelakovic et al, 2012). Antioxidant supplements may be beneficial, however, for prevention of age-related macular degeneration (AMD). In the Age Related Eye Disease Study (AREDS), high-dose vitamin C (500 mg),

TABLE 12-3 Populations Potentially at Risk for Nutrient Deficiencies

At-Risk Population or Life Cycle Stage	Nutrients of Concern that Could Potentially be Corrected by Supplementation
Those living in poverty (especially children)	Iron, calcium, magnesium, folate, vitamins A, B_6, C, D, and E
Women taking oral contraceptives	Zinc, folic acid, B_6, and B_{12}
Adolescent women	Iron and calcium
Pregnant women	Iron and folic acid
Elders	B_{12} and vitamin D, multiple micronutrients
Vegans	B_{12}
Those following a calorie-restricted, allergy-restricted diet	Multiple nutrients
People with dark pigmented skin	Vitamin D
People with malabsorption (IBD, gastric bypass)	Multiple nutrients
Those with genetic predisposition to nutrient deficiencies (i.e., MTHFR or vitamin D receptor mutations)	Folate, B_{12}, vitamin D
Smokers	Vitamin C
Alcoholics	Folate and thiamin

Reference: Position of the American Dietetic Association: Nutrient supplementation, *J Acad Nutr Diet* 109:2073-2085, 2009.

vitamin E (400 IU), beta carotene (15 mg), and zinc (80 mg) had a significant reduction in the risk of developing AMD after taking the antioxidant supplements for 6.3 years. The effects were still present after a 10-year follow-up (Chew et al, 2013). For the majority of people, it is probably best to get antioxidants and phytonutrients by eating a variety of plant-based foods, including fruits, vegetables, herbs, spices, nuts, seeds, legumes, and whole grains.

Potentially At-Risk Populations

Although dietary supplement use is most common among people who are least likely to have a nutrient deficiency, the Academy of Nutrition and Dietetics has identified several populations and life cycle stages that potentially could benefit from dietary supplements (ADA, 2009). Table 12-3 outlines potentially at risk populations. Clinicians should be aware of these at-risk subgroups and complete a nutrition assessment to determine the need for supplementation on an individual basis if nutrition status cannot be improved by dietary changes alone.

DIETARY SUPPLEMENT REGULATION

Dietary supplements (DS) are regulated by two government agencies, The Food and Drug Administration (FDA), which oversees safety concerns, and the Federal Trade Commission (FTC), which oversees advertising, label, and health claims. Before 1994, dietary supplements existed in limbo under the general, but unspecified, regulation of the FDA. The **Dietary Supplement Health and Education Act of 1994 (DHEA)** defined DS under the category of food and explicitly removed them from consideration as drugs or dietary additives. This was seen as a victory to the dietary supplement industry and consumers; they had become accustomed to

open access in ability to manufacture and purchase dietary supplements.

Dietary Supplement regulation set forth by DSHEA includes the following (Dickinson, 2011; FDA/DSHEA, 2014):

- **Generally recognized as safe (GRAS)** status to all supplements produced before October 15, 1994. This allows manufacturers to continue to sell all of the products that were on the market at the time DSHEA was passed. Any company that introduces a new dietary supplement must send notification and safety information to the FDA 75 days before selling the supplement.
- A supplement facts panel that defines how ingredients must be listed on the label. See Figure 12-2 for an example of a dietary supplement label.
- Structure function claims vs. health claims: Supplement companies are no longer allowed to list disease states or make specific health claims on a DS label. A **structure function claim** allows for a description that includes a structure or function of the body or a stage of life. "Supports strong bones" is an allowable structure function claim; "Prevents osteoporosis" is not. The label must also include the disclaimer, "This statement has not been evaluated by the Food and Drug Administration. This product is not intended to diagnose, treat, cure or prevent any disease." Opponents of DSHEA feel that structure function claims are too similar to drug claims and encourage DS to be used like drugs. By contrast, a **health claim** can mention a disease state as long as it has met the significant scientific agreement standard of the FDA and can exist on foods and dietary supplements. For example, "soluble fiber from foods such as oat bran, as part of a diet low in saturated fat and cholesterol, may reduce the risk of heart disease." The FDA has approved only a limited number of health claims (Food and Drug Administration [FDA], 2003).

Supplement Facts

Serving Size 1 Capsule

Amount Per Capsule	% Daily Value
Calories 20	
Calories from Fat 20	
Total Fat 2 g	3%*
Saturated Fat 0.5 g	3%*
Polyunsaturated Fat 1 g	†
Monounsaturated Fat 0.5 g	†
Vitamin A 4250 IU	85%
Vitamin D 425 IU	106%
Omega-3 fatty acids 0.5 g	†

* Percent Daily Values are based on a 2,000 calorie diet.
† Daily Value not established.

Ingredients: Cod liver oil, gelatin, water, and glycerin.

FIGURE 12-2 A dietary supplement facts label per Food and Drug Administration regulation as defined under the Dietary Supplement Health Education Act. (From http://www.fda.gov/ucm/groups/fdagov-public/documents/image/ucm070717.gif Accessed June 19, 2015.)

- Disseminating product literature: DS manufacturers and retailers are no longer able to display product information or technical data sheets next to products because they can mislead consumers and make DS appear to be drugs.
- Because a wide variety of DS are available, including some hormones and megadose vitamins, it is up to consumers to be educated about the DS they choose to consume. The National Institutes of Health founded the Office of Dietary Supplements (ODS) in 1994 to fund research and disseminate credible information on DS to consumers. On this government website, consumers can find basic consumer information, technical data sheets about dietary supplements and herbs, and FDA warnings.
- Good manufacturing procedures (GMPs) were adopted in 2007 and went into full enforcement in 2010. According to the GMPs, manufacturers of DS must meet minimum standards for production and are subject to random audits. The GMPs regulate the design and construction of manufacturing plants, maintenance and cleaning procedures, manufacturing procedures, quality control procedures, testing of materials, handling of consumer complaints, and maintaining records (Food and Drug Administration [FDA], 2010).

Under DSHEA, DS are regulated only for safety and not for efficacy. Manufacturers are beholden to follow the regulatory laws governing dietary supplements; however, they do not have to send any premarket notification to the FDA except for structure function claims and safety documentation for **new dietary ingredients (NDIs)** that were not used before 1994. The FDA randomly inspects more than 300 DS manufacturers per year. According to the Director of Dietary Supplement Programs at the FDA, almost two-thirds of the companies audited in 2012 were found to not be in compliance with the federal GMPs, and warning letters were sent to one-third of those companies inspected (Trine, 2012). The most common noncompliance issues were failure to test products for identity, potency and purity, and contamination with non-approved dietary ingredients or pharmaceutical drugs. The FDA is increasing its auditing program every year. With repeated audits, many of the noncompliant companies will be forced to comply or shut down, which will help ensure increased safety in the industry. For now, health care providers should recommend dietary supplements only from reputable companies.

Ensuring Dietary Supplement Safety

Under DSHEA, the FDA bears the burden of proving a supplement is unsafe. This can be a challenging task once a product is released onto the market. To date, only two dietary supplements have been banned by the FDA over safety issues, *Ephedra sinica* in 2004, and dimethylamylamine (DMAA) in 2013. Both have been linked to cardiovascular toxicity and death. The most common supplements with health and safety concerns are those used for weight loss, performance enhancement (ergogenic aids), and sexual dysfunction (Food and Drug Administration [FDA], 2010). These supplements have the highest risk of contamination and adulteration with unapproved dietary ingredients and pharmaceutical drugs, especially when purchased from obscure retailers and the Internet. Internet sales of DS is the fastest-growing retail market and is also the hardest to regulate. Consumers can find banned supplements easily on the Internet.

In December 2006 the Dietary Supplement and Nonprescription Drug Consumer Protection Act was signed into law, requiring mandatory reporting by manufacturers and retailers of known serious **adverse events (AEs)** related to dietary supplement and over-the-counter (OTC) medications (Frankos, 2010). Serious adverse events include a life-threatening event, incapacitation, hospitalization, a birth defect, or death. These must be reported to the FDA MedWatch website and can be filed by an individual, health care provider, or industry representative. In addition, supplement manufacturers are required by law to have contact information on supplement bottles. Adverse event reports are forwarded to the Center for Food Safety and Applied Nutrition, where they are further evaluated by qualified reviewers (Frankos, 2010). Health care providers and consumers are not mandatory reporters under the law but are strongly encouraged to report adverse events.

Between 2008 and 2011 the FDA and poison control centers received almost 13,000 adverse event reports related to DS. Of those 71% were considered serious adverse events. During that same time, the FDA logged 2.7 million adverse drug events, of which 63% were considered serious (Government Accountability Office, 2013). It is estimated that many adverse events from taking supplements are not being reported or are not being reported correctly. Common barriers from consumers include downplaying the significance, not knowing where or how to report, and embarrassment (Food and Drug Administration [FDA], 2012). After 9 years of tracking (2004-2013), the CDC released a report indicating that an estimated 23,000 emergency department visits per year could be attributed to dietary supplements. Among young adults aged 20-34, the most common supplements causing adverse events were for weight loss and energy (ergogenic aids) and the most common symptoms were tachycardia, chest pain and palpitations. For adults 65 and older, adverse events were mostly attributed to choking on micronutrient pills. 20% of dietary supplement related emergency visits were for unsupervised children who ingested dietary supplements (Geller A, et all, 2015). Health care providers who wish to stay abreast of alerts from the FDA can subscribe to the MedWatch email list on the FDA website. The Office of Dietary Supplements website is another resource for information about current warnings and recalls as well as consumer tips for buying and taking dietary supplements safely.

Botanical supplements are increasing in popularity, and some have the likelihood for producing adverse events, especially when taken in combination products and in concentrated form. Most of the common herbs used in the United States do not pose a great risk for a **drug nutrient interaction** (DNI). Of the herbs most commonly used, St. John's wort is the most problematic and has been shown to reduce efficacy of many drugs, including antiretrovirals for HIV, antirejection medications for organ transplants, oral contraceptives, cardiac medications, chemotherapy, and cholesterol medications. Two other herbs have been shown to have a high risk for DNI, including goldenseal (*Hydrastis canadensis*) and black pepper (*Piper nigrum*), although black pepper is only a problem in supplemental form and not in amounts commonly found in food (Gurley et al, 2012).

In recent years the Office of Dietary Supplements has worked collaboratively with several organizations and experts to develop a **Dietary Supplement Label Database** of dietary supplements used in the United States. Because the database provides specific information on the nutrient, herbal, or other constituents contained in a supplement, it allows clinicians to assess more accurately the appropriate use of select supplements by their patients. (See Figure 12-3). The database includes dietary supplement label information for more than

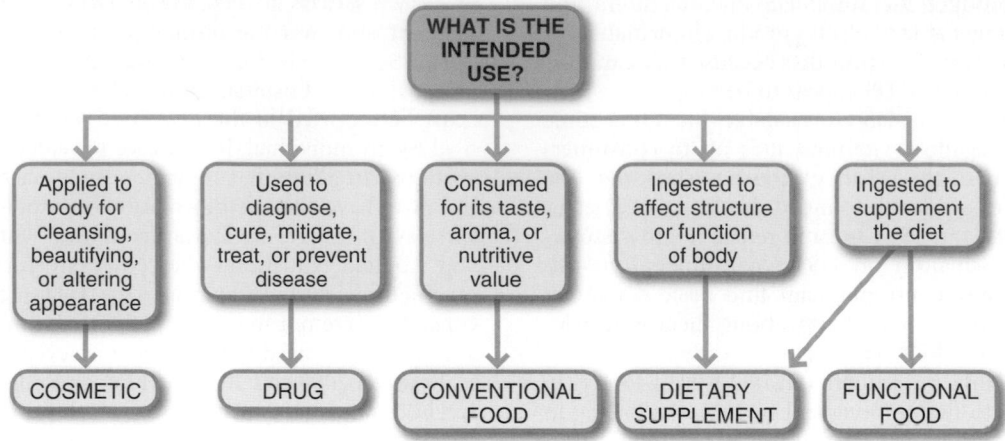

FIGURE 12-3 Use of dietary supplementation in clinical practice requires use of a credible resource for evaluation and application. (From Thomson CA, Newton T: Dietary supplements: evaluation and application in clinical practice, *Topics Clin Nutr* 20(1):32, 2005. Reprinted with permission.)

17,000 supplements, including the structure and function claims. The Office of Dietary Supplements (www.ods.od.nih. gov) offers Supplement Fact Sheets containing information about dietary supplements that is linked to PubMed, allowing clinicians access to peer-reviewed information on use in human trials, adverse events associated with use, and information regarding the mechanism of action. The subscription databases, Natural Standard (www.naturalstandard.com) and the Natural Medicines Comprehensive Database (www. naturaldatabase.com), offer similar information.

Third Party Certification

The FDA and FTC have primary jurisdiction for ensuring dietary supplements are safe and do not have misleading advertising. With 85,000 products on the market, this is a daunting task. Because supplement manufacturers are audited randomly, it is not easy for consumers to know whether a company is truly following good manufacturing procedures (GMPs). Several private companies offer **third party certification** in the supplement industry. Consumer Lab is a well-known subscription-based company that randomly pulls supplements from store shelves to test them for potency, identity, and purity. Subscribers to the Consumer Lab website are able to access reports that reference specific brands (Consumer Labs, 2015). The U.S. Pharmacopeia (USP) (USP, 2015) the National Sanitation Foundation (NSF) (NSF, 2015) and the Therapeutic Goods Association (TGA) (TGA, 2015) each certify supplement companies for compliance with federal GMPs. Once verified, companies can display a stamp on their supplement labels that signifies the products have been third party certified. In addition, NSF offers a "Certified for Sport" certification for supplements that are used by competitive athletes to ensure they are not contaminated with illegal substances (NSF, 2015).

The **Codex Alimentarius Commission (Codex)** is an agency with international significance. It was created in 1963 by two U.N. organizations, the Food and Agriculture Organization and the World Health Organization, to protect the health of consumers and to ensure fair practices in international food trade. Codex participants work on the development of food standards, codes of practice, and guidelines for products such as

dietary supplements. Codex standards and guidelines are developed by committees from 180 member countries, where they voluntarily review and provide comments on standards at several stages in the development process (Crane, 2010).

Quality Issues in Dietary Supplements

Not all dietary supplements are high quality. As discussed previously, many manufacturers are not in full compliance with DSHEA, which means many substandard and contaminated products are on the market. Many of the mainstream brands in health food stores and major retail outlets are likely safe. Products bought off the Internet and from obscure retailers may be adulterated and/or may not meet label claim. What determines quality in a supplement must go beyond the safety issues to address the quantity, formulations, and quality of all ingredients used.

Quantity of Ingredients

Many MVMs contain **megadoses** of nutrients, which greatly exceed the RDA and may or may not be appropriate for each individual consumer. Some individuals may benefit from high doses of certain nutrients because of genetic variations in enzyme function or other pharmacologic effects of megadoses. Examples include increased need for folic acid with an MTHFR gene variant or reduction in triglycerides with megadoses of niacin (Ames et al, 2002; Boden et al, 2014).

It is important to assess for upper limits, especially when patients are taking multiple sources of nutrients. Most water-soluble vitamins do not have overt toxicity at high doses with the exception of niacin (flushing, prickly heat, and liver irritation in some people) and pyridoxine (reversible neuropathy). Fat-soluble vitamins can become toxic more quickly, such as vitamin A (hepatotoxicity and teratogenicity) and vitamin D (nephrolithiasis, calcification of soft tissue). Often vitamin A is listed in its provitamin form, beta carotene, which does not pose the same health risks at high doses.

Minerals can become toxic more easily than vitamins, so they often are not formulated using megadoses. In some cases, people may take a megadose of a mineral for a limited time, such as zinc for the common cold. To ensure patient safety, it is important to coordinate care with a physician when a patient is taking a megadose of a mineral. Although it is not a megadose, the FDA limits potassium content in dietary supplements to 99 mg because of the prevalence of chronic kidney disease.

Formulations

Dietary supplements come in many formulations, including capsules, tablets, gels, chewables, liquids, and powders. The form a consumer selects has to do with convenience, preference, and affordability. Supplement powders can be added easily to foods and beverages, but most have added sugars to increase palatability. Chewable and liquid supplements often are missing multiple nutrients to increase taste appeal, so it is important to assess the label to ensure it meets the patient's needs.

Tablets tend to be more compressed than capsules and require fewer number of pills to achieve the optimal dosage. Capsules tend to be easier to swallow but less concentrated than tablets. Gelatin capsules may not be suitable for vegetarians. Some companies make vegetarian capsules out of vegetable cellulose to accommodate vegetarian consumers. Other nutrient forms that may not be suitable for vegetarian clients include cholecalciferol (often from fish oil or lambswool) and vitamin A/retinol (also usually from fish oil). Vegetarian formulations usually contain ergocalciferol and beta carotene as alternatives.

Excipients

Excipients are extra ingredients added to dietary supplements to increase bulk, mask "off flavors," add color, and improve compressibility and flow through machinery. To assess whether a dietary supplement is right for an individual, it is important to consider the quality of the excipients used. Some contain allergens and potentially unfavorable ingredients such as hydrogenated oils and artificial colors. When choosing a dietary supplement, it is important to read the label for quantity and quality of active ingredients and excipients.

Vitamins

Most vitamins in dietary supplements are similar across brands with the exception of B_6 (pyridoxine), B_{12} (cyanocobalamin), folate (folic acid), and vitamin E. Some formulations contain active, methylated, or phosphorylated forms of these nutrients such as in active B_6: pyridoxyl 5′-phosphate, active B_{12}: methylcobalamin, and active folate: methyltetrahydrofolate. Individuals with genetic polymorphisms, nervous system disorders, increased oxidative stress, or impaired digestion may benefit from the increased bioavailability of these nutrients; however, research is limited on their widespread need and efficacy. In addition, the active forms tend to be more expensive (Head et al, 2006; Hendren, 2013).

Vitamin E can be made synthetically or extracted naturally from soybean oil, sunflower oil, or other vegetable oils. Natural vitamin E (d-alpha tocopherol) is more expensive but has a greater bioavailability than synthetic vitamin E (dl-alpha tocopherol) (Azzi et al, 2000). High-quality vitamin E products usually contain mixed tocopherols in addition to the d-alpha tocopherol, which is thought to mimic more closely what one would get from eating a food source of vitamin E. Some tocopherols, especially gamma tocopherol, has been studied for its cardioprotective effects (Liu et al, 2003).

Minerals

Chelated minerals bound to an amino acid or a Krebs cycle intermediary are considered the most easily absorbed form of a mineral supplement and most similar to how a mineral would exist in food. Examples of chelates include citrate, bisglycinate, succinate, aspartate, and picolinate. Quality differences exist between companies that produce chelated minerals. A mineral must be bonded covalently to its ligand to be considered a bioavailable "true chelate" (Albion, 2014). Chelated minerals are best for elders and people with low stomach acid and compromised digestion and can be taken on an empty stomach. Ionic mineral preparations such as carbonates and oxides should be taken with food, especially protein, to increase absorption (Straub, 2007).

ASSESSMENT OF DIETARY SUPPLEMENT USE IN PATIENTS

Health care professionals should be aware that patients typically do not report their use of botanicals or other dietary supplements. Therefore practitioners must inquire specifically about the use of supplements by their patients. To facilitate disclosure, health care providers should approach patients in an open-minded, nonjudgmental manner. Key questions to ask are summarized in Box 12-3. Ideally, patients should be encouraged to bring all of their dietary supplements and medications into the clinic to be evaluated. In this way the health care provider can review doses (including those above the upper limit [UL]), forms, frequency of use, rationale for use, side effects, and the patient-perceived efficacy of each supplement (American Dietetic Association [ADA], 2009; National Institutes of Health/Office of Dietary Supplements [NIH/ODS], 2015). This should be done on a regular basis. It is particularly important that dietary supplement use be reviewed before surgery because some dietary supplements and botanicals alter the rate of blood coagulation. Box 12-4 provides specific recommendations regarding the discontinuation of dietary supplements before surgery to avoid complications associated with prolonged bleeding time. In addition, patients on blood-thinning medications may have to be monitored for a potential interaction with these supplements (American College of Surgeons, 2014).

For assessing patients for dietary supplement use using the nutrition care process, potential diagnosis and intervention codes are shown in Box 12-5.

Recommendation and Sale of Dietary Supplements

Many health care professionals are uncomfortable recommending dietary supplements. Clinical guidelines for recommending and selling dietary supplements have been published previously by the Academy of Nutrition (Thompson et al, 2002). Dietitians and nutritionists who recommend dietary supplements must take the initiative to develop their knowledge, skills, and resources to provide accurate and safe recommendations. The Academy has developed *The Academy Scope of Practice Decision Tool: A Self-Assessment Guide* for dietetics providers; it is available through the Academy website. It can be used to assess competence and scope of practice as defined by training, place of employment, and state of residence (Academy of Nutrition and Dietetics [AND], 2015). It is advisable to use this tool before beginning any new practice, including recommending or selling dietary supplements.

When recommending dietary supplements to clients, clinicians should use an evidence- or science-based approach and document thoroughly in the patient's medical chart. Documentation should include the supplement name, dosage, form, duration of use, and a short description of supporting evidence. Each provider is responsible to cross-check for contraindications and potential drug nutrient interactions (DNIs) and document any risks in the patients' medical chart. See Box 12-6 for guidelines

BOX 12-3 Evaluating Dietary Supplement Use: The Patient–Health Care Provider Information Exchange

Ask

- What dietary supplements are you taking (type: vitamin, mineral, botanical, amino acid, fiber)?
- Why are you taking these dietary supplements? Include review of patient's medical diagnosis and symptoms for reasons why he or she may be taking supplements (e.g., osteoarthritis, heart disease, high blood pressure, PMS, loss of memory, fatigue).
- How long have you been taking these dietary supplements?
- What dose or how much are you taking? For each, include supplement form and manufacturer.
- With what frequency are you taking each supplement?
- Where were the supplements purchased (e.g., health food store, Internet, health care provider)?
- Who recommended the supplement (e.g., media, physician, nurse, dietitian, alternative medicine practitioner, friend, family)?

Evaluate

- Dietary intake (including intake of fortified foods and beverages, and nutritional and sports bars)
- Health status and health history—include lifestyle habits (e.g., smoking, alcohol, exercise)
- Biochemical profile, laboratory data
- Prescribed and OTC medications
- Clinical response to supplements
- Adverse events, symptoms

Educate

- Scientific evidence of benefit and effectiveness
- Potential interaction with foods, nutrients, and medications or other dietary supplements
- Appropriate dose, brand, and chemical form; duration of supplementation; appropriate follow-up
- Quality of products, manufacturers, good manufacturing practices (USP, Consumer Labs)
- Mechanism of action of the primary active ingredient
- Appropriate storage of the dietary supplement
- Administration instructions: With or without food? Potential food-supplement interactions?
- Awareness and reporting of any side effects or adverse events, symptoms
- Recommend necessary dietary changes to support needs. Food should come first.

Document

- List specific supplements and brand names of each supplement being taken.
- Record batch number from bottle in case of an adverse event.
- Record patient perception and expected level of compliance.
- Monitor efficacy and safety, including health outcomes and adverse effects.
- Record medication-supplement or supplement-supplement interactions.
- Plan for follow-up.

From Practice Paper of the American Dietetic Association: Dietary supplements, *J Am Diet Assoc* 105(3):466, 2005. Reprinted with permission.

BOX 12-4 Dietary Supplements that Affect Blood Clotting and Should be Discontinued 10 To 14 Days Before Surgery or Certain Medical Tests

Ajoene, birch bark, cayenne, Chinese black tree fungus, cumin, evening primrose oil, feverfew, garlic, ginger, *Ginkgo biloba*, ginseng, grapeseed extract, milk thistle, omega-3 fatty acids, onion extract, St. John's wort, turmeric, vitamins C and E

Reference: American College of Surgeons. College of Education: *Medication and Surgery Before Your Operation* (website): http://www.facs.org/patienteducation/medications.html. Accessed January 31, 2014.

for choosing dietary supplements and botanical products and Box 12-7 for information about usage, dosage, and safety of some of the most commonly used dietary supplements.

Resources for Clinicians

As awareness of dietary supplement use expands within the health care community, the number of evidence-based resources available to clinicians also is growing considerably. Clinicians should have access to online and print resources that are updated at regular intervals. Resources that provide reference to the original research are preferable. A list of evidence-based resources can be found at the end of the chapter. In addition, accessing available medical literature is advised, given that there are a growing number of studies being published in peer-reviewed literature.

Text continued on page 12-17

BOX 12-5 International Dietetics and Nutrition Terminology (IDNT) that Applies to the Documentation of Dietary Supplement use Among Patients

Assessment Terminology: Food and Nutrient Intake, Medication and Complementary and Alternative Medicine Use and Knowledge, Beliefs and Attitudes

Diagnosis Terminology: Inadequate bioactive substance intake (NI-4.1), Excessive bioactive substance intake (NI-4.2), Increased nutrient needs (NI5.1), Decreased nutrient needs (NI-5.4), Imbalance of nutrients (NI-5.5), Less than optimal intake of types of fats (NI-5.6.3), Less than optimal intake of types of proteins or amino acids (NI-5.7.3), Inadequate fiber intake (NI-5.8.6), Inadequate vitamin intake (specify) (NI-5.9.1), Excessive vitamin intake (specify) (NI-5.9.2) Inadequate mineral intake (specify) (NI-5.10.1), Excessive mineral intake (specify) (NI-5.10.2), Predicted suboptimal nutrient intake (specify) (NI-5.11.1), Predicted excessive nutrient intake (specify) (NI-5.11.2), Impaired nutrient utilization (NC-2.1), Altered nutrition related laboratory values (specify) (NC 2.2), Food medication interaction (NC-2.3), Predicted food-medication interaction (NC-2.4), Food and nutrition related knowledge deficit (NB-1.1), Unsupported beliefs and attitudes about food or nutrition related topics (NB-1.2), Limited adherence to nutrition related recommendations (NB-1.6)

Intervention Terminology: Vitamin and mineral supplements (specify) (ND-3.2), Bioactive substance management (specify) (ND-3.3), Nutrition related medication management: Nutrition related complementary/alternative medicine (ND-6.3), Nutrition education (specify) (E-1), Nutrition counseling (specify) (C-1), Collaboration and referral of nutrition Care (RC-1)

BOX 12-6　Guidelines For Choosing Dietary Supplements and Botanical Products

- Ensure the supplement is appropriate for the individual patient based on state of health, dietary deficiency, and scientific evidence.
- Consider multiple sources of dietary supplements including fortified foods, bars, cereals, and beverages to ensure patients are not exceeding safe intake limits.
- Check for potential drug nutrient interactions and be aware of side effects and contraindications. For example, fish oil can reduce blood clotting in high doses and antioxidant supplements can inhibit the effects of some chemotherapy drugs.
- Investigate the quality of the manufacturer to ensure a quality product. Look for companies that have third party certification (NSF, USP), or well-known companies with a longstanding reputation for quality. Check Consumer Labs or the FDA warning letters website for documented problems (www.fda.gov/ICECI/EnforcementActions/WarningLetters).

- Use the dietary supplement label to obtain important information, including the following:
  - Product identity (including scientific or botanical names), form, and dosage
  - Allergy information in case the patient has a dietary restriction. Excipients (inactive ingredients) are often the source of allergens or unwanted ingredients.
  - A lot number, which is helpful if problems arise because it allows the product to be tracked through each stage of the manufacturing process
  - An expiration date
- After determining that a manufacturer and its product meet these standards, compare prices among products of similar quality. Prices can vary widely.

National Institutes of Health, Office of Dietary Supplements. *Dietary Supplements: What You Need to Know.* http://ods.od.nih.gov/HealthInformation/DS_WhatYouNeedToKnow.aspx. *Accessed June 19, 2015;* Position of the American Dietetic Association: Nutrient Supplementation, *J Acad Nutr Diet.* 109:2073-2085, 2009.

BOX 12-7　Popular Dietary Supplements and Their Efficacy

Supplement	Benefits	Dosage	Potential Contraindications	Quality Considerations
Vitamins				
Vitamin B_6	Effective for hereditary sideroblastic anemia, pyridoxine-dependent seizures; Likely effective for hyperhomocysteinemia, age related macular degeneration, hypertension, calcium oxalate kidney stones, pregnancy induced nausea and vomiting	Most supplemental doses are 5 mg-50 mg/day. 25 mg q 8 hours for pregnancy induced nausea and vomiting. Doses up to 200 mg/day have been used for carpel tunnel, but close monitoring is recommended.	Doses up to 200 mg/day appear to be tolerated by most people, although high doses can cause hypotension and reversible neuropathy.	Available as pyridoxine and pyridoxyl 5'-phosphate (active form). People with genetic polymorphisms, nervous system disorders, increased oxidative stress, or impaired digestion may benefit from the active form.
Vitamin B_{12}	Effective for pernicious anemia and B_{12} deficiency. Likely effective for hyperhomocysteinemia, Possibly effective for age related macular degeneration	Doses in supplements are often in megadoses due to lack of toxicity. Can be taken orally and injected. Common dosage range is 2.4- 1000 mcg/day.	Most risk is associated with intravenous forms, not oral forms. People with pernicious anemia will not benefit from oral dosing.	Available as cyanocobalamin or methylcobalamin (active form). Active form may be beneficial for those with genetic polymorphisms, nervous system disorders, increased oxidative stress, or impaired digestion.
Vitamin C	Effective for scurvy; Likely effective for iron absorption enhancement; Possibly effective for age related macular degeneration, cancer prevention, common cold prevention and treatment, complex regional pain syndrome, hypertension, osteoarthritis, sunburn	Doses vary widely but usually range from 100 mg-2000 mg/day; Divided doses for larger amounts.	Safe at lower doses and in amounts found in foods. Higher doses can cause diarrhea and gastrointestinal cramping. Greater than 500 mg is contraindicated for those who have a history of calcium oxalate kidney stones.	Mineral ascorbates (buffered vitamin C) may be better tolerated than ascorbic acid.
Vitamin D	Effective for familial hypophosphatemia, hypoparathyroidism, osteomalacia, psoriasis, renal osteodystrophy and rickets. Likely effective for corticosteroid induced osteoporosis, fall prevention in older adults, osteoporosis. Possibly effective for prevention of cancer, dental caries, multiple sclerosis, respiratory tract infections, Rheumatoid arthritis and obesity.	Dose is usually based on individual serum levels and can vary from person to person. Optimal serum level is considered to be 30-50 nmol/L. In research, doses range from 400 IU to 50,000 IU/day. The UL is 4,000 IU (100 mcg)/day.	Exceeding the UL and elevated serum concentrations are associated with calcification of soft tissues (damage to the heart, blood vessels, and kidney), and increased risk for kidney stones. Risk may be increased in postmenopausal women who also take supplemental calcium. Best to coordinate care with primary care provider and monitor blood levels.	Cholecalciferol (D_3) is the most common supplement and is usually sourced from fish or sheep (lanolin). Ergocalciferol (D_2) is suitable for vegetarians and vegans.

Continued

BOX 12-7 Popular Dietary Supplements and Their Efficacy—cont'd

Supplement	Benefits	Dosage	Potential Contraindications	Quality Considerations
Vitamins				
Vitamin E	Effective for vitamin E deficiency. Possibly effective for slowing cognitive decline in Alzheimer's disease, improving response to erythropoietin in hemodialysis, reducing cisplatin induced neurotoxicity and pain in rheumatoid arthritis, prevention of dementia, dysmenorrhea, PMS, Parkinson's disease and radiation induced fibrosis and increasing muscle strength in the elderly.	Most supplements are between 50 and 2000 IU. Most common dose is 200-400 IU/day. Higher doses used therapeutically.	Doses above 400 IU/day may increase risk for bleeding, prostate cancer, and have prooxidant effects.	D-alpha tocopherol is the natural form of vitamin E and dl- alpha tocopherol is the synthetic form. Natural forms with mixed tocopherols, specifically gamma tocopherol, may have cardioprotective effects.
Folic acid	Effective for folate deficiency. Likely effective for hyperhomocysteinemia, methotrexate toxicity, and neural tube defects. Possibly effective for age related macular degeneration, depression, hypertension	RDA level is recommended in most people, although those with MTHFR variant or chronic conditions may need higher levels (200 mcg-5 mg/day has been used). Coordinate care with physician for megadose amounts.	Caution with folate supplementation in those at risk for colon cancer.	Supplemental sources have greater bioavailability than folate in food. People with a MTHFR variant may have increased need for folate. Activated form, methylenetetrahydrofolate is also used.
Minerals				
Calcium	Effective for dyspepsia, hyperkalemia, and renal failure (as a phosphate binder). Likely effective for osteoporosis and premenstrual syndrome. Possibly effective for reducing risk of colorectal cancer, hypercholesterolemia, hypertension and prevention of weight gain.	500-1000 mg/day is a typical dose. Do not exceed the UL.	High doses can increase risk for kidney stones, cardiovascular disease, and constipation. Caution in patients with hyperparathyroidism.	Chelated forms such as citrate and malate are better absorbed than carbonate unless taken with a meal. Coadministration with vitamin K may be helpful to reduce risk of hypercalcemia except in those taking blood-thinning medications
Chromium	Effective for chromium deficiency. Possibly effective for reducing blood sugar in diabetes, decreasing LDL cholesterol and triglycerides.	Studies have used 150-1000 mcg/day. Adequate intakes have thought to be 25-35 mcg/day for adults. No UL has been established.	Trivalent chromium is found in appropriate dietary supplements. Poor quality brands may contain hexavalent chromium, which is toxic and linked to cancer. Caution in those with diabetes, renal impairment. Higher doses may cause dermatitis and/or gastrointestinal irritation.	Chromium picolinate is the most common form and is thought to be well absorbed.
Iron	Effective for anemia. Possibly effective for ACE Inhibitor induced cough, cognitive function, heart failure	RDA is recommended unless blood work indicates increased need. Needs increase in pregnancy. Vegetarians may need higher levels because of decreased bioavailability from plant foods. 4-6 mg/kg /day or 60-120 mg/day for those with anemia.	Do not exceed the UL except with coordination of care with a physician. Excessive iron intake can cause nausea, constipation, and black stools and may increase the risk of heart disease.	Chelated iron (citrate, bisglycinate) may be better tolerated and cause less gastrointestinal side effects.
Magnesium	Effective for constipation, dyspepsia, pre-eclampsia and eclampsia. IV forms are effective for cardiac arrhythmia and asthma. Magnesium is often used in fibromyalgia and migraine headache, but the results are mixed.	Typical dose is 100-500 mg/day. Exceeding the UL from supplements (350 mg/day) is not recommended because of potential for diarrhea.	The most common side effects with high doses are diarrhea, bloating, and reduction in blood pressure. Serious side effects are a risk with IV magnesium, including hypotension, nausea, and ataxia.	Similar to calcium, chelated forms such as citrate, bisglycinate, and amino acid chelate may be better absorbed and tolerated than oxide form.
Selenium	Possibly effective for autoimmune thyroiditis and dyslipidemia. Often used as an antioxidant supplement to support glutathione production.	DRI is between 55-70 mcg/day although most supplemental doses are in the 100-200 mcg range. Exceeding the UL of 400 mcg/day is not recommended.	Gastrointestinal symptoms, nausea and vomiting, are most common with high doses. Acute toxicity may impair liver, kidney, and cardiac function.	Brazil nuts are an excellent source of selenium. Selenium and vitamin E have a synergistic effect and are best taken together.

BOX 12-7	**Popular Dietary Supplements and Their Efficacy—cont'd**			
Supplement	**Benefits**	**Dosage**	**Potential Contraindications**	**Quality Considerations**
Minerals				
Zinc	Likely effective for diarrhea and Wilson's disease. Possibly effective for acne, age related macular degeneration, anemia, anorexia nervosa, attention deficit hyperactivity disorder, burns, common cold, dandruff, depression, diabetic foot ulcers, diaper rash, halitosis, gingivitis, herpes simplex virus, muscle cramps, radiation mucositis, osteoporosis, peptic ulcers, pressure ulcers, sickle cell disease, vitamin A deficiency, warts	Doses vary depending on condition. 15-45 mg/day range is common. Much higher doses sometimes given for wound healing short term. Coordination of care recommended.	Mostly nontoxic below the UL of 40 mg/day in adults. High Zn intake can deplete copper and can cause nausea, dermatitis, and copper deficient anemia.	Take Zn supplements with copper to prevent depletion of copper.
Other Supplements				
Alpha lipoic acid	Possibly effective for atherosclerosis, cardiovascular disease, hypertension, and pneumonia. Often used to treat neuropathy with success.	Doses used in research are 600, 1200, and 1800 mg/day for up to 2 years. 5% topical preparation for skin aging	Doses over 600 mg/day can cause nausea, vomiting and vertigo and may interfere with some chemotherapy. In patients with cardiovascular disease, high doses can cause angina, blood pressure changes, and arrhythmia. Can reduce blood glucose in diabetes. Caution with hypoglycemia	Bioactive form is R-ALA. Some quality issues exist with production, so ensure a quality brand. Helps to regenerate vitamin C, E, and glutathione
Arginine	Possibly effective for angina, erectile dysfunction, hypertension, necrotizing enterocolitis (NEC), peripheral artery disease, post surgery recovery and pre-eclampsia.	Therapeutic dose range is thought to be from 400-6,000 mg/day. There is no tolerable upper limit and higher doses (up to 30 g/day) have been used. Coordination of care recommended	High doses may increase bleeding in those on warfarin, may lower blood sugar and blood pressure. Caution in those with history of myocardial infarction or cancer	No special production or quality control issues with arginine. L-arginine is the active form.
Beta-glucan	Likely effective for hyperlipidemia. Possibly effective for allergic rhinitis (hayfever), cancer survival, and postoperative infection.	3 g beta-glucan/day (from oats) per the FDA as a cholesterol lowering food. In supplements, 2-16 g/day is common dosing for hyperlipidemia.	Generally well tolerated with few side effects. May cause mild gastrointestinal symptoms in some. Can lower blood pressure and blood sugar	Found widely in plant-based foods, especially oats and mushrooms.
Coenzyme Q10 (Ubiquinone)	Possibly effective for age related macular degeneration, congestive heart failure, diabetic neuropathy, HIV/AIDS, Hypertension, Ischemic reperfusion injury, migraine headache, and Parkinson's disease.	Doses vary from 30 mg-600 mg/day.	Very few side effects reported other than mild nausea, headache, and skin itching. May decrease blood pressure Caution with people on blood-thinning medications	Oil-based preparations may be better absorbed.
Creatine	Possibly effective for athletic performance enhancement (muscle mass and muscle strength).	Usually taken as a loading dose (0.3 g/kg/day) followed by a maintenance dose (0.03 g/kg/day). Doses up to 30 g have been taken safely short term.	Considered safe for healthy people Increased fluid needs when taking creatine Caution with kidney disease especially if taking NSAIDs Increased symptoms of anxiety and depression have been noted.	Usually sold as creatine monohydrate
DHEA *Dehydroepiandrosterone*	Possibly effective for aging skin and depression. Mixed results in studies on use in adrenal insufficiency, chronic fatigue syndrome, fibromyalgia, HIV/AIDS, osteoporosis, physical performance, sexual dysfunction, weight loss. Most doctors treat with DHEA based on individual lab values.	Dose should be recommended by a physician and based on laboratory results. Doses range from 5-450 mg/day.	May increase estrogen and testosterone and risk for cancer May increase acne, facial hair growth, and cause other hormonal side effects Avoid with hormone blockers such as tamoxifen. Multiple contraindications	7 Keto DHEA is a metabolite of DHEA that is not converted into estrogen or testosterone and is thought to be a safer alternative to DHEA.

Continued

BOX 12-7 Popular Dietary Supplements and Their Efficacy—cont'd

Supplement	Benefits	Dosage	Potential Contraindications	Quality Considerations
Other Supplements				
Fish oil	Effective for hypertriglyceridemia. Likely effective for cardiovascular disease. Possibly effective for age related macular degeneration, asthma, atherosclerosis, attention deficit hyperactivity disorder, cachexia, heart failure, hypertension, psoriasis, Raynaud's syndrome, Rheumatoid arthritis, stroke. Conflicting evidence for depression, inflammatory bowel disease, autism	1-4 g/day of EPA and DHA combined Up to 3 g/day is considered GRAS	More than 3 g/day EPA/DHA may increase risk for bleeding, bruising, and elevation in blood sugar Caution with people on blood-thinning medications and those with diabetes	Molecular distilled fish oil is considered the best quality. For vegetarians, flaxseed oil may also be beneficial. Use cold pressed oil in dark bottles or refrigerate.
Glucosamine	Likely effective for osteoarthritis; Conflicting or insufficient evidence to rate effectiveness for interstitial cystitis and temporomandibular (TMJ) disorders	Typical dose for joint conditions is 1500 mg/day taken in 2-3 divided doses Lower doses of 400-1000 mg/day have been used for other conditions.	Considered to be a safe supplement for most people Most is sourced from shellfish, so may be an allergen in some High doses can disrupt blood sugar metabolism in those with diabetes. Caution in those with renal dysfunction or in those taking warfarin	Most research has been done on glucosamine sulfate form, although glucosamine hydrochloride has also been used with success. Glucosamine is often sold in combination with chondroitin for added benefit.
Glutamine	Possibly effective for use in burn patients, bone marrow transplants, burns, critical illness (trauma), AIDS wasting, oral mucositis and improve nitrogen balance in surgery. Conflicting evidence for use in diarrhea, inflammatory bowel disease and short bowel syndrome.	5-30 g/day orally is a typical dose. Doses in IV or TPN in the critically ill may be higher.	Considered safe Many drugs deplete body stores of glutamine.	Take separately from food (especially protein) for maximal absorption.
Melatonin	Likely effective for delayed sleep phase syndrome, and sleep disorders; Possibly effective for insomnia, benzodiazepine withdrawal, jet lag, improved tumor regression in chemotherapy	500 mcg – 5 mg/day have been used in research. 3 - 5 mg/day is the most common dose.	Generally regarded as safe for use up to 3 months and is even tolerated in neonates. Most common side effects are headache, nausea, and drowsiness. May lower blood pressure and disrupt hormone balance	Usually taken 30 minutes before bed
N-Acetyl Cysteine	Effective for acetaminophen toxicity and tracheostomy care. Can be used as a mucolytic. Possibly effective for angina, bronchitis, bipolar disorder, COPD, hyperlipidemia, hyperhomocysteinemia, prevention of cardiovascular events in end stage renal disease. Often used to support glutathione production	400-600 mg/day for respiratory infections Most common dose is between 600-1200 mg/day for a variety of conditions Much higher dose for acetaminophen poisoning	Well tolerated at usual doses with little evidence of toxicity Very high doses are associated with nausea, vomiting, diarrhea, skin flushing, tachycardia, dizziness, headache, and zinc malabsorption May increase bleeding time in those on anticoagulants	No special considerations except to use a quality product
Probiotics (lactobacillus acidophilus and bifidobacteria)	Likely effective for rotaviral diarrhea. Possibly effective for anti-biotic associated diarrhea, atopic dermatitis (eczema), clostridium difficile diarrhea, chemotherapy induced diarrhea, constipation, Helicobacter pylori inflammation, infantile colic, irritable bowel syndrome, pouchitis, respiratory tract infections, travelers diarrhea, ulcerative colitis	Dosage varies and is measured in colony forming units (CFU's). Range is 1-450 billion CFU depending on the disease condition and therapeutic goal.	May be contraindicated in the immune suppressed, those with central line placement, and in those on hemodialysis due to risk of sepsis May cause diarrhea in high doses	Refrigeration is important to preserve quality in most products.

BOX 12-7	**Popular Dietary Supplements and Their Efficacy—cont'd**			
Supplement	**Benefits**	**Dosage**	**Potential Contraindications**	**Quality Considerations**
Herbs				
Chamomile *Matricaria recutita* (Gernam Chamomile)	Possibly effective for anxiety, colic, diarrhea, dyspepsia, and oral mucositis.	250-500 mg/day in capsules or 1-4 cups/day as tea	Generally recognized as safe. Caution in those with allergy to ragweed or asteraceae family	Ensure correct plant is used. German chamomile is the most common.
Cinnamon *Cinnamomum cassia*	Conflicting evidence for diabetes and for use topically as a mosquito repellant	Typical dose is 1-6 g/day in capsules or 1 teaspoon/day in food. 5% cream used topically as a mosquito repellant.	Generally safe Caution in people with diabetes or blood sugar dysregulation or in those with impaired liver function. May enhance blood-thinning effects of warfarin	Cassia cinnamon is thought to be more biologically active than Ceylon cinnamon.
Cranberry *Vaccinium macrocarpon*	Possibly effective for urinary tract infection, (prevention and treatment). Preliminary evidence for reducing urinary odor and improve symptoms in benign prostatic hyperplasia (BPH).	As juice: 1 ounce cranberry concentrate or 10 ounces cranberry cocktail (sweetened). As capsules: 300-500 mg twice/day	Generally safe. Caution with sugar in juice for diabetics, may increase calcium oxalate kidney stones	Blueberries have similar constituents and may be similarly beneficial.
Echinacea angustifolia, pallida and purpurea	Possibly effective for the common cold and for vaginal candidiasis. Insufficient evidence for influenza and otitis media	Can be taken as a capsule, tablet, tea or tincture. Doses vary and are dependent on the variety used and preparation.	Caution in people with allergy to Asteraceae family (daisy, sunflower), and those on immunosuppressive medications	Sometimes standardized to contain a specific amount of echinacoside or cichoric acid
Garlic *Allium sativum*	Possibly effective for atherosclerosis, colorectal cancer, gastric ulcer, hypertension, reduced number of tick bites, and topical treatment of ringworm and athletes foot. Conflicting evidence for hyperlipidemia, common cold	2-5 g fresh garlic, 0.4-1.2 g dried powder, 2-5 mg oil, or 300-1000 mg extract to deliver 2-5 mg allicin (active constituent) per day. One clove fresh garlic has also been used	Generally well tolerated. Higher doses may cause gastric irritation, body odor and decreased blood pressure. Caution with those who are taking blood thinners.	Comes in many forms in supplements. Those that preserve allicin content may be more effective. Aged extracts have shown benefits as well because of the multitude of sulfur compounds present.
Ginkgo biloba	Possibly effective for cognitive function, dementia, generalized anxiety disorder, and schizophrenia, premenstrual syndrome, peripheral vascular disease, vertigo, glaucoma, and diabetic retinopathy.	80-240 mg standardized extract and 3-6 mg of a 40 mg/mL liquid extract in 2-3 divided doses per day has been used. 30-40 mg in a tea bag has also been used.	Generally considered safe except in high-risk patients. Ginkgo can reduce blood pressure, decrease blood sugar, and cause mild gastrointestinal discomfort in some. Some reports of dizziness and sedation	Ginkgo leaf preparations are the most commonly used. Often standardized to 24% ginkgoflavone glycosides and 6% terpenes
Green tea *Camellia sinensis*	Likely effective for hypercholesterolemia and mental alertness. Possibly effective for coronary artery disease, hypotension, osteoporosis. Conflicting evidence for cancer prevention, cardiovascular disease, obesity.	Epigallocatechin (EGCG) epicatechin gallate, and epicatechin levels vary when taken as tea. 3 cups daily is a common dosage. Standardized extracts (60-97% polyphenols) of 200-500 mg/day are common for a variety of conditions. 10% topical cream for skin aging and acne.	Well tolerated in most people. Most side effects come from the caffeine content (nervousness, anxiety, sleeplessness, and increased blood pressure). Use with caution in patients with psychiatric or cardiovascular conditions.	Decaffeinated versions are available to eliminate caffeine side effects.
Kava Kava *Piper methysticum*	Possibly effective for anxiety; Insufficient evidence for benzodiazepine withdrawal, insomnia and menopausal anxiety.	60-400 mg standardized extract per day	Typical therapeutic doses are tolerated by most. Significant evidence of liver injury in the literature. Caution in people with liver disease. Chronic use can cause dry, scaly skin and photosensitivity.	Often standardized to contain 30% to 70% kavalactones. May be best to start at lower doses and titrate up
Milk thistle *Silybum marianum*	Although it is commonly used to reduce inflammation and fibrosis in liver disease, there is conflicting and insufficient evidence for alcohol related liver disease, amanita mushroom poisoning, cirrhosis, and hepatitis induced liver damage.	160-1200 mg/day based on condition treated. Take as divided doses.	Low toxicity risk. Can cause a mild laxative effect if taken in large amounts. Rare risk of allergic reaction. May lower blood sugar. May mildly inhibit CYP 34A, 2C19 and 2D6 cytochrome enzymes	Often standardized to contain 70% to 80% silymarin. Tea preparation is not recommended because of poor water solubility. Whole, ground milk thistle seeds can be added to food.

Continued

BOX 12-7   Popular Dietary Supplements and Their Efficacy—cont'd

Supplement	Benefits	Dosage	Potential Contraindications	Quality Considerations
Herbs				
Red Yeast Rice (RYR) *Monascus purpureus*	Likely effective for hyperlipidemia. Possibly effective for cardiovascular disease and HIV/AIDS related dyslipidemia. Preliminary evidence for use in non alcoholic fatty liver disease (NAFLD).	The most common dose is between 600- 2400 mg/day. It is estimated that average intake of naturally occurring RYR in Asia is 14-55 g/day.	Limited data on adverse events. Side effects appear to be similar to those with low-dose statin medications (headache, gastrointestinal discomfort, and muscle pain). May increase serum liver enzyme levels.	Contains naturally occurring lovastatin (Monacolin K). Dosing is difficult because of natural variations in products. It is illegal in the United States to standardize Monocolin K levels in supplements.
Saw palmetto *Serenoa repens*	Conflicting evidence for use in benign prostatic hyperplasia (BPH). Insufficient evidence for use in androgenic alopecia, neurogenic bladder and prostate cancer.	1-2 g of ground, dried berries, 2-4 ml tincture (1:4) three times per day or 160 mg four times per day	Well tolerated in most people. Studies show low risk for allergy or herb drug interactions. Some reports of mild gastrointestinal side effects. May have estrogenic effects.	Berries have the active constituents (sterols and fatty acids). Tea preparations may be ineffective due to lipophilic nature.
St Johns Wort *Hypericum perforatum*	Likely effective for mild to moderate depression. Possibly effective for menopausal symptoms, somatization disorder. Conflicting or insufficient evidence for anxiety, obsessive compulsive disorder, premenstrual syndrome, seasonal affective disorder. Can be used topically for wound healing.	Typical dose is 300-450 mg three times per day	Has the most drug nutrient interactions of any common herb. Inhibit CYP 34A, 2C19 and 2C9 cytochrome enzymes and the P-glycoprotein (P-gp) transporter. Reduces the effectiveness of immunosuppressive, antiretroviral, cardiovascular, and oral contraceptive medications among others. Can cause photosensitivity	Typically standardized at 0.3% hypericin
Turmeric *Curcuma longa*	Possibly effective for osteoarthritis. Insufficient or conflicting evidence for Alzheimer's disease, colorectal cancer, Crohn's disease, irritable bowel syndrome, rheumatoid arthritis, ulcerative colitis.	500 mg-2 g curcumin per day depending on disease condition Higher doses taken in divided doses	Safe in amounts eaten in food Higher doses can lower blood pressure and blood sugar and increase risk of bleeding. Caution in those with liver and gall bladder diseases and in those taking blood-thinning medications	May be best absorbed when taken with food, especially a meal that contains fat Curcumin supplements bound to phosphatidyl choline may be better absorbed.

Popular Dietary Supplements and Their Efficacy According to the Natural Medicines Database https://naturalmedicines.therapeuticresearch.com. Accessed June 19, 2015.

CLINICAL CASE STUDY

Ellen is a 60-year-old female who was referred from her primary care provider for evaluation of her dietary supplements. Medical history includes hypertension, hypercholesterolemia, osteopenia, mild depression, and memory problems. Two years ago, she had angioplasty (PTCA) with a stent placement in her coronary artery. Ellen is a retired school teacher, married, and has two grown children. Her neighbor works in a supplement store and recommended some herbs and supplements to address Ellen's health concerns.

At the initial consult Ellen reports she is taking the following supplements: calcium carbonate 1200 mg/d, garlic (*Allium sativum*) 500 mg/d, *Ginkgo biloba* 240 mg/d, and St. John's wort (*Hypericum perforatum*) 900 mg/d. Her prescription medications include warfarin, simvastatin, sertraline, and atenolol.

Height: 64" Weight 165 lbs BMI: 28.4

Blood pressure readings: 134/92, 140/95 "This is higher than it usually is" Ellen reports.

Recent labs:
  Total cholesterol: 284 mg/dl
  HDL: 36 mg/dl
  LDL: 140 mg/dl
  Prothrombin times (INR) has been inconsistent lately.

Typical dietary intake includes the following:

Breakfast: Total cereal with milk and calcium fortified orange juice for breakfast

Lunch: Frozen entrée—beef and broccoli with rice and a diet coke

Snack: Strawberry yogurt and pretzels, coffee with milk

Dinner: Meatloaf, mashed potatoes with gravy and carrots. Glass of red wine.

Dessert: Chocolate ice cream, coffee with milk

Questions to consider:

1. Using the Office of Dietary Supplements Fact sheets (ODS website), identify what each dietary supplement Ellen is taking is used for and if it has good evidence to support use.
2. List any potential drug nutrient interactions (DNI) Ellen may have with her current concomitant use of medications and dietary supplements.
3. Looking at Ellen's labs, is there any evidence she may be having a drug nutrient interaction (DNI)?
4. Does Ellen need to be taking a calcium supplement? Are there any potential risks with taking 1200 mg/day with a positive history of cardiovascular disease (CVD)?
5. Write a PES statement for your top concern based on your assessment.

USEFUL WEBSITES

Free Sites

Dietary Supplements Labels Database
http://dietarysupplements.nlm.nih.gov/dietary

Drug Interactions Checker
http://www.drugs.com/drug_interactions.php

Linus Pauling Micronutrient Information Center
http://lpi.oregonstate.edu/infocenter/

Medscape Drug Interaction Checker
http://reference.medscape.com/drug-interactionchecker

MedWatch
http://www.fda.gov/medwatch/

National Center for Complementary and Integrative Health
https://nccih.nih.gov

Natural Products Association
http://www.npainfo.org/

Office of Dietary Supplements
http://ods.od.nih.gov/Health_Information/Health_Information.
aspx

Subscription Sites

Cochrane Database Review
http://www.cochranelibrary.com

Consumer Lab
http://www.consumerlab.com/

Dietitians in Integrative and Functional Medicine (DIFM) practice group through the Academy of Nutrition
http://integrativerd.org/

Natural Medicines Database (formerly Natural Standard and Natural Medicines Comprehensive Database)
https://naturalmedicines.therapeuticresearch.com

Institute for Functional Medicine
http://www.functionalmedicine.org

Text/Print

Skidmore-Roth L: *Mosby's handbook of herbs and natural supplements,* ed 4, St Louis, 2010, Elsevier.

Sarubin-Fragakis A, Thompson C: *The health professionals guide to popular dietary supplements,* ed 3, Chicago, 2007, American Dietetic Association.

Talbot SM, Hughes K: *The health professionals guide to dietary supplements,* Baltimore, 2007, Lippincott Williams.

Resources for Herbal Medicine

American Botanical Council (ABC)
http://cms.herbalgram.org/herbstream/library/homePage/

American Herbalists Guild
http://www.americanherbalistsguild.com/

American Herbal Products Association
http://www.ahpa.org/

Dr. Duke's Phytochemical and Ethnobotanical Database
http://www.ars-grin.gov/duke/

REFERENCES

Academy of Nutrition and Dietetics (2013). *Academy scope of practice decision tool: a self-assessment guide* (website). http://www.andjrnl.org/article/S2212-2672(13)00359-6/pdf. Accessed June 19, 2015.

Albion Human Nutrition (2015). *Research notes* (website). http://www.albion-humannutrition.com/research-notes?start=1. Accessed October 30, 2014.

American College of Surgeons, College of Education. (2012). *Medication and surgery before your operation* (website). http://www.facs.org/patienteducation/medications.html. Accessed January 31, 2014.

American Herbalists Guild. (2015). *What is herbal medicine?* (website). http://www.americanherbalistsguild.com/herbal-medicine-fundamentals. Accessed June 19, 2015.

Ames BN, Elson-Schwabe H, Silver EA: High dose vitamin therapy stimulates variant enzymes with decreased coenzyme binding affinity (increased Km): relevance to genetic disease and polymorphisms, *Am J Clin Nutr* 75:616, 2002.

Azzi A, Stocker A: Vitamin E: non-antioxidant roles, *Progr Lipid Research* 39:231, 2000.

Bailey RL, Fulgoni VL 3rd, Keast DR, et al: Do dietary supplements improve micronutrient sufficiency in children and adolescents? *J Pediatr* 161:837, 2012.

Bailey RL, Gahche JJ, Miller PE, et al: Why US adults use dietary supplements, *JAMA Intern Med* 173(5):355, 2013.

Barnes PM, Bloom B, Nahin RL: Complementary and alternative medicine use among adults and children: United States, 2007, *Natl Health Stat Report* 10(12):1, 2008.

Birdee GS, Phillips RS, Davis RB, et al: Factors associated with pediatric use of complementary and alternative medicine, *Pediatrics* 125:249, 2010.

Bjelakovic G, Nikolova D, Gluud LL, et al: Antioxidant supplements for prevention of mortality in healthy participants and patients with various diseases, *Cochrane Database Syst Rev* 3:CD007176, 2012. doi: 10.1002/14651858.CD007176.pub2.

Boden WE, Sidhu MS, Toth PP: The therapeutic role of niacin in dyslipidemia management, *J Cardiovasc Pharmacol Ther* 19(2):141, 2014.

Centers for Disease Control and Prevention: *National health interview survey,* 2012. http://www.cdc.gov/nchs/nhis/nhis_2012_data_release.htm. Accessed January 22, 2014.

Chew EY, Clemons TE, Agrón E, et al: Long-term effects of vitamins C and E, β-carotene, and zinc on age-related macular degeneration: AREDS report no. 35, *Ophthalmology* 120(8):1604, 2013.

Consumer Labs: *Reviews of supplements and health products* (website). http://www.consumerlab.com. Accessed June 19, 2015.

Crane NT, Nalubola R, Schneeman BO: The role and relevance of Codex in Nutrition Standards, *J Am Diet Assoc* 110:672, 2010.

Dickinson A: History and overview of DSHEA, *Fitoterapia* 82:5, 2011.

Food and Drug Administration Regulatory Information (2009). *The dietary supplement health and education act* (website). http://www.fda.gov/RegulatoryInformation/Legislation/FederalFoodDrugandCosmeticActFDCAct/SignificantAmendmentstotheFDCAct/ucm148003.htm. Accessed January 29, 2014.

Food and Drug Administration: *Claims that can be made for conventional foods and dietary supplements* (website), 2003. http://www.fda.gov/Food/IngredientsPackagingLabeling/LabelingNutrition/ucm111447.htm. Accessed January 27, 2014.

Food and Drug Administration: *Guidance for industry: current good manufacturing practice in manufacturing, packaging, labeling, or holding operations for dietary supplements; small entity compliance guide* (website), 2010. http://www.fda.gov/food/guidanceregulation/guidancedocumentsregulatoryinformation/dietarysupplements/ucm238182.htm. Accessed January 27, 2014.

Food and Drug Administration (2015). *Q and A on dietary supplements: what is a dietary supplement?* (website). http://www.fda.gov/Food/DietarySupplements/QADietarySupplements/default.htm#what_is. Accessed October 15, 2015.

Food and Drug Administration: *Tainted products marketed as dietary supplements potentially dangerous* (website), 2010. http://www.fda.gov/NewsEvents/Newsroom/PressAnnouncements/ucm236967.htm. Accessed January 27, 2014.

Food and Drug Administration: *Reports received and reports entered into FAERS by year* (website), 2012. http://www.fda.gov/Drugs/GuidanceComplianceRegulatoryInformation/Surveillance/AdverseDrugEffects/ucm070434.htm. Accessed June 19, 2015.

Ford D, Raj S, Batheja RK, et al: American dietetic association: standards of practice and standards of professional performance for registered dietitians (competent, proficient, and expert) in integrative and functional medicine glossary of terms, *J Am Diet Assoc* 111(6):902, 2011.

Fortmann SP, Burda BU, Senger CA, et al: *Vitamin, mineral and multivitamin supplements for the primary prevention of cardiovascular disease and cancer: a systematic evidence review for the U.S. preventive services task force*, Rockville, MD, 2013, Agency for Healthcare Research and Quality (US). Report No.: 14-05199-EF-1.

Frankos VH, Street DA, O'Neill RK: FDA regulation of dietary supplements and requirements regarding adverse event reporting, *Clin Pharmacol Ther* 87:239, 2010.

Fulgoni VL, Keast DR, Bailey RL, et al: Foods, fortificants, and supplements: where do Americans get their nutrients? *J Nutr* 141(10):1847, 2011.

Gahche J, Bailey R, Burt V, et al: *Centers for disease control and prevention. Dietary supplement use among US adults and children has increased since NHANESIII* (website). http://www.cdc.gov/nchs/data/databriefs/db61.pdf. Accessed January 22, 2014.

Geller A, Shehab N, Weidle N, et al. Emergency department visits for adverse events related to dietary supplements. NEJM 373(16):1531, 2015.

Government Accountability Office: *Dietary supplements: FDA may have opportunities to expand its use of reported health problems to oversee products* (website), 2013. http://www.gao.gov/assets/660/653113.pdf. Accessed October 15, 2015.

Gurley BJ: Pharmacokinetic herb-drug interactions (Part 1): origins, mechanisms, and the impact of botanical dietary supplements, *Planta Medica* 78:1478, 2012.

Gurley BJ, Fifer EK, Gardner Z: Pharmacokinetic herb-drug interactions (Part 2): drug interactions involving popular botanical dietary supplements and their clinical relevance, *Planta Medica* 78:1490, 2012.

Harris PE, Cooper KL, Relton C, et al: Prevalence of complementary and alternative medicine (CAM) use by the general population: a systematic review, *Int J Clin Prac* 66(10):924, 2012.

Head KA: Peripheral neuropathy: pathogenic mechanisms and alternative therapies, *Alt Med Rev* 11(14):294, 2006.

Hendren RL: Autism: biomedical complementary treatment approaches, *Child Adolesc Psychiatric Clin N Am* 22:443, 2013.

Horrigan B, Lewis S, Abrams D, et al: *Integrative medicine in America. How integrative medicine is being practiced in clinical centers across the United States. The Bravewell Collaborative* (website), 2012. http://www.bravewell.org/current_projects/mapping_field/. Accessed January 22, 2014.

Institute for Functional Medicine: *What is functional medicine?* (website). http://www.functionalmedicine.org/about/whatisfm. Accessed January 21, 2014.

Krebs-Smith S, Guenther PM, Subar AF, et al: Americans do not meet federal dietary recommendations, *J Nutr* 140(10):1832, 2010.

Lindstrom A, Ooyen C, Lynch ME, et al: Herb supplement sales increase 5.5% in 2012: herb supplement sales rise for 9th consecutive year, *Herbal Gram* 99:60, 2013.

Liu M, Wallmon A, Olsson-Mortlock C, et al: Mixed tocopherols inhibit platelet aggregation in humans: potential mechanisms, *Am J Clin Nutr* 77(3):700, 2003.

Murphy SP, White KK, Park SY, et al: Multivitamin-multimineral supplements' effect on total nutrient intake, *Am J Clin Nutr* 85(1):S280, 2007.

National Center for Complementary and Integrative Health (2008). *Complementary, alternative, or integrative health: what's in a name?* (website). http://nccam.nih.gov/health/whatiscam. Accessed June 19, 2015

National Institutes of Health (2015). Office of Dietary Supplements: *Multivitamin/mineral supplements fact sheet for healthcare professionals* (website). http://ods.od.nih.gov/factsheets/MVMS-HealthProfessional/. Accessed June 19, 2015.

National Institutes of Health State-of-the-science conference statement: multivitamin/mineral supplements and chronic disease prevention, *Ann Intern Med* 145:364, 2006.

National Institutes of Health, Office of Dietary Supplements (2011). *Dietary supplements: what you need to know* (website). http://ods.od.nih.gov/HealthInformation/DS_WhatYouNeedToKnow.aspx. Accessed June 19, 2015.

National Institutes of Health, Office of Dietary Supplements: *Dietary supplement label database* (website), 2015. http://ods.od.nih.gov/Research/Dietary_Supplement_Label_Database.aspx. Accessed June 19, 2015.

Neuhouser ML, Wassertheil-Smoller S, Thomson C, et al: Multivitamin use and risk of cancer and cardiovascular disease in the women's health initiative cohorts, *Arch Intern Med* 169(3):294, 2009.

NSF International (2015). *Services by industry: dietary supplements* (website). http://www.nsf.org/services/by-industry/dietary-supplements. Accessed June 19, 2015.

NSF International (2015). *Services by industry: sports supplement screening-certified for sport* (website). http://www.nsf.org/services/by-industry/dietary-supplements/sports-supplement-screening. Accessed June 19, 2015.

Peregoy JA, Clarke TC, Jones LI, et al: Regional variation in use of complementary health approaches by US adults, *NCHS Data Brief* (146):1, 2014.

Marra MV, Boyar AP: Position of the American Dietetic Association: nutrient supplementation, *J Acad Nutr Diet* 109:2073, 2009.

Straub DA: Calcium supplementation in clinical practice: a review of forms, doses, and indications, Nutr Clin Pract 22(3):286, 2007.

Therapeutic Goods Administration (2015). *Complementary medicines* (website). https://www.tga.gov.au/complementary-medicines. Accessed June 19, 2015.

Thompson C, Diekman C, Fragakis AS, et al: Guidelines regarding the recommendation and sale of dietary supplements, *J Am Diet Assoc* 102(8):1158, 2002.

Trine T: *Dietary supplements: manufacturing troubles widespread, FDA inspections show*, June 30, 2012, Chicago Tribune (serial online). http://articles.chicagotribune.com/2012-06-30/news/ct-met-supplement-inspections-20120630_1_dietary-supplements-inspections-american-herbal-products-association. Accessed January 27, 2014.

US Pharmacopeia (2015). *USP dietary supplement standards* (website). http://www.usp.org/dietary-supplements/overview. Accessed June 19, 2015.

13

Food and Nutrient Delivery: Nutrition Support[1]

Carol S. Ireton-Jones, PhD, RDN, LD, CNSC, FAND, FASPEN,
Mary Krystofiak Russell MS, RDN, LDN, FAND

KEY TERMS

advance directives
bolus enteral feeding
catheter
central parenteral nutrition (CPN)
closed enteral system
computerized provider order entry (CPOE)
durable medical equipment (DME) provider
enteral nutrition (EN)
essential fatty acid deficiency (EFAD)
extended dwell catheter
French size
gastrointestinal decompression
gastrojejunostomy

gastric residual volume (GRV)
hang time
hemodynamic stability
home enteral nutrition (HEN)
home parenteral nutrition (HPN)
intermittent enteral feeding
multiple lumen tube
nasoduodenal tube (NDT)
nasogastric tube (NGT)
nasojejunal tube (NJT)
open enteral system
osmolality
osmolarity
parenteral nutrition (PN)

percutaneous endoscopic gastrostomy (PEG)
percutaneous endoscopic jejunostomy (PEJ)
peripheral parenteral nutrition (PPN)
peripherally inserted central catheter (PICC or PIC)
polymeric enteral formula
rebound hypoglycemia
refeeding syndrome
sentinel event
total nutrient admixture (3-in-1)
transitional feeding

Nutrition support is the delivery of formulated enteral or parenteral nutrients for the purpose of maintaining or restoring nutritional status. **Enteral nutrition (EN)** refers to nutrition provided through the gastrointestinal tract (GIT) via a **catheter** or a tube or stoma that delivers nutrients distal to the oral cavity. **Parenteral nutrition (PN)** is the provision of nutrients intravenously.

RATIONALE AND CRITERIA FOR APPROPRIATE NUTRITION SUPPORT

When patients cannot or will not eat enough to support their nutritional needs for more than a few days, nutrition support should be considered as part of the integrated care plan. Using the GIT (EN) vs. using PN alone helps preserve the intestinal mucosal barrier function and integrity. In critically ill patients, feeding the GIT has been shown to attenuate the catabolic response and preserve immunologic function (McClave et al, 2009). Research shows less septic morbidity, fewer infectious complications, and significant cost savings in critically ill adult patients who received EN vs. PN. There is limited evidence that EN vs. PN affects hospital length of stay (LOS), but an impact on mortality has not been demonstrated (Academy of Nutrition and Dietetics [AND], Evidence Analysis Library [EAL],

2012). A recent study found no significant difference in 30-day mortality in critically ill adults who received nutrition support by the parenteral or the enteral route (Harvey et al, 2014).

A variety of diseases and conditions may result in the need for nutrition support (Table 13-1). PN should be used in patients who are or will become malnourished and who do not have sufficient gastrointestinal function to be able to restore or maintain optimal nutritional status (McClave et al, 2009). EN should be considered when an individual has a functional GIT and is unable or unwilling to consume sufficient nutrients to meet his or her estimated needs. Figure 13-1 presents an algorithm for selecting appropriate routes for EN and PN. Although these guidelines provide ideas, the choice of the most optimal method of nutrition support can be challenging. For example, the small bowel feeding access for EN may not be available in every health care setting. In such a case, PN may be the only realistic option for provision of nutrition support. PN may be used temporarily until adequate gastrointestinal function to support EN or oral intake returns, or PN may be used to supplement EN or oral intake to meet needs effectively for energy, protein, and other key nutrients. "Transitional Feeding," described later in the chapter, refers to the provision of nutrition support via two or more methods, until nutrition adequacy is reached via oral intake alone.

Although specific nutrition support regimens may be standardized for specific disease states or courses of therapy, each patient presents a unique challenge. Nutrition support frequently

---

[1]Sections of this chapter were written by Janice L. Raymond, MS, RDN, CSG for the previous edition of this text.

TABLE 13-1 Conditions That May Require Nutrition Support

Recommended Route of Feeding	Condition	Typical Disorders
Enteral nutrition	Inability to eat	Neurologic disorders (dysphagia)
		Facial trauma
		Oral or esophageal trauma
		Congenital anomalies
		Respiratory failure (on a ventilator)
		Traumatic brain injury
		Comatose state
		GI surgery (e.g., esophagectomy)
	Inability to eat enough	Hypermetabolic states such as with burns
		Cancer
		Heart failure
		Congenital heart disease
		Impaired intake after orofacial surgery or injury
		Anorexia nervosa
		Failure to thrive
		Cystic fibrosis
	Impaired digestion, absorption, metabolism	Severe gastroparesis
		Inborn errors of metabolism
		Crohn's disease
		Short bowel syndrome with minimum resection
		Pancreatitis
Parenteral nutrition	Gastrointestinal incompetency	Short bowel syndrome—major resection
		Severe acute pancreatitis with intolerance to enteral feeding
		Severe inflammatory bowel disease
		Small bowel ischemia
		Intestinal atresia
		Severe liver failure
		Persistent postoperative ileus
		Intractable vomiting/diarrhea refractory to medical management
		Distal high-output fistulas
		Severe GI bleeding
	Critical illness with poor enteral tolerance or accessibility	Multi-organ system failure
		Major trauma or burns
		Bone marrow transplantation
		Acute respiratory failure with ventilator dependency and gastrointestinal malfunction
		Severe wasting in renal failure with dialysis
		Small bowel transplantation, immediate after surgery

McClave SA et al: Guidelines for the provision and assessment of nutrition support therapy in the adult critically ill patient, *J Parenter Enteral Nutr* 33:277, 2009.
GI, Gastrointestinal.

must be adapted to address unanticipated developments or complications. An optimal treatment plan requires interdisciplinary collaboration that is aligned closely with the comprehensive plan of patient care. In rare cases, nutrition support may be warranted but physically impossible to implement. In other situations, nutrition support may be possible but not warranted because it presents an unacceptable risk or is not indicated because of the prognosis or the patient's right to self-determination.

In all cases, it is important to prevent errors in ordering, delivery, and monitoring of nutrition support to prevent undesirable risks or outcomes (sentinel events) such as an unexpected death, serious physical injury with loss of limb or function, or psychologic injury (Joint Commission, 2014). A computerized provider order entry (CPOE) system allows prescribers to enter an order directly into a computer, often aided by decision-support technology to help facilitate accuracy and clinical effectiveness (Bankhead et al, 2009).

ENTERAL NUTRITION

By definition, *enteral* implies using the GIT, usually via a feeding tube with the tip in the stomach or small bowel. The location of nutrient administration and type of enteral access device are selected after the patient is determined to be a candidate for EN. (The process for determining whether an individual is a candidate for EN is described later.) Enteral access selection depends on the (1) anticipated length of time enteral feeding will be required, (2) degree of risk for aspiration or tube displacement, (3) patient's clinical status, (4) adequacy of digestion and absorption, (5) patient's anatomy (e.g., after previous surgical resection or in extreme obesity), and (6) whether future surgical intervention is planned.

Feeding tubes may be referred to by their French size, which is a measure of the outer tube diameter. One French unit is 0.33 mm. A French size of 5 to 12 typically is considered "small bore," and a French size of more than 14 is considered "large bore."

ENTERAL NUTRITION ACCESS

Short-Term Enteral Nutrition Support
Nasogastric Access

Nasogastric tubes (NGTs) are used most commonly to access the GIT, for gastric decompression, medication delivery, and/or feeding. They are appropriate only for those patients who require short-term (no more than 3 to 4 weeks) EN. Typically, the tube is inserted at the bedside by a nurse or physician (or a registered dietitian with appropriate clinical privileges) and passed through the nose into the stomach (Figure 13-2). Polyurethane or silicone tubes of various diameters, lengths, and design features may be used, depending on formula characteristics and feeding requirements. These tubes are soft, flexible, and often well tolerated by patients. Tube placement is verified by aspirating gastric contents in combination with auscultation of air insufflation into the stomach or by radiographic confirmation of the tube tip location. Techniques for placing a tube are described by Metheny and Meert (2004).

NGT feedings are provided by bolus administration or by intermittent or continuous infusions (see Administration later in this chapter). Patients with normal gastrointestinal function are often fed via this route, which takes advantage of normal digestive, hormonal, and bactericidal processes in the stomach. Rarely, complications occur (Box 13-1).

Gastric Versus Small-Bowel Access

Placement of a feeding tube into the stomach is more straightforward and far less time consuming than placing a tube into the small bowel, so gastric feedings generally are initiated

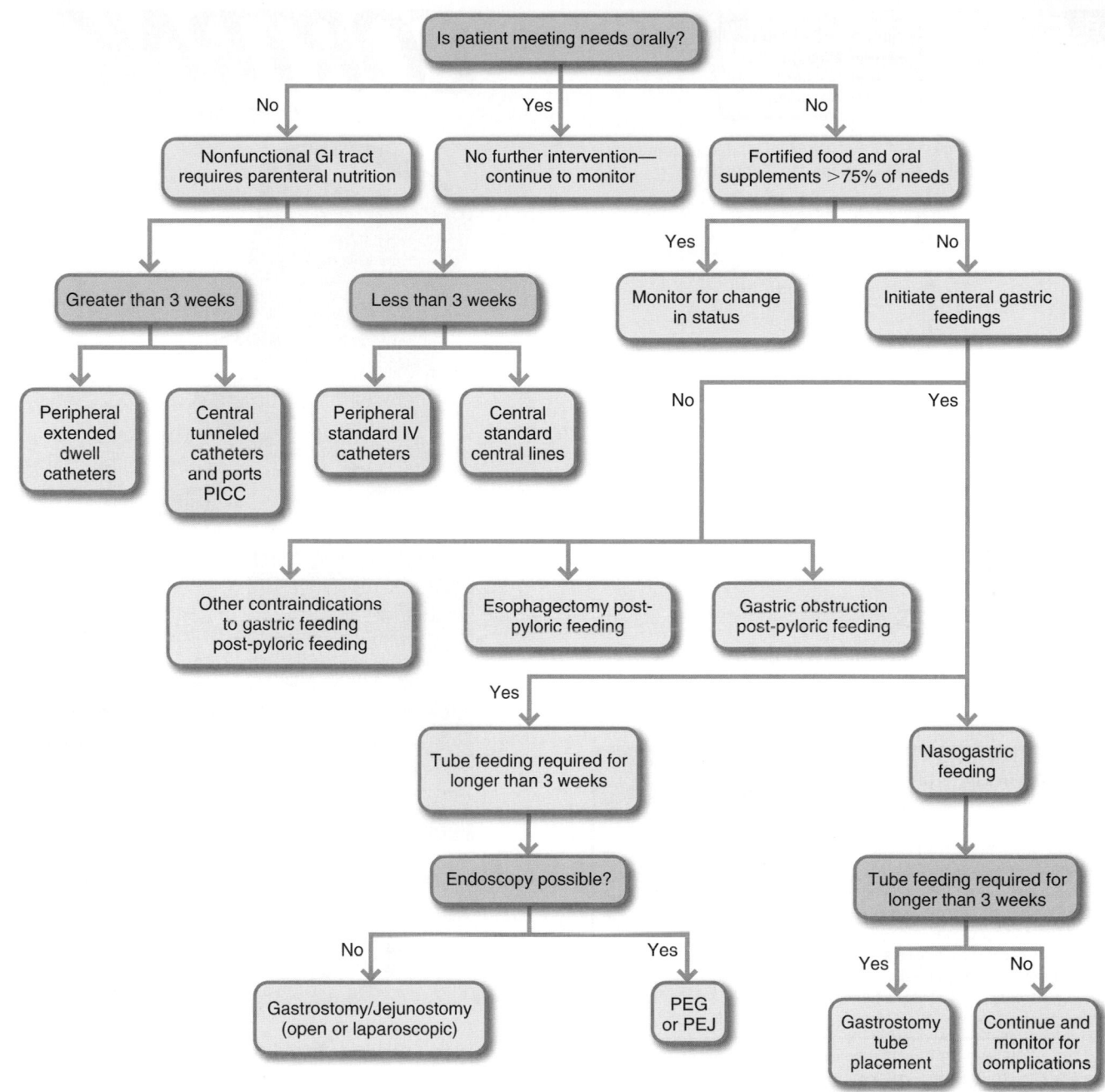

FIGURE 13-1 Algorithm for route selection for nutrition support.

more quickly. However, ease of access is only one consideration. Critically ill patients, including those who have undergone surgery, or suffered a head injury or major intra-abdominal trauma, may not tolerate gastric feeding (see Chapter 38).

Signs and symptoms of intolerance to gastric feeding include, but are not limited to, the following:
- Abdominal distention and discomfort
- Vomiting
- Persistent diarrhea

Some clinicians believe that intragastric feeding increases the risk of aspiration pneumonia; the data on this subject are not totally clear (Bankhead et al, 2009; McClave et al, 2009).

Nasoduodenal or Nasojejunal Access

Patients who do not tolerate gastric feedings and require relatively short-term enteral nutrition support will benefit from placement of a nasoduodenal tube (NDT) or a nasojejunal tube (NJT), described by the point at which the tube tip terminates. These tubes may be placed with endoscopic or fluoroscopic guidance (Figure 13-3, *A*); using a computer guidance system (Figure 13-3, *B*); or intraoperatively as part of a surgical procedure.

In some cases, a feeding tube may be placed intragastrically with the goal of migration into the duodenum by peristalsis; this process is unlikely to result in desired location of the feeding tube tip and inevitably delays initiation of appropriate EN. Spontaneous migration never achieves jejunal tip placement.

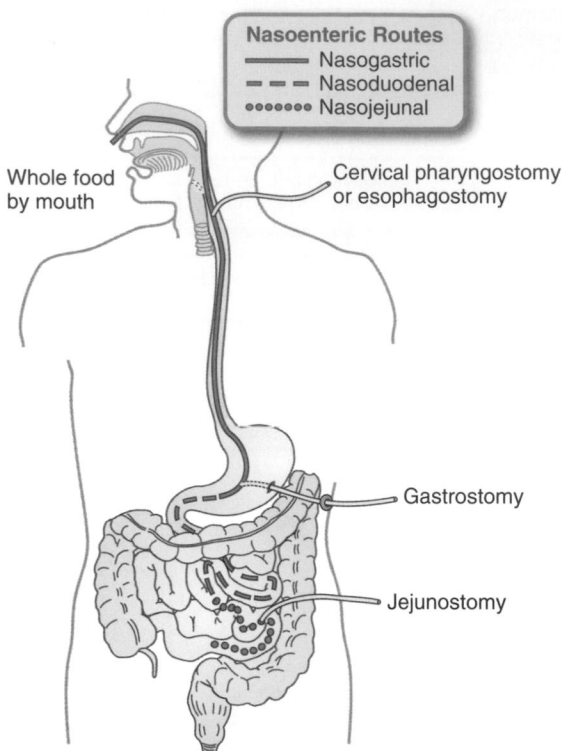

FIGURE 13-2 Diagram of enteral tube placement.

BOX 13-1   Potential Complications of Nasoenteric Tubes

Esophageal strictures
Gastroesophageal reflux resulting in aspiration pneumonia
Tracheoesophageal fistula
Incorrect position of the tube leading to pulmonary injury
Mucosal damage at the insertion site
Nasal irritation and erosion
Pharyngeal or vocal cord paralysis
Rhinorrhea, sinusitis, otitis media
Ruptured gastroesophageal varices in hepatic disease
Ulcerations or perforations of the upper gastrointestinal tract and airway

Adapted from McClave SA et al: Guidelines for the provision and assessment of nutrition support therapy in the adult critically ill patient, *J Parenter Enteral Nutr* 33:277, 2009; Cresci G: Enteral access. In Charney P, Malone A: *Pocket guide to enteral nutrition,* ed 2, Chicago, 2013, AND, p 62.

Long-Term Enteral Access

Gastrostomy or Jejunostomy

When EN is required for more than 3 to 4 weeks, a surgically or endoscopically placed gastrostomy or jejunostomy feeding tube should be considered for overall patient comfort (Figure 13-4) and to minimize nasal and upper GIT irritation (see Box 13-1). Such a tube may be placed during a required surgical or endoscopic procedure to maximize efficiency and cost effectiveness.

Percutaneous endoscopic gastrostomy (PEG) or **percutaneous endoscopic jejunostomy (PEJ)** is a nonsurgical technique for placing a tube directly into the stomach through the abdominal wall, using an endoscope and local anesthesia. The

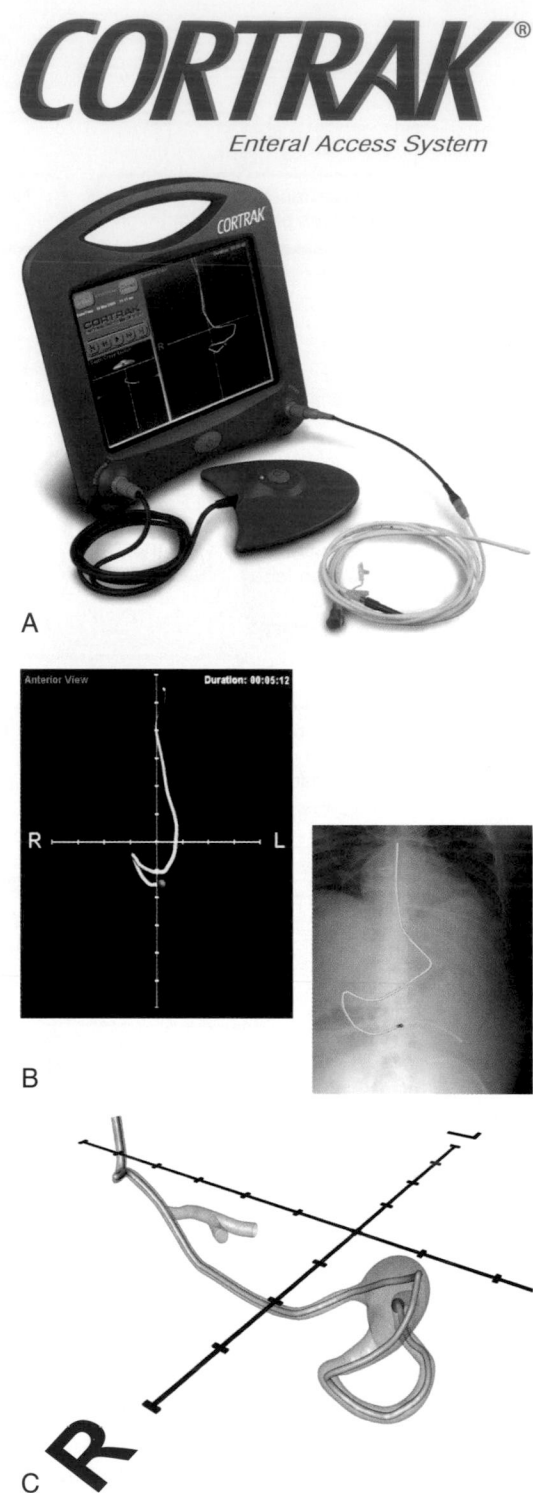

FIGURE 13-3 Computerized Cortrak tube feeding placement system. **A,** CORTRAK System; **B,** CORTRAK anterior view compared with abdominal radiograph; **C,** 3-Dimensional graphic representation of a CORTRAK feeding tube in post pyloric position. (Used with permission from CORPAK MedSystems.)

tube is guided from the mouth into the stomach or the jejunum and brought out through the abdominal wall. The short procedure time and limited anesthesia requirements have contributed to making it a very common method of feeding tube placement.

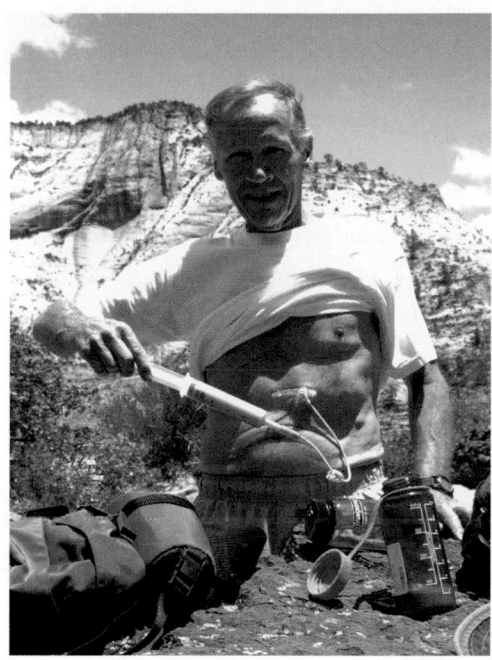

FIGURE 13-4 A man with a gastrostomy tube out hiking. (From Oley Foundation, Albany, NY: www.oley.org. Accessed December 2014.)

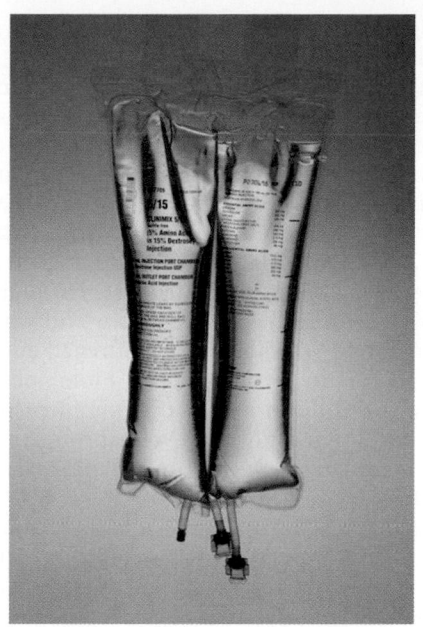

FIGURE 13-5 Baxter Clinimix Compounding System. (Image provided by Baxter Healthcare Corporation. CLINIMIX is a trademark of Baxter International Inc.)

Tubes placed by PEG (note the PEG is the procedure, not the tube, although clinicians commonly refer to "PEGs" as the tube) are generally large bore (or French size), facilitating administration of medications and reducing the incidence of clogging. These tubes may be connected to a short piece of tubing used to infuse a bolus feeding or connect to a bag of prepared formula. Some tubes placed by PEG are flush to the skin, or "low profile." These tubes, also known as "buttons," are a good choice for children and adults with dementia who may be likely to pull out a tube that protrudes from the skin. Active individuals, and those who prefer a sleeker profile under clothing, also may opt for this type of tube. Figure 13-5 shows a component from a skin level balloon G-tube kit, designed to improve patient comfort and increase the length of time the G-tube may remain in place. To prevent the accidental parenteral infusion of enteral formula, a universal connector that is incompatible with IV equipment has been developed. Figure 13-5 shows a silicone G-tube with a purple connector, which is incompatible with a Luer lock syringe or an IV connection. This innovation, recently made the industry standard, is designed to reduce the risk of accidental connection or infusion. During the placement procedure, if the color of the device changes, the operator will immediately see that the tube is malpositioned and must be removed immediately.

A tube placed by PEG may be converted to a **gastrojejunostomy** using fluoroscopy or endoscopy by threading a small-bore tube through the larger tube into the jejunum.

Other Minimally Invasive Techniques

High-resolution video cameras have made percutaneous radiologic and laparoscopic gastrostomy and jejunostomy enteral access an option for patients in whom endoscopic procedures are contraindicated. Using fluoroscopy, a radiologic technique, tubes can be guided visually into the stomach or the jejunum and then brought out through the abdominal wall to provide the access route for enteral feedings. Laparoscopic or fluoroscopic techniques offer alternative options for enteral access.

Gastrojejunal dual tubes, used for early postoperative feeding, are available for endoscopic or surgical placement. These tubes are designed for patients in whom prolonged **gastrointestinal decompression** (removal of the contents of the stomach through a nasogastric tube) is anticipated. The **multiple lumen tube** has one lumen for decompression and one to feed into the small bowel.

Formula Content and Selection

More than 75 enteral formulas, marketed for a wide variety of clinical conditions and indications, are currently available (Charney and Malone, 2013):
- Enteral formulas are classified as (1) standard, (2) chemically defined (elemental); or (3) specialized (marketed for specific clinical conditions or diseases). A significant variety of formulas are available in each of these categories. Health care organizations, including hospitals and long-term care organizations, typically develop a formulary of products to be used within the facility. Selection of an enteral formula for a specific patient should involve consideration of the patient's:
  - Nutrient needs
  - GIT function
  - Clinical status

In the past, **osmolality** was considered key to EN tolerance, and belief was widespread that EN formulas should be the same osmolality as body fluids (290 mOsm/kg). However, studies in the mid-1980s showed that patients tolerate feedings across a wide range of osmolality, and clinical experience of many clinicians has reinforced those study results. Cost of the formula and its availability after discharge from the hospital or other facility can be of significant concern to facility administrators, clinicians, patients, and families.

Formulas often are classified based on protein or overall macronutrient composition. Most patients with a variety of clinical conditions tolerate standard (**polymeric**) **enteral formulas** intended to meet the nutritional requirements of healthy individuals, and by extension patients with a variety of medical conditions. The formulas contain intact macronutrients, 1 to 2 kcal/ml, are lactose free, and may be used as oral supplements as well as for enteral feeding. The higher nutrient density (1.5 to 2 kcal/ml) formulas are useful when fluid restriction is required (cardiopulmonary, renal, and/or hepatic dysfunction), and for patients with intolerance to typical feeding volume. Products intended to supplement oral diets may be used for EN in some cases; these products are flavored and may contain simple sugars to enhance palatability. See Appendix 24.

The manufacture and labeling of enteral formulas are regulated by the Food and Drug Administration (FDA), which classifies enteral formulas as medical foods (a subclassification of foods for special dietary use). As such, these products are exempt from specific nutrition labeling requirements in the Code of Federal Regulations. The products must be labeled as "intended to be used under medical supervision" (FDA, 2014).

Manufacturers are not obligated to register enteral products with the FDA or obtain FDA approval before placing them on the market. Many enteral nutrition formulas lack rigorous scientific evidence to support their specific composition, and their marketing materials are not subject to the rigorous standards used for prescription drugs. Evaluation of the efficacy of enteral nutrition products and the statements made in marketing materials and by company representatives requires the attention of qualified RDNs. Claims of pharmacologic effects must be evaluated using clinical evidence before a decision is made to use a specific product (Box 13-2).

Blenderized (Homemade) Tube Feedings

Tube feedings made from common ingredients such as eggs, sugar, and wine have been used since the 1500s, and blenderized tube feedings (BTF) were used in the United States throughout the first half of the twentieth century (Vassilyadi, 2013). Clinicians often are concerned about nutritional adequacy, food safety, and the additional burden preparation of BTF places on the caregivers (Malone, 2005). Advantages of BTF may include cost effectiveness (because commercial formulas may not be covered by insurance), health benefits from using whole foods, and ability to tailor the formula exactly to patient needs. The social bond between the caregiver who prepares the feeding (possibly from foods served to the rest of the family) and the patient also is cited as a strong driver for BTF use.

BTF are contraindicated for patients who are immunocompromised, for infusion through tubes smaller than 10 French, for continuous feeding (unless the formula hangs for ≤2 hours), if fluid restriction of less than 900 ml/day is required, in cases of multiple food allergies, and if a jejunostomy tube (JT)is used (Novak, 2009). Some state regulations prohibit use of BTF in long-term care facilities (see *New Directions:* Pureed by Gastrostomy Tube – the PBGT Diet).

BOX 13-2 Factors to Consider when Choosing an Enteral Formula

Ability of the formula to meet the patient's nutrient requirements
Caloric and protein density of the formula (i.e., kcal/ml, g protein/ml, ml fluid/L)
Gastrointestinal function
Sodium, potassium, magnesium, and phosphorus content of the formula, especially for patients with cardiopulmonary, renal, or hepatic failure
Form and amount of protein, fat, carbohydrate, and fiber in the formula relative to the patient's digestive and absorptive capacity
Cost effectiveness of formula
Patient compliance
Cost-to-benefit ratio

✴ NEW DIRECTIONS

Pureed by Gastrostomy Tube – the PBGT Diet

by Therese O'Flaherty MS, RD, CSP, LD

The Pureed by Gastrostomy (G) Tube (PBGT) Diet is a specialized, nutritionally balanced blended food feeding given by G-tube. It was originally designed to decrease or eliminate symptoms of retching and gagging which can be a complication of a Nissen Fundoplication surgery. In addition to improving tolerance of bolus feeds for individuals who are volume sensitive, the PBGT diet is also used by families seeking an alternative to commercial formulas.

The goals of the PBGT diet are to:
- Decrease frequency of GT feedings and transition from drip feedings
- Meet all nutritional and fluid requirements
- Improve weight gain, growth, and overall nutritional status
- Encourage increased opportunities for oral intake
- Improve and sustain quality of life for individuals and their families

The PBGT diet is different from the usual blended tube feeding in that it is calculated and formulated by a registered dietitian nutritionist (RDN) to provide an individual with complete nutrition through small, calorie-dense gastrostomy tube boluses, thereby eliminating the need and cost for a feeding pump. In addition to the easier preparation of the PBGT, special attention is also given to the variety of foods, nutrient content, cost, and ease of the 5-10 minute bolus administration (Pentiuk, et all 2011).

The use of Stage 2 infant foods promotes consistency in the viscosity of the diet, provides availability and affordability, and eliminates the need for an expensive blender. They can be premeasured, and individually sealed in containers that can be easily used in formula rooms within hospitals if allowed by hospital policy. Families can be educated on the easy preparation method and proper storage, along with additional fluid and vitamin and mineral supplementation guidelines (O'Flaherty, et al 2011; O'Flaherty, 2015).

Protein

The amount of protein in available commercial enteral formulas varies from 6% to 25% of total kilocalories. The protein typically is derived from casein, whey, or soy protein isolate. Standard formulas provide intact protein, whereas elemental formulas contain di- and tripeptides and amino acids, which are absorbed more easily. Specialized formulas (for hepatic or renal failure or in cases of multiple, severe allergies) may include crystalline amino acids.

Specific amino acids may be added to some enteral formulas. Branched chain amino acids are used in formulas for patients with severe hepatic disease, and arginine has been added to formulas marketed for critically ill patients. (See Chapter 38 for further discussion.)

Carbohydrate

Carbohydrate content in enteral formulas varies from 30% to 85% of kilocalories. Corn syrup solids typically are used in standard formulas. Sucrose is added to flavored formulas that are meant for oral consumption. Hydrolyzed formulas contain carbohydrate from cornstarch or maltodextrin.

Carbohydrate or fiber that cannot be processed by human digestive enzymes is added frequently to enteral formulas. Fibers are classified as water soluble (pectins and gums) or water insoluble (cellulose or hemicellulose). The effectiveness of different fibers added to enteral formulas in treating GIT symptoms of critically ill patients is controversial. The Adult Critical Illness guidelines, in the Evidence Analysis Library of the Academy of Nutrition and Dietetics (AND, EAL, 2012) suggests that the RDN "consider using soluble fiber to prevent and/or manage diarrhea."

Fructooligosaccharides (FOS), which are prebiotics, have been added to enteral formulas, often in combination with a source of dietary fiber, for more than 15 years. FOS have been shown to stimulate the production of beneficial bifidobacteria, and when combined with dietary fiber may produce beneficial changes in colonic pH, fecal microbiota, and short-chain fatty acid concentrations. Animal models provide evidence that FOS may help to achieve colonization resistance against *Clostridium difficile*. Use of FOS in individuals with irritable bowel syndrome (IBS) may worsen symptoms transiently; some studies have suggested that these adverse symptoms may abate with consistent FOS use (Charney and Malone, 2013).

All commercially available enteral formulas are lactose free, because lactase insufficiency is common in acutely ill patients.

Lipid

Lipid content of enteral formulas varies from 1.5% to 55% of the total kilocalories. In standard formulas, lipid as corn, sunflower, safflower, or canola oil provides between 15% and 30% of the total kilocalories. Elemental formulas contain minimal amounts of fat, typically in the form of medium-chain triglycerides (MCTs) rather than long-chain (LCTs) triglycerides.

Most of the fat in standard enteral formulas is in the form of LCTs and MCTs. Some formulas contain "structured lipids," which are a mix of LCTs and MCTs and contain properties of both. Most of the LCTs found in structured lipids are omega-3 fatty acids (such as eicosapentaenoic acid and docosahexanoic acid); these omega-3 fatty acids may have anti-inflammatory effects (see Chapter 3). Structured lipids are absorbed more readily and better tolerated than LCT/MCT combinations (Malone, 2005).

MCTs do not require bile salts or pancreatic lipase for digestion and are absorbed directly into the portal circulation. The percentage of fat as MCT in enteral formulas varies from 0 to 85%. Approximately 2% to 4% of daily energy intake from linoleic and linolenic acid is necessary to prevent essential fatty acid deficiency (EFAD). MCTs do not provide linoleic or linolenic acids; the clinician must ensure that patients who receive high MCT enteral formulas receive linoleic and linolenic acids from other sources.

Vitamins, Minerals, and Electrolytes

Most, but not all, available formulas provide the dietary reference intakes (DRIs) for vitamins and minerals in a volume that may be administered to most patients. Because the DRIs are intended for healthy populations, not specifically for individuals (whether healthy or acutely or chronically ill), it is difficult to know for certain whether the vitamin and mineral provision from these formulas is adequate. Formulas intended for patients with renal or hepatic failure are intentionally low in vitamins A, D, and E, sodium, and potassium. Conversely, disease-specific formulas often are supplemented with antioxidant vitamins and minerals and marketed to suggest that these additions improve immune function or accelerate wound healing. Definitive studies demonstrating these effects are not available.

Electrolyte content of enteral formulas is typically modest compared with the oral diet. Patients who experience large electrolyte losses (e.g., because of diarrhea, fistula, emesis) likely will require electrolyte supplementation.

Fluid

Adult fluid needs often are estimated at 1 ml of water per kilocalorie consumed, or 30 to 35 ml/kg of usual body weight. Patients fed exclusively by EN may receive insufficient fluid (water) to meet their needs, especially when concentrated formulas are used. Insufficient fluid intake along with a high-fiber product may lead to a number of undesirable consequences, including inadequate urine output, constipation, and formation of a fiber bezoar (a hard ball of hair or vegetable fiber that may develop within the stomach of humans). All sources of fluid, including feeding tube flushes, medications, and intravenous fluids, should be considered when assessing a patient's fluid intake relative to his or her needs.

Standard (1 kcal/ml) formulas contain approximately 85% water by volume; concentrated (2 kcal/ml) formulas contain only approximately 70% water by volume. Additional water (as flushes and for additional hydration) may be necessary.

Administration

EN may be administered as a bolus, intermittent, or continuous feeding. Selection of the optimal method should be based on the patient's clinical status, living situation, and quality-of-life considerations. One method may serve as a transition to another method as the patient's status changes.

In a closed enteral system the container or bag is prefilled with sterile liquid formula by the manufacturer and is "ready to feed" after connecting to the patient's feeding access. In an open enteral system, the contents of formula cans or packages are poured into a separate, empty container or bag and then connected to the feeding access.

Hang time is the length of time an enteral formula hanging at room temperature is considered safe for delivery to the patient. Most facilities allow a 4-hour hang time for a product in an open system and 24 to 48 hours for products in closed system (depending on the manufacturer's directions).

Bolus

Syringe bolus enteral feedings may be optimal for patients with adequate gastric emptying who are clinically stable (see Figure 13-4). Administered over 5 to 20 minutes, these feedings are more convenient and less expensive than pump or gravity bolus feedings and should be encouraged when tolerated. A 60-ml syringe may be used to infuse the formula. If bloating or abdominal discomfort develops, the patient should wait 10 to 15 minutes before infusing the remainder of formula allocated for that feeding. Patients with normal gastric function generally tolerate 500 ml or more of formula per feeding; therefore, three or four bolus feedings per day typically provide their daily nutritional requirements. However some people, especially the elderly, may not be able to tolerate such large boluses and need a regimen of smaller, more frequent feedings. Formula at room temperature may be better tolerated than cold formula; however, food safety must be the primary consideration. Follow label directions for storing partially used cans of formula.

Intermittent and Cyclic

Quality-of-life issues are often the reason for the initiation of intermittent enteral feedings, and cyclical regimens allow mobile patients to enjoy an improved quality of life by offering time "off the pump" and more autonomy than do continuous infusions. They are initiated to allow time for treatments, therapies, and activities. Intermittent feedings can be given by pump or gravity drip. Gravity feeding is accomplished by pouring formula into a feeding bag that is equipped with a roller clamp. The clamp is adjusted to the desired drips per minute. A typical daily feeding schedule is four to six feedings, each administered over 20 to 60 minutes. Formula administration is initiated at 100 to 150 ml per feeding and increased incrementally as tolerated. Patients who most often succeed with this regimen are motivated, organized, alert, and mobile. Cyclic feeding also allows for a period of time away from the tube feeding. This feeding regimen is a good choice for patients who are receiving physical therapy or participate in other activities that make being tethered to a feeding apparatus inconvenient. A typical daily feeding schedule is 90 to 125 ml per hour of formula administered over 18 to 20 hours. This type of feeding often is used in transition to oral feedings and often is done at night to avoid feeding during meal times.

Continuous

Continuous infusion of EN requires a pump. This method is appropriate for patients who do not tolerate the volume of infusion used with the bolus, cyclical or intermittent methods. Patients with compromised gastrointestinal function because of disease, surgery, cancer therapy, or other physiologic impediments are candidates for continuous feedings. Patients with a feeding tube tip in the small intestine should be fed only by continuous or cyclic infusion. (Use of bolus or gravity feeding in these patients is strongly discouraged, although anecdotal verbal reports of use of both have been shared by some providers.) The feeding rate goal, in milliliters per hour, is set by dividing the total daily volume by the number of hours per day of administration. Full strength feeding is started at one quarter to one half of the hourly goal rate and advanced every 8 to 12 hours to the final volume. Dilution of formulas is not necessary and can lead to underfeeding. High osmolality formulas may require more time to achieve tolerance and should be advanced conservatively.

One possible drawback to continuous feedings is when the patient requires medication be given on an empty stomach. For example, when administering phenytoin (Dilantin) it is recommended that tube feedings be stopped before and after administration. The times vary by situation and medication (see Chapter 8).

Enteral pumps available today are small and easy to handle. Many pumps run for up to 8 hours on battery power, with a "plug-in" option, allowing flexibility and mobility for the patient. Pump sets typically include bags and tubing compatible with proper pump operation. Feeding bags should be labeled in accordance with the A.S.P.E.N. Enteral Nutrition Practice Guidelines and should include information on the name of the formula and its concentration, the date and time the bag was filled, and the initials of the health care provider who hung the feeding.

Monitoring and Evaluation
Monitoring for Complications

Box 13-3 provides a comprehensive list of complications associated with EN. Many complications can be prevented or managed with careful patient monitoring.

Aspiration, a common concern for patients receiving EN, is also a controversial topic. Many experts believe that aspiration

---

BOX 13-3 Complications of Enteral Nutrition

Access
Leakage from ostomy/stoma site
Pressure necrosis/ulceration/stenosis
Tissue erosion
Tube displacement/migration
Tube obstruction/occlusion

Administration
Microbial contamination
Enteral misconnections or misplacement of tube, causing infection, aspiration pneumonia, peritonitis, pulmonary or venous infusion
Regurgitation
Inadequate delivery for one or more reasons

Gastrointestinal
Constipation
Delayed gastric emptying/elevated gastric residual volume
Diarrhea
 Osmotic diarrhea, especially if sorbitol is present in liquid drug preparations
 Secretory
Distention/bloating/cramping
Formula choice/rate of administration
Intolerance of nutrient components
Maldigestion/malabsorption
Nausea/vomiting

Metabolic
Drug-nutrient interactions
Glucose intolerance/hyperglycemia/hypoglycemia
Dehydration/overhydration
Hypernatremia/hyponatremia
Hyperkalemia/hypokalemia
Hyperphosphatemia/hypophosphatemia
Micronutrient deficiencies (notably thiamin)
Refeeding syndrome

Data from Russell M: Complications of enteral feedings. In Charney P, Malone A, editors: *Pocket guide to enteral nutrition*, ed 2, Chicago, 2013, AND, p 170.

of throat contents and saliva is as much as or more important than aspiration of formula. To minimize the risk of aspiration, patients should be positioned with their heads and shoulders above their chests during and immediately after feeding (Bankhead et al, 2009; McClave et al, 2009).

Significant disagreement exists about the value of **gastric residual volumes (GRV)** as an indicator of EN tolerance. GRV procedures are not standardized and checking GRV does not protect patients from aspiration. GRV does not have to be checked regularly in patients who are stable on a feeding regimen and those who have a long history on tube feedings. In critically ill tube-fed patients the best methods for reducing the risk of aspiration include elevation of the head of the bed, continuous subglottic suctioning, and oral decontamination (Bankhead et al, 2009; McClave et al, 2009).

In the presence of gastroparesis, doses of a promotility drug may increase gastrointestinal transit, improve EN delivery, and improve feeding tolerance (McClave et al, 2009).

Diarrhea is a common EN complication, often related to the antibiotic therapy, colonic bacterial overgrowth, and gastrointestinal motility disorders associated with acute and critical illness. Hyperosmolar medications such as magnesium-containing antacids, sorbitol-containing elixirs, and electrolyte supplements also contribute to diarrhea. Adjustment of medications or administration methods may reduce or eliminate the diarrhea. FOS, pectin, guar gum, bulking agents, and antidiarrheal medications also can be beneficial. (Care must be taken to avoid clogging the feeding tube when using bulking agents or pectin.) A predigested formula may be useful but is rarely the best "first line" option, because the formula is often not the cause of the diarrhea.

Constipation is a concern with EN, particularly among bed-bound patients who receive long-term feedings. Fiber-containing formulas or stool-bulking medication may be helpful; daily provision of adequate fluid is important. Narcotic pain relievers slow GIT activity; iron supplements can cause constipation. Diarrhea may coexist with constipation, usually when there is also a fecal impaction because the liquid stool can get past the impaction.

Monitoring for Tolerance and Nutrient Intake Goals

Monitoring the patient's *actual* (not prescribed) intake and tolerance is necessary to ensure that all nutrition goals are achieved and maintained. Monitoring of metabolic and gastrointestinal tolerance, hydration status, weight, and lean body mass is extremely important (Box 13-4). The development and use of practice guidelines, institutional protocols, and standardized ordering procedures are helpful to ensure optimal, safe monitoring of EN (McClave et al, 2009).

During routine patient care, time commonly is lost from the prescribed feeding schedule as a result of issues such as NPO status for medical procedures, clogged tubes, dislodged or misplaced tubes, and perceived or actual gastrointestinal intolerance. The result of "held" feedings is always inadequate nutrition with the risk of new or worsening malnutrition. Adjustment in the tube feeding regimen must be made. For example, if tube feedings are being turned off for 2 hours every afternoon for physical therapy, the feeding rate on the feeding should be increased and the feeding time decreased to accommodate the therapy schedule.

BOX 13-4 Monitoring the Patient Receiving Enteral Nutrition

Abdominal distention and discomfort
Confirm proper tube placement and maintain head of bed >30 degrees (daily)
Change feeding delivery container and tubing (daily)
Fluid intake and output (daily)
Gastric residual volume if appropriate
Signs and symptoms of edema or dehydration (daily)
Stool frequency, volume, and consistency (daily)
Weight (at least three times/wk)
Nutritional intake adequacy (daily)
Clinical status/physical examination (daily)
Serum electrolytes, blood urea nitrogen, creatinine, (daily till stable, then 2 to 3 times/wk)
Serum glucose, calcium, magnesium, phosphorus (daily till stable, then weekly)

Data from McClave SA et al: Guidelines for the provision and assessment of nutrition support therapy in the adult critically ill patient, *J Parenter Enteral Nutr* 33:277, 2009.
Shelton M: Monitoring and evaluation of enteral feedings. In Charney P, Malone A: *Pocket guide to enteral nutrition*, ed 2, Chicago, 2013, AND, p 153.

PARENTERAL NUTRITION

PN provides nutrients directly into the bloodstream intravenously. PN is indicated when the patient or individual is unable or unwilling to take adequate nutrients orally or enterally. PN may be used as an adjunct to oral or EN to meet nutrient needs. Alternatively, PN may be the sole source of nutrition during recovery from illness or injury or may be a life-sustaining therapy for patients who have lost the function of their intestine for nutrient absorption. As any type of nutrition support other than oral is invasive, it is important to evaluate ethical issues if the patient is terminal or has a short life expectancy (Barrocas et al, 2010).

Getting Started with Parenteral Nutrition

After the patient has been deemed to require nutrition support via the parenteral route, the clinician must choose between central and peripheral access. *Central access* refers to catheter tip placement in a large, high-blood-flow vein such as the superior vena cava; this is **central parenteral nutrition (CPN)**. **Peripheral parenteral nutrition (PPN)** refers to catheter tip placement in a small vein, typically in the hand or forearm.

The osmolarity of the PN solution dictates the location of the catheter; central catheter placement allows for the higher caloric PN formulation and therefore greater osmolarity (Table 13-2). The use of PPN is limited: it is short-term therapy and therefore has a minimum effect on nutritional status because the type and amount of fluids that can be provided peripherally are limited and most often do not fully meet nutrition requirements. Volume-sensitive patients such as those with cardiopulmonary, renal, or hepatic failure are not good candidates for PPN. PPN may be appropriate when used as a supplemental feeding or in transition to enteral or oral feeding, or as a temporary method to begin feeding when central access has not been initiated. Calculation of the osmolarity of a parenteral solution is important to ensure venous tolerance. **Osmolarity**, or mOsm/ml, is used to

TABLE 13-2 Osmolarity of Nutrients in PN Solutions

Nutrient	Osmolarity (mOsm/ml)	Sample Calculations
Dextrose 5%	0.25	500 ml = 125 mOsm
Dextrose 10%	0.505	500 ml = 252 mOsm
Dextrose 50%	2.52	500 ml = 1260 mOsm
Dextrose 70%	3.53	500 ml = 1765 mOsm
Amino acids 8.5%	0.81	1000 ml = 810 mOsm
Amino acids 10%	0.998	1000 ml = 998 mOsm
Lipids 10%	0.6	500 ml = 300 mOsm
Lipids 20%	0.7	500 ml = 350 mOsm
Electrolytes	Varies by additive	
Multitrace elements	0.36	5 ml = 1.8 mOsm
Multivitamin concentrate	4.11	10 ml = 41 mOsm

Data from RxKinetics: *Calculating Osmolarity of an IV Admixture* (website): http://www.rxkinetics.com/iv_osmolarity.html. Accessed December 2014.

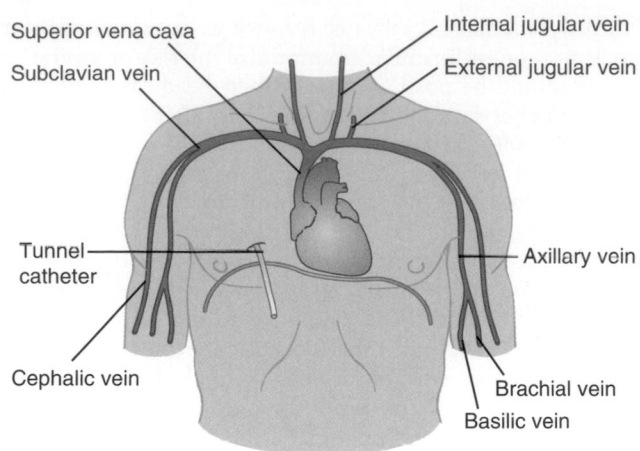

FIGURE 13-6 Venous sites from which the superior vena cava may be assessed.

calculate IV fluids rather than osmolality, which is used for body fluids.

Access

Peripheral Access

Peripheral parenteral nutrition (PPN) solutions of up to 800 to 900 mOsm/kg of solvent can be infused through a routine peripheral intravenous angiocatheter placed in a vein in good condition (Gura, 2009). Most often, PPN solutions are provided through catheters called *midline* or *midclavicular catheters,* depending on their position. They are not central catheters. Extended dwell catheters, which can remain at the original site for 3 to 6 weeks, require a vein large enough to advance the catheter 5 to 7 inches into the vein. These catheters make PPN a more feasible option in patients with veins large enough to tolerate the catheter for more than 2 to 3 days.

Short-Term Central Access

Catheters used for CPN ideally consist of a single lumen. If central access is needed for other reasons, such as hemodynamic monitoring, drawing blood samples, or giving medications, multiple-lumen catheters are available. To reduce the risk of infection, the catheter lumen used to infuse CPN should be reserved for that purpose only. Catheters are inserted most commonly into the subclavian vein and advanced until the catheter tip is in the superior vena cava, using strict aseptic technique. Alternatively, an internal or external jugular vein catheter can be used with the same catheter tip placement. However, the motion of the neck makes this site much more difficult for maintaining the sterility of a dressing. Radiologic verification of the tip site is necessary before infusion of nutrients can begin. Strict infection control protocols should be used for catheter placement and maintenance. Figure 13-6 shows alternative venous access sites for CPN; femoral placement is also possible.

A **peripherally inserted central catheter (PICC)** may be used for short- or moderate-term infusion in the hospital or in the home. This catheter is inserted into a vein in the antecubital area of the arm and threaded into the subclavian vein with the catheter tip placed in the superior vena cava. Trained nonphysicians can insert a PICC, whereas placement of a tunneled catheter is a surgical procedure. All catheters must have

radiologic confirmation of the placement of the catheter tip before initiating any infusion.

Long-Term Central Access

A commonly used long-term catheter is a "tunneled" catheter. This single- or multiple-lumen catheter is placed in the cephalic, subclavian, or internal jugular vein and fed into the superior vena cava. A subcutaneous tunnel is created so that the catheter exits the skin several inches from its venous entry site. This allows the patient to care for the catheter more easily as is necessary for long-term infusion. Another type of long-term catheter is a surgically implanted port under the skin where the catheter normally would exit at the end of the subcutaneous tunnel. A special needle must access the entrance port. Ports can be single or double; an individual port is equivalent to a lumen. Both tunneled catheters and PICCs can be used for extended therapy in the hospital or for home infusion therapy. Care of long-term catheters requires specialized handling and extensive patient education.

Parenteral Solutions

Protein

Commercially available standard PN solutions contain all essential amino acids and only some of the nonessential amino acids. Nonessential nitrogen is provided principally by the amino acids alanine and glycine, usually without aspartate, glutamate, cysteine, and taurine. Specialized solutions with adjusted amino acid content that contain taurine are available for infants, for whom taurine is thought to be conditionally essential.

The concentration of amino acids in PN solutions ranges from 3% to 20% by volume. Thus a 10% solution of amino acids supplies 100 g of protein per liter (1000 ml). The percentage of a solution usually is expressed at its final concentration after dilution with other nutrient solutions. The caloric content of amino acid solutions is approximately 4 kcal/g of protein provided. Protein needs are calculated based on the nutrition assessment data related to disease, injury, or clinical/nutrition status and range between 15% to 20% of total energy intake (Mueller et al, 2011).

Carbohydrates are supplied as dextrose monohydrate in concentrations ranging from 5% to 70% by volume. The dextrose monohydrate yields 3.4 calories per gram. As with amino acids, a 10% solution yields 100 g of carbohydrates per liter of solution. The use of carbohydrates (100 g daily for a 70-kg person) ensures that protein is not catabolized for energy during conditions of normal metabolism.

Maximum rates of carbohydrate administration should not exceed 5 to 6 mg/kg/min in critically ill patients. When PN solutions provide 15% to 20% of total calories as protein, 20% to 30% of total calories as lipid, and the balance from carbohydrate (dextrose), infusion of dextrose should not exceed this amount. Excessive administration can lead to hyperglycemia, hepatic abnormalities, or increased ventilatory drive (see Chapter 34).

Lipids

Lipid emulsions provide calories and essential fatty acids in PN to avoid essential fatty acid deficiency. Lipid emulsions, currently on the market in the United States, available in 10%, 20%, and 30% concentrations, are composed of aqueous suspensions of soybean oil with egg yolk phospholipid as the emulsifier. Lipid emulsions containing egg phospholipids should not be used when a patient has an egg allergy. No safflower oil emulsions have been available in the United States in recent years. Intralipid (Fresenius Kabi, FDA approved 1975, marketed by Baxter Healthcare), Nutrilipid (BBraun, FDA approved but not marketed in the United States), and Liposyn III (Hospira, FDA approved but not marketed in the United States) are soybean oil emulsions.

Approximately 10% of calories per day from soybean based fat emulsions provide the 2% to 4% of calories from linoleic acid required to prevent EFAD. Administration should not exceed 2 g of lipid emulsion per kilogram of body weight per day, although recommendations of 1 to 1.5 g/kg are more common. Triglyceride levels should be monitored. When they exceed 400, the lipid infusion should be discontinued.

A 10% lipid emulsion contains 1.1 kcal/ml, whereas a 20% emulsion contains 2 kcal/ml. Providing 20% to 30% of total calories as lipid emulsion should result in a daily dosage of approximately 1 g of fat per kilogram of body weight. For critically ill patients who receive sedation in a lipid emulsion, these calories should be included in the nutrient intake calculations to avoid overfeeding or underfeeding (Drover et al, 2010). Diprivan (propofol) is an example of a sedation/anesthesia agent administered as an injectable infusion in a lipid emulsion providing approximately 1.1 kcal/ml infused. In the hospital, lipid is infused during 24 hours when mixed with the dextrose and amino acids. Alternatively, lipids can be provided separately by infusion via an infusion pump. Providing 20% to 30% of total calories as lipid emulsion should result in a daily dosage of approximately 1 g of fat per kilogram of body weight. In the hospital, lipid is infused during 24 hours when mixed with the dextrose and amino acids. Alternatively, lipids can be provided separately by infusion via an infusion pump. For adult patients receiving PN at home **or home parenteral nutrition (HPN)**, the PN most often is infused during 10 to 12 hours per day with the lipid as part of the PN solution. It may be infused as a daily component of the home parenteral nutrition (HPN) or a few times per week.

Alternative forms of lipids are available that contain varying levels of omega-6 polyunsaturated fatty acids as indicated earlier but also contain omega-3 fatty acids and monounsaturated fat. Lipid sources other than soybean or safflower oil including coconut, olive, and fish oil are used (Waitzberg et al, 2006). ClinOleic/Clinolipid (Baxter Healthcare, FDA approved but not

marketed in the United States) is a new lipid emulsion that contains 80% olive oil and 20% soybean oil as well as egg phosphatides for emulsion. It provides essential fatty acids and contains 2 kcal/ml and should be dosed similarly at 1 to 1.5 g/kg to prevent any risk of EFAD. A lipid emulsion containing soybean oil, medium-chain triglycerides, olive oil, and fish oil (SMOFlipid, Fresenius Kabi–not FDA approved) is available outside the United States and has been shown to be safe and efficacious in healthy subjects and patients as compared with a standard soybean oil emulsion. The results of the clinical studies indicate that SMOFlipid is safe and well tolerated. Because of the multiple lipid types in the emulsion, the plasma fatty acid pattern demonstrated a rise in EPA- and DHA-derived lipid mediators and maintenance of an adequate vitamin E status.

Omegaven (Fresenius Kabi, not FDA approved, available in the United States for compassionate use only) is a fish oil–based lipid emulsion. Proposed benefits of fish oil lipid emulsion, as well as those that contain medium-chain triglycerides, include decreased inflammatory effects and less immunosuppression (Manzanares et al, 2014). Careful attention to the caloric load as well as the adequacy of essential fatty acids is important when these lipids are used. In a study of surgical patients who received one of four different intravenous lipid emulsions: medium-chain triglycerides/long-chain triglycerides (soybean oil; MCT/LCT), olive/soybean oil (olcic), long-chain triglycerides (soybean oil; LCT), or structured lipids, all were well tolerated and safe (Puiggros, 2009). The authors did note the serum fatty acid levels were similar to the pattern of fatty acids in the administered lipid emulsion. In addition, those who received the olive oil–based lipid emulsion had favorable changes in serum lipid levels. All lipid emulsions should be administered through a 1.2 micron filter set.

Electrolytes, Vitamins, Trace Elements

General guidelines for daily requirements for electrolytes are given in Table 13-3, for vitamins in Table 13-4, and for trace elements in Table 13-5. Parenteral solutions also represent a significant portion of total daily fluid and electrolyte intake. Once a solution is prescribed and initiated, adjustments for proper fluid and electrolyte balance may be necessary, depending on the stability of the patient. The choice of the salt form of electrolytes (e.g., chloride, acetate) affects acid-base balance.

Parenterally administered multivitamin and mineral preparations are designed to meet most patient's needs. These levels may be inadequate in some situations when additional

TABLE 13-3 Daily Electrolyte Requirements During Total Parenteral Nutrition—Adults

Electrolyte	Standard Intake/Day
Calcium	10-15 mEq
Magnesium	8-20 mEq
Phosphate	20-40 mmol
Sodium	1-2 mEq/kg + replacement
Potassium	1-2 mEq/kg
Acetate	As needed to maintain acid-base balance
Chloride	As needed to maintain acid-base balance

From McClave SA et al: Guidelines for the provision and assessment of nutrition support therapy in the adult critically ill patient, *JPEN J Parenter Enteral Nutr* 33:277, 2009.

TABLE 13-4 **Adult Parenteral Multivitamins: Comparison of Guidelines and Products**

Vitamin	NAG-AMA Guidelines	FDA Requirements	MVI-12	MVI-13 (Infuvite) Baxter
A (retinol)	3300 units (1 mg)	3300 units (1 mg)	3300 units (1 mg)	3300 units (1 mg)
D (ergocalciferol cholecalciferol)	200 units (5 mcg)	200 units (5 mcg)	200 units (5 mcg)	200 units (5 mcg)
E (mcg-tocopherol)	10 units (10 mg)	10 units (10 mg)	10 units (10 mg)	10 units (10 mg)
B_1 (thiamin)	3 mg	6 mg	3 mg	6 mg
B_2 (riboflavin)	3.6 mg	3.6 mg	3.6 mg	3.6 mg
B_3 (nlacinamide)	40 mg	40 mg	40 mg	40 mg
B_5 (dexpanthenol)	15 mg	15 mg	15 mg	15 mg
B_6 (pyridoxine)	4 mg	6 mg	4 mg	6 mg
B_{12} (cyanocobalamin)	5 mcg	5 mcg	5 mcg	5 mcg
C (ascorbic acid)	100 mg	200 mg	100 mg	200 mg
Biotin	60 mcg	60 mcg	60 mcg	60 mcg
Folic acid	400 mcg	600 mcg	400 mcg	600 mcg
K		150 mcg	0	150 mcg

Vanek V et al: A.S.P.E.N. position paper: recommendations for changes in commercially available parenteral multivitamin and multi-trace element products, *Nutr Clin Prac* 27:440, 2012.
AMA, American Medical Association; *FDA,* U.S. Food and Drug Administration; *MVI-12* and *MVI-13,* multivitamin supplements; *NAG,* National Advisory Group.

TABLE 13-5 **Daily Trace Element Supplementation for Adult Parenteral Formulations**

Trace Element	Intake
Chromium	10-15 mcg
Copper	0.3-0.5 mg
Manganese	60-100 mcg
Zinc	2.5-5.0 mg
Selenium	20-60 mcg

individual supplementation is required (Vanek et al, 2012). Patients receiving PN as their sole source of nutrition should receive added multivitamins and trace elements daily and be monitored closely, especially those who are critically ill (Sriram and Lonchyna, 2009). Monitoring of manganese and chromium status is recommended for patients receiving PN for longer than 6 months (Buchman et al, 2009).

Iron is not normally part of parenteral infusions because it is not compatible with lipids and may enhance certain bacterial growth. In addition, care must be taken to ensure that a patient can tolerate the separate iron infusion. When patients receive iron on an outpatient basis, the first dose should be done in a controlled setting (such as an outpatient infusion suite) to observe for any reactions that the patient may experience.

One of the challenges in PN in the last 5 years has been the occurrence of drug shortages that have affected micro- and macronutrients, including intravenous lipid emulsion, multivitamins, multitrace elements, and electrolytes including phosphorous. Patients in the hospital, at home, and in long-term care receiving not only parenteral nutrition but also other intravenous and injectable therapies have been affected. This problem is expected to be ongoing, and therefore clinicians should be aware of alternative products as well as methods to allocate safely products in short supply.

Fluid

Fluid needs for PN or EN are calculated similarly. Maximum volumes of CPN rarely exceed 3 L, with typical prescriptions of 1.5 to 3 L daily. In critically ill patients, volumes of prescribed CPN should be coordinated closely with their overall care plan.

The administration of other medical therapies requiring fluid administration, such as intravenous medications and blood products, necessitates careful monitoring. Patients with cardiopulmonary, renal, and hepatic failure are especially sensitive to fluid administration. For HPN, higher volumes may be best provided in separate infusions. For example, if additional fluid is required as a result of high output by the patient, then a liter bag of intravenous fluid containing minimal electrolytes may be infused during a short time during the day if the PN is infused overnight. See Appendix XX on calculating PN prescriptions.

Compounding Methods

PN prescriptions historically have required preparation or compounding by competent pharmacy personnel under laminar airflow hoods using aseptic techniques. Hospitals may have their own compounding pharmacy or may purchase PN solutions that have been compounded outside the hospital in a central location and then returned to the hospital for distribution to individual patients. A third method of providing PN solutions is to use multichamber bag technology, whereby solutions are manufactured in a quality-controlled environment using good manufacturing processes. PN solutions of two chamber bags contain amino acids (with or without electrolytes) and dextrose and are available in multiple formulas with varying amounts of dextrose and amino acids, making them suitable for CPN or PPN infusion. Some multichamber bag formulas may contain lipids in a third chamber; however, these are not currently available in the United States but are available in Europe and Canada. They contain conservative amounts of electrolytes or may be electrolyte free. These products have a shelf life of 2 years and do not have to be refrigerated unless the product covering has been opened to reveal the infusion bag. They do not contain vitamins or trace elements that may be added to the solutions; therefore the clinician must add vitamins/minerals to the patients' treatment plan to avoid any deficiencies. Institutions frequently use standardized solutions, which are compounded in batches, thus saving labor and lowering costs; however, flexibility for individualized compounding should be available when warranted (Ayers et al, 2014).

Prescriptions for PN are compounded in two general ways. One method combines all components except the fat emulsion, which is infused separately. The second method combines the lipid emulsion with the dextrose and amino acid solution and is referred to as a total nutrient admixture or 3-in-1 solution. The PN Safe Practices Guidelines provide clinicians with information on many techniques and procedures that enhance safety and prevent mistakes in the preparation of PN (Boullata et al, 2014).

A number of medications, including antibiotics, vasopressors, narcotics, diuretics, and many other commonly administered drugs, can be compounded with PN solutions. In practice this occurs infrequently because it requires specialized knowledge of physical compatibility or incompatibility of the solution contents. The most common drug additives are insulin for persistent hyperglycemia and histamine-2 antagonists to avoid gastroduodenal stress ulceration. One other consideration is that the PN usually is ordered 24 hours before its administration, and patient status may have changed.

Administration

The methods used to administer PN are addressed after the goal infusion rate has been established. For critically ill and hospitalized patients, a 24-hour infusion rate is used. However, for patients transitioning to a long term or lifetime of receiving PN, infusion rate should be decreased to 10- to 12-hour cycle per day to complete activities of daily living and improve quality of life. Nevertheless, general considerations as listed in Box 13-5 can be applied to almost any protocol.

Continuous Infusion

Parenteral solutions usually are initiated below the goal infusion rate via a volumetric pump and then increased incrementally over a 2- or 3-day period to attain the goal infusion rate. Some clinicians start PN based on the amount of dextrose, with initial prescriptions containing 100 to 200 g daily and advancing over a 2- or 3-day period to a final goal. With high dextrose concentrations, abrupt cessation of CPN should be avoided, particularly if the patient's glucose tolerance is abnormal. If CPN is to be stopped, it is prudent to taper the rate of infusion in an unstable patient to prevent rebound hypoglycemia, low blood sugar levels resulting from abrupt cessation. For most stable patients this is not necessary.

Cyclic Infusion

Individuals who require PN at home benefit from a cyclic infusion; this entails infusion of PN for 8- to 12-hour periods, usually at night. This allows the person to have a free period of 12 to 16 hours each day, which may improve quality of life. The goal cycle for infusion time is established incrementally when a higher rate of infusion or a more concentrated solution is required. Cycled infusions should not be attempted if glucose intolerance or fluid tolerance is a problem. The pumps used for home infusion of PN are small and convenient, allowing mobility during daytime infusions. Administration time may be decreased because of patient ambulation and bathing, tests or other treatments, intravenous administration of medications, or other therapies.

Monitoring and Evaluation

As with enteral feeding, routine monitoring of PN is necessary more frequently for the patient receiving PN in the hospital. For

---

BOX 13-5 Nutrition Care Process for Enteral and Parenteral Nutrition

Assessment
1. Clinical status, including medications
2. Fluid requirement
3. Route of administration
4. Energy (kcal) requirement
5. Protein requirement
6. Carbohydrate/lipid considerations
7. Micronutrient considerations
8. Formula selection or PN solution considerations
   A. Concentration (osmolarity)
   B. Protein content
   C. Carbohydrate/lipid content
   D. Micronutrient content
   E. Special formula considerations
9. Calculations
   A. Energy: use kcal/ml formula
   B. Protein: use g/1000 ml
   C. Fat and micronutrient considerations: units/1000 ml
   D. Fluid considerations: extra water, IV fluids (including medications)

Nutrition Diagnosis
1. Identify the problems affecting oral nutritional intake.
2. Identify problems related to access or administration of tube feedings.
3. Write PES statements. These may include inadequate or excess infusion of enteral or parenteral nutrition, or other nutrition diagnoses.

Intervention
1. Each problem should have an intervention and a way to evaluate it.
2. Recommend what method and how to begin feedings.
3. Recommend how to advance feedings.
4. Determine how fluids will be given in adequate amounts.
5. Calculate final feeding prescription.

Monitoring and Evaluation
1. Describe clinical signs and symptoms to monitor for feeding tolerance.
2. List laboratory values and other measurements to be monitored.
3. Determine how feeding outcomes will be evaluated.

IV, Intravenous; *PES,* problem, etiology, and signs and symptoms; *PN,* parenteral nutrition.

---

patients receiving HPN, initial monitoring is done on a weekly basis or less frequently as the patient becomes more stable on PN. Monitoring is done not only to evaluate response to therapy but also to ensure compliance with the treatment plan.

COMPLICATIONS

Infection

The primary complication associated with PN is infection (Box 13-6). Therefore strict adherence to protocols and monitoring for signs of infection such as chills, fever, tachycardia, sudden hyperglycemia, or elevated white blood cell count are necessary. Monitoring of metabolic tolerance is also critical. Electrolytes, acid-base balance, glucose tolerance, renal function, and cardiopulmonary and hemodynamic stability (maintenance of adequate blood pressure) can be affected by PN and should be monitored

BOX 13-6 Parenteral Nutrition Complications

Mechanical Complications

Air embolism
Arteriovenous fistula
Brachial plexus injury
Catheter fragment embolism
Catheter misplacement
Cardiac perforation
Central vein thrombophlebitis
Endocarditis
Hemothorax
Hydromediastinum
Hydrothorax
Pneumothorax or tension pneumothorax
Subcutaneous emphysema
Subclavian artery injury
Subclavian hematoma
Thoracic duct injury

Infection and Sepsis

Catheter entrance site
Catheter seeding from bloodborne or distant infection
Contamination during insertion
Long-term catheter placement
Solution contamination

Metabolic Complications

Dehydration from osmotic diuresis
Electrolyte imbalance
Essential fatty acid deficiency
Hyperosmolar, nonketotic, hyperglycemic coma
Hyperammonemia
Hypercalcemia
Hyperchloremic metabolic acidosis
Hyperlipidemia
Hyperphosphatemia
Hypocalcemia
Hypomagnesemia
Hypophosphatemia
Rebound hypoglycemia on sudden cessation of PN in patient with unstable glucose levels
Uremia
Trace mineral deficiencies

Gastrointestinal Complications

Cholestasis
Gastrointestinal villous atrophy
Hepatic abnormalities

Adapted from McClave SA et al: Guidelines for the provision and assessment of nutrition support therapy in the adult critically ill patient, *J Parenter Enteral Nutr* 33:277, 2009.

TABLE 13-6 Inpatient Parenteral Nutrition Monitoring (Critical/Acute Care)

VARIABLE TO BE MONITORED	SUGGESTED FREQUENCY	
	Initial Period*	Later Period*
Weight	Daily	Weekly
Serum electrolytes	Daily	1-2/wk
Blood urea nitrogen	3-wk	Weekly
Serum total calcium or ionized Ca⁺, inorganic phosphorus, magnesium	3-wk	Weekly
Serum glucose	Daily	3-wk
Serum triglycerides	Weekly	Weekly
Liver function enzymes	3-wk	Weekly
Hemoglobin, hematocrit	Weekly	Weekly
Platelets	Weekly	Weekly
WBC count	As indicated	As indicated
Clinical status	Daily	Daily
Catheter site	Daily	Daily
Temperature	Daily	Daily
I&O	Daily	Daily

McClave SA et al: Guidelines for the provision and assessment of nutrition support therapy in the adult critically ill patient, *J Parenter Enteral Nutr* 33:277, 2009.
I&O, Intake and output; *WBC,* white blood cell.
Initial period is that period in which a full glucose intake is being achieved. *Later period* implies that the patient had achieved a steady metabolic state. In the presence of metabolic instability, the more intensive monitoring outlined under initial period should be followed.
I&O refers to all fluids going into the patient: oral, intravenous, medication; and all fluid coming out: urine, surgical drains, exudates.

REFEEDING SYNDROME

Patients who require enteral or PN therapies may have been eating poorly before initiating therapy because of the disease process and may be moderately to severely malnourished. Aggressive administration of nutrition, particularly via the intravenous route, can precipitate refeeding syndrome with severe, potentially lethal electrolyte fluctuations involving metabolic, hemodynamic, and neuromuscular problems. Refeeding syndrome occurs when energy substrates, particularly carbohydrate, are introduced into the plasma of anabolic patients (Parrish, 2009).

Proliferation of new tissue requires increased amounts of glucose, potassium, phosphorus, magnesium, and other nutrients essential for tissue growth. If intracellular electrolytes are not supplied in sufficient quantity to keep up with tissue growth, low serum levels of potassium, phosphorus, and magnesium develop. Low levels of these electrolytes are the hallmark of refeeding syndrome, especially hypokalemia. Carbohydrate metabolism by cells also causes a shift of electrolytes to the intracellular space as glucose moves into cells for oxidation. Rapid infusion of carbohydrate stimulates insulin release, which reduces salt and water excretion and increases the chance of cardiac and pulmonary complications from fluid overload.

Patients starting on PN who have received minimal nutrition for a significant period should be monitored closely for electrolyte fluctuation and fluid overload. A review of baseline laboratory values, including glucose, magnesium, potassium, and phosphorus should be completed and any abnormalities corrected before initiating nutrition support, particularly PN. Conservative amounts of carbohydrate and adequate amounts

carefully. Table 13-6 lists parameters that should be monitored routinely.

The CPN catheter site is a potential source for introduction of microorganisms into a major vein. Protocols to prevent infection vary and should follow Centers for Disease Control Prevention guidelines (Naomi et al, 2011). Catheter care and prevention of catheter-related bloodstream infections are of utmost importance in the hospital and alternate settings. These infections not only are costly but also may be life-threatening. Catheter care is dictated by the site of the catheter and the setting in which the patient receives care.

of intracellular electrolytes should be provided. The initial PN formulation usually should contain 25% to 50% of goal dextrose concentration and be increased slowly to avoid the consequences of hypophosphatemia, hypokalemia, and hypomagnesemia. PN compatibilities must be assessed when very low levels of dextrose are provided with higher levels of amino acids and electrolytes. The syndrome also occurs in enterally fed patients, but less often because of the effects of the digestive process.

In managing the nutrition care process, refeeding syndrome is an undesirable outcome that requires monitoring and evaluation. Most often, the nutrition diagnosis may be "excessive carbohydrate intake" or "excessive infusion from enteral or parenteral nutrition" in the undernourished patient. Thus, in the early phase of refeeding, nutrient prescriptions should be moderate in carbohydrate and supplemented with phosphorus, potassium, and magnesium.

TRANSITIONAL FEEDING

All nutrition support care plans strive to use the GIT when possible, either with EN or by a total or partial return to oral intake. Therefore patient care plans frequently involve transitional feeding, moving from one type of feeding to another, with several feeding methods used simultaneously while continuously administering estimated nutrient requirements. This requires careful monitoring of patient tolerance and quantification of intake from parenteral, enteral, and oral routes. Most experts advise that initial oral diets be low in simple carbohydrates and fat, as well as lactose free. These provisions make digestion easier and minimize the possibility of osmotic diarrhea. Attention to individual tolerance and food preferences also helps maximize intake. During the transition stage from HPN to HEN or an oral diet, careful attention should be paid to assuring multivitamin and mineral adequacy. This may require laboratory assessment of micronutrients if a deficiency is suspected.

Parenteral to Enteral Feeding

To begin the transition from PN to EN, introduce a minimal amount of enteral feeding at a low rate of 30 to 40 ml/hr to establish gastrointestinal tolerance. When there is severe gastrointestinal compromise, predigested formula to initiate enteral feedings may be better tolerated. Once formula has been given during a period of hours, the parenteral rate can be decreased to keep the nutrient levels at the same prescribed amount. As the enteral rate is increased by 25 to 30 ml/hr increments every 8 to 24 hours, the parenteral prescription is reduced accordingly. Once the patient is tolerating about 75% of nutrient needs by the enteral route, the PN solution can be discontinued. This process ideally takes 2 to 3 days; however, it may become more complicated, depending on the degree of gastrointestinal function. At times the weaning process may not be practical, and PN can be stopped sooner, depending on overall treatment decisions and likelihood for tolerance of enteral feeding.

Parenteral to Oral Feeding

The transition from parenteral to oral feeding ideally is accomplished by monitoring oral intake and concomitantly decreasing the PN to maintain a stable nutrient intake. Approximately 75% of nutrient needs should be met consistently by oral intake before the PN is discontinued. The process is less predictable than the transition to enteral feeding. Variations include the patient's appetite, motivation, and general well-being. It is important to continue monitoring the patient for adequate oral intake once PN has been stopped and to initiate alternate nutrition support if necessary. Generally patients are transitioned from clear liquids to a diet that is low in fiber and fat and is lactose free. It takes several days for the GIT to regain function; during that time, the diet should be composed of easily digested foods.

Special nutrient needs may be employed, especially when transitioning a patient with gastrointestinal disorders such as short bowel syndrome. Specialized nutrients, optimized drug therapy, and nutrition counseling should be comprehensive to improve outcome. Some PN patients may not be able to discontinue PN fully but may be able to use PN less than 7 days per week, necessitating careful attention to nutrient intake. A skilled registered dietitian nutritionist (RDN) can coordinate diet and PN needs for this type of patient.

Enteral to Oral Feeding

A stepwise decrease also is used to transition from EN to oral feeding. It is effective to move from continuous feeding to a 12- and then an 8-hour formula administration cycle during the night; this reestablishes hunger and satiety cues for oral intake during daytime. In practice, oral diets often are attempted after inadvertent or deliberate removal of a nasoenteric tube. This type of interrupted transition should be monitored closely for adequate oral intake. Patients receiving EN who desire to eat and for whom it is not contraindicated can be encouraged to do so. A transition from liquids to easy-to-digest foods may be necessary during a period of days. Patients who cannot meet their needs by the oral route can be maintained by a combination of EN and oral intake.

Oral Supplements

The most common types of oral supplements are commercial formulas meant primarily to augment the intake of solid foods. They often provide approximately 250 kcal/8 oz or 240-ml portion and approximately 8 to 14 g of intact protein. Some products have 360 or 500 or as much as 575 kcal in a can. There are different types of products for different disease states.

Fat sources are often long-chain triglycerides, although some supplements contain MCTs. More concentrated and thus more nutrient-dense formulas are also available. A variety of flavors, consistencies, and modifications of nutrients are appropriate for various disease states. Some oral supplements provide a nutritionally complete diet if taken in sufficient volume.

The form of carbohydrate is a key factor to patient acceptance and tolerance. Supplements with appreciable amounts of simple carbohydrate taste sweeter and have higher osmolalities, which may contribute to gastrointestinal intolerance. Individual taste preferences vary widely, and normal taste is altered by certain drug therapies, especially chemotherapy. Concentrated formulas or large volumes can contribute to taste fatigue and early satiety. Thus oral nutrient intake and the intake of prescribed supplements should be monitored.

Oral supplements that contain hydrolyzed protein and free amino acids such as those developed for patients with renal, liver, and malabsorptive diseases tend to be mildly to markedly unpalatable, and acceptance by the patient depends on motivation. Formulas for renal and liver disease in particular may lack sufficient vitamins and minerals and are not nutritionally complete and therefore useful only to the specific population.

Although commercially available modular supplements are used most commonly for convenience, modules of protein, carbohydrate, or fat or commonly available food items can produce highly palatable additions to a diet. As examples, liquid or powdered milk, yogurt, tofu, or protein powders can be used to enrich cereals, casseroles, soups, or milk shakes. Thickening agents are now used to add variety, texture, and aesthetics to pureed foods, which are used when swallowing ability is limited (see Chapter 40). Imagination and individual tailoring can increase oral intake, avoiding the necessity for more complex forms of nutrition support.

NUTRITION SUPPORT IN LONG-TERM AND HOME CARE

Long-Term Care

Long-term care (LTC) generally refers to a skilled nursing facility but includes subacute care for the purpose of rehabilitation that often can take several weeks or even months. Health care provided in this environment focuses on quality of life, self-determination, and management of acute and chronic disease. Indications for EN and PN are generally the same for older patients as for younger adults and varies according to the age, gender, disease state, and most importantly, the care goals of the individual. PN and EN often are provided to these facilities by offsite pharmacies that specialize in LTC. These providers may employ dietitians and specially trained nurses to assist the facilities with education and training on PEN.

Oral supplements have gained widespread use in this LTC over the last two decades, again for convenience. However, they appear to have detrimental effects, and real food always should be attempted first. See Chapter 19 for a discussion of the Dining Standards for Long Term Care that have been endorsed by 12 professional organizations. A major goal in the Dining Standards is the elimination of canned nutrition supplements.

Advance directives are legal documents that residents use to state their preferences about aspects of care, including those regarding the use of nutrition support. These directives may be written in any setting, including acute or home care but are especially useful in LTC to guide interventions on behalf of long-term care residents when they are no longer able to make decisions (Barrocas et al, 2010).

Differentiation between the effects of advanced age versus malnutrition is an assessment challenge for dietitians working in long-term care (see Chapter 20). This is an area of active research, as is the influence that nutrition support has on the quality of life among long-term care residents. Studies generally show that use of nutrition support in older adults is beneficial, especially when used in conjunction with physical activity. Patients who are actively pursuing physical therapy are good candidates for nutrition support. However, when there is a terminal illness or condition, starting nutrition support may have no advantage and may prolong suffering in some cases. Dietitians can be strong patient advocates in end-of-life decisions and should be involved in writing and implementing the policies in their institutions.

BOX 13-7 Considerations When Deciding on Home Nutrition Support

Sanitation of the home environment to preserve the patient's health and reduce risk of infection

Potential for improvement in quality of life and nutritional status

The financial and time commitment needed by patient or family; potential loss of income outside the home in some cases

Ability to understand the techniques for administration of the product and safe use of all equipment and supplies

Any physical limitations that prevent the implementation of HEN or HPN therapy

Capacity for patient or caregiver to contact medical services when needed

HEN, Home enteral nutrition; *HPN,* home parenteral nutrition.

Home Care

Home enteral nutrition (HEN) or home parenteral nutrition (HPN) support usually entails the provision of nutrients or formulas, supplies, equipment, and professional clinical services. Resources and technology for safe and effective management of long-term enteral or parenteral therapy are widely available for the home care setting. Although home nutrition support has been available for more than 30 years, few outcome data have been generated. Because mandatory reporting requirements do not exist in the United States for patients receiving home nutrition support, the exact number of patients receiving this support is unknown.

The elements needed to implement home nutrition successfully include identification of appropriate candidates and a feasible home environment with responsive caregivers, a choice of a suitable nutrition support regimen, training of the patient and family, and a plan for medical and nutritional follow-up by the physician as well as by the home infusion provider (Box 13-7). These objectives are best achieved through coordinated efforts of an interdisciplinary team (see *Clinical Insight:* Home Tube Feeding—Key Considerations).

Patients receiving HEN may receive supplies only, or formula and supplies with or without clinical oversight by the provider. Many enteral patients receive services from a durable medical equipment (DME) provider that may or may not provide clinical services. A home infusion provider provides intravenous therapies, including home PN, intravenous antibiotics, and other therapies. Home nursing agencies may be associated with a DME company or a home infusion agency to provide nursing services to home EN or PN patients. Often the patient's reimbursement source for home therapy plays a major role in determining the type of home infusion provider. In fact, reimbursement is a key component of a patient's ability to receive home therapy of any kind and should be evaluated early in the care plan so that appropriate decisions can be made before discharge or initiating a therapy.

Companies that provide home infusion services for EN or PN may be private or affiliated with acute care facilities. Criteria for selecting a home care company to provide nutrition support should be based on the company's ability to provide ongoing monitoring, patient education, and coordination of care. When a patient is receiving home EN or PN, it is important to determine whether the provider has an RDN on staff or access to the services of a RDN. The RDN is uniquely qualified not only to provide oversight and monitoring for the patient while receiving EN or PN but also to provide the appropriate nutrition

CLINICAL INSIGHT

Home Tube Feeding—Key Considerations

What Is the Best Kind of Tube?

In general, nasal tubes should be avoided because they are more difficult to manage, clog easily, are easily dislodged, and over time can cause tissue irritation and even erosion. PEG tubes are now the most common and preferred method for home tube feedings. They can be either low profile (flat to the abdomen), button-type tubes, or they can have a short piece of tubing attached through the abdomen and into the stomach. The button tubes require some manual dexterity to access and can be difficult to use for patients who are very obese. **Percutaneous endoscopic jejunostomy (PEJ)** tubes are best for patients who require postpyloric feedings as a result of intolerance of gastric feeding, but PEJ feedings require a pump, which severely limits mobility of the patient.

What Is the Best Method of Administration?

Bolus feeding is the easiest administration method and generally should be tried first. It should be started slowly at half of an 8-oz can four to six times a day. If bolus feeding is not tolerated, gravity feeding is a second option. It does require a bag and pole but can be accomplished fairly quickly and requires less manual dexterity than bolus feeding.

Pump feeding is sometimes necessary when a patient requires small amounts of formula delivered slowly. Although it is well tolerated, it has major implications for a patient at home because even the simplest pump is often viewed as "high tech." Its use greatly limits mobility, and, like any piece of equipment, it can break and interrupt feeding schedules.

What Is the Best Way to Educate the Patient and Caregiver?

- Directions should be written in common measurements such as cups, tablespoons, and cans rather than milliliters.
- The enteral nutrition regimen should be as simple as possible; use whole cans of formula rather than partial cans.
- Additives to the feedings should be minimized to avoid confusion and clogging of the feedings tubes.
- Provide clear directions for gradually increasing to the goal feeding rate.
- Provide clear directions for water flushing of the tube and for additional water requirements to prevent dehydration.
- Discuss common problems that may come up and provide guidance for resolving them.
- Make sure that the patient or caregiver can demonstrate understanding of the feeding process by either explaining it or by doing it.

---

counseling and food suggestions when the patient transitions between therapies (Fuhrman et al, 2009).

Ethical Issues

Whether to provide or withhold nutrition support is often a central issue in "end-of-life" decision making. For patients who are terminally ill or in a persistent vegetative state, nutrition support can extend life to the point that issues of quality of life and the patient's right to self-determination come into play. Often surrogate decision makers are involved in treatment decisions. The nutrition support clinician has a responsibility to know whether documentation, such as a living will regarding the patient's wishes for nutrition support, is in the medical record and whether counseling and support resources for legal and ethical aspects of patient care are available to the patient and his or her significant others (Barrocas et al, 2010).

CLINICAL CASE STUDY

A 24-year-old has newly diagnosed type 1 diabetes mellitus and Crohn's disease. She recently had surgery for removal of one third of her ileum. She is 75% of her usual weight, which is 125 lb; she is 65 inches tall. She requires specialized nutrition support for several months until her body adapts to the shortened bowel.

Nutrition Diagnostic Statements

- Involuntary weight loss related to poor intake, surgery, and pain during flare-up of Crohn's disease as evidenced by 25% weight loss.
- Inadequate oral food and beverage intake related to recent ileal resection as evidenced by 75% of usual weight and need for artificial nutrition.

Nutrition Care Questions

1. What immediate nutrition support method would be recommended?
2. What long-term nutrition support plan is likely to be designed?
3. What specialty products, if any, may be beneficial?
4. What parameters would you monitor to determine tolerance and response to the nutrition plan?

USEFUL WEBSITES

Academy of Nutrition and Dietetics—Evidence Analysis Library (member/subscription access only)
http://andevidencelibrary.com
American Society for Parenteral and Enteral Nutrition
http://www.nutritioncare.org/
European Society for Parenteral and Enteral Nutrition
http://www.espen.org
Infusion Nurses Society
http://www.ins1.org
Medscape—Integrated Med Information
http://www.medscape.com/
Oley Foundation
http://www.oley.org/

REFERENCES

Academy of Nutrition and Dietetics (AND), Evidence Analysis Library (EAL): *Critical illness guidelines*, 2012. http://andevidencelibrary.com/topic.cfm?cat=4800. Accessed December 2014.

Ayers P, Adams S, Boullata J, et al: A.S.P.E.N. parenteral nutrition safety consensus recommendations, *JPEN J Parenter Enteral Nutr* 38:296–333, 2014.

Bankhead R, Boullata J, Brantley S, et al: Enteral nutrition practice recommendations, *JPEN J Parenter Enteral Nutr* 33:122–167, 2009.

Barrocas A, Geppert C, Durfee SM, et al: A.S.P.E.N. ethics position paper, *Nutr Clin Pract* 25:672–679, 2010.

Boullata JI, Gilbert K, Sacks G, et al: A.S.P.E.N. clinical guidelines: parenteral nutrition ordering, order review, compounding, labeling, and dispensing, *JPEN* J Parenter Enteral Nutr 38:334–377, 2014.

Buchman AL, Howard LJ, Guenter P, et al: Micronutrients in parenteral nutrition: too little or too much? The past, present, and recommendations for the future, *Gastroenterology* 137(Suppl 5):S1–S6, 2009.

Charney P, Malone A: *Pocket guide to enteral nutrition*, ed 3, Chicago, 2013, Academy of Nutrition and Dietetics.

DeChicco R, Seidner DL, Brun C, et al: Tip position of long-term central venous access devices used for parenteral nutrition, *JPEN J Parenter Enteral Nutr* 31:382–387, 2007.

Drover JW, Cahill NE, Kutsogiannis J, et al: Nutrition therapy for the critically ill surgical patient: we need to do better! *JPEN* J Parenter Enteral Nutr 34:644–652, 2010.

Food and Drug Administration (FDA): *Medical foods guidance documents & regulatory information,* 2014. http://www.fda.gov/Food/GuidanceRegulation/GuidanceDocumentsRegulatoryInformation/MedicalFoods/. Accessed December 2014.

Fuhrman MP, Galvin TA, Ireton-Jones CS, et al: Practice paper of the American Dietetic Association: home care- opportunities for food and nutrition professionals, *J Am Diet Assoc* 109:1092–1100, 2009.

Gura KM: Is there still a role for peripheral parenteral nutrition? *Nutr Clin Pract* 24:709–717, 2009.

Harvey SE, Parrott F, Harrison DA, et al: Trial of the route of early nutritional support in critically ill adults, *N Engl J Med* 371:1673–1684, 2014.

Joint Commission: *Sentinel event policy and procedures.* 2014. http://www.jointcommission.org/Sentinel_Event_Policy_and_Procedures/. Accessed December 2014.

Kumpf VJ et al: Parenteral nutrition formulations: Preparation and ordering. In R. Merritt (Ed.), *The A.S.P.E.N. Nutrition Support Practice Manual.* 2nd ed. American Society for Parenteral and Enteral Nutrition: Silver Springs, MD, 2005.

Malone A: Enteral formula selection: a review of selected product categories. In Parish CR, editor: *Nutrition issues in gastroenterology, Series #28, Practical Gastroenterology,* 2005. http://www.medicine.virginia.edu/clinical/departments/medicine/divisions/digestive-health/nutrition-support-team/nutrition-articles/MaloneArticle.pdf. Accessed December 2014.

Manzanares W, Dhaliwal R, Jurewitsch B, et al: Parenteral fish oil lipid emulsion in the critically ill: a systematic review and meta-analysis, *JPEN* J Parenter Enteral Nutr 38:20–28, 2014.

McClave SA, Martindale RG, Vanek VW, et al: Guidelines for the provision and assessment of nutrition support therapy in the adult critically ill patient: Society of Critical Care Medicine (SCCM) and American Society for Parenteral and Enteral Nutrition (A.S.P.E.N.), *JPEN* J Parenter Enteral Nutr 33:277–316, 2009. http://www.ncbi.nlm.nih.gov/pubmed/?term=McCarthy%20M%5BAuthor%5D&cauthor=true&cauthor_uid=19398613.

Metheny NA, Meert KL: Monitoring tube feeding placement, *Nutr Clin Pract* 19:487–495, 2004.

Mueller C, Compher C, Ellen DM, et al: A.S.P.E.N. clinical guidelines: nutrition screening, assessment, and intervention in adults, *JPEN J Parenter Enteral Nutr* 35:16–24, 2011.

Naomi P, Mary Alexander RN, Lillian AB, et al: *2011 Guidelines for the prevention of intravascular catheter-related infections,* 2011. http://www.cdc.gov/hicpac/bsi/bsi-guidelines-2011.html. Accessed December 2014.

Novak P, Wilson KF, Ausderau K, et al: The use of blenderized tube feedings, *Infant Child Adolesc Nutr* 1:21–23, 2009.

O'Flaherty T, Santoro K, Pentiuk S: Calculating and preparing a pureed-gastrostomy tube (PBGT) diet for pediatric patients with retching and gagging post-fundoplication, *Infant Child Adolesc Nutr* 3:361–364, 2011.

O'Flaherty T: Use of a pureed by gastrostomy tube diet (PBGT) to promote oral intake: Review and case study, *Support Line* 37:21, 2015.

Parrish CR: The refeeding syndrome in 2009: prevention is the key to treatment, *J Support Oncol* 7:20–21, 2009.

Pentiuk SP, O'Flaherty T, Santoro K, et al: Pureed by gastrostomy tube diet improves gagging and retching in children with fundoplication, *JPEN J Parenter Enteral Nutr* 35:375–379, 2011.

Puiggros C, Sánchez J, Chacón P, et al: Evolution of lipid profile, liver function, and pattern of plasma fatty acids according to the type of lipid emulsion administered in parenteral nutrition in the early postoperative period after digestive surgery, *J Parenter Enteral Nutr* 33:501–512, 2009.

Sriram K, Lonchyna V: Micronutrient supplementation in adult nutrition therapy: practical considerations, *Nutr Clin Prac* 33:548–562, 2009.

Vanek V, Borum P, Buchman A, et al: A.S.P.E.N. position paper: recommendations for changes in commercially available parenteral multivitamin and multi-trace element products, *Nutr Clin Prac* 27:440–491, 2012.

Vassilyadi, F, Panteliadou AK, Panteliadis C: Hallmarks in the history of enteral and parenteral nutrition: from antiquity to the 20th century, *Nutr Clin Prac* 28:209–217, 2013.

Waitzberg DL, Torrinhas RS, Jacintho TM: New parenteral lipid emulsions for clinical use, *JPEN J Parenter Enteral Nutr* 30:351–367, 2006.

14

Education and Counseling: Behavioral Change

Karen Chapman-Novakofski, PhD, RDN, LDN

KEY TERMS

alignment
ambivalence
behavior change
behavior modification
cognitive behavioral therapy (CBT)
cultural competency
discrepancy
double-sided reflection
empathy

health belief model (HBM)
health literacy
maleficence
motivational interviewing (MI)
negotiation
normalization
peer educator
PRECEDE-PROCEED model
reflective listening

reframing
self-efficacy
self-management
self-monitoring
social cognitive theory (SCT)
social-ecological model
stages of change
theory of planned behavior (TPB)
transtheoretical model (TTM)

Key factors in changing nutrition behavior are the person's awareness that a change is needed and the motivation to change. Nutrition education and nutrition counseling provide information and motivation, but they do differ. *Nutrition education* can be individualized or delivered in a group setting; it is usually more preventive than therapeutic, and there is a transmission of knowledge. *Counseling* is used most often during medical nutrition therapy, one-on-one. In the one-on-one setting, the nutritionist sets up a transient support system to prepare the client to handle social and personal demands more effectively while identifying favorable conditions for change. The goal of nutrition education and nutrition counseling is to help individuals make meaningful changes in their dietary behaviors.

BEHAVIOR CHANGE

Although there are differences between education and counseling as intervention techniques, the distinctions are not as important as the desired outcome, behavior change. Behavior change requires a focus on the broad range of activities and approaches that affect the individual choosing food and beverages in his or her community and home environment. Behavior modification implies the use of techniques to alter a person's behavior or reactions to environmental cues through positive and negative reinforcement, and extinction of maladaptive behaviors. In the context of nutrition, education and counseling can assist the individual in achieving short-term or long-term health goals.

Factors Affecting the Ability to Change

Multiple factors affect a person's ability or desire to change, the educator's ability to teach new information, and the counselor's ability to stimulate and support small changes. Financial constraints, unstable living environments, inadequate family or social support, insufficient transportation, and low literacy are some of the socioeconomic factors that may be barriers for obtaining and maintaining a healthy diet. With a population that is culturally diverse, it is imperative to appreciate the differences in beliefs or understanding that may lead to the inability to change.

Physical and emotional factors also make it hard to change, especially for seniors. Older adults need education and counseling programs that address low vision, poor hearing, limited mobility, decreased dexterity, and memory problems or cognitive impairments (Kamp et al, 2010). Expectations of the food preparer, time restraints, routines, preferences, and roles within the family also may hinder changes in food intake (Brown and Wenrich, 2012). For children, barriers include taste, ease of eating, and competing foods that may be available that are less healthy (Nicklas et al, 2013). Across all ages are issues of how culture affects what foods are eaten and how and perceptions about education, counseling, health, and health care (see Chapters 9 and 11).

MODELS FOR BEHAVIOR CHANGE

Changing behavior is the ultimate goal for nutrition counseling and education. Providing a pamphlet or a list of foods can reinforce information, but it usually does nothing to change eating behavior. Because so many different factors influence what someone eats, nutritionists have been learning from behavioral scientists to identify and intervene based on mediators of people's eating behavior. Health professionals can support individuals in deciding what and when to change by using a variety of health behavior

TABLE 14-1	**Overview of Behavior Theories Used in Nutrition Education and Counseling**
Health Belief Model (HBM)	Perceived susceptibility: An individual's belief regarding the chance that he or she may get a condition or disease Perceived severity: An individual's belief of how serious a condition and its consequences are Perceived benefits: An individual's belief in the positive effects of the advised action in reducing the risk or the seriousness of a condition Perceived barriers: An individual's belief about the tangible and psychologic costs of the advised action Self-efficacy: An individual's belief that he or she is capable of performing the desired action Cues to action: Strategies to activate one's readiness to change a behavior
Social Cognitive Theory (SCT)	Personal factors: Outcome expectations, self-efficacy, reinforcements, impediments, goals and intentions, relapse prevention Behavioral factors: Knowledge and skills, self-regulation and control, and goal setting Environmental factors: Include imposed, selected, and created environments
Theory of Planned Behavior (TPB)	Subjective norms: The people who may influence the patient Attitudes: What the patient thinks about the behavior Perceived control: How much control the patient has to change things that affect the behavior Behavioral intention: Whether the patient plans to perform the behavior
Transtheoretical Model (TM), or Stages of Change Model	Precontemplation: The individual has not thought about making a change. Contemplation: The individual has thought about making a change but has done no more than think about it. Preparation: The individual has taken some steps to begin to make the desired change. Action: The individual has made the change and continues it for less than 6 months. Maintenance: The individual has continued the behavior for longer than 6 months. Termination: The individual no longer thinks about the change; it has become a habit.

theories. Some of the most common theories for behavior change are listed in Table 14-1, with examples described in the following paragraphs.

Health Belief Model

The **health belief model (HBM)** focuses on a disease or condition, and factors that may influence behavior related to that disease (Rosenstock, 1974). The HBM has been used most with behaviors related to diabetes and osteoporosis, focusing on barriers to and benefits of changing behaviors (James et al, 2012; Plawecki and Chapman-Novakofski, 2013).

Social Cognitive Theory

Social cognitive theory (SCT) represents the reciprocal interaction among personal, behavioral, and environmental factors (Bandura, 1977, 1986). This theory is extensive and includes many variables; some of the most important to counseling include self-efficacy, goal setting, and relapse prevention (Poddar et al, 2012).

Theory of Planned Behavior

The **theory of planned behavior (TPB)** and the reasoned action approach are based on the concept that intentions predict behavior (Ajzen, 1991; Fishbein and Ajzen, 2010). Intentions are predicted by attitudes, subjective norms (important others), and perceived control. This theory is most successful when a discrete behavior is targeted (e.g., vegetable intake) but has also been used for healthy diet consumption (Sheats et al, 2013).

Transtheoretical Model of Change

The **transtheoretical model (TTM)**, or **stages of change** model, has been used for many years to alter addictive behaviors and often is described as "tailored education." TTM describes behavior change as a process in which individuals progress through a series of six distinct stages of change, as shown in Figure 14-1 (Prochaska and Norcross, 2001). The value of the TTM is in determining the individual's current stage, then using change processes matched to that stage (Mochari-Greenberger et al, 2010).

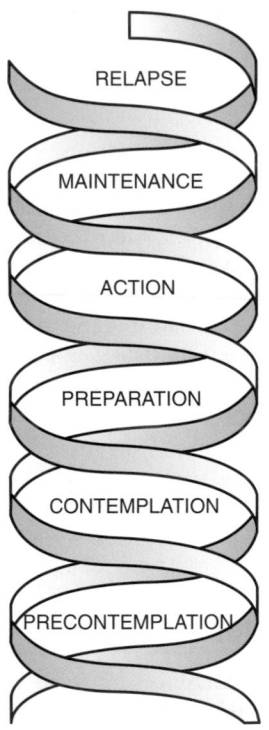

FIGURE 14-1 A model of the stages of change. In changing, a person progresses up these steps to maintenance. If relapse occurs, he or she gets back on the steps at some point and works up them again.

MODELS FOR COUNSELING STRATEGIES

Cognitive behavior therapy (CBT) focuses on identifying and changing erroneous perceptions of the self, environment, and behavioral consequences. CBT often identifies behavior and thoughts that have a negative impact on desired behavioral goals and apply strategies to change those. CBT counselors can help clients explore troubling themes, strengthen their coping skills, and focus on their well-being (Beck, 2011).

CBT often is used for obesity interventions and eating disorders as well as a range of psychologic and psychiatric disorders (Cooper et al, 2010; Murphy et al, 2010).

Motivational interviewing (MI) has been used in a variety of conditions to encourage clients to identify discrepancies between how they would like to behave and how they are behaving and then motivate them to change. The following are principles used in MI to enhance behavior change (Johnston and Stevens, 2013).

Expressing Empathy

The nutrition counselor should demonstrate empathy for what a client feels, rather than giving advice. As clients review situations in their lives and the lack of time for dietary changes, the nutrition counselor will hear ambivalence. On the one hand, clients want to make changes; on the other hand, they want to pretend that change is not important.

Developing Discrepancy

An awareness of consequences is important. Identifying the advantages and disadvantages of modifying a behavior, or developing discrepancy, is a crucial process in making changes.

> Client: I want to follow the new eating pattern, but I just can't afford it.
> Nutrition counselor: Let's look at your diet record and discuss some healthy, low-cost changes.

Rolling with Resistance (Legitimation, Affirmation)

Rolling with resistance involves inviting new perspectives without imposing them. The client is a valuable resource in finding solutions to problems. Perceptions can be shifted, and the nutrition counselor's role is to help with this process. For example, a client who is wary of describing why she is not ready to change may become much more open to change if she sees openness to her resistive behaviors. When it becomes okay to discuss resistance, the rationale for its original existence may seem less important.

> Client: I just feel that my level of enthusiasm for following the diet is low. It all seems like too much effort.
> Nutrition counselor: I appreciate your concerns. At this point in following a new diet, many people feel the same way. Tell me more about your concerns and feelings.

Supporting Self-Efficacy

Belief in one's own capability to change is an important motivator. The client is responsible for choosing and carrying out personal change. However, the nutrition counselor can support self-efficacy by having the client try behaviors or activities while the counselor is there.

> Client: I just don't know what to buy once I get to the grocery store. I end up with hamburger and potato chips.
> Nutrition counselor: Let's think of one day's meals right now. Then we can make a grocery list from that.

MODELS FOR EDUCATIONAL PROGRAM DEVELOPMENT

The **PRECEDE-PROCEED model** is a participatory health program planning model that has been used in a variety of health topics communities to optimize positive outcomes. PRECEDE consists of four planning phases represented in its acronym for

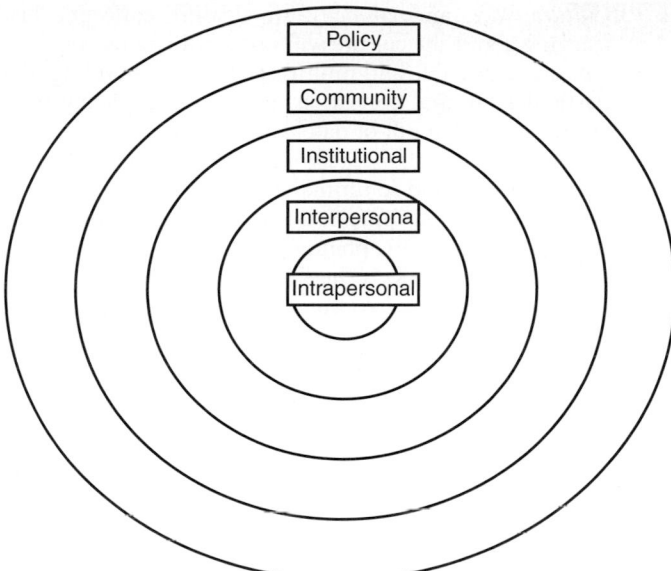

FIGURE 14-2 The intrapersonal, interpersonal, institutional, community, and policy levels of the social-ecological model.

predisposing, reinforcing, enabling, constructs in education/ecological diagnosis and evaluation. This reflects the needs assessment and participatory planning of the educational program. PROCEED's acronym stands for **P**olicy, **R**egulatory, and **O**rganizational **C**onstructs in **E**ducational and **E**nvironmental **D**evelopment and provides a framework for program implementation and evaluation (Green et al, 1980). This model has been applied to a number of nutrition education programs (Kattelmann et al, 2014; Walsh et al, 2014).

The social-ecological model (Sallis and Owen, 2015) (Figure 14-2) can be applied to health promotion and disease prevention programs by addressing interventions at each stage of the model: intrapersonal, interpersonal, institutional, community, and policy levels (Fitzgerald et al, 2013).

SKILLS AND ATTRIBUTES OF THE NUTRITION EDUCATOR OR COUNSELOR

Cultural Competency

The medical community was one of the first to promote cultural competency and, although there is no agreement on its exact definition, it is fair to say it involves cultural sensitivity or awareness. Learning about different cultures is important; however, memorizing attributes commonly thought to reflect a certain culture can lead to stereotyping. A preferred approach is to develop skills in eliciting the learner's perceptions, skills, and literacy as an individual (Stein, 2009).

Gregg et al (2006) define the following five tenets as the basis for cultural competency:

- Understanding the role of culture. Learning the skills to elicit patients' individual beliefs and interpretations and to negotiate conflicting beliefs is important to good patient care, regardless of the social, ethnic, or racial backgrounds of the patient.
- Learning about culture and becoming "culturally competent" is not a panacea for health disparities.

- *Culture, race,* and *ethnicity* are distinct concepts. Just learning about the culture will not eliminate racism.
- Culture is mutable and multiple; any understanding of a particular cultural context is always incompletely true, always somewhat out of date, and partial.
- Context is critical. Because culture is so complex, so shape-shifting, and so ultimately inseparable from its social and economic context, it is impossible to consider it as an isolated or static phenomenon.

Multicultural awareness is the first step toward establishing rapport and becoming a competent nutrition educator or counselor. It is important to evaluate one's own beliefs and attitudes and become comfortable with differences among racial, ethnic, or religious beliefs, culture, and food practices (see *Clinical Insight:* The Counselor Looks Within). Heightening awareness of personal biases and increasing sensitivity allow the counselor to be more effective in understanding what the client may need to move forward.

Educating or counseling with cultural competency should acknowledge surface and deep structure. Surface structure includes such things as language and foods (see Chapter 11). Deep structure includes psychologic or social beliefs and the context of the intervention.

Language is the primary surface structure issue that is addressed. Although knowing several languages can be an asset, many counselors rely on translators. Unofficial translators, such as family or friends, are not usually a good choice because of a lack of understanding of nutrition and health. Using professional translators is also not without limitations in that the educator must understand the client and the interpreter. The educator should maintain contact with the client and explain the role of the interpreter (Mossavar-Rahmani, 2007). When working with clients who have limited ability to speak and understand English, always use common terms, avoiding slang and words with multiple meanings. Always speak directly to the client, even when using a translator, and watch the client for nonverbal responses during the translation.

Effective communication in education or counseling should encompass not only language but also deeper structure issues, such as the role of the individual within a group, and how or why certain foods are prepared (Broyles et al, 2011). Spatial relationships vary among cultures and among individuals. Movements such as gestures, facial expressions, and postures are often the cause of confusion and misinterpretations in intercultural communication. Rules regarding eye contact are usually complex and vary according to issues such as gender, distance apart, and social status (see *Clinical Insight:* Body Language and Communication Skills).

CLINICAL INSIGHT
The Counselor Looks Within

Before entering a counseling relationship and after reflecting on the session, the nutritionist should look inward and consider any factors that affect his or her own thinking and how they may affect the client. The nutritionist should reflect on ethical issues, such as the autonomy of the client, and beneficence versus **maleficence** (harm). An example may be when a female client decides not to set goals for her blood glucose levels and not to learn the amounts of carbohydrates in foods (autonomy). These choices serve as barriers to the benefit the counselor would make in teaching these **self-management** tools (beneficenco) and the need for nonmaleficence (do no harm). Whenever clients decide a behavior change is not right for them, the counselor's role is not to force the issue but to encourage its future consideration.

CLINICAL INSIGHT
Body Language and Communication Skills

Active listening forms the basis for effective nutrition counseling. There are two aspects to effective listening: nonverbal and verbal. Nonverbal listening skills consist of varied eye contact, attentive body language, a respectful but close space, adequate silence, and encouragers. Eye contact is direct yet varied. Lack of eye contact implies that the counselor is too busy to spend time with the client. When the counselor leans forward slightly and has a relaxed posture and avoids fidgeting and gesturing, the client will be more at ease. Silence can give the client time to think and provide time for the counselor to contemplate what the client has said. Nodding one's head in agreement can be a positive encourager, leading to more conversation. Moving forward slightly toward the client is an encourager that allows for more positive interaction.

When developing interventions that are culturally competent, the clinician can use the PRECEDE-PROCEED model to provide the framework to guide appreciation for the target audience's surface and deep structure culture (DePue et al, 2010).

Asking Questions

Qualities of good counselors and educators include empathy, positive regard, and genuineness, as well as knowledge of nutritional sciences. For counseling, there also should be periods of information gathering. For information gathering, open-ended questions are most effective when they elicit more discussion. Questions that do not often lead to effective discussion include data questions (e.g., "What did you eat …?") and knowledge questions that often elicit a defensive response (e.g., "Can you tell me about low-fat diets?").

Open-ended questions allow the client to express a wider range of ideas, whereas closed questions can help in targeting concepts and eliminating tangential discussions. For the person who is not ready to change, targeted discussions around difficult topics can help focus the session. The nutritionist asks questions that must be answered by explaining and discussing, not by one-word answers. This is particularly important for someone who is not ready to change, because it opens the discussion to problem areas that keep the client from being ready. The following statements and questions are examples that create an atmosphere for discussion:

- "We are here to talk about your dietary change experiences to this point. Could you start at the beginning and tell me how it has been for you?"
- "What are some things you would like to discuss about your dietary changes so far? What do you like about them? What don't you like about them?"

Framing the optimal discussion question is not easy and requires the counselor to be self-reflective on which questions were successful. Teaching counseling skills has included simulated patient-counselor scenarios with a standardized patient. A tool for evaluating has been developed called the Feedback on Counseling Using Simulation (FOCUS) instrument (Henry and Smith, 2010). Verbal and nonverbal communication is important; for the latter, maintaining an appropriate facial expression and using affirmative gestures seem to be important (Collins et al, 2010).

Building Rapport

It may be difficult to build rapport with some clients. Someone who appears hostile, unusually quiet, or dismissive may have more success with either a different nutritionist or someone with whom he or she has background in common. In those cases, working with a peer educator may be most effective. The peer educator ideally should share similarities with the target population in terms of age or ethnicity and have primary experience in the nutrition topic (e.g., has breastfed her infant). Peer educators are usually community health workers or paraprofessionals. The Expanded Food and Nutrition Education Program (EFNEP) has demonstrated the effectiveness and cost efficiency of peer educators (Dollahite et al, 2008). In prenatal or WIC clinics, breastfeeding peer counselors are often highly effective in helping new mothers with their questions and concerns (Pérez-Escamilla et al, 2008).

Reflective Listening

Nutrition counselors listen and try to tag the feelings that surface as a client is describing difficulties with an eating pattern. Listening is not simply hearing the words spoken by the client and paraphrasing them. Figure 14-3 shows a nutrition counselor listening reflectively to her client.

Reflective listening involves a guess at what the person feels and is phrased as a statement, not a question. By stating a feeling, the nutrition counselor communicates understanding. The following are three examples of listening reflectively:

Client: I really do try, but I am retired and my husband always wants to eat out. How can I stay on the right path when that happens?

Nutrition counselor: You feel frustrated because you want to follow the diet, but at the same time you want to be spontaneous with your husband. Is this correct?

Client: I feel like I let you down every time I come in to see you. We always discuss plans and I never follow them. I almost hate to come in.

Nutrition counselor: You are feeling like giving up. You haven't been able to modify your diet, and it is difficult for you to come into our visits when you haven't met the goals we set. Is this how you are feeling? (reflective listening) Can you think of a specific time when you feel that you had an opportunity to achieve your plan, but didn't?

Client: Some days I just give up. It is on those days that I do very badly in following my diet.

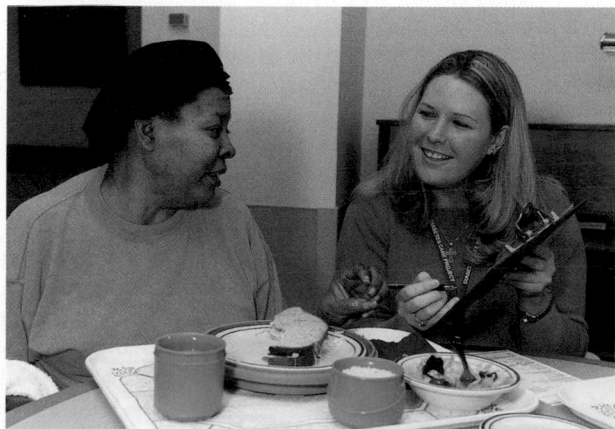

FIGURE 14-3 This nutrition counselor is using reflective listening techniques with her client.

Nutrition counselor: You just lose the desire to try to eat well on some days and that is very depressing for you. Do I have that right? (rephrasing) Are those days when something in particular has happened?

Affirming

Counselors often understand the idea of supporting a client who is very depressed about their eating style, but does not put those thoughts into words. When the counselor affirms someone, there is alignment and normalization. During alignment, the counselor tells the client that he or she understands these difficult times. Normalization means telling the client that he or she is perfectly within reason and that it is normal to have such reactions and feelings. The following statements indicate affirmation:

- "I know that it is hard for you to tell me this. But thank you."
- "You have had amazing competing priorities. I feel that you have done extremely well, given your circumstances."
- "Many people I talk with express the same problems. I can understand why you are having difficulty."

Summarizing

The nutrition counselor periodically summarizes the content of what the client has said by covering all the key points. Simple and straightforward statements are most effective, even if they involve negative feelings. If conflicting ideas arise, the counselor can use the strategy exemplified by the statement, "On the one hand you want to change, but love those old eating patterns." This helps the client recognize the dichotomy in thinking that often prevents behavior change.

ASSESSMENT RESULTS: CHOOSING FOCUS AREAS

Health and Nutrition Literacy

Low health literacy, or the ability to understand health information well enough to make informed decisions, is common among older adults, minorities, and those who are medically underserved or have a low socioeconomic status (Health Resources and Services Administration, 2010). This problem can lead to poor management of chronic health conditions, as well as low adherence to recommendations. Useful resources available from the Agency on Healthcare Research and Quality are *Rapid Estimate of Adult Health Literacy in Medicine* (REALM) and *Short Assessment of Health Literacy for Spanish Adults* (SAHLSA-50) (Agency on Healthcare Research and Quality, 2014). Nutrition-targeted evaluation measures include the Newest Vital Sign, which focuses on a nutrition facts label (Rowlands et al, 2013) and the Nutrition Literacy Assessment Instrument, which evaluates several components, including understanding of nutrition and health, macronutrients, household food measurement, food labels and numeracy, and food groups (Gibbs and Chapman-Novakofski, 2013). Relying on the client's educational attainment provides some guidance, but asking the client to repeat explanations in his or her own words also can help the nutrition educator evaluate the client's level of understanding.

Assessing Readiness to Change

One purpose of assessment is to identify the client's stage of change and to provide appropriate help in facilitating change. The assessment should be completed in the first visit if possible.

If conversation extends beyond the designated time for the session, the assessment steps should be completed at the next session. The nutritional assessment requires gathering the appropriate anthropometric, biochemical, clinical, dietary, and economic data relating to the client's condition (see Chapters 4 and 7). The nutritional diagnosis then focuses on any problems related to food or nutrient intake (see Chapter 10).

Determining present eating habits provides ideas on how to change in the future. It is important to review the client's eating behavior, to identify areas needing change, and to help the client select goals that will have the most effect on health conditions. For instance, if the nutrition diagnosis includes excessive fat intake (nutrient intake NI-51.2), inappropriate intake of food fats (NI-51.3), excessive energy intake (NI-1.5), inadequate potassium intake (NI-55.1), food- and nutrition-related knowledge deficit (nutrition behavior NB-1.1), and impaired ability to prepare foods or meals (NB-2.4), the counselor may have to focus on the last diagnosis before the others. If all other diagnoses are present except impaired ability to prepare foods or meals (NB-2.4), the nutritionist may want to have a discussion about whether excessive fat intake, inappropriate intake of types of food fats, or excessive energy intake are more appealing or possible for the client to focus on first.

Once the nutrition diagnosis is selected for intervention, it is important to assess readiness for change. Using a ruler that allows the client to select his or her level of intention to change is one method of allowing client participation in the discussion. The counselor asks the client, "On a scale of 1 to 12, how ready are you right now to make any new changes to eat less fat? (1 = not ready to change; 12 = very ready to change)." The nutritionist may use this method with each nutrition diagnosis to help the client decide where to focus first.

Three possibilities for readiness exist: (1) not ready to change; (2) unsure about change; (3) ready to change. These three concepts of readiness have condensed the six distinct stages of change described in this chapter to assist the counselor in determining the level of client readiness. There are many concepts to remember, and readiness to change may fluctuate during the course of the discussion. The counselor must be ready to move back and forth between the phase-specific strategies. If the client seems confused, detached, or resistant during the discussion, the counselor should return and ask about readiness to change. If readiness has lessened, tailoring the intervention is necessary. Not every counseling session has to end with the client's agreement to change; even the decision to think about change can be a useful conclusion.

COUNSELING APPROACHES AFTER THE ASSESSMENT

Not-Ready-to-Change Counseling Sessions

In approaching the "not-ready-to-change" stage of intervention, there are three goals: (1) facilitate the client's ability to consider change, (2) identify and reduce the client's resistance and barriers to change, and (3) identify behavioral steps toward change that are tailored to each client's needs. At this stage identifying barriers from the HBM in Table 14-1, the influence of subjective norms and attitudes (TPB), or personal and environmental factors (SCT) that may have negative influences on the intention to change can be helpful. To achieve these goals, several communication skills are important to master: asking open-ended questions, listening reflectively, affirming the patient's statements, summarizing the patient's statements, and eliciting self-motivational statements.

The four communication strategies (asking open-ended questions, listening reflectively, affirming, and summarizing) are important when eliciting self-motivational statements. The goal here is for the client to realize that a problem exists, that concern results, and that positive steps in the future can be taken to correct the problem. The goal is to use these realizations to set the stage for later efforts at dietary change. Examples of questions to use in eliciting self-motivational feeling statements follow.

Problem Recognition
- "What things make you think that eating out is a problem?"
- "In what ways has following your diet been a problem?"

Concern
- "How do you feel when you can't follow your diet?"
- "In what ways does not being able to follow your diet concern you?"
- "What do you think will happen if you don't make a change?"

Intention to Change
- "The fact that you're here indicates that at least a part of you thinks it's time to do something. What are the reasons you see for making a change?"
- "If you were 100% successful and things worked out exactly as you would like, what would be different?"
- "What things make you think that you should keep on eating the way you have been?" And in the opposite direction, "What makes you think it is time for a change?"

Optimism
- "What encourages you that you can change if you want to?"
- "What do you think would work for you if you decided to change?"

Clients in this "not-ready-to-change" category have already told the counselor they are not doing well at making changes. Usually if a tentative approach is used by asking permission to discuss the problem, the client will not refuse. One asks permission by saying, "Would you be willing to continue our discussion and talk about the possibility of change?" At this point, it is helpful to discuss thoughts and feelings about the current status of dietary change by asking open-ended questions:
- "Tell me why you picked _____ on the ruler." (Refer to previous discussion on the use of a ruler.)
- "What would have to happen for you to move from a _____ to a _____ (referring to a number on the ruler)? How could I help get you there?"
- "If you did start to think about changing, what would be your main concern?"

To show real understanding about what the client is saying, it is beneficial to summarize the statements about his or her progress, difficulties, possible reasons for change, and what has to be different to move forward. This paraphrasing allows the client to rethink his or her reasoning about readiness to change. The mental processing provides new ideas that can promote actual change.

Ending the Session

Counselors often expect a decision and at least a goal-setting session when working with a client. However, it is important in

NEW DIRECTIONS

Counseling and Educating Online

More counselors and educators are turning to online connections with their clients and target audiences. Although all the basics of counseling and education remain the same, there are additional issues to consider when online. If clients are recording food intake and physical activity through mobile technology, the frequency of monitoring and providing feedback must be considered. Although many best practices in nutrition education include the use of mobile technology, development and maintenance of the website or app in a constantly changing technological world must be addressed. Short message service (SMS) usually does not require a data plan for mobile phones, but clinicians should check with clients about their mobile plans so as not to increase monthly charges. Other online ways to reach clients include social media platforms, blogs, and recipe apps and websites. However, Health Insurance Portability and Accountability Act (HIPAA) regulations and confidentiality should be considered.

this stage to realize that traditional goal setting will result in feelings of failure on the part of the client and the nutritionist. If the client is not ready to change, respectful acknowledgment of this decision is important. The counselor may say, "I can understand why making a change right now would be very hard for you. The fact that you are able to indicate this as a problem is very important, and I respect your decision. Our lives do change, and, if you feel differently later on, I will always be available to talk with you. I know that, when the time is right for you to make a change, you will find a way to do it." When the session ends, the counselor lets the client know that the issues will be revisited after he or she has time to think. Expression of hope and confidence in the client's ability to make changes in the future, when the time is right, is beneficial. Arrangements for follow-up contact can be made at this time.

With a client who is not ready to change, it is easy to become defensive and authoritarian. At this point, it is important to avoid pushing, persuading, confronting, coaxing, or telling the client what to do. It is reassuring to a nutritionist to know that change at this level often occurs outside the office. The client is not expected to be ready to do something during the visit (see *New Directions:* Counseling and Educating Online).

UNSURE-ABOUT-CHANGE COUNSELING SESSIONS

The only goal in the "unsure-about-change" session is to build readiness to change. This is the point at which changes in eating behavior can escalate. This "unsure" stage is a transition from not being ready to deal with a problem eating behavior to preparing to continue the change. It involves summarizing the client's perceptions of the barriers to a healthy eating style and how they can be eliminated or circumvented to achieve change. Heightened self-efficacy may provide confidence that goals can be achieved. A restatement of the client's self-motivational statements assists in setting the stage for success. The client's ambivalence is discussed, listing the positive and negative aspects of change. The nutritionist can restate any statements that the client has made about intentions or plans to change or to do better in the future.

One crucial aspect of this stage is the process of discussing thoughts and feelings about current status. Use of open-ended questions encourages the client to discuss dietary change progress

and difficulties. Change is promoted through discussions focused on possible reasons for change. The counselor might ask the question, "What would need to be different to move forward?"

This stage is characterized by feelings of ambivalence. The counselor should encourage the client to explore ambivalence to change by thinking about the "pros" and "cons." Some questions to ask are:

- "What are some of the things you like about your current eating habits?"
- "What are some of the good things about making a change?"
- "What are some of the bad things about making a change?"

By trying to look into the future, the nutrition counselor can help a client see new and often positive scenarios. As a change facilitator, the counselor helps to tip the balance away from being ambivalent about change toward considering change by guiding the client to talk about what life may be like after a change, anticipating the difficulties as well as the advantages. An example of an opening to generate discussion with the client might be: "I can see why you're unsure about making changes in your eating habits. Imagine that you decided to change. What would that be like? What would you want to do?" The counselor then summarizes the client's statements about the "pros" and "cons" of making a change and includes any statements about wanting, intending, or planning to change.

The next step is to negotiate a change. The negotiation process has three parts. The first is setting goals. Set broad goals at first and hold more specific nutritional goals until later. "How would you like things to be different from the way they are?" and "What would you like to change?"

The second step in negotiation is to consider options. The counselor asks about alternative strategies and options and then asks the client to choose from among them. This is effective because, if the first strategy does not work, the client has other choices. The third step is to arrive at a plan, one that has been devised by the client. The counselor touches on the key points and the problems, and then asks the client to write down the plan.

To end the session the counselor asks about the next step, allowing the client to describe what may occur next in the process of change. The following questions provide some ideas for questions that may promote discussion:

- "Where do you think you will go from here?"
- "What do you plan to do between now and the next visit?"

RESISTANCE BEHAVIORS AND STRATEGIES TO MODIFY THEM

Resistance to change is the most consistent emotion or state when dealing with clients who have difficulty with dietary change. Examples of resistance behaviors on the part of the client include contesting the accuracy, expertise, or integrity of the nutrition counselor; or directly challenging the accuracy of the information provided (e.g., the accuracy of the nutrition content). The nutrition counselor may even be confronted with a hostile client. Resistance also may surface as interrupting, when the client breaks in during a conversation in a defensive manner. In this case the client may speak while the nutrition counselor is still talking without waiting for an appropriate pause or silence. In another, more obvious manner, the client may break in with words intended to cut off the nutrition counselor's discussion.

When clients express an unwillingness to recognize problems, cooperate, accept responsibility, or take advice, they may be denying a problem. Some clients blame other people for their problems (e.g., a wife may blame her husband for her inability to follow a diet). Other clients may disagree with the nutrition counselor when a suggestion is offered, but they frequently provide no constructive alternative. The familiar "Yes, but ..." explains what is wrong with the suggestion but offers no alternative solution.

Clients try to excuse their behavior. A client may say, "I want to do better, but my life is in turmoil since my husband died 3 years ago." An excuse that was once acceptable is reused even when it is no longer a factor in the client's life.

Some clients make pessimistic statements about themselves or others. This is done to dismiss an inability to follow an eating pattern by excusing poor compliance as just a given resulting from past behaviors. Examples are, "My husband will never help me" or "I have never been good at sticking with a goal. I'm sure I won't do well with one now."

In some cases, clients are reluctant to accept options that may have worked for others in the past. They express reservations about information or advice given. "I just don't think that will work for me." Some clients express a lack of willingness to change or an intention not to change. They make it very clear that they want to stop the dietary regimen.

Often clients provide evidence that they are not following the nutrition counselor's advice. Such clues include using a response that does not answer the question, providing no response to a question, or changing the direction of the conversation.

These types of behavior can occur within a counseling session as clients move from one stage to another. They are not necessarily stage-specific, although most are connected with either the "not ready" or "unsure-about-change" stages. A variety of strategies are available to assist the nutrition counselor in dealing with these difficult counseling situations. These strategies include reflecting, double-sided reflection, shifting focus, agreeing with a twist, emphasizing personal choice, and reframing. Each of these options is described in the following paragraphs.

Reflecting

In reflecting, the counselor identifies the client's emotion or feeling and repeats it. This allows the client to stop and reflect on what was said. An example of this type of counseling is, "You seem to be very frustrated by what your husband says about your food choices."

Double-Sided Reflection

In double-sided reflection, the counselor uses ideas that the client has expressed previously to show the discrepancy between the client's current words and the previous ones. For example:

Client: I am doing the best I can. (Previously this client stated that she sometimes just gives up and doesn't care about following the diet.)
Nutrition counselor: On the one hand you say you are doing your best, but on the other hand I recall that you said you just felt like giving up and didn't care about following the

diet. Do you remember that? How was that point in time different than now?

Shifting Focus

Clients may hold onto an idea that they think is getting in the way of their progress. The counselor may question the feasibility of continuing to focus on this barrier to change when other barriers may be more appropriate targets. For example:

Client: I will never be able to follow a low–saturated fat diet as long as my grandchildren come to my house and want snacks.
Nutrition counselor: Are you sure that this is really the problem? Is part of the problem that you like those same snacks?
Client: Oh, you are right. I love them.
Nutrition counselor: Could you compromise? Could you ask your grandchildren which of this long list of low–saturated fat snacks they like and then buy them?

Agreeing with a Twist

This strategy involves offering agreement, then moving the discussion in a different direction. The counselor agrees with a piece of what the client says but then offers another perspective on his or her problems. This allows the opportunity to agree with the statement and the feeling but then to redirect the conversation onto a key topic.

For example:

Client: I really like eating out, but I always eat too much, and my blood sugars go sky high.
Nutrition counselor: Most people do like eating out. Now that you are retired it is easier to eat out than to cook. I can understand that. What can we do to make you feel great about eating out so that you can still follow your eating plan and keep your blood glucose values in the normal range?`

Reframing

With reframing, the counselor changes the client's interpretation of the basic data by offering a new perspective. The counselor repeats the basic observation that the client has provided and then offers a new hypothesis for interpreting the data. For example:

Client: I gave up trying to meet my dietary goals because I was having some difficulties when my husband died, and I have decided now that I just cannot meet those strict goals.
Nutrition counselor: I remember how devastated you were when he died and how just cooking meals was an effort. Do you think that this happened as a kind of immediate response to his death and that you might have just decided that all of the goals were too strict at that time? (Pause)
Client: Well, you are probably right.
Nutrition counselor: Could we look at where you are now and try to find things that will work for you now to help you in following the goals we have set?

These strategies help by offering tools to ensure that nutrition counseling is not ended without appropriate attempts to turn difficult counseling situations in a more positive direction.

Ending the Session

Counselors always should emphasize that any future action belongs to the client, that the advice can be taken or disregarded. This emphasis on personal choice (autonomy) helps clients avoid feeling trapped or confined by the discussion. Belief in the ability to change through his or her own decisions is an essential and worthy goal. A sense of self-efficacy reflects the belief about being capable of influencing events and choices in life. These beliefs determine how individuals think, feel, and behave. If people doubt their capabilities, they will have weak commitments to their goals. Success breeds success, and failure breeds a sense of failure. Having resilience, positive role models, and effective coaching can make a significant difference.

READY-TO-CHANGE COUNSELING SESSIONS

Setting goals

The major goal in the "ready-to-change" session is to collaborate with the client to set goals that include a plan of action. The nutrition counselor provides the client with the tools to use in meeting nutrition goals. This is the stage of change that most often is assumed when a counseling session begins. To erroneously assume this stage means that inappropriate counseling strategies set the stage for failure. Misaligned assumptions often result in lack of adherence on the part of the client and discouragement on the part of the nutritionist. Therefore, it is important to discuss the client's thoughts and feelings about where he or she stands relative to the current change status. Use of open-ended questions helps the client confirm and justify the decision to make a change and in which area. The following questions may elicit information about feelings toward change:

- "Tell me why you picked _____ on the ruler."
- "Why did you pick (nutrition diagnosis 1) instead of (other nutrition diagnoses)?"

In this stage, goal setting is extremely important. Here the counselor helps the client set a realistic and achievable short-term goal: "Let's do things gradually. What is a reasonable first step? What may be your first goal?"

Action Plan

After goal setting, an action plan is set to assist the client in mapping out the specifics of goal achievement. Identifying a network to support dietary change is important. What can others do to help?

Early identification of barriers to adherence is also important. If barriers are identified, plans can be formed to help eliminate these roadblocks.

Many clients fail to notice when their plan is working. Clients can be asked to summarize their plans and identify markers of success. The counselor then documents the plan for discussion at future sessions and ensures that the clients also have their plans in writing. The session should close with an encouraging statement and reflection about how the client identified this plan personally. Indicate that each person is the expert about his or her own behavior. Compliment the client on carrying out the plan. Some ways to express these ideas to clients are the following:

- "You are working very hard at this, and it's clear that you're the expert about what is best for you. You can do this!"
- "Keep in mind that change is gradual and takes time. If this plan doesn't work, there will be other plans to try."

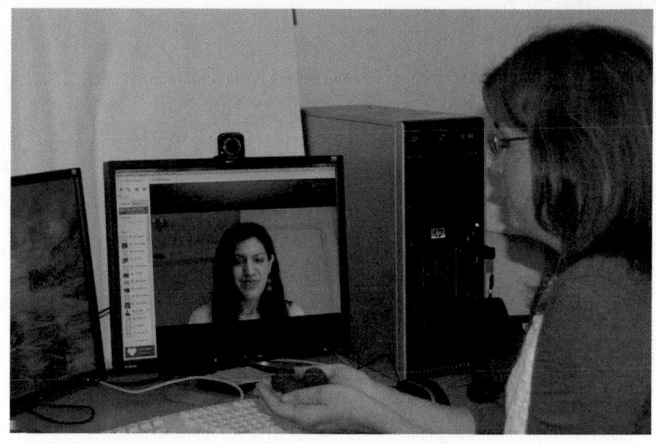

FIGURE 14-4 This client is connecting with her nutrition counselor using Skype to discuss how she is doing with her eating behavior changes.

The key point for this stage is to avoid telling the client what to do. Clinicians often want to provide advice. However, it is critical that the client express ideas of what will work best: "There are a number of things you could do, but what do you think will work best for you?" The next contact may be in person, online, or by phone.

Following up with clients by phone or online has become a popular counseling method for many nutritionists (Figure 14-4). When behavior and counseling theories are combined with phone counseling, the results have been effective in managing weight, type 2 diabetes, and hypertension (Eakin et al, 2009; Kim et al, 2010). Online weight reduction programs also have been successful, especially when the websites are interactive and communication with counselors is available (Krukowski et al, 2009).

EVALUATION OF EFFECTIVENESS

Counseling

Clinicians and educators must evaluate their services. Just completing the counseling process with clients does not mean that outcomes will match the goals. A review of literature related to behavior change theories and strategies used in nutrition counseling reported the following (Spahn et al, 2010):

1. Strong evidence supports the use of CBT in facilitating modification of targeted dietary habits, weight, and cardiovascular and diabetes risk factors.
2. MI is a highly effective counseling strategy, particularly when combined with CBT.
3. Few studies have assessed the application of the TTM or SCT on nutrition-related behavior change.
4. Self-monitoring, meal replacements, and structured meal plans are effective; financial reward strategies are not.
5. Goal setting, problem solving, and social support are effective strategies.
6. Research is needed in more diverse populations to determine the most effective counseling techniques and strategies.

Educational Programs

The LOGIC model often is used to evaluate a program's effectiveness. The most simple version includes inputs (resources or investments into a program), outputs (activities, services and events), and outcomes (behavior change of individuals, group or communities), although some include multiple levels within these three broad categories. The LOGIC model has guided evaluation of national nutrition programs as well as educational programs at the individual level, such as a video program to improve dietary habits of children (Beasley et al, 2012).

SUMMARY

For nutrition education and counseling efforts to be effective, skills must be developed by the educator or counselor, the characteristics of the target audience or client must be assessed, a behavioral theory should be incorporated, and evaluation of the process and outcomes should be completed.

CLINICAL CASE STUDY

Mrs. Lee is originally from mainland China. She has been living in your area for several years and has numerous health problems, including high blood pressure and glaucoma. You have been asked to counsel her about making changes in her diet. Because her vision is poor, she will not be able to use printed materials that you have in your office that have been translated into Chinese.

Nutrition Diagnostic Statement

Impaired ability to prepare food and meals related to inability to see as evidenced by client report and history of glaucoma

Nutrition Care Questions

1. What steps should you take to make her comfortable with this session?
2. Should you invite family members to attend the counseling session? Why or why not?
3. What tools may be useful to help Mrs. Lee understand portions or types of food that she should select?
4. Would a supermarket tour be useful? Why or why not?
5. What other types of information will be needed to help Mrs. Lee?

USEFUL WEBSITES

American Counseling Association
http://www.counseling.org/
Cultural Competency
http://www.thinkculturalhealth.org/
Motivational Interviewing
http://www.motivationalinterviewing.org/
National Cancer Institute. Theory at a Glance. A Guide for Health Promotion Practice
http://www.cancer.gov/cancertopics/cancerlibrary/theory.pdf
Office of Minority Health
http://minorityhealth.hhs.gov/
Society for Nutrition Education and Behavior
http://www.sneb.org/
University of Wisconsin. LOGIC Model in Program Planning and Evaluation
http://www.uwex.edu/ces/pdande/evaluation/evallogicmodel.html

REFERENCES

Agency on Healthcare Research and Quality (AHRQ): *Health literacy measurement tools.* http://www.ahrq.gov/populations/sahlsatool.htm, 2014. Accessed January 3, 2015.

Ajzen I: The theory of planned behavior, *Organ Behav Hum Decis Process* 50:179, 1991.

Bandura A: *Social foundations of thought and action*, Englewood Cliffs, NJ, 1986, Prentice-Hall.

Bandura A: *Social learning theory*, New York, 1977, General Learning Press.

Beasley N, Sharma S, Shegog R, et al: The quest to Lava Mountain: using video games for dietary change in children, *J Acad Nutr Diet* 112:1334, 2012.

Beck JS: *Cognitive behavior therapy: basics and beyond*, ed 2, New York, 2011, Guilford Press.

Brown JL, Wenrich TR: Intra-family role expectations and reluctance to change identified as key barriers to expanding vegetable consumption patterns during interactive family-based program for Appalachian low-income food preparers, *J Acad Nutr Diet* 112:1188, 2012.

Broyles SL, Brennan JJ, Burke KH, et al: Cultural adaptation of a nutrition education curriculum for Latino families to promote acceptance, *J Nutr Educ Behav* 43(4 Suppl 2):S158, 2011.

Collins LG, Schrimmer A, Diamond J, et al: Evaluating verbal and non-verbal communication skills, in an ethnogeriatric OSCE, *Patient Educ Couns* 83:158, 2011.

Cooper Z, Doll HA, Hawker DM, et al: Testing a new cognitive behavioural treatment for obesity: a randomized controlled trial with three-year follow-up, *Behav Res Ther* 48:706, 2010.

DePue JD, Rosen RK, Batts-Turner M, et al: Cultural translation of interventions: diabetes care in American Samoa, *Am J Public Health* 100:2085, 2010.

Dollahite J, Kenkel D, Thompson CS: An economic evaluation of the expanded food and nutrition education program, *J Nutr Educ Behav* 40:134, 2008.

Eakin E, Reeves M, Lawler S, et al: Telephone counseling for physical activity and diet in primary care patients, *Am J Prev Med* 36:142, 2009.

Fishbein M, Ajzen I: *Predicting and changing behavior: the reasoned action approach*, New York, 2010, Psychology Press (Taylor & Francis).

Fitzgerald N, Morgan KT, Slawson DL: Practice paper of the Academy of Nutrition and Dietetics abstract: the role of nutrition in health promotion and chronic disease prevention, *J Acad Nutr Diet* 113:983, 2013.

Gibbs H, Chapman-Novakofski K: Establishing content validity for the Nutrition Literacy Assessment Instrument (NLAI), *Prev Chronic Dis* 10:E109, 2013.

Green LW, et al: *Health education planning: a diagnostic approach*, Mountain View, Calif, 1980, Mayfield.

Gregg J, Saha S: Losing culture on the way to competence: the use and misuse of culture in medical curriculum, *Acad Med* 81:542, 2006.

Health Resources and Services Administration (HRSA): *Health literacy.* http://www.hrsa.gov/healthliteracy/. 2010. Accessed January 3, 2015.

Henry BW, Smith TJ: Evaluation of the FOCUS (Feedback on Counseling Using Simulation) instrument for assessment of client-centered nutrition counseling behaviors, *J Nutr Educ Behav* 42:57, 2010.

James DC, Pobee JW, Oxidine D, et al: Using the health belief model to develop culturally appropriate weight-management materials for African-American women, *J Acad Nutr Diet* 112:664, 2012.

Johnston CA, Stevens BE: Motivational interviewing in the health care setting, *Am J Lifestyle Med* 7:246, 2013.

Kamp B, Wellman NS, Russell C: Position of the American Dietetic Association, American Society for Nutrition, and Society for Nutrition Education: food and nutrition programs for community-residing older adults, *J Nutr Educ Behav* 42:72, 2010.

Kattelmann K, Bredbenner CB, White AA, et al: The effects of young adults eating and active for health (YEAH): a theory-based web-delivered intervention, *J Nutr Educ Behav* 46(Suppl 6):S27, 2014.

Kim Y, Pike J, Adams H, et al: Telephone intervention promoting weight-related health behaviors, *Prev Med* 50:112, 2010.

Krukowski RA, West DS, Harvey-Berino J: Recent advances in internet-delivered, evidence-based weight control programs for adults, *J Diabetes Sci Technol* 3:184, 2009.

Mochari-Greenberger H, Terry MB, Mosca L: Does stage of change modify the effectiveness of an educational intervention to improve diet among family members of hospitalized cardiovascular disease patients? *J Am Diet Assoc* 110:1027, 2010.

Mossavar-Rahmani Y: Applying motivational enhancement to diverse populations, *J Am Diet Assoc* 107:918, 2007.

Murphy R, Straebler S, Cooper Z, et al: Cognitive behavioral therapy for eating disorders, *Psychiatr Clin North Am* 33:611, 2010.

Nicklas TA, Jahns L, Bogle ML, et al: Barriers and facilitators for consumer adherence to the dietary guidelines for Americans: the HEALTH study, *J Acad Nutr Diet* 113:1317, 2013.

Pérez-Escamilla R, Hromi-Fiedler A, Vega-López S, et al: Impact of peer nutrition education on dietary behaviors and health outcomes among Latinos: a systematic literature review, *J Nutr Educ Behav* 40:208, 2008.

Plawecki K, Chapman-Novakofski K: Effectiveness of community intervention in improving bone health behaviors in older adults, *J Nutr Gerontol Geriatr* 32:145, 2013.

Poddar KH, Hosig KW, Anderson-Bill ES, et al: Dairy intake and related self-regulation improved in college students using online nutrition education, *J Acad Nutr Diet* 12:1976, 2012.

Prochaska JO, Norcross JC: Psychotherapy: theory, research, practice, *Training* 38:443, 2001.

Rosenstock IM: The health belief model and preventive health behavior, *Health Educ Behav* 2:354, 1974.

Rowlands G, Khazaezadeh N, Oteng-Ntim E, et al: Development and validation of a measure of health literacy in the UK: the newest vital sign, *BMC Pub Health* 13:116, 2013.

Sallis JF, Owen N: Ecological models of health behavior. In Glanz, K et al (Eds): Health Behavior: Theory, Research, and Practice, 5th Ed., San Francisco, Jossey-Bass, John Wiley and Sons, Inc, 2015, p 43-64.

Sheats JL, Middlestadt SE, Ona FF, et al: Understanding African American women's decisions to buy and eat dark green leafy vegetables: an application of the reasoned action approach, *J Nutr Educ Behav* 45:676, 2013.

Spahn JM, Reeves RS, Keim KS, et al: State of the evidence regarding behavior change theories and strategies in nutrition counseling to facilitate health and food behavior change, *J Am Diet Assoc* 110:879, 2010.

Stein K: Navigating cultural competency: in preparation for an expected standard in 2010, *J Am Diet Assoc* 109:1676, 2009.

Walsh J, White AA2, Kattelmann KK: Using PRECEDE to develop a weight management program for disadvantaged young adults, *J Nutr Educ Behav* 46:S1, 2014.

PART III

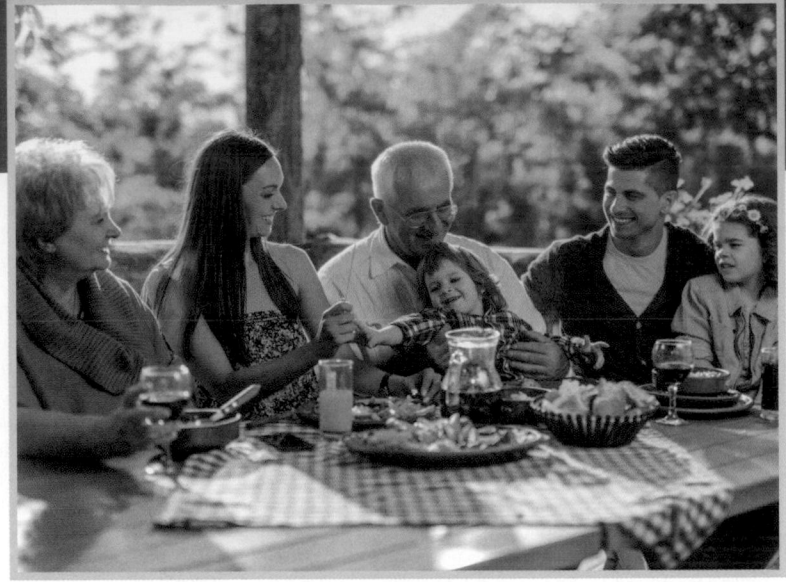

Nutrition in the Life Cycle

The importance of nutrition throughout the life cycle cannot be refuted. However, the significance of nutrition during specific times of growth, development, and aging is becoming increasingly appreciated.

Health professionals have recognized for quite some time the effects of proper nutrition during pregnancy on the health of the infant and mother, even after her childbearing years. However looking at "nutrition in the womb" encompasses not only maternal health history and nutrition but also paternal nutrition and the health of sperm before conception. "Fetal origin" has far more lifelong effects on the new life than originally thought.

Establishing good dietary habits during childhood lessens the possibility of inappropriate eating behavior later in life. Although the influence of proper nutrition on morbidity and mortality usually remains unacknowledged until adulthood, dietary practices aimed at preventing the degenerative diseases that develop later in life should be instituted in childhood.

During early adulthood many changes begin that lead to the development of chronic disease, the so called diseases of aging, years later. Many of these changes can be accelerated or slowed over the years, depending on the genetic makeup of the individual, quality of the nutritional intake, the health of the gut, and the function of the immune system.

With the rapid growth of the population of older adults has evolved a need to expand the limited nutrition data currently available for these individuals. Although it is known that energy needs decrease with aging, little is known about whether requirements for specific nutrients increase or decrease. Identifying the unique nutritional differences among the various stages of aging is becoming even more important.

15

Nutrition for Reproductive Health and Lactation

Jean T. Cox, MS, RD, LN and Virginia H. Carney, MPH, RDN, LDN, IBCLC, RLC, FILCA, FAND

KEY TERMS

amylophagia
assisted reproductive technology (ART)
baby-led weaning
colostrum
conception
congenital anomalies
developmental origins of health and disease (DOHaD)
fetal alcohol syndrome (FAS)
fetal origins of disease
foremilk
galactogogue
geophagia

gestational diabetes mellitus (GDM)
gestational hypertension
gravida
HELLP syndrome
hindmilk
hyperemesis gravidarum (HG)
intrauterine fetal demise (IUFD)
intrauterine growth restriction (IUGR)
lactogenesis I
lactogenesis II
let-down
macrosomia
mature milk

Montgomery glands
mother-led weaning
nausea and vomiting in pregnancy (NVP)
neural tube defects (NTDs)
oxytocin
pagophagia
perinatal mortality
pica
postpartum depression (PPD)
preeclampsia
prolactin
ptyalism gravidarum
transitional milk

Optimal nutrition during pregnancy, which includes adequate amounts of all of the required vitamins, minerals, and energy-providing macronutrients, actually begins preconceptually. Because developing fetuses depend solely on the transfer of substrates from their host, there is simply no other means to acquire nutrition in utero. The cliché that the "fetus is the perfect parasite" implies fetuses take all they require at the expense of the host. However, at some point nutritional deficiency can result in premature labor, relieving the host of an ongoing nutritional debt. After birth, quality nutrition during lactation continues the process of providing nutritional building blocks for normal cerebral development, and growth of all body organs in the neonate.

This time period—growing a new human being—sets the stage for the health of future generations. The quality and quantity of nourishment to the developing zygote, then fetus, then neonate, then adult emerge as one explanation for diseases that manifest in adulthood. This concept is known as fetal origins of disease or developmental origins of health and disease (DOHaD) (Guéant et al, 2013; Monk et al, 2013).

PRECONCEPTION AND FERTILITY

Reproductive Readiness and Fertility

The focus on preconceptual nutrition and health is important for women and men. Infertility affects 10% to 12% of U.S.

couples of reproductive age, and extremes in body mass index (BMI) in either partner may be one cause. Women with a BMI less than 20 have an increased risk of anovulation. Men and women have increased rates of subfertility when overweight or obese; weight loss and increased physical activity may be helpful (Simon, 2014). Box 15-1 lists additional risk factors for birth defects.

Dietary changes have been shown to decrease ovulatory disorders and improve fertility. Vitamin D deficiency in men and women can be associated with infertility (Pludowski et al, 2013). For women, vitamin D deficiency may be associated with insulin resistance and metabolic syndrome in polycystic ovary syndrome (PCOS); for men it is associated with lower testosterone levels and lower sperm quality. However, in both cases, neither causality nor ability to treat has yet been demonstrated. Calcium has been shown to be important in males for spermatogenesis, sperm motility, hyperactivation, and acrosome (area of the sperm that contains digestive enzymes to break down the outer layers of the ovum) reactions. Healthier sperm counts are associated with optimal dietary zinc, folic acid, and antioxidants, as well as avoidance of tobacco and alcohol (Gaur et al, 2010). Recommendations for improved male fertility include eating a higher fiber, lower glycemic index (including high-fat dairy products and monounsaturated fats, but reducing trans fats) and lower animal protein diet, in addition to obtaining iron from plant sources, consuming a multivitamin daily, and being moderately physically active (Simon, 2014). Oxidative stress is associated with impaired spermatogenesis. However, the evidence for a supplementation

Sections of this chapter were written by Miriam Erick, MS, RDN, CDE, LDN for previous editions of this text.

BOX 15-1 Potential Risk Factors for Development of Birth Defects

Assisted reproductive technologies (ART)
Genetic alterations
Gene-environmental interactions, such as maternal smoking
Hypoxia during pregnancy
Infection during pregnancy (bacterial, parasitic, viral)
In utero exposure to toxins or heavy metals (lawn chemicals, formaldehyde, endocrine disruptors, agricultural products, pesticides, carbon monoxide, radiation, mercury, lead)
Maternal medical conditions (diabetes, hypothyroidism, phenylketonuria)
Maternal medication or substance exposure (including but not restricted to isotretinoin, phenytoin, carbamazepine, triamterene, trimethoprim, warfarin, and radioactive iodine), illicit recreational substances, alcohol
Nutrient deficits during early pregnancy (iodine, vitamin B_{12}, vitamin D, vitamin A, vitamin K, copper, zinc, folic acid, choline)
Obesity
Older mother or father

TABLE 15-1 Examples of Nutrients Likely Important in the Periconceptual Period: Preconception Through Organogenesis

System or Function	Nutrients
Brain and nervous system	Iron, zinc, iodine, LCPUFA, vitamins A, B_6, B_{12}, folic acid, copper, protein, selenium
Placental function and structure	Iron, LCPUFA, vitamins E, C, B_{12}, zinc, selenium, copper, omega-3 PUFA, folate
Inflammation and immune function	Vitamins A, D, zinc, fatty acids
Oxidative stress	Vitamins C, E, B_6, B_{12}, folic acid
Embryogenesis	Vitamins A, B_6, B_{12}, folic acid, zinc

Adapted from Cetin I et al: Role of micronutrients in the periconceptional period, *Hum Reprod Update* 16:80, 2010; Monk C et al: Research review: maternal prenatal distress and poor nutrition —mutually influencing risk factors affecting infant neurocognitive development, *J Child Psychol Psychiatry* 54:115, 2013; Ramakrishnan U et al: Effect of women's nutrition before and during early pregnancy on maternal and infant outcomes: a systematic review, *Paediatr Perinat Epidemiol* 26:285, 2012.
LCPUFA, Long chain polyunsaturated fatty acids; *PUFA,* polyunsaturated fatty acids.

benefit appears weak and inconsistent. The optimal types and dosages of the specific antioxidants are not yet known, and individuals also may exhibit variable responses (Mora-Esteves and Shin, 2013). On the other hand, supplementation is not likely to be harmful, assuming it is at levels of the RDA or less. Whether supplements are as effective as a diet rich in antioxidants is unknown.

Preconceptual guidance is based on findings that many women enter pregnancy with suboptimal nutritional status, including obesity, and with low intakes of long-chain polyunsaturated fatty acids (LCPUFA), protein, zinc, iron, and choline (Monk et al, 2013). Although current public health recommendations primarily promote folic acid supplementation, many other nutrients are also important in the periconceptual period. Optimal intakes are associated with lower risk of growth restricted babies (low birth weight [LBW] or small-for-gestational age [SGA]) or preterm births (Ramakrisnan et al, 2012; see Table 15-1). Thus a preconceptual multivitamin-multimineral supplement may confer more benefit than single supplements for a pregnant woman, or gravida.

Preconception educational programs for both parents are promoted, but evidence of benefit is inconsistent. However, it appears that nutrition interventions are more effective in promoting change than those targeting smoking and alcohol cessation (Temel et al, 2013).

Toxins

Screening women for alcohol, tobacco (including e-cigarettes), and recreational drug use is critical and also may be important for occupational toxin exposure. In vitro studies, using first trimester placental villous cells from terminated pregnancies transplanted to a nutrient medium, demonstrate poor placental growth and function, including lower taurine transport to the fetus, when the fetus is exposed to high amounts of alcohol in early pregnancy (Lui et al, 2014). Women may be at risk for entering pregnancy with toxic levels of mercury, and the types of fish eaten should be discussed. (see *Focus On*: Omega-3 Fatty Acids in Pregnancy and Lactation). The effect of maternal caffeine intake on infertility often is debated. No increased risk of miscarriage has been seen with caffeine consumption less than 200 mg/day, but data are conflicting for higher intakes (ACOG, 2010; see Appendix 39).

◎ FOCUS ON

Omega-3 Fatty Acids in Pregnancy and Lactation

Our ancestors likely consumed a diet with equal amounts of omega-3 and omega-6 fatty acids. American diets currently are estimated to contain much higher levels of omega-6 than omega-3 fatty acids. This dramatic change in the ratio is thought to affect overall disease prevalence, as well as pregnancy outcome. However, there is no evidence that the absolute amounts of essential fatty acids provided by any culture are inadequate for the placenta, fetus, or infant growth (Lauritzen and Carlson, 2011).

Fatty acids are found in all cell membranes; the fetal brain contains equal amounts of omega-6 (arachidonic acid) and omega-3 (docosahexaenoic acid [DHA]). Arachidonic acid intake is seldom limited. The omega-3s, primarily eicosapentaenoic acid (EPA) and DHA, are important for fetal neurodevelopment, vasodilation, reduced inflammation, and thrombosis inhibition. Although EPA is thought to be beneficial, the separate effects have not yet been tested because purified EPA supplements are only recently available.

DHA is important for the growth development of the fetal central nervous system and the retina. It is speculated that DHA may be helpful regarding birth weight and gestational length, as well as maternal depression, but the results of supplementation trials have been mixed (Carlson et al, 2013). There may be a slight benefit with supplementation on infant visual and neural development, as well as infant immune function and lowered risk of food allergy (Larqué et al, 2012).

There is selective and preferential transfer of DHA across the placenta (Lauritzen and Carlson, 2011). Fetal DHA accretion is highest in the last half of pregnancy, reaching 30 to 45 mg/day in the last trimester (Koletzko et al, 2007), primarily to the brain and adipose tissue, and in the first few months of life. DHA must be mobilized from maternal stores or the prenatal diet must include adequate amounts of preformed DHA. Transfer rates are highly variable and are lower among women with obesity, preeclampsia, hypertension, and diabetes (type 1, type 2, and GDM) (Lauritzen and Carlson, 2011). Women who smoke and have growth restricted fetuses also have lower transfer rates. It is thought that short interconceptual periods may cause a mother to enter a subsequent pregnancy depleted.

An average daily intake of 200 mg DHA during pregnancy and lactation currently is recommended (Koletzko et al, 2007), but studies are underway testing the benefit of larger amounts (Carlson et al, 2013). Current intakes are often far lower. Intakes of up to 1 g/day of DHA or 2.7 g/day of total omega-3 PUFAs appear safe (Koletzko et al, 2007). The main food source of DHA is fatty, cold-water fish, and a couple of meals per week of low-mercury fish during pregnancy appear to provide adequate amounts of DHA. Those fish that are low in methylmercury but high in DHA include salmon, sardines, trout, herring, anchovies, and mackerel (not King mackerel). Caviar and brains (do not use where prion contamination is of concern) are also particularly high in DHA. Others also may be used, depending on local availability and acceptability of safe sources.

Vegetable sources of omega-3 fats (alpha-linolenic acid [ALA]) include flaxseeds and nuts, especially walnuts, but the conversion rate to DHA is usually very low. Other options to increase the DHA content in the diet of pregnant and lactating women include the consumption of DHA fortified eggs, but other fortified foods contain very little DHA. Foods labeled as fortified with omega-3s likely contain ALA.

Any pregnant woman allergic to fish should seek an algal source of supplemental DHA. However, this contains only DHA. It is currently unknown if EPA or other components (e.g., other fatty acids, vitamin D, iodine, and selenium) are also important (Oken et al, 2013). Fish oil supplements contain EPA and DHA, although better long-term outcomes are seen with fish consumption than with supplements. In general, fish contain more DHA than EPA (although there is variability between species)

and fish oil supplements contain more EPA than DHA. (Kris-Etherton et al, 2009). Caution is advised, though, with the fish liver oils (such as cod liver oil) because of high preformed vitamin A levels.

The breastfed infant obtains DHA through maternal milk when the mother eats sufficient quantities of foods containing DHA. If the exclusively breastfeeding mother is not consuming fish or DHA supplements, a DHA supplement can be given to the infant. Most infant formulas are fortified with DHA.

There is no DRI for either EPA or DHA in the United States and the intake levels that provide benefit still have to be determined. The benefit of maternal supplementation has not been proven as of yet and there are potential epigenetic effects that must also be considered. Maternal fish consumption is associated with better child neurodevelopment, at least in observational studies subject to confounding. Perhaps supplementation is merited only for those women with very low intakes of LCPUFAs and/or for the premature infants who had insufficient time to accumulate enough.

Promoting a variety of safe seafood choices is preferable. Women have consumed less fish since the mercury advisories were issued (Oken et al, 2013); they should be reassured that fish can be eaten safely as a good protein source as long as care is taken in choosing and preparing the fish (see Box 15-9). If at least some of the high DHA sources are chosen, pregnancy outcomes, as well as infant neurodevelopment and visual acuity, may improve. In addition, if women eat these fish during pregnancy, they are also likely to continue eating them postpartum, improving the child's DHA accretion that continues after birth.

Exposure of men and women to environmental chemicals, including pesticides, heavy metals, and organic solvents, is associated with an increased time to pregnancy. However, most studies are plagued with important confounders (age, smoking, alcohol use, parity, use of contraceptives, underlying disease) and causality cannot be determined; it is also unknown whether men and women have different susceptibility to the effects of environmental toxins. The strongest evidence of adverse effect is with pesticide and lead exposure. Pesticide exposure affects semen quality and increases risk of sterility (ACOG, 2013d; see Table 15-2).

A father's regular preconceptual smoking is associated with DNA damage to the sperm. Smoking also increases the risk that his child will have acute lymphoblastic leukemia, but the absolute risk is still very small, raising it from 27 per million births to 34 per million births (Van der Zee et al, 2013). Habitual alcohol

TABLE 15-2 Examples of Reproductive Health Effects of Prenatal Exposure to Environmental Contaminants

Chemicals	Exposure Sources and Pathways	Reproductive or Developmental Health Effects
Pesticides	Pesticides are applied in large quantities in agricultural, community, and household settings. In 2001, more than 1.2 billion pounds of active ingredients were used in the United States. Pesticides can be ingested, inhaled, and absorbed by the skin. The pathways of pesticide exposure include food, water, air, dust, and soil.	Impaired cognitive development Impaired neurodevelopment Impaired fetal growth Increased susceptibility to testicular cancer Childhood cancer
Solvents	Examples include benzene, toluene, xylene, styrene, 1-bromopropane, 2-bromopropane, perchloroethylene, and trichloroethylene. Solvents include some of the highest production volume chemicals in the United States. They are used in plastics, resins, nylon, synthetic fibers, rubber, lubricants, dyes, detergents, drugs, pesticides, glues, paints, paint thinners, fingernail polish, lacquers, detergents, printing and leather tanning processes, insulation, fiberglass, food containers, carpet backing, and cleaning products. Solvents are a component of cigarette smoke. Exposure is primarily through breathing contaminated air.	Fetal loss Miscarriage
Toluene	Exposure occurs from breathing contaminated air at the workplace, in automobile exhaust, some consumer products, paints, paint thinners, fingernail polish, lacquers, and adhesives.	Decreased fetal and birth weight Congenital malformations
Phthalates	Phthalates are synthetically derived. They are used in a variety of consumer goods, such as medical devices, cleaning and building materials, personal care products, cosmetics, pharmaceuticals, food processing, and toys. Exposure occurs through ingestion, inhalation, and dermal absorption.	Reduced masculine play in boys Reduced anogenital distance Shortened gestational age Impaired neurodevelopment in girls
Lead	Occupational exposure occurs in battery manufacturing and recycling, smelting, car repair, welding, soldering, firearm cleaning and shooting, and stained glass ornament and jewelry production. Nonoccupational exposure occurs in older homes where lead-based paints were used, water pipes, imported ceramics and pottery, herbal remedies, traditional cosmetics, hair dyes, contaminated soil, toys, and costume jewelry.	Alterations in genomic methylation Intellectual impairment Increased likelihood of allergies

Continued

TABLE 15-2   Examples of Reproductive Health Effects of Prenatal Exposure to Environmental Contaminants—cont'd

Chemicals	Exposure Sources and Pathways	Reproductive or Developmental Health Effects
Mercury	Mercury from coal-fired power plants is the largest man-made source of mercury pollution in the United States. Primary human exposure is by consumption of contaminated seafood.	Reduced cognitive performance Impaired neurodevelopment
Polychlorinated biphenyls	Polychlorinated biphenyls were used as industrial insulators and lubricants. They were banned in the 1970s but are persistent in the aquatic and terrestrial food chains, resulting in exposure by ingestion.	Development of attention deficit and hyperactivity disorder-associated behavior Increased body mass index Reduced IQ
Air pollutants	Common air pollutants include carbon monoxide, lead, ground-level ozone, particulate matter, nitrogen dioxide, and sulfur dioxide. Air pollution arises from a variety of sources, including motor vehicles, industrial production, energy (coal) production, wood burning, and small local sources, such as dry cleaners.	Low birth weight Birth defects
Cigarette smoke	Cigarette smoke exposure includes active smoking, passive smoking, or both.	Miscarriage Intrauterine growth restriction, low birth weight, and preterm delivery Decreased semen quality
Perchlorate	Perchlorate is used to produce rocket fuel, fireworks, flares, and explosives and also can be present in bleach and some fertilizers. Sources of exposure are contaminated drinking water, food, and other nonwater beverages. Infants also may be exposed through breast milk.	Altered thyroid function
Perfluorochemicals	Perfluorochemicals are widely used man-made organofluorine compounds with many diverse industrial and consumer product applications. Examples are perfluorooctane sulfonate and perfluorooctanate, which are used in cookware products with nonstick surfaces and in packaging to provide grease, oil, and water resistance to plates, food containers, bags, and wraps that come into contact with food. They persist in the environment. Occupational exposure and general population exposure occurs by inhalation, ingestion, and dermal contact.	Reduced birth weight
Polybrominated diphenyl ethers	These include flame retardant materials that persist and bioaccumulate in the environment. They are found in furniture, textiles, carpeting, electronics, and plastics that are mixed into but not bound to foam or plastic.	Impaired neurodevelopment Premature delivery, low birth weight, and stillbirth
Bisphenol A	Bisphenol A is a chemical intermediate for polycarbonate plastic and resins. It is found in food, consumer products, and packaging. Exposure occurs through inhalation, ingestion, and dermal absorption	Recurrent miscarriage Aggression and hyperactivity in female children
Formaldehyde	Formaldehyde is used in the production of wood adhesives, abrasive materials, and other industrial products and in clinical laboratories and embalming. It is found in some germicides, fungicides, insecticides, and personal care products. Routes of exposure are oral, dermal, and inhaled.	Spontaneous abortion Low birth weight
Antineoplastic drugs	This class of chemotherapy drugs presents an occupational exposure for nurses and other health care professionals.	Spontaneous abortion Low birth weight
Anesthetic gases	Anesthetic gases are administered by inhalation in health care settings and veterinary care. Occupational exposure is a risk for nurses, physicians, dentists, veterinarians and, other health care professionals who work in settings where anesthetic gases are used.	Congenital anomalies Spontaneous abortion
Ethylene oxide	Ethylene oxide is used to sterilize heat-sensitive medical items, surgical instruments, and other objects that come into contact with biologic tissues. Occupational exposure is a risk in some health care settings, particularly sterilization units. Exposure is through inhalation.	Spontaneous abortion and pregnancy loss Preterm and postterm birth

consumption may be associated with reduced semen quality and changes in testosterone and sex hormone-binding globulin levels. Although higher intakes are of more concern, even five drinks per week have been associated with a reduced sperm count and concentration, as well as a reduction in the percentage of spermatozoa with normal morphology (Jensen, 2014).

Obesity and Endocrine Conditions

Preconceptual obesity raises risk for men and women. In men, elevated BMI is associated with lower success with in vitro fertilization (IVF). Maternal prepregnant obesity is correlated with lower rates of conception, higher rates of congenital anomalies, and lower live birth rates (Merhi et al, 2013). Obesity affects ovulation, oocyte development, embryo development, endometrial development, implantation, and pregnancy loss. Those with known diabetes and hypothyroidism, as well as hypertension, should be in good control before conception. Although weight loss improves fertility for women, it has less effect on fertility in men (see *Focus On:* Special Case of Obesity).

Special Case of Obesity

The rates of obesity have increased dramatically in industrialized and, to a lesser extent, in developing countries (see Chapter 21).

Among women with obesity, rates of conception are lower and **congenital anomalies** (neural tube defects [NTDs], cardiovascular anomalies, oral clefts, anorectal atresia, hydrocephaly, limb reductions) occur more frequently and are detected less often prenatally than in the general population. Rates of NTDs increase with the degree of obesity; for severely obese women, rates are more than triple that for women with normal weight. Supplementation with folic acid is not as protective for these women, but the benefit of supplementing with more than 400 mcg folic acid/day has not been studied (Tenenbaum-Gavish and Hod, 2013).

During pregnancy, women with obesity have an exaggerated response to the normal physiologic changes. Genetic, hormonal, and biochemical environments are altered, influencing fetal growth and organ development. Women who enter pregnancy with a BMI greater than 30 have a higher risk of spontaneous abortion (SAB, i.e., miscarriage), **intrauterine fetal demise (IUFD)** or stillbirth, and increased risk of gestational diabetes, hypertension, or preeclampsia (ACOG, 2013a; Tenenbaum-Gavish and Hod, 2013), with the risk of many complications increasing linearly (Nelson et al, 2010). Normal fetal growth patterns are disrupted. Risk is increased for macrosomia, birth injury (shoulder dystocia, brachial plexus injury, fetal hypoxia), and childhood obesity, but there are also significant rates of growth restricted babies and preterm deliveries. These women are more likely to have intrapartum, operative, and postoperative complications, and their infants are more likely to require admission to the NICU. Women with obesity are also less likely to initiate and sustain breastfeeding.

Although excessive gestational weight gain is common among overweight or obese women and this weight gain is associated with similar increased risks, the prepregnant BMI is the more important factor. Weight loss before pregnancy is recommended (Tenenbaum-Gavish and Hod, 2013), and women who have undergone bariatric surgery are less likely to develop gestational diabetes, hypertension, preeclampsia, or to have a macrosomic infant.

How maternal obesity mediates poor maternal and fetal outcomes is not clear (Tenenbaum-Gavish and Hod, 2013). There are likely genetic and fetal-maternal interactions. It was thought that exposure to hyperglycemia was the main predictor, but it is now recognized that other factors are also important, including hypertriglyceridemia, insulin and insulin resistance, androgens, leptin, and increased blood pressure. Obesity, with low levels of adiponectin, is associated with increased fetal growth. The normal two-fold to threefold increases in serum cholesterol and free fatty acid levels during pregnancy are exaggerated in obese women. Triglycerides do not pass through the placenta easily, but there is increased placental transfer of metabolites and an increase in fetal fat deposits with obesity. Altered placental development or function, leading to increased amino acid transfer, contributes to a fetal hyperinsulinemic state. In addition, obesity is associated with tissue-specific changes in mitochondrial function and elevated oxidative stress. High lipid levels also may cause epigenetic changes in lipid sensing and metabolism genes. Obesity may also alter the regulation of appetite, satiety, and adipocyte maturation of the fetus.

These babies born to obese mothers also have permanently altered body weight-regulating mechanisms and there are changes in the hypothalamus, pancreatic islet cells, and adipose tissue (Tenenbaum-Gavish and Hod, 2013). They are more likely to have obesity, hypertension, and diabetes as adults. They also have increased rates of neurodevelopmental disorders and autism spectrum disorders if exposed to diabetes, hypertension, and obesity in utero.

Polycystic ovary syndrome (PCOS) affects up to 10% of women of reproductive age (Usadi and Legro, 2012). These ovarian cysts alter the testosterone-estrogen balance, resulting in insulin resistance and infertility. Recent recommendations suggest that 5% to 10% weight loss is preferred to the use of metformin for ovulation induction in patients with PCOS (Usadi and Legro, 2012; see Chapter 31).

A healthy diet and exercise program helps parents prepare for an optimal pregnancy outcome, with the goal of achieving normal weight before conception. However, although preconceptual intervention is recommended, it is seldom achieved because half of pregnancies in the United States are unplanned. In addition, advances in assisted reproductive technology (ART) mean that "parents" may be egg or sperm donors or surrogate mothers. The preconceptual health of these "parents" is likely also important but the impact is unknown.

CONCEPTION

Conception involves a complex series of endocrine events in which a healthy sperm fertilizes a healthy ovum (egg) within 24 hours of ovulation. Conception does not guarantee successful pregnancy outcome, and it is estimated that 41% to 70% fail, depending on the timing and sensitivity of the pregnancy test (Kwak-Kim et al, 2010).

The Carnegie Stages are a system used to describe predictable embryonic changes and developmental milestones. As noted in Table 15-3, as well as in Table 15-1 and Box 15-1, optimal conditions, including the absence of hostile factors and optimal status of many nutrients, are thought to be critical preconceptually and during organogenesis.

PREGNANCY

Physiologic Changes of Pregnancy
Blood Volume and Composition

Blood volume expands by nearly 50% by the end of pregnancy, with wide variability among women. This increased blood volume results in decreased levels of hemoglobin, serum albumin, other serum proteins, and water-soluble vitamins, primarily after the end of the first trimester. In contrast, serum concentrations of fat-soluble vitamins and other lipid fractions such as triglycerides, cholesterol, and free fatty acids increase to ensure sufficient transport to the fetus. A compilation of laboratory values by trimester is available, and selected values are listed in Table 15-4. However, wide individual variability makes determination of an inadequate intake or a deficient nutrient state difficult. Normal hematocrit and hemoglobin values change by trimester and cutpoints increase with altitude and smoking status, as shown in Table 15-5 (CDC, 1998).

Cardiovascular and Pulmonary Function

Increased cardiac output accompanies pregnancy, and cardiac size increases by 12%. Blood pressure, primarily diastolic, decreases during the first two trimesters because of peripheral vasodilation but may return to prepregnancy values in the third trimester. Mild lower extremity edema is a normal condition of pregnancy resulting from the pressure of the expanding uterus on the inferior vena cava.

Maternal oxygen requirements increase and the threshold for carbon dioxide lowers, making the pregnant woman feel dyspneic. Adding to this feeling of dyspnea is the growing uterus pushing the diaphragm upward. Compensation results from more efficient pulmonary gas exchange and larger chest diameter.

TABLE 15-3   The Carnegie Stages of Human Gestation Through 16 Weeks Postovulation

Carnegie Stage (time postovulation)	Structure Size	Highlighted Developmental Events with Selected Potential Nutrient Implications
Stage 1 Fertilization (1 day)	0.1-0.15 millimeters (mm); smaller than the size of a pencil point	Fertilization begins when the sperm penetrates the oocyte. This requires the sperm, which can survive up to 48 hours, to travel 10 hours up the female reproductive track. Then the sperm must successfully penetrate the zona pellucida, a tough membrane surrounding the egg, a process that takes approximately 20 minutes. Once the fertilization is successful, the structure now becomes a zygote. This is the end of the fertilization process. **Optimal amounts of folate** are needed for cell division and formation of DNA.
Stage 2 First Cell Division (1.5-3 days)	0.1-0.2 mm	Zygote begins to divide. Division begins to occur approximately every 20 hours. When cell division generates a mass of approximately 16 cells, the zygote now becomes a morula, a mulberry shaped structure. The newly created morula leaves the fallopian tube and enters the uterine cavity 3-4 days after fertilization.
Stage 3 Early Blastocyst (4 days)	0.1-0.2 mm	The morula enters the uterus and cell division continues. A cavity (hole), known as a blastocele, forms in the middle of the morula. Cells are flattening and compacting inside this cavity. The zona pellucida remains the same size as it was after fertilization, with the cavity in the center. The entire structure is now called a blastocyst. Two cell types are forming: embryoblasts, on the inside of the blastocele, and trophoblasts, on the outside portion of the blastocele.
Stage 4 Implantation Begins (5-6 days)	0.1-0.2 mm	Pressure from the blastocele expanding in the middle of the blastocyst against the rigid wall of the zona pellucida creates a "hatching" of the blastocyst from this zona pellucida. Separation of the embryoblasts and trophoblasts is complete. The outer layer of trophoblast cells secretes an enzyme that erodes the epithelial lining of the uterus so the blastocyst can implant. Trophoblast cells also secrete hCG, which stimulates the corpus luteum (the yellow glandular mass in the ovary formed by an ovarian follicle that has matured and discharged its ovum) to continue progesterone production, important in maintaining the blood-rich uterine lining. Progesterone is also later produced by the placenta. Five days is the latest that an IVF embryo would be transferred. **Consider vitamin D.**
Stage 5 Implantation Complete (7-12 days)	0.1-0.2 mm	Trophoblast cells continue to destroy cells of the uterine lining, creating blood pools and stimulating new capillaries to grow. This begins the growth of the placenta. The blastocyst inner cell mass differentiates into the epiblast (top layer of cells, becoming the embryo and the amniotic cavity) and the hypoblast (lower layer of cells, becoming the yolk sac). Ectopic pregnancies are those that do not implant in the uterus at this time, eventually becoming a life-threatening problem.
Stage 6 Primitive Streak (13 days)	0.2 mm	Placental formation: Chorionic villi "fingers" form, anchoring the embryo to the uterus. Blood vessels begin appearing. Stalk formation: The embryo is attached to the developing placenta by a stalk, which later becomes part of the umbilical cord. Gastrulation: A narrow line of cells, called the *primitive streak*, appears on the surface of the two-layered embryonic disc. Cells migrate in, with bilateral symmetry, from the outer edges of the disc to the primitive streak and begin to form 3 layers: the ectoderm (top layer of the embryonic disc that will later form skin, hair, lenses of the eye, lining of the internal and external ear, nose, sinuses, mouth, anus, tooth enamel, pituitary and mammary glands, and all parts of the nervous system), the mesoderm (middle cell layer that will later form muscles, bones, lymphatic tissue, spleen, blood cells, heart, lungs, reproductive, and excretory systems), and the endoderm (inner cell layer that will later form the lining of the lungs, the tongue, tonsils, urethra and associated glands, the bladder, and the digestive tract). **Consider vitamins A, E, C, copper, and DHA.**
Stage 7 Neurulation (16 days)	0.4 mm	Gastrulation continues, forming the three-layered embryonic disc. Neural crest cells originate at the top of the neural tube and migrate extensively throughout the embryo, differentiating into many cell types, including neurons, glial cells, pigmented cells of the epidermis, epinephrine-producing cells of the adrenal glands, and various skeletal and connective tissues of the head. Fetal alcohol syndrome results from disruption of the migration of neural crest cells. **Consider vitamins A, E, folic acid, choline, zinc, selenium, DHA, and antioxidants.**
Stage 8 (17-19 days)	1-1.5 mm	The embryonic area is now shaped like a pear, with the head region broader than the tail. The ectoderm has thickened to form the neural plate. The edges rise, forming the concave neural groove. This groove is the precursor of the embryo's nervous system, one of the first organs to develop. Blood cells are already developed and begin to form channels alongside the epithelial cells that are also forming. *Sonic hedgehog (Shh)* is one of three genes that are now secreted from the notochord (rod-shaped body composed of mesoderm cells). These genes encode for signaling molecules involved in patterning processes during embryogenesis, including the development of cerebral neurons, the separation of the single eye field into two bilateral fields, hair growth, and limb development. A repression of Shh by the notochord initiates pancreatic development. **Consider vitamin B_{12}, omega-3 fatty acids, folate, and choline.**

TABLE 15-3   The Carnegie Stages of Human Gestation Through 16 Weeks Postovulation—cont'd

Carnegie Stage (time postovulation)	Structure Size	Highlighted Developmental Events with Selected Potential Nutrient Implications
Stage 9 Appearance of Somites (19-21 days)	1.5-2.5 mm	Embryo looks like a peanut with a larger head end compared with the tail end. One to three pairs of somites (mesoderm tissue that looks like "bumps") are now present, with every ridge, bump, and recess indicating cellular differentiation. The head fold rises on either side of the primitive streak. Endocardial (muscle) cells begin to fuse and form into the early embryo's two heart tubes. Secondary blood vessels now appear in the chorion/placenta. Hematopoietic cells (forming blood cells) and endothelial cells (forming blood vessels) appear on the yolk sac simultaneously. **Consider folic acid, copper, and iron.**
Stage 10 (21-23 days)	1.5-3.0 mm	At this time, the embryo looks like an old fashioned key-hole with a big oval top, with an ear of corn in the bottom two thirds of the structure. Rapid cell growth elongates the embryo and expands the yolk sac. By the end of this stage, 4-12 somite pairs can exist. Cells that will become the eyes and ears appear. Neural folds begin to rise and fuse, "zippering" the neural tube closed. Failure of this closure results in a neural tube defect, including anencephaly and spina bifida, which varies in severity depending on location and extent of the area left open. The two endocardial tubes fuse into one. This heart tube takes on an S-shaped form and cardiac muscle contraction begins. **Consider folate, B$_6$, B$_{12}$, choline, vitamin A, zinc, and methionine.**
Stage 11 (23-25 days)	2.5-3.0 mm	Embryo has a modified S-curve shape with a bulb-like tail and a stalk connecting to the developing placenta. Somites increase to 20 pairs, at which point the forebrain is completely closed. The primitive tubal heart is beating and peristalsis begins. **Consider Vitamin A.**
Stage 12 (25-27 days)	3-5 mm	Embryo now has a C-shape. Brain and spinal cord are the largest tissue in the embryo. Face is becoming apparent, eyes and ears are beginning to form. Heart valves and septa may become apparent. Blood system is developing. Blood cells follow the surface of the yolk sac (where they originated), then move along the central nervous system to the chorionic villi, part of the maternal blood system. Liver cells are beginning to form, before the rest of the digestive system. Upper limb buds appear. **Consider vitamin A, folic acid, choline, methionine, and zinc.**
Stage 13 (26-30 days)	4-6 mm; size of the head of a pencil eraser	More than 30 somite pairs are now evident, precursors of multiple organ systems. First thin surface layer of skin appears to cover the embryo. Back muscles and ribs begin to form. The digestive epithelium layer begins to differentiate, eventually developing into the liver, lung, stomach, and pancreas.
Stage 14 (31-35 days)	5-7 mm	Brain and head are growing rapidly, sections of the brain and spinal cord wall are becoming differentiated. The eye is developing and the nasal plate can be detected. The adenohypophyseal pouch, later developing into the anterior pituitary, is defined. The esophagus is forming and lung sacs appear. Ureteric buds and the metanephros, later developing into the kidney, appear. Upper limbs elongate and innervation begins. **Consider LCPUFA (especially DHA and AA), protein, zinc, iron, choline, copper, iodine, vitamin A, and folate.**
Stage 15 (35-38 days)	7-9 mm	Brain is still larger than the trunk. Maxillary and mandibular arches are more prominent. The stomodeum, the depression in the ectoderm that will develop into the mouth and oral cavity, appears. Retinal pigment may appear in the optic cup. Symmetric and separate nasal pits appear as depressions in the nasal disc. Future cerebral hemispheres are distinct. Blood flowing through the atrioventricular canal is now divided into left and right streams. Handplate, forearm, arm, and shoulder may now be discerned in the upper limb bud. Lower limb bud begins to develop and innervation begins.
Stage 16 (37-42 days)	9-11 mm	Hindbrain, responsible for heart regulation, breathing, and muscle movements, begins to develop. Future lower jaw is now visible. Nasal pits rotate to face ventrally as head widens. Cardiac tube begins to develop. Mammary gland tissue begins to mature. Mesentery, the tissue that attaches the intestines to the rear abdominal wall and supplies them with blood, nerves, and lymphatics, is now defined. Hands begin to develop. Thigh, leg, and foot areas can now be distinguished. **Consider vitamin A.**
Stage 17 (42-44 days)	10-13 mm	Jaw and facial muscles are developing. The nasofrontal groove becomes distinct. An olfactory bulb (sense of smell) forms in the brain. Teeth buds (without a clear cell arrangement) begin to form. Heart separates into four distinct chambers. The diaphragm forms and the pituitary gland, trachea, larynx, and bronchi begin to form. Intestines begin to develop within the umbilical cord, later migrating to the abdomen when there is space. Primitive germ cells arrive at the genital area, responding to genetic instructions on whether they develop into female or male genitals. Digital rays are apparent on feet and hands. **Consider vitamin K.**

Continued

TABLE 15-3   The Carnegie Stages of Human Gestation Through 16 Weeks Postovulation—cont'd

Carnegie Stage (time postovulation)	Structure Size	Highlighted Developmental Events with Selected Potential Nutrient Implications
Stage 18 (44-48 days)	11-14 mm	Body appears more like a cube. Eyelids begin to develop, eyes are pigmented. Nipples appear on the chest. Kidneys begin to produce urine. Ossification of the skeleton begins. **Consider calcium, phosphorus, magnesium, vitamins A, D, and K.** See Box 15-2.
Stage 19 (48-51 days)	13-18 mm	Semicircular canals are forming in the inner ear, enabling a sense of balance and body position. Gonads are forming. Knee and ankle locations are now apparent, joints are more distinct. Toes are nearly completely notched and toenails begin to appear. Bone cartilage begins to form a more solid structure. Muscles develop and strengthen.
Stage 20 (51-53 days)	15-20 mm	Spontaneous movement begins. Nose is fully formed. Anal membrane is perforated. Testes or ovaries, as well as toes, are distinguishable.
Stage 21 (53-54 days)	17-22 mm	Eyes are well developed but have not yet migrated forward from the side of the head. External ears have not yet migrated up. Tongue is developing. Intestines begin to recede into the abdominal cavity. Failure to recede may result in either *gastroschisis* or *omphalocele*.
Stage 22 (54-56 days)	19-24 mm	Development of multiple organs continues. Upper lip now fully formed. The brain can signal muscle movement. Limbs begin to ossify (replacing cartilage with bone), starting in the upper limbs. **Consider the bone nutrients.** See Box 15-2.
Stage 23 Embryonic Period Ends (56-60 days)	23-26 mm	Head is erect and round. External ear is completely developed. Retina is fully pigmented. Eyelids begin to unite and are half closed. Taste buds begin to form. Bones of the palate begin to fuse. Primary teeth are at cap state (cells are now arranged and look like a cap). Upper and lower limbs are well formed; fingers and toes no longer webbed. Intestines continue to migrate from the umbilical cord into the body cavity. Layers of rather flattened cells (precursors to the surface layer of skin) replace the thin ectoderm. **Consider vitamins A, D, and K, calcium, phosphorus, magnesium, protein, and omega-3 fatty acids.**
(61-68 days, approximately 10 weeks)	31-42 mm	Basic brain structure is complete and the brain mass is rapidly growing. Sockets for all 20 teeth are formed in the gum line. Face has human appearance. Vocal cords form and the fetus can make sounds. Fetus develops reflexes. Digestive track muscles can function and practice contraction. Nutrient-extracting villi line the folded intestines. The liver begins to secrete bile (thick, brown-green liquid containing bile salts, bile pigments, cholesterol, and inorganic salts), which is stored in the gallbladder. The thyroid and pancreas are fully developed. The pancreas produces insulin. Genitalia are not yet fully formed. Fingernails begin growing. Skin is very sensitive. **Consider folate, omega-3 fatty acids, vitamins D, A, choline, Bs, protein, zinc, iron, copper, and iodine.**
(12 weeks)	Length: crown-rump length 61 mm (almost 2.5 inches) Weight: 8-14 g (0.3-0.5 oz)	Fetus begins to move around as muscle and nervous systems continue to develop. Heartbeat can be detected. Sucking muscles develop, salivary glands begin to function. Sweat glands and body hair begin to grow. Scalp hair pattern is discernible. Fetus inhales and exhales amniotic fluid, essential for the development of the air sacs in the lungs. Spleen is fully functional, removing old red blood cells and producing antibodies.
(Approximately 14 Weeks)	Length: 80-104 mm (3.2-4.1 inches) Weight: 25 g (almost 1 oz)	Bones continue to form, muscles strengthen. Eyes face more forward and ears are near their final position. Torso is growing rapidly, increasing its proportion to the head. Limbs are well developed. Toenails begin to grow. Heart pumps 25 quarts of blood/day (by the time of delivery it will be 300 quarts/d). Breathing, swallowing, and sucking are all becoming more developed. **Consider vitamin A, protein, and the bone nutrients.** See Box 15-2.
(16 weeks)	Length: 109-117 mm (4.3-4.6 inches) Weight: 80 g (approximately 2.8 oz)	The placenta is now the size of the fetus. The umbilical cord system grows and thickens, with the blood providing nourishment to the fetus through considerable force. 7.5 oz (250 ml) of amniotic fluid surround the conceptus. Eyes and ears are in correct positions. Fetus can blink, ears stand out from head. Fingerprints and toe prints develop. Circulation is completely functional. Meconium, the product of cell loss, digestive secretions, and swallowed amniotic fluid, begins to accumulate in the intestines. Nerves are being coated with myelin, a fatty substance that speeds nerve cell transmission and insulates them for uninterrupted impulses. **Consider omega-3 fatty acids, iron, vitamin A, and cholesterol.**

Adapted from *The Visible Embryo* (website): http://www.visembryo.com/. Accessed November 2014.

AA, Arachidonic acid; *DNA,* deoxyribonucleic acid; *hCG,* human chorionic gonadotropin; *LCPUFA,* long chain polyunsaturated fatty acids, *DHA,* docosahexaenoic acid.

TABLE 15-4 Selected Reference Ranges for Nutrient Levels in Nonpregnant and Pregnant Women, by Trimester

Component	Nonpregnant Adult	First Trimester	Second Trimester	Third Trimester
Albumin, g/dl	4.1-5.3	3.1-5.1	2.6-4.5	2.3-4.2
Protein, total, g/dl	6.7-8.6	6.2-7.6	5.7-6.9	5.6-6.7
Cholesterol, total, mg/dl	< 200	141-210	176-299	219-349
Triglycerides, mg/dl	< 150	40-159	75-382	131-453
Vitamin A (retinol), mcg/dl	20-100	32-47	35-44	29-42
Vitamin B_{12}, pg/ml	279-966	118-438	130-656	99-526
Vitamin C, mg/dl	0.4-1.0	Not reported	Not reported	0.9-1.3
Vitamin D, 25 hydroxy, ng/ml	14-80	18-27	10-22	10-18
Vitamin E, mcg/ml	5-18	7-13	10-16	13-23
Folate, red blood cell, ng/ml	150-450	137-589	94-828	109-663
Calcium, total, mg/dl	8.7-10.2	8.8-10.6	8.2-9.0	8.2-9.7
Copper, mcg/dl	70-140	112-199	165-221	130-240
Ferritin, ng/ml	10-150	6-130	2-230	0-116
Hemoglobin, g/dl	12-15.8	11.6-13.9	9.7-14.8	9.5-15.0
Hematocrit, %	35.4-44.4	31.0-41.0	30.0-39.0	28.0-40.0
Magnesium, mg/dl	1.5-2.3	1.6-2.2	1.5-2.2	1.1-2.2
Selenium, mcg/L	63-160	116-146	75-145	71-133
Zinc, mcg/dl	75-120	57-88	51-80	50-77

Adapted from Abbassi-Ghanavati M et al: Pregnancy and laboratory studies: a reference table for clinicians, *Obstet Gynecol* 114:1326, 2009.

TABLE 15-5 Maximum Hemoglobin and Hematocrit Values for Prenatal Anemia Diagnosis

Trimester	Hemoglobin Cutpoints at Sea Level	Hematocrit Cutpoints at Sea Level
First	< 11.0 g/dl	< 33.0 %
Second	< 10.5	< 32.0
Third	< 11.0	< 33.0
Altitude adjustments: must be added to the above cutpoints for accurate diagnosis		
3000-3999 feet	+0.2 g/dl	+0.5 %
4000-4999	+0.3	+1.0
5000-5999	+0.5	+1.5
6000-6999	+0.7	+2.0
7000-7999	+1.0	+3.0
8000-8999	+1.3	+4.0
9000-9999	+1.6	+5.0
10,000-11,000	+2.0	+6.0
Cigarette smoking: may be added to the above cutpoints for accurate diagnosis		
0.5 - < 1.0 pack per day	+0.3 g/dl	+1.0 %
1.0 - < 2.0 packs per day	+0.5	+1.5
≥ 2.0 packs per day	+0.7	+2.0
All smokers	+0.3 g/dl	+1.0 %

Adapted from Centers for Disease Control and Prevention: Recommendations to prevent and control iron deficiency in the United States, *MMWR Recomm Rep* 47:1, 1998.

Gastrointestinal Function

During pregnancy the function of the gastrointestinal (GI) tract changes in several ways that affect nutritional status. Gums may bleed more easily because of increased blood flow. In the first trimester nausea and vomiting may occur, followed by a return of appetite that may be ravenous (see Nausea and Vomiting, Hyperemesis Gravidarum, and Ptyalism). Cravings for and aversions to foods are common (see Cravings, Aversions, and Pica). Increased progesterone concentration relaxes the uterine muscle to allow for fetal growth while also decreasing GI motility with

BOX 15-2 Bone Nutrients

Protein

Forms organic matrix, for collagen, production of hormones, growth factors

Minerals

Boron: Considered to have minor role in bone function
Calcium: Main bone-forming mineral; 99% in skeleton
Copper: Functions in lysyl oxidase, an enzyme essential for cross-linking of collagen fibrils
Fluoride: Can replace hydroxyl groups in hydroxyapatite to form less soluble fluoroapatite
Iron: Cofactor in enzyme involved in collagen bone matrix synthesis, cofactor in 25-hydroxycholecalciferol hydroxylase
Magnesium: 60% of this mineral is in bone; it has an indirect role in ATP metabolism
Manganese: For biosynthesis of mucopolysaccharides in bone matrix, cofactor for several enzymes in bone tissue
Phosphorus: Essential bone-forming mineral
Zinc: For osteoblastic activity, collagen synthesis, alkaline phosphatase activity

Fat-Soluble Vitamins

Vitamin A: Essential in bone remodeling process: osteoblasts and osteoclasts have receptors for retinoic acid
Vitamin D: Maintains calcium levels
Vitamin K: Cofactor for gamma carboxylation of glutamic acid residues, including osteocalcin, the noncollagenous protein of bone

Water-Soluble Vitamins

Folic acid: Coenzyme mediating variety of reactions critical to nucleic and amino acid metabolism critical to bone development
Riboflavin: Needed to convert vitamin B_6 and folate into active forms
Vitamin B_6: Essential cofactor for enzyme ornithine decarboxylase; osteoblast NADPH concentrations, essential for Vitamin K
Vitamin B_{12}: Osteoblast function; cofactor for osteoblast-related proteins (bone alkaline phosphatase and osteocalcin); iron metabolism
Vitamin C: Hydroxylation of lysine, proline; linking of collagen fibril; stimulates alkaline phosphatase for osteoblast formation

ATP, Adenosine triphosphate; *NADPH,* nicotinamide adenine dinucleotide phosphate.
Adapted from Palacios C: The role of nutrients in bone health, from A to Z, *Crit Rev Food Sci Nutr* 46:621, 2006.

increased reabsorption of water. This often results in constipation. In addition, a relaxed lower esophageal sphincter and pressure on the stomach from the growing uterus can cause regurgitation and gastric reflux (see Heartburn).

Gallbladder emptying becomes less efficient because of the effect of progesterone on muscle contractility. Constipation, dehydration, and a low-calorie diet are risk factors for gallstone development. During the second and third trimesters, the volume of the gallbladder doubles and its ability to empty efficiently is reduced. Bile composition also changes, becoming more sludge-like, increasing the intrinsic risk of gallstones.

Metabolic Responses

The metabolism of macronutrients changes during pregnancy. This response varies between normal weight women and obese women (see Table 15-6).

Renal Function

The glomerular filtration rate (GFR) increases by 50% during pregnancy, although the volume of urine excreted each day is not increased. Renal plasma flow increases because of the increased GFR with lower serum creatinine and blood urea nitrogen concentrations. Renal tubular resorption is less efficient than in the nonpregnant state, and glucosuria, because of increased GFR, may occur, along with increased excretion of water-soluble vitamins and amino acids. Small amounts of glucosuria increase the risk for urinary tract infections.

Placenta and Uterine Environment

The fetus is not provided nutrients and oxygen through the placenta until after blood flow is established through the umbilical cord, around 10 weeks' gestation. Before that, nourishment is through the endometrium and uterine gland secretions, the contents of which are poorly understood (Bloomfield, 2011).

The placenta produces several hormones responsible for regulating fetal growth and the development of maternal support tissues. It is the conduit for exchange of nutrients, oxygen, and waste products. Placental insults compromise the ability to nourish the fetus, regardless of how well nourished the mother is. These insults can be the result of poor placentation from early pregnancy or small infarcts associated with preeclampsia or other hypertensive disorders.

A small placenta has a smaller surface area of placental villi, with a reduced functional capacity, often resulting in intrauterine growth restriction (IUGR). However, the placenta also has the ability to respond to a poor environment. For example, women affected by the World War II Dutch famine in their first trimesters had larger placentas, resulting in normal weight infants (Belkacemi et al, 2010). Although the efficiency of the placenta to support fetal growth varies, exhibiting morphologic and functional adaptations with varying environmental conditions, the fetus is also more than just a passive recipient of nutrients from the placenta (Fowden et al, 2009). Fetal and maternal endocrine changes signal nutrient availability and match the rate of fetal growth to the nutrient supply.

A less-than-optimal environment in utero can lead to a mismatch between available nutrients and the genetically determined fetal drive for growth. The goal is to support a healthy environment through a proper balance of nutrients and the avoidance of teratogens (see *Clinical Insight:* High-Risk Pregnancies with Nutritional Components).

CLINICAL INSIGHT

High-Risk Pregnancies with Nutritional Components

Approximately 10% of all pregnancies are considered "high risk," meaning there is a maternal preexisting complication or a situation that antedates pregnancy or presents in the current gestation that puts the mother or the fetus at risk for a poor outcome. Many of these may include nutritional concerns as well. Women who present with the following issues need increased medical surveillance and nutrition assessment to ensure the most favorable outcomes, controlled medical costs, and the fewest complications.

Anemias: microcytic or macrocytic
Cardiovascular issues: maternal cardiac structural defects, preexisting cardiovascular disease
Endocrine issues: polycystic ovary syndrome, thyroid disease, gestational diabetes, type 1 or 2 diabetes
Functional alterations: deafness, blindness, paralysis, paraplegia, quadriplegia
Gastrointestinal issues: food allergies, celiac disease, Crohn's disease, ulcerative colitis, postbariatric surgery, gallstones
Hyperemesis gravidarum
Hypertension: preexisting, pregnancy-induced, preeclampsia
Infections: HIV and AIDS, malaria, dental disease, intestinal parasites
Maternal genetic diseases or mental retardation
Medical problems: lupus, myasthenia gravis, cystic fibrosis, pancreatitis, phenylketonuria, cancer, sickle cell disease
Multiple fetuses
Obesity: BMI ≥30
Pica
Psychiatric: eating disorders, depression, bipolar disorders, Munchausen syndrome, suicidal ideation, substance abuse
Respiratory issues: asthma, tuberculosis, adult respiratory distress disorder
Surgeries: cancers, gallbladder, appendectomy, trauma
Young age - teenagers

AIDS, Acquired immune deficiency syndrome; *HIV,* human immunodeficiency virus.

TABLE 15-6 Metabolic Changes During Pregnancy for Women of Normal Weight and Obese

Component	Normal Weight	Obese
Fat deposition with gestational weight gain	Gestational fat gain is primarily accumulated centrally, both subcutaneous and visceral fat. Visceral accumulation may increase as pregnancy progresses.	Locations are similar, amount may be less
Lipid metabolism	50% to 80% increase in basal fat oxidation and in response to glucose, marked hyperlipidemia	Hyperlipidemia is exaggerated
Amino acid metabolism	Protein synthesis increases in the second (15%) and third (25%) trimesters	Unknown, but limited evidence suggests anabolic response may be impaired
Glucose metabolism, insulin resistance	Improved fasting glucose levels, glucose tolerance and insulin sensitivity in early pregnancy, then insulin sensitivity decreases 50% to 70% by third trimester	Early fasting glucose improves less if at all, more insulin resistance, which increases serum levels of all macronutrients

Adapted from Nelson SM et al: Maternal metabolism and obesity: modifiable determinants of pregnancy outcome, *Human Reprod Update* 16:255, 2010.

All nutrients are thought to be important, although some are better studied than others. Table 15-1 lists some potential functions, however, in reality more complex interactions involving multiple functions, are likely. For example, multiple nutrients are involved in the creation of bone (see Box 15-2) and brain (see Table 15-7). When either macro- or micronutrients are lacking, the timing of the deficit is important in predicting the impact of that insult (Monk et al, 2013; Wu et al, 2012a).

Effects of Nutritional Status on Pregnancy Outcome
Fetal Growth and Development

In the early 1900s U.S. women with poor nutritional status had adverse pregnancy outcomes with hemorrhage at delivery, prolonged labor, and LBW infants, conditions still of concern today in many developing countries. During World War II, the effects of severe food deprivation on previously well-nourished Dutch populations were explored. Higher rates of miscarriage (spontaneous abortion, "SAB"), stillbirths, neonatal deaths, and congenital malformations were noted in offspring born to women who conceived during the famine; surviving infants were smaller if exposed to famine late in gestation (Roseboom et al, 2011). Similar findings have been found in other countries as well. In addition, individuals may be at higher risk of undernutrition because of preexisting medical conditions or because of either physical or cultural limitations on food availability.

Even if a mother is not starving, the developing fetus may be unable to obtain optimal nutrients from a host who is compromised nutritionally, resulting in growth restriction. The causes of IUGR are many and include maternal, fetal, and placental factors (see Box 15-3). Infants born LBW (<2500 g) and especially very low birth weight (<1500 g) are at higher risk for **perinatal mortality** (infant death occurring

---

TABLE 15-7   Key Nutrients for Fetal and Neonatal Brain Development

Nutrient	Function in Brain Development	Negative Effect of Deficiency
Long-chain polyunsaturated fatty acids, primarily DHA and AA	Cell membrane formation, myelin, synaptosomes, intracellular communication, signal transduction	Neurodevelopment, visual development
Protein	Neuronal and glial structural proteins, synaptic structures and numbers, neurotransmitter peptide production, especially in cerebellum, hippocampus, and cerebral cortex	Overall central nervous system growth, neurodevelopment
Zinc	Cofactor in enzymes mediating protein and nucleic biochemistry, growth, gene expression, neurotransmitters, especially affecting cerebellum, limbic system, cerebral cortex, temporal lobe, frontal lobe	Attention, motor development delays, short-term memory, brain growth
Iron	Myelination, dendritogenesis, synaptogenesis, neurotransmission, especially in the hippocampus, striatum, frontal cortex	Global intelligence, general motor development, neurodevelopment, attention, memory, language, auditory recognition
Choline	Methylation, myelin, neurotransmitters, especially affecting hippocampus, septum, striatum, anterior neocortex, midposterior neocortex	Visual spatial and auditory memory in rodents (no information yet available for humans)
Copper	Iron transport, antioxidant activity, neurotransmitter synthesis, neuronal and glial energy metabolism, especially affecting cerebellum	Motor control, cognitive function
Iodine	Thyroid synthesis, neuronal synthesis, myelination	Cognitive function
Vitamin A	Structural development, antioxidant	Visual function
Folate	One-carbon metabolism	Neural tube development

Adapted from Monk C et al: Research review: maternal prenatal distress and poor nutrition—mutually influencing risk factors affecting infant neurocognitive development, *J Child Psychol Psychiatry* 54:115, 2013.

BOX 15-3   Potential Causes of Intrauterine Growth Restriction (IUGR)

Maternal Factors

Medical conditions: chronic hypertension, preeclampsia (early in gestation), diabetes, systemic lupus erythematosus, chronic kidney disease, inflammatory bowel disease, severe lung disease, cancer, hyperemesis gravidarum

Infections: syphilis, toxoplasmosis, cytomegalovirus, rubella, hepatitis B, herpes simplex virus 1 or 2, HIV-1, *Helicobacter pylori*, malaria

Malnutrition: low prepregnant weight, small maternal size, poor weight gain (especially in the last half of pregnancy), obesity (especially if combined with weight loss), nutrient deficiencies, including protein, vitamins A, Bs, C, folic acid, zinc, calcium, iron, recent history of pregnancy, high parity, multiple pregnancy, history of IUGR, active eating disorders

Social conditions: very young age; poverty; lack of food because of war, famine, natural disasters (earthquake, tsunami); physical or mental abuse; substance abuse (cigarettes, alcohol, heroin, cocaine); exposure

to teratogens; exposure to therapeutic medications (antimetabolites, warfarin, phenytoin)

Fetal Factors

Genetic: race, ethnicity, sex, genetic disorders

Parity: first baby often weighs less than subsequent siblings

Chromosomal anomalies: chromosomal deletions, trisomy 13, 18, 21

Congenital malformations: anencephaly, gastrointestinal atresia, Potter syndrome, pancreatic agenesis

Placental Factors

Placental insufficiency: reduced blood flow, impaired transfer of nutrients

Anatomic problems: multiple infarcts, aberrant cord insertions, umbilical vascular thrombosis and hemangiomas, premature placental separation, small placenta

Adapted from Alisi A et al: Intrauterine growth retardation and nonalcoholic fatty liver disease in children, *Int J Endocrinol* 2011:269853, 2011; Wu G et al: Biological mechanisms for nutritional regulation of maternal health and fetal development, *Paediatr Perinat Epidemiol* 26:4, 2012a.

between 28 weeks' gestation and 4 weeks postpartum). Babies who are born LBW may suffer from necrotizing enterocolitis, respiratory distress syndrome, intraventricular hemorrhage, cerebral palsy, or retinopathy of prematurity (see Chapter 42).

In addition to fetal growth restriction, any adverse maternal condition, including poor nutritional status, puts the fetus at risk for being delivered prematurely. Associated with prematurity is increased neonatal morbidity and mortality, especially if the baby is also growth restricted. Preterm rates are rising in developed countries and are higher in the United States than in Europe (Bloomfield, 2011). In the United States, rates are highest among non-Hispanic black women, and it is unclear if early fetal developmental programming is playing a role. Preterm rates are higher with ART, among both singletons and twins.

Oxidative stress, metabolic stress, and inflammation may be important in increasing risk of preterm delivery, and it appears that periconceptual malnutrition is more important than nutrition later in pregnancy. Although obesity does not predict optimal nutrition, it is somewhat protective for preterm delivery. However, prepregnant underweight, combined with low weight gain during pregnancy, has an additive effect on preterm and LBW risk. Even for those women of normal weight, low weight gain doubles the risk of preterm delivery; weight loss triples the risk (Bloomfield, 2011). Those women who are still growing or who have eating disorders may have competition for nutrients. Supplementation with macronutrients may be helpful, but there are no preconceptual studies. For many micronutrients, including omega-3 polyunsaturated fatty acids (PUFAs), folic acid, iron, vitamin C, vitamin D, calcium, magnesium, and zinc, it is unclear whether supplementation during pregnancy provides an acute beneficial effect or whether long-term stores are more important (Bloomfield, 2011).

Particular toxins may increase the risk of prematurity. One study found nearly double the risk of preterm delivery if women consumed more than four servings of diet soda per day (Bloomfield, 2011), although that finding has been disputed (La Vecchia, 2013). Licorice (glycyrrhiza glabra root) blocks the enzyme that inactivates cortisol, and the effect on preterm risk is dose-related. Similar results are seen when mother is exposed to psychological stress (see *Clinical Insight:* Stress During Pregnancy). The role of paternal nutrition in preterm risk is unexplored (Bloomfield, 2011).

The effect of poor maternal nutrition or exposure to toxins may follow the infant for decades. A very preterm, growth-restricted baby may suffer permanent brain damage. Neural tube defects (NTDs) may cause lifelong problems with mobility and bodily functions. Fetal alcohol syndrome (FAS) is a major cause of mental retardation and learning disorders. However, even those babies who are born with no apparent defects may suffer increased risk of chronic diseases because of a less-than-optimal prenatal environment. See Figure 15-1 for a summary of the effects of maternal malnutrition.

Epigenetic Effects

Compromises in structural or cognitive potential may not be evident when an infant is born but may manifest later in life. A child with IUGR, often resulting from maternal hypertension or severe malnutrition or anemia, may have permanent

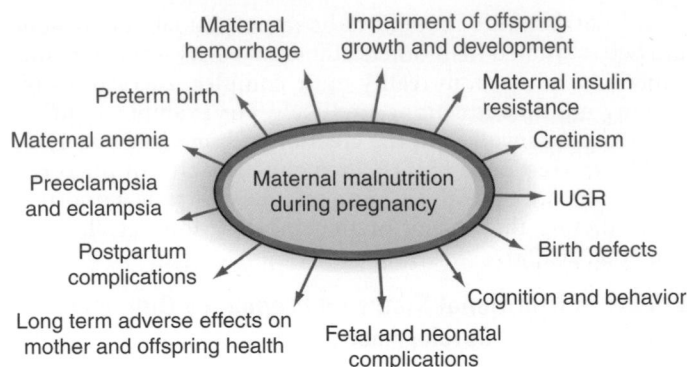

FIGURE 15-1 Major negative effects of maternal malnutrition (both under- and overnutrition) on mother and infant.

mild neurodevelopmental cognitive abnormalities. Babies born preterm or growth restricted are more likely to have a higher risk of obesity, type 2 diabetes, and cardiovascular disease (CVD) later in life. Those babies exposed to the Dutch famine early in gestation were at highest risk of CVD and had double the risk for schizophrenia, whereas those exposed midpregnancy were three times more likely to develop microalbuminuria and decreased creatinine clearance, as well as having an increased risk for obstructive airway disease (Roseboom et al, 2011).

Girls born preterm are more likely to deliver preterm with their own pregnancies and more likely to develop anorexia nervosa (Bloomfield, 2011). Immune function, learning ability, mental health, cancer, and aging are likely affected by LBW. Functional neural pathways controlling appetite and satiety likely develop in the third trimester, so preterm infants may experience disruptions in their development.

Those babies born large for gestational age (LGA) or exposed to hyperglycemia or maternal obesity are at increased risk of chronic diseases, likely through multiple mechanisms (see *Focus On:* Special Case of Obesity).

Birth weight may not be the only predictor for the propensity for adult disease. Exposure to high folate during pregnancy is associated with insulin resistance and obesity in later life if combined with low vitamin B_{12} levels (DelCurto et al, 2013), and increased rates of cancer are associated with supraphysiologic intakes of methyl donors (Milagro et al, 2013; see Chapter 5). Maternal and paternal nutritional imbalances are likely to increase the risk of metabolic syndrome (DelCurto et al, 2013).

Exposure to endocrine-disrupting chemicals may modify gene expression and the effects, including increased risk of obesity, insulin resistance, and type 2 diabetes, may be nonlinear (i.e., low doses may be more harmful than high doses) (Barouki et al, 2012). In one study, mothers who ate an unbalanced high-protein diet (1 pound red meat/day, no carbohydrate) during late pregnancy produced offspring who experienced higher cortisol levels when exposed to stress as adults (Bloomfield, 2011).

This developmental plasticity can be helpful. However, when there is a mismatch between in utero programming and the later environment, the risk of chronic disease rises. Whether the fetus develops a thrifty phenotype or whether harm is caused by overcompensation later with catch-up growth is unknown. Altered organ structure, cell numbers, and metabolic functioning appear important (Koletzko et al, 2012). See Chapter 5 for more information.

Exposure of the embryo or fetus to specific maternal nutrients, as well as environmental contaminants, can turn the imprinting genes that control growth and development on or off, but the amounts, timing, and effects are still being investigated. Paternal nutrient imbalance and gene-environment interactions are also likely important (Barouki et al, 2012; DelCurto et al, 2013). Although DOHaD originally focused on undernutrition, overnutrition also is being studied. Effects of macro- and micronutrients, as well as phytonutrients and hypoxia, are being examined, primarily through animal studies so far, and the ideal maternal and paternal diet for epigenetic effects has not yet been established (Vanhees et al, 2014).

New research also is focusing on the grandchildren of people affected by the Dutch famine (Roseboom et al, 2011) to document the long-term epigenetic effects. Preliminary results show that under- and overnutrition are important issues, but there are differences in response by sex, and the timing of the insult matters (Vanhees et al, 2014). The preconceptual nutritional role in altering the epigenome has yet had little attention, although animal research shows components of a preconceptual diet may resolve toxicant epigenetic changes (Owen et al, 2013). Maternal and paternal nutritional status, as well as that of previous generations, are likely important in affecting, and being affected by, genetic variations (see Chapter 5).

Nutrient Requirements During Pregnancy

Nutrition during pregnancy often is equated with weight gain because weight is most easily and consistently measured. However, the increased need for nutrients to support adequate fetal growth is greater than the limited additional energy needed, and maternal weight gain is not necessarily predictive of health outcomes, especially for heavier women. The U.S. DRIs are found on the inside front cover, and estimated requirements vary between countries (see Table 15-8).

Energy

Additional energy is required during pregnancy to support the metabolic demands of pregnancy and fetal growth. Metabolism increases by an average of 15% in the singleton pregnancy, but with wide variability, especially in the third trimester. The DRI for energy increases by only 340 kcal/day during the second trimester and by 452 kcal/day in the third trimester. If maternal weight gain is within the desirable limits, the range of acceptable energy intakes varies widely, given individual differences in energy output and basal metabolic rate. Modifying intakes to achieve recommended weight gain (see Pregnancy Weight Gain Recommendations) is more useful than calculating caloric requirements.

Exercise. Energy expended in voluntary physical activity is the largest variable in overall energy expenditure. Physical activity increases energy expenditure proportional to body weight. However, most pregnant women compensate for increased weight gain by slowing their work and movement pace; thus total daily energy expenditure may not be substantially greater than before pregnancy.

The American College of Obstetricians and Gynecologists (ACOG) recommends at least 30 minutes of moderate intensity exercise on most, if not all, days for pregnant women without contraindications. Short duration strenuous exercise appears unconcerning, but the impact of long duration strenuous exercise

on the fetus is unknown (Szymanski and Satin, 2012). Excessive exercise, combined with inadequate energy intake, may lead to suboptimal maternal weight gain and poor fetal growth. Therefore a pregnant woman should always discuss exercise with her health practitioner. Although there is limited evidence that exercise helps modify gestational weight gain, there is also no evidence of harm.

Protein

Additional protein is required to support the synthesis of maternal and fetal tissues. This demand increases throughout gestation and is maximized during the third trimester. The protein RDA of 0.8 g/kg current body weight/day for pregnant women (46 g for someone with a prepregnant weight of 126 pounds) in the first half of pregnancy is the same as that for the nonpregnant women. Needs increase in the second half to 1.1 gm/kg/day, which would be 71 g/day only for that same reference woman who is also gaining weight appropriately. For many women, the protein requirement is higher. For each additional fetus, at least another 25 g/day of protein is recommended, but because protein is also used as an energy source, the total may be as much as 175 g/day for the normal-weight woman carrying a twin gestation who is consuming 3500 kcal/day (Goodnight and Newman, 2009). The World Health Organization (WHO) uses slightly different calculations in their 2007 report; 0.83 g/kg/day as a baseline protein requirement with additional recommended intakes of + 0.7 g/day (first trimester), + 9.6 g/day (second trimester), or + 31.2 g/day (third trimester) to support a total 13.8 kg weight gain, although some researchers recommend the older (1985) and more conservative guidelines (additional intakes of 1.2, 6.1, and 10.7 g/day respectively, averaged to an additional 6 g/day throughout pregnancy added to the prepregnant value) (Millward, 2012).

Protein deficiency during pregnancy has adverse consequences, including poor fetal growth. Protein also is involved in the synthesis of hormones and neurotransmitters. Limited intakes of protein and energy usually occur together, making it difficult to separate the effects of energy deficiency from those of protein deficiency. Although most women in the United States likely eat more than enough protein, there are some for whom particular attention must be paid, including those consuming a vegetarian diet, those who are still growing themselves, or those who are pregnant with multiples.

The optimal balance of protein to total calories has yet to be determined and recommendations, as well as intakes, vary across cultures (Blumfield and Collins, 2014). Caution is advised when considering very high protein supplements. Intakes at the high end of the acceptable macronutrient distribution ranges (AMDR) (i.e., 30% to 35% of calories from protein) have been associated with an increased risk of adverse outcomes in some studies (Millward, 2012). Current U.S. practice often targets protein intakes at 20% of total calories, possibly higher for multiples. WHO recommends 23% of calories from protein (Millward, 2012). Supplementation, if necessary, should be done with food rather than with protein supplements. For example, someone consuming 2240 kcal from 6 cups/day of 2% milk, 8 oz of meat, six servings of starch, three vegetable servings, two fruit servings, and six fat servings gets 23% of her calories from protein (128 g). If using skim milk, the total is 1970 kcal with 26% from protein. *Text continued on page 256*

TABLE 15-8 Global DRIs for Pregnant Women (PW) and Women Who Are Breastfeeding (BF)

[Ranges vary with age, time period (pregnancy trimesters, early vs late lactation), degree of lactation (full vs partial), maternal fat stores, well-nourished vs undernourished, and nutrient bioavailability.]

Nutrient	United States, Canada (1) PW	United States, Canada (1) BF	United Kingdom (2) PW	United Kingdom (2) BF	Italy (3) PW	Italy (3) BF	German Group (4) PW	German Group (4) BF	Nordic Group (5) PW	Nordic Group (5) BF	France (6) PW	France (6) BF	Spain (7) PW	Spain (7) BF	WHO (8) PW	WHO (8) BF
Calories, added to baseline	340-452	330-400	191	330	350-460	330	255	285-635	96-525	478-669					85-475	460-675
Protein, g (baseline estimates vary by country)	71 (a) Base + 0.3 g/kg current body weight/d	71 (a) Base + 0.5 g/kg/d	51 (a) Base + 6 g/d	51 (a) Base + 8-11 g/d	Base + 1-29 g/d	Base + 13-19 g/d	58	63	10%-20% kcal	10%-20% kcal					Base + 0.7-31.2 g/d	Base + 12.5-19 g/d
Fat, g			PUFA 6.5% kcal	PUFA 6.5% kcal	LCPUFA 5%-10% kcal	LCPUFA 5%-10% kcal			PUFA 5%-10% kcal	PUFA 5%-10% kcal					PUFA 6%-11% kcal	PUFA 6%-11% kcal
Linoleic acid, g	13	13			ω-6 4%-8% kcal	ω-6 4%-8% kcal	ω-6 2.5% kcal	ω-6 2.5% kcal	5% kcal EFA (ω-6 + ω-3)	5% kcal EFA (ω-6 + ω-3)					ω-6 2.5%-9% kcal	ω-6 2.5%-9% kcal
Alpha-linolenic acid, g	1.4	1.3			ω-3 0.5%-2.0% kcal	ω-3 0.5%-2.0% kcal	ω-3 0.5% kcal	ω-3 0.5% kcal	5% kcal EFA (ω-6 + ω-3)	5% kcal EFA (ω-6 + ω-3)					ω-3 0.5-2.0% kcal	ω-3 0.5-2.0% kcal
DHA, mg					100-200	100-200	200	200	200	200	250 DHA + 250 EPA	250 DHA + 250 EPA			200 DHA, 300 DHA + EPA	200 DHA, 300 DHA + EPA
Carbohydrate, g	175	210	50% kcal	50% kcal	45%-60% kcal	45%-60% kcal			45%-60% kcal	45%-60% kcal					55% kcal	55% kcal
Fiber, g	28	29	12-24	12-24	12.6-16.7/1000 kcal	12.6-16.7/1000 kcal			25-35	25-35						
Water, total, liter	3.0	3.8			2.2-2.3	2.6-2.7	2.36	2.71								
Vitamin A mcg RAE	750-770	1200-1300	610	950	700	1000	1100	1500	800	1100	700	950	700	950	800	850
Thiamin, mg	1.4	1.4	0.8-0.9	0.9-1.0	1.4	1.4	1.2	1.4	1.5	1.6	1.8	1.8	1.2	1.4	1.4	1.5
Riboflavin, mg	1.4	1.6	1.4	1.6	1.7	1.8	1.5	1.6	1.6	1.7	1.6	1.8	1.6	1.7	1.4	1.6
Niacin, mg NE	18	17	12-14	14-16	22	22	15	17	17	20	16	15	15	16	18	17
Vitamin B$_6$, mg	1.9	2.0	1.0-1.2	1.0-1.2	1.9	2.0	1.9	1.9	1.4	1.5	2.0	2.0	1.5	1.6	1.9	2.0
Folate, mcg DFE	600	500	300	260	600	500	550	450	500	500	400	400	500	400	600	500
Vitamin B$_{12}$, mcg	2.6	2.8	1.2-1.5	1.7-2.0	2.6	2.8	3.5	4.0	2.0	2.6	2.6	2.8	2.2	2.6	2.6	2.8
Pantothenic acid, mg	6	7			6	7	6	6			5	7	6	7	6	7
Biotin, mcg	30	35			35	35	30-60	30-60					30	35	30	35
Inositol, mcg											50	55				
Choline, mg	450	550														

Southeast Asia (9)		Philippines (10)		Japan (11)		Korea (12)		India (13)		Australia, New Zealand (14)		Mexico (15)		Venezuela (16)	
PW	BF	PW	BF	PW	BF	PW	BF	PW	BF	PW	BF	PW	BF	PW	BF
360-475	505-675	300	500	50-450	350	340-450	320	350	520-600	334-454	478-502			263	500
46-67	52-81	66	76-81	50-80	70-75	45-80	70-75	82.2	70.2-77.9	58-60 (a) = 1-1.02 g/kg/d	63-67 (a) = 1.1 g/kg/d	Base + 6-11 g/d	Base + 11-16 g/d	70-86	70-89
								30	30						
				< 11	< 10	ω-6 4-8% kcal	ω-6 4-8% kcal			10	12	ω-6 5-8% kcal	ω-6 5-8% kcal		
				1.9	1.7	ω-3 1% kcal	ω-3 1% kcal			1.0	1.2	ω-3 1-2% kcal	ω-3 1-2% kcal		
										110-115 DHA + EPA + DPA	140-145 DHA + EPA + DPA				
				50%-70% kcal	50%-70% kcal	55%-70% kcal	55%-70% kcal					130-175	120-210	56%-69% kcal	56%-69% kcal
				> 17	> 17	25	25			25-28	27-30	25-30	25-30	20-40	20-40
		1 ml/kcal + 300 ml	1 ml/kcal + 750-1000 ml			2.2-2.3	2.7-2.8			2.4-3.1	2.9-3.5				
800	850	800	900	650-780	1100-1150	670-720	1090-1140	800	950	700-800	1100	640	1100	800	1300
1.4	1.5	1.4	1.5	1.1-1.4	1.3-1.4	1.5	1.5	1.2-1.6	1.2-1.7	1.4	1.4	1.2	1.2	1.4	1.5
1.4	1.6	1.7	1.7	1.2-1.7	1.6-1.8	1.6	1.6	1.4-2.0	1.4-2.1	1.4	1.6	1.2	1.3	1.4	1.5
18	17	18	17	11-13	14-16	18	19	14-18	15-20	18	17	15	15	18	17
		1.9	2.0	1.9-2.1	1.4-1.6	2.2	2.2	2.5	2.5	1.9	2.0	1.4	1.6	1.9	2.0
600	500	600	500	480	340	600	550	500	300	600	500	750	650	600	500
		2.6	2.8	2.8	3.2	2.6	2.8	1.2	1.5	2.6	2.8	2.6	2.8	2.6	2.8
				6-7	6-7	6-7	7-8			5	6	6	7	6	7
				52	55	25-30	30-35			30	35			30	35
										415-440	525-550			450	550

Continued

TABLE 15-8 Global DRIs for Pregnant Women (PW) and Women Who Are Breastfeeding (BF)—cont'd

Nutrient	United States, Canada (1) PW	BF	United Kingdom (2) PW	BF	Italy (3) PW	BF	German Group (4) PW	BF	Nordic Group (5) PW	BF	France (6) PW	BF	Spain (7) PW	BF	WHO (8) PW	BF
Vitamin C, mg	80-85	115-120	45-50	65-70	100	130	110	150	85	100	120	130	80	100	55	70
Vitamin D, mcg	15	15	10	10	15	15	20	20	10	10	10	10	10	10	5	5
Vitamin E, mg	15	19			12	15	13	17	10	11	12	12	15	19	7.5	7.5
Vitamin K, mcg	75-90	75-90			140	140	60	60			45	45	90	90	55	55
Boron, mg																
Calcium, mg	1000-1300	1000-1300	700-800	1250-1350	1000	1000	1000-1200	1000-1200	900	900	1000	1000	1000	1200	1200	1000
Chloride, g	2.3	2.3	2.5	2.5	2.3	2.3	0.83	0.83					2.3	2.3		
Chromium, mcg	29-30	44-45			30	45	30-100	30-100			60	55	30	45		
Copper, mg	1.0	1.3	0.8-1.2	1.1-1.5	1.2	1.6	1.0-1.5	1.0-1.5	1.0	1.3	2.0	2.0	1.1	1.4		
Fluoride, mg	3.0	3.0			3.0	3.0	3.1	3.1			2.0	2.0	3.0	3.0		
Iodine, mcg	220	290	130-140	130-140	220	290	230 (b), 200 (c)	260 (b), 200 (c)	175	200	200	200	175	200	250	250
Iron, mg	27	9-10	14.8	14.8	27	11	30	20	(d)	15	30	10	25	15	(d)	10-30
Magnesium, mg	350-400	310-360	270-300	320-350	240	240	310	390	280	280	400	390	360	360	220	270
Manganese, mg	2.0	2.6			2.5	3.1	2.0-5.0	2.0-5.0					2.0	2.6		
Molybde-num, mcg	50	50			50	50	50-100	50-100					50	50		
Phosphorus, mg	700-1250	700-1250	550-625	990-1065	700	700	800-1250	900-1250	700	900	800	850	800	990		
Potassium, g	4.7	5.1	3.1-3.5	3.1-3.5	3.9	3.9	2.0	2.0	3.1	3.1			3.1	3.1	3.51	3.51
Selenium, mcg	60	70	45-60	60-75	55	70	30-70	30-70	60	60	60	60	55	70	26-30	35-42
Sodium, g	1.5	1.5	1.6	1.6	1.5	1.5	0.55	0.55					1.5	1.5	<2.0	<2.0
Zinc, mg	11-12	12-13			11	13	10	11	9	11	14	19	10	12	3.4-20	4.3-19

DFE, Dietary folate equivalent; *DHA,* docosahexaenoic acid; *DPA,* docosapentaenoic acid; *EFA,* essential fatty acids; *EPA,* eicosapentaenoic acid; *LCPUFA,* long-chain polyunsaturated fatty acids; *NE,* niacin equivalent; *PUFA,* polyunsaturated fatty acids; *RAE,* retinol activity equivalent.

(a) only for a woman at reference weight
(b) Germany, Austria
(c) Switzerland, WHO
(d) needs supplementation

(1) United States and Canada: Otten JJ et al: *Dietary reference intakes: the essential guide to nutrient requirements,* Washington, DC, 2006, Institute of Medicine of the National Academies, National Academies Press.
(2) United Kingdom: British Nutrition Foundation: *Nutrient Requirements* (website): http://www.nutrition.org.uk/nutritionscience/nutrients/nutrient-requirements, 2012. Accessed December 2014; Scientific Advisory Committee on Nutrition: *Dietary Reference Values for Energy,* 2011 (website): http://www.sacn.gov.uk/pdfs/sacn_dietary_reference_values_for_energy.pdf, 2011. Accessed December 2014.
(3) Italy: Società Italiana di Nutrizione Umana: *Livelli di assunzione di riferimento di nutrienti ed energia per la popolazione italiana,* 2012 (website): http://www.sinu.it/documenti/20121016_LARN_bologna_sintesi_prefinale.pdf, 2012. Accessed November 2014.
(4) German Group (Germany, Austria, Switzerland): *Deutsche Gesellschaft für Ernährung e.V.:* Referenzwerte für die nährstoffzufuhr (website): http://www.dge.de/modules.php?name=Content&pa=showpage&pid=3. Accessed February 2014.
(5) Nordic Group (Norway, Sweden, Finland, Denmark, Faroe Islands, Iceland, Greenland, Åland): *Norden:* Nordic nutrition recommendations, 2012 (website): http://norden.diva-portal.org/smash/record.jsf?pid=diva2%3A704251&dswid=2786, 2014. Accessed November 2014.
(6) France: *Nutrition Expertise:* Tables ANC (website): http://www.nutrition-expertise.fr/mineraux/119-tableaux-anc.html, 2013. Accessed December 2014.
(7) Spain: Guíasy herramientas: ingestas dietéticas de referencia (IDR) para la población Española, *Act Diet* 14:196, 2010.
(8) WHO: *World Health Organization (WHO):* Dietary recommendations (website): http://www.who.int/nutrition/publications/nutrientrequirements/en/, 2014. Accessed February 2014; World Health Organization (WHO), UNICEF: Reaching optimal iodine nutrition in pregnant and lactation women and young children, 2007 (website): http://www.who.int/nutrition/publications/WHOStatement__IDD_pregnancy.pdf, 2007. Accessed December 2014.

Southeast Asia (9)		Philippines (10)		Japan (11)		Korea (12)		India (13)		Australia, New Zealand (14)		Mexico (15)		Venezuela (16)	
PW	*BF*	*PW*	*BF*	*PW*	*BF*	*PW*	*BF*	*PW*	*BF*	*PW*	*BF*	*PW*	*BF*	*PW*	*BF*
80	95	80	105	110	150	110	135	60	80	55-60	80-85	138	128	70	90
5	5	5	5	5-7	6-8	10	10			5	5	5	5	10	10
		12	16	6.5-7.0	9.5-10	9-10	12-13			7-8	11-12	13	17	10	12
		51	51	60-65	60-65	65	65			60	60	75	75	65	65
						2.5-3.0	2.5-3.0								
1000	1000	800	750	650-800	650-800	930-1180	1020-1270	1200	1200	1000-1300	1000-1300	1000	1000	1100-1300	1100-1300
		At least 0.75	At least 0.75			2.3	2.3								
				30	30					30	45	26	42		
				0.8-0.9	1.3-1.4	0.87-1.0	1.19-1.32			1.2-1.3	1.4-1.5	0.75	1.15	2.2	2.2
		2.5	2.5							3.0	3.0	2.45	2.45	3.0	3.0
200	200	200	200	240-250	270-280	220-240	310-330			220	270	195	265	200	200
(d)	15-20	27-38	27-30	8.5-25	8.5-12.5	23-27	13-17	35	25	27	9-10	28	17-25	30	15
		205	250	310-340	270-300	320-380	280-340	310	310	350-400	310-360	285	250	400	360
		2.0	2.6	3.5	3.5	3.5	3.5			5	5				
				20-25	23-28					50	50				
		700	700	900-1100	900-1100	700-900	700-900			1000-1250	1000-1250	1250	700	700	700
		At least 2.0	At least 2.0	2.0-2.1	2.4-2.5	3.5	3.9			2.8	3.2				
26-30	35-42	35	40	30	45	54-64	60-70			65	75	55	65	65	75
		At least 0.5	At least 0.5	0.6	0.6	1.5	1.5			0.46-0.92	0.46-0.92				
5.5-10.0	7.2-9.5	5.1-9.6	11.5	11	12	9.5-11.5	12-14	12	12	10-11	11-12	14	16	15	19

(9) Southeast Asia: Barba CVC, Cabrera MIZ: Recommended dietary allowances harmonization in Southeast Asia, *Asia Pac J Clin Nutr* 17:405, 2008.

(10) Philippines: Food and Nutrition Research Institute, Department of Science and Technology: Recommended energy and nutrient intakes for Filipinos, 2002, powerpoint presentation. Correspondence with author.

(11) Japan: National Institute of Health and Nutrition: Dietary reference intakes for Japanese, 2010 (website).http://www.nih.go.jp/eiken/english/research/pdf/dris2010_eng.pdf, 2011. Accessed February 2014.

(12) Korea: *Korean Nutrition Society:* Dietary reference intakes for Koreans, 2010 (website):http://image.campushomepage.com/users/knsweb/ssugi513/DRIs/2010KDRIs_open_final.pdf. Accessed February 2014.

(13) India: *Indian Council of Medical Research, National Institute of Nutrition:* Nutrient requirements and recommended dietary allowances for Indians, 2010 (website): http://icmr.nic.in/final/RDA-2010.pdf, 2009. Accessed February 2014.

(14) Australia and New Zealand: *Australian National Health and Medical Research Council (NHMRC), New Zealand Ministry of Health:* Nutrient reference values for Australia and New Zealand (website): https://www.nrv.gov.au/nutrients. Accessed November 2014.

(15) Mexico: *Recomendaciones para la ingestión de nutrimentos* (website): http://www.slideshare.net/MPPGLuno/recomendaciones-10179041. Accessed February 2014.

(16) Venezuela: *Instituto Nacional de Nutrición:* Valores de referencia de energia y nutrientes para la pobación Venezolana, 2000 (website): http://www.scribd.com/doc/53061105/Valores-de-Referencia-de-Energia-y-Nutrientes-para-la-Poblacion-Venezolana-Revision-2000-INN. Accessed February 2014.

Carbohydrates

The RDA for carbohydrates increases slightly, helping maintain appropriate blood glucose and prevent ketosis. Intakes may be greater in women consuming more calories, but careful carbohydrate choices are needed to include all the daily nutrients for pregnancy. Priority should be given to complex carbohydrates from whole grains, fruits, and vegetables rather than just simple sugars, including refined liquid sugars, whether natural (juices) or industrially produced (soda).

Fiber

Daily consumption of whole-grain breads and cereals, leafy green and yellow vegetables, and fresh and dried fruits should be encouraged to provide additional minerals, vitamins, and fiber. The DRI for fiber during pregnancy is 14 g/day/1000 kcal and, if met, will help a great deal in managing the constipation that often accompanies pregnancy.

Lipids

As with nonpregnant women, there is no DRI for total lipids during pregnancy. The amount of fat in the diet should depend on energy requirements for proper weight gain. However, recommendations for omega-6 PUFA (linoleic acid) and omega-3 PUFA (alpha-linolenic acid) increase slightly. Although not a DRI, the recommended intake of docosahexaenoic acid (DHA) is 200 mg/day and can be met by one to two portions of fish per week (Koletzko et al, 2007) (see *Focus On:* Omega-3 Fatty Acids in Pregnancy and Lactation).

Vitamins

All vitamins and minerals are needed for optimal pregnancy outcome. In some instances requirements may be met through diet; for others a supplement, started preconceptually, is often necessary. Many, but not all, vitamin and mineral recommendations increase with pregnancy, but the magnitude of the increase varies by nutrient (see the DRI tables on the inside cover).

Folic Acid. The RDA for dietary folate equivalents increases to support maternal erythropoiesis, DNA synthesis, and fetal and placental growth. Low folate levels are associated with miscarriages, LBW, and preterm birth. Early maternal folate deficiency is associated with an increased incidence of congenital malformations, including NTDs (including spina bifida and anencephaly), and possibly orofacial clefts and congenital heart defects (Guéant et al, 2013; Obeid et al, 2013). Approximately 3000 new cases of NTDs occur in the United States annually (CDC, 2014a).

Because more than half of all U.S. pregnancies are unplanned, and the neural tube closes by 28 days of gestation, before most women realize they are pregnant, the Centers for Disease Control and Prevention (CDC) recommends that all women of childbearing age in anticipation of pregnancy increase their intake of folic acid by 400 mcg/day, the synthetic version that is available in supplements and fortified foods, especially some breakfast cereals (CDC, 2014a). The U.S. Preventive Services Task Force (USPSTF) recommends 400 to 800 mcg/day of folic acid preconceptually. Women who have had a previous NTD-affected pregnancy should consume 400 mcg/day when not planning to conceive; those planning pregnancy should consider 4000 mcg/day (4 mg/day) from 1 month before to 3 months after conception (CDC, 2014a). These higher doses should be taken as a separate supplement and not as part of a multiple vitamin supplement to avoid excess intakes of other nutrients in the multivitamin. Although this level is recommended by many medical providers, the lower dose may be equally beneficial. Supplementation recommendations vary by country (Talaulikar and Arulkumaran, 2011), and some evidence suggests that, although the 800 mcg dose achieves recommended blood levels in 4 weeks, the 400 mcg dose requires 8 to 12 weeks to reach these levels (Berti et al, 2011). Also available is synthetic 5-methyltetrahydrofolate, the primary circulating form of folate proposed to be better used, especially by those with polymorphisms (see Chapter 5), and without the detrimental rise in unmetabolized folic acid. However, its role in preventing NTDs or other birth defects is untested in clinical trials (Obeid et al, 2013).

Red blood cell folate levels exceeding 906 nmol/L (400 ng/ml) have been associated with the fewest NTDs (Obeid et al, 2013). Natural folate is less bioavailable and has not been shown to raise blood levels as well as the synthetic folic acid or to lower the risk of NTDs. Although theoretically natural folate could be effective, 6 to 12 cups of raw spinach (more than 2 cups cooked) daily is the bioequivalent level of natural folate that is found in one bowl of fortified breakfast cereal.

Women who are obese or who smoke, consume alcohol moderately or heavily, or use recreational drugs are at risk for marginal folate status, as are those with malabsorption syndromes or genetic differences related to methylation and the metabolic use of dietary folate, including the estimated 11% of the U.S. population with the MTHFR 677 C to T variation (Caudill, 2010). European prevalence is estimated to be 10% to 22% (Obeid et al, 2013). Although increased folate intake is helpful, added riboflavin also may be beneficial (see Chapters 5 and 7). Women using antiseizure medications must be monitored closely when starting folic acid because it can reduce their seizure control (see Chapter 8).

Enriched grain products in the United States are fortified with folic acid and are estimated to provide an average 200 mcg/day, with resulting higher blood folate levels and reduced (19% to 54%) NTD rates (Caudill, 2010). Because NTD rates remain higher among the Hispanic population in the United States, targeted fortification of corn masa flour has been proposed. However, grain fortification also exposes the entire population to extra folic acid, which is potentially undesirable; in some countries, folic acid fortification is not practiced.

Possible adverse effects include masking of vitamin B_{12} deficiency, tumor promotion, epigenetic hypermethylation, interference with antifolate treatments, and an increase in miscarriages and multiple births. Widespread problems have not been seen. However, high intakes of folic acid also have potential epigenetic effects, but data are fragmentary and sometimes conflicting. Caution is advised with the use of pharmacologic doses (Milagro et al, 2013). For example, although some studies have seen no negative effects on DNA methylation at doses up to 4000 mcg/day (Crider et al, 2011), other studies have found that in the context of low vitamin B_{12} status, supplementing pregnant women with just 500 mcg/day was associated with an increased risk of offspring adiposity and insulin resistance at age 6 (Yajnik et al, 2008).

On the other hand, adequate folic acid in the second trimester may decrease inflammation, and folate status is associated inversely with the severity of bacterial vaginosis, a documented risk factor for preterm delivery (Dunlop et al, 2011). Murine studies have found that the negative effect of maternal exposure to bisphenol A is effectively neutralized by maternal supplementation with folic acid, betaine, and choline (Guéant et al, 2013). Supplementation with methyl donors, such as folic acid, also may reduce the harmful effects of fumonisin (a mycotoxin produced by *Fusarium* molds that grow on agricultural commodities, especially corn, that has been associated with increased risk of NTDs) contamination and of a father's exposure to dioxins (Guéant et al, 2013).

An estimated 50% to 70% (not 100%) of NTDs could be prevented with the periconceptual use of 400 mcg folic acid/day (CDC, 2014a). Optimal levels of other methyl donors (B_2, B_6, B_{12}, and choline) may also lower the risk of NTDs and improve birth weight.

Vitamin B_6. Pyridoxine functions as a cofactor for many decarboxylase and transaminase enzymes, especially those involved in amino acid metabolism. Although this vitamin catalyzes a number of reactions involving neurotransmitter production, it is not known whether this function is involved in the relief of nausea and vomiting. Because meat, fish, and poultry are good dietary sources, deficiency is not common, and routine prenatal vitamins contain sufficient amounts (Hovdenak and Haram, 2012). Regarding nausea and vomiting, standard doses of 25 mg three times per day have questionable efficacy but do not appear to be dangerous.

Vitamin B_{12}. Cobalamin is required for enzyme reactions and for generation of methionine and tetrahydrofolate; it is important in growth and development, including immune function (Wu et al, 2012a). Vitamin B_{12} is naturally found exclusively in foods of animal origin, so vegetarians, especially vegans, are at risk for dietary vitamin B_{12} deficiency and should consume fortified foods or supplements. Also at risk are those people with malabsorption, including those with Crohn's disease involving the terminal ileum, women who have had gastric bypass surgery, and those using proton pump inhibitor medications (see Chapter 8) (People taking metformin also may be at risk). Deficiencies in folate and vitamin B_{12} have been related to depression in adults. Inadequate amounts of folate and B_{12} may affect negatively infant cognitive and motor development as well as increase risk of NTDs and inadequate fetal growth.

Choline. Choline is needed for structural integrity of cell membranes, cell signaling, and nerve impulse transmission and is a major source of methyl groups. Choline and folate are metabolically interrelated; both support fetal brain development and lower risk of NTDs and orofacial clefts (Zeisel, 2013). Choline also appears to be important in placental functioning and may affect maternal and fetal responses to stress.

The DRI for choline increases slightly during pregnancy. Genetic variations and concurrent intakes of folate and methionine may affect requirements, and de novo synthesis may not meet fetal and maternal needs (Zeisel, 2013). Choline-rich foods include milk, meat, and eggs (see Table 15-9), and women not eating these foods may need supplementation. Many popular prenatal supplements do not contain choline and those that do contain very little. Large supplemental doses may cause gastrointestinal discomfort, but a small study using 750 mg during pregnancy did not identify adverse effects (Zeisel, 2013).

Vitamin C. The DRI for vitamin C increases during pregnancy and may be even higher for those who smoke, abuse alcohol or drugs, or regularly take aspirin. Daily consumption of good food sources should be encouraged. Low plasma levels are associated with preterm labor (Dror and Allen, 2012), possibly

TABLE 15-9	Choline Content of Selected Foods	
Food	**Serving Size**	**Choline (mg)**
Eggs		
Egg, whole	1 large	146.9
Egg, white	1 large	0.4
Egg, yolk	1 large	139.4
Fish		
Fish, Atlantic cod	3 oz	71.1
Fish, pink salmon	3 oz	96.4
Shrimp	3 oz	115.1
Oysters, Eastern	3 oz	110.5
Meats		
Beef chuck	3 oz	93.7
Beef liver	3 oz	362.1
Beef kidneys	3 oz	436.2
Beef brains	3 oz	417.3
Beef heart	3 oz	194.5
Pork loin	3 oz	65.7
Chicken, dark meat	3 oz	84.2
Chicken, light meat	3 oz	72.5
Chicken liver	3 oz	277.8
Turkey, dark meat	3 oz	76.8
Turkey, light meat	3 oz	59.3
Milk		
Milk, whole	1 cup	34.9
Milk, skim	1 cup	39.2
Cheese, cheddar	1.5 oz	7.0
Others		
Soybeans, mature, roasted	1 oz	35.2
Peanuts, dry roasted	1 oz	15.7
Mushrooms, shiitake, cooked	½ cup	26.7
Mushrooms, white, cooked	½ cup	15.9
Broccoli, cooked	½ cup	31.3
Bread, white	1 slice	4.1
Bread, whole wheat	1 slice	8.7

Adapted from *United States Department of Agriculture, Nutrient Data Labs:* USDA food composition tables, release 26 (website): http://ndb.nal.usda.gov/ndb/search/list, 2014. Accessed January 2014.

because of its antioxidant function or its role in collagen synthesis. However supplemental vitamin C is not recommended for the prevention of premature rupture of membranes (PROM). Supplementation with vitamin C (1000 mg) along with vitamin E (400 IU) also is not recommended for prevention of preeclampsia (ACOG, 2013e) and actually may increase risk of gestational hypertension and PROM (Dror and Allen, 2012). Vitamin C is actively transported across the placenta, so there is also potential for excessive levels in the fetus (Dror and Allen, 2012).

Vitamin A. Vitamin A is critical during periods of rapid growth, important in cellular differentiation, ocular development, immune function, and lung development and maturity, as well as gene expression (Wu et al, 2012a). Low vitamin A levels are associated with IUGR and increased risk of maternal and neonatal mortality. Malformations are seen in animals exposed to deficiencies, but confirmation of human malformations has not been established. However, among women positive for human immunodeficiency virus (HIV), improved vitamin A status is associated with improved birth weight possibly by improving immunity (Hovdenak and Haram, 2012).

Excess preformed vitamin A is teratogenic. Supplementation is usually not necessary and is often limited to 5000 IU/day, although doses up to 10,000 IU/day are not associated with increased risk of malformations (Hovdenak and Haram, 2012). The acne medication isotretinoin is a vitamin A analog, and exposed infants are at extremely high risk for fetal anomalies and miscarriages. Women should stop its use for at least 1 month before conception. Beta-carotene is not associated with birth defects. Although no cases have been seen, theoretically someone eating liver could consume as much preformed vitamin A as has been associated with fetal anomalies, so large amounts of liver, liver pâté, and liverwurst or braunschweiger are not recommended in the first trimester.

Vitamin D. According to the IOM, vitamin D requirements do not increase during pregnancy; intakes of 600 IU/day (15 mcg/day) are sufficient when considering bone health. The few dietary sources of vitamin D are salmon and other fatty fish, as well as some fortified breakfast cereals and mushrooms exposed to UV light. Not all dairy products are fortified, but liquid milk (if sold interstate) is a good source, usually containing 100 IU/8 oz (see Appendix Table 51 and *Clinical Insight: Vitamin D: How Much Sun is Needed?*).

CLINICAL INSIGHT

Vitamin D: How Much Sun Is Needed?

Skin exposure is the best source of vitamin D, but the amount of sun exposure that is necessary is difficult to predict. For example, a Caucasian with light skin at 42° N (latitude for Boston or Chicago) can satisfy her vitamin D requirements by exposing arms and legs to sunlight (at noon on a clear day) for 5 to 15 minutes 2 to 3 times/week in the summertime. On the other hand, people living north of 35° N (or south of 35° S) can produce almost no vitamin D in the winter months. A person's age, BMI, and skin pigmentation, the use of sunscreen, clothing style, the time of day, season of the year, latitude, altitude, and weather conditions all matter (Holick, 2014). See Appendix 51 for apps for estimating sun exposure requirements and vitamin D in foods.

Vitamin D deficiency is recognized increasingly in dark-skinned and veiled women living in latitudes where sun exposure is low. Women who are at risk of entering pregnancy with low vitamin D levels also include those with BMI more than 30, those with fat malabsorption, and those with high use of sunblock, along with poor dietary intake. Screening for vitamin D status is advised for those women (ACOG, 2011).

Severe vitamin D deficiency is associated with congenital rickets and newborn fractures and also may manifest as seizures (ACOG, 2011), although it is unknown if calcium insufficiency also plays a role (Brannon and Picciano, 2011). There is concern that low maternal vitamin D status may negatively affect fetal bone accrual. However, small studies have shown that although maternal supplementation can increase cord blood levels, there is no effect on fetal calcium, phosphorus, parathyroid hormone (PTH), or skeletal parameters (Kovacs, 2012). A recent study found no association between maternal vitamin D status and her offspring's bone mineral content at ages 9 to 10 years (Lawlor et al, 2013).

Vitamin D metabolism changes in pregnancy, with the conversion of 25(OH)D to 1,25(OH)$_2$D drastically increased (Pludowski et al, 2013). 1,25(OH)$_2$D levels are three times nonpregnant levels by 12 weeks and keep rising throughout the pregnancy, depending on 25(OH)D availability. These levels are not associated with hypercalciuria or hypercalcemia and appear to be driven by the pregnancy itself rather than by increasing vitamin D-binding protein levels. Mechanisms are still unknown but likely include an uncoupling of renal 1-alpha-hydroxylase from feedback control and upregulating it twofold to fivefold for reasons other than calcium homeostasis (Kovacs, 2012). It is assumed that high 1,25(OH)$_2$D values increase delivery of vitamin D to tissues and may modulate innate and adaptive immunity. Vitamin D may be important in regulating gene expression and in promoting successful implantation (Wu et al, 2012a). It also may have a role in preventing preeclampsia, preterm delivery, gestational diabetes, bacterial vaginosis, and the need for cesarean delivery. In addition, it may be involved in the development of the infant's immune function and development of allergy, and other developmental programming (Brannon and Picciano, 2011), including risk of type 1 diabetes (Kovacs, 2012). However, associations are inconclusive, often contradictory, confounded, and lack causality. Although supplementation raises maternal vitamin D levels, it has not been positively associated with improved obstetric outcomes (Kovacs, 2012).

Optimal serum levels of 25(OH)D during pregnancy are not yet known but must be at least 20 ng/ml (50 nmol/L) for bone health (ACOG, 2011). Other experts suggest at least 32 ng/ml (80 nmol/L) for pregnancy, but increased risk of growth restriction at levels exceeding 70 nmol/L and child eczema at levels exceeding 75 nmol/L also have been reported (Brannon and Picciano, 2011). Research is active and ongoing. Vitamin D supplementation may be needed to reach desired serum concentrations, although there is insufficient evidence to recommend routine supplementation. A dosage of 1000 to 2000 IU/day of vitamin D appears safe (ACOG, 2011). Although some researchers have found no hypercalciuria with 4000 IU/day (the UL), caution is advised; only spot checks of urine were done, not 24-hour urine collections, and there was no long-term follow-up on kidney stone formation rates (Kovacs, 2012). Very high supplementation ($\geq$1000 mcg = 40,000 IU/day) has been associated with hypercalcemia, and although vitamin D does not appear to be teratogenic, some animal data suggest the need for concern (Roth, 2011). The potency of vitamin D supplements is variable; many contain less than the labeled amounts (LeBlanc et al, 2013).

Vitamin E. Vitamin E requirements do not increase. Although deficiency is speculated to cause miscarriage, preterm birth, preeclampsia, and IUGR, vitamin E deficiency specifically has not yet been reported in human pregnancy. Vitamin E is an important lipophilic antioxidant, but supplementation of vitamin E (along with vitamin C) is not an effective strategy for preventing preeclampsia nor does it reduce risk of fetal or neonatal loss, SGA, or preterm delivery. Supplementation actually may be proinflammatory, preventing the switch from Th1 cytokines (proinflammatory) to Th2 cytokines (antiinflammatory) that is normal during pregnancy (Hovdenak and Haram, 2012; see Appendix 49 for food sources of vitamin E).

Vitamin K. Although vitamin K requirements do not increase during pregnancy, usual diets often do not provide sufficient vitamin K as most food sources (e.g., dark leafy green vegetables) are not consumed in recommended amounts. Vitamin K has an important role in bone health as well as in coagulation homeostasis, so adequate amounts during pregnancy are vital (see Chapter 24). Vitamin K deficiency has been reported in women who have had hyperemesis gravidarum,

Crohn's disease, or gastric bypass. See Appendix 50 for sources of vitamin K.

Minerals

Calcium. Hormonal factors strongly influence calcium metabolism in pregnancy. Human placental lactogen modestly increases the rate of maternal bone turnover, and although estrogen inhibits bone resorption, accretion and resorption increase. Maternal absorption of calcium across the gut doubles during pregnancy (Olausson et al, 2012). PTH often drops in North American and European women consuming adequate calcium. In areas with lower calcium diets that are also rich in phytates, PTH levels stay the same or increase; more research is necessary on the limitations of maternal response when intakes are marginal or low (Olausson et al, 2012). These changes maintain maternal serum calcium levels and promote calcium retention to meet progressively increasing fetal skeletal demands for mineralization. Fetal hypercalcemia and subsequent endocrine adjustments ultimately stimulate the mineralization process.

The net effects of pregnancy and lactation on the maternal skeleton are not yet clear. Bone mineral is mobilized during pregnancy and replenished starting in later lactation. The degree of bone changes varies considerably by site and also between individuals; it appears that genetics, endocrine responses, and nutritional factors are important. No prospective studies have examined whether there is increased risk of osteoporosis later in life attributed to pregnancy or lactation; retrospective studies are inconsistent. Higher intakes are associated with improved calcium balance when intakes are low, but some evidence suggests that supplementation may temporarily disrupt the process of adaptation to habitually low intakes (Olausson et al, 2012).

Approximately 30 g of calcium is accumulated during pregnancy, primarily in the fetal skeleton (25 g), but there is wide variation. The remainder is stored in the maternal skeleton, held in reserve for the calcium demands of lactation. Most fetal accretion occurs during the last half of pregnancy, increasing from 50 mg/day at 20 weeks to 330 mg/day at 35 weeks (Olausson et al, 2012). There is conflicting evidence regarding whether maternal calcium intake affects a child's long-term accretion.

In addition to its role in bone formation, low calcium intake is associated with increased risk of IUGR and preeclampsia (Hovdenak and Haram, 2012). Calcium also is involved in many other processes, including blood clotting, intracellular proteolysis, nitric oxide synthesis, and has a role in regulating uterine contractions (Wu et al, 2012a).

The requirement for calcium during pregnancy does not increase. However, many women enter pregnancy with low intakes and often need encouragement to increase consumption of calcium-rich foods. Dairy products are the most common sources of dietary calcium.

Milk, including extra dry milk powder, can be incorporated into foods. One-third cup of dried skim milk is equivalent to 1 cup of fluid milk. Small amounts can be added to liquid milk; much more can be added to foods with stronger flavors. Although most of the dry milk sold in the United States is nonfat, powdered whole milk is also available in the ethnic food sections of grocery stores. Yogurt is often well accepted, and using plain nonfat yogurt with fruit and minimal added sugar can maximize nutrients without providing as many extra calories. Greek yogurt, although higher in protein, may contain less calcium than regular yogurt. Although cheese can be used, often the higher calories from fat become a limiting factor. Lactose intolerance can be managed (see Chapter 28).

Soy milks are fortified with calcium, but this often precipitates to the bottom of the container. It is difficult to reincorporate the sludge, with the milk containing only 31% of the labeled amount without shaking, 59% with shaking (Heaney and Rafferty, 2006). The fortificant should be calcium carbonate for best absorption. Other drinks, including enriched rice, coconut, and nut milks, are often low in protein, and caution is advised. Regarding vegetable sources of calcium, the concern is one of quantity and bioavailability (see Table 15-10 and Appendix 51).

Care should be taken when considering the use of calcium supplements. Overconsumption of calcium through food is not common; however, elevated serum calcium levels also can result from excess antacid ingestion if the UL is exceeded (see Heartburn).

Copper. Diets of pregnant women are often marginal in copper, and requirements rise slightly in pregnancy. In addition to primary deficiency from genetic mutation (Menkes disease),

TABLE 15-10 Comparison of Absorbable Calcium with 1 cup Milk

Food	Calcium Content	Fractional Absorption	Estimated Absorbed Calcium	Amount Needed to Equal 1 c Milk
Milk	300 mg/c	32.1%	96.3 mg	1.0 cup
Beans, pinto	44.7 mg/0.5 c*	26.7	11.9	4.05 cups, cooked*
Beans, red	40.5 mg/0.5 c	24.4	9.9	4.85 cups
Beans, white	113 mg/0.5 c	21.8	24.7	1.95 cups
Bok choy	79 mg/0.5 c	53.8	42.5	1.15 cups
Broccoli	35 mg/0.5 c	61.3	21.5	2.25 cups
Cheddar cheese	303 mg/1.5 oz	32.1	97.2	1.5 oz
Chinese mustard greens	212 mg/0.5 c	40.2	85.3	0.55 cup
Chinese spinach	347 mg/0.5 c	8.36	29.0	1.65 cups
Kale	61 mg/0.5 c	49.3	30.1	1.6 cups
Spinach	115 mg/0.5 c	5.1	5.9	8.15 cups
Sweet potatoes	44 mg/0.5 c	22.2	9.8	4.9 cups
Tofu with calcium	258 mg/0.5 c	31.0	80.0	0.6 cup
Yogurt	300 mg/c	32.1	96.3	1.0 cup

* All vegetables are cooked portions.
Adapted from Weaver CM et al: Choices for achieving adequate dietary calcium with a vegetarian diet, *Am J Clin Nutr* 70:543s, 1999.

secondary deficiency from increased zinc or iron intake, certain drugs, and gastric bypass surgery is also of concern. Copper deficiency alters embryo development; induced copper deficiency has been shown to be teratogenic. There is decreased activity of cuproenzymes, increased oxidative stress, altered iron metabolism, abnormal protein crosslinking, decreased angiogenesis, and altered cell signaling (Uriu-Adams et al, 2010). Copper interacts with iron, affecting neurocognitive and neurobehavioral development. Although not commonly included in prenatal supplements, it is recommended that copper be supplemented when zinc and iron are given during pregnancy (Uriu-Adams et al, 2010).

Fluoride. The role of fluoride in prenatal development is controversial, and fluoride requirements do not increase during pregnancy. Development of primary dentition begins at 10 to 12 weeks' gestation. From the sixth to the ninth month, the first four permanent molars and eight of the permanent incisors are forming. Thus 32 teeth are developing during gestation. Controversy involves the extent to which fluoride is transported across the placenta and its value in utero in the development of caries-resistant permanent teeth (see Chapter 25). Most bottled water does not contain fluoride.

Iodine. Iodine is part of the thyroxine molecule, with a critical role in the metabolism of macronutrients, as well as in fetal neuronal myelination and gene expression (Wu et al, 2012a). Because the thyroid hormone synthesis increases 50% during pregnancy, iodine requirements also increase (Stagnaro-Green and Pearce, 2012). Severe iodine deficiency is associated with increased risk of miscarriage, congenital anomalies, fetal goiter, and stillbirth, as well as prematurity, poor fetal growth, and decreased IQ. Infant cretinism, although rare in the United States, is a significant public health problem; iodine deficiency is the most common cause of preventable mental retardation in the world (Leung et al, 2013).

Worldwide, many people are at risk for iodine deficiency caused by low intake of seafood or by consuming produce grown in iodine-deficient soils, especially if eating locally and consuming goitrogens or exposed to perchlorate contamination. An estimated 70% of the world population has access to iodized salt (Pearce et al, 2013). Salt iodization is voluntary in the United States and Canada; iodized salt rarely is used in processed foods, the primary source of dietary sodium, and must be labeled if used. Kosher salt and sea salt do not naturally contain iodine. Women should be encouraged to use iodized salt when cooking at home and to limit the intake of processed foods made with uniodized salt.

Median urinary iodine values in the United States have declined, mainly because of the reduction of iodine in dairy and bread products, such that 35% of U.S. women of childbearing age now have urinary iodine values suggesting mild iodine deficiency or insufficiency (Leung et al, 2013). Similar reductions have been seen in women in other developed countries as well (Pearce et al, 2013).

Although the effects of severe iodine deficiency on fetal brain development are well established, the effects of milder deficits are not as clear. Results of supplementation studies are mixed regarding thyroid function and the neurodevelopment of children, but children of women with mild to moderate deficiency demonstrate better neurocognitive scores if mothers were supplemented starting very early in pregnancy, that is, by 4 to 6 weeks' gestation (Leung et al, 2013). Current research is studying the effect of iodine supplementation on obstetric outcomes and long-term child development (Stagnaro-Green and Pearce, 2013).

Because of the concern that a subset of the population may be at risk for mild deficiency, the American Thyroid Association now recommends that women receive 150 mcg/day during pregnancy and lactation as potassium iodide, given the variability of iodine content in kelp and seaweed (Leung et al, 2013; Stagnaro-Green and Pearce, 2012). However, only half the prenatal supplements in the United States contain iodine, and the content is highly variable.

High iodine levels are also of concern, potentially causing the same symptoms as low levels. There is concern about the safety of iodine supplementation in areas of iodine sufficiency, but the problems appear to be temporary (Pearce et al, 2013). However, congenital hypothyroidism resulting from high prenatal intake of seaweeds has been documented (Nishiyama et al, 2004). The iodine content is variable, but kombu and kelp often contain extremely high levels, and ingesting even very small amounts may be problematic (Teas et al, 2004). Very high breastmilk iodine levels also have been seen among Korean women ingesting the customary brown seaweed soup postpartum (Rhee et al, 2011), and it is not recommended for those whose babies are preterm.

As a reminder, postpartum thyroiditis affects an estimated 5.4% of all women (Stagnaro-Green and Pearce, 2012). Thyroiditis can manifest as either hyper- or hypothyroidism, and both can affect breastmilk production (see Chapter 32).

Iron. The RDA for iron nearly doubles in pregnancy. An estimated 42% of pregnant women worldwide have iron deficiency anemia, with wide regional variability. Although prevalence is highest in developing countries, an estimated 33% of low-income pregnant women in the United States are anemic in the third trimester (Murray-Kolb, 2011).

Inadequate iron consumption may lead to poor hemoglobin production, followed by compromised delivery of oxygen to the uterus, placenta, and developing fetus. Iron deficiency anemia (IDA) is associated with IUGR, preterm delivery, increased fetal and neonatal mortality, and if severe (hemoglobin <9 g/dl), with complications during delivery (Lee and Okam, 2011). IDA also is associated with increased fetal cortisol production and oxidative damage to fetal erythrocytes (Hovdenak and Haram, 2012). Early iron deficiency affects fetal brain development and the regulation of brain function in multiple ways (see Table 15-7). Neonatal iron deficiency can result if the mother is extremely iron deficient, but maternal hypertension and therefore restricted blood flow, as well as maternal smoking and prematurity, also increase the risk. Infants of mothers with diabetes are also more likely to develop iron deficiency because of increased fetal demands. These changes result in long-term neurobehavioral impairments affecting temperament, interactions with others, learning, and memory and also may result in genomic changes (Georgieff, 2011).

Maternal effects of IDA include fatigue, dyspnea, light-headedness, and poor exercise tolerance. Prenatal weight gain is likely to be low. Mother is at risk of increased blood loss with uterine atony during delivery, thus increasing her risk of needing a blood transfusion. Wound healing and immune function are impaired. She is more likely to suffer from postpartum depression, poor maternal/infant interaction, and impaired lactation. There is some evidence that negative alterations in cognition, emotions, quality of life, and behavior may occur before overt IDA is reached, but the degree of iron deficiency associated with negative consequences remains unknown (Murray-Kolb, 2011). Treatment during pregnancy improves maternal iron status postpartum and also is associated with improved infant development (Murray-Kolb, 2011).

Plasma volume increases 50% from baseline, and normal erythrocyte volume increases by 20% to 30% in pregnancy (Lee and Okam, 2011). This marked increase in the maternal blood supply during pregnancy, as well as fetal needs, greatly increases the demand for iron. The estimated total requirement for pregnancy is 1190 mg, but with the cessation of menses, the average net deficit is 580 mg (Lee and Okam, 2011). Added to her normal requirements, a pregnant woman often needs to absorb 17 mg/day; normal absorption is often 1 to 2 mg/day from a normal diet, and 3 to 5 mg/day if the diet contains high-iron foods (Lee and Okam, 2011). Most accretion occurs after the twentieth week of gestation, when maternal and fetal demands are greatest. Those at highest risk of IDA are women with inadequate iron stores, including those with short interconceptual periods, poor habitual intakes, those with impaired absorption, including those with a history of bariatric surgery or chronic use of antacids, those who have experienced red cell destruction from malaria or excessive blood loss from heavy menstrual flow or prior hookworm infections.

A first trimester serum ferritin level may be assessed and if less than 20 mcg/L, supplementation may be necessary (Lee and Okam, 2011). However, checking red blood cell indices on the complete blood count (CBC) (see Chapter 7) is often adequate. Hemoglobin and hematocrit values decrease in the second trimester (see Table 15-5); not decreasing is a sign of poor blood volume expansion, associated wth increasing risk of a growth-restricted infant, preterm delivery, and stillbirth (Luke, 2015). Serum values should increase again in the third trimester for best outcomes, but often this rise is not seen and intervention is merited. If anemia does not improve with iron therapy (i.e., an increase of 1 g hemoglobin or 3% in hematocrit by 4 weeks [CDC, 1998]), it is advised to check vitamins B_6, B_{12}, and folate status, although many other nutrients, including protein, cobalt, magnesium, selenium, zinc, copper, vitamins A and C, lipids, and carbohydrate, also may play a role (Lee and Okam, 2011; Mechanick et al, 2013; Wu et al, 2012a).

Because many women do not enter pregnancy with sufficient iron stores to cover the physiologic needs of pregnancy, iron supplementation (usually as a ferrous salt) often is prescribed, but the amount of elemental iron contained varies by the preparation (ODS iron 2014). The iron in the supplement already is reduced (i.e., ferrous rather than ferric), so taking the supplement with water is effective and consuming it with juice is not necessary. As with all nonheme sources, supplements should not be taken with coffee, tea, or milk to optimize absorption; iron supplements should be taken separately from the prenatal vitamins. Absorption is best if taken on an empty stomach, but tolerance is often worse. Multiple supplements should be taken separately from each other to maximize absorption, but diminishing absorption is seen with increasing dosage, so tolerance of side effects should be balanced against need. Enteric-coated and delayed-release preparations produce fewer side effects, but because they are not well absorbed they are not recommended. Parenteral iron is also available. Although it will promote a faster response, it also is associated with more potential complications. However, newer, safer preparations are now available (Lee and Okam, 2011).

Iron supplementation is controversial. CDC and WHO recommend early iron supplementation to lower the risk of LBW. The U.S. Preventive Services Task Force (USPSTF) recently reported that, while supplementation may improve maternal iron status, the evidence supporting routine supplementation to improve either maternal or infant clinical outcomes is inconclusive (Cantor et al, 2015). ACOG recommends screening everyone and supplementing those with documented IDA. However, for those at risk of chronic iron overload, including those with hemochromatosis and beta-thalassemia, iron supplementation may not be recommended. Iron supplements may cause oxidative damage and may exacerbate inflammation; overtreatment of IDA is now thought to be associated with preterm delivery, IUGR, and GDM (Hovdenak and Haram, 2012; see Chapter 3 for other examples of oxidative damage). Intermittent supplementation (one to two times per week) may be effective (Kaiser and Campbell, 2014). In addition, iron supplements are extremely dangerous for small children. Doses as little as 36 mg elemental iron/kg body weight have been lethal (ODS, 2014), so mothers must be reminded to keep supplements out of the reach of children.

Because of the concerns with iron supplementation, including compliance, safety, and effectiveness, emphasizing dietary sources of iron is necessary. The best sources of iron are red meats (see Box 15-4) because of their heme content, and many

---

BOX 15-4 Comparison of Selected Iron Sources

Serving sizes for meats are all 3 oz. Ranges depend on the type of animal or the cut of meat.

Excellent Sources of Iron

Spleen	6.26-33.46 mg
Bear	9.12 mg
Liver	4.34-25.95 mg limit in first trimester
Braunschweiger/liverwurst	5.44-9.53 mg limit in first trimester
Octopus	8.11 mg
Oysters	5.70-7.83 mg
Mussels	5.71 mg
Blood sausage	5.44 mg
Kidneys	4.5-10.54 mg
Heart	3.67-7.68 mg

Good Sources of Iron

Horse	4.28 mg
Antelope	3.57 mg
Deer/Venison	2.85-4.26 mg
Goat	3.17 mg
Elk	2.84-3.47 mg
Gizzards	2.71-3.13 mg
Bison	2.45-4.13 mg
Sardines	1.95-2.48 mg
Beef	1.44-3.20 mg
Tongue	1.78 4.24 mg
Clams	2.39 mg
Lamb	1.52-2.38 mg
Shrimp	1.81 mg

Fair Sources of Iron

Breakfast cereals that say "iron fortified"	9-18 mg/ serving
Chitterlings (intestines)	1.25 mg
Stomach	0.56-1.05 mg
Pork	0.54-1.57 mg
Leg and thigh of chicken or turkey	0.44-1.35 mg
Tuna	0.55-1.39 mg
Breast of chicken or turkey	0.37-0.97 mg

Adapted from United States Department of Agriculture (USDA), Nutrient Data Labs: *USDA food composition tables, release 27* (website): http://ndb.nal.usda.gov/ndb/search/list, 2015. Accessed June 2015.

organ meats may contain even higher levels of iron. It is important to limit the amount of liver and liver products (pâté, liverwurst, braunschweiger) in the first trimester because of their high vitamin A contents.

Vegetable sources, containing only nonheme iron, are less well absorbed, and volume may become the limiting factor, especially late in pregnancy. Absorption can be enhanced by eating them with ascorbic acid or a little meat.

Women who follow vegetarian diets should pay particular attention to iron and try to prevent having their hematocrit drop so far that it cannot recover sufficiently. Followers of Jehovah's Witness also must pay close attention to their iron levels. Because they choose not to receive blood transfusions, these women should receive nutrition counseling on high-iron foods early in pregnancy, with reinforcement as the pregnancy continues.

Magnesium. Magnesium functions as an enzyme cofactor and activator. The full-term fetus accumulates 1 g of magnesium during gestation, and maternal deficiency may interfere with fetal growth and development, including possible teratogenesis (Hovdenak and Haram, 2012). Recommendations for magnesium increase slightly during pregnancy. Magnesium sulfate is sometimes used to treat women with preeclampsia. Maternal magnesium deficiency has been speculated to play a part in increased risk for SIDS, but prospective supplementation trials have not been done. Optimal magnesium levels may be beneficial in helping prevent leg cramps (see Edema and Leg Cramps). However, too few data are available to give supplementation recommendations (Hovdenak and Haram, 2012). See Appendix 50 for good dietary sources.

Phosphorus. Phosphorus is found in a variety of foods, and deficiency is rare if one is able to eat normally. Requirements do not rise with pregnancy. However, low phosphorus levels, indicative of "refeeding syndrome," have been found in women experiencing severe vomiting or other situations resulting in starvation. Hypophosphatemia can be life threatening because phosphorus is important in energy metabolism as a component of adenosine triphosphate (ATP) and must be replenished promptly.

Selenium. Selenium functions as an antioxidant and is important for reproduction. Low selenium status is associated with recurrent miscarriages, preeclampsia, and IUGR. The DRI increases slightly during pregnancy, but there are no evidence-based recommendations for supplementation (Hovdenak and Haram, 2012). Excess selenium intake is also of concern, especially if women eat locally from areas where soil selenium contents are high. There are no known areas in the United States or Canada with recognized cases of selenosis.

Sodium. The hormonal milieu of pregnancy affects sodium metabolism. Increased maternal blood volume leads to increased glomerular filtration of sodium; compensatory mechanisms maintain fluid and electrolyte balance.

Rigorous sodium restriction stresses the renin-angiotensin-aldosterone system. Although moderation in the use of salt and other sodium-rich foods is appropriate for the general population, aggressive restriction is usually unwarranted in pregnancy, and the use of diuretics in pregnant women with edema is not recommended. Normal intakes are often much higher than the DRI, which does not increase during pregnancy. ACOG recommends that sodium intake should not be restricted below 2300 mg/day (ACOG, 2013e). Use of iodized salt should be encouraged, but processed food consumption, the source of more than 75% of

dietary sodium in the United States, should be limited because of the noniodized salt content.

Zinc. Zinc is critical for growth and development, and requirements rise during pregnancy. A zinc-deficient diet does not result in effective mobilization of zinc stored in the maternal skeletal muscle and bone; therefore a compromised zinc status develops rapidly. Zinc is part of 100 enzymes related to the metabolism of macronutrients (Hovdenak and Haram, 2012). It provides a structural function in many tissues, including some proteins involved in gene expression. Deficiency is highly teratogenic, leading to congenital malformations, including anencephaly and possibly oral clefts. Even a mild zinc deficiency may lead to impaired fetal growth and brain development, as well as impaired immune function. Women with untreated low zinc levels associated with acrodermatitis enteropathica have increased risk of miscarriage, fetal growth restriction, hypertension, preeclampsia, preterm delivery, and intrapartum hemorrhage.

Zinc is widely available and good sources include red meat, seafood, whole grains, and some fortified breakfast cereals (see Appendix 53). Extra supplementation exceeding that found in prenatal vitamins usually is not required but may be necessary for women with gastrointestinal disorders that affect absorption. Overt deficiency is rare in the United States, but rates are higher where the main staple foods are high in phytates (i.e., the unrefined cereals), and women following a vegetarian diet may experience low zinc bioavailability. High levels of iron supplementation may inhibit zinc absorption if both are taken without food (Kaiser and Campbell, 2014).

Pregnancy Weight Gain Recommendations
General Weight Gain Recommendations

With a singleton gestation, less than half of the total weight gain of a normal-weight pregnant woman resides in the fetus, placenta, and amniotic fluid. The remainder is in maternal reproductive tissues (breast tissues and uterus), interstitial fluid, blood volume, and maternal adipose tissue. Increased subcutaneous fat in the abdomen, back, and upper thigh serves as an energy reserve for pregnancy and lactation. The normal distribution of weight is illustrated in Figure 15-2.

Recommended weight gains to support a healthy pregnancy vary by prepregnant BMI and are summarized in Table 15-11. Designed for women living in healthy environments, the Institute of Medicine (IOM) balanced the risk of adverse birth outcomes with the mother's risk of postpartum weight retention. Insufficient gain, especially if also associated with prepregnant

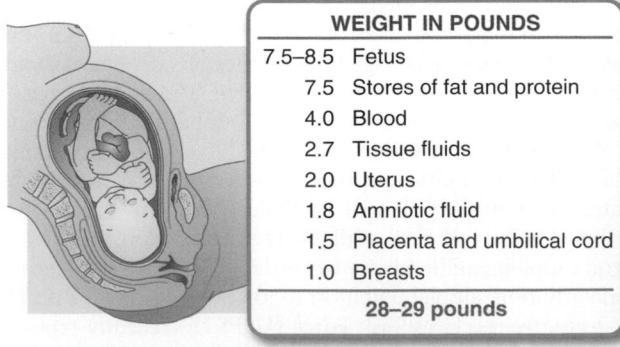

WEIGHT IN POUNDS	
7.5–8.5	Fetus
7.5	Stores of fat and protein
4.0	Blood
2.7	Tissue fluids
2.0	Uterus
1.8	Amniotic fluid
1.5	Placenta and umbilical cord
1.0	Breasts
28–29 pounds	

FIGURE 15-2 Distribution of weight gain during pregnancy.

TABLE 15-11 U.S. Institute of Medicine (IOM) Prenatal Weight Gain Goals

Prepregnant Weight Category	Total Singleton Weight Gain	Rates of Gain in 2nd and 3rd Trimesters for Singletons* Mean/week (Range)	Total Twins Weight Gain (Provisional guidelines)
Underweight BMI < 18.5	28-40 lb [12.5-18 kg]	1 lb (1-1.3) [0.51 kg (0.44-0.58)]	Insufficient information available for guideline
Normal weight BMI 18.5-24.9	25-35 lb [11.5-16 kg]	1 lb (0.8-1) [0.42 kg (0.35-0.50)]	37-54 lb [17-25 kg]
Overweight BMI 25.0-29.9	15-25 lb [7-11.5 kg]	0.6 lb (0.5-0.7) [0.28 kg (0.23-0.33)]	31-50 lb [14-23 kg]
Obese BMI ≥ 30.0	11-20 lb [5-9 kg]	0.5 lb (0.4-0.6) [0.22 kg (0.17-0.27)]	25-42 lb [11-19 kg]

* Calculations assume a first trimester gain for singleton pregnancy of 1-3 kg (2.2-6.6 lb) for women who are underweight, normal weight, or overweight and 0.5–2 kg (1.1-4.4 lb) for those who are in the obese category.

Adapted from Rasmussen KM et al: Recommendations for weight gain during pregnancy in the context of the obesity epidemic, *Obstet Gynecol* 116:1191, 2010; Rasmussen KM, Yaktine AL: *Weight gain during pregnancy: reexamining the guidelines,* Washington, DC, 2009, IOM, NRC.

underweight, is associated with increased risk of SGA babies and spontaneous preterm deliveries. Excessive gain often results in LGA babies, with increased risk during delivery. Excessive gain is also the strongest predictor of later maternal obesity. Outcomes are best when women gain within the recommended ranges. However, less than one third of pregnant women do so, and most (especially those who are overweight or obese) gain too much, although a significant proportion of underweight women gain too little (Siega-Riz and Gray, 2013).

Height and, ideally, prepregnant weight should be measured, not asked, to determine prepregnant BMI. Women need guidance on target weight gains. One third try to keep the same weight or even lose weight during pregnancy (Rasmussen and Yaktine, 2009). Weight gain should be monitored as a way to evaluate progress and to intervene when necessary. The pattern of weight gain is also important; higher rates of weight gain in the second trimester are associated with higher birth weight, especially among women whose prepregnant BMI is less than 26 (Rasmussen and Yaktine, 2009). Maternal weight gain plotted on the appropriate grid is an effective teaching tool. See Figure 15-3 for weight gain grids for singleton pregnancies.

Weight loss during pregnancy should be discouraged. There are no intervention studies documenting benefit (Furber et al, 2013). As adipose tissue is mobilized, semivolatile organic compounds may be released (see *Clinical Insight: What's in That Fat When You Lose It* in Chapter 21). Because of the accelerated starvation characteristic of pregnancy, women are more likely to develop ketonemia and ketonuria after a 12- to 18-hour fast, with ketone levels higher than in nonpregnant women. Although the fetus has a limited ability to metabolize ketones, these compounds may adversely affect fetal brain development (Rasmussen and Yaktine, 2009). In addition, mobilized protein stores, increased free fatty acids, urinary nitrogen excretion, and lower plasma glucose, insulin, and gluconeogenic amino acids have been seen, resulting in increased risk of IUGR and preterm birth (Furber et al, 2013; Rasmussen et al, 2010).

The IOM guidelines are based on observational, not interventional, data. Thus many countries do not advocate either a particular weight gain or even routine weighing after determining the prepregnant BMI status. Although there are many small intervention studies, large trials are not yet available. It also must be noted that it is unclear whether maternal weight gain itself is a critical variable or whether it is a marker for nutritional status. Even so, tracking weight gain is useful and when variation from normal patterns is noted, more questions should be asked.

Obesity Weight Gain Recommendations

Pregravid obesity is described as class I (BMI 30 to 34.9), class II (BMI 35 to 39.9), and class III (BMI at least 40). The IOM's weight gain recommendation of 11 to 20 pounds does not distinguish between these classes (Rasmussen and Yaktine, 2009). Optimal gestational weight gains for these groups are not yet known and research continues, with some evidence that lower gains, or even loss, can be managed successfully as individuals may balance intakes well enough to avoid ketonemia (Rasmussen et al, 2010). Overweight, and therefore overnutrition, is not the same as good quality nutrition and, in fact, obesity is associated with lower serum levels of carotenoids; vitamins C, D, B_6, K; folate; iron; and selenium (Saltzman and Karl, 2013). Individual guidance and clinical judgment, including optimizing nutrient intakes and encouraging exercise, is necessary, and fetal growth must be monitored (ACOG, 2013a). Although weight gain targets may be too high for some women, some evidence suggests that the risk of preterm delivery, IUGR, and perinatal mortality all increase if the weight gain is too restrictive; long-term effects also must be considered.

Postbariatric Surgery. The prevalence of obesity has resulted in an increase in bariatric surgeries. Although prepregnancy weight loss may improve fertility, it has the potential to provide a suboptimal uterine environment for the developing fetus. Pregnancy should be delayed for at least 12 to 18 months (Mechanick et al, 2013; Usadi and Legro, 2012), and adequate nutrient supplementation is essential. Which nutrients are most likely to be deficient will be determined by the type of surgery and the nutritional status since that surgery (see Chapter 21). ACOG recommends evaluating iron, calcium, vitamins B_{12}, D, and folate, and supplementing if necessary (ACOG, 2013a). Other deficiencies, although potentially severe, are more sporadic (Saltzman and Karl, 2013). If anemia does not respond to treatment, vitamin B_{12}, folate, protein, copper, selenium, and zinc should be assessed (Mechanick et al, 2013).

An optimum nutrient prescription and caloric requirement for pregnant women after bariatric surgery has not been determined and must be individualized. These women may have more difficulty eating enough if they have had a restrictive procedure and the gastric band may have to be adjusted. Those with bypass procedures may have malabsorptive problems.

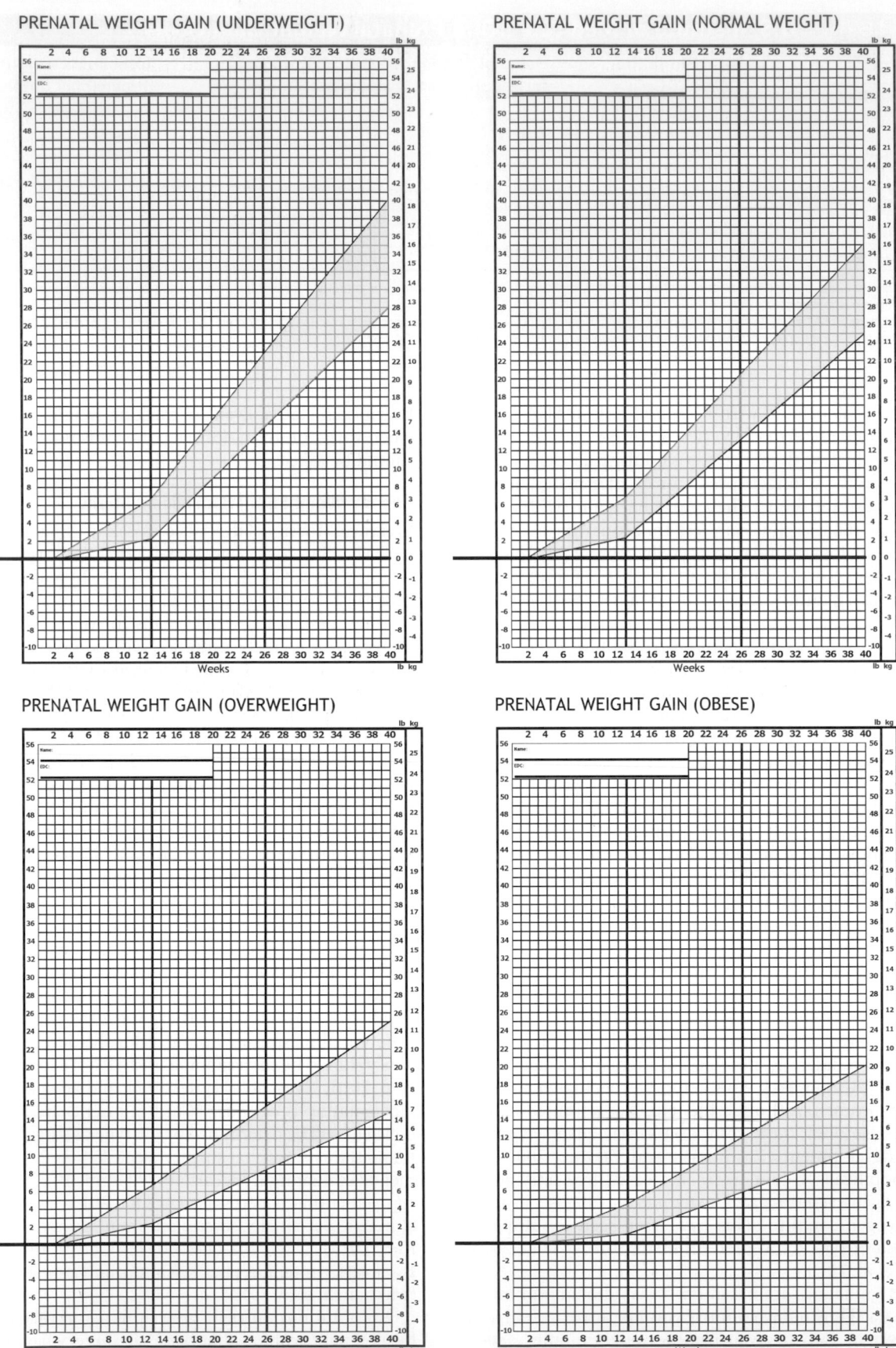

FIGURE 15-3 Desirable weight gain during singleton pregnancy for a woman whose prepregnant weight (BMI) category is a) underweight, b) normal weight, c) overweight, or d) obese. (Adapted from Rasmussen KM et al (2010): Recommendations for weight gain during pregnancy in the context of the obesity epidemic. *Obstetrics & Gynecology* 116:1191.)

Those experiencing dumping syndrome may require glucose monitoring rather than trying to use the glucola to diagnose gestational diabetes. In addition, women with a history of bariatric surgery may be less willing to gain enough weight after having invested so much in losing it, so guidance with reassurance and support may be necessary (see Chapter 21).

Women who have had bariatric surgery often have successful pregnancy outcomes, with lower rates of gestational diabetes, hypertension, preeclampsia, and macrosomia than seen among obese women who have not undergone bariatric surgery (ACOG, 2013a). However, they also may have higher risk of fetal growth restriction, shorter gestational length, and possibly increased rates of perinatal mortality (Johansson et al, 2015). If women have had Roux-en-Y or biliopancreatic diversion surgery, with or without the duodenal switch, they also have higher risk of fetal malformations (Pelizzo et al, 2014).

Multiple Births

The incidence of multiple births in the United States is rising because of the increased use of fertility drugs and ART, age at conception, and obesity rates among pregnant women. Multifetal gestations cause significant maternal physiologic adaptations beyond the usual pregnancy changes, including increased plasma volume, metabolic rate, and increased insulin resistance (Goodnight and Newman, 2009).

These infants have a greater risk of preterm delivery with accompanying IUGR or LBW than do singletons. Adequate maternal weight gain, especially early in pregnancy, has been shown to be particularly important; a rule of thumb is to target a 24-pound gain by 24 weeks for twins (Goodnight and Newman, 2009). The IOM guidelines for twins are provisional but are now delineated by prepregnant BMI (see Table 15-11).

The optimal nutrient requirements for twins and higher-order multiples are not yet known but are certainly higher than for singleton pregnancies. One nutritional plan for twins is summarized in Table 15-12 but may have to include iodine and choline as well; newer evidence cautions against high doses of vitamins C and E (see Hypertension and nutrient sections) (ACOG, 2013e; Hovdenak and Haram, 2012). Because of a greater need for nutritional density in the diet, it is recommended that only 40% of calories come from carbohydrate, with 20% from protein, and 40% from fat (Goodnight and Newman, 2009).

For those pregnant with triplets or other higher-order multiples, there is limited information available, but best practice advice does exist (Luke and Eberlein, 2011; Luke, 2015). Mean gestational weight gain for triplets is 45 to 51 pounds (20.5 to 23 kg) at 32 to 34 weeks; for quadruplets, it is 46 to 68 pounds (20.8 to 31 kg) at 31 to 32 weeks (Rasmussen and Yaktine, 2009).

Adolescent Pregnancy

Public health initiatives have helped reduce the incidence of teen pregnancies overall, but it continues as a major problem in the United States among some minority groups (CDC, 2014b). Risk factors for poor outcome in pregnant adolescents are listed in Box 15-5.

Increased rates of LBW and preterm delivery are especially common among those who are very young and underweight, for whom there may be competition for nutrients between the mother and the fetus (see Chapter 18). Poor outcomes are also common in obese teens who become pregnant. Many teens enter pregnancy with suboptimal nutritional status, especially

for iron, calcium, and folic acid. In one study, women in the United States who gave birth as teens were more likely to be overweight or obese as adults (Chang et al, 2013).

Improved dietary practices can be one of the most important factors for the pregnant teen. In counseling young mothers, the nutrition professional must be aware of the teen's psychosocial and literacy levels, her economic status and level of independence, as well as her cultural environment, all of which may influence her food choices.

TABLE 15-12 Nutrient Recommendations for Women Pregnant with Twins

Nutrient	Twins	Comments
Calories	Underweight: 4000 kcal Normal: 3000-3500 kcal Overweight: 3250 kcal Obese: 2700-3000 kcal	Estimated needs are 40-45 kcal/kg. Monitor weight gain and modify calories to meet target weight goals.
Protein	Underweight: 200 g Normal: 175 g Overweight: 163 g Obese: 150 g	Target 20% of calories from protein. Choose concentrated sources as space becomes limiting.
Carbohydrate	Underweight: 400 g Normal: 350 g Overweight: 325 g Obese: 300 g	Encourage low glycemic choices.
Fat	Underweight: 178 g Normal: 156 g Overweight: 144 g Obese: 133 g	Encourage healthy fats.
Vitamin D	1000 IU/day	Assessment of maternal levels should be considered in first and early third trimesters to allow alterations in the supplemental dose, especially important if the mother is on bed rest.
Vitamin C	500-1000 mg/day	This is half of the UL of 1800-2000 mg/day. See more recent cautions.
Vitamin E	400 mg/day	This is half of the UL of 800-1000 mg/day. See more recent cautions.
Zinc	15 mg/day (T1); 30mg/day (T2-3)	Diet alone may not be enough. Supplementation may be required.
Iron	30 mg/day as part of 1 multivitamin/day (T1), 2 multivitamins/day (T2 and T3)	Twin gestation requirement is likely double that of singletons. Higher intakes may be needed for treatment of anemia.
Folic acid	1000 mcg/day	
Calcium	1500 mg/day (T1); 2500 mg (T2-3)	UL: 2500 mg/day, consider limiting if there is a history of kidney stones.
Magnesium	400 mg/day (T1); 800 mg/day (T2-3)	
DHA + EPA	300-500 mg/day	

Adapted from Goodnight W, Newman R: Optimal nutrition for improved twin pregnancy outcome, *Obstet Gynecol* 114:1121, 2009.
DHA, Docosahexaenoic acid; *EPA*, eicosapentaenoic acid; *T*, trimester; *UL*, tolerable upper limit.

BOX 15-5 Risk Factors for Poor Pregnancy Outcome in Teenagers

- Young maternal age
- Pregnancy less than 2 years after onset of menarche
- Poor nutrition and low prepregnancy weight
- Preexisting anemia
- Inappropriate weight gain (too low and too high)
- Obesity
- Sexually transmitted disease or infection
- Substance abuse: smoking, drinking, and drugs
- Poverty
- Lack of social support
- Low educational level
- Rapid repeat pregnancies
- Lack of access to age-appropriate prenatal care
- Late entry into the health system
- Unmarried status
- Unstable housing, shelter living, homelessness

Complications and Nutritional Implications

Many of the following complications follow from the normal hormonal changes during the pregnancy. These changes cause the gastrointestinal transit time to slow so that more nutrients are available to the fetus. However, that causes more nausea and vomiting, constipation, and heartburn. Although normal, these complications can be uncomfortable and potentially dangerous but can be managed.

Constipation and Hemorrhoids

Pregnant women become constipated if they fail to consume adequate water and fiber. Women who are treated with ondansetron for nausea and vomiting often experience severe constipation. Compression of the pelvic floor by the fetus, as well as straining during stooling (Valsalva), increases the risk for hemorrhoids. Increased consumption of fluids and fiber-rich foods (see Appendix 41), including dried fruits (especially prunes), usually controls these problems. Some women also may require a bulking type of stool softener.

Cravings, Aversions, and Pica

Most women change their diets during their pregnancies as a result of medical advice, cultural beliefs, or changes in food preference and appetite. Food avoidances may not reflect a mother's conscious choice but may include smell adversity caused by enhanced perception of aromas, a heightened gag response, getting ill while eating or smelling a particular food, or altered gastric comfort.

Cravings and Aversions. Cravings and aversions are powerful urges toward or away from foods, including foods about which women experience no unusual attitudes when not pregnant. In the United States, the most commonly craved foods are sweets and dairy products, or foods that can be eaten quickly. The most common aversions reported are to alcohol, coffee, other caffeinated drinks, and meats. However, cravings and aversions are not limited to any particular food or food groups, and they vary widely across cultures.

Pica. Consumption of nonfood substances (pica) during pregnancy most often involves geophagia (consumption of dirt or clay), amylophagia (laundry starch or corn starch), or pagophagia (ice). Other substances include paper, burnt matches, stones or gravel, charcoal, bleach, cigarette ashes, baking soda, soap, tires, and coffee grounds. Although some of the common substances are of little concern, others are dangerous to the mother. The local poison control center can give guidance on which require immediate intervention.

Pica is common in pregnancy, and the incidence of pica in the United States is estimated to be 14% to 44%, with wide variability (Scolari Childress and Myles, 2013). Pica is not limited to any one geographic area, race, culture, or social status, but there are cultural components related to the substances chosen and the acceptability of disclosure. Preferred substances often are imported from home countries, including dirt or clay and blocks of magnesium carbonate.

The cause of pica is poorly understood. One theory suggests that pica relieves nausea and vomiting, although pica often appears later in pregnancy when nausea and vomiting are not so prevalent. One hypothesis is that it is due to a deficiency of an essential nutrient, most often iron, but zinc, calcium, and potassium also have been mentioned (Cardwell, 2013). Although it is hypothesized that the craving causes one to eat the nonfood substance that contains the missing nutrients, that is seldom the case. Pica also can be a craving for smell or texture as well as taste. Taste perceptions often change, but whether that is associated with lower zinc levels is not known.

Malnutrition can be a consequence of pica when nonfood substances displace essential nutrients in the diet. Starch in excessive amounts contributes to obesity and can negatively affect glucose control. Large intakes of baking soda can raise blood pressure and extreme doses (1 box/day) have caused rhabdomyolysis and cardiomyopathy (Scolari Childress and Myles, 2013). Excessive intakes of baking powder can mimic preeclampsia. Substances may contain toxic compounds or heavy metals, including lead, parasites, or other pathogens. The absorption of iron or other minerals may be disrupted. Excessive geophagia can result in intestinal obstruction or perforation (Young, 2011).

Recommending stopping a pica often fails, either because of the physiologic drive or the cultural perception that not complying with the craving will cause harm to the fetus. Rather than insisting on cessation, resulting only in less willingness to admit the pica, a more productive approach is to offer a better alternative. Allowing the mother to continue to smell the wet dirt, but trading its consumption for a burned tortilla, toast, or jicama often is successful. Pica often is associated with iron deficiency anemia, but whether the pica is a result, a cause, or a marker of other concurrent deficiencies is unknown. However, treatment with very high iron foods often decreases the cravings.

Diabetes Mellitus

Gestational diabetes mellitus (GDM), carbohydrate intolerance with onset or recognition during pregnancy, encompasses two distinct groups; those who have unrecognized preexisting diabetes and those for whom the pregnancy precipitates the carbohydrate intolerance (ACOG, 2013c).

Women with risk factors for type 2 diabetes (including but not limited to a history of GDM, known impaired glucose metabolism, and BMI ≥ 30) should be screened early in pregnancy using standard diagnostic criteria (ACOG, 2013c; ADA, 2014; see Chapter 30). According to the American Diabetes Association (ADA), those women identified with diabetes in the first trimester should be given a diagnosis of overt diabetes rather than GDM (ADA, 2014).

Women identified by early screening, as well as those with known preexisting diabetes (either type 1 or 2), should be referred to a Certified Diabetes Educator (CDE) and/or a diabetes management team. Fetuses of mothers with poorly controlled diabetes at conception are at risk for multiple congenital anomalies.

As pregnancy progresses and insulin resistance increases, GDM resulting from the pregnancy may appear. GDM rates in the United States are 5% to 6% of the prenatal population (NIH, 2013), but the prevalence can be much greater in high-risk groups, including women with a high BMI, advanced maternal age, and personal and family history (first-degree relative with diabetes). Rates are higher among African American, Asian, Hispanic, Native American, and Pacific Islander women compared with non-Hispanic white women (ACOG, 2013c).

A diagnosis of GDM is associated with increased risk of gestational hypertension and of preeclampsia, as well as increased risk of type 2 diabetes and cardiovascular disease later in life. Fetal implications include hyperinsulinemia, macrosomia (often defined as a baby weighing more than 4000 g), and, therefore, increased risk of delivery complications, including shoulder dystocia and cesarean delivery. The neonate is more likely to require admission to NICU and to experience respiratory distress syndrome and metabolic complications, including hyperbilirubinemia and hypoglycemia. Infant iron levels may be lower because of overgrowth and therefore increased demand (Monk et al, 2013); other nutrients also may be low. Fetal programming, with increased longterm risk of obesity and type 2 diabetes, is also of concern.

Although some practitioners believe that GDM may represent the early stages of type 2 diabetes, others feel that women should not be labeled at all with a GDM diagnosis. However, treatment for GDM is merited, because it lowers the risk by 40% for gestational hypertensive disorders, reduces the risk of macrosomia, and therefore reduces the risk of shoulder dystocia from 3.5% to 1.5% (NIH, 2013).

The diagnostic criteria for GDM are controversial. Historically, the United States and other countries have used a twostep process, whereas the World Health Organization (WHO) has advocated a one-step approach. Cutoffs and testing protocols vary. Table 15-13 summarizes current practice. Recently the International Association of the Diabetes and Pregnancy Study Groups (IADPSG) advocated for a universal one-step approach developed from the Hyperglycemia and Adverse Pregnancy Outcomes (HAPO) trials. The HAPO study was the first to correlate glucose values with pregnancy outcomes; all other protocols were designed to identify women at risk of developing type 2 diabetes later in life. Because only one elevated value is diagnostic, using the more liberal IADPSG criteria results in a twofold to threefold increase in the number of people defined as having GDM, arriving at a national prevalence of 15% to 20% (NIH, 2013).

Because of the increased cost to the medical system and the patient, increased patient stress with likely increased interventions, combined with concern that treatment may not be as beneficial for those at the lower glucose levels, a National Institutes of Health (NIH) consensus committee concluded there is currently insufficient evidence to recommend changing to the IADPSG approach (NIH, 2013).

The ADA and ACOG recommend screening all pregnant women for GDM (unless already identified with diabetes) at 24 to 28 weeks (ACOG, 2013c; ADA, 2014). Only those with an abnormal result on the 1-hour screen receive the 3-hour diagnostic test. ACOG recommends that the choice of a screening cutpoint and the choice of diagnostic tests (using the Carpenter and Coustan criteria if testing serum or plasma, or the National Diabetes Data Group criteria if testing plasma), be guided by local community GDM prevalence rates (ACOG, 2013c).

As with preexisting diabetes, those women with GDM should be followed carefully during pregnancy and managed by a diabetes team that includes a CDE. See Chapter 30 for diet and exercise recommendations, including target glucose values. Medications may be necessary to manage blood sugars; insulin and some oral hypoglycemic agents (e.g., metformin and glyburide) can be used. Long-term use of metformin is associated with decreased vitamin B_{12} levels, but its use only in late pregnancy has not been shown to be problematic for maintenance of normal B_{12} levels (Gatford et al, 2013).

Women with GDM should be screened for persistent diabetes at 6 to 12 weeks postpartum, and at least every 3 years for

TABLE 15-13 Screening and Diagnosis of Gestational Diabetes Mellitus (GDM) at 24-28 Weeks' Gestation: Blood Glucose Thresholds and Testing Protocols

Approach	Fasting mg/dl	1-hour mg/dl	2-hour mg/dl	3-hour mg/dl	Source
Two Step: universal screening; only those ≥ cutoff need diagnostic test					
Screening: (nonfasting)					
50 g glucose load		130, 135, or 140			
Diagnosis: (fasting)					
100 g load, 2 values ≥	95	180	155	140	Carpenter and Coustan
100 g load, 2 values ≥	105	190	165	145	National Diabetes Data Group
75 g load, 1 value ≥	95	191	160		Canadian Diabetes Association
One Step: universal testing					
Diagnosis: (fasting)					World Health
75 g load, 1 value ≥	92-125 *	180	153-199 *		Organization (WHO)**
75 g load, 1 value ≥	92	180	153		International Association of the Diabetes and Pregnancy Study Groups

* Values above these cutpoints are considered diagnostic of diabetes mellitus in pregnancy rather than GDM, as is a random plasma value of ≥ 200 mg/dl with diabetes symptoms.

** Considered diagnostic of GDM when found any time during the pregnancy.

Adapted from National Institutes of Health consensus development conference statement: diagnosing gestational diabetes mellitus, March 4-6, 2013, *Obstet Gynecol* 122:358, 2013; World Health Organization: *Diagnostic Criteria and Classification of Hyperglycaemia First Detected in Pregnancy* (website): http://apps.who.int/iris/bitstream/10665/85975/1/WHO_NMH_MND_13.2_eng.pdf?ua=1. Accessed July 2015.

diabetes or prediabetes, using nonpregnancy diagnostic criteria (ADA, 2014; see Chapter 30).

Eating Disorders

The rates of eating disorders during pregnancy are 1% for anorexia nervosa and slightly more for bulimia, with the prevalence likely underestimated (Cardwell, 2013). Anorexia and bulimia are associated with increased risk of miscarriage, birth defects, hyperemesis, IUGR, and micronutrient deficiencies, as well as postpartum depression and impaired infant bonding. For those with binge eating, excessive weight gain, macrosomia, and increased cesarean rates are seen. Those that purge may have caries or fractured teeth severe enough that they cannot chew meat.

The effect of pregnancy on the individual with an eating disorder varies, but 70% may show improvement, especially with purging behaviors (Harris, 2010). However, symptoms often are exacerbated after delivery; pregnancy will not cure the eating disorder. In fact, in some cases the newborn is seen as "too fat," to the point of restricting food, administering suppositories or enemas, or inducing vomiting. A team approach to treating the mom is helpful in those cases.

For the woman with an eating disorder, pregnancy may be particularly frightening because of the loss of control and disturbed body image. Anorexia can be diagnosed during pregnancy. Substance abuse, as well as the use of laxatives or diet pills, may be coping mechanisms; insulin has been used as a purging mechanism. Women may fear being weighed and may need reassurance that the nausea and vomiting of pregnancy is not necessarily a resurgence of purging. Fatigue, irritability, and depression may be due to starvation. These pregnant women should be treated with particular care, including focusing on healthy eating for optimal fetal growth and development (see Chapter 22).

Edema and Leg Cramps

Mild physiologic edema is usually present in the third trimester and should not be confused with the pathologic, generalized edema associated with preeclampsia. Normal edema in the lower extremities is caused by the pressure of the enlarging uterus on the vena cava, obstructing the return of blood flow to the heart. When a woman reclines on her side, the mechanical effect is removed, and extravascular fluid is mobilized and eventually eliminated by increased urine output. No dietary intervention is required, assuming her protein intake is adequate. If, however, her urine is dark and/or she has swelling in her hands, increased fluid intake is recommended.

Increased fluid intake also is recommended for leg cramps. Women should be advised to stretch with their toes pointing back toward their bodies rather than away from them. The literature is conflicting about the benefit of magnesium supplementation for treatment of pregnancy-related leg cramps (Garrison et al, 2012). Caution is advised against large intakes of supplements.

Heartburn

Gastric esophageal reflux is common during the latter part of pregnancy and often occurs at night. The pressure of the enlarged uterus on the intestines and stomach, along with the relaxation of the esophageal sphincter, may result in regurgitation of stomach contents into the esophagus. Relief measures may include eating smaller meals, limiting caffeine, carbonated beverages, tomatoes, citrus, fat, and spicy foods, and staying upright for at least 3 hours after a meal, but interventions have not been evaluated for effectiveness (Kaiser and Campbell, 2014). Using more pillows at night also may help (see Chapter 27).

Although heartburn medicines can be used, they are not benign and use should be limited. Taking excessive calcium carbonate can lead to life-threatening milk-alkali syndrome (hypercalcemia, renal sufficiency, and metabolic alkalosis). The UL of 2500 mg of elemental calcium (food plus supplements) should be observed. If a couple of calcium carbonate tablets (two regular strength Tums contain 400 mg calcium; two ultra-strength tablets provide 800 mg) do not resolve the heartburn, switching to those containing magnesium may be beneficial. Proton pump inhibitors may reduce the bioavailability of many nutrients, including vitamins C, B_{12}, and nonheme iron (see Chapter 8). The use of antacids also potentially can increase the risk of food allergies by impeding gastric protein digestion, but whether that translates into a higher risk of food allergy or asthma for the child is unclear.

Hypertension

Hypertension observed during pregnancy may be preexisting or observed for the first time. Elevated blood pressure that is first diagnosed in pregnancy may be relatively benign. However, a rise in blood pressure, accompanied by other changes listed in this chapter, can be a sign that preeclampsia is developing, a progressive, systemic problem with high morbidity and mortality for mother and fetus. Although delivery resolves the problem for most, some women develop hypertension after delivery.

Chronic hypertension predates pregnancy and is associated with fetal growth restriction. Avoidance of severe hypertension is a goal, but the optimal blood pressure during pregnancy for someone with preexisting hypertension is unclear (see Chapter 33). Appropriate weight gain, a modified DASH diet (see Appendix 33), and regular aerobic exercise for those without complications are recommended. Although excessive sodium should be reduced, intake should not be less than 2300 mg/day (ACOG, 2013e). Calcium supplementation for those with low calcium intakes may be helpful. Some antihypertensive medications can be used during pregnancy but may have to be modified during breastfeeding.

Gestational hypertension is defined as elevated blood pressure that appears after 20 weeks, but without proteinuria or other findings. Some women (at least 25%) go on to develop preeclampsia; others have no risk except the elevated blood pressure (ACOG, 2013e). They are treated the same as those with chronic hypertension and monitored for worsening of symptoms. Gestational hypertension may predict increased risk for future hypertension. Optimal periconceptual nutrition, including focus on folate, sodium, calcium, potassium, iron, copper, and zinc intakes, is important (Tande et al, 2013).

Some women who develop hypertension during pregnancy develop preeclampsia. Risk factors include women who are primiparous, have a personal or family history of preeclampsia, chronic hypertension, obesity, type 1 or 2 diabetes, chronic renal disease, history of thrombophilia, systemic lupus erythematosus, multifetal pregnancy, IVF, and maternal age of more than 40 years (ACOG, 2013e). Paternal factors also likely play a role; risk increases with advanced paternal age, paternal obesity, and family history of early-onset CVD. Risk of preeclampsia is less likely in subsequent pregnancies with the same partner than when the mother is pregnant with a new partner. Paternal genes also may be important; increased risk for preeclampsia is seen if the man has fathered a preeclamptic pregnancy or if he was born of a preeclamptic pregnancy (Dekker et al, 2011). Maternal smoking reduces the risk by 35% (ACOG, 2013e), but if preeclampsia occurs, the severity increases (Trogstad et al, 2011).

Preeclampsia involves dysfunction of multiple organ systems. It is dynamic, progressive, and once evident, is not reversible and delivery is needed because it is potentially fatal for mother and baby. Growth restriction is common and babies are often also premature in an effort to avoid the mother progressing to eclampsia (new onset grand mal seizures) or HELLP syndrome (hemolysis, elevated liver enzymes, and low platelets), which have high rates of maternal morbidity and mortality. Those women with superimposed preeclampsia onto chronic hypertension (13% to 40% of women) have much worse consequences (ACOG, 2013e). Women with preeclampsia that develops near term have double the risk of CVD later in life; the risk of CVD is nearly 10-fold for those who must be delivered at less than 34 weeks because of preeclampsia (Roberts and Bell, 2013).

Preeclampsia has been defined by elevated blood pressure and proteinuria, but newer guidelines now recommend not waiting for the proteinuria to appear. Box 15-6 summarizes diagnostic criteria designed to facilitate earlier diagnosis and therefore earlier treatment.

The causes of preeclampsia are under intense investigation. It appears to be a two-stage process, with a poorly perfused placenta (from failed remodeling of the maternal spiral arteries) being the root cause (ACOG, 2013e). Reduced perfusion and increased velocity of blood perfusing the intervillous spaces alters placental function and leads to maternal disease through oxidative and endoplasmic reticulum stress and inflammation, as well as modified endothelial function and angiogenesis. The second-stage, called *maternal syndrome*, is a cascade of events; what links the hypoxic placenta and the maternal syndrome is unclear and possibly involves oxidative stress (Roberts and Bell, 2013). The hypertension and proteinuria are only a small part of the syndrome; reduced perfusion of any organ in the body can lead to hemorrhage and necrosis. Not all women with inadequate placental perfusion develop preeclampsia; a woman's underlying disease (e.g., diabetes, hypertension), lifestyle (e.g., obesity, activity, sleep), genetics, and environmental conditions (e.g., air pollution) may affect the maternal response (Roberts and Bell, 2013). The inflammatory response is accentuated in preeclampsia. Predictive tests are being studied but are not ready for clinical use (ACOG, 2013e). It is now thought that preeclampsia is actually a syndrome of many diseases with subsets of pathophysiology and varied contributions of maternal and placental factors (Roberts and Bell, 2013; Trogstad et al, 2011).

Prevention of preeclampsia has not yet been effective, although daily low-dose aspirin may be beneficial (ACOG, 2013e). Vitamin C and E supplements do not prevent occurrence of preeclampsia or adverse outcomes and may be associated with increased risk of gestational hypertension and LBW (ACOG, 2013e; Hovdenak and Haram, 2012). Calcium supplementation may help reduce symptom severity if a mother's baseline calcium intake has been less than 600 mg/day (ACOG, 2013e). There is insufficient evidence to provide guidance on fish oil, garlic, or vitamin D supplementation. Protein and calorie restriction for obese women does not reduce the risk of either gestational hypertension or preeclampsia and may increase the risk of IUGR. Neither bed rest nor salt restriction appear to reduce risk, but the trials may have been too small. Diuretics are not recommended. Moderate exercise (30 minutes/day) is recommended as during normal pregnancy, but it is unclear whether it can help reverse the endothelial dysfunction and prevent adverse pregnancy outcomes. Obesity, leptin, insulin, and free fatty acids appear to affect various stages of preeclampsia. Endothelial cell disorder from placental ischemia and hypoxia appear important. An imbalance of angiogenic factors, immune factors, inflammation, endothelin (a protein that constricts blood vessels), nitric oxide, oxidative and endoplasmic reticulum stress, the stress response gene hemeoxygenase and its catalytic product carbon monoxide, and the effect of statins are being studied.

For those women with a history of preeclampsia, weight loss, increased physical activity, and optimization of blood glucose levels and nutrient intakes preconceptually are recommended. During pregnancy, helping women maintain a normal rate of weight gain, with optimal calcium intake and fruits and vegetables (antioxidants), may be beneficial. Encourage notifying the medical provider immediately if there is a sudden onset of face or hand swelling, persistent headaches, seeing spots or changes in eyesight, pain in the upper right quadrant or stomach, nausea and vomiting in the second half of pregnancy, rapid weight gain, or difficulty breathing.

Although delivery resolves the preeclampsia for most, a subset of women have a worsening of preeclampsia after delivery; others may first develop preeclampsia postpartum, including HELLP. Pain medications may have to be modified. Blood pressure may be labile for months but usually normalizes by 1 year postpartum. Postpartum hypertension may predict future chronic hypertension (ACOG, 2013e).

BOX 15-6   Preeclampsia Diagnostic Criteria

Elevated blood pressure
 Confirmed ≥160 or ≥110 for anyone (confirmed over a few minutes) or ≥140 or ≥90 after 20 weeks (confirmed over 4 hours) if previously normal

AND

Proteinuria
 ≥300 mg/24-hour urine collection, an extrapolated amount from a timed collection, protein/creatinine ratio ≥0.3, or dipstick reading of 1+ if no other quantitative methods are available

OR

Elevated blood pressure
 Confirmed ≥160 or ≥110 for anyone (confirmed over a few minutes) or ≥140 or ≥90 after 20 weeks (confirmed over 4 hours) if previously normal

AND

New onset of any of the following:
 Thrombocytopenia: platelets <100,000/microliter
 Renal insufficiency: serum creatinine >1.1 mg/dl or doubling of serum creatinine concentration in absence of other renal disease
 Impaired liver function: elevated liver transaminases to twice normal blood concentrations
 Pulmonary edema
 Cerebral or visual symptoms

Adapted from American College of Obstetricians and Gynecologists (ACOG): *Hypertension in Pregnancy* (website): http://www.acog.org/Resources_And_Publications/Task_Force_and_Work_Group_Reports/Hypertension_in_Pregnancy, 2013e. Accessed December 2013.

Nausea and Vomiting, Hyperemesis Gravidarum, and Ptyalism

Morning sickness, nausea and vomiting in pregnancy (NVP), affects 50% to 90% of all pregnant women during the first trimester and usually resolves by 20 weeks' gestation (Clark et al, 2012). The cause of NVP is unclear but likely includes a genetic predisposition, combined with changes in human chorionic gonadotropin (hCG), estrogen, and progesterone levels. It may be mediated through the vestibuloocular reflex pathway (Fejzo et al, 2012). Those pregnant with a female fetus, multiple fetuses, or a molar pregnancy (sperm fertilizes an empty egg, resulting in no embryo but a placenta that develops into an abnormal mass of cells) are more likely to suffer with either NVP or hyperemesis gravidarum, as are those with hyperthyroid disorders, gastrointestinal disorders, preexisting diabetes, or a psychiatric illness. Maternal age more than 30 years and smoking are protective, but paternal smoking increases risk (Fejzo et al, 2012). NVP is associated with more favorable pregnancy outcomes, including fewer birth defects, reduced risk of miscarriage, preterm delivery or stillbirth, and greater birth weight.

Treatment for NVP involves managing the symptoms. Motion, loud noises, bright lights, and adverse climate conditions may trigger the nausea. Fortunately, most women with NVP are functional, able to work, do not lose weight, and are helped by simple dietary measures. Although many dietary and lifestyle recommendations have not been evaluated in the literature (Kaiser and Campbell, 2014), ginger (1 g/day divided in four doses) reduces the severity of symptoms of NVP better than vitamin B_6 but not the number of vomiting episodes (Medscape, 2014). However women on anticoagulation therapy, those with duodenal ulcers, or those at risk for intestinal obstruction should avoid ginger use. Other therapies suggested include eating crackers or potato chips, sucking on special lollipops, drinking red raspberry leaf tea, or wearing elastic or electronic wrist bands. Noise reduction, acupuncture, and hypnosis also can be helpful. Stopping the prenatal vitamins may help, but women should continue the supplemental folic acid if possible. Various antinausea medications are also available, with different modes of action.

Small, frequent snacks of carbohydrate foods reduce nausea for some, whereas protein foods may help others (Erick, 2014). Some women do not tolerate odors; some are bothered by hot foods and may prefer foods that are cold or at least at room temperature. Smelling lemons may help block noxious odors. Avoiding hunger by eating more frequently often helps, as does separating dry foods from liquids. Avoiding highly spiced foods or bitter foods is helpful for some; for others taste sensitivity decreases and strong flavors are craved. Women should avoid odors or situations that trigger symptoms and should eat whatever reduces the nausea sensation. Unfortunately, there is no cure-all. However, reminding the mother that this is a good sign for the pregnancy (i.e., the body is responding as it should), and that it *will* end, often reassures her and lowers the worry and stress, thus helping with the nausea.

When early pregnancy is characterized by excessive vomiting and weight loss (often >5% prepregnant weight), fluid and electrolyte imbalances can occur. Here, "morning sickness" becomes hyperemesis gravidarum (HG), and prevalence is 0.3% to 3% of pregnancies (Clark et al, 2012). Risk factors are the same as those with NVP; recurrence risk is high, but not 100% (Fejzo et al, 2012).

Complications of HG vary but include poor fetal growth, preterm delivery, and increased risk of fetal loss with gestational malnutrition. Chondrodysplasia punctata resulting from maternal vitamin K deficiency has been documented (Erick, 2014), as have permanent neurobehavioral and neuroendocrine abnormalities in exposed fetuses.

Maternal complications may include splenic avulsion (spleen is torn from its normal location, resulting in an emergency situation due to excessive bleeding), esophageal rupture, diaphragmatic tears, Valsalva retinopathy, acute renal failure, rhabdomyolysis, and delirium, as well as maternal posttraumatic stress syndrome and high risk of pregnancy termination when management of HG fails (Erick, 2014; Fejzo et al, 2012). Difficulty producing breastmilk and bonding also may have to be addressed.

Hospitalization for nutrition support and hydration usually is indicated for HG. Management goals include appropriate weight gain for pregnancy, correction of fluid and electrolyte deficits, avoidance of ketosis, control of HG symptoms, and achievement of nitrogen, vitamin, and mineral balance.

Because pregnancy is a condition of accelerated starvation, refeeding syndrome is seen often. Phosphorus, magnesium, and potassium must be evaluated daily because low levels may result in cardiac irregularities and respiratory failure (see Chapter 13). Another potentially serious complication is Wernicke's encephalopathy, with at least 63 cases being reported worldwide (Di Gangi et al, 2012). Caused by maternal vitamin deficiencies, including thiamin depletion, there is no consensus on early diagnosis, treatment, or prevention (see Chapter 29). The classic triad of nystagmus and ophthalmoplegia, mental status changes, and ataxia has been found in only 16% of known cases; women in 60% of cases displayed ocular symptoms, 83% had cerebellar changes, and 52% had memory impairment (Di Gangi et al, 2012). Symptoms are often vague and nonspecific, including headaches, fatigue, abdominal discomfort, irritability, and inability to concentrate. Wernicke's encephalopathy is associated with a 37% fetal loss rate and can progress to Korsakoff syndrome, with chronic maternal memory impairment (Clark et al, 2012). Thiamin blood levels are not useful for diagnosis; thiamin is given intravenously, and a presumptive diagnosis is made if the patient responds (Di Gangi et al, 2012). Correcting deficiencies of niacin and magnesium also may be helpful.

In HG, enteral nutrition has variable effectiveness. Women with severe emesis and retching have often dislodged tubes and are sometimes reluctant for replacement. During hospitalization, frequent nursing checks on tube placement add to sleep deprivation issues, which have not been fully appreciated (Erick, 2014). Parenteral nutrition is used if the GI tract is not accessible or if enteral nutrition is not tolerated.

Women historically have been reassured that even with HG the fetus is protected, using adequate birth weight as evidence. However, given the results of the Dutch famine studies, it is known that birth weight does not necessarily predict long-term health and that there are consequences of early malnutrition, even if later resolved (Erick, 2014; Roseboom et al, 2011). HG merits aggressive attention and treatment.

Some women develop ptyalism gravidarum, or excess saliva. Salivary output can be substantial, up to 500 to 1000 ml/day, and can be a source of lost electrolytes (Cardwell, 2013). It may interfere with swallowing, the sense of taste, sleep, and speech but does not appear dangerous for the fetus. Antihistamines may be helpful.

Oral Health

Good oral health is important throughout one's lifetime, including during pregnancy (see Chapter 25). Pregnant women can receive dental care while pregnant, with some qualifications; the National Maternal and Child Oral Health Resource Center provides guidance. Although periodontal infection is associated with preterm birth and LBW, treatment does not appear to lower that risk. However, optimal maternal oral hygiene may lower the amount of *Streptococcus mutans* transmitted to the infant through sharing spoons or licking pacifiers, thus lowering or delaying the risk of childhood caries. During pregnancy, increased inflammatory response to dental plaque causes gingivae to swell and bleed more easily. Rinsing with salt water (1 tsp salt in 1 cup warm water) can help soothe the irritation. Erosion of enamel may occur with increased exposure to gastric acid from vomiting or gastric reflux. Rinsing with a baking soda solution (1 tsp baking soda in 1 cup water) may help neutralize the acid (ACOG, 2013b).

Preexisting Medical Conditions

Many women begin pregnancy with preexisting conditions that can complicate the pregnancy and modify nutrient requirements and appropriate food sources, as well as the supplementation that is necessary. As an example, celiac disease adversely affects fertility for men and women, and the absorption of nutrients often is impaired (Freeman, 2010). Women with celiac disease have increased risk of miscarriages and premature deliveries. Some prenatal supplements may contain gluten or wheat binders and should be avoided (see Chapter 28). Women with inflammatory bowel disease may have low serum vitamin B_{12} levels if there is damage to the intestines. Women with HIV infection may have higher energy needs and the interaction of nutrients with medications may have to be considered. Immigrant women may suffer with active malaria, which invades the placenta, or gastrointestinal parasites, which can decrease nutrient intakes and increase nutrient losses. Women with preexisting depression are at risk for poor pregnancy outcome and postpartum depression, putting the mother and her newborn at risk if she is unable to function optimally.

Women also may develop conditions resulting from the pregnancy that need particular attention, including HG, gallstones, or intrahepatic cholestatis of pregnancy. She also may be involved in a motor vehicle accident or other trauma that requires special care or even time in an ICU. In all cases, the needs of the mother and the fetus must remain paramount. Although guidance is available for some conditions, strong evidence-based recommendations are lacking.

Food Safety During Pregnancy

Although a pregnant woman is no more likely to be exposed to pathogens than a nonpregnant woman, she and her fetus may be at higher risk of suffering negative consequences from foodborne illnesses. In addition, because metabolically active tissues may be more susceptible to the action of toxins, along with the potential long-term effects of fetal exposure to suboptimal conditions, a pregnant woman often has questions regarding the safety of common foods and nonnutritive substances. Those food safety issues of most concern vary between populations. Box 15-7 summarizes general food safety guidelines.

BOX 15-7 General Food Safety Guidelines

Clean
- Wash hands thoroughly with soap and water, especially before and after handling food, and after using the bathroom, changing diapers, or handling pets. Do not touch mucous membranes after handling meats.
- Wash cutting boards, dishes, utensils, and countertops with hot water and soap. Washing utensils, including cutting boards, in the dishwasher is preferable.
- Rinse raw fruits and vegetables thoroughly under running water, even if the skin will not be eaten.
- Do not wash or rinse meat and poultry.

Separate to Avoid Cross Contamination
- Separate raw meat, poultry, and seafood from ready-to-eat foods when shopping, preparing, and storing foods.
- Use one cutting board for raw meat, poultry, and seafood and another one for fresh fruits and vegetables.
- Place cooked food on a clean plate. The unwashed plate that held raw meat, poultry, or seafood, may be contaminated.

Cook to Proper Temperature
- Cook foods thoroughly. Use a food thermometer to check the temperature. (Color is not a reliable indicator of meat doneness.) Examples include the following:
  - Beef, pork, veal, lamb large cuts (steaks, roasts, and chops): 145° F + 3-minute rest
  - Fish: 145° F
  - Beef, pork, veal, lamb ground meats: 160° F
  - Egg dishes: 160° F
  - Turkey, chicken, duck (whole animal, pieces, ground): 165° F

- Cook eggs until firm.
- Reheat leftovers to at least 165° F and sauces, gravies, and soups should be boiled.

Chill to Avoid the Danger Zone
- Refrigerator should register at 40° F or below and the freezer at 0° F. Check the temperature periodically with an appliance thermometer.
- Limit the time foods are in the danger zone, the range of temperatures at which bacteria can grow quickly, usually between 40° F and 140° F.
- Defrost (and marinate) foods in the refrigerator, not on the kitchen counter.
- Refrigerate or freeze perishables (foods that can spoil or become contaminated by bacteria if left unrefrigerated) promptly.
- Use ready-to-eat, perishable foods (dairy, meat, poultry, seafood, produce) as soon as possible.
- 2-hour rule: discard perishable foods left out at room temperature for more than 2 hours. If it is a hot day (more than 90° F), shorten the time to 1 hour.

Avoid High-Risk Foods
- Avoid unpasteurized milks, including goat milk, and foods made of unpasteurized milks. Even if soft cheeses are pasteurized, hard cheeses are safer.
- Avoid raw or undercooked meats, poultry, eggs, fish, or seafood.
- Avoid unpasteurized fruit or vegetable juices. Unpasteurized juice must be boiled (full rolling boil) for at least 1 minute.
- Avoid raw or undercooked sprouts, including alfalfa, clover, mung bean, and radish. Cooked sprouts are lower risk.
- Do not open bulging cans.
- Boil home-canned foods for 20 minutes.
- Pay attention to food recalls. This is not the time to gamble.

Adapted from Cox JT, Phelan ST: Food safety in pregnancy, part 1: putting risks into perspective, *Contemporary Ob/Gyn* 54:44, 2009a; United States Department of Health and Human Services (USDHHS): *Checklist Of Foods To Avoid During Pregnancy* (website): http://www.foodsafety.gov/poisoning/risk/pregnant/chklist_pregnancy.html, 2014. Accessed January 2014.

However, caution is advised to not overestimate the risk of food contamination in pregnancy or the amount of control that an individual has in lowering that risk. It is critical to avoid the impression that a healthy baby is guaranteed if parents do everything right and that the mother is to blame if anything goes wrong. In addition, it is becoming increasingly apparent that maternal psychological stress is also harmful to the pregnancy (see *Clinical Insight:* Stress During Pregnancy).

CLINICAL INSIGHT

Stress During Pregnancy

Prenatal psychological stress is associated with shorter gestations and lower birth weights. Stress also appears to interact with poor nutrition to negatively affect fetal neurocognitive development, especially the hippocampus and memory functioning, using the same mechanisms as infectious stress (Monk et al, 2013).

All nutrients are important for neuronal and glial cell growth and development. Stress alters the metabolism of many nutrients (protein, glucose, zinc, iron, choline, folate), but not others (LCPUFA, copper, iodine, vitamin A), and some nutrients (LCPUFA, protein, zinc, iron, choline) have a role in the stress response (Monk et al, 2013).

Distress can induce insulin resistance and proinflammatory cytokines, diverting amino acids to gluconeogenesis and energy production rather than protein production (Monk et al, 2013). Stress also raises the risk of hypertension, increasing uterine artery resistance and lowering nutrient delivery to the fetus (Monk et al, 2013). Risk of autism and schizophrenia may increase, but the timing of the insult may affect the response (Marques et al, 2013).

Maternal and fetal immune systems communicate bidirectionally, and the fetal immune system (innate and adaptive) can be disrupted with maternal stress, as well as by exposure to toxins and malnutrition. This disruption may be sufficient to affect a child's response to vaccines but there is no consensus on the timeframe of vulnerability or on the mechanisms (Marques et al, 2013).

When studying infant neurocognitive development, psychological stress and nutritional status must be studied together to examine their synergistic effects and optimal intervention strategies (Monk et al, 2013).

Often issues of psychological stress arise in the course of discussing food intake and weight gain. They would include, but are not limited to, catastrophic life events, verbal or physical abuse, unemployment, and food insecurity, as well as anxiety about the pregnancy itself. A referral to a mental health professional for evaluation and treatment is warranted (Kaiser and Campbell, 2014).

Alcohol

Abundant evidence from animal studies and human experience associates maternal alcohol consumption with teratogenicity. Features of fetal alcohol syndrome (FAS) include a specific pattern of abnormalities (see Figure 15-4). Alcohol has been shown to alter gene expression; changes involve proteins associated with central nervous system development, organ morphogenesis, immunologic responses, endocrine function, and skeletal, cardiovascular, and cartilage development.

Use of alcohol during pregnancy has been associated with an increased rate of miscarriage, placenta abruption, LBW, and cognitive compromise. Although there is individual variability, problems appear to be more severe with successive pregnancies, especially with binging, intoxication, and in older mothers. Drinking at least one drink per day is associated with a five-fold

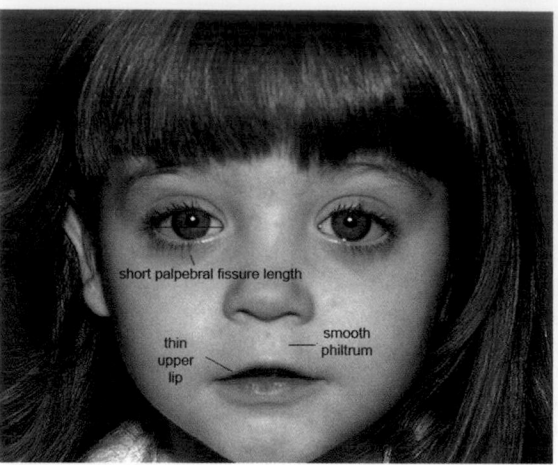

FIGURE 15-4 Child presents with all three facial features that are diagnostic for fetal alcohol syndrome. (Copyright 2016, Susan Astley PhD, University of Washington.)

increased risk of LBW and two-fold risk of preterm delivery (Cox and Phelan, 2009b). The cognitive and behavioral deficits seen with moderate intake can affect later school performance. For lower intakes of alcohol there is less consistency in the negative findings, but the evidence is too weak to say that any level of alcohol intake is safe.

ACOG, the American Academy of Pediatrics (AAP), and the March of Dimes, recommend that alcohol not be used during pregnancy, because no safe threshold has been identified. Reduced-alcohol wines and beers do contain small amounts of alcohol and also are contraindicated. Despite the multiple warnings of fetal injury caused by alcohol, some women continue to drink in pregnancy and they should be offered assistance. However, for those women who are fearful of the alcohol they consumed early in pregnancy, possibly before realizing they were pregnant, reassurance is advised.

Allergens

Restriction of the maternal diet during pregnancy and lactation is not advised as a strategy to lower the risk of infant food allergies (Joneja, 2012). The mother should avoid her own allergens during pregnancy and lactation but should eat a variety of other foods, including the father's allergenic foods, so that the fetus and neonate can adapt. Regarding peanuts, studies have shown the child has a slightly increased risk of developing peanut sensitization if a mother eats peanuts more than twice a week, but avoidance by the mother appears to be associated with even higher risk (Fleischer et al, 2013). The mother is encouraged to breastfeed exclusively; foods should be added carefully, but delaying introduction of solid foods past 6 months provides no benefit. Use of probiotics by the mother or child may be beneficial, but type, timing, and dose are unknown (see Chapter 26).

Artificial Sweeteners

Research on the safety of artificial sweeteners is limited, but the FDA has deemed the following safe for use in moderation, including during pregnancy and lactation: saccharin, acesulfame-K, sucralose, aspartame, neotame, advantame, steviol glycosides from stevia leaves, and extracts from monk fruit.

Food additives, including artificial sweeteners, are tested for short- and long-term toxicity; reproductive effects, including teratogenicity; and any adverse effects on an animal's reproductive organs or systems, any birth defects, and genetic toxicity (Rulis and Levitt, 2009). From that data, a safety factor is applied, usually 1/100th of the dose in which any problems have been seen. The resulting value is the Acceptable Daily Intake (ADI), defined as the estimated amount of a food additive that someone can safely consume on average every day over a lifetime without any appreciable health risk. Except for advantame, stevia, and monk fruit, all too new for ADIs to have been determined, current intakes of the other sweeteners listed here are well below these ADI levels (Kroger et al, 2006; Shankar et al, 2013; see Chapter 30).

Saccharin (Sweet'N Low, Sweet Twin, Sugar Twin, Necta Sweet) crosses the placenta (Cohen-Addad et al, 1986) and may accumulate in the fetus and in breastmilk, but adverse effects on the fetus and infant have not been seen. It has been delisted as a human carcinogen (Kroger et al, 2006; Shankar et al, 2013).

Acesulfame-K (Sunett, Sweet One) consumption by pregnant women is classified as safe, even without long-term studies during human pregnancy. It often is used in conjunction with other artificial sweeteners. It is said to not be metabolized in humans (Kroger et al, 2006), but in mice it can appear in the amniotic fluid and breastmilk after an oral infusion (Zhang et al, 2011).

Sucralose (Splenda, Nevella), a carbohydrate derived from sucrose, appears to pass through the GI track relatively unchanged, is not bioreactive, and does not bioaccummulate (Shankar et al, 2013) and therefore is assumed to have little effect on pregnancy and lactation. It has not been found to be teratogenic in animal studies.

Aspartame (Equal, NutraSweet, Natra Taste) is metabolized to phenylalanine, aspartic acid, and methanol in the GI track. Studies have shown no significant effect on fertility, conception rates, embryo toxicity, fetotoxicity, or teratogenesis at the levels tested in animals (London, 1988). Its use during pregnancy and lactation has not been found to increase risk of brain tumors in children (Shankar et al, 2013). The aspartic acid does not cross the placenta in monkeys, and the methanol content is less than that of many fruit juices (Kroger et al, 2006; London, 1988). Although it is not absolutely contraindicated for women with phenylketonuria (PKU) or for women breastfeeding an infant with PKU, it must be counted as a phenylalanine source. High circulating concentrations of phenylalanine are known to damage the fetal brain (see Chapter 43). Neotame is also a source of phenylalanine and aspartic acid but, because it is much sweeter, the amounts consumed are negligible and do not have to be counted (Kroger et al, 2006). The newly approved advantame is also a source of phenylalanine but at such low concentrations that it also does not need to be counted (FDA, 2014). There are no human reproductive studies on advantame, but it is sweeter than neotame, so very small amounts would likely be consumed.

Both stevia and monk fruit are plant-derived sweeteners considered GRAS in their purified forms. Stevia (Pure Via, Truvia, SweetLeaf), has not been found to affect fetal development, at least with short-term use. *Stevia rebaudiana* traditionally has been used by the indigenous populations of Paraguay for fertility control (Ulbricht et al, 2010). Animal studies have suggested that steviol glycosides may have adverse effects on the male reproductive system, but there are no confirming studies in humans (Kroger et al, 2006; Ulbricht et al, 2010). Caution is advised when used by pregnant or lactating women, or for use longer than 2 years, because of insufficient evidence of safety (Ulbricht et al, 2010). There is little information on the excretion of Rebaudioside A (the refined preparation of the active ingredient, now considered GRAS) and the other plant components, including steviol glycosides, into breastmilk, so caution is advised when nursing a newborn or a preterm infant. For the extracts of *Siraitia grosvenorii*, known as Swingle fruit, Luo Han Guo, or monk fruit, there is no information available for pregnancy or lactation.

Artificial sweeteners often are found in foods with low nutrient content. Intakes may have to be limited so as not to displace the more valuable, nutrient dense foods. Although average intakes are well below the ADI, an assessment of the diet is warranted to identify those women who may be ingesting multiple sources of artificial sweeteners. If intakes are high, alternatives should be offered.

Bisphenol-A, Phthalates, and Other Environmental Toxins

Bisphenol-A (BPA), an endocrine disruptor, is associated with recurrent miscarriages and may affect thyroid function in humans, especially in the fetus. Its function at the cellular level is still being investigated but there is evidence in mice that it acts similar to diethylstilbestrol (DES) (ACOG, 2013d). Phthalates are associated with shortened gestational length and developmental disruptions. BPA and phthalates, along with 20 other chemicals, are associated with increased risk of weight gain, insulin resistance, and type 2 diabetes later in life after developmental exposure (Barouki et al, 2012). See Table 15-2 for more examples.

There are calls to limit the use of BPA, phthalates, and other environmental toxins. Although recommendations can be made to avoid specific plastics and canned foods (BPA is used as a lining material), most people also have high exposure through air, dust, and personal care products (Sathyanarayana et al, 2013), and changing behavior does not necessarily reduce risk. In addition, having a plastic labeled "BPA free" does not ensure safety. Most plastics under stress (exposure to boiling water, ultraviolet rays in sunlight, or microwaving) release estrogenic chemicals that may be of more concern than those plastics containing BPA (Yang et al, 2011).

Although it is known that exposure to environmental toxins can have long-term effects, it is unknown whether the effects vary by gender or life stage. It is also unknown how the placenta mediates exposure to toxins (ACOG, 2013d; Bloomfield, 2011). The effects may be nonlinear; low doses can be more harmful than high doses (Barouki et al, 2012). There are also potential effects on gene expression. ACOG is calling for better research on the reproductive effects of environmental toxins and societal change regarding exposure to these toxins (ACOG, 2013d).

Much of the effect of these chemicals may be during organogenesis, so reducing preconceptual exposure is likely to be most productive. Raising concerns with a mother later in pregnancy without actually being able to change outcomes would not be helpful.

Caffeine and Energy Drinks

Caffeine crosses the placenta and increases maternal catecholamines, but it appears that intakes of less than 200 mg/day are not associated with increased risk of miscarriages or preterm birth (ACOG, 2010). It does not decrease uterine blood flow or oxygenation. However, although there is no clear evidence of harm, the evidence also does not follow the expected dose-response curve, so the effect cannot be determined definitively. Caffeinated beverages are not considered to be of high nutritional quality, and moderation is encouraged. See Appendix 39 for caffeine food sources.

Energy drinks are not recommended during pregnancy. In addition to the high caffeine and sugar contents they contain, these drinks often have high levels of added nutrients and herbal products that have not been evaluated for safety during pregnancy (Procter and Campbell, 2014).

Lead

Contaminants in food are the exception rather than the rule in the United States, but they do occur. In high concentrations, they can pass across the placenta to the fetus (see Figure 15-5). Lead contamination is associated with increased risk of miscarriage, gestational hypertension, IUGR, preterm delivery, and impaired neurobehavioral development.

In addition to old paint chips, poorly glazed dishware (often imported) and leaded crystal decanters may contain high amounts of lead. Pregnant women should avoid using dolomite as a calcium supplement; the seashells or sea coral often contain heavy metals, including lead, the result of dumping industrial wastes in the oceans. Imported candies from many areas, including Mexico, India, China, and Hong Kong have also been found to contain lead (see http://www.cdph.ca.gov/data/documents/fdbliclic07.pdf).

Listeria monocytogenes

Listeria monocytogenes affects 1600 Americans each year and, with a 21% case fatality rate, is the third leading cause of death resulting from food poisoning (CDC, 2013). Pregnant women are 10 times more likely than other healthy adults to become infected with *Listeria* spp.; rates among U.S. Hispanic women are 24 times higher than the general population (CDC, 2013). It is a known cause of miscarriage (10% to 20%), preterm birth (50%), or stillbirth (11%) (Adams Waldorf and McAdams, 2013) and can cause neonatal meningitis, sepsis, and pneumonia. It may only cause flu-like symptoms in the mother and can mimic a urinary tract infection, but many women have no symptoms. Most cases of listeriosis are associated with sporadic contamination rather than epidemics (CDC, 2013). Fetal transmission is not inevitable, and outcomes are worse if infection occurs early in the pregnancy (Cox and Phelan, 2009a).

Listeria is a soilborne bacteria; infection results from eating contaminated foods of animal origin and raw produce. Because it can also be airborne, can tolerate high salt environments, and grows in moist environments at refrigeration temperatures, raw milk, smoked seafood, frankfurters, pâté, soft cheeses (especially if made with unpasteurized milk), and uncooked meats are likely sources. Because of improvements in processing, the risk of contamination in packaged cold cuts is now one fifth that of retail-sliced meats (Batz, 2011). Recommendations to reduce risk include using only pasteurized food products and heating precooked meat products to steaming (see Box 15-8).

Mercury and Polychlorinated Biphenyls (PCBs)

Methylmercury contamination is known to affect fetal neural development disproportionately. It crosses the placenta and blood-brain barrier and accumulates in the fetus; cord blood levels are 70% higher than maternal levels (Cox and Phelan, 2009b).

Traces of methylmercury are found in most fish, but concentrations are highest in those fish that are large and predatory. Although advisories are specific to local conditions, the U.S. EPA and FDA currently recommend that all women of

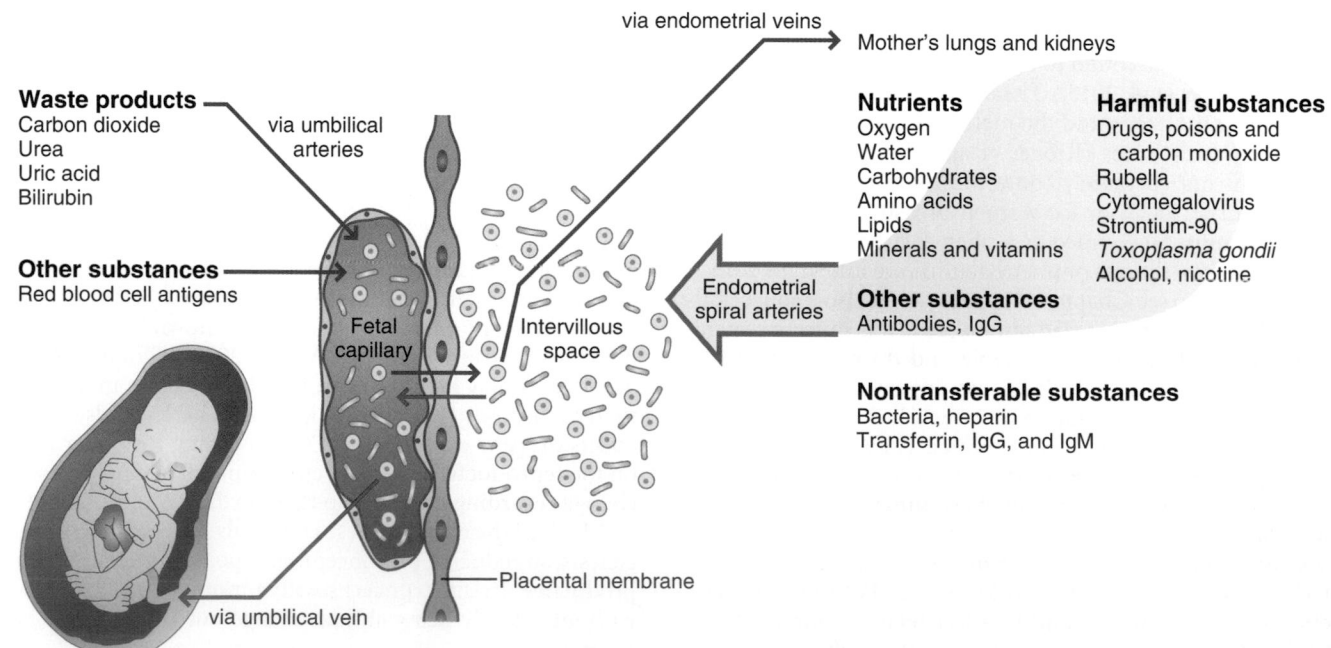

FIGURE 15-5 Transfer of substances across the placental membrane. *Ig*, Immunoglobulin.

BOX 15-8 *Listeria* Guidelines

Follow the general safety guidelines in Box 15-7, including the following:

- Avoid cross contamination with the fluid from hot dog packages.
- Keep raw meats separated from vegetables, cooked foods, and ready-to-eat foods.
- Wash vegetables thoroughly.
- Eat perishable and ready-to-eat foods (dairy, meat, poultry, seafood, produce) as soon as possible. Check for "use by" dates once/week and throw out food that has passed. Follow recommended storage times for foods.
- Wipe up spills immediately. Clean the refrigerator regularly with hot water and mild liquid detergent, rinse.

Choose lower risk foods.

- Avoid unpasteurized milk or any foods made from raw milks.
- Make sure soft cheeses (feta, Brie, Camembert, blue-veined, or Mexican style "queso blanco," "queso fresco," or Panela) are made with pasteurized milk.
- Do not eat hot dogs, luncheon meats, or deli meats unless reheated to steaming (165° F). Meats may be chilled afterward. As an alternative, cooked meats or canned meats (salmon, chicken, tuna) may be used for sandwiches.
- Do not eat refrigerated pâtés or meat spreads. Canned or shelf-stable versions may be eaten.
- Do not eat ham salad, chicken salad, or seafood salad made at the store. Instead, make them at home following general food safety guidelines.
- Do not eat refrigerated smoked seafood unless it is in a cooked dish (165° F). This includes smoked salmon, trout, whitefish, cod, tuna, and mackerel. They are often labeled "nova-style," "lox," "kippered," "smoked," or "jerky." They are found in the refrigerated section or sold at the deli counter. Canned or shelf-stable versions may be eaten.

Adapted from Cox JT, Phelan ST: Food safety in pregnancy, part 1: putting risks into perspective, *Contemporary Ob/Gyn* 54:44, 2009a; United States Department of Health and Human Services (USDHHS): *Checklist of Foods to Avoid During Pregnancy* (website): http://www.foodsafety.gov/poisoning/risk/pregnant/chklist_pregnancy.html, 2014. Accessed January 2014.

childbearing age avoid the consumption of those fish that surpass 1 ppm methylmercury. The methylmercury accumulates in the lean tissue, so cooking methods do not affect the mercury content of the fish (see *Focus On:* Childhood Methylmercury Exposure and Toxicity in Chapter 17).

Not everyone has found long-term problems with methylmercury consumption (Van Wijngaarden et al, 2013). Research shows that selenium can form selenoproteins that may mitigate the harmful effects of mercury and other heavy metals. The selenium and mercury contents of fish and shellfish are now being characterized worldwide (Burger and Gochfeld, 2013). However, although some have promoted a selenium:mercury ratio as a better way to characterize risk, that may be premature. Selenium appears to protect against mercury toxicity only up to a limit, and excess selenium also can be highly toxic.

Fish also can be a source of polychlorinated biphenyls (PCBs), and prenatal exposure has been associated with child neurologic deficits (Cox and Phelan, 2009b). Although no longer produced, PCBs still remain in the water systems. Although PCBs can be absorbed through the skin and lungs, they primarily enter the body from ingestion of contaminated fatty fish. Farmed and wild ocean fish can contain PCBs, but fresh water fish from the Great Lakes are often of more concern.

PCBs readily pass through the placenta and breastmilk; pregnant and nursing women should avoid eating fish from water known to be highly contaminated with PCBs. For fish from other areas, they should be cooked to minimize the ingestion of the fat and the skin should not be eaten.

Regarding wild versus farmed salmon, there is controversy. Farmed Atlantic salmon is higher in contaminants (PCBs, dioxins, PBDEs, and some pesticides) than wild Pacific salmon, but it also contains higher levels of omega-3s than wild Pacific salmon. Although no data are specific to pregnancy, researchers conclude that the benefit (lives saved from coronary disease) from North and South American farmed sources outweighs the risk (lives lost to cancer) and is on par with the wild sources (Cox and Phelan, 2009b).

Local fresh waters and, therefore, fish also may be contaminated. Questions regarding methylmercury, PCBs, and other contaminants should be directed to state natural resource departments.

Most fish and seafood are low in methylmercury, and a few are particularly high in DHA (see *Focus On:* Omega-3 Fatty Acids in Pregnancy and Lactation). Fish may carry pathogens as well and all fish and seafood should be well cooked (see Box 15-9).

Other Foodborne Pathogens and Probiotics

Brucella spp., *Salmonella* spp., and *Campylobacter jejuni* are also of particular concern for pregnant women (Procter and Campbell, 2014). Prompt diagnosis of brucellosis and maternal antibiotic treatment can save the life of the fetus. Transmission of *Brucella* spp. through breastmilk also has been reported. Cases of fetal sepsis and multiorgan failure, leading to death, have been reported with nontyphoidal *Salmonella*. *Salmonella typhi*, the bacteria that cause typhoid fever, and *Campylobacter jejuni* can cross the placenta and infect the fetus, causing miscarriage, stillbirth, or preterm labor (Dean and Kendall, 2012; see Chapter 9).

For a discussion of the issues regarding the microbiome, see *Clinical Insight:* The Microbiome During Pregnancy and Lactation.

BOX 15-9 Fish Safety Guidelines

- Do not eat shark, tilefish (also called golden or white snapper), king mackerel, or swordfish.
- Albacore ("white") tuna should be limited to 6 oz/week. Limit marlin, orange roughy, and large tuna, often used in sushi or as tuna steaks.
- Other cooked fish and seafood may be eaten, up to 12 oz/week. See *Focus On:* Omega-3 Fatty Acids in Pregnancy and Lactation for recommended choices.
- Avoid refrigerated seafood products unless cooked before eating (165° F).
- Avoid raw or undercooked fish and seafood, including sushi and shellfish. All fish and shellfish should be cooked to 145° F.
- Observe local advisories regarding mercury and other contaminants. (For access to your state's or territory's advisories, see: http://fishadvisoryonline.epa.gov/General.aspx. Accessed October 2015.)

Adapted from Cox JT, Phelan ST: Food safety in pregnancy, part 2: what can I eat, doctor? *Contemporary Ob/Gyn* 54:24, 2009b; United States Department of Health and Human Services (USDHHS): *Checklist of Foods to Avoid During Pregnancy* (website): http://www.foodsafety.gov/poisoning/risk/pregnant/chklist_pregnancy.html, 2014. Accessed January 2014.

CLINICAL INSIGHT

The Microbiome During Pregnancy and Lactation

Probiotics are being investigated for potential benefit during pregnancy. Long-term effects include the influence on offspring immunity, including the potential prevention of atopic disorders. Probiotics also may play a role in early life programming, affecting the ability to metabolize macronutrients and maintain energy balance. In addition, effects on the pregnancy are also being investigated, including the lowered risk of preterm birth and preeclampsia, and improvement of glucose metabolism, lipid profiles, inflammation, and gestational weight gain (Lindsay et al, 2013). The abilities of the human microbiome to sequester toxic metals, degrade pesticides and carcinogens, and to lower blood pressure and serum cholesterol levels are also under investigation.

Although preliminary studies show probiotic use is associated with reduced rates of preeclampsia and GDM, these studies are few and small, with variable types and amounts of organisms being used (Lindsay et al, 2013). For most, interventions have been studied only in women with normal weights, although there are ongoing studies among overweight and obese women.

General guidelines cannot yet be made. It is now known that the fetus is not sterile and that microbes move from the maternal to the fetal environment from her GI track as well as vaginally (Prince et al, 2014). Transfer of bacteria to amniotic fluid could cause inflammation and therefore preterm delivery. Particular concern is raised for those women with immune suppression or dysfunction, as well as those with abnormalities in the gastrointestinal mucosal barrier. However, so far probiotics appear safe when used by healthy people.

During lactation, the milk microbiome may contribute to short- and long-term infant health and also to mammary health. Mammary dysbiosis often leads to acute, subacute, or subclinical mastitis. This condition may be resistant to antibiotics and could lead to undesired early weaning. New research providing selected lactobacilli strains isolated from breast milk show potential in treating this painful condition so that the continuation of successful breastfeeding is not jeopardized (Fernandez et al, 2012).

BOX 15-10   *Toxoplasma* Guidelines

- Follow the general food safety guidelines from Box 15-7.
- Freeze meats for several days before cooking.
- Wash hands after handling raw meats.
- Cook meats to at least 150° F + 3-minute rest (whole cuts), 160° F (ground meats, wild game), or 165° F (poultry). These temperatures may be higher than the USDA recommends for other pathogens. Do not sample meat until it is cooked. Meats that are smoked, cured in brine, or dried may still be infectious.
- Raw oysters, mussels, and clams should not be eaten.
- Keep children's sandboxes covered when not in use.
- Wear gloves when gardening or handling sand from a sandbox. Wash hands thoroughly afterward.
- Peel or thoroughly wash fruits and vegetables before eating.
- Avoid unpasteurized milk, including goat's milk.
- Do not drink water from the environment unless it is boiled.
- Keep your cats indoors. Do not feed them raw or undercooked meats or unpasteurized milks.
- Clean the litter box daily. If possible, have someone else change the litter box. If not, wear gloves and wash hands with soap and warm water afterward.
- Do not adopt a new cat while pregnant nor handle strays, especially kittens.
- Control rodents and other potential intermediate hosts.
- If butchering wild game or venison, bury the organs so that wild cats cannot eat them and spread the infection.

Adapted from Cox JT, Phelan ST: Food safety in pregnancy, part 1: putting risks into perspective, *Contemporary Ob/Gyn* 54:44, 2009a; Jones JL, Dubey JP: Foodborne toxoplasmosis, *Clin Infect Dis* 55:845, 2012.

Toxoplasma gondii

Toxoplasma gondii is a parasite that may cross the placenta, causing miscarriage, fetal death, chorioretinitis, and long-term neurologic and neurocognitive deficits for baby. Rates of congenital toxoplasmosis in the United States are unknown (it is not a reportable disease) but are estimated at 400 to 4000 cases/year (Cox and Phelan, 2009a). Although present in all countries, the prevalence varies considerably; highest rates of congenital toxoplasmosis are found in some countries in South America, the Middle East, and Africa (Torgerson and Mastroiacovo, 2013).

Symptoms are often mild, flu-like, and unrecognized, although people with immunosuppression can have chorioretinitis and encephalitis (Torgerson and Mastroiacovo, 2013). Clinical toxoplasmosis is rare in the United States, and 90% of pregnant women who are infected have no noticeable symptoms (Cox and Phelan, 2009a). However, even without maternal symptoms, the fetus can become infected. Overall transmission rates appear to be 20% to 50% but vary by trimester (Cox and Phelan, 2009a). Although transmission is lowest in the first trimester, the severity is also highest. The risk of passing the parasite to the fetus is reduced greatly if the mother has been previously exposed and is already seropositive. Although some countries (including France and Austria) routinely screen pregnant women, this is not standard practice in the United States.

Commonly women are encouraged to not handle used kitty litter when pregnant, because the cat is the definitive host for *Toxoplasma*. However, a cat passes the oocysts for only a few weeks in its lifetime. In addition, these oocysts are infective only after being exposed to the environment for at least a day; if the litter box is changed daily, there is little danger, even if the cat were infected and passing the eggs. Cats should be kept indoors and not fed raw meat.

Because the oocysts can live in the environment for years, water, dust, and garden soil can also be contaminated. Fruits and vegetables must be washed and contaminated water should not be ingested. Gloves should be used when gardening.

Meats and milks also can be infected with tissue cysts, and it is estimated that up to half the cases of toxoplasmosis occur with handling or eating undercooked or raw infected meats, especially wild game and those meats labeled "free-range" or organic (Jones and Dubey, 2012). Oysters, clams, and mussels can be contaminated through water runoff. Unpasteurized goat milk is also a known source, as are homemade cured, dried, and smoked meats. The injected salt solution that often is used in pork and chicken will kill tissue cysts, as may freezing the meat for a few days. To kill the parasite, meats must be cooked well (see Box 15-10).

Guide for Eating During Pregnancy

Recommended Food Intake

The increased nutrient requirements of pregnancy can often be met by following the Daily Food Guide (see Table 15-14). The USDA Daily Food Plan for Moms can be used interactively online. Although it can be a starting point, it is designed for those women with uncomplicated pregnancies. In addition, unless very nutrient-dense foods are chosen, it is likely to be deficient in iron, vitamin D, vitamin E, choline, potassium, and DHA (CNPP, 2013). Box 15-11 provides a summary of nutritional care. Weight gain and fetal growth should be monitored and the plan modified as needed.

TABLE 15-14 Daily Food Guide: Recommended Servings for a Woman Pregnant with a Singleton or Lactating

Food Group	PREGNANT WOMAN (NORMAL WEIGHT, < 30 MINUTES EXERCISE/WEEK)			LACTATING WOMAN (NO FORMULA SUPPLEMENTATION)		Serving Sizes (1)
	First Trimester	Second Trimester	Third Trimester	Early Lactation (0-6 mos)	Later Lactation (6+ mos)	
Total daily calories	1800	2200	2400	2130	2200	
Meat and beans, oz	5	6	6.5	7	6	1 oz = 1 oz meat , poultry, or fish, 1 egg, 1/4 c beans, ½ oz nuts, ¼ c tofu
Milk products, cups	3	3	3	3-4	3	1 c = 1 c milk or yogurt, 1.5 oz hard cheese, 2 c cottage cheese
Breads, grains, oz – half should be whole grains	6	7	8	8	9	1 oz = 1 slice bread, ½ c cooked starch, 1 c RTE cereal
Fruits and Vegetables (cups)	4	5	5	6	6	1 c = 1 c raw or cooked fruit or vegetable, ½ c dried fruit, 2 c leafy vegetables
Vitamin C rich	1	1	1	1	1	
Beta-carotene rich	1	1	1	1	1	
Folate rich	1	1	1	1	1	
Others	1	2	2	3	3	
Fats and oils, tsp	6	7	8	8	8	Included are those foods naturally high in fats, including olives, avocados, and nuts
Extras, calories	290	360	410	330	400	High fat or sugar foods or higher amounts of foods from the other groups
Beverages	10 c water/day (watch urine color)			8-12 glasses water or other beverage (drink to satisfy thirst)		8 oz.

(1) See the ChooseMyPlate website for more examples.
RTE, Ready to eat.
Adapted from *American College of Obstetricians and Gynecologists (ACOG):* Nutrition during Pregnancy. Patient Education Pamphlet AP001, September 2012; USDA: Choose My Plate food groups. http://www.choosemyplate.gov/food-groups/, 2014. Accessed February 2014.

BOX 15-11 Summary of Nutritional Care During Pregnancy

1. Include a variety of foods, focusing on nutrient dense food choices
2. Energy intake to allow for appropriate weight gain
3. Protein intake to meet nutritional needs, approximately an additional 25 g/day; additional 25 g/day/fetus if pregnant with more than one fetus. This often requires 20% of energy intake from protein
4. DHA from fatty fish (low in methylmercury) twice a week
5. Mineral and vitamin intakes to meet the recommended daily allowances. Folic acid supplementation is often required; iron supplementation may be necessary
6. Sodium intake that is not excessive but not <2300 mg/day. Iodized salt is recommended
7. Sufficient fluid intake to produce dilute urine, usually at least 2 L/day
8. Alcohol omitted
9. Omission of toxins and nonnutritive substances from food, water, and environment as much as possible

Fluids

Drinking 8 to 10 glasses of quality fluid daily, mainly water, is encouraged. The DRI for fluid increases slightly during pregnancy, but a woman's body size as well as climatic conditions are important considerations. Adequate hydration improves the overall sense of well-being. Frequent urination is often a complaint from pregnant women; however, optimal hydration reduces risks for urinary tract infections, kidney stones, and constipation and dehydration can cause uterine irritability. Women often have to be reminded to pay attention to their intake of liquids, using urine color after the first morning void as a guide.

Nutrient Supplementation During Pregnancy

Supplementation of a mother's diet during pregnancy may take the form of additional energy, protein, fatty acids, vitamins, or minerals that exceed her routine daily intake. The more compromised the nutritional status of the woman, the greater the benefit for pregnancy outcome with improved diet and nutrient supplementation. The goal is to consume the necessary nutrients as food, taking advantage of the likely beneficial synergistic effects and including phytonutrients or other bioactive compounds whose effects are not yet fully appreciated. However, judicious use of supplements is needed with undernourished women, teenage mothers, women with substance abuse, women with a short interval between pregnancies, women with a history of delivering a LBW infant, and those pregnant with multiple fetuses. Preconceptual supplementation is recommended for folic acid and may be warranted for other nutrients as well.

Pregnant women at nutritional risk are encouraged to enroll in the Special Supplemental Nutrition Program for Women, Infants, and Children (WIC), under the auspices of the U.S. Department of Agriculture (USDA). The WIC program serves eligible pregnant women, breastfeeding (until 1 year postpartum) and nonbreastfeeding postpartum women (until 6 months postpartum), as well as infants and children (up to age 5; see Chapter 9). For women, "nutritional risk" criteria may include anemia, poor gestational weight gain, and inadequate diet, as well as a variety of preexisting medical conditions. WIC provides targeted supplemental foods, nutrition education and breastfeeding support, as well as health care referrals. Outcome studies show improved birth weights and higher mean gestational ages in infants born to WIC participants.

Many pregnant women have limited knowledge regarding the nutrients in the supplements they have been advised to purchase. The composition of multivitamin-multimineral supplements varies, and formulations change frequently (see Table 15-15). It is

TABLE 15-15   Comparison of Selected Prenatal Supplements

THE TOTAL NUTRIENT CONTENT IS SUPPLIED BY THE NUMBER OF RECOMMENDED TABLETS OR GUMMIES NOTED FOR EACH OF THE SUPPLEMENTS LISTED

Nutrient	1 Tablet/ Day	1 Tablet/ Day	1 Tablet/ Day	3 Tablets/Day	2 Gummies/Day	6 Tablets/Day	Child's Chewable: 1 Tablet/ Day
Vitamin A, IU	4000, all beta-carotene	2675, all retinyl palmitate	4000, acetate, beta-carotene	5000, all beta-carotene + 3 mg mixed carotenoids	4000, all retinyl palmitate	5000, beta-carotene, palmitate	3000, 33% beta-carotene
Vitamin D, IU	400	200	400	1000	400	1000	600
Vitamin E, IU	30	22.5	22	30	15	30 mg	30
Vitamin K, mcg				80		100	
Vitamin B₁ (thiamin), mg	1.8	1.4	1.84	4.0		30	1.5
Vitamin B₂ (riboflavin), mg	1.7	1.4	3	5.0		35	1.7
Vitamin B₃ (niacin), mg	20	18	20	20	20	40	15
Pantothenic acid, mg				10		60	10
Vitamin B₆, mg	2.6	1.9	10	5	2.5	20	2
Vitamin B₁₂, mcg	8	2.6	12	30	8	60	6
Folic acid, mcg	800	600	1000	600	800	1000	400
Vitamin C, mg	120	55	120	60	30	250	60
Choline, mg					10	120	
Biotin, mcg				300		600	40
Inositol, mg						20	
PABA, mg						10	
Calcium, mg	200			75		1000	100
Chromium, mcg				100		200	
Copper, mg		1.15	2	0.75		1.5	2
Iodine, mcg		250		90		150	150
Iron, mg	28	27	27	18		30	18
Magnesium, mg				15		500	
Manganese, mg				2			
Molybdenum, mcg				20		50	
Phosphorus, mg							
Potassium, mg						50	
Selenium, mcg		30		50		200	
Sodium, mg							10
Zinc mg	25	10	25	7.5	3.8	15	12
Omega-3 fish oil					50 mg DHA, 15 mg other omega-3 PUFAs		

TABLE 15-15 Comparison of Selected Prenatal Supplements—cont'd

	THE TOTAL NUTRIENT CONTENT IS SUPPLIED BY THE NUMBER OF RECOMMENDED TABLETS OR GUMMIES NOTED FOR EACH OF THE SUPPLEMENTS LISTED						
Nutrient	**1 Tablet/ Day**	**1 Tablet/ Day**	**1 Tablet/ Day**	**3 Tablets/Day**	**2 Gummies/Day**	**6 Tablets/Day**	**Child's Chewable: 1 Tablet/ Day**
Enzymes						"Digestive support" - protease, amylase, lipase, betaine	
Probiotics				Lactobacillus casei, L. plantarum, L. salivarius, L. acidophilus, L. rhamnosus, Streptococcus thermophilus, Bifidobacterium bifidus, B. infantis, B. longum, B. breve.		Lactobacillus sporogenes – 30 million	
Foods, herbs				Brown rice, oats, blueberries, prunes, blackberries, flame raisins, raspberries, dandelion leaf, rose hips, lavender, lemon balm, peppermint, cloves, broccoli, cauliflower, kale, daikon radish, cabbage, mustard		80 mg lemon bioflavonoids, 10 mg rutin, spirulina, alfalfa, chlorella, red raspberry, chamomile, ginger	

DHA, Docosahexaenoic acid; *PUFAs,* polyunsaturated fatty acids.

important to read the label on prenatal supplements—some are much more complete than others, and some include ingredients in addition to the vitamins and minerals. Women often need advice on local, suitable choices. Look for those that contain the USP, Consumer Labs, or NSF seals of approval for quality (not safety or effectiveness). A balanced prenatal supplement should contain 400 to 800 mcg of folic acid and also should contain iron unless contraindicated. Copper is recommended if the supplement also contains zinc or iron (Uriu-Adams et al, 2010). It should contain 150 mcg of iodine in the form of potassium iodide, not kelp or seaweed (Leung et al, 2013). Although some contain DHA, at least as much benefit can come from including high DHA fish regularly in the diet (see *Focus On:* Omega-3 Fatty Acids in Pregnancy and Lactation).

Those supplements containing levels much higher than the DRI are not recommended because of known teratogenic effects (e.g., preformed vitamin A), as well as potential epigenetic effects. Some contain many additional ingredients, including herbal preparations, many of which have not been evaluated for safety during pregnancy.

As a reminder, prenatal multivitamins-multiminerals may be more critical when a woman's nutritional status is at risk. For others, they may be used as insurance but should not be used as a substitute for eating well. Whether prenatal multivitamin-multimineral supplements are necessary for women living in affluent societies is debated, but their use is common. For women living in low- and middle-income conditions, prenatal supplementation has been associated with better birth outcomes (Hovdenak and Haram, 2012).

Nutrition Education

Nutrition intervention, including medical nutrition therapy (MNT), has been effective in improving the maternal diet, reducing the risk of anemia in late pregnancy, and improving gestational weight gain, thus lowering the risk of preterm birth, improving infant head circumference size, and birth weight (Girard and Olude, 2012). For low-income recipients, results are enhanced if education is combined with balanced energy and protein supplementation and/or micronutrient supplements.

Regarding the effectiveness of MNT on curbing excessive maternal weight gain, results are mixed. Many types of interventions are effective for some groups but not others and studies are ongoing, but dietary interventions appear to be more effective than those focusing on physical activity (Thangaratinam et al, 2012). Women should be given appropriate guidance on the weight gain, as well as nutrient intakes, expected. Although energy needs increase slightly, the mother is not "eating for two." Helping a mother find acceptable concentrated sources of nutrients and minimizing the intake of high-calorie, low-nutrient foods is likely to reassure the woman who starts the pregnancy overweight or obese and/or is gaining excessively. Most likely to be effective are more intense and frequent interventions (Nelson et al, 2010) with personalized advice (Kaiser and Campbell, 2014); just giving printed materials is likely to not be beneficial.

MNT is known to be helpful during pregnancy. However, to be most effective, dietitians and nutritionists must consider all current issues. A pregnant woman may have poor weight gain but also low iron levels; foods that address both issues should be used. She may have low calcium intake but also have GDM, thus modifying how she is counseled. She may have cultural practices that could affect her nutritional status (e.g., veiling and vitamin D). She may have preexisting medical conditions that must be managed, including carrying parasitic infections common in her home country. She may develop issues during pregnancy (e.g., anemia, gallstones, or GDM) but also may find medical issues that are not directly related to the pregnancy (e.g., cancer or a Crohn's disease flare-up). She may experience trauma from a motor vehicle accident or physical abuse that could require an ICU admission. All nutritional issues must be balanced, often with little research data to give firm guidance. One should give the best advice known but be open to changes as the evidence becomes available.

In addition, cultural aspects of counseling also must be kept in mind (see Chapter 14). A woman's perceived risk of abnormal weight gain may differ from the U.S. norm. Childrearing, including pregnancy and lactation, usually has strong cultural components, and it is advisable to understand the beliefs and customs of the population groups being served. Although each individual does not necessarily follow, or may not even be aware of, all the beliefs held in the culture, they may color a person's response to nutritional suggestions. For example, a woman coming from a culture that believes that cleft lip and palate are caused by seeing an eclipse may rely on the safety pin over her abdomen to protect her and may therefore be less concerned about taking her folic acid supplements. A Vietnamese woman who is fearful of drinking cold orange juice immediately postpartum because of the negative effect it will have on the skin years later may be willing to warm the juice, put sugar in it, or eat kiwis for vitamin C instead. A woman from Mexico who believes that you must comply with a craving or something will be missing from the baby, will be afraid to NOT eat the dirt she is craving. However, she may be willing to smell the wet dirt and eat a burned tortilla, thus complying with the craving but ingesting something that is not likely to be contaminated. She may believe that "vitamins make you hungry" and so will stop taking her prenatal supplements if she feels, or has been told, she is gaining too much weight.

Families often need to be reassured that low-fat and nonfat milks contain the same levels of protein, calcium, and vitamin D as the whole milk (i.e., they are not watered down milk and therefore dangerous for pregnancy). Immigrants from countries where tap water is not potable need to be reassured that it is treated in the United States and is safe to drink, and that bottled water is not only more expensive but also often does not contain fluoride. On the other hand, an immigrant may be fearful of the prenatal care in the United States, when she is not routinely screened for *Toxoplasma gondii*, as is the standard of care at home.

Cultural differences are not apparent just with immigrants. Women who are vegetarians may need nutritional guidance regarding protein, iron, calcium, and vitamin B_{12}, especially as volume of food becomes the limiting factor later in the pregnancy. Followers of Jehovah's Witness need advice on high-iron foods to lower their risk of needing a blood transfusion. Those who practice different dietary patterns during holidays, including fasting, may need guidance on how to minimize the impact of that change on the developing fetus. Someone working nights may need ideas on how to distribute her meals to optimize glucose control.

Pregnant women are adult learners and relevant, simple, concrete messages are most effective, especially if they are memorable and motivational (Girard and Olude, 2012). All people should be counseled with sensitivity, reinforcing those practices that are particularly helpful and modifying only those practices that may be harmful. One must investigate atypical dietary patterns and food sources to best fit the customs of the patient. Cultural differences should not be ignored or rejected outright. If there are some that must be modified now, it is best to explain why, how, and for how long. Otherwise, the guidance of grandmothers and cultural history will likely prevail.

Pregnancy is a time of great impact. Although historically the goal had just been a full-term, full-size newborn, now the focus has expanded to include ensuring someone biologically predisposed to be healthy from birth to old age (ACOG, 2013d). It is often a time when a mother is very receptive to doing her best for her child. Eating more fruits and vegetables, lean meats, low-fat milks, and whole grains while minimizing excess fat, sugar, and salt intakes will likely improve maternal health and birth outcomes in the short term. Animal research is showing high maternal intakes of fats and sugars during pregnancy and lactation results in altered development of the central reward system in offspring, leading to excessive intakes of these foods postnatally (Mennella, 2014). In addition, human research has demonstrated that flavors familiar to the infant, from exposure through the amniotic fluid and breastmilk, are more likely to be accepted by that child when first offered, thus increasing the chance that he or she will consume it. Although this may be important nutritionally, exposure to a variety of flavors early in life when the developing brain has heightened sensitivity to environmental influences also appears to facilitate acceptance of novel foods later (Mennella, 2014). Eating better during pregnancy helps develop better food habits for the mother and the rest of her family that, hopefully, will carry on past the current pregnancy, improving the entire family's health. In addition, she is likely to be having positive epigenetic effects, improving the health of future generations.

POSTPARTUM PERIOD = PRECONCEPTUAL PERIOD

Reproductive health concerns do not end at delivery. For many women, the postpartum period can be considered a preconceptual period. Excess postpartum weight retention is associated with increased risk of GDM and hypertension during a subsequent pregnancy, even in normal- and underweight women who gain appropriately in that subsequent pregnancy (Bogaerts et al, 2013). Nutrition and exercise counseling should continue postpartum, with the goal of returning the mother to her prepregnant weight within 6 to 12 months and achieving normal BMI before attempting another pregnancy (ACOG, 2013a). Medical issues, including GDM, must be resolved or appropriately treated before a subsequent pregnancy.

Nutrient stores also have to be replenished, and short interpregnancy intervals (less than 12 to 18 months) are associated with increased risk of miscarriage, preterm delivery, IUGR or LBW, stillbirth, and early neonatal death (Wendt et al, 2012; Wu et al, 2012a). The nutritional demands of breastfeeding also must be considered, and for those in areas with limited resources, it may take at least 1 year to recover. Even in high-income countries, LBW risk increases if the interpregnancy interval is less than 6 months (Wendt et al, 2012), and a significant proportion of low-income women in the United States are still iron deficient 2 years after delivery (Bodnar et al, 2002). Other nutrients also may be depleted for an extended period, including folate, vitamin A, and DHA. An antioxidant-rich diet may lower oxidative stress and improve pregnancy outcomes. Inflammation is also thought to play a role in increased risk with short interconceptual periods (Wendt et al, 2012), and those women who have no nonpregnant, nonlactating time may be at particular risk.

Current theory is that preconceptual nutrition is as critical as nutrition during pregnancy and for many nutrients, likely more critical because of their role in placental formation and organogenesis (see Preconception and Fertility).

LACTATION

Exclusive breastfeeding is unequivocally the preferred method of infant feeding for the first 6 months of life. Many professional health organizations have endorsed this recommendation, including the Academy of Nutrition and Dietetics, the AAP, ACOG, the American Academy of Family Practitioners, Healthy People 2020, the WIC program, the U.S. Surgeon General, and the U.S. Breastfeeding Committee. These organizations recommend breastfeeding throughout the first year and beyond, as long as mutually desired by mother and child; the WHO encourages breastfeeding throughout the second year of life. Breastfeeding offers protection from gastrointestinal and other infections and serves as a critical source of energy and nutrients during illness, reducing mortality among malnourished children. The development of strong immune and digestive systems in breastfed babies is thought to be due to the development of beneficial bacteria in the baby's gut, providing a healthy gut microbial population.

Mothers should be encouraged to breastfeed for as long as possible, even if it is not the full year. Nutrition from breastmilk and the protection from illness it provides are unmatched by any other substitute. Women should be supported in their decision to breastfeed for any length of time, whether it is for just 2 weeks, 2 years, or longer. Breastmilk continues to provide nutrition and immunities throughout the time the mother is lactating. Many women face barriers that may prevent them from breastfeeding for as long as they would like, so support from the health care system along with family members and the community is necessary for mothers to reach their goals (see Figure 15-6).

There are many health benefits for mother and child, as shown in Box 15-12. A recent study examined the racial and socioeconomic disparities in infant feeding, noting that higher rates of breastfeeding are seen in families in which the mother is older, married, with a higher education and income. Longterm health outcomes of breastfed infants and their non-breastfed siblings

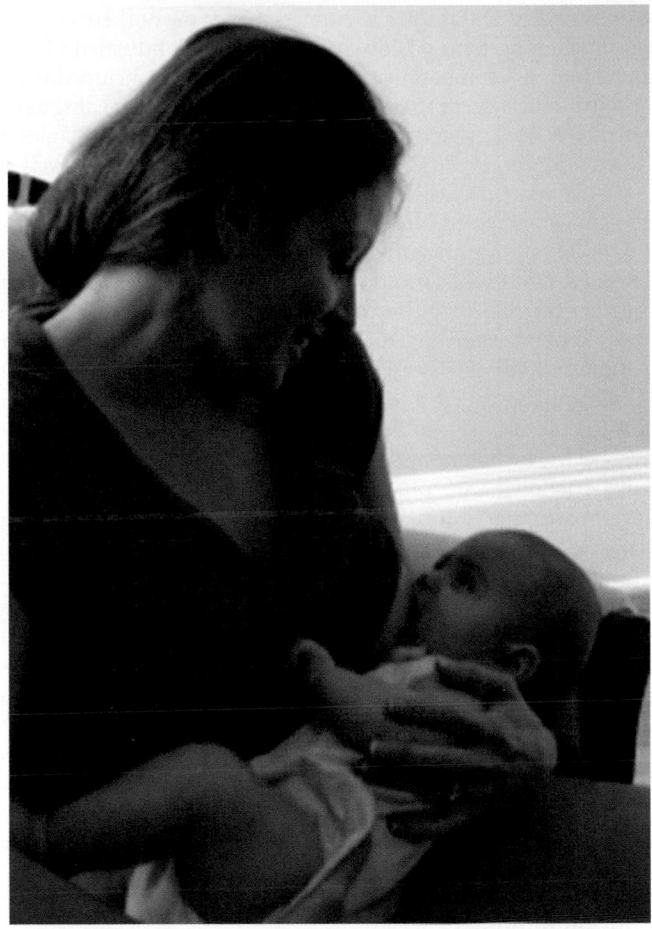

FIGURE 15-6 A nursing mother and her infant enjoy the close physical and emotional contact that accompanies breastfeeding. (Courtesy Robert Raab.)

BOX 15-12 Benefits of Breastfeeding

For Infant

Decreases Incidence and Severity of Infectious Diseases

Bacterial meningitis
Bacteremia
Diarrhea
Infant botulism
Necrotizing enterocolitis
Otitis media
Respiratory tract infection
Septicemia
Urinary tract infection

Decreases Rates of Other Diseases

Asthma
Celiac disease
Crohn's disease
Food allergies
Hodgkin disease
Hypercholesterolemia
Leukemia
Lymphoma
Overweight and obesity
Sudden infant death syndrome
Types 1 and 2 diabetes

Other Benefits

Promotes analgesia during painful procedures (heel stick for newborns)
Promotes enhanced performance on cognitive development tests
Promotes mother-child bonding
Promotes ready acceptance of solid foods

For Mother

Decreases menstrual blood loss
Decreases postpartum bleeding
Decreases risk of hormonal (breast and ovarian) cancers
Promotes earlier return to prepregnancy weight
Increases child spacing
Promotes rapid uterine involution
Decreases need for insulin in mothers with diabetes
Decreases risk of postmenopausal hip fracture and osteoporosis

For Society

Reduces health care costs
Decreases costs to public programs (i.e., WIC)
Prevents excess lost wages resulting from employee absenteeism for sick children
Supports greener environment

Reference: American Academy of Pediatrics and American College of Obstetricians and Gynecologists: *Breastfeeding handbook for physicians*, Elk Grove Village, Ill, 2006, American Academy of Pediatrics.

were compared and researchers noted that many of these children had similar long-term positive outcomes as their breastfed siblings or children in a comparative group. The authors concluded that a supportive breastfeeding environment and not breastfeeding alone contributes to long-term positive health outcomes of children (Colen and Ramey, 2014). Studies also have shown that levels of C-reactive protein (CRP), a key biomarker of inflammation and a predictor of increased cardiovascular and metabolic disease risk in adulthood, are significantly lower among individuals who were breast fed. Decreased concentrations corresponded to the duration of earlier breastfeeding. Researchers conclude that the longer the duration of breastfeeding, the less inflammation and lower risk for heart and metabolic diseases later in life (McDade et al, 2014).

In 1991 the WHO and the United Nations Children's Fund adopted the Baby-Friendly Hospital Initiative, a global effort to increase the incidence and duration of breastfeeding. To become "baby-friendly," a hospital must demonstrate to an outside review board that it implements the "Ten Steps to Successful Breastfeeding," a guideline for mother-baby management in the hospital; see Box 15-13.

The *Surgeon General's Call to Action to Support Breastfeeding* 2011 report states that breastfeeding should be promoted to all women in the United States and supported by clinicians, employers, communities, researchers, and government leaders. All are encouraged to commit to enabling mothers to meet their personal goals for breastfeeding. However, too many mothers are still not able to reach these goals. Improvement of support systems is needed for mothers to overcome challenges and barriers so often in the way of successful breastfeeding. Excess health risks associated with not breastfeeding can be found in Box 15-14.

Contraindications

Contraindications to breastfeeding are rare, but a few conditions warrant at least a temporary interruption from either direct feeding from the breast or from feeding breastmilk. Breastfeeding is contraindicated for infants with classic galactosemia, and for mothers who have active untreated tuberculosis, are positive for human T-cell lymphotropic virus type 1 or 2, have brucellosis, use drugs of abuse (without medical supervision), have

---

BOX 15-14   Excess Health Risks Associated with Not Breastfeeding

Outcome Excess Risk* (%) Among full-term infants		Comparison Groups
Acute ear infections (otitis media)	100	EFF‡ vs. EBF§ for 3 or 6 mos
Eczema (atopic dermatitis)	47	EBF <3 mos vs. EBF ≥3 mos
Diarrhea and vomiting (gastrointestinal infection)	178	Never BF¶ vs. ever BF
Hospitalization for lower respiratory tract diseases in the first year	257	Never BF vs. EBF ≥4 mos
Asthma, with family history	67	BF <3 mos vs. ≥3 mos
Asthma, no family history	35	BF <3 mos vs. ≥3 mos
Childhood obesity	32	Never BF vs. ever BF
Type 2 diabetes mellitus	64	Never BF vs. ever BF
Acute lymphocytic leukemia	23	Never BF vs. >6 mos
Acute myelogenous leukemia	18	Never BF vs. >6 mos
Sudden infant death syndrome	56	Never BF vs. ever BF
Among preterm infants		
Necrotizing enterocolitis	138	Never BF vs. ever BF
Among mothers		
Breast cancer	4	Never BF vs. ever BF (per year of breastfeeding)
Ovarian cancer	27	Never BF vs. ever BF

*The excess risk is approximated by using the odds ratios reported in the referenced studies.
‡*EFF,* Exclusive formula feeding.
§*EBF,* Exclusive breastfeeding.
¶*BF,* Breastfeeding.
Adapted from U.S. Department of Health and Human Services: *The Surgeon General's Call to Action to Support Breastfeeding,* Washington, DC, 2011, Office of the Surgeon General.

HIV (in the United States), or who take certain medications (i.e., antimetabolites and chemotherapeutic agents).

A mother should not breastfeed with active herpes simplex lesions on her breast; however, expressed milk can be used without concern. If a mother develops varicella 5 days before through 2 days after delivery, she should be separated from her infant but can provide her expressed milk to the infant. Mothers acutely infected with H1N1 influenza should separate themselves from their infants while febrile, but again, can provide their expressed milk for feedings (AAP, 2012). The use of most radioactive isotopes requires temporary cessation of breastfeeding, ranging from 6 hours to up to 1 month (Hale, 2012). Women undergoing procedures using these types of medications should consult with their health care provider to determine the specific drug used so that adequate time is allowed for clearance, but no more time than is necessary so that breastfeeding can be resumed. Clearance time varies between drugs; expressing and discarding breastmilk can help preserve milk production if extended cessation is necessary.

CDC advises women in the United States who have HIV to refrain from breastfeeding to avoid postnatal transmission to their infants through their breastmilk. Because sanitary conditions for safe use of infant formula are available in the United States, experts believe the morbidity risk can be kept to a minimum. However, in developing countries where sanitary conditions are not as prevalent, and the rate of mortality in the infant from infectious diseases and malnutrition are high, the

---

BOX 15-13   Baby-Friendly Hospital Initiative: Ten Steps to Successful Breastfeeding

1. Have a written breastfeeding policy that is routinely communicated to all health care staff.
2. Train all health care staff in the skills necessary to implement this policy.
3. Inform all pregnant women about the benefits and management of breastfeeding.
4. Help the mother initiate breastfeeding within a half-hour of birth.
5. Show mothers how to breastfeed and how to maintain lactation, even if they are separated from their infants.
6. Give newborn infants no food or drink other than breast milk unless medically indicated.
7. Practice rooming-in; allow mothers and infants to remain together 24 hours a day.
8. Encourage breastfeeding on demand.
9. Give no artificial teats or pacifiers (also called dummies or soothers) to breastfeeding infants.
10. Foster the establishment of breastfeeding support groups and refer mothers to them on discharge from the hospital or clinic.

Adapted from Randolph L et al: Baby Friendly Hospital Initiative feasibility study: final report. Healthy Mothers, Healthy Babies National Coalition Expert Work Group, Alexandria, Virginia, 1994, HMHB.

health risks of not breastfeeding must be considered. In addition, in areas where HIV is prevalent, exclusively breastfeeding for the first 3 months has been shown to reduce the risk of infants acquiring HIV compared with infants who receive a mixed diet of human milk and other foods, including infant formula. Six months of exclusive breastfeeding while the mother receives antiretroviral therapy has been shown to significantly reduce the postnatal acquisition of HIV (AAP, 2012).

Nutritional Requirements of Lactation

Despite the fact that breastfeeding increases the need for energy and some nutrients, human milk is made from maternal nutrient stores, so well-nourished mothers need not worry that the quality of their breastmilk will suffer from an imperfect diet. Breastmilk remains perfect for the infant even in cases of hardship and famine. Only in rare cases when mothers experience long-term, severe nutritional deficiency is their breastmilk affected. An excuse to not choose breastfeeding based on the fact that a woman enjoys drinking coffee or tea, or an occasional alcoholic beverage, is unwarranted.

Unless a vitamin-mineral deficiency is identified, or the mother has a restricted diet, dietary supplements are not necessary. A diet including a variety of foods, adequate in calories, should provide the woman with all the nutrients she needs. Despite this fact, many clinicians recommend the continued use of a prenatal vitamin/mineral supplement for the duration of lactation (AAP, 2012).

Increased prolactin receptors in the breast and therefore higher maternal prolactin levels develop with early suckling stimulation and milk removal, a process enhanced with increased frequency of breastfeeding in the early neonatal period. The maternal response to her infant's hunger cues will stimulate her milk supply, averaging about 8 to 12 breastfeeds over 24 hours in the first 2 to 3 weeks. The belief that more milk is made with increased fluid consumption is misguided because the body will excrete excessive fluid to maintain electrolyte balance. This actually may result in a decrease of milk production. Concern for the mother's hydration and her ability to produce an adequate milk supply is only valid during extreme conditions such as severe drought or famine. Insufficient milk supply can be as much of a problem in well-nourished as well as poorly nourished women; cross-cultural studies show it to be unrelated to maternal nutrition status. Poor maternal nutrition may affect the quantity, but not quality, of mothers' milk (Lawrence and Lawrence, 2011). Although a mother's milk maintains its quality even when nutrient intake is suboptimal, the woman feels the effects of eating poorly, possibly affecting her immune system, and feeling tired with less energy. A nutritious dietary intake helps her cope with the everyday demands of caring for a new infant.

Milk composition varies according to the mother's diet. For example, the fatty acid composition of a mother's milk reflects her dietary intake. In addition, milk concentrations of selenium, iodine, and some of the B vitamins reflect the maternal diet. Breastmilk of *extremely malnourished* mothers has been shown to have lower levels of various nutrients, reflecting the foods she has available to eat. One must remember that milk composition varies widely in the concentration of macronutrients within and between individual mothers. Several factors, including length of pregnancy, mother's diet, stage of lactation, duration of a feeding, and the time of day the feeding takes place, can affect the composition of human milk. Protein levels tend to fall in the early postpartum period, whereas the fat component of the milk initially may decrease and eventually increase in concentration over time. During an individual feeding, fat content typically increases significantly and can result in a much higher caloric content in the milk toward the end of the feeding (Khan et al, 2013). Fat content also may be higher when the interval between breastfeedings is closer together. When the infant "cluster feeds," the milk available in the breast is higher in fat content. When more time is allowed between feedings, the breasts fill with milk with higher water content. At the next feeding, the infant may not be able to consume all the milk available and ends up taking mainly low-fat milk.

Energy

Milk production is 80% efficient: production of 100 ml of milk (approximately 75 kcal) requires an 85-kcal expenditure (Lawrence and Lawrence, 2011). During the first 6 months of lactation, average milk production is 750 ml/day (about 24 oz), with a range of 550 to more than 1200 ml/day. Because production is a function of the frequency, duration, and intensity of infant suckling, infants who feed well are likely to stimulate the production of larger volumes of milk.

The DRI for energy during lactation is 330 kcal greater during the first 6 months of lactation and 400 kcal greater during the second 6 months of lactation over that for a nonpregnant woman. However, considering milk production usually drops to an average of 600 ml/day (approximately 20 oz/day) after other foods are introduced into the infant's diet, ingested calorie levels may have to be adjusted for the individual woman who wishes to avoid weight gain. A mother is able to draw approximately 100 to 150 kcal/day from pregnancy fat stores.

Healthy breastfeeding women can lose as much as 1 pound per week and still supply adequate milk to maintain their infants' growth. The combination of diet and exercise together, or diet alone can help women to lose weight after childbirth (Amorim Adegboye and Linne, 2013). In a study of 68 adolescent mothers and 64 adult mothers, postpartum weight loss in both groups was significantly greater in those who were exclusively breastfeeding (EBF) compared with those who did not EBF. Moreover, the infants of the mothers continued to grow according to the 2006 WHO growth standards despite their mothers' weight loss (Sámano et al, 2013). However, milk production has been shown to decrease in mothers whose intakes are suboptimal (less than 1500 to 1800 calories/day) (West and Marasco, 2009). Mothers are advised to wait until breastfeeding is well established (approximately 2 months) before consciously trying to lose weight so that an adequate milk supply can be established. Appropriate fluid intake (such as drinking for thirst) and adequate rest also are recommended. A slow weight loss of no more than about 5 pounds per month supports more permanent weight loss as well as allows for adequate energy and nutrition for new motherhood.

Protein

The DRI suggests an additional 25 g of protein a day for lactation, or 71 g of protein a day, based on an RDA of 1.1 gm/kg/day of a woman's body weight. Clinical judgment is necessary with protein recommendations because 71 g/day may be too low in an overweight woman and too high for the woman with a lower BMI. Women with surgical delivery and women who enter pregnancy with poor nutritional status may need additional protein. The average protein requirement for lactation is estimated from milk composition data and the mean daily volume of 750 mL, assuming 70% efficiency in the conversion of dietary protein to milk protein.

Breastmilk has a whey:casein ratio of 90:10 early in lactation, which changes to 80:20 as an average, and to 60:40 as the baby gets older. It is speculated that this ratio makes breastmilk more digestible. In contrast, the whey:casein ratio of cow's milk protein is 18:82. Cow's milk–based infant formula varies among commercial manufacturers, ranging from 18:82 whey:casein, to 52:48 whey:casein, and even up to 100% whey (see Chapter 16).

Carbohydrates

The RDA for carbohydrate is designed to provide enough calories in the diet for adequate volumes of milk and to maintain an adequate energy level during lactation. This may have to be adjusted depending on activity of the mother and the amount of breastfeeding. The woman with poor gestational weight gain may require more carbohydrates.

The principal carbohydrate in human milk is lactose; however, there is no evidence that maternal intake of carbohydrates affects the level of lactose in her milk.

Lipids

Dietary fat choices by the mother can increase or decrease specific fatty acids in her milk, but not the total amount of fat in the milk. Severe restriction of energy intake results in mobilization of body fat, and the milk produced has a fatty acid composition resembling that of the mother's body fat.

There is no DRI for total lipids during lactation because it depends on the amount of energy required by the mother to maintain milk production. The recommended amounts of specific omega-6 and omega-3 LCPUFAs during lactation vary little from pregnancy; they are crucial for fetal and infant brain development. One to two servings of fish per week meet this need (herring, canned light tuna, salmon). Mothers should avoid eating predatory fish to prevent excessive levels of dietary mercury (pike, marlin, mackerel, and swordfish) (AAP, 2012). Intake of trans fats should be kept to a minimum by the nursing mother so that the potential for their appearance in her breastmilk is reduced. See *Focus On:* Omega-3 Fatty Acids in Pregnancy and Lactation for more information about including DHA in the maternal diet.

Human milk contains 10 to 20 mg/dl of cholesterol, resulting in an approximate consumption of 100 mg/day, which has been determined to be essential to the diet of the infant. The amount of cholesterol in milk does not reflect the mother's diet and decreases over time as lactation progresses.

Vitamins and Minerals

Vitamin D. The vitamin D content of milk is related to maternal vitamin D intake as well as environmental conditions. Numerous case reports document marginal or significant vitamin D deficiency in infants of lactating women who are veiled, dark skinned, with BMI of more than 30, who use sunscreens heavily, or who live in latitudes with decreased sun exposure. Women with lactose intolerance who do not drink vitamin D–fortified milk or take a vitamin supplement may be at higher risk for vitamin D deficiency. Hypocalcemic rickets, including cases of dilated cardiomyopathy, have been reported in the United States in breastfed, dark-skinned infants (Brown et al, 2009).

Because of reports of clinical rickets, the AAP recommends that all breastfed infants receive 400 IU (10 mcg) of vitamin D as a daily supplement starting at birth, allowing him or her to easily achieve vitamin D sufficiency. Canada recommends 800 IU/day for adults living north of 45° N latitude, but the mother may need much higher doses (100 mcg or 4000 IU/ day) to achieve normal 25(OH)D concentrations and vitamin D adequacy in her exclusively breastfed infant. Because the antirachitic activity of human milk is low (5-80 IU/L), the lactating mother requires a significant amount of vitamin D daily from food or UV exposure. Maternal circulation allows transfer of the parent compound, Vitamin D3 itself, and not circulating 25(OH)D, into human milk. Although maternal baseline circulating 25(OH)D level may be adequate, it cannot be assumed that the vitamin D activity of her milk is adequate for the infant. Because of the binding affinity to vitamin D binding protein, the circulating half-life of 25(OH)D is 3-4 weeks, while that of vitamin D3 is just 12-24 hours; the reduced affinity of vitamin D3 allows the unbound vitamin D3 to diffuse across cell membranes from blood into the milk. In order for levels for vitamin D to be sustained in both the maternal circulation as well as the milk supply, a daily dose of Vitamin D is required. Recent studies have shown that a daily maternal intake of 6400 IU of vitamin D is safe, and allows a mother to produce milk that will provide adequate amounts of vitamin D to her exclusively breastfed nursling, without additional supplementation directly to the infant (Hollis, 2015).

Calcium. Although breastfeeding mothers should be encouraged to meet their DRI for calcium from their diet, the calcium content of breastmilk is not related to maternal intake, and there is no convincing evidence that maternal change in bone mineral density is influenced by calcium intake across a broad range of intakes up to 1600 mg/day. A recent study evaluated calcium intakes of 33 Gambian lactating women during two different lactational time periods. The study found that even with suboptimal intakes, the bone mineral mobilization during lactation was recovered after lactation. They concluded that successive periods of long lactation are not associated with progressive skeletal depletion (Sawo et al, 2013).

Iodine. Adequate breastmilk iodine levels are particularly important for proper neurodevelopment in nursing infants, and required intakes are nearly double nonpregnant values. Iodine concentrations in breastmilk are considered to be adequate to meet infants' iodine nutritional needs in areas where food sources are adequate. However, mothers living in iodine-deficient areas, especially if also consuming goitrogens or exposed to perchlorate contamination, may produce milk with iodine concentrations insufficient to meet the needs of the infant. As mentioned earlier, hyper- and hypo-thyroidism can affect breastmilk production, and so mothers should choose food sources of iodine, such as iodized salt, dairy foods, seafood, and breads made with iodide. Recent recommendations from the American Academy of Pediatrics state that lactating women should ensure a daily intake of 290 mcg of iodide, which generally requires supplementation of 150 mcg/day.

Zinc. The requirements for zinc during lactation are greater than those during pregnancy. Breastmilk provides the only dietary source of zinc for exclusively breastfed infants, and it remains a potentially important source of zinc for children beyond infancy who continue to breastfeed. In the process of normal lactation, the zinc content of breastmilk drops dramatically during the first few months from 2 to 3 mg/day to 1 mg/day by the third month after birth. Zinc supplementation has not been found to affect concentrations in the breastmilk of women in developed countries but may increase the zinc content of the milk of women in developing countries with suboptimal zinc status (Sazawal et al, 2013).

Vitamin B_{12} and the Vegan Mother. For lactating mothers who follow a strict vegan diet without any animal products, a vitamin B_{12} supplement is recommended strongly. The milk of a vegan mother can be severely deficient in vitamin B_{12}, leading to a deficiency in her infant which, if not treated, can lead to growth failure and permanent damage to the nervous system. Nursing mothers who follow a strict vegetarian diet should have their infant's B_{12} levels monitored.

Sodium. Sodium intake during lactation should be controlled with the inclusion of a diet composed of foods high in nutritional value, which are naturally lower in sodium. Although there is no specific recommendation or restriction for sodium in the diet of breastfeeding mothers, a relationship has been established between the sodium intake of mothers and breastfeeding success. A recent study examined whether maternal salt preference may facilitate breastfeeding. The investigators found that mothers with a preference for a low salt intake had higher rates of successful breastfeeding beyond day 7 compared with mothers with high salt preference. Mothers with high salt preference had the shortest exclusive breastfeeding duration up to postnatal day 25 (Verd et al, 2010). Future studies are warranted to determine exactly what effect maternal sodium intake has on the success of breastfeeding.

Fluids

A nursing mother may feel a need to drink simply because of increased fluid output when breastfeeding her infant. She should drink to thirst but not feel she must force fluids, which is not beneficial and may cause discomfort. The beverage of choice is water; however, water is the main component of many beverages and can be used as such in the body.

Caffeine. Caffeine is acceptable in moderate amounts (less than 300 mg daily, see Appendix 39) and does not present a problem for the healthy full-term infant. If the mother is nursing a preterm infant, however, the baby may be particularly sensitive to large intakes of caffeine. In this case the mother is advised to observe her infant closely for signs of overstimulation, such as being unusually fussy or not being able to settle easily. If so, the mother should adjust her caffeine intake accordingly. It may take a few days after reducing caffeine intake for mother to notice a difference in the baby's symptoms. There is no evidence that caffeine affects milk supply, although if a baby is overstimulated, he may not nurse well, which could lead to dysfunctional breastfeeding and eventually a lowered maternal milk supply.

Alcohol. No safe amount of alcohol has been established for the nursing mother, but recommendations include limiting intake to 0.5 g alcohol/kg maternal body weight (AAP, 2012). For a 60-kg mother, this equals approximately 2 oz liquor, 8 oz wine, or two beers per day. Peak alcohol levels occur in about ½ to 1 hour after drinking, although this varies among women depending on mother's body composition. There is no need for a mother to express and discard her milk after taking 1 to 2 drinks, thinking this will speed the elimination of alcohol from the milk, unless it is for her own comfort. As blood alcohol decreases, so does alcohol concentration in the milk. Mothers should be discriminatory about any alcohol intake when nursing a premature, young, or sick baby because this baby would be affected much more than the older, more mature baby. In addition, mothers should consider their ability to care for their children when under the influence of alcohol. If occasional alcohol intake occurs, moderation is advised at all times for breastfeeding mothers.

See Table 15-14 and Box 15-15 for summaries of nutritional care during lactation.

Physiology and Management of Lactation

Mammary gland growth during menarche and pregnancy prepares the woman for lactation. Hormonal changes in pregnancy markedly increase breast, areola, and nipple size as well as

---

> **BOX 15-15 Summary of Nutritional Care During Lactation**
>
> 1. Include a variety of foods, focusing on nutrient dense food choices.
> 2. Energy intake to allow for maintaining health and well-being; calorie level no less than 1800 kcal/day. Intentional weight loss not advised before breastfeeding is well established (approximately 2 months).
> 3. Protein intake to meet nutritional needs, approximately an additional 25 g/day from base level prepregnancy. This often requires 20% of energy intake from protein.
> 4. DHA from fatty fish (low in methylmercury) twice a week.
> 5. Mineral and vitamin intakes to meet the recommended daily allowances (usually met from a variety of foods in the diet). Supplements as directed from health care provider.
> 6. Drink to thirst; have beverages readily available during nursing and when expressing breastmilk.
> 7. If desired, alcoholic beverages can be consumed on occasion, in moderation. Not recommended with preterm, very young, or sick infants.
> 8. Omission of toxins and nonnutritive substances from food, water, and environment as much as possible.

significantly increase ducts and alveoli and influence mammary growth. Late in pregnancy the lobules of the alveolar system are maximally developed, and small amounts of colostrum may be released for several weeks before term and for a few days after delivery. After birth there is a rapid drop in circulating levels of estrogen and progesterone accompanied by a rapid increase in prolactin secretion, setting the stage for a copious milk supply.

The usual stimulus for milk production and secretion is suckling. Subcutaneous nerves of the areola send a message via the spinal cord to the hypothalamus, which in turn transmits a message to the pituitary gland, where the anterior and posterior areas are stimulated. Prolactin from the anterior pituitary stimulates alveolar cell milk production, as shown in Figure 15-7. Women who have diabetes, who are obese, who are stressed during

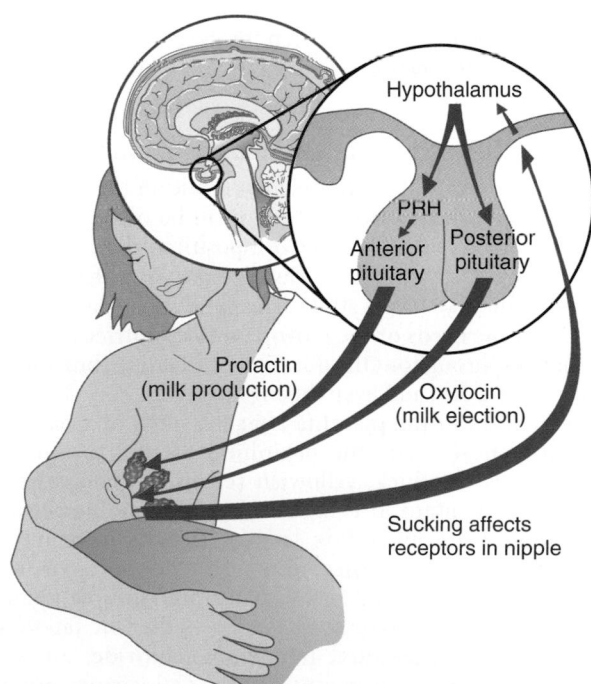

FIGURE 15-7 Physiology of milk production and the let-down reflex. *PRH,* Pituitary-releasing hormone.

delivery, or who have retained placental fragments in the uterus are at risk for delayed milk production (i.e. when signs of lactogenesis are absent 72 hours after birth).

Oxytocin from the posterior pituitary stimulates the myoepithelial cells of the mammary gland to contract, causing movement of milk through the ducts and lactiferous sinuses, a process referred to as let-down. "Let-down" is highly sensitive. Oxytocin may be released by visual, tactile, olfactory, and auditory stimuli; and even by thinking about the infant. Oxytocin secretion also can be inhibited by pain, emotional and physical stress, fatigue, and anxiety.

Prenatal Breastfeeding Education

The advantages of breastfeeding should be presented throughout the childbearing years. During pregnancy, counseling on the risks of formula feeding and the process of lactation should be provided to women so that they can make an informed decision about how they will feed their baby and so that they understand how to achieve successful breastfeeding. Prenatal breastfeeding education is recommended strongly for women and their partners. The emotional support provided by the mother's partner contributes heavily to the success of the breastfeeding experience.

During this time the mother should identify a support person to call upon after breastfeeding begins. Because initiation and establishment of breastfeeding can seem intense and full of challenges for new mothers, it is wise for her to know whom to turn to when questions or concerns arise. A knowledgeable family member or health professional, a doula, or childbirth educator can provide the encouragement so often needed for a mother in the early postpartum period. Prenatal breastfeeding counseling with regular follow-up after delivery has shown to have a positive effect on early initiation and sustained exclusive breastfeeding, especially among primiparous mothers, with group counseling having even more beneficial impact than individual counseling (Rai et al, 2014). When more complicated problems are identified, an International Board Certified Lactation Consultant (IBCLC) can intervene, which may mean the difference between early weaning and a successful breastfeeding experience.

Stages of Milk and Variations in Composition

Human milk varies in nutritional composition throughout the maternal lactational period and seems to be more sensitive to maternal factors such as body composition, diet, and parity during later lactation than during the first few months (Lawrence and Lawrence, 2011). This fluid is constantly changing to meet the needs of the growing infant; nutrient composition changes throughout the duration of lactation, but also over the course of a day, and even during a feeding.

The delivery of the placenta after the birth of a baby triggers lactogenesis I, or the beginning of milk production. Colostrum is the thick, yellowish secretion that is the first feeding for the infant. It is higher in protein and lower in fat and carbohydrate, including lactose, than mature milk. It facilitates the passage of meconium (first stool of neonate), is high in antioxidants, and is lower in water-soluble vitamins than mature milk. Colostrum is also higher in fat-soluble vitamins, protein, sodium, potassium, chloride, zinc, and immunoglobulins than mature milk. Colostrum provides approximately 20 kcal/oz and is a rich source of antibodies. It is considered the baby's first immunization.

Transitional milk begins to be produced approximately 2 to 5 days after delivery until around 10 to 14 days postpartum. During this stage of lactogenesis II, this white, creamy milk is produced in much greater quantities than colostrum, and breasts become larger and firmer. This is the time when mothers feel their milk "come in." It is important for mothers to breastfeed often during this stage (8 to 12 times/day) to avoid engorgement and allow proper emptying of the breast by the infant. This also ensures adequate fluid and nutrition for the baby during this time. This period is an extremely important time to bring in a full milk supply, which can be established by the infant only with unrestricted access to breastfeeding.

Mature milk is the final stage of milk production and usually begins to appear near the end of the second week after childbirth. Foremilk, the first milk released during a breastfeed, is high in water content to meet the baby's hydration needs. It is low in calories but high in water-soluble vitamins and protein. This milk is thinner, sometimes with a bluish color, and resembles skim milk when first released from the breast.

As the baby nurses during a breastfeed, the milk becomes creamier, indicating a higher fat content. This milk, high in fat-soluble vitamins and other nutrients, is called hindmilk. It provides satiety and the calories to ensure growth in the baby. It is important for the mother to allow the infant to empty the first breast at each feeding to obtain this hindmilk, before offering the other breast. This way, the baby is assured of obtaining the complete nutrition available from the mother's milk. Hindmilk is released as the breast is emptied and signals to the baby that a feeding is over. This mechanism helps the infant to learn when to end a feeding and may contribute to the prevention of overeating and subsequently becoming overweight later in life. The longer the mother goes between feedings, the more foremilk will be stored in the breast; however, when feedings are closer together, the baby receives more hindmilk in each feeding. Babies need a balanced diet, with sufficient amounts of foremilk and hindmilk for proper growth and development.

As the mother progresses during the lactational stage of motherhood, her breasts return to her prepregnancy size and may appear somewhat softer and smaller than earlier. This does not indicate a lower milk supply, but only her body's adjustment to established breastfeeding. A woman continues to produce nutritious mature milk, as well as enjoy the emotional and immunologic benefits, for as long as she breastfeeds. Exclusive breastfeeding is recommended for the first 6 months, followed by continued breastfeeding as complementary foods are introduced, with continuation of breastfeeding for 1 year or longer, as mutually desired by mother and child (AAP, 2012).

As mentioned previously, breastmilk is a dynamic fluid, changing throughout the lactational period of the mother. Breastmilk continues to provide an infant with needed amounts of essential nutrients well beyond the first year of life, especially protein, fat, and most vitamins. Breastfed infants tend to gain less weight and usually are leaner than are formula-fed infants in the second half of infancy, which does not seem to be the result of nutritional deficits, but rather infant self-regulation of energy intake. The nutrients most likely to be limiting in the diets of breastfed infants after 6 months of exclusive breastfeeding are minerals, such as iron, zinc, and calcium. These nutrients are readily available through an age-appropriate diet consisting of meats, whole grains, dairy foods, fruits, and vegetables.

During growth spurts, or times of rapid infant development—typically around 2 weeks, again at 4 to 6 weeks, and anytime between 3 and 6 months—babies may increase their desire to nurse to meet caloric needs. If allowed to do so, this triggers an increase in the mother's prolactin level, and after a few days, she will begin to make more milk. If supplements are introduced at these times to satisfy the infant's hunger, the mother will not have the advantage of increased stimulation from the infant's suckling and will not be able to keep up her supply to meet the baby's nutritional needs. Many mothers do not understand this concept of "supply and demand" and unintentionally may sabotage their breastfeeding relationship.

Initiation of Breastfeeding

Breastfeeding is a learned skill for mother and her infant. The baby should be put to breast soon after birth (within the first 30 to 60 minutes) and remain in direct skin-to-skin contact until the first feed is accomplished (AAP, 2012). Within 48 to 96 hours after birth the breasts become fuller and firmer as the milk volumes increase.

Exclusively breastfed babies do not need additional water because 87% of breastmilk is water. However, cases of hypernatremic dehydration in babies caused by suboptimal breastfeeding do occur. Most cases are due to lack of support for mothers who feel intimidated and overwhelmed at delivery, lack breastfeeding education, and are unaware of the consequences of dehydration. Extreme heat or hot weather also may increase the need for more frequent breastfeeding to avoid dehydration. The consequence of hypernatremic dehydration can be permanent brain damage or death. Therefore it is vital that an experienced health care professional evaluate the breastfeeding within 3 to 5 days after birth; problems identified can be addressed and a plan of care can be implemented (AAP, 2012).

During the first days and weeks of breastfeeding, mothers should feed on demand or "on cue." Watching and listening to the infant guides a mother to know when to offer a feeding. When a mother responds to her infant's hunger cues, nursing "on demand," she provides the quantity the baby needs, as long as supplements are avoided, and pacifiers are not used to "mask" the baby's hunger. A newborn's stomach is very small and holds only about a teaspoon or two of fluid at a time, matching the small amount of colostrum available from the mother. The colostrum is very easily absorbed, and that is why the infant will give frequent cues to his mother that he is hungry again. As a newborn's stomach enlarges over the next few days and weeks, so does the mother's milk supply as long as no supplement has interfered with this process of supply and demand. Extra bottle feedings can stretch the infant's stomach so that the supply the mother has available can no longer satisfy the baby. This situation may cause a mother to feel that she does not have enough milk and has failed at breastfeeding, and possibly unnecessarily cause her to wean. It is common to breastfeed 8 to 12 times a day while the breastmilk is increasing and an adequate supply is being established. After breastfeeding has been fully established after the first few weeks, lactating women may begin to feel the strong tingling sensation in the breasts caused by oxytocin release, signaling the let-down reflex. (See earlier explanation.) This sensation automatically causes a sudden release of milk from the breasts. If this occurs when the mother is not available for her baby, firm pressure on the breasts stops milk from flowing.

As breastfeeding continues, mothers begin to settle into a pattern of feeding that is comfortable and relaxed. Although each mother-baby couplet is different, most babies become more efficient at the breast and are able to take in more milk at a feeding time, as much as several ounces in just a few minutes. This allows the feedings to become less frequent and take less time. When breastfeeding is total nourishment for the baby, some feeds may be short just to satisfy a baby's thirst, and others may last 20 to 30 minutes if the baby is very hungry. This is no cause for worry, as long as the mother continues to respond to the infant's cues. Parents should be educated about this process so that they do not get discouraged or think that the intense feeding schedule that is common in the early weeks will last for the entire breastfeeding experience.

Practice, patience, and perseverance are necessary for successful breastfeeding, along with a strong support system for the mother, including family, friends, health care personnel, her workplace, and the community around her (see Box 15-13). With learned hand expression or the help of an effective breast pump, the mother is able to express and store her milk for later use when she is away from her infant. Pump rentals or purchase may be covered by insurance or available through the WIC program. See Box 15-16 for a summary of tips for success in breastfeeding.

Breastfeeding by Women with Diabetes. Women who have insulin-dependent diabetes may experience "lactation hypoglycemia" as they increase their breastfeeding sessions. Plasma glucose levels in the lactating diabetic mother are lower because of maternal stores being used for milk production. The daily maternal insulin requirement is usually lower in these women, and frequent glucose monitoring must be emphasized to ensure safety for the mother and baby. Because newborns of mothers with diabetes frequently are admitted to the NICU for closer observation, more support should be offered to these mothers to ensure breastfeeding success.

Breastfeeding Preterm and Sick Infants. Breastmilk for a preterm infant is not only beneficial but also absolutely necessary to ensure protection from infection and other illnesses (see

---

BOX 15-16 Tips for Breastfeeding Success

During your pregnancy:
- Enroll in the WIC program, if eligible.
- Attend a breastfeeding class.
- Read about breastfeeding.
- Get 1 to 2 good nursing bras.
- Find a supportive person that can help you.

In the hospital:
- Let doctors and nurses know that you plan to breastfeed.
- Do not use any bottles or pacifiers.
- Breastfeed during the first hour after birth.
- Keep baby in room with you 24 hours/day.
- Ask for lactation consultant (IBCLC) to help with correct latch.
- Breastfeed every 2 to 3 hours.
- Hold baby skin-to-skin to bond with baby and increase milk supply.
- If doctor orders supplementation, use expressed breastmilk.
- If you and your baby are separated because of illness, ask for a breast pump.

During the first 2 to 3 weeks at home:
- Don't give bottles or a pacifier.
- Breastfeed every 2 to 3 hours, at least 8 times a day.
- Make sure baby latches onto the breast correctly.
- Continue skin-to-skin care whenever possible.
- Watch for 6 to 8 wet and 2 to 3 messy diapers daily by end of first week.
- For questions or concerns, call the WIC Lactation Specialist or an IBCLC.
- See baby's doctor at 4 to 5 days of age for a weight check.
- If enrolled in WIC, see nutritionist to obtain nutritious foods for yourself!

Chapter 42). A mother may be overwhelmed when her baby is delivered before the due date or is admitted to the NICU for any reason. If the baby is not strong enough for effective breastfeeding, professional help should be used so that the mother can begin milk expression, and her milk can be available for the infant's nutrition.

A mother may find that she is totally dependent on the breast pump for several days, weeks, or even months. During this time, it is important for the mother (and father) to employ skin-to-skin care of their baby to allow appropriate stimulation of prolactin production in mother for her milk supply to be maintained. This connection with her newborn also assists in the bonding process, so important in the development of a healthy, loving relationship, which is challenged by the unfortunate situation in which the mother and her family find themselves. The mother will continue to need support and encouragement throughout the baby's hospitalization, and even more so when discharge gets closer. The total transfer of care to the parents can be an even bigger challenge, and they will need much guidance and follow-up to ensure breastfeeding is successful.

In the case of adoption, a devastating prognosis, or infant death, the mother can prepare herself for a gradual decrease in her milk supply to allow for her physical health. Any milk she has in storage can be donated to a human milk bank (see Focus On: *What Is a Human Milk Bank?* in Chapter 42). This will give her comfort in knowing that the milk she produced and saved for her own baby will not be wasted but be used for another infant who may need it. Again, much support and guidance from knowledgeable professionals is necessary during these trying times.

Breastfeeding Multiples. Breastfeeding twins, triplets, or more is certainly challenging, but possible. A mother who plans to breastfeed multiples will most likely need assistance, especially in the early days. If the babies are healthy and brought home soon after birth, she can begin breastfeeding them right away and establish her milk supply with the help of at least two babies instead of one. This means a greater milk supply will be available if she responds to their hunger cues, just like with a singleton. She will be busier, no doubt, and feeding multiples during the first few weeks will be intense, to say the least. If the mother is determined to establish a good breastmilk supply early on and has the household help she needs, she can be successful. If, however, the infants are sick and must remain hospitalized for a while, she needs to use an effective breast pump to bring in her milk supply and should make her expressed breastmilk available for the babies' nutrition. A lactation consult with an IBCLC is strongly recommended in such cases.

See Table 15-16 for a summary of common problems that breastfeeding mothers may encounter, with ways to prevent or remedy these situations.

Galactogogues

Low milk supply is a common concern among breastfeeding mothers. Whether real or perceived, mothers throughout the ages have turned to herbal remedies and medications to assist them in increasing their milk supply. Because milk supply is determined mainly by emptying the breasts regularly and effectively, this should be the first action taken to promote milk production. However, sometimes because of the effects of maternal or infant illness and hospitalization or separation because of work or school, a mother may find that despite her efforts, her milk supply is faltering. Galactogogues also have been used in cases of adoption or relactation (re-establishing a milk supply after weaning). **Galactagogues**, or milk production stimulants, can be classified as medications, herbals, or foods—each with its own results. Herbals must be used with caution as many contain chemical substances that may be dangerous to the infant. A lactation consultant or herbalist who is knowledgeable about their use in breastfeeding mothers should be consulted before using them. Standard recommended doses should not be exceeded (Hale, 2012).

Table 15-17 provides a list of common galactogogues along with possible side effects and contraindications. Medications

---

TABLE 15-16 Management of Breastfeeding Difficulties

Problem	Approaches
Inverted nipples	Breast shells with appropriate backing can be used during the last trimester of pregnancy. Before feeding the infant, roll the nipple gently between the fingers until erect. May use breast pump for 1-2 minutes before latching baby to bring nipple out.
Breast engorgement	Soften breasts/nipple by expressing a small amount of milk or use reverse pressure softening technique; allow baby to nurse frequently and/or express with hand or pump after feeding to relieve engorgement. Use cool compresses to ease pain after breastfeeding. Raw cabbage leaves placed on breasts for a few minutes every few hours may help to reduce swelling. Approved oral antiinflammatory medication may be used for pain.
Poor latch	Ensure proper positioning at breast; encourage baby to take a "mouth-full" of breast into his mouth; use nipple shield as last resort (use only with professional guidance).
Baby's mouth not open wide enough	Before feeding, depress the infant's lower jaw with one finger as the nipple is guided into the mouth. Elicit wide-open mouth from baby tickling upper lip with nipple.
Sore nipples	Strive for proper latch (possible temporary use of nipple shields with professional guidance); for pain relief: approved nipple ointment, breast shells with appropriate backing if extremely sensitive, hydrogel pads, approved pain meds. Check for ankyloglossia, fungal infection, or improperly fitting pump flange.
Baby sucks poorly	Stimulate sucking motions by pressing upward under the baby's chin. Use breast massage to express milk in baby's mouth and stimulate suck/swallow. Rule out infant/maternal physical or medical issues.
Baby demonstrates rooting but does not grasp the nipple; eventually cries in frustration	Interrupt the feeding, comfort the infant; the mother should take time to relax before trying again. Place baby in a comfortable position facing the breast. Express a few drops of milk on the nipple to entice the baby to latch.
Baby falls asleep while nursing	Mother may be able to awaken the infant by holding baby upright using skin-to-skin (when possible), rubbing baby's back, talking to baby, or providing similar quiet stimuli; another effort at feeding can then be made. If the baby falls asleep again, the feeding should be postponed. Use breast massage to encourage milk to flow more rapidly and stimulate infant to suck/swallow.

TABLE 15-16   Management of Breastfeeding Difficulties—cont'd

Problem	Approaches
Plugged ducts	Firm fingertip massage in area of plug. Warm compresses before/during feedings on affected area. Frequent emptying of breast. Point baby's tongue in direction of plugged duct. Lecithin supplement may help to prevent reoccurrence.
Mastitis	Signs of infection: breast is red and tender. Possible maternal fever, malaise. Maternal antibiotics may be indicated; call physician. Continue to breastfeed as comfort allows; frequent emptying of breasts with breastfeeding or expression. Breastmilk is safe for baby. Maternal rest recommended.
Thrush	Treatment must include mother and baby to prevent cross-infection/reinfection. Wash hands meticulously; sterilize items in contact with mother's breasts or baby's mouth or diaper area. Keep nipples dry. Approved nipple ointment for mother and oral medication (antifungal) for infant indicated—call physician. Breastmilk is safe for baby. Continue to treat at least 1 week after symptoms are gone to prevent return of infection. Some natural remedies may help: vinegar rinses on nipples and baby's diaper area, garlic supplements, probiotics/acidophilus, Echinacea, grapefruit seed extract—consult physician or lactation consultant.
Raynaud's Nipple vasospasms	Ensure proper latch to prevent worsening of symptoms. Keep nipples warm; lambswool bra pads may be helpful. May apply dry heat immediately after nursing. Use approved pain medication as needed; consider calcium channel blocker. Avoid caffeine, nicotine, and other vasoconstrictive drugs.
Perceived low milk supply	Offer breast frequently to allow infant to stimulate milk supply as desired; practice skin-to-skin care to stimulate prolactin production; express milk after/between feedings; avoid pacifiers and bottle supplementation unless advised by health care professional. Good nutrition, rest, and stress management is also advised. Watch for signs of adequate infant output (frequent wet diapers; appropriate bowel movements). Monitor baby's weight for reassurance of adequate maternal milk supply/infant intake.
True low milk supply	Ensure infant is latched correctly for maximum comfort & effectiveness; offer both breasts at every feeding—switch sides a few times during a feeding session for extra stimulation; avoid pacifiers and bottles; increase breast emptying by nursing or expression (length and frequency)—8-12 times/day; use pump for a few minutes after a breastfeed; when pumping, continue for 5 minutes after milk stops flowing to elicit additional let down; include pumping session between 1 and 5 A.M. when milk production is highest; use high-quality electric double pump (consider renting hospital grade pump); massage breast while pumping; always use correct flange size; use skin-to-skin care at each nursing session; rest/adequate nutrition/hydration; manage stress. Consider galactogogues (natural herbs or medication)—only with medical supervision (see Table 15-17). Supplementation may be necessary (human milk preferred, possibly using supplementer at breast, cup, syringe, dropper).

Consult with physician and IBCLC (International Board Certified Lactation Consultant) for expert advice.

TABLE 15-17   Common Galactogogues

Class of Galactogogue	Specific Substance	Comments
Medications	Domperidone (Motilium)	Raises prolactin and proven useful as a galactogogue; few CNS effects such as depression. Recommended dosage: 10-20 mg orally 3-4 times daily.
	Metoclopramide (Reglan/Maxeran/Maxolon)	Raises prolactin and proven useful as a galactogogue; side effects may include diarrhea, sedation, gastric upset, nausea, extrapyramidal symptoms, severe depression. Recommended dosage: 10-15 mg orally 3 times daily.
Herbals	Fenugreek (Trigonella foenum graecum)	Strong reputation as an effective galactogogue, but undocumented. Side effects include maple syrup odor in urine and sweat (mother and baby); may cause diarrhea, hypoglycemia, dyspnea. Not to be taken during pregnancy. Recommended dosage: 2-3 capsules orally 3 times daily (no more than 6 grams per day).
	Milk Thistle (Silybum marianum/Silymarin)	Reputation as a galactagogue, but undocumented. Side effects include occasional mild GI side effects, increased clearance of metronidazole. Suggested dosage: 420 mg daily or 2-6 cups tea/day.
	Cooking herbs: anise, blackseed, caraway, coriander, dill, fennel Nonfood herbs: alfalfa, blessed thistle, nettle, goats rue, red clover, shatavari	Historical and cultural uses as galactogogues; effectiveness undocumented. Assumed to be safe with recommended dosages (varies with specific herbs), although strengths of herbal product ingredients may vary depending on particular plant used and how processed; caution is advised for use during pregnancy. Some companies make special blends for breastfeeding mothers.
Foods/beverages	Grains, nuts, seeds: oats (not instant), barley, brown rice, beans, sesame, almonds Fruits/Vegetables: dark green leafy vegetables, apricots, dates, figs, cooked green papaya Soups made from Torbangun or Mulunggay leaves	Historical and cultural uses as galactogogues; effectiveness undocumented. Recommended daily intake not documented.

Adapted from Marasco L: Inside track: increasing your milk supply with galactogogues, *J Hum Lact* 24:455, 2008; Hale TW: *Medications and mother's milk*, ed 15, Amarillo, Tex, 2012, Hale Publishing; Academy of Breastfeeding Medicine Protocol Committee (ABM): ABM Clinical Protocol #9: Use of Galactogogues in initiating or augmenting the rate of maternal milk secretion, *Breastfeeding Med* 6:41, 2011.

used to increase a mother's milk supply must be prescribed by the mother's health care provider. Lactating women always should let the baby's health care provider know if anything is taken to increase milk supply. Although traditional use of galactogogues suggests safety and possible efficacy, the mechanisms of action for most herbals have not been proven (ABM, 2011). Despite some traditional beliefs, beer and other alcoholic beverages do not increase milk supply and should not be used for this purpose.

Sustaining Maternal Milk Supply and Preservation of Successful Breastfeeding

Insufficient milk supply is rarely a problem for the well-fed, well-rested, and unstressed mother who stays in close contact with her baby. Sucking stimulates the flow of milk; thus feeding on demand should supply ample amounts of milk to the infant. Skin-to-skin care also can benefit the mother and baby by stimulating prolactin production in the mother while keeping the baby comforted and familiar with the mother. In the early days, indications of sufficient milk supply are that the baby continues to gain weight and length steadily, has at least six to eight wet diapers daily, and has frequent stools. Refer to Table 15-16 for tips on increasing milk supply.

Occasionally, however, breastfeeding complications can interfere with success. Figure 15-8 illustrates potential problems in the mother or the infant that should be investigated if the mother feels that her milk supply is dropping or the baby is showing signs of slow growth. The cause of the problem must be identified and corrected to preserve the breastfeeding relationship and maintain the infant's growth and development. Professional assistance is available to identify and correct any complications that may interfere with successful breastfeeding. An IBCLC can be found at birth hospitals or centers, pediatric hospitals, maternal-child clinics, physicians' offices, and private practices.

Sometimes the infant may show intolerance (i.e., fussiness, loose stools) to something the mother has ingested. The mother is advised to temporarily eliminate suspected irritants until a later time when the baby is older and the gastrointestinal track more mature. Many times food sensitivity is outgrown after a few weeks or months. Any food may be the culprit, including cow's milk protein (casein fraction), cruciferous vegetables, carbonated drinks, or even spicy foods. When suspicious foods are removed from the mother's diet, it is important to assess the nutritional quality of her diet and supplement appropriately.

Concerns During Lactation
Transfer of Drugs and Toxins into Human Milk

Almost all drugs taken by the mother appear in her milk to some degree. The amount that usually transfers is small and only rarely does the amount transferred into the mother's milk result in clinically relevant doses in the infant. Many factors influence how medications transfer into human milk: milk/plasma ratio, molecular weight of the drug, and the protein binding and lipid solubility of the drug. Once a drug has been ingested by the infant through the mother's milk, it must travel through the baby's gastrointestinal tract before absorption. There are many processes here that may disallow the drug actually to be metabolized in the infant's system. Caution is recommended especially for mothers who are nursing premature or ill infants as they are at a higher risk of the effects of even small amounts of medications that may come through maternal milk (Hale, 2012).

Many mothers have discontinued breastfeeding because of their need for a medication, when in fact there was a good chance that the drug could have been taken without risk to the baby. It is likely that medications penetrate into colostrum more than in mature milk, although even during this time, the amounts the baby is exposed to are very low. When the medication increases in the mother's plasma, it also increases in her milk. When the medication level falls in the mother's plasma, equilibrium is sought in the mother's milk, which drives the medication back into her plasma for elimination (Hale, 2012).

Centrally active drugs (anticonvulsants, antidepressants, antipsychotics) frequently penetrate milk in elevated levels based

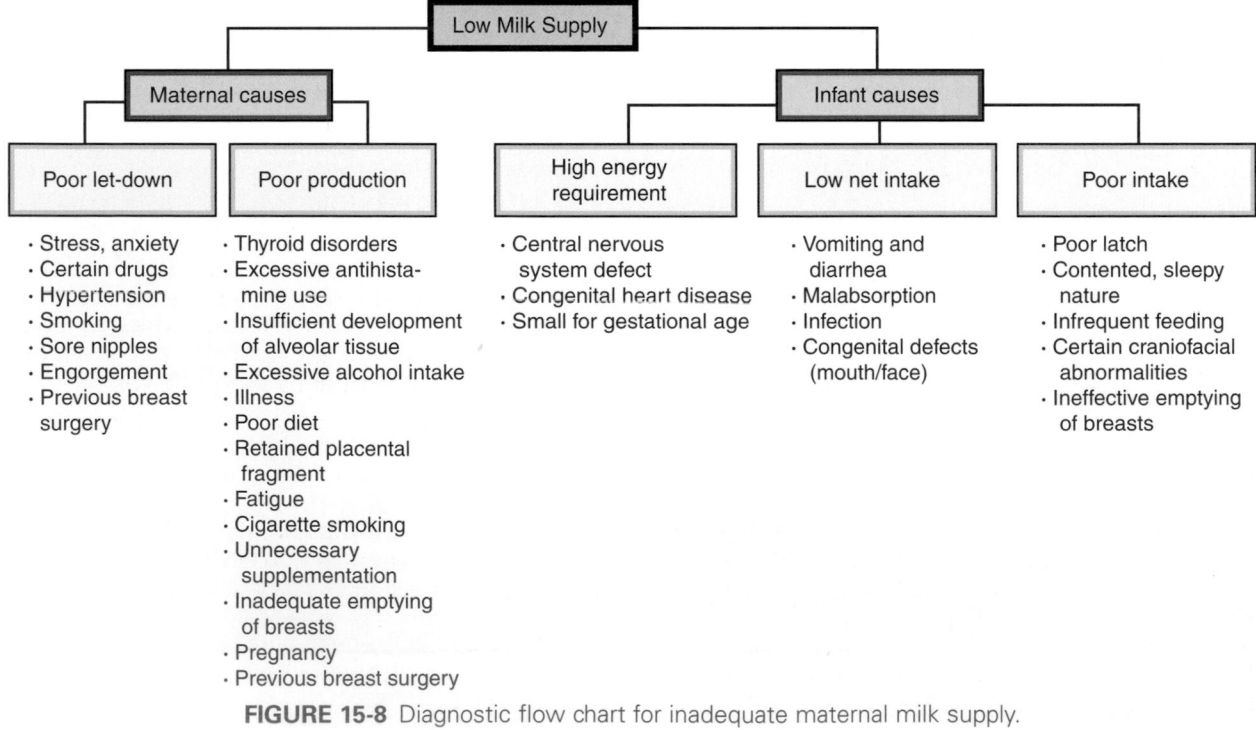

FIGURE 15-8 Diagnostic flow chart for inadequate maternal milk supply.

merely on their physiochemistry. When sedation, depression, or other CNS effects are experienced by the mother when taking the medication, it is likely to penetrate the milk and cause similar effects in the infant. These drugs must be used with caution, and the mother should always discuss risk-benefits of breastfeeding and her need for such medications with her health care provider.

Maternal Substance Abuse. According to the AAP, maternal substance abuse is not a categorical contraindication to breastfeeding. If a mother is well nourished and negative for HIV, even if narcotic-dependent, she should be encouraged to breastfeed as long as she is supervised in a methadone maintenance program (AAP, 2012; ABM and Jansson, 2009). Breastfeeding still provides the many immunologic, nutritional, and bonding advantages over artificial feeding. Very little methadone is transferred into breastmilk; however, studies are mixed reporting how breastfeeding should be managed in the mother-infant dyad to lessen the risk for neonatal abstinence syndrome (Dryden et al, 2009; Isemann et al, 2011). Growth parameters in the child should be monitored to ensure adequate development, but breastfeeding should continue to be encouraged as long as these measures are within the normal range. The long-term effect of methadone exposure beyond the neonatal period is relatively unknown. Studies have shown samples of blood and breastmilk up to 1 year show low concentrations of methadone, justifying the recommendation that mothers continue to breastfeed (Hudak et al, 2012). If a mother decides to discontinue breastfeeding, weaning slowly over 3 to 4 weeks helps to protect the infant from withdrawal symptoms.

The AAP and ACOG have provided information regarding the transfer of drugs and other chemicals into human milk (AAP, 2006). Websites that can provide more information include the AAP (www.aap.org), Lactmed (http://toxnet.nlm.nih.gov/newtoxnet/lactmed.htm), and the Infant Risk Center (www.infantrisk.com).

Environmental Toxins. There is concern about environmental toxins entering the milk of a lactating mother; however, at this time there are no established "safe" levels to aid in clinical interpretation. Despite any pollutants that may be found in human milk, the benefits of breastfeeding far outweigh the risks posed by any contaminants that may be found there. Nonetheless, mothers should take care not to allow any unnecessary exposure to pesticides and other harsh chemicals, as well as limit intake of animal fat, which can contain higher amounts of environmental contaminants. This helps safeguard against unwanted substances in human milk.

In the past, mothers were told not to lose too much weight too fast after pregnancy because it was thought that a rapid weight loss could possibly accelerate the release of toxins stored in a woman's body fat. However, this has not been proven to be true. Nonetheless, slow, steady weight loss during the postpartum period is recommended to allow a healthy return to prepregnancy weight with greater likelihood of keeping the weight off.

Overweight or Obesity

Overweight or obese lactating women can restrict their energy intake (once the milk supply is well-established) by 500 kcal per day by decreasing consumption of foods high in fat and simple sugars, but they must increase their intake of foods high in calcium, vitamin D, vitamin A, vitamin C, and omega-3 fats to provide key nutrients for their milk supply. The lactational period can be used as a time to allow natural slow weight loss in these mothers by taking advantage of the caloric demands of breastfeeding. The nutritional status of lactating women who have previously undergone gastric bypass surgery requires close attention, because suboptimal levels of iron, vitamin A, vitamin D, vitamin K, folate, and calcium have been reported (see Chapter 21).

Women with higher prepregnant BMI values also warrant extra lactation support to prevent early weaning and to reach their breastfeeding goals. Research has shown that although intentions of the obese woman to breastfeed may be strong, there can be many psychosocial determinants that may influence her commitment and ability to initiate or continue nursing her infant. Obese women also have shown to have delayed lactogenesis II, the sudden increase in volume a few days after delivery, which could be a risk factor in not establishing a milk supply. Although obese women experience lower rates of successful breastfeeding, the association between maternal obesity and breastfeeding outcomes has not been explained fully (Hauff et al, 2014).

Exercise and Breastfeeding

The breastfeeding mother should be encouraged to resume an exercise routine a few weeks after delivery and after lactation is well established. Aerobic exercise at 60% to 70% of maximum heart rate has no adverse effect on lactation; infants gain weight at the same rate, and the mother's cardiovascular fitness improves. Exercise also improves plasma lipids and insulin response in lactating women (Lovelady, 2011).

Mothers may be reluctant to exercise because of concerns of how this affects their breastmilk and consequently the growth of their infants. Moderate aerobic exercise (45 minutes/day, 5 days/week) has not been shown to affect milk volume or its composition. Mothers who incorporate diet and exercise into their routines in an effort to lose weight during the postpartum period also have been studied and have shown no ill effects on the growth of their infants (Daley et al, 2012; Lovelady, 2011).

Breast Augmentation

Breast augmentation, a procedure in which an implant is inserted into the breast to enlarge it, is a common elective breast procedure. Periareolar and transareolar incisions can cause lactation insufficiency. These mothers should be encouraged to breastfeed, and their infants monitored for appropriate weight gain. Other means of augmentation, in which implants are placed between breast tissue and the chest wall, usually have no effect on the woman's ability to produce a full milk supply.

Reduction Mammoplasty

Reduction mammoplasty often is recommended for women with extremely large breasts who suffer from back, shoulder, or neck pain or poor body image. In lactating women who have had this surgery there are wide variations in milk production, from a little to full production, depending on the amount of tissue removed and the type of surgical incision. These mothers also should be encouraged to breastfeed and be given anticipatory guidance and support; their infants should be monitored closely for appropriate weight gain.

Postpartum Depression

Postpartum depression (PPD) may be one of the most underdiagnosed obstetric complications in the United States. PPD leads to numerous negative consequences affecting the mother and child, including increased costs of medical care, inappropriate medical care, child abuse and neglect, discontinuation of breastfeeding, and family dysfunction. All this adversely affects early brain development in the infant (Earls, 2010), which could possibly lead to future problems.

Although effective treatment is available, fewer than half of mothers with this condition are recognized or seek help. PPD has been found to be lower in breastfeeding mothers (Xu et al, 2014). Because breastfeeding triggers the release of the hormone oxytocin, many women report feeling calm and relaxed while they are nursing. When breastfeeding is successful and things are going well, with maintenance of a good milk supply without complications, and baby is gaining appropriate weight, the breastfeeding relationship can ward off feelings of loneliness, emptiness, or failure—-common feelings in PPD. A higher circulating oxytocin level sustains a sense of calm and allows a mother to cope with the everyday stresses of new motherhood. Conversely, when things are not going well, when complications of breastfeeding and new motherhood become overwhelming, many new mothers experience signs of the "blues," which can escalate into full PPD. The "baby blues," affecting 70% to 80% of all new mothers (APO, 2014), is short lived, does not impair functioning, and can be treated with reassurance and emotional support. PPD, however, is characterized by a major depressive episode within 1 month after delivery, and is experienced in 10% to 15% of women after giving birth. Symptoms are restlessness, anxiety, fatigue, and a sense of worthlessness. Some new mothers worry they will hurt themselves or their babies. Unlike the "baby blues," PPD does not go away quickly. A mother with diagnosed PPD usually requires a more intensive approach to treatment (USDHHS, 2014).

Diet quality and overall nutritional status may affect the risk of postpartum depression (Procter and Campbell, 2014). Many dietary components are being investigated regarding their role in minimizing PPD, including omega-3 fatty acids, folate, vitamins B_2, B_6, B_{12}, D, calcium, iron, and selenium. However, there is little evidence of benefit from supplementation. Mawson and Wang recently proposed that high levels of vitamin A compounds may be in part responsible for maternal PPD, and that breastfeeding offers protection against PPD by maintaining endogenous retinoids below a threshold concentration. Women accumulate retinoids in the liver and the breast during pregnancy in preparation of providing vitamin A to their infants. Because prolonged lactation reduces maternal stores of retinoids, this also provides a natural means of reducing potentially toxic concentrations in the mother (Mawson and Wang, 2013).

When early signs of PPD are present, and a mother stops breastfeeding, even more severe depression can affect the mother. Oxytocin levels fall abruptly, and a mother's feelings of failure may become even more pronounced. It is critical for families to be aware and for health care providers to screen for early symptoms of PPD not only to prevent more serious symptoms of the disease but also to protect and preserve the breastfeeding relationship. Maternal-child health care providers must prepare mothers and families for expected breastfeeding challenges, advocate for a supportive environment in birthing hospitals, and promote breastfeeding as the cultural norm in the community so that the breastfeeding relationship is successfully established early in the postpartum period (Olson et al, 2014).

PPD can affect milk production, let-down, and the ability to maintain an adequate milk supply for the baby. The elevated levels of cortisol present in PPD may delay lactogenesis II. When the blues turns into a more serious form of PPD, the establishment of a healthy bond between mother and child may be affected, jeopardizing the breastfeeding relationship and potentially leading to early weaning (Wu et al, 2012b).

Medical treatment for PPD while breastfeeding includes medications such as Zoloft, Paxil, and Prozac. These should be taken immediately after a feeding to allow the maximum time for drug clearance from milk before the next feeding. Also, the mother can express and discard her milk collected when peak serum levels of the drug are present. Monoamine oxidase (MAO) inhibitors are contraindicated for treatment of PPD if the mother is breastfeeding (Hale, 2012; see Chapter 8).

Birth Control and Breastfeeding

Many women begin to think about birth control shortly after delivery and while they are breastfeeding a new baby. The mother must consider the effects of the birth control method on her nursling, as well as how it may affect her milk supply.

The Lactation Amenorrhea Method (LAM) does not involve any device or medication and is completely safe for breastfeeding mothers. LAM is an important modern contraceptive method that, when practiced correctly, has a 98% effectiveness rate 6 months postpartum (Fabic and Choi, 2013). It must be emphasized that the method is effective ONLY when three conditions are met: (1) the infant is less than 6 months old, (2) the mother is amenorrheic, and (3) the mother is fully breastfeeding (baby not receiving anything other than milk at the breast, meeting all sucking needs at the breast without a pacifier). Mothers must be very attentive to the inclusion of all these factors if they are dependent on this method to prevent pregnancy. As soon as one of these parameters is absent, the mother is advised that she should employ an additional form of birth control if pregnancy is still not desirable.

Birth control methods using a combination of progestin and estrogen come in several different forms: combination birth control pill, monthly injections, patch, and the vaginal ring. Although progestin and estrogen are approved by the AAP for use in breastfeeding mothers, it is possible that estrogen-containing contraceptives may affect a mother's milk supply and therefore a progestin-only medication (minipill) may be a better choice, at least until 6 months postpartum. A longer lasting form of progestin-only birth control is the Depo-Provera ("depo") shot that lasts at least 12 weeks but may be effective even up to a year.

There are concerns that Latina women with a history of gestational diabetes taking the minipill or depo shot as a means of birth control may be at a higher risk of developing chronic diabetes (Kjos et al, 1998). This is especially the case when the depo shot is taken when other risk factors are present, including increased baseline diabetes risk, weight gain during use, and high baseline triglycerides or during breastfeeding (Xiang et al, 2006). Latina women with a history of GDM may need to consider another form of birth control other than progestin-only medications; combination oral contraceptives (COC) do not seem to increase the risk of type 2 diabetes, however, these are not recommended during lactation because of the negative effect on maternal milk supply.

A progestin-only IUD such as Mirena may have fewer side effects on a mother's milk supply. This product delivers hormones directly to the lining of the uterus, leading to only a slight increase in serum progesterone levels, less than with the minipill. The birth control implant (Norplant, Implanon) is another choice for women who wish to choose progestin-only means of birth control. The implant can last up to 5 years. Women are warned they may want to consider the pill form before using a longer-lasting form of birth control in case they are susceptible to a drop in milk supply even with progestin-only pills. This allows them to stop the pills and choose another birth control method (i.e., LAM or barrier) so that they do not have to wait for the effects of the progestin to wear off. No effect on infant growth has been noted with these medications, but for those who may be concerned about the unknown, barrier methods of birth control, an IUD without hormones (Para-Gard), or LAM, ensure that no drug is secreted in breastmilk.

One other form of birth control pill, meant to be used as a last resort (breastfeeding or not), is the so-called "morning-after pill." These are also available in a combination of estrogen and progestin (Preven, Ovral), or the progestin-only form (Plan B, Plan B One-Step). Mothers should consult with their health care providers or lactation consultants if a drop in milk supply is noticed. This may be just a short-lived, temporary condition, but close follow-up can ensure that this is the case. The AAP has approved this medication for use during breastfeeding, although it should be used only in rare circumstances.

Breastfeeding during Pregnancy

Mothers may discover they are pregnant while they are still nursing a young baby or child. If the pregnancy is normal and healthy, it is considered safe to continue to breastfeed throughout the pregnancy. A mother need not worry that her milk will be any less nutritious for her nursling. She may be concerned that the act of breastfeeding will interfere with her pregnancy, but that is not a valid concern unless she experiences a difficult pregnancy and is at risk for early labor. If she has been told to avoid intercourse by her physician, this also may indicate that she should stop breastfeeding since the release of oxytocin is involved in both. Earlier in pregnancy, the amount of oxytocin normally released during breastfeeding is not usually enough to cause the cervix to open.

Increased fatigue and nausea early in pregnancy may be challenging for the expectant mother; however, if breastfeeding continues, rest and a concerted effort to maintain good nutritional intake is a must. Sore nipples are also common early in pregnancy and may be the first sign to the mother that she is pregnant. She may need to employ methods of dealing with nipple tenderness (i.e., distraction, pain management techniques) to get through this period of time if breastfeeding is to continue. Because the quantity of the milk may decrease and the taste of the milk may change early during pregnancy, the nursling may reject breastfeeding altogether and self-wean. A mother may need to encourage her baby to continue to breastfeed if desired, especially if the baby is very young and still dependent on her milk for the majority of his or her nutritional intake.

Tandem Nursing

Tandem nursing is when the mother breastfeeds siblings who are not twins. As soon as the placenta is delivered, the mother will begin to produce colostrum once again. The mother should ensure that the new baby always has priority to this because it provides the protection the newborn needs. Sometimes mothers find that the nursing toddler is a help to her by preventing or relieving engorgement. In fact, with the stronger suck and intake of the toddler, the mother may begin to overproduce for the newborn. If she develops a strong let-down reflex releasing a large quantity of milk when the newborn first latches, it may cause coughing and choking. In this case the mother may want to express a small amount of milk before latching her newborn, or simply allow the toddler to nurse for a few minutes first.

Concerns of hygiene are unwarranted when a mother is nursing two siblings. The small bumps on the areola called

Montgomery glands produce a natural oil that cleans, lubricates, and protects the nipple during pregnancy and breastfeeding. This oil contains an enzyme that kills bacteria so that both children are protected. In addition, more immunities will be passed on through the breastmilk itself. If, however, the mother or one child develops thrush, she is advised to limit each child to one breast temporarily.

An older baby who has weaned prior to the birth of a new sibling may express interest in breastfeeding again. Handling this situation is a delicate one and calls for special attention to the older child, whether or not the mother decides to offer the breast again.

Weaning

Weaning begins at the first introduction of anything other than mother's milk. As a breastmilk substitute or solid foods begin to be offered to the baby, the weaning process has begun. Although breastfed babies tend to accept a variety of solid foods well, because of the fact that they already have been introduced to different flavors of food through their mother's milk, this does not mean that the infant is ready to stop breastfeeding. Breastmilk is recommended for the infant throughout at least the first year of life as stated previously, and even through the second year of life by some authorities (WHO, 2013). A mother may choose to allow baby-led weaning, which simply means she will offer breastfeeding for as long as the baby is interested. If a baby seems to be losing interest in breastfeeding while still very young (i.e., younger than 12 months), the mother can try various methods of encouraging him to continue to breastfeed, such as ensuring a good position at the breast, and cutting out any bottles or foods so that more nutrition will be offered through breastfeeding. An older baby may be distracted easily during nursing sessions; a quiet, darkened room may help to keep the baby focused on nursing, and get him back on track with breastfeeding regularly. Human milk remains a nutritious fluid for as long as it is produced by the mother; however, the breastfeeding relationship changes as the baby gets older. Babies may show a lack in desire to breastfeed at different ages, depending on many factors. As the child grows, breastfeeding becomes less of a nutritional need but more of a need for the psychological bond with their mother. Older infants may be happy to nurse three to four times a day, and toddlers may show interest only every now and then.

Some mothers may choose mother-led weaning, which is when the mother encourages the baby to stop breastfeeding. She may begin to offer other foods or beverages when the baby wants to nurse, or try to distract the baby in other ways. If this method is used, the mother should ensure that the baby's emotional needs are met because this could be a trying time for mother and child. The decision is up to the mother, and her decision should be supported, although if at all possible, she should be encouraged to provide her milk throughout the first year for her health of that of her baby.

Return to Work or School

A mother's return to work or school can be a major challenge for continued successful breastfeeding; however, it is possible and encouraged. If a nursing mother returns to work or school, it is best to wait until breastfeeding is going well and a good milk supply has been established. Babies placed in child care experience a higher chance of becoming ill

TABLE 15-18 Storage of Human Milk for Healthy Full-term Infants

STORING FRESH BREASTMILK

Location	Temperature	Maximum Time	Comments
Outside refrigerator	Room temperature (60° F-85° F)	3-4 hours (optimal) 6-8 hours (maximum)	Containers should be covered; discard leftover milk within 1-2 hours after feeding
Small cooler with blue-ice pack	59°F	24 hours	Ice packs should be in contact with containers; keep cooler closed—open only when needed
Refrigerator	≤39°F	≤72 hours (optimal) 5-8 days (maximum)	Keep milk in rear of refrigerator for maximal cooling
Freezer	≤0°F	≤6 months (optimal) ≤12 months (maximum)	Store in back of freezer for constant temperature

STORING THAWED BREASTMILK

	Room temperature (60° F-85° F)	Refrigerator (≤39° F)	Freezer
Thawed breastmilk	≤1-2 hours (optimal) ≤3-4 hours (maximum)	24 hours	Do not refreeze

Adapted from USDHHS, Office on Women's Health: *Breastfeeding: Pumping and Milk Storage* (website): http://www.womenshealth.gov/breastfeeding/pumping-and-milk-storage/, 2014. Accessed February 2014.

when exposed to other children; however, breastmilk offers protection against germs the child is likely to be exposed to in these environments.

An exclusive diet of human milk continues to provide optimal nutrition through the baby's first 6 months. After that time, when appropriate solid foods are introduced into the baby's diet, mother's milk is the milk of choice at least through the baby's first year, and even beyond. The mother also experiences rewards if she is able to continue to breastfeed after her return to work or school. This helps to maintain an emotional connection with her baby because she will be reminded physically throughout the day of the need to express milk from her breasts. She also can continue to preserve the breastfeeding relationship with her baby when at home. Because of the advance in quality of breast pumps on the market today, mothers are able to express milk and maintain their supply effectively and comfortably. See Table 15-18 for breastmilk storage guidelines for healthy full-term infants and Table 15-19 for guidelines for hospitalized infants.

Many mothers are able to obtain breast pumps using their health insurance or through the WIC program. Federal and state laws also offer protection for the lactating worker so that she is ensured a private, clean space (other than a restroom) to express her milk while away from her baby. Mothers should talk to school personnel or their work supervisor before their maternity leave so that a plan is in place upon her return, and so that all parties involved will have an understanding of what to expect. A woman who expresses her milk regularly throughout the day with an effective pump can maintain a full milk supply for as long as she desires while at work or school full time. A mother facing this situation can find more help with this by discussing any questions or challenges with a lactation professional.

TABLE 15-19 Human Milk Storage Recommendations for Hospitalized Infants

Storage Method	Recommended Storage Time
Freezer (home unit combined with refrigerator)	3 months
Freezer (-20° C, -4° F)	6-12 months
Freezer (-70° C, -94° F)	≥12 months
Refrigerator (4° C, 40° F), fresh milk	48-96 hours*
Refrigerator (4° C, 40° F), thawed milk	24 hours
Refrigerator (4° C, 40° F) fortified milk	24 hours
Refrigerator (4° C, 40° F), thawed pasteurized donor milk	48 hours
Cooler with ice packs (15° C, 59° F), fresh milk	24 hours
Room temperature (25° C, 77° F)	<4 hours

Adapted from Academy of Nutrition and Dietetics: *Infant feedings: guidelines for preparation of human milk and formula in health care facilities*, ed 2, 2011, ADA.
*Applies to fresh milk unit-dosed at time of expression when expressed under clean conditions before infant feeding.

Common Nutrition Diagnosis Statements in Pregnant or Lactating Women

Limited access to food related to low income and misunderstanding of the use of WIC vouchers as evidenced by other family members using the WIC foods in the household

Obesity related to frequent meals and snacking during pregnancy as evidenced by weight gain of 30 pounds in second trimester

Intake of unsafe foods related to storing fresh milk on the counter as evidenced by home visit by social worker and discussions with client

Inconsistent carbohydrate intake related to management of gestational diabetes as evidenced by nutritional history of skipping breakfast and sometimes lunch

Abnormal gastrointestinal function related to heartburn as evidenced by complaints of reflux after every meal and excessive use of antacids

Inadequate food and beverage intake related to irregular income as evidenced by discussion about migrant status and the challenges during pregnancy

Breastfeeding difficulty related to frequent nipple soreness as evidenced by mother's hesitancy to continue nursing her 6-month-old

Food- and nutrition-related knowledge deficit of breastfeeding management related to frequent infant crying and slow infant weight gain as evidenced by a mother's report of keeping baby on a strict feeding schedule

Undesirable food choices as related to mother's desire for rapid weight loss while breastfeeding as evidenced by dietary recall showing excessive intake of diet drinks and low calorie food items.

CLINICAL CASE STUDY 1

Carol is a 34-year-old woman who was pregnant recently for the first time, but the baby had anencephaly and died at birth. She has a sister who has spina bifida and an older brother who had a stroke when he was 14. Carol has now been tested and found to have a genetic defect known as a 677C>T polymorphism in the methylenetetrahydrofolate reductase (MTHFR) gene.

Of course, she and her husband were devastated with the loss of their first child, but they also very much want to be parents. She has gone to genetic counseling but is also coming to you to find out what she can do to lower the chances that this happens again. She is worried about using the traditional prenatal vitamin-mineral supplement because she has been cautioned that she is unable to metabolize folic acid from diet and supplements.

Nutrition Diagnostic Statement

Altered nutrient (folic acid) metabolism related to a genetic alteration as evidenced by positive results for C>T in the MTHFR gene and family history of spina bifida and stroke

Nutrition Care Questions

1. What advice would you give Carol about any special dietary changes?
2. Carol knows that there is a special prenatal vitamin-mineral supplement available but does not know how to obtain it. How will you help Carol find this supplement?
3. What are the risks for a successful pregnancy outcome if Carol cannot find this special prenatal supplement?
4. What other concerns do you have regarding her pregnancy?

CLINICAL CASE STUDY 2

Cecilia is 3 months postpartum after a normal labor and full-term delivery. She tells you that she is exclusively breastfeeding her baby about eight times a day but is very tired and is not getting much sleep because her baby always seems fussy between feedings—day and night. She has been determined to lose her "baby weight" and for the past 6 weeks, she has been restricting her caloric intake to around 1200 calories/day, including approximately six diet drinks every day. She reports that the pediatrician told her that the baby's weight gain has slowed over the past month and she would like her to begin supplementing the baby with formula. She is hesitant to do this because her goal is to continue breastfeeding exclusively until the baby is 6 months old, and then possibly continue until at least the baby's first birthday.

Nutrition Diagnostic Statement

Difficulty breastfeeding related to poor maternal dietary intake as evidenced by mother's report of inappropriate diet and baby's poor weight gain

Nutrition Care Questions

1. What would you tell Cecilia regarding her concern about losing her "baby weight"?
2. What would you tell her to do to improve her dietary intake?
3. How would you address her baby's fussiness and inadequate weight gain?
4. What advice would you give her to preserve her breastfeeding and achieve her breastfeeding goals?

USEFUL WEBSITES

Academy of Breastfeeding Medicine
www.bfmed.org
American Academy of Pediatrics
www.aap.org/breastfeeding

Breastfeeding After Breast Reduction
www.bfar.org
Breastfeeding Online (Jack Newman, MD)
www.breastfeedingonline.com
Food Safety for Pregnant Women
http://www.foodsafety.gov/risk/pregnant
International Lactation Consultant Association
www.ilca.org
Kelly Mom: evidence-based breastfeeding and parenting
www.kellymom.com
Lactation Education Resources
www.lactationtraining.com
La Leche League
www.lalecheleague.org
National Maternal and Child Oral Health Resource Center
www.mchoralhealth.org/
Natural Medicines Comprehensive Database: "Natural Medicines used during Pregnancy and Lactation"
http://naturaldatabase.therapeuticresearch.com/ce/ceCourse.aspx?cs=SCAMEL&st=2&li=1&pc=08%2D23&cec=1&pm=5&&AspxAutoDetectCookieSupport=1.
United States Breastfeeding Committee
www.usbreastfeeding.org
United States Department of Agriculture; Daily Food Plan for Moms
http://www.choosemyplate.gov/supertracker-tools/daily-food-plans/moms.html
United States Fish Consumption Advisories
http://www.epa.gov/mercury
United States Lactation Consultant Association
www.uslca.org
Wellstart International
www.wellstart.org
Women's Health: Breastfeeding
http://www.womenshealth.gov/breastfeeding
World Alliance for Breastfeeding Action (WABA)
http://www.waba.org.my/

REFERENCES

Academy of Breastfeeding Medicine Protocol Committee (ABM): ABM Clinical Protocol #9: use of galactogogues in initiating or augmenting the rate of maternal milk secretion, *Breastfeed Med* 6:41, 2011.

Academy of Breastfeeding Medicine Protocol Committee (ABM), Jansson LM: ABM Clinical Protocol #21: Guidelines for breastfeeding and the drug-dependent woman, *Breastfeed Med* 4:225, 2009.

Adams Waldorf KM, McAdams RM: Influence of infection during pregnancy on fetal development, *Reproduction* 146:R151, 2013.

American Academy of Pediatrics (AAP), Section on Breastfeeding: Breastfeeding and the use of human milk, *Pediatrics* 129:e827, 2012.

American Academy of Pediatrics (AAP), American College of Obstetricians and Gynecologists: *Breastfeeding handbook for physicians*, Elk Grove Village, Il, 2006, American Academy of Pediatrics.

American College of Obstetricians and Gynecologists: ACOG committee opinion No. 549: Obesity in pregnancy, *Obstet Gynecol* 121:213, 2013a.

American College of Obstetricians and Gynecologists: ACOG committee opinion No. 462: Moderate caffeine consumption during pregnancy, *Obstet Gynecol* 116:467, 2010.

American College of Obstetricians and Gynecologists: ACOG committee opinion No. 495: Vitamin D: screening and supplementation during pregnancy, *Obstet Gynecol* 118:197, 2011.

American College of Obstetricians and Gynecologists Women's Health Care Physicians, Committee on Health Care for Underserved Woman: ACOG committee opinion No. 569: Oral health care during pregnancy and through the lifespan, *Obstet Gynecol* 122:417, 2013b.

American College of Obstetricians and Gynecologists ACOG: Practice bulletin No. 137: Gestational diabetes mellitus, *Obstet Gynecol* 122: 406, 2013c.

American College of Obstetricians and Gynecologists: *Exposure to Toxic Environmental Agents, Companion Document,* 2013d. http://www.acog.org/~/media/Committee%20Opinions/Committee%20on%20Health%20Care%20for%20Underserved%20Women/ExposuretoToxic.pdf. Accessed December 2014.

American College of Obstetricians and Gynecologists: *Hypertension in Pregnancy, November 2013,* 2013e. http://www.acog.org/Resources_And_Publications/Task_Force_and_Work_Group_Reports/Hypertension_in_Pregnancy. Accessed December 2013.

American Diabetes Association (ADA): Standards of medical care in diabetes – 2014, *Diabetes Care* 37(Suppl 1):S14, 2014.

American Pregnancy Organization (APO): *Baby Blues,* 2014. http://american-pregnancy.org/firstyearoflife/babyblues.htm. Accessed December 2014.

Amorim Adegboye AR, Linne YM: Diet or exercise, or both, for weight reduction in women after childbirth, *Cochrane Database Syst Rev* 7:CD005627, 2013.

Barouki R, Gluckman PD, Grandjean P, et al: Developmental origins of non-communicable disease: implications for research and public health, *Environ Health* 11:42, 2012.

Batz MB, Hoffman S, Morris JG: *Ranking the Risks: the 10 Pathogen-food Combinations with the Greatest Burden on Public Health,* 2011. https://folio.iupui.edu/bitstream/handle/10244/1022/72267report.pdf. Accessed October 2015.

Belkacemi L, Nelson DM, Desai M, et al: Maternal undernutrition influences placental-fetal development, *Biol Reprod* 83:325, 2010.

Berti C, Biesalski HK, Gärtner R, et al: Micronutrients in pregnancy: current knowledge and unresolved questions, *Clin Nutr* 30:689, 2011.

Bloomfield FH: How is maternal nutrition related to preterm birth? *Annu Rev Nutr* 31:235, 2011.

Blumfield ML, Collins CE: High-protein diets during pregnancy: healthful or harmful for offspring? *Am J Clin Nutr* 100:993, 2014.

Bodnar LM, Cogswell ME, Scanlon KS: Low income postpartum women are at risk of iron deficiency, *J Nutr* 132:2298, 2002.

Bogaerts A, Van den Bergh BR, Ameye L, et al: Interpregnancy weight change and risk for adverse perinatal outcome, *Obstet Gynecol* 122:999, 2013.

Brannon PM, Picciano MF: Vitamin D in pregnancy and lactation in humans, *Annu Rev Nutr* 31:89, 2011.

Brown J, Nunez S, Russell M, et al: Hypocalcemic rickets and dilated cardio-myopathy: case reports and review of the literature, *Pediatr Cardiol* 30:818, 2009.

Burger J, Gochfeld M: Selenium and mercury molar ratios in commercial fish from New Jersey and Illinois: variation within species and relevance to risk communication, *Food Chem Toxicol* 57:235, 2013.

Cantor AG, Bougatsos C, Dana T, et al: Routine iron supplementation and screening for iron deficiency anemia in pregnancy: a systematic review for the U.S. Preventive Services Task Force, *Ann Intern Med* 162:566, 2015.

Cardwell MS: Eating disorders during pregnancy, *Obstet Gynecol Surv* 68: 312, 2013.

Carlson SE, Colombo J, Gajewski BJ, et al: DHA supplementation and pregnancy outcomes, *Am J Clin Nutr* 97:808, 2013.

Caudill MA: Folate bioavailability: implications for establishing dietary recommendations and optimizing status, *Am J Clin Nutr* 91:S1455, 2010.

Center for Nutrition Policy and Promotion (CNPP): *Nutrients in 2010 USDA Food Patterns at All Calorie Levels,* 2013. http://www.cnpp.usda.gov/sites/default/files/usda_food_patterns/Nutrientsin2010USDAFoodPatternsatAll-CalorieLevels.pdf. Accessed December 2014.

Centers for Disease Control and Prevention (CDC): *Facts About Folic Acid,* 2014a. http://www.cdc.gov/ncbddd/folicacid/about.html. Accessed December 2014.

Centers for Disease Control and Prevention (CDC): *Recommendations to Prevent and Control Iron Deficiency in the United States,* 1998. http://www.cdc.gov/mmwr/pdf/rr/rr4703.pdf. Accessed December 2014.

Centers for Disease Control and Prevention (CDC): *Teen Pregnancy,* 2014b. http://www.cdc.gov/teenpregnancy/. Accessed December 2014.

Centers for Disease Control and Prevention (CDC): Vital signs: Listeria illnesses, deaths, and outbreaks—United States, 2009-2011, *MMWR Morb Mortal Wkly Rep* 62:448, 2013.

Chang T, Choi H, Richardson CR, et al: Implications of teen birth for overweight and obesity in adulthood, *Am J Obstet Gynecol* 209:110e1, 2013.

Clark SM, Costantine MH, Hankins GD, Review of NVP and HG and early pharmacotherapeutic intervention, *Obstet Gynecol Int* 2012:252676, 2012.

Cohen-Addad N, Chatterjee M, Bekersky I, et al: In utero-exposure to saccharin: a threat? *Cancer Lett* 32:151, 1986.

Colen CG, Ramey DM: Is breast truly best? Estimating the effects of breast-feeding on long-term child health and wellbeing in the United States using sibling comparisons, *Soc Sci Med* 109:55, 2014.

Cox JT, Phelan ST: Food safety in pregnancy, part 1: putting risks into perspective, *Contemporary Ob Gyn* 54:44, 2009a.

Cox JT, Phelan ST: Food safety in pregnancy, part 2: what can I eat, doctor? *Contemporary Ob Gyn* 54:24, 2009b.

Crider KS, Quinlivan EP, Berry RJ, et al: Genomic DNA methylation changes in response to folic acid supplementation in a population-based intervention study among women of reproductive age, *PLoS One* 6:e28144, 2011.

Daley AJ, Thomas A, Cooper H, et al: Maternal exercise and growth in breast-fed infants: a meta-analysis of randomized controlled trials, *Pediatrics* 130:108, 2012.

Dean J, Kendall P: *Food Safety During Pregnancy, Fact Sheet No. 9.372,* 2012. http://www.ext.colostate.edu/pubs/foodnut/09372.pdf. Accessed December 2014.

Dekker G, Robillard PY, Roberts C: The etiology of preeclampsia: the role of the father, *J Reprod Immunol* 89:126, 2011.

DelCurto H, Wu G, Satterfield MC: Nutrition and reproduction: links to epigenetics and metabolic syndrome in offspring, *Curr Opin Clin Nutr Metab Care* 16:385, 2013.

Di Gangi S, Gizzo S, Patrelli TS, et al: Wernicke's encephalopathy complicating hyperemesis gravidarum: from the background to the present, *J Matern Fetal Neonatal Med* 25:1499, 2012.

Dror DK, Allen LH: Interventions with vitamins B6, B12 and C in pregnancy, *Paediatr Perinat Epidemiol* 26:55, 2012.

Dryden C, Young D, Hepburn M, et al: Maternal methadone use in pregnancy: factors associated with the development of neonatal abstinence syndrome and implications for healthcare resources, *BJOG* 116:665, 2009.

Dunlop AL, Kramer MR, Hogue CJ, et al: Racial disparities in preterm birth: an overview of the potential role of nutrient deficiencies, *Acta Obstet Gynecol Scand* 90:1332, 2011.

Earls MF, Committee on Psychosocial Aspects of Child and Family health American Academy of Pediatrics: Incorporating recognition and management of perinatal and postpartum depression into pediatric practice, *Pediatrics* 126:1032, 2010.

Erick M: Hyperemesis gravidarum: a case of starvation and altered sensorium gestosis (ASG), *Med Hypotheses* 82:572, 2014.

Fabic MS, Choi Y: Assessing the quality of data regarding use of the lactational amenorrhea method, *Stud Fam Plann* 44:205, 2013.

Fejzo MS, Ching C, Schoenberg FP, et al: Change in paternity and recurrence of hyperemesis gravidarum, *J Matern Fetal Neonatal Med* 25:1241, 2012.

Fernandez I, Arroyo R, Espinosa I, et al: Probiotics for human lactational mastitis, *Beneficial Microbes* 5:169, 2012.

Fleischer DM, Spergel JM, Assa'ad AH, et al: Primary prevention of allergic disease through nutritional interventions, *J Allergy Clin Immunol Pract* 1:29, 2013.

Food and Drug Administration (FDA): *How sweet it is: All about sugar substitutes,* 2014. http://www.fda.gov/ForConsumers/ConsumerUpdates/ucm397711.htm. Accessed December 2014.

Fowden AL, Sferruzzi-Perri AN, Coan PM, et al: Placental efficiency and adaptation: endocrine regulation, *J Physiol* 587:3459, 2009.

Freeman HJ: Reproductive changes associated with celiac disease, *World J Gastroenterol* 16:5810, 2010.

Furber CM, McGowan L, Bower P, et al: Antenatal interventions for reducing weight in obese women for improving pregnancy outcome, *Cochrane Database Syst Rev* 1:CD009334, 2013.

Garrison SR, Allan GM, Sekhon RK, et al: Magnesium for skeletal muscle cramps, *Cochrane Database Syst Rev* 9:CD009402, 2012.

Gatford KL, Houda CM, Lu ZX, et al: Vitamin B12 and homocysteine status during pregnancy in the metformin in gestational diabetes trial: responses to maternal metformin compared with insulin treatment, *Diabetes Obes Metab* 15:660, 2013.

Gaur DS, Talekar MS, Pathak VP: Alcohol intake and cigarette smoking: impact of two major lifestyle factors on male infertility, *Indian J Pathol Microbiol* 53:35, 2010.

Georgieff MK: Long-term brain and behavioral consequences of early iron deficiency, *Nutr Rev* 69:S43, 2011.

Girard AW, Olude O: Nutrition education and counseling provided during pregnancy: effects on maternal, neonatal and child health outcomes, *Paediatr Perinat Epidemiol* 26:191, 2012.

Goodnight W, Newman R, Newman R, Society of Maternal-Fetal Medicine: Optimal nutrition for improved twin pregnancy outcome, *Obstet Gynecol* 114:1121, 2009.

Guéant JL, Namour F, Guéant-Rodriguez RM, et al: Folate and fetal programming: a play in epigenomics? *Trends Endocrinol Metab* 24:279, 2013.

Hale TW: *Medications and mothers' milk*, ed 15, Amarillo, Tx, 2012, Hale Publishing.

Harris AA: Practical advice for caring for women with eating disorders during the perinatal period, *J Midwifery Womens Health* 55:579, 2010.

Hauff LE, Leonard SA, Rasmussen KM: Associations of maternal obesity and psychosocial factors with breastfeeding intention, initiation, and duration, *Am J Clin Nutr* 99:524, 2014.

Heaney RP, Rafferty K: The settling problem in calcium-fortified soybean drinks, *J Am Diet Assoc* 106:1753, 2006.

Holick MF: Sunlight, ultraviolet radiation, vitamin D and skin cancer: how much sunlight do we need? *Adv Exp Med Biol* 810:1, 2014.

Hollis BW, Wagner CL, Howard CR, et al: Maternal versus infant vitamin D supplementation during lactation: A randomized controlled trial, Pediatrics 136:625, 2015.

Hovdenak N, Haram K: Influence of mineral and vitamin supplements on pregnancy outcome, *Eur J Obstet Gynecol Reprod Biol* 164:127, 2012.

Hudak ML, Tan RC, COMMITTEE ON DRUGS, et al: Neonatal drug withdrawal, *Pediatrics* 129:e540, 2012.

Isemann B, Meinzen-Der J, Akinbi H: Maternal and neonatal factors impacting response to methadone therapy in infants treated for neonatal abstinence syndrome, *J Perinatol* 31:25, 2011.

Jensen TK, Gottschau M, Madsen JO, et al: Habitual alcohol consumption associated with reduced semen quality and changes in reproductive hormones; a cross-sectional study among 1221 young Danish men, *BMJ Open* 4:e005462, 2014.

Johansson K, Cnattingius S, Näslund I, et al: Outcomes of pregnancy after bariatric surgery, *N Engl J Med* 372:814, 2015.

Joneja JM: Infant food allergy: where are we now? *JPEN J Parenter Enteral Nutr* 36(Suppl 1):S49, 2012.

Jones JL, Dubey JP: Foodborne toxoplasmosis, *Clin Infect Dis* 55:845, 2012.

Kaiser LL, Campbell CG: *Practice paper of the Academy of Nutrition and Dietetics: Nutrition and lifestyle for a healthy pregnancy outcome*, 2014. http://www.eatright.org/Members/content.aspx?id=6442481526. Accessed December 2014.

Khan S, Prime DK, Hepworth AR, et al: Investigation of short-term variations in term breast milk composition during repeated breast expression sessions, *J Hum Lact* 29:196, 2013.

Kjos SL, Peters RK, Xiang A, et al: Contraception and the risk of type 2 diabetes mellitus in Latina women with prior gestational diabetes mellitus, *JAMA* 280:533, 1998.

Koletzko B, Cetin I, Brenna JT, et al: Dietary fat intakes for pregnant and lactation women, *Br J Nutr* 98:873, 2007.

Koletzko B, Brands B, Poston L, et al: Early nutrition programming of long-term health, *Proc Nutr Soc* 71:371, 2012.

Kovacs CS: The role of vitamin D in pregnancy and lactation: insights from animal models and clinical studies, *Annu Rev Nutr* 32:97, 2012.

Kris-Etherton PM, Grieger JA, Etherton TD: Dietary reference intakes for DHA and EPA, *Prostaglandins Leukot Essent Fatty Acids* 81:99, 2009.

Kroger M, et al: Low-calorie sweeteners and other sugar substitutes: a review of the safety issues, *Compr Rev Food Sci Food Saf* 5:35, 2006.

Kwak-Kim J, Park JC, Ahn HK, et al: Immunological modes of pregnancy loss, *Am J Reprod Immunol* 63:611, 2010.

Larqué E, Gil-Sánchez A, Prieto-Sánchez MT, et al: Omega 3 fatty acids, gestation and pregnancy outcomes, *Br J Nutr* 107(Suppl 2):S77, 2012.

Lauritzen L, Carlson SE: Maternal fatty acid status during pregnancy and lactation and relation to newborn and infant status, *Matern Child Nutr* 7:41, 2011.

La Vecchia C: Low-calorie sweeteners and the risk of preterm delivery: results from two studies and a meta-analysis, *J Fam Plann Reprod Health Care* 39:12, 2013.

Lawlor DA, Wills AK, Fraser A, et al: Association of maternal vitamin D status during pregnancy with bone-mineral content in offspring: a prospective cohort study, *Lancet* 381:2176, 2013.

Lawrence RA, Lawrence RM: *Breastfeeding: a guide for the medical profession*, ed 7, Maryland Heights, Mo, 2011, Elsevier Mosby.

LeBlanc ES, Perrin N, Johnson JD Jr, et al: Over-the-counter and compounded vitamin D: is potency what we expect? *JAMA Intern Med* 173:585, 2013.

Lee AI, Okam MM: Anemia in pregnancy, *Hematol Oncol Clin N Am* 25:241, 2011.

Lessen R, Kavanaugh K: Position of the Academy of Nutrition and Dietetics: Promoting and Supporting Breastfeeding, J Acad Nutr Diet 115:444, 2015.

Leung AM, Pearce EN, Braverman LE: Sufficient iodine intake during pregnancy: just do it, *Thyroid* 23:7, 2013.

Lindsay KL, Walsh CA, Brennan L, et al: Probiotics in pregnancy and maternal outcomes: a systematic review, *J Matern Fetal Neonatal Med* 26:772, 2013.

London RS: Saccharin and aspartame. Are they safe to consume during pregnancy? *J Reprod Med* 33:17, 1988.

Lovelady C: Balancing exercise and food intake with lactation to promote post-partum weight loss, *Proc Nutr Soc* 70:181, 2011.

Lui S, Jones RL, Robinson NJ, et al: Detrimental effects of ethanol and its metabolite acetaldehyde, on first trimester human placental cell turnover and function, *PLoS One* 9:e87328, 2014.

Luke B: Nutrition for multiples, *Clin Obstet Gynecol* 58:585, 2015.

Luke B, Eberlein T: *When you're expecting twins, triplets, or quads*, ed 3, New York, 2011, Harper.

Marques AH, O'Connor TG, Roth C, et al: The influence of maternal prenatal and early childhood nutrition and maternal prenatal stress on offspring immune system development and neurodevelopmental disorders, *Front Neurosci* 7:120, 2013.

Mawson AR, Xueyuan W: Breastfeeding, retinoids, and postpartum depression: a new theory, *J Affective Disorders* 150:1129, 2013.

McDade TW, Metzger MW, Chyu L, et al: Long-term effects of birth weight and breastfeeding duration on inflammation in early adulthood, *Proc Biol Sci* 281:20133116, 2014.

Mechanick JI, Youdim A, Jones DB, et al: Clinical practice guidelines for the perioperative nutritional, metabolic, and nonsurgical support of the bariatric surgery patient—2013 update: cosponsored by American Association of Clinical Endocrinologists, the Obesity Society, and American Society for Metabolic and Bariatric Surgery, *Endocr Pract* 19:337, 2013.

Medscape: *Nausea and Vomiting: What CAM Options Are Viable?* 2014. http://www.medscape.com/viewarticle/818872. Accessed December 2014.

Mennella JA: Ontogeny of taste preferences: basic biology and implications for health, *Am J Clin Nutr* 99:S704, 2014.

Merhi ZO, Keltz J, Zapantis A, et al: Male adiposity impairs clinical pregnancy rate by in vitro fertilization without affecting day 3 embryo quality, *Obesity* 21:1608, 2013.

Milagro FI, Mansego ML, De Miguel C, et al: Dietary factors, epigenetic modifications and obesity outcomes: progresses and perspectives, *Mol Aspects Med* 34:782, 2013.

Millward DJ: Identifying recommended dietary allowances for protein and amino acids: a critique of the 2007 WHO/FAO/UNU report, *Br J Nutr* 108(Suppl 2):S3, 2012.

Monk C, Georgieff MK, Osterholm EA: Research review: maternal prenatal distress and poor nutrition—mutually influencing risk factors affecting infant neurocognitive development, *J Child Psychol Psychiatry* 54:115, 2013.

Mora-Esteves C, Shin D: Nutrient supplementation: improving male fertility fourfold, *Semin Reprod Med* 31:293, 2013.

Murray-Kolb LE: Iron status and neuropsychological consequences in women of reproductive age: what do we know and where are we headed? *J Nutr* 141:S747, 2011.

National Institutes of Health (NIH) consensus development conference statement: diagnosing gestational diabetes mellitus, March 4-6, 2013, *Obstet Gynecol* 122:358, 2013.

Nelson SM, Matthews P, Poston L: Maternal metabolism and obesity: modifiable determinants of pregnancy outcome, *Human Reprod Update* 16:255, 2010.

Nishiyama S, Mikeda T, Okada T, et al: Transient hypothyroidism or persistent hyperthyrotropinemia in neonates born to mothers with excessive iodine intake, *Thyroid* 14:1077, 2004.

Obeid R, Holzgreve W, Pietrzik K: Is 5-methyltetrahydrofolate an alternative to folic acid for the prevention of neural tube defects? *J Perinat Med* 41:469, 2013.

Office of Dietary Supplements (ODS), National Institute of Health (NIH): *Dietary Supplement Fact Sheet: Iron*, 2014. http://ods.od.nih.gov/factsheets/Iron-HealthProfessional/. Accessed December 2014.

Oken E, Guthrie LB, Bloomingdale A, et al: A pilot randomized controlled trial to promote healthful fish consumption during pregnancy: the Food for Thought Study, *Nutr J* 12:33, 2013.

Olausson H, Goldberg GR, Laskey MA, et al: Calcium economy in human pregnancy and lactation, *Nutr Res Rev* 25:40, 2012.

Olson T, Holtslander L, Bowen A: Mother's milk, mother's tears, breastfeeding with postpartum depression, *Clin Lact* 5:9, 2014.

Owen CM, Goldstein EH, Clayton JA, et al: Racial and ethnic health disparities in reproductive medicine: an evidence-based overview, *Semin Reprod Med* 31:317, 2013.

Pearce EN, Andersson M, Zimmermann MB: Global iodine nutrition: where do we stand in 2013? *Thyroid* 23:523, 2013.

Pelizzo G, Calcaterra V, Fusillo M, et al: Malnutrition in pregnancy following bariatric surgery: three clinical cases of fetal neural defects, *Nutr J* 13:59, 2014.

Pludowski P, Holick MF, Pilz S, et al: Vitamin D effects on musculoskeletal health, immunity, autoimmunity, cardiovascular disease, cancer, fertility, pregnancy, dementia and mortality—a review of recent evidence, *Autoimmun Rev* 12:976, 2013.

Prince AL, Antony KM, Ma J, et al: The microbiome and development: a mother's perspective, *Semin Reprod Med* 32:14, 2014.

Procter SB, Campbell CG: Position of the Academy of Nutrition and Dietetics: Nutrition and lifestyle for a healthy pregnancy outcome, *J Acad Nutr Diet* 114:1099, 2014.

Rai PL, Sharma N, Gaur A, et al: Effect of counseling on breast feeding practices, *Indian J Child Health* 1:54, 2014.

Ramakrishnan U, Grant F, Goldenberg T, et al: Effect of women's nutrition before and during early pregnancy on maternal and infant outcomes: a systematic review, *Paediatr Perinat Epidemiol* 26:285, 2012.

Rasmussen KM, Abrams B, Bodnar LM, et al: Recommendations for weight gain during pregnancy in the context of the obesity epidemic, *Obstet Gynecol* 116:1191, 2010.

Rasmussen KM, Yaktine AL: *Weight gain during pregnancy: reexamining the recommendations*, Washington, DC, 2009, Institute of Medicine, National Research Council.

Rhee SS, Braverman LE, Pino S, et al: High iodine content of Korean seaweed soup: a health risk for lactating women and their infants? *Thyroid* 21:927, 2011.

Roberts JM, Bell MJ: If we know so much about preeclampsia, why haven't we cured the disease? *J Reprod Immunol* 99:1, 2013.

Roseboom TJ, Painter RC, van Abeelen AF, et al: Hungry in the womb: what are the consequences? Lessons from the Dutch famine, *Maturitas* 70:141, 2011.

Roth DE: Vitamin D supplementation during pregnancy: safety considerations in the design and interpretation of clinical trials, *J Perinatol* 31:449, 2011.

Rulis AM, Levitt JA: FDA's food ingredient approval process: safety assurance based on scientific assessment, *Regul Toxicol Pharmacol* 53:20, 2009.

Saltzman E, Karl JP: Nutrient deficiencies after gastric bypass surgery, *Annu Rev Nutr* 33:183, 2013.

Sámano R, Martínez-Rojano H, Godínez Martínez E, et al: Effects of breastfeeding on weight loss and recovery of pregestational weight in adolescent and adult mothers, *Food Nutr Bull* 34:123, 2013.

Sathyanarayana S, Alcedo G, Saelens BE, et al: Unexpected results in a randomized dietary trial to reduce phthalate and bisphenol A exposures, *J Expo Sci Environ Epidemiol* 23:378, 2013.

Sawo Y, Jarjou LM, Goldberg GR, et al: Bone mineral changes after lactation in Gambian women accustomed to a low calcium intake, *Euro J Clin Nutr* 67:1142, 2013.

Sazawal S, Black RE, Dhingra P, et al: Zinc supplementation does not affect the breast milk zinc concentration of lactation women belonging to low socioeconomic population, *J Hum Nutr Food Sci* 1:1014, 2013.

Scolari Childress KM, Myles T: Baking soda pica associated with rhabdomyolysis and cardiomyopathy in pregnancy, *Obstet Gynecol* 122:495, 2013.

Shankar P, Ahuja S, Sriram K: Non-nutritive sweeteners: review and update, *Nutrition* 29:1293, 2013.

Siega-Riz AM, Gray GL: Gestational weight gain recommendations in the context of the obesity epidemic, *Nutr Rev* 71(Suppl 1):S26, 2013.

Simon J: Promoting fertility via optimal nutrition: nutrition in infertility prevention and management, *Women's Health Report* 2:1, 2014.

Stagnaro-Green A, Pearce EN: Iodine and pregnancy: a call to action, *Lancet* 382:292, 2013.

Stagnaro-Green A, Pearce E: Thyroid disorders in pregnancy, *Nat Rev Endocrinol* 8:650, 2012.

Szymanski LM, Satin AJ: Strenuous exercise during pregnancy: is there a limit? *Am J Obstet Gynecol* 207:179e1, 2012.

Talaulikar VS, Arulkumaran S: Folic acid in obstetric practice: a review, *Obstet Gynecol Surv* 66:240, 2011.

Tande DL, Ralph JL, Johnson LK, et al: First trimester dietary intake, biochemical measures, and subsequent gestational hypertension among nulliparous women, *J Midwifery Womens Health* 58:423, 2013.

Teas J, Pino S, Critchley A, et al: Variability of iodine content in common commercially available edible seaweeds, *Thyroid* 14:836, 2004.

Temel, S et al: Evidence-based preconceptional lifestyle interventions, Epidemiologic Rev, 36:19, 2013.

Tenenbaum-Gavish K, Hod M: Impact of maternal obesity on fetal health, *Fetal Diagn Ther* 34:1, 2013.

Thangaratinam S, Rogozinska E, Jolly K, et al: Effects of interventions in pregnancy on maternal weight and obstetric outcomes: meta-analysis of randomised evidence, *BMJ* 344:e2088, 2012.

Torgerson PR, Mastroiacovo P: The global burden of congenital toxoplasmosis: a systematic review, *Bull World Health Organ* 91:501, 2013.

Trogstad L, Magnus P, Stoltenberg C: Pre-eclampsia: risk factors and causal models, *Best Pract Res Clin Obstet Gynaecol* 25:329, 2011.

Ulbricht C, Isaac R, Milkin T, et al: An evidence-based systematic review of stevia by the Natural Standard Research Collaboration, *Cardiovasc Hematol Agents Med Chem* 8:113, 2010.

United States Department of Health and Human Services (USDHHS), Office on Women's Health: *Postpartum Depression*, 2014. http://womenshealth.gov/mental-health/illnesses/postpartum-depression.html. Accessed December 2014.

Uriu-Adams JY, Scherr RE, Lanoue L, et al: Influence of copper on early development: prenatal and postnatal considerations, *Biofactors* 36:136, 2010.

Usadi RS, Legro RS: Reproductive impact of polycystic ovary syndrome, *Curr Opin Endocrinol Diabetes Obes* 19:505, 2012.

Van der Zee B, de Wert G, Steegers EA, et al: Ethical aspects of paternal preconception lifestyle modification, *Am J Obstet Gynecol* 209:11, 2013.

Vanhees K, Vonhögen IG, van Schooten FJ, et al: You are what you eat, and so are your children: the impact of micronutrients on the epigenetic programming of offspring, *Cell Mol Life Sci* 71:271, 2014.

Van Wijngaarden E, Thurston SW, Myers GJ, et al: Prenatal methyl mercury exposure in relation to neurodevelopment and behavior at 19 years of age in the Seychelles Child Development Study, *Neurotoxicol Teratol* 39:19, 2013.

Verd S, Nadal-Amat J, Gich I, et al: Salt preference of nursing mothers is associated with earlier cessation of exclusive breastfeeding, *Appetite* 54:233, 2010.

Wendt A, Gibbs CM, Peters S, et al: Impact of increasing inter-pregnancy interval on maternal and infant health, *Paediatr Perinat Epidemiol* 26:239, 2012.

West D, Marasco L: *The breastfeeding mother's guide to making more milk*, New York, 2009, McGraw Hill.

World Health Organization (WHO): *Infant and Young Child Feeding*, 2013. http://www.who.int/mediacentre/factsheets/fs342/en/. Accessed December 2014.

Wu G, Imhoff-Kunsch B, Girard AW: Biological mechanisms for nutritional regulation of maternal health and fetal development, *Paediatr Perinat Epidemiol* 26:4, 2012a.

Wu Q, Chen HL, Xu XJ: Violence as a risk factor for postpartum depression in mothers: a meta-analysis, *Arch Womens Ment Health* 15:107, 2012b.

Xiang AH, Kawakubo M, Kjos SL, et al: Long-acting injectable progestin contraception and risk of type 2 diabetes in Latino women with prior gestational diabetes mellitus, *Diabetes Care* 29:613, 2006.

Xu F, Li Z, Binns C, et al: Does infant feeding method impact on maternal mental health? *Breastfeed Med* 9:215, 2014.

Yajnik CS, Deshpande SS, Jackson AA, et al: Vitamin B12 and folate concentrations during pregnancy and insulin resistance in the offspring: the Pune Maternal Nutrition Study, *Diabetologia* 51:29, 2008.

Yang CZ, Yaniger SI, Jordan VC, et al: Most plastic products release estrogenic chemicals: a potential health problem that can be solved, *Environ Health Perspect* 119:989, 2011.

Young SL: *Craving earth: understanding pica, the urge to eat clay, starch, ice, and chalk*, New York, 2011, Columbia University Press.

Zeisel SH: Nutrition in pregnancy: the argument for including a source of choline, *Int J Womens Health* 5:193, 2013.

Zhang GH, Chen ML, Liu SS, et al: Effects of mother's dietary exposure to acesulfame-K in pregnancy or lactation on the adult offspring's sweet preference, *Chem Senses* 36:763, 2011.

16

Nutrition in Infancy

Kelly N. McKean, MS, RDN, CSP, CD
Mari O. Mazon, MS, RDN, CD

KEY TERMS

arachidonic acid (ARA)
casein
casein hydrolysate
catch-up growth
colostrum
docosahexaenoic acid (DHA)

early childhood caries (ECC)
electrolytically reduced iron
growth channel
lactalbumin
lactoferrin
lag-down growth

oligosaccharides
palmar grasp
pincer grasp
renal solute load
secretory immunoglobin A (sIgA)
whey proteins

During the first 2 years of life, which are characterized by rapid physical and social growth and development, many changes occur that affect feeding and nutrient intake. The adequacy of infants' nutrient intakes affects their interaction with their environment. Healthy, well-nourished infants have the energy to respond to and learn from the stimuli in their environment and to interact with their parents and caregivers in a manner that encourages bonding and attachment.

PHYSIOLOGIC DEVELOPMENT

The length of gestation, the mother's prepregnancy weight, and the mother's weight gain during gestation determine an infant's birth weight. After birth, the growth of an infant is influenced by genetics and nourishment. Most infants who are genetically determined to be larger reach their growth channel, a curve of weight and length or height gain throughout the period of growth, at between 3 and 6 months of age. However, many infants born at or below the tenth percentile for length may not reach their genetically appropriate growth channel until 1 year of age; this is called catch-up growth. Infants who are larger at birth and who are genetically determined to be smaller grow at their fetal rate for several months and often do not reach their growth channel until 13 months of age. This phenomenon during the first year of life is called lag-down growth.

Growth in infancy is monitored with the routine collection and monitoring of anthropometric data, including weight, length, head circumference, and weight-for-length for age. These are plotted on the appropriate World Health Organization (WHO) growth chart shown in Appendices 4, 5, 8, and 9. The WHO growth charts are used for the first 2 years of life and consist of a series of percentile curves that show the distribution of body measurements in infants and children in optimal growth conditions. When the anthropometric data are plotted on the growth charts, the percentiles rank the infant by showing what percentage of the reference population the infant would equal or exceed. For example, a 7-month-old infant girl who has a weight-for-age at the 75th percentile weighs the same or more than 75% of the reference population for 7-month-old girls and weighs less than 25% of the same population. It is important to monitor growth trends over time and not focus on one measurement.

Infants may lose approximately 7% of their body weight during the first few days of life, but their birth weight usually is regained by the seventh to tenth day. Weight loss of more than 10% in the newborn period indicates need for further assessment regarding adequacy of feeding. Growth thereafter proceeds at a rapid but decelerating rate. Infants usually double their birth weight by 4 to 6 months of age and triple it by the age of 1 year. The amount of weight gained by the infant during the second year approximates the birth weight. Infants increase their length by 50% during the first year of life and double it by 4 years. Total body fat increases rapidly during the first 9 months, after which the rate of fat gain tapers off throughout the rest of childhood. Total body water decreases throughout infancy from 70% at birth to 60% at 1 year. The decrease is almost all in extracellular water, which declines from 42% at birth to 32% at 1 year of age.

The stomach capacity of infants increases from a range of 10 to 20 ml at birth to 200 ml by 1 year, enabling infants to consume more food at a given time and at less frequent intervals as they grow older. During the first weeks of life, gastric acidity decreases and for the first few months remains lower than that of older infants and adults. The rate of emptying is relatively slow, depending on the size and composition of the meal.

Fat absorption varies in the neonate. Human milk fat is well absorbed, but butterfat is poorly absorbed, with fecal excretions of 20% to 48%. The fat combinations in commercially prepared infant formula are well absorbed. The infant's lingual and gastric lipases hydrolyze short- and medium-chain fatty acids in the

Sections of this chapter were written by Cristine M. Trahms, MS, RD, CD, FADA

stomach. Gastric lipase also hydrolyzes long-chain fatty acids and is important in initiating the digestion of triglycerides in the stomach. Most long-chain triglycerides pass unhydrolyzed into the small intestine, where they are broken down by pancreatic lipase. The bile salt–stimulated lipase present in human milk is stimulated by the infant's bile salts and hydrolyzes the triglycerides in the small intestine into free fatty acids and glycerol. Bile salts, which are effective emulsifiers when combined with monoglycerides, fatty acids, and lecithin, aid in the intestinal digestion of fat.

The activities of the enzymes responsible for the digestion of disaccharides—maltase, isomaltase, and sucrase—reach adult levels by 28 to 32 weeks' gestation. Lactase activity (responsible for digesting the disaccharide in milk) reaches adult levels by birth. Pancreatic amylase, which digests starch, continues to remain low during the first 6 months after birth. If the infant consumes starch before this time, increased activity of salivary amylase and digestion in the colon usually compensate.

The neonate has functional but physiologically immature kidneys that increase in size and concentrating capacity in the early weeks of life. The kidneys double in weight by 6 months and triple in weight by 1 year of age. The last renal tubule is estimated to form between the eighth fetal month and the end of the first postnatal month. The glomerular tuft is covered by a much thicker layer of cells throughout neonatal life than at any later time, which may explain why the glomerular filtration rate is lower during the first 9 months of life than it is in later childhood and adulthood. In the neonatal period the ability to form acid, urine, and concentrate solutes is often limited. The renal concentrating capacity at birth may be limited to as little as 700 mOsm/L in some infants. Others have the concentrating capacity of adults (1200 to 1400 mOsm/L). By 6 weeks, most infants can concentrate urine at adult levels. Renal function in a normal newborn infant is rarely a concern; however, difficulties may arise in infants with diarrhea or those who are fed formula that is too concentrated (Butte et al, 2004).

NUTRIENT REQUIREMENTS

Nutrient needs of infants reflect rates of growth, energy expended in activity, basal metabolic needs, and the interaction of the nutrients consumed. Balance studies have defined minimum acceptable levels of intakes for a few nutrients, but for most nutrients the suggested intakes have been extrapolated from the intakes of normal, thriving infants consuming human milk. The dietary reference intakes (DRIs) for infants are shown in the inside front cover.

Energy

Full-term infants who are breast-fed to satiety or who are fed a standard infant formula generally adjust their intake to meet their energy needs when caregivers are sensitive to the infants' hunger and satiety cues. An effective method for determining the adequacy of an infant's energy intake is to monitor carefully gains in weight, length, head circumference, and weight-for-length for age and plot these data on the WHO growth charts shown in Appendix Tables 4, 5, 8, and 9. During the first year a catch-up or lag-down period in growth may occur.

If infants begin to experience a decrease in their rate of weight gain, do not gain weight, or lose weight, their energy and nutrient intake should be monitored carefully. If the rate of growth in length decreases or ceases, potential malnutrition, an undetected disease, or both should be investigated thoroughly.

If the weight gain proceeds at a much more rapid rate than growth in length, the energy concentration of the formula, the quantity of formula consumed, and the amount and type of semisolid and table foods offered should be evaluated. The activity level of the infant also should be assessed. Infants who are at the highest end of the growth charts for weight-for-length, or who grow rapidly in infancy, tend to be at greater risk for obesity later in life (Druet et al, 2012).

The equations to calculate the estimated energy requirement (EER) for infants 0 to 12 months of age are in Table 16-1. The EER includes the total energy expenditure plus energy needed for growth for healthy infants with normal growth (see Chapter 2).

Protein

Protein is needed for tissue replacement, deposition of lean body mass, and growth. Protein requirements during the rapid growth of infancy are higher per kilogram of weight than those for older children or adults (see Table 16-2). Recommendations for protein intake are based on the composition of human milk, and it is assumed that the efficiency of human milk use is 100%.

Infants require a larger percentage of total amino acids as essential amino acids than do adults. Histidine seems to be an essential amino acid for infants, but not for adults, and tyrosine, cystine, and taurine may be essential for premature infants (see Chapter 42).

Human milk or infant formula provides the major portion of protein during the first year of life. The amount of protein in human milk is adequate for the first 6 months of life, even though the amount of protein in human milk is considerably less than in infant formula. From 6 months of age the diet should be supplemented with additional sources of high-quality protein, such as yogurt, strained meats, or cereal mixed with formula or human milk.

Infants may not receive adequate protein if their formula is excessively diluted for a prolonged period, or if they have multiple food allergies and are placed on a restricted diet without appropriate medical or nutritional supervision (see Chapter 26).

TABLE 16-1   Equations for Calculating Estimated Energy Requirement (EER) for Infants

Age	Calculation
0-3 months	(89 × Weight of infant [kg] − 100) + 175
4-6 months	(89 × Weight of infant [kg] − 100) + 56
7-12 months	(89 × Weight of infant [kg] − 100) + 22

From Institute of Medicine: *Dietary reference intakes for energy, carbohydrate, fiber, fat, fatty acids, cholesterol, protein, and amino acids,* Washington, DC, 2002/2005, The National Academies Press.

TABLE 16-2   Protein Dietary Reference Intakes (DRIs) for Infants

Age	Grams/Day	Grams/Kilogram/Day
0-6 months	9.1	1.52
6-12 months	11	1.2

From Institute of Medicine: *Dietary reference intakes for energy, carbohydrate, fiber, fat, fatty acids, cholesterol, protein, and amino acids,* Washington, DC, 2002/2005, The National Academies Press.

Lipids

The current recommendation for infants younger than 1 year of age is to consume a minimum of 30 g of fat per day. This quantity is present in a normal intake of human milk and infant formulas. Significantly lower fat intakes (e.g., with skim-milk feedings) may result in an inadequate total energy intake. An infant may try to correct the energy deficit by increasing the volume of milk ingested but usually cannot make up the entire deficit this way.

Human milk contains the essential fatty acids linoleic acid and alpha-linolenic acid, as well as the longer-chain derivatives arachidonic acid (ARA) ($C20:4\omega-6$) and docosahexaenoic acid (DHA) ($C22:6\omega-3$). They are found in a wide range of concentrations in human milk, depending on the maternal diet (see Chapter 15 - *Focus On:* Omega-3 Fatty Acids in Pregnancy and Lactation). Infant formulas are supplemented with linoleic acid and alpha-linolenic acid, from which ARA and DHA are derived. Except for a few specialty products, standard formulas for term infants in the United States now also are supplemented with ARA and DHA, although there are no regulatory requirements for their inclusion.

Linoleic acid, which is essential for growth and dermal integrity, should provide 3% of the infant's total energy intake, or 4.4 g/day for infants younger than 6 months of age and 4.6 g/day for infants 7 months to 1 year of age. In human milk 5% of the kilocalories and 10% in most infant formulas are derived from linoleic acid. Smaller amounts of alpha-linolenic acid should be included. The current recommendation for alpha-linolenic acid is 0.5 g/day during the first year of life.

The concentration of DHA in human milk varies, depending on the amount of DHA in the mother's diet. DHA and ARA are the major omega-3 and omega-6 long-chain polyunsaturated fatty acids (LCPUFAs) of neural tissues, and DHA is the major fatty acid of the photoreceptor membranes of the retina. Some studies suggest that supplementation of DHA and ARA positively affects visual acuity and psychomotor development, especially in premature infants. However, other studies have shown no differences in cognitive development later in childhood between supplemented and unsupplemented infants (Willatts et al, 2013). The American Academy of Pediatrics (AAP) has not taken an official stand on the addition of LCPUFAs to infant formula. The Academy of Nutrition and Dietetics (AND) recommends that infants who are not breast-fed receive infant formula that contains DHA and ARA (ADA, 2007).

Carbohydrates

Carbohydrates should supply 30% to 60% of the energy intake during infancy. Approximately 40% of the energy in human milk and 40% to 50% of the energy in infant formulas is derived from lactose or other carbohydrates. Although rare, some infants cannot tolerate lactose and require a modified formula in their diet (see Chapters 28 and 43).

Botulism in infancy is caused by the ingestion of *Clostridium botulinum* spores, which germinate and produce toxin in the bowel lumen. Infant botulism has been associated with eating the carbohydrate honey that contains the bacterial spores. Light and dark corn syrups also have been reported to contain the spores, although cases of infant botulism have not been linked to corn syrup. The spores are extremely resistant to heat treatment and are not destroyed by current methods of processing. Thus honey and corn syrup should not be fed to infants younger than 1 year of age because they have not yet developed the immunity required to resist botulism spore development.

Water

The water requirement for infants is determined by the amount lost from the skin and lungs and in the feces and urine, in addition to a small amount needed for growth. The recommended total water intake for infants, based on the DRIs, is 0.7 L/day for infants up to 6 months and 0.8 L/day for infants 6 to 12 months of age. Note that total water includes all water contained in food, beverages, and drinking water. Fluid recommendations per kilogram of body weight are shown in Table 16-3.

Because the renal concentrating capacity of young infants may be less than that of older children and adults, they may be vulnerable to developing a water imbalance. Under ordinary conditions, human milk and formula that is properly prepared supply adequate amounts of water. However, when formula is boiled, the water evaporates and the solutes become concentrated; therefore boiled milk or formula is inappropriate for infants. In very hot, humid environments, infants may require additional water. When losses of water are high (e.g., vomiting and diarrhea), infants should be monitored carefully for fluid and electrolyte imbalances.

Water deficits result in hypernatremic dehydration and its associated neurologic consequences (e.g., seizures, vascular damage). Hypernatremic dehydration has been reported in breast-fed infants who lose greater than 10% of their birth weight in the first few days of life (Leven and MacDonald, 2008). Because of the potential for hypernatremic dehydration, careful monitoring of volume of intake, daily weights, and hydration status (e.g., number of wet diapers) in all newborns is warranted.

Water intoxication results in hyponatremia, restlessness, nausea, vomiting, diarrhea, and polyuria or oliguria; seizures also can result. This condition may occur when water is provided as a replacement for milk, the formula is excessively diluted, or bottled water is used instead of an electrolyte solution in the treatment of diarrhea.

Minerals
Calcium

Breast-fed infants retain approximately two thirds of their calcium intake. The recommended adequate intake (AI), the mean intake, is based on calcium intakes in healthy breast-fed infants. The AI for infants 0 to 6 months of age is 200 mg/day; for infants 6 to 12 months of age the AI is 260 mg/day; formulas are enhanced accordingly.

Fluoride

The importance of fluoride in preventing dental caries has been well documented. However, excessive fluoride may cause dental fluorosis, ranging from fine white lines to entirely chalky teeth (see Chapter 25). To prevent fluorosis, the tolerable upper in-

TABLE 16-3 **Maintenance Fluid Requirements of Infants and Children**	
Body Weight	**Fluid Requirement**
0-10 kg	100 ml/kg
11-20 kg	1000 ml + 50 ml/kg for each kg >10 kg
>20 kg	1500 ml + 20 ml/kg for each kg >20 kg

take level for fluoride has been set at 0.7 mg/day for infants up to 6 months and 0.9 mg/day for infants 6 to 12 months of age. Fluoride concentration of 0.7 ppm (0.7 mg/L) in drinking water has been proposed as being optimal for safety and caries prevention (AND, 2012). Fluoride content of water supplies can be obtained through local public health departments or water utilities. Fluoride containing toothpaste should be used sparingly – just a smear on a toothbrush (AAPD, 2015).

Human milk is very low in fluoride. Infants who exclusively consume infant formula reconstituted with fluoridated water may be at increased risk of developing mild fluorosis (CDC, 2013). Using water that is free of or low in fluoride, which are waters labeled "purified," "demineralized," "deionized," "distilled," or "produced through reverse-osmosis," may decrease this risk. Other dietary sources of fluoride during infancy include commercially prepared infant cereals and wet pack cereals processed with fluoridated water. Fluoride supplementation is not recommended for infants younger than 6 months of age, and after 6 months of age is recommended only if an infant is at high risk of developing dental caries and drinks insufficiently fluoridated water (AND, 2012). After tooth eruption it is recommended that fluoridated water be offered several times per day to breast-fed infants, those who receive cow's milk, and those fed formulas made with water that contains less than 0.3 mg of fluoride/L (AAP, 2014b).

Iron

Full-term infants are considered to have adequate stores of iron for growth up to a doubling of their birth weight. This occurs at approximately 4 months of age in full-term infants and much earlier in prematurely born infants. Recommended intakes of iron increase according to age, growth rate, and iron stores. At 4 to 6 months of age, infants who are fed only human milk are at risk for developing a negative iron balance and may deplete their reserves by 6 to 9 months. Iron in human milk is highly bioavailable; however, breast-fed infants should receive an additional source of iron by 4 to 6 months of age (AAP, 2012). For breast-fed term infants, the AAP recommends iron supplementation of 1 mg/kg/day starting at 4 months of age and continuing until appropriate complementary foods have been introduced (Baker and Greer, 2010). Complementary foods high in iron include strained meats and iron-fortified infant cereals. In addition, by 6 months of age offering one serving of vitamin C-rich foods per day enhances iron absorption from nonheme sources. Formula-fed infants receive adequate iron from formula. Cow's milk is a poor source of iron and should not be given before 12 months of age.

Iron deficiency and iron deficiency anemia are common health concerns for the older infant. Between 6 and 24 months of age, because of rapid growth, iron requirements per kilogram of body weight are higher than at any other period of life. Risk factors associated with a higher prevalence of iron deficiency anemia include low birth weight, low intake of iron-rich complementary foods, high intake of cow's milk, low socioeconomic status, and immigrant status.

Monitoring iron status is important because of the long-term cognitive effects of iron deficiency in infancy. There is consistent association between iron deficiency anemia in infancy and long-lasting poor cognition, developmental deficits, and behavioral performance (Domellöf et al, 2014). Thus it is important dietary advice reaches high-risk groups to prevent these significant long-term effects.

Zinc

Newborn infants are immediately dependent on a dietary source of zinc. Zinc is better absorbed from human milk than from infant formula. Human milk and infant formulas provide adequate zinc (0.3 to 0.5 mg/100 kcal) for the first year of life. Other foods (e.g., meats, cereals) should provide most of the zinc required during the second year. Infants who are zinc deficient can exhibit growth retardation (Cole and Lifshitz, 2008) (see Appendix 53).

Vitamins

Vitamin B$_{12}$

Milk from lactating mothers who follow a strict vegan diet may be deficient in vitamin B$_{12}$, especially if the mother followed the regimen for a long time before and during her pregnancy. Vitamin B$_{12}$ deficiency also has been diagnosed in infants breast-fed by mothers with pernicious anemia (Roumeliotis et al, 2012) (see Chapter 32). Symptoms of vitamin B$_{12}$ deficiency include lethargy, hypotonia, developmental regression, vomiting, and diarrhea.

Vitamin D

The vitamin D content of breast milk is correlated directly to the vitamin D status of the mother. Studies of lactating mothers who were supplemented with anywhere from 2000 IU to 6400 IU of vitamin D per day achieved sufficient vitamin D status in their exclusively breast-fed infants without directly supplementing the infant (Uriu-Adams et al, 2013). However, the current RDA for vitamin D for lactating mothers is 600 IU per day, and the tolerable upper limit is 4000 IU per day. Coupled with the AAP's recommendation to keep all infants under the age of 6 months out of direct sunlight, exclusively and partially breast-fed infants are at high risk for vitamin D deficiency (Balk, 2011). For the prevention of rickets and vitamin D deficiency, the AAP recommends a minimum vitamin D intake of 400 IU per day shortly after birth for all infants. All breast-fed infants need a vitamin D supplement of 400 IU per day. Formula-fed infants who consume less than 1000 ml of formula per day also need supplementation (Wagner and Greer, 2008).

There appears to be a higher risk of rickets among unsupplemented, breast-fed infants and children with dark skin (Uriu-Adams et al, 2013). Because a variety of environmental and family lifestyle factors can affect sunlight exposure and absorption of vitamin D, the AAP recommendations to provide supplemental vitamin D are appropriate for all infants. Supplementation up to 800 IU of vitamin D per day may be needed for infants at higher risk, such as premature infants, dark-skinned infants and children, and those who reside in northern latitudes or at higher altitudes (Misra et al, 2008).

The Food and Drug Administration (FDA) states that some droppers that come with liquid vitamin D supplements could hold more than the 400 IU per day recommended by the AAP. Thus it is important that parents or caregivers provide only the recommended amount. Excessive vitamin D can cause nausea and vomiting, loss of appetite, excessive thirst, frequent urination, constipation, abdominal pain, muscle weakness, muscle and joint aches, confusion, fatigue, or damage to kidneys (see Appendix 45).

Vitamin K

The vitamin K requirements of the neonate need special attention. Deficiency may result in bleeding or hemorrhagic disease of the newborn. This condition is more common in breast-fed infants than in other infants because human milk contains only 2.5 mcg/l of vitamin K, whereas cow's milk–based formulas contain approximately 20 times this amount. All infant formulas contain a minimum of 4 mcg of vitamin K per 100 kcal of formula. The AI for infants is 2 mcg/day during the first 6 months and 2.5 mcg/day during the second 6 months of life. This can be supplied by mature breast milk, although perhaps not during the first week of life. For breast-fed infants, vitamin K supplementation is necessary during that time to considerably decrease the risk for hemorrhagic disease. Most hospitals require that infants receive an injection of vitamin K as a prophylactic measure shortly after birth.

Supplementation

Vitamin and mineral supplements should be prescribed only after careful evaluation of the infant's intake. Commercially prepared infant formulas are fortified with all necessary vitamins and minerals; therefore formula-fed infants rarely need supplements. Breast-fed infants need additional vitamin D supplementation shortly after birth, and iron by 4 to 6 months of age (see *Focus On:* Vitamin and Mineral Supplementation Recommendations for Full-Term Infants). Chapter 42 discusses the feeding of premature or high-risk infants and their special needs.

◎ FOCUS ON

Vitamin and Mineral Supplementation Recommendations for Full-Term Infants

Vitamin D

Supplementation shortly after birth of 400 IU/day for all breast-fed infants and infants consuming less than 1000 ml (33 oz) of vitamin D–fortified formula each day

Vitamin K

Supplementation soon after birth to prevent hemorrhagic disease of the newborn

Iron

Breast-Fed Infants

Approximately 1 mg/kg/day by 4 to 6 months of age, preferably from supplemental foods, and only iron-fortified formulas for weaning or supplementing breastmilk

Formula-Fed Infants

Only iron-fortified formula during the first year of life

Modified from American Academy of Pediatrics Committee on Nutrition: *Pediatric nutrition,* ed 7, Elk Grove Village, Ill, 2014, American Academy of Pediatrics, 2014.

MILK

Human Milk

Human milk is unquestionably the food of choice for the infant. Its composition is designed to provide the necessary energy and nutrients in appropriate amounts. It contains specific and nonspecific immune factors that support and strengthen the immature immune system of the newborn and thus protect the body against infections. Human milk also helps prevent diarrhea and otitis media (AAP, 2012). Allergic reactions to human milk protein are rare. Moreover, the closeness of the mother and infant during breast-feeding facilitates attachment and bonding (see Fig 15-6) and breast milk provides nutritional benefits (e.g., optimal nourishment in an easily digestible and

bioavailable form), decreases infant morbidity, provides maternal health benefits (e.g., lactation amenorrhea, maternal weight loss, some cancer protection), and has economic and environmental benefits (ADA, 2009; see Chapter 15).

During the first few days of life, a breastfeeding infant receives colostrum, a yellow, transparent fluid that meets the infant's needs during the first week. It contains less fat and carbohydrate, but more protein and greater concentrations of sodium, potassium, and chloride than mature milk. It is also an excellent source of immunologic substances.

Note that breastfeeding may not be appropriate for mothers with certain infections or those who are taking medications that may have untoward effects on the infant. For example, a mother who is infected with human immunodeficiency virus can transmit the infection to the infant, and a mother using psychotropic drugs or other pharmacologic drugs may pass the medication to the infant through her breastmilk (AAP, 2012; see Chapter 15).

The Academy of Nutrition and Dietetics (AND) and the AAP support exclusive breastfeeding (EBF) for the first 6 months of life and then breastfeeding supplemented by complementary foods until at least 12 months (AAP, 2012; Lessen and Kavanaugh, 2015). It is important to note the ages of the infants in these recommendations; adding other foods at too young of an age decreases breastmilk intake and increases early weaning. There is some evidence that early introduction of complementary foods increases the chances of picky eating behavior (Shim et al, 2011). Healthy Children 2020 objectives propose to support breastfeeding among mothers of newborn infants (see *Focus On:* Healthy Children 2020 Objectives: Nourishment of Infants).

◎ FOCUS ON

Healthy Children 2020 Objectives: Nourishment of Infants

Healthy People 2020 is a comprehensive set of health objectives for the United States to achieve during the second decade of the twenty-first century. Healthy People 2020 identifies a wide range of public health priorities and specific, measurable objectives. The objectives have 42 focus areas, one of which is Maternal, Infant, and Child Health. The objectives related to nourishment of infants are as follows:

GOAL: Improve the health and well-being of women, infants, children, and families.

Objective: Increase the proportion of infants who are breast-fed to 81.9% in the early postpartum period, to 60.6% at 6 months, and to 34.1% at 1 year of age. Increase the proportion of infants that are exclusively breast-fed to 46.2% through 3 months of age and 25.5% through 6 months of age.

Objective: Reduce the proportion of breast-fed newborns who receive formula supplementation within the first 2 days of life to 14.2%.

GOAL: Promote health and reduce chronic disease risk through the consumption of healthful diets and achievement and maintenance of healthy body weights.

Objective: Eliminate very low food security among children.

Objective: Reduce iron deficiency among children ages 1 to 2 years to less than 14.3%.

GOAL: Prevent and control oral and craniofacial diseases, conditions, and injuries and improve access to preventive services and dental care.

Objective: Reduce the proportion of young children with dental caries in their primary teeth.

The complete text of the Healthy People 2020 Objectives can be found at www.healthypeople.gov/2020/topicsobjectives2020/default.aspx

Composition of Human and Cow's Milk

The composition of human milk is different from that of cow's milk; for this reason, unmodified cow's milk is not recommended for infants until at least 1 year of age. Both provide approximately 20 kcal/oz; however, the nutrient sources of the energy are different. Protein provides 6% to 7% of the energy in human milk and 20% of the energy in cow's milk. Human milk is 60% **whey proteins** (mainly lactalbumins) and 40% casein; by contrast, cow's milk is 20% whey proteins and 80% casein. **Casein** forms a tough, hard-to-digest curd in the infant's stomach, whereas **lactalbumin** in human milk forms soft, flocculent, easy-to-digest curds. Taurine and cystine are present in higher concentrations in human milk than in cow's milk; these amino acids may be essential for premature infants. Lactose provides 42% of the energy in human milk and only 30% of the energy in cow's milk.

Lipids provide 50% of the energy in human and whole cow's milk. Linoleic acid, an essential fatty acid, provides 4% of the energy in human milk and only 1% in cow's milk. The cholesterol content of human milk is 10 to 20 mg/dl compared with 10 to 15 mg/dl in whole cow's milk. Less fat is absorbed from cow's milk than from human milk; a lipase in human milk is stimulated by bile salts and contributes significantly to the hydrolysis of milk triglycerides.

All of the water-soluble vitamins in human milk reflect maternal intake. Cow's milk contains adequate quantities of the B-complex vitamins, but little vitamin C. Human milk and supplemented cow's milk provide sufficient vitamin A. Human milk is a richer source of vitamin E than cow's milk.

The quantity of iron in human and cow's milk is small (0.3 mg/L). Approximately 50% of the iron in human milk is absorbed, whereas less than 1% of the iron in cow's milk is absorbed. The bioavailability of zinc in human milk is higher than in cow's milk. Cow's milk contains three times as much calcium and six times as much phosphorus as human milk, and its fluoride concentration is twice that of human milk.

The much higher protein and ash content of cow's milk results in a higher **renal solute load**, or amount of nitrogenous waste and minerals that must be excreted by the kidney. The sodium and potassium concentrations in human milk are about one third those in cow's milk, contributing to the lower renal solute load of human milk. The osmolality of human milk averages 300 mOsm/kg, whereas that of cow's milk is 400 mOsm/kg.

Antiinfective Factors

Human milk and colostrum contain antibodies and antiinfective factors that are not present in infant formulas. **Secretory immunoglobulin A (sIgA)**, the predominant immunoglobulin in human milk, plays a role in protecting the infant's immature gut from infection. Breastfeeding should be maintained until the infant is at least 3 months of age to obtain this benefit.

The iron-binding protein **lactoferrin** in human milk deprives bacteria of iron and thus slows their growth. Lysozymes, which are bacteriolytic enzymes found in human milk, destroy the cell membranes of bacteria after the peroxides and ascorbic acid that are also present in human milk have inactivated them. Human milk enhances the growth of the bacterium *Lactobacillus bifidus*, which produces an acidic gastrointestinal (GI) environment that interferes with the growth of certain pathogenic organisms. Because of these antiinfective factors, the incidence of infections is lower in breast-fed infants than in formula-fed infants.

The Microbiome and Probiotics and Prebiotics

Colonization with nonpathogenic microbiota is important for infant health and probably affects health in later life. By the time a mother weans her infant, the baby's GI tract has established its normal flora or microbiome. This ecosystem in early life is influenced by such factors as mode of birth, environment, diet, and use of antibiotics (Marques et al, 2010).

Probiotics are microorganisms that, when administered as an oral supplement or as part of food, may confer health benefits to the host by changing the gut microbiome. Prebiotics are nondigestible food ingredients that promote the growth of the gut's bacteria. Studies have looked at the effects of postnatal probiotic supplementation on the prevention of atopic disease such as asthma, eczema, and allergic rhinitis. Results have been mixed, depending on the strain of probiotics used, and whether the mother also was supplemented during pregnancy (Elazab et al, 2013). Evidence is emerging that supplementing term infants with the probiotic *Lactobacillus reuteri* (*L. reuteri*) may decrease their risk of colic, gastroesophageal reflux, and constipation (Indrio et al, 2014). However, supplementation with *L. reuteri* does not appear to be effective in treating colic. In fact, a well-controlled study found no reduction in crying or fussiness in colicky infants receiving the probiotic. Interestingly the formula-fed infants who were given *L. reuteri* actually fussed more than formula-fed infants given placebo (Sung et al, 2014). The effectiveness of supplemental probiotic use is still under study. Although probiotics have been found generally to be safe, their content is not regulated (Van den Nieuwboer et al, 2014). Similar caution should be used as when using other nutrition supplements.

Human milk contains prebiotics in the form of **oligosaccharides**, which by some estimates can be as much as 12 to 15 g/L (Jeurink et al, 2013). The addition of short-chain gluco-oligosaccharides and long-chain fructo-oligosaccharides to infant formula results in gut microflora more similar to those of human milk-fed infants (Oozeer et al, 2013). The AAP has no official stance on the addition of probiotics or prebiotics to infant formula; however, some infant formulas in the United States are now supplemented with probiotics or prebiotics. The addition of oligosaccharides to infant formula has been deemed to be of no major concern in Europe (Thomas et al, 2010).

Formulas

Infants who are not breast-fed usually are fed a formula based on cow's milk or a soy product. Many mothers also may choose to offer a combination of breastmilk and formula feedings. Those infants who have special requirements receive specially designed products.

Commercial formulas made from heat-treated nonfat milk or a soy product and supplemented with vegetables fats, vitamins, and minerals are formulated to approximate, as closely as possible, the composition of human milk. They provide the necessary nutrients in an easily absorbed form. The manufacture of infant formulas is regulated by the FDA through the Infant Formula Act (Nutrient Requirements for Infant Formulas, 1985). By law, infant formulas are required to have a nutrient level that is consistent with these guidelines (see Table 16-4). Refer to individual manufacturers' websites to obtain the most accurate information and compare the composition of various infant formulas and feeding products.

Formulas are also available for older infants and toddlers. However, typically "older infant" formulas are unnecessary unless toddlers are not receiving adequate amounts of infant or table foods.

TABLE 16-4 Nutrient Levels in Infant Formulas as Specified by the Infant Formula Act

Specified Nutrient Component	Minimum Level Required (per 100 kcal of energy)
Protein (g)	1.8
Fat (g)	3.3
Percentage of calories	30
Linoleic acid (mg)	300
Percentage of calories	2.7
Vitamin A (IU)	250
Vitamin E (IU)	0.7
Vitamin D (IU)	40
Vitamin K (mcg)	4
Thiamin (mcg)	40
Riboflavin (mcg)	60
Niacin (mcg)	250
Ascorbic acid (mg)	8
Pyridoxine (mcg)	35
Vitamin B_{12} (mcg)	0.15
Folic acid (mcg)	4
Biotin (mcg) (non-milk–based formulas only)	1.5
Pantothenic acid (mcg)	300
Choline (mg) (non-milk–based formulas only)	7
Inositol (mg) (non-milk–based formulas only)	4
Calcium (mg)	60
Phosphorus (mg)	30
Iron (mg)	0.15
Zinc (mg)	0.5
Magnesium (mg)	6
Manganese (mcg)	5
Sodium (mg)	20
Potassium (mg)	80
Iodine (mcg)	5
Chloride (mg)	55
Copper (mcg)	60

From Food and Drug Administration: Nutrient requirements for infant formulas, Final Rule (21 CFR 107), *Fed Reg* 50:45106, 1985.

The declining prevalence of anemia in infants is credited to the use of iron-fortified formula. The AAP recommends iron-fortified formulas for all formula-fed infants. The widespread theory that iron-fortified formula may cause constipation, loose stools, colic (severe abdominal pain), and spitting up has not been confirmed by clinical studies (AAP, 1999).

Various products are available for infants who cannot tolerate the protein in cow's milk–based formulas. Soy-based infant formulas are recommended for (1) infants in vegetarian families, and (2) infants with galactosemia or hereditary primary lactase deficiency. Soy formulas are not recommended for children known to have protein allergies because many infants who are allergic to cow's milk protein also develop allergies to soy protein (Bhatia and Greer, 2008; see Chapter 26).

Infants who cannot tolerate cow's milk–based or soy products can be fed formulas made from a **casein hydrolysate**, which is casein that has been split into smaller components by treatment with acid, alkali, or enzymes. These formulas do not contain lactose. For infants who have severe food protein intolerances and cannot tolerate hydrolysate formulas, free amino acid–based formulas are available. Other formulas are available for children with problems such as malabsorption or metabolic disorders (e.g., phenylketonuria) (see Box 26-9 in Chapter 26).

Soy-based formulas are under regular scrutiny. Full-term infants ingesting soy formulas grow and absorb minerals as well as infants fed cow's milk–based formulas, but they are exposed to several thousand times higher levels of phytoestrogens and isoflavones. The biologic effect of these elevated isoflavone levels on long-term infant development is not yet clear (National Toxicology Program, 2010). Mental, psychomotor, and language development have been found to be similar in infants fed soy-based formula compared with infants fed breastmilk and cow's milk-based formula (Andres et al, 2012). Soy-based formulas are not recommended for preterm infants because of the increased risk for osteopenia (Bhatia and Greer, 2008).

The protein in soy infant formula is soy protein isolate supplemented with L-methionine, L-carnitine, and taurine. Contaminants include phytates, which bind minerals and niacin; and protease inhibitors, which have antitrypsin, antichymotrypsin, and antielastin properties. Aluminum from mineral salts is found in soy infant formulas at concentrations of 600 to 1300 ng/ml, levels that exceed aluminum concentrations in human milk of 4 to 65 ng/ml. This does not appear to put term infants with normal renal function at risk of developing aluminum toxicity (Bhatia and Greer, 2008).

Whole Cow's Milk

Some parents may choose to transition their infant from formula to fresh cow's milk before 1 year of age. However, the AAP Committee on Nutrition has concluded that infants should not be fed whole cow's milk during the first year of life (AAP, 2014a). Infants who are fed whole cow's milk have been found to have lower intakes of iron, linoleic acid, and vitamin E, and excessive intakes of sodium, potassium, and protein. Cow's milk may cause a small amount of GI blood loss.

Low-fat (1% to 2%) and nonfat milk are also inappropriate for infants during the first 12 months of life. The infants may ingest excessive amounts of protein in large volumes of milk in an effort to meet their energy needs, and the decreased amount of essential fatty acids may be insufficient for preventing deficiency (AAP, 2014a). Substitute or imitation milks such as soy, rice, oat, or nut milks are also inappropriate during the first year of life. When introduced, only pasteurized cow milk and milk products should be offered (AAP, 2014a).

Formula Preparation

Commercial infant formulas are available in ready-to-feed forms that require no preparation, as concentrates prepared by mixing with equal parts of water, and in powder form that is designed to be mixed with 2 oz of water per level scoop of powder.

Infant formulas should be prepared in a clean environment. All equipment, including bottles, nipples, mixers, and the top of the can of formula, should be washed thoroughly. Formula may be prepared for up to a 24-hour period and refrigerated. Formula for each feeding should be warmed in a hot water bath. Microwave heating is not recommended because of the risk of burns from formula that is too hot or unevenly heated. Any formula offered and not consumed at that feeding should be discarded and not reused later, because of bacterial contamination from the infant's mouth.

FOOD

Dry infant cereals are fortified with electrolytically reduced iron, which is iron that has been fractionated into small particles for improved absorption. Four level tablespoons of cereal provide approximately 5 mg of iron, or approximately half the amount the infant requires. Therefore infant cereal is usually the first food added to the infant's diet. In recent years, concern has been raised about the arsenic content in rice. The Food and Drug Administration (FDA) has determined the arsenic content in rice and rice products, such as infant rice cereal, is too low to cause any immediate or short-term adverse health effects. The FDA recommends offering infants a variety of grains and to avoid the excessive intake of any one food (FDA, 2013).

Strained and "junior" vegetables and fruits provide carbohydrates and vitamins A and C. Vitamin C is added to numerous jarred fruits and all fruit juices. In addition, tapioca is added to several of the jarred fruits. Milk is added to the creamed vegetables, and wheat is incorporated into the mixed vegetables.

Most strained and junior meats are prepared with water. Strained meats, which have the highest energy density of any of the commercial baby foods, are an excellent source of high-quality protein and heme iron.

Numerous dessert items are also available such as puddings and fruit desserts. The nutrient composition of these products varies, but all contain excess energy in the form of sugar and modified cornstarch or tapioca starch. Most infants do not need this excess energy.

Various commercially prepared foods and organically grown products are available for infants. See *Clinical Insight: Is Organic Produce Healthier?* in Chapter 9 for a discussion of organic foods. These products vary widely in their nutrient value. Foods for infants should be thoughtfully selected to meet their nutritional and developmental needs.

Mothers who would like to make their own infant food can do so easily by following the directions in Box 16-1. Home-prepared foods generally are more concentrated in nutrients than commercially prepared foods because less water is used. Salt and sugar should not be added to foods prepared for infants.

FEEDING

Early Feeding Patterns

Because milk from a mother with an adequate diet is designed uniquely to meet the needs of the human infant, breastfeeding for the first 6 months of life is recommended strongly. Most chronic medical conditions do not contraindicate breastfeeding.

A mother should be encouraged to nurse her infant immediately after birth. Those who care for and counsel parents during the first postpartum days should acquaint themselves with ways in which they can be supportive of breastfeeding. Ideally, counseling and preparation for breastfeeding starts in the last few months or weeks of pregnancy (see Chapter 15).

Regardless of whether infants are breast-fed or formula fed, they should be held and cuddled during feedings. Once a feeding rhythm has been established, infants become fussy or cry to indicate they are hungry, whereas they often smile and fall asleep when they are satisfied (see Table 16-5). Infants, not adults, should establish the feeding schedules. Initially, most infants feed every 2 to 3 hours; by 2 months of age most feed every 4 hours. By 3 to 4 months of age infants have usually matured enough to allow the mother to omit night feedings.

BOX 16-1 Directions for Home Preparation of Infant Foods

1. Select fresh, high-quality fruits, vegetables, or meats.
2. Be sure that all utensils, including cutting boards, grinder, knives, and other items, are thoroughly cleaned.
3. Wash hands before preparing the food.
4. Clean, wash, and trim the food in as little water as possible.
5. Cook the foods until tender in as little water as possible. Avoid overcooking, which may destroy heat-sensitive nutrients.
6. Do not add salt or sugar. Do not add honey to food intended for infants younger than 1 year of age.*
7. Add enough water for the food to be easily puréed.
8. Strain or purée the food using an electric blender, a food mill, a baby food grinder, or a kitchen strainer.
9. Pour purée into an ice cube tray and freeze.
10. When the food is frozen hard, remove the cubes and store in freezer bags.
11. When ready to serve, defrost and heat in a serving container the amount of food that will be consumed at a single feeding.

Clostridium botulinum spores, which cause botulism, have been reported in honey; young infants do not have the immune capacity to resist this infection.

TABLE 16-5 Hunger and Satiety Behaviors in Infants

Approximate Age	Hunger Cue	Satiety Cue
Birth through 5 months	Wakes and tosses Sucks on fist Fusses or cries Opens mouth while feeding to show wants more	Falls asleep Turns head away Seals lips together Decreases rate of sucking or stops sucking Purses lips, bites nipple, or spits nipple out or smiles and lets go
4 months through 6 months	Fusses or cries Smiles, coos, gazes at caregiver during feeding Moves head toward spoon Tries to swipe food toward mouth	Distracted or pays more attention to surroundings Turns head away Bites nipple or spits it out Decreases rate of sucking or stops sucking Obstructs mouth with hands
5 months through 9 months	Reaches for food Points to food	Rate of feeding slows down Pushes food away Keeps mouth tightly closed Changes posture Uses hands more actively
8 months through 11 months	Gets excited when food is presented Reaches for food Points to food	Clenches mouth shut Pushes food away Rate of feeding slows down Shakes head to say "no more" Plays with utensils, throws utensils
10 months through 12 months	Expresses desire for specific food with words or sounds	Hands bottle or cup to caregiver Shakes head to say "no more" Sputters with tongue and lips

Modified from U.S. Department of Agriculture: *Infant Nutrition and Feeding: a Guide for Use in the WIC And CSF Programs* (website): http://www.nal.usda.gov/wicworks/Topics/FG/CompleteIFG.pdf, 2009. Accessed December 2014.

Bisphenol A (BPA) is a chemical that was present in many hard plastic bottles, such as baby bottles and reusable cups, and metal food and beverage containers, including canned liquid infant formula. Concern has been raised about the potential effects of BPA on the brain, behavior, and prostate gland in fetuses, infants, and young children. Since 2012, U.S. manufacturers have stopped producing BPA-containing bottles and infant feeding cups for the U.S. market. BPA has not been used in packaging for infant formula in the United States since 2013 (FDA, 2014).

Development of Feeding Skills

At birth, infants coordinate sucking, swallowing, and breathing, and are prepared to suckle liquids from the breast or bottle but are not able to handle foods with texture. During the first year, typical infants develop head control, the ability to move into and sustain a sitting posture, and the ability to grasp, first with a palmar grasp and then with a refined pincer grasp (see Figure 16-1, *B*). They develop mature sucking and rotary chewing abilities and progress from being fed

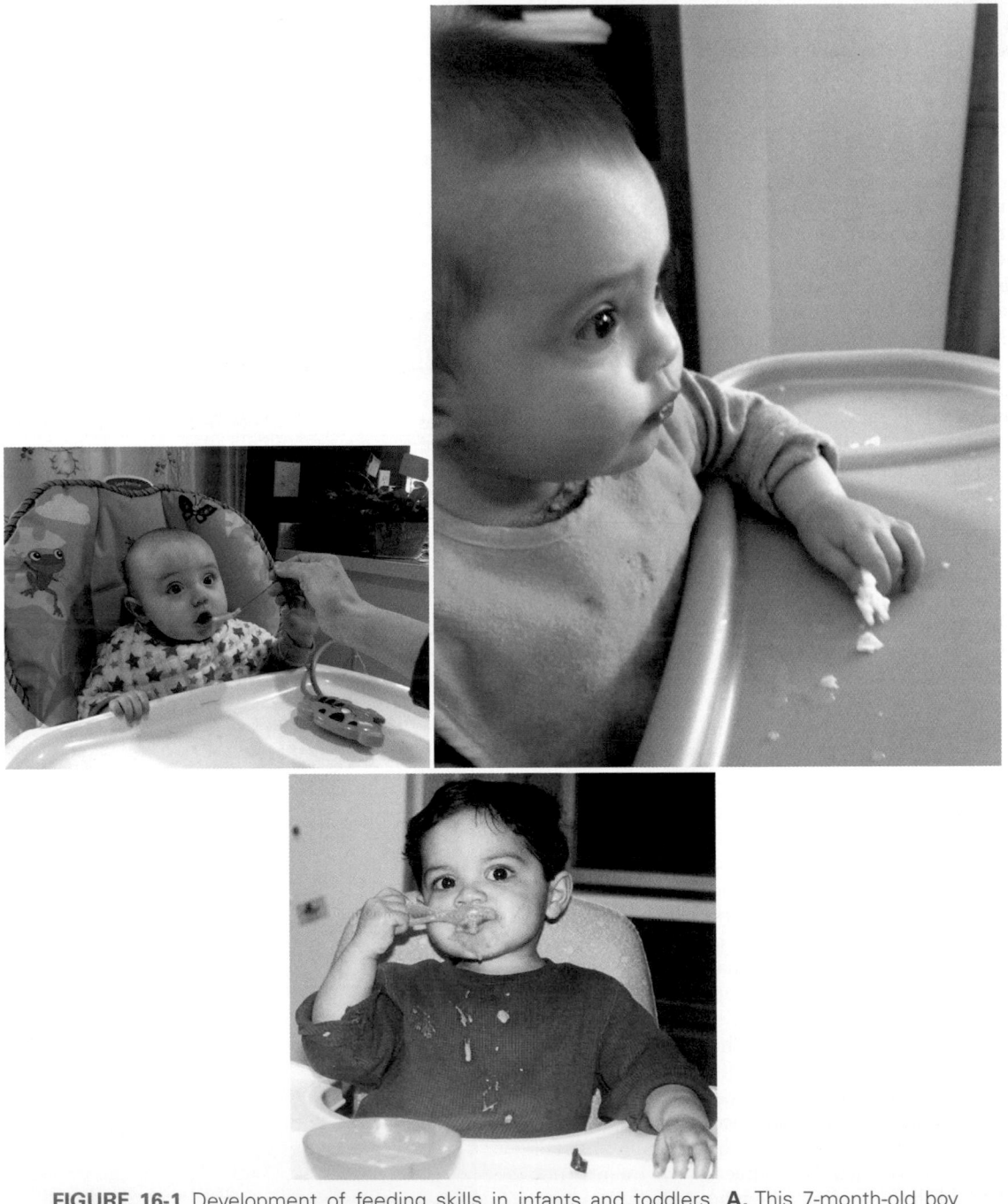

FIGURE 16-1 Development of feeding skills in infants and toddlers. **A,** This 7-month-old boy shows the beginnings of involvement with feeding by anticipating the spoon. **B,** This 8-month-old girl is using a refined pincer grasp to pick up her food. **C,** This 19-month-old boy is beginning to use his spoon independently, although he is not yet able to rotate his wrist to keep food on it.

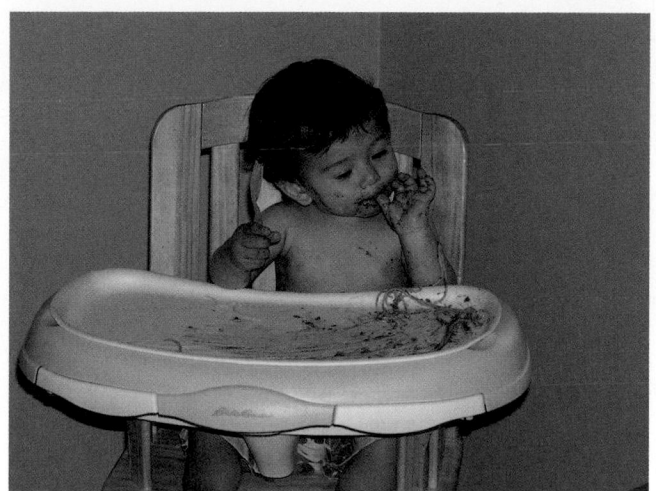

FIGURE 16-2 This 14-month-old boy is learning to self-feed; it's normal to be messy.

to feeding themselves using their fingers. In the second year, they learn to feed themselves independently with a spoon (see Figure 16-2).

Addition of Semisolid Foods

Developmental readiness and nutrient needs are the criteria that determine appropriate times for the addition of various foods. During the first 4 months of life, the infant attains head and neck control, and oral motor patterns progress from a suck to a suckling to the beginnings of a mature sucking pattern. Puréed foods introduced during this phase are consumed in the same manner as are liquids, with each suckle being followed by a tongue-thrust swallow. Table 16-6 lists developmental landmarks and their indications for semisolid and table food introduction.

Between 4 and 6 months of age, when the mature sucking movement is refined and munching movements (up-and-down chopping motions) begin, the introduction of strained foods is appropriate. Infant cereal usually is introduced first. To support developmental progress, cereal is offered to the infant from a spoon, not combined with formula in a bottle (see Figure 16-1, *A*). Thereafter various commercial or home-prepared foods may be offered. The sequence in which these foods are introduced is not important; however, it is important that one single ingredient food (e.g., peaches, not peach cobbler, which has many ingredients) be introduced at a time. Introducing a single new food at a time at 2- to 7-day intervals enables parents to identify any allergic responses or food intolerances. Introducing vegetables before fruits may increase vegetable acceptance.

Infants demonstrate their acceptance of new foods by slowly increasing the variety and quantity of solids they accept. Breast-fed infants seem to accept greater quantities than do formula-fed infants. Dietary flavors from the maternal diet transfer through breastmilk and may facilitate the introduction of new foods in breast-fed infants (Hausner et al, 2008). Parents who thoughtfully offer a variety of nourishing foods are more likely to provide a well-balanced diet and help their children learn to accept more flavors.

As oral-motor maturation proceeds, an infant's rotary chewing ability develops, indicating a readiness for more textured foods such as well-cooked mashed vegetables, casseroles, and pasta from the family menu. Learning to grasp—with the palmar

---

TABLE 16-6   Feeding Behaviors: Developmental Landmarks During the First 2 Years of Life

Developmental Landmarks	Change Indicated	Examples of Appropriate Foods
Tongue laterally transfers food in the mouth Shows voluntary and independent movements of the tongue and lips Sitting posture can be sustained Shows beginning of chewing movements (up and down movements of the jaw)	Introduction of soft, mashed table food	Tuna fish; mashed potatoes; well-cooked, mashed vegetables; ground meats in gravy and sauces; soft, diced fruit such as bananas, peaches, and pears; flavored yogurt
Reaches for and grasps objects with palmar grasp Brings hand to mouth	Finger feeding (large pieces of food)	Oven-dried toast, teething biscuits; cheese sticks (should be soluble in the mouth to prevent choking)
Voluntarily releases food (refined digital [pincer] grasp)	Finger feeding (small pieces of food)	Bits of cottage cheese, dry cereal, peas, and other bite-size vegetables; small pieces of meat
Shows rotary chewing pattern	Introduction of food of varied textures from family menu	Well-cooked, chopped meats and casseroles; cooked vegetables and canned fruit (not mashed); toast; potatoes; macaroni, spaghetti; peeled ripe fruit
Approximates lips to rim of the cup	Introduction of cup for sipping liquids	
Understands relationship of container and its contents	Beginning of self-feeding (though messiness should be expected)	Food that when scooped adheres to the spoon, such as applesauce, cooked cereal, mashed potatoes, cottage cheese, yogurt
Shows increased movements of the jaw Shows development of ulnar deviation of the wrist	More skilled at cup and spoon feeding	Chopped fibrous meats, such as roast and steak; raw vegetables and fruit (introduced gradually)
Walks alone	May seek food and obtain food independently	Mixed textures, food from the family meal; foods of high nutritional value
Names food, expresses preferences; prefers unmixed foods Goes on food jags Appetite appears to decrease		Balanced food choices, with child permitted to develop food preferences (parents should not be concerned that these preferences will last forever)

Reference: Trahms CM, Pipes P: *Nutrition in infancy and childhood,* ed 6, New York, 1997, McGraw-Hill.

TABLE 16-7 Suggested Ages for the Introduction of Semisolid and Table Foods

Food	AGE (MO)		
	4-6	6-8	9-12
Iron-fortified cereals for infants	Add		
Vegetables		Add strained.	Gradually eliminate strained foods and introduce table foods.
Fruits		Add strained.	Gradually eliminate strained foods; introduce chopped, well-cooked, or canned foods.
Meats		Add strained or finely chopped table meats.	Decrease the use of strained meats; increase the varieties of table meats offered.
Finger foods, such as arrowroot biscuits, oven-dried toast		Add foods that can be secured with a palmar grasp.	Increase the use of small finger foods as the pincer grasp develops.
Well-cooked mashed or chopped table foods prepared without added salt or sugar			Add and introduce use of spoon.

Modified from Trahms CM, Pipes P: *Nutrition in infancy and childhood,* ed 6, New York, 1997, McGraw-Hill.

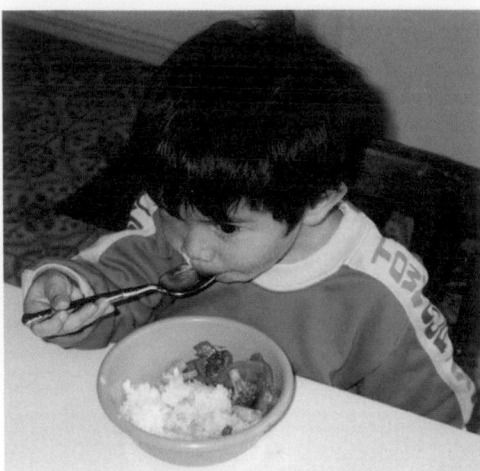

FIGURE 16-3 This 2-year-old is skilled at self-feeding because he has the ability to rotate his wrist and elevate his elbow to keep food on the spoon.

grasp, then with an inferior pincer grasp, and finally with the refined pincer grasp—indicates a readiness for finger foods such as oven-dried toast, arrowroot biscuits, or cheese sticks (see Figure 16-1, *B*). Table 16-7 presents recommendations for adding foods to an infant's diet. Foods with skins or rinds and foods that stick to the roof of the mouth (e.g., hot dogs, grapes, nut butters) may cause choking and should not be offered to young infants.

During the last quarter of the first year, infants can approximate their lips to the rim of the cup and can drink if the cup is held for them. During the second year they gain the ability to rotate their wrists and elevate their elbows, thus allowing them to hold the cup themselves and manage a spoon (see Figure 16-1, *C*). They are very messy eaters at first (see Figure 16-2), but by 2 years of age most typical children skillfully feed themselves (see Figure 16-3).

Weaning from Breast or Bottle to Cup

The introduction of solids into an infant's diet begins the weaning process in which the infant transitions from a diet of only breastmilk or formula to a more varied one. Weaning should proceed gradually and be based on the infant's rate of growth and developmental skills. Weaning foods should be chosen carefully to complement the nutrient needs of the infant, promote appropriate nutrient intake, and maintain growth.

Many infants begin the process of weaning with the introduction of the cup at approximately 6 to 9 months of age and complete the process when they are able to ingest an adequate

amount of milk or formula from a cup at 18 to 24 months of age. Parents of infants who are breast-fed may choose to transition the infant directly to a cup or have an intermittent transition to a bottle before the cup is introduced.

Early Childhood Caries

Dental caries is the most common chronic disease of childhood (AAP, 2014c). **Early childhood caries (ECC),** or "baby bottle tooth decay" is a pattern of tooth decay that involves the upper anterior and sometimes lower posterior teeth. ECC is common among infants and children who are allowed to bathe their teeth in sugar (sucrose or lactose) throughout the day and night. If infants are given sugar-sweetened beverages or fruit juice in a bottle during the day or at bedtime after teeth have erupted, the risk of dental caries increases (see Chapter 25).

To promote dental health, infants should be fed and burped and then put to bed without milk, juice, or food. Juice should not be introduced into the diet before 6 months of age. Juice should be limited to 4 to 6 oz/day for infants and young children and offered to children only from a cup (AAP, 2013). Parents and caregivers can be taught effective oral health practices for infants, not only by dentists but also by other paraprofessionals (MacIntosh et al, 2010).

Feeding Older Infants

As maturation proceeds and the rate of growth slows down, infants' interest in and approach to food changes. Between 9 and 18 months of age most reduce their breastmilk or formula intake. They can become finicky about what and how much they eat.

In the weaning stage infants have to learn many manipulative skills, including the ability to chew and swallow solid food and use utensils. They learn to tolerate various textures and flavors of food, eat with their fingers, and then feed themselves with a utensil. Very young children should be encouraged to feed themselves (see *Clinical Insight:* A New Look at the Food Practices of Infants and Toddlers).

CLINICAL INSIGHT

A Look at the Food Practices of Infants and Toddlers

The Feeding Infants and Toddlers Study was a national random sample of more than 2500 infants and toddlers from 4 to 24 months of age and their mothers.

- Assuming that a variety of nutritious foods are offered to infants and toddlers, parents and caregivers should encourage self-feeding without concern for compromising energy intake and nutrient adequacy (Carruth et al, 2004b).
- Parents and caregivers should offer a variety of fruits and vegetables daily; sweets, desserts, sweetened beverages, and salty snacks should be offered only occasionally. Because family food choices influence the foods offered to infants, family-based approaches to healthy eating habits should be encouraged (Fox et al, 2004).
- By 24 months of age, 50% of toddlers were described as picky eaters. When offering a new food, caregivers must be willing to provide 8 to 15 repeated exposures to enhance acceptance of that food (Carruth et al, 2004a).
- Infants and toddlers have an innate ability to regulate energy intake. Parents and caregivers should understand the cues of hunger and satiety and recognize that coercive admonitions about eating more or less food can interfere with the infant's or toddler's innate ability to regulate energy intake (Fox et al, 2006).
- On average, infants and toddlers were fed seven times per day, and the percentage of children reported to be eating snacks increased with age. Snack choices for infants and toddlers could be improved by delaying the introduction of and limiting foods that have a low nutrient content and are energy dense (Skinner et al, 2004).

At the beginning of a meal, children are hungry and should be allowed to feed themselves; when they become tired, they can be helped quietly. Emphasis on table manners and the fine points of eating should be delayed until they have the necessary maturity and developmental readiness for such training.

The food should be in a form that is easy to handle and eat. Meat should be cut into bite-size pieces. Potatoes and vegetables should be mashed so that they can be eaten easily with a spoon. Raw fruits and vegetables should be in sizes that can be picked up easily. In addition, the utensils should be small and manageable. Cups should be easy to hold, and dishes should be designed so that they do not tip over easily.

Type of Food

In general, children prefer simple, uncomplicated foods. Food from the family meal can be adapted for the child and served in child-size portions. Children younger than 6 years of age usually prefer mild-flavored foods. Because a young child's stomach is small, a snack may be required between meals. Fruit, cheese, crackers, dry cereal, fruit juices, and milk contribute nutrients and energy. Children ages 2 to 6 years often prefer raw instead of cooked vegetables and fruits.

Infants should be offered foods that vary in texture and flavor. Infants who are accustomed to many kinds of foods are less likely to limit their variety of food choices later. To add variety to an infant's diet, vegetables and fruits can be added to cereal feedings. It is important to offer various foods and not allow the infant to continue consuming a diet consisting of one or two favorite foods. Older infants generally reject unfamiliar foods the first time they are offered. When parents continue to offer small portions of these foods without comment, infants become familiar with them and often accept them. It may take 8 to 15 repeated exposures before acceptance of the food (Carruth et al, 2004a). It is important that fruit juice does not replace more nutrient-dense foods. If excessive amounts of juice are consumed, children may fail to thrive.

Serving Size

The size of a serving of food offered to a child is very important. At 1 year of age infants eat one third to one half the amount an adult normally consumes. This proportion increases to one half an adult portion by the time the child reaches 3 years of age and increases to about two thirds by 6 years of age. Young children should not be served a large plateful of food; the size of the plate and the amount should be in proportion to their age. A tablespoon (not a heaping tablespoon) of each food for each year of age is a good guide to follow. Serving less food than parents think or hope will be eaten helps children eat successfully and happily. They will ask for more food if their appetite is not satisfied.

Forced Feeding

Children should not be forced to eat; instead, the cause for the unwillingness to eat should be determined. A typical, healthy child eats without coaxing. Children may refuse food because they are too inactive to be hungry or too active and overtired. To avoid overfeeding and underfeeding, parents should be responsive to the cues for hunger and satiety offered by the infant. A child who is fed snacks or given a bottle too close to mealtime (within 90 minutes) is not hungry for the meal and may refuse it.

Parents who support the development of self-feeding skills respond to the infant's need for assistance and offer encouragement for self-feeding; they also allow the infant to initiate and guide feeding interactions without excessive pressure on the infant for neatness in self-feeding or amount of food consumed. If a child refuses to eat, the family meal should be completed without comment, and the plate should be removed. This procedure is usually harder on the parent than on the child. At the next mealtime, the child will be hungry enough to enjoy the food presented.

Eating Environment

Young children should eat their meals at the family table; it gives them an opportunity to learn table manners while enjoying meals with a family group. Sharing the family fare strengthens ties and makes mealtime pleasant. However, if the family meal is delayed, the children should receive their meals at the usual time. When children eat with the family, everyone must be careful not to make unfavorable comments about any food. Children are great imitators of the people they admire; thus, if the father or older siblings make disparaging remarks about squash, for example, young children are likely to do the same.

The Bright Futures materials and guidelines (www.bright futures.org/nutrition/) provide information and support to families as they guide their children to healthy eating habits and nourishment.

CLINICAL CASE STUDY

Ethan is an 8-month-old male who was born vaginally at 37 weeks' gestational age. The pregnancy and delivery were uncomplicated. This was his mother's second pregnancy. Ethan's brother, who is now 4 years old, was born prematurely at 27 weeks' gestational age.

Ethan's mother is concerned that Ethan is underweight and not eating enough food. Ethan was born small for gestational age and weighed less than 5 lb at birth. His weight and length percentiles have since increased: His weight has followed the 5th percentile for age and his length has followed roughly the 50th percentile for age since 2 months of age. His weight-for-length has consistently been between the 2nd and 5th percentiles.

Ethan's mother offers him Similac Advance formula mixed at standard dilution (1 scoop of powder mixed with 2 oz. water) 6 to 8 times daily. Ethan's mother has a hard time reading Ethan's hunger cues. She is so concerned about his growth that she offers him a bottle frequently, every 1½ to 2 hours. He consumes 26 to 30 ounces (780 to 900 ml) of formula daily. She offers him homemade purées of fruits or vegetables mixed with grains twice a day; he eats a couple of tablespoons at a time. When she feels he has not eaten enough food, she offers him a bottle.

Nutrition Diagnostic Statement

Food- and nutrition-related knowledge deficit related to age-inappropriate frequency of formula feeding as evidenced by formula offered every 1½ to 2 hours

Nutrition Care Questions

1. What additional information is needed to get an accurate assessment of this infant's intake?
2. When you assess Ethan's growth, what are your expectations for his growth rate? Do you have concerns about his rate of growth?
3. What is a typical eating pattern for an infant Ethan's age? Is Ethan's eating pattern appropriate? Comment on his food and formula intake.
4. How would you assess Ethan's readiness for more textured foods? For self-feeding?

Other Common Nutrition Diagnostic Statements in Infants:

Inadequate energy intake related to mother diluting formula to save money as evidenced by slowed growth pattern and small head circumference

Underweight related to dietary restrictions to address multiple food allergies without medical supervision as evidenced by decrease of weight-for-length from the 50th percentile to the 25th percentile over 1 month

Inadequate vitamin B_{12} intake related to exclusively breast-fed by vegan mother without vitamin supplementation as evidenced by serum B_{12} levels below normal range and lethargy

Excessive oral intake related to using foods to soothe baby as evidenced by weight-for-length at the 95th percentile for age

USEFUL WEBSITES

American Academy of Pediatrics
www.aap.org/
Bright Futures: Nutrition in Practice
www.brightfutures.org/nutrition/
CDC and WHO Growth Charts
www.cdc.gov/growthcharts/
Healthy People 2020: Objectives for Improving Health
www.healthypeople.gov/
University of Washington Assuring Pediatric Nutrition in the Hospital and Community
http://depts.washington.edu/nutrpeds/

REFERENCES

Academy of Nutrition and Dietetics (AND), Palmer CA, Gilbert JA: Position of the Academy of Nutrition and Dietetics: the impact of fluoride on health, *J Acad Nutr Diet* 112:1443–1453, 2012.

American Academy of Pediatric Dentistry (AAPD): *Reference Manual, Clinical Guidelines, Guideline on fluoride therapy*, 36:171, 2015. http://www.aapd.org/media/Policies_Guidelines/G_fluoridetherapy.pdf. Accessed July 28, 2015.

American Academy of Pediatrics (AAP), Committee on Infectious Diseases and Committee on Nutrition: Consumption of raw or unpasteurized milk and milk products by pregnant women and children, *Pediatrics* 133:175–179, 2014a.

American Academy of Pediatrics (AAP), Committee on Nutrition: *Pediatric nutrition*, ed 7, Elk Grove Village, Ill, 2014b, American Academy of Pediatrics.

American Academy of Pediatrics (AAP), Section on Breastfeeding: Breastfeeding and the use of human milk, *Pediatrics* 129:e827–e841, 2012.

American Academy of Pediatrics (AAP), Section on Oral Health: Maintaining and improving the oral health of young children, *Pediatrics* 134:1224–1229, 2014c.

American Dietetic Association, Kris-Etherton PM, Innis S: Position of the American Dietetic Association and Dietitians of Canada: dietary fatty acids, *J Am Diet Assoc* 107:1599–1611, 2007.

Andres A, Cleves MA, Bellando JB, et al: Developmental status of 1-year-old infants fed breast milk, cow's milk formula, or soy formula, *Pediatrics* 129:1134–1140, 2012.

Baker RD, Greer FR, Committee on Nutrition American Academy of Pediatrics: Diagnosis and prevention of iron-deficiency anemia in infants and young children (0-3 years of age), *Pediatrics* 126:1040–1050, 2010.

Balk SJ: American Academy of Pediatrics, Council on Environmental Health and Section and Dermatology: technical report—ultraviolet radiation: a hazard to children and adolescents, *Pediatrics* 20:1358, 2011.

Bhatia J, Greer F, American Academy of Pediatrics Committee on Nutrition: Use of soy proteinbased formulas in infant feeding, *Pediatrics* 121:1062–1068, 2008.

Carruth BR, Ziegler PJ, Gordon A, et al: Prevalence of picky eaters among infants and toddlers and their caregivers' decisions about offering a new food, *J Am Diet Assoc* 104:S57–S64, 2004a.

Carruth BR, Ziegler PJ, Gordon A, et al: Developmental milestones and self-feeding behaviors in infants and toddlers, *J Am Diet Assoc* 104:S51–S56, 2004b.

Centers for Disease Control and Prevention (CDC): *Overview: Infant Formula and Fluorosis*, 2013. http://www.cdc.gov/fluoridation/safety/infant_formula.htm. Accessed December 2014.

Cole CR, Lifshitz F: Zinc nutrition and growth retardation, *Pediatr Endocrinol Rev* 5:889–896, 2008.

Domellöf M, Braegger C, Campoy C, et al: Iron requirements of infants and toddlers, *J Pediatr Gastroenterol Nutr* 58:119–129, 2014.

Druet C, Stettler N, Sharp S, et al: Prediction of childhood obesity by infancy weight gain: an individual level meta-analysis, *Paediatr Perinat Epidemiol* 26:19–26, 2012.

Elazab N, Mendy A, Gasana J, et al: Probiotic administration in early life, atopy, and asthma: a meta-analysis of clinical trials, *Pediatrics* 132:e666–e676, 2013.

Food and Drug Administration (FDA): *Bisphenol A (BPA): Use in Food Contact Application*, 2014. http://www.fda.gov/Food/IngredientsPackagingLabeling/FoodAdditivesIngredients/ucm064437.htm#regulations. Accessed December 2014.

Food and Drug Administration (FDA): *FDA Statement on Testing and Analysis of Arsenic in Rice and Rice Products*, 2013. http://www.fda.gov/Food/FoodborneIllnessContaminants/Metals/ucm367263.htm. Accessed December 2014.

Fox MK, Pac S, Devaney B, et al: Feeding infants and toddlers study: What foods are infants and toddlers eating? *J Am Diet Assoc* 104:S22–S30, 2004.

Fox MK, Devaney B, Reidy K, et al: Relationship between portion size and energy intake among infants and toddlers: evidence of self-regulation, *J Am Diet Assoc* 106:S77–S83, 2006.

Hausner H, Bredie WL, Mølgaard C, et al: Differential transfer of dietary flavour compounds into human breast milk, *Physiol Behav* 98:118–124, 2008.

Indrio F, Di Mauro A, Riezzo G, et al: Prophylactic use of a probiotic in the prevention of colic, regurgitation, and functional constipation: a randomized clinical trial, *JAMA Pediatr* 168:228–233, 2014.

Jeurink PV, van Esch BC, Rijnierse A, et al: Mechanisms underlying immune effects of dietary oligosaccharides, *Am J Clin Nutr* 98:S572–S577, 2013.

Lessen R, Kavanaugh K: Position of the Academy of Nutrition and Dietetics: Promoting and Supporting Breastfeeding, *J Acad Nutr Diet* 115:444, 2015.

Leven LV, MacDonald PD: Reducing the incidence of neonatal hypernatraemic dehydration, *Arch Dis Child* 93:811, 2008.

MacIntosh AC, Schroth RJ, Edwards J, et al: The impact of community workshops on improving early childhood oral health knowledge, *Pediatric Dent* 32:110–117, 2010.

Marques TM, Wall R, Ross RP, et al: Programming infant gut microbiota: influence of dietary and environmental factors, *Curr Opin Biotechnol* 21(2):149–156, 2010.

Misra M, Pacaud D, Petryk A, et al: Vitamin D deficiency in children and its management: review of current knowledge and recommendations, *Pediatrics* 122:398–417, 2008.

National Toxicology Program (NTP): *Final NTP brief on soy infant formula*, Washington, DC, 2010, US Department of Health and Human Services.

Oozeer R, van Limpt K, Ludwig T, et al: Intestinal microbiology in early life: specific prebiotics can have similar functionalities as human milk oligosaccharides, *Am J Clin Nutr* 98:S561–S571, 2013.

Roumeliotis N, Dix D, Lipson A: Vitamin B12 deficiency in infants secondary to maternal causes, *CMAJ* 184:1593–1598, 2012.

Shim JE, Kim J, Mathai RA, et al: Associations of infant feeding practices and picky eating behaviors of preschool children, *J Am Diet Assoc* 111:1363–1368, 2011.

Skinner JD, Ziegler P, Pac S, et al: Meal and snack patterns of infants and toddlers, *J Am Diet Assoc* 104:S65–S70, 2004.

Sung V, Hiscock H, Tang ML, et al: Treating infant colic with the probiotic Lactobacillus reuteri: double blind, placebo controlled randomized trial, *BMJ* 348:g2107, 2014.

Thomas DW, American Academy of Pediatrics Committee on Nutrition, American Academy of Pediatrics Section on Gastroenterology, Hepatology, and Nutrition, et al: Probiotics and prebiotics in pediatrics, *Pediatrics* 126:1217–1231, 2010.

Uriu-Adams JY, Obican SG, Keen CL: Vitamin D and maternal and child health: overview and implications for dietary requirements, *Birth Defects Res C Embryo Today* 99:24–44, 2013.

Van den Nieuwboer M, Claassen E, Morelli L, et al: Probiotic and synbiotic safety in infants under two years of age, *Beneficial Microbes* 5:45–60, 2014.

Wagner CL, Greer FR, American Academy of Pediatrics Section on Breastfeeding, et al: Prevention of rickets and vitamin D deficiency in infants, children, and adolescents, *Pediatrics* 122:1142–1152, 2008.

Willatts P, Forsyth S, Agostoni C, et al: Effects of long-chain PUFA supplementation in infant formula on cognitive function in later childhood, *Am J Clin Nutr* 98:S536–S542, 2013.

17

Nutrition in Childhood

Beth Ogata, MS, RDN, CD, CSP, Sharon A. Feucht, MA, RDN, CD, Betty L. Lucas, MPH, RDN, CD

KEY TERMS

adiposity rebound
catch-up growth
failure to thrive (FTT)

food jags
growth channels
growth deficiency

pediatric undernutrition
primarily wasted
stunted growth

The period that begins after infancy and lasts until puberty often is referred to as the *latent* or *quiescent* period of growth—a contrast to the dramatic changes that occur during infancy and adolescence. Although physical growth may be less remarkable and proceed at a steadier pace than it did during the first year, these preschool and elementary school years are a time of significant growth in the social, cognitive, and emotional areas.

GROWTH AND DEVELOPMENT

Growth Patterns

The rate of growth slows considerably after the first year of life. Increments of change are small compared with those of infancy and adolescence; weight typically increases an average of 1.6 to 3.3 kg (3½ to 7 lb) per year until the child is 9 or 10 years old. Then the rate increases, signaling the approach of puberty. Height increase increments average 5 to 9 cm (2 to 3½ inches) per year until the individual growth spurt seen in puberty.

Growth is generally steady and slow during the preschool and school age years, but it can be erratic in individual children, with periods of no growth followed by growth spurts. These patterns usually parallel similar changes in appetite and food intake. For parents, periods of slow growth and poor appetite can cause anxiety, leading to mealtime struggles.

Body proportions of young children change significantly after the first year. Head growth is minimal, trunk growth slows substantially, and limbs lengthen considerably, all of which create more mature body proportions. Walking and increased physical activity of the now-erect child lead to the legs straightening and increased muscle strength in the abdomen and back.

The body composition of preschool and school age children remains relatively constant. Fat gradually decreases during the early childhood years, reaching a minimum between 4 and 6 years of age. Children then experience the **adiposity rebound**, or increase in body fatness in preparation for the pubertal growth spurt. Earlier adiposity rebound has been associated with increased adult body mass index (BMI) (Williams and Goulding, 2009). Sex differences in body composition become increasingly apparent: boys have more lean body mass per

centimeter of height than girls. Girls have a higher percentage of weight as fat than boys, even in the preschool years, but these differences in lean body mass and fat do not become significant until adolescence.

Assessing Growth

A complete nutrition assessment includes the collection of anthropometric data. This includes length or stature, weight, and weight-for-length or BMI, all of which are plotted on the recommended growth charts (see Appendixes 4 through 11). Other measurements that are less commonly used but that provide estimates of body composition include upper-arm circumference and triceps or subscapular skin folds. Care should be taken to use standardized equipment and techniques for obtaining and plotting growth measurements. Charts designed for birth to 24 months of age are based on length measurements and nude weights, whereas charts used for 2- to 20-year-olds are based on stature (standing height) and weight with light clothing and without shoes (see Chapter 7).

The proportion of weight to length or height is a critical element of growth assessment. This parameter is determined by plotting the weight-for-length on the WHO birth to 24-month growth charts or calculating BMI, and plotting it on the 2- to 20-year-old CDC growth charts. Growth measurements obtained at regular intervals provide information about an individual's growth pattern. One-time measurements do not allow for interpretation of growth status. Growth channels are not well established until after 2 years of age. Children generally maintain their heights and weights in the same **growth channels** during the preschool and childhood years, although rates of growth can vary within a selected period.

Regular monitoring of growth enables problematic trends to be identified early and intervention initiated so that long-term growth is not compromised. Weight that increases rapidly and crosses growth channels may suggest the development of obesity (Figure 17-1). Lack of weight gain over a period of months or weight loss may be a result of undernutrition, an acute illness, an undiagnosed chronic disease, or significant emotional or family problems (Figure 17-2). However, many

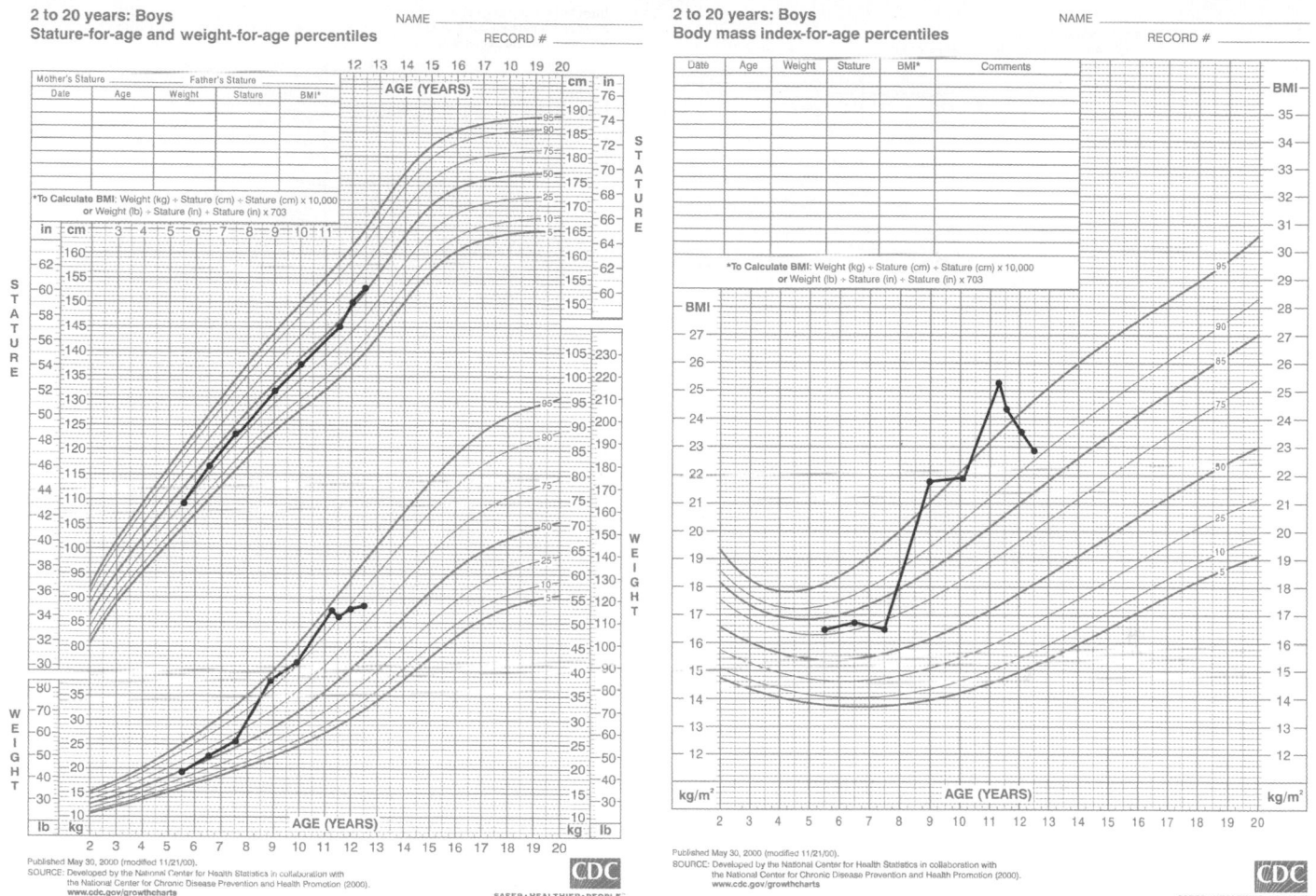

FIGURE 17-1 Growth chart and BMI chart for an 8-year-old boy who gained excessive weight after having leg surgery and being immobilized in a body cast for 2 months. The surgery and immobilization were followed by a long period of stress caused by family problems. At the age of 11 years, he became involved in a weight management program. (Source of growth charts only: Centers for Disease Control and Prevention: Growth Charts [website]: http://www.cdc.gov/growthcharts/, 2014. Accessed December 2014.)

children are evaluated by health care professionals only when they are ill, so growth evaluation and development may not be a focus of care.

Catch-Up Growth

A child who is recovering from an illness or undernutrition and whose growth has slowed or ceased experiences a greater than expected rate of recovery. This recovery is referred to as catch-up growth, a period during which the body strives to return to the child's normal growth channel. The degree of growth suppression is influenced by the timing, severity, and duration of the precipitating cause, such as a severe illness or prolonged nutritional deprivation.

Initial studies supported the thesis that malnourished infants who did not experience immediate catch-up growth would have permanent growth retardation. However, studies of malnourished children from developing countries who subsequently received adequate nourishment, as well as reports of children who were malnourished because of chronic disease such as celiac disease or cystic fibrosis, have shown that these children caught up to their normal growth channels after the first year or two of life when their disease was managed.

The nutritional requirements for catch-up growth depend on whether the child has overall stunted growth (height and weight are proportionally low) and is chronically malnourished, or is primarily wasted, meaning that the weight deficit exceeds the height deficit. With renourishment, expectations for weight gain vary. A chronically malnourished child may not be expected to gain more than 2 to 3 g/kg/day, whereas a child who is primarily wasted may gain as much as 20 g/kg/day.

Nutrient requirements, especially for energy and protein, depend on the rate and stage of catch-up growth. For instance, more protein and energy are needed during the initial period of very rapid weight gain and for those in whom lean tissue is the major component of the weight gain. In addition to energy, other nutrients are important, including vitamin A, iron, and zinc.

Current growth parameters are used to evaluate the child's weight in relation to age and stature and to estimate a "desirable" or goal weight. Formulas are then used to estimate the minimum and maximum energy needed for catch-up growth. After a child who is wasted catches up in weight, dietary management must change to slow the weight gain velocity and avoid

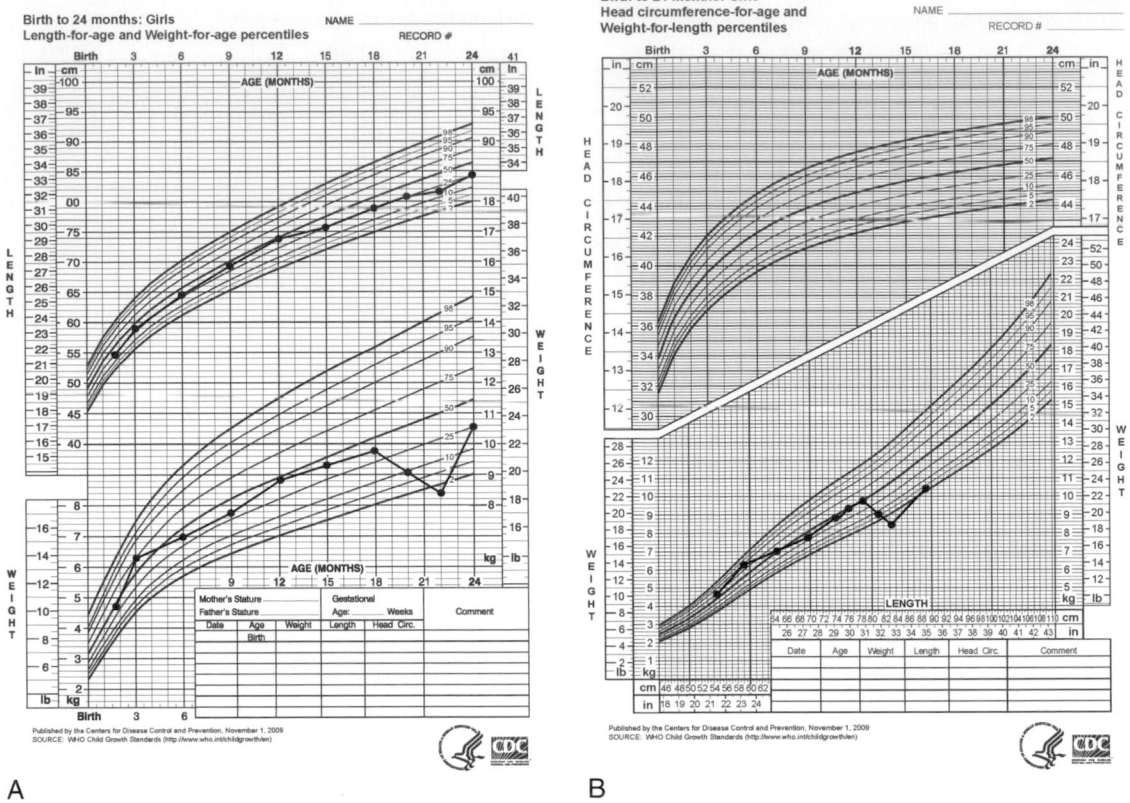

A   B

FIGURE 17-2 Growth charts for a 2-year-old girl who experienced significant weight loss during a prolonged period of diarrhea and feeding problems. After being diagnosed with celiac disease, she began following a gluten-free diet and entered a period of catch-up growth. (Source of growth charts only: Centers for Disease Control and Prevention: *Growth Charts* [website]: http://www.cdc.gov/growthcharts/, 2014. Accessed December 2014.)

excessive gain. The catch-up in linear growth peaks approximately 1 to 3 months after treatment starts, whereas weight gain begins immediately.

NUTRIENT REQUIREMENTS

Because children are growing and developing bones, teeth, muscles, and blood, they need more nutritious food in proportion to their size than do adults. They may be at risk for malnutrition when they have a poor appetite for a long period, eat a limited number of foods, or dilute their diets significantly with nutrient-poor foods.

The dietary reference intakes (DRIs) are based on current knowledge of nutrient intakes needed for optimal health. (See inside front cover.) Most data for preschool and school age children are values interpolated from data on infants and adults. The DRIs are meant to improve the long-term health of the population by reducing the risk of chronic disease and preventing nutritional deficiencies. Thus, when intakes are less than the recommended level, it cannot be assumed that a particular child is inadequately nourished.

Energy

The energy needs of healthy children are determined by basal metabolism, rate of growth, and energy expenditure of activity. Dietary energy must be sufficient to ensure growth and spare protein from being used for energy, while not allowing excess

weight gain. Suggested intake proportions of energy are 45% to 65% as carbohydrate, 30% to 40% as fat, and 5% to 20% as protein for 1- to 3-year-olds, with carbohydrates the same for 4- to 18-year-olds, 25% to 35% as fat, and 10% to 30% as protein.

The DRIs for estimated energy requirement (EER) are average energy requirements based on life-stage groupings for healthy individuals of normal weight. Toddlers 13 through 35 months are grouped together; for older children the EERs are divided by sex and age (3 to 8 years and 9 to 18 years). The EER includes the total energy expenditure plus energy needed for growth (see Chapter 2). The DRIs are applied to child nutrition programs and other guidelines (Otten et al, 2006). Box 17-1 provides examples of determining EER for two children. On an individual basis, it can be useful to estimate energy requirements using kilocalories per kilogram of weight or per centimeter of height.

Protein

The need for protein decreases from approximately 1.1 g/kg in early childhood to 0.95 g/kg in late childhood (Table 17-1). Protein intake can range from 5% to 30% of total energy, depending on age. Protein deficiency is uncommon in American children, partly because of the cultural emphasis on high-protein foods. National surveys show that less than 3% of children fail to meet the recommended dietary allowance. Children who are most at risk for inadequate protein intake are those on strict vegan diets,

BOX 17-1   Determining Estimated Energy Requirements

(Examples using data from Box 2-1, Chapter 2)
1. For 13- to 35-month-old children:

$$EER \ (kcal) = (89 \times wt \ [kg]) - 100 + 20$$

An 18-month-old boy has a length of 84 cm and weighs 12.5 kg

$$EER \ (kcal) = (89 \times 12.5) - 100 + 20$$

$$EER \ (kcal) = 1113 - 100 + 20$$

$$EER \ (kcal) = 1033$$

2. For girls 3 through 8 years:

$$EER \ (kcal) = 135.3 - ([30.8 \times age \ in \ yrs] + PA \times ([10 \times wgt \ in \ kg] + [934 \times hgt \ in \ m]) + 20$$

A 6½-year-old girl is 112 cm tall, weighs 20.8 kg, and has moderate activity (PA coefficient of 1.31)

$$EER \ (kcal) = 135.3 - (30.8 \times 6.5) + 1.31 \times ([10 \times 20.8] + [934 \times 1.12]) + 20$$

$$EER \ (kcal) = 135.3 - 200.2 + 1.31 \times (208 + 1046.1) + 20$$

$$EER \ (kcal) = 135.3 - 200.2 + 1642.9 + 20$$

$$EER \ (kcal) = 1598$$

EER, Estimated energy requirement; *PA*, physical activity.

TABLE 17-1   Protein Dietary Reference Intakes (DRIs) for Children Through Age 13 Years

Age	Grams/Day*	PROTEIN Grams/Kilogram/Day
1-3 yr	13 g/day	1.05 g/kg/day
4-8 yr	19 g/day	0.95 g/kg/day
9-13 yr	34 g/day	0.95 g/kg/day

*Recommended dietary allowance for reference individual (g/day).

those with multiple food allergies, or who have limited food selections because of fad diets, behavioral problems, or inadequate access to food.

Minerals and Vitamins

Minerals and vitamins are necessary for normal growth and development. Insufficient intake can cause impaired growth and result in deficiency diseases. The DRIs are listed inside the front cover.

Iron

Children between 1 and 3 years of age are at risk for iron deficiency anemia, which can affect development. The rapid growth period of infancy is marked by an increase in hemoglobin and total iron mass. National Health and Nutrition Examination Survey (NHANES) data indicate that children with prolonged bottle feeding and those of Mexican American descent are at highest risk for iron deficiency (Moshfegh et al, 2005). Recommended intakes must factor in the absorption rate and quantity of iron in foods, especially those of plant origin.

Calcium

Calcium is needed for adequate mineralization and maintenance of growing bone in children. The RDA for calcium for children 1 to 3 years old is 700 mg/day, for children 4 to 8 years it is 1000 mg/day, and for those 9 to 18 years it is 1300 mg per day. Actual need depends on individual absorption rates and dietary factors such as quantities of protein, vitamin D, and phosphorus. Because milk and other dairy products are primary sources of calcium, children who consume limited amounts of these foods are often at risk for poor bone mineralization. Other calcium-fortified foods such as soy and rice milks and fruit juices are also good sources (see Appendix 46).

Zinc

Zinc is essential for growth; a deficiency results in growth failure, poor appetite, decreased taste acuity, and poor wound healing. Because the best sources of zinc are meat and seafood, some children may regularly have low intakes (see Appendix 53). Diagnosis of zinc deficiency, especially marginal deficiency, may be difficult because laboratory parameters, including plasma, serum erythrocyte, hair, and urine, are of limited value in determining zinc deficiency. There is a positive influence of zinc supplementation on growth and serum zinc concentrations.

Vitamin D

Vitamin D is needed for calcium absorption and deposition of calcium in the bones; other functions within the body, including prevention of chronic diseases such as cancer, cardiovascular disease, and diabetes, are important areas of current investigation. Because this nutrient also is formed from sunlight exposure on the skin, the amount required from dietary sources depends on factors such as geographic location and time spent outside (see Appendix 45).

The DRI for vitamin D for infants is 400 IU (10 mcg) per day and for children is 600 IU (15 mcg) per day. Vitamin D-fortified milk is the primary dietary source of this nutrient, and breakfast cereals and nondairy milks often are fortified with vitamin D (see Appendix 45). Dairy products such as cheese and yogurt, however, are not always made from fortified milk. Milks other than cow milk (e.g., goat, soy, almond, or rice) may not be fortified with vitamin D. For young children the current DRI for vitamin D is higher than what may be consumed from a typical diet. Supplementation may be needed after a careful assessment or measurement of vitamin D status. It is becoming more common to measure serum 25(OH) vitamin D in children; however, there is some controversy regarding what constitutes optimal levels (Rovner and O'Brien, 2008).

Vitamin-Mineral Supplements

Forty percent of preschool children are given a multivitamin-mineral supplement; this percentage decreases in older children (Butte et al, 2010; Picciano et al, 2007). Families with more education, health insurance coverage, and higher incomes generally have higher rates of supplement use, although these may not be the families who are at greatest risk for having inadequate diets.

Evidence shows that fluoride can help prevent dental caries. If a community's water supply is not fluoridated, fluoride supplements are recommended from 6 months until 16 years of age. However, individual family practices should be assessed, including the child's primary source of fluids (e.g., drinking water, juices, or other beverages) and fluoride sources from child care, school, toothpaste, and mouthwash (see Chapter 25).

The AAP does not support giving healthy children routine supplements of any vitamins or minerals other than fluoride. However, children at risk for inadequate nutrition who may benefit include those (1) with anorexia, inadequate appetite, or who consume fad diets; (2) with chronic disease (e.g., cystic fibrosis, inflammatory bowel disease, hepatic disease); (3) from food-deprived families or who suffer parental neglect or abuse; (4) who participate in a dietary program for managing obesity; (5) who consume a vegetarian diet without adequate dairy products; (6) with faltering growth (failure to thrive); (7) with developmental disabilities.

Children who routinely take a multiple vitamin or a vitamin-mineral supplement usually do not experience negative effects if the supplement contains nutrients in amounts that do not exceed the DRIs, especially the tolerable upper intake level. However, some nutrients can be "missed" by general multiple vitamin supplements. Although many children consume less than the recommended amount of calcium, children's vitamin-mineral supplements typically do not contain significant amounts of calcium. For example, among children ages 2 to 18 years who took supplements, one third did not meet recommendations for calcium and vitamin D intakes even with supplements. In addition, supplement use was associated with increased prevalence of excessive intakes of iron, zinc, vitamin A, and folic acid (Bailey et al, 2012). In addition, an analysis of supplements marketed for infants and children indicated that available supplements do not necessarily meet recommendations for intake; for some nutrients, not enough is provided, and for others, the supplements provide excessive amounts (Madden et al, 2014). Children should not take megadoses, particularly of the fat-soluble vitamins because large amounts can result in toxicity. Careful evaluation of each pediatric supplement is suggested because many types are available but incomplete. Because many vitamin-mineral supplements look and taste like candy, parents should keep them out of reach of children to avoid excessive intake of nutrients such as iron.

Complementary nutrition therapies are becoming more common for children, especially for those with special health care needs such as children with Down syndrome, autism spectrum disorder (ASD), or cystic fibrosis (see Chapters 34 and 44). As part of the nutrition assessment, practitioners should inquire as to the use of these products and therapies, be knowledgeable about their efficacy and safety, and help families determine whether they are beneficial and how to use them (see Chapter 12).

PROVIDING AN ADEQUATE DIET

The development of feeding skills, food habits, and nutrition knowledge parallels the cognitive development that takes place in a series of stages, each laying the groundwork for the next. Table 17-2 outlines the development of feeding skills in terms of Piaget's theory of child psychology and development.

Intake Patterns

Children's food patterns have changed over the years. Although they drink less milk, more of it is low-fat or nonfat milk. The total fat as a percent of energy intake has decreased, but remains above recommendations of 25% to 40% of total

---

TABLE 17-2   Feeding, Nutrition, and Piaget's Theory of Cognitive Development

Developmental Period	Cognitive Characteristics	Relationships to Feeding and Nutrition
Sensorimotor (birth-2 yr)	Neonate progresses from autonomic reflexes to a young child with intentional interaction with the environment and the beginning use of symbols. Food is used primarily to satisfy hunger, as a medium to explore the environment, and as an opportunity to practice fine motor skills.	Progression involves advancing from sucking and rooting reflexes to the acquisition of self-feeding skills.
Preoperational (2-7 yr)	Thought processes become internalized; they are unsystematic and intuitive. Use of symbols increases. Reasoning is based on appearances and happenstance. The child's approach to classification is functional and unsystematic. The child's world is viewed egocentrically.	Eating becomes less the center of attention and is secondary to social, language, and cognitive growth. Food is described by color, shape, and quantity, but the child has only a limited ability to classify food into "groups." Foods tend to be categorized into "like" and "don't like." Foods can be identified as "good for you," but reasons why they are healthy are unknown or mistaken.
Concrete operational (7-11 yr)	The child can focus on several aspects of a situation simultaneously. Cause-and-effect reasoning becomes more rational and systematic. The ability to classify, reclassify, and generalize emerges. A decrease in egocentrism permits the child to take another's view.	The child begins to realize that nutritious food has a positive effect on growth and health but has a limited understanding of how or why. Mealtimes take on a social significance. The expanding environment increases the opportunities for influences on food selection; for example, peer influence increases.
Formal operational (11 yr and beyond)	Hypothetical and abstract thought expand. The child's understanding of scientific and theoretical processes deepens.	The concept of nutrients from food functioning at physiologic and biochemical levels can be understood. Conflicts in making food choices may be realized (i.e., knowledge of the nutritious value of foods may conflict with preferences and nonnutritive influences).

energy intake depending on age. More energy comes from snacks, and portion sizes have increased. In addition, more food is consumed in environments other than the home (Nicklas and Hayes, 2008). Foods with low nutrient density (soft drinks, baked and dairy desserts, sweeteners, and salty snacks) often displace nutrient-dense foods. National food intake studies of children and adolescents indicate that most of their diets do not meet the national recommendations for food groups.

Like physical growth patterns, food intake patterns are not smooth and consistent. Although subjective, appetites usually follow the rate of growth and nutrient needs. By a child's first birthday, milk consumption begins to decline. In the next year vegetable intake decreases; intakes of cereals, grain products, and sweets increase. Young children often prefer softer protein sources instead of meats that are harder to chew.

Changes in food consumption are reflected in nutrient intakes. The early preschool years show a decrease in calcium, phosphorus, riboflavin, iron, and vitamin A compared with infancy. Intakes of most other key nutrients remain relatively stable. During the early school years, a pattern of consistent and steadily increased intakes of most nutrients is seen until adolescence. In healthy children a wide variability of nutrient intake is seen at any age. Children are most likely to consume inadequate amounts of calcium, vitamin D, fiber, and potassium (Bailey et al, 2010; Kranz et al, 2012). However, clinical signs of malnutrition in American children are rare.

Factors Influencing Food Intake

Numerous influences, some obvious and others subtle, determine the food intake and habits of children. Habits, likes, and dislikes are established in the early years and carried through to adulthood. The major influences on food intake in the developing years include family environment, societal trends, the media, peer pressure, and illness or disease.

Family Environment

For toddlers and preschool children the family is the primary influence in the development of food habits. In young children's immediate environment, parents and older siblings are significant models. Food attitudes of parents can be strong predictors of food likes and dislikes and diet complexity in children of primary school age. Similarities between children's and their parents' food preferences are likely to reflect genetic and environmental influences (Savage et al, 2007).

Contrary to common belief, young children do not have the innate ability to choose a balanced, nutritious diet; they can choose one only when presented with nutritious foods. A positive feeding relationship includes a division of responsibility between parents and children. The parents and other adults are to provide safe, nutritious, developmentally appropriate food as regular meals and snacks. The children decide how much, if any, they eat (Eneli et al, 2008).

Eating together at family meals is becoming less common, partly because of family schedules, more time eating in front of a screen, and the decreasing amount of time devoted to planning and preparing family meals. School age children and adolescents who eat more dinners with their families consume more fruits and vegetables, less soda, and fewer fried foods than those who rarely eat dinner with their families (Larson et al, 2007). Family meals have other influences, including a positive influence on nutrition beliefs and possibly prevention of overweight (Chan and Sobal, 2011).

The atmosphere around food and mealtime also influences attitudes toward food and eating. Unrealistic expectations for a child's mealtime manners, arguments, and other emotional stress can have a negative effect. Meals that are rushed create a hectic atmosphere and reinforce the tendency to eat too fast. A positive environment is one in which sufficient time is set aside to eat, occasional spills are tolerated, and conversation that includes all family members is encouraged (Figure 17-3).

Societal Trends

Because almost three fourths of women with school age children are employed outside the home, children may eat one or more meals at a child care center or school. In these settings all children should have access to nutritious meals served in a safe and sanitary environment that promotes healthy growth and development (Benjamin Neelon et al, 2011; Bergman and Gordon, 2010). Because of time constraints, family meals may include more convenience or fast foods. However, having a mother who is employed outside the home does not seem to affect children's dietary intakes negatively. Food service in group settings such as child care centers, Head Start programs, preschool programs, and in elementary schools is regulated by federal or state guidelines. Many facilities and some in-home child care centers may participate in the U.S. Department of Agriculture (USDA) Child and Adult Care Food Program. However, the quality of meals and snacks can vary greatly; parents should investigate food service when considering child care options. In addition to providing children with optimal nutrients, a program should offer food that is appealing, safely prepared, and appropriate, incorporating cultural and developmental patterns (Benjamin Neelon et al, 2007).

Approximately one in five American children lives in a family with an income below the poverty line; in 2012 nearly 16 million children lived in poverty (DeNavas-Walt et al, 2013). The increasing numbers of single-parent households predominantly headed by women have lower incomes and less money for all expenses, including food, than households headed by men. This

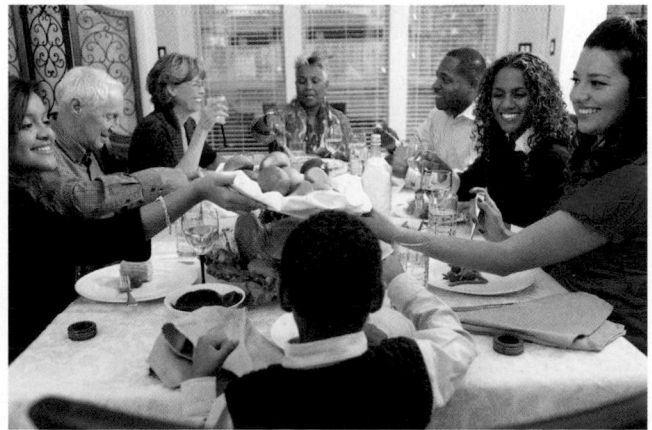

FIGURE 17-3 Three generations of a family share a meal. Eating together gives meals a place of prominence in the home—meals that will not be replaced with fast foods eaten on the run. (From Photo©istock.com.)

phenomenon makes these families increasingly vulnerable to multiple stressors such as marginal health and nutritional status partly because of lack of jobs, child care, adequate housing, and health insurance.

In 2013, 11.3% of U.S. households experienced food insecurity. Federal food and nutrition assistance programs (including National School Lunch, Food Stamp Program, and Special Supplemental Nutrition Program for Women, Infants and Children [WIC]) provided benefits to about 60% of food-insecure households (Coleman-Jensen, et al , 2013; see Chapter 9). The food stamp allotment for families, based on the USDA Thrifty Food Plan, does not provide adequate funds to purchase food based on the government's nutrition guidelines, especially when labor is considered (Davis and You, 2010). Food insecurity also increases the risk for children younger than age 3 years to be iron-deficient with anemia. Studies suggest that intermittent hunger in American children is associated with increased developmental risk (see *Focus On:* Childhood Hunger and Its Effect on Behavior and Emotions) (Rose-Jacobs et al, 2008). Even marginal food insecurity, which is often thought not to be an indicator of nutrition risk in adults, is associated with adverse health outcomes in children (Cook et al, 2013).

◎ FOCUS ON

Childhood Hunger and Its Effect on Behavior and Emotions

It is well accepted that malnourished children are less responsive, less inquisitive, and participate in less exploratory behavior than well-nourished children. Specific nutrient deficiencies such as iron deficiency anemia also can result in a decreased ability to pay attention and poorer problem-solving skills. Less clear is the effect of periodic hunger or food insecurity on a child's behavior and functioning. With recent federal welfare reform legislation and economic downturns, an increasing number of children from low-income families are at risk for limited food resources (Stang and Bayerl, 2010).

In the 1990s the Community Childhood Hunger Identification Project conducted surveys using standardized questions and large, rigorously selected samples to categorize families as "hungry," "at risk for hunger," or "not hungry" (Kleinman et al, 1998). It was estimated that each year 8% of children younger than 12 years of age in the United States experienced prolonged periods in which they had insufficient food. Data from 2012 indicated that 10% of U.S. households with children were food-insecure. In 2012, 49.0 million people in the United States lived in food-insecure households; 15.9 million of those people (11.3%) were children (Food and Research Action Center, 2014). A longitudinal study following approximately 21,000 children from kindergarten through third grade found that persistent food insecurity was predictive of impaired academic outcomes, poorer social skills, and a tendency to increased BMI (Ryu and Bartfeld, 2012).

Although these studies have limitations because of other factors that may affect a child's functioning (e.g., stress, family dysfunction, or substance abuse), a correlation exists between children's lack of sufficient food and their behavioral and academic functioning. As future studies provide more evidence of this relationship, it will be clear that social policies must ensure the provision of children's basic needs for optimal growth and development.

Media Messages

Food is marketed to children using a variety of techniques, including television advertising, in-school marketing, sponsorship, product placement, Internet marketing, and sales promotion. Television advertising and in-school marketing are regulated to some degree. By the time the average American child graduates from high school, he or she has watched 15,000 hours of television and spent 11,000 hours in the classroom. In a sample of television advertising to children, more than 40% of commercials were for food. Of these, 80% to 95% were for items high in saturated fat, trans fat, sugar, and sodium (Powell et al, 2013).

Screen time can be detrimental to growth and development because it encourages inactivity and passive use of leisure time. Television viewing and its multiple media cues to eat have been suggested as a factor contributing to excessive weight gain in school age children and adolescents, especially when there is a television in the child's bedroom (Gilbert-Diamond et al, 2014). Increases in hours of television viewing are associated with rising BMIs in boys and girls, with females also affected by watching DVDs/videos and electronic games. For those already at risk with higher BMIs, limits on uneducational viewing may be part of intervention strategies (Falbe et al, 2013).

The types of food eaten during television viewing can contribute to increased dental caries resulting from the continued exposure of the teeth to dense carbohydrate- and sugar-laden foods (Ghimire and Rao, 2013). Children ages 2 to 11 are viewing less food-related advertising than in the past, with the largest decrease in ads for sweet foods; foods shown are still high in saturated fat, sodium, and/or sugar (Powell et al, 2011).

Preschool children are generally unable to distinguish commercial messages from regular programs. In fact, they often pay more attention to the commercials. As children get older, they gain knowledge about the purpose of commercial advertising and become more critical of its validity but are still susceptible to the commercial message. Media literacy education programs teach children and adolescents about the intent of advertising and media messages and how to evaluate and interpret their obvious and subtle influences. Comprehensive and consistent regulation approaches plus monitoring the use of the most common persuasive marketing techniques (premium offers, promotional characters, nutrition- and health-related claims, taste and fun appeal) is suggested (Jenkin et al, 2014).

Significant decreases have occurred in beverage and food vending in schools, but both forms of sales still occur. Elementary-age students often are given coupons to encourage their families to purchase food, whereas those in upper grades may be exposed to in-school exclusive beverage contracts and other types of marketing (Terry-McElrath et al, 2014). The USDA has established nutrition standards for snack foods and beverages available for sale in schools but does not address food marketing. Standards that can be enforced are still needed to clarify the nutrition content of all foods and beverages marketed in school settings.

Fortunately, some media messages are beneficial. For example, public health messages about eating fish versus the risks of acquiring mercury are important. (See *Focus On:* Childhood Methylmercury Exposure and Toxicity: Media Messaging.)

Peer Influence

As children grow, their world expands and their social contacts become more important. Peer influence increases with age and affects food attitudes and choices. This may result in a sudden refusal of a food or a request for a currently popular food. Decisions about whether to participate in school meals may be made more on the basis of friends' choices than on the menu. Such behaviors are developmentally typical. Positive behaviors such as a willingness to try new foods can be reinforced. Parents

Childhood Methylmercury Exposure and Toxicity: Media Messaging

Mercury toxicity can cause neurologic problems, which can lead to cognitive and motor deficits. Toxicity related to prenatal exposure is documented, and there is evidence that postnatal exposure is dangerous as well (Myers et al, 2009; Oken and Bellinger, 2008). Exposure to mercury can occur through environmental contact and eating contaminated foods. Methylmercury, the most toxic form of mercury, accumulates in fish.

Public health agencies have looked at balancing the benefits of minimizing exposure to this neurotoxin with the risk of limiting intake of docosahexaenoic acid (DHA) and eicosapentaenoic acid (EPA) as well as a source of high biologic value protein. DHA and EPA are essential omega-3 fatty acids and have received much attention because of their importance in cognitive and vision development and their cardiovascular benefits (Mahaffey et al, 2008). In addition, fish advisories are available in certain states. The U.S. Environmental Protection Agency's (EPA) reference dose for methylmercury is based on body weight: 0.1 mcg/kg/day. For a 20-kg child, this is approximately 14 mcg/week (U.S. EPA, 2004). The methylmercury content of 3 ounces of albacore tuna is approximately 29.7 mcg, canned light tuna approximately 10 mcg, and fresh or frozen salmon approximately 1.2 mcg. The Food and Drug Administration (FDA) and EPA have made recommendations for fish intake by young children:

- Do not eat shark, swordfish, king mackerel, or tilefish because they contain high levels of mercury.
- Eat up to 12 oz (two average meals) a week of a variety of fish and shellfish that are lower in mercury.
- Five of the most commonly eaten fish that are low in mercury are shrimp, canned light tuna, salmon, pollock, and catfish.
- Another commonly eaten fish, albacore ("white") tuna has more mercury than canned light tuna. So, when choosing two meals of fish and shellfish, eat up to 6 ounces (one average meal) of albacore tuna per week, but only 3 ounces for a child.
- Check local advisories about the safety of fish caught by family and friends in local lakes, rivers, and coastal areas. If no advice is available, eat up to 6 ounces (3 oz for a child) per week of fish caught from local waters, but do not consume any other fish during that week.
- Follow these same recommendations when feeding fish and shellfish to young children, but serve smaller portions.

Revised fish consumption guidelines from U.S. EPA and FDA are expected in 2016. See: http://www2.epa.gov/fish-tech/epa-fda-advisory-mercury-fish-and-shellfish. Accessed November 2015.

must set limits on undesirable influences but also must be realistic; struggles over food are self-defeating.

Illness or Disease

Children who are ill usually have a decreased appetite and limited food intake. Acute viral or bacterial illnesses are often short-lived but may require an increase in fluids, protein, or other nutrients. Chronic conditions such as asthma, cystic fibrosis, or chronic renal disease may make it difficult to obtain sufficient nutrients for optimal growth. Children with these types of conditions are more likely to have behavior problems relating to food. Children requiring special diets (e.g., those who have diabetes or phenylketonuria) not only have to adjust to the limits of foods allowed but also have to address issues of independence and peer acceptance as they grow older. Some rebellion against the prescribed diet is typical, especially as children approach puberty.

Feeding Preschool Children

From 1 to 6 years of age children experience vast developmental progress and acquisition of skills. One-year-old children primarily use fingers to eat and may need assistance with a cup. By 2 years of age, they can hold a cup in one hand and use a spoon well but may prefer to use their hands at times. Six-year-old children have refined skills and are beginning to use a knife for cutting and spreading.

As the growth rate slows after the first year of life, appetite decreases, which often concerns parents. Children have less interest in food and an increased interest in the world around them. They can develop **food jags,** which can be periods when foods that were previously liked are refused, or there are repeated requests to eat the same food meal after meal. This behavior may be attributable to boredom with the usual foods or may be a means of asserting newly discovered independence. Parents may have concerns with their child's seemingly irrational food behavior. Struggles over control of the eating situation are fruitless; no child can be forced to eat. This period is developmental and temporary (Figure 17-4).

A positive feeding relationship includes a division of responsibility between parents and children. Young children can choose a balanced nutritious diet if presented with nutritious foods. The parents and other adults provide safe, nutritious, developmentally appropriate food as regular meals and snacks; and the children decide how much, if any, they eat (Satter, 2000). Parents maintain control over what foods are offered and have the opportunity to set limits on inappropriate behaviors. Neither rigid control nor a laissez-faire approach is likely to succeed. Parents and other care providers should continue to offer a variety of foods, including the child's favorites, and not make substitutions a routine.

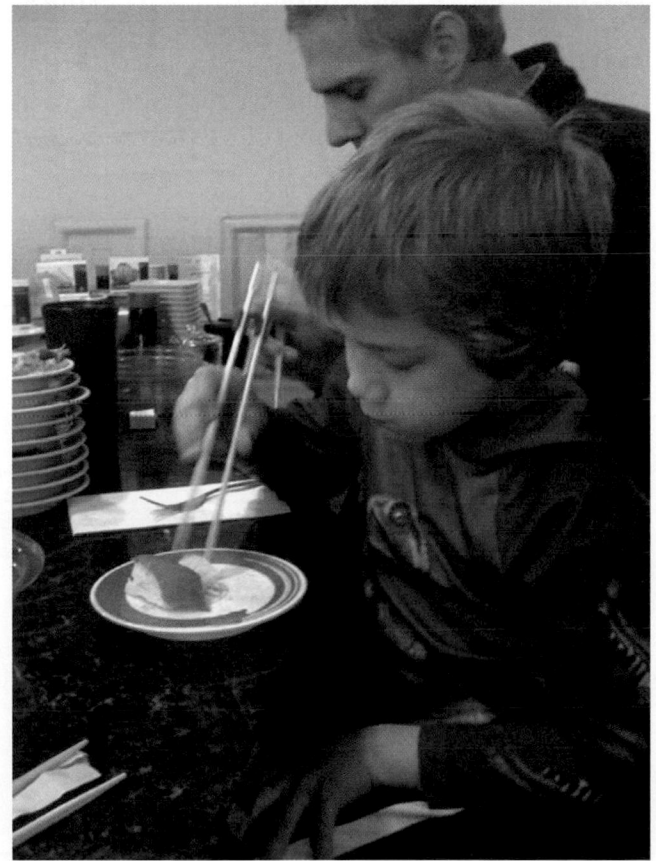

FIGURE 17-4 Use of alternative eating utensils can increase a preschooler's interest in trying new foods and development of fine motor skills.

With smaller stomach capacities and variable appetites, preschool children should be offered small servings of food four to six times a day. Snacks are as important as meals in contributing to the total daily nutrient intake. Carefully chosen snacks are those dense in nutrients and least likely to promote dental caries. A general rule of thumb is to offer 1 tablespoon of each food for every year of age and to serve more food according to the child's appetite. Table 17-3 is a guide for food and portion size.

Senses other than taste play an important part in food acceptance by young children. They tend to avoid food with extreme temperatures, and some foods are rejected because of odor rather than taste. A sense of order in the food presentation often is preferred; many children do not accept foods that touch each other on the plate, and mixed dishes or casseroles with unidentifiable foods are not popular. Broken crackers may go uneaten, or a sandwich may be refused because it is "cut the wrong way."

The physical setting for meals is important. Children's feet should be supported, and chair height should allow a comfortable reach to the table at chest height. Sturdy, child-size tables and chairs are ideal, or a high chair or booster seat should be used. Dishes and cups should be unbreakable and heavy enough to resist tipping. For very young children, a shallow bowl is often better than a plate for scooping. Thick, short-handled spoons and forks allow for an easier grasp.

Young children do not eat well if they are tired; this should be considered when meal and play times are scheduled. A quiet activity or rest immediately before eating is conducive to a relaxed, enjoyable meal. However, children also need active, large-motor activities and time in the fresh air to stimulate a good appetite.

Fruit juices and juice drinks are common beverages for young children; they frequently replace water and milk in children's diets. In addition to altering the diet's nutrient content, excessive intake of fruit juice can result in carbohydrate malabsorption and chronic, nonspecific diarrhea. This suggests that juices, especially apple and pear, should be avoided when using liquids to treat acute diarrhea. For children with chronic diarrhea, a trial of restricting fruit juices may be warranted before more costly diagnostic tests are done.

When children aged 2 to 11 years consume 100% juice, their diets have significantly higher intakes of energy, carbohydrates, vitamins C and B_6, potassium, riboflavin, magnesium, iron, and folate, and significantly lower intakes of total fat, saturated fatty acids, discretionary fat, and added sugar; this 100% juice intake does not correlate with overweight later (Nicklas et al, 2008). However, excess juice intake (12 to 30 oz/day) by young children may decrease a child's appetite, resulting in decreased food intake and poor growth. Here, a reduction in juice intake results in improved growth (American Academy of Pediatrics [AAP], Committee on Nutrition, 2001). Fruit juice intake should be

TABLE 17-3 Suggested Portion Sizes for Children*

These suggestions are not necessarily appropriate for all children (and may be inappropriate for some children with medical conditions that greatly affect nutrient needs). They are intended to serve as a general framework that can be individualized based on a child's condition and growth pattern.

	1- to 3-Year-Olds	4- to 6-Year-Olds	7- to 12-Year-Olds	Comments
Grain Products	Bread: ½ to 1 slice Rice, pasta, potatoes: ¼ to ½ cup Cooked cereal: ¼ to ½ cup Ready-to-eat cereal: ¼ to ½ cup Tortilla: ½ to 1	Bread: 1 slice Rice, pasta, potatoes: ½ cup Cooked cereal: ½ cup Ready-to-eat cereal: ¾ to 1 cup Tortilla: 1	Bread: 1 slice Rice, pasta, potatoes: ½ cup Cooked cereal: ½ cup Ready-to-eat cereal: 1 cup Tortilla: 1	Include whole grain foods and enriched grain products.
Vegetables	Cooked or pureed: 2-4 tablespoons Raw: few pieces, if child can chew well	Cooked or pureed: 3-4 tablespoons Raw: few pieces	Cooked or pureed: ½ cup Raw: ½ to 1 cup	Include one green leafy or yellow vegetable for vitamin A, such as spinach, carrots, broccoli, or winter squash.
Fruit	Raw (apple, banana, etc.): ½ to 1 small, if child can chew well Canned: 2-4 Tablespoons Juice: 3-4 ounces	Raw (apple, banana, etc.): ½ to 1 small, if child can chew well Canned: 4-8 tablespoons Juice: 4 ounces	Raw (apple, banana, etc.): 1 small Canned: ¾ cup Juice: 5 ounces	Include one vitamin C–rich fruit, vegetable, or juice, such as citrus juices, an orange, grapefruit sections, strawberries, melon in season, a tomato, or broccoli.
Milk and Dairy Products	Milk, yogurt, pudding: 2-4 ounces Cheese: ¾ ounce	Milk, yogurt, pudding: ½ to ¾ cup Cheese: 1 ounce	Milk, yogurt, pudding: 1 cup Cheese: 1½ ounces	
Meat, Poultry, Fish, Other Protein	Meat, poultry, fish: 1-2 ounces Eggs: ½ to 1 Peanut butter: 1 Tablespoon Cooked dried beans: 4-5 Tablespoons	Meat, poultry, fish: 1-2 ounces Eggs: 1-2 Peanut butter: 2 Tablespoons Cooked dried beans: 4-8 Tablespoons	Meat, poultry, fish: 2 ounces Eggs: 2 Peanut butter: 3 Tablespoons Cooked dried beans: 1 cup	

Modified from Lowenberg ME: Development of food patterns in young children. In Trahms CM, Pipes P: *Nutrition in infancy and childhood,* ed 6, St Louis, 1997, WCB/McGraw-Hill and Harris; Harris AB et al: *Nutrition strategies for children with special needs,* 1999, USC University Affiliated Program, Los Angeles.

*This is a guide to a basic diet. Fats, oils, sauces, desserts, and snack foods provide additional energy to meet the needs of a growing child. Foods can be selected from this pattern for meals and snacks.

limited to 4 to 6 oz/day for children 1 through 6 years of age and 8 to 12 oz/day (in two servings) for older children and adolescents (AAP, 2014).

Large volumes of sweetened beverages, combined with other dietary and activity factors, may contribute to overweight in a child. High intake of fructose, especially from sucrose and high-fructose corn syrup in processed foods and beverages, may lead to increased plasma triglycerides and insulin resistance. In several studies, low calcium intake and obesity have been correlated with high intake of sugar-sweetened beverages in preschool children (Keller et al, 2009; Lim et al, 2009). High milk and low sweetened-beverage intake is associated with improved nutrient intake, including calcium, potassium, magnesium, and vitamin A (O'Neil et al, 2009). Children should be offered milk, water, and healthy snacks throughout the day instead of sugar-sweetened choices.

Excess sodium is another concern. An increase in sodium or salt intake results in an increase in systolic blood pressure and diastolic blood pressure (Bergman et al, 2010). A reduction in the use of processed foods may be warranted for children with elevated blood pressure. The Dietary Approaches to Stop Hypertension (DASH) diet is useful for all age groups because it increases potassium, magnesium, and calcium in relation to sodium intake (see Appendix 26).

Meal time in group settings is an ideal opportunity for nutrition education programs focused on various learning activities around food (Figure 17-5). Experiencing new foods, participating in simple food preparation, and planting a garden are activities that develop and enhance positive food habits and attitudes.

Feeding School Age Children

Growth from ages 6 to 12 years is slow but steady, paralleled by a constant increase in food intake. Children are in school a greater part of the day; and they begin to participate in clubs, organized sports, and recreational programs. The influence of peers and significant adults such as teachers, coaches, or sports idols increases. Except for severe issues, most behavioral problems connected with food have been resolved by this age, and children enjoy eating to alleviate hunger and obtain social satisfaction.

School age children may participate in the school lunch program or bring a lunch from home. The National School Lunch Program (NSLP), established in 1946, is administered by the

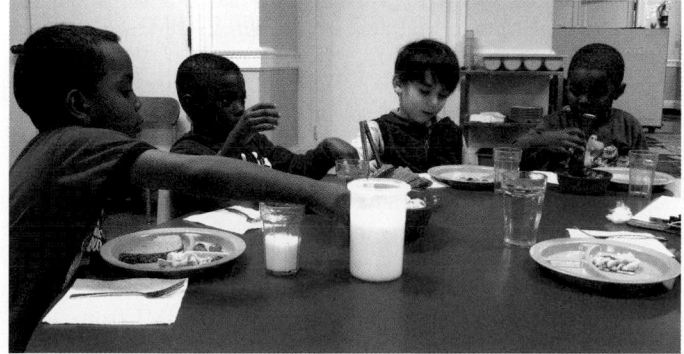

FIGURE 17-5 Children who eat with each other in an appropriate environment often eat more nutritiously and try a wider variety of foods than when eating alone or at home. (Courtesy of Ana Raab.)

USDA. Children from low-income families are eligible for free or reduced-price meals. In addition, the School Breakfast Program (SBP), begun in 1966, is offered in approximately 85% of the public schools that participate in the lunch program. The USDA also offers the Afterschool Snacks and Summer Food Service for organized programs, the Fresh Fruit and Vegetable Program in selected schools, and the Special Milk program for children not participating in school lunch (see Chapter 9).

Guidelines for the meals provided by the NSLP and SBP are based on the Institute of Medicine (IOM) report, School Meals, Building Blocks for Healthy Eating and legislated by the 2010 Healthy, Hunger-Free Kids Act (IOM, 2009; McGuire, 2009). In addition to guidelines to align meals patterns with the Dietary Guidelines and to address other childhood health concerns, the Act makes resources and technical assistance available. Nutrition standards for the NSLP and SBP that follow the IOM recommendations and made significant changes to meal patterns were published in 2012 (Food and Nutrition Service, 2012).

Efforts have been made to decrease food waste by altering menus to accommodate student preferences, allowing students to decline one or two menu items and offering salad bars. Efforts to increase participation in school lunch require consistent messages that support healthful eating.

School wellness policies were required by the school year 2006 to 2007 in institutions participating in school lunch and school breakfast programs. The school, including the administration, teachers, students, and food service personnel, in cooperation with families and the community, are encouraged to work together to support nutrition integrity in the educational setting (Bergman et al, 2010).

Consumption of school meals also is affected by the daily school schedule and the amount of time allotted for children to eat. When recess is scheduled before lunch rather than after, intake is better. A Montana "Recess Before Lunch" pilot study documented improvement in the mealtime atmosphere and students' behavior. Discipline problems on the playground, in the lunchroom, and in the classroom decreased (Montana Office of Public Instruction, 2010).

Children who require a special diet because of certain medical conditions such as diabetes, celiac disease, or documented food allergy are eligible for modified school meals. Children with developmental disabilities are eligible to attend public school from ages 3 to 21 years, and some of them need modified school meals (e.g., meals that are texture modified, or with increased or decreased energy density). To receive modified meals, families must submit written documentation by a medical professional of the diagnosis, meal modification, and rationale. For children receiving special education services, the documentation for meals and feeding can be incorporated as objectives in a child's individual education plan (IEP) (see Chapter 44).

Studies of lunches packed at home indicate that they usually provide fewer nutrients but less fat than school lunch meals. Favorite foods tend to be packed, so children have less variety. Food choices are limited to those that travel well and require no heating or refrigeration. A typical well-balanced lunch brought from home could include a sandwich with whole-grain bread and a protein-rich filling; fresh vegetables, fruit, or both; low-fat milk; and possibly a cookie, a graham cracker, or another simple dessert. Food safety measures (e.g., keeping perishable foods well chilled) must be observed when packing lunches for school.

Today many school age children are responsible for preparing their own breakfasts. It is not uncommon for children to skip this meal altogether, even children in the primary grades. Children who skip breakfast tend to consume less energy and other nutrients than those who eat breakfast (Wilson et al, 2006). Reviews of the effects of breakfast on cognition and school performance indicate a positive association between breakfast and school performance (Adolphus et al, 2013) (see *Focus On:* Breakfast: Does It Affect Learning?).

◎ FOCUS ON

Breakfast: Does It Affect Learning?

The educational benefits of school meal programs and especially the role of breakfast in better school performance have been debated and discussed for decades. Overall, breakfast consumption has been associated with better on-task classroom behavior (i.e., attention in class, and engagement in learning activities) regardless of nutritional and/or socioeconomic status. A literature review indicates associations between school performance and breakfast consumption, especially among children who were at nutritional risk (i.e., had wasted and stunted growth) and or were from low socioeconomic backgrounds (Adolphus et al, 2013). School-based breakfast experiments in 9- to 11-year-old and 6- to 8-year-old children found similar positive results with breakfast consumption (i.e., enhanced short-term memory, better spatial memory, and improved processing of complex visual stimuli), but other reports are less supportive (Adolphus et al, 2013). These studies suggest that brain functioning is sensitive to short-term variations in nutrient availability. A short fast may impose greater stress on young children than on adults, resulting in metabolic alterations as various homeostatic mechanisms work to maintain circulating glucose concentrations.

In addition to potential positive effects on academic performance, breakfast contributes significantly to the child's overall nutrient intake. These studies underscore the potential benefits—not only for low-income and at-risk children but also for all school children—of a breakfast at home or school meal programs that include breakfast. In the 2012 to 2013 school year, 10.8 million low-income children, or 51.9%, participated in a school breakfast program on an average day (FRAC, 2014). This is an increase from about 42 out of 100 children in 2002 to 2003.

Snacks are commonly eaten by school age children, primarily after school and in the evening. As children grow older and have money to spend, they tend to consume more snacks from vending machines, fast-food restaurants, and neighborhood grocery stores. Families should continue to offer wholesome snacks at home and support nutrition education efforts in the school. In most cases, good eating habits established in the first few years help children through this period of decision making and responsibility. Developing and supporting programs and policies that ensure access to better-quality food, larger quantities of food, and better living conditions for low-income children help to reduce health disparities where present.

Nutrition Education

As children grow, they acquire knowledge and assimilate concepts. The early years are ideal for providing nutrition information and promoting positive attitudes about all foods. This education can be informal and take place in the home with parents as models and a diet with a wide variety of foods. Food can be used in daily experiences for the toddler and preschooler and to promote the development of language, cognition, and self-help behaviors (i.e., labeling; describing size, shape, and color; sorting; assisting in preparation; and tasting).

More formal nutrition education is provided in preschools, Head Start programs, and public schools. Some programs such as Head Start have federal guidance and standards that incorporate healthy eating and nutrition education for the families involved. Nutrition education in schools is less standard and frequently has minimum or no requirements for inclusion in the curriculum or the training of teachers. Recommendations include policies in schools promoting coordination between nutrition education; access to and promotion of child nutrition programs; and cooperation with families, the community, and health services (Bergman et al, 2010).

Teachers attempting to teach children nutrition concepts and information should take into account the children's developmental level. The play approach, based on Piaget's theory of learning, is one method for teaching nutrition and fitness to school age children. Activities and information that focus on real-world relationships with food are most likely to have positive results. Meals, snacks, and food preparation activities provide children opportunities to practice and reinforce their nutrition knowledge and demonstrate their cognitive understanding. Involving parents in nutrition education projects can produce positive outcomes that are also beneficial in the home. Many written and electronic resources on nutrition education for children exist, such as at the National Center for Education in Maternal and Child Health.

NUTRITIONAL CONCERNS

Overweight and Obesity

Overweight and obesity among children is a significant public health problem. The prevalence of obesity and overweight increased rapidly in the 1990s and 2000s, plateaued between 2007 to 2008 and 2009 to 2010 and may be decreasing during the first part of the 2010 decade. Obesity rates in some populations, for example Hispanic and non-Hispanic white children and adolescents, are continuing to increase.

The most recent NHANES (2011 to 2012) reported an obesity (BMI-for-age above the 95th percentile) prevalence of 16.9% in children ages 2 to 19 years, and high BMI (BMI-for-age above the 85th percentile) prevalence of 31.8%, relatively unchanged from rates in 2003 to 2004. For children 2 to 5 years of age, the prevalence of obesity decreased from 14% in 2003 to 2004 to 8.4 in 2011 to 2012 (Ogden et al, 2012).

The Expert Committee report suggests the following terms to describe risk based on BMI: *obesity* as BMI-for-age at or above the 95th percentile and *overweight* as BMI-for-age between the 85th and 94th percentiles (Barlow and Committee, 2007). Determining whether growing children are obese is difficult. Some excess weight may be gained at either end of the childhood spectrum; the 1-year-old toddler and the prepubescent child may weigh more for developmental and physiologic reasons, but this extra weight is often not permanent. BMI, a useful clinical tool for screening for overweight, has limitations in determining obesity because of variability related to sex, race, body composition, and maturation stage.

The CDC growth charts allow tracking of BMI from age 2 into adulthood; thus children can be monitored periodically, and intervention provided when the rate of BMI change is excessive. The BMI charts show the **adiposity rebound**, which normally occurs in children between 4 and 6 years of age (see Appendices 12 and 16). Children whose adiposity rebound occurs before 5½ years of age are more likely to weigh more as adults than those whose adiposity rebound occurs after 7 years of age. The timing of the adiposity rebound and excess fatness in adolescence are two critical factors in the development of obesity in childhood, with the latter being the most predictive of adult obesity and related morbidity (Williams and Goulding, 2009).

Although genetic predisposition is an important factor in obesity development, the increases in the prevalence of overweight children cannot be explained by genetics alone. Factors contributing to excess energy intake for the pediatric population include ready access to eating and food establishments, eating tied to sedentary leisure activities, children making more food and eating decisions, larger portion sizes, and decreased physical activity. In addition, American children snack three times a day, with chips, candy, and other low-nutrient foods providing more than 27% of their daily energy intake; this contributes 168 kcal per day (Piernas and Popkin, 2010).

Inactivity plays a major role in obesity development, whether it results from screen time, limited opportunities for physical activity, or safety concerns that prevent children from enjoying free play outdoors. Although increased television viewing and computer and handheld game use have been associated with childhood overweight, a review suggests that the greater risk of overweight is related to television viewing plus a low activity level (Ritchie et al, 2005). The need to use automobiles for short trips limits children's opportunities to walk to local destinations, a phenomenon particularly relevant to children in the suburbs.

Obesity in childhood is not a benign condition, despite the popular belief that overweight children will outgrow their condition. The longer a child has been overweight, the more likely the child is to be overweight or obese during adolescence and adulthood. Consequences of overweight in childhood include psychosocial difficulties such as discrimination, a negative self-image, depression, and decreased socialization. Many overweight children have one or more cardiovascular risk factors such as hyperlipidemia, hypertension, or hyperinsulinemia (Daniels, 2009). An even more dramatic health consequence of overweight is the rapid increase in the incidence of type 2 diabetes in children and adolescents, which has a serious effect on adult health, development of other chronic diseases, and health care costs (see Chapter 30).

The AAP has developed guidelines for overweight screening and assessment for children from age 2 through adolescence (Barlow and Committee, 2007). In addition to growth parameters, other important information includes dietary intake and patterns, previous growth patterns, family history, physical activity, and family interactions. The U.S. Preventive Services Task Force (USPSTF) recommends obesity screening for 6- to 18-year-olds and referral to treatment programs, if appropriate (USPSTF, 2010).

A 2010 paper described a lower prevalence of obesity among children who were exposed to the following routines: regularly eating the evening meal as a family, obtaining adequate nighttime sleep, and having limited screen-viewing time (Anderson and Whitaker, 2010). Interventions for obesity in children have had limited effect on the childhood obesity problem, especially for black, Hispanic, and Native American populations. Success is most likely to result from programs that include comprehensive behavioral components such as family involvement, dietary modifications, nutrition information, physical activity, and behavioral strategies (Barlow and Committee, 2007). Incorporating behavioral intervention in obesity treatment improves outcomes and is most effective with a team approach. Depending on the child, goals for weight change may include a decrease in the rate of weight gain, maintenance of weight, or, in severe cases, gradual weight loss (see Chapter 21). An individualized approach should be tailored to each child, with minimum use of highly restrictive diets or medication, except if there are other significant diseases and no other options.

Intervention strategies require family involvement and support. Incorporating motivational interviewing and stages of change theory into the comprehensive program will likely be more successful (see Chapter 14). Changes to address overweight should include the child's input, with choices and plans that modify the family's food and activity environment, not just the child's. Adequate energy and other nutrients are needed to ensure maintenance of height gain velocity and nutrient stores. The hazards of treating overweight children too aggressively include alternate periods of undereating and overeating, feelings of failure in meeting external expectations, ignoring internal cues for appetite and satiation, feelings of deprivation and isolation, an increased risk for eating disorders, and a poor or an increasingly poor self-image.

Some children with special health care needs, such as those with Down syndrome, Prader-Willi syndrome, short stature, and limited mobility, are at increased risk for being overweight. Their size, level of activity, and developmental status must be considered when estimating energy intake and providing dietary guidance to their families (see Chapter 44).

Prevention of childhood obesity is an important public health priority in the United States. The Institute of Medicine (IOM) has published recommendations that target families, health care professionals, industry, schools, and communities (IOM, 2012). The recommendations include schools (improved nutritional quality of food sold and served, increased physical activity, wellness education), industry (improved nutrition information for consumers, clear media messages), health care professionals (tracking BMI, providing counseling for children and families), and communities and government (better access to healthy foods, improved physical activity opportunities). Schools are a natural environment for obesity prevention, which can include nutrition and health curricula, opportunities for physical education and activity, and appropriate school meals. Efforts have resulted in school nutrition policies that limit the kinds of products sold in vending machines and food and beverages sold for fundraising. Cross-sectional data indicate that policies that limit the sale of competitive foods and beverages (foods sold outside the school meal programs) are associated with changes in consumption and availability of foods. More research is needed to understand long-term health effects of these policies (Chriqui et al, 2014). More research also is needed to develop effective prevention strategies that address the needs of diverse populations.

Families are essential for modeling food choices, healthy eating, and leisure activities for their children. Parents influence children's environment by choosing nutrient-rich foods, having family meals (including breakfast), offering regular snacks, and spending time together in physical activity, all of which can be critical in overweight prevention. Reducing sedentary behaviors can increase energy expenditure and reduce prompts to eat; the AAP recommends limiting television and video time to no more than 2 hours per day (Krebs and Jacobson, 2003). Parents exerting too much control over their child's food intake or promoting a restrictive diet may cause children to be less able to self-regulate and more likely to overeat when the opportunity is available (Ritchie et al, 2005). Health professionals should support positive parenting within the child's developmental level.

Underweight and Failure to Thrive

Weight loss, lack of weight gain, or failure to thrive (FTT) can be caused by an acute or chronic illness, a restricted diet, a poor appetite (resulting from constipation, medication, or other issues), feeding problems, neglect, or a simple lack of food. Some experts prefer the terms pediatric undernutrition or growth deficiency. Infants and toddlers are most at risk for poor growth, often as a result of prematurity, medical conditions, developmental delays, inadequate parenting, or a combination of these. Dietary practices also can contribute to poor growth, including food restrictions in preschool children stemming from parents' concerns about obesity, atherosclerosis, or other potential health problems.

A careful assessment is critical and must include the social and emotional environment of the child and any physical findings. If neglect is documented to be a contributing factor, health professionals are obligated to report the case to the local child protective services. Because of the complexity of growth failure, an interdisciplinary team is ideal for assessments and interventions.

The provision of adequate energy and other nutrients and nutrition education should be one part of an overall interdisciplinary plan to assist children and their families. Attempts should be made to increase children's appetites and modify the environment to ensure optimal intake. Frequent small meals and snacks should be offered at regular times, using developmentally appropriate, nutrient-dense foods. This optimizes the smaller stomach capacity of the young child and provides structure and predictability for the eating environment. Families should receive support for positive parent-child interactions, with respect for the division of responsibility in feeding and avoidance of any pressure or coercion on the child's eating. Severe malnutrition may require carefully planned interventions and close monitoring to prevent refeeding syndrome.

Chronic constipation can result in poor appetite, diminished intake, and FTT. Ensuring adequate fluid and fiber intake can help relieve constipation, improve appetite, and eventually promote weight gain. Because the fiber intake of children is often low, especially in children who are picky eaters, fiber intake always should be addressed in the evaluation. Fiber can be increased by adding legumes, fruits (especially dried fruits), vegetables, high-fiber breakfast cereals, bran muffins, or all of these to the diet.

Iron Deficiency

Iron deficiency is one of the most common nutrient disorders of childhood. The highest prevalence of anemia in children occurs in those younger than 2 years of age. Iron deficiency is less of a problem among older preschool and school age children.

Infants with iron deficiency, with or without anemia, tend to score lower on standardized tests of mental development and pay less attention to relevant information needed for problem solving. Poorer cognitive performance and delayed psychomotor development have been reported in infants and preschool children with iron deficiency. Deficiency can have long-term consequences, as demonstrated by poorer performance on developmental tests in late childhood and early adolescence (Lozoff et al, 2007). Iron intake should be considered during assessments of

individual diets and in policy decisions intended to address the nutrition needs of low-income, high-risk children.

In addition to growth and the increased physiologic need for iron, dietary factors also play a role. For example, a 1-year-old child who continues to consume a large quantity of milk and excludes other foods may develop anemia. Some young preschool children do not eat much meat, so most of their iron is consumed in the nonheme form from fortified cereals, which is absorbed less efficiently (see Chapter 32).

Dental Caries

Nutrition and eating habits are important factors affecting oral health. An optimal nutrient intake is needed to produce strong teeth and healthy gums. The composition of the diet and an individual's eating habits (e.g., dietary carbohydrate intake, eating frequency) are significant factors in the development of dental caries (see Chapter 25).

Allergies

Food allergies during infancy and childhood are more likely when a child has a family history of allergies. Allergic symptoms are seen most often as respiratory or gastrointestinal responses as well as skin responses but may include fatigue, lethargy, and behavior changes. There can be confusion about over the definitions of *food allergy, food intolerance,* and *food sensitivity,* and some tests for food allergies are unspecific and equivocal. See Chapter 26 for management of food allergies in children.

Attention Deficit Hyperactivity Disorder

ADHD is one of the most common disorders of childhood. It usually is diagnosed first in childhood and often lasts into adulthood. ADHD is defined by academic or behavioral problems and symptoms of inattention, hyperactivity, or impulsivity that are inappropriate for a child's developmental level. The diagnosis is based on information about the child's behavior at home, school, and other settings. Various dietary factors have been suggested as a cause of this disorder, including artificial flavors and colors, sugar, altered fatty acid metabolism, and allergies. Several studies have suggested that artificial food colors and a food preservative, sodium benzoate, were associated with some negative behaviors in both those children with a diagnosis of ADHD and some children who did not have this diagnosis. However, for a complete answer, more evidence is needed (Bateman, 2004; McCann, et al, 2007). Research looking at the effects of artificial food colors and sodium benzoate, exposure to pesticides, and fatty acid supplementation are ongoing (Rytter et al, 2015). Sugar shows no effect on behavior or cognition in most children with ADHD. See Chapter 44 for further discussion of ADHD.

Autism Spectrum Disorder

Autism spectrum disorder (ASD) affects 1 in 68 children. All children should receive developmental screening in early childhood during routine well child visits and specifically at 18 and 24 months of age. If significant delays or concerns are noted in social interaction, communication, and behavior a more comprehensive diagnostic evaluation is needed (see Chapter 44).

These concerns can affect nutrient intake and eating behaviors if a child accepts only specific foods, refuses new or unfamiliar foods, or has increased hypersensitivities (e.g., to texture, temperature, color, and smell) or difficulty making transitions. Children with ASD often refuse fruits and vegetables and may eat only a few foods from the other food groups. Although most children have normal growth parameters, their restricted diets make them at risk for marginal or inadequate nutrient intake. They may be resistant to taking a vitamin-mineral supplement, even though they could benefit from one.

Popular nutrition advice for children with ASD includes elimination diets (e.g., gluten-free or casein-free), essential fatty acid supplements, large doses of vitamins, and other alternative therapies. Despite anecdotal reports of benefits, few well-designed controlled studies have been done to test the effectiveness of these interventions, and currently there is no strong evidence of benefits (Dosman et al, 2013). Behavioral nutrition interventions may increase the types of food accepted at home and school. If families want to try alternative dietary therapies, nutrition professionals can help them ensure that the child's diet is adequate and any supplements are safe (see Chapter 12).

PREVENTING CHRONIC DISEASE

The roots of chronic adult diseases such as heart disease, cancer, diabetes, and obesity are often based in childhood—a phenomenon that is particularly relevant to the increasing rate of obesity-related diseases such as type 2 diabetes. To help decrease the prevalence of chronic conditions in Americans, government and nonprofit agencies have been promoting healthy eating habits for children. Their recommendations include the Dietary Guidelines for Americans, the USDA MyPlate, the National Cholesterol Education Program (NCEP), and the National Cancer Institute Dietary Guidelines (see Chapter 11).

Cardiovascular Health

Compared with their counterparts in many other countries, American children and adolescents have higher blood cholesterol levels and higher intakes of saturated fatty acids and cholesterol. Early coronary atherosclerosis begins in childhood and adolescence. Risk factors include family history, breastfeeding and perinatal factors, nutrition and diet, physical activity, tobacco exposure, hypertension, hyper- and dyslipidemia, overweight and obesity, and diabetes. These were explored by an expert panel (National Heart Lung and Blood Institute, 2011); selected recommendations with nutrition implications are briefly summarized as follows:

For most healthy children limiting total fat to 30% of total energy, saturated fat to 7% to 10%, and dietary cholesterol to 300 mg/day is recommended. Use of fat-free milk is appropriate for most children ages 2 years and older. A balanced energy intake, increased intake of fruits and vegetables, and limiting "extra calories" to 5% to 15% total intake also is recommended for most children. Fiber intake of at least "age + 5 grams" (e.g., for a 4-year-old, 4 + 5 = 9 g per day) or 14 g fiber/1000 kilocalories is suggested.

For children with dyslipidemia, who are overweight or obese, or who have "risk factor clustering" or high-risk medical conditions, the Expert Panel recommends consideration of the Cardiovascular Health Integrated Lifestyle Diet (CHILD-1) as the first stage in dietary change (National Heart Lung and Blood Institute, 2012). This is a DASH-style pattern with emphasis on fat-free/low-fat dairy and increased intake of fruits and vegetables.

For all children, the approach to modifying risk factors, especially related to dietary fat intake, should be individualized (see Chapter 33).

Calcium and Bone Health

Osteoporosis prevention begins early by maximizing calcium retention and bone density during childhood and adolescence, when bones are growing rapidly and are most sensitive to diet and the important effects of physical activity (see Chapter 24). However, mean dietary intakes of calcium are lower than the AI, with 20% to 30% of pubertal girls having intakes less than 500 mg/day. One longitudinal study of white children from infancy to 8 years of age found that bone mineral content was positively correlated with intake of protein and several minerals, suggesting that many nutrients are related to bone health in children (Bounds et al, 2005). Because food consumption surveys show that children are drinking more soft drinks and noncitrus juices and less milk, education is needed to encourage young people to consume an appropriate amount of calcium from food sources and possibly supplements (see Appendix 46).

Fiber

Education about dietary fiber and disease prevention has mainly been focused on adults, and only limited information is available on the dietary fiber intake of children. Dietary fiber is needed for health and normal laxation in children. National survey data indicate that preschool children consume a mean of 11 to 12 g/day of dietary fiber; school age children consume approximately 13 to 14 g/day (U.S. Department of Agriculture, 2012). This is lower than the DRI for children, which is based on the same 14 g/1000 kcal as adults because of lack of scientific evidence for the pediatric population (Otten et al, 2006). Generally, higher fiber intakes are associated with more nutrient-dense diets in young children (Kranz et al, 2012).

The Gut Microbiome

The gut microbiome is an emerging topic in nutrition, including pediatric nutrition. It is clear that dietary and other factors affect the number and type of bacteria that colonize the gut. Factors that can affect the gut microbial community include dietary fiber, prebiotics, probiotics, and the use of antibiotic medication (see Chapter 1).

The gut bacteria profile seems to be associated with short- and long-term health outcomes. In addition to effects on GI disorders, research continues to explore the relationship between the gut microbiome and short- and long-term health outcomes, including obesity, inflammation, and cancers (Peregrin, 2013).

Physical Activity

A decreased level of physical activity in children has been noted for several decades. Participation in school physical education programs has declined over time and generally decreases with increasing age. Regular physical activity not only helps control excess weight gain but also improves strength and endurance, enhances self-esteem, and reduces anxiety and stress. Activity, combined with an optimal calcium intake, is associated with increased bone mineral density in children and adolescents. Current physical activity recommendations for those ages 6 through 17 years of age are 60 minutes or more of physical activity every day with the majority at a moderate or vigorous aerobic intensity. Children and adolescents should do vigorous intensity activity at least 3 days per week and include muscle-strengthening and bone-strengthening activity on at least 3 days per week. Information regarding activities that will meet these recommendations and are appropriate for children is available (U.S. Department of Health and Human Services, 2008). Screen time (active games, exercise or dance videos, or TV exercise programs) can be a beneficial source of activity for youth. Three in 10 youth ages 9 to 18 engaged in at least 1 hour of active screen time weekdays, and 4 in 10 youth did the same on weekends (Wethington et al, 2013). MyPlate's *Eat Smart to Play Hard* materials promote the recommendation for 60 minutes of physical activity each day (Figure 17-6). The Dietary Guidelines for Americans and MyPlate also have been applied to children and their parents (www.chooseMyPlate.gov/kids).

CLINICAL CASE STUDY

Brian is a 7-year, 4-month-old male who gained 15 pounds during the past school year. His height is 50½ inches, and his weight is 75 pounds. Brian moved to a new home and began a new school a year ago after his parents' divorce. After-school care has been provided by a retired neighbor, who loves to bake for Brian. He has few friends in the neighborhood, and his main leisure activities have been watching television and playing video games. When he gets bored, he often looks for a snack. His mother reports that they often rely on take-out and fast-food meals because of the time constraints of her full-time job, and she has gained weight herself. She recently started an aerobics class with a friend and is interested in developing healthier eating habits for herself and Brian.

After joint sessions with Brian and his mother, the following goals were identified by the family: (1) explore after-school care at the local community center, which has a physical activity component; (2) alter grocery and menu selection to emphasize the MyPlate and low-fat choices while still meeting the family's time and resource constraints; (3) begin to incorporate physical activities (Brian identified swimming and bicycling as things he would like to do) on the weekends; and (4) limit television and video games to no more than 2 hours daily.

After 4 months, Brian has enrolled in the local community center's afterschool program and participates in organized soccer and "pick-up" basketball. Weekends are a challenge. Brian and his mother have not yet incorporated physical activity into their weekend routine, and Brian finds it tough to limit screen time to 2 hours on the weekends. Brian has lost 4 pounds and is taller; he is 51 inches tall and weighs 66 pounds.

Nutrition Diagnostic Statement

Overweight/obesity as evidenced by BMI-for-age above the 95th percentile or more related to infrequent physical inactivity, large amounts of sedentary activity, and estimated excessive energy intake.

Nutrition Care Questions

1. Calculate and plot Brian's BMI over time. Discuss the changes.
2. What recommendations should be made to prevent Brian and his mother from resuming their old habits?
3. What other activities can Brian try to help him avoid or reduce the tendency to eat when he is not hungry?
4. What would you suggest to promote a positive feeding relationship between Brian and his mother, considering his age and level of development?
5. What recommendations can you make to decrease Brian's energy intake and make it more consistent with MyPlate recommendations? Consider ideas to alter Brian's favorite recipes (e.g., his favorite meal is fried chicken with gravy, mashed potatoes, and ice cream), select healthy options from take-out or fast-food options, and modifications to snack options.
6. Are there any nutrient-related concerns because Brian's diet is being altered to help with weight management? Or because of his age? Or other factors?

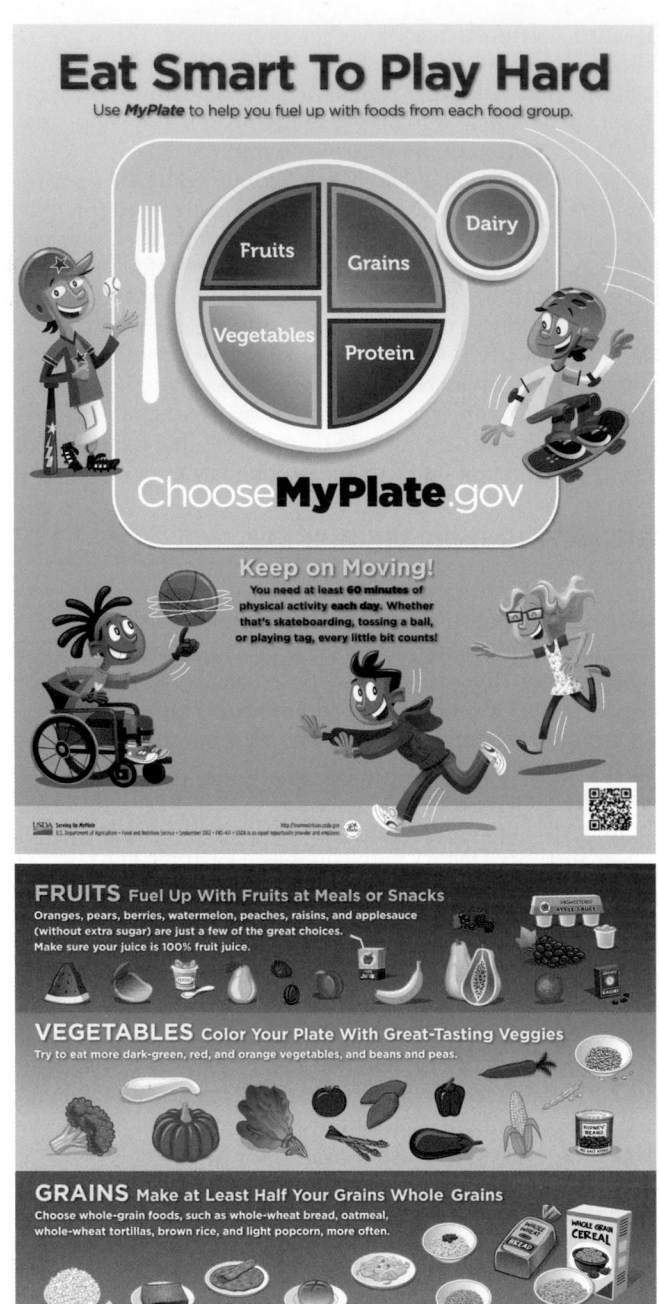

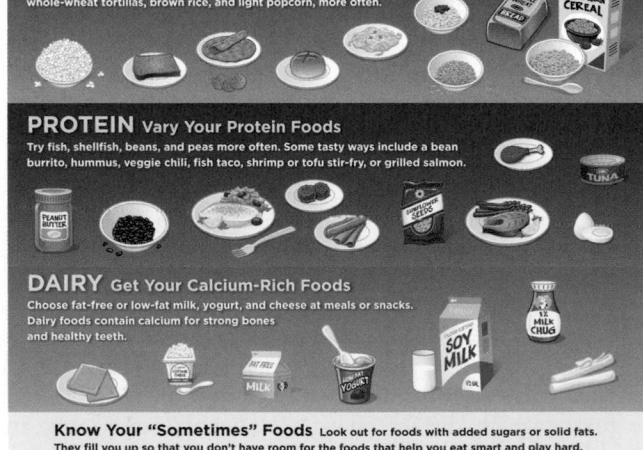

FIGURE 17-6 Eat smart to play hard. (From United States Department of Agriculture: *Eat Smart to Play Hard* (website): http://www.fns.usda.gov/sites/default/files/eatsmartminiposter.pdf, 2012. Accessed December 2014.)

USEFUL WEBSITES

Bright Futures in Practice: Nutrition
www.brightfutures.org/nutrition/
Growth Charts
www.cdc.gov/growthcharts/
Guidelines for Physical Activity
www.health.gov/paguidelines/guidelines
MyPlate Food Guidance System
www.chooseMyPlate.gov
National Center for Education in Maternal and Child Health
www.ncemch.org

The National Center for Education in Maternal and Child Health's MCH Library
www.mchlibrary.info/KnowledgePaths/kp_childnutr.html
Nutrition and Physical Activity
www.cdc.gov/nccdphp/dnpa/
Pediatric Nutrition Practice Group—Academy of Nutrition and Dietetics
www.pnpg.org/
USDA Food and Nutrition Service—School Meals
www.fns.usda.gov/cnd

REFERENCES

Adolphus K, Lawton CL, Dye L: The effects of breakfast on behavior and academic performance in children and adolescents, *Front Hum Neurosci* 7:425, 2013.

American Academy of Pediatrics: *Pediatric nutrition*, ed 7, Elk Grove, Ill, 2014, American Academy of Pediatrics.

Anderson SE, Whitaker RC: Household routines and obesity in US preschool-aged children, *Pediatrics* 125:420, 2010.

Bailey RL, Fulgoni VL III, Keast DR, et al: Do dietary supplements improve micronutrient sufficiency in children and adolescents? *J Pediatr* 161: 837, 2012.

Bailey RL, Dodd KW, Goldman JA, et al: Estimation of total usual calcium and vitamin D intakes in the United States, *J Nutr* 140:817, 2010.

Barlow SE, Committee E: Expert committee recommendations regarding the prevention, assessment, and treatment of child and adolescent overweight and obesity: summary report, *Pediatrics* 120(Suppl 4):S164, 2007.

Bateman B, Warner JO, Hutchinson E, et al: The effects of a double blind, placebo controlled, artificial food colourings and benzoate preservative challenge on hyperactivity in a general population sample of preschool children, *Arch Dis Child* 89:506, 2004.

Benjamin Neelon SE, Briley ME, American Dietetic Association: Position of the American Dietetic Association: benchmarks for nutrition in child care, *J Am Diet Assoc* 111:607, 2011.

Bergman EA, Gordon RW, American Dietetic Association: Position of the American Dietetic Association: local support for nutrition integrity in schools, *J Am Diet Assoc* 110:1244, 2010.

Bounds W, Skinner J, Carruth BR, et al: The relationship of dietary and life-style factors to bone mineral indexes in children, *J Am Diet Assoc* 105: 735, 2005.

Butte NF, Fox MK, Briefel RR, et al: Nutrient intakes of US infants, toddlers, and preschoolers meet or exceed dietary reference intakes, *J Am Diet Assoc* 110(Suppl 12):S27, 2010.

Chan JC, Sobal J: Family meals and body weight. Analysis of multiple family members in family units, *Appetite* 57:517, 2011.

Chriqui JF, Pickel M, Story M: Influence of school competitive food and beverage policies on obesity, consumption, and availability: a systematic review, *JAMA Pediatr* 168:279, 2014.

Coleman-Jensen A, Nord M, Singh A: *Household Food Security in the United States in 2012, ERR-155*, Washington, DC, 2013, US Department of Agriculture, Economic Research Service.

Committee on Accelerating Progress in Obesity Prevention; Food and Nutrition Board; Institute of Medicine: *Accelerating Progress in Obesity Prevention: Solving the Weight of the Nation*, 2012, National Academies Press.

Committee on Nutrition, American Academy of Pediatrics: The use and misuse of fruit juice in pediatrics, *Pediatrics* 107:1210, 2001.

Cook JT, Black M, Chilton M: Are food insecurity's health impacts underestimated in the U.S. population? Marginal food security also predicts adverse health outcomes in young U.S. children and mothers, *Adv Nutr* 4:51, 2013.

Daniels SR: Complications of obesity in children and adolescents, *Int J Obes (Lond)* 33(Suppl 1):S60, 2009.

Davis GC, You W: The Thrifty Food Plan is not thrifty when labor cost is considered, *J Nutr* 140:854, 2010.

DeNavas-Walt C, Proctor BD, Smith JC: *US Census Bureau, current population reports, P60 245, income, poverty, and health insurance coverage in the United States: 2012*, Washington, DC, 2013, US Government Printing Office.

Dosman C, Adams D, Wudel B, et al: Complementary, holistic, and integrative medicine: autism spectrum disorder and gluten-and casein-free diet, *Pediatr Rev* 34(10):e36, 2013.

Eneli IU, Crum PA, Tylka TL: The trust model: a different feeding paradigm for managing childhood obesity, *Obesity (Silver Spring)* 16:2197, 2008.

Expert Panel on Integrated Guidelines for Cardiovascular Health and Risk Reduction in Children and Adolescents, National Heart Lung and Blood Institute: Expert panel on integrated guidelines for cardiovascular health and risk reduction in children and adolescents: summary report, *Pediatrics* 128(Suppl 5):S213, 2011.

Falbe J, Rosner B, Willett WC, et al: Adiposity and different types of screen time, *Pediatrics* 132:e1497, 2013.

Food and Nutrition Service (FNS) USDA: Nutrition standards in the National School Lunch and School Breakfast Programs. Final rule, *Fed Regist* 77:4088, 2012.

Food Research and Action Center (FRAC): *School Breakfast Scorecard: 2012-2013 School Year*, 2014. http://frac.org/pdf/School_Breakfast_Scorecard_SY_2012_2013.pdf. Accessed December 2014.

Ghimire N, Rao A: Comparative evaluation of the influence of television advertisements on children and caries prevalence, *Glob Health Action* 6:20066, 2013.

Gilbert-Diamond D, Adachi-Mejia AM, McClure AC, et al: Association of a television in the bedroom with increased adiposity gain in a nationally representative sample of children and adolescents, *JAMA Pediatr* 168: 427, 2014.

Glickman D: *Accelerating progress in obesity prevention: solving the weight of the nation*, Washington, DC, 2012, National Academies Press.

Jenkin G, Madhvani N, Signal L, et al: A systematic review of persuasive marketing techniques to promote food to children on television, *Obes Rev* 15:281, 2014.

Keller KL, Kirzner J, Pietrobelli A, et al: Increased sweetened beverage intake is associated with reduced milk and calcium intake in 3- to 7-year-old children at multi-item laboratory lunches, *J Am Diet Assoc* 109:497, 2009.

Kleinman RE, Murphy JM, Little M, et al: Hunger in children in the United States: potential behavioral and emotional correlates, *Pediatrics* 101:E3, 1998.

Kranz S, Brauchla M, Slavin JL, et al: What do we know about dietary fiber intake in children and health? The effects of fiber intake on constipation, obesity, and diabetes in children, *Adv Nutr* 3:47, 2012.

Krebs NF, Jacobson MS: American Academy of Pediatrics Committee on Nutrition. Prevention of pediatric overweight and obesity, *Pediatrics* 112:424, 2003.

Larson NI, Neumark-Sztainer D, Hannan PJ, et al: Family meals during adolescence are associated with higher diet quality and healthful meal patterns during young adulthood, *J Am Diet Assoc* 107:1502, 2007.

Lim S, Zoellner JM, Lee JM, et al: Obesity and sugar-sweetened beverages in African-American preschool children: a longitudinal study, *Obesity (Silver Spring)* 17:1262, 2009.

Lozoff B, Corapci F, Burden MJ, et al: Preschool-aged children with iron deficiency anemia show altered affect and behavior, *J Nutr* 137:683, 2007.

Madden MM, DeBias D, Cook GE, et al: Market analysis of vitamin supplementation in infants and children: evidence from the dietary supplement label database, *JAMA Pediatr* 168:291, 2014.

Mahaffey KR, Clickner RP, Jeffries RA, et al: Methylmercury and omega-3 fatty acids: co-occurrence of dietary sources with emphasis on fish and shellfish, *Environ Res* 107:20, 2008.

McCann D, Barrett A, Cooper A, et al: Food additives and hyperactive behavior in 3-year-old and 8/9-year-old children in the community: a randomized, double-blinded, placebo-controlled trials, *Lancet* 370:1560, 2007.

McGuire S: Institute of Medicine. 2009. School meals: building blocks for healthy children, Washington, DC: the National Academies Press, *Adv Nutr* 2:64, 2011.

Montana Office of Public Instruction: *The Montana Office of Public Instruction School Nutrition Pilot Project - A recess before lunch policy in four Montana schools*, 2010. http://opi.mt.gov/PDF/SchoolFood/RBL/RBLPilot.pdf. Accessed May 2010.

Moshfegh A, Goldman J, Cleveland L, et al: *What we eat in America, NHANES 2001-2002: usual nutrient intakes from food compared to dietary reference intakes*, Washington, DC, 2005, US Department of Agriculture, Agricultural Research Service.

Myers GJ, Thurston SW, Pearson AT, et al: Postnatal exposure to methyl mercury from fish consumption: a review and new data from the Seychelles Child Development Study, *Neurotoxicology* 30:338, 2009.

National Heart, Lung and Blood Institute (NHIBI): Expert panel on integrated guidelines for cardiovascular health and risk reduction in children and adolescents summary report, *Pediatrics* 128(Suppl 5):S213, 2012, NIH Publication number 12-7486A.

Nicklas TA, O'Neil CE, Kleinman R: Association between 100% juice consumption and nutrient intake and weight of children aged 2 to 11 years, *Arch Pediatr Adolesc Med* 162:557, 2008.

Nicklas TA, Hayes D, American Dietetic Association: Position of the American Dietetic Association: nutrition guidance for healthy children ages 2 to 11 years, *J Am Diet Assoc* 108:1038, 1046, 2008.

Ogden CL, Carroll MD, Kit BK, et al: Prevalence of obesity and trends in body mass index among US children and adolescents, 1999-2010, *JAMA* 307:483, 2012.

Oken E, Bellinger DC: Fish consumption, methylmercury and child neurodevelopment, *Curr Opin Pediatr* 20:178, 2008.

O'Neil CE, Nicklas TA, Liu Y, et al: Impact of dairy and sweetened beverage consumption on diet and weight of a multiethnic population of head start mothers, *J Am Diet Assoc* 109:874, 2009.

Otten JJ, Hellwig JP, Meyers LD, eds. *DRI, dietary reference intakes: the essential guide to nutrient requirements*, Washington, DC, 2006, National Academies Press.

Peregrin T: The inside tract: what RDs need to know about the gut microbiome, *J Acad Nutr Diet* 113:1019, 2013.

Picciano MF, Dwyer JT, Radimer KL, et al: Dietary supplement use among infants, children, and adolescents in the United States, 1999-2002, *Arch Pediatr Adolesc Med* 161:978, 2007.

Piernas C, Popkin BM: Trends in snacking among U.S. children, *Health Aff (Millwood)* 29(3):398, 2010.

Powell LM, Schermbeck RM, Chaloupka FJ: Nutritional content of food and beverage products in television advertisements seen on children's programming, *Child Obes* 9:524, 2013.

Powell LM, Schermbeck RM, Szczypka G, et al: Trends in the nutritional content of television food advertisements seen by children in the United States: analyses by age, food categories, and companies, *Arch Pediatr Adolesc Med* 165:1078, 2011.

Ritchie LD, Welk G, Styne D, et al: Family environment and pediatric overweight: what is a parent to do? *J Am Diet Assoc* 105(5 Suppl 1):S70, 2005.

Rose-Jacobs R, Black MM, Casey PH, et al: Household food insecurity: associations with at-risk infant and toddler development, *Pediatrics* 121:65, 2008.

Rovner AJ, O'Brien KO: Hypovitaminosis D among healthy children in the United States: a review of the current evidence, *Arch Pediatr Adolesc Med* 162:513, 2008.

Heilskov Rytter MJ, Andersen LB, Houmann T, et al: Diet in the treatment of ADHD in children – A systematic review of the literature, *Nord J Psychiatry* 69(1):1, 2015.

Ryu JH, Bartfeld JS: Household food insecurity during childhood and subsequent health status: the early childhood longitudinal study—kindergarten cohort, *Am J Public Health* 102(11):e50, 2012.

Satter E: *Child of mine: feeding with love and good sense*, Berkeley, 2000, Publishers Group West.

Savage JS, Fisher JO, Birch LL: Parental influence on eating behavior: conception to adolescence, *J Law Med Ethics* 35:22, 2007.

Stallings VA, Suitor CW, Taylor CL, editors; Committee on Nutrition Standards for National School Lunch and Breakfast Programs; Food and Nutrition Board; Institute of Medicine: *School Meals: Building Blocks for Healthy Children*, 2010, National Academies Press.

Stang J, Bayerl CT, American Dietetic Association: Position of the American Dietetic Association: child and adolescent nutrition assistance programs, *J Am Diet Assoc* 10:791, 2010.

Terry-McElrath YM, Turner L, Sandoval A, et al: Commercialism in US Elementary and Secondary School Nutrition Environments: trends from 2007 to 2012, *JAMA Pediatr* 168:234, 2014.

U.S. Department of Agriculture Agricultural Research Service: *Nutrient Intakes from Food: Mean Amounts Consumed per Individual, by Gender and Age, What We Eat in America, NHANES 2009-2010*, 2012. www.ars.usda.gov/ba/bhnrc/fsrg. Accessed January 2014.

U.S. Department of Health and Human Services (DHHS): *2008 physical activity guidelines for Americans*, 2008. http://www.health.gov/paguidelines/. Accessed December 2014.

U.S. Environmental Protection Agency (US EPA): *What You Need to Know About Mercury in Fish and Shellfish*, 2004. http://www.epa.gov/waterscience/fish/advice/index.html. Accessed December 2014.

U.S. Preventive Services Task Force: *Screening for obesity in children and adolescents*, Rockville, MD, 2010, Agency for Healthcare Research and Quality.

Wethington H, Sherry B, Park S, et al: Active screen time among US youth aged 9-18 years, 2009, *Games Health J* 2:362, 2013.

18

Nutrition in Adolescence

Nicole Larson, PhD, MPH, RDN, LD, Jamie S. Stang, PhD, MPH, RDN
and Tashara Leak, PhD, RDN

KEY TERMS

adolescence	menarche	sexual maturity rating (SMR)
body image	peak height gain velocity	Tanner staging
disordered eating	physiologic anemia of growth	thelarche
growth spurt	pubarche	
gynecologic age	puberty	

Adolescence is one of the most exciting yet challenging periods in human development. Generally thought of as the period of life that occurs between 12 and 21 years of age, adolescence is a period of tremendous physiologic, psychologic, and cognitive transformation during which a child becomes a young adult. The gradual growth pattern that characterizes early childhood changes to one of rapid growth and development, affecting physical and psychosocial aspects of health. Changes in cognitive and emotional functioning allow teens to become more independent as they mature. Peer influence and acceptance may become more important than family values, creating periods of conflict between teens and parents. Because all of these changes have a direct effect on the nutrient needs and dietary behaviors of adolescents, it is important that health care providers develop a full understanding of how these developmental changes of adolescence can affect nutritional status.

GROWTH AND DEVELOPMENT

Puberty is the period of rapid growth and development during which a child physically develops into an adult and becomes capable of reproduction. It is initiated by the increased production of reproductive hormones such as estrogen, progesterone, and testosterone and is characterized by the outward appearance of secondary sexual characteristics, such as breast development in females and the appearance of facial hair in males.

Psychologic Changes

Adolescence often is depicted as a time of irrational behavior. The physical growth of puberty transforms the teen body into an adult-like form, leading adults to believe that adolescent development is complete. However, the social and emotional development of adolescence lags behind. The mismatch between how teens look and how they act may lead adults to deduce that the adolescent is "not acting his or her age." The rebellion that is associated with the teen years is actually the manifestation of their search for independence and a sense of

autonomy. Food can be, and often is, used as a means of exerting autonomy. Adolescents may choose to become vegetarian as a way to differentiate themselves from their meat-eating parents or to express their moral and ethical concerns over animal welfare or the environment.

Cognitive and emotional development may vary greatly among adolescents, with some adolescents maturing faster than others. In general, adolescence is a time of impulsivity as a result of slow development in regions of the brain that govern cognitive control combined with a heightened reward response. Cognitive ability, including abstract reasoning, expands during adolescence; however, teens are more likely to base decisions on emotional as opposed to rational contexts (Blakemore and Robbins, 2012; Steinberg, 2010). Psychosocial development can affect health and nutritional status in many ways, including the following:

- Preoccupation with body size, body shape, and body image (the mental self-concept and perception of personal body size), resulting from the rapid growth and development that has occurred, may lead to dieting and possibly disordered eating behaviors
- Diminishing trust and respect for adults as authority figures, including nutrition and health professionals
- Strong influence of peers, especially around areas of body image and appearance, with the influence of a few select peers becoming more important than that of large groups as adulthood approaches
- More pronounced social, emotional, and financial independence, leading to increased independent decision making related to food and beverage intake
- Significant cognitive development as abstract reasoning is nearly complete and egocentrism decreases; however, teens may still revert to less complex thinking patterns when they are stressed
- Developed future orientation, which is required to understand the link between current behavior and chronic health risks

- Development of social, emotional, financial, and physical independence from family as teens leave home to attend college or seek employment
- Development of a core set of values and beliefs that guides moral, ethical, and health decisions

The psychosocial development of adolescents has a direct bearing on the foods and beverages they choose. Food choices are more likely to be based on taste, cost, and peer behaviors than on health benefits because these influences satisfy a teen's innate preference for immediate reward. Nutrition education and counseling methods that focus on how adolescents look, such as improving skin appearance or promoting hair growth, are most likely to be effective with young teens because these reinforce emotional influences.

Sexual Maturity

Sexual maturity rating (SMR), also known as Tanner staging, is used to assess clinically the degree of sexual maturation during puberty (Tanner, 1962). Among males, SMR is based on genital and pubic hair development (see Figure 18-1 and Table 18-1). Among females SMR is assessed by breast and pubic hair development. SMR is measured through a series of five stages, with stage 1 marking prepubertal development and stage 5 marking

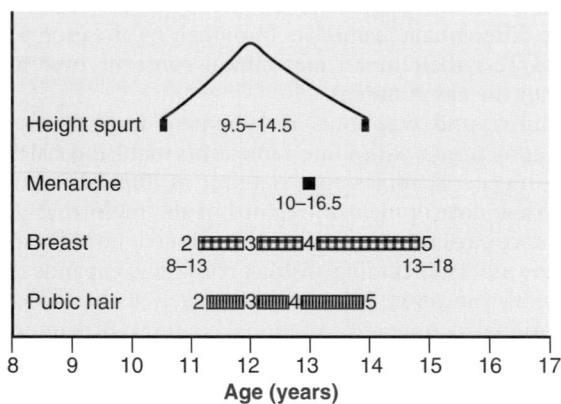

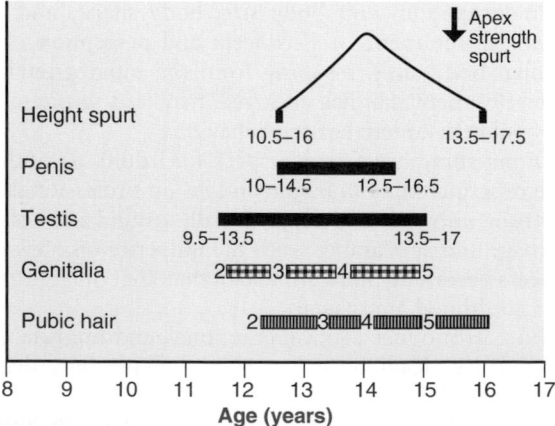

FIGURE 18-1 Sequence of events during puberty in females *(upper chart)* and males *(lower chart)*. Breast, genitalia, and pubic hair development are numbered 2 to 5 based on the Tanner developmental stages. (From Marshall WA, Tanner JM: Variations in the pattern of pubertal changes in males, *Arch Dis Child* 45:13, 1970.)

the completion of physical growth and development (see Appendix Tables 12 and 13). The five stages of SMR correlate with other markers of growth and development during puberty, such as alterations in height, weight, body composition, and endocrine functioning. A thorough understanding of the relationship between physical growth and development and SMR enables health care professionals to assess an adolescent's potential for future growth.

In general, females enter puberty earlier than males. An example of ethnic variation in female development is shown in data from the National Health and Nutrition Examination Study III (NHANES III). The data suggest that most non-Hispanic black and Mexican American females reach breast development stage 2 (thelarche) at 9.6 years of age, 8 months earlier than non-Hispanic white females (Rosenfield et al, 2009). Racial and ethnic differences in maturation are also seen for pubic hair stage 3 (pubarche), which occurs earlier among most non-Hispanic black females (10.6 years) compared with Mexican American and white females (11.6 years). Most females enter puberty at least 2.5 years earlier than their male counterparts, with Mexican American youth showing the greatest gender variance in age at pubarche (Rosenfield et al, 2009).

Data from NHANES III also suggest variation in the timing of pubarche among males of different racial and ethnic backgrounds (Rosenfield et al, 2009). The median age among non-Hispanic white and black males (12.3 and 12.5 years) is approximately 6 months earlier than among Mexican American males (13.2 years).

Adolescent females with a body mass index (BMI) in the 85th percentile or higher are four times more likely to have reached thelarche by age 8 and twice as likely by 9.6 years of age than normal weight females (Rosenfield et al, 2009). Excessive body weight plays a larger role in the timing and duration of puberty among females than among males (Pinkney et al, 2014).

Menarche, the onset of menses or menstruation, often is considered the hallmark of puberty among females (at 12.5 years in the average girl). However, the onset of menses can occur anywhere between the ages of 8 and 17 years (Tanner, 1962; Rosenfield et al, 2009). The median age of menarche is 12.1 years for black, 12.3 years for Mexican American, and 12.6 years for white females (Rosenfield et al, 2009).

Excessive body weight among females is associated with earlier onset of puberty and earlier menses among females of all racial and ethnic groups. Females with a BMI in the 85th percentile or higher are four times as likely to have experienced menses by 10.6 years of age. The timing of menarche increases micronutrient requirements among females; thus it is imperative that the timing of menarche be evaluated during a full nutrition assessment.

In summary, puberty may begin earlier but last longer for nonwhite females (Rosenfield et al, 2009). Although racial and ethnic differences in the age of pubarche occur among males, the differences are not as pronounced. No significant relationship between weight status and pubarche is observable among males.

Linear Growth

The velocity of physical growth during adolescence is much higher than that of early childhood (see Figure 18-2). On average, adolescents gain approximately 20% of their adult height during puberty. There is a great deal of variability in the timing

TABLE 18-1 Ratings of Sexual Maturation*

	Pubic Hair	Genitalia	Corresponding Changes
Males			
Stage 1	None	Prepubertal	
Stage 2	Small amount at outer edges of pubis, slight darkening	Beginning penile enlargement Testes enlarged to 5-ml volume Scrotum reddened and changed in texture	Increased sweat gland activity
Stage 3	Covers pubis	Penis longer Testes enlarged to 8-10 ml Scrotum enlarged	Voice changes Faint mustache and facial hair Axillary hair Beginning of peak height gain velocity (growth spurt of 6-8 inches)
Stage 4	Adult type, does not extend to thighs	Penis wider and longer Testes enlarged to 12 ml Scrotal skin darker	End of peak height gain velocity More facial hair Darker hair on legs Voice deeper Possibly severe acne
Stage 5	Adult type, spreads to thighs	Adult penis Testes enlarged to 15 ml	Significantly increased muscle mass
Females			
Stage 1	None	No change from childhood	
Stage 2	Small amount, downy, on medial labia	Breast buds	Increased sweat gland activity Beginning of peak height gain velocity (growth spurt of 3-5 inches)
Stage 3	Increased, darker, curly	Larger, but no separation of the nipple and the areola	End of peak height gain velocity Beginning of acne Axillary hair
Stage 4	More abundant, coarse texture	Larger Areola and nipple form secondary mound	Possibly severe acne Menarche begins
Stage 5	Adult, spreads to medial thighs	Adult distribution of breast tissue, continuous outline	Increased fat and muscle mass

Modified from Tanner JM: *Growth at adolescence,* ed 2, Oxford, 1962, Blackwell Scientific Publications.
*See Appendixes 12 and 13.

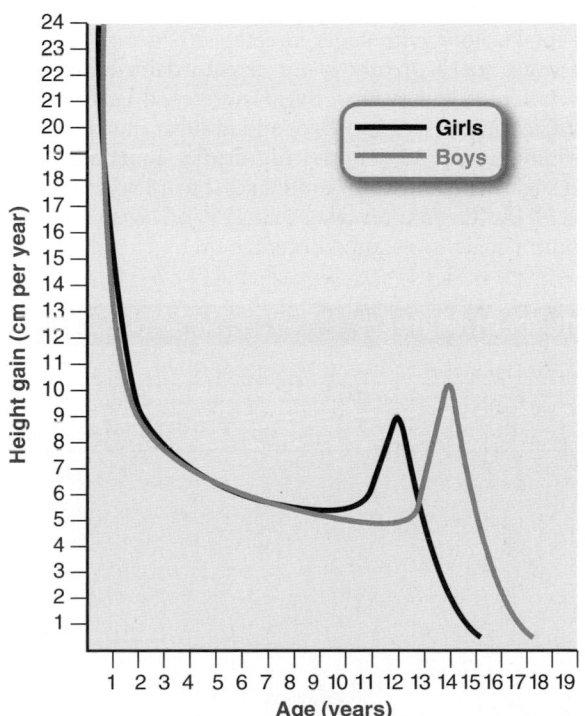

FIGURE 18-2 Typical individual velocity curves for supine length or height in males and females. Curves represent the growth velocity of the typical boy and girl at any given age.

and duration of growth among adolescents as illustrated in Figure 18-3 by a group of 13-year-old males.

Linear growth occurs throughout the 4 to 7 years of pubertal development in most teens; however, the largest percentage of height is gained during an 18- to 24-month period commonly referred to as the **growth spurt**. The fastest rate of growth during the growth spurt is labeled the **peak height gain velocity**. Although growth slows after the achievement of sexual maturity, linear growth and weight acquisition continue into the late teens for females and early 20s for males and young men. Most females gain no more than 2 to 3 inches after menarche, although females who have early menarche tend to grow more after its onset than do those having later menarche. Longitudinal data suggest that the velocity of linear growth among males may be reduced or delayed by the prolonged use of stimulant medications such as those for attention deficit hyperactivity disorder (ADHD). These effects are most pronounced among 14- to 16-year-old males, with a dose-response pattern noted. Stimulant medication use among females is not as well studied, and thus it is not clear if this phenomenon also occurs among girls (Poulton et al, 2013).

Increases in height are accompanied by increases in weight during puberty. Teens gain 40% to 50% of adult body weight during adolescence. The majority of weight gain coincides with increases in linear height. However, it should be noted that teens may gain more than 15 pounds after linear growth has ceased. Changes in body composition accompany changes in weight and height. Males gain twice as much lean tissue as females, resulting in differentiation in percent body fat and lean body mass.

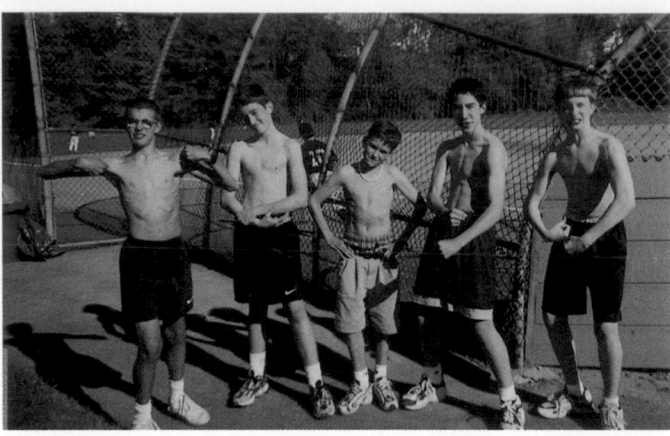

FIGURE 18-3 These males are all 13 years old, but their energy needs vary according to their individual growth rates.

Body fat levels increase from prepuberty averages of 15% for males and 19% for females, to 15% to 18% in males and 22% to 26% in females. Differences in lean body mass and body fat mass affect energy and nutrient needs throughout adolescence and differentiate the needs of females from those of males.

NUTRIENT REQUIREMENTS

The dietary reference intakes (DRIs) for adolescents are listed by chronologic age and gender (see inside front cover). Although the DRIs provide an estimate of the energy and nutrient needs for an individual adolescent, actual need varies greatly between teens as a result of differences in body composition, degree of physical maturation, and level of physical activity. Therefore health professionals should use the DRIs as a guideline during nutritional assessment but should rely on clinical judgment and indicators of growth and physical maturation to make a final determination of an individual's nutrient and energy requirements.

Energy

Estimated energy requirements (EERs) vary greatly among males and females because of variations in growth rate, body composition, and physical activity level (PAL). EERs are calculated using an adolescent's gender, age, height, weight, and PAL, with an additional 25 kilocalories (kcal) per day added for energy deposition or growth (Institute of Medicine [IOM], 2006). To determine adequate energy intake, physical activity assessment is required. The energy requirements allow for four levels of activity (sedentary, low active, active, and very active), which reflect the energy expended in activities other than the activities of daily living. Tables 18-2 and 18-3 show the EER for each activity level based on PALs.

Adequacy of energy intake for adolescents is assessed best by monitoring weight and BMI. Excessive weight gain indicates that energy intake is exceeding energy needs, whereas weight loss or a drop in BMI below an established percentile curve suggests that energy intake is inadequate to support the body's needs. Groups of adolescents who are at elevated risk for inadequate energy intake include teens who "diet" or frequently restrict caloric intake to reduce body weight; individuals living in food-insecure households, temporary housing, or on the street; adolescents who frequently use alcohol or illicit drugs, which may reduce appetite or replace food intake; and teens with chronic health conditions such as cystic fibrosis, Crohn's disease, or muscular dystrophy.

Recent concerns about excessive energy intake among youth have centered on intake of solid fats and added sugars. The mean daily intake of solid fats and added sugars among young people ages 12 to 18 years represents 34% of total energy consumption or approximately 740 kcal (Slining and Popkin, 2013). Solid fats account for a greater proportion of these empty calories with about 18% of total energy consumption coming from solid fats and 15% of total energy coming from added sugars. The main food and beverage sources of solid fats are milk, grain-based desserts, pizza, cheese, processed meats, and fried potatoes. Grain-based desserts are also a main source of added sugar intake along with sugar-sweetened beverages, candy, and other sweet snacks, ready-to-eat cereals, dairy-based desserts, and sweeteners and syrups. Sugar-sweetened beverages are of particular concern as a source of added sugar intake; soft drinks contribute nearly 30% and fruit drinks contribute 15% of added sugars consumed by youth ages 2 to 18 years (Keast et al, 2013). NHANES data revealed that 77% of 12- to 18-year-olds consume a sugar-sweetened beverage on a given day (Han and

TABLE 18-2   Estimated Energy Requirements for Adolescent Males

			ESTIMATED ENERGY REQUIREMENTS (KCAL/DAY)			
Age	Reference Weight (kg [lb])	Reference Height (m [in])	Sedentary PAL*	Low Active PAL*	Active PAL*	Very Active PAL*
9	28.6 (63.0)	1.34 (52.8)	1505	1762	2018	2334
10	31.9 (70.3)	1.39 (54.7)	1601	1875	2149	2486
11	35.9 (79.1)	1.44 (56.7)	1691	1985	2279	2640
12	40.5 (89.2)	1.49 (58.7)	1798	2113	2428	2817
13	45.6 (100.4)	1.56 (61.4)	1935	2276	2618	3038
14	51.0 (112.3)	1.64 (64.6)	2090	2459	2829	3283
15	56.3 (124)	1.70 (66.9)	2223	2618	3013	3499
16	60.9 (134.1)	1.74 (68.5)	2320	2736	3152	3663
17	64.6 (142.3)	1.75 (68.9)	2366	2796	3226	3754
18	67.2 (148)	1.76 (69.3)	2383	2823	3263	3804

Data from Institute of Medicine, Food and Nutrition Board: *Dietary reference intakes for energy, carbohydrate, fiber, fat, fatty acids, cholesterol, protein, and amino acids*, Washington, DC, 2002, National Academies Press.

PAL, Physical activity level.

*PAL categories, which are based on the amount of walking per day at 2-4 mph, are as follows: *sedentary,* no additional activity; *low active,* 1.5-2.9 miles/day; *active,* 3-5.8 miles/day; and *very active,* 7.5-14 miles/day (see Table 2-3).

TABLE 18-3   Estimated Energy Requirements for Adolescent Females

Age	Reference Weight (kg [lb])	Reference Height (m [in])	ESTIMATED ENERGY REQUIREMENTS (KCAL/DAY)			
			Sedentary PAL*	Low Active PAL*	Active PAL*	Very Active PAL*
9	29.0 (63.9)	1.33 (52.4)	1390	1635	1865	2248
10	32.9 (72.5)	1.38 (54.3)	1470	1729	1972	2376
11	37.2 (81.9)	1.44 (56.7)	1538	1813	2071	2500
12	40.5 (89.2)	1.49 (58.7)	1798	2113	2428	2817
13	44.6 (91.6)	1.51 (59.4)	1617	1909	2183	3640
14	49.4 (108.8)	1.60 (63)	1718	2036	2334	3831
15	52.0 (114.5)	1.62 (63.8)	1731	2057	2362	2870
16	53.9 (118.7)	1.63 (64.2)	1729	2059	2368	2883
17	55.1 (121.4)	1.63 (64.2)	1710	2042	2353	2871
18	56.2 (123.8)	1.63 (64.2)	1690	2024	2336	2858

Data from Institute of Medicine, Food and Nutrition Board: *Dietary reference intakes for energy, carbohydrate, fiber, fat, fatty acids, cholesterol, protein, and amino acids,* Washington, DC, 2002, National Academies Press.

PAL, Physical activity level.

*PAL categories, which are based on the amount of walking per day at 2-4 mph are as follows: sedentary, no additional activity; low active, 1.5-2.9 miles/day; active, 3-5.8 miles/day; and very active, 7.5-14 miles/day (see Table 2-3).

Powell, 2013). The proportion of energy from solid fats and added sugars is similar for foods and beverages obtained from stores (33%), schools (32%), and fast-food restaurants (35%) (Poti et al, 2014).

Counseling related to excessive energy intakes among adolescents should focus on intake of discretionary calories, especially those from added sweeteners consumed through soft drinks and candy and from solid fats consumed through snack foods and fried food. Tips should be provided for selecting nutrient-dense foods and beverages at all locations where teens spend their time.

Protein

During adolescence protein requirements vary with degree of physical maturation. The DRIs for protein intake are estimated to allow for adequate pubertal growth and positive nitrogen balance (IOM, 2006). Table 18-4 illustrates the protein requirements for adolescents. Actual protein needs are best determined based on a per kilogram of body weight method during puberty to account for differences in rates of growth and development among teens.

Insufficient protein intake is uncommon in the U.S. adolescent population. However, as with energy intake, food security issues, chronic illness, frequent dieting, and substance use may compromise protein intakes among adolescents. Teens who follow vegan or macrobiotic diets are also at elevated risk for inadequate protein intake.

TABLE 18-4   Protein: Estimated Average Requirements and Recommended Dietary Allowances for Adolescents

Age (yr)	EAR (g/kg/day)	RDA (g/kg/day)
9-13	0.76	0.95 or 34 g/day*
14-18 Males	0.73	0.85 or 52 g/day*
14-18 Females	0.71	0.85 or 46 g/day*

Data from Institute of Medicine, Food and Nutrition Board: *Dietary reference intakes for energy, carbohydrate, fiber, fat, fatty acids, cholesterol, protein, and amino acids,* Washington, DC, 2002, National Academies Press.

EAR, Estimated average requirement; *RDA,* recommended dietary allowance.

*Based on average weight for age.

When protein intake is inadequate, alterations in growth and development are seen. In the still-growing adolescent, insufficient protein intake results in delayed or stunted increases in height and weight. In the physically mature teen, inadequate protein intake can result in weight loss, loss of lean body mass, and alterations in body composition. Impaired immune response and susceptibility to infection also may be seen.

Carbohydrates and Fiber

Carbohydrate requirements of adolescents are estimated to be 130 g/day (IOM, 2006). The requirements for carbohydrates, as for most nutrients, are extrapolated from adult needs and should be used as a starting point for the determination of an individual adolescent's actual need. Teens who are very active or actively growing need additional carbohydrates to maintain adequate energy intake, whereas those who are inactive or have a chronic condition that limits mobility, may require fewer carbohydrates. Whole grains are the preferred source of carbohydrates because these foods provide vitamins, minerals, and fiber. Intake of carbohydrate is adequate in most teens; data from the 2009 to 2010 What We Eat in America survey, a component of the NHANES, suggest that average daily intakes of carbohydrate are 335 g for teenage males and 242 g for females (U.S. Department of Agricultural [USDA], Agricultural Research Service [ARS], 2012b).

However, fiber intakes of youth are low because of poor intake of whole grains, fruits, and vegetables. The adequate intake (AI) values for fiber intake among adolescents are 31 g/day for males 9 to 13 years old, 38 g/day for males 14 to 18 years old, and 26 g/day for 9- to 18-year-old females (IOM, 2006). These values are derived from calculations that suggest that an intake of 14 g/1000 kcal provides optimal protection against cardiovascular disease (CVD) and cancer (IOM, 2006). Adolescents who require less energy intake because of activity restrictions may have needs that are lower than the AI values.

What We Eat in America survey data suggest that average daily intakes of fiber are 16.4 g for teenage males and 12.6 g for females (USDA, ARS, 2012b). The disparities between fiber recommendations and actual intakes suggest that more emphasis must be placed on educating adolescents about optimal sources of carbohydrates, including whole grains, fruits, vegetables, and legumes.

Fat

DRI values for total fat intake have not been established for adolescents. Instead it is recommended that total fat intakes not exceed 30% to 35% of overall energy intake, with no more than 10% of calories coming from saturated fatty acids. Specific recommendations for intakes of omega-6 and omega-3 fatty acids have been set in an attempt to ensure that teens consume adequate essential fatty acids to support growth and development, as well as to reduce chronic disease risk later in life. The AI for omega-6 polyunsaturated fatty acids (linoleic acid) is 12 g/day for 9- to 13-year-old males, 10 g/day for 9- to 13-year-old females, 16 g/day for 14- to 18-year-old males, and 11 g/day for 14- to 18-year-old females. Estimated requirements for omega-3 polyunsaturated fatty acids (alpha-linolenic acid) among teens are 1.2 g/day for 9- to 13-year-old males, 1 g/day for 9- to 13-year-old females, 1.6 g/day for 14- to 18-year-old males, and 1.1 g/day for 14- to 18-year-old females (IOM, 2006).

Minerals and Vitamins

Micronutrient needs of youth are elevated during adolescence to support physical growth and development. The micronutrients involved in the synthesis of lean body mass, bone, and red blood cells are especially important during adolescence. Vitamins and minerals involved in protein, ribonucleic acid, and deoxyribonucleic acid synthesis are needed in the greatest amounts during the growth spurt. Needs decline after physical maturation is complete; however, the requirements for vitamins and minerals involved in bone formation are elevated throughout adolescence and into adulthood, because bone density acquisition is not completed by the end of puberty.

In general, adolescent males require greater amounts of most micronutrients during puberty, with the exception of iron. Micronutrient intakes during adolescence are often inadequate among some subgroups of teens, especially among females. Data from the National Growth and Health Study, which followed a cohort of more than 2300 girls over 10 years, suggest that the majority of teenage girls have inadequate intakes of calcium, magnesium, potassium, and vitamins D and E (Moore et al, 2012). The proportion of girls with inadequate intakes tends to increase with age. What We Eat in America survey data also can be used to monitor the adequacy of micronutrient intakes among U.S. adolescents. Compared with DRI recommendations this survey data suggests intakes of vitamin E and calcium are often too low among males and females (see Tables 18-5 and 18-6) (USDA, ARS, 2012b).

Calcium

Because of accelerated muscular, skeletal, and endocrine development, calcium needs are greater during puberty and adolescence than during childhood or the adult years. Bone mass is acquired at much higher rates during puberty than any other time of life. In fact, females accrue approximately 37% of their total skeletal mass from ages 11 to 15 years, making adolescence a crucial time for osteoporosis prevention (IOM, 2011).

The RDA for calcium is 1300 mg for all adolescents with an upper level intake of 3000 mg/day (IOM, 2011). Calcium intake declines with age during adolescence, especially among females. Research suggests that high soft drink consumption in the adolescent population contributes to low calcium intake by displacing milk consumption (Ranjit et al, 2010). Interventions to promote calcium consumption among youth should be initiated early and focus not only on increasing dairy product intake

TABLE 18-5 Mean Intakes of Select Nutrients Compared with DRIs: Adolescent Males

	Mean Intake	9- to 13-year-old RDA/AI	14- to 18-year-old RDA/AI
Vitamin A (mcg RAE)	647	600	700
Vitamin E (mg)	7.8	11	15
Thiamin (mg)	1.98	0.9	1.2
Riboflavin (mg)	2.41	0.9	1.3
Niacin (mg)	29.9	12	16
Vitamin B$_6$ (mg)	2.31	1	1.3
Folate (μg DFE)	639	300	400
Vitamin B$_{12}$ (μg)	6.30	1.8	2.4
Vitamin C (mg)	87.7	45	75
Phosphorus (mg)	1640	1250	1250
Magnesium (mg)	299	240	410
Iron (mg)	17.6	8	11
Zinc (mg)	13.9	8	11
Calcium (mg)	1260	1300	1300
Sodium (mg)	4211	1500	1500
Fiber (g)	16.4	31	38

Data sources: U.S. Department of Agriculture (USDA), Agricultural Research Service (ARS): *Nutrient Intakes from Food: Mean Amounts Consumed per Individual, by Gender and Age, What We Eat in America, NHANES 2009-2010* (website): www.ars.usda.gov/ba/bhnrc/fsrg, 2012. Accessed December 30, 2013.

AI, Adequate intake; *DRI*, dietary reference intake; *RDA*, recommended dietary allowance.

TABLE 18-6 Mean Intakes of Select Nutrients Compared with DRIs: Adolescent Females

	Mean Intake	9- to 13-year-old Female RDA/AI	14- to 18-year-old Females RDA/AI
Vitamin A (mcg RAE)	516	600	700
Vitamin E (mg)	6.5	11	15
Thiamin (mg)	1.41	0.9	1
Riboflavin (mg)	1.72	0.9	1
Niacin (mg)	20.0	12	14
Vitamin B$_6$ (mg)	1.53	1	1.2
Folate (μg DFE)	502	300	400
Vitamin B$_{12}$ (μg)	4.01	1.8	2.4
Vitamin C (mg)	77.8	45	65
Phosphorus (mg)	1192	1250	1250
Magnesium (mg)	224	240	360
Iron (mg)	12.9	8	15
Zinc (mg)	9.3	8	9
Calcium (mg)	948	1300	1300
Sodium (mg)	2958	1500	1500
Fiber (g)	12.6	26	26

Data sources: US Department of Agriculture (USDA), Agricultural Research Service (ARS): *Nutrient Intakes from Food: Mean Amounts Consumed per Individual, by Gender and Age, What We Eat in America, NHANES 2009-2010* (website): www.ars.usda.gov/ba/bhnrc/fsrg, 2012. Accessed December 2013.

AI, Adequate intake; *DRI*, dietary reference intake; *RDA*, recommended dietary allowance.

but also on decreasing intakes of soft drinks and increasing intakes of calcium-rich foods such as fortified orange juice and ready-to-eat cereals, enriched breads and other grains, dark leafy green vegetables, and tofu prepared with calcium sulfate.

Iron

Iron requirements are increased during adolescence to support the deposition of lean body mass, increase in red blood cell volume, and need to replace iron lost during menses among females. Iron needs are highest during periods of active growth among all teens and are especially elevated after the onset of menses in adolescent females. The DRI for iron among females increases from 8 mg/day before age 13 (or before the onset of menses) to 15 mg/day after the onset of menses (IOM, 2006). Among adolescent males recommended intakes increase from 8 to 11 mg/day, with higher levels required during the growth spurt. Iron needs remain elevated for women after age 18 but fall back to prepubescent levels in men once growth and development are completed (IOM, 2006).

Median intakes of iron among adolescents in the United States are less than desirable. Increased needs for iron, combined with low intakes of dietary iron, place adolescent females at risk for iron deficiency and anemia. Rapid growth may temporarily decrease circulating iron levels, resulting in **physiologic anemia of growth**. Other risk factors for iron deficiency anemia are listed in Box 18-1. During adolescence, iron deficiency anemia may impair the immune response, decrease resistance to infection, and decrease cognitive functioning and short-term memory (see Appendix 49).

Folic Acid

The DRI for folate intake among teens is 300 mcg/day for 9- to 13-year-old males and females, increasing to 400 mcg/day for 14- to 18-year-olds (IOM, 2006). The need for folate increases during later adolescence to support accretion of lean body mass and to prevent neural tube defects among females of reproductive age. Food sources of folate should include naturally occurring folate, found in dark green leafy vegetables and citrus fruit, and folic acid found in fortified grain products (see Appendix 40).

BOX 18-1   Risk Factors for Iron Deficiency

Inadequate Iron Intake/Absorption/Stores

Vegetarian eating styles, especially vegan diets
Macrobiotic diet
Low intakes of meat, fish, poultry, or iron fortified foods
Low intake of foods rich in ascorbic acid
Frequent dieting or restricted eating
Chronic or significant weight loss
Meal skipping
Substance abuse
History of iron-deficiency anemia
Recent immigration from developing country
Special health care needs

Increased Iron Requirements and Losses

Heavy or lengthy menstrual periods
Rapid growth
Pregnancy (recent or current)
Inflammatory bowel disease
Chronic use of aspirin, nonsteroidal antiinflammatory drugs (e.g., ibuprofen), or corticosteroids
Participation in endurance sports (e.g., long-distance running, swimming, cycling)
Intensive physical training
Frequent blood donations
Parasitic infection

Reprinted with permission from Stang J, Story M, editors: *Guidelines for adolescent nutrition services,* Minneapolis, 2010, Center for Leadership Education and Training in Maternal and Child Nutrition, Division of Epidemiology and Community Health, School of Public Health, University of Minnesota.

Average intakes of folate reported in the 2009 to 2010 What We Eat in America survey suggest that adolescent females are at greater risk for inadequate intake than are males (USDA, ARS, 2012b). This is a cause for concern among adolescent females who have achieved menses and are sexually active, as having adequate folic acid status before conception is important for the prevention of birth defects such as spina bifida (see Chapter 15).

Vitamin D

Vitamin D plays an important role in facilitating calcium and phosphorus absorption and metabolism, which has important implications for bone development during adolescence (IOM, 2011). The current recommended dietary allowance (RDA) for vitamin D requirements among adolescents is 600 IU/day (IOM, 2011). Natural food sources of vitamin D include cod liver oil and fatty fish and milk is fortified to 100 IU per 8-ounce serving. Vitamin D also can be synthesized by the exposure of skin to sunlight (vitamin D_2) or ingested through supplements in the form of vitamin D_2 or D_3 (see Appendix 45). Activation of these biologically inert forms begins in the liver where 25-hydroxyvitamin D (25-OH-D) is formed. The second step occurs in the kidneys, where 25-OH-D is converted to the biologically active form, 1,25-dihydroxyvitamin D (calcitriol), which exerts its action in the small intestine and bone to raise serum calcium and phosphorus levels. Despite its important role, calcitriol has limited value as a marker of vitamin D status because it has a half-life of only 4 hours; a serum level of 25-OH-D is the most accurate measure of vitamin D stores.

A recent IOM report concluded that a serum 25-OH-D level of 20 ng/ml covers the requirement of 97.5% of the population (IOM, 2011). However, it is recommended that individuals at risk for vitamin D deficiency maintain a higher level of 30 ng/ml (Holick et al, 2011).

Based on these guidelines, there is a prevalence of vitamin D deficiency among U.S. adolescents. Among youth ages 12 to 19 years, approximately one third have serum 25-OH-D levels below 10 ng/ml and three quarters have levels below 30 ng/ml (Ganji et al, 2012). There also have been noted declines in vitamin D status over the past two decades. NHANES data collected during the preceding few decades established that serum 25-OH-D levels decreased by 15% to 16% (Ganji et al, 2012). The reductions were especially obvious among non-Hispanic black participants and those in the highest BMI quintile.

Several factors may contribute to the recent increases and prevalence of vitamin D deficiency (Ma and Gordon, 2012). Increased use of topical sunblock lotions has been advocated to prevent premature aging of the skin and some skin cancers, but its use also decreases vitamin D synthesis. Some evidence suggests that individuals with a higher BMI more readily sequester cutaneous vitamin D in adipose tissue, making it less bioavailable. Further, overweight youth may be less likely to engage in regular physical activity outdoors and thus have less exposure to sunlight. Other risk factors for vitamin D deficiency include malabsorption syndromes such as cystic fibrosis, long-term use of medications which increase its catabolism (e.g., corticosteroids), lactose intolerance or milk allergy, having darkly pigmented skin, and residence at northern geographic latitudes where youth may spend little time outdoors during colder months. Low vitamin D intake is an important health risk for adolescents and deserves attention during nutrition assessment, education, and intervention (see Appendix 55).

Supplement Use by Adolescents

The consumption of moderate portions of a wide variety of foods is preferred to nutrient supplementation as a method for obtaining adequate nutrient intake. Despite this recommendation, studies show that adolescents do not consume nutrient-dense foods and usually have inadequate intakes of many vitamins and minerals; thus supplements may be beneficial for many teens (Keast et al, 2013; Moore et al, 2012). National surveys show that 28% of adolescents report using vitamin or mineral supplements (Dwyer et al, 2013). The adolescents most likely to use supplements are those in good health with a higher household income and health insurance.

The use of herbal and other nonvitamin, nonmineral dietary supplements is not well documented. National data suggest that 5% of adolescents consume nonvitamin, nonmineral supplements; however, this estimate is based on parental report and the actual prevalence of use is likely higher as adolescents may not disclose all supplement use to their parents (Wu et al, 2013). Echinacea, fish oil, and combination herbal pills are the most commonly taken herbal supplements. Adolescents most likely to use nonvitamin, nonmineral supplements are those who report non-Hispanic white race, a higher household income, activity limitations resulting from chronic health conditions, long-term prescription use, or relatively heavy use of physician services. Many adolescent athletes also use or may consider the use of dietary supplements to improve sport performance (see Chapter 23). The short- and long-term effects of such nonnutritional supplement use by adolescents are not known. Health professionals should screen adolescents for supplement use and should counsel them accordingly (see Chapter 12).

FOOD HABITS AND EATING BEHAVIORS

Food habits of concern that are seen more frequently among teens than other age groups include irregular consumption of meals, excessive snacking, eating away from home (especially at fast-food restaurants), dieting, and meal skipping. Many factors contribute to these behaviors, including decreasing influence of family, increasing influence of peers, exposure to media, employment outside the home, greater discretionary spending capacity, and increasing responsibilities that leave less time for teens to eat meals with their families. Most adolescents are aware of the importance of nutrition and the components of a healthy diet; however, they may have many barriers to overcome.

Teens perceive taste preferences, hectic schedules, the cost and accessibility of different foods, and social support from family and friends to be key factors that affect their food and beverage choices (Berge et al, 2012; Gellar et al, 2012). For example, parents may positively influence the food and beverage choices of teens by modeling healthy eating habits, selecting healthy foods for family meals, encouraging healthy eating, and setting limits on the consumption of unhealthy snack foods. Friends influence each other through modeling and shared activities, such as eating out at fast-food restaurants and purchasing snacks at convenience stores near school.

Developmentally, many teens lack the ability to associate current eating habits with future disease risk. Teens often are more focused on "fitting in" with their peers. They adopt health behaviors that demonstrate their quest for autonomy and make them feel more like adults such as drinking alcohol, smoking, and engaging in sexual activity. Nutrition education and counseling should focus on short-term benefits, such as improving school performance, looking good, and having more energy. Messages should be positive, developmentally appropriate, and concrete. Specific skills such as choosing water or milk over sugar-sweetened drinks, ordering broiled rather than fried meats, and choosing baked rather than fried snack chips are key concepts to discuss.

Irregular Meals and Snacking

Meal skipping is common among adolescents. Meal skipping increases throughout adolescence as teens try to sleep longer in the morning, try to lose weight through calorie restriction, and try to manage their busy lives. Breakfast is the most commonly skipped meal. National data suggest that one quarter of adolescents (12 to 19 years) skip breakfast on a given day (USDA, ARS, 2012a). Breakfast skipping has been associated with poor health outcomes, including higher BMI; poorer concentration and school performance; and increased risk of inadequate nutrient intake (De la Hunty et al, 2013; Hoyland et al, 2009). Adolescents who skip breakfast tend to have a higher intake of added sugars and poorer intake of key nutrients (e.g., calcium, vitamin A) compared with those who eat breakfast, especially when the breakfast meal is composed of healthy foods that may be fortified such as ready-to-eat cereal (Deshmukh-Tasker et al, 2010).

Teens who skip meals often snack in response to hunger instead of eating a meal. Most teens (92% of males, 94% of females) consume at least one snack per day, and the majority of teens who report snacking consume two or more snacks per day (USDA, ARS, 2012c). Snack foods consumed by teens are often high in added fats, sweeteners, and sodium. Soft drinks and other sugar-sweetened beverages are consumed commonly, accounting for a substantial proportion of daily caloric intake and representing an important source of caffeine consumption (see *Focus On:* Caffeine and Substance Use by Teens). Teens consume a daily average of 286 calories from sugar-sweetened beverages, and 16% report heavy consumption of 500 or more calories (Han and Powell, 2013). Frequent snacking may promote higher total energy intake and a higher proportion of energy provided by added and total sugars (Larson and Story, 2013). However, national data indicate that snacks also make positive contributions to intake of key nutrients. For example, 2009-2010 NHANES data for male and female adolescents indicate that foods and beverages consumed at snack occasions provide 17% to 20% of folate intake, 27% to 35% of vitamin C intake, 17% to 19% of vitamin D intake, 23% to 26% of calcium intake, and 18% to 21% of iron intake (USDA, ARS, 2012d). Because snacks are prevalent and often consumed in place of meals, teens should be encouraged to make healthy choices when choosing these snack foods and beverages. Box 18-2 provides ideas for healthy snacks or meal alternatives for teens.

Fast Foods and Convenience Foods

Convenience foods include foods and beverages from vending machines, canteens, school stores, fast-food restaurants, and convenience stores. As adolescents spend considerable amounts of time in and around schools, convenience foods available at school and in the surrounding neighborhood are likely to influence their eating patterns. National data indicate vending machines are available in 72% of middle schools and 87% of high schools (Fox et al, 2012). One in five middle schools and

BOX 18-2 Teen-Friendly Healthy Snacks

Nonfat yogurt layered with berries and granola
Instant oatmeal made with skim milk and sliced fruit
Pudding made with skim milk
Glass of skim milk with a teaspoon of chocolate or strawberry syrup
Soft pretzel topped with mustard or salsa
Sliced apples dipped in peanut butter or fat-free caramel dip
Whole-wheat English muffins topped with low-fat cream cheese and diced fresh vegetables
Mini-bagel topped with one tablespoon of peanut butter or almond butter
Air-popped popcorn
Whole-wheat pita wedges topped with 1-2 tablespoons of hummus
String cheese and crackers containing no trans fat
Baked tortilla chips with bean dip or salsa
Baked potato topped with salsa or broccoli and melted low-fat cheese
Graham crackers containing no trans fat
Frozen yogurt or juice bars
Fruit drink spritzer (half juice and half seltzer water)
Trail mix (dried fruit with nuts and seeds)
Baby carrots and low-fat ranch dressing
Low-fat granola bars
Mini-rice cakes or popcorn cakes
Tortilla wraps filled with slices of turkey, cheese, lettuce, and tomato

Adapted with permission from Stang J, Story M, editors: *Guidelines for adolescent nutrition services,* Minneapolis, 2010, Center for Leadership Education and Training in Maternal and Child Nutrition, Division of Epidemiology and Community Health, School of Public Health, University of Minnesota.

◎ FOCUS ON

Are Teenagers Who Consume Energy Drinks More Likely to Become Substance Abusers?

Three out of four adolescents consume caffeine on a given day, mostly from soft drinks, tea, and coffee (Branum et al, 2014). Although average caffeine intake among adolescents does not exceed the recommended daily limit of 100 mg, energy drinks are becoming increasingly popular, and the amount of caffeine in these drinks is not regulated by the Food and Drug Administration (FDA) (Branum et al, 2014; Seifert et al, 2011). The FDA has imposed a limit on caffeine of 71 mg per 12-ounce serving for soft drinks, whereas energy drinks have been found to contain nonnutritive stimulants (e.g., caffeine, guarana, taurine) in amounts that range from 2.5 to 171 mg per ounce (Terry-McElrath et al, 2014). Of further concern, recent evidence suggests that energy drink users are more likely than their peers to report alcohol, cigarette, and illicit drug use.

The relationship between energy drink consumption and substance abuse was explored using a 2010-2011 survey. In this survey data were collected from a nationally representative sample of 21,995 secondary school students (grades 8, 10, and 12) who were participating in the Monitoring the Future study (Terry-McElrath et al, 2014). Students self-reported how many energy drinks they consumed on an average day. Substance use data was also self-reported, including frequency of alcohol, cigarette, marijuana, and amphetamine use in the past 30 days. Energy drink consumption was related to greater use of each substance for students in all grades. This research suggests that certain groups of adolescents may be particularly likely to consume energy drinks and to be substance users, and nutrition educators should inform parents and adolescents about the masking effects of caffeine in energy drinks on alcohol- and other substance-related impairments.

approximately one quarter of all high schools have a school store where students can purchase food or beverages (Fox et al, 2012). In addition, middle schools and high schools often have a fast-food restaurant or convenience store within walking distance (Forsyth et al, 2012). Fast-food restaurants and convenience stores are socially acceptable places for teens to eat, spend time with their friends, and even work.

Convenience foods tend to be low in vitamins, minerals, and fiber, but high in calories, added fat, sweeteners, and sodium. National data suggest that 46% of adolescents (12 to 18 years) consume at least one item from a fast-food restaurant, and 44% to 55% consume at least one convenience food item at school on a given day (Fox et al, 2009; Poti et al, 2014). Few teens are willing to stop purchasing convenience foods; the low price, convenient access, and taste appeal to them. Instead of asking teenagers to not eat these foods, health professionals should counsel them on how to make healthy choices and work with schools to implement the U.S. Department of Agriculture nutrition standards for convenience foods sold in schools (see Figure 18-4). Counseling teens with concrete guidelines that are easy to remember, such as choosing snacks or vending and fast-food options with fewer than 5 g of fat per serving, can be particularly effective. Teens also can be encouraged to check labels to determine whether foods are made from whole grains or are high in added sweeteners or sodium.

Family Meals

The frequency with which adolescents eat meals with their families decreases with age (Child Trends, 2013). Nearly half of 12- to 14-year-olds eat meals with their families at least 6 days per week compared with just more than one third of 15- to 17-year-olds. Adolescents who eat meals with their families

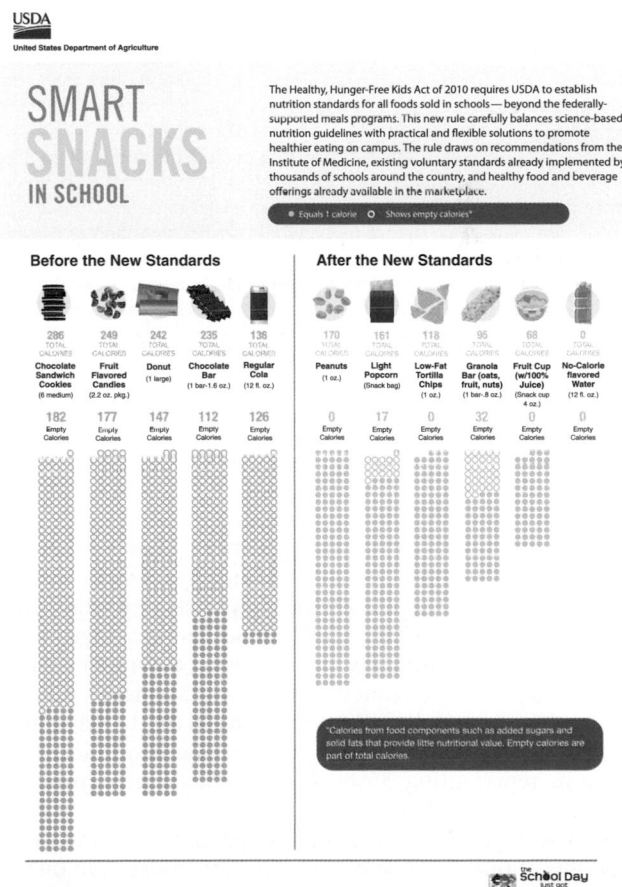

FIGURE 18-4 Smart Snacks in School: U.S. Department of Agriculture nutrition standards for convenience foods sold in schools.

have been found to have better academic performance and to be less likely to engage in risky behaviors such as drinking alcohol and smoking compared with peers who do not frequently engage in family meals (Neumark-Sztainer et al, 2010).

Developing healthful eating patterns at family meals during adolescence may improve the likelihood that individuals will choose to consume nutritious foods in adulthood and possibly also protect them from the future development of overweight (Berge et al, 2015; Fulkerson et al, 2014). Family meals not only allow for more communication between teens and their parents but also provide an ideal environment during which parents can model healthy food and beverage choices and attitudes toward eating. Teens who eat at home more frequently have been found to consume fewer soft drinks and more calcium-rich foods, fruit, and vegetables (Fulkerson et al, 2014; Larson et al, 2013) (see *Focus On: Family Meals and Nutritional Benefits for Teens*).

◎ FOCUS ON

Family Meals and Nutritional Benefits for Teens

When teens regularly share dinners with their families, they are more likely to have diets of higher nutritional quality, and some evidence suggests the practice may protect them against the future development of overweight in young adulthood (Berge et al, 2015; Fulkerson et al, 2014). However, different schedules and difficulty finding time to eat together are common barriers to sharing the evening meal. One recent study examined whether there are similar benefits associated with eating breakfast together (Larson et al, 2013). Students at 20 public middle schools and high schools in the Minneapolis-St. Paul metropolitan area of Minnesota were surveyed about their dietary practices and how often they have a family meal at breakfast and at dinner. Approximately 71% of students at these schools qualified for free or reduced-price school meals and 81% represented a racial/ethnic background other than non-Hispanic white. Among these students, family breakfast meals occurred on average less often than family dinners (1.5 breakfast meals versus 4.1 dinner meals per week) and less than 10% of students ate together daily with "all or most" of their family at breakfast. However, participation in more frequent family breakfast meals was linked to several markers of better diet quality (e.g., more fruits, whole grains, and fiber) as well as lower risk for overweight. These associations were found while accounting for family dinner frequency as well as structural and organizational characteristics of families and thus suggest, when it is not always possible to eat dinner together, coming together for other meals such as breakfast can provide benefits. Health professionals should encourage families to eat together at breakfast as well as at dinner, and provide supports for addressing challenges such as lack of time, food security, and limited food preparation skills.

Media and Advertising

Marketing to teenagers has become a multi-billion dollar business, as the nation's largest food and beverage companies spend $1.8 billion per year to market their products to youth (Federal Trade Commission [FTC], 2012). Food and beverage companies promote their products to youth using a number of different techniques (e.g., contests, product placements, sponsorships, celebrity endorsements, viral marketing) and multiple platforms; however, television is the dominant advertising medium, representing 35% of all youth-directed marketing expenditures (FTC, 2012).

American youth spend 7.5 hours per day with media and, given the amount of time they spend using more than one medium at a time, they are exposed to more than 10.5 hours of media content (Rideout et al, 2010). Outside of school work, on an average day, youth spend 4.5 hours watching television and movies, 2.5 hours listening to the radio or recorded music,

1.5 hours using a computer, 1.2 hours playing video games, and 38 minutes reading magazines or books. The majority of youth (71%) have a television, and 33% have Internet access in their bedroom. As the time that youth spend with media has increased, so has the ability for advertisers to influence their eating behaviors (Rideout et al, 2010). Teenagers (12 to 17 years) view an estimated 14 television advertisements for food products on an average day (Powell et al, 2010). Despite some recent evidence of improvement in the nutritional quality of advertised products, most viewed food advertisements are for products high in fat, sugar, or sodium, and fast-food restaurant advertisements are the most frequently viewed food advertisements at an average of four per day (Powell et al, 2010, 2013). In addition, the majority of the nation's largest food and beverage companies market their products to youth online (FTC, 2012). Media literacy education can and should be taught to teens to assist them in determining the accuracy and validity of media and advertising messages.

Dieting and Body Image

Body image concerns are common during adolescence. Many teens describe themselves as being overweight despite being of normal weight, signifying a disturbance in their body image. Poor body image can lead to weight control issues and dieting. The Youth Risk Behavior Surveillance System data from 2011 show that 46% of U.S. high school students were attempting to lose weight. The prevalence of dieting was higher among female (61%) than male (32%) students. Hispanic females had the highest prevalence of dieting at 66%, followed by white females (61%), black females (55%), Hispanic males (40%), white males (29%), and black males (27%) (Eaton et al, 2012).

Eating nutrient-dense foods (e.g., skim milk, fruits, and vegetables) to limit calories and getting regular exercise can be viewed as healthy weight loss behaviors when used in moderation and can be a starting point for nutrition education and counseling to improve eating behaviors. However, not all dieting behaviors have the potential to improve health. High-risk dieting practices are used by many teens and carry with them the risk of poor nutritional status and increased risk for **disordered eating** (see Chapter 22). Fasting, or refraining from eating for more than 24 hours, was practiced by 17% of female and 7% of male U.S. high school students in the past month as a means of dieting (Eaton et al, 2012). Furthermore, 6% of females and 4% of males had used diet pills to lose weight; the prevalence of this behavior was highest among Hispanic students and increased with age. The use of purging methods, including vomiting and laxative or diuretic use, was reported by 6% of females and 3% of males. White and Hispanic students were more likely to report purging behaviors than African American students.

NUTRITION SCREENING, ASSESSMENT, AND COUNSELING

The American Academy of Pediatrics recommends that adolescents have an annual health screening to address priority issues, including physical growth and development, social and academic competence, emotional well-being, risk reduction (e.g., for substance use, sexually transmitted infections), and violence and injury prevention (Hagan et al, 2008). The supervision of physical growth and development should involve an assessment of nutrition risk and the provision of anticipatory guidance.

Nutrition screening should include the assessment of height, weight, and BMI to determine weight status; evaluation for the presence of iron deficiency anemia (females only); review of oral health behaviors (e.g., regular dental visits, intake of high-sugar foods); and assessment of physical fitness and media use (Holt et al, 2011). Anticipatory guidance should further address healthy eating behaviors and building a positive body image.

Weight, height, and BMI should be plotted using the Centers for Disease Control and Prevention (CDC) National Center for Health Statistics BMI tables to determine appropriateness of weight for height (see Appendix Tables 6, 7, 10, and 11). A BMI below the fifth percentile may signal the presence of chronic or metabolic disease, growth failure, or an eating disorder. A BMI at or above the 85th percentile, but below the 95th percentile, indicates that an adolescent is overweight, whereas a BMI at or above the 95th percentile indicates the presence of obesity. All BMI values that indicate the presence of overweight should be corroborated with a direct measure of body fat to determine that excessive fat, or obesity, is truly indicated (see Chapter 7).

When nutrition screening indicates the presence of nutritional risk, a full assessment should be conducted. Nutrition assessment should include a complete evaluation of food intake through a 24-hour recall, dietary records, or brief food frequency questionnaire (see Chapter 4). The adequacy of energy, fiber, macronutrients, and micronutrients should be determined, as well as excessive intake of any dietary components such as sodium or sweeteners. Nutritional assessments also should include an evaluation of the nutritional environment, including parental, peer, school, cultural, and personal lifestyle factors. The attitude of the adolescent toward food and nutrition is important; helping them overcome their perceived barriers to eating well is an essential component of nutrition counseling.

Teens who live in food-insecure households, temporary housing, or shelters, or who have run away from home are at especially high nutritional risk, as are adolescents who use alcohol and street drugs. It is important that health professionals working with high-risk teens develop partnerships with community-based food assistance programs to ensure that youth have access to a steady, nutritious food supply. Homeless teens, as well as those living in temporary shelters, benefit from nutrition counseling focusing on lightweight, low-cost, prepackaged foods that do not require refrigeration or cooking facilities. Dried fruit, nuts, granola bars, cereal bars, tuna in pouches, and meat jerky are foods that should be available for runaway or homeless teens.

Education and counseling should be tailored to meet any specific nutrition diagnoses identified during the assessment. A teen who has been found to be overweight with type 2 diabetes requires a different type and intensity of counseling than a teen who has been diagnosed with iron deficiency anemia. Knowledge, attitude, and behavior must be addressed when guiding adolescents toward acquiring healthful food habits. For a plan to succeed the adolescent must be willing to change; therefore an assessment of a teenager's desire to change is essential. Encouraging the desire to change usually requires much attention (see Chapter 14).

Information can be provided in various settings ranging from the classroom to the hospital (see Figure 18-5). The clinician must understand the change process and how to communicate it meaningfully. Parents may be included in the process and are encouraged to be supportive. Recommended eating plans based on recommended energy intakes for adolescents are shown in Table 18-7.

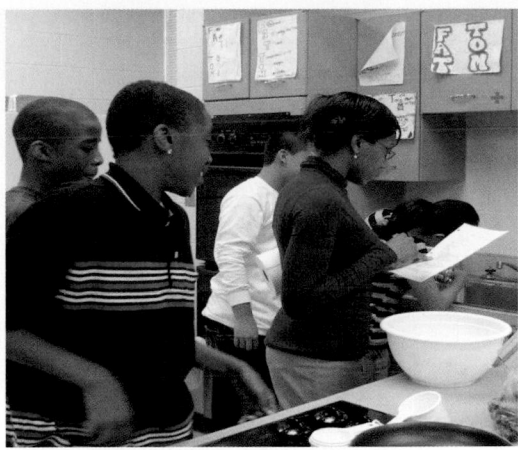

FIGURE 18-5 Teenagers who help to prepare safe, nutritious meals become engaged in the healthy eating process.

SPECIAL CONCERNS

Vegetarian Dietary Patterns

As adolescents mature, they begin to develop autonomous social, moral, and ethical values. These values may lead to vegetarian eating practices because of concerns about animal welfare, the environment, or personal health. Concerns about body weight also motivate some adolescents to adopt a vegetarian diet because it is a socially acceptable way to reduce dietary fat. Recent data confirm that adolescents who consume vegetarian diets are less likely to be overweight or obese than their omnivorous peers (Robinson-O'Brien et al, 2009). Well-planned vegetarian diets that include a variety of legumes, nuts, and whole grains can provide adequate nutrients for teens who have completed the majority of their growth and development (Craig et al, 2009).

Vegetarian diets that become increasingly more restrictive should be viewed with caution, because this may signal the development of disordered eating, with the vegetarian diet used as a means to hide a restriction of food intake (Craig et al, 2009). Teen males and females who adopt vegetarian dietary patterns have been found to use more high-risk weight control behaviors, especially vomiting, to lose weight (Robinson-O'Brien et al, 2009). This increased risk for unhealthy weight control behaviors seems to persist even after the vegetarian eating style is discontinued, suggesting that although the issues are related, vegetarian diets likely do not cause disordered eating and instead may serve as an early symptom.

Vegetarian adolescents often have high intakes of iron, vitamin A, and fiber and low intakes of dietary cholesterol. Vegetarian diets that include eggs or dairy products are consistent with the Dietary Guidelines for Americans and can meet the DRIs for all nutrients. A sample eating plan to assist vegetarian teens in achieving adequate energy and nutrient intakes is listed in Table 18-8.

Vegan and macrobiotic diets, which do not include animal products of any kind, do not provide natural sources of vitamin B_{12} and may be deficient in calcium, vitamin D, zinc, iron, and long-chain omega-3 fatty acids (Craig et al, 2009). Therefore vegan adolescents must choose foods fortified with these nutrients or take a daily multivitamin-mineral supplement. Adolescents and their caregivers should be instructed on the planning of well-balanced vegetarian diets and fortified foods that can prevent potential nutrient deficiencies.

TABLE 18-7　Recommended Number of Servings for Adolescents Ages 13 and 16 Years Based on Activity Level*

	Grains (oz-eq/day)	Whole Grains (oz-eq/day)[†]	Vegetables (cups/day)	Fruit (cups/day)	Dairy (cups/day)	Seafood (oz/week)	Meat, poultry, eggs (oz/week)	Nuts, seeds, soy products (oz/week)	Oils (g/day)
Males									
13 Years									
Sedentary	6	3	2.5	2	3	8	26	4	27
Moderately Active	7	3.5	3	2	3	9	29	4	29
Active	9	4.5	3.5	2	3	10	31	5	34
16 Years									
Sedentary	8	4	3	2	3	10	31	5	31
Moderately Active	10	5	3.5	2.5	3	11	34	5	36
Active	10	4	4	2.5	3	11	34	5	51
Females									
13 Years									
Sedentary	5	3	2	1.5	3	8	24	4	22
Moderately Active	6	3	2.5	2	3	8	26	4	27
Active	7	3.5	3	2	3	9	29	4	29
16 Years									
Sedentary	6	3	2.5	1.5	3	8	24	4	24
Moderately Active	6	3	2.5	2	3	8	26	4	27
Active	8	4	3	2	3	10	31	5	31

Adapted from the U.S. Department of Agriculture (USDA): *Dietary Guidelines for Americans, 2010* (website): http://www.cnpp.usda.gov/DGAs2010-PolicyDocument.htm. Accessed December 30, 2013.

oz-eq, one ounce-equivalent is: 1 slice (1 ounce) of bread; 1 ounce uncooked pasta or rice; ½ cup cooked rice, pasta, or cereal; 1 tortilla (6″ diameter); 1 pancake (5″ diameter); 1 ounce ready-to-eat cereal (about 1 cup cereal flakes)

*Activity level categories are defined as follows: *sedentary,* a lifestyle that includes only the light physical activity associated with typical day-to-day life; *moderately active,* a lifestyle that includes physical activity equivalent to walking about 1.5 to 3 miles per day at 3 to 4 miles per hour, in addition to the light physical activity associated with typical day-to-day life; and *active,* a lifestyle that includes physical activity equivalent to walking more than 3 miles per day at 3 to 4 miles per hour, in addition to the light physical activity associated with typical day-to-day life.

[†]Number of servings of whole grains are not in addition to but are included in the number of servings of grains.

Acne

The appearance of acne most often peaks during adolescence and affects 80% to 90% of U.S. teens (Burris et al, 2013). Effective treatment for the condition is important because acne can significantly affect quality of life and in some cases lead to social withdrawal, anxiety, or depression (Burris et al, 2013). Research suggesting the potential value of incorporating medical nutrition therapy in the treatment of acne continues to emerge. For example, a recent study among 250 young adults (ages 18 to 25) in New York City found evidence that dietary factors may influence or aggravate acne development by comparing the self-reported usual dietary patterns of participants who reported no or mild acne to those with moderate to severe acne (Burris et al, 2014). Young adults with moderate to severe acne reported higher glycemic index diets, including more added sugars, total sugars, milk servings, saturated fat, and trans fatty acids and fewer servings of fish. The majority of all participants (58%) additionally reported the perception that diet aggravates or influences their acne.

The evidence from this study combined with other epidemiologic, observational, and experimental research does not demonstrate that diet causes acne but indicates it may aggravate or influence the condition to some degree (Burris et al, 2013). Medical nutrition therapy as an adjunct to dermatology therapy may be beneficial for some young people with acne.

However, a number of questions remain that must be addressed by additional research before the efficacy and clinical relevance of diet therapy can be established and evidence-based guidelines developed to guide dietitian nutritionist in practice.

Currently, the most reasonable approach to practice is to approach each young person with acne on an individual basis to determine whether dietary counseling may be beneficial. The evidence base most consistently supports guiding individuals with acne toward a healthful, low-glycemic load diet that is low in saturated fat and high in whole grains, fruit, and vegetables (see Chapter 30 and Appendix 37). An additional dietary intervention that may similarly offer multiple health benefits is to recommend increasing consumption of omega-3 fatty acids (see Appendix 34). As long as intake of calcium and vitamin D are sufficient, it may further be beneficial to recommend a diet lower in dairy but as yet the quantity of milk necessary to exacerbate acne has not been established.

Disordered Eating and Eating Disorders

An estimated 10% to 20% of teens engage in disordered eating behaviors, such as binge-purge behavior, compensatory exercise, laxative and diuretic abuse, and binge eating (Neumark-Sztainer et al, 2012). These behaviors do not occur with enough regularity

TABLE 18-8   Recommended Number of Servings for Vegetarian Adolescents Ages 13 and 16 Years Based on Activity Level*

	Grains (oz-eq/ day)	Vegetables (cups/day)	Fruit (cups/day)	Dairy (cups/day)	Eggs (oz-eq/week)	Beans and peas (oz-eq/ week)	Nuts and seeds (oz-eq/week)	Soy products (oz-eq/week)	Oils (g/day)
Males									
13 Years									
Sedentary	6	2.5	2	3	4	10	13	12	19
Moderately Active	7	3	2	3	4	10	15	13	21
Active	9	3.5	2	3	5	11	16	14	25
16 Years									
Sedentary	8	3	2	3	5	11	16	14	22
Moderately Active	10	3.5	2.5	3	5	12	17	15	26
Active	10	4	2.5	3	5	12	17	15	41
Females									
13 Years									
Sedentary	5	2	1.5	3	4	9	12	11	15
Moderately Active	6	2.5	2	3	4	10	13	12	19
Active	7	3	2	3	4	10	15	13	21
16 Years									
Sedentary	6	2.5	1.5	3	4	9	12	11	17
Moderately Active	6	2.5	2	3	4	10	13	12	19
Active	8	3	2	3	5	11	16	14	22

Adapted from the U.S. Department of Agriculture (USDA): *Dietary Guidelines for Americans, 2010* (website): http://www.cnpp.usda.gov/DGAs2010-PolicyDocument.htm. Accessed December 30, 2013.

oz-eq, one ounce-equivalent is: 1 slice (1 ounce) of bread; 1 ounce uncooked pasta or rice; ½ cup cooked rice, pasta, or cereal; 1 tortilla (6″ diameter); 1 pancake (5″ diameter); 1 ounce ready-to-eat cereal (about 1 cup cereal flakes)

*Activity level categories are defined as follows: *sedentary,* a lifestyle that includes only the light physical activity associated with typical day-to-day life; *moderately active,* a lifestyle that includes physical activity equivalent to walking about 1.5 to 3 miles per day at 3 to 4 miles per hour, in addition to the light physical activity associated with typical day-to-day life; and *active,* a lifestyle that includes physical activity equivalent to walking more than 3 miles per day at 3 to 4 miles per hour, in addition to the light physical activity associated with typical day-to-day life.

or frequency to be diagnosed as an eating disorder, but may still have significant health implications for teens. Symptoms that may signal the presence of disordered eating behaviors include recurring gastrointestinal complaints, amenorrhea, or unexplained weight loss. Overweight females have been found to be twice as likely to engage in disordered eating behaviors. A screening for disordered eating can easily be done and should include questions about body dissatisfaction, fear of weight gain, frequency of dieting and fasting, use of laxatives and diuretics, use of diet pills, fear of certain foods (e.g., foods containing fat or sugar), vomiting, bingeing, and compensatory exercise.

Eating disorders occur in adolescent females and males and across all socioeconomic, racial, and ethnic groups (see Chapter 22). In general, anorexia nervosa is characterized by a dangerously low body weight, preoccupation with thinness, and restrictive dietary behaviors. Bulimia nervosa is characterized by a body weight that is close to normal, episodes of uncontrollable eating (bingeing), and efforts to eliminate calories or food from the body (purging). Binge eating disorder is characterized by frequent, recurrent episodes of binge eating and loss of control over eating. Although prevalence rates are difficult to estimate, national data suggest that bulimia nervosa and binge eating disorder are somewhat more common than anorexia nervosa (Ozier et al, 2011).

Diagnostic criteria for eating disorders provided by the *Diagnostic and Statistical Manual of Mental Disorders,* 5th edition, must be used judiciously with adolescents because of issues surrounding normal growth and development (American Psychiatric Association [APA], 2013). The wide variability in the rate, timing, and velocity of height and weight gain during normal puberty; the absence of menstrual periods in early puberty combined with the unpredictability of menses soon after menarche; and the cognitive inability to understand abstract concepts can make application of the diagnostic criteria challenging in adolescents. Adolescents are particularly vulnerable to the complications of eating disorders. The effect of malnutrition on linear growth, brain development, and bone acquisition can be persistent and irreversible. Yet with early and aggressive treatment, adolescents have the potential for a better outcome than adults who have had the disease longer (Steinhausen, 2008).

Overweight and Obesity

Overweight and obesity in adolescence have short- and long-term health consequences. Adolescents who are overweight and particularly those with more severe obesity are at higher risk for hyperlipidemia, hypertension, insulin resistance, and type 2 diabetes compared with normal weight peers (Kelly et al, 2013). Epidemiologic studies of obesity and disease risk demonstrate an increased risk of premature mortality and morbidity from diabetes, hypertension, coronary heart disease, stroke, asthma, and polycystic ovary syndrome among individuals who were overweight or obese during adolescence (Reilly and Kelly, 2011).

Adolescent weight status is evaluated based on BMI (weight/height² [kg/m2]) as shown in Appendices 7 and 11. Among 12- to 19-year-olds in the United States, the prevalence of overweight, characterized by a BMI higher than the 85th percentile, is 32.6% (Ogden et al, 2012). The prevalence of obesity (BMI of at least the 95th percentile) is 17.1%, and it is estimated that severe obesity (120% of the 95th percentile) afflicts 4% to 6% of youth (Kelly et al, 2013; Ogden et al, 2012). Obesity is a complex, multifactorial health issue that is influenced by genetics, metabolic efficiency, PAL, dietary intake, and environmental and psychosocial factors (see Chapter 21). Adolescents who are found to be overweight should have a fasting lipid profile completed and should be assessed for additional risk factors for chronic disease, such as personal history of hypertension, hyperlipidemia, tobacco use, and family history of hypertension, early cardiovascular death, stroke, hyperlipidemia, and type 2 diabetes mellitus (Krebs et al, 2007). If risk factors are noted, aspartate aminotransferase and alanine aminotransferase measurements to assess liver function should be obtained as well.

A fasting glucose level should be drawn on any overweight adolescent with two or more risk factors for CVD, or with a family history of diabetes. Obese teens should undergo the same laboratory assessments as overweight children, with the addition of microalbumin/creatinine or microalbumin/creatinine ratio. Additional assessments for conditions such as sleep apnea, orthopedic disorders, polycystic ovary disease, and hormonal abnormalities should be performed based on presenting symptoms.

Recent guidelines for adolescent overweight and obesity suggest a staged care treatment process (see Box 18-3) based on a teen's BMI, age, motivation, and the presence of comorbid conditions (Hoelscher et al, 2013). Four stages are recommended, with progress through the stages based on age, biologic development, level of motivation, weight status, and success with previous stages of treatment. Advancing to the next stage of treatment may be recommended if insufficient progress is made to improve weight status or resolve comorbid conditions after 3 to 6 months.

Concern has been expressed regarding the use of bariatric surgery in adolescents. Recommendations for bariatric surgery suggest that it can be justified only by the combination of severe obesity and the existence of comorbid medical conditions (Kelly et al, 2013). Difficulty in complying with dietary restrictions after surgery may lead to complications such as dumping syndrome after high carbohydrate intake, voluntary excessive food intake, digestion of meat affected in a gastrojejunal anastomosis,

---

BOX 18-3   Staged Care Treatment for Overweight and Obesity

Four treatment stages are recommended, with progress through the stages based on the adolescent's age, biologic development, level of motivation, weight status, and success with previous stages of treatment. Advancing to the next stage of treatment may be recommended if insufficient progress is made to improve weight status or resolve comorbid conditions after 3 to 6 months.

Stage 1 is appropriate for overweight adolescents with no comorbid conditions and/or SMR of 4 or less. This stage of obesity treatment consists of general nutrition and physical activity advice and can be provided by a single health care provider, including physicians, nurses, and dietitians who have training in pediatric weight management. Weight loss should be monitored monthly by the provider and not exceed 1 to 2 pounds per week. Achieve 1 hour of moderate-to-vigorous physical activity each day. Limit daily screen time to no more than 2 hours.

Guidelines for Stage 1
- Remove television and other forms of screen media from the bedroom.
- Consume five fruit and vegetable servings per day, but limit intake of juice.
- Limit eating occasions away from home with the exception of school meals.
- Participate in family meals on most days of the week.
- Consume at least three meals per day rather than frequently snacking.
- Eat mindfully, only when hungry and only until satiated.
- Reduce consumption of most energy-dense foods and beverages and eliminate consumption of sugar-sweetened beverages.
- Select appropriate portion sizes when eating at home and away from home.

Stage 2 includes the same concepts as Stage 1, but provides more structure. This stage of obesity treatment can be provided by a single health care provider with training in motivational counseling. However, referrals for additional services such as physical therapy or counseling may be necessary for some adolescents. Stage 2 treatment is considered successful if weight maintenance or weight loss of up to two pounds per week is achieved. Assessment of progress should be monitored monthly.

Guidelines for Stage 2
- Monitor food and beverage intake through daily food and exercise journals or record books.

- Set goals for food and physical activity behavior changes and monitor progress toward goals.
- Limit time spent with screen media to no more than 60 minutes per day.
- Follow a structured meal plan with scheduled meal and snack times.
- Plan and monitor physical activity to ensure 60 minutes of moderate-to-vigorous activity is achieved each day.
- Reinforce successful lifestyle changes through the use of age-appropriate, nonfood rewards such as tickets to a local event or museum, jewelry, clothing, or music.

Stage 3 is more structured than Stage 2. Youth with a BMI at or above the 99th percentile for age and gender may start treatment in Stage 3. Treatment services are provided by a multidisciplinary team that includes a physician or pediatric nurse practitioner, a counselor (psychologist or social worker), a registered dietitian/nutritionist, and an exercise physiologist or physical therapist. Stage 3 treatment is considered successful when BMI no longer exceeds the 85th percentile for age and gender; however, weight loss should be monitored to not exceed 2 pounds per week. If no improvement is seen after 3 to 6 months, or if comorbid conditions worsen, it is recommended that treatment advance to stage 4.

Guidelines for Stage 3
- The treatment program provides at least 50 hours and ideally more than 70 hours of intervention within 2 to 6 months.
- A family component and an adolescent-only component are offered.
- A highly structured meal plan is developed and monitored.
- A highly structured physical activity plan is developed and monitored.
- A formal behavior modification program is instituted by a counselor, with parent involvement as appropriate.

Stage 4 treatment is a tertiary care service and is reserved for severely obese adolescents or those who have a BMI at or above the 95th percentile for age and gender and who have significant comorbidities that require concerted intervention. This treatment stage is available only in clinical settings that employ a full range of health professionals who are trained specifically in the behavioral and medical management of pediatric obesity.

Guidelines for Stage 4
- Intensive dietary regimens, such as meal replacement, protein-sparing modified fasts, oral medication
- Bariatric surgery may be used

Adapted from Spear B et al: Recommendations for treatment of child and adolescent overweight and obesity, Pediatrics 120:S254, 2007 and U.S. Preventative Services Task Force; Barton M: Screening for Obesity in Children and Adolescents: U.S. Preventive Services Task Force Recommendation Statement, Pediatrics 125:361, 2010.

and B vitamin deficiencies caused by poor compliance with vitamin-mineral supplementation (see Chapter 21).

Hyperlipidemia and Hypertension

Hyperlipidemia and hypertension, risk factors for CVD, are apparent in adolescence and have been shown to be predictive of CVD risk in later life. Components of a health screening assessment aimed at the identification and prevention of risk for CVD and other chronic diseases are listed in Table 18-9. Table 18-10 lists the classification criteria for the diagnosis of hyperlipidemia among youth. National data suggest that one in five adolescents 12 to 19 years old has elevated blood lipid levels

TABLE 18-9	Suggested Health Screening Schedule for Health Promotion and Chronic Disease Prevention	
Risk Factor	**Ages 12-17 Years**	**Ages 18-21 Years**
Family history of premature cardio-vascular disease	• Update previous family history at each visit. • Provide dietary counseling and referral based on family history as necessary.	• Assess changes in family history at least annually. • Provide dietary counseling and referral based on family history as necessary.
Eating behaviors and patterns	• Assess diet using appropriate methods. • Provide education and counseling as needed.	• Review eating behaviors and provide education to improve dietary intake and nutritional status.
Growth and weight status	• Weigh and measure teen at each visit. Plot height, weight, and BMI. Review with adolescent and parent(s). • If adolescent is overweight, provide Step 1 counseling to adolescent and parent(s) and schedule follow-up visit. • If adolescent is obese, provide Step 2 counseling and refer to a comprehensive weight management program.	• Weigh and measure client at each visit. Calculate BMI based on height and weight measurements. • If overweight or obese, thoroughly assess diet and physical activity patterns and provide counseling as appropriate. • If overweight or obese, refer to primary health provider for full health assessment.
Blood lipids	• Refer adolescent with family history of premature heart disease, family history of dyslipidemia, or those who are overweight/obese to primary care provider and request a blood lipid panel. • Review blood lipid levels with adolescent and parent(s). Provide nutrition counseling as appropriate. • If adolescent is overweight, provide dietary counseling in accordance with Step 1. • If adolescent is obese, provide dietary counseling in accordance with Step 2 and refer to comprehensive weight management program. • The addition of plant sterols or stanols at no more than 2 g/day can be recommended for teens with familial hyperlipidemia. • If dietary management is not effective, refer to primary care provider for physical examination and management of dyslipidemia by medication as needed.	• Refer adolescent with family history of premature heart disease, family history of dyslipidemia, or those who are overweight/obese to primary care provider and request a blood lipid panel. • Review blood lipid levels with adolescent and parent(s). Provide nutrition counseling as appropriate. • If client is overweight or obese, provide dietary counseling as appropriate and refer to weight management program. • The addition of plant sterols or stanols at no more than 2 g/day can be recommended for clients with familial hyperlipidemia. • If dietary management is not effective, refer to primary care provider for physical examination and management of dyslipidemia by medication as needed.
Blood pressure	• Review blood pressure results with adolescent and parent(s). • Provide counseling in accordance with the DASH diet. Request follow-up visit. • If adolescent is overweight, provide dietary counseling in accordance with Step 1. • If adolescent is obese, provide dietary counseling in accordance with Step 2 and refer to comprehensive weight management program. • If dietary management is not effective, refer to primary care provider for physical examination and management of hypertension by medication as needed.	• Review blood pressure results with client. • Provide counseling in accordance with the DASH diet. Request follow-up visit. • If client is overweight or obese, provide dietary counseling as appropriate and refer to weight management program. • If dietary management is not effective, refer to primary care provider for physical examination and management of hypertension by medication as needed.
Diabetes	• Refer adolescent with family history of diabetes, signs of acanthosis nigricans, symptoms consistent with diabetes or those who are overweight/obese to a primary care provider and request a fasting blood glucose. • Review fasting blood glucose levels with adolescent and parent(s). Provide nutrition counseling as appropriate. • If adolescent is overweight, provide dietary counseling in accordance with Step 1. • If adolescent is obese, provide dietary counseling in accordance with Step 2 and refer to comprehensive weight management program.	• Refer client with family history of diabetes, signs of acanthosis nigricans, symptoms consistent with diabetes or those who are overweight/obese to primary care provider and request a fasting blood glucose. • Review fasting blood glucose levels with client. Provide nutrition counseling as appropriate. • If client is overweight or obese, provide dietary counseling and refer to comprehensive weight management program.
Physical activity	• Review physical activity pattern and behaviors with adolescent and parent(s). • Reinforce need for 60 min or more of moderate-to-vigorous physical activity per day. • Reinforce limiting sedentary and screen time to no more than 2 hours per day.	• Review physical activity pattern and behaviors with client. • Reinforce need for 60 min or more of moderate-to-vigorous physical activity each day. • Reinforce limiting sedentary and screen time to no more than 2 hours per day.

Adapted from U.S. Department of Health and Human Services (USDHHS), National Institutes of Health (NIH), National Heart, Lung and Blood Institute (NHLBI): *Expert panel on integrated guidelines for cardiovascular health and risk reduction in children and adolescents. Summary report,* NIH Publication No 12-7486A, October 2012.

TABLE 18-10   **Classification Criteria for the Diagnosis of Hyperlipidemia in Adolescents (10- to 19-years-old)***

	Acceptable	Borderline	Unacceptable
Total cholesterol (mg/dl)	≤170	170-199	≥200
LDL cholesterol (mg/dl)	<110	110-129	≥130
Non-HDL cholesterol (mg/dl)	<120	120-144	>145
HDL cholesterol (mg/dl)	>45	40-45	<40
Triglycerides (mg/dl)	<90	90-129	>130
Apolipoprotein A-1 (mg/dl)	>120	115-120	<115
Apolipoprotein B (mg/dl)	<90	90-109	>110

Adapted from U. S. Department of Health and Human Services (USDHHS), National Institutes of Health (NIH), National Heart, Lung and Blood Institute (NHLBI): *Expert panel on integrated guidelines for cardiovascular health and risk reduction in children and adolescents. Summary report,* NIH Publication No 12-7486A, October 2012.
HDL, High-density lipoprotein; *LDL,* low-density lipoprotein.
*Based on the average of two measurements.

(CDC, 2010). The prevalence of hyperlipidemia among adolescents varies according to adolescent weight status from 14% among normal weight to 22% among overweight and 43% among obese teens. The prevalence of low high-density lipoprotein (HDL) cholesterol and high triglyceride levels appeared to increase with age. Adolescent males were almost three times more likely to have low HDL cholesterol levels compared with females at any age. These youth are considered candidates for therapeutic lifestyle counseling with emphasis on nutrition and physical activity intervention.

The National Heart, Lung and Blood Institute (NHLBI) has recommended that all youth with elevated blood lipids be referred to a registered dietitian or nutritionist for medical nutrition therapy. The dietary recommendations for youth up to 21 years of age with elevated low-density lipoprotein (LDL) cholesterol are listed in Box 18-4, and those for elevated triglycerides and non-HDL cholesterol are listed in Box 18-5.

BOX 18-4   **Dietary Recommendations for Elevated Low-Density Lipoprotein Cholesterol in Adolescents**

- Limit total fat intake to no more than 25% to 30% of calories.
- Limit saturated fat intake to no more than 7% of calories.
- Dietary cholesterol intake should not exceed 200 mg/day.
- Plant sterol esters and/or stanol esters can replace usual fat intake up to 2 g/day for children with familial hypercholesterolemia.
- Up to 12 g of psyllium fiber can be added to the diet each day as cereal enriched with psyllium.
- At least 1 hour of moderate to vigorous exercise should be obtained daily.
- Sedentary and/or screen time should be limited to less than 2 hours each day.

Adapted from U.S. Department of Health and Human Services, National Institutes of Health, National Heart, Lung and Blood Institute: *Expert panel on integrated guidelines for cardiovascular health and risk reduction in children and adolescents. Summary report,* NIH Publication No 12-7486A, October 2012.

BOX 18-5   **Dietary Recommendations for Adolescents with Elevated Triglyceride or Non-High-Density Lipoprotein Cholesterol Levels**

- Limit total fat intake to no more than 25% to 30% of calories.
- Limit saturated fat intake to no more than 7% of calories.
- Reduce intake of added and natural sugars in the diet.
- Replace simple carbohydrates with complex carbohydrate and whole grains.
- Avoid sugar-sweetened beverages.
- Increase the intake of fish high in omega-3 fatty acids.

Adapted from U.S. Department of Health and Human Services, National Institutes of Health, National Heart, Lung and Blood Institute: *Expert panel on integrated guidelines for cardiovascular health and risk reduction in children and adolescents. Summary report,* NIH Publication No 12-7486A, October 2012.

National screening criteria for blood pressure levels among adolescents are listed in Tables 18-11and 18-12. Teenagers 17 years of age and younger are determined to have prehypertension if their average blood pressure readings fall between the 90th and 94th percentiles. Hypertension is diagnosed when the average of three blood pressure measurements exceed the 95th percentile for age, gender, and height.

Dietary counseling and weight management are integral components of hypertension treatment. The Dietary Approaches to Stop Hypertension (DASH) eating pattern has been shown to be effective in reducing blood pressure in many individuals (see Chapter 33 and Appendix 26). In addition to the DASH diet, teens with elevated blood pressure should be counseled to reduce sodium intake to less than 2000 mg/day and to achieve and maintain a healthy body weight.

The NHLBI has developed the CHILD 1 (Cardiovascular Health Integrated Lifestyle Diet) diet and nutrition guidelines which integrate dietary approaches to prevent hypertension, hyperlipidemia, and obesity (see Table 18-13). These guidelines include the DASH dietary guidelines as well as recommendations for upper limits for total and saturated fatty acids and dietary cholesterol intake. The CHILD 1 guidelines recommend the avoidance of sweetened beverages, limiting juice intake and increasing fiber intake to a level of 14 g/1000 kcal.

Metabolic syndrome is not well defined in the adolescent population, and therefore it is not consistently considered a separate risk factor for CVD. Rather it is considered to be a clustering of risk factors that, taken together, signal a need to intensify the depth and breadth of prevention measures that are recommended. It is estimated that between 2.0% and 9.4% of all U.S. adolescents have metabolic syndrome; the rates are much higher among obese teens, in whom they are estimated at 12.4% to 44.2% (U.S. Department of Health and Human Services [USDHHS], National Institutes of Health [NIH], NHLBI, 2012).

Diabetes

The exact prevalence of diabetes among adolescents is not known. Approximately 215,000 people under the age of 20 have diabetes, with the majority of the cases being type 1 diabetes (CDC, 2011). The CDC estimates that type 1 diabetes occurs in 1.7 per 1000 youth (younger than 19 years old) in the United States. Type 2 diabetes can be hard to detect in adolescents

TABLE 18-11 90th and 95th Percentiles for Blood Pressure for Adolescent Males by Height Percentiles

Age (years)	HEIGHT PERCENTILES* BP†	SYSTOLIC BP (MM HG)							DIASTOLIC BP (MM HG)						
		5%	10%	25%	50%	75%	90%	95%	5%	10%	25%	50%	75%	90%	95%
10	90th	111	112	114	115	117	119	119	73	73	74	75	76	77	78
	95th	115	116	117	119	121	122	123	77	78	79	80	81	81	82
11	90th	113	114	115	117	119	120	121	74	74	75	76	77	78	78
	95th	117	118	119	121	123	124	125	78	78	79	80	81	82	82
12	90th	115	116	118	120	121	123	123	74	75	75	76	77	78	79
	95th	119	120	122	123	125	127	127	78	79	80	81	82	82	83
13	90th	117	118	120	122	124	125	126	75	75	76	77	78	79	79
	95th	121	122	124	126	128	129	130	79	79	80	81	82	83	83
14	90th	120	121	123	125	126	128	128	75	76	77	78	79	79	80
	95th	124	125	127	128	130	132	132	80	80	81	82	83	84	84
15	90th	122	124	125	127	129	130	131	76	77	78	79	80	80	81
	95th	126	127	129	131	133	134	135	81	81	82	83	84	85	85
16	90th	125	126	128	130	131	133	134	78	78	79	80	81	82	82
	95th	129	130	132	134	135	137	137	82	83	83	84	85	86	87
17	90th	127	128	130	132	134	135	136	80	80	81	82	83	84	84
	95th	131	132	134	136	138	139	140	84	85	86	87	87	88	89

From National High Blood Pressure Education Program Working Group on High Blood Pressure in Children and Adolescents: Fourth report on the diagnosis, evaluation, and treatment of high blood pressure in children and adolescents, *Pediatrics* 114:555, 2004. This supplement is a work of the U.S. government, published in the public domain by the American Academy of Pediatrics. Available at http://pediatrics.aappublications.org/content/114/Supplement_2/555.full.pdf.

BP, Blood pressure.

*Height percentile determined by standard growth curves.

†Blood pressure percentile determined by a single measurement.

TABLE 18-12 90th and 95th Percentiles for Blood Pressure for Adolescent Females by Height Percentiles

Age (years)	HEIGHT PERCENTILES* BP†	SYSTOLIC BP (MM HG)							DIASTOLIC BP (MM HG)						
		5%	10%	25%	50%	75%	90%	95%	5%	10%	25%	50%	75%	90%	95%
10	90th	112	112	114	115	116	118	118	73	73	73	74	75	76	76
	95th	116	116	117	119	120	121	122	77	77	77	78	79	80	80
11	90th	114	114	116	117	118	119	120	74	74	74	75	76	77	77
	95th	118	118	119	121	122	123	124	78	78	78	79	80	81	81
12	90th	116	116	117	119	120	121	122	75	75	75	76	77	78	78
	95th	119	120	121	123	124	125	126	79	79	79	80	81	82	82
13	90th	117	118	119	121	122	123	124	76	76	76	77	78	79	79
	95th	121	122	123	124	126	127	128	80	80	80	81	82	83	83
14	90th	119	120	121	122	124	125	125	77	77	77	78	79	80	81
	95th	123	124	125	126	127	129	129	81	81	81	82	83	84	84
15	90th	120	121	122	123	125	126	127	78	78	78	79	80	81	81
	95th	124	125	126	127	129	130	131	82	82	82	83	84	85	86
16	90th	121	122	123	124	126	127	128	78	78	79	80	81	81	82
	95th	125	126	127	128	130	131	132	82	82	83	84	85	85	86
17	90th	122	122	123	125	126	127	128	78	79	79	80	81	81	82
	95th	125	126	127	129	130	131	132	82	83	83	84	85	85	86

From National High Blood Pressure Education Program Working Group on High Blood Pressure in Children and Adolescents: Fourth report on the diagnosis, evaluation, and treatment of high blood pressure in children and adolescents, *Pediatrics* 114:555, 2004. This supplement is a work of the U.S. government, published in the public domain by the American Academy of Pediatrics. Available at http://pediatrics.aappublications.org/content/114/Supplement_2/555.full.pdf.

BP, Blood pressure.

*Height percentile determined by standard growth curves.

†Blood pressure percentile determined by a single measurement.

because they may show no symptoms and even when they do, differentiating between type 1 and type 2 can be difficult. Adolescents who are diagnosed with type 2 diabetes usually have a strong family history for diabetes and are obese. Recommendations for type 2 diabetes screening are listed in Box 18-6. The risk of type 2 diabetes among adolescents varies among racial/ethnic groups with 15- to 19-year-old American Indian youth having the highest rates (4.5/1000 among all U.S. American Indian youth; 50.9/1000 among Pima Indian youth). The prevention of type 2 diabetes includes following the CHILD 1 dietary guidelines and additional physical activity at a level to reduce body weight (USDHHS, NIH, NHLBI, 2012).

TABLE 18-13 Cardiovascular Health Integrated Lifestyle Diet (CHILD 1) Recommendations, Ages 11 to 21 Years

Fat-free unflavored milk should be the primary beverage consumed.

Sugar-sweetened beverages should be limited or avoided.

Water intake should be encouraged.

A range of 25% to 30% of daily energy needs should come from total fatty acids.

No more than 8% to 10% of daily energy needs should come from saturated fatty acids.

Monounsaturated and polyunsaturated fatty acids should provide no more than 20% of daily energy intake.

Trans fatty acids should be avoided.

Dietary cholesterol intake should not exceed 300 mg/day.

Foods high in dietary fiber should be encouraged.

A goal of 14 g of dietary fiber per 1000 kcal should be encouraged.

Intake of naturally sweetened juices (no added sugar) should be limited to 4 to 6 oz/day.

Sodium intake should be limited.

Breakfast should be eaten each day.

Family meals should be encouraged.

Fast food meals should be limited.

The use of the Dietary Approaches to Stop Hypertension eating plan should be encouraged.

Energy intake should be based on estimated energy requirements and adjusted for growth and physical activity as needed.

Adapted from U.S. Department of Health and Human Services (USDHHS), National Institutes of Health (NIH), National Heart, Lung and Blood Institute (NHLBI): *Expert panel on integrated guidelines for cardiovascular health and risk reduction in children and adolescents. Summary report*, NIH Publication No 12-7486A, October 2012.

BOX 18-6 Recommendations for Screening Adolescents for Type 2 Diabetes Mellitus

Youth who are overweight or obese and exhibit two of the following risk factors are at high risk:

- First- or second-degree relative with a history of type 2 diabetes
- Member of a racial/ethnic group considered at higher risk (American Indian, African American, Latino, Asian American/Pacific Islander)
- Dyslipidemia
- Hypertension
- Acanthosis nigricans
- Polycystic ovary syndrome

Screening should begin at age 10 or the onset of puberty, whichever occurs first.

Screening should occur every 2 years.

Adapted from U.S. Department of Health and Human Services, National Institutes of Health, National Heart, Lung and Blood Institute: *Expert panel on integrated guidelines for cardiovascular health and risk reduction in children and adolescents. Summary report*, NIH Publication No 12-7486A, October 2012.

Physical Activity

National recommendations for physical activity suggest that all youth should be active at least 60 minutes each day, including participation in vigorous activity at least 3 days each week (USDHHS, Physical Activity Guidelines Steering Committee, 2008). In addition, muscle-strengthening and bone-strengthening activities should each be included in the 60 minutes of physical activity at least three times a week. However, many youths do not meet these recommendations. Only half of U.S. high school students report being physically active for at least 60 minutes per day on 5 days or more per week, with males nearly twice as likely to meet these recommendations as females (Eaton et al, 2012).

Teenage athletes have unique nutrient needs. Adequate fluid intake to prevent dehydration is especially critical for young athletes. Young adolescents are at higher risk for dehydration because they produce more heat during exercise but have less ability to transfer heat from the muscles to the skin. They also sweat less, which decreases their capacity to dissipate heat through the evaporation of the sweat (see Chapter 23).

Athletes who participate in sports that use competitive weight categories or emphasize body weight are at elevated risk for the development of disordered eating behaviors. A concern among female athletes is the female athlete triad relationship, a constellation of low body weight and inadequate body fat levels, amenorrhea, and osteoporosis (see Chapter 23). The female athlete triad may lead to premature bone loss, decreased bone density, increased risk of stress fractures, and eventual infertility (Javed, 2013). Nutrition assessment and education for teenage athletes should focus on obtaining adequate energy, macronutrients, and micronutrients to meet the needs for growth and development and to maintain a healthy body weight. The use of anabolic agents (such as steroids or insulin) and other ergogenic supplements also should be included in nutrition screening. Survey data suggest the use of muscle-enhancing substances should be a concern for adolescent males and females; one study found that steroids were used by 6% of males and 5% of females, whereas other substances such as creatine and growth hormone were used by 10% of males and 5% of females (Eisenberg et al, 2012).

Pregnancy

Although birth rates among females 15 to 19 years have declined over the past few decades and reached a low of 29.4 births per 1000 adolescents in 2012, adolescent pregnancy remains a significant public health issue (Hamilton et al, 2013). Adolescent females who become pregnant are at particularly high risk for nutritional deficiencies because of elevated nutrient needs. Pregnant adolescents with a gynecologic age (the number of years between the onset of menses and current age) of less than 4 and those who are undernourished at the time of conception have the greatest nutritional needs. As with adult women, pregnant teens require additional folic acid, iron, zinc, and other micronutrients to support fetal growth (see Chapter 15). Calcium and vitamin D are also important nutrients in pregnancy, because both are necessary for growth and development of the adolescent mother and fetus (Young et al, 2012). Pregnant teens should have a full nutrition assessment done early in pregnancy to determine any nutrient deficiencies and to promote adequate weight gain. Weight gain recommendations for pregnancy are listed in Table 15-11 in Chapter 15. Referral to appropriate food assistance programs such as the Special Supplemental Nutrition Program for Women, Infants and Children is an important part of prenatal nutrition education.

CLINICAL CASE STUDY

Cherise is an 18-year-old girl and high school senior who saw a nurse at the school-based clinic. While taking her medical history, the school nurse noted that Cherise had frequent headaches and fatigue. Cherise's blood pressure reading fell into the 92nd percentile. The school nurse referred her to a local community clinic for a more thorough evaluation.

A physician's assistant (PA) at the community clinic took a social history and performed a physical examination on Cherise. An SMR stage of 5 was noted. The PA noted that Cherise's BMI was at the 94th percentile for her age and gender. Her blood pressure registered at the 94th percentile. The family history revealed a strong family history of cardiovascular disease, diabetes and renal disease. Cherise thought her father may be taking medication for his cholesterol and blood pressure, but reported no health issues for her mother. No signs of acanthosis nigricans were noted on the physical examination.

Laboratory results show that Cherise had elevated total, non-HDL, and LDL cholesterol levels along with a marginally low HDL level. The liver enzyme and blood glucose values were at the upper end of normal. A referral was made for Cherise to see a registered dietitian/nutritionist for diet and exercise counseling.

The outpatient dietitian/nutritionist (RDN) reviewed Cherise's medical history, confirmed her family history of cardiovascular disease, and measured her height and weight. Cherise's BMI value plotted at the 94th percentile. The RDN completed a 24-hour dietary recall with Cherise, beginning with the last thing she had eaten that day and working backward to facilitate a complete and accurate recall. The RDN also inquired about usual dietary patterns and physical activity as well as the presence of any food allergies/intolerances and avoidances.

Cherise reported that she usually skipped breakfast because she didn't have time to eat in the morning, but she often buys a caramel macchiato from the school store at 7:15 AM. The first food Cherise ate most days was usually a snack from the vending machine at 10:30 AM, which consisted of a granola bar or a bag of chips and a juice drink. Occasionally she would purchase a la carte lunches of tacos or a burger, but generally she skipped lunch. Cherise was out of school at 2 pm each day, at which time she went to work as a clothing sales clerk at the local mall. She had a half-hour break in the late afternoon or early evening, when she would go to the food court for dinner. Her evening meal usually consisted of one to two slices of pepperoni pizza, two tacos, or one to two pieces of fried chicken with a soft drink. About half of the time she also ordered fries or nachos. When Cherise returned home from work at 10:15 PM, she usually had a snack of ice cream, tortilla chips, spicy cheese puffs, or microwave popcorn while doing her homework. A large glass of juice or lemonade usually accompanied her snack. On weekends, Cherise worked as many hours at the mall as she could, often meeting friends for pizza or fast food on her nights off. Her physical activity consisted of walking between the house and bus stop in the morning and evening, walking around school between classes and being on her feet in the evenings at her sales job.

The RDN counseled Cherise regarding a healthy diet and physical activity. A follow-up visit was scheduled 4 weeks in the future.

Cherise did not return to see the RDN for her follow-up appointment and did not keep her follow-up appointments with the PA. Five months later, she returned to see the PA at which time her health status was reassessed. Cherise's blood pressure was still at the 94th percentile and her BMI now at the 95th percentile,. When questioned about her dietary habits and physical activity, Cherise reported that she had tried to follow the recommendations of the RDN but found it hard because of time constraints. She reported that she wanted to lose weight and thought she could do this because she would graduate in a few weeks and would have more time to devote to exercise and cooking. The PA suggested she see the RDN again for more dietary and physical activity counseling.

The RDN reviewed the previous dietary recommendations with Cherise and suggested she attend the clinic's 12-week weight management program. Cherise attended the first five sessions of the program, then stopped. She had lost 12 pounds during the five sessions. Several months later Cherise was once again seen by the PA. Her blood pressure continued to be elevated and her BMI was plotted at the 94th percentile. When questioned about the weight loss program, Cherise reported that her mother had changed jobs and lost her health insurance benefits, so she could no longer participate in the program. The RDN connected Cherise with the local YMCA, which offered a weight management program for adults on a sliding fee scale. Five months later Cherise's BMI was assessed at 26.8 and a weight loss of 19 pounds from previous levels was noted.

Nutrition Diagnostic Statements

1. Excessive energy intake as evidenced by dietary history and BMI at 94th %tile. (NI-1.3)
2. Excessive fat intake as evidenced from dietary history. (NI – 5.6.2)
3. Obesity as evidenced by BMI of 94th %tile. (NC 3.3.1)
4. Limited adherence to nutrition-related recommendations as evidenced by BMI up 1%tile at followup visit. (NB-1.6)

Nutrition Care Questions

1. How would you classify Cherise's blood pressure based on the reading at the school nurses office?
2. How would you classify Cherise's weight based on the readings at the first visit at the community clinic? Based on this classification, what laboratory tests would you order to be consistent with the NHLBI recommendations?
3. What type of diet should the RDN recommend Cherise follow, based on her blood pressure, weight and laboratory results?
4. What specific strategies would be beneficial for the RDN to recommend to Cherise regarding improving her dietary intake?
5. What strategies would you recommend for Cherise to change her level of physical activity?
6. Based on the staged treatment recommendations for weight, what type of program would the RDN recommend for Cherise?

USEFUL WEBSITES

American Academy of Pediatrics: Media and Children
http://www.aap.org/en-us/advocacy-and-policy/aap-health-initiatives/Pages/Media-and-Children.aspx
American Alliance for Health, Physical Education, Recreation and Dance (Society of Health and Physical Educators, SHAPE America)
http://www.shapeamerica.org
American School Health Association
www.ashaweb.org
Bright Futures
www.brightfutures.org
Centers for Disease Control and Prevention
www.cdc.gov

Let's Move!
www.letsmove.gov
National Collegiate Athletics Association
www.ncaa.org
National Eating Disorder Association
www.nationaleatingdisorders.org
School Nutrition Association
www.schoolnutrition.org
U.S. Department of Agriculture: Choose MyPlate
www.choosemyplate.gov
Vegetarian Resource Group
www.vrg.org

REFERENCES

American Psychiatric Association: *Diagnostic and statistical manual of mental disorders*, ed 5, Arlington, VA, 2013, American Psychiatric Association. www.dsm.psychiatryonline.org. Accessed January 10, 2014.

Berge JM, Arikian A, Doherty WJ, et al: Healthful eating and physical activity in the home environment: results from multi-family focus groups, *J Nutr Educ* 44:123, 2012.

Berge JM, Wall M, Hsueh TF, et al: The protective role of family meals for youth obesity: 10-year longitudinal associations, *J Pediatr* 166:296, 2015.

Blakemore SJ, Robbins TW: Decision-making in the adolescent brain, *Nat Neurosci* 15:1184, 2012.

Branum AM, Rossen LM, Schoendorf KC: Trends in caffeine intake among U.S. children and adolescents, *Pediatrics* 133:386, 2014.

Burris J, Rietkerk W, Woolf K: Acne: the role of medical nutrition therapy, *J Acad Nutr Diet* 113:416, 2013.

Burris J, Rietkerk W, Woolf K: Relationships of self-reported dietary factors and perceived acne severity in a cohort of New York young adults, *J Acad Nutr Diet* 114:384, 2014.

Centers for Disease Control and Prevention: *National diabetes fact sheet: national estimates and general information on diabetes and prediabetes in the United States, 2011* (website), 2011. http://www.cdc.gov/diabetes/pubs/pdf/ndfs_2011.pdf. Accessed February 2, 2013.

Centers for Disease Control and Prevention: Prevalence of abnormal lipid levels among youths—United States, 1999–2006, *MMWR Morb Mortal Wkly Rep* 59(2):29, 2010.

Child Trends: *Family meals: indicators on children and youth* (website), 2013. http://www.childtrends.org/wp-content/uploads/2012/09/96_Family_Meals.pdf. Accessed December 23, 2013.

Craig WJ, Mangels AR, American Dietetic Association: Position of the American Dietetic Association: vegetarian diets, *J Am Diet Assoc* 109:1266, 2009.

De la Hunty A, Gibson S, Ashwell M: Does regular breakfast cereal consumption help children and adolescents stay slimmer? A systematic review and meta-analysis, *Obes Facts* 6:70, 2013.

Deshmukh-Taskar PR, Nicklas TA, O'Neil CE, et al: The relationship of breakfast skipping and type of breakfast consumption with nutrient intake and weight status in children and adolescents: the National Health and Nutrition Examination Survey 1999-2006, *J Am Diet Assoc* 110:869, 2010.

Dwyer J, Nahin RL, Rogers GT, et al: Prevalence and predictors of children's dietary supplement use: the 2007 National Health Interview Survey, *Am J Clin Nutr* 97:1331, 2013.

Eaton DK, Kann L, Kinchen S, et al: Youth risk behavior surveillance—United States, 2011, *MMWR Surveill Summ* 61(4):1, 2012.

Eisenberg ME, Wall M, Neumark-Sztainer D, et al: Muscle-enhancing behaviors among adolescent girls and boys, *Pediatrics* 130:1019, 2012.

Federal Trade Commission: *A review of food marketing to children and adolescents: follow-up report*, Washington, DC, 2012, Federal Trade Commission.

Forsyth A, Wall M, Larson N, et al: Do adolescents who live or go to school near fast-food restaurants eat more frequently from fast-food restaurants? *Health Place* 18:1261, 2012.

Fox MK, Gordon A, Nogales R, et al: Availability and consumption of competitive foods in US public schools, *J Am Diet Assoc* 109:S57, 2009.

Fox MK: *School nutrition dietary assessment study IV, Volume I: school food service operations, school environments, and meals offered and served*, Alexandria, VA, 2012, U.S. Department of Agriculture, Food and Nutrition Service, Office of Research and Analysis.

Fulkerson JA, Larson N, Horning M, et al: A review of associations between family or shared meal frequency and dietary and weight status outcomes across the lifespan, *J Nutr Educ Behav* 46:2, 2014.

Ganji V, Zhang X, Tangpricha V: Serum 25-hydroxyvitamin D concentrations and prevalence estimates of hypovitaminosis D in the U.S. population based on assay-adjusted data, *J Nutr* 142:498, 2012.

Gellar L, Druker S, Osganian SK, et al: Exploratory research to design a school nurse-delivered intervention to treat adolescent overweight and obesity, *J Nutr Educ Behav* 44:46, 2012.

Hagan JF, editors: *Bright futures: guidelines for health supervision of infants, children, and adoelscents*, ed 3, Elk Grove Village, Il, 2008, American Academy of Pediatrics.

Hamilton BE, Martin JA, Ventura JS: *Natl Vital Stat Rep 62:3: Births: preliminary data for 2012* (website), 2013. http://www.cdc.gov/nchs/data/nvsr/nvsr62/nvsr62_03.pdf. Accessed February 1, 2014.

Han E, Powell LM: Consumption patterns of sugar-sweetened beverages in the United States, *J Acad Nutr Diet* 113:43, 2013.

Hoelscher DM, Kirk S, Ritchie L, et al: Position of the Academy of Nutrition and Dietetics: interventions for the prevention and treatment of pediatric overweight and obesity, *J Acad Nutr Diet* 113:1375, 2013.

Holick MF, Binkley NC, Bischoff-Ferrari HA, et al: Evaluation, treatment, and prevention of vitamin D deficiency: an Endocrine Society clinical practice guidelines, *J Clin Endocrinol Metab* 96:1911, 2011.

Holt K, editors: *Bright futures nutrition*, ed 3, Elk Grove Village, Il, 2011, American Academy of Pediatrics.

Hoyland A, Dye L, Lawton CL: A systematic review of the effect of breakfast on the cognitive performance of children and adolescents, *Nutr Res Rev* 22:220, 2009.

Institute of Medicine (IOM): *Dietary reference intakes: the essential guide to nutrient requirements*, Washington, DC, 2006, National Academies Press.

Institute of Medicine (IOM): *Dietary reference intakes for calcium and vitamin D*, Washington, DC, 2011, The National Academies Press.

Javed A, Tebben PJ, Fischer PR, et al: Female athlete triad and its components: toward improved screening and management, *Mayo Clin Proc* 88:996, 2013.

Keast DR, Fulgoni VL 3rd, Nicklas TA, et al: Food sources of energy and nutrients among children in the United States: National Health and Nutrition Examination Survey 2003–2006, *Nutrients* 5:283, 2013.

Kelly AS, Barlow SE, Rao G, et al: Severe obesity in children and adolescents: identification, associated health risks, and treatment approaches: a scientific statement from the American Heart Association, *Circulation* 128:1689, 2013.

Krebs NF, Himes JH, Jacobson D, et al: Assessment of child and adolescent overweight and obesity, *Pediatrics* 120(Suppl 4):S193, 2007.

Larson N, MacLehose R, Fulkerson JA, et al: Eating breakfast and dinner together as a family: associations with sociodemographic characteristics and implications for diet quality and weight status, *J Acad Nutr Diet* 113:1601, 2013.

Larson N, Story M: A review of snacking patterns among U.S. children and adolescents: what are the implications of snacking for weight status? *Child Obes* 9:104, 2013.

Ma NS, Gordon CM: The truth about vitamin D and adolescent skeletal health, *Adolesc Med State Art Rev* 23:457, 2012.

Moore LL, Singer MR, Qureshi MM, et al: Food group intake and micronutrient adequacy in adolescent girls, *Nutrients* 4:1692, 2012.

Neumark-Sztainer D, Larson NI, Fulkerson JA, et al: Family meals and adolescents: what have we learned from Project EAT (Eating Among Teens), *Public Health Nutr* 13:1113, 2010.

Neumark-Sztainer D, Wall MM, Larson N, et al: Secular trends in weight status and weight-related attitudes and behaviors in adolescents from 1999 to 2010, *Prev Med* 54:77, 2012.

Ogden CL, Carroll MD, Kit BK, et al: Prevalence of obesity and trends in body mass index among US children and adolescents, 1999–2010, *JAMA* 307:483, 2012.

Ozier AD, Henry BW, American Dietetic Association: Position of the American Dietetic Association: nutrition intervention in the treatment of eating disorders, *J Am Diet Assoc* 111:1236, 2011.

Pinkney J, Streeter A, Hosking J, et al: Adiposity, chronic inflammation and the prepubertal decline of sex hormone binding globulin in children: evidence for associations with the timing of puberty, *J Clin Endocrin Met* 99:3224, 2014.

Poti JM, Slining MM, Popkin BM: Where are kids getting their empty calories? Stores, schools, and fast-food restaurants each played an important role in empty calorie intake among US children during 2009-2010, *J Acad Nutr Diet* 114:908, 2014.

Poulton AS, Melzer E, Tait PR, et al: Growth and pubertal development of adolescent boys on stimulant medication for attention deficit hyperactivity disorder, *Med J Aust* 198:29, 2013.

Powell L, Harris JL, Fox T: Food marketing expenditures aimed at youth: putting the numbers in context, *Am J Prev Med* 45:453, 2013.

Powell L, Szczypka G, Chaloupka FJ: Trends in exposure to television food advertisements among children and adolescents in the United States, *Arch Pediatr Adolesc Med* 164:794, 2010.

Ranjit N, Evans MH, Byrd-Williams C, et al: Dietary and activity correlates of sugar-sweetened beverage consumption among adolescents, *Pediatrics* 126:e754, 2010.

Reilly JJ, Kelly J: Long-term impact of overweight and obesity in childhood and adolescence on morbidity and premature mortality in adulthood: systematic review, *Int J Obes* 35:891, 2011.

Rideout VJ, Henry J: *Generation M2: media in the lives of 8- to 18-year-olds*, Menlo Park, CA, 2012, Kaiser Family Foundation.

Robinson-O'Brien R, Perry CL, Wall MM, et al: Adolescent and young adult vegetarianism: better dietary intake and weight outcomes but increased risk of disordered eating behaviors, *J Am Diet Assoc* 109:648, 2009.

Rosenfield RL, Lipton RB, Drum ML: Thelarche, pubarche and menarche attainment in children with normal and elevated body mass index, *Pediatrics* 123:84, 2009.

Seifert SM, Schaechter JL, Hershorin ER, et al: Health effects of energy drinks on children, adolescents, and young adults, *Pediatrics* 127:511, 2011.

Slining MM, Popkin BM: Trends in intakes and sources of solid fats and added sugars among U.S. children and adolescents: 1994–2010, *Pediatr Obes* 8:307, 2013.

Steinberg L: *Adolescence*, ed 9, 2010, McGraw-Hill Higher Education.

Steinhausen HC: Outcome of eating disorders, *Child Adolesc Psych Clin N Am* 18:225, 2009.

Tanner J: *Growth at adolescence*. Oxford, 1962, Blackwell Scientific Publications.

Terry-McElrath YM, O'Malley PM, Johnston LD: Energy drinks, soft drinks, and substance use among United States secondary school students, *J Addict Med* 8:6, 2014.

U.S. Department of Agriculture (USDA), Agricultural Research Service (ARS): *Breakfast: percentages of selected nutrients contributed by foods eaten at breakfast, by gender and age. What we eat in America, NHANES 2009-2010* (website), 2012a. www.ars.usda.gov/ba/bhnrc/fsrg. Accessed December 23, 2013.

U.S. Department of Agriculture (USDA), Agricultural Research Service (ARS): *Nutrient Intakes from food: mean amounts consumed per individual, by gender and age. What we eat in America, NHANES 2009–2010* (website), 2012b. www.ars.usda.gov/ba/bhnrc/fsrg. Accessed December 29, 2013.

U.S. Department of Agriculture (USDA), Agricultural Research Service (ARS): *Snacks: distribution of snack occasions, by gender and age. What we eat in America, NHANES 2009–2010* (website), 2012c. www.ars.usda.gov/ba/bhnrc/fsrg. Accessed December 23, 2013.

U.S. Department of Agriculture (USDA), Agricultural Research Service (ARS): Snacks: percentages of selected nutrients contributed by foods eaten at *snack occasions, by gender and age. What we eat in America, NHANES 2009–2010* (website), 2012d. www.ars.usda.gov/ba/bhnrc/fsrg. Accessed December 23, 2013.

U.S. Department of Health and Human Services (USDHHS), National Institutes of Health (NIH), National Heart, Lung and Blood Institute (NHLBI): *Expert panel on integrated guidelines for cardiovascular health and risk reduction in children and adolescents*, October 2012. Summary report. NIH Publication No 12-7486A.

U.S. Department of Health and Human Services (USDHHS), Physical Activity Guidelines Steering Committee: *2008 physical activity guidelines for Americans* (website), 2008. www.health.gov/paguidelines. Accessed February 1, 2014.

Wu CH, Wang CC, Kennedy J: The prevalence of herb and dietary supplement use among children and adolescents in the United States: results from the 2007 National Health Interview Survey, *Complement Ther Med* 21: 358, 2013.

Young BE, McNanley TJ, Cooper EM, et al: Maternal vitamin D status and calcium intake interact to affect fetal skeletal growth in utero in pregnant adolescents, *Am J Clin Nutr* 95:1103, 2012.

19

Nutrition in the Adult Years

Judith L. Dodd, MS, RDN, LDN, FAND

KEY TERMS

consumer price index (CPI)
detoxification
food desert
food security
functional foods
health-related quality of life (HRQOL)

isoflavones
metabolic syndrome
nutritional genomics
phytochemicals
phytoestrogens
phytonutrients

prebiotics
premenstrual syndrome (PMS)
probiotics
wellness

This chapter emphasizes the background and tools for encouraging adults to set nutrition-related lifestyle goals that promote positive health and reduce risk factors. Other chapters of this text provide a focus on the present and potential role of medical nutrition therapy (MNT) on prevention and intervention for major chronic diseases and conditions that affect food and nutrition choices in the adult years, such as cardiovascular disease (CVD), diabetes, cancer, weight control, and osteoporosis. Added to these are health-related conditions such as arthritis, Alzheimer's disease, renal disease, and inflammatory-related conditions, which research is indicating may have a link to lifestyle and food and nutrition choices. Although these links are mentioned here, other chapters and ongoing research provide the core of information. The focus of this chapter is that the adult years are a time for nutrition and dietetics professionals to be leaders and team members helping adults achieve and maintain positive health. The goals for Healthy People 2010 and 2020 provide the framework (Centers for Disease Control and Prevention [CDC], 2011c, 2013b). The evidence is convincing that decisions for a healthy lifestyle must be early in life to build the road for health promotion and disease prevention (Academy of Nutrition and Dietetics [AND], 2013b).

SETTING THE STAGE: NUTRITION IN THE ADULT YEARS

This chapter focuses on nutrition and food-related behaviors for the years after adolescence but before one is deemed an "older adult," often defined as age 65, based on traditional retirement age. Admittedly this is a wide range of ages, and, like all population groups, the adult years are heterogeneous. The description of what constitutes being an "older adult" is in constant flux as people change their retirement age, as life expectancy projections are adjusted and as medical science and lifestyle alterations extend life spans and opportunities for an optimum quality of life. A life expectancy of 80 and above is a reality backed up by Centers for Disease Control statistics with life expectancy in 2013 at 78.8 (CDC, 2013a). Evidence

continues to indicate that the adult years set the framework for quality of life as well as life expectancy. Nutrition and food-related behaviors are key factors, and the earlier prevention becomes the goal, the better the outcome (AND, 2013b).

The dietary reference intakes (DRIs) on the inside cover of this text provide an overview of the nutrient recommendations for age groups under the DRI umbrella. Staying current on changes in DRI is a critical part of the dietetics and nutrition professionals tools because changes are made as research is validated (Institute of Medicine [IOM], National Academy of Sciences [NAS], 1984-2004). Nutrient needs in the adult life cycle are similar but, as in all life stages, are affected by gender, state of health, genetics, medications, and lifestyle choices such as eating behaviors, smoking, and activity. These are markers, determined through assessment, that a nutrition and health professional can use to determine this population's needs. Other markers are less evident and include the adult's perceptions of quality of life and motivation in the areas of nutrition and health.

When the objectives are prevention and behavior change, such markers become critical. Research continues to indicate that positive changes at any age and lifestyle behaviors can make a difference in total health and life expectancy. Making these changes early in life, rather than later, and maintaining them throughout the adult years should be goals. Genetics always has been a consideration in assessment of nutrition status and life potential, but the evolving science of nutritional genomics has become an important marker in nutrition and dietetics practice (AND, 2014b).

SETTING THE STAGE: MESSAGES

A first step for nutrition and dietetics professionals is to recognize that many adults are prime targets for nutrition and health information that offers positive guidance that is understandable and implementable. However, this translates into growing evidence that adults can be willing targets for misinformation and guidance based on promises and quick-fixes rather than evidence-based MNT. Rebekah Nagler, PhD, studied the potential role of consumer reaction to what appeared to be contradictory nutrition information or guidance. According to Nagler, confusion and backlash may make people more likely to ignore not only the contradictory information but also the widely accepted nutritional advice such as eating more fruits and vegetables. Nagler also noted that those with the greatest exposure to contradictory information expressed the most confusion with nutrition (Nagler, 2014).

As with any group, adults must be approached with strategies and guidance that fit their health and education needs as well as their capability to implement them. An appreciation that research constantly is altering and changing should be firmly fixed in the minds of the messenger (the nutrition professional) and the receiver (the patient or client). It is the role of the nutrition professional to verify messaging, separating current evidence based messages from those based on preliminary or single studies. What is reported as news or guidance to the consumer may appear to be contradictory to current practice when in fact the basis is preliminary research rather than evidence based.

The challenge to nutrition and dietetics professionals is staying current on research and guidelines while acknowledging the potential motivations of their audience or clients and their sources of their information. In a technologically savvy world with instant access to nutrition and health advice by self-proclaimed as well as credentialed professionals, this becomes even more of a challenge.

The Academy of Nutrition and Dietetics (AND, formerly American Dietetic Association, or ADA) Trends surveys have set the stage for communication. These surveys included a representative sampling of adult Americans with a focus on food, nutrition, and activity messages and consumers' reactions to these messages. Because this survey was conducted every 2 years for 12 years and was repeated in 2008 and 2011, Trends provides a snapshot of evolving attitudes about the importance of nutrition, activity, and sources of information. Trends 2008 indicated that respondents noted they were making positive steps to meeting nutrition and activity guidelines (AND, 2008). The 2011 snapshot indicated a slight drop in the number of respondents who already had made changes or identified that they should make changes. Many of the remaining questions provided clues that for some adults, reaching health goals was difficult (AND, 2011).

Like the Trends information, other surveys support the idea that adults are seeking nutrition information and using it to make positive lifestyle changes but are finding that making these changes is a challenge. Time, lack of willpower, apparent mixed messages, and identifying the efficacy of the messages are cited as barriers (International Food Information Council [IFIC], 2013). The 2015 IFIC Foundation Food and Health Survey continued with identifying barriers and noted that consumer confusion is emerging as a key concern. Of interest is the remark that consumers are wanting to hear "what to eat" rather than what to avoid (IFIC, 2015). Although women continue to lead men in these efforts, the influence of men is growing in such areas as wellness initiatives, meal planning, and shopping with health in mind. According to the ADA/AND's Trends survey, half of consumers believe they are already doing what they can to achieve balanced nutrition and a healthy diet. Younger adults were less likely than older adults to rate diet and nutrition as "very important," whereas exercise and physical activity were rated as important across the life cycle. Reasons for not adjusting their diet or exercise patterns were satisfaction with their current health and nutrition status and concerns they would have to eliminate foods they like. For those interested in changing their beliefs and behaviors, time limitations, lack of practical information, and unclear guidelines were noted (AND, 2008, 2011).

Another helpful tool for reaching adults is to review the influences of behavior and knowledge on nutrition and health. A review of the health and nutrition information in the media reinforces the idea that nutrition and health information is popular. However, consumers are selective about their personal concerns and their source of information. The International Food Information Council (IFIC) Foundation Food and Health Surveys 2013 and 2015 noted that more than half of Americans state they are trying to lose weight and reported making changes in the types and amounts of food eaten. Changes included eating more fruits and vegetables (82%), drinking more water or low- or no-calorie beverages(76%), including more whole grains (70%), reducing the choice of foods higher in sugar or added sugars (69%) , and consuming smaller portions (68%). The 2015 study also indicated a move away from processed foods especially in higher income groups (IFIC, 2013, 2014, 2015).

The interest in nutrition and in food continues to be evident in the adult years. Popular literature demonstrates a growing interest in cooking, cookbooks, supermarket RDs, grocery store and farm-to-table events, and other "foodie" behavior (see Box 19-1).

Messages regarding the potential benefits and risks of certain foods and nutrients are being heard by consumers. These include messages on the negative effect of saturated fat, trans fatty acids, and sodium. According to Elizabeth Sloan, there is a re-orienting of priorities and behaviors that puts healthfulness as a major driver for both the consumer and the producer. More consumers are looking for "healthful foods" thus increasing the demand for creating and marketing foods that fit this image (Sloan, 2010). Food companies are changing products to reflect a more health-promoting choice, and restaurants are following this lead. However, a study on energy and sodium contents of menu items in U.S. chain restaurants concluded that industry marketing that indicated healthier options was balanced by

---

BOX 19-1 Buying the Dream

A cadre of "foodies" is developing at all age levels but is a tracked trend in the millennials; those who reached adulthood around the year 2000. Evidence of this phenomenon includes the sale of cookbooks, the number of chef and other food-centered shows on television and the Internet, and even the types of food now offered in restaurants. This interest in food has reached the big screen and TV reruns with the movie "Julie and Julia" in 2009 and "Chef" in 2014. There are Internet sites that advise on how to publish your own cookbook and many apps to download on your phone or computer related to food and nutrition. The social media site, Pinterest, has an overwhelming number of users interested in food, recipes and food culture. Popular high-end grocery stores are hiring RDN's to do store tours and cooking classes. Farm cooperatives are hiring outreach staff who may also be dietitians. Check your local area for the list of cooking classes, community kitchens, supermarket RDNs, and food demonstrations, or take a look at the number of cookbooks, food and recipe links accessible from the Web. The challenge to the nutrition and food professional is to be a player and aim to be a leader.

simultaneous less-healthy changes in menu choices. For example, as lower-calorie options were offered, the appetizer menu added more fried foods to dip in high-sodium sauces with the featured drinks. The conclusion was there was no meaningful change in energy and sodium content in main entrées in a 1-year (2010-2011) time period (Wu and Sturm, 2014).

The nutrition and dietetics professional can be a positive influence in advocating and educating for meaningful and real changes in the food supply with a focus on prevention. However, there must be a consumer-driven effort to support these changes. To be a leader, or at least a player, the nutrition and dietetics professional must be aware of community resources and influences, available food sources, and changing food behaviors.

INFORMATION SOURCES

Where consumers get their information is another factor to consider. The source and the appeal of the message affect how realistic and meaningful information is to the consumer. However, the scientific value and the application of evidence-based information vary. To the adult consumer, the promise of specific benefit is more important than the standard "it's good for you" message, and the scientific validity of the message may not be the determining point.

Sources of information have continued to change. Traditional print sources continue to decline as digital and electronic sources increase. The 2013 Trends study noted a gain in consumers use of the internet for information of +16 points, bringing the Internet into a position similar to magazines (see Box 19-2).

Use of phones for digital applications, or "apps," is a growing trend and so is creating, marketing, and evaluating apps. The Academy of Nutrition and Dietetics website includes ratings on apps for nutrition and dietetics as do other sites aimed at professionals and consumers. Future studies likely will look at the Internet and related links as major information sources (AND, 2014a).

Regarding believable human sources of nutrition information, health professionals, including registered dietitians, doctors, and nurses, continue to be rated as the most credible (IFIC, 2014, 2015). However, when consumers were asked about the factors that affect their willingness to believe new food and health information, others in their environment including family and friends were named as potential influencers (see Box 19-3).

Surveys have shown an increase in the number of consumers familiar with My Plate and in those who use food labels, shelf information, and other tools (AND, 2011; IFIC, 2013, 2014, 2015). Popular literature indicates a growing segment of the population interested in food, cooking, cookbooks, and "foodie" behavior. The Nutrition Facts Panel and other label information influence nutrition and food decisions, but there may be gaps in the interpretation. The growing lists of ingredients, unknown terminology, changing ingredients, and even the format can make these tools less useful. Changes in the format and content of labels as well as front-of-package systems have been

BOX 19-2 Consumer Sources of Information

Television (67%)
Magazines (41%)
Internet (41%)

AND, 2011.

BOX 19-3 Consumer's Trusted Sources of Health Information

Personal Healthcare Professionals	70%
Friend or Family Member	34%
US Government Agencies	26%
Food Expert on TV	24%
Health, food and Nutrition bloggers	24%
Farmer	18%
Food company or manufacturer	7%

IFIC, 2015 Food & Health Survey.

discussed for at least 10 years and are a work in progress to be released in 2015. Changes in portion size, the Nutrition Facts panel, and the front-of-package/label claims should be appearing in 2015 (U.S. Department of Health and Human Services [USDHHS] 2015; Healthfinder, January 24, 2014; Food and Drug Administration [FDA], 2014). Studies continue to indicate that consumers will use labels and would welcome a reliable front-of-package system. However, barriers continue to be related to developing a more universal system and providing the support and education important for knowledgeable consumer use (IOM, Label 2011). Although the movement for more labeling on menus has met with mixed reactions, forthcoming regulations will require additional labeling (Wu and Strum, 2014). All of these efforts are additional pieces of what is a developing puzzle that involves actions at the state and regional level as well as from federal sources. A continuing theme is the need for an overall consumer-related valid message based on current evidence-based tools that are understandable. Also critical to the effort is credentialed food, nutrition, and health professionals who can guide consumers to sources they can easily use to validate information.

Nutrition Information and Education for Adults

Mainstream adults in reasonable health frequently are ignored as a unique segment of the population who can benefit from nutrition assessment and education. Preventive strategies are likely to be targeted to address the formative years of prenatal, infancy, childhood, adolescence, and young adulthood. The older adult group is likely to be targeted with health intervention strategies and quality-of-life messages. However, the population group in the middle of the continuum, the adult age 25 to approximately 65, is likely to be segmented in reference to a disease state, a life event, or a lifestyle choice. For example, adults are targeted as having or being at risk for diabetes or heart disease, in need of a medication, being pregnant, or being an athlete.

The adult who is not pregnant, an athlete, or "sick," but who seeks guidance on normal nutrition or prevention of disease may be directed toward diets for chronic disease or weight loss. Such information may be a good fit when the information is based on science, but it can miss the mark on overall prevention goals. Fortunately, the guidance provided by such groups as the American Heart Association (AHA), the Academy of Nutrition and Dietetics (AND), the American Diabetes Association (ADA), and the American Cancer Society (ACS) tend to mirror the Dietary Guidelines for Americans 2010 (DGA) (USDHHS, 2010). These guidelines will continue to change with the updating of the DGA (FDA, 2015). The overall focus on diet with evolving guidelines is to emphasize quality of food choices including a message of the role of choices of "healthy fats" (NIH, Fat 2015). Another change that will affect how the DGA will be implemented both by consumers and food producers will be the elimination of trans fats as ingredients (Health.Gov 2015).

The AHA released prevention guidelines in 2006 with a focus on improving overall health and achieving improved cardiovascular health of all Americans by 20% by 2020 (Lloyd-Jones, 2010). In November 2013 the AHA, along with the American College of Cardiology (ACC) and The National Heart, Lung, and Blood Institute (NHLBI), released four guidelines based on evidence-based reviews sponsored by NHLBI (see Chapter 33). The ACC/AHA recommendations are for a diet high in vegetables, fruits, whole grains, low-fat poultry, fish, non-tropical vegetable oils, nuts and low-fat dairy and low in sweets, sugar sweetened beverages and red meat. The DASH diet pattern or USDA food pattern (MyPlate) is recommended to achieve this diet (Eckel 2013). The 2015 DGA is consistent with the AHA/ACC and also emphasizes increasing the intake of vegetables and fruit to meet the MyPlate guidance of half the plate. A 2015 study by the Produce for Better Health Foundation noted that fruit and vegetable consumptions has declined 7% over five years (from 2009 -2014). Adults 18-44 were cited as an agegroup (along with children of all ages) as a population group showing this decrease. (PBH, 2015) Nutrition messages related to consumption of fat, choices of fat sources, and of vegetables and fruit are ones that are likely to frame the guidance provided by groups such as the American Heart Association.

Guidelines for diabetes prevention continue to be related to healthy lifestyle guidelines of the DGA (see Chapter 30). A 2014 study indicated that research will continue to explore obesity and overweight. In a Danish study the link to being obese or overweight was a factor but there was a time difference noted. The presence of overweight or obese for several years was the identified risk factor rather than the BMI or amount of weight. This led to the conclusion that focusing on small weight reduction for the total population may be more beneficial than concentrating on weight loss targeted to high-risk individuals (Vistisen et al, 2014).

Adults are prime targets for information on chronic disease prevention and weight management. However, the messages may appear to be conflicting or less sensational than advice promising quick solutions. Determining adults' likely source of information can help the professional be the leader in delivering a validated message.

Health education and public health programs, along with improved research and care, have contributed to changes in morbidity and mortality of the adult population (CDC, 2013). U.S. adults are on a path to positive change, moving from knowledge to action (CDC, 2013). Nutrition assessment is a critical component of MNT and guidance for prevention. The nutrition and dietetics professional should either lead or be a part of lifestyle management teams. These professionals can link MNT to food, economic and social choices and can frame the guidance to be useful and achievable. Nutrition education, communication, and assessment skills add other dimensions to the goal of moving adults to action. Adults in the awareness and action stages are likely to be looking for answers, often short-term fixes or reversals of a health problem rather than more realistic long-term behavior changes. For example, adults may want to know where carbohydrates fit into the total diet and whether there are "better carbs." What's the message on "good" or any fat now that trans fats have been almost banned?

What is a "healthy" or "unhealthy" food or diet? Should I be buying organically grown or locally grown foods? What should I do about sodium? These are questions best addressed by skilled nutrition and dietetics professionals who can provide valid current information that answers the short-term questions but builds on long-term solutions.

Guidance based on science generally addresses total diet and lifestyle rather than single nutrients or foods. The concepts of *healthful eating, nutrient density,* and *nutritious food* are being debated by food and nutrition professionals as science and technology move the discussions along. The idea of expressing nutrient density using food labels is a major discussion point. Unfortunately, food and nutrition debates and new research findings, often meant to clarify the evidence, are fodder for media coverage, adding to the confusion and perception of mixed messages.

However, adults, as already mentioned, are a population group with the interest and the ability to seek out their own resources and answers. A search for information on choosing foods for health can result in evidence-based information such as the DGA, as well as questionable guidance based on single studies or product promotion. The combination of marketing and electronic media makes it easier to mix science with speculation and outright untruths. Adults with an interest in improving the nutritional quality of their diet may end up with unreliable advice pointing to quick-fix solutions.

The Wellness Years and Food Security

The adult years span a broad range chronologically and are complicated by physiologic, developmental, and social factors. Along with their genetic and social history, adults have accumulated the results of behaviors and risks from environmental factors. These factors shape the heterogeneity of the adult years. Nonetheless, the adult years are an ideal time for positive health promotion and disease prevention messages. In the transitions from early to middle adulthood, health and wellness may take on a new importance. This may be the result of a life event or education (an epiphany) that triggers awareness that being well and staying well are important. Examples include learning the results of a screening for blood pressure, cholesterol, or diabetes; facing the reality of death; the self-reflection that occurs when personal health or that of a peer or family member is in crisis; or realizing that clothes do not fit as well as they should. Regardless of the reason, the concept of wellness takes on a new meaning, and these events are teachable moments.

The Wellness Councils of America (WELCOA) describes wellness as a process that involves being aware of better health and actively working toward that goal (WELCOA, 2009). With this mindset, a state of wellness can exist at any age and can start at any point in a person's life course. Wellness is more than physical health and well-being. A state of well-being includes mental and spiritual health and encompasses the ability of a person to move through Maslow's Hierarchy of Needs (Maslow, 1970).

The ability to address nutrition needs requires food security (i.e., access to a safe, acceptable, and adequate source of food). Part of the issue of food security is quantity and part is quality. According to USDA data, in 2012, 85.5% of U.S. households were food secure, unchanged from 2011. Of the remaining population, 14.5% (17.6 million households) were reported as food insecure (United States Department of Agriculture [USDA], 2014b). The Food Research and Action Center (FRAC) offers similar figures, which identifies food security as a major issue in the United States (Feeding America, 2014a).

http://feedingamerica.org/how-we-fight-hunger/programs-and-services/public-assistance-programs/supplemental-nutrition-assistance-program/snap-myths-realities.aspx 2013.

The current economic climate has put added emphasis on food security or access and potential population inequalities. Hispanic, Native Americans, and African Americans in all age groups are more likely to live in poverty than Caucasians and Asian Americans. Native Americans and Alaska Natives have the highest rate of poverty in the United States (U.S. Census Bureau). The highest levels of food insecurity are reported to be in African American, Native American, and Hispanic households (Coleman-Jensen et al, 2013).

The issue of quantity as well as quality and acceptability are a part of the food security discussion. It is often more expensive to eat healthy foods than less healthy, high-calorie foods. Access is a part of this. However, limited skills in the areas of wise food purchasing and food preparation coupled with limited food and equipment resources further complicate a person's ability to follow advice for a healthy lifestyle. This emphasizes the need for adult consumer education in basic food skills. Eligibility for participation in the Supplemental Nutrition Assistance Program (SNAP), formerly known as food stamps (see Box 19-4), is based on income level and aims to alleviate food insecurity. The program includes some money for nutrition education (USDA, 2014c). SNAP, like other food and nutrition assistance programs, is being reviewed and altered to not only increase access but also increase the nutrition quality and types of food offered. The fact that SNAP is a program that serves the working poor as well as those who are unemployed often is overlooked. One in 5 children will rely on SNAP at some point in their lives (see Chapter 9).

Food insecurity frames the need for guidance from nutrition and dietetics professionals on food access, acceptability, and use.

Quality of Life and Work-Life Balance

Perceptions of personal health (mental and physical) relate to views on wellness and perceptions of quality of life. **Health-related quality of life (HRQOL)** is a concept used to measure the effects of current health conditions on a person's everyday life. To capture this and create a tool for professionals, the CDC measures population HRQOL perceptions, including the perception of "feeling healthy." Using HRQOL, one can learn about how adults relate their health to their daily performance. Americans report feeling "unhealthy" approximately 6 days a month and "healthy" or "full of energy" approximately 19 days a month; adults with the lowest income levels and more chronic diseases report more "unhealthy" days (CDC, 2011b, 2012b, 2012c). Similarly adults are being urged to set a goal of "work-life" balance. This is not a new concept and fits into the need for stress reduction and relaxation as a part of a healthy lifestyle. However, the idea of balancing work time with leisure also can be a part of the reasons adults use for not exercising, not cooking, for eating on the run, ignoring nutrition guidelines, or skipping meals. Leisure time can be interpreted as screen time, inactivity while watching activity, or social interaction, all of which are sedentary and may be accompanied by eating and drinking. Regardless of the reasons and the interpretations, the idea of work-life balance is a message that is receiving social media time and is an issue that often is related to multitasking and multiple roles adults are assuming (see Figure 19-1). In the concept of wellness or prevention, there is a mental health link as well as a potential block to leading a health-promoting lifestyle, not only for adults but also for their associates, family members, and others in their sphere of influence. The pros and cons and the potential health benefits are a topic for worksites and for dietetic and nutrition professionals (National Institutes of Health [NIH], Office of Human Resources, 2014).

The adult years offer unique opportunities to evaluate health status, build on positive factors, and change the negative factors that affect quality of life. Because adults are teachers, coaches, parents, caregivers, and worksite leaders, targeting the wellness-related attitudes and behaviors of adults potentially can have a multiplier effect. A positive wellness focus may influence the health of not only the adult but also those in his or her sphere of influence.

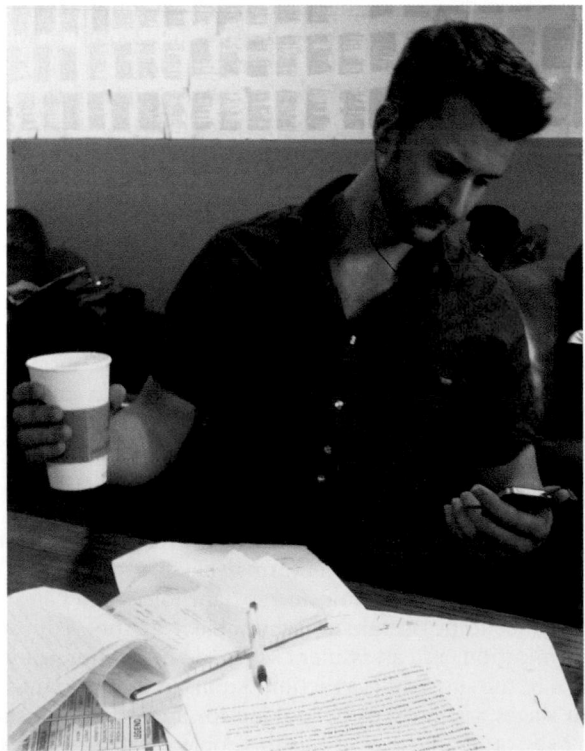

FIGURE 19-1 Eating quickly without attention, when stressed or when multitasking often results in poor nutritional intake in the adult years. (Copyright 2011 Photos.com a division of Getty Images. All rights reserved.)

LIFESTYLE HEALTH RISK FACTORS

Lifestyle choices, including activity, lay the framework for health and wellness. The health of people living in the United States has continued to improve in part because of education that has led to lifestyle changes. Life expectancy has continued to increase (projected at 78.7 years), and the morbidity and mortality rates from heart disease, cancer, and stroke have dropped (CDC, 2013a). Overall life expectancy for the African American population is 3.8 years less than that of the Caucasian population. This disparity is reported to be related to higher death rates from heart disease, cancer, homicide, diabetes, and perinatal conditions (CDC, 2013e).

These statistics point the way for increased emphasis on prevention and intervention initiatives in minority populations.

Even when the emphasis is on wellness and prevention, there is a strong link to risk factors that influence morbidity and mortality. In the United States the leading causes of death and debilitation among adults include (1) heart disease, (2) cancer, (3) chronic lower respiratory diseases, (4) cerebrovascular disease, (5) accidents (unintentional injuries), (6) Alzheimer's disease, (7) diabetes, and (8) nephritis, nephrotic syndrome, and nephrosis (CDC, 2014b). Chronic diseases, including heart disease, stroke, cancer, and diabetes, are among the most costly and preventable of all health problems and account for one third of the years of potential life lost before age 65 and for 75% of the nation's medical care costs (CDC, 2014b). The information quoted is for all adults, but when adjusting for age, the leading causes of death for young adults 18 to 44 are related to preventable causes, with suicide and homicide in the top three causes for adults under 34 years of age (CDC, 2013c). These health issues also have direct links to diet and lifestyle and to life cycle status. Accidents or unintentional injuries play a different role in younger adults. Accidents are the fifth leading cause of death and debilitation among all adults but moves up to first place for adults under 44 with emphasis on ages 25 to 44 (CDC, 2012e). Presumably the other leading causes of death, involving chronic diseases and those more diet related, can be important prevention teaching points at younger ages. Add to the list osteoporosis and new links to such health issues as Alzheimer's disease or arthritis as health problems that affect health care costs and loss of quality of life and that have a potential lifestyle and nutrition link (CDC, 2014d).

Overweight and obesity is either a precursor or complication in all of these diseases. The prevalence of overweight, as measured by a body mass index (BMI) of 25 or more, has increased at all ages but appears to be holding steady and even showing slight decline. It is important when looking at the overall health of adults to consider elevated BMI as a major risk factor but to move to the next phase of total assessment to identify the health profile. Hypertension, hyperlipidemia, and elevated blood glucose often are seen together with or without obesity, known as the metabolic syndrome (see Chapter 30). Increasing numbers of obese and overweight adults have been linked to an increase in the number of cases of metabolic syndrome. There is a genetic link to this syndrome but lifestyle is a major issue. Evidence suggests that it is possible to delay or control the risk factors associated with metabolic syndrome with lifestyle changes, including health-promoting diet and exercise patterns, with the help of health professionals (NIH, NHLBI, 2011).

Obesity and overweight directly link with calorie imbalance. An estimated less than half of U.S. adults participate in regular physical activity, with one fourth reporting no activity. Many health risks in the adult years, including coronary artery disease, certain types of cancer, hypertension, type 2 diabetes, depression, anxiety, and osteoporosis have a relationship with lack of participation in regular physical activity and poor eating behaviors. One cannot achieve positive health without a combination of physical activity and food choices that fit personal needs for energy balance and nutrition. Note the emphasis on *personal* needs.

On the other end of the weight spectrum is chronic underweight, frequently accompanied by undernutrition. Anorexia nervosa is the extreme condition, found in both genders across the age span. An unhealthy weight or unhealthy concern about body weight not only affects overall health but in women also can affect fertility and the ability to conceive.

HEALTH DISPARITIES AND ACCESS TO CARE

Implementation of the Healthy People 2020 goals are based in part on eliminating disparities that increase the health risks for affected populations. Such disparities are related to inadequate access to a safe and affordable food supply and health care based on race, ethnicity, gender, education, income level, and geographic location. Inadequate access to care is a disparity that has a major effect on a person's wellness. Chronic diseases and obesity have been shown to be more of a burden to racial minorities and women (CDC, 2013e, 2014b). There is a higher incidence of heart disease, diabetes, and obesity or overweight in low-income, African American, and Hispanic populations (CDC, 2013e). These same population groups have limited access to preventive care, nutrition education, and guidance (USDHHS, 2011).

The Affordable Healthcare Act was passed by Congress and signed into law on March 23, 2010, by President Obama. After a Supreme Court decision on June 28, 2012, the interpretation of the law began (see Chapter 10). Implementation began slowly with a goal of access to affordable care by all. Preventive care is highlighted. For current progress, check the Health and Human Services website at http://www.hhs.gov/healthcare/ (USDHHS, 2014).

World Health

The problems associated with chronic diseases are similar in other countries (World Health Organization [WHO], 2009). Also cited are human immunodeficiency virus, acquired immune deficiency syndrome, tuberculosis, and tropical diseases as barriers to global achievement of positive health status. Eight United Nation Millennium Development Goals seek to reduce the number of people who suffer from hunger and to increase access to safe water and sanitation (WHO, 2009). However, obesity has been cited as being of epidemic proportions globally, with at least 2.8 million people dying each year as a result of being overweight or obese.

WHO: Key Facts

- Worldwide obesity has nearly doubled since 1980.
- In 2008 more than 1.4 billion adults, 20 and older, were overweight. Of these more than 200 million men and nearly 300 million women were obese.
- 35% of adults aged 20 and over were overweight in 2008, and 11% were obese.
- 65% of the world's population live in countries where overweight and obesity kills more people than underweight.
- More than 40 million children under the age of 5 were overweight or obese in 2012.

This condition, once associated with higher-income countries, is now listed by WHO as prevalent in low and middle income countries. The growing international problem of obesity is a point for consideration and involvement (WHO Media Center, 2014).

Access to a safe and affordable food supply goes beyond the borders of the United States. The quality and quantity of that food and lifestyle factors are concerns that require more than provision of food. A newer and growing emphasis on food lifestyles is identifying "food deserts." CDC defines food deserts as areas that lack access to affordable fruits, vegetables, whole grains, low-fat dairy, and other foods that make up the full range of a healthy diet (CDC, 2012d). USDA expands the definition with a focus on limited access to supermarkets, supercenters, and other sources of affordable and *healthy* foods, noting it can occur in rural or urban settings. Knowing the potential of access to healthy foods, the limitations, and working to expand this access is a critical part of assisting adults and families in meeting nutrition goals. The USDA Food Access Research Atlas is a starting point for nutrition and dietetic professionals.

Emphasis: Women's Health

The reproductive years constitute a significant stage of a woman's life. Many issues that affect the health of women are related to the monthly hormonal shifts associated with menses. Osteoporosis, heart disease, and some cancers are disease states that are affected by specific hormones. Pregnancy and breastfeeding have an effect on a woman's health (see Chapter 15). Breastfeeding helps control weight, lower the risk for diabetes, and improves bone health. Therefore encouraging women to breastfeed is a potential prevention strategy for the future health of the mother and her infant.

Shifts of estrogen and progesterone hormones trigger the female reproductive cycle and affect health. Associated with menses is a complex set of physical and psychologic symptoms known as premenstrual syndrome (PMS). Reported symptoms vary but are described as general discomfort, anxiety, depression, fatigue, breast pain, and cramping. Such symptoms are reported to occur approximately 1 week to 10 days before the onset of menses and increase in severity into menses. Currently, there is no single cause or intervention identified for PMS. Hormone imbalance, neurotransmitter synthesis defects, and low levels of certain nutrients (i.e., vitamin B_6 and calcium) have been implicated (NIH, Office of Dietary Supplements [ODS], 2011). A diet high in sodium and refined carbohydrates has been implicated, but the evidence is not complete enough to make recommendations (NIH, ODS, 2007). A greater emphasis on a plant-based diet of whole grains, fruits, vegetables, lean or low-fat protein sources, and low-fat dairy or soy beverages is a reasonable intervention and may cause relief in some women. Exercise and relaxation techniques have been reported as lessening the symptoms.

When menses end, either because of age or surgical removal of reproductive organs, women have unique health and nutrition concerns. Perimenopause and menopause generally begin in the late forties. However, genetics, general health, and the age that menses began can alter the timing of this marker. Typically, estrogen production decreases around age 50, when endogenous estrogen circulation decreases approximately 60%. The effects include a cessation of menses and the loss of the healthful benefits of estrogen. Even after the ovaries cease production,

a weaker form of estrogen continues to be produced by the adrenal glands, and some is stored in adipose tissue (Barrett-Connor and Laughlin, 2005).

As estrogen decreases, symptoms associated with menopause may occur. The onset of menopause and the reported side effects vary. Some women experience a gradual decline in the frequency and duration of menses, whereas others experience an abrupt cessation. The symptoms most often reported include low energy levels and vasomotor symptoms (hot flashes). Bone, heart, and brain health are affected. The decrease in circulating estrogen limits the body's ability to remodel bones, resulting in a decrease of bone mass. Lower levels of circulating estrogen also affect blood lipid levels, increasing total cholesterol and low-density lipoprotein cholesterol levels and decreasing high-density lipoprotein (HDL) levels. Brain function, particularly memory, also is affected; negative changes may be alleviated somewhat with hormone therapy (MacLennan et al, 2006).

Managing menopause promotes emphasis on plant-based foods for the benefits of phytoestrogens, soluble fiber, and other components. Having sufficient calcium, vitamin D, vitamin K, and magnesium, and using the DRI as the guideline are important for protecting bone health. Although soy (isoflavones) continues to be rumored by the popular press as a way to control hot flashes, current research is not definitive. A recent study in American women published online in *Menopause* found that only women who are able to produce the soy metabolite equol get relief from hot flashes by eating soy (Newton et al, 2014). Of 357 study participants 34% were equol producers. The authors warned that a readily available test for the metabolite must be developed, and more randomized studies are needed to be able to make any recommendations that soy be a treatment for hot flashes.

Heart disease, cancer, and stroke continue to be the leading causes of death in women (CDC, 2014e). Again, although genetics are a factor, lifestyle is a major predictor and complicating factor.

Weight is a risk factor for heart disease and some cancers. Weight gain is an issue for women, with a 35% prevalence of obesity in American women aged 20 to 74 years compared with 33% in the same aged men. One-half of non-Hispanic African American women and two-fifths of Hispanic women are obese, compared with one-third of non-Hispanic white women (CDC, 2014a). Physical activity with aerobic endeavors and resistance and weight-bearing exercise is protective for bone, cardiovascular, and emotional health. The key nutrition message is one of balanced food intake with nutrient dense foods that are low in fat. However, once again personal assessment and tailoring to meet individual needs are a critical part of success in weight loss and maintenance.

Emphasis: Men's Health

The leading causes of death among American men include heart disease, prostate and lung cancers, and unintentional injuries. For the adult man, a diet that supports reducing the risk for heart disease is especially important because men develop heart disease at a younger age than women. Regular exercise and activity are important. Along with contributing to cardiovascular health, weight-bearing exercise has a positive effect on bone health.

Another issue in adult men is iron intake. Unless adult men are diagnosed with iron deficiency anemia and require additional iron, they should not seek additional iron from multivitamin or mineral supplements, enriched sports drinks, or energy bars. Excessive iron intake is problematic because it is an oxidant in the body; men and postmenopausal women do not have menstruation, pregnancy, or lactation to get rid of excess iron. A certain percentage of men carry the genetic variant for hemochromatosis and iron overload, and in this situation iron is particularly dangerous (see Chapter 32).

Like women, today's male population also is affected by obesity and the risk factors that come with excess weight such as diabetes, heart disease, and orthopedic problems. The American Cancer Society reports that one in seven men will have prostate cancer in his lifetime but only one in 36 will die of this disease. Obesity may play a role in these cancers. Some studies indicate that foods high in lycopene, an antioxidant found in tomatoes and other fruits and vegetables, may provide a protective role in lowering the risk factors for developing prostate cancer. Although this is still being studied, it is an emerging area for nutrition and diet in lowering risk factors and an area for dietetic and nutrition professionals to continue to explore. Such factors as how the food high in lycopene is prepared may have an effect on the usefulness of the lycopene (American Cancer Society, 2014).

INTERVENTIONS, NUTRITION, AND PREVENTION

Adults are in the ideal life-cycle phase for health promotion and disease prevention nutrition advice because of the combination of life experience and influence. This group has the potential to shape personal lifestyle choices and influence others. The tools are in place, including the DGA, My Plate, and the Nutrition Facts panel on food labels.

The vegetarian diet or a more plant-based diet and the Mediterranean diet have become popular with health and nutrition professionals and the public. Alternative patterns and resources support those who choose to be vegetarian or vegan (AND, 2009b). Both patterns are more plant based and support the recommendations of the Dietary Guidelines for Americans.

Implementation of positive choices and moving people along the continuum of a healthy lifestyle are other issues. Studies indicate consumers are aware of the concerns associated with lifestyle and diet but have a limited interest in making sustainable changes (IFIC, 2013). Consumers are aware of the implied promises for good health that come with messages from the media, friends, and health professionals; however, they are unlikely to move from awareness to action without motivation stronger than a message or promise. One perception of consumers is that eating healthful foods means giving up foods they like or having to eat foods that do not have the taste they prefer (AND, 2011). A total diet approach of making gradual changes of food and lifestyle choices may help. The Small Steps: Big Rewards Program is an example of such an approach with a goal of preventing type 2 diabetes (NIH, National Diabetes Education Program, 2006). America on the Move is another program that emphasizes achievable goals while maintaining calorie balance through small changes (America on the Move, 2014).

The steps to prevention and health promotion, even when small, are personal responsibilities that cannot be legislated. Americans have many choices: what and where they eat, where they receive their information, and what they include or exclude from their lifestyle. Adults value choice and food selection is a right, even if it leads to poor health, chronic disease, or

death. Some messages are directed at reaching adults where they live and work. For the working adult populations, much of the day is tied to a work site. There are increasing efforts in the private and public sectors to promote positive work site nutrition-related behaviors and programs.

FOOD TRENDS AND PATTERNS

Where one eats, who prepares it, and how much is consumed are patterns of behavior and choice. There is no stereotypic "adult" lifestyle. Adults may be single or partnered, with or without children, and working outside the home or at home. The sit-down family meals at home have given way to eating on the run, take-out, and drive-through. Too little time for planning or preparation and limited cooking skills can lead to reliance on processed foods, speed-scratch cooking (combining processed with fresh ingredients), or more food prepared out of the home. Today's economic climate and changing dietary recommendations present new challenges. The nutrient-dense approach is essential (Miller et al, 2009). Reaching men and women with an understandable and relevant message, especially heads of households or gatekeepers, is critical.

The consumer price index (CPI) estimates that Americans spend more than 52% of their food dollars away from home. This is an amount that has continued to increase and that fluctuates by month. The CPI for food measures the average change over time in the prices paid by urban consumers, using a representative market basket of consumer goods and services. The Economic Research Service (ERS) of the USDA follows these expenditures and manages the data set. This is a valuable resource for monitoring expenditures and planning for meaningful interventions (USDA, 2014a).

Changing food patterns and the use of more processed and purchased foods can result in an increase in dietary sodium, fat, and sweeteners and a decrease in use of basic foods such as fruits, vegetables, and whole grains. Portion sizes (either the amount presented or the amount eaten) replace serving sizes (what is recommended as a serving by the DGA or other source), as others determine what is considered a "meal" or "snack." Portions have continued to increase in size, as evidenced from using the tool "Portion Distortion" available at http://hp2010.nhlbihin.net/portion/keep.htm.

Dietary changes have affected nutrition and already are reflected in the current concerns for weight and nutrient imbalances. The DGA 2010 and My Plate (see Chapter 11) can be viewed as attempts to put more emphasis on basic foods that are nutrient dense rather than calorie dense and on total amounts of foods per day rather than numbers of servings. The most current information is reflected in the information used to shape the 2010 DGAs, but stay tuned as the 2015 DGA evolve guidance will change (Health.Gov, 2015).

Based on 2010 studies adult diets are likely to be higher in total fat than the 30% of total calories recommended in the 2010 DGA and include a predominance of carbohydrates as added sugar and refined grains. Fruit and vegetable guidelines are not being met, although increases are being noted. Although chicken and fish servings have increased, animal sources outweigh plant-based protein sources. Health guidelines continue to move in the direction of increasing plant-based foods. Key nutrients that may be in short supply are calcium, magnesium, and potassium; the antioxidants vitamins A, C, and E; and vitamin D (USDHHS, 2010). Accessing information building to the

2015 DGA (Scientific Report of the 2015 DGA Advisory Committee) will give a clearer picture (Health.gov, 2015).

NUTRITIONAL SUPPLEMENTATION

The position of the Academy of Nutrition and Dietetics (formerly the American Dietetic Association) is that the best nutritional strategy for promoting optimal health and reducing the risk of chronic disease is to choose wisely a variety of nutrient-rich foods. Additional nutrients from fortified foods and supplements help people meet their nutritional needs as specified by science-based nutrition standards such as the DRI (AND, 2009a). In making this statement, the Academy puts food first but leaves the door open for those with specific nutrient needs, identified through assessment by a dietetics or health professional, to be nutritionally supplemented.

Traditionally, one thinks of vitamins and minerals, fiber, and protein as nutrient supplements, generally in a pill, capsule, or liquid form. The DRIs are the standards used with most adults. However, food fortification is another form of nutrient supplementation. The level of fortified foods (such as "energy bars," "sports drinks," smoothies, or ingredients for fortification) in the marketplace puts another layer of potential nutrient sources in the mix with traditional supplements. Less traditional supplements such as herbals and other natural dietary "enhancers" are added to the array of supplements available to consumers. Information continues to build on the safety of some of the ingredients used to fortify or supplement. Examples include the 2014 report on the safety of caffeine added to foods and supplements and the ongoing updates from the NIH, Office of Dietary Supplements, and National Center for Alternative and Complementary Medicine (IOM, 2014; NIH, 2014; NIH, NCACM, 2012).

Either because of choice, access, or health-related issues, Americans may not meet the dietary recommendations for promoting optimal health. Several segments of the adult population fall into high-risk groups who are unlikely to meet their nutrient needs because of life stage (e.g., pregnancy), alcohol or drug dependency, food insecurity, chronic illness, recovery from illness, or choosing a nutritionally restrictive diet or lifestyle. Other persons with special needs include those with food allergies or intolerances that eliminate major food groups, persons using prescription drugs or therapies that change the way the body uses nutrients, those with disabilities that limit their ability to enjoy a varied diet, and those who are just unable or unwilling because of time or energy to prepare or consume a nutritionally adequate diet. These adults potentially need a nutritional supplement (AND, 2009a; AND, 2013b; see Chapter 12).

FUNCTIONAL FOODS

Adults interested in attaining and maintaining wellness are frequently interested in altering dietary patterns or choosing foods for added health benefits. The desire for fewer calories and multiple health benefits, especially when children are in the home, is driving the growth in the U.S. functional foods market. Sloan described this drive for real-food solutions, for "healthy" foods as a reminder to consumers of the long-term value of staying healthy (Sloan, 2012). Eight of ten Americans are making an effort to eat healthfully, and 42% are concerned about the nutrient content of the foods they buy. One result is an increase in sales of functional foods and beverages. Sloan notes that young adults, ages 18 to 24, are the top users of functional foods and beverages. This increase in sales of these foods and beverages is related to the search for healthier foods from familiar staples with better health profiles as well as options for individual nutrients (Sloan, 2012).

In a 2013 position paper on functional foods, the Academy of Nutrition and Dietetics noted all food is functional at some level, but there is growing evidence of components in food beyond traditional nutrients (AND, 2013a). Examples of large classes of functional foods are fruits and vegetables, including legumes, flax seeds, whole grains, the oils of fish, certain spices, yogurt, nuts, and soy. These are examples of foods believed to have benefits beyond their usual nutrient value (AND, 2013a; IFIC, 2011). Functional foods can include whole foods as well as those that are fortified, enriched, or enhanced by the addition of food components or nutrients. The potential benefit for health is when these foods are consumed as part of a varied diet on a regular basis.

Providing this information to the segment of the adult population who is looking for ways to enhance health not only gains the adults' attention but also takes nutrition guidance to a higher level. Research continues to provide information on dietary patterns and components of foods that may have added benefits for health. Helping to lower blood cholesterol or control blood sugar, serving as an antioxidant or scavenger against harmful components, promoting a healthy gastrointestinal tract, or stimulating activity of detoxification enzyme systems in the liver are examples of benefits being reported and researched for validity (see *Focus On:* Eating to Detoxify).

◎ FOCUS ON

Eating To Detoxify

By Sheila Dean, DSc, RDN, CDE, and L. Kathleen Mahan, RDN, MS

Detoxification, or "detox," is an elusive term because it does not always mean the same thing to everyone. However, the scientific meaning for detoxification, also referred to as biotransformation, is simply the elimination of anything that is toxic or foreign to the body. Detoxification can become impaired for a variety of reasons, including poor diet, drug-induced nutrient depletion, intestinal permeability, and genetic variations that may predispose a person to poor detoxification ability.

As a result, current thinking on eating to detoxify for optimal health is based on a system of choosing foods to protect, maintain, and renew the body. The body is protected from xenobiotics (compounds foreign to the body) by natural barriers, including the GI system, the lungs, and the skin. When compounds that are potentially harmful or unknown cross these barriers, the body's detoxification systems, which are series of metabolic reactions, go into play, with the result of decreasing the negative impact of the xenobiotics, drugs, or toxins.

Toxins may be of external origin (also referred to as xenobiotics or exogenous toxins), such as chemicals and pollutants in the air, water, food additives, or drugs. They also may be generated internally (also referred to as endogenous toxins), as the end-products from the metabolism of hormones, bacterial byproducts, and other complex molecules. The prolonged presence of these molecules can have damaging effects on tissues or lead to undesirable imbalances.

The detoxification (also referred to as biotransformation) process occurs in two classical steps —named Phase 1 and Phase 2—each involving a battery of enzymes of broad specificity. Specifically, Phase 1 reactions are

FOCUS ON—cont'd

Eating To Detoxify

catalyzed by the cytochrome P450 (CYP450) supergene family of isoenzymes, which have very broad substrate specificity. The products generated from Phase 1 reactions are often highly volatile and reactive intermediate metabolites and/or reactive oxygen species, which may cause tissue damage. The reactions in Phase 2 generally involve conversion or conjugation of the intermediate metabolites of Phase 1. This process is facilitated by the addition of a host of nutrients including various amino acids, methyl donors, and glutathione, a tripeptide consisting of glutamic acid, cysteine, and glycine, and which acts as a powerful antioxidant. The Phase 2 reactions that require the above-mentioned nutrients include glucuronidation, sulfation, methylation, acetylation, glutathione conjugation, and amino acid conjugation to the reactive site of the final products that are then eliminated. In some cases, a toxin may be converted directly via Phase 1 or Phase 2. Although both phases have different characteristics, it is essential that they function in balance with one another to minimize the presence of intermediate metabolites and carry through an effective detoxification.

Although as much as 75% of detoxification activity occurs in the liver, much of the remainder takes place in the intestinal mucosa wall. Still, an additional small percentage occurs in other tissues. Although the liver is thought of as the detoxification site, it makes sense that the intestine also plays an important role in detoxification, because the gastrointestinal lining provides the initial physical barrier to the largest load of xenobiotics.

The potential power of these systems to protect the body is demonstrated by a closer look at the major barrier, the gut. More than half the body's lymphoid tissue surrounds the digestive tract. Gut-associated lymphoid tissue (GALT) generates almost 70% of the body's antibodies and contains the greatest number of lymphocytes in the body. It is the GALT immunoglobulins that prevent absorption of bacteria and viruses. Secretory immunoglobulin A (sIgA) is a part of the major immune system of the gut and has been reported to directly deactivate enzymes and toxins from bacteria such as *Escherichia coli*.

The mechanisms for the food and nutrient link to detoxification are being explored, but it is suggested that phytochemicals are involved, along with more traditional nutrients that build and support the enzyme systems. Isothiocyanates such as sulforaphanes found in cruciferous vegetables; organosulfuric compounds in garlic, onions, and other members of the allium family; and the components present in prebiotics (nondigestible food products that stimulate the growth of bacteria already present in the colon) are examples of food choices that can affect detoxification in prevention and healing. In addition, the use of probiotics has been suggested as a helpful dietary addition for improving barrier activity, immune health, and gut function (Martin et al, 2014).

Foods and phytochemicals that boost detoxification include the following:
- At least one cup of cruciferous vegetables (cabbage, broccoli, collards, kale, Brussels sprouts) daily for their Phase II enzyme promoting effect
- A few cloves of garlic, which also promote Phase II enzymes
- Epigallocatechin gallate (EGCG) from regular or decaffeinated green tea
- Fresh vegetable juices, including carrots, celery, cilantro, beets, parsley, and ginger
- Herbal teas containing a mixture of burdock root, dandelion root, ginger root, licorice root, sarsaparilla root, cardamom seed, cinnamon bark, and other herbs
- High-quality, sulfur-containing foods—eggs or whey protein, garlic, onions
- Limonene in citrus peels, caraway, and dill oil
- Bioflavonoids in grapes, berries, and citrus fruits that promote Phase I enzymes
- Dandelion greens to help liver detoxification, improve the flow of bile, and increase urine flow

- Celery to increase the flow of urine and aid in detoxification
- Cilantro which may help remove heavy metals
- Rosemary, which has carnosol, a potent booster of detoxification enzymes
- Curcuminoids (turmeric and curry) for their antioxidant and antiinflammatory action
- Chlorophyll in dark green leafy vegetables and in wheat grass

Putting It All Together with the Functional Medicine "4R" Program

There is a growing awareness that understanding the cause of disease at the genetic-molecular-environmental level may be just as important if not more important than disease classification. Functional medicine, an evidence-based biology systems approach, addresses this concept of underlying cause and root cause solutions. In essence, functional medicine assessment is concerned with understanding the antecedents, triggers, and mediators of dysfunction that give rise to molecular imbalances underlying the signs and symptoms of disease (Lyon, 2010).

The following is a brief adaptation of the "4R Program" that the Institute for Functional Medicine pioneered for the management of chronic disease by targeting detoxification and improving GI function.

1. REMOVE: What does this person need to have removed for healthy detoxification?

   Remove focuses on eliminating pathogenic bacteria, viruses, fungi, parasites, and other environmentally derived toxic substances from the GI tract. Dietary modification is important, because foods to which a person is intolerant or allergic can exacerbate GI dysfunction and stimulate immune and inflammatory responses systemically.

2. REPLACE: What does this person need to have replaced to support normal detoxification?

   Replace refers to the replenishment of enzymes and other digestive factors lacking or in limited supply in an individual's GI environment. GI enzymes that may need to be replaced include proteases, lipases, and saccharidases normally secreted by cells of the GI tract or by the pancreas. Other digestive factors that may require replenishment include betaine hydrochloride and intrinsic factor, normally produced by parietal cells in the stomach wall.

3. REINOCULATE: What does this person need to support or reestablish a healthy balance of microflora?

   Reinoculate refers to the reintroduction of desirable bacteria, or "probiotics," into the intestine to reestablish microflora balance and to limit proliferation of pathogenic bacteria and candida. Probiotics serve a variety of functions in the GI tract: they synthesize various vitamins, produce short chain fatty acids necessary for colonic cell growth and function, degrade toxins, prevent colonization by pathogens, improve epithelial and mucosal barrier function, and alter immune-regulation via stimulation of secretory IgA or reduction in TNF-alpha.

4. REGENERATE (or REPAIR): What does this person need to support healing?

   Regenerate refers to providing support for the healing and regeneration of the GI mucosa. Part of the support for healing comes from removing insults that continually reinjure or irritate the mucosa, promoting the return and growth of healthy microflora. L-glutamine supplementation also has been found useful in restoring GI mucosal integrity.

   Using this type of functional medicine approach may allow for a more precise and clear evaluation of all the information available to create a systematic, effective, and functional nutrition care plan for an individual that can potentially significantly alter the trajectory of health maintenance over time.

Hyman M: Systems Biology, Toxins, Obesity, and Functional Medicine in Managing Biotransformation: The metabolic, genomic, and detoxification balance points, Proceedings from the 13th International Symposium of The Institute for Functional Medicine, Gig Harbor, Wash, 2006, Institute for Functional Medicine,.

Liska DJ, Lukaczer D: Gut dysfunction and chronic disease: the benefits of applying the 4R GI restoration program, *ANSR-Appl Nutr Sci Rep* 1:1-8, 2001.

Lyon M, Bland J, Jones DS: Clinical approaches to detoxification and biotransformation. In Jones DS, editor: *Textbook of functional medicine*, Gig Harbor, 2010, Institute for Functional Medicine.

Martin R et al: Gut ecosystem: how microbes help us, *Benef Microb* 28:1-15, 2014.

As a first step, adults who have no major health problems that would restrict food choices can benefit from guidance on meeting the recommendations of My Plate and the DGA. This guidance is based on increasing the intake of fruits, vegetables (including legumes), grains (with emphasis on whole grains), and seeds and nuts—some of the same foods known to have components that go beyond the benefits associated with major nutrients. Most of these components that are considered dietary enhancers are associated with plant foods.

Phytochemicals or **phytonutrients** (from the Greek word *phyto*, meaning "plant") are biologically active and naturally occurring chemical components in plant foods. In plants, phytochemicals act as natural defense systems for their host and offer protection against microbial invasions or infections. They also provide color, aroma, and flavor, with more than 2000 plant pigments identified (see Figure 19-2). These include flavonoids, anthocyanins, and carotenoids. Functional foods have become a favorite topic of the consumer press who often exaggerates the benefit of the food (see *Focus On: Chocolate: A Functional Food?*). As part of human consumption, phytonutrients can have antioxidant, detoxification, and antiinflammatory functions in the body.

Soy is another example of a food with value beyond quality protein but like others, research is still being collected and evaluated. The potential health benefits of soy products or components of soy include the potential of reducing the risk for heart disease and certain types of cancer and reducing vasomotor symptoms (hot flashes) in menopausal females. Note that soy itself, as a plant, has no cholesterol and is a source of **isoflavones**, a **phytoestrogen** or plant estrogen. In 1999 the Food and Drug Administration (FDA) approved a food label claim for soy, addressing its potential role in reducing the risk

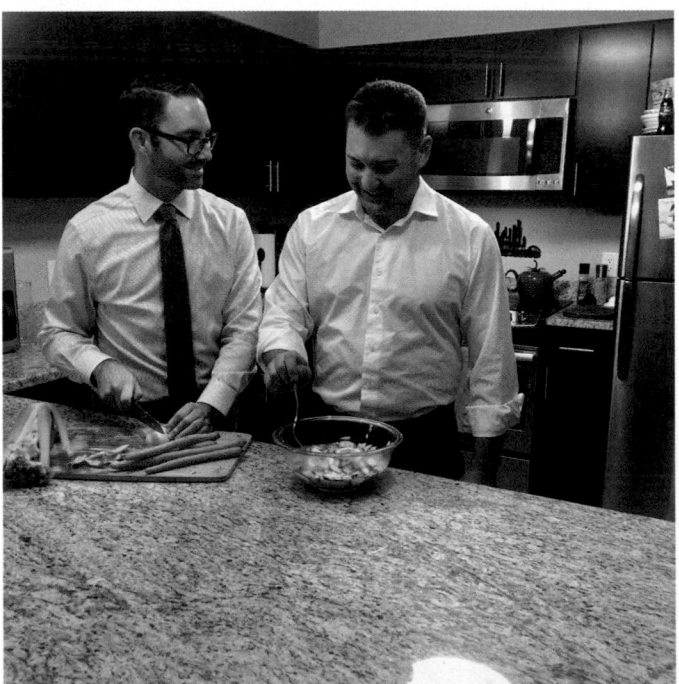

FIGURE 19-2 Cooking at home can be the best way to eat balanced and nutritious meals but can also be the most challenging during the adult years due to busy schedules.

FOCUS ON

Chocolate: A Functional Food?

What is there to hate about chocolate? Some people are allergic to it and some do not enjoy the flavor, but many people enjoy eating it. Chocolate can be considered a healthy food, as long as it is eaten in moderation. White chocolate is generally the cocoa butter portion with added sugar and flavorings and does not possess the same health benefits as milk or dark chocolate. Some facts about chocolate are the following:

- Chocolate is a plant food, made from beans harvested from a cocoa tree. Once the beans are removed from a pod, they are fermented, dried, roasted, and then ground. This produces a liquid, which is pressed to separate the cocoa butter from the solids. The end result is a cake that is then ground to make cocoa powder.
- Cocoa butter contains saturated fat, but research indicates the effect on blood cholesterol is neutral and may even be positive. However, it is a calorie source.
- Chocolate is a source of flavonoids, naturally occurring compounds that serve as antioxidants. Known as polyphenols, these are the same antioxidants found in tea, red wine, and some fruits and vegetables. These compounds give chocolate its rich color as well as potential health benefits. Dark chocolate has the most flavonoids.
- It is believed flavonoids help the body repair damage to the many cells and may even provide a protective shield. The cocoa in chocolate has a similar effect on blood vessels as taking small doses of aspirin. That is something to consider if you are on certain medications.
- Chocolate is also a source of plant sterols, B vitamins, magnesium, and potassium, all with potential heart health benefits.
- Chocolate can potentially improve mood because cocoa is believed to have a positive effect on boosting endorphin and serotonin levels in the brain.
- There are some potential negatives along with the potential of an allergic reaction:
  Cocoa is a source of oxalates. For some this can be a trigger for certain types of kidney stones.
  Caffeine is present in chocolate with dark chocolate taking the lead and milk chocolate at about one third the amount of the dark chocolate. This is a stimulant with varying effects based on your health and the amount consumed.
  Dark chocolate is a source of tyramine, also present in red wine, some fermented and aged foods. Still under investigation but worth noting is the potential for triggering migraine headaches.
  Chocolate is often in foods with excessive calories. Added sugar and fat in popular chocolate desserts, candies, and beverages bring to light the ongoing theme....keep the portions real for your personal needs.

of heart disease (FDA, 1999). This was reevaluated in 2013 when FDA Model guidelines noted the following:

1. 25 grams of soy protein a day, as part of a diet low in saturated fat and cholesterol, may reduce the risk of heart disease.
2. Diets low in saturated fat and cholesterol that include 25 g of soy protein a day may reduce the risk of heart disease (FDA, 2013).

The American Heart Association continues to note the positive influences of soy with a low saturated fat, low-cholesterol diet most recently on blood pressure, but the AHA has not updated statements dating back to 2006. The statement in 2006 noted there was no position after the results of a review of 22 randomized trials on the effect of soy protein with isoflavones on serum cholesterol (Sacks et al, 2006). The committee noted that soy protein and isoflavones have not been shown to lessen vasomotor symptoms of menopause and show no significant effects on HDL cholesterol or triglyceride levels. Foods that fit the FDA label claim for soy protein have a positive nutrition profile by virtue of the label requirements. Soy provides quality protein and provide an alternative for those limiting their animal protein intake. Soy can be used to displace animal protein and help lower intake of saturated fat, but soy is not recommended as a therapy to reduce LDL cholesterol or other cardiovascular risk factors (Lichtenstein et al, 2006). Whole soy foods continue to be a reasonable part of a diet with a role in disease prevention and health promotion (Messina et al, 2009). In addition, moderate amounts of soy foods can be part of a balanced diet even for cancer survivors (Maskarinec, 2005). The ACS concludes that cancer survivors may safely consume up to three servings daily (American Cancer Society, 2014; McCullough, 2012).

One cannot address dietary guidance without considering the issues of functional components and functional foods. Rather than isolating and promoting food components, current thinking supports the emphasis on food as a package and as a first source for nutrients and potential enhancers (see Figure 19-2). In the big picture it is the person's health status, lifestyle choices, and genetics that form his or her potential for wellness, but dietary enhancement is a tool that gains attention and helps the person move forward on the wellness continuum.

HEALTHY FOOD AND WATER SYSTEMS AND SUSTAINABILITY

This chapter began with a note that community nutrition is a constantly evolving and growing area of practice with the broad focus of serving the population at large with a thrust to be proactive and responsive to the needs of the community. Today's community and the community needs differ, but regardless of environmental, social, angeographic variations, a goal of nutrition and dietetics professionals is to promote and sustain access to a safe, affordable, and health-promoting food sources. In 2014 The Academy of Nutrition and Dietetics issued Standards of Professional Performance that addressed building and supporting sustainable, resilient, and healthy food and water systems (AND, 2014c). These standards are meant to provide guidance to Registered Dietitian Nutritionists beyond the usual safety standards. This paper identifies *sustainability* as the ability to maintain the system for the long term. *Resilience* encompasses the concept that a system can withstand interruptions. A practical example of resilience is that standards are in place for access to health-supporting and safe food and water even after a flood, natural disaster, or funding interruption. The sustainability is rooted in how the system is built, guided, and nourished. Public and private programs and resources are critical components but must meet the tests of resiliencyto be sustainable to meet funding requirements. The safety, adequacy, and quality of the food and water supply along with energy sources are components that build the sustainability and the resiliency. The nutrition and dietetics professional can be a major player but must have the expertise and competency as well as the initiative to build as well as promote standards and conditions in which people can reach the goal of being healthy.

ADULT HEALTH NEXT STEPS

The objectives for this chapter are to introduce direction for the well adult. This is a segment of the population who already may be a candidate for MNT, but the intent is to focus on resources for prevention and wellness. The 2013 position of the Academy of Nutrition and Dietetics, The Role of Nutrition in Health Promotion and Chronic Disease Prevention, is a rallying point. In this position the statement is made that primary prevention is the most affordable method to prevent chronic disease (AND, 2013b). Prevention strategies may include MNT because the line between being "healthy" and being "well" relates to control, maintenance, and for the adult, taking personal responsibility for setting a path as early as possible in the life cycle.

CLINICAL CASE STUDY

Aileen is a 28-year-old woman who lives in an urban neighborhood with her husband and 12-year-old daughter. She is 5 ft, 10 in tall and currently weighs 165 pounds. In the past 2 years she has gained 10 pounds. At a recent neighborhood health fair at the YMCA, Aileen's blood glucose and blood pressure screening results were higher than they had been a year ago but were still in a good range. She has a family history of heart disease and diabetes and recognizes that her weight gain is an issue. Both she and her husband work full time, and blending their schedules with that of their daughter is hectic. Aileen does all the cooking and shopping, they have a kitchen with a range, oven, microwave, and refrigerator/freezer. She describes her food shopping habits as chaotic and last minute, often stopping at the local convenience store. They eat out (fast food or take out) for most lunches and at least two dinners a week. They have no regular activity or exercise. They have the minimum health insurance with a large copayment; thus they do not have an ongoing health care routine.

Aileen made an appointment with a locally based health care source. She asked for dietary counseling and was asked to bring a 1-day food recall for the registered dietitian. She reported the following: breakfast: egg and sausage on a bagel, coffee; midmorning: low-fat snack bar from vending machine with coffee; lunch: double burger with cheese on a bun and large fries, ketchup, and extra pickles, diet soda; dinner: frozen dinner that included chicken, rice, and corn. She had an iceberg lettuce salad with diet ranch dressing "to add something green." Beverage was a diet soda. During the evening she had a dish of chocolate ice cream and sweet tea. She reports that in her coffee she likes two packets of sugar and some nondairy creamer.

Nutrition Diagnostic Statements

1. Physical inactivity related to lifestyle issues as evidenced by no regular physical activity and a 10-lb weight gain.
2. Undesirable food choices related to high fat and low fruit and vegetable intake as evidenced by diet history revealing high-fat foods at every meal and an average of one fruit or vegetable each day. Sodium level questionable.

Nutrition Care Questions

1. What lifestyle factors and nutrition triggers are likely to be identified by the dietitian?
2. What foods should Aileen consider including in her diet to build a prevention-related meal plan?
3. Plan a meal pattern and two sample meals that illustrate your recommendations, including at least one at-home and away-from-home breakfast, lunch, and dinner.

USEFUL WEBSITES

American Diabetes Association
http://www.diabetes.org/

American Heart Association
http://www.heart.org/HEARTORG/
American Cancer Society
http://www.cancer.org.
America on the Move
https://aom3.americaonthemove.org/default.aspx
Academy of Nutrition and Dietetics (Formerly the American Dietetic Association)
http://www.eatright.org/
Centers for Disease Control and Prevention Health
http://www.cdc.gov/women/
http://www.cdc.gov/men/
http://www.cdc.gov/nchs/hdi.htm
Dietary Guidelines for Americans
http://www.dietaryguidelines.gov
Food and Agriculture Organization
http://www.fao.org/
Healthy People 2020
http://www.healthypeople.gov/hp2020/Objectives/TopicAreas.aspx
Institute of Medicine
http://www.iom.edu/
Institute of Food Technology
http://www.ift.org/
International Food Information Council Food Insights
http://www.foodinsight.org/food-research.aspx
National Institutes of Health (NIH) Office of Dietary Supplements
http://ods.od.nih.gov/
U.S. Department of Agriculture: Agricultural Research Service
http://www.ars.usda.gov/
U.S. Department of Agriculture: MyPlate
http://www.chooseMyPlate.gov/
U.S. Department of Health and Human Services
http://www.hhs.gov/
http://hp2010.nhlbihin.net/portion/keep.htm. Portion Sizes
http://www.hhs.gov/healthcare/index.html. Healthcare
Wellness Councils of America
http://www.welcoa.org/
World Health Organization
http://www.who.int/topics/en/ http://www.who.int/mediacentre/en/

REFERENCES

Academy of Nutrition and Dietetics (AND): *Consumer and lifestyle app reviews* (website), 2014a. http://www.eatright.org/appreviews/. Accessed February 2014.

Academy of Nutrition and Dietetics (AND), Crowe KM, Francis C: Position of the academy of nutrition and dietetics: functional foods, *J Acad Nutr Diet* 113:1096, 2013a.

Academy of Nutrition and Dietetics (AND), Camp KM, Trujillo E: Position of the academy of nutrition and dietetics: nutritional genomics, *J Acad Nutr Diet* 114:299, 2014b.

Academy of Nutrition and Dietetics (AND), Slawson DL, Fitzgerald N, et al: Position of the academy of nutrition and dietetics: the role of nutrition in health promotion and chronic disease prevention, *J Acad Nutr Diet* 113:972, 2013b.

Tagtow A, Robien K, Bergquist E, et al: Academy of Nutrition and Dietetics (AND): standards of professional performance for registered dietitian nutritionists (competent, proficient, and expert) in sustainable, resilient, and healthy food and water systems, *J Acad Nutr Diet* 114:475, 2014c.

Academy of Nutrition and Dietetics (AND), formerly the American Dietetic Association: *Nutrition and you: trends 2008* (website), 2008. http://www.eatright.org/. Accessed January 2014.

Academy of Nutrition and Dietetics (AND), formerly the American Dietetic Association: *Nutrition and you: trends 2011* (website), 2011. http://www.eatright.org/. Accessed January 2014.

Academy of Nutrition and Dietetics (AND), formerly the American Dietetic Association, Marra MV, Boyar AP: Position of the American Dietetic Association: nutrient supplementation, *J Am Diet Assoc* 109:2073, 2009a.

Academy of Nutrition and Dietetics (AND), formerly the American Dietetic Association, Craig WJ, Mangels AR: Position of the American Dietetic Association: vegetarian diets, *J Am Diet Assoc* 109:1266, 2009b. http://www.eatright.org/search.aspx?search=vegetarian. Accessed January 2014.

America on the move (website), 2014. https://aom3.americaonthemove.org/. Accessed February 2014.

American Cancer Society: www.cancer.org. Accessed February 2014.

Barrett-Connor E, Laughlin GA: Hormone therapy and coronary artery calcification in asymptomatic postmenopausal women: the Rancho Bernardo Study, *Menopause* 12:40, 2005.

Breslow RA, Guenther PM, Juan W, et al: Alcoholic beverage consumption, nutrient intakes and diet quality in the US adult population, 1999-2006 *J Am Diet Assoc* 110:551, 2010.

Centers for Disease Control and Prevention (CDC): *10 leading causes of death by age group, United States—2012* (website). http://www.cdc.gov/injury/wisqars/pdf/leading_causes_of_death_by_age_group_2012-a.pdf. Accessed November 2014.

Centers for Disease Control and Prevention (CDC): *Adult obesity facts* (website), 2014a. http://www.cdc.gov/obesity/data/adult.html. Accessed January 2014.

Centers for Disease Control and Prevention (CDC): *Chronic disease prevention and health promotion* (website), 2014b. http://www.cdc.gov/nccdphp/overview.htm. Accessed January 2014.

Centers for Disease Control and Prevention (CDC): *FastStats A to Z* (website), 2011a. http://www.cdc.gov/nchs/fastats/. Accessed January 2014.

Center for Disease Control and Prevention (CDC): *FastStats: death and mortality* (website), 2014c. http://www.cdc.gov/nchs/fastats/deaths.htm. Accessed November 29, 2014.

Centers for Disease Control and Prevention (CDC): *FastStats: life expectancy* (website), 2013a. http://www.cdc.gov/nchs/fastats/lifexpec.htm. Accessed January 2014.

Centers for Disease Control and Prevention (CDC): *Health, United States 2013* (website), 2014d. http://www.cdc.gov/nchs/hus.htm. Accessed January 2014.

Centers for Disease Control and Prevention (CDC): *Health-related quality of life (HRQOL)* (website), 2012b. http://www.cdc.gov/hrqol/. Accessed January 2014.

Centers for Disease Control and Prevention (CDC): *Health-related quality of life (HRQOL): CDC's healthy days measures used in the America's health ranking* (website), 2012c. http://www.cdc.gov/hrqol/featured-items/healthy-days.htm. Accessed January 2014.

Centers for Disease Control and Prevention (CDC): *Health-related quality of life (HRQOL): key findings* (website), 2011b. http://www.cdc.gov/hrqol/key_findings.htm. Accessed January 2014.

Centers for Disease Control and Prevention (CDC): *Healthy people 2010 final review* (website), 2013b. http://www.cdc.gov/nchs/healthy_people/hp2010/hp2010_final_review.htm. Accessed January 2014.

Centers for Disease Control and Prevention (CDC): *Healthy people 2020* (website), 2011c. http://www.cdc.gov/nchs/healthy_people/hp2020.htm. Accessed January 2014.

Centers for Disease Control and Prevention (CDC): *Heart disease facts* (website), 2014e. http://www.cdc.gov/heartdisease/facts.htm. Accessed January 2014.

Centers for Disease Control and Prevention (CDC): *A look inside food deserts* (website), 2012d. http://www.cdc.gov/Features/FoodDeserts/. Accessed December 12, 2014.

Centers for Disease Control and Prevention (CDC): *National vital statistics report: death: leading causes 2010* (website), 2013c. http://www.cdc.gov/nchs/data/nvsr/nvsr62/nvsr62_06.pdf. Accessed January 2014.

Centers for Disease Control and Prevention (CDC): *National vital statistics report: deaths: preliminary data for 2011* (website), 2012e. http://www.cdc.gov/nchs/data/nvsr/nvsr61/nvsr61_06.pdf. Accessed January 2014. www.cdc.gov/.../pdf/leading_causes_of_death_by_age_group_2011-a.pdf

Centers for Disease Control and Prevention (CDC): *National vital statistics report: deaths: final data for 2010* (website), 2013d. http://www.cdc.gov/nchs/data/nvsr/nvsr61/nvsr61_04.pdf. Accessed January 2014.

Centers for Disease Control and Prevention (CDC): *NCHS data brief: what did cause of death contribute to racial differences in life expectancy in the United States in 2010?* (website), 2013e. http://www.cdc.gov/nchs/data/databriefs/db125.htm. Accessed January 2014.

Centers for Disease Control and Prevention (CDC): *Vital and health statistics series 10:259: summary health statistics for the US population: national health interview survey, 2012* (website), 2013f. http://www.cdc.gov/nchs/data/series/sr_10/sr10_259.pdf. Accessed January 2014.

Coleman-Jensen A, Nord M, Singh A: *Household food security in the United States in 2012.* USDA. http://www.ers.usda.gov/publications/err-economic-research-report/err155.aspx. Economic Research Report 155:41, 2013. Accessed January 2014.

Eckel RH, Jakicic JM, Ard JD, et al: 2013 AHA/ACC guideline on lifestyle management to reduce cardiovascular risk: a report of the American College of Cardiology/American Heart Association Task Force on Practice Guidelines, *Circulation* 129(25 Suppl 2):S76, 2013.

Feeding America: *The state of hunger in America* (website), 2014a. http://www.feedingamerica.org/hunger-in-america/news-and-updates/press-room/press-releases/the-state-of-hunger-in-america.html. Accessed January 2014.

Feeding America: *Supplemental nutrition assistance programs (SNAP)* (website), 2014b. http://feedingamerica.org/how-we-fight-hunger/programs-and-services/public-assistance-programs/supplemental-nutrition-assistance-program/snap-myths-realities.aspx. Accessed May 2014.

Food and Drug Administration: *FDA cuts trans fats from processed food,* June 2015. http://www.fda.gov/downloads/ForConsumers/ConsumerUpdates/UCM451467.pdf. Accessed June 2015.

Food and Drug Administration: *Nutrition facts label: 20 and evolving* (website), 2014. http://www.fda.gov/forconsumers/consumerupdates/ucm334749.htm#proposed. Accessed January 2014.

Food and Drug Administration: *Code of federal regulations (Title 21:2) Revised April 1, 2013. Food labeling health claims. Soy protein and the risk of heart disease.* http://www.fda.gov/forconsumers/consumerupdates/ucm334749.htm#proposed. Accessed January 2014. http://www.fda.gov/Food/IngredientsPackagingLabeling/LabelingNutrition/ucm2006873.htm

Harold JG, Jessup M: ACC/AHA special report: new ACC/AHA prevention guidelines: building a bridge to even stronger guideline collaborations, *Circulation* 128:2852, 2013.

Health.Gov: *Scientific Report of the 2015 dietary guidelines for Americans Advisory Committee.* (website). http://www.health.gov/dietaryguidelines/2015-scientific-report. Accessed June 2015.

Institute of Medicine (IOM): *Caffeine in Food and Dietary Supplements: Examining Safety- Workshop Summary* (website), 2014. http://www.iom.edu/Reports/2014/Caffeine-in-Food-and-Dietary-Supplements-Examining-Safety.aspx. Accessed January 2014.

Institute of Medicine (IOM), National Academy of Sciences (NAS): *Dietary reference intake (DRI) series*, Washington, DC, 1998–2004, National Academies Press.

Institute of Medicine (IOM): *Examination of front-of-package nutrition rating systems and symbols* (website), 2011. http://www.iom.edu/Activities/Nutrition/NutritionSymbols.aspx. Accessed January 2014.

International Food Information Council (IFIC): *Background on functional foods* (website), 2011. http://www.foodinsight.org/Resources/Detail.aspx?topic=Background_on_Functional_Foods. Accessed January 2014.

International Food Information Council (IFIC): *2013 IFIC foundation food and health survey*, Washington, DC, 2013. http://www.foodinsight.org/. Accessed January 2014.

International Food Information Council (IFIC): *2014 Food and health survey*, Washington, DC, 2014. http://www.foodinsight.org. Accessed May 2014.

International Food Information Council (IFIC): *2015 Food and health survey*, Washington, DC, 2015. http://www.foodinsight.org. Accessed June 2015.

Lichtenstein AH, American Heart Association Nutrition Committee, Appel LJ, et al: Diet and lifestyle recommendations revision 2006: a scientific statement from the American Heart Association Nutrition Committee, *Circulation* 114:82, 2006.

Lloyd-Jones DM, Hong Y, Labarthe D, et al: Defining and setting national goals for cardiovascular health promotion and disease reduction, *Circulation* 121:586, 2010.

MacLennan AH, Henderson VW, Paine BJ, et al: Hormone therapy, timing of initiation, and cognition in women older than 60 years: the REMEMBER pilot study, *Menopause* 13:28, 2006.

Maskarinec G: Commentary: soy foods for breast cancer survivors and women at high risk for breast cancer, *J Am Diet Assoc* 105:1524, 2005.

Maslow A: *Motivation and personality*, ed 2, New York, 1970, Harper.

McCullough M: *The bottom line on soy and breast cancer risk, American Cancer Society*, 2012. http://www.cancer.org/cancer/news/expertvoices/post/2012/08/02/the-bottom-line-on-soy-and-breast-cancer-risk.aspx. Accessed January 2014.

Messina M, Watanabe S, Setchell KD: Report on the 8th international symposium on the role of soy in health promotion and chronic disease prevention and treatment, *J Nutr* 139:S796, 2009.

Miller GD, Drewnowski A, Fulgoni V, et al: It is time for a positive approach to dietary guidance using nutrient density as a basic principle, *J Nutr* 139:1198, 2009.

Nagler RH: Outcomes associated with media exposure to contradictory nutrition messages. *J Health Commun* 19:24, 2014.

National Institutes of Health (NIH), National Center for Complementary and Alternative Medicine (NCCAM): *Soy* (website), 2012. http://nccam.nih.gov/health/soy/ataglance.htm. Accessed February 2014.

National Institutes of Health (NIH), National Diabetes Education Program: *Small steps. Big rewards. Prevent type 2 diabetes campaign* (website), 2006. http://ndep.nih.gov/partners-community-organization/campaigns/SmallStepsBigRewards.aspx. Accessed February 2014.

National Institutes of Health (NIH), National Heart, Lung and Blood Institute (NHLBI): *What is metabolic syndrome?* (website), 2011. http://www.nhlbi.nih.gov/health/health-topics/topics/ms/. Accessed January 2014.

National Institutes of Health (NIH), HealthDay: *Fat no longer the focus of new U.S. dietary guidelines.* June 2015. http://www.nlm.nih.gov/medlineplus/news/fullstory_153294.html. Accessed June 2015.

National Institutes of Health (NIH), Office of Dietary Supplements (ODS): *Dietary supplement fact sheet: B6* (website), 2011. http://ods.od.nih.gov/factsheets/vitaminb6.asp. Accessed January 2014.

National Institutes of Health (NIH), Office of Dietary Supplements (ODS): *Dietary supplements: what you need to know* (website), 2014. http://ods.od.nih.gov/. Accessed January 2014.

National Institutes of Health (NIH), Office of Human Resources: *Work/life at NIH* (website), 2014. http://hr.od.nih.gov/workingatnih/worklife. Accessed February 2014.

Newton KM, et al: A cross-sectional study of equol producer status and self-reported vasomotor symptoms, *Menopause* 2014.

Produce for Better Health: *State of the plate*, 2015. http://pbhfoundation.org/pdfs/about/res/pbh_res/State_of_the_Plate_2015_WEB_Bookmarked.pdf. Accessed June 2015.

Sacks F, Lichtenstein A, Van Horn L, et al: Soy protein, isoflavones, and cardiovascular health: an American Heart Association Science Advisory for Professionals from the Nutrition Committee, *Circulation* 113:1034, 2006.

Sloan AE: Top 10 functional food trends, *Food Technol* 68, 2012.

Sloan AE: What, when and where America eats, *Food Technol* 64, 2010.

U.S. Department of Agriculture (USDA), Economic Research Service (ERS): *Food CPI and expenditures* (website), 2014a. http://www.ers.usda.gov/data-products/food-price-outlook/summary-findings.aspx. Accessed January 2014.

U.S. Department of Agriculture (USDA), Economic Research Service (ERS): *Food security status of US households in 2013* (website), 2014b. http://www.ers.usda.gov/topics/food-nutrition-assistance/food-security-in-the-us/key-statistics-graphics.aspx#foodsecure. Accessed February 2014.

U.S. Department of Agriculture (USDA), Economic Research Service (ERS): *Supplemental nutrition assistance program SNAP* (website), 2014c.

http://www.ers.usda.gov/topics/food-nutrition-assistance/supplemental-nutrition-assistance-program-(snap).aspx. Accessed January 2014.

U.S. Department of Health and Human Services (USDHHS): *Building healthier communities by investing in prevention* (website), 2011. http://www.hhs.gov/healthcare/facts/factsheets/2011/09/prevention02092011.html. Accessed January 2014.

U.S. Department of Health and Human Services (USDHHS): *Dietary guidelines for Americans, 2010.* ed 7, Washington, DC, December 2010, US Government Printing Office.

U.S. Department of Health and Human Services (USDHHS): *Healthcare HHS. gov/healthcare,* 2014. http://www.hhs.gov/healthcare/index.html. Accessed January 2014.

U.S. Department of Health and Human Services (USDHHS): *A key to choosing healthful foods using the nutrition facts on the food label.* May, 2015. http://www.nutrition.gov/shopping-cooking-meal-planning/food-labels. Accessed June, 2015.

U.S. Department of Health and Human Services (USDHHS): *Healthfinder.gov. FDA wants to update food labels,* January 24, 2014. http://www.healthfinder.gov. Accessed January 2014.

U.S. Department of Health and Human Services (USDHHS): *Breastfeeding* (website), www.womenshealth.gov/breastfeeding. Accessed February 2014.

Vistisen D, Witte DR, Tabák AG, et al: Patterns of obesity development before the diagnosis of type 2 diabetes: the Whitehall II cohort study, *PLOS Med* 11:e1001602, 2014.

Wellness Councils of America (WELCOA): *The 7 benchmarks of success, Omaha, NE* (website), 2009. www.welcoa.org/services/build/welcoas-seven-benchmarks/. Accessed January 2014.

World Health Organization (WHO): *10 Facts on obesity* (website), 2013a. http://www.who.int/features/factfiles/obesity/en/index.html. Accessed February 2014.

World Health Organization (WHO): *Media centre: overweight and obesity* (website), 2014. http://www.who.int/mediacentre/factsheets/fs311/en/. Accessed November 29, 2014.

World Health Organization (WHO): *Progress on health-related millennium development goals (MDGs), Copenhagen.* (website), 2009. http://www.who.int/whosis/whostat/2009/en/index.html. Accessed January 2014.

World Health Organization (WHO): *World health statistics 2013 Geneva* (website), 2013b. http://www.who.int/gho/publications/world_health_statistics/EN_WHS2013_Full.pdf. Accessed January 2014.

Wu HW, Sturm R: Changes in the energy and sodium content of main entrees in US Chain Restaurants from 2010 to 2011, *J Acad Nutr Dietet* 114:209, 2014.

20

Nutrition in Aging

Nancy S. Wellman, PhD, RDN, FAND
Barbara J. Kamp, MS, RDN

KEY TERMS

achlorhydria
activities of daily living (ADLs)
age-related macular degeneration (AMD)
cataract
constipation
dysgeusia
dysphagia
functionality
geriatrics
gerontology

glaucoma
home- and community-based services (HCBS) waivers
hyposmia
instrumental activities of daily living (IADLs)
long-term services and supports (LSS)
Minimum Data Set (MDS)
polypharmacy
pressure ulcers
presbycusis

quality of life
Resident Assessment Instrument (RAI)
sarcopenia
sarcopenic obesity
sedentary death syndrome (SeDS)
senescence
skilled nursing facility (SNF)
supercentenarians
xerostomia

THE OLDER POPULATION

Population aging, now a global phenomenon, is no longer limited to developed, higher-income countries. The World Health Organization's Global Forum on Innovations for Ageing Populations describes how quickly the older population is growing even in low- and middle-income countries and that over the next 40 years, developing countries will be home to about 80% of older adults worldwide (World Health Organization [WHO], 2013).

Today, one in seven Americans is age 65 or older. They are living longer, healthier, and more functionally fit lives than ever before. Figure 20-1 shows older adults involved in physical activities. Those born today can expect to live an average of 80 years. Women who reach age 65 can expect to live an additional 20.4 years, and men, 17.8 years. By the year 2050 the population older than age 65 will grow from approximately 44 million to 84 million, increasing from 14% to 21% of the population. The fastest-growing segment is those older than age 85, currently 6 million and increasing to 18 million in 2050. Members of minority groups also will increase from 21% to more than 39% of the older population (Colby and Ortman, 2014; Ortman et al, 2014) (see Figures 20-2 and 20-3).

By 2056, the total U.S. population 65 years and over is projected to become larger than the population under 18 years (Colby and Ortman, 2014). Even sooner, more than half of the states will double their older-than-65 population by 2030, when the oldest of the baby boomer generation enter their 80s. By 2030 the number of older adults will exceed the number of school-age children in 10 or more states—Florida, Pennsylvania, Vermont, Wyoming, North Dakota, Delaware, New Mexico, Montana, Massachusetts, and West Virginia. A few years ago no state had more people older than age 65 than those younger than 18. Growth in the older-than-65 population will equal 3.5 times the U.S. growth as a whole. This demographic shift has enormous social, economic, and political implications (Ortman et al, 2014).

Women live longer than men. The older-than-65 female/male ratio is 129:100; it increases to 200:100 among those older than age 85. More than 71% of older men are married, whereas only 45% of older women are married (Ortman et al, 2014). Almost half (45%) of women over age 75 live alone; thus more men die married and most women die unmarried.

Classification

Everyone knows people older than themselves, but those considered "old" depends a lot on one's own age. Youngsters consider their 20- or 30-something parents old. Today gray hair color, wrinkles, retirement, or age 65 no longer defines *old*. Yet qualifying as an "older adult" is based on the minimum eligibility age of 65 in many federal programs. The U.S. Census Bureau uses a stratified system to define this generation-spanning age group; those aged 65 to 74 are the *young old*; 75 to 84, *old*; and 85 or older, *oldest old*. Some consider today's *new old* to be those in their 90s. The more than 100,000 centenarians alive today are no longer considered unique, and many of them still live independently (see *Focus On:* Centenarians . . . Life in the Blue Zone).

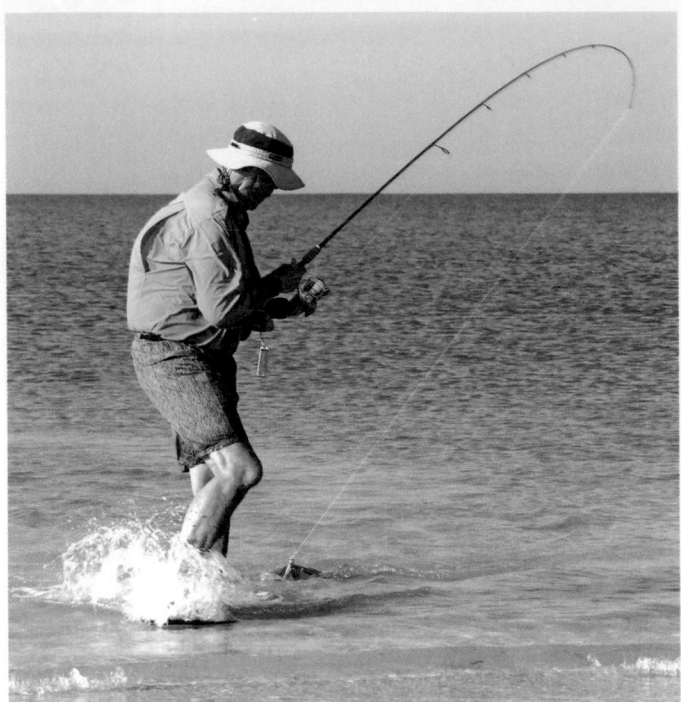

FIGURE 20-1 Active older adult fishing at 70.

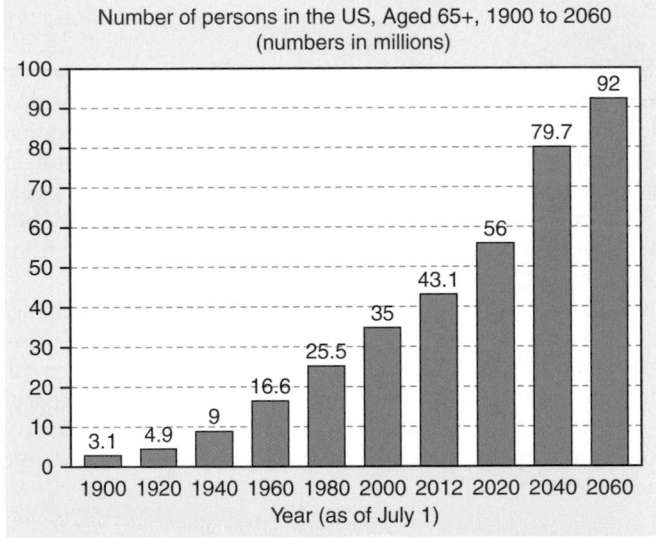

FIGURE 20-2 Population ages 65 and older: 2000 to 2060.

GERONTOLOGY + GERIATRICS = THE SPECTRUM OF AGING

Gerontology is the study of normal aging, including factors in biology, psychology, and sociology. **Geriatrics** is the study of the chronic diseases frequently associated with aging, including diagnosis and treatment. Although medical nutrition therapy commonly has been practiced in hospitals and long-term care facilities, nutrition services have moved out of hospitals and into homes and communities where the focus is on health promotion, risk reduction, and disease prevention.

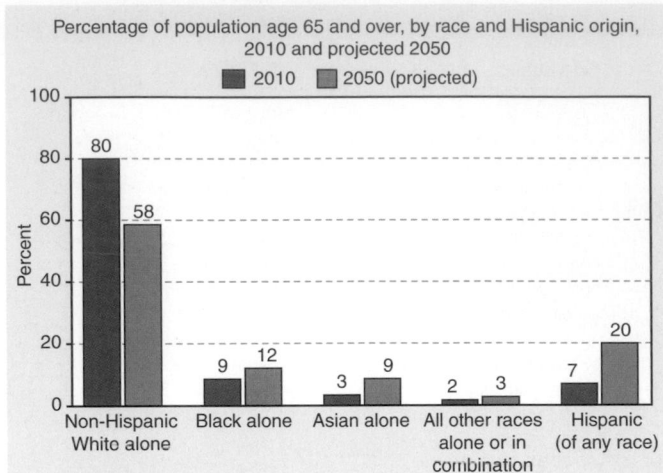

FIGURE 20-3 Population age 65 and over, by race and Hispanic origin, 2010 and projected 2050. Note: The term *non-Hispanic white alone* is used to refer to people who reported being white and no other race and who are not Hispanic. The term *black alone* is used to refer to people who reported being black or African American and no other race, and the term *Asian alone* is used to refer to people who reported only Asian as their race. The use of single-race populations in this chart does not imply that this is the preferred method of presenting or analyzing data. The U.S. Census Bureau uses a variety of approaches. The race group "All other races alone or in combination" includes American Indian and Alaska Native alone; Native Hawaiian and Other Pacific Islander alone; and all people who reported two or more races. Reference population: These data refer to the resident population. (*U.S. Census Bureau:* 2010 Census Summary File 1; Table 4. http://www.census.gov/prod/cen2010/doc/sf1.pdf, 2011. Accessed December 31, 2014.)

NUTRITION IN HEALTH PROMOTION AND DISEASE PREVENTION

In aging adults, nutrition care is not limited to disease management or medical nutrition therapy but has broadened to have a stronger focus on healthy lifestyles and disease prevention. Without increased emphasis on better diets and more physical activity at all ages, health care expenditures will rise exorbitantly as the population ages. Thus it is never too late to emphasize nutrition for health promotion and disease prevention. Older Americans, more than any other age group, want health and nutrition information and are willing to make changes to maintain their independence and quality of life. They often need help in improving self-care behaviors. They want to know how to eat healthier, exercise safely, and stay motivated.

Nutrition may include three types of preventive services. In *primary prevention,* the emphasis is on nutrition in health promotion and disease prevention. Pairing healthy eating with physical activity is equally important.

Secondary prevention involves risk reduction and slowing the progression of chronic nutrition-related diseases to maintain functionality and quality of life. *Functionality* as related to strength and mobility is perceived as a positive way to discuss fitness versus disability and dependence. Many community

FOCUS ON

Centenarians . . . Life in the Blue Zone

By Janice M. Raymond, CSG, RD, MS

Centenarians are the fastest growing segment of older adults in the United States and in other developed nations, including Japan. The worldwide estimate of centenarians is 450,000. The U.S. Census Bureau estimates for 2009 there are about 65,000 centenarians and more than 1 million by 2050. As with the aging population as a whole, women represent 85% of the long lived. A new group of individuals older than age 110, **supercentenarians**, have sufficient numbers to merit dedicated research.

What is known about extremely long-lived individuals? Centenarians generally have delays in functional decline. They also tend to either never develop a chronic disease or develop one late in life. Much has been written about longevity in the southern Japanese prefecture of Okinawa. The ongoing Okinawa Centenarian Study suggests that low caloric intake may produce fewer destructive free radicals. This intake plus an active lifestyle, natural ability to combat the stresses of life, and a genetic predisposition favor a healthy, functional, longer life.

The National Institute on Aging has identified communities around the world where people are living longer and living measurably better. They called these areas, where people reach the age of 100 at rates 10 times greater than in the United States, the *Blue Zones*. One such community is Okinawa. Others include the Nicoya Peninsula in Costa Rica and Sardinia in Italy. Residents of Loma Linda in California boast the longest life spans in America. They found that these groups had common characteristics related to food: very little animal protein and four to six servings of fruits, vegetables, legumes, and nuts. However, eating wisely is only part of what seems to be a prescription for long life. The people of these communities don't smoke and make regular low-intensity exercise part of their daily routine (e.g., gardening, walking). They are people who can articulate their purpose in life, are spiritually fulfilled, and have strong social networks.

In the New England Centenarian Study, independent function to at least age 90 is a predominant feature. Other important factors are that few centenarians are obese, they rarely smoke, and they consume little or no alcohol. At least 50% of centenarians have first-degree relatives or grandparents who also achieved very old age, and many have exceptionally old siblings.

TABLE 20-1 Predetermination and Accumulated Damage Theories on Aging

Theory	Description
Predetermination: Built-in mechanism determines when aging begins and time of death	
Pacemaker theory	"Biologic clock" is set at birth, runs for a specified time, winds down with aging, and ends at death.
Genetic theory	Life span is determined by heredity.
Rate of living theory	Each living creature has a finite amount of a "vital substance," and, when it is exhausted, the result is aging and death.
Oxygen metabolism theory	Animals with the highest metabolisms are likely to have the shortest life spans.
Immune system theory	Cells undergo a finite number of cell divisions that eventually cause deregulation of immune function, excessive inflammation, aging, and death.
Accumulated damage: Systemic breakdown over time	
Crosslink/glycosylation theory	With time, proteins, DNA and other structural molecules in the body make inappropriate attachments, or crosslinks, to each other, leading to decreased mobility, elasticity, and cell permeability.
Wear-and-tear theory	Years of damage to cells, tissues, and organs eventually take their toll, wearing them out and ultimately causing death.
Free radical theory	Accumulated, random damage caused by oxygen radicals slowly cause cells, tissues, and organs to stop functioning.
Somatic mutation theory	Genetic mutations caused by oxidizing radiation and other factors accumulate with age, causing cells to deteriorate and malfunction.
Telomere length	Telomeres protect and cap linear chromosome ends. Short telomeres have been associated with many age-related conditions.

dining centers funded through the Older Americans Act (OAA) Nutrition Programs attract participants through new fitness programs.

In *tertiary prevention*, care/case management and discharge planning often involve chewing and appetite problems, modified diets, and functional limitations. Complex cases often are influenced by nutrition issues that must be addressed; care managers can benefit from consulting with dietitians. In some circumstances dietitians are the case managers.

THEORIES ON AGING

Gerontologists study aging and have diverse theories about why the body ages. No single theory can fully explain the complex processes of aging (American Federation for Aging Research, 2011). A good theory integrates knowledge and tells how and why phenomena are related. Broadly, theories can be grouped into two categories: predetermined (genetic) and accumulated damage. A loss of efficiency comes about as some cells wear out, die, or are not replaced. Identification of the mechanisms that affect aging could lead to interventions that slow or alter aging. Most likely several theories explain the heterogeneity in older populations (see Table 20-1).

PHYSIOLOGIC CHANGES

Aging is a normal biologic process. However, it involves some decline in physiologic function. Organs change with age. The rates of change differ among individuals and within organ systems. It is important to distinguish between normal changes of aging and changes caused by chronic disease such as atherosclerosis.

The human growth period draws to a close at approximately age 30, when senescence begins. **Senescence** is the organic process of growing older and displaying the effects of increased age. Disease and impaired function are not inevitable parts of aging. Nevertheless, certain systemic changes occur as part of growing older. These changes result in varying degrees of efficiency and functional decline. Factors such as genetics, illnesses, socioeconomics, and lifestyle determine how aging progresses for each person. Indeed, one's outward expression of age may or may not reflect one's chronologic age, and ageist stereotypes should be eliminated (see Figure 20-1). Examples of active older adults include those surf fishing at 70, skiing expert slopes at 75, cycling 25 miles at 85, and playing league tennis at 90.

Body Composition

Body composition changes with aging. Fat mass and visceral fat increase, whereas lean muscle mass decreases. **Sarcopenia**, the loss of muscle mass, strength, and function, can be age related and can significantly affect an older adult's quality of life by decreasing mobility, increasing risk for falls, and altering metabolic rates (Dam et al, 2014). Sarcopenia accelerates with a decrease in physical activity, but weight-bearing exercise can slow its pace. Although inactive persons have faster and greater losses of muscle mass, sarcopenia also is found in active older individuals to a lesser degree. The criteria to make a diagnosis of sarcopenia are evolving and must be validated. The evidence-based cutpoints for weakness are grip strength less than 26 kg for men and less than 16 kg for women, and for low lean mass, appendicular lean mass adjusted for body mass index less than 0.789 for men and less than 0.512 for women. Further research using these cutpoint criteria is needed, especially in populations with high rates of functional limitations (Studenski et al, 2014). The proposed term "skeletal muscle function deficit" best describes the variety of muscular conditions that contribute to clinically meaningful mobility impairment (Correa-de-Araujo and Hadley, 2014). All losses are important because of the close connection between muscle mass and strength. By the fourth decade of life, evidence of sarcopenia is detectable, and the process accelerates after approximately age 75. Prevention strategies deserve emphasis because of the strong relationships of sarcopenia to functional decline, disability, hospitalization, institutionalization, and mortality (Litchford, 2014).

Sarcopenic obesity is the loss of lean muscle mass in older persons with excess adipose tissue. Together the excess weight and decreased muscle mass exponentially compound to further decrease physical activity, which in turn accelerates sarcopenia. An extremely sedentary lifestyle in obese persons is a major detractor from quality of life.

Sedentary lifestyle choices can lead to sedentary death syndrome (SeDS), a phrase coined by The President's Council on Physical Fitness. It describes the life-threatening health problems caused by a sedentary lifestyle. *Sedentary lifestyle* can be defined as a level of inactivity below the threshold of the beneficial health effects of regular physical activity or, more simply, burning fewer than 200 calories in physical activity per day. *The Surgeon General's Vision for a Healthy and Fit Nation 2010* emphasizes health consequences of inactivity as greater risk for cardiovascular disease (CVD), hypertension, diabetes, dyslipidemia, obesity, overweight, and even death (U.S. Department of Health and Human Services [USDHHS], 2010).

Few older adults achieve the minimum recommended 30 or more minutes of moderate physical activity on 5 or more days per week. About 42% of those aged 65 to 74 and 29% of those 75 and older reported that they engaged in regular leisure-time physical activity (Colby and Ortman, 2014). Inactivity is more common in older people than younger people; women often report no leisure-time activity. The American College of Sports Medicine (ACSM) position emphasizes that all older adults should engage in regular physical activity and avoid an inactive lifestyle (ACSM, 2009). The Centers for Disease Control and Prevention (CDC) quantifies the amount of exercise older adults need and the National Institute on Aging (NIA) has a guide for physical activity (CDC, 2013; NIA, 2010).

Taste and Smell

Sensory losses affect people to varying degrees, at varying rates, and at different ages (Benelam, 2009; Schiffman, 2009). Genetics, environment, and lifestyle are part of the decline in sensory competence. Age-related alterations to the sense of taste, smell, and touch can lead to poor appetite, inappropriate food choices,

and lower nutrient intake. Although some dysgeusia (altered taste), loss of taste, or hyposmia (decreased sense of smell) are attributable to aging, many changes are due to medications. Dysgeusia has been shown to be predictive of mortality in the elderly. Other causes include conditions such as Bell's palsy; head injury; diabetes; liver or kidney disease; hypertension; neurologic conditions, including Alzheimer's disease and Parkinson's disease; and zinc or niacin deficiency. Untreated mouth sores, tooth decay, poor dental or nasal hygiene, and cigarette smoking also can decrease these senses. Olfactory dysfunction is related to mortality (Jayant et al, 2014).

Because taste and smell sensation thresholds are higher, older adults may be tempted to overseason foods, especially to add more salt, which may have a negative effect in many older adults. Because taste and smell stimulate metabolic changes such as salivary, gastric acid, and pancreatic secretions and increases in plasma levels of insulin, decreased sensory stimulation may impair these metabolic processes as well.

Hearing and Eyesight

Hearing loss is the third most prevalent chronic condition in older Americans, it is the number one communicative disorder of the aged: between 25% and 40% of the population aged 65 years or older is hearing impaired (National Institute in Deafness and Other Communicative Disease [NIDCD], 2013b). The most common type of hearing loss is presbycusis (NIDCD, 2013a). This loss is usually greater in the high-pitched tonal range (e.g., telephone ring). The cumulative effect of exposure to daily noises such as traffic, construction, loud music, noisy office, and machines causes a change to the inner ear complex. The change occurs slowly over time, and sufferers may not be aware of the loss. The prevalence of presbycusis rises with age, ranging from 40% to 60% in patients older than 75 years to more than 80% in patients older than 85 years.

Some vitamins may play a part in hearing loss. Vitamin B_{12}, a nutrient often found to be deficient in the diets of older adults, has been associated with increased ringing in the ears, presbycusis, and reduced auditory brainstem response. Vitamin D may have an effect on hearing loss because of the role it plays in calcium metabolism, fluid and nerve transmission, and bone structure.

Age-related macular degeneration (AMD) is a disease of the retina that affects central vision and can lead to blindness in older people. AMD is the leading cause of legal blindness in Americans age 65 and older. It affects more than 1.75 million individuals in the United States. It is expected to increase to more than 5 million by 2050 (American Optometric Association [AOA], 2014). Smoking, race (it is more common in Caucasians), and family history are known risk factors (Chew et al, 2014; National Eye Institute, 2014). As the population ages, AMD is becoming a more significant public health problem. AMD occurs when the macula, the center part of the retina, degrades. The result is central vision loss. The macular pigment is composed of two chemicals, lutein and zeaxanthin. A diet rich in fruits and vegetables may help delay or prevent the development of AMD. Zinc also has been shown to decrease the risk of developing AMD. Micronutrition supplementation often is used in the treatment of AMD (Aslam et al, 2014). Finally, correcting obesity and smoking are modifiable factors that can reduce progression of AMD.

Presbyopia is a loss of elasticity in the crystalline lens that causes an inability to focus clearly at close distances and results in the need for reading glasses. This becomes apparent around the fourth decade of life (AOA, 2014). As it worsens, poor vision interferes with shopping, cooking, and eating.

Glaucoma is damage to the optic nerve resulting from high pressure in the eye. It is the second most common cause of vision loss, affecting approximately 3 million Americans. Hypertension, diabetes, and CVD increase the risk of glaucoma.

A cataract is a clouding of the lens of the eye. Approximately half of Americans 65 and older have some degree of clouding of the lens. The most common treatment is surgery; the clouded lens is removed and replaced with a permanent prosthetic lens. A diet high in antioxidants, such as beta carotene, selenium, resveratrol, and vitamins C and E, may delay cataract development. Studies show that a high sodium intake may increase risk of cataract development. Ultraviolet (UV) radiation exposure is related directly to 5% of worldwide cataracts. When the UV index is 3 and above, protective sunglasses are recommended.

Immunocompetence

As immunocompetence declines with age, immune response is slower and less efficient. Changes occur at all levels of the immune system, from chemical alterations within the cells to differences in the kinds of proteins found on the cell surface and even to mutations to entire organs. The progressive decline in T-lymphocyte function and cell-mediated immunity contributes to the increased infection and cancer rates seen in aging populations. The mechanisms of age-related changes in immune function are not fully understood but likely depend on environmental factors and lifestyle choices that affect overall immune function. Maintaining good nutritional status promotes good immune function.

Oral

Diet and nutrition can be compromised by poor oral health (see Chapter 25). Tooth loss, use of dentures, and xerostomia (dry mouth) can lead to difficulties in chewing and swallowing. Decreases in taste sensation and saliva production make eating less pleasurable and more difficult. Oral diseases and conditions are common among Americans who grew up without the benefit of community water fluoridation and other fluoride products. However, the percentage of Americans age 65 and older who are missing all of their natural teeth (edentulous) fell from 28% in 2000 to 2003 to 26% during 2004 to 2007. Missing, loose, or decayed teeth or poor-fitting, painful dentures are common problems that make it difficult to eat some foods. People with these mouth problems often prefer soft, easily chewed foods and avoid some nutritionally dense options such as whole grains, fresh fruits and vegetables, and meats.

The nutrition-related consequences of taking five or more medications or over-the-counter drugs daily (polypharmacy) are significant. More than 400 commonly used medications can cause dry mouth (see Chapter 8). Preparing foods that are moisture-rich such as hearty soups and stews, adding sauces, and pureeing and chopping foods can make meals easier to eat. In addition, those with poor oral health may benefit from fortified foods with increased nutrient density (see *Focus On: Food First!*).

Gastrointestinal

Some gastrointestinal (GI) changes may be age related. Rather than ascribing any of these disorders to aging, the true clinical cause should be determined. GI changes can negatively affect a person's nutrient intake, starting in the mouth. Dysphagia, a dysfunction in swallowing, commonly is associated with neurologic diseases and dementia. It increases the risk for aspiration pneumonia, an infection caused by food or fluids entering the lungs (see Chapter 34). Thickened liquids and texture-modified foods can help people with dysphagia eat safely (see The National Dysphagia Diet, Appendix 28, and appropriate levels of texture modification in Chapter 40).

Gastric changes also can occur. Decreased gastric mucosal function leads to an inability to resist damage such as ulcers, cancer, and infections. Gastritis causes inflammation and pain, delayed gastric emptying, and discomfort. These affect the bioavailability of nutrients such as calcium and zinc and increase the risk of developing a chronic deficiency disease such as osteoporosis.

Achlorhydria is the insufficient production of stomach acid. Approximately 30% of those older than age 50 have achlorhydria (Plummer, 2004). Sufficient stomach acid and intrinsic factor are required for the absorption of vitamin B_{12}. Although substantial amounts are stored in the liver, B_{12} deficiency does occur. Symptoms, often misdiagnosed because they mimic Alzheimer's disease or other chronic conditions, include extreme fatigue, dementia, confusion, and tingling and weakness in the arms and legs (see Chapter 40). It has become common practice to use calcium carbonate antacids as a way to supplement calcium intake. This is contraindicated in the elderly who are already at risk of inadequate gastric acid.

The incidence of diverticulosis increases with age. Half of the population older than age 60 develops it, but only 20% of them have clinical manifestations. The most common problems with diverticular disease are lower abdominal pain and diarrhea (see Chapter 28).

Constipation is defined as having fewer bowel movements than usual, having difficulty or excessive straining at stool, painful bowel movements, hard stool, or incomplete emptying of the bowel. It is one of the most common disorders in the U.S. population, and its prevalence increases with age. Primary causes include insufficient fluids, lack of physical activity, and low intake of dietary fiber. Studies have also shown distinct physiologic changes affecting colonic motility occur in older people. They include myenteric dysfunction, increased collagen deposits in the left colon, reduced inhibitory nerve input to the colon's muscle layer, and increased binding of plasma endorphins to intestinal receptors.

Diminished anal sphincter pressure or degeneration of the internal anal sphincter and loss of rectal wall elasticity are age-related changes. Constipation also is caused by some medications commonly used in older people such as narcotics and antidepressants that actually slow intestinal transit. Diuretics can cause decreased stool moisture, another contributing factor in constipation (see Chapters 7 and 8).

Cardiovascular

Cardiovascular disease (CVD), including heart disease and stroke, is the leading cause of death in both genders in all racial and ethnic groups and not necessarily a disease of aging. CVD age-related changes are extremely variable and are affected by environmental influences such as smoking, exercise, and diet. Changes include decreased arterial wall compliance, decreased maximum heart rate, decreased responsiveness to beta-adrenergic stimuli, increased left ventricle muscle mass, and slowed ventricular relaxation. Often the end result of hypertension and artery disease is chronic heart failure. One in nine hospital admissions in the United States include the diagnosis of heart failure. A low-sodium diet and fluid restriction are integral to the treatment of this condition. These necessary diet restrictions in conjunction with other side effects of heart failure often lead to decreased nutrient consumption. See Chapter 33 for discussion of the multifaceted approach required to manage CVD in older adults.

Renal

Age-related changes in renal function vary tremendously. Some older adults experience little change, whereas others can have devastating, life-threatening change. On average glomerular filtration rate, measured in creatinine clearance rates, declines by approximately 8 to 10 ml/min/1.73m2 per decade after age 30 to 35. The resulting increase in serum creatinine concentrations should be considered when determining medication dosages. The progressive decline in renal function can lead to an inability to excrete concentrated or dilute urine, a delayed response to sodium deprivation or a sodium load, and delayed response to an acid load. Renal function is also affected by dehydration, diuretic use, and medications, especially antibiotics (see Chapter 35).

Neurologic

There can be significant age-related declines in neurologic processes. Cognition, steadiness, reaction time, coordination, gait, sensations, and daily living tasks can decline as much as 90% or as little as 10%. On average, the brain loses 5% to 10% of its weight between the ages of 20 and 90, but most, if not all, neurons are functional until death unless a specific pathologic condition is present (Galvin and Sadowsky, 2012).

It is important to make the distinction between normal, age-related decline and impairment from conditions such as dementia, a disease process (Galvin and Sadowsky, 2012). Memory difficulties do not necessarily indicate dementia, Alzheimer's disease, Parkinson's disease, or any mental disorder (see Chapters 40 and 41). Many changes in memory can be attributed to environmental factors, including stress, chemical exposure, and poor diet rather than to physiologic processes. Urinary tract infections are associated with changes in cognition that mimic dementia but are reversible with treatment (Beveridge et al, 2011). However, even mild cognitive impairment may affect eating, chewing, and swallowing, thus increasing the risk of malnutrition (Lopes da Silva et al, 2012).

Pressure Ulcers

Pressure ulcers, formerly called bedsores or decubitus ulcers, develop from continuous pressure that impedes capillary blood flow to skin and underlying tissue. Several factors contribute to the formation of pressure ulcers, but impaired mobility, poor circulation, obesity, and urinary incontinence are key. Older adults with neurologic problems, those heavily sedated, and those with dementia are often unable to shift positions to alleviate pressure. Paralysis, incontinence, sensory losses, and rigidity can contribute to the problem. Notably malnutrition (inadequate protein) and undernutrition (inadequate energy intake) set the stage for its development and can delay wound healing. The escalating chronic nature of pressure

ulcers in non-ambulatory or sedentary elderly requires vigilant attention to nutrition.

Several classification systems describe pressure ulcers. The four stages of pressure ulcers, based on the depth of the sore and level of tissue involvement, are described in Table 20-2. As wound nutrition tends to equal whole-body nutrition, coordinated efforts of a multidisciplinary treatment team are important. Nutrition recommendations for the treatment of pressure ulcers are as follows (Doley, 2010; Thomas, 2014; Thomas and Burkemper, 2013):

- Optimize protein intake with a goal of 1.2 to 1.5 g/kg/day. Providing protein beyond 1.5 g/kg/day may cause dehydration without increasing protein synthesis. Also, there is no likely benefit from the administration of specific amino acids.
- Meet calorie requirements at 30 to 35 kcal/kg/day.
- Assess the effect of medications on wound healing and supplement if indicated.
- Replace micronutrients if depleted—routine supplementation is not warranted. There are no demonstrated benefits from supertherapeutic doses of vitamin C and zinc.

QUALITY OF LIFE

Quality of life is a general sense of happiness and satisfaction with one's life and environment. Health-related quality of life is the personal sense of physical and mental health and the ability to react to factors in the physical and social environments. To assess health-related quality of life, common measures and scales, either general or disease-specific, can be used. Because older age often is associated with health problems and decrease in functionality, quality-of-life issues become relevant.

Depression

Psychologic changes often manifest as depression, and its extent can vary widely from person to person. Among older persons depression often is caused by other conditions such as heart disease, stroke, diabetes, cancer, grief, or stress. Depression in older people frequently is undiagnosed or misdiagnosed because symptoms are confused with other medical illnesses. Untreated depression can have serious side effects for older adults. It diminishes the pleasures of living, including eating; it can exacerbate other medical conditions; and it can compromise immune function. It is associated with decreased appetite, weight loss, and fatigue. Nutritional care plays an important role in addressing this condition (see Chapter 41). Providing nutrient- and calorie-dense foods, additional beverages, texture-modified foods, and favorite foods at times when people are most likely to eat the greatest quantity can be very effective. In that comorbidities lead to polypharmacy and concern regarding drug-drug interactions, providers may choose to omit antidepressants, which leaves the depression untreated.

Given the untoward consequences of unintentional weight loss with aging and the lack of FDA-approved medications for appetite stimulation in older adults, food and nutritional interventions along with the treatment of underlying conditions that contribute to weight loss, such as poor dentition, deserve greater attention. One, antidepressant mirtazapine (Remeron) has helped increase appetite and weight gain in depressed elderly patients. With appropriate monitoring for side effects,

TABLE 20-2   Pressure Ulcer Stages

Suspected Deep Tissue Injury

Purple or maroon localized area of discolored intact skin or blood-filled blister caused by damage of underlying soft tissue from pressure or shear. The area may be preceded by tissue that is painful, firm, mushy, boggy, warmer, or cooler compared with adjacent tissue.

Deep tissue injury may be difficult to detect in individuals with dark skin tones. Evolution may include a thin blister over a dark wound bed. The wound may further evolve and become covered by thin eschar. Evolution may be rapid, exposing additional layers of tissue even with optimal treatment.

Stage I

Intact skin with non-blanchable redness of a localized area, usually over a bony prominence. Darkly pigmented skin may not have visible blanching; its color may differ from the surrounding area. The area may be painful, firm, soft, warmer, or cooler compared with adjacent tissue. Stage I may be difficult to detect in individuals with dark skin tones. May indicate "at-risk" persons (a heralding sign of risk).

Stage II

Partial thickness loss of dermis presenting as a shallow open ulcer with a red pink wound bed without slough. May also present as an intact or open or ruptured serum-filled blister.

Presents as a shiny or dry, shallow ulcer without slough or bruising. This stage should not be used to describe skin tears, tape burns, perineal dermatitis, maceration, or excoriation.

Bruising indicates suspected deep tissue injury

Stage III

Full-thickness tissue loss. Subcutaneous fat may be visible but bone, tendon, or muscle are not exposed. Slough may be present but does not obscure the depth of tissue loss. May include undermining and tunneling.

The depth of a stage III pressure ulcer varies by anatomic location. The bridge of the nose, ear, occiput, and malleolus do not have subcutaneous tissue, and stage III ulcers can be shallow. In contrast, areas of significant adiposity can develop extremely deep stage III pressure ulcers. Bone and tendon are not visible or directly palpable.

Stage IV

Full-thickness tissue loss with exposed bone, tendon, or muscle. Slough or eschar may be present on some parts of the wound bed, often include undermining and tunneling.

The depth of a stage IV pressure ulcer varies by anatomic location. The bridge of the nose, ear, occiput, and malleolus do not have subcutaneous tissue, and these ulcers can be shallow. Stage IV ulcers can extend into muscle and supporting structures (e.g., fascia, tendon, or joint capsule), making osteomyelitis possible. Exposed bone or tendon is visible or directly palpable.

Unstageable

Full-thickness tissue loss in which the base of the ulcer is covered by slough (yellow, tan, gray, green, or brown) or eschar (tan, brown, or black) in the wound bed. Until enough slough or eschar is removed to expose the base of the wound, the true depth, and therefore stage, cannot be determined. Stable (dry, adherent, intact without erythema or fluctuance) eschar on the heels serves as "the body's natural (biologic) cover" and should not be removed.

National Pressure Ulcer Advisory Panel, European Pressure Ulcer Advisory Panel and Pan Pacific Pressure Injury Alliance, The Prevention and Treatment of Pressure Ulcers: Quick Reference Guide, 2014 http://www.npuap.org/wp-content/uploads/2014/08/Updated-10-16-14-Quick-Reference-Guide-DIGITAL-NPUAP-EPUAP-PPPIA-16Oct2014.pdf

mirtazapine may be a drug of choice for older persons experiencing weight loss and depression (Rudolph, 2009).

Food and nutrition contribute to one's physiologic, psychologic, and social quality of life. A measure of nutrition-related quality of life has been proposed to document quality-of-life outcomes for individuals receiving medical nutrition therapy. Effective strategies to improve eating and thereby improve nursing home residents' quality of life are well established but could be more widely implemented (Bernstein et al, 2012) (see *New Directions: Culture Change*).

✳ NEW DIRECTION

Culture Change

Janice L. Raymond, MS, RD, CSG

Culture Change in Long-Term Care

Pioneer Network was formed in 1997 by a small group of prominent professionals (including dietitians) working in long-term care to advocate for person-directed care. This group called for a radical change in the culture of aging so that when our grandparents, parents—and ultimately we—go to a nursing home or other community-based setting, it is to thrive, not to decline. This movement, away from institutional provider-driven models to more humane consumer-driven models that embrace flexibility and self-determination, has come to be known as the *long-term care culture change movement*. The belief is that the quality of life and living for older Americans is rooted in a supportive community and cemented by relationships that respect each individual regardless of age, medical condition, or limitations.

The mission of the Pioneer Network is to

- Create communication, networking, and learning opportunities
- Build and support relationships and community
- Identify and promote transformations in practice, services, public policy, and research
- Develop and provide access to resources and leadership

Values and Principles

- Know each person.
- Each person can and does make a difference.
- Relationship is the fundamental building block of a transformed culture.
- Respond to spirit, as well as mind and body.
- Risk taking is a normal part of life.
- Put person before task.
- All elders are entitled to self-determination wherever they live.
- Community is the antidote to institutionalization.
- Do unto others as you would have them do unto you.
- Promote the growth and development of all.
- Shape and use the potential of the environment in all its aspects: physical, organizational, psycho/social/spiritual.
- Practice self-examination, searching for new creativity and opportunities for doing better.
- Recognize that culture change and transformation are not destinations but a journey, always a work in progress. https://www.pioneernetwork.net/

Functionality

Functionality and *functional status* are terms used to describe physical abilities and limitations in, for example, ambulation. **Functionality**, the ability to perform self-care, self-maintenance, and physical activities, correlates with independence and quality of life. Disability rates among older adults are declining, but the actual number considered disabled is increasing as the size of the aging population grows. Limitations in **activities of** daily living (ADLs) (toileting, bathing, eating, dressing) and instrumental activities of daily living (IADLs) such as managing money, shopping, telephone use, travel in community, housekeeping, preparing meals, taking medications correctly, and other individual self-performance skills needed in everyday life, are used to monitor physical function (Federal Interagency Forum on Aging-Related Statistics, 2012).

Many nutrition-related diseases affect functional status in older individuals. Inadequate nutrient intake may hasten loss of muscle mass and strength, which can have a negative effect on performing ADLs. Among the older adults who have one or more nutrition-related chronic diseases, impaired physical function may cause greater disability, with increased morbidity, nursing home admissions, or death.

Frailty and Failure to Thrive

The four syndromes known to be predictive of adverse outcomes in older adults that are prevalent in patients with frailty or "geriatric failure to thrive" include impaired physical functioning, malnutrition, depression, and cognitive impairment. Symptoms include weight loss, decreased appetite, poor nutrition, dehydration, inactivity, and impaired immune function. Interventions should be directed at easily remediable contributors in the hope of improving overall functional status. Optimal management requires a multidisciplinary multifaceted approach. Occupational therapists and speech therapists are essential to comprehensive care management. Nutrition interventions, especially those rectifying protein-energy malnutrition (PEM), are essential but often difficult to implement in an older person who is disinterested in eating. Because overall diet quality has been shown to be associated inversely with prevalent and future frailty status in a large cohort of community-living older men, more attention to the total dietary intakes when advancing age is critical (Galvin and Sadowsky, 2012). Liberalization of overly restrictive diet prescriptions is often key to improving calorie intake and dietary quality (American Dietetic Association [ADA], 2010).

Weight Maintenance
Obesity

The prevalence of obesity in all ages has increased during the past 25 years in the United States; older adults are no exception. Obesity rates are greater among those ages 65 to 74 than among those age 75 and older. Obesity is a major cause of preventable disease and premature death. Both are linked to increased risk of coronary heart disease; type 2 diabetes; endometrial, colon, postmenopausal breast, and other cancers; asthma and other respiratory problems; osteoarthritis; and disability (Flicker et al, 2010). Obesity causes a progressive decline in physical function, which may lead to increased frailty. Overweight and obesity can lead to a decline in IADLs.

Weight loss therapy that maintains muscle and bone mass is recommended for obese older adults because it improves physical function and quality of life and reduces the multiple medical complications associated with obesity. Lifestyle changes that include diet, physical activity, and behavior modification techniques are the most effective. The goals of weight loss and management for adults are the same for the general population and should include prevention of further weight gain, or reduction of body weight, and maintenance of long-term weight loss (see Chapter 21).

Weight loss of 10% of total body weight over 6 months should be the initial goal. After that, strategies for maintenance should be implemented. Dietary changes include an energy deficit of 500 to 1000 kcal/day. Calorie restriction should not be less than 1200 kcal/day. It is critical for the older adult on a calorie-restricted diet to meet nutrient requirements. This may necessitate the use of a multivitamin or mineral supplement as well as nutrition education.

Being overweight after age 70 may be health protective. A study reviewed data from two long-term studies and found that adults who were overweight averaged a 13% lower risk of death from any cause over 10 years, compared with those who were normal weight (Flicker et al, 2010). Those who were underweight were 76% more likely to die (see later in this chapter), although the obese had the same mortality risk as those of normal weight. The researchers concluded that the BMI thresholds for overweight and obese may be overly restrictive for older adults. Notably, the researchers also found that being sedentary increased the risk of death in men by 28%; in women, the risk was doubled.

Underweight and Malnutrition

The actual prevalence of underweight among older adults is low; women older than age 65 are three times as likely as their male counterparts to be underweight (Winter et al, 2014). However, many older adults are at risk for undernutrition and malnutrition (Federal Interagency Forum on Aging-Related Statistics, 2012). Among those hospitalized, 40% to 60% are malnourished or at risk for malnutrition, 40% to 85% of nursing home residents have malnutrition, and 20% to 60% of home care patients are malnourished. Many community-residing older persons consume fewer than 1000 kcal/day, an amount not adequate to maintain good nutrition. Some causes of undernutrition include medications, depression, decreased sense of taste or smell, poor oral health, chronic diseases, dysphagia, and other physical problems that make eating difficult. Social causes may include living alone, inadequate income, lack of transportation, and limitations in shopping for and preparing food.

Health care professionals frequently overlook protein-energy malnutrition (PEM). The physiologic changes of aging, as well as changes in living conditions and income, contribute to the problem. Symptoms of PEM often are attributed to other conditions, leading to misdiagnosis. Some common symptoms are confusion, fatigue, and weakness. Older adults with low incomes, who have difficulty chewing and swallowing meat, who smoke, or engage in little or no physical activity are at increased risk of developing PEM.

Strategies to decrease PEM include increased caloric and protein intake. The Practice Paper for dietitians provides a variety of approaches that can be used in residential facilities (ADA, 2010). In a long-term care clinical setting oral medical nutrition supplements and enteral feedings may be considered but should be the last resort. Reliance on medical nutritional supplements actually may affect the elderly negatively. It is important that people continue to smell and chew real food.

In community settings older adults should be encouraged to eat energy-dense and high-protein foods. Federal food and nutrition services are also available for the many who reside at home (see sections below) (See *Focus On: Food First!*). Diet restrictions should be liberalized to offer more choices (ADA, 2010). Simple practical approaches, such as adding gravies and creams, can increase calories and soften foods for easier chewing.

Food First!

Digna Cassens, MHA, RDN

There are many reasons for practitioners to consider changing from the use of commercially manufactured nutritional supplements to nutrient-dense real food. Although commercial nutritional supplements are convenient to use and provide high calories and high protein, people like to eat food and drink fluids that taste good, provide a variety of flavors, and are familiar to them. Food is more than a can of soy protein with added vitamins and minerals, it is culture, tradition, and part of life celebrations. The smell of food and appearance on a plate is part of the overall eating experience.

Fortified foods at meals and snack time in lieu of commercially prepared supplements can satisfy the most demanding palate because they can be flexible and individualized. Virtually any food can be calorie enhanced; many can be protein enhanced.

Fortified food programs have been known by a variety of names: Every Bite Counts, Nutrition Intervention Program, Enhanced Food Program, Super Foods, or Food Fortification Program. Today, thanks to the Dining Practice Standards published in 2011 and adopted by the Centers for Medicare and Medicaid, **Food First!** is the term of choice for this approach. Traditionally, fortified food programs have focused on adding calories and protein to a couple of foods on the menu each day. For example, cream is added to hot cereal and powdered milk is added to milk (double-strength milk). This approach can lead to lack of variety and food fatigue. A program approach to fortifying food will provide more flexibility and ultimately be more successful.

Modified from www.flavorfulfortifiedfood.com.

NUTRITION SCREENING AND ASSESSMENT

Simple and easy-to-use nutrition screening tools have been validated (Skipper et al, 2012). However, the physical and metabolic changes of aging can yield inaccurate results. Examples are anthropometric measurements: height and weight, and BMI. A meta-analysis of BMI and all-cause mortality concluded that being overweight was not associated with an increased risk of mortality in older populations. The mortality risk increased in underweight older people, those with a BMI of less than 23 (Winter et al, 2014).

With aging, fat mass increases and height decreases as a result of vertebral compression. An accurate height measure may be difficult in those unable to stand up straight, the bed bound, those with spinal deformations such as a dowager's hump, and those with osteoporosis. Measuring arm span or knee height may give more accurate measurements (see Appendix 15). BMIs based on questionable heights are inaccurate. Clinical judgment is needed for accuracy.

The Mini Nutritional Assessment (MNA) includes two forms: a screening Short Form (MNA-SF) and the full assessment (Kaiser et al, 2009). The validated MNA-SF is the most widely used screening method to identify malnutrition in non-institutionalized older adults (see Figure 4-5). It includes six questions and a body mass index (BMI) evaluation, or a calf circumference if a BMI is not possible. The MNA-SF is being used as a screening assessment tool in long-term care and is especially useful in the short stay units.

NUTRITION NEEDS

Many older adults have special nutrient requirements because aging affects absorption, use, and excretion of nutrients (Bernstein et al, 2012). The dietary reference intakes (DRIs) separate the cohort of people age 50 and older into two groups, ages 50 to 70 and 71 and older. Based on the Healthy Eating Index, older Americans need to a) increase their intakes of whole grains, dark green and orange vegetables, legumes, and milk; b) choose more nutrient-dense forms of foods, that is, foods low in solid fats and free of added sugars; and c) lower their intake of sodium and saturated fat. Other studies show that older persons have low intakes of calories, total fat, fiber, calcium, magnesium, zinc, copper, folate, and vitamins B_{12}, C, E, and D. Box 20-1 lists the Key Recommendations for Older Adults as specified in the *2010 Dietary Guidelines for Americans*. A *MyPlate for Older Adults* that corresponds to the *2010 Guidelines* is available online (Lichtenstein, 2014).

The Mifflin-St. Jeor energy equation can be used to assess calorie needs in healthy older adults (see Chapter 2). The DRI tables (see Table 20-3 and inside cover) also can be used. DRIs for energy suggest 3067 kcal/day for men and 2403/day for

---

BOX 20-1 Dietary Guidelines for Americans 2010

Key Recommendations for Older Adults

- **Maintain calorie balance over the lifetime to achieve and sustain a healthy weight.** Healthy eating patterns limit intake of sodium, solid fats, added sugars, and refined grains. Increased physical activity and reduced time spent in sedentary behaviors are also desired.
- **Focus on consuming nutrient-dense foods and beverages.** A healthy eating pattern emphasizes nutrient-dense foods and beverages. Select fat-free or low-fat milk and milk products, seafood, lean meats and poultry, eggs, beans and peas, and nuts and seeds. Choose vegetables, fruits, whole grains, and milk and milk products for more potassium, dietary fiber, calcium, and vitamin D as nutrients of concern. Eat a variety of vegetables, especially dark-green and red and orange vegetables, beans and peas. Consume at least half of all grains as whole grains.
- **Nutrient needs should be met primarily through consuming foods.** When needed, fortified foods and dietary supplements may be useful in providing one or more nutrients that otherwise might be consumed in less than recommended amounts. Consume foods fortified with vi-

tamin B_{12}, such as fortified cereals, or dietary supplements. Two eating patterns that are beneficial are Vegetarian adaptations and the DASH (Dietary Approaches to Stop Hypertension) Eating Plan.
- **A healthy eating pattern should prevent foodborne illness.** Four basic food safety principles (Clean, Separate, Cook, and Chill) work together to reduce the risk of foodborne illnesses. In addition, some foods (such as milks, cheeses, and juices that have not been pasteurized, and undercooked animal foods) pose high risk for foodborne illness and should be avoided.
- **Use alcohol in moderation.** If alcohol is consumed, it should be consumed in moderation—up to one drink per day for women and two drinks per day for men—and only by adults of legal drinking age.
- Individuals should meet the following recommendations as part of a healthy eating pattern while staying within their calorie needs.
- Information on the type and strength of evidence supporting the Dietary Guidelines recommendations can be found at http://www.nutritionevidencelibrary.gov.

U.S. Department of Health and Human Services, U.S. Department of Agriculture: *Dietary Guidelines for Americans, 2010*, ed 7, Washington, DC, 2010, U.S. Government Printing Office.

TABLE 20-3 Nutrient Needs Change with Aging

Nutrient	Changes with Aging	Practical Solutions
Energy	Basal metabolic rate decreases with age because of changes in body composition. Energy needs decrease ~3% per decade in adults.	Encourage nutrient-dense foods in amounts appropriate for caloric needs.
Protein 0.8 g/kg minimum	Minimal change with age but research is not conclusive. Requirements vary with chronic disease, decreased absorption, and synthesis.	Protein intake should not be routinely increased; excess protein could unnecessarily stress aging kidneys.
Carbohydrates 45%-65% total calories Men 30 g fiber Women 21 g fiber	Constipation may be a serious concern for many.	Emphasize complex carbohydrates: legumes, vegetables, whole grains, fruits to provide fiber, essential vitamins, minerals. Increase dietary fiber to improve laxation especially in older adults.
Lipids 20%-35% total calories	Heart disease is a common diagnosis.	Overly severe restriction of dietary fats alters taste, texture, and enjoyment of food; can negatively affect overall diet, weight, and quality of life. Emphasize healthy fats rather restricting fat.
Vitamins and minerals	Understanding vitamin and mineral requirements, absorption, use, and excretion with aging has increased but much remains unknown.	Encourage nutrient-dense foods in amounts appropriate for caloric needs. Oxidative and inflammatory processes affecting aging reinforce the central role of micronutrients, especially antioxidants.
Vitamin B_{12} 2.4 mg	Risk of deficiency increases because of low intakes of vitamin B_{12}, and decline in gastric acid, which facilitates B_{12} absorption.	Those 50 and older should eat foods fortified with the crystalline form of vitamin B_{12} such as in fortified cereals or supplements.
Vitamin D 600-800 IU*	Risk of deficiency increases as synthesis is less efficient; skin responsiveness as well as exposure to sunlight decline; kidneys are less able to convert D_3 to active hormone form. As many as 30%-40% of those with hip fractures are vitamin D insufficient.	Supplementation may be necessary and is inexpensive. A supplement is indicated in virtually all institutionalized older adults.
Folate 400 μg	May lower homocysteine levels; possible risk marker for atherothrombosis, Alzheimer's disease, and Parkinson's disease	Fortification of grain products has improved folate status. When supplementing with folate, must monitor B_{12} levels.
Calcium 1200 mg	Dietary requirement may increase because of decreased absorption; only 4% of women and 10% of men age 60 and older meet daily recommendation from food sources alone.	Recommend naturally occurring and fortified foods. Supplementation may be necessary. However, in older women, high intakes may be occurring with supplements.
Potassium 4700 mg	Potassium-rich diet can blunt the effect of sodium on blood pressure.	Recommend meeting potassium recommendation with food, especially fruits and vegetables.
Sodium 1500 mg	Risk of hypernatremia caused by dietary excess and dehydration Risk of hyponatremia caused by fluid retention	Newer evidence based on direct health outcomes is inconsistent with the recommendation to lower dietary sodium in the general population, including older adults, to 1500 mg per day. More research is needed.†
Zinc Men 11 mg Women 8 mg	Low intake associated with impaired immune function, anorexia, loss of sense of taste, delayed wound healing, and pressure ulcer development.	Encourage food sources: lean meats, oysters, dairy products, beans, peanuts, tree nuts, and seeds.
Water	Hydration status can easily be problematic. Dehydration causes decreased fluid intake, decreased kidney function, increased losses caused by increased urine output from medications (laxatives, diuretics). Symptoms: electrolyte imbalance, altered drug effects, headache, constipation, blood pressure change, dizziness, confusion, dry mouth and nose	Encourage fluid intake of at least 1500 ml/day or 1 ml per calorie consumed. Risk increases because of impaired sense of thirst, fear of incontinence, and dependence on others to get beverages. Dehydration is often unrecognized; it can present as falls, confusion, change in level of consciousness, weakness or change in functional status, or fatigue.

* National Research Council: *Dietary Reference Intakes for Calcium and Vitamin D*, Washington, DC, 2011, The National Academies Press.
†National Research Council: *Sodium intake in populations: assessment of evidence*, Washington, DC, 2013, The National Academies Press.

women 18 years; subtract 10 kcal/day for men and 7 kcal/day for women for each year of age older than 19 years.

The DRIs are not specific for protein in older adults. After age 65, the minimum protein requirement is 1 g protein/kg of body weight with newer evidence supporting up to 1.2 gm/kg. In those individuals with impaired renal function or long-standing diabetes, 0.8 g/kg to 1.0 g/kg may be more appropriate. Protein distribution evenly throughout the day with no single serving exceeding 30 g should be a goal.

MEDICARE BENEFITS

The federal Medicare program covers most of the health care costs of those 65 and older and persons with disabilities. However, this federally funded health insurance program does not cover the entire cost of residential/institutional long-term care. A portion of payroll taxes and monthly premiums deducted from Social Security payments finance Medicare.

Medicare benefits are provided in four parts. *Part A* covers inpatient hospital care, some skilled nursing care, hospice care, and some home health care costs for limited periods of time. It is premium free for most citizens. *Part B* has a monthly premium that helps pay for doctors, outpatient hospital care, and some other care not covered by Part A (physical and occupational therapy, for example). *Part C* allows private insurers, including health maintenance organizations (HMOs) and preferred provider organizations (PPOs), to offer health insurance plans to Medicare beneficiaries. These must provide the same benefits the original Medicare plan provides under Parts A and B. Part C HMOs and PPOs also may offer additional benefits, such as dental and vision care. *Part D* provides prescription drug benefits through private insurance companies.

The **2010 Affordable Care Act** (see Chapter 10) changed Medicare to include an annual wellness visit and a personalized prevention assessment and plan with no copayment or deductible. Prevention services include referrals to education and preventive counseling or community-based interventions to address risk factors. Thus expansion of medical nutrition therapy reimbursement for registered dietitians/nutritionists is likely. It will cover therapy considered reasonable and necessary for the prevention of an illness or disability as well as a broader array of nutrition counseling for chronic conditions. More universal access to nutrition services has implications for aging healthier and promoting quality of life and independence.

Medicaid, for qualified low-income individuals, finances a variety of long-term care services via multiple mechanisms, including Medicaid State Plans and home and community-based services (HCBS) waivers, Section 1915 (c). Both provide service to nursing home–appropriate older adults to help prevent or decrease nursing home or institutionalization. States may offer an unlimited variety of services under this waiver. These programs may provide traditional medical services (dental, skilled nursing) and nonmedical services (meal delivery, case management, environmental modifications). States have the discretion to choose the number of older persons served and the services offered.

Program of All-Inclusive Care for the Elderly (PACE) is a comprehensive managed care system for people over 55 who are nursing home eligible and who meet low income criteria. The program is funded through Medicare and Medicaid. Coordinated preventive, primary, acute and long-term care services allow older adults to remain in their homes for as long as possible (Thomas and Burkemper, 2013). The PACE model is based on the belief that it is better for the well-being of older adults with chronic care needs to be served in the community whenever possible. PACE is multidisciplinary and includes dietitian services. There are more than 100 PACE Programs nationwide.

PACE Programs and HCBS waiver reflect federal commitments to delay or avoid nursing home placement whenever possible. The U.S. Administration on Aging is now under the new umbrella of the U.S Administration on Community Living. Terms such as "aging in community," "communitarian alternatives," "age-friendly living," "care circles," and especially "long-term services and supports" (LSS) (versus "long-term *care*") are indicative of the transformations taking place in the more positive approaches to aging (Bernstein et al, 2012; Rudolph, 2009).

NUTRITION SUPPORT SERVICES

U.S. Department of Health and Human Services Older Americans Act (OAA) Nutrition Program

The OAA Nutrition Program is the largest, most visible, federally funded community-based nutrition program for older persons (Lloyd and Wellman, 2015). Primarily a state-run program, it has few federal regulations and considerable variation in state-to-state policies and procedures. This nutrition program provides congregate and home-delivered meals (usually 5 days per week), nutrition screening, education, and counseling, as well as an array of other supportive and health services. Although frequently called *meals on wheels,* that term accurately refers *only* to the home-delivered meals. Participants are poorer, older, sicker, frailer, more likely to live alone, be members of minority groups, and live in rural areas. The OAA Nutrition Program, available to all persons age 60 and older regardless of income, successfully targets those in greatest economic and social need, with particular attention to low-income minorities and rural populations. Unfortunately, the program reaches fewer than 5% of older Americans, and those are served an average of fewer than three meals per week because of budget constraints. However, if all states had increased by 1% the number of adults age 65 and older who received home-delivered meals in 2009, total annual savings to states' Medicaid programs could have exceeded $109 million (Thomas and Mor, 2013). The savings would come from decreased Medicaid spending on those with low care needs because they would no longer require nursing home care. The Nutrition Program has neither received the research or evaluation attention that a program its size deserves nor the growth in federal funding to keep pace with inflation and the growing numbers of older adults (Wellman, 2010).

More than half of the OAA annual budget supports the nutrition program, which provides about 224 million congregate and home-delivered meals to 2.5 million older adults annually (U.S. Administration on Aging, 2014). Home-delivered meals have grown to more than 61% of all meals served; almost half of the programs have waiting lists. To receive home-delivered meals, an individual must be assessed to be homebound or otherwise isolated. Home-delivered meal recipients are especially frail; half are at high nutrition risk or are malnourished and approximately one third qualify as nursing home appropriate.

At congregate sites, the nutrition program provides access and linkages to other community-based services. It is the primary source of food and nutrients for many program participants and presents opportunities for active social engagement and meaningful volunteer roles.

For the majority of program participants, the meal provides half or more of their total food for the day. Thus participants have higher daily intakes of key nutrients than similar nonparticipants. The meals are nutritionally dense per calorie and each meal supplies more than 33% of the recommended dietary allowances (an OAA requirement) and provides 40% to 50% of daily intakes of most nutrients (Lloyd and Wellman, 2015). Otherwise, inadequate nutrient intake affects approximately 37% to 40% of community-dwelling individuals 65 years of age and older (Lloyd and Wellman, 2015).

The OAA Nutrition Program is closely linked to **home- and community-based services (HCBS)** through cross-referrals within the Aging Network. Because older adults are being discharged earlier from hospitals and nursing homes, many require a care plan that includes home-delivered meals and other nutrition services (e.g., nutrition screening, assessment, education, counseling, and care planning). Many states are creating programs to provide necessary medical, social, and supportive HCBS, including home-delivered meals, nutrition education, and counseling services. States are being encouraged to help older adults and people with disabilities live in their homes and fully participate in their communities by the new U.S. Administration for Community Living (ACL). Its role is to build the capacity of the national aging and disability networks to better serve older persons, caregivers, and individuals with disabilities.

USDA Food Assistance Programs

Several U.S. Department of Agriculture (USDA) food and nutrition assistance programs are available to older adults (Kamp et al, 2010). All USDA programs are means tested (i.e., recipients must meet income criteria). Several of these programs, for example, the Supplemental Nutrition Assistance Program (SNAP, formerly food stamps), are discussed in Chapter 9.

Commodity Supplemental Food Program

The Commodity Supplemental Food Program (CSFP) strives to improve the health of low-income Americans by supplementing their diets with nutritious USDA commodity foods. It provides food and administrative funds to states, but not all are enrolled. In states, CSFP administration may be located in diverse sites such as public health, nutrition services, or agriculture departments. Eligible populations include adults age 60 and older with incomes less than 130% of the poverty level. Local CSFP agencies determine eligibility, distribute the foods, and provide nutrition education. The food packages do not provide a complete diet but may be good sources of nutrients frequently lacking in low-income diets.

Seniors Farmers' Market Nutrition Program

The Seniors Farmers' Market Nutrition Program (SFMNP) is administered by state departments of agriculture, aging and disability services, health and human service, markets, public health, state units on aging, or state food and nutrition services. SFMNP provides coupons to low-income older individuals to purchase fresh, unprepared foods at farmers' markets, roadside stands, and community-supported agriculture programs. It provides eligible older adults with local, seasonal access to fresh fruits, vegetables, and fresh-cut herbs as well as nutrition education and information.

Medicaid and Nutrition Services

The Social Security Act suggests seven core HCBS waiver program services: case management, homemaker services, home health aide services, personal care services, adult day health, rehabilitation, and respite care. Nutrition service is not a core Medicaid service. Older persons who are eligible for nursing home placement are not usually able to shop for food, store food safely, or plan and prepare nutritionally appropriate meals. Thus a strong argument can be made to fund all or some meals and nutrition services based on health and nutrition risk criteria. However, not all states include meals or nutrition services among the specified benefits available through Medicaid waivers. Approved nutrition services include home-delivered meals, nutrition risk reduction counseling, and in some cases, nutritional supplements.

COMMUNITY AND RESIDENTIAL FACILITIES FOR OLDER ADULTS

The report *Long-term Care Services in the United States* found that about 58,500 paid, regulated long-term care services providers served about 8 million people (Harris-Kojetin et al, 2013). Long-term care services were provided by 4800 adult day services centers, 12,200 home health agencies, 3700 hospices, 15,700 nursing homes, and 22,200 assisted living and similar residential care communities. Each day, there are more than 273,200 participants enrolled in adult day services centers, 1,383,700 residents in skilled nursing facilities (SNFs), and 713,300 residents in residential care communities; in 2011, about 4,742,500 patients received services from home health agencies, and 1,244,500 patients received services from hospices.

People move to residential facilities, generally known as assisted living, when they can no longer safely live alone because they have some cognitive impairment requiring supervision or need help with ADLs because of immobility. Care is provided in ways that promote maximum independence and dignity. Assisted living care's annual cost is about half that of nursing homes (MetLife Mature Market Institute, 2012). Residents are encouraged to maintain active social lives with planned activities, exercise classes, religious and social functions, and field trips directed by the facilities. These communities are now required in some states to provide therapeutic diets but in those states without such regulation residents have difficulty getting special requirements met.

Comprehensive state regulations for food and nutrition services in assisted living care is not yet widespread, but there is early consensus of what should be regulated (Chao et al, 2009). Emphasizing that food and nutrition matter at every age, it is essential that support for nutrition and quality of life extend beyond food availability and safety. Dietitian expertise is needed for nutrition assessment and care planning to meet special needs such as type and amounts of macronutrients and micronutrients, texture modifications, and quality of food choices and presentation.

Only about 3% or 1.4 million older adults live in the approximately 15,700 nursing homes (Harris-Kojetin et al, 2013). The percentage of the population that lives in nursing homes increases dramatically with age, especially for those older than age 85. However, the overall percentage has declined since 1990, likely because of healthier aging, the federal cost-containment policy to delay residential placement in nursing homes by providing more aging services in the community, as well as the increased availability and use of hospice. The percentage increases dramatically with age, ranging from 1% for persons age 65 to 74 years to 3% for persons age 75 to 84 years and 10% for persons age 85. The average annual cost is $90,500 (MetLife Mature Market Institute, 2012).

SNFs are federally regulated by the Centers for Medicare and Medicaid Services; assisted living centers, by each state. More residents are in SNFs for short-stay, postacute care; thus more comprehensive medical nutrition therapy is now needed. Nutritional care is directed toward identifying and responding to changing physiologic and psychologic needs over time that protect against avoidable decline.

The culture change movement in long-term care has led to the creation of the Dining Practice Standards (DPS). The DPS were published by the Pioneer Network's Dining Clinical Task Force and have been endorsed by CMS and over a dozen professional groups, including the AND. They provide evidence-based support for resident-centered dining, for liberalized diets, for the use of real food rather than medical nutritional supplements, and for the incorporation of these standards into the CMS survey process.

In 1987 Congress passed reform legislation as part of the Omnibus Reconciliation Act (OBRA) to improve the quality of care in SNFs by strengthening standards that must be met for Medicare/Medicaid reimbursement. Since that time SNFs have been required by CMS to conduct periodic assessments to determine the residents' needs; to provide services that ensure residents maintain the highest practical physical, mental, and psychologic well-being; and to ensure that no harm is inflicted. This is accomplished using the **Minimum Data Set (MDS)**, which is part of the federally mandated process for clinical assessment of residents of LTC facilities licensed under Medicare or Medicaid. Section K of the MDS is specific to nutrition and is generally the responsibility of the dietitian to complete but can be done by nursing staff (see Figure 20-4). This form documents "triggers" that may place a resident at nutrition risk and therefore requires an intervention. This assessment must be done at admission and if there is a significant change in the resident's condition such as weight loss or skin breakdown. Reassessment is required quarterly and annually. The entire process is known as the **Resident Assessment Instrument (RAI)**. It provides the individual assessment of each resident's functional capabilities and helps identify problems and develop a care plan.

High nutrition risk individuals must be identified and assessed monthly by the dietitian. High risk is defined as:

- Significant weight loss defined as 5% of body weight in 1 month or 10% of body weight in 6 months
- Nutrition support (tube feedings or parenteral nutrition)
- Dialysis patients
- Wounds or pressure ulcers

Section K	**Swallowing/Nutritional Status**

K0100. Swallowing Disorder

Signs and symptoms of possible swallowing disorder

↓ Check all that apply

☐	A. **Loss of liquids/solids from mouth when eating or drinking**
☐	B. **Holding food in mouth/cheeks or residual food in mouth after meals**
☐	C. **Coughing or choking during meals or when swallowing medications**
☐	D. **Complaints of difficulty or pain with swallowing**
☐	Z. **None of the above**

K0200. Height and Weight - While measuring, if the number is X.1 - X.4 round down; X.5 or greater round up

☐☐ inches	A. **Height** (in inches). Record most recent height measure since admission
☐☐☐ pounds	B. **Weight** (in pounds). Base weight on most recent measure in last 30 days; measure weight consistently, according to standard facility practice (e.g., in a.m. after voiding, before meal, with shoes off, etc.)

K0300. Weight Loss

Enter Code ☐	**Loss of 5% or more in the last month or loss of 10% or more in last 6 months** 0. **No** or unknown 1. **Yes, on** physician-prescribed weight-loss regimen 2. **Yes, not on** physician-prescribed weight-loss regimen

K0500. Nutritional Approaches

↓ Check all that apply

☐	A. **Parenteral/IV feeding**
☐	B. **Feeding tube** - nasogastric or abdominal (PEG)
☐	C. **Mechanically altered diet** - require change in texture of food or liquids (e.g., pureed food, thickened liquids)
☐	D. **Therapeutic diet** (e.g., low salt, diabetic, low cholesterol)
☐	Z. **None of the above**

K0700. Percent Intake by Artificial Route - Complete K0700 only if K0500A or K0500B is checked

Enter Code ☐	A. **Proportion of total calories the resident received through parenteral or tube feeding** 1. **25% or less** 2. **26-50%** 3. **51% or more**
Enter Code ☐	B. **Average fluid intake per day by IV or tube feeding** 1. **500 cc/day or less** 2. **501 cc/day or more**

FIGURE 20-4 The Minimum Data Set, Section K version 3.0. (From the Centers for Medicare & Medicaid Services, Baltimore, MD.)

CLINICAL CASE STUDY

MF is an 86-year-old Caucasian female resident in a skilled nursing facility with unintentional weight loss. She was admitted 3 months ago from the hospital after a hip fracture. She had been residing in an independent living facility for several years. She reports she has been eating poorly because of difficulty moving around, being generally uncomfortable, and states, "If I am not active I don't need to eat so much." Intake is less than 50% of regular diet. No problems chewing or swallowing are noted after a speech language pathologist's evaluation. Admission weight was 112 pounds; current weight is 95 pounds. Self-reported height is 5'3"; Hgb/Hct, normal; total cholesterol, 135; and Mini Nutrition Assessment score, 5. Hip scans show slow fracture healing and no improvement in bone density; currently she is being supplemented with calcium 1000 mg/day and vitamin D 600 IU/day. Blood pressure, 128/80 with furosemide (Lasix); other medications are lorazepam (Ativan), fentanyl transdermal patch (Duragesic), senna (Senokot-S), docusate (Colace), and mirtazapine (Remeron).

Nutrition Diagnostic Statement

Unintentional weight loss related to food intake of less than 50% of meals with limited physical activity as evidenced by weight loss of 17 lb.

Nutrition Case Study Questions

1. Comment on the appropriateness of and use for each medication. Would you suggest any changes or additional medications?
2. What strategies could you use to help improve this resident's food and fluid intake?
3. What suggestions are appropriate to promote fracture healing and increase bone density?
4. Do you suspect that this client is constipated? What would you recommend in terms of food choices to deal with this?

USEFUL WEBSITES

Administration on Aging
http://www.aoa.gov
Administration for Community Living
www.acl.org
American Association of Retired Persons
http://www.aarp.org
American Geriatrics Society
http://www.americangeriatrics.org
American Society on Aging
http://www.asaging.org/
Centers for Medicare and Medicaid Services
http://www.cms.hhs.gov/
Meals on Wheels Association of America
http://www.mowaa.org/
Mini Nutritional Assessment
http://www.mna-elderly.com/default.html
National Association of Nutrition and Aging Services Programs
http://www.nanasp.org
National Institute on Aging
http://www.nih.gov/nia
National Institutes of Health Senior Health
http://nihseniorhealth.gov/
National Study of Long-Term Care Providers (NSLTCP)
http://www.cdc.gov/nchs/nsltcp.htm
Older Americans Act Nutrition Program
http://www.aoa.gov/AoARoot/AoA_Programs/HCLTC/Nutrition_Services/index.aspx
Pioneer Network
www.pioneernetwork.net

REFERENCES

Academy of Nutrition and Dietetics Position: Food and nutrition for older adults: promoting health and wellness, *J Acad Nutr Diet* 112:1255, 2012. http://www.eatright.org/About/Content.aspx?id=8374. Accessed 1 July 2014.

American College of Sports Medicine (ACSM): Position stand: Exercise and physical activity for older adults, *Med Sci Sports Exerc* 41:1510, 2009.

American Dietetic Association (ADA): Individualized nutrition approaches for older adults in health care communities, *J Am Diet Assoc* 110:1549, 2010.

American Dietetic Association, American Society for Nutrition, and Society for Nutrition Education: Joint Position. Food and nutrition programs for community-residing older adults, *J Am Diet Assoc* 110:463, 2010. http://www.eatright.org/About/Content.aspx?id=6442451115. Accessed 1 July 2014.

American Federation for Aging Research: *InfoGuide to Theories on Aging*, 2011. http://www.afar.org/infoaging/biology-of-aging/theories-of-aging. Accessed December 30, 2014.

American Optometric Association (AOA): *Glossary of All Eye & Vision Conditions Presbyopia*, 2014. http://www.aoa.org/patients-and-public/eye-and-vision-problems/glossary-of-eye-and-vision-conditions/presbyopia. Accessed December 30, 2014.

Aslam T, Delcourt C, Holz F, et al: European survey on the opinion and use of micronutrition in age-related macular degeneration: 10 years on from the Age-Related Eye Disease Study, *Clin Ophthalmol* 8:2045, 2014.

Benelam B: Satiety and the anorexia of ageing: review, *Br J Comm Nurs* 14:332, 2009.

Centers for Disease Control and Prevention (CDC): *The State of Aging and Health in America 2013*, 2013. http://www.cdc.gov/features/agingandhealth/state_of_aging_and_health_in_america_2013.pdf. Accessed December 30, 2014.

Bernstein M, Munoz N, Academy of Nutrition and Dietetics: Position of the Academy of Nutrition and Dietetics: food and nutrition for older adults: promoting health and wellness, *J Acad Nutr Diet* 112:1255, 2012.

Beveridge LA, Davey PG, Phillips G, et al: Optimal management of urinary tract infections in older people, *Clin Interv Aging* 6:173, 2011.

Centers for Disease Control and Prevention: *The State of Aging and Health in America 2013*, Atlanta, GA, 2013, US Dept of Health and Human Services. http://www.cdc.gov/features/agingandhealth/state_of_aging_and_health_in_america_2013.pdf. Accessed 1 July 2014.

Chao SY, Dwyer JT, Houser RF, et al: What food and nutrition services should be regulated in assisted-living facilities for older adults? *J Am Diet Assoc* 109:1048, 2009.

Chew EY, Clemons TE, Agrón E, et al: Ten-year follow-up of age-related macular degeneration in the Age-Related Eye Disease Study: AREDS Report No. 36, *JAMA Ophthalmol* 132:272, 2014.

Colby SL, Ortman JM: *The Baby Boom Cohort in the United States: 2012 to 2060*, 2014. http://www.census.gov/prod/2014pubs/p25-1141.pdf. Accessed December 30, 2014.

Correa-de-Araujo R, Hadley E: Skeletal Muscle Function Deficit: a new terminology to embrace the evolving concepts of sarcopenia and age-related muscle dysfunction, *J Gerontol A Biol Sci Med Sci* 69:591, 2014.

Dam TT, Peters KW, Fragala M, et al: An evidence-based comparison of operational criteria for the presence of sarcopenia, *J Gerontol A Biol Sci Med Sci* 69:584, 2014.

Doley J: Nutrition management of pressure ulcers, *Nutr Clin Prac* 25:50, 2010.

Federal Interagency Forum on Aging-Related Statistics: *Older Americans 2012: key indicators of well-being*, Washington, DC, 2012, U.S. Government Printing Office.

Flicker L, McCaul KA, Hankey GJ, et al: Body mass index and survival in men and women aged 70 to 75, *J Am Geriatr Soc* 58:234, 2010.

Galvin JE, Sadowsky CH: Practical guidelines for the recognition and diagnosis of dementia, *J Am Board Fam Med* 25:367, 2012.

Harris-Kojetin L, Sengupta M, Park-Lee E, et al: *Long-term care services in the United States: 2013 overview*, Hyattsville, 2013, National Center for Health Statistics.

Jayant M, Wroblewski KE, Kern DW, et al: Olfactory dysfunction predicts 5-year mortality in older adults, *PLoS One* 9:e107541, 2014, doi:10.1371/journal.pone.0107541.

Kaiser MJ, Bauer JM, Ramsch C, et al: Validation of the mini nutritional assessment short-form (MNA®-SF): a practical tool for identification of nutritional status, *J Nutr Health Aging* 13:782, 2009.

Kamp BJ, Wellman NS, Russell C: Position of the American Dietetic Association, American Society for Nutrition, and Society for Nutrition Education: Food and nutrition programs for community-residing older adults, *J Am Diet Assoc* 110:463, 2010.

Lichtenstein AL: *MyPlate for Older Adults*, 2014. http://www.nutrition.tufts.edu/research/myplate-older-adults. Accessed December 31, 2014.

Litchford MD: Counteracting the trajectory of frailty and sarcopenia in older adults, *Nutr Clin Pract* 29:428, 2014.

Lloyd JL, Wellman NS: Older Americans Act Nutrition Programs: a community based Nutrition Program helping older adults remain at home, *J Nutr Geron Geratric* 34:90, 2015.

Lopes da Silva S, Vellas B, Elemans S, et al: Plasma nutrient status of patients with Alzheimer's disease: systematic review and meta-analysis, *Alzheimers Dement* 10:485, 2012.

MetLife Mature Market Institute: *Market Survey of Long-Term Care Costs: The 2012 MetLife Market Survey of Nursing Home, Assisted Living, Adult Day Services, and Home Care Costs*, 2012. www.MatureMarketInstitute.com. Accessed December 31, 2014.

National Eye Institute (NEI), National Institute of Health (NIH): *Age-Related Macular Degeneration*. https://www.nei.nih.gov/eyedata/amd.asp. Accessed December 30, 2014.

National Institute on Deafness and Other Communicative Disorders (NIDCD), National Institutes of Health (NIH): *Age-Related Hearing Loss*, 2013a. http://www.nidcd.nih.gov/health/hearing/Pages/presbycusis.aspx. Accessed December 30, 2014.

National Institute in Deafness and Other Communicative Disease (NIDCD), National Institutes of Health (NIH): *Hearing Loss and Older Adults*, 2013b. http://www.nidcd.nih.gov/health/hearing/pages/older.aspx. Accessed December 30, 2014.

National Institute on Aging (NIA): *Exercise & Physical Activity: Your Everyday Guide from the National Institute on Aging*, 2010. http://www.nia.nih.gov/health/publication/exercise-physical-activity/introduction. Accessed December 30, 2014.

National Research Council: *Nutrition and healthy aging in the community: workshop summary*, Washington, DC, 2012, The National Academics Press.

Ortman JM, Velkoff VA, Hogan H: *An Aging Nation: The Older Population in the United States*, 2014. http://www.census.gov/prod/2014pubs/p25-1140.pdf?eml=gd&utm_medium=email&utm_source=govdelivery. Accessed December 30, 2014.

Plummer N: The unseen epidemic: the linked syndromes of achlorhydria and atrophic gastritis, *Townsend Letter Doctors Patients* 252:89, 2004.

Rudolph DM: Appetite stimulants in long term care: a literature review, *Internet J Adv Nur Practice* 11:1, 2009.

Schiffman SS: Effects of aging on the human taste system, *Ann NY Acad Sci* 1170:725, 2009.

Shikany JM: Macronutrients, diet quality, and frailty in older men, *J Gerontol A Biol Sci Med Sci* 69:695, 2014.

Simmons J, Atkins A, editors: Aging in community, *Generations* 37:4, 2014.

Skipper AL, Ferguson M, Thompson K, et al: Nutrition screening tools: an analysis of the evidence, *J Parenter Enteral Nutr* 36:292, 2012.

Studenski S, Peters KW, Alley De, et al: The FNIH Sarcopenia Project: rationale, study description, conference recommendations, and final estimates, *J Gerontol A Biol Sci Med Sci* 69:547, 2014.

Thomas DR: Role of nutrition in the treatment and prevention of pressure ulcers, *Nutr Clin Pract* 29:466, 2014.

Thomas DR, Burkemper NM: Aging skin and wound healing, *Clin Geriatr Med* 29(2):xi, 2013.

Thomas KS, Mor V: Providing more home-delivered meals is one way to keep older adults with low care needs out of nursing homes, *Health Aff* 32:1796, 2013.

U.S. Administration on Aging: *Nutrition Services (OAA Title IIIC)*. http://www.aoa.gov/AoARoot/AoA_Programs/HCLTC/Nutrition_Services/index.aspx. Accessed December 31, 2014.

U.S. Department of Health and Human Services (USDHHS): *The Surgeon General's Vision for a Healthy and Fit Nation*, Rockville, Md, 2010, USDHHS, Office of the Surgeon General.

Wellman NS: Aging at home: more research on nutrition and independence, please, *Am J Clin Nutr* 91:1151, 2010.

Winter JE, MacInnis RJ, Wattanapenpaiboon N, et al: BMI and all-cause mortality in older adults: a meta-analysis, *Am J Clin Nutr* 99:875, 2014.

World Health Organization (WHO): *Report: WHO Global Forum on Innovations for Ageing Populations*, 2013. http://www.who.int/kobe_centre/publications/GFIAP_report.pdf?ua=1, 2013. Accessed December 30, 2014.

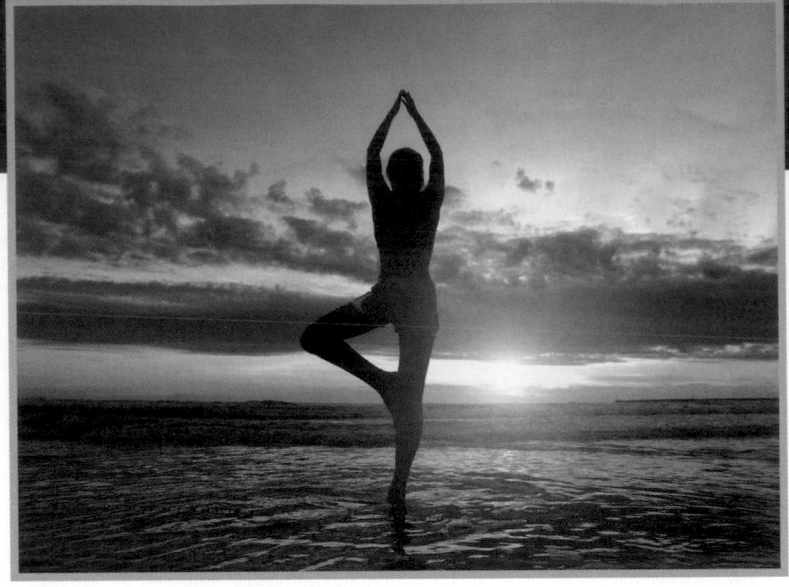

PART IV

Nutrition for Health and Fitness

The chapters in this section reflect the evolution of nutritional science, from the identification of nutrient requirements and the practical application of this knowledge to the concepts that relate nutrition, to the prevention of chronic and degenerative diseases, and to optimization of health and performance.

The relationship between nutrition and dental disease has long been recognized. In more recent decades the possibility of reducing the incidence of osteoporosis by emphasizing appropriate nutrition has accumulated supportive evidence. Medical research now shows the role of nutrition on gene expression; dietary intake can turn on or turn off the inflammatory process, a key factor in disease onset and management.

Weight management and exercise form the basis for a great deal of nutrition in health, fitness, and disease prevention. Understanding the role of nutrition in sports and in optimizing performance has led to dietary and exercise practices generally applicable to a rewarding, healthy lifestyle.

The opportunities for members of an affluent society to choose from a great variety of foods has led to an overabundant intake of energy for many individuals. Efforts to reduce body weight, widely pursued with varying degrees of enthusiasm and diligence, are often disheartening, making the knowledge presented here so important. Frustration with dieting and stress often lead to eating disorders, which are increasing in frequency and require attention and understanding from the nutrition professional.

21

Nutrition in Weight Management

Lucinda K. Lysen, RDN, RN, BSN
Donna A. Israel, PhD, RDN, LPC, FADA, FAND

KEY TERMS

abdominal fat
activity thermogenesis (AT)
adipocyte
adipocytokines or adipokines
adiposity rebound
android fat distribution
bariatric surgery
body mass index (BMI)
brown adipose tissue (BAT)
comorbidities
essential fat
fat mass
fat-free mass (FFM)
gastric banding
gastric bypass
gastroplasty
ghrelin
gynoid fat distribution
hormone-sensitive lipase (HSL)

hyperphagia
hyperplasia
hypertrophy
hypophagia
incretin
insulin
laparoscopic sleeve gastrectomy (LSG)
lean body mass (LBM)
leptin
lifestyle modification
lipogenesis
lipoprotein lipase (LPL)
liposuction
metabolic syndrome (MetS)
morbid obesity
night-eating syndrome (NES)
nonalcoholic fatty liver disease
   (NAFLD)

nonexercise activity thermogenesis
   (NEAT)
nutritional genomics
obesity
obesogen
overweight
sensory-specific satiety
set point theory
storage fat
semivolatile organic compounds
   (SVOCs)
underweight
vagus nerve
very low–calorie diet (VLCD)
visceral adipose tissue (VAT)
white adipose tissue (WAT)
yo-yo effect

Body weight is the sum of bone, muscle, organs, body fluids, and adipose tissue. Some or all of these components are subject to normal change as a reflection of growth, reproductive status, variation in physical activity, and the effects of aging. Consistent body weight is orchestrated by neural, hormonal, and chemical mechanisms as well as individual genetic polymorphisms that balance energy intake and expenditure within fairly precise limits. Abnormalities of these complex mechanisms can result in weight fluctuations.

On one end of the weight spectrum is underweight. Although the inability to gain weight can be a primary problem, low body weight is usually secondary to a disease state, an eating disorder, or a psychiatric disorder. In the elderly or in children, unintentional weight loss can be especially detrimental and should be addressed early to prevent malnutrition or other undesirable consequences. Most crucial is the in utero development of the fetus. Babies deprived of nutrition before birth and who have low birth weight may be primed for accelerated growth after birth when exposed to a nutrient-rich environment (which often consists of infant formula). Furthermore, inadequate passage of nutrients across the placenta and low birth weight eventually can lead to an increased risk of developing obesity and diabetes (Apovian, 2011).

On the other end of the spectrum and more common, are the conditions of overweight and obesity.

BODY WEIGHT COMPONENTS

Body weight often is described in terms of its composition, and different models have been advanced to estimate body fat. Assessment of body composition is discussed in detail in Chapter 7. Traditionally, a two-compartment model divides the body into fat mass, the fat from all body sources including the brain, skeleton, and adipose tissue, and fat-free mass (FFM), which includes water, protein, and mineral components (see Figure 21-1). The proportions of FFM are relatively constant from person to person.

Although *FFM* often is used interchangeably with the term lean body mass, it is not exactly the same. Lean body mass (LBM) is muscle. LBM is higher in men than in women, increases with exercise, and is lower in older adults. It is the major determinant of the resting metabolic rate (RMR).

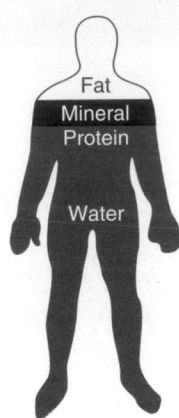

FIGURE 21-1 The components of fat-free mass in the body.

It follows that a decrease in LBM could hinder the progress of weight loss. Therefore, to achieve long-term weight loss, the loss of fat mass while maintaining FFM is desirable. Water, which makes up 60% to 65% of body weight, is the most variable component of LBM, and the state of hydration can induce fluctuations of several pounds.

Body Fat

Total body fat is the combination of "essential" and "storage" fats, usually expressed as a percentage of total body weight that is associated with optimum health. Muscle and even skeletal mass adjust to some extent to support the burden of adipose tissue.

Essential fat, necessary for normal physiologic functioning, is stored in small amounts in the bone marrow, heart, lung, liver, spleen, kidneys, muscles, and the nervous system. In men, approximately 3% of body fat is essential. In women, essential fat is higher (12%) because it includes body fat in the breasts, pelvic regions, and thighs that supports the reproductive process.

Storage fat is the energy reserve, primarily as triglycerides (TGs), in adipose tissue. This fat accumulates under the skin and around the internal organs to protect them from trauma. Most storage fat is "expendable." The fat stores in adipocytes are capable of extensive variation. This allows for the changing requirements of growth, reproduction, aging, environmental and physiologic circumstances, the availability of food, and the demands of physical activity. Total body fat (essential fat plus storage fat) as a percentage of body weight associated with the average individual is between 18% and 24% for men and 25% and 31% for women. On the other extreme, "elite fit" men are as low as 2% to 5% body fat and women 10% to 13% (Digate Muth, 2014).

Adipose Tissue Composition

Adipose tissue exerts a profound influence on whole-body homeostasis. Adipose tissue is located primarily under the skin, in the mesenteries and omentum, and behind the peritoneum. This is often referred to as visceral adipose tissue (VAT). Although it is primarily fat, adipose tissue also contains small amounts of protein and water. White adipose tissue (WAT) stores energy as a repository for TGs, cushions abdominal organs, and insulates the body to preserve heat. Carotene gives it

a slight yellow color. Brown adipose tissue (BAT) can be found in a substantial proportion of adults in small amounts as well as in infants. Unlike WAT, BAT is made of small droplets and many more iron containing mitochondria, which makes it brown. In adults, it plays a role in controlling energy expenditure. In newborns, it provides body heat. Although WAT stores energy, BAT helps regulate body temperature by regulating heat (Apovian, 2011). It is found mainly in scapular and subscapular areas.

Adipocyte Size and Number

The mature fat cell (adipocyte) consists of a large central lipid droplet surrounded by a thin rim of cytoplasm, which contains the nucleus and the mitochondria. These cells can store fat equal to 80% to 95% of their volume. Gains in weight and adipose tissue occur by increasing the number of cells, the size of cells as lipid is added, or a combination of the two.

Hyperplasia (increased number of cells) occurs as a normal growth process during infancy and adolescence. Cell number increases in lean and obese children into adolescence, but the number increases faster in obese children. In teens and adults, increases in fat cell size are more common, but hyperplasia also can occur after the fat content of existing cells has reached capacity.

During normal growth, the greatest percentage of body fat (approximately 25%) is set by 6 months of age. In lean children, fat cell size then decreases; this decrease does not occur in obese children. At the age of 6 years in lean children, adiposity rebound occurs, especially in girls, with an increase in body fat. An early adiposity rebound occurring before five and a half years old is predictive of a higher level of adiposity at 16 years of age and in adulthood; a period of later rebound is correlated with normal adult weight (Rolland-Cachera, 2005).

With hypertrophy (increased cell size), fat depots can expand as much as 1000 times at any age, as long as space is available. In a classic study Bjorntorp and Sjostrom (1971) demonstrated, using weight loss as a result of trauma, illness, or starvation, that fat cell size decreases but cell numbers remain the same. Although weight loss of any amount in severely obese individuals improves basic adipocyte physiology, a weight loss of at least 5% is required to decrease fat cell size (Varady et al, 2009).

Fat Storage

Most depot fat comes directly from dietary TGs. The fatty acid composition of adipose tissue mirrors the fatty acid composition of the diet. Even excess dietary carbohydrate and protein are converted to fatty acids in the liver by the comparatively inefficient process of lipogenesis. Under normal conditions, little dietary carbohydrate is used to produce adipose tissue; three times more energy is required to convert excess energy from carbohydrate to fat storage compared with dietary fat.

Semivolatile organic compounds (SVOCs) accumulate in adipose tissues from exposure to toxins, chemicals, and pesticides. When adipose tissue is mobilized during weight loss, SVOCs are released (see *Clinical Insight:* What's in That Fat When You Lose It?). The effect of SVOCs on the developing fetal brain is not yet known (see Chapter 15), which adds to the health concern about obese pregnant women who lose weight.

Lipoprotein Lipase

Dietary TG is transported to the liver by chylomicrons. Endogenous TGs, synthesized in the liver from free fatty acids (FFA) travel as part of very low–density lipoprotein particles. The enzyme **lipoprotein lipase (LPL)** moves lipid from the blood into the adipose cell, by hydrolyzing TGs into free fatty acids and glycerol. Glycerol proceeds to the liver; fatty acids enter the adipocyte and are reesterified into TGs. When needed by other cells, TGs are hydrolyzed once again to fatty acids and glycerol by **hormone-sensitive lipase (HSL)** within the adipose cell; they then are released into the circulation.

Hormones affect LPL activity in different adipose tissue regions. Estrogens stimulate LPL activity in the gluteofemoral adipocytes, and thus promote fat storage in this area for childbearing and lactation. In the presence of sex steroid hormones, a normal distribution of body fat exists. With a decrease in sex steroid hormones—as occurs with menopause or gonadectomy—central obesity tends to develop.

REGULATION OF BODY WEIGHT

Neurochemicals, body fat stores, protein mass, hormones, and postingestion factors play a role in regulating intake and weight. Regulation takes place on a short-term and a long-term basis. Short-term regulation governs consumption of food from meal to meal; long-term regulation is controlled by the availability of adipose stores and hormone responses.

Metabolic Rate and Voluntary Activity

The resting metabolic rate (RMR) (see Chapter 2) explains 60% to 70% of total energy expenditure. RMR declines with age or with restriction of energy intake. When the body suddenly is deprived of adequate energy from involuntary or deliberate starvation, the body conserves energy by dropping its RMR as rapidly as 15% in 2 weeks.

Activity thermogenesis (AT) is the energy expended in voluntary activity, the most variable component of energy expenditure. Under normal circumstances physical activity accounts for 15% to 30% of total energy expenditure. However, all activity counts. **Nonexercise activity thermogenesis (NEAT)** is the energy expended for all activity that is not sleeping, eating, or sports-like exercise. It includes going to work, typing, doing yard work, toe-tapping, even fidgeting (see Chapter 2). NEAT and a sedentary lifestyle may have profound importance in weight management. NEAT varies as much as 2000 kcal/day between individuals (Levine, 2007). To reverse obesity, individual strategies should promote standing and ambulating for 2.5 hours per day and should also reengineer work, school, and home environments to support a more active lifestyle (Levine, 2007).

Short- and Long-Term Regulation

Short-term controls are concerned primarily with factors governing hunger, appetite, and satiety. Satiety is associated with the postprandial state when excess food is being stored. Hunger is associated with the postabsorptive state when those stores are being mobilized. Physical triggers for hunger are much stronger than those for satiety; it is easier to override the signals for satiety.

When either overfeeding or underfeeding occurs, younger individuals exhibit spontaneous **hypophagia** (undereating) or **hyperphagia** (overeating) accordingly. Older individuals do not have the same responsiveness; they are more vulnerable to unexplained weight losses or gains because they are unable to control spontaneous, short-term changes in food intake.

Long-term regulation seems to involve a feedback mechanism in which a signal from the adipose mass is released when "normal" body composition is disturbed, as when weight loss occurs. **Adipocytokines or adipokines** are proteins released by the adipose cell into the bloodstream that act as signaling molecules. Younger persons have more responsiveness to this feedback than older adults do (see Table 21-1 and *Focus On: Signals from a Host of Hormones*).

Set Point Theory

Fat storage in non-obese adults appears to be regulated in a manner that preserves a specific body weight. In animals and humans, deliberate efforts to starve or overfeed are followed by a rapid return to the original body weight, a "set point." According to the **set point theory**, body weight remains remarkably stable from internal regulatory mechanisms that are genetically determined. Emerging evidence from the bariatric surgery experience suggests that this drastic approach to weight loss may result in a new set point by altering anatomy and physiology (Farias 2011). More research is needed to establish definitively that there is a set point for weight.

TABLE 21-1   Regulatory Factors Involved in Eating and Weight Management

Brain Neurotransmitters	Characteristics and Function
Norepinephrine and dopamine	Released by the SNS in response to dietary intake; mediates the activity of areas in the hypothalamus that govern feeding behavior. Fasting and semi-starvation lead to decreased SNS activity and increased adrenal medullary activity with a consequent increase in epinephrine, which fosters substrate mobilization. Dopaminergic pathways in the brain play a role in the reinforcement properties of food.
Serotonin, neuropeptide Y, and endorphins	Decreases in serotonin and increases in neuropeptide Y have been associated with an increase in carbohydrate appetite. Neuropeptide Y increases during food deprivation; it may be a factor leading to an increase in appetite after dieting. Preferences and cravings for sweet, high-fat foods observed among obese and bulimic patients involve the endorphin system.
CRF	Involved in controlling adrenocorticotropic hormone release from the pituitary gland; CRF is a potent anorexic agent and weakens the feeding response produced by norepinephrine and neuropeptide Y. CRF is released during exercise.
Orexin (hypocretin)	Orexin is a neurotransmitter produced by the hypothalamus that has a weak resemblance to secretin produced in the gut and is an appetite stimulant and central regulator of glucose and energy homeostasis.

Gut Hormones	Characteristics and Function
Incretins	Gastrointestinal peptides increase the amount of insulin released from the beta cells of the pancreas after eating, even before blood glucose levels become elevated. They also slow the rate of absorption by reducing gastric emptying and may directly reduce food intake. Incretins also inhibit glucagon release from the alpha cells of the pancreas. (See GLP-1 and GIP.)
CCK	Released by the intestinal tract when fats and proteins reach the small intestine, receptors for CCK have been found in the gastrointestinal tract and the brain. CCK causes the gallbladder to contract and stimulates the pancreas to release enzymes. At the brain level, CCK inhibits food intake.
Bombesin	Released by enteric neurons; reduces food intake and enhances the release of CCK.
Enterostatin	A portion of pancreatic lipase involved specifically with satiety after the consumption of fat.
Adiponectin	An adipocytokine secreted by the adipose tissue that modulates glucose regulation and fatty acid catabolism. Levels of this hormone are inversely correlated with BMI. The hormone plays a role in metabolic disorders such as type 2 diabetes, obesity, and atherosclerosis. Levels drop after gastric bypass surgery for up to 6 months (Couce et al, 2006).
Glucagon	Increased secretion of glucagon is caused by hypoglycemia, increased levels of norepinephrine and epinephrine, increased plasma amino acids, and cholecystokinin. Decreased secretion of glucagon occurs when insulin or somatostatin is released.
Apolipoprotein A-IV	Synthesized and secreted by the intestine during lymphatic secretion of chylomicrons. After entering the circulation, a small portion of apolipoprotein A-IV enters the CNS and suppresses food consumption.
Fatty acids	Free fatty acids, triglycerides, and glycerol are factors that also affect uptake of glucose by peripheral tissues.
GLP-1 and GIP	Released by intestinal mucosa in the presence of meals rich in glucose and fat; stimulate insulin synthesis and release; GLP-1 decreases glucagon secretion, delays gastric emptying time, and may promote satiety; examples of incretin hormones.
Insulin	Acts in the CNS and the periphery nervous system to regulate food intake. Insulin is involved in the synthesis and storage of fat. Impaired insulin activity may lead to impaired thermogenesis. It is possible that obese persons with insulin resistance or deficiency have a defective glucose disposal system and a depressed level of thermogenesis. The greater the insulin resistance, the lower the thermic effect of food. Fasting insulin levels increase proportionately with the degree of obesity; however, many obese persons demonstrate insulin resistance because of a lack of response by insulin receptors, impaired glucose tolerance, and associated hyperlipidemia. These sequelae can usually be corrected with weight loss.
Leptin	An adipocytokine secreted by the adipose tissue, correlated with percent of body fat. Primary signal from energy stores; in obesity loses the ability to inhibit energy intake or to increase energy expenditure (Enriori et al, 2006). Compared with men, women have significantly higher concentrations of serum leptin.
Resistin	An adipocytokine expressed primarily in adipocytes; antagonizes insulin action (Goldstein and Scalia, 2007).
Ghrelin	Produced primarily by the stomach; acts on the hypothalamus to stimulate hunger and feeding. Ghrelin levels are highest in lean individuals and lowest in the obese. Increased levels are seen in people who are dieting, and suppressed levels are noted after gastric bypass, possibly counteracted by adiponectin (Couce et al, 2006).
PYY$_{3-06}$	Secreted by endocrine cells lining the small bowel and colon in response to food; a "middle man" in appetite management. PYY seems to work opposite from ghrelin; it induces satiety.
IL-6 and TNF-α	Both are gut hormones. Cytokines secreted by adipose tissue and participate in metabolic events. Impair insulin signals in muscle and liver. Levels are proportional to body fat mass (Thomas and Schauer, 2010).
Oxytomodulin	Secreted from L-cells in small intestine in response to a meal. Exerts its biologic effects through activation of GLP-1 and glicentin-related pancreatic peptide (GRPP) (Bray and Bouchard, 2014).
GLP-2	Produced in the L-cells of small intestines and in neurons of CNS. Is an intestinal growth factor. Inhibits gastric emptying and acid secretion while stimulating intestinal blood flow. Decreases gastric acid secretion and gastric emptying and increases mucosal growth (Bray and Bouchard, 2014).
FGF-21	Expressed in the liver and secreted mainly during faster and after feeding a ketongenic diet. Can decrease body weight without affecting food intake. Increases insulin sensitivity, decreases gluconeogenesis, and increases glucose uptake in adipocytes (Bray and Bouchard, 2014).

TABLE 21-1 Regulatory Factors Involved in Eating and Weight Management—cont'd

Other Hormones	Characteristics and Function
Thyroid hormones	Modulate the tissue responsiveness to the catecholamines secreted by the SNS. A decrease in triiodothyronine lowers the response to SNS activity and diminishes adaptive thermogenesis. Women should be tested for hypothyroidism, particularly after menopause. Weight regain after weight loss may be a function of a hypometabolic state; energy restriction produces a transient, hypothyroid, hypometabolic state.
Visfatin	An adipocytokine protein secreted by visceral adipose tissue that has an insulin-like effect; plasma levels increase with increasing adiposity and insulin resistance.
Adrenomedullin	A new regulatory peptide secreted by adipocytes as a result of inflammatory processes.

BMI, Body mass index; *CCK,* cholecystokinin; *CNS,* central nervous system; *CRF,* corticotropin-releasing factor; *GIP,* glucose-dependent insulinotropic peptide; *GLP-1,* glucagon-like peptide 1; *IL-6,* interleukin-6; *PYY3-36.* peptide YY_{3-36}; *SNS,* sympathetic nervous system; *TNF-α.* tumor necrosis factor alpha.
See below for addition of gut hormones to chart.
Couce ME et al: Is ghrelin the culprit for weight loss after gastric bypass surgery? A negative answer, *Obes Surg* 16:870, 2006; Enriori JP et al: Leptin resistance and obesity, *Obesity* 14(Suppl 5):254S, 2006; Goldstein BJ, Scalia R: Adipokines and vascular disease in diabetes, *Curr Diab Rep* 7:25, 2007; Stevens JM, Vidal-Puig AJ: An update on visfatin/pre-B cell colony-enhancing factor, an ubiquitously expressed, illusive cytokine that is regulated in obesity, *Curr Opin Lipidol* 17:128, 2006; Thomas S, Scahauer P: Bariatric surgery and the gut hormone response, *Nutr Clin Pract* 25:175, 2010.
Bray GA, Bouchard C: Handbook of obesity, ed 3, Boca Raton, Fla, 2014, CRC Press.

◎ FOCUS ON

Signals from a Host of Hormones

A host of hormones—insulin, leptin, adiponectin, and ghrelin, among others—communicate with the hypothalamus to control a person's intake and weight. These regulatory hormones govern feeding in response to signals originated in affected body tissues.

Insulin controls the amount of glucose in the blood by moving it into the cells for energy. Leptin, which is produced mainly by fat cells, contributes to long-term fullness by sensing the body's overall energy stores. Adiponectin is also made by fat cells and apparently helps the body respond better to insulin by boosting metabolism. Ghrelin, the hunger hormone, tells the brain when the stomach is empty, prompting hunger pangs and a drop in metabolism.

The stomach communicates with the brain via the vagus nerve, part of the autonomic nervous system that travels from the brain to the stomach. When filled with food or liquid, the stomach's stretch receptors send a message to the brain indicating satiety. Gastric bypass surgery reduces the stomach to the size of an egg, and triggers a sharp drop in ghrelin levels, which lessens hunger and oral intake (Blackburn, 2008). Unfortunately, traditional dieting tends to boost ghrelin levels.

WEIGHT IMBALANCE: OVERWEIGHT AND OBESITY

Overweight occurs as a result of an imbalance between food consumed and physical activity. Obesity is a complex issue related to lifestyle, environment, and genes. Environmental and genetic factors have a complex interaction with psychologic, cultural, and physiologic influences. Over the years, many hypotheses have evolved to explain why some people become fat and others remain lean, and why it is so difficult for reduced-obese persons to maintain weight loss. No single theory can completely explain all manifestations of obesity or apply consistently to all persons.

Prevalence

Until recently, the United States has had the highest prevalence of obesity among the developed nations. However, increases in the prevalence of overweight and obesity have been observed throughout the world. For example, the number of overweight individuals in Germany is now the same percentage as the United States (English, Scharioth, 2011). The international trend often is called "globesity."

The estimates of overweight and obesity among adults and children are based on measured weights and heights from the National Health and Nutrition Examination Survey (NHANES), conducted by the National Center for Health Statistics, Center for Disease Control and Prevention (see Figure 21-2). In the United States the 2009 to 2010 findings were that an estimated one third of adults and almost 20% of children were obese. The prevalence of obesity remains higher among African American and Hispanic populations (see *New Directions:* Organizing to Solve the Childhood Obesity Problem "Within a Generation").

✴ NEW DIRECTIONS

Organizing to Solve the Childhood Obesity Problem "Within a Generation"

Because the number of obese children in the United States has tripled since 1980, and obesity now rivals smoking as the largest cause of preventable death and disease, a new foundation was launched in the spring of 2010 to address this serious epidemic of childhood obesity (Ogden et al, 2010). This foundation, Partnership for a Healthier America, has as its mission the simple concept that children should have good, nutritious food to eat and the chance to be physically active every day to become healthy adults.

The objectives of the partnership are to support the national goal of solving the childhood obesity challenge "within a generation" set by First Lady Michelle Obama, who also serves as Honorary Chair of the organization. The Partnership brings together the public and private sectors, organizations, business and thought leaders, the media, and states and local communities to make meaningful and measurable commitments for fighting childhood obesity. The plan has four pillars:

- Offering parents the tools and information they need to make healthy choices for their children
- Introducing healthier food into the nation's schools
- Ensuring that all families have access to healthy, affordable food in their communities
- Increasing opportunities for children to be physically active, both in and out of school

The partnership will support, unite, and inspire families from every corner of the United States to implement and sustain the 4 pillar plan. The initiative was started with the *Let's Move!* Campaign. www.letsmove.gov/

The White House Task Force on Childhood Obesity—Report to the President "Solving the Problem of Childhood Obesity within a Generation" (Task Force on Childhood Obesity, Domestic Policy Council, 2010) can be accessed at www.nj.gov/health/fhs/shapingnj/pdf/wh_obesity_report.pdf.

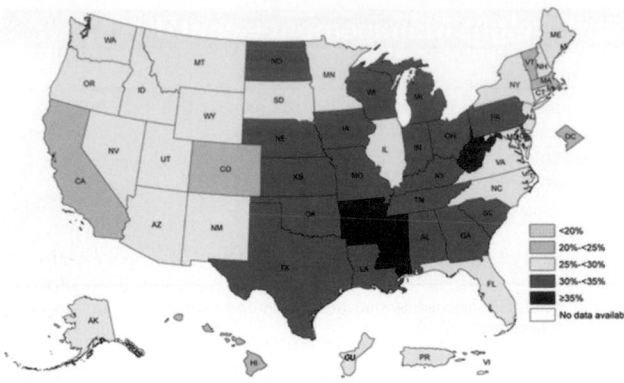

FIGURE 21-2 CDC Obesity Prevalence Map Prevalence of obesity among U.S. adults in 2013. (Centers for Disease Control and Prevention [CDC] Behavioral Risk Factor Surveillance System Survey, 2013.)

In February 2014 a researcher for the CDC reported to the media around the world that among children 2 to 5 years old, there had been a broad decline in the obesity epidemic. The drop emerged from a major federal health survey that experts stated was the "gold standard for evidence." Theories emerged as to why the decline happened; possibly children were consuming less refined sugar, or maybe the decline was due to the fact that more women were breastfeeding their children. However, criticism followed that the sample size was too small to validate the results (CDC, 2014; Ogden, 2010). Combined with media sensationalism, the news mistakenly sent a message that early childhood obesity numbers were finally reversing themselves when, indeed, they are not.

Genetics

Many hormonal and neural factors involved in weight regulation are determined by heredity and genetics. These include short-term and long-term "signals" that determine satiety and feeding activity. Small defects in their expression or interaction could contribute significantly to weight gain. **Nutritional genomics** is the study of the interactions between dietary components and the instructions in a cell or genome, and the resulting changes in metabolites that affect gene expression (Camp and Trujillo, 2014) (see Chapter 5).

The number and size of fat cells, regional distribution of body fat, and RMR also are influenced by genes. Studies of twins confirm that genes determine 50% to 70% of the predisposition to obesity (Prentice, 2005). Although numerous genes are involved, several have received much attention—the *Ob* gene, the *adiponectin (ADIPOQ)* gene, the "fat mass and obesity associated" gene or *FTO* gene, and the *beta3*-adrenoreceptor gene. The *Ob* gene produces leptin. Mutations in the *Ob* gene, leptin receptor (LEPR), or *ADIPOQ* genes can result in obesity or **metabolic syndrome (MetS)**, especially if the person's diet provides too much saturated fat (Ferguson et al, 2010). The *beta3-adrenoreceptor* gene, located primarily in the adipose tissue, is thought to regulate RMR and fat oxidation in humans. The *FTO* gene predisposes individuals to diabetes by its effect on body mass (Frayling et al, 2007).

Nutritional or lifestyle choices can activate or deactivate these obesity-triggering genes. Thus the "formula" for successful long-term weight management is likely to require the behavioral application of individual genetics. Deoxyribonucleic acid

(DNA) tests can provide predictions about an individual's response to a particular diet (see *Clinical Insight*: Low Fat vs Low Carb: The Answer May Be in Your Genes).

CLINICAL INSIGHT

Low Fat vs Low Carb: The Answer May Be in Your Genes

While eating a low-fat diet is generally a successful strategy for weight loss and weight maintenance because of the lower calorie content, your genes may have an effect. Genetic studies now show that, for example, a person identified as obesogenic from a high-carbohydrate diet will not be as successful on a lower-fat diet as a person identified as obesogenic from high-fat diet and vice versa (Collins, 2010). However, because genetic testing is complicated, the AND Position Statement states that only advanced qualified health professionals should be interpreting the results.

In a study that did not consider genetics, researchers studied 19 obese adults in a metabolic unit (Hall 2015). They found that when given isocaloric diets, the low-fat diet resulted in more fat loss than the low-carbohydrate diet. This occurred despite the fact that only the carbohydrate-restricted diet led to decreased insulin secretion. Ultimately both diets, along with the 60 minutes per day of exercise resulted in weight loss.

Through the examination of genetic markers known to affect metabolism, exercise, and energy within the human body (expressed in organs such as the brain, stomach, muscle, pancreas, and fat tissue), insight is given into how a person processes nutrients. DNA testing provides an analysis of how the body responds to exercise and performance and gives strategies to help a person reach and maintain a healthy weight based on his or her genes (see Chapter 5).

Inadequate Physical Activity

Lack of exercise and a sedentary lifestyle, compounded by chronic overeating, are also causes of weight gain. The sedentary nature of society is a factor in the growing problem of obesity. Fewer people are exercising, and more time is being spent in low-energy, screen-watching activities such as watching television or movies, using a computer or smartphone, playing video games, and sitting in cars driving to work or events.

Inflammation

Adipose tissue actively causes secretion of a wide range of pro- and anti-inflammatory cytokines that are influenced by single-nucleotide polymorphisms in the cytokine genes. Effects include insulin insensitivity, hyperlipidemia, muscle protein loss, and oxidant stress (Grimble, 2010). Scientists have found a direct relationship between obesity and inflammatory diseases such as cardiovascular disorders, some cancers, and type 2 diabetes (Bueno et al, 2014).

Metabolic signals are triggered in the hypothalamus of obese individuals, laying the groundwork for chronic inflammation and tissue damage during a prolonged period. In mice fed a high-fat diet, the "master switch" of inflammation turns on the hypothalamus. In humans, chronic overeating "flips on" the inflammation switch, leading to weight gain and insulin resistance. In insulin-resistant individuals on a weight-loss diet, and using the drug ezetimibe (Zetia), there is a reduction in hepatic steatosis and inflammatory markers with weight loss (Chan et al, 2010).

A combined approach of diet and drug use is likely to improve health outcomes. A simple dietary change to an anti-inflammatory diet and lifestyle changes can alter obesity-related inflammation. Genotypic factors influence the effectiveness of immunonutrients; antioxidants and omega-3 polyunsaturated fatty acids decrease the intensity of the inflammatory process (Grimble, 2010) (For discussion of inflammation, see Chapter 3).

Medication Usage and Weight Gain

Although weight gain can be due to disease, therapists always should consider the possibility that the patient's medication may be contributing. This often is seen with diabetes medications, and psychotropic, antidepressant, steroid, and antihypertensive medications. The use of such medications must be considered carefully, and alternative ones with less deleterious effects selected when possible (see Chapter 8 and Appendix 23).

Sleep, Stress, and Circadian Rhythms

Shortened sleep alters the endocrine regulation of hunger and appetite. Hormones that affect appetite take over and may promote excessive energy intake. Thus recurrent sleep deprivation can modify the amount, composition, and distribution of food intake and may contribute to the obesity epidemic. It is estimated that more than 50 million Americans suffer from sleep deprivation. Others may have shift work or exposure to bright light at night, increasing the disruption of circadian rhythms and enhancing the prevalence of adiposity (Garaulet et al, 2010).

There is also a relationship between sleep, disrupted circadian rhythm, genes, and the metabolic syndrome. Stress is another factor. The cortisol hormone is released when an individual is under stress, and stimulates insulin release to maintain blood glucose levels in the "fight-or-flight" response. Thus an increase in appetite occurs. Chronic stress with constantly elevated cortisol levels can also lead to appetite changes.

Cortisol levels are typically high in the early morning and low around midnight. Individuals with **night-eating syndrome (NES)** have a delayed circadian rhythm of meal intake as a result of genetically programmed neuroendocrine factors, including altered cortisol levels (Stunkard and Lu, 2010).

Taste, Satiety, and Portion Sizes

Food and its taste elements evoke pleasure responses. The endless variety of food available at any time at a reasonable cost can contribute to higher calorie intake; people eat more when offered a variety of choices than when a single food is available. Normally, as foods are consumed, they become less desirable; this phenomenon is known as **sensory-specific satiety**. Overriding this principle is the "all-you-can-eat buffet," in which the diner reaches satiety for one food but has many choices for the "next course." Although sensory-specific satiety can promote the intake of a varied and nutritionally balanced diet, it can also lead to overconsumption.

Leptin is a hormone, made by fat cells, that decreases appetite. **Ghrelin** is a hormone that increases appetite and plays a role in body weight. Levels of leptin, the appetite suppressor, are lower in normal weight individuals and higher in the obese. However, many obese people seem to build up a resistance to the appetite-suppressing effects of leptin.

Active overeating is partly the result of excessive portion sizes that are now accepted as normal. The portions and calories that restaurants and fast-food outlets offer in one meal often exceed a person's energy needs for the entire day. Frequent intake of energy-dense food also can be problematic.

Obesogens

Obesogens are chemical compounds foreign to the body that act to disrupt the normal metabolism of lipids, ultimately resulting in fatness and obesity (Grün and Blumberg, 2006). Obesogens can be called "endocrine disruptors" in that they alter lipid homeostasis and fat storage, change metabolic set points, disrupt energy balance, or modify the regulation of satiety and appetite to promote accumulation of fat and obesity. Examples of suspected obesogens in the environment and food supply are bisphenol A (BPA) and phthalates, which are found in many plastics used in food packaging and which migrate into foods processed or stored in them (Grün, 2010) (see *Clinical Insight*: What's in that Fat When You Lose It?).

Viruses and Pathogens

In the last two decades, at least 10 adipogenic pathogens have been identified, including viruses, scrapie agents (spongiform encephalopathies from sheep or goats), bacteria, and gut microflora. Whether "infectobesity" is a relevant contributor to the obesity epidemic remains to be determined. A human adenovirus, adenovirus-36, is capable of inducing adiposity in experimentally infected animals by increasing the replication, differentiation, lipid accumulation, and insulin sensitivity in fat cells and reduces leptin secretion and expression (van Ginnekin et al, 2009).

Gut Microflora and Diet

Research has identified a strong and complex relationship between the microflora population of the gut and food absorption. The microbes *firmicutes* and *bacteriodetes,* normally found in gut flora, are believed to have a symbiotic relationship, acting as either fattening or slimming microbiota, dependent on the person's nutritional status, food intake, and ability to absorb food. Firmicutes bacteria tend to be much more efficient at nutrient breakdown and calorie absorption than bacteriodetes, and therefore contribute to calorie absorption and the development and maintenance of obesity in individuals. A higher number of bacteriodetes, on the other hand, may help to make or keep people lean. Weight loss, then, it appears would require a higher number of bacteriodetes and a lower number of firmicutes. A number of theories attempt to explain how this complicated process works, the ecologic relationship between the two, and ways to manipulate it continue to evolve (Krajmalnik-Brown et al, 2012).

Assessment

Overweight is a state in which the weight exceeds a standard based on height. **Obesity** is a condition of excessive fatness, either generalized or localized. Overweight and obesity usually parallel each other, but it is possible to be overweight according to standards but not be "overfat" or obese. It is also possible to have excessive fatness and yet not be overweight.

Body Fatness and Circumference Measurements

Assessing body fatness or "adiposity" is explained in detail in Chapter 7. Clinically practical assessment tools are (1) the **body mass index (BMI)** or W/H², in which W = weight in kg and H = height in meters, (2) the waist circumference, (3) the neck circumference, (4) the waist-to-hip ratio, (4) waist-to-height ratio and the (5) the neck-to-waist ratio, all of which are detailed in Chapter 7.

The NIH guidelines classify individuals with a BMI of 25 as overweight and those with a BMI of 30 or more as obese (see Table 21-2). Optimal BMI for longevity varies with race, gender, and age. BMI that increases over time has a substantial effect on health outcomes (see Appendix 18).

Waist circumference of more than 40 inches in men and more than 35 inches in women signifies increased risk, equivalent to a BMI of 25 to 34. When waist circumference and percentage of fat are both high, they are significant predictors of heart failure and other risks associated with obesity. Waist circumference is a strong correlate of insulin sensitivity index in older adults; measurement of waist circumference is helpful to assess disease risk (Racette et al, 2006). Waist/hip ratio (WHR) is a measurement in which a ratio of more than 0.8 for women and 1 for men is also associated with high risk for cardiovascular events (see Chapter 7).

Deurenberg Equation

The Deurenberg equation using the BMI, age, and gender of an individual to determine body fatness is as follows (Deurenberg and Deurenberg-Yap, 2003):

$$\% \text{ body fat} = (1.2 \times \text{BMI}) + (0.23 \times \text{age in yrs})$$
$$- (10.8 \times G) - 5.4$$

$$G = 1 \text{ for male; } G = 0 \text{ for female}$$

For example if BMI = 28, age = 21 years and G = female:

$$\% \text{ body fat} = (1.2 \times 28) + (0.23 \times 21) - (10.8 \times 0) - 5.4$$
$$= 33.6 + 4.83 - 0 - 5.4$$
$$= 33\%$$

A body fat percentage of 20% to 25% or more in a male and 25% to 32% or more in a female usually is considered to be excessive and associated with the metabolic and health risks of obesity.

A Body Shape Index

Measuring BMI historically has been the most common way to assess body fat and a person's risk of weight-related health problems. Because BMI measures body fat through a formula using height and weight only, it does not account for where the weight is concentrated. Athletes, for example, could weigh more from muscle mass, and their BMI would be higher because of it. As a result, Dr. Nir Krakauer, an engineer and professor at New York University, developed A Body Shape Index (ABSI), incorporating waist circumference (WC) as well as height and weight into one formula to determine mortality rates. ABSI has been found to be a better mortality predictor, because of the added evaluation of abdominal fat via WC, which, with age, turns from brown to white fat and becomes a measure of central adiposity as well as body shape (Krakauer and Krakauer, 2014).

Health Risks and Longevity

In general, obesity can be viewed as metabolically unhealthy. Chronic diseases such as heart disease, type 2 diabetes, hypertension, stroke, gallbladder disease, infertility, sleep apnea, hormonal cancers, and osteoarthritis tend to worsen as the degree of obesity increases (see Figure 21-3).

A subset of obese persons who are metabolically normal seems to exist. This subgroup, the metabolically healthy obese (MHO), has good levels of insulin sensitivity, and absence of diabetes, dyslipidemia and hypertension. (Boonchaya-anant and Apovian, 2014). However, they are the exception and not the rule. Estimates using mortality data from the NHANES surveys show that thousands of deaths are related to obesity. Moderately high BMI in adolescence is correlated with premature death in younger and middle-age women (van Dam et al, 2006). Increased adiposity and reduced physical activity are strong independent risk factors for death in women.

A huge study of more than 100,000 U.S. men and women age 50 and older who took part in the 9-year Cancer Prevention Study II Nutrition Cohort found that obesity is linked to death. Those individuals with very large waists (at least 47 inches in men and 43 inches in women) had twice the risk of mortality compared with those with small waists (35 inches or less for men and 30 inches or less for women). This was true at all BMIs but was strongest in women of normal weight, indicating the danger of waistline, abdominal, or visceral fat (Jacobs et al, 2010).

Several large studies have determined that the optimal BMI with the least risk for mortality is a BMI of 23 to 24.9. BMI above or below this range seems to increase mortality risk (Adams et al, 2006; Jee et al, 2006). The optimal range for longevity appears to be within the range of 20.5 to 24.9.

Nonalcoholic fatty liver disease (NAFLD) is associated with obesity and may progress to end-stage liver disease (see Chapter 29). Obesity is also a risk factor for cancer, infertility, poor wound healing, and poor antibody response to hepatitis B vaccine. Thus the costs of obesity are staggering. Health economists estimate costs of overweight and obesity to account for nearly 10% of total annual U.S. medical expenditures. The Internal Revenue Service issued a rule in 2002 qualifying obesity as a disease, allowing taxpayers to claim weight loss expenses as a medical deduction if undertaken to treat an existing disease.

The U.S. government recognizes the immense effect of obesity on the health and financial well-being of its citizens. In June 2013 the American Medical Association (AMA) finally recognized obesity as a disease classification in its own entity (AMA, 2013). Healthy People 2020 objectives also identify the implications of overweight and obesity (see Chapter 9). The objectives include targets to increase the proportion of adults who are at a healthy weight and to reduce the proportion of adults, children, and adolescents who are obese. Overweight adolescents often become obese adults; obese individuals are at increased risk for comorbidities of type 2 diabetes, hypertension, stroke, certain cancers, infertility, and other conditions.

TABLE 21-2 **Classification of Overweight and Obesity**	
Classification	**Body Mass Index (kg/m²)**
Underweight	<18.5
Normal	18.5-24.9
Overweight	25.0-29.9
Obesity, class I	30.0-34.9
Obesity, class II	35.0-39.9
Extreme obesity, class III	>40

From National Institutes of Health, National Heart, Lung, and Blood Institute: Clinical guidelines on the identification, evaluation, and treatment of overweight and obesity in adults after Mennce report, NIH Publication No. 98-4083, 1998.

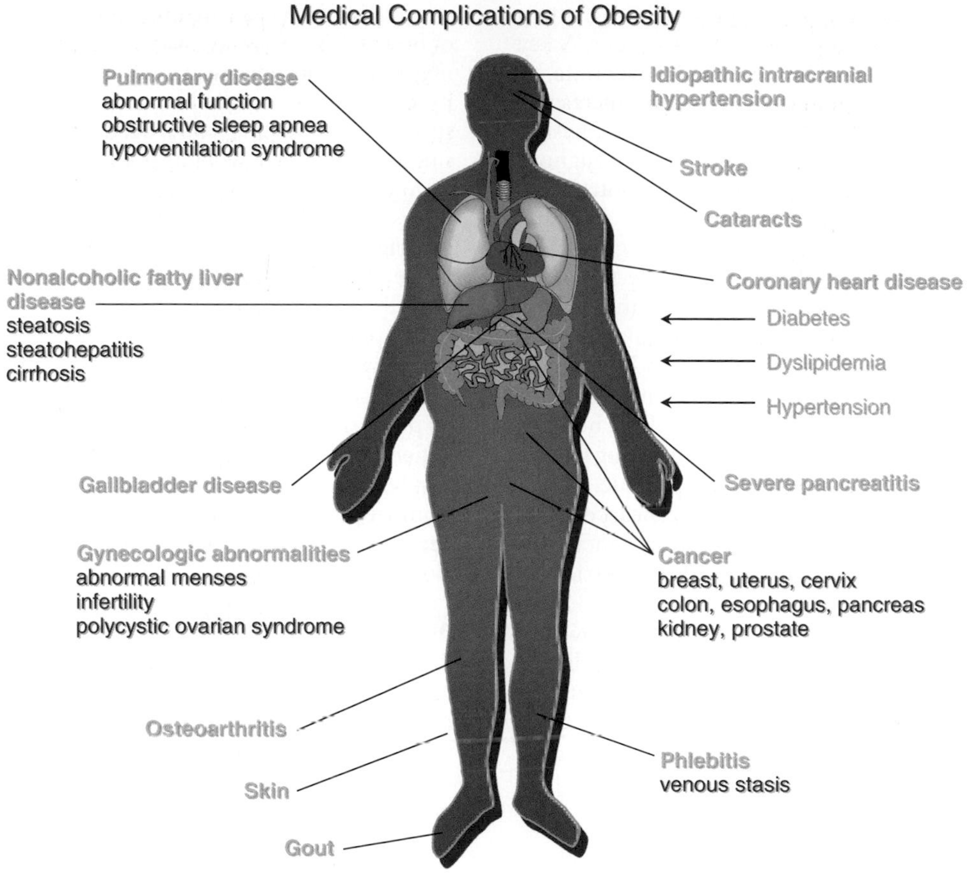

Medical Complications of Obesity

FIGURE 21-3 The medical complications of obesity are extensive. (Reprinted with permission from Delichatsios HK: Obesity assessment in the primary care office, Harvard Medical School. 23rd Annual International Conference-Practical approaches to the treatment of obesity, Boston, June 18-20 2009, GL Blackburn, course director.)

Fat Deposition and the Metabolic Syndrome

Regional patterns of fat deposit are controlled genetically and differ between and among men and women. Two major types of fat deposition currently are recognized: excess subcutaneous truncal-abdominal fat (the apple-shaped **android fat distribution**) and excess gluteofemoral fat in thighs and buttocks (the pear-shaped **gynoid fat distribution**). The android shape is more common among men. Gynoid fat deposition in women during child-bearing years is utilized to support the demands of pregnancy and lactation. Women with the gynoid type of obesity do not develop the impairments of glucose metabolism in those with an android deposition (Wajchenberg 2013). Postmenopausal women more closely follow the male pattern of abdominal fat stores, sometimes referred to as "belly fat."

Abdominal fat is an indicator of fat surrounding internal organs or visceral fat. According to a major study done through the Brigham and Women's Hospital in Boston over 7 years and including more than 3000 people (Framingham Study patients were used), those with higher amounts of abdominal fat, versus fat in other parts of body, were found to have higher risks of cancer and heart disease (Britton et al, 2013). Many other reputable scientific studies have been performed, validating the findings repeatedly.

Reports on methods to lose abdominal or "belly" fat (reputable and unorthodox ones) have targeted the media in the recent past. Data from smaller studies show that the Mediterranean diet, with a concentration on monounsaturated fat intake, appears to have a positive effect on diminishing belly fat; however, adequate protein intake, combined with a reduction in saturated fats, refined sugar, and calories, plus an increase in physical activity, still appear to remain the key to overall loss of body fat (Doheny, 2014).

Visceral obesity, or excessive **visceral adipose tissue (VAT)** under the peritoneum and in the intraabdominal cavity, is correlated highly with insulin resistance and diabetes. Individuals diagnosed with the metabolic syndrome (MetS) have three or more of the following abnormalities: waist circumference of more than 102 cm (40 in) in men and more than 88 cm (35 in) in women, serum TGs of at least 150 mg/dl, high-density lipoprotein (HDL) level less than 40 mg/dl in men and less than 50 mg/dl in women, blood pressure 135/85 mm Hg or higher, or fasting glucose 100 mg/dl or higher. Increased visceral fat is a risk factor for coronary artery disease, dyslipidemia, hypertension, stroke, type 2 diabetes, and MetS (Wajchenberg 2013). By the same token, VAT and low cardiorespiratory fitness (CRF) levels are associated with a deteriorated cardiometabolic risk profile. Achieving a low level of VAT and a high level of CRF is an important target for cardiometabolic health (Rhéaume et al, 2011).

Calorie Restriction and Longevity

Balancing energy intake and energy expenditure is the basis of weight management throughout life. **Lifestyle modification,** and becoming aware of eating behavior triggers to manage them more effectively, is vital for permanent change to occur. A key recommendation is to prevent gradual weight gain over time, by making small decreases in overall caloric intake and increasing physical activity. Patterns of healthful eating and regular physical activity should begin in childhood and continue throughout adulthood. The aging process with a lower RMR introduces special challenges. Energy balance is maintained by adjusting energy intake and physical activity to prevent weight gain.

Prolonged calorie restriction (CR) increases life span and slows aging in animals. The apparent generality of the longevity-increasing effects of CR has prompted speculation that similar results could be obtained in humans. Two biomarkers of longevity—fasting insulin level and body temperature—have been noted to be decreased by prolonged CR in humans (Heilbronn et al, 2006). Proponents of CR for anti-aging believe that cutting calorie intake reduces aging and chronic disease development. In rodents with Alzheimer's disease, heart disease, and stroke, decreased deterioration of nerves and increased nerve creation also was demonstrated with calorie restriction. (Mayo Clinic, 2010).

Whether CR can slow the aging process in humans, however, remains an important question (Fontana, 2009). Unless clinical studies provide clear evidence of its utility, the wider use of CR in the human population cannot be justified, based on current data. On the other hand, the randomization of humans to CR may not be ethical, making it difficult to study its effect on individuals (Adomaityte et al, 2014).

Weight Discrimination

Widespread bias and discrimination based on weight have been documented in education, employment, and health care. Like other forms of prejudice, this stems from a lack of understanding of the chronic disease of obesity and its medical consequences. The vast majority of the U.S. does not consider obesity a protected class and therefore weight-based employment discrimination does not have a basis for a legal claim (Pomeranz JL 2013). Overweight children experience adverse social, educational, and psychologic consequences as a result of weight bias. There are automatic negative associations for obese people among health professionals, exercise science students, and obese individuals themselves. It is essential to break down the barriers caused by ignorance and indifference. Patient support groups help to correct the negative effect of this type of discrimination.

MANAGEMENT OF OBESITY IN ADULTS

The management of obesity has evolved over the years. Initially, clinicians focused entirely on weight loss, and little was known about weight maintenance. Treatment also has evolved. Years ago, an energy-restricted diet was the only treatment. Eventually, lifestyle modifications were added. The importance of developing physical activity behaviors is recognized as an essential ingredient for weight maintenance during and after weight loss. Today, a chronic disease-prevention model incorporates lifestyle interventions and interdisciplinary therapies from physicians, dietitians, exercise specialists, and behavior therapists.

Goals of Treatment

The goal of obesity treatment should focus on weight management and attaining the best weight possible in the context of overall health. Achieving an "ideal" body weight or percentage of body fat is not always realistic; under some circumstances, it may not be appropriate at all. Depending on the type and severity of the obesity and the age and lifestyle of the individual, successfully reducing body weight varies from being relatively simple to being virtually impossible.

Maintaining present body weight or achieving a moderate loss is beneficial. Obese persons who lose even small amounts of weight (5% to 10% of initial body weight) are likely to improve their blood glucose, blood pressure, and cholesterol levels.

Despite the recognition that modest weight loss is beneficial and may be more achievable, obese persons usually have self-defined goal weights that differ considerably from that suggested by professionals. Therefore, health professionals must help their patients accept more modest, realistic weight loss goals. For example, actuarial tables support no benefit and possible harm from weight loss after age 65. In fact, in the obese elderly, sarcopenia (loss of muscle mass) is the greatest predictor of disability along with the inability to perform daily activities.

Rate and Extent of Weight Loss

Reduction of body weight involves the loss of protein and fat in amounts determined to some degree by the rate of weight reduction. A drastic reduction in calories resulting in a high rate of weight loss can mimic the starvation response. Tissue response to starvation is one of adaptation to an anticipated period of deprivation. The classic starvation studies done by Keys (1950) found that during the first 10 days of a fast and after depletion of glycogen stores, approximately 8% to 12% of the energy expenditure is from protein, and the balance is from fat. As starvation progresses, up to 97% of energy expenditure is from stored TGs. Metabolic aberrations during starvation include bradycardia, hypotension, dry skin and hair, easy fatigue, constipation, nervous system abnormalities, depression, and even death.

Mobilizing fat, with more than twice the kilocalories of protein, is more efficient and also spares vital LBM. Steady weight loss over a longer period favors reduction of fat stores, limits the loss of vital protein tissues, and avoids the sharp decline in RMR that accompanies rapid weight reduction. Calorie deficits that result in a loss of approximately 0.5 to 1 lb per week for persons with a BMI of 27 to 35, and 1 to 2 lb per week for those with BMIs greater than 35, should continue for approximately 6 months for a reduction of 10% of body weight (Academy of Nutrition and Dietetics [AND], formerly the American Dietetic Association [ADA], 2010). For the next 6 months the focus changes from weight loss to weight maintenance. After this phase, further weight loss may be considered.

Even with the same caloric intake, rates of weight reduction vary. Men reduce weight faster than women of similar size because of their higher LBM and RMR. The heavier person expends more energy than one who is less obese and loses faster on a given calorie intake than a lighter person. Many obese persons who fail to lose weight on a diet actually consume more energy than they report and overestimate their physical activity levels.

Lifestyle Modification

Behavior modification is the cornerstone of lifestyle intervention. It focuses on restructuring a person's environment, nutrient intake, and physical activity by using goal setting, stimulus control, cognitive restructuring, and relapse prevention. It also provides feedback on progress and places the responsibility for change and accomplishment on the patient.

Stimulus control involves modification of (1) the settings or the chain of events that precede eating, (2) the kinds of foods consumed when eating does occur, and (3) the consequences of eating. Patients are taught to slow their rate of eating to become mindful of satiety cues, and reduce food intake. Strategies such as putting down utensils between bites, pausing during meals, and chewing for a minimum number of times are some ways to slow the eating process.

Problem solving is the process of defining the intake problem, generating possible solutions, evaluating and choosing the best solution, implementing the new behavior, evaluating outcomes, and reevaluating alternative solutions if needed.

Cognitive restructuring teaches patients to identify, challenge, and correct the negative thoughts that frequently undermine their efforts to lose weight and keep it off. A cognitive therapy program that underscores the inextricable connection between emotions and eating, and how to manage that connection successfully using positive long-term mental strategies has been developed and found useful (Beck et al, 2011).

Self-monitoring with daily records of place and time of food intake, as well as accompanying thoughts and feelings, helps identify the physical and emotional settings in which eating occurs. Physical activity typically is recorded in minutes or calories expended. Self-monitoring also gives clues to the occurrence of relapses and consequent guilt and how they can be prevented.

A comprehensive program of lifestyle modification produces a loss of approximately 10% of initial weight in 16 to 26 weeks, as revealed by a review of recent randomized controlled trials (RCTs), including the Diabetes Prevention Program. Long-term weight control is facilitated by continued patient-therapist contact, whether provided in person or by telephone, mail, text messaging, or email. Multiple strategies for behavioral therapy often are needed (AND, 2010).

Technology shows promise as a delivery mechanism. Email and phone consults appear to be viable methods for contact and support as part of structured behavioral weight loss programs. Future treatment methods may include augmenting behavioral interventions with specific stimulus controls, self-monitoring with mobile device apps, pharmacotherapy, targeted educational interventions from the Internet, meal replacements, and telephone interventions. Nontraditional behavioral interventions for children and culturally sensitive interventions for racial and ethnic minority populations are needed.

Dietary Modification Recommendations

Weight loss programs with any degree of success integrate food-choice changes with exercise, behavior modification, nutrition education, and psychologic support. When these approaches fail to bring about the desired reduction in body fat, medication may be added. For **morbid obesity** (BMI of 40 or greater), surgical intervention may be required.

Weight loss programs should combine a nutritionally balanced dietary regimen with exercise and lifestyle modification. Selecting the appropriate treatment strategy depends on the goals and health risks of the patient. Treatment options include the following:

- A low calorie, macronutrient adjusted eating plan, increased physical activity, and lifestyle modification

- A low calorie macronutrient adjusted eating plan, increased physical activity, lifestyle modification, and pharmacotherapy
- Surgery plus an individually prescribed eating regimen, physical activity, and lifestyle modification program
- Prevention of weight regain through energy intake and output balance
- Mindset interventions

Restricted-Energy Diets

A balanced, restricted-energy diet is the most widely prescribed method of weight reduction. The diet should be nutritionally adequate except for energy, which is decreased to the point at which fat stores must be mobilized to meet daily energy needs. A caloric deficit of 500 to 1000 kcal daily usually meets this goal. The energy level varies with the individual's size and activities, usually ranging from 1200 to 1800 kcal daily. Regardless of the level of CR, healthful eating should be taught and recommendations for increasing physical activity should be included.

The low-calorie diet should be individualized for carbohydrates (50% to 55% of total kilocalories), using sources such as vegetables, fruits, beans, and whole grains. Generous protein, approximately 15% to 25% of kilocalories, is needed to prevent conversion of dietary protein to energy. Fat content should not exceed 30% of total calories. Extra fiber is recommended to reduce caloric density, to promote satiety by delaying stomach-emptying time, and to decrease to a small degree the efficiency of intestinal absorption.

Calculating fat as a percentage of calories is useful. A simple rule is to divide ideal calorie level by 4 for a 25% fat intake (e.g., an 1800-kcal intake needs 450 kcal from fat, or, at approximately 9 kcal/g, approximately 50 g of fat). Giving the person the option to distribute fat grams throughout the day makes the approach more appealing, involves the person in the process, and decreases energy intake without hunger. Total calories also must be considered.

Alcohol and foods high in sugar should be limited to small amounts for palatability. Alcohol makes up 10% of the diet for many regular drinkers and contributes 7 kcal/g. Heavy drinkers who consume 50% or more of daily calories from alcohol may have a depressed appetite, whereas moderate users tend to gain weight with the added alcohol calories. Habitual use of alcohol may result in lipid storage, weight gain, or obesity (see Chapter 29).

Artificial sweeteners and fat substitutes improve the acceptability of limited food intakes for some people. There is no evidence that using artificial sweeteners reduces food intake or enhances an individual's weight loss.

Vitamin and mineral supplements that meet age-related requirements usually are recommended when there is a daily intake of less than 1200 kcal for women, and 1800 kcal for men, or when it is difficult to choose foods that will meet all nutrient needs at the restricted energy intake.

Formula Diets and Meal Replacement Programs

Formula diets are commercially prepared, ready-to-use, portion-controlled meal replacements. These meal replacements - drinks, prepackaged meals or entrees, or meal bars - can be found over the counter (OTC) in drug stores, supermarkets, and franchised weight loss centers, or in a clinical setting. The goal with use of these foods is to provide structure and replace other higher calorie foods. Per serving, most meal replacements include 10 to 20 g of protein, various amounts of carbohydrate, 0 to 10 g of fat, up to 5 g of fiber, and 25% to 30% of recommended dietary allowances for vitamins and minerals. Usually drinks or shakes are milk (casein or whey), pea protein, rice protein, or soy based, are high in calcium, and have 150 to 250 kcal per 8 oz. They are frequently ready to use, portion controlled, or are made with a purchased powder. People who have difficulty with self-selection or portion control may use meal replacements as part of a comprehensive weight management program. Substituting one or two daily meals or snacks with meal replacements is a successful weight loss and weight maintenance strategy (AND, 2010).

Commercial Programs

Millions of Americans turn to commercial weight loss or self-help programs in search of permanent weight loss. The more calorie-restricted programs usually are supervised medically in a health care setting. The programs vary considerably but the majority are books or internet-based programs that are not medically supervised (see Table 21-3). Some require the use of proprietary prepackaged low-fat meals. Prepackaged diets appeal to some people because they allow them to avoid making choices about food. Some provide classes on self-introspection, behavior modification, and nutrition.

Use of the Internet has spawned a new generation of commercial programs. The importance of a tailored approach was the conclusion of an RCT comparing an Internet-based tailored weight management program with an information-only Internet weight management program based in an integrated health care setting (Rothert et al, 2006).

With the exception of Weight Watchers, there is not strong evidence to support the use of the major commercial and self-help weight loss programs. The reported results are probably a best-case scenario because many studies do not control for high attrition rates. More controlled trials are needed to assess the efficacy and cost effectiveness of commercial programs. Thus it is important to evaluate all weight loss programs for sound nutritional practices. Consumers are savvy, and many programs have begun to report data on dropout or success rates, as well as weight maintenance.

Extreme Energy Restriction and Fasting

Extreme energy-restricted diets provide fewer than 800 kcal per day, and starvation or fasting diets provide fewer than 200 kcal per day. Fasting is seldom prescribed as a treatment; however, it frequently is invoked as a part of religious or protest regimen or in a personal effort to lose weight. Under these circumstances it is seldom continued long enough to produce the serious neurologic, hormonal, and other side effects that accompany prolonged starvation. More than 50% of the rapid weight reduction is fluid, which often leads to serious hypotension. Accumulation of uric acid can precipitate episodes of gout; gallstones also can occur. Also, as fat stores diminish, molecules are released that can affect further weight loss (see *Clinical Insight:* What's in That Fat When You Lose It?). Sometimes what starts as extreme energy restriction to lose weight leads to more disordered eating patterns (see Chapter 22).

Very Low–Calorie Diets

Diets providing 200 to 800 kcal are classified as very low–calorie diets (VLCDs). Little evidence suggests that an intake of fewer than 800 calories daily is of any advantage. An example of a significant exception to this would be the hospitalized patient on a metabolic unit who is monitored carefully, is less than 65 years old, and has a condition such as congestive heart

---

TABLE 21-3 Popular Weight Loss Diets*
Atkins Diet
Belly Fat Cure
Blood Type Diet
Biggest Loser Diet
Caveman (Paleo) Diet
Detox Diets
The Diet Solution
Dr. Oz Ultimate Diet
Glycemic Index Diet
HCG Diet
Jenny Craig
LA Weight Loss
Mayo Clinic Diet
Medifast Diet
NutriSystem Diet
South Beach Diet
Volumetrics Diet
Weight Watchers
Zone Diet

*For a complete description of these diets and discussion of studies supporting their use see the following websites:
http://health.usnews.com/best-diet/best-weight-loss-diets?page=3
http://www.webmd.com/diet/evaluate-latest-diets

failure secondary to obesity. In such a case, the immediacy of rapid weight loss is considered life saving.

Most VLCDs are hypocaloric, but relatively rich in protein (0.8 to 1.5 g/kg IBW per day). They are designed to include a full complement of vitamins, minerals, electrolytes, and essential fatty acids, but not calories, and they are usually given for a period of 12 to 16 weeks. Their major advantage is rapid weight loss. Because of potential side effects, prescription of these diets is reserved for persons with a BMI of more than 30 for whom other diet programs with psychotherapy have been unsuccessful. Occasionally VLCDs may be indicated for persons with a BMI of 27 to 30 who have one or more comorbidities, or other risk factors.

The VLCD that first became popular in the early 1970s resulted in several deaths; however, improved protein formulations have increased acceptability and safety for those with morbid obesity. VLCDs can lead to an increase of urinary ketones that interfere with the renal clearance of uric acid, resulting in increased serum uric acid levels or gout. Higher serum cholesterol levels resulting from mobilization of adipose stores pose a risk of gallstones. Additional adverse reactions include cold intolerance, fatigue, lightheadedness, nervousness, euphoria, constipation or diarrhea, dry skin, anemia, and menstrual irregularities; some of these are related to triiodothyronine (thyroid) deficiency (see Chapter 31).

Even though there are significantly greater weight losses with VLCDs in the short term, there are no significant differences in the weight losses in the long term (Tsai and Wadden, 2006). Thus there rarely seems to be reason to recommend these VLCDs over more moderate CR. For those who have lost weight on a VLCD, limiting dietary fat intake and maintaining physical activity are important factors for the prevention of weight regain. To promote better weight loss, patients should limit their fat intake to less than 30% of calories and increase activity levels.

Popular Diets and Practices

Each year, new approaches to weight loss find their way to the consumer through the popular press and media. Some of the programs are sensible and appropriate, whereas others emphasize fast results with minimum effort. Some of the proposed diets would lead to nutritional deficiencies over an extended period; however, the potential health risks are seldom realized because the diets usually are abandoned after a few weeks (see *Focus On:* Eating Like a Caveman). Diets that emphasize fast results with minimum effort encourage unrealistic expectations, setting the dieter up for failure, subsequent guilt, and feelings of helplessness about managing the weight problem.

Online commercial diet programs have grown dramatically in the past decade. A programmed approach, for people on the run who carry their phones and computers, with a product line offered and accessibility to counselors and health professionals, has made the business of diets a multibillion dollar industry. One-on-one and group online counseling, phone access to discuss weight loss progress and setbacks, and delivery of "to-your-door" foods and meals are some of the enticing aspects of joining these programs. Consumers continue to need proper guidance to separate the good, sound diet programs

EATING LIKE A CAVEMAN

The Paleo diet, also called the caveman diet or stone age diet, claims that eating like our prehistoric ancestors will make us leaner and less likely to get diabetes, heart disease, cancer, and other health-related problems. It is a high-protein, high-fiber eating plan that promises weight loss without reducing calories. Because our ancestors were hunters and gatherers (not farmers), the diet eliminates processed foods, dairy, refined sugar, potatoes, and salt and refined vegetable oils such as canola oil. Calorie counting is eliminated. The rationale for the diet rests with the belief that lean meat and high-fiber fruits and vegetables will provide the feeling of fullness and create a lack of desire to overeat.

Foods allowed include lean meats, fresh fish, fruits, vegetables, eggs, seeds, nuts, and some oils such as olive and coconut.

The diet appears adequate with the exceptions of calcium and vitamin D. These should be supplemented. The Paleo diet has been shown to be of benefit in some studies that compared it to the Mediterranean diet and low fat-high carbohydrate diets (Lindeberg, 2007). A 2-year randomized trial also found benefit in obese postmenopausal women (Mellberg, 2013).

from the bad. The diets are described at many websites (see Table 21-3).

The low-carbohydrate, high-fat diet restricts carbohydrates to less than 20% of calories (and often less than 10% in the beginning), and fat constitutes 55% to 65% of calories, with protein making up the balance. Protein obtained from animal sources means that fat, saturated fat, and cholesterol intakes are high. These diets feature high ketone production and do suppress appetite, at least initially. The initial rapid weight loss from diuresis is secondary to the carbohydrate restriction. Examples of severe carbohydrate-restricted diets include Dr. Atkin's New Diet Revolution and The Paleo Diet.

The Zone Diet and The South Beach Diet restrict carbohydrates to no more than 40% of total calories, with fat and protein each providing 30% of total calories. This diet composition is claimed to keep insulin in check, which is blamed for fat storage. The diet includes generous amounts of fiber and fresh fruits and vegetables. There is attention to the kind of fat, with emphasis on monounsaturated and polyunsaturated fat and limitation of saturated fat. Weight loss ensues not because insulin is kept in a narrow range, but because calories are restricted.

Very low fat diets contain less than 10% of calories from fat, such as the original Dr. Dean Ornish's Program for Reversing Heart Disease and The Pritikin Program. These diets produce rapid weight loss because they are very restrictive. A more popular variation limits fat to 20% of total energy intake. Because fat provides more than two times the energy per gram as protein or carbohydrate (9 kcal versus 4 kcal), limiting fat is the most efficient way to decrease calories.

Moderate-fat, balanced-nutrient reduction diets contain 20% to 30% of calories from fat, 15% to 20% of calories from protein, and 55% to 60% of calories from carbohydrate. *Volumetrics,* a program in this category, focuses on the energy density of foods (Rolls et al, 2005). Foods high in water content have a low energy density. These include fruits, vegetables, low-fat milk, cooked grains, lean meats, poultry, fish, and beans. Low water–containing foods that are energy dense, such as potato chips, crackers, and fat-free cookies, are restricted.

The U.S. Department of Agriculture (USDA) supported a scientific review of popular diets to assess their efficacy for weight loss and weight maintenance, as well as their effect on metabolic parameters, mental well-being, and reduction of chronic disease. A summary is shown in Table 21-4. See Table 21-5 for popular nutritional supplements used for weight loss.

Physical Activity

Physical activity is the most variable component of energy expenditure (see Chapter 2). Increases in energy expenditure through exercise and other forms of physical activity are important components of interventions for weight loss and its maintenance. By increasing LBM in proportion to fat, physical activity helps to balance the loss of LBM and reduction of RMR that inevitably accompany intentional weight reduction. Other positive side effects of increased activity include strengthening cardiovascular integrity, increasing sensitivity to insulin, and expending additional energy and therefore calories.

Adequate levels of physical activity appear to be 60 to 90 minutes daily, as recommended by the USDA. This is also the amount of activity reported by those in the National Weight Control Registry (NWCR) who have kept off at least 10% of their weight for at least a year. Overweight and obese adults should gradually increase to these levels of physical activity. There is evidence that, even if an overweight or obese adult is unable to achieve this level of activity, significant health benefits can be realized by participating in at least 30 minutes of daily activity of moderate intensity (AND, 2010). Therefore it is important to target these levels of physical activity to improve health-related outcomes and to facilitate long-term weight control.

Aerobic and resistance training should be recommended. Resistance training increases LBM, adding to the RMR and the ability to use more of the energy intake, and it increases bone mineral density, especially for women (see Chapter 24). Aerobic exercise is important for cardiovascular health through elevated RMR, calorie expenditure, energy deficit, and loss of fat. In addition to the physiologic benefits of exercise are relief of boredom, increased sense of control, and improved sense of well-being. The whole family can get involved in pleasurable activities (see Figure 21-4).

The recommendations for exercise from the American College of Sports Medicine differ for weight loss vs weight maintenance. Physical activity <150 minutes/week has a minimal effect on weight loss. Physical activity >150 minutes/week usually results in modest weight loss (defined as ~2-3 kg), with physical activity between 225 and 420 minutes/week resulting in the greatest weight loss (5 to 7.5 kg). While research on maintaining weight indicates that moderately vigorous physical activity of 150 to 250 minutes per week at an energy equivalent of ~1200 to 2,000 kilocalories per week (about 12 to 20 miles per week of jogging or running) is sufficient to prevent weight gain (Donnelly 2009).

Pharmaceutical Management

Appropriate pharmacotherapy can augment diet, physical activity, and behavior therapy as treatment for patients with a BMI of 30 or higher or patients with 27 or higher who

TABLE 21-4	**Results of U.S. Department of Agriculture Scientific Review of Popular Diets**
Area	**Finding**
Weight loss	Diets that reduce caloric intake result in weight loss; all popular diets result in short-term weight loss if followed.
Body composition	All low-calorie diets result in a loss of body fat. In the short term, high-fat, low-carbohydrate ketogenic diets cause a greater loss of body water than body fat.
Nutritional adequacy	• High-fat, low-carbohydrate diets are low in vitamins E and A, thiamin, B_6, and folate; and the minerals calcium, magnesium, iron, and potassium. They are also low in dietary fiber. • Very-low-fat diets are low in vitamins E and B_{12} and the mineral zinc. • With proper food choices, a moderate-fat, balanced nutrient–reduction diet is nutritionally adequate.
Metabolic parameters	• Low-carbohydrate diets cause ketosis and may significantly increase blood uric acid concentrations. • Blood lipid levels decline as body weight decreases. • Energy restriction improves glycemic control. • As body weight declines, blood insulin and plasma leptin levels decrease. • As body weight declines, blood pressure decreases.
Hunger and compliance	No diet was optimal for reducing hunger.
Effect on weight maintenance	Controlled clinical trials of high-fat, low-carbohydrate, low-fat, and very-low-fat diets are lacking; therefore no data are available on weight maintenance after weight loss or long-term health benefits or risk.

From Freedman M et al: Popular diets: a scientific review, *Obes Res* 9(Suppl 1):1S, 2001.

also have significant risk factors or disease. These agents can decrease appetite, reduce absorption of fat, or increase energy expenditure. As with any drug treatment, physician monitoring for efficacy and safety is necessary. Pharmacotherapy is not a "magic pill"; dietitians should collaborate with other health professionals regarding the use of Food and Drug Administration (FDA)–approved pharmacotherapy. Not all individuals respond, but for patients who do respond, weight loss of approximately 2 to 20 kg can be expected usually during the first 6 months of treatment. Medication without lifestyle modification is less effective.

Medications currently available can be categorized as central nervous system (CNS) acting agents and non–CNS-acting agents. The CNS-acting agents fall into the categories of catecholaminergic agents, serotoninergic agents, and combination catecholaminergic-serotoninergic agents. Common side effects of CNS-acting agents are dry mouth, headache, insomnia, and constipation. As of April, 2015, five long-term weight loss drugs were listed as approved by the FDA (FDA, 2015). They are: orlistat (Xenical), locaserin (Beliviq), phentermine topiramate (Qysmia), naltrexone-buproprion (Contrav), and liraglude (Saxenda) (see Table 21-5 for mechanisms of action and common side effects of prescription weight loss drugs).

Catecholaminergic drugs act on the brain, increasing the availability of norepinephrine. Drug Enforcement Agency Schedule II anorexic agents such as amphetamines have a

TABLE 21-5 Nonprescription Weight Loss Products

Product	Claim	Effectiveness	Safety
Alli: OTC version of prescription drug orlistat (Xenical)	Decreases absorption of dietary fat	Effective; weight loss amounts typically less for OTC versus prescription	FDA investigating reports of liver injury, pancreatitis
Bitter orange	Increases calories burned	Insufficient reliable evidence to rate	Possibly unsafe
Chitosan	Blocks absorption of dietary fat	Insufficient reliable evidence to rate	Possibly safe
Chromium	Increases calories burned, decreases appetite, and builds muscle	Insufficient reliable evidence to rate	Likely safe
CLA	Reduces body fat and builds muscle	Possibly effective	Possibly safe
Country mallow (heartleaf)	Decreases appetite and increases calories burned	Insufficient reliable evidence to rate	Likely unsafe and banned by FDA
Ephedra (Ma Huang)	Decreases appetite	Possibly effective	Likely unsafe and banned by FDA
Green tea extract	Increases calorie and fat metabolism and decreases appetite	Insufficient reliable evidence to rate	Possibly safe
Guar gum	Blocks absorption of dietary fat and increases feeling of fullness	Possibly ineffective	Likely safe
Hoodia	Decreases appetite	Insufficient reliable evidence to rate	Insufficient information
Senna	Cathartic; causes diarrhea	Insufficient reliable evidence	Likely unsafe
Raspberry ketones	Increases lipolysis	No human studies	Likely unsafe especially for hypertensives
Qsymia, by qualified G	Phentermine increases metabolism for short term and topiramate for long term	Human studies indicate short and long term success for majority.	Not for the pregnant, caution with stroke/heart disease, glaucoma
Garcinia Cambogia	Blocks enzymes from in body which convert glucose to fat. Also increases serotonin in brain, limiting appetite and providing extra energy	Contradictory evidence	Reports of liver damage associated

Adapted from Natural Medicines in the Clinical Management of Obesity, Natural Medicines Comprehensive Database (website): http://naturaldatabase.therapeuticresearch.com:80/ce/ceCourse.aspx?s=ND&cs=&pc=09%2D32&cec=1&pm=. Accessed April 19, 2011; Scott GN: *Is raspberry ketone effective for weight loss?* http://www.medscape.com/viewarticle/775741, 2012. Accessed January 19, 2015.
CLA, Conjugated linoleic acid; *FDA,* Food and Drug Administration; *OTC,* over the counter.

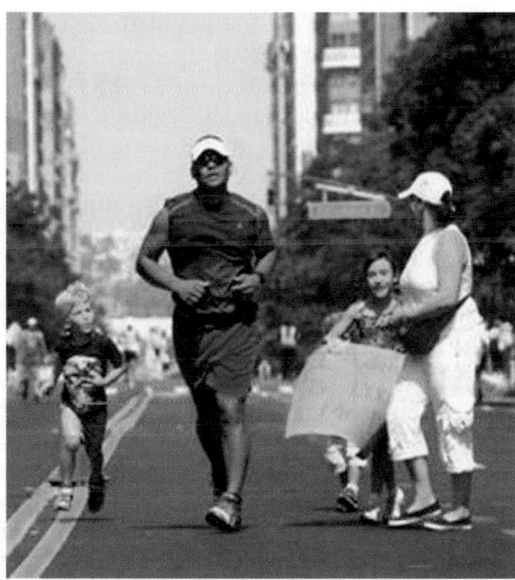

FIGURE 21-4 Jogging is an excellent aerobic activity for the whole family. (Photo printed with permission from Dr. David Rivera, 2010.)

high potential for abuse and are not recommended for obesity treatment.

Serotoninergic agents act by increasing serotonin levels in the brain. Two drugs in this category, fenfluramine (commonly used in combination with phentermine, known as "fen-phen") and dexfenfluramine, were removed from the market in 1997 after concerns were raised regarding the possible side effects of cardiac valvulopathy, regurgitation, and primary pulmonary hypertension.

The mode of action of the weight loss drug orlistat is unusual in that it inhibits gastrointestinal lipase, which reduces approximately one third the amount of fat that is absorbed from food. Depending on the fat content of a person's diet, this lowered absorption can represent 150 to 200 kcal/day. With lowered fat-soluble vitamin absorption, supplements typically are recommended, separated from the drug dosage by 2 hours or more. A weight loss of 3 to 5 kg in orlistat-treated patients is common. Side effects are gastrointestinal: oily spotting, fecal urgency, and flatus with discharge. Health benefits include reduced low-density lipoprotein (LDL) cholesterol and elevated HDL cholesterol, improved glycemic control, and reduced blood pressure.

Other drugs targeting weight loss and obesity through the CNS pathway or peripheral adiposity signals are in early phase clinical trials. Orexin is an appetite stimulant produced by the hypothalamus. Orexin is also known as hypocretin (Tsuneki et al, 2012). The FDA-approved, OTC weight loss product Alli contains 50% of the prescription dose of orlistat and Qsymia, which is a combination of two FDA-approved drugs, phentermine and topiramate, in an extended-release formulation. OTC and natural weight-loss products hold varying degrees of efficacy (see Table 21-6).

Other Nonsurgical Approaches

The non-diet paradigm maintains that the body will attain its natural weight if the individual eats healthfully, becomes attuned to hunger and satiety cues, and incorporates physical activity. This approach focuses on achieving health rather than attaining a certain weight. Advocates for this approach promote

TABLE 21-6   Prescription Drugs Approved for Obesity Treatment*

Weight Loss Drug	Approved for	How it works	Common side effects
Orlistat Sold as Xenical by prescription; over-the-counter version sold as Alli	Xenical: adults and children ages 12 and older Alli: adults only	Blocks some of the fat that you eat, keeping it from being absorbed by your body	Stomach pain, gas, diarrhea, and leakage of oily stools Note: Rare cases of severe liver injury reported. Should not be taken with cyclosporine.
Lorcaserin Sold as Belviq	Adults	Acts on the serotonin receptors in the brain. This may help you eat less and feel full after eating smaller amounts of food.	Headaches, dizziness, feeling tired, nausea, dry mouth, cough, and constipation. Should not be taken with selective serotonin reuptake inhibitors (SSRIs) and monoamine oxidase inhibitor (MAOI) medications
Phentermine-topiramate Sold as Qsymia	Adults	A mix of two drugs: phentermine (suppresses your appetite and curbs your desire to eat) and topiramate (used to treat seizures or migraine headaches). May make you feel full and make foods taste less appealing.	Tingling of hands and feet, dizziness, taste alterations (particularly with carbonated beverages), trouble sleeping, constipation, and dry mouth Note: Sold only through certified pharmacies. May lead to birth defects. Do not take Qsymia if you are pregnant or planning a pregnancy.
Other appetite suppressant drugs (drugs that curb your desire to eat), which include phentermine benzphetamine diethylpropion phendimetrazine Sold under many names	Adults	Increase chemicals in the brain that affect appetite. Make you feel that you are not hungry or that you are full. Note: Only FDA approved for a short period of time (up to 12 weeks).	Dry mouth, difficulty sleeping, dizziness, headache, feeling nervous, feeling restless, upset stomach, diarrhea, and constipation

*Note: Metformin, used for type 2 diabetes, is a prescription drug which has been used by physicians as an "off-label" treatment of obesity. Historically, health care providers have had some leverage in how they may prescribe drugs approved by the FDA. For example, in treating obesity, a qualified health care provider may prescribe a drug approved for treating another medical problem, prescribe two or more drugs at the same time, and/or prescribe a drug for a longer period of time than approved by the FDA.
Adapted from www.niddk.nih.gov Mar 3, 2014.

size acceptance and respect for the diversity of body shapes and sizes. Given the evidence that a 5% to 10% loss of initial weight can result in health benefits, that many persons set weight loss goals that are unrealistic, and that fat discrimination continues to plague society, this approach may help some persons to develop a better relationship with food and a healthier perspective about their bodies.

Bariatric Surgery

Bariatric surgery is at this point considered the only long-term effective treatment for extreme or class III obesity with a BMI of 40 or greater, or a BMI of 35 or greater with comorbidities. Approximately 179,000 surgeries are done annually in the United States (Beebe 2015). Gastroplasty or stomach restricting procedures, decrease the amount of food entering the gastrointestinal tract. Other surgical procedures, such as Roux-en-Y, are restrictive and cause malabsorption because they also prevent food from being absorbed from the gastrointestinal tract.

Before any extremely obese person is considered for surgery, failure of a comprehensive program that includes CR, exercise, lifestyle modification, psychologic counseling, and family involvement must be demonstrated. *Failure* is defined as an inability of the patient to reduce body weight by one third and body fat by one half, and an inability to maintain any weight loss achieved. Such patients have intractable morbid obesity and should be considered for surgery.

If surgery is chosen, the patient is evaluated extensively with respect to physiologic and medical complications, psychologic problems such as depression or poor self-esteem, and motivation. Counseling sharply improves the outcomes for

dieting and drug therapy in this population (Wadden and Sarwer, 2006). Postoperative follow-up requires evaluation at regular intervals by the surgical team and a registered dietitian nutritionist (RDN). In addition, behavioral or psychologic support is necessary. Studies indicate some positive physiologic changes in liver fibrosis, BMI, branched chain amino acid production and reversal of insulin-induced increases in brain glucose metabolism (Abdennour et al, 2014; Tuulari et al, 2013).

Gastric Bypass, Gastroplasty, Gastric Banding, and the Sleeve Gastrectomy

Gastroplasty and gastric bypass procedures reduce the amount of food that can be eaten at one time and produce early satiety (see Figure 21-5). The new stomach capacity may be as small as 30 ml or approximately 2 tablespoons. After surgery the patient's diet progresses from clear liquid, to full liquid, to puree, soft, and finally to a regular diet as tolerated, with emphasis on protein intake (see Table 21-7). The results of gastric surgery are more favorable than those from the intestinal bypass surgery practiced during the 1970s. On average, the reduction of excess body weight after gastric restriction surgery correlates to approximately 30% to 40% of initial body weight. In addition to the greater absolute weight loss observed, the gastric bypass tends to have sustainable results with significant resolution of hypertension, type 2 diabetes mellitus, osteoarthritis, back pain, dyslipidemia, cardiomyopathy, nonalcoholic steatohepatitis, and sleep apnea. However, late complications may be seen, such as vitamin deficiencies, electrolyte problems, or even intestinal failure. Patients should be nutritionally assessed regularly (see Appendices 21 and 22).

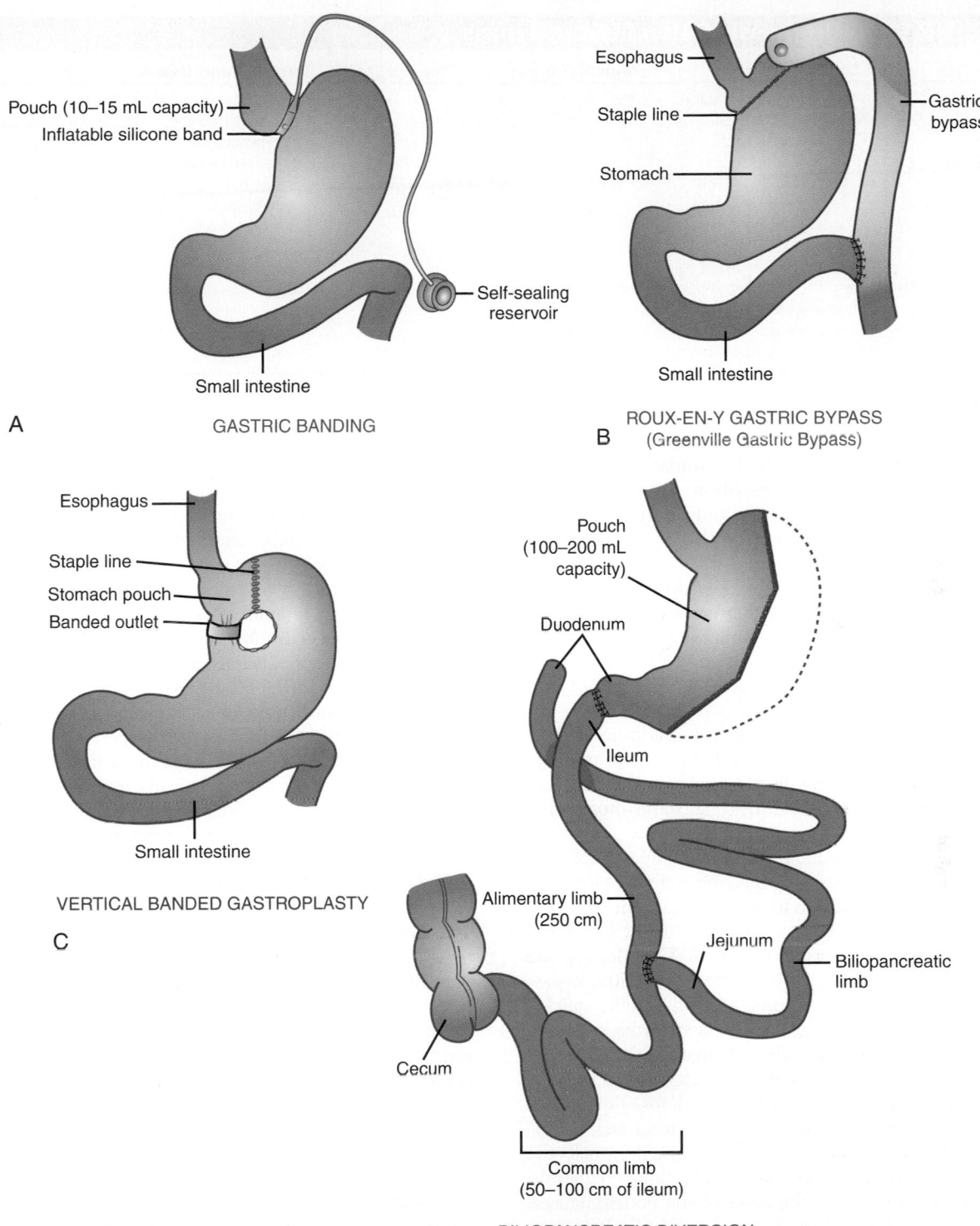

FIGURE 21-5 Bariatric surgeries. New diagram from Dietitians in Nutrition Support newsletter Support Line, June, 2014, P 10, Vol 6, No. 3. Academy of Nutrition and Dietetics.

TABLE 21-7   Diet Progression After Gastric Bypass

Phases of Diet	Total Quantity	Typical Progression after Surgery	Sample Food Items
Liquid diet	NPO 1-2 days post surgery for stomach healing then no more than ½ cup total	2-3 days after surgery	Plain and flavored waters, broth, unsweetened juices, diet gelatin, noncarbonated noncaffeinated diet drinks, strained cream soups
Semisolids and pureed diet	Gradually increase from ½ cup to no more than 1cup total	Day 4-5 up to 4 weeks as semi-solids are tolerated	Blenderized or pureed soft meats, fish, chicken, turkey; pureed fruits and tender vegetables; hot cereals cooked in milk; yogurt
Soft foods	Meals should be from ¾ cup to no more than 1 cup total 3 × per day	Up to 8 weeks	Foods that can be mashed with a fork, such as ground or finely diced meats, canned or soft, fresh fruit, and cooked vegetables
Regular small meals and snacks	No more than 1 cup total; meat should be no more than 2 oz 48-64 oz water not at meals and multivitamin daily is necessary	6 weeks and beyond	Firmer foods without being pureed. Avoid popcorn, nuts, meats with gristle, dried fruits, vegetables and fruits that are stringy or coarse, sodas, bread, seeds, granola.

Adapted from Mayo Clinic: *Gastric Bypass Diet: What to Eat after the Surgery* (website): http://www.mayoclinic.com/health/gastric-bypass-diet/my00827, 2011. Accessed April 7, 2014.

Gastroplasty reduces the size of the stomach by applying rows of stainless-steel staples to partition the stomach and create a small gastric pouch, leaving only a small opening (0.8 to 1 cm) into the distal stomach. This opening may be banded by a piece of mesh to prevent it from enlarging during the years after surgery. Vertical-banded gastroplasty is the most popular of these surgeries. In the lap-band procedure, also called **gastric banding**, the band creating the reduced stomach pouch can be adjusted so that the opening to the rest of the stomach can be made smaller or enlarged. The band, filled with saline, has a tube exiting from it to the surface of the belly just under the skin; this allows for the injection of additional fluid or reduction of fluid into the lap band. Patients who undergo the banding procedures usually do not require folic acid, iron, or vitamin B_{12} replacements, but nutritional status monitoring on a regular basis is still recommended.

Gastric bypass involves reducing the size of the stomach with the stapling procedure but then connecting a small opening in the upper portion of the stomach to the small intestine by means of an intestinal loop. The original operation in the late 1960s evolved into the Roux-en-Y gastric bypass (RYGB). Because use of the lower part of the stomach is omitted, the gastric bypass patient may have dumping syndrome as food empties quickly into the duodenum (see Chapter 27). The tachycardia, sweating, and abdominal pain are so uncomfortable that they motivate the patient to make the appropriate behavioral changes and refrain from overeating. However, patients tend to choose liquids and weight loss can then be deterred by drinking too much calorically dense liquid like milk shakes and soft drinks. Eventually the pouch expands to accommodate 4 to 5 oz at a time. Frequently, gastric bypass surgery leads to bloating of the pouch, nausea, and vomiting. A postsurgical food record noting the tolerance for specific foods in particular amounts helps in devising a program to avoid these episodes.

Up to 16% of patients may experience postoperative complications (Beebe 2015). These include anastomotic leaks, strictures, perforation, gastric fistulas, bowel obstructions, wound infections, respiratory failure and intractable nausea and vomiting. Additionally, bypass surgery places an individual at high risk for malnutrition that requires lifelong follow-up and monitoring by the multidisciplinary team. Nutritional status should be frequently evaluated by an RDN. Monitoring should include an assessment of total body fat loss, potential anemia, and deficiencies of potassium, magnesium, folate, and vitamin B_{12}. Ice-cube pica and iron deficiency anemia are possible (Kushner and Shanta Retelny, 2005). Supplementation is necessary. An adult vitamin-mineral supplement (one liquid or chewable tablet twice daily) containing 1200 to 1500 mg calcium citrate, 400 to 2000 IU vitamin D, 500 mcg vitamin B_{12}, 400 mg folic acid, and 65 to 80 mg elemental iron with vitamin C is suggested (Kuluck et al, 2010; Snyder-Marlow et al, 2010).

The **laparoscopic sleeve gastrectomy (LSG)** initially was used for patients with a BMI greater than 60 as a precursor to RYGB, but it is now used as a stand-alone procedure and currently is the most popular bariatric surgery in the U.S. A sleeve is created by cutting the antrum of the stomach away from the pylorus and forming a pouch around a bougie on the side of the lesser curvature of the stomach. This reduces the stomach capacity by about 80% through the removal of the fundus and body (Mechanick et al, 2013). Complications associated with the LSG can include gastric bleeding, stenosis, leak, and reflux. After resection, the greater curvature of the stomach can bleed. Treatment involves transfusion and possibly an additional laparoscopy to reinforce the bleeding area with sutures. Each case requires the surgeon's expertise to decide if a patient can resume oral intake, will need nutrition support such as enteral feedings through a jejunostomy tube, or may require parenteral nutrition. Occasionally, RYGB is necessary to resolve reflux complications (Weiner et al, 2011) (see Figure 21-5).

Liposuction

Liposuction (or liposculpture) involves aspiration of fat deposits by means of a 1- to 2-cm incision through which a tube is fanned out into the adipose tissue. The most successful operations are performed on younger persons with only small amounts of fat to be removed, where the elastic properties of the skin are able to allow tightening over the aspirated areas. It is not usually a weight-reduction technique, but rather a cosmetic surgery because usually only approximately 5 lb of fat are removed at a time. Deaths, severe infections, cellulitis, and hemorrhage have occurred with liposuction surgeries.

COMMON PROBLEMS IN OBESITY TREATMENT

The prognosis for maintaining reduced body weight is typically poor. Continued dieting, with repeated ups and downs, leads gradually to a net increase in body fat and thus to a health risk for hyperlipidemia, hypertension, diabetes, and even osteoarthritis. Women having bariatric surgery have had lower serum (25-OH vit D) and higher parathyroid hormone (PTH). The major determinant of (25-OH vit D) and PTH was weight. Hyperparathyroidism in obesity did not indicate vitamin D insufficiency. Low (25-OH vit D) was not associated with comorbid conditions, apart from osteoarthritis (Grethen et al, 2011).

Maintaining Reduced Body Weight

Energy requirements for weight maintenance after weight reduction appear to be 25% lower than at the original weight. The net effect is that reduced-obese persons are faced with the necessity of maintaining a reduced energy intake, even after the desired weight has been lost. Whether this reduced intake must be maintained indefinitely is not known.

The NWCR consists of more than 5000 individuals who have been successful in long-term weight loss maintenance. The purpose of establishing the NWCR is to identify the common characteristics of those who succeed in long-term weight loss maintenance. There is very little similarity in how these individuals lost weight, but there are some common behaviors they all have for keeping the weight off. Lifestyle modification and a sense of self-efficacy appear to be essential. To maintain weight loss, NWCR participants report the following:

1. Eating a relatively low-fat (24%) diet
2. Eating breakfast almost every day
3. Weighing themselves regularly, usually once per day to once per week
4. Engaging in high levels (60 to 90 minutes per day) of physical activity

A national weight loss registry is contributing to our understanding of those tactics that lead to long term success. Dietary restriction of fat, frequent self-weighing and ongoing leisure time physical activity were factors associated with maintaining weight loss (Thomas, 2014). Support groups are valuable for obese persons who are maintaining a new lower weight; they help individuals facing similar problems. Two self-help support groups are Overeaters Anonymous and Take Off Pounds Sensibly. These groups are inexpensive, continuous, include a "buddy system," and encourage participation on a regular basis, or as often as needed. Weight Watchers programs offer free lifelong maintenance classes for those who have reached and are maintaining their goal weights.

Interestingly, boring and monotonous diets can provide the strategy for reducing food intake. Diets that are repetitious (without change from meal to meal) are a useful consideration for controlling intake, because people tend to overeat when they have many mealtime choices. This can be a particular problem in a society where 1 in 3 meals is eaten away from home. Reliance on restaurants and vending trucks or machines generally offer many options, most high in calories (see *Focus On:* Restaurant and Vending Machine Nutrition Labeling).

Overall, a common sense approach is needed. Some phrases can be shared with individuals who are trying to maintain their weight loss, including the following:

1. The best diet is "don't buy it."
2. "Easy does it"—use moderation at all meals.
3. "Don't drink your calories."
4. Keep the "extras" to no more than 200 kcal per day.

FOCUS ON

Restaurant and Vending Machine Nutrition Labeling

DeeAnna Wales VanReken, MS, RDN, CD

When President Obama signed the Affordable Care Act into law in 2010, restaurant labeling laws were included as part of the legislation for health care reform (Federal Register, 2014). This public health effort has been proposed with the intent of providing consumers with the appropriate tools to make nutritious choices when dining out. The ruling will apply to chain restaurants, retail food businesses, and vending machines with 20 or more locations or units (FDA, 2014b).

The law mandates that all participants list the calorie content of menu items directly on the menu or provide the information from nutrition labels that may not be visible in vending machines. Further, if a vending machine consumer requests it, other nutrition data must also be available to them in writing. These data include total calories, fat, saturated fat, cholesterol, sodium, total carbohydrates, sugars, fiber, and total protein (FDA, 2014b). The FDA also has developed a colorful info-graphic to demonstrate basic facts about the new law, which may be posted in restaurants or on vending machines to help consumers understand the changes (FDA, 2014a).

Although it is not required, those with *fewer* than 20 restaurant locations or vending machines may also register voluntarily with the FDA to meet federal requirements. Although some businesses are already in compliance, restaurants will have until December 2015 and vending machines until December 2016 to fulfill the labeling agreement (FDA, 2014b). For more information, including exclusions, children's menus, and timing of implementation of these laws, visit www.fda.gov.

Plateau Effect

A common experience for the person in a weight reduction program is arrival at a weight plateau, when weight remains at the same level for a long period. Eventually weight loss halts completely. One theory is that interim plateaus reflect a reduction of lipid in individual adipocytes to some level that signals metabolic adjustment and weight maintenance. Another theory is that there is a release of toxins from adipose tissue that acts as an endocrine disruptor and inflammatory agent and affects subsequent weight loss. To move out of this phase usually requires an increase in activity level or a change in food choices to include more fruits and vegetables which are naturally higher in detoxifying phytochemicals (see *Clinical Insight:* What's in That Fat When You Lose It?).

Any weight loss—whether fast or slow—results in a loss of the extra muscle that has developed to support the excess adipose tissue. Because this extra LBM has contributed to an increase in metabolic rate, RMR decreases as LBM is lost. The fact that RMR decreases rapidly at the onset of a weight-reduction diet, by as much as 15% within 2 weeks, indicates that other adaptations to the lower weight and the threat of deprivation are taking place.

Other factors join to decrease RMR and limit effectiveness of the restricted energy intake. A decrease in the total kilocalories ingested results in a decrease in total energy expenditure. Because a body that weighs less requires less energy expenditure to move around, the cost of physical activity is also less. A state of equilibrium eventually is reached at which the energy intake is equal to energy expenditure. Unless a change is made in either nutritional intake or physical activity, weight loss stops at this point.

Weight Cycling

Repeated bouts of weight loss and regain, known as weight cycling or the yo-yo effect, occurs in men and women and is common in overweight and normal weight individuals. The effect of weight cycling appears to result in increased body fatness and weight, with the end of each cycle. There are metabolic and psychologic effects that are undesirable.

WEIGHT MANAGEMENT IN CHILDREN AND ADOLESCENTS

About one third of U.S. children ages 2 to 19 are overweight or obese (Ogden et al, 2010). Obese children are often the targets of discrimination. Childhood obesity increases the risk of obesity in adulthood. For the child who is obese after 6 years of age, the probability of obesity in adulthood is significantly greater, if either the mother or the father is obese.

The BMI tables for determining childhood obesity are available for use by health care practitioners (see Appendices 7 and 11). Children whose BMI is greater than the 85th percentile are six times more likely to be overweight later (Nader et al, 2006). In addition, children who have growth failure and undernutrition in utero or in the early years of life tend to become overweight in later childhood with subsequent risks of elevated blood pressure, lipid, and glucose levels (Stein et al, 2005). Obesity that begins in childhood tends to lead to hypertension, elevated LDL cholesterol, and TGs in adults (Thompson et al, 2007).

Children or adolescents with a body mass index (BMI) in the 85th percentile or higher with complications of obesity, or with a BMI in the 95th percentile or higher with or without complications, should be carefully assessed for genetic, endocrinologic, and psychologic conditions, and secondary complications such as hypertension, dyslipidemias, type 2 diabetes, sleep apnea, and orthopedic problems. If the complications cause serious morbidity and require rapid weight loss, referral to a pediatric obesity specialist may be necessary. Otherwise, parent and child readiness to make changes should be evaluated and eating and activity patterns carefully assessed.

Once assessment is complete, treatment can begin. The primary goal of treatment is to achieve healthy eating and activity, not to achieve an IBW. For children 7 years of age and younger, the goal is prolonged weight maintenance or slowing of the rate of weight gain, which allows for a gradual decline in BMI as children grow in height. This is an appropriate goal in the absence of any secondary complication of obesity. However, if secondary complications are present, children in this age group may benefit from weight loss if their BMI is at the 95th percentile or higher. For children older than 7 years, prolonged weight maintenance is appropriate if their BMI is between the 85th and 95th percentile and if they have no secondary complications. If a secondary complication is present, or if the BMI is at the 95th percentile or above, weight loss (about 1 lb per month) is advised.

If the weight appropriate for the child or teen's anticipated adult height has already been reached, maintenance at that weight should be the lifetime goal. The child who already exceeds an optimal adult weight can safely experience a slow weight loss of 10 to 12 pounds per year until the optimal adult weight is reached. Balanced micronutrient intake for children includes 45% to 60% of kilocalories from carbohydrates, 25% to 40% from fat, and 10% to 35% from protein. New directions

in childhood obesity research since the turn of the twenty-first century have uncovered 25 (OH)D deficiency (defined as a level less than or equal to 57 nmol/L or 20 ng/ml). This has been manifested by a lack of sun exposure and the increase in use of sunscreen—blocking the skin's absorption of ultraviolet light. Low vitamin D is predominant in obese children. The accompanying proinflammatory association with diabetes and atherogenic pathways has prompted recommendations to test kindergarten and first grade children. Children with low levels of vitamin D could have the systemic inflammatory mediators and reduced insulin sensitivity pathways inhibited by vitamin D supplementation (Reyman et al, 2014).

The child or adolescent who needs to reduce weight requires attention from family and health professionals. This attention should be directed to all the areas mentioned previously, with family modification of eating habits and increased physical activity. The program should be long term, over the entire growth period and perhaps longer (see Box 18-3: Staged Care Treatment for Overweight and Obesity in Chapter 18).

Inactivity often is coupled with sedentary hobbies, excessive TV watching, or prolonged sitting in front of a computer or game screen. However, there is a new theory that physical inactivity appears to be the result of fatness rather than its cause (Metcalf et al, 2011). This requires further research but does suggest that factors other than inactivity may be more important in obesity development in children (see *New Directions:* Organizing to Solve the Childhood Obesity Problem "Within a Generation").

WEIGHT IMBALANCE: EXCESSIVE LEANNESS OR UNINTENTIONAL WEIGHT LOSS

Almost eclipsed by the attention focused on obesity is the need for some people to gain weight. The term underweight is applicable to those who are 15% to 20% or more below accepted weight standards. Because underweight is often a symptom of disease, it should be assessed medically. A low BMI (less than 18.5) is associated with greater mortality risk than that of individuals with optimal BMI (18.5 to 24.9), especially with aging and in the elderly. Undernutrition may lead to under functioning of the pituitary, thyroid, gonads, and adrenals. Other risk factors include loss of energy and susceptibility to injury and infection, as well as a distorted body image and other psychologic problems (see Chapter 22).

Cause

Underweight or unintentional weight loss can be caused by (1) inadequate oral food and beverage intake, with insufficient quantities to match activity; (2) excessive physical activity, as in the case of compulsive athletic training; (3) inadequate capacity for absorption and metabolism of foods consumed; (4) a wasting disease that increases the metabolic rate and energy needs, as in cancer, acquired immune deficiency syndrome (AIDS), or hyperthyroidism; or (5) excess energy expenditure during psychologic or emotional stress (see Chapter 22).

Assessment

Assessing the cause and extent of underweight before starting a treatment program is important. A thorough history and pertinent medical tests usually determine whether underlying disorders are causing the underweight. From anthropometric data such as arm muscle and fat areas, it is possible to determine whether health-endangering underweight really exists (see Appendices 21 and 22). Assessment of body fatness is useful, especially in dealing with the patient who has an eating disorder (see Chapter 7 and Appendix 21). Biochemical measurements indicate whether malnutrition accompanies the underweight (see Chapter 7).

Management

Any underlying cause of unintentional weight loss or low BMI must be the first priority. A wasting disease or malabsorption requires treatment. Nutrition support and dietary changes are effective, along with treatment of the underlying disorder (see Table 21-8).

If the cause of the underweight is inadequate oral food and beverage intake, activity should be modified and psychologic counseling initiated if necessary.

Appetite Enhancers

The FDA has approved orexigenic agents that include corticosteroids, cyproheptadine, loxiglumide (cholecystokinin antagonist), megestrol acetate, mirtazapine, dronabinol, oxoglutarate, anabolic agents (testosterone or Anadrol), oxandrin, and growth hormone. Use of orexigenic agents for weight loss in seniors is saved for those whose conditions are refractory to usual treatments. One third of older adults, especially women, exhibit weight loss in combination with depression. Mirtazapine is an effective antidepressant that is well tolerated and increases appetite. It is particularly effective in elderly patients with dementia-related weight loss (Fox et al, 2009). Dronabinol is used for chemotherapy-induced nausea and vomiting in cancer and AIDS patients; it has been shown to induce weight gain in patients with dementia.

High-Energy Diets

A careful history may reveal inadequacies in dietary habits and nutritional intakes. Meals should be scheduled and relaxed instead of hastily planned or quickly eaten. The underweight person frequently must be encouraged to eat, even if not hungry. The secret is to individualize the program with readily available foods that the individual really enjoys, with a plan for regular eating times throughout the day. In addition to meals, snacks are usually necessary to adequately increase the energy intake. High-calorie liquids taken with meals or between meals are often effective in those who have loss of appetite or early satiety. Everyday foods can be fortified to increase the calories and protein (see *Focus On:* Food First! in Chapter 20).

The energy distribution of the diet should be approximately 30% of the kilocalories from fat, with the majority from monounsaturated or polyunsaturated sources and at least 12% to 15% of the kilocalories from protein. A basic vitamin and mineral supplement may be encouraged. In addition to an intake according to estimated energy requirements for the present weight, 500 to 1000 extra kilocalories per day should be planned. If 2400 kcal maintains the current weight, 2900 to 3400 kcal would be required for weight gain.

The intake should be increased gradually to avoid gastric discomfort, discouragement, electrolyte imbalances, and heart dysfunction. Step-up plans are outlined in Table 21-9. In underweight children, nonnutritional factors, insufficient caloric intake, excessive nutrient losses, and abnormal energy metabolism may contribute to growth failure and morbidity. Thus adequate nutritional support should be an integral part of the management plan. Lipid-based nutrient supplements are fortified products that are often ready-to-use therapeutic foods or highly concentrated supplements that can be administered at "point of service" or emergency settings (Chaparro and Dewey, 2010).

TABLE 21-8   Nutrition Management of Unintentional Weight Loss

Concern	Tips
Anxiety, stress, depression	Antidepressants can help; monitor choice to be sure they do not contribute to weight loss.
Cancer	Gastrointestinal cancers are especially detrimental. Some treatments and medications can cause loss of appetite, as can the cancer itself.
Celiac disease	Ensure that all gluten-containing foods and ingredients are eliminated from the diet.
Changes in activity level or dietary preparation methods	Avoid skipping meals; prepare foods with high energy density.
Diabetes, new onset	See a physician; monitor medications and meals accordingly.
Dysphagia or chewing difficulties	Alter food and liquid textures accordingly to improve chewing and swallowing capability.
Hyperthyroidism	Too much thyroxine can cause weight loss.
Inflammatory bowel disease	Check medications and treatments to determine whether new choices are in order.
Intestinal ischemia	See a physician.
Medications	Some medications can cause weight loss; check with physician; add snacks or enhanced meals if needed.
Nausea and vomiting	Infections, other illnesses, hormonal changes, and some medications cause nausea and vomiting; small, frequent meals are useful; serve liquids between meals instead of with meals to reduce fullness.
Pancreatitis and cystic fibrosis	Monitor for sufficiency of pancreatic enzyme replacement.

CLINICAL CASE STUDY

Maria is a 45-year-old Latina woman who has tried numerous weight loss programs. She has followed strict diets and has never exercised in previous weight loss attempts. She takes several cardiac medications, none of which she can remember. Her blood pressure is 160/90, she is 5 ft 4 in, and she weighs 195 lb. Her lowest body weight was 130 lb at age 30, maintained for 2 years. Maria mentioned that she tried numerous diets while a teenager, when she weighed 170 lb for 3 years. What guidelines would you offer to Maria at this time?

Nutrition Diagnostic Statements

1. Limited adherence to nutrition-related recommendations related to multiple failed weight loss attempts as evidenced by no change in weight
2. Overweight and obesity related to excessive energy intake as evidenced by weight 70 lb over desirable weight

Nutrition Care Questions

1. How would you address the concern about medications?
2. What types of exercise would you be likely to discuss?
3. Which macro- and micronutrients would you discuss with Maria (e.g., total fat, saturated fat, sodium, potassium, calcium)?
4. How would you bring up exercise and what would you recommend for Maria?
5. What would be the goals of her treatment?

TABLE 21-9 Suggestions for Increasing Energy Intake

Additional Foods		kcal	Protein (g)
Plus 500 kcal (Served Between Meals)			
A. 1 c dry cereal		110	2
1 banana		80	
1 c whole milk		159	8
1 slice toast		60	2
1 T peanut butter		86	4
	Total	495	16
B. 8 saltine crackers		99	3
1 oz cheese		113	7
1 c ice cream		290	6
	Total	502	16
C. 6 graham cracker squares		165	3
2 T peanut butter		172	8
1 c orange juice		122	
2 T raisins		52	
	Total	511	11
Plus 1000 kcal (Served Between Meals)			
A. 8 oz fruit flavored whole milk yogurt		240	9
1 slice bread		60	2
2 oz cheese		226	14
1 apple		87	
¼ of 14-inch cheese pizza		306	16
1 small banana		81	1
	Total	1000	42
B. Instant breakfast with whole milk		280	15
1 c cottage cheese		239	31
½ c pineapple		95	
1 c apple juice		117	3
6 graham cracker squares		165	
1 pear		100	1
	Total	996	50
Plus 1500 kcal (Served Between Meals)			
A. 2 slices bread		120	4
2 T peanut butter		172	8
1 T jam		110	
4 graham cracker squares		110	2
8 oz fruit-flavored whole milk yogurt		240	9
¾ c roasted peanuts		628	28
1 c apricot nectar		143	1
	Total	1523	52
B. 1 baked custard		285	13
Instant breakfast with whole milk		280	15
1 c dry cereal		110	2
1 banana		80	
1 c whole milk		159	8
1 c orange juice		122	
1 bagel		165	6
2 T cream cheese		199	
2 T jam		110	
	Total	1510	44

USEFUL WEBSITES

America on the Move
http://www.americaonthemove.org
American Obesity Association
http://www.obesity.org/
American Society of Bariatric Surgery
http://www.asmbs.org/

Calorie Restriction Society International
www.crsociety.org
International Association for the Study of Obesity
http://www.iaso.org/
International Obesity Task Force
http://www.iotf.org
Let's Move!
www.letsmove.gov/
National Heart, Lung, and Blood Institute: Identification, Evaluation, and Treatment of Overweight and Obesity in Adults
http://www.nhlbi.nih.gov/guidelines/obesity/ob_home.htm
National Weight Control Registry
www.nwcr.ws
Obesity Week
http://obesityweek.org
The Obesity Society
http://www.naaso.org
Treat Obesity Seriously
http://www.treatobesityseriously.org
Shape Up America!
http://www.shapeup.org/
Weight Control Network: National Institute of Diabetes and Digestive and Kidney Disease
http://win.niddk.nih.gov/

REFERENCES

Academy of Nutrition and Dietetics (AND), formerly the American Dietetic Association (ADA): *Evidence-Based Nutrition Practice Guidelines on Adult Weight Management, Dietary Intervention Algorithm* (website): www.adaevidencelibrary.com/topic.cfm?cat=2849, 2006. Accessed July 20, 2010.

Adams KF et al: Overweight, obesity, and mortality in a large prospective cohort of persons 50 to 71 years old, *N Engl J Med* 355:763, 2006.

Adomaityte J et al: Anti-aging diet & supplements: fact or fiction? *Nutr Clin Pract* 29:844, 2014.

American Academy of Pediatrics Press Release: *Kids and Vitamin D Deficiency,* October 17, 2012.

American Medical Association Press Release: *AMA Adopts New Policies,* June 18, 2013.

Apovian, C: Is the secret in the strands?, Proceedings of the 25th International Conference of Practical Approaches to the Treatment of Obesity, *Harvard Medical School,* June 16-18, 2011, p. 407-411.

Barouki R: Linking long-term toxicity of xeno-chemicals with short-term biological adaptation, *Biochimie* 92:1222, 2010.

Beck JS et al: *Cognitive therapy: the basics and beyond,* ed 2, New York, 2011, Guilford.

Beebe ML, Crowley N: Can hypocaloric, high-protein nutrition support be used in complicated bariatric patients to promote weight loss?, NCP 30:522, 2015.

Björntorp P, Sjöström L: Number and size of adipose fat cells in relation to metabolism in human obesity, *Metabolism* 20:703, 1971.

Blackburn GL: *Break through your set point,* New York, 2008, Harper-Collins.

Boonchayan-anant P and Apovian C: Metabolically healthy obesity —does it exist? *Curr Atheroscler Rep,* 16:441, 2014.

Bray GA, Bouchard C: *Handbook of obesity,* ed 3, Boca Raton, Fla, 2014, CRC Press.

Britton K et al: Abdominal fat linked to raised heart, cancer risks, *J Am Coll Cardio,* July 10, 2013.

Bueno AC et al: A novel ADIPOQ mutation impairs assembly of high molecular weight, *J Clin Endocrinol Metab* 99;E683, 2014.

Camp KM, Trujillo E: Position of the Academy of Nutrition and Dietetics: nutritional genomics, *J Acad Nutr Diet* 114:299, 2014.

Centers for Disease Control and Prevention (CDC): *Overweight and Obesity Trends, 2007* (website): www.cdc.gov/nccdphp/obesity/trend/index.htm. Accessed May 12, 2010.

Chan DC et al: Effect of ezetimibe on hepatic fat, inflammatory markers, and apolipoprotein B-100 kinetics in insulin-resistant obese subjects on a weight loss diet, *Diabetes Care* 33:1134, 2010.

Chaparro CM, Dewey KG: Use of lipid-based nutrient supplements (LNS) to improve the nutrient adequacy of general food distribution rations for vulnerable sub-groups in emergency settings, *Matern Child Nutr* 6(Suppl 1):1S, 2010.

Collins F: *The language of life: DNA and the revolution in personalized medicine*, New York, 2010, HarperCollins.

Couce ME et al: Is ghrelin the culprit for weight loss after gastric bypass surgery? A negative answer, *Obes Surg* 16:870, 2006.

Deurenberg P, Deurenberg-Yap M: Validity of body composition methods across ethnic population groups, *Acta Diabetol* 40(Suppl 1):S246, 2003.

Doheny K: Mediterranean diet linked to heart health. Healthy Day News. WebMD. Oct 14, 2014.

Donnelly, Blair SN, et al:American College of Sports Medicine Position Stand. Appropriate physical activity intervention strategies for weight loss and prevention of weight regain for adults, *Med Sci Sports Exerc* 41:459, 2009

English C, Scharioth N: *Half of Germans Are Overweight and Obese* (website): http://www.gallup.com/poll/150359/half-germans-obese-overweight.aspx, 2011. Accessed January 19, 2015.

Enriori JP et al: Leptin resistance and obesity, *Obesity* 14(Suppl 5):254S, 2006.

Farias MM, Cuevas AM, Rodriguez F: Set-Point theory and obesity, *Metab Syndr Relat Disord*, 9:85, 2011.

Federal Register: Food Labeling: *Nutrition Labeling of Standard Menu Items in Restaurants and Similar Retail Food Establishments* (website): https://www.federalregister.gov/regulations/0910-AG57/food-labeling-nutrition-labeling-of-standard-menu-items-in-restaurants-and-similar-retail-food-estab>, 2014 (Accessed 11.28.14).

Ferguson JF et al: Gene-nutrient interactions in the metabolic syndrome: single nucleotide polymorphisms in ADIPOQ and ADIPOR1 interact with plasma saturated fatty acids to modulate insulin resistance, *Am J Clin Nutr* 91:794, 2010.

Food and Drug Administration (FDA): *FDA Approves Orlistat for Over-the-Counter Use, 2009* (website): http://www.fda.gov/NewsEvents/Newsroom/PressAnnouncements/2007/ucm108839.htm, 2013. Accessed January 19, 2015.

Food and Drug Administration: *Infographic: Calories Now on the Menu* (website): http://www.fda.gov/downloads/Food/IngredientsPackagingLabeling/LabelingNutrition/UCM423991.pdf. Accessed November 28, 2014.

Food and Drug Administration: *Menu and Vending Machines Labeling Requirements* (website): http://www.fda.gov/Food/IngredientsPackagingLabeling/LabelingNutrition/ucm217762.htm>, 2014b. Accessed November 28, 2014.

Fontana L: *Calorie restriction, endurance exercise, and successful aging*, 62nd Annual Scientific Meeting of the Gerontological Society of America, Atlanta, Ga, November 21, 2009.

Fox CB et al: Megestrol and mirtazapine for the treatment of unplanned weight loss in the elderly, *Pharmacotherapy* 29:4, 2009.

Frayling TM et al: A common variant in the FTO gene is associated with body mass index and predisposes to childhood and adult obesity, *Science* 316:889, 2007.

Garaulet M et al: The chronobiology, etiology and pathophysiology of obesity, *Int J Obes (Lond)* 34:1667, 2010.

Goldstein BJ, Scalia R: Adipokines and vascular disease in diabetes, *Curr Diab Rep* 7:25, 2007.

Grethen E et al: Vitamin D and Hyperparathyroidism in Obesity, *J Clin Endocrinol Metab* 96:1320, 2011.

Grimble RF: The true cost of in-patient obesity: impact of obesity on inflammatory stress and morbidity, *Proc Nutr Soc* 69:511, 2010.

Grün F: Obesogens, *Curr Opin Endocrinal Diabetes Obes* 17:453, 2010.

Grün F, Blumberg B: Environmental obesogens: organotins and endocrine disruption via nuclear receptor signaling, *Endocrinology* 147(Suppl 6):S50, 2006.

Hall KD et al: Calorie for calorie, dietary fat restriction results in more body fat loss than carbohydrate restriction in people with obesity, *Cell Metabolism* 22:1, 2015

Heilbronn LK et al: Effect of 6-month calorie restriction on biomarkers of longevity, metabolic adaptation, and oxidative stress in overweight individuals: a randomized, controlled trial, *JAMA* 295:1539, 2006.

Hyman M: *Systems biology, toxins, obesity, and functional medicine*. The Proceedings From the Institute of Medicine (IOM), Food and Nutrition Board: *Dietary reference intakes for energy, carbohydrate, fiber, fat, fatty acids, cholesterol, protein, and amino acids*, Washington, DC, 2002, National Academies Press.

Jacobs EJ et al: Waist circumference and all-cause mortality in a large US cohort, *Arch Intern Med* 170:1293, 2010.

Jee SH et al: Body-mass index and mortality in Korean men and women, *N Engl J Med* 355:779, 2006.

Krajmalnik-Brown R et al: Effect of gut microbes on nutrient absorption and energy regulation, *Nutr Clin Pract* 27:201, 2012.

Krakauer NY, Krakauer JC: Dynamic association of mortality hazards with body shape, *PLoS One* 9:e88793, 2014.

Kuluck D et al: The bariatric surgery patient: a growing role for registered dietitians, *J Am Diet Assoc* 110:593, 2010.

Kushner RF, Shanta Retelny V: Emergence of pica (ingestion of non-food substances) accompanying iron deficiency anemia after gastric bypass surgery, *Obes Surg* 15:1491, 2005.

La Merrill M et al: Toxicological Function of Adipose Tissue: Focus on persistent organic pollutants, *Environ Health Perspect* 121:162, 2013.

Levine JA: Nonexercise activity thermogenesis—liberating the life-force, *J Intern Med* 262:273, 2007.

Lindeberg S et al: A Paleolithic diet improves glucose tolerance more than a Mediterranean diet in individuals with ischemic heart disease, *Diabetologia* 50:1795, 2007

Li R: Polymorphisms of angiotensinogen and angiotensin-converting enzyme associated with lower extremity arterial disease in the health, aging and body composition study, *J Hum Hypertens* 21:673, 2007.

Mayo Clinic: *Calorie Restriction for Anti-aging* (website): http://www.mayoclinic.com/, Accessed April 16, 2010.

Mechanick JI et al: Clinical practice guidelines for the perioperative nutritional, metabolic, and non-surgical support of the bariatric surgery patient—2013 update: co-sponsored by American Association of Clinical Endocrinologists, the Obesity Society, and American Society of Metabolic and Bariatric Surgery, *Surg Obes Relat Dis* 9:159, 2013.

Mellberg C et al: Long term effects on a Paleolithic-type diet in obese menopausal women: a 2-year randomized trial, *Euro J of Clin Nutr*, 68:350, 2014.

Metcalf BS et al: Fatness leads to inactivity, but inactivity does not lead to fatness: a longitudinal study in children (EarlyBird 45), *Arch Dis Child* 96:942, 2011.

Nader PR et al: Identifying risk for obesity in early childhood, *Pediatrics* 118:e594, 2006.

Ogden CL et al: Prevalence of high body mass index in US children and adolescents, 2007-2008, *J Am Med Assoc* 303:242, 2010.

Pasarica M, Dhurandhar NV: Infectobesity: obesity of infectious origin, *Adv Food Nutr Res* 52:61, 2007.

Pomeranz JL, Puhl RM: New developments in the law for obesity and discrimination protection, *Obesity* 21:469, 2013.

Prentice AM: Early influences on human energy regulation: thrifty genotypes and thrifty phenotypes, *Physiol Behav* 86:640, 2005.

Racette SB et al: Abdominal adiposity is a stronger predictor of insulin resistance than fitness among 50-95 year olds, *Diabetes Care* 29:673, 2006.

Reyman M et al: Vitamin D deficiency in childhood obesity is associated with high levels of circulating inflammatory mediators, and low insulin sensitivity, *Int J Obes (Lond)* 38(1):46, 2014.

Rhéaume C et al: Contributions of Cardiorespiratory Fitness and Visceral Adiposity to Six-Year Changes in Cardiometabolic Risk Markers in Apparently Healthy Men and Women, *J Clin Endocrinol Metab* 96:1462, 2011.

Rolland-Cachera MF: Rate of growth in early life: a predictor of later health? *Adv Exp Med Biol* 569:35, 2005.

Rolls BJ et al: Provision of foods differing in energy density affects long-term weight loss, *Obes Res* 13:1052, 2005.

Rothert K et al: Web-based weight management programs in an integrated health care setting: a randomized controlled trial, *Obesity* 14:266, 2006.

Snyder-Marlow G et al: Nutrition care for patients undergoing laparoscopic sleeve gastrectomy for weight loss, *J Am Diet Assoc* 110:600, 2010.

Stein AD et al: Childhood growth and chronic disease: evidence from countries undergoing nutrition transition, *Matern Child Nutr* 1:177, 2005.

Stunkard A, Lu XY: Rapid changes in night eating: considering mechanisms, *Eat Weight Disord* 15:e2, 2010.

Task Force on Childhood Obesity, Domestic Policy Council: *Solving the Problem of Childhood Obesity Within a Generation—White House Task Force on Childhood Obesity—Report to the President,* May, 2010.

Thomas JG, Bond DS et al, Weight-loss maintenance for 10 years in the National Weight Control Registry, *Am J Prev Med* 46:17, 2014.

Thompson DR et al: Childhood overweight and cardiovascular disease risks: the National Heart, Lung and Blood Institute Growth and Health Study, *J Pediatr* 150:18, 2007.

Tremblay A et al: Thermogenesis and weight loss in obese individuals: a primary association with organochlorine pollution, *Int J Obes Relat Metab Disord* 28:936, 2004.

Tsai AG, Wadden TA: The evolution of very-low-calorie diets: an update and meta-analysis, *Obesity* 14:1283, 2006.

Tsuneki H et al: Role of orexin in the central regulation of glucose and energy homeostasis, *Endocr J* 59:365, 2012.

Tuulari JJ et al: Weight loss after bariatric surgery reverses insulin-induced increases in brain glucose metabolism of the morbidly obese, *Diabetes* 62:2747, 2013.

van Dam RM et al: The relationship between overweight in adolescence and premature death in women, *Ann Intern Med* 145:91, 2006.

van Ginnekin V et al: Infectobesity: viral infections (especially with human adenovirus-36: Ad-36) may be a cause of obesity, *Med Hypotheses* 72:383, 2009.

Varady KA et al: Degree of weight loss required to improve adipokine concentrations and decrease fat cell size in severely obese women, *Metabolism* 58:1096, 2009.

Wadden T, Sarwer DB: Behavioral assessment of candidates for bariatric surgery: a patient-oriented approach, *Surg Obes Relat Dis* 2:171, 2006.

Wajchenberg BL: Subcutaneous and visceral adipose tissue: their relation to the metabolic syndrome, *Endocrine Reviews* 21:6, 2013.

Weiner RA et al: Failure of laparoscopic sleeve gastrectomy—further procedure? *Obes Facts* 4 (Suppl 1):42, 2011.

22

Nutrition in Eating Disorders

Janet E. Schebendach, PhD, RDN,
Justine Roth, MS, RDN

KEY TERMS

anorexia nervosa (AN)
binge
binge eating disorder (BED)
bulimia nervosa (BN)
cognitive-behavioral therapy (CBT)

Diagnostic and Statistical Manual of
   Mental Disorders, 5th Edition
   (DSM-5)
other specified feeding or eating
   disorder

purging
refeeding syndrome (RFS)
Russell's sign

Feeding and eating disorders (EDs) are characterized by a persistent disturbance of eating or eating-related behavior that results in significantly impaired physical health and psychosocial functioning. Diagnostic criteria (see Box 22-1) are published in the ***Diagnostic and Statistical Manual of Mental Disorders, fifth edition (DSM-5)*** (American Psychiatric Association [APA], 2013). Revised DSM-5 criteria are available for anorexia nervosa (AN), bulimia nervosa (BN), and binge eating disorder (BED); new criteria have been established for avoidant/restrictive food intake disorder, other specified feeding or eating disorder, pica, and rumination disorder. However, a commonly referred to disorder is not yet clinically defined (see *Clinical Insight: Orthorexia*).

CLINICAL INSIGHT

Orthorexia

Orthorexia refers to the fixation on foods to be perfect and clean. The disorder is categorized by compulsive dieting and adherence to very strict food rules, often leading to a major disruption in one's ability to take part in everyday life (Mathieu, 2005). Steven Bratman, author of *Health Food Junkies* (Bratman and Knight, 2000), coined the term and described the disorder as an "unhealthy obsession with eating healthy food." The Greek word *ortho* refers to "correct or right," so unlike anorexia or bulimia, in which foods are often restricted or binged on, orthorexia often leads to individuals consuming food only if they believe it is wholesome and pure.

Orthorexia is not a clinically defined eating disorder and is not included in the DSM-5. Little research has been done on its prevalence rates to date. However, preliminary studies have shown prevalence rates of 6.9 % for the general population and, interestingly, 35% to 58% in high-risk groups such as health care professionals (Varga et al, 2013). The desire to eat "healthy" foods is not orthorexia, rather it is an obsession with these types of foods combined with the social isolation and disordered behaviors that become dangerous, possibly leading to the development of a diagnosed eating disorder.

Anorexia Nervosa

Essential features of anorexia nervosa (AN) include persistent energy intake restriction; intense fear of gaining weight or of becoming fat or persistent behavior that interferes with maintenance of appropriate weight; and a disturbance in self-perceived weight or shape. Two diagnostic subtypes are restrictive eating only and restrictive eating interspersed with purging, and crossover between the subtypes is possible over the course of illness. The DSM-5 is the first to allow clinicians to document a severity rating for a case of AN: mild, moderate, severe, and extreme. Severity ratings are differentiated based on current body mass index (BMI, adults) or BMI percentile (children/adolescents); however, the rating may be increased at the clinician's discretion to reflect clinical symptoms, degree of functional disability, and the need for supervision. In the general population, lifetime prevalence of AN is approximately 1% in women and less than 0.5% in men (Hay et al, 2014). Presentation typically occurs during adolescence or young adulthood, but prepubertal and late-onset (after age 40) cases have been described. Although AN occurs across culturally and socially diverse populations, increased prevalence occurs in postindustrialized, high-income countries. Within the United States, prevalence appears to be comparatively low among Latinos, African Americans, and Asians; however, presentation of weight concerns among individuals with eating disorders may vary substantially across cultural and ethnic groups. Risk and prognostic factors associated with this disorder include genetic, physiologic, environmental, and temperamental characteristics (see Table 22-1). The crude mortality rate is approximately 5% per decade with death attributed to medical complications directly related to AN or suicide (APA, 2013).

Bulimia Nervosa

Essential features of bulimia nervosa (BN) include recurrent episodes of binge eating followed by inappropriate compensatory behaviors in an effort to prevent weight gain; and self-evaluation

BOX 22-1   American Psychiatric Association (DSM-5) Diagnostic Criteria

Anorexia Nervosa (AN)

A. Restriction of energy intake relative to requirements, leading to a significantly low body weight in the context of age, sex, developmental trajectory, and physical health. *Significantly low weight* is defined as a weight that is less than minimally normal, or for children and adolescents, less than that minimally expected.

B. Intense fear of gaining weight or of becoming fat, or persistent behavior that interferes with weight gain, even though at a significantly low weight.

C. Disturbance in the way in which one's body weight or shape is experienced, undue influence of body weight or shape on self-evaluation, or persistent lack of recognition of the seriousness of the current low body weight.

Specify whether:

1. Restricting type: During the last 3 months, the individual has not engaged in recurrent episodes of binge eating or purging behavior (i.e., self-induced vomiting or the misuse of laxatives, diuretics, or enemas). This subtype describes presentations in which weight loss is accomplished primarily through dieting, fasting, and/or excessive exercise.

2. Binge-eating/purging type: During the last 3 months, the individual has engaged in recurrent episodes of binge eating or purging behavior (i.e., self-induced vomiting or the misuse of laxatives, diuretics, or enemas).

Specify current severity:

The minimum level of severity is based, for adults, on current body mass index (BMI) (see below) or, for children and adolescents, on BMI percentile. The ranges below are derived from World Health Organization categories for thinness in adults; for children and adolescents, corresponding BMI percentiles should be used. The level of severity may be increased to reflect clinical symptoms, the degree of functional disability, and the need for supervision.

Mild: BMI ≥17 kg/m^2

Moderate: BMI 16-16.99 kg/m^2

Severe: BMI 15-15.99 kg/m^2

Extreme: BMI <15 kg/m^2

Bulimia Nervosa (BN)

A. Recurrent episodes of binge eating at least once a week for three months. An episode of binge-eating is characterized by both of the following:

1. Eating, in a discrete period of time (e.g., within any 2-hour period), an amount of food that is definitely larger than what most individuals would eat in a similar period of time under similar circumstances.

2. A sense of lack of control over eating during the episode (e.g., a feeling that one cannot stop eating or control what or how much one is eating).

B. Recurrent inappropriate compensatory behaviors in order to prevent weight gain, such as self-induced vomiting; misuse of laxatives, diuretics, or other medications; fasting; or excessive exercise.

C. The binge eating and inappropriate compensatory behaviors both occur, on average, at least once a week for 3 months.

D. Self-evaluation is unduly influenced by body shape and weight.

E. The disturbance does not occur exclusively during episodes of anorexia nervosa.

Specify current severity:

The minimum level of severity is based on the frequency of inappropriate compensatory behaviors (see below). The level of severity may be increased to reflect other symptoms and the degree of functional disability.

Mild: An average of 1-3 episodes of inappropriate compensatory behaviors per week.

Moderate: An average of 4-7 episodes of inappropriate compensatory behaviors per week.

Severe: An average of 8-13 episodes of inappropriate compensatory behaviors per week.

Extreme: An average of 14 or more episodes of inappropriate compensatory behaviors per week.

Binge Eating Disorder (BED)

A. Recurrent episodes of binge eating. An episode of binge-eating is characterized by both of the following:

1. Eating, in a discrete period of time (e.g., within any 2-hour period), an amount of food that is definitely larger than what most individuals would eat in a similar period of time under similar circumstances.

2. A sense of lack of control over eating during the episode (e.g., a feeling that one cannot stop eating or control what or how much one is eating).

B. The binge-eating episodes are associated with three (or more) of the following:

1. Eating more rapidly than normal.

2. Eating until feeling uncomfortably full.

3. Eating large amount of food when not physically hungry.

4. Eating alone because of feeling embarrassed by how much one is eating.

5. Feeling disgusted with oneself, depressed, or very guilty afterward.

C. Marked distress regarding binge eating is present.

D. The binge eating occurs, on average, at least once a week for 3 months.

E. The binge eating is not associated with the recurrent use of inappropriate compensatory behavior as in bulimia nervosa and does not occur exclusively during the course of bulimia nervosa or anorexia nervosa.

Specify current severity:

The minimum level of severity is based on the frequency of episodes of binge eating (see below). The level of severity may be increased to reflect other symptoms and the degree of functional disability.

Mild: 1-3 binge-eating episodes per week.

Moderate: 4-7 binge-eating episodes per week.

Severe: 8-13 binge-eating episodes per week.

Extreme: 14 or more binge-eating episodes per week.

Other Specified Feeding and Eating Disorder

This category applies to presentations in which symptoms characteristic of a feeding and eating disorder that cause clinically significant distress or impairment in social, occupational, or other important areas of functions predominate but do not meet the full criteria for any of the disorders in the feeding and eating disorders diagnostic class. The other specified feeding and eating disorder category is used in situations in which the clinician chooses to communicate the specific reason that the presentation does not meet the criteria for any specific feeding and eating disorder. This is done by recording "other specified feeding or eating disorder" followed by the specific reason (e.g., "bulimia nervosa of low frequency"). Examples of presentations that can be specified using the "other specified" designation include the following:

1. Atypical anorexia nervosa: All of the criteria for anorexia nervosa are met, except that despite significant weight loss, the individual's weight is within or above the normal range.

2. Bulimia nervosa (of low frequency and/or limited duration): All of the criteria from bulimia nervosa are met, except that the binge eating and inappropriate compensatory behaviors occur, on average, less than once a week and/or for less than 3 months.

3. Binge eating disorder (of low frequency and/or limited duration): All of the criteria for binge eating disorder are met, except that the binge eating occurs, on average, less than once a week and/or for less than 3 months.

4. Purging disorder: Recurrent purging behavior to influence weight or shape (e.g., self-induced vomiting; misuse of laxatives, diuretics, or other medications) in the absence of binge eating.

5. Night eating syndrome: Recurrent episodes of night eating, as manifested by eating after awakening from sleep or by excessive food consumption after the evening meal. There is awareness and recall of the eating. The night eating is not better explained by external influences such as changes in the individual's sleep-wake cycle or by local social norms. The night eating causes significant distress and/or impairment in functioning. The disordered pattern of eating is not better explained by binge eating disorder or another mental disorder, including substance use, and is not attributable to another medical disorder or to the effect of medication.

BOX 22-1 American Psychiatric Association (DSM-5) Diagnostic Criteria—cont'd

Unspecified Feeding or Eating Disorder

This category applies to presentations in which symptoms characteristic of a feeding and eating disorder that cause clinically significant distress or impairment in social, occupational, or other important areas of functioning predominate but do not meet the full criteria for any of the disorders in the feeding and eating disorders diagnostic class. The unspecified feeding and eating disorder category is used in situations in which the clinician chooses *not* to specify the reason that the criteria are not met for a specific feeding and eating disorder, and includes presentations in which there is insufficient information to make a more specific diagnosis (e.g., in emergency room settings).

Avoidant/Restrictive Food Intake Disorder

A. An eating or feeding disturbance (e.g., apparent lack of interest in eating or food; avoidance based on the sensory characteristics of food; concern about aversive consequences of eating) as manifested by persistent failure to meet appropriate nutritional and/or energy needs associated with one (or more) of the following: 1. Significant weight loss (or failure to achieve expected weight gain or faltering growth in children). 2. Significant nutritional deficiency. 3. Dependence on enteral feeding or oral nutritional supplements. 4. Marked interference with psychosocial functioning.

B. The disturbance is not better explained by lack of available food or by an associated culturally sanctioned practice.

C. The eating disturbance does not occur exclusively during the course of anorexia nervosa or bulimia nervosa, and there is no evidence of a disturbance in the way in which one's body weight or shape is experienced.

D. The eating disturbance is not attributable to a concurrent medical condition or not better explained by another mental disorder. When the eating disturbance occurs in the context of another condition or disorder, the severity of the eating disturbance exceeds that routinely associated with the condition or disorder and warrants additional clinical attention.

Pica

A. Persistent eating of nonnutritive, nonfood substances over a period of at least 1 month.

B. The eating of nonnutritive, nonfood substances is inappropriate to the developmental level of the individual.

C. The eating behavior is not part of a culturally supported or socially normative practice.

D. If the eating behaviors occurs in the context of another mental disorder (e.g., intellectual disability [intellectual developmental disorder], autism spectrum disorder, schizophrenia) or medical condition (including pregnancy), it is sufficiently severe to warrant additional clinical attention.

Rumination Disorder

A. Repeated regurgitation of food over a period of at least 1 month. Regurgitated food may be re-chewed, re-swallowed, or spit out.

B. The repeated regurgitation is not attributable to an associated gastrointestinal or other medical condition (e.g., gastroesophageal reflux, pyloric stenosis).

C. The eating disturbance does not occur exclusively during the course of anorexia nervosa, bulimia nervosa, binge eating disorder, or avoidant/restrictive food intake disorder.

D. If the symptoms occur in the context of another mental disorder (e.g., intellectual disability [intellectual developmental disorder] or another neurodevelopmental disorder), they are sufficiently severe to warrant additional clinical attention.

American Psychiatric Association: Diagnostic and Statistical Manual of Mental Disorders, ed 5, Arlington, Va, 2013, American Psychiatric Association.

TABLE 22-1 Risk and Prognostic Factors Associated with Anorexia Nervosa and Bulimia Nervosa

Diagnosis	Temperament	Environment	Genetic and Physiologic
AN	Obsessional traits in childhood	Cultures/settings that value thinness	First-degree biological relative with AN, BN, bipolar disorder, or depressive disorder
	Anxiety disorders	Occupations/avocations that encourage thinness, e.g., modeling, elite athletics	Higher concordance rates in monozygotic vs. dizygotic twins
			Functional imaging studies indicate a range of brain abnormalities but unclear if changes are primary anomalies or secondary to malnutrition
BN	Weight concerns	Internalization of thin body ideal	Childhood obesity
	Low self-esteem	Increased weight concerns	Early pubertal maturation
	Depressive symptoms	Childhood sexual abuse	Familial transmission
	Social anxiety disorder	Childhood physical abuse	Genetic vulnerabilities
	Overanxious disorder of childhood		

American Psychiatric Association: Diagnostic and Statistical Manual of Mental Disorders, Fifth Edition, Arlington, VA, American Psychiatric Association, 2013.

that is unduly influenced by body shape and weight (APA, 2013). A binge consumption is an episode of uncontrollable eating of an excessive amount of food. Inappropriate compensatory mechanisms include self-induced vomiting, misuse of laxatives, diuretics, other medications (e.g., thyroid hormone), fasting, and excessive exercise. An individual may employ one or more methods. The DSM-5 includes four levels of severity ratings based on frequency of inappropriate compensatory behaviors: mild, moderate, severe, extreme. Although the default level of severity is based on the frequency of these episodes, the level of severity may be increased at the clinician's discretion to reflect other symptoms and the degree of functional disability. Lifetime prevalence of BN is approximately 2% in women and 0.5% in men (Hay et al, 2014). Initial presentation typically occurs during adolescence or young adulthood; prepubertal and late onset (after age 40) cases are uncommon. Diagnostic crossover from BN to AN occurs in 10% to 15% of cases. However, individuals who cross over to AN commonly revert back to BN, and some experience multiple crossovers between these disorders. BN occurs at similar frequencies in industrialized countries (APA, 2013). The prevalence of BN is similar among ethnic groups (APA, 2013). Risk and prognostic factors associated with BN include genetic, physiologic, environmental, and temperamental characteristics (see Table 22-1). BN is associated with a significantly elevated risk for mortality (all-cause and suicide) with a crude mortality rate of approximately 2% per decade (APA, 2013).

Binge Eating Disorder

A major change in the DSM-5 is the official recognition of binge eating disorder (BED) as a clinical disorder. Although BED was included in the DSM-IV (APA, 2000), those criteria were established only for research purposes. The essential feature of BED is recurrent episodes of binge eating without inappropriate compensatory measures (such as purging) intended to prevent weight gain. BED diagnostic criteria include four levels of severity ratings (mild, moderate, severe, and extreme) that are based on the frequency of binge episodes. The level of severity may be increased at the clinician's discretion to reflect other symptoms as well as the degree of functional disability. The lifetime prevalence of BED is approximately 3.5% in women and 2% in men (Hay et al, 2014). BED occurs at similar frequencies in most industrialized countries. In the United States prevalence rates appear comparable among Caucasians, Latinos, Asians, and African Americans. BED is more prevalent among individuals seeking weight loss treatment than in the general population. Crossover from BED to other eating disorders is uncommon. Binge eating disorder appears to run in families, which may reflect additive genetic influences (APA, 2013); less is known about temperamental and environmental risk and prognostic factors.

Other Specified Feeding or Eating Disorder

Other specified feeding or eating disorder applies to atypical AN (restrictive eating in the presence of normal weight), atypical BN and atypical BED (episodes are less frequent or of limited duration), purging disorder (i.e., recurrent purging in the absence of binge eating), and night eating syndrome. Treatment of subclinical AN, BN, and BED is similar to that used for full criteria presentation, but the frequency of therapeutic interventions and the treatment setting may differ. Patients with a purging disorder and night eating syndrome often benefit from psychotherapeutic approaches used in the treatment of BN and BED.

CLINICAL CHARACTERISTICS AND MEDICAL COMPLICATIONS

Although EDs are classified as psychiatric illnesses, they are associated with significant medical complications, morbidity, and mortality. Numerous physiologic changes result from the dysfunctional behaviors associated with AN, BN, and BED. Some are minor changes related to excessive or inadequate nutrient intake; some are pathologic alterations with long-term consequences; a few represent potentially life-threatening conditions.

Anorexia Nervosa

Initially, individuals with AN may simply appear underweight. As the disease progresses, patients appear increasingly cachectic and prepubescent in their appearance (see Figure 22-1). Common physical findings at this stage include lanugo (i.e., a soft,

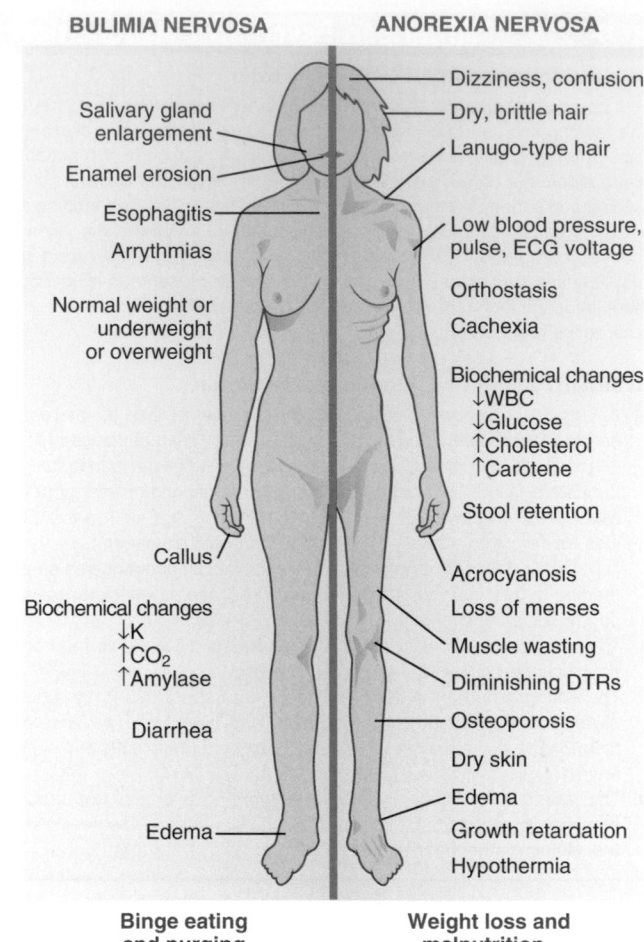

FIGURE 22-1 Physical and clinical signs and symptoms of bulimia nervosa and anorexia nervosa. *DTRs,* Deep tendon reflexes; *ECG,* electrocardiogram; *WBC,* white blood cell.

downy hair growth on the face and extremities), dry skin and hair, cold intolerance, cyanosis of the extremities, edema, and primary or secondary amenorrhea. The degree of symptomatology varies person to person and with duration of illness; for example, some women with anorexia never experience amenorrhea; others exhibit cold intolerance even before weight loss is significant.

Cardiovascular complications may include bradycardia, orthostatic hypotension, cardiac arrhythmias, and pericardial effusion. Protein-energy malnutrition (PEM) with resultant loss of lean body mass is associated with reduced left ventricular mass and systolic dysfunction; however, cardiac function is largely reversible with nutritional rehabilitation and weight restoration. Baseline deficiencies in thiamin, phosphorus, and magnesium levels in very malnourished patients may exacerbate during early refeeding and heart failure may ensue (Winston, 2012). For this reason extremely malnourished patients must be monitored closely during nutritional restoration.

Gastrointestinal complications secondary to starvation include delayed gastric emptying, decreased small bowel motility, and constipation. Complaints of abdominal bloating and a prolonged sensation of abdominal fullness complicate the refeeding process. A protocol for management of constipation during refeeding may be necessary (see Figure 22-2).

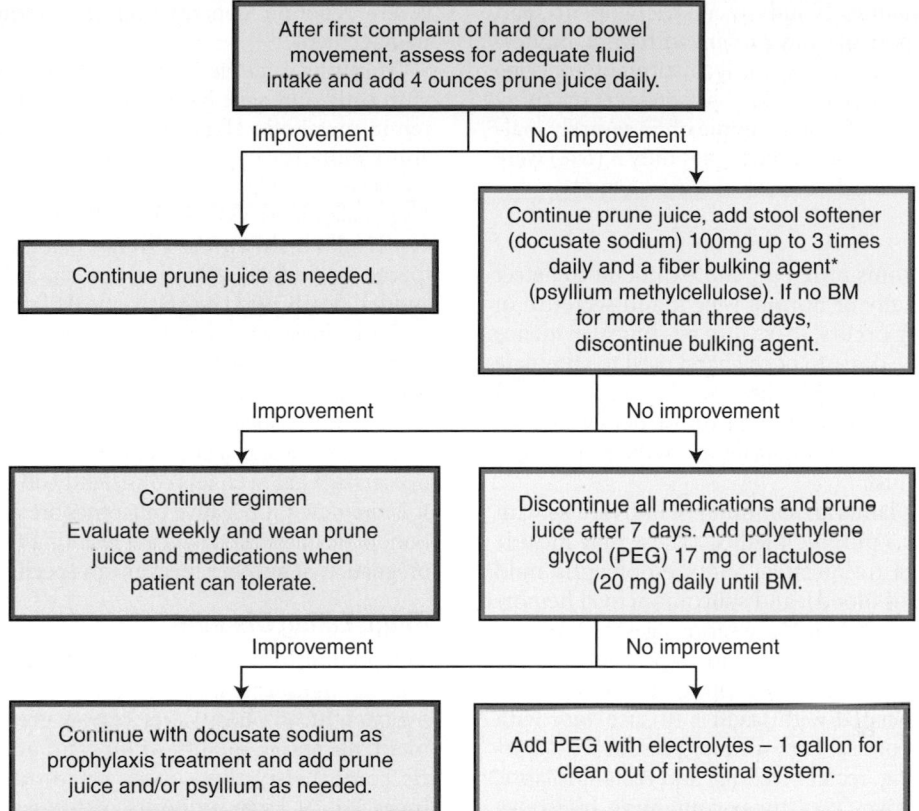

The over use of laxatives is common and are used to control weight or offset the effects of binge eating. Laxatives are among the most commonly abused substances in this population with prevalence rates ranging from 10-60% (Tozzi et al, 2006). Because of the high prevalence of laxative use it is important to be cautious when treating constipation in these individuals. Prophylactic measures during refeeding or weaning from laxative abuse may include the use of prune juice, a stool softner (docusate sodium) or a bulking agent (psyllium methylcellulose.) An example of a treatment plan for an individual in an inpatient setting is presented above. This treatment approach may be modified when treating someone with less severe eating disorder symptoms to include the addition of high fiber foods and an increase in fluid intake.

(1) Tozzi F et.al. Features associated with laxative abuse in individuals with eating disorders. Psychosom Med 68:470,2006.

FIGURE 22-2 Algorithm for treatment of constipation in eating disorders in an inpatient treatment setting.

Bone loss occurs frequently and bone mineral density (BMD) findings consistent with osteopenia in early illness, and osteoporosis later in the course of disease, have been described. Hormonal adaptations aimed at decreasing energy expenditure during periods of chronic energy restriction cause an uncoupling of bone formation and resorption that results in decreased bone mass (Fazeli and Klibanski, 2014). A number of therapies have been investigated to treat low bone mass in AN (i.e., oral contraceptives, physiologic estrogen replacement, insulin-like growth factor I, androgen replacement, and bisphosphonates); however, none result in normalization of BMD, and the effect of treatment on risk of fracture is unknown (Fazeli and Klibanski, 2014). Bone density of males with AN actually may be worse than their female counterparts (Mehler et al, 2011).

Women with AN have thyroid hormones levels consistent with the nonthyroidal illness syndrome: thyroxin (T_4) and triiodothyronine (T_3) are low or low normal, reverse T_3 is elevated, and thyroid-stimulating hormone (TSH) is normal. This syndrome is likely an adaptive response to conserve energy during chronic undernutrition, and these abnormalities usually normalize with refeeding (Fazeli and Klibanski, 2014).

Hepatic changes are generally asymptomatic and self-limiting, but rare cases of severe liver damage and liver failure have been reported. Abnormalities in liver function tests may occur before refeeding and improve during nutritional rehabilitation or arise during the course of refeeding. When this occurs during refeeding, it is suggested that increased carbohydrate intake stimulates increased insulin secretion causing lipogenesis and fatty changes in the liver (Winston, 2012).

Renal complications include renal insufficiency, decreased renal concentrating ability, increased urine output, proteinuria, and hematuria. In general, these symptoms ameliorate with adequate hydration and treatment of malnutrition (Campbell and Peebles, 2014).

Hematologic abnormalities include anemia, leukopenia, and thrombocytopenia. AN patients may present with mild, moderate, or severe anemia that is frequently attributed to bone marrow failure. Iron deficiency anemia is, however, relatively uncommon (Cleary et al, 2010). In a sample of 53 severely malnourished AN patients, 83% were anemic, but only 3 (6%) were iron deficient (Sabel et al, 2013).

Bulimia Nervosa

Clinical signs and symptoms of BN are more difficult to detect because patients are usually of normal weight and secretive in behavior. When vomiting occurs, there may be clinical evidence such as (1) scarring of the dorsum of the hand used to stimulate the gag reflex, known as Russell's sign (see Figure 22-3); (2) parotid gland enlargement; and (3) erosion of dental enamel with increased dental caries resulting from the frequent presence of gastric acid in the mouth.

Gastrointestinal complaints are common in individuals with BN who use vomiting as a purging method. These may include sore throat, dysphagia, gastrointestinal reflux, esophagitis, mild hematemesis (vomiting of blood), and subconjunctival hemorrhage (Brown and Mehler, 2013). More serious gastrointestinal complications include Mallory-Weiss esophageal tear, rare occurrence of esophageal rupture, and acute gastric dilation or rupture. Symptoms associated with laxative misuse vary with type, dose, and duration of use. Patients may present with diarrhea, abdominal cramping, rectal bleeding, and rectal prolapse. Abuse of stimulant laxatives (i.e., those containing bisacodyl, cascara, or senna) can damage intestinal nerve fibers in the bowel wall, whereby the colon becomes increasingly dependent on these stimulants to propulse fecal material; this results in cathartic colon syndrome (Brown and Mehler, 2012). Cessation of laxatives, particularly of the stimulant type, may result in

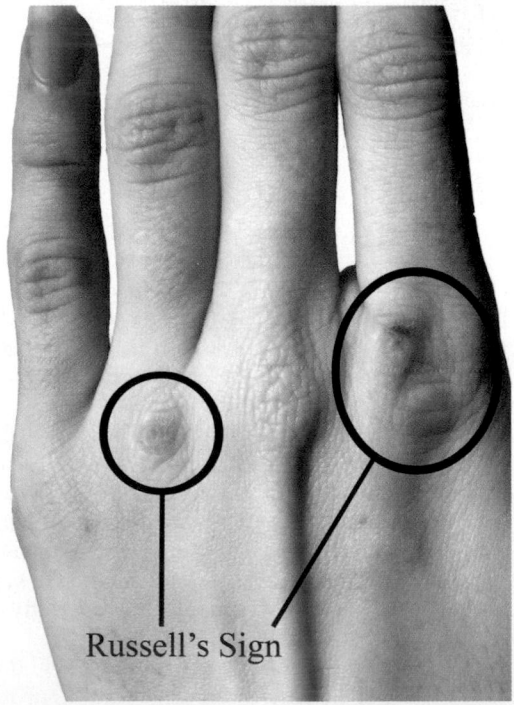

Russell's Sign

FIGURE 22-3 Russell's sign: calluses on the knuckles or the back of the hand resulting from repeated self-induced vomiting over a long period of time.

severe rebound constipation that requires ongoing medical management.

Vomiting, laxative misuse, and diuretic misuse are associated with fluid and acid-base imbalances. Hypokalemic, hypochloremic metabolic alkalosis occurs in patients who vomit and abuse diuretics; hypokalemic, hyperchloremic metabolic acidosis occurs in patients who abuse laxatives (Winston, 2012). Hypokalemia is associated with increased risk of atrial and ventricular arrhythmias (Trent et al, 2013). Patients who abuse ipecac to induce vomiting are at risk for cardiomyopathy, sudden death, and congestive heart failure (Trent et al, 2013).

Individuals with BN may experience menstrual irregularity, leading to the mistaken belief that they are unable to conceive. Thus unplanned pregnancy can occur, with the possibility of negative outcomes such as lower birthweight and a smaller head circumference (Koubaa et al, 2013). An association between BN and miscarriage has been less consistently observed (Linna et al, 2013). It is unknown if negative outcomes are associated with malnutrition, inadequate prenatal care resulting from delayed detection of pregnancy, or another mechanism specific to bulimic behavior.

Binge Eating Disorder

The predominant feature of BED is episodes of excessive eating. In many cases, but not all, this binge eating results in overweight or obesity, yet causes greater functional impairment, decreased quality of life, and greater levels of psychiatric comorbidity than obesity without BED (Wilson, 2011). Ingestion of large amounts of food may cause considerable upper and lower gastrointestinal distress. Symptoms include abdominal pain, fullness, delayed gastric emptying, bloating, acid regurgitation, heartburn, dysphagia, nausea, diarrhea, constipation, hard or loose and watery stools, fecal urgency, fecal incontinence, and anal blockage. It may be difficult to sort out physical complications of BED that are independent of body weight status. For example, metabolic syndrome is common in obese patients with BED (Barnes et al, 2011).

TREATMENT APPROACH

Treatment of EDs requires a multidisciplinary approach that includes psychiatric, psychologic, medical, and nutrition interventions, ideally provided at a level of care appropriate to the severity of the illness. Levels of care offered by facilities in the United States include inpatient hospitalization, residential treatment, partial or day hospitalization, intensive outpatient treatment, and outpatient treatment. Treatment guidelines and policy statements on the necessary components of treatment are available from the American Psychiatric Association (APA, 2006; APA, 2012), the Society for Adolescent Health and Medicine (SAHM, 2015), the American Academy of Pediatrics (Rosen and American Academy of Pediatrics Committee on Adolescence, 2010), the Academy of Nutrition and Dietetics (Ozier et al, 2011), and the Royal Australian and New Zealand College of Psychiatrists (Hay et al, 2014).

Inpatient treatment can be provided on a psychiatric or medical unit of a general or specialty hospital and a behavioral protocol developed specifically for the management of eating-disordered patients is highly recommended. Residential treatment programs also provide 24-hour care but are less likely to admit the medically or psychiatrically unstable patient because of their location outside of a hospital setting. Partial and day hospital programs typically provide 6 to 8 hours of specialized multidisciplinary treatment for 5 to 7 days per week, depending on an individual patient's need for supervision, and decreasing as improvement occurs. Intensive outpatient treatment programs provide several hours of multidisciplinary care each week. This may be scheduled in the late afternoon or early evening so that the patient can attend after school or work. The least intensive form of treatment is outpatient care, with separate psychotherapist, doctor, and dietitian nutritionist appointments. Because providers may be in more than one physical location, effective outpatient care will require ongoing, coordinated effort.

Standard guidelines use a variety of factors in determining the recommended care level, but the ultimate decision should be made by the health care professionals based on individual needs.

PSYCHOLOGIC MANAGEMENT

EDs are complex psychiatric illnesses that require psychologic assessment and ongoing treatment. Evaluation of the patient's cognitive and psychologic stage of development, family history, family dynamics, and psychopathologic condition is essential for the development of a comprehensive psychosocial treatment program.

The long-term goals of psychosocial interventions in AN are (1) to help patients understand and cooperate with their nutritional and physical rehabilitation, (2) to help patients understand and change behaviors and dysfunctional attitudes related to their EDs, (3) to improve interpersonal and social functioning, and (4) to address psychopathologic and psychologic conflicts that reinforce or maintain eating-disordered behaviors.

In the acute stage of illness, malnourished AN patients are obsessive and negativistic, making it difficult to conduct formal psychotherapy. It therefore is recommended that intensive, highly structured psychologic therapies be initiated after the medical and cognitive effects of acute starvation have been stabilized (Hay et al, 2014). Behavior modification protocols that link privileges and "rewards" (e.g., physical activity vs. bed rest, off-unit passes, visits from friends and family) to targeted weight gain and food intake goals are used commonly during inpatient or residential treatment (Attia and Walsh, 2009). Once acute malnutrition has been corrected and weight restoration is underway, the AN patient is more likely to benefit from psychotherapy. Psychotherapy can help the patient understand and change core dysfunctional thoughts, attitudes, motives, conflicts, and feelings related to his or her ED. Associated psychiatric conditions, including deficits in mood, impulse control, and self-esteem, as well as relapse prevention, should be addressed in the psychotherapeutic treatment plan.

No consensus has been reached on the best overall approach to psychotherapy in AN. Studies suggest that family-based therapy (FBT) is the first-line treatment for adolescents less than 19 years of age with duration of illness less than 3 years (Hay et al, 2014). If FBT is contraindicated, then enhanced cognitive behavioral therapy (CBT-E) may be an effective option for the adolescents (Dalle Grave et al, 2013). In adults with AN, CBT-E may be the best choice. FBT and CBT-E are specialized therapies that require highly trained psychotherapists. If FBT and CBT-E are unavailable, then individualized psychotherapy provided by a therapist with experience in the management of eating disorders should be initiated.

Cognitive behavioral therapy (CBT) is structured present-oriented psychotherapy that combines behavioral and cognitive

principles. It directs the client toward modifying dysfunctional thinking and behavior (see Chapter 14). It is thought to be the best therapy option for adults with BN; however, interpersonal therapy (IPT) has also demonstrated benefits (Kass et al, 2013). Dialectical behavioral therapy (DBT), a skill-based therapy that focuses on mindfulness, distress tolerance, emotion regulation, and interpersonal effectiveness, may be helpful in BN cases in which comorbid psychiatric disorders (e.g., depression and mood disorders, personality disorders, and substance abuse disorders), self-injurious behaviors (e.g., cutting), and greater impulsivity are manifested (Berg and Wonderlich, 2013). In some instances, an antidepressant medication (typically a selective serotonin reuptake inhibitor [SSRI] such as fluoxetine) is prescribed adjunctive to psychotherapy. Technology-based interventions using smartphone applications are currently being tested in this population.

A variety of psychologic and pharmacologic interventions are used to treat BED (Wilson, 2011). CBT and IPT are efficacious treatments, with total remission of binge eating reported in greater than 50% of cases at 1-, 2-, and 5-year follow-ups. Behavioral weight loss treatment and guided self-help (using CBT-based manuals) have been used with varying degrees of success (Wilson, 2011). Pharmacotherapy with antidepressant and antiepileptic agents is less effective than psychotherapy, and when combined with psychotherapy, medications fail to augment the treatment response (Wilson, 2011).

Several validated psychologic instruments and questionnaires are available for the assessment of patients with EDs. Self-report measures may be used for screening purposes, whereas structured interviews often are used to confirm the diagnosis, or assess response to treatment. Representative instruments include the Eating Attitudes Test (Eat-26), Eating Disorder Inventory, Eating Disorder Examination, Eating Disorders Questionnaire, and the Yale-Brown-Cornell Eating Disorder Scale (APA, 2006). The SCOFF (Morgan et al, 1999), a brief and effective screening tool that is easy to administer and score, is highlighted in Box 22-2.

NUTRITION MANAGEMENT

Roles and responsibilities of the registered dietitian nutritionist (RDN) in the treatment of individuals with eating disorders include assessment, intervention, monitoring, evaluation, and care coordination. Although AN, BN, and BED have different presenting features, similarities exist in the assessment and management of these disorders.

Nutrition Assessment

Nutrition assessment should include a thorough diet history, as well as the evaluation of biochemical, energy metabolism, and anthropometric markers of nutritional status.

BOX 22-2   The SCOFF Questionnaire

1. Do you make yourself **Sick** because you feel uncomfortably full?
2. Do you worry you have lost **Control** over how much you eat?
3. Have you recently lost more than **One** stone (14 lb) in a 3-month period?
4. Do you believe yourself to be **Fat** when others say you are too thin?
5. Would you say that **Food** dominates your life?

*Two or more "yes" answers suggest the presence of an eating disorder. From Morgan JF, Reid F, Lacey JH: *BMJ* 4:1467, 1999.

Diet History

The diet history should include assessment of energy; macronutrient, micronutrient, and fluid intakes; energy density; diet variety; and an evaluation of eating attitudes, behaviors, and habits (see Chapter 4). Patients with a shorter duration of illness should be queried about their premorbid diet and eating habits as this may be a useful benchmark by which to gauge recovery.

Anorexia Nervosa

Patients with restricting type AN typically eat fewer than 1000 kcal/day. Patients with binge-purge type AN have more variable diet patterns, and energy intake should be assessed across the spectrum of restriction and binge eating. The early literature often described AN patients as carbohydrate "phobic" (Russell, 1967). Recent studies report a restriction of dietary fat, with intakes substantially less than 30% of calories (Schebendach et al, 2008). Percent of calories contributed by protein may be in the average to above-average range, but adequacy of protein intake becomes marginalized as caloric intake decreases. A vegetarian diet may affect the adequacy of high-biologic value protein intake.

Inadequate calories, limited diet variety, and poor food group representation increase risk for deficient micronutrient intakes. In general, micronutrient intake parallels macronutrient intake; thus AN patients who consistently restrict dietary fat are at greater risk for diets that are deficient in essential fatty acids and fat-soluble vitamins. Based on a 30-day diet history, Hadigan et al (2000) found that more than 50% of 30 AN patients failed to meet Recommended Dietary Allowances (RDA) for vitamin D, calcium, folate, vitamin B_{12}, magnesium, copper, and zinc (see inside front cover for DRIs). Abnormal fluid balance is common, and the diet history should query patients about types, amounts, and rationale for fluid intake. Some individuals restrict fluid intake because they find it difficult to tolerate feelings of fullness afterward; others drink excessive amounts to feel full and suppress appetite. Extremes in fluid restriction or ingestion may require monitoring of urine specific gravity and serum electrolytes. Many AN patients consume excessive amounts of artificially sweetened beverages and artificial sweeteners. Use of these products should be addressed during the course of nutrition therapy.

Bulimia Nervosa

Chaotic eating, ranging from restriction to normal eating to binge eating, makes it difficult to assess total energy intake in BN. The caloric content of a binge, the degree of caloric absorption after a purge, and the extent of calorie restriction between binge episodes must be evaluated. Patients with BN assume that vomiting is an efficient mechanism for eliminating calories consumed during binge episodes; however, this is a common misconception. In a study of the caloric content of foods ingested and purged in a feeding laboratory, it was determined that, as a group, BN subjects consumed a mean of 2131 kcal during a binge and vomited only 979 kcal afterward (Kaye et al, 1993). As a rule of thumb, RDNs can estimate that approximately *50% of energy consumed during a binge is retained.*

In a similar manner, patients misusing laxatives believe that catharsis will prevent the absorption of food and calories; however, laxatives do not act on the small intestine, where the majority of absorption occurs. In a laboratory study that was conducted by Bo-Linn et al (1983), two BN participants ate a standardized diet and took their regular daily dose of laxatives (35 and 50 tablets, accordingly). Results indicated that despite outputs of 4 to 6 L of diarrhea per day, these participants

---

BOX 22-3 Determination of Average Daily Energy Intake in the Individual with BN

1. Keep a record of patient intake for 7 days.
2. Out of the 7 days determine the number of nonbinge days (which may include restrictive and normal intake days)
3. Approximate the total caloric content for the week.
4. Determine the number of binge days.
5. Determine the approximate caloric content of the binge days and then deduct 50% of the caloric content of binges that are purged (vomited).
6. Finally, average the caloric intake over the 7-day period. Determination of this average energy intake, as well as the range of intake, will be useful information for the assessment process.

---

decreased calorie absorption by only 12%. Because of day-to-day variability, a 24-hour recall is not a particularly useful assessment tool. To assess energy intake, it is helpful to estimate daily food consumption over the course of a week using the method outlined in Box 22-3.

Nutrient intake in BN patients varies with the cycle of binge eating and restriction, and it is likely that overall diet quality and micronutrient intake is inadequate. A 14-day dietary intake study of 50 BN patients revealed that at least 50% of participants consumed less than two thirds of the recommended dietary allowance (RDA) for calcium, iron, and zinc on nonbinge days. Furthermore, 25% of participants still had inadequate intakes of zinc and iron when overall intake (i.e., binge and nonbinge days) was assessed (Gendall et al, 1997). Even when the diet appears adequate, nutrient loss occurs secondary to purging, thus making it difficult to assess true adequacy of nutrient intake. Use of vitamin and mineral supplements also should be determined but, once again, retention after purging must be considered.

Eating Behavior

Characteristic attitudes, behaviors, and eating habits seen in AN and BN are shown in Box 22-4. Food aversions, common in this population, include red meat, baked goods, desserts, full-fat dairy products, added fats, fried foods, and caloric beverages. Patients with EDs often incorrectly regard specific foods or groups of foods as absolutely "good" or absolutely "bad." Irrational beliefs and dichotomous thinking about food choices should be identified and challenged throughout the treatment process.

In the assessment process, the RDN may discover unusual or ritualistic behaviors the patient practices, such as ingestion of food in an atypical manner or with nontraditional utensils; unusual food combinations; or the excessive use of spices, vinegar, lemon juice, and artificial sweeteners. Meal spacing and length of time allocated for a meal also should be determined. Many patients save their self-allotted food ration until late in the day; others are fearful of eating past a certain time of day.

Many AN patients eat in an excessively slow manner, often playing with their food and cutting it into small pieces. This is sometimes regarded as a tactic to avoid food intake, but it also may be an effect of starvation (Keys et al, 1950). Time limits for meal and snack consumption frequently are incorporated into behavioral treatment plans and family-based therapy.

Many BN patients eat quickly, reflecting their difficulties with satiety cues. In addition, BN patients may identify foods they fear will trigger a binge episode. The patient may have an all-or-nothing approach to "trigger" foods. Although the patient may

BOX 22-4 **Assessment of Eating Attitudes, Behaviors, and Habits**

1. Eating attitudes
   A. Food aversions
   B. Safe, risky, forbidden foods
   C. Magical thinking
   D. Binge trigger foods
   E. Ideas on appropriate amounts of food
   F. Refusal to eat a food item that does not have a nutrition facts label
2. Eating behaviors
   A. Ritualistic behaviors
   B. Unusual food combinations
   C. Atypical use of condiments (e.g., mustard, lemon juice, vinegar) and seasonings (e.g., black pepper)
   D. Atypical use of eating utensils and use of utensils to consume a finger food (e.g., using a knife and fork to eat a muffin)
   E. Excessive use of artificial sweeteners
3. Eating habits
   A. Intake pattern
      (1) Number of meals and snacks
      (2) Time of day, including times when eating may be restricted (e.g., patients will not permit themselves to eat before or after a certain time in the day).
      (3) Duration of meals and snacks
      (4) Eating environment—where and with whom
      (5) How consumed—sitting or standing or while looking at a screen
   B. Food group avoidance; particularly those with higher energy density
   C. Diet variety from all food groups, including those with a low energy density content
   D. Fluid consumption:
      Restricted vs. excessive
      Types: caloric, noncaloric, beverage water

prefer avoidance, assistance with reintroduction of controlled amounts of these foods at regular times and intervals is helpful.

Patients may feel a sense of shame about particular food and eating practices, so these behaviors may not be identified during the initial assessment period. The assessment process continues during subsequent meetings and, in some cases, will not be complete until the RDN has observed the patient during a meal time.

Biochemical Assessment

The marked cachexia of AN may lead one to expect many biochemical indices of malnutrition (see Chapter 7), but this is rarely the case. Compensatory mechanisms are remarkable, and laboratory abnormalities may not be observed until the illness is far advanced.

Significant alterations in visceral protein status are uncommon in AN. Indeed, adaptive phenomena that occur in chronic starvation are aimed at the maintenance of visceral protein metabolism at the expense of the somatic compartment. Although serum albumin is usually normal, when hypoalbuminemia does occur, it is associated with a poorer prognosis (Winston, 2012). A low baseline transferrin concentration that improves with weight restoration may occur. A low serum prealbumin level may be associated with the development of serious complications of refeeding (i.e., hypophosphatemia and hypoglycemia) in extremely underweight individuals (Guadiani et al, 2014) (see Appendix 22).

Despite typical consumption of a very low-fat, low-cholesterol diet, malnourished AN patients often manifest elevated total cholesterol, LDL cholesterol, and HDL cholesterol levels (Winston, 2012). Although the cause is unclear and cardiovascular risk is uncertain, the bulk of available evidence suggests that lipid abnormalities improve or normalize after recovery and a low-fat, low-cholesterol diet is not warranted during the weight restoration process. If hyperlipidemia predates the development of AN, or a strong family history of hyperlipidemia is identified, the patient can be reassessed after nutritional rehabilitation. Lipid profiles routinely are included in laboratory assessments; however, a fasting lipid profile is not warranted until the patient is restored to a healthy and stable body weight.

Individuals with BN also may have elevated lipid levels, but the validity of the test must be questioned if the patient is actively binge eating. Furthermore, some BN patients cannot comply with the abstinence period required for a fasting lipid profile. Patients with BN eat chaotically, consuming a high-fat, high-calorie diet during binge episodes, and a low-fat, low calorie diet during intermittent periods of restriction. An inaccurate lipid profile may lead to the unnecessary prescription of a low-fat, low-cholesterol diet, which in turn may exacerbate binge eating episodes and reinforce an all-or-nothing approach to eating. If hyperlipidemia predates the development of BN, or if a strong family history of hyperlipidemia is identified, the patient should be reassessed after eating behavior and diet are stabilized (see Chapter 33).

Hypoglycemia results from a deficit of precursors that are needed for gluconeogenesis and glucose production. Patients with mild hypoglycemia are often asymptomatic; however, severe hypoglycemia is associated with increased risk of the refeeding syndrome (Gaudiani et al, 2014) and hospitalization may be warranted (Winston, 2012; see Chapter 13).

Vitamin and Mineral Deficiencies

Despite obviously deficient diets, surprisingly few studies address biochemical markers of micronutrient status in patients with eating disorders. The decreased need for micronutrients in a catabolic state, possible use of vitamin supplements, and the selection of micronutrient-rich foods may afford some degree of protection in low weight patients; however, the shift from catabolic to anabolic processes may precipitate micronutrient deficiencies during refeeding and weight restoration. Zinc, copper, vitamin C, vitamin A, riboflavin, and vitamin B_6 deficiencies have been reported in AN. Thiamin deficiency, prevalent among low-weight AN patients, is exacerbated by increased carbohydrate intake during refeeding, and a thiamin supplement may be warranted (Winston, 2012). Given that assays for some vitamins and trace elements may not always be readily available, and that the relationship between blood concentrations and whole-body status is unclear, it may be more practical to prescribe a prophylactic vitamin/mineral supplement during refeeding and weight restoration (Winston, 2012).

Hypercarotenemia, attributed to mobilization of lipid stores, catabolic changes caused by weight loss, and metabolic stress, may occur in AN; excessive dietary intake of carotenoids is less likely. Hypercarotenemia resolves during weight restoration and measurement of serum carotene levels is unnecessary.

Iron requirements are decreased in AN secondary to amenorrhea and the overall catabolic state. At treatment onset, the hemoglobin level may be falsely elevated as a result of dehydration resulting in hemoconcentration. Malnourished patients may also have fluid retention, and associated hemodilution may falsely lower the hemoglobin level. In severely malnourished AN patients, iron use may be blocked. Loss of lean tissue results in decreased red blood cell mass. Iron released from red cell mass is bound to ferritin and stored. Saturated ferritin-bound iron stores increase the risk of unbound iron that may result in cell damage, and use of iron supplements should be avoided at this phase of treatment (Royal College of Psychiatrists, 2005). During nutrition rehabilitation, ferritin-bound iron is taken out of storage; this is generally adequate to meet the need for cellular repair and increased red blood cell mass. Patients should, however, be periodically reassessed for depletion of their reserve and the possible need for supplemental iron later in treatment.

Zinc deficiency may result from inadequate energy consumption and transition to a vegetarian diet. Although zinc deficiency may be associated with altered taste perception and weight loss, there is no evidence that deficiency causes or perpetuates symptoms of AN. Supplemental zinc is purported to enhance food intake and weight gain in AN patients, but there is limited evidence to support this claim (Lock and Fitzpatrick, 2009).

Inadequate calcium and vitamin D intakes are reported in AN (Marzola et al, 2013). Although these nutrients contribute to healthy bone development, their role in the cause and treatment of bone loss appears to be minimal (Fazeli and Klibanski, 2014; Mehler et al, 2011). Dual x-ray absorptiometry (DXA) to determine the degree of impaired bone mineralization is recommended in AN (see Chapters 7 and 24).

Laboratory values are not always accurate in assessing micronutrient deficiencies because blood values in many cases do not reflect the full extent of depletion of total body nutrient stores.

Fluid and Electrolyte Balance

Vomiting and laxative and diuretic use can result in significant fluid and electrolyte imbalances in patients with EDs (Trent et al, 2013). Laxative use may result in hypokalemia, and diuretic use may result in hypokalemia and dehydration. Vomiting is associated with dehydration, hypokalemia, and alkalosis with hypochloremia. Hyponatremia, another serious complication, occurs less frequently.

Urine concentration is decreased and urine output is increased in semistarvation. Edema may occur in response to malnutrition and refeeding. An increase in extracellular water frequently occurs in AN patients with a BMI less than 15 to 16 kg/m^2 (Rigaud et al, 2010). Although fluid retention generally dissipates with refeeding, a moderate sodium-restricted diet (4 to 5 g NaCl/day) may be helpful (Rigaud et al, 2010). Depletion of glycogen and lean tissue is accompanied by obligatory water loss that reflects characteristic hydration ratios. For example, the obligatory water loss associated with glycogen depletion may be in the range of 600 to 800 ml. Varying degrees of fluid intake, ranging from restricted to excessive, may affect electrolyte values in patients with eating disorders (see Chapter 6).

Energy Expenditure

Resting energy expenditure (REE) is characteristically low in malnourished AN patients (Kosmiski et al, 2014). Weight loss, decreased lean body mass, energy restriction, and decreased leptin levels have been implicated in the pathogenesis of this hypometabolic state. Refeeding increases and normalizes REE in AN patients. An exaggerated diet-induced thermogenesis (DIT) also has been reported during the course of refeeding, and this may pose metabolic resistance to weight gain during the course of nutritional rehabilitation in patients with AN (Kosmiski et al, 2014).

Patients with BN can have unpredictable metabolic rates. Intermittent periods of dietary restraint may result in a hypometabolic rate. However, binge eating followed by purging can increase the metabolic rate secondary to a preabsorptive release of insulin that activates the sympathetic nervous system.

Baseline and follow-up measurements of REE are useful during the nutritional rehabilitation process (Mehler et al, 2010), but access to indirect calorimetry equipment often is limited. Handheld calorimeters are readily available but data on their accuracy in this patient population are limited (Hipskind et al, 2011; see Chapter 2).

Anthropometric Assessment

Patients with AN have protein-energy malnutrition, characterized by significantly depleted adipose and somatic protein stores but a relatively intact visceral protein compartment. These patients meet the criteria for a diagnosis of severe protein-energy malnutrition. A goal of nutritional rehabilitation is restoration of body fat and fat-free mass. Although these compartments do regenerate, the extent and rate vary.

Body composition studies of eating disordered patients have used underwater weighing, dual-energy x-ray absorptiometry (DXA) equipped with body composition software, and skinfold thicknesses. Imaging techniques such as CT and MRI also have been used to obtain detailed measurements of specific regions or tissues (e.g., visceral adipose fat) or fat infiltration of tissues. Most methodologies are limited to the research setting. Bioelectrical impedance analysis (BIA) is more clinically available, but shifts in intracellular and extracellular fluid compartments in patients with severe EDs may affect the accuracy of body fat estimate (see Chapter 7 and Appendix 22).

Careful assessment and routine monitoring of body weight and stature are critical in the clinical management of patients with EDs. In AN, weight gain and then maintenance is necessary for recovery. In BN, cessation of binge eating and purging episodes is the immediate goal. In BED, cessation of binge eating is the immediate goal, and weight loss is a secondary objective.

When individual body composition data are not available, estimates of appropriate weight ranges are a substandard option. Typical methods historically used by RDNs, such as Metropolitan Life Insurance Company tables and the Hamwi method provide widely varying and empirically unsupported results.*

Use of BMI has become increasingly accepted in the management of AN patients (see Chapter 7 and Appendix 18). Four categories of BMI severity ratings, based on the World Health Organization categories for thinness in adults, have been incorporated into the DSM-5 (APA, 2013). For children and adolescents, BMI percentiles with corresponding thinness cutoffs should be used (Cole et al, 2007).

Delayed growth and stunting can occur in AN, and growth records should be obtained to determine whether linear growth has deviated from premorbid height curves. If stunting has occurred, calculation of the weight deficit should be based on the premorbid height percentile.

Because puberty and peak height velocity occur later in males than females, boys are more vulnerable to the impact of

---

*Hamwi Method for women: 100 lb for the first 5 feet of height plus 5 lb per inch for every inch over 5 feet plus 10% for a large frame and minus 10% for a small frame. For men: 106 lb for the first 5 feet of height plus 6 lb per inch for every inch over 5 feet plus 10% for a large frame and minus 10% for a small frame.

malnutrition on growth and development (Nicholls et al, 2011). Pubertal ratings (e.g., Tanner stages, see Appendices 12 and 13), a baseline bone age x-ray, growth history (i.e., carefully plotted growth charts), and parental height measurements provide information about actual versus expected development. In all age groups, height should be measured carefully using a stadiometer rather than a scale-anchored measuring rod (see Appendix 14).

The height, weight, and BMI percentile tables of the NCHS can be used to assess boys and girls up to 20 years of age (see Appendices 6, 7, 10, and 11). Expected body weight in adolescents also can be determined from weight-for-stature (defined as the median weight by sex, age, and height group) tables recently derived from NHANES II data by Golden et al (2012).

Rate of weight gain in AN may be affected by hydration status, glycogen stores, metabolic factors, and changes in body composition (see Box 22-5). Rehydration and replenished glycogen stores contribute to weight gain during the first few days of refeeding. Thereafter, weight gain results from increased lean and fat stores. A general assumption is that someone has to increase or decrease caloric intake by 3500 kcal to cause a 1-lb change in body weight, but the true energy cost depends on the type of tissue gained. More energy is required to gain fat versus lean tissue, but weight gain may be a mix of fat and lean tissues.

In adult women with AN, short-term weight restoration has been associated with a significant increase in truncal fat and central adiposity; this distribution, however, appears to normalize within 1 year of weight maintenance (Mayer et al, 2009). Short-term weight restoration in adolescent females has been associated with and without central adiposity (de Alvaro et al, 2007; Franzoni et al, 2013).

In hospitalized AN patients, an early morning, preprandial, gowned body weight measurement should be obtained every 1 to 2 days. Before weigh-in the patient should void, and urine specific gravity should be checked for dehydration or fluid loading.

BOX 22-5 Factors Affecting Rate of Weight Gain in Anorexia Nervosa

1. Fluid balance
   A. Polyuria seen in semistarvation
   B. Edema
      (1) Starvation
      (2) Refeeding
   C. Hydration ratios in tissues
      (1) Glycogen: 3-4:1
      (2) Protein stores: 2-3:1
2. Metabolic rate
   A. Resting energy expenditure (REE): Low weight: REE 30%-40% below predicted value for height, weight, age, gender
      Refeeding: progressive increases in REE
      Weight restoration: REE normalizes
   B. Postprandial energy expenditure (PPEE)
      Under normal metabolic conditions: PPEE approx. 10% greater than REE
      In AN: PPEE may be 30%-40% greater than REE
      Duration of exaggerated response varies among individuals
   C. Respiratory quotient
3. Energy cost of tissue gained
   A. Lean body mass (early to midtreatment)
   B. Adipose tissue (mid- to late treatment)
4. Previous obesity associated with decreased metabolic resistance to weight gain
5. Physical activity: volitional vs. fidgeting

If the patient claims to be unable to provide a urine specimen, the physician should examine the patient to see whether the bladder is full. Patients may resort to deceptive tactics (water loading, hiding heavy objects on their person, and withholding urine and bowel movements) to make a mandated weight goal.

On an outpatient basis, a gowned weight should be obtained on the same scale, at approximately the same time of day, at least once a week in early treatment. Before informing a patient of his or her weight or weight goals, the RDN should consult with the other members of the treatment team about the pros and cons of this information on the patient's recovery.

MEDICAL NUTRITION THERAPY AND COUNSELING

Treatment of an ED may begin at one of five levels of care: outpatient, intensive outpatient, partial or day treatment, inpatient, or residential. The registered dietitian nutritionist (RDN) is an essential part of the treatment team at all levels of care; roles and responsibilities of caring for individuals with eating disorders are summarized in Table 22-2.

In AN, the chosen level of care is determined by the severity of malnutrition, degree of medical and psychiatric instability, duration of illness, growth failure, and ability to manage recovery in the home. In some instances, treatment begins on an inpatient unit but is stepped down to a less intensive level of care as weight restoration progresses. In other instances, treatment begins on an outpatient basis; however, if progress is absent or considered inadequate, care is stepped up to a more intensive level.

In BN, treatment typically begins and continues on an outpatient basis. On occasion a BN patient may be directly admitted to an intensive outpatient or day treatment program. However, inpatient hospitalization is relatively uncommon and generally is of short duration and for the specific purpose of fluid and electrolyte stabilization.

Anorexia Nervosa

Guidelines for MNT for AN are summarized in Box 22-6. Goals for nutrition rehabilitation include restoration of body weight and normalization of eating patterns and behaviors. Although MNT is an essential component of treatment, guidelines are based largely on clinical experience rather than scientific evidence.

Weight restoration is essential for recovery. The medically unstable, severely malnourished, or growth-retarded patient typically requires supervised weight gain in a specialized hospital unit or residential ED treatment program. Treatment programs often have three phases to the weight restoration process: weight stabilization and prevention of further weight loss, weight gain, and weight maintenance. Although the duration of these phases vary, the weight restoration process is typically the longest and is obviously influenced by the patient's state of malnutrition.

Treatment typically includes a targeted rate of expected weight gain. The APA recommends a weight gain of 2 to 3 lb/week during inpatient or residential treatment (APA, 2006); however, others consider this rate too conservative (SAHM, 2015, Garber et al, 2012; Katzman, 2012; Kohn et al, 2011).

Initial calorie prescriptions, and subsequent caloric adjustments, are also not widely agreed upon. Convention has been to "start low and advance slow" and to prescribe initial diets in the range of 30 to 40 kcal/kg of body weight per day (approximately 1000 to 1600 kcal/day) (APA, 2006), but this approach recently has been challenged. Whitelaw et al (2010) safely initiated weight gain using a meal-based diet that provided approximately

TABLE 22-2 Roles and Responsibilities of Registered Dietitian Nutritionists Caring for individuals with Eating Disorders

Nutrition Assessment:	Specific Activities:

Identify nutrition problems that relate to medical and physical condition, including eating disorder symptoms and behaviors.	Eating patterns
	Core eating attitudes
	Core attitudes regarding body weight and shape
	Assess behavioral-environmental symptoms:
	  Food restriction
	  Binge eating
	  Preoccupation
	  Rituals
	  Secretive eating
	  Affect and impulse control
	  Vomiting or other purging behaviors
	  Excessive exercise
	Anthropometric assessment:
	  Perform anthropometric measurements
	  Obtain height and weight history
	  Complete growth chart
	  Assess growth patterns and maturation in patients
	  ≤ age 20 years
	Interpret biochemical data and assess risk of refeeding syndrome
	Apply diagnosis, plan intervention, coordinate with treatment team

Nutrition Intervention: Calculate and monitor energy and macronutrient intake to establish expected rates of weight change, and body composition and health goals. Guide goal setting to normalize eating patterns for nutrition rehabilitation and weight restoration or maintenance as appropriate.	Ensure diet quality, regular eating pattern, increased amount and variety of foods, normal perceptions of hunger and satiety, provide suggestions about supplement use Provide a structured meal plan Provide psychological support and positive reinforcement Counsel patients and caregivers on food selection with consideration given to individual preferences, health history, physical factors, psychological factors, and resources
Nutrition Monitoring & Evaluation: Monitor nutrient intake and adjust as needed.	Monitor rate of weight gain Upon weight restoration, adjust food plan for weight maintenance Communicate progress with the treatment team Adjust treatment plan as needed
Care Coordination: Provide counsel to team about protocols to maximize tolerance of feeding regimen or nutrition recommendations, guidance about supplements to ensure maximum absorption, minimize drug nutrient interactions, and referral for continuation of care as needed.	Work collaboratively with the treatment team, delineate roles and tasks, communicate nutrition needs across treatment settings (i.e., inpatient, day patient, outpatient) Function as a resource and educator for other health care professionals and family members Advocate for evidence-based treatment and access to care
Advanced Training: Seek specialized training in other counseling techniques, such as cognitive behavioral therapy, dialectical behavioral therapy, and motivational interviewing.	Use advanced knowledge and skills relating to nutrition Seek supervision and case consultation from a licensed health professional to gain and maintain proficiency in eating disorders treatment

Adapted from: Ozier AD, Henry BW: Position of the American Dietetic Association: Nutrition intervention in the treatment of eating disorders. *J Acad Nutr Diet*, 111: 1236, 2011.

1900 kcal/day. Kohn et al (2011) initiated refeeding using a 40% carbohydrate continuous NG tube feeding diet that provided a minimum of 2000 kcal/day. Golden et al (2013) safely fed hospitalized adolescents on a 1400 to 2000 kcal/day diet. After the baseline calorie prescription is implemented, progressive increases in caloric intake are needed to promote continued weight gain. This increase may be provided in increments of 100 kcal/day (for severely malnourished patients) to 500 kcal/day (for medically stable patients).

Risk of life-threatening complications associated with the refeeding syndrome (RFS) may present during the first few weeks of nutritional rehabilitation. Manifestations include fluid and electrolyte imbalance; cardiac, neurologic, and hematologic complications; and sudden death. Risk for the development of RFS may depend more on the degree of malnutrition rather than caloric intake and rate of weight gain (Agostino et al, 2013; Garber et al, 2012; Golden et al, 2013; Kohn et al, 2011; Whitelaw et al, 2010). A position statement of the Society for Adolescent Health and Medicine (2014) suggests that physicians should have a high index of suspicion for the development of refeeding hypophosphatemia when severely malnourished adolescents (less than 70% median BMI) are admitted to the hospital for nutritional rehabilitation; guidelines for the interpretation of laboratory findings and phosphate replacement regimes in adolescents are provided. The National Institute for Health and Clinical Excellence (NICE) Guidelines have established two sets of criteria for the identification of adults at high risk for RFS (NICE, 2009).

At-risk individuals must be monitored carefully with daily measurements of serum phosphorus, potassium, and magnesium for the first 5 to 7 days of refeeding, and every other day for several weeks thereafter. Supplemental phosphorus, magnesium, and potassium may be given orally or intravenously. In some instances, prophylactic supplementation is provided to high-risk individuals; in other cases, supplementation is based on serum levels. Thiamin (B_1) supplementation may be required at the onset and throughout the course of nutritional rehabilitation. Plasma glucose levels must be closely monitored for hypo- and hyperglycemia (Boateng et al, 2010).

BOX 22-6 Guidelines for Medical Nutrition Therapy for Anorexia Nervosa

1. Caloric prescription
   A. Initial prescription
      Typically in the range of 30 to 40 kcal/kg/day (approx. 1000-1600 kcal/day)
      Higher caloric prescriptions require careful assessment and ongoing monitoring for symptoms associated with the refeeding syndrome.
      Types of feedings: whole foods, liquid supplements, tube feedings; TPN is rarely indicated.
   B. Controlled weight gain phase:
      Progressive increases in kcal prescription (e.g., 100 kcal to 200 kcal increments) to promote controlled weight gain (inpatients: 2-3 lb/wk; outpatients: minimum of 1 lb/wk)
   C. Late treatment weight gain phase:
      70 to 100 kcal/kg/day
      Approx. 3000 to 4000 kcal/day for females
      Approx. 4000 to 4500 kcal/day for males
      If a larger energy prescription is required, the patient must be evaluated for vomiting, discarding food, excessive exercise, exaggerated postprandial thermogenesis.
   D. Weight maintenance phase:
      Adults: 40 to 60 kcal/kg/day
      Children and adolescents: adjust prescription to promote normal growth and development.
2. Macronutrient intake
   A. Protein
      15% to 20% kcal
      Minimum intake = RDA in g/kg ideal body weight
      Promote high biologic value sources; avoid vegetarian diets
   B. Carbohydrate
      50% to 55% kcal
      Decrease carbohydrate to 40% kcal if patient has an elevated blood glucose level or symptoms associated with the refeeding syndrome.
      Provide insoluble fiber for treatment of constipation.
   C. Fat
      Hospitalized/day treatment patients: 30% kcal from fat
      Outpatients: progressively increase dietary fat until a 30% fat kcal diet is attained.
      Include sources of essential fatty acids
3. Micronutrient intake:
   A. 100% RDA multivitamin/mineral supplement.
   B. Avoid supplemental iron: during initial phase of refeeding and if patient is constipated.
   C. Assess need for additional thiamin supplement.
   D. Assess need for additional calcium supplementation.
4. Energy density
   A. Promote intake of energy dense foods and beverages
   B. If nutrient intake is assessed by computer analysis, calculate a Dietary Energy Density Score (DEDS): DEDS = kcal intake divided by weight (g) of food and beverage
      Goal for DEDS: $\geq$ 1.0
5. Diet variety
   A. Promote intake of a wide variety of foods and beverages within all food groups.
   B. Pay particular attention to the variety of complex carbohydrates, caloric beverages, and added fats.

RDA, Recommended dietary allowance.

Later in the course of weight restoration, caloric prescriptions in the range of 70 to 100 kcal/kg of body weight per day (approximately 3000 to 4000 kcal/day) may be needed, and male patients may require as much as 4000 to 4500 kcal/day (APA, 2006). Changes in REE, DIT, and the type of tissue gained contribute to high energy requirements. Patients who require extraordinarily high energy intakes should be questioned or observed for discarding of food, vomiting, exercising, and excessive physical activity, including fidgeting.

After the goal weight is attained, the caloric prescription may be slowly decreased to promote weight maintenance. Weight maintenance requirements are generally higher than expected and are usually in the range of 2200 to 3000 kcal/day. Caloric prescriptions may remain at higher levels in adolescents with the potential for continued growth and development.

AN patients receiving care in less structured environments, such as an outpatient treatment program or a private nutrition practice, may be challenging and resistant to following formalized meal plans. A practical approach may be the addition of 200 to 300 calories per day to the patient's typical (baseline) energy intake; however, the RDN must be mindful that these patients tend to overestimate their energy intake (Schebendach et al, 2012).

Once the energy prescription is calculated, a reasonable distribution of macronutrients must be determined. Patients may express multiple food aversions. Extreme avoidance of dietary fat is common, but continued omission will make it difficult to provide concentrated sources of energy needed for weight restoration. A dietary fat intake of at least 30% of calories is recommended. This can be accomplished easily when AN patients are treated on inpatient units or in day hospital programs. On an outpatient basis, however, small, progressive increases in the dietary fat prescription may elicit more cooperation and less

resistance. Although some patients will accept small amounts of added fat (such as salad dressing, mayonnaise, or butter), many do better when the fat content is less obvious (as in cheese, peanut butter, granola, and snack foods). Encouraging the gradual change from fat-free products (fat-free milk) to low-fat products (1% or 2% milk) and finally to full-fat items (whole milk) is also acceptable to some patients.

A protein intake in the range of 15% to 20% of total calories is recommended. To ensure adequacy the minimum protein prescription should equal the RDA for age and sex in gram per kilogram (g/kg) ideal body weight (see inside front cover). Vegetarian diets often are requested but should be discouraged during the weight restoration phase of treatment.

Carbohydrate intakes in the range of 50% to 55% of calories are generally well tolerated. A lower carbohydrate diet (e.g., 40% of calories) may be indicated for a hyperglycemic patient. Constipation is a common problem in early treatment, and food sources of insoluble fiber may be beneficial (see Appendix 35 and Figure 22-2).

Although vitamin and mineral supplements are not universally prescribed, the potential for increased needs during the later stages of weight gain must be considered. Prophylactic prescription of a vitamin and mineral supplement that provides 100% of the RDA may be reasonable, but iron supplementation may be contraindicated early in treatment (Royal College of Psychiatrists, 2005). Owing to the increased risk of low BMD, calcium and vitamin D–rich foods should be encouraged; there is no consensus on the use of calcium and vitamin D supplements in this population.

Delayed gastric emptying and resultant early satiety with complaints of abdominal distention and discomfort after eating are common in AN. In early treatment intake is generally low and can be tolerated in three meals per day. However, as the caloric prescription increases, between-meal feedings become essential. The addition of an afternoon or evening snack may relieve the physical discomfort associated with larger meals, but some patients express feelings of guilt for "indulging" between meals. Commercially available, defined-formula liquid supplements containing 30 to 45 calories per fluid ounce often are prescribed once or twice daily. Patients are fearful that they will become accustomed to the large amount of food required to meet increased caloric requirements; thus use of a liquid supplement is appealing because it can easily be discontinued when the goal weight is attained. The consumption of meals, snacks, and liquid supplements must be supervised.

Claims of lactose intolerance, food allergies, and gluten sensitivity complicate the refeeding process. These may be legitimate or simply a covert means of limiting food choice. To the extent possible, all claims should be verified by prior or current medical testing. Lactose intolerance secondary to malnutrition may occur but typically resolves during the course of weight restoration. If medically warranted, lactose-free whole milk products and the prescription of an oral enzyme supplement before meals and snacks can be easily accommodated.

Food allergies and a gluten-free diet are far more challenging. Many patients claim to be vegetarians; however, the adoption of this dietary practice usually occurs in close proximity to the onset of AN. Many treatment programs prohibit vegetarian diets during the weight restoration phase of treatment; others allow a lacto-ovo vegetarian diet. The relationship of social, cultural, and family influences and religious beliefs relative to the patient's vegetarian status must be explored.

Institutions vary with respect to their menu-planning protocol. In some institutions the meal plan and food choices are fixed initially without patient input; as treatment progresses and weight is restored, the patient generally assumes more responsibility for menu planning. In other inpatient programs the patient participates in menu planning from the beginning of treatment. Some institutions have established guidelines that the patient must comply with to maintain the "privilege" of menu planning. Guidelines may require a certain type of milk (e.g., whole versus low-fat) and the inclusion of specific types of foods such as added fats, animal proteins, desserts, and snacks. A certain number of servings from the different food groups may be prescribed at different calorie levels.

Meal planning methods vary among treatment programs but data to suggest that one method is superior to another is lacking. Some programs use food group exchanges, others customize their approach. Regardless of the method, AN patients find it difficult to make food choices and plan menus. The RDN can be extremely helpful in providing a structured meal plan and guidance in the selection of nutritionally adequate meals and a varied diet. In a study of recently weight-restored, hospitalized AN patients, those who selected more energy-dense foods and a diet with greater variety had better treatment outcomes during the 1-year period immediately after hospital discharge, and this effect was independent of total caloric intake (Schebendach et al, 2008).

In an outpatient setting, the treatment team has less control over energy intake, food choice, and macronutrient distribution. Under these circumstances the RDN must use counseling skills to begin the process of developing a plan for nutritional rehabilitation. AN patients are typically precontemplative and, at best, ambivalent about making changes in eating behavior, diet, and body weight; some are defiant and hostile on initial presentation. Motivational interviewing and cognitive behavior

therapy techniques may be useful in the nutrition counseling of AN patients (Ozier et al, 2011); the reader is referred to Fairburn (2008) for a thorough review of CBT techniques.

Effective nutritional rehabilitation and counseling must ultimately result in weight gain and improved eating attitudes and behaviors. A comprehensive review of nutrition counseling techniques can be found in Chapter 14 and in Herrin and Larkin (2013) and Stellefson Myers (2006).

Bulimia Nervosa

Guidelines for MNT in BN are summarized in Box 22-7. BN is described as a state of dietary chaos characterized by periods of uncontrolled, poorly structured eating, followed by periods of restrained food intake. The RDN's role is to help develop a reasonable plan of controlled eating while assessing the patient's tolerance for structure.

During the initial onset of BN, much of the patient's eating and purging behavior is aimed at weight loss. Later in the process, the behaviors may be habitual and out of control. Even if the patient is legitimately overweight, immediate goals must be interruption of the binge-and-purge cycle, restoration of normal eating behavior, and stabilization of body weight. Attempts at dietary restraint for the purpose of weight loss typically exacerbate binge-purge behavior in BN patients.

Patients with BN have varying degrees of metabolic efficiency, which must be taken into account when prescribing the baseline diet. Assessment of REE along with clinical signs of a hypometabolic state, such as a low T3 level and cold intolerance,

---

BOX 22-7 Guidelines for Medical Nutrition Therapy of Bulimia Nervosa

1. Caloric prescription for weight maintenance
   A. If metabolic rate appears normal, provide DRI for energy (approximately 2200-2400 kcal/day).
   B. If there is evidence of a hypometabolic rate:
      Start at 1500 to 1600 kcal/day
      Increase diet in 100 to 200 kcal increments until DRI for energy is attained (approximately 2000-2400 kcal/day)
   C. Monitor body weight and adjust caloric prescription for weight maintenance.
   D. Avoid low calorie diets as these may exacerbate bingeing and purging behaviors.
2. Macronutrients
   A. Protein
      (1) 15% to 20% kcal
      (2) Minimum: RDA in g/kg of ideal body weight
      (3) High biological value sources
   B. Carbohydrate
      (1) 50% to 55% kcal
      (2) Provide insoluble fiber sources for treatment of constipation
   C. Fat
      (1) 30% kcal
      (2) Provide source of essential fatty acids
3. Micronutrients
   A. 100% RDA multivitamin/mineral supplement
   B. Avoid supplemental iron if patient is constipated
4. Energy density
   A. Provide foods with a range of energy densities
   B. Provide an overall diet with an energy density of approximately 1.0
5. Diet variety
   A. Promote intake of a wide variety of foods and beverages within all food groups

DRI, Dietary reference intake; *RDA,* recommended dietary allowance.

are useful in determining the caloric prescription. If a low metabolism is suspected, a caloric prescription of 1600 to 1800 calories daily is a reasonable place to start; however, this prescription should be titrated upwards, in 100 to 200 calorie increments, to stimulate the metabolic rate. Ultimately, a weight maintenance diet of 2200 to 2400 kcal/day is attainable and well tolerated. If a patient is willing and able to provide a detailed diet history or a 7-day food record, the initial caloric prescription can also be calculated by the method described in Box 22-3.

Body weight should be monitored with a goal of stabilization; however, BN patients need a great deal of encouragement to follow weight maintenance versus weight loss diets. They must be reminded that attempts to restrict caloric intake may only increase the risk of binge eating and that their pattern of restrained intake followed by binge eating has not facilitated weight loss in the past.

A balanced macronutrient intake is essential for the provision of a regular meal pattern. This should include sufficient carbohydrates to prevent craving and adequate protein and fat to promote satiety. In general, a balanced diet providing 50% to 55% of the calories from carbohydrate, 15% to 20% from protein, and approximately 30% from fat is reasonable.

Adequacy of micronutrient intake relative to the caloric prescription, macronutrient distribution, and diet variety should be assessed. A multivitamin and mineral preparation may be prescribed to ensure adequacy, particularly in the initial phase of treatment.

Bingeing, purging, and restrained intake often impair recognition of hunger and satiety cues. The cessation of purging behavior coupled with a reasonable daily distribution of calories at three meals and prescribed snacks can be instrumental in strengthening these biologic cues. Many patients with BN are afraid to eat earlier in the day because they are fearful that these calories will contribute to caloric excess if they binge later. They also may digress from their meal plans after a binge, attempting to restrict intake to balance out the binge calories. Patience and support are essential in this process of making positive changes in their eating habits.

CBT is the most studied therapeutic intervention for the treatment of BN (Hay et al, 2014). When applied to an ED, CBT is typically a 20-week intervention that consists of three distinct and systematic phases of treatment: (1) establishing a regular eating pattern, (2) evaluating and changing beliefs about shape and weight, and (3) preventing relapse. When the BN patient is receiving CBT, the RDN can be instrumental in helping the patient establish a regular meal pattern (phase 1). However, the RDN and the psychotherapist must maintain active communication to avoid overlap in the counseling sessions. If the BN patient is engaged in a type of psychotherapy other than CBT, the RDN should incorporate more CBT skills into the nutrition counseling sessions (Herrin and Larkin, 2013). See Fairburn (2008) for guidance on CBT techniques.

Patients with BN are typically more receptive to nutrition counseling than AN patients and less likely to present in the precontemplation stage of change. Suggested strategies for nutrition counseling at the precontemplation, contemplation, preparation, action, and maintenance stages are given in Table 22-3 (see Chapter 14).

Binge Eating Disorder

Strategies for treatment of BED include nutrition counseling and dietary management, individual and group psychotherapy, and medication. Some treatment programs focus primarily on nutrition counseling and weight loss. Behavioral weight loss therapy may be effective in attaining weight loss in the short term, but not

TABLE 22-3 Counseling Strategies Using the Stages of Change Model in Eating Disorders

Stage of Change	Counseling Strategies
Precontemplation	Establish rapport.
	Assess nutrition knowledge, beliefs, attitudes.
	Conduct thorough review of food likes and dislikes, safe and risky foods, forbidden foods (assess reason), binge and purge foods.
	Assess physical, anthropometric, metabolic status.
	Assess level of motivation.
	Use motivational interviewing techniques.
	Decisional balance: weigh costs and benefits of maintaining current status versus costs and benefits of change.
Contemplation	Identify behaviors to change; prioritize.
	Identify barriers to change.
	Identify coping mechanisms.
	Identify support systems.
	Discuss self-monitoring tools: food and eating behavior records.
	Continue motivational interviewing technique.
Preparation	Implement nutrition-focused CBT.
	Implement self-monitoring tools: food and eating behavior records.
	Determine list of alternative behaviors to bingeing and purging.
Action	Develop a plan of healthy eating.
	Reinforce positive decision making, self-confidence, and self-efficacy.
	Promote positive self-rewarding behaviors.
	Develop strategies for handling impulsive behaviors, high-risk situations, and "slips."
	Continue CBT.
	Continue self-monitoring.
Maintenance and relapse	Identify strategies; manage high-risk situations.
	Continue positive self-rewarding behaviors.
	Reinforce coping skills and impulse-control techniques.
	Reinforce relapse prevention strategies.
	Determine and schedule follow-up sessions needed for maintenance and reinforcement of positive changes in eating behavior and nutrition status.

Modified from Stellefson Myers E: *Winning the war within: nutrition therapy for clients with anorexia or bulimia nervosa*, Dallas, 2006, Helm Publishing.
CBT, Cognitive behavioral therapy.

the longer term (Wilson, 2011). Other treatment programs focus primarily on reduction of binge episodes rather than weight loss. Self-acceptance, improved body image, increased physical activity, and better overall nutrition are also goals of treatment in BED. Guided self-help CBT (Fairburn, 1995) is an effective treatment option (Striegel-Moore et al, 2010).

Monitoring Nutritional Rehabilitation

Guidelines for patient monitoring are indicated in Box 22-8. The health professional, patient, and family must be realistic about treatment, which is often a long-term process. Although outcomes may be favorable, the course of treatment is rarely smooth, and clinicians must be prepared to monitor progress carefully.

Nutrition Education

Patients with EDs may appear knowledgeable about food and nutrition. Despite this, nutrition education is an essential

BOX 22-8   Patient Monitoring

1. Body weight
   A. Establish treatment goal weight
   B. Determine:
      (1) Acceptable rate of weight gain in AN
      (2) Maintenance weight in BN
   C. Children and adolescents:
      (1) Plot weight on NCHS weight-for-age growth chart
      (2) Determine weight percentile
   D. Monitor weight:
      (1) Inpatient and partial hospitalization
         a. Frequency: Inpatient: daily or every other day; partial hospitalization: varies with diagnosis, age of patient, phase of treatment (i.e., daily, several times per week, once per week)
         b. Gowned
         c. Morning weight
         d. Preprandial
         e. Post void
         f. Same scale
         g. Check urine specific gravity if fluid loading is suspected
         h. Additional random weight checks if fluid loading is suspected
      (2) Outpatient treatment:
         a. Once every 1-2 weeks in early treatment, less frequently in mid- to late treatment
         b. Gowned
         c. Post void
         d. Same time of day
         e. Same scale
         f. Check urine specific gravity if fluid loading is suspected
2. Height
   A. Measure baseline height using a stadiometer
   B. Children and adolescents:
      (1) Plot height on NCHS stature-for-age growth chart
      (2) Determine height percentile
      (3) Assess for growth impairment
      (4) Monitor height every 1 to 2 months in patients with growth potential
3. Body mass index (BMI):
   A. Adults: calculate BMI
   B. Children and adolescents:
      (1) Calculate BMI
      (2) Plot BMI on NCHS body mass index-for-age percentile chart
      (2) Determine median BMI (50th percentile BMI for age and sex)
      (3) Calculate percent median BMI [(current BMI/median BMI) x 100]
      (4) Determine BMI z score
4. Outpatient diet monitoring
   A. Anorexia nervosa
      Daily food record to include:
      (1) Food
      (2) Fluid: caloric, noncaloric, alcohol
      (3) Artificial sweeteners
      (4) Eating behavior: time, place, how eaten, with whom
      (5) Dietary energy density
      (6) Diet variety
   B. Bulimia nervosa
      Daily food record to include:
      (1) Food
      (2) Fluid: caloric, noncaloric, alcohol
      (3) Artificial sweeteners
      (4) Eating behavior: time, place, how eaten, with whom
      (5) Emotions and feelings when eating
      (6) Foods eaten at a binge
      (7) Time and method of purge
      (8) Dietary energy density
      (9) Diet variety
      (10) Exercise

AN, Anorexia nervosa; *BN,* bulimia nervosa; *NCHS,* National Center for Health Statistics.

component of their treatment plan. Indeed, some patients spend significant amounts of time reading nutrition-related information, but their sources may be unreliable, and their interpretation potentially distorted by their illness. Malnutrition may impair the patient's ability to assimilate and process new information. Early and middle adolescent development is characterized by the transition from concrete to abstract operations in problem solving and directed thinking, and normal developmental issues must be considered when teaching adolescents with EDs (see Chapter 18).

Nutrition education materials must be assessed thoroughly to determine whether language and subject matter are bias free and appropriate for AN and BN patients. For example, literature provided by many health organizations promotes a low-fat diet and low-calorie lifestyle for the prevention and treatment of chronic disease. This material is in direct conflict with a treatment plan that encourages increased caloric and fat intake for the purpose of nutritional rehabilitation and weight restoration.

Although the interactive process of a group setting may have advantages, these topics can also be effectively incorporated into individual counseling sessions. Topics for nutrition education are suggested in Box 22-9.

Prognosis

The course and outcome of AN are highly variable. Some individuals fully recover, some have periods of recovery followed by

BOX 22-9   Topics for Nutrition Education

Guidelines for recovery: energy, macronutrient, vitamin, mineral, and fluid intakes
Impact of malnutrition on adolescent growth and development
Physiologic and psychological consequences of malnutrition
Set-point theory and the determination of a healthy body weight
Impact of energy restriction on the metabolic rate
Ineffectiveness of vomiting, laxatives, and diuretics in long-term weight control
Causes of bingeing and purging, and techniques to break the cycle
Changes in body composition that occur during weight restoration
Exercise and energy balance
What does "healthy eating" mean to you?
Challenging food rules
Emotional undereating and overeating
Intuitive eating: how to get in touch with hunger and satiety cues
Meal planning strategies for recovery and maintenance of a healthy body weight
Social and holiday dining
Interpreting food labels
Strategies for food shopping

relapse, and others are chronically ill for many years (APA, 2013). Although approximately 70% of individuals with BN achieve remission, those who have not achieved remission after 5 years of illness may demonstrate a chronic course (Keel and Brown, 2010).

CLINICAL CASE STUDY 1

Anorexia Nervosa

Melissa has just been admitted to an inpatient hospital unit. She is 19 years old and reports the onset of anorexia nervosa at 12 years of age. Upon admission, Melissa's weight is 68 lb, and her height is 61 inches.

Patient began menses early at the age of 11, and because of adolescent developmental changes reported feeling uncomfortable in her body. At this time she was 58 inches and weighed 100 lb (between 50th and 75th percentile). She learned she could restrict through seeing her mom diet at home and began counting her calories. She would aim for less than 1000 calories per day and began walking for 30 to 60 minutes daily. After 6 months, halfway through her sixth grade year, Melissa had dropped to 82 pounds and did not grow in height during this time; she remained at the 25th percentile and stopped menstruating. Melissa's parents began worrying and started to adapt a Maudsley/family-based therapy approach of eating at home in which she ate all of her meals at home with them. She would continue to restrict at school and exercise as much as she could. By the age of 17 Melissa had gained back some weight and graduated from high school, weighing 105 lb with a height of 62 inches (10th percentile for weight and 10th to 25th for height).

After her first year away at college, Melissa began restricting again, this time down to approximately 500 calories per day. Her typical daily intake now is 1 cup coffee in the morning with an apple. For lunch she has salad from the dining hall with 3 ounces of sliced turkey on it and a ½ cup of brown rice with balsamic vinegar. For dinner she has two pieces of laughing cow cheese with steamed vegetables from the dining hall. If she gets hungry at night, she will have an individual bag of fat-free popcorn. She also reports 60 to 90 minutes of walking or running per day around campus or at the gym. Since her first onset of menses, Melissa was getting her period on average 2 to 3 times per year. It has now been 1 year since her last period (age 18). Melissa denies any purging or laxative abuse.

Since being in the hospital, Melissa has struggled with eating 100% of her planned meals. She reports fearing any foods high in fat such as cheese, fried foods, desserts of any kind, meat, oils, and potato chips. Melissa is refusing to drink regular milk as well. The nursing staff on the unit told you that Melissa has been consuming approximately 50% to 60% of her 1800 kcal meal plan and has not taken any of the recommended supplements.

Medical history: amenorrhea, hypokalemia

Current medications: MVI with trace minerals, thiamine daily

Inpatient calorie prescription: 1800 kcal/day

B/P: 89/58

Pulse: 58

Laboratory Values:

Test	Result	Reference Range
Sodium	**129**	135-147 mEq/L
Potassium	**3.3**	3.5-5.2 mEq/L
Chloride	**94**	95-107 mEq/L
Calcium	**8.2**	8.7-10.7 mg/dL
CO_2	**32**	22- 29 mmol/L
Glucose	65	60- 69 mg/dl (fasting)
BUN	**23**	8-21 mg/dl
Creatinine	**1.2**	0.65-1.00 mg/dl
Phosphorous	3.2	2.5-4.6 mg/dl
Magnesium	2.2	1.7-2.3
Cholesterol	**240**	<200

Nutrition Diagnostic Statement

Underweight related to abnormal eating pattern as evidenced by a restrictive caloric intake and excessive exercise in the setting of being below 75% IBW.

Questions

1. List the essential criteria for the diagnosis of anorexia nervosa.
2. What are some behavioral or psychologic treatment approaches that could be used to help Melissa?
3. What are the significant physical findings from a nutrition-focused physical examination of Melissa? What are some other symptoms commonly seen in anorexia nervosa?
4. Assess Melissa's laboratory values and indicate what other values also may be altered in her condition.
5. What is Melissa's goal weight? How would you calculate that?
6. What are some typical reasons why Melissa may be avoiding food and losing weight?
7. What are common complications to assess for when monitoring refeeding syndrome?
8. What would be a safe and appropriate rate of weight gain for Melissa in the inpatient hospital setting?

CLINICAL CASE STUDY 2

Bulimia Nervosa

Kristin is a 34-year-old female who has come to see you in your outpatient private practice. Her chief complaint is that she feels "out of control and wants to stop bingeing."

Kristin currently is employed as a marketing director at a company in New York City. She describes her life to be very stressful: working approximately 50 to 55 hours per week in the office and has several social engagements in the evenings. She reports an "unhealthy" relationship with food since she was a teenager, when she was a "yoyo dieter" and would take various diet pills to lose weight. Her weight as a teenager fluctuated between slightly underweight and normal. Kristin began to purge in college after some of her friends introduced her to the idea of vomiting. Later after moving to New York and becoming stressed with life events, she began to purge more often after what she describes as "binges."

Currently Kristin reports skipping breakfast most days but has a large cup of coffee, black with 5 packets of artificial sweetener. She has a snack around 10 AM of a handful of almonds and sometimes a fruit. She usually goes to the gym during her lunch hour, where she does 45 to 55 minutes of cardio. For lunch Kristin has two hardboiled eggs, a piece of toast, and diet coke. A few times per week after client lunches Kristin feels stressed that she ate "fear foods," so she binges on cookies or candy and afterward purges in her private bathroom. In the afternoon Kristin usually has another coffee or diet coke and a protein bar. After work Kristin goes home with plans of eating a normal dinner but, after ordering take out from the local Chinese, Italian, or sushi restaurant, binges on approximately 2000 to 3000 calories worth of food before purging.

Kristin has a hard time at social events that occur several times a week and binges or purges after them as well. In total Kristin estimates she is binge/purging five times per week, sometimes twice per day. Kristin is frustrated with the binge/purge cycle she is caught in and is requesting guidance for a meal plan.

Medical history: Dental caries requiring three root canals and two implants; irritable bowel syndrome with constipation

Current medications: Fluoxetine 40 mg, Colace 100 mg once daily

Height: 5'5", weight: 138 lb

Continued

CLINICAL CASE STUDY 2

Bulimia Nervosa—cont'd

Laboratory data:

Test	Result	Reference Range
Sodium	139	135-147 mEq/L
Potassium	**3.3**	3.5-5.2 mEq/L
Chloride	**94**	95-107 mEq/L
Calcium	8.2	8.7-10.7 mg/dl
CO2	29	22-29 mmol/L
Glucose	85	60-99 mg/dl (fasting)
BUN	15	8-21 mg/dL
Creatinine	**1.2**	0.65-1.00 mg/dl
Phosphorous	3.6	2.5-4.6 mg/dl
Magnesium	2.2	1.7-2.3
Amylase	105	25-100 units/L
Cholesterol	**210**	<200 mg/dl
Bicarbonate	**16.5**	18.0-23.0 mmol/L

Nutrition Diagnostic Statement

Disordered eating pattern related to bingeing and purging as evidenced by a pattern of restrictive eating, bingeing and then self-induced vomiting.

Questions

1. What are the medical complications Kristin is experiencing secondary to her bingeing and purging? What are some others she could develop if she does not stop?
2. Discuss which laboratory values are abnormal.
3. What are your main goals for nutrition therapy while working with Kristin?
4. How might you approach meal planning with Kristin?
5. How might you help Kristin talk about her fear foods and set goals for including them in her diet without bingeing on them?
6. What techniques would be helpful for Kristin to challenge her urges to binge and purge during stressful work situations?

USEFUL WEBSITES

Academy for Eating Disorders: For Professionals Working in the Area of Eating Disorders

http://www.aedweb.org

National Association of Anorexia Nervosa and Associated Disorders

http://www.anad.org

National Eating Disorders Association

http://www.nationaleatingdisorders.org

REFERENCES

Agostino H, Erdstein J, et al: Shifting paradigms: continuous nasogastric feeding with high caloric intakes in anorexia nervosa, *J Adolesc Health* 53:590, 2013.

American Psychiatric Association (APA): *Diagnostic and statistical manual of mental disorders*, ed 5, Arlington, VA, 2013, APA Press.

American Psychiatric Association (APA): *Practice guidelines for the treatment of patients with eating disorders*, ed 3, Washington, DC, 2006, APA Press.

American Psychiatric Association (APA): *Guide watch*, Washington DC, 2012, APA Press.

American Psychiatric Association (APA): *Diagnostic and statistical manual for mental disorders*, ed 4, Washington, DC, 2000, APA Press, text revision.

Attia A, Walsh BT: Behavioral management for anorexia nervosa, *N Engl J Med* 360:500, 2009.

Barnes RD, Boeka AG, et al: Metabolic syndrome in obese patients with binge-eating disorder in primary care clinics: a cross-sectional study, *Prim Care Companion CNS Disord* 13:PCC.10m01050, 2011.

Berg KC, Wonderlich SA: Emerging psychological treatments in the field of eating disorders, *Curr Psychiatry Rep* 15:407, 2013.

Boateng AA, Sriram K, et al: Refeeding syndrome: treatment considerations based on collective analysis of literature case reports, *Nutrition* 26:156, 2010.

Bo-Linn GW, Santa Ana CA, et al: Purging and calorie absorption in bulimic patients and normal women, *Ann Intern Med* 99:14, 1983.

Bratman S, Knight D: *Heath food junkies: overcoming the obsession with healthful eating*, New York, 2000, Broadway Books.

Brown CA, Mehler PS: Medical complications of self-induced vomiting, *Eat Disord* 21:287, 2013.

Brown CA, Mehler PS: Successful "detoxing" from commonly utilized modes of purging in bulimia nervosa, *Eat Disord* 20:312, 2012.

Campbell K, Peebles R: Eating disorders in children and adolescents: state of the art review, *Pediatrics* 134:582, 2014.

Cleary BS, Gaudiani JL, et al: Interpreting the complete blood count in anorexia nervosa, *Eat Disord* 18:132, 2010.

Cole TJ, Flegal KM, et al: Body mass index cut offs to define thinness in children and adolescents: international survey, *BMJ* 335:194, 2007.

Dalle Grave, Calugi S, et al: Enhanced cognitive behaviour therapy for adolescents with anorexia nervosa: an alternative to family therapy? *Behav Res Ther* 51:R9, 2013.

de Alvaro MT, Muñoz-Calvo MT, et al: Regional fat distribution in adolescents with anorexia nervosa: effect of duration of malnutrition and weight recovery, *Eur J Endocrinol* 157:473, 2007.

Fairburn CG: *Cognitive behavior therapy and eating disorders*, New York, 2008, Guilford Press.

Fairburn CG: *Overcoming binge eating*, New York, 1995, Guilford Press.

Fazeli PK, Klibanski A: Bone metabolism in anorexia nervosa, *Curr Osteoporos Rep* 12:82, 2014.

Franzoni E, Ciccarese F, et al: Follow-up of bone mineral density and body composition in adolescents with restrictive anorexia nervosa: role of dual-energy X-ray absorptiometry, *Eur J Clin Nutr* 68:247, 2013.

Garber AK, Michihata N, et al: A prospective examination of weight gain in hospitalized adolescents with anorexia nervosa on a recommended refeeding protocol, *J Adolesc Health* 50:24, 2012.

Gaudiani JL, Sabel AL, et al: Low prealbumin is a significant predictor of medical complications in severe anorexia nervosa, *Int J Eat Disord* 47:148, 2014.

Gendall KA, Sullivan PE, et al: The nutrient intake of women with bulimia nervosa, *Int J Eat Disord* 21:115, 1997.

Golden NH, Yang W, et al: Expected body weight in adolescents: comparison between weight-for-stature and BMI methods, *Pediatrics* 130:e1607, 2012.

Golden NH, Keane-Miller C, et al: Higher caloric intake in hospitalized adolescents with anorexia nervosa is associated with reduced length of stay and no increased rate of refeeding syndrome, *J Adolesc Health* 53:573, 2013.

Hadigan CM, Anderson EJ, et al: Assessment of macronutrient and micronutrient intake in women with anorexia nervosa, *Int J Eating Disord* 28:284, 2000.

Hay P, Chinn D, et al: Royal Australian and New Zealand College of Psychiatrists clinical practice guidelines for the treatment of eating disorders, *Aust N Z J Psychiatry* 48:977, 2014.

Herrin M, Larkin M: *Nutrition counseling in the treatment of eating disorders*, ed 2, New York, 2013, Routledge.

Hipskind P, Glass C, et al: Do handheld calorimeters have a role in assessment of nutrition needs in hospitalized patients? A systematic review of literature, *Nutr Clin Pract* 26:426, 2011.

Kass AE, Kolko RP, et al: Psychological treatments for eating disorders, *Curr Opin Psychiatry* 26:549, 2013.

Katzman DK: Refeeding hospitalized adolescents with anorexia nervosa: is "start low, advance slow" urban legend or evidence based? *J Adolesc Health* 50:1, 2012.

Kaye WH, Weltzin TE, et al: Amounts of calories retained after binge eating and vomiting, *Am J Psychiatry* 150:969, 1993.

Keel PK, Brown TA: Update on course and outcome in eating disorders, *Int J Eat Disord* 43:195, 2010.

Keys A: *The biology of human starvation*, vol 1 and 2, Minneapolis, 1950, University of Minnesota Press.

Kohn MR, Madden S, et al: Refeeding in anorexia nervosa: increased safety and efficiency through understanding the pathophysiology of protein calorie malnutrition, *Curr Opin Pediatr* 23:390, 2011.

Kosmiski L, Schmiege SJ, et al: Chronic starvation secondary to anorexia nervosa is associated with an adaptive suppression of resting energy expenditure, *J Clin Endocrinol Metab* 99:908, 2014.

Koubaa S, Hällström T, et al: Retarded head growth and neurocognitive development in infants of mothers with a history of eating disorders: longitudinal cohort study, *BJOG* 120:1413, 2013.

Linna MS, Raevuori A, et al: Reproductive health outcomes in eating disorders, *Int J Eat Disord* 46:826, 2013.

Lock JD, Fitzpatrick KK: Anorexia nervosa, *BMJ Clin Evid* 2009: 1011, 2009.

Marzola E, Nasser JA, et al: Nutritional rehabilitation in anorexia nervosa: review of the literature and implications for treatment, *BMC Psychiatry* 13:290, 2013.

Mathieu J: What is orthorexia? *J Am Diet Assoc* 105:1510, 2005.

Mayer LE, Klein DA, et al: Adipose tissue distribution after weight restoration and weight maintenance in women with anorexia nervosa, *Am J Clin Nutr* 90:1132, 2009.

Mehler PS, Cleary BS, et al: Osteoporosis in anorexia nervosa, *Eat Disord* 19:194, 2011.

Morgan JF, Reid F, et al: The SCOFF questionnaire: assessment of a new screening tool for eating disorders, *BMJ* 319:1467, 1999.

National Institute for Health and Clinical Excellence (NICE): *Guideline for the management of refeeding syndrome (adults)*. ed 2. 2009. United Kingdom: NHS Foundation Trust.

Nicholls D, Hudson L, et al: Managing anorexia nervosa, *Arch Dis Child* 96:977, 2011.

Ozier AD, Henry BW, et al: Position of the American Dietetic Association: nutrition intervention in the treatment of eating disorders, *J Am Diet Assoc* 111:1236, 2011.

Riguad D, Boulier A, et al: Body fluid retention and body weight change in anorexia nervosa patients during refeeding, *Clin Nutr* 29:749, 2010.

Rosen DS, American Academy of Pediatrics Committee on Adolescence: Identification and management of eating disorders in children and adolescents, *Pediatrics* 126:1240, 2010.

Royal College of Psychiatrists: *Guidelines for the nutritional management of anorexia nervosa, council report CR130* (website), 2005. http://www.rcpsych.ac.uk/files/pdfversion/cr130.pdf. Accessed January 11, 2015.

Russell GF: The nutritional disorder in anorexia nervosa, *J Psychosom Res* 11:141, 1967.

Sabel AL, Gaudiani JL, et al: Hematological abnormalities in severe anorexia nervosa, *Ann Hematol* 92:605, 2013.

Schebendach JE, Porter KJ, et al: Accuracy of self-reported energy intake in weight-restored patients with anorexia nervosa compared with obese and normal weight individuals, *Int J Eat Disord* 45:570, 2012.

Schebendach JE, Mayer LE, et al: Dietary energy density and diet variety as predictors of outcome in anorexia nervosa, *Am J Clin Nutr* 87:810, 2008.

Society for Adolescent Health and Medicine (SAHM), Golden NH, et al: Position paper of the Society for Adolescent Health and Medicine: medical management of restrictive eating disorders in adolescents and young adults, *J Adolesc Health* 56:121, 2015.

Society for Adolescent Health and Medicine (SAHM): Refeeding hypophosphatemia in hospitalized adolescents with anorexia nervosa: a position statement of the Society for Adolescent Health and Medicine, *J Adolesc Health* 55:455, 2014.

Stellefson Myers E: *Winning the war within: nutrition therapy for clients with eating disorders*, ed 2, Dallas, 2006, Helm Publishing.

Striegel-Moore RH, Wilson GT, et al: Cognitive behavioral guided self-help for the treatment of recurrent binge eating, *J Consult Clin Psychol* 78:312, 2010.

Trent SA, Moreira ME, et al: ED management of patients with eating disorders, *Am J Emerg Med* 31:859, 2013.

Varga M, Dukay-Szabó S, Túry F, et al: Evidence and gaps in the literature on orthorexia nervosa, *Eat Weight Disord* 18:103, 2013.

Whitelaw M, Gilbertson H, et al: Does aggressive refeeding in hospitalized adolescents with anorexia nervosa result in increased hypophosphatemia? *J Adolesc Heath* 46:577, 2010.

Wilson TG: Treatment of binge eating disorder, *Psychiatr Clin North Am* 34:773, 2011.

Winston AP: The clinical biochemistry of anorexia nervosa, *Ann Clin Biochem* 49:132, 2012.

23

Nutrition in Exercise and Sports Performance

Lisa Dorfman, MS, RDN, CSSD, LMHC, FAND

KEY TERMS

actomyosin
adenosine diphosphate (ADP)
adenosine triphosphate (ATP)
aerobic metabolism
anabolic effects
anaerobic metabolism
androgenic effects
anorexia athletica (AA)
athletic energy deficit (AED)
creatine phosphate (CP)
dehydroepiandrosterone (DHEA)
eating, exercise, body image (EEBI)
  disorders

ergogenic aid
fat adaptation strategy
female athlete triad (FAT)
glycemic index
glycogen
glycogen loading (glycogen supercompensation)
glycogenolysis
glycolysis
high-intensity interval training (HIIT)
hypohydration
human growth hormone (HGH)
lactic acid

mitochondria
muscle dysmorphia (MD)
myoglobin
nutrition periodization
oxidative phosphorylation
pseudoanemia
respiratory exchange ratio (RER)
reactive oxygen species (ROS)
sports anemia
The Athlete's Plate
thermoregulation
Vo_2max

Athletic performance is the culmination of genetics, proper training, adequate nutrition, hydration, desire, and rest. Understanding sport-specific physiologic requirements for training and competition is integral to obtaining sufficient energy, optimal levels of macronutrients and micronutrients, and adequate levels of fluids. Healthy eating habits and the use of supplements and sports foods may be necessary to support energy needs for training hard, achieving performance goals, and reducing the incidence of illness and injury. Energy and fuel requirements for training and competition also have to adapt for recovery between training sessions to reduce the risk of illness or injury and maintain appropriate body composition (International Olympic Committee [IOC], 2011).

AN INTEGRATIVE APPROACH TO WORKING WITH ATHLETES

To advance the practice of dietitians working with fitness-minded individuals, cross-disciplinary training provides a broader and more comprehensive understanding and application of the dietary needs for individuals who exercise. Exercise nutrition is not limited to exercise physiology or nutrition but considers six core areas of study including the role of optimal overall health and longevity, optimal growth, peak physiologic function, energy balance and body composition, nutrition enhancement, and safety.

Genetics and individualized differences, exercise environments, and life stress also can affect the athlete's tolerance of specific nutrients. To prevent nutrient deficiencies, dietitians must integrate anthropometric, biochemical, and dietary data and feedback from athletes to determine whether additional factors such as gut dysbiosis, food allergies or intolerances, dietary preferences or aversions, or disease processes may affect the overall absorption, assimilation, digestions, biotransformation, and transport of specific macronutrients, micronutrients, or fluids and ultimately affect performance potential.

A comprehensive understanding of the relationship between optimal nutrition and exercise science also enables dietitians and nutrition practitioners to appreciate the importance of ensuring adequate nutrition for active individuals and to critically evaluate the validity of claims concerning nutritional supplements and special dietary modifications to enhance physique, physical performance, and exercise training responses.

BIOENERGETICS OF PHYSICAL ACTIVITY

Exercise nutrition requires essential elements from food to fuel muscle contractions, build new tissue, preserve lean muscle mass, optimize skeletal structure, repair existing cells, maximize oxygen transport, maintain favorable fluid and electrolyte balance, and regulate metabolic processes.

The human body must be supplied continuously with energy to perform its many complex functions. Three metabolic systems supply energy for the body: one dependent on oxygen (oxidative phosphorylation or aerobic metabolism) and the other two independent of oxygen (creatine phosphate and anaerobic glycolysis or anaerobic metabolism). The use of one system over the other depends on the duration, intensity, and type of physical activity.

Adenosine Triphosphate: Ultimate Energy Source

Regardless of the energy system used to generate power for exercise, the body relies on a continuous supply of fuel through adenosine triphosphate (ATP), found within the mitochondria of the body. The energy produced from the breakdown of ATP provides the fuel that activates muscle contraction. The energy from ATP is transferred to the contractile filaments (myosin and actin) in the muscle, which form an attachment of actin to the cross-bridges on the myosin molecule, thus forming actomyosin. Once activated the myofibrils slide past each other and cause the muscle to contract.

Although ATP is the main currency for energy in the body, it is stored in limited amounts. In fact, only approximately 3 oz of ATP is stored in the body at any one time (McArdle et al, 2013). This provides only enough energy for several seconds of exercise, and yet ATP must be resynthesized continually to provide a constant energy source. When ATP loses a phosphate, thus releasing energy, the resulting adenosine diphosphate (ADP) is combined enzymatically with another high-energy phosphate from creatine phosphate (CP) to resynthesize ATP. The concentration of high-energy CP in the muscle is five times that of ATP.

Creatine kinase is the enzyme that catalyzes the reaction of CP with ADP and inorganic phosphate. This is the fastest and most immediate means of replenishing ATP, and it does so without the use of oxygen (anaerobic). Although this system has great power, it is time-limited because of the limited concentration of CP found in the muscles (see Creatine later in the chapter).

The energy released from this ATP-CP system will support an all-out exercise effort of only a few seconds, such as in a power lift, tennis serve, or sprint. If the all-out effort continues for longer than 8 seconds, or if moderate exercise is to proceed for longer periods, an additional source of energy must be provided for the resynthesis of ATP. The production of ATP carries on within the muscle cells through either the anaerobic or aerobic pathways.

Anaerobic or Lactic Acid Pathway

The next energy pathway for supplying ATP for more than 8 seconds of physical activity is the process of glycolysis. In this pathway the energy in glucose is released without the presence of oxygen. Lactic acid is the end product of glycolysis. Without the production of lactic acid, glycolysis would shut down. The coenzyme called nicotinic acid dehydrogenase (NAD) is in limited supply in this pathway. When NAD is limited, the glycolytic pathway cannot provide constant energy. By converting pyruvic acid to lactic acid, NAD is freed to participate in further ATP synthesis. The amount of ATP furnished is relatively small; the process is only 30% efficient. This pathway contributes energy during an all-out effort lasting up to 60 to 120 seconds. Examples are a 440-yard sprint and many sprint-swimming events.

Although this process provides immediate protection from the consequences of insufficient oxygen, it cannot continue indefinitely. When exercise continues at intensities beyond the body's ability to supply oxygen and convert lactic acid to fuel, lactic acid accumulates in the blood and muscle, lowers the pH to a level that interferes with enzymatic action, and causes fatigue. Lactic acid can be removed from the muscle, transported into the bloodstream, and converted to energy in muscle, liver, or brain. Otherwise, it is converted to glycogen. Conversion to

glycogen occurs in the liver and to some extent in muscle, particularly among trained athletes.

The amount of ATP produced through glycolysis is small compared with that available through aerobic pathways. Substrate for this reaction is limited to glucose from blood sugar or the glycogen stored in the muscle. Liver glycogen contributes but is limited.

Aerobic Pathway

Production of ATP in amounts sufficient to support continued muscle activity for longer than 90 to 120 seconds requires oxygen. If sufficient oxygen is not present to combine with hydrogen in the electron transport chain, no further ATP is made. Thus the oxygen furnished through respiration is of vital importance. Here, glucose can be broken down far more efficiently for energy, producing 18 to 19 times more ATP. In the presence of oxygen, pyruvate is converted to acetyl coenzyme A (CoA), which enters the mitochondria. In the mitochondria acetyl CoA goes through the Krebs cycle, which generates 36 to 38 ATP per molecule of glucose (see Figure 23-1).

Aerobic metabolism is limited by the availability of substrate, a continuous and adequate supply of oxygen, and the availability of coenzymes. At the onset of exercise and with the increase in exercise intensity, the capability of the cardiovascular system to supply adequate oxygen is a limiting factor, and this is largely due to the level of conditioning. The aerobic pathway provides ATP by metabolizing fats and proteins. A large amount of acetyl CoA, which enters the Krebs cycle and provides enormous amounts of ATP, is provided by beta-oxidation of fatty acids. Proteins may be catabolized into acetyl CoA or Krebs cycle intermediates, or they may be directly oxidized as another source of ATP.

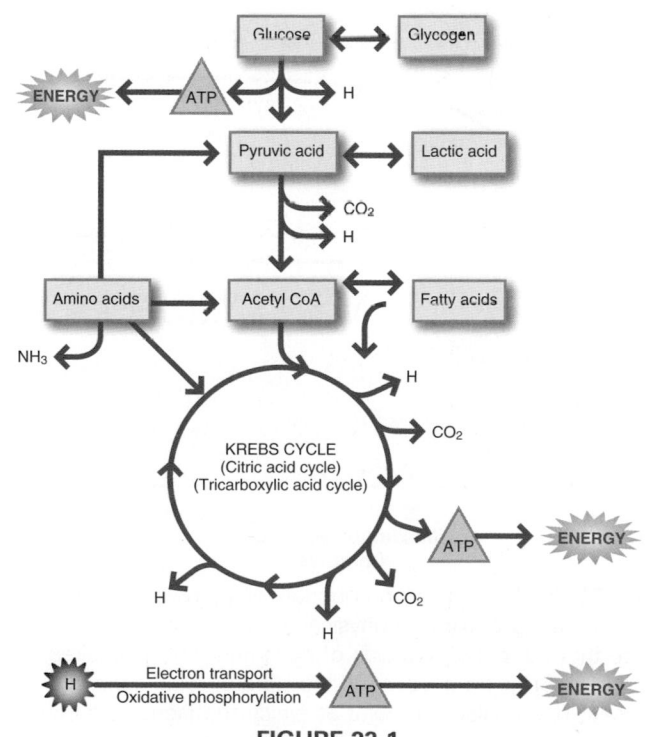

FIGURE 23-1

Energy Continuum

A person who is exercising may use one or more energy pathways. For example, at the beginning of any physical activity, ATP is produced anaerobically. As exercise continues, the lactic acid system produces ATP for exercise. If the person continues to exercise and does so at a moderate intensity for a prolonged period, the aerobic pathway will become the dominant pathway for fuel. On the other hand, the anaerobic pathway provides most of the energy for short-duration, high-intensity exercise such as sprinting; the 200-meter swim; or high-power, high-intensity moves in basketball, football, or soccer. However, all of the ATP-generating pathways are turned on at the onset of exercise.

The production of ATP for exercise is on a continuum that depends on the availability of oxygen. Other factors that influence oxygen capabilities and thus energy pathways are the capacity for intense exercise and its duration. These two factors are inversely related. For example, an athlete cannot perform high-power, high-intensity moves over a prolonged period. To do this, he or she would have to decrease the intensity of the exercise to increase its duration (see Figure 23-2).

The aerobic pathway cannot tolerate the same level of intensity as duration increases because of the decreased availability of oxygen and accumulation of lactic acid. As the duration of exercise increases, power output decreases. The contribution of energy-yielding nutrients must be considered also. As the duration of exercise lengthens, fats contribute more as an energy source. The opposite is true for high-intensity exercise; when intensity increases, the body relies increasingly on carbohydrates as substrate.

FUELS FOR CONTRACTING MUSCLES

Protein, fat, and carbohydrate are possible sources of fuel for ATP generation and therefore muscle contraction. The glycolytic pathway is restricted to glucose, which can originate in dietary carbohydrates or stored glycogen, or it can be synthesized from the carbon skeletons of certain amino acids through the process of gluconeogenesis. The Krebs cycle is fueled by three-carbon fragments of glucose; two-carbon fragments of fatty acids; and carbon skeletons of specific amino acids, primarily alanine and the branched-chain amino acids. All these substrates can be used during exercise; however, the intensity and duration of the exercise determine the relative rates of substrate use.

Intensity

The intensity of the exercise is important in determining what fuel will be used by contracting muscles. High-intensity, short-duration exercise has to rely on anaerobic production of ATP. Because oxygen is not available for anaerobic pathways, only glucose and glycogen can be broken down anaerobically for fuel. When glycogen is broken down anaerobically, it is used 18 to 19 times faster than when broken down aerobically. Persons who are performing high-intensity workouts or competitive races may run the risk of running out of muscle glycogen before the event or exercise is done as a result of its high rate of use.

Sports that use the anaerobic and aerobic pathways also have a higher glycogen-use rate and, like anaerobic athletes, athletes in these sports also run the risk of running out of fuel before the race or exercise is finished. Sports such as basketball, football, soccer, tennis and swimming are good examples; glycogen usage is high because of the intermittent bursts of high-intensity sprints and running drills. In moderate-intensity sports or exercise such as jogging, hiking, aerobic dance, gymnastics, cycling, and recreational swimming, approximately half of the energy for these activities comes from the aerobic breakdown of muscle glycogen, whereas the other half comes from circulating blood glucose and fatty acids.

Moderate- to low-intensity exercise such as walking is fueled primarily by the aerobic pathway; thus a greater proportion of fat can be used to create ATP for energy. Fatty acids cannot supply all the ATP during high-intensity exercise because fat cannot be broken down fast enough to provide the energy. Also, fat provides less energy per liter of oxygen consumed than does glucose (4.65 kcal/L of O_2 versus 5.01 kcal/L of O_2). Therefore when less oxygen is available in high-intensity activities, there is a definite advantage for the muscles to be able to use glycogen because less oxygen is required.

In general, glucose and fatty acids provide fuel for exercise in proportions depending on the intensity and duration of the exercise and the fitness of the athlete. Exertion of extremely high intensity and short duration draws primarily on reserves of ATP and CP. High-intensity exercise that continues for more than a few seconds depends on anaerobic glycolysis. During exercise of low-to-moderate intensity (60% of maximum oxygen uptake [Vo_2max]), energy is derived mainly from fatty acids. Carbohydrate becomes a larger fraction of the energy source as intensity increases until, at an intensity level of 85% to 90% Vo_2max, carbohydrates from glycogen are the principal energy source, and the duration of activity is limited (see Figure 23-3).

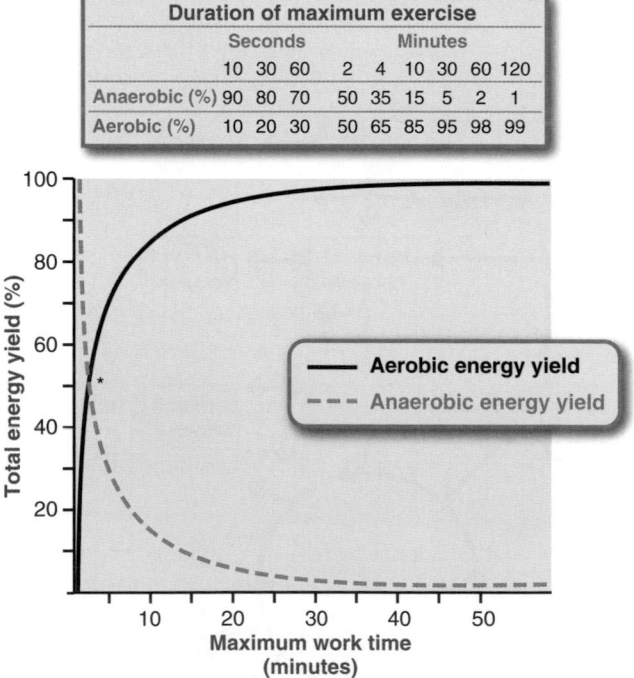

Duration of maximum exercise								
	Seconds			Minutes				
	10	30	60	2	4	10	30	60	120
Anaerobic (%)	90	80	70	50	35	15	5	2	1
Aerobic (%)	10	20	30	50	65	85	95	98	99

FIGURE 23-2 Relative contribution of aerobic and anaerobic energy during maximum physical activity of various durations. Note that 90 to 120 seconds of maximum effort requires 50% of the energy from each of the aerobic and anaerobic processes. This is also the point at which the lactic acid pathway for energy production is at its maximum.

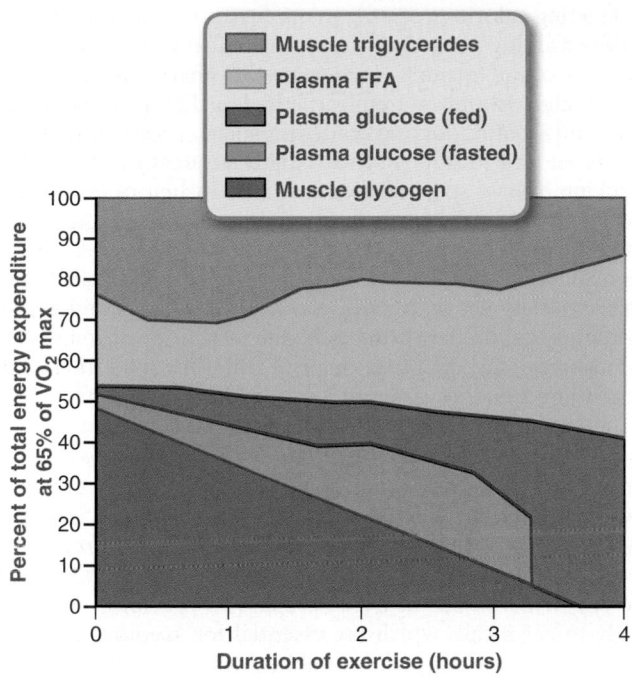

FIGURE 23-3 Principle Energy Source and Exercise Duration.

Duration

The duration of a training session determines the substrate used during the exercise bout. For example, the longer the time spent exercising, the greater the contribution of fat as the fuel. Fat can supply up to 60% to 70% of the energy needed for ultraendurance events lasting 6 to 10 hours. As the duration of exercise increases, the reliance on aerobic metabolism becomes greater, and a greater amount of ATP can be produced from fatty acids. However, fat cannot be metabolized unless a continuous stream of some carbohydrates is also available through the energy pathways. Therefore muscle glycogen and blood glucose are the limiting factors in human performance of any type of intensity or duration.

Effect of Training

The length of time an athlete can oxidize fatty acids as a fuel source is related to the athlete's conditioning, as well as the exercise intensity. In addition to improving cardiovascular systems involved in oxygen delivery, training increases the number of mitochondria and the levels of enzymes involved in the aerobic synthesis of ATP, thus increasing the capacity for fatty acid metabolism. Increases in mitochondria with aerobic training are seen mainly in the type IIA (intermediate fast-twitch) muscle fibers. However, these fibers quickly lose their aerobic capacity with the cessation of aerobic training, reverting to the genetic baseline.

These changes from training result in a lower **respiratory exchange ratio (RER)**, (also called respiratory quotient [RQ]), which is RQ = CO_2 eliminated / O_2 consumed; lower blood lactate and catecholamine levels, and a lower net muscle glycogen breakdown at a specific power output. These metabolic adaptations enhance the ability of muscle to oxidize all fuels, especially fat.

NUTRITIONAL REQUIREMENTS OF EXERCISE

Energy

The most important component of successful sport training and performance is to ensure adequate calorie intake to support energy expenditure and maintain strength, endurance, muscle mass, and overall health. Energy and nutrient requirements vary with age, gender, weight, height, training/sport type, frequency, intensity, and duration; typical diet, diet history, history of restrictive and disordered eating; endocrine and environmental conditions such as heat, cold, and altitude. Estimating energy intake is challenging to accomplish, especially in sports that are less well studied (Driskell and Wolinsky, 2011).

Individuals who participate in an overall fitness program (i.e., 30 to 40 min/day, three times per week) can generally meet their daily nutritional needs by following a normal diet providing 25 to 35 kcal/kg/day or roughly 1800 to 2400 calories a day. However, energy requirements for athletes training 90 minutes a day has been suggested to be 45 to 50 kcal/kg/day, and in certain sports even more.

For example, the 50-kg athlete engaging in more intense training of 2 to 3 hours/day five to six times a week or high-volume training of 3 to 6 hours in one to two workouts per day 5 to 6 days a week may expend up to an additional 600 to 1200 calories a day above and beyond REE, thus requiring 50 to 80 kcal/kg/day or roughly 2500 to 4000 kcal/day. For elite athletes or heavier athletes, daily calorie needs can reach 150 to 200 kcal/kg, or roughly 7500 to 10,000 calories a day, depending on the volume and intensity of different training phases.

Estimation of Energy Requirements

Resting metabolic rate (RMR) or resting energy expenditure (REE) can be measured using indirect calorimetry or estimated by using predictive equations. Indirect calorimetry involves using a hand-held device such as the MedGem calorimeter or metabolic cart typically used in exercise physiology or research settings to measure a person's oxygen consumption to determine RMR or basal metabolic rate (BMR). Measuring RMR or BMR is more accurate than using prediction equations.

Predictive equations are used to estimate RMR/BMR when technical equipment, such as a metabolic cart, is not available. The Cunningham equation has been shown to be the best predictor of RMR or REE for active men and women followed by the Harris Benedict equation (Rodriguez et al, 2009). DeLorenzo developed an equation that also has been shown to be accurate specifically with male strength and power athletes such as those in water polo, judo, and karate (Academy of Nutrition and Dietetics [AND], 2014; DeLorenzo et al, 1999).

If the sports dietitian has body composition data including percent body fat, the REE can be calculated as shown in Box 23-1.

Once REE has been calculated, the total energy expenditure (TEE) can be estimated using energy expenditure from physical activity. Because metabolic equipment is expensive, requires considerable training to use, and is not practical outside

---

BOX 23-1 Calculating RMR from Body Composition Data

RMR (calories/day) = 500 + (22 x Lean Body Mass in kilograms)
RMR = resting metabolic rate
LBM = lean body mass

research settings, indirect methods can be employed and include heart rate monitors, pedometers, or accelerometers. Other indirect methods are to use a daily activity factor as a base to which is added calories expended in exercise, which are calculated by multiplying the calories expended per minute of exercise times the amount of time spent in that activity, known as METS, metabolic equivalent of task (Driskell and Wolinsky, 2011; see Chapter 2).

Heart rate monitoring to estimate energy expenditure is based on the assumption that there is a linear relationship between heart rate and oxygen consumption (VO_2). Pedometers measure ambulatory distance covered, which is a limitation of the method because it does not consider other types of physical activities such as weight lifting, cycling, or yoga. Accelerometers have the advantage of measuring all activities, are easy to wear, and can give feedback for long periods of time. Other personal fitness devices have been developed in recent years, although no method is as accurate as measuring directly with a metabolic cart.

A method for calculating total energy expenditure using activity factors provided is shown in Box 23-2.

BOX 23-2 Calculating Daily Energy Requirements for Athletes

Cunningham Formula

RMR or REE (resting energy expenditure in kcalories/day) = 500 + [22 x Lean Body Mass (LBM) in kilograms (kg)]

For example:

175-pound (79.5kg) athlete with 10% body fat

Kg of fat = weight = 79.5 kg x .10 = 7.9 kg fat.

Lean body mass = total weight - fat weight = 79.5 – 7.9 = 71.6 kg of LBM

REE = 500 + (22 x 71.6kg LBM) = 2075 calories.

To Determine EEPA—Energy Expended for Physical Activity

Can use:

Calories expended in a day using: http://www.cdc.gov/nccdphp/dnpa/physical/pdf/PA_Intensity_table_2_1.pdf

Or

Can use:

Specific caloric expenditures for different weights using: http://www.nutribase.com/exercala.htm.

Or

Can multiply REE by the activity factor using:

1.200 = sedentary (little or no exercise)

1.375 = lightly active (about 30 minutes of moderate training, 1 to 3 days/week)

1.550 = moderately active (45 minutes of moderate training, 3 to 5 days/week)

1.725 = very active (training for 1 hour, 6 to 7 days/week)

1.900 = extra active (very hard training, including weight lifting, 2-3 days/week)

To continue the example:

The EEPA for this 175-pound athlete who is training hard would be the following:

REE (2075 kcalories) x activity factor (1.9) = 3942 *total* kcalories for BEE and EEPA

To continue the example:

Thermic effect of food (TEF) = the total kcalories for REE and EEPA x 10% = 3942 x0.1 = 394 kcalories

Total daily energy requirements = total kcalories (3942)+ TEF (394 kcalories) = 4336 kcalories.

Total daily energy requirements = 4336 kcalories

Thompson J, Manore MM. Predicted and measured resting metabolic rate of male and female endurance athletes. *J Am Diet Assoc.* 1996 Jan; 96(1):30-4.

Meeting caloric needs for many fitness-minded or elite, intensely training individuals can be a challenge regardless of the accuracy of the formulas used to predict energy needs.

For high school and college athletes, disruptive sleep patterns and accommodating academic, social, and training schedules often lead to skipped meals, high frequency of unplanned snacking, use of sport shakes and bars in lieu of whole food meals, and late-night snacking while studying, or socializing online or with friends. Adult athletes with family and work responsibilities are also meal challenged when juggling daily training schedules with carpools, work deadlines, and accommodating children's eating schedules, which ultimately can compromise the quantity, quality, and timing of meals and greatly affect energy, strength levels, and overall health.

In elite athletes, consuming enough food at regular intervals without compromising performance is challenging, particularly when athletes are traveling abroad, are at the mercy of airport food, foreign food schedules, unfamiliar training facilities, delays, and unforeseen events such as weather-postponed game and competition schedules. All athletes regardless of age and lifestyle demands can be better prepared by packing snacks and ready-to-eat meals, which are essential for keeping energy intakes adequate to support overall health and performance.

Meeting the daily energy needs and the appropriate macronutrient distribution for active individuals may necessitate the use of sports bars, drinks, and convenience foods and snacks in addition to whole foods and meals. Dietitian nutritionists should stay open minded and be flexible in accommodating lifestyles and eating behaviors when designing meal plans for maximum sport performance.

WEIGHT MANAGEMENT

Although lean body mass has been associated with positive health benefits, negative health outcomes are associated with excessive loss or gain of body mass. Although weight classifications in sports such as youth and sprint football, wrestling, lightweight crew, and boxing were designed to ensure healthy, safe, and equitable participation, few published and widely accepted weight and body composition standards exist, and the governing organizations for these sports have no mandated weight control practices. Only sprint football and wrestling consider the components of an athlete's weight and body composition as well as the safety considerations for achieving and maintaining that body size.

In 1997 specific rules and guidelines were implemented by the NCAA to ensure safe weight control practices in wrestling, applied early in the competitive season and conducted on a regular basis to ensure prevention of dehydration and other weight-cutting behaviors. In 2006 the National Federation of State High School Associations adopted similar standards for determining body weights, although they are not accepted or enforced universally.

Weight Loss

In efforts to maximize performance or meet weight criteria determined by specific sports whether it is in the case of "making a lower weight" in sports such as martial arts, sailing, rowing, or wrestling, or reaching a higher weight for power lifting, football, or baseball, many athletes alter normal energy intake to either gain or lose weight. Although such efforts are sometimes appropriate, weight reduction or weight gain programs may involve elements of risk, especially when the pressure to lose or gain weight is expected in an unrealistically short amount of time. For some young athletes achievement of an unrealistically low weight or conversely a high weight with the use of weight gainer or other supplements can jeopardize growth and development.

The goal weight of an athlete should be based on optimizing health and performance and be determined by the athlete's best previous performance weight and body composition. Adequate time should be allowed for a slow, steady weight loss of approximately 1 to 2 pounds each week over several weeks. Weight loss should be achieved during off-season or preseason when competition is not a priority. A weight loss planning guide can be found online at the *AND Sports Nutrition Care Manual*.

The National Athletic Trainers Association (NATA) suggests the lowest safe weight should be calculated at no lower than the weight determined by the low reference body fat composition delineated by sex and age. The lowest safe weight can be defined as the lowest weight sanctioned by the governing body at which a competitor may compete (Turocy et al, 2011).When no standard exists, participants would be required to remain above a certain minimal body fat. The highest safe weight should be calculated using a value no higher than the highest end of the range satisfactory for health: 10% to 22% body fat in males and 20% to 32% in females (Turocy et al, 2011; see Table 23-1).

Weight Gain

To accomplish a healthy weight gain of lean muscle tissue, 500 to 1000 additional calories per day can be added in addition to strength training, which will dually increase muscle strength. The rate of weight gain depends on the athlete's genetic make-up, degree of positive energy balance, number of rest and recovery sessions a week, and exercise type.

WEIGHT MANAGEMENT AND AESTHETICS

Disordered Eating

Although drive, perfection, and attention to detail are the hallmarks of talented athletes, they are also some of the personality traits associated with the development of eating disorders (see Chapter 22). Disordered eating behaviors among athletes can be difficult to detect given the tendencies of athletes to maintain rigid nutritional requirements, follow intense training schedules, and push through fatigue and pain.

Disordered eating behaviors specifically in athletes have been termed **anorexia athletica (AA)**, where the ultimate goal is to perform at one's best as opposed to thinness in and of itself being the goal. Athletes who are more vulnerable to AA are those who participate in "lean-build" sports, such as cross country running, swimming, gymnastics, cheerleading, dance, yoga, and wrestling, who may think they need to be a certain

weight or body type, often far less than what it is realistic to attain and maintain to be competitive. This desire to be unrealistically light or lean may lead to restrictive eating, bingeing and purging, and excessive training far beyond what is required for their sport.

Female Athlete Triad

Chronic dieting by female athletes can lead to the **female athlete triad (FAT)**, which consists of three interrelated health disorders: low energy availability with or without an eating disorder, osteoporosis, and amenorrhea. The prevalence of FAT for athletes participating in lean-requiring versus non–lean-requiring sports has been shown to range from 1.5% to 6.7% and from 0% to 2.0% respectively (Gibbs et al, 2013). For example, it has been shown that student and professional female dancers consume only 70% to 80% of the Recommended Dietary Allowance (RDA) for total daily energy intake (Mountjoy et al, 2014).

Also known as **athletic energy deficit (AED)**, this low-energy intake can lead to an increase in bone fractures and lifelong consequences for the bone and reproductive health of developing adolescent girls. Evidence suggests it is energy availability that regulates reproductive function in women, not exercise or body composition, and that ensuring adequate calorie intake is imperative to the overall health of the athletic woman (De Souza et al, 2014). Low energy intake paired with ovarian suppression or amenorrhea has been associated with poor athletic performance.

Muscle Dysmorphia

Although many studies suggest females are more susceptible to disordered eating behaviors than males, results from descriptive data from project EAT (Eating Amongst Teens) revealed that males who consider themselves in a weight-related sport are comparative to females in the same category. In fact, as the media's portrayal of the male physique has been increasingly muscular and unattainable, men have become more dissatisfied with their bodies and more vulnerable to **eating, exercise, and body image (EEBI) disorders**.

Muscle dysmorphia (MD), also known as "bigorexia"or reverse anorexia nervosa (AN), is a disorder in which individuals are preoccupied with their bodies not being muscular enough or big enough. It is marked by symptoms that are similar to and the opposite of anorexia nervosa symptomatology (see Chapter 22).

AA and MD experience grossly distorted perceptions of their bodies, which in the case of MD, often leads to maladaptive eating, exercise and substance use behaviors, including preoccupation with diet and excessively high protein intakes. In addition there is anabolic steroid, diet pill, caffeine, and over-the-counter supplement abuse, especially of those reputed for fat burning, ergogenic, or thermogenic effects. Last, the athlete exercises excessively, especially weight lifting, in an attempt to increase body satisfaction and attain the "perfect" lean and muscular physique. As with other EEBI, MD can lead to social, occupational, and relationship impairments (see Box 23-3).

Research suggests that this preference for a muscular physique is already evident in boys as young as 6 years old and may affect up to 95% of college-age American men who are dissatisfied with some aspect of their body and up to 25% of college men engaging in negative body talk (Engeln et al, 2013; Murray et al, 2012).

TABLE 23-1 Body Fat (%) Standards by Sex and Age		
Body Fat Standard	**Males**	**Females**
Lowest reference body fat for adults	5	12
Lowest reference body fat for adolescents	7	14
Healthy body fat ranges	10-22	20-32

BOX 23-3 Body Image and Eating Disorders in Athletes

Anorexia Athletica

Exercising beyond the requirements for good health
Obsessive dieting; fear of certain foods
Obsessive or compulsive exercising; overtraining
Individual won't eat with teammates, tries to hide dieting
Stealing time from work, school, and relationships to exercise
Focusing on challenge and forgetting that physical activity can be fun
Defining self-worth in terms of performance
Rarely or never being satisfied with athletic achievements
Always pushing on to the next challenge
Justifying excessive behavior by defining self as an athlete or insisting that the behavior is healthy
Desire to keep losing more pounds despite already low body weight
Mood swings; angry outbursts
Menstrual periods stop
REF: http://www.eatingdisordersonline.com/explain/anorexiathleticasigns.php

Muscle Dysphoria

Primarily male eating disorder
Getting bigger is on the mind constantly. This includes thinking about diet, working out, or appearance
See themselves as looking small or "puny" even though they typically appear normal or very muscular to others
Constant concerns with body fat percentage
Hide physique with baggy clothing since never feel "good enough" and is source of shame
Workouts take precedence over other significant events or time spent with family and friends
Fear that missing one workout session will set them back or stymie progress
Workout even when injured
Common to abuse anabolic steroids to enhance their appearance
Missing workout or eating a "forbidden" food item can trigger extreme anxiety and crush self-esteem
Individual might add additional workout sessions, skip meals, or use some means to punish themselves for diet cheating
Frequently accompanying symptoms of depression
REF: http://www.eatingdisordersonline.com/lifestyle/general/recognizing-muscle-dysmorphia-bigorexia

TABLE 23-2 A Nutrition Periodization Program

Cycle	Training Goal/Dietary Recommendation
Preseason training	Preparation load cycles followed by recovery cycles
	Higher or lower energy needs depending on weight goals
	Greater protein needs for lean muscle mass development
Competitive season	Peak cycles with recovery; energy needs depending on expenditure; higher carbohydrate needs to support high intensity competition; protein and fat needs relative to weight maintenance, recovery and overall health
Postseason training	Active rest-transition cycle of conditioning and recovery; energy to support but not exceed needs; emphasis on more lax dietary guidelines for mental and emotional competitive break

Nutrition periodization is a term to describe dietary modification to match specific training patterns during in and off seasons as well as pre- and postcompetition periods, which are marked by different nutritional needs (Driskell and Wolinsky, 2011). Periodization involves different training cycles, including load, recovery peak, and conditioning that are implemented according to the athlete's sports demands and competition schedules (Driskell and Wolinsky, 2011; see Table 23-2).

Strategies and Tools for Eating Guides in Athletes

According to the United States Olympic Committee (USOC), sports dietitians, and other sports nutrition experts, keeping guidelines simple for athletes is imperative for compliance. See http://www.outsideonline.com/fitness/nutrition/The-Secret-Food-of-Athletes.html.

The USOC dietitians created **The Athlete's Plate** as a guide for eating for athletes based on easy, moderate, and hard training regimens (see Figure 23-4). This tool helps athletes who play a sport for more than 5 hours a week modify servings and portion sizes from each food group based on their training (Mettler et al, 2010).

CARBOHYDRATE

Carbohydrates are one of two main fuels used for sport activity. The first source of glucose for the exercising muscle is its own glycogen store. When this is depleted, **glycogenolysis** and then gluconeogenesis (both in the liver) maintain the glucose supply. The relationship between carbohydrate intake, muscle glycogen content, and endurance exercise capacity is well documented, and it has become widely accepted that a high-carbohydrate diet before combined with carbohydrate supplementation during prolonged submaximal exercise can postpone the development of muscular fatigue and enhance performance (Burke, 2010).

During endurance exercise that exceeds 90 minutes, such as marathon running, muscle glycogen stores become progressively smaller. When they drop to critically low levels, high-intensity exercise cannot be maintained. In practical terms the athlete is exhausted and must either stop exercising or drastically reduce the pace. Athletes often refer to this as "hitting the wall."

MACRONUTRIENTS

According to the position of the Academy of Nutrition and Dietetics (AND), Dietitians of Canada, and the American College of Sports Medicine, most recreational athletes do not need to eat a diet that is substantially different than the U.S. Dietary Guidelines for Americans to perform optimally (Rodriguez et al, 2009; see Chapter 11). Individuals engaging in a general fitness program typically can meet their macronutrient needs by consuming a normal diet of 45% to 55% of calories from carbohydrates (3 to 5 g/kg/day), 10% to 15% from protein (0.8 to 1 g/kg/day), and 25% to 35% from fat (0.5 to 1.5 g/kg/day).

Nutrition Periodization

Athletes involved in moderate- to high-volume training need greater amounts of carbohydrates, protein, and fat to meet macronutrient needs. The composition of the athlete's diet is dependent on training phase: preseason, season, off season; sport type including intensity and duration of training; and weight and body composition goals.

Specific macronutrient recommendations should be used when counseling a competitive or elite athlete to maximize performance, a concept known as **nutrition periodization**.

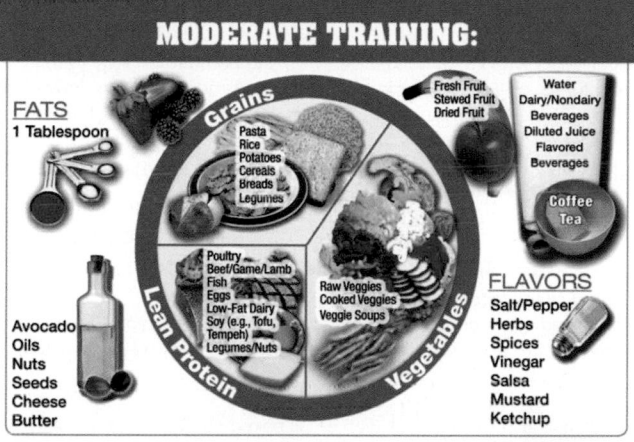

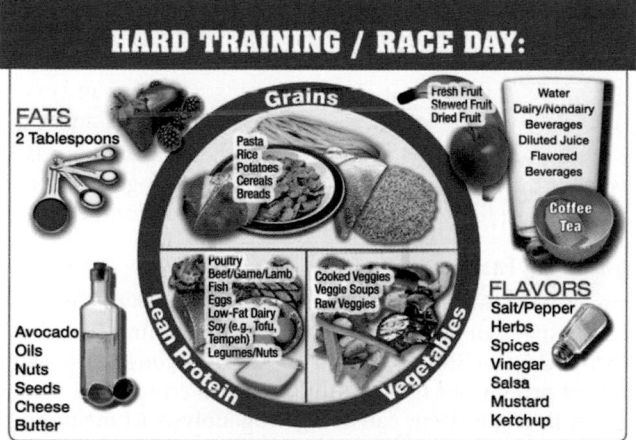

FIGURE 23-4 The athlete's plate adjusted to type of training and competition.

Glycogen depletion also may be a gradual process, occurring over repeated days of heavy training, in which muscle glycogen breakdown exceeds its replacement, as well as during high-intensity exercise that is repeated several times during competition or training. For example, a distance runner who averages 10 miles per day but does not take the time to consume enough

carbohydrates in his or her diet, or the swimmer who completes several interval sets at maximum oxygen consumption within hours can deplete glycogen stores rapidly.

Historically, a high-carbohydrate or glycogen loading (glycogen supercompensation) diet was used to guide athletes to enhance maximize glycogen stores and be able to continue endurance performance, but this approach has its benefits and drawbacks (McArdle et al, 2013).

Traditionally, the 7-day carbohydrate-loading approach combined muscle-specific depletion training with a low-carbohydrate diet for 4 days followed by a high-carbohydrate diet and little to no training for 3 days before competition. Normal muscle typically contains about 1.7 g glycogen per 100 g of muscle; supercompensation packs up to 5 g glycogen per 100 g of muscle. Although this may be beneficial for the endurance athlete training or competing over 60 minutes, it has not been shown to benefit those in higher-intensity, shorter-duration activities. The negative effects of the additional weight of 2.7 g of water for each gram of glycogen can be a hindrance to performance, making it a heavy fuel. A modified approach of gradual exercise tapering along with more modified increases in carbohydrate intake may minimize the negative outcomes associated with classical loading (McArdle et al, 2013).

Effects of Training Low, Competing High

Recent studies have investigated the impact of short-term, 1- to 2-week diet-training interventions that increase endogenous muscle glycogen and lipids and alter patterns of substrate utilization during exercise. Otherwise known as the fat adaptation strategy or "train low" approach, well-trained endurance athletes consume a high-fat, low-CHO diet for up to 2 weeks while undertaking their normal training and then immediately follow this by a high-carbohydrate diet and tapering of exercise 1 to 3 days before an endurance event. Research suggests that this nutritional periodization approach can increase the rate of fat oxidation while attenuating the rate of muscle glygenolysis during submaximal exercise.

Carbohydrate Recommendations

The amount of carbohydrate required depends on the athlete's total daily energy expenditure, type of sport, gender, and the environmental conditions, with the ultimate goal of providing adequate energy for performance and recovery, and a protein sparing effect.

Recommendations should provide for daily carbohydrate intake in grams relative to body mass and allow flexibility for the athlete to meet these targets within the context of energy needs and other dietary goals. Carbohydrate intake of 5 to 7 g/kg/day can meet general training needs, and 7 to 10 g/kg/day will likely suffice for endurance athletes, although elite athletes training 5 to 6 hours a day may need as much as 12 g/kg/day or a range of 420 to 720 g of carbohydrates a day for the 60-kg athlete (AND, 2014; Driskell and Wolinsky, 2011).

Carbohydrates are especially important not only as an overall contributor to meeting daily calorie needs but also as ergogenic aids in a more time-specific approach, also known as nutritional periodization, designed to enhance and maximize performance for competition, especially more than 90 minutes in length. However, a recent meta-analysis suggests that the impact of carbohydrates on performance is subject to debate as numerous studies use fasting subjects and time-to-exhaustion test modes, which may offer a less-convincing picture, especially with an exercise session lasting less than 70 minutes (Colombani et al, 2013).

Types of Carbohydrate

Even though the effects of different sugars on performance, substrate use, and recovery have been studied extensively, the optimal type of carbohydrate for the athlete is still subject to debate by sports performance experts (Colombani et al, 2013). The glycemic index (GI) represents the ratio of the area under the blood glucose curve resulting from the ingestion of a given quantity of carbohydrate and the area under the glucose curve resulting from the ingestion of the same quantity of white bread or glucose (see Appendix 37).

Studies concerning whether the GI of carbohydrate in the preexercise meal affects performance have been performed primarily in athletes in endurance sports, and are inconclusive. In one study, high-glycemic and low-glycemic carbohydrate solutions demonstrated similar performance outcome when consumed during a long distance run (Bennett et al, 2012). A preexercise low-glycemic index meal was shown to diminish increases in stress hormones and accelerate recovery. Another study also showed that compared with fasting, low- and high-GI foods consumed 3 hours before and halfway through prolonged, high-intensity intermittent exercise improved repeated sprint performance (Little et al, 2009).

Food Timing

Pre-Training Carbohydrates

The pretraining or preevent meal serves two purposes: (1) it keeps the athlete from feeling hungry before and during the exercise, and (2) it maintains optimal levels of blood glucose for the exercising muscles. A preexercise meal can improve performance compared with exercising in a fasted state. Athletes who train early in the morning before eating or drinking risk developing low liver glycogen stores, which can impair performance, particularly if the exercise regimen involves endurance training.

Carbohydrate meals before exercise can enhance liver glycogen stores. In addition to allowing for personal preferences and psychologic factors, the preevent meal should be high in carbohydrate, nongreasy, and readily digested. Fat should be limited because it delays gastric emptying time and takes longer to digest. A meal eaten 3½ to 4 hours before competition should be limited to 25% of the kilocalories from fat. Closer to the event, the fat content should be less than 25% (see Box 23-4).

Exercising with a full stomach may cause indigestion, nausea, and vomiting. Thus the pregame meal should be eaten 3 to 4 hours before an event and should provide 200 to 350 g of carbohydrates (4 g/kg) (Driskell and Wolinsky, 2011). Allowing time for partial digestion and absorption provides a final addition to muscle glycogen, additional blood sugar, and also relatively complete emptying of the stomach. To avoid gastrointestinal (GI) distress, the carbohydrate content of the meal should be reduced when the meal is close to the exercise time. For example, 4 hours before the event it is suggested that the athlete consume 4 g of carbohydrate per kilogram of body weight, whereas 1 hour before the competition the athlete would consume 1 g of carbohydrate per kilogram of body weight.

Commercial liquid formulas providing an easily digested high-carbohydrate fluid are popular with athletes and probably leave the stomach faster. Foods high in fiber, fat, and lactose cause GI distress for some (e.g., bloating, gas, or diarrhea) and

---

BOX 23-4   Examples of Pre-Event Meals and Snacks

For athletes who compete in events such as track or swimming meets or soccer, basketball, volleyball, and wrestling tournaments all day, nutritious, easy-to-digest food and fluid choices may be a challenge. The athlete should consider the amount of time between eating and performance when choosing foods during all-day events. Suggested pre-competition menus include the following:

1 hr. or Less Before Competition—About 100 kcal
One of these choices:
Fresh fruit such as a banana or orange slices
Half of a sports or breakfast bar
½ plain bagel or English muffin
Crackers such as rice crackers, saltines or Melba toast
Small box of plain cereal such as Kashi, Kind, Krispies, or Flakes
8-12 oz. of a sports drink such as Body Armor, Gatorade

2 to 3 Hours Before Competition—About 300-400 kcal
One of these choices:
½ of turkey sandwich on white bread with baked chips
½ bagel with low-sugar jelly and 1 banana
2 pancakes with lite or sugar-free syrup and berries
32 fluid oz. of a sports drink such as Body Armor, Gatorade, PowerBar, Endurance Sports Drink or 32 oz. endurance drink with protein such as UCAN, Endurox, or Accelerade
1 low-sugar smoothie with berries, banana, and 1 scoop (< or = 20 gm), of protein, either plant-based, whey or egg whites
1 sports energy bar, 1 cup sports drink, 1 cup water

3 to 4 Hours Before Competition—About 700 kcal
One of these selections:
Scrambled egg whites with white toast/low-sugar jam and banana
1 bagel with fat free or low-fat cream cheese and low-sugar jelly and 1 banana
1 6-in turkey sub on Italian bread with lettuce, tomato, and mustard
1 3-oz grilled chicken breast with small baked potato, roll, and water
2 cups plain pasta with 1 plain roll
1 can of low fat sport shake with no more than 25 g protein, 1 sports bar, 1 banana, water

---

should be avoided before competition. Athletes should always use what works best for them by experimenting with foods and beverages during practice sessions and planning ahead to ensure they have these foods available when they compete.

Pre-training Fasting

Some athletes either rise too early for workouts to consume a meal or snack or feel nauseous when consuming food before exercise. Overnight fasts of 8 to 10 hours or longer are normal for most people, but not for athletes. An overnight fast causes a drop in liver glycogen, causing glycogenolysis to maintain the supply of glucose to the brain. Although a modest fall in blood sugar may not affect the average individual, it may affect the physical and cognitive performance of athletes fasting longer than 12 to 24 hours. Although some evidence suggests a metabolic advantage of endurance training in a fasted state to increase fat oxidation in trained muscles, other evidence supports the intake of nutrients, primarily carbohydrates, before, during, and after training sessions (Van Proeyen et al, 2011).

Training Fuel During Exercise

Carbohydrates consumed during endurance exercise lasting longer than 1 hour ensure the availability of sufficient amounts

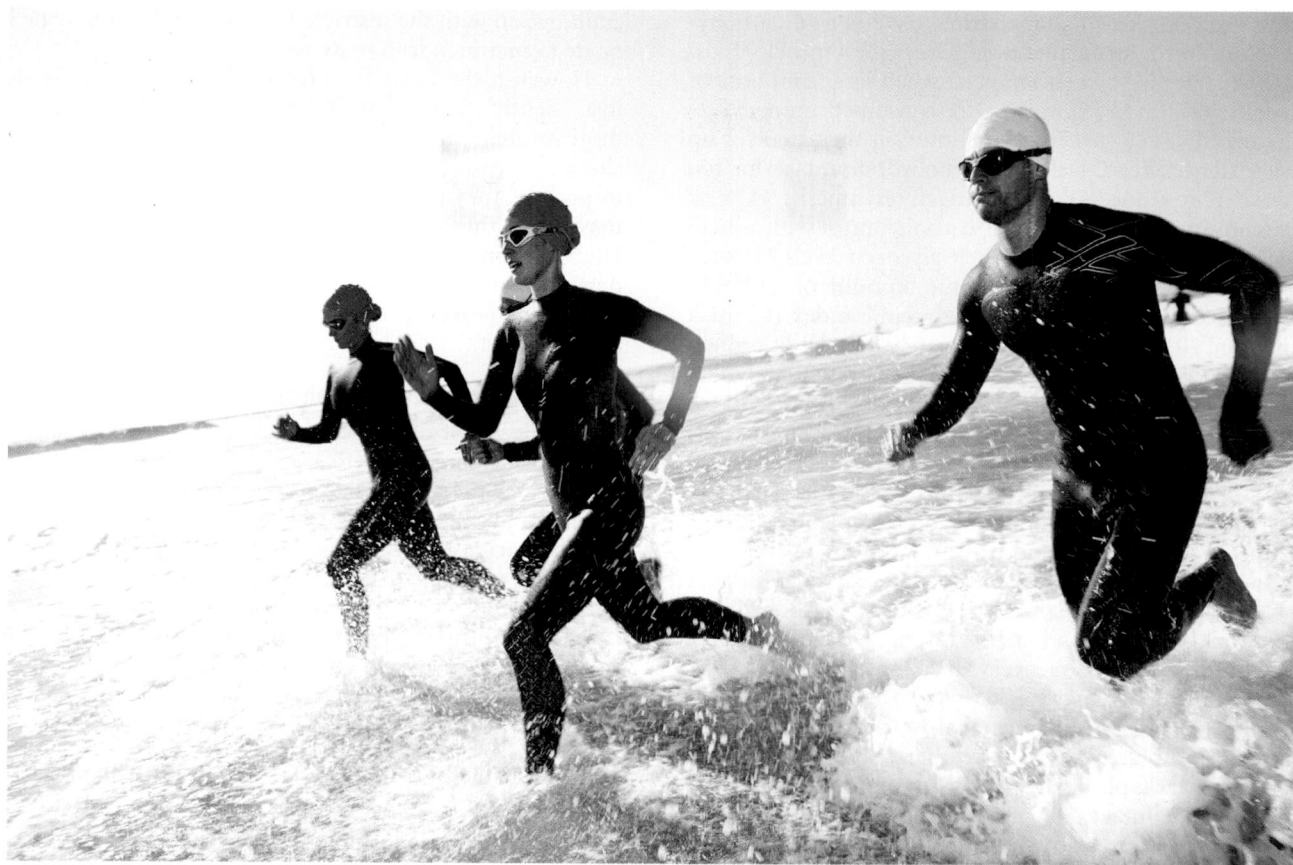

FIGURE 23-5 A triathlon is a high-intensity endurance sport during which both carbohydrates and fats are used as fuels, the amount depending on the speed and length of the event. (Photo©istock. com).

of energy during the later stages of exercise, improve performance, and enhance feelings of pleasure during and after exercise (Driskell and Wolinsky, 2011). Carbohydrate feedings may not prevent fatigue but may delay it. During the final minutes of exercise, when muscle glycogen is low and athletes rely heavily on blood glucose for energy, their muscles feel heavy, and they must concentrate to maintain exercise at intensities that are ordinarily not stressful when muscle glycogen stores are full. Glucose ingestion during exercise also has been shown to spare endogenous protein and carbohydrates in fed cyclists without glycogen depletion; thus consuming an exogenous carbohydrate during endurance exercise helps to maintain blood glucose and improve performance (McArdle et al, 2013). (See Figure 23-5).

The type of carbohydrates consumed may affect performance during exercise. Recent research suggests that compared with water, a solution containing fructose attenuates thermoregulatory responses compared with glucose (Suzuki et al, 2014). However, the form of carbohydrate consumed does not seem to matter physiologically. Some athletes prefer to use a sports drink, whereas others prefer to eat a solid or gel and drink water.

If a sports drink with carbohydrates is consumed during exercise, the rate of carbohydrate ingestion should be approximately 25 to 30 g every 30 minutes, an amount equivalent to 1 cup of a 4% to 8% carbohydrate solution taken every 15 to 20 minutes. This ensures that 1 g of carbohydrate is delivered to the tissues per minute at the time fatigue sets in. It is unlikely that a carbohydrate concentration of less than 5% is enough to help performance, but solutions with a concentration greater than 10% often are associated with abdominal cramps, nausea, and diarrhea.

Combining protein and carbohydrates in a sport fluid or snack also may improve performance, muscle protein synthesis and net balance, and recovery. Amino acids ingested in small amounts, alone or in conjunction with carbohydrates before or after exercise, appear to improve net protein balance, and may stimulate protein synthesis during exercise and postexercise recovery (AIS, 2014).

Postworkout and Recovery Fuel

Dietary strategies that can enhance recovery from the negative effects of exercise can help promote effective physiologic adaptation, muscle conditioning after exercise, and enable a faster return to training. The resulting improvement in training efficiency may lead to significant performance benefits and sport career longevity by supporting repetitive training and competition and helping to maintain immune status and long-term health (Lynch, 2013).

On average, only 5% of the muscle glycogen used during exercise is resynthesized each hour after exercise. Accordingly, at least 20 hours are required for complete restoration after exhaustive exercise, provided approximately 600 g of carbohydrates are consumed during that time. The highest muscle glycogen synthesis rates have been reported when large amounts of carbohydrates—1 to 1.85 g/kg/hr—are consumed immediately after exercise and at 15- to 60-minute intervals thereafter for up to 5 hours after exercise. Delaying carbohydrate intake for too long after exercise reduces muscle glycogen resynthesis.

Apparently the consumption of carbohydrates with a high glycemic index results in higher muscle glycogen levels 24 hours after exercise compared with the same amount of carbohydrates provided as foods with a low glycemic index (Cermak and van Loon, 2013). Adding approximately 5 to 9 g of protein with every 100 g of carbohydrate eaten after exercise may further increase glycogen resynthesis rate, provide amino acids for muscle repair, and promote a more anabolic hormonal profile (Sousa et al, 2014).

Many athletes find it difficult to consume food immediately after exercise. Usually when body or core temperature is elevated, appetite is depressed, and it is difficult to consume carbohydrate-rich foods. Many athletes find it easier and simpler to drink their carbohydrates, ingest easy-to-eat, carbohydrate-rich foods such as fruit pops, bananas, oranges, melon, or apple slices, or consume a sports recovery shake or bar.

Sports supplements may include the easy-to-carry, easy-to-consume, and easy-to-digest meal-replacement powders, ready-to-drink supplements, energy bars, and energy gels. These products are typically fortified with 33% to 100% of the Dietary Reference Intakes (DRIs) for vitamins and minerals, provide varying amounts and types of carbohydrates, protein, and fat, and are ideal for athletes on the run. They provide a portable, easy-to-consume food that can be used pericompetitively, while traveling, at work, in the car, or throughout the day at multievent meets such as in track and field, swimming, diving, or gymnastics.

Many fitness-minded and athletic individuals use these products, generally recognized as safe, as a convenient way to enhance their diets. However, if they are substituted in the place of whole foods on a regular basis, they can deprive the athlete of a well-balanced diet. They also may contain excesses of sugars, fats, and protein and banned substances such as herbs, stimulants, and other botanicals prohibited by United States Anti-Doping Agency (USADA) in and out of competition.

PROTEIN

The protein needs of athletes have been debated. The current RDA is 0.8 g/kg bodyweight, and the acceptable macronutrient distribution range for protein for people 18 years and older is 10% to 35% of total calories. Factors affecting the protein needs of athletes include age, gender, lean body mass, fitness level, training regimen, and phase of competition.

Nitrogen balance studies in endurance athletes suggest a range of 1.2 g/kg to 1.4 g/kg/day, and for strength athletes 1.2 to 1.7 g/kg/day for protein intake, with the higher end of the range recommended early in the competitive season (Phillips, 2012).

Reports of food intake in athletes and nonathletes consistently indicate that protein represents from 12% to 20% of total energy intake or 1.2 to 2 g/kg/day. The exception to the rule is small, active women who may consume a low-energy intake in conjunction with their exercise or training program. Although these women may consume close to the RDA for protein in conjunction with the restricted energy intake, it may be inadequate to maintain lean body mass.

However, the need for protein during exercise is elevated just slightly above that for sedentary persons. Consuming more protein than the body can use is not necessary and should be avoided. When athletes consume diets that are high in protein, they compromise their carbohydrate status, which may affect their ability to train and compete at peak levels. High protein intakes also can result in diuresis and potential dehydration. Protein foods are often also high in fat, and consumption of excess protein can create difficulty in maintaining a low-fat diet.

Protein Needs for Resistance Exercise

Protein needs for resistance exercise involve maintenance (minimum protein required to accomplish nitrogen equilibrium) and the need for increasing lean tissue (positive nitrogen balance). Strategies to increase the concentration and availability of amino acids after resistance exercise such as timing of snacks and meals continue to be an area of ongoing research (Aguirre et al, 2013).

Dietary protein intake also may have a beneficial role in exercise recovery by attenuating impairments in endurance performance, which accompany intensified periods of training.

Type, Timing, and Amount of Protein for Muscle Hypertrophy

Still a hot topic among athletes and in the sports nutrition community, many factors appear to contribute to overall muscle hypertrophy. Nutritional factors that control protein synthesis during exercise are not well understood, leaving experts in discord about the type, amount, and timing of meals to enhance protein synthesis and muscle hypertrophy.

Resistance training (RT) and diet consistently appear to play a role in post-workout muscle protein synthesis. The metabolic basis for muscle growth appears to be a balance between muscle protein synthesis (MPS) and prevention of catabolism, especially the balance of myofibrillar protein or contractile protein synthesis, in which dietary protein plus exercise plays an important role. Resistance training enhances the anabolism by 40% to 100% over and above resting levels and dietary protein response for up to 24 hours when protein is consumed immediately before and at least within 24 hours after (Tipton and Phillips, 2013). This higher combined rate of protein synthesis after exercise has been shown to occur in young and elderly men.

Research suggests the anabolic response to resistance exercise, and protein ingestion works just as well with whole food proteins as with nutritional supplement proteins, although convenience often makes the difference because taking a high-protein shake or bar to training is more practical than carrying a chicken breast.

Between 20 and 25 g of a high-quality protein maximizes the response of MPS after resistance exercise, whereas no difference occurs between the ingestion of 20 g of protein and 40 g, suggesting that more is not better, at least in young, resistance-trained males. Preworkout ingestion of essential amino acids also appears to enhance the MPS response. However, more protein may be required to maximize the response of MPS when less than optimal protein sources (complete vs. noncomplete) are used in older individuals (Tipton and Phillips, 2013).

Although the inclusion of carbohydrates does not seem to have an impact on protein synthesis, it may have an impact on the prevention of breakdown. Fat content of postworkout fuel also may have a positive impact as in one study, whole milk enhanced synthesis more than skim milk did (Tipton and Phillips, 2013).

For athletes interested in muscle hypertrophy, it appears that neither the type nor the amount of protein matters if the day's total amount is within the recommended range for resistance-training athletes of 1.2 to 2 g of protein per kilogram of body weight. Research shows that a minimum of 30 g of high-quality protein at each meal that contains 2.5 g leucine per meal will optimally stimulate protein synthesis. Recent preliminary evidence suggests that leucine in addition to omega-3 fatty acid supplementation may help reduce muscle loss for acutely injured athletes (Tipton, 2013).

FAT

Even though maximum performance is impossible without muscle glycogen, fat also provides energy for exercise. Fat is the most concentrated source of food energy, supplying 9 kcal/g. Essential fatty acids are necessary for cell membranes, skin health, hormones, and transport of fat-soluble vitamins. The body has total glycogen stores (muscle and liver), equaling approximately 2600 calories, whereas each pound of body fat supplies about 3500 calories. This means that an athlete weighing 74 kg (163 lb) with 10% body fat has 16.3 lb of fat and thus carries energy worth about 57,000 calories depending on his or her metabolism. Even if this number is individualized, and not known accurately, it is still far more calories than that supplied by the athlete's glycogen stores.

Fat is the major, if not most important, fuel for light- to moderate-intensity exercise. Although fat is a valuable metabolic fuel for muscle activity during longer aerobic exercise and performs many important functions in the body, more than the usual recommended amount of fat is not indicated. In addition, athletes who consume a high-fat diet may consume fewer calories from carbohydrate, which may be detrimental to short-term performance.

The distribution of substrate in the diet also determines which substrate is used during an exercise bout. If an athlete is consuming a high-carbohydrate diet, he or she will use more glycogen as fuel for the exercise. If the diet is high in fat, more fat will be oxidized as a fuel source. Fat oxidation rates decline after the ingestion of a high-fat diet, partly because of adaptations at the muscle level, greater utilization of fat, and decreased glycogen stores as a result of lower carbohydrate intakes. Fasting longer than 6 hours optimizes fat oxidation; however, the ingestion of carbohydrates in the hours before or at the beginning of an exercise session augments the rate of fat oxidation significantly compared with fasting all the way up to the race (Volek et al, 2014; Yeo et al, 2011).

Exercise intensity and duration are important determinants of fat oxidation. Fat oxidation rates decrease when exercise intensity becomes high. A high-fat diet has been shown to compromise high-intensity performance even when a high-fat diet regimen is followed by carbohydrate loading before high-intensity performance (McArdle et al, 2013). The mode and duration of exercise also can affect fat oxidation; running increases fat oxidation more than cycling (Rosenkilde et al, 2013).

Fats, Inflammation, and Sports Injury

When athletes are injured, they want to heal and get back to training as soon as possible. Specific foods at the right time can help to provide energy for rehabilitation, rebuild strength, and ensure a complete, healthy, and faster recovery.

Stress to muscle leads to inflammation, bruising, and tissue breakdown. Failure to decrease inflammation can lead to scar tissue, poor mobility, and delayed recovery times. The inflammatory stage is affected by foods, especially by the types of dietary fat consumed. A diet high in trans fats, saturated fats, and some omega-6 vegetable oils has been shown to promote inflammation, whereas a diet high in monounsaturated fat and essential omega-3 fats has been shown to be anti-inflammatory (see Chapter 3 and Appendix 31). Monounsaturated fats such as olive, peanut, canola, and sesame oils as well as avocado oil also inhibit and reduce inflammation by interfering with proinflammatory compounds such as leukotrienes, which are produced naturally by the body. Diets supplemented with omega-3 fats have been shown to reduce postexercise delayed-onset muscle soreness and inflammation and promote healing (Jouris et al, 2011). There is also evidence to suggest a strong connection between omega-3 status and neuroprotection and supplementation to accelerate recovery from traumatic brain injury, including concussion (Michael-Titus and Priestley, 2014).

Supplemental omega-3 fat has been recommended during the inflammation stage after injury, especially when the diet is deficient. However, some concern exists regarding the sources of omega-3 fat supplements and fish oils, because some have been found to be contaminated with mercury and polychlorinated biphenyls (PCBs), toxins dangerous to humans (see *Focus On*: Omega-3 Fatty Acids in Pregnancy and Lactation in Chapter 15).

Fruits and vegetables are also good sources of alpha linolenic acid (ALA), an omega-3 fatty acid. However, the conversion in the body of ALA to the more active forms of omega-3 fatty acids, DHA and EPA, is very low. Plant-based foods rich in ALA include flaxseeds, chia seeds, walnuts, almonds, and tofu. Wheat germ, free-range beef, poultry, and some eggs are also good sources of omega-3 fats when the animals are fed omega-3 rich food (see Appendix 34).

FLUID

Maintaining fluid balance requires the constant integration of input from hypothalamic osmoreceptors and vascular baroreceptors so that fluid intake matches or modestly exceeds fluid loss (McArdle et al, 2013). Proper fluid balance maintains blood volume, which in turn supplies blood to the skin for body temperature regulation. Because exercise produces heat, which must be eliminated from the body to maintain appropriate temperatures, regular fluid intake is essential. Any fluid deficit that is incurred during an exercise session can potentially compromise the subsequent exercise bout.

The body maintains appropriate temperatures by **thermoregulation**. As heat is generated in the muscles during exercise, it is transferred via the blood to the body's core. Increased core temperature results in increased blood flow to the skin; in cool to moderate ambient temperatures, heat is then transferred to the environment by convection, radiation, and evaporation.

Environmental conditions have a large effect on thermoregulation. When ambient temperatures range from warm to hot, the body must dissipate the heat generated from exercise, as well as the heat absorbed from the environment. When this occurs, the body relies solely on the evaporation of sweat to maintain appropriate body temperatures. Thus maintaining hydration becomes crucial when ambient temperatures reach or exceed 36° C (96.8° F). The hotter the temperature, the more important sweating is for body-heat dissipation. Exercise in the heat also affects blood flow and alters the stress response, with modest changes in circulating leukocytes and cytokines. A critical threshold for elevation of body temperature is 6° F (3.5° C), above which the systemic inflammatory response leads to heatstroke.

Humidity affects the body's ability to dissipate heat to a greater extent than air temperatures. As humidity increases, the rate at which sweat evaporates decreases, which means more sweat drips off the body without transferring heat from the body to the environment. Combining the effects of a hot, humid environment with a large metabolic heat load produced during exercise taxes the thermoregulatory system to its maximum. Ensuring proper and adequate fluid intake is key to reducing the risk of heat stress.

Fluid Balance

Body fluid balance is regulated by mechanisms that reduce urinary water and sodium excretion, stimulate thirst, and control the intake and output of water and electrolytes. In response to dehydration, antidiuretic hormone (ADH or vasopressin) and the renin-angiotensin II–aldosterone system increase water and sodium retention by the kidneys and provoke an increase in thirst. These hormones maintain the osmolality, sodium content, and volume of extracellular fluids and play a major role in the regulation of fluid balance (see Chapter 6).

Water losses throughout the course of the day include those from sweat and the respiratory tract, plus losses from the kidneys and GI tract. When fluid is lost from the body in the form of sweat, plasma volume decreases and plasma osmolality increases. The kidneys, under hormonal control, regulate water and solute excretion in excess of the obligatory urine loss. However, when the body is subjected to hot environments, hormonal adjustments occur to maintain body function. Some of these adjustments include the body's conservation of water and sodium and the release of ADH by the pituitary gland to increase water absorption from the kidneys. These changes cause the urine to become more concentrated, thus conserving fluid and making the urine a dark gold color. This feedback process helps to conserve body water and blood volume.

At the same time, aldosterone is released from the adrenal cortex and acts on the renal tubules to increase the resorption of sodium, which helps maintain the correct osmotic pressure. These reactions also activate thirst mechanisms in the body. However, in situations in which water losses are increased acutely, such as in athletic workouts or competition, the thirst response can be delayed, making it difficult for athletes to trust their thirst to ingest enough fluid to offset the volume of fluid lost during training and competition. A loss of 1.5 to 2 L of fluid is necessary before the thirst mechanism kicks in, and this level of water loss already has a serious effect on temperature control. *Athletes need to rehydrate on a timed basis rather than as a reaction to thirst, and it should be enough to maintain the preexercise weight.*

Imbalance between fluid intake and fluid loss during prolonged exercise may increase the risk for dehydration. Dehydration may enhance the development of hyperthermia, heat exhaustion, and heat stroke.

Men appear to have higher sweat rates that may lead to more fluid loss during exercise compared with women. Studies also have shown that men have higher plasma sodium levels and a higher prevalence of hypernatremia than women after prolonged exercise, which suggests larger fluid losses in men. In contrast, it also is reported that women have an increased risk for overdrinking, which could lead to exercise-associated hyponatremia. This was demonstrated in a recent endurance study that compared female and male walkers. The study demonstrated a significantly larger change in body mass in men than in women, a higher incidence of dehydration in the men (27% of the men vs. 0% of the women showed postexercise hypernatremia), and a significantly lower fluid intake and higher fluid loss in the men compared with females (Eijsvogels et al, 2013).

In one study, approximately 66% of collegiate athletes, more men than women, were found to be dehydrated pretraining, which may be due to individual hydration habits, lack of hydration before early morning practices, or lack of knowledge regarding proper hydration before and after training (Volpe et al, 2009).

Although for years, studies have shown that substantial fluid and body mass losses greater than 2% of total body weight were related to an impaired exercise performance, a recent study shows otherwise (Wall et al, 2013). High-intensity prolonged exercise may increase the discrepancy between fluid intake and losses. In one study, increased body temperature and dehydration up to 3% in well-trained male cyclists, had no effect on a 25-km cycling time-trial performance in hot conditions in well-trained men who were blinded to their hydration status (Wall et al, 2013).

Daily Fluid Needs

Fluid intake recommendations for sedentary individuals vary greatly because of the wide disparity in daily fluid needs created by body size, physical activity, and environmental conditions. The DRI for water and electrolytes identifies the adequate intake for water to be 3.7 L/day for men (130 oz/day, 16 cups of fluid/day) and 2.7 L/day for women (95 oz/day, approximately 12 cups/day) (Institute of Medicine [IOM], 2005). Approximately 20% of the daily water need comes from water found in fruits and vegetables; the remaining 80% is provided by beverages, including water, juice, milk, coffee, tea, soup, sports drinks, and soft drinks. When individuals work, train, and compete in warm environments, their fluid needs can increase greatly, and this should be appreciated (McArdle et al, 2013).

Fluid Replacement

Controversy exists among experts as to how to assess fluid needs because there is no scientific consensus regarding the best method to assess hydration status. Recreational sports typically result in hypotonic fluid losses, which increase relative concentrations of blood and urine. Field measures to assess body hydration status include body mass measurements, urine specific gravity and color, and taste sensation. Each has its limitations (McArdle et al, 2013).

Several position statements and recommendations are published by a variety of professional organizations that address fluid and electrolyte replacement before, during, and after exercise. A summary of these recommendations can be found in Box 23-5.

BOX 23-5 Summary of Guidelines for Proper Hydration

General Guidelines

Monitor fluid losses: Weigh in before and after practice, especially during hot weather and the conditioning phase of the season.

Do not restrict fluids before, during or after the event.

Do not rely on thirst as an indicator of fluid losses.

Drink early and at regular intervals throughout the activity.

Do not consume alcohol before, during, or after exercise because it may act as a diuretic and prevent adequate fluid replenishment.

Discourage caffeinated beverages a few hours before and after physical activity because of their diuretic effect.

Before Exercise

Drink approximately 400 to 600 mL (14 to 22 oz) of water or sports drink 2 to 3 hr before the start of exercise.

During Exercise

Drink 150 to 350 mL (6 to 12 oz) of fluid every 15 to 20 min, depending on race speed, environmental conditions, and tolerance; no more than 1 C (8 to 10 oz) every 15 to 20 min, although individualized recommendations must be followed.

After Exercise

Drink 25% to 50% more than existing weight loss to ensure hydration 4 to 6 hours after exercise.

Drink 450 to 675 mL (16 to 24 oz) of fluid for every pound of body weight lost during exercise.

If an athlete is participating in multiple workouts in 1 day, then 80% of fluid loss must be replaced before the next workout.

Electrolyte Replacement

Sodium: 0.5 to 0.7 g/L in activity longer than 1 hour to enhance palatability and the drive to drink, to reduce the risk of hyponatremia and to minimize risk of muscle cramps.

TABLE 23-3 Comparison of the Sweat Electrolyte Losses* and Sports Drink Content

Electrolyte	Sweat Loss mg/L	Standard Sport Drink mg/L	Endurance Specific Sport Drink mg/L
Sodium	900-2600	230-1700	800-1110
Potassium	150	80-125	390-650
Magnesium	8.3-14.2	0	10-815
Chloride	900-1900	0	390-1550
Calcium	28	0-100	24-275
Iron	0.1-0.4	0	0
Phosphorus	40	0	0
Zinc	0.36-0.48	0	0—5

*Dependent on exercise duration, intensity, ambient temperature, hydration status before and during exercise

Baker A: Nutrition for Sports 22: Sweat mineral losses. http://www.arniebakercycling.com/pubs/Free/NS%20Sweat.pdf>. Accessed January 13, 2015; Kenefick RW, Cheuvront SN: Hydration for recreational sport and physical activity, *Nutr Rev* 70 (Suppl 2):S137, 2012.

When possible, fluid should be consumed at rates that closely match sweating rate. It appears that plain water is not the best beverage to consume after exercise to replace the water lost as sweat. Although specific recommendations differ slightly, the intent is to keep athletes well hydrated (Kenefick and Cheuvront, 2012).

Electrolytes

The replacement of electrolytes as well as water is essential for complete rehydration (see Table 23-3).

Sodium

It is important to include sodium in fluid-replacement solutions, especially with excessive intake of plain water (McArdle et al, 2013) for events lasting more than 2 hours; sodium should be added to the fluid to replace losses and to prevent hyponatremia. Rehydration with water alone dilutes the blood rapidly, increases its volume, and stimulates urine output. Blood dilution lowers sodium and the volume-dependent part of the thirst drive, thus removing much of the drive to drink and replace fluid losses.

The potential benefits of temporary hyperhydration with sodium salts are important. Sodium losses can contribute to heat cramping, especially among football players. In fact, in one study, 75% of National Football League teams use pregame hyperhydration with intravenous fluid to prevent muscle cramps.

Besides individual variations, the intensity and duration of workouts appear to play a role in the amount of sodium lost.

Water-soluble electrolytes such as sodium can move rapidly across the proximal intestines. During prolonged exercise lasting more than 4 to 5 hours, including sodium in replacement fluids increases palatability and facilitates fluid uptake from the intestines. Sodium and carbohydrate are actively transported from the lumen to the bloodstream.

Water replacement in the absence of supplemental sodium can lead to decreased plasma sodium concentrations. As plasma sodium levels fall below 130 mEq/L, symptoms can include lethargy, confusion, seizures, or loss of consciousness. Exercise-induced hyponatremia may result from fluid overloading during prolonged exercise over 4 hours. Hyponatremia is associated with individuals who drink plain water in excess of their sweat losses or who are less physically conditioned and produce a saltier sweat.

Potassium

As the major electrolyte inside the body's cells, potassium works in close association with sodium and chloride in maintaining body fluids, as well as generating electrical impulses in the nerves, muscles, and heart. Potassium balance is regulated by aldosterone and its regulation is precise. Although aldosterone acts on sweat glands to increase the resorption of sodium, potassium secretion is unaffected. Loss of potassium from skeletal muscle has been implicated in fatigue during athletic events. There is little loss of potassium through sweat; loss of 32 to 48 mEq/day does not appear to be significant and is easily replaced by diet.

Fluid Absorption

The speed at which fluid is absorbed depends on a number of different factors, including the amount, type, temperature, and osmolality of the fluid consumed and the rate of gastric emptying. Because glucose is absorbed actively in the intestines, it can markedly increase sodium and water absorption. A carbohydrate-electrolyte solution enhances exercise capacity by elevating blood sugar, maintaining high rates of carbohydrate oxidation, preventing central fatigue, and reducing perceived exertion (Lynch, 2013).

Early studies indicate that water absorption is maximized when luminal glucose concentrations range from 1% to 3% (55 to 140 mM); however, most sports drinks contain two to three times this quantity without causing adverse GI symptoms. To determine the concentration of carbohydrate in a sports drink, the grams of carbohydrate or sugar in a serving are divided by the weight of a serving of the drink, which is usually 240 g, the approximate weight of 1 cup of water. A 6% carbohydrate drink contains 14 to 16 g of carbohydrate per 8 oz (1 cup).

Cold water is preferable to warm water because it attenuates changes in core temperature and peripheral blood flow, decreases sweat rate, speeds up gastric emptying, and is absorbed more quickly. In one recent study, sweating response was influenced by water temperature and voluntary intake volume. Cool tap water at 60° F appeared to replace fluids better in dehydrated individuals compared with warmer fluids (Hosseinlou et al, 2013).

Burton showed that, although ingestion of cold beverages is preferable, an ergogenic benefit was also seen from the effect of ice slush ingestion and mouthwash on thermoregulation and endurance performance in the heat (Burdon et al, 2013). Another study compared ice slush to cold water in moderately active males while running and showed prolonged time to exhaustion and reduced rectal temperature, supporting possible sensory and psychologic effects of ice slush beverages either consumed or used as a mouthwash. Precooling with an ice slushy solution also may have more beneficial effects over cold fluid ingestion during exercise and performance (Dugas, 2011).

Children

Children differ from adults in that, for any given level of dehydration, their core temperatures rise faster than those of adults, probably because of a greater number of heat-activated sweat glands per unit skin area than in adolescents or adults. Children sweat less even though they achieve higher core temperatures. Sweat composition also differs between children and adults: adults have higher sodium and chloride concentrations but lower lactate, hydrogen, and potassium concentrations. Children also take longer to acclimate to heat than adolescents and adults (McArdle et al, 2013).

Because young children do not drink enough when offered fluids freely during exercise in hot and humid climates, and because they participate in physical activities less than 60 minutes in duration, often little attention is paid to their hydration.

Children who participate in sports activities must be taught to prevent dehydration by drinking above and beyond thirst and at frequent intervals, such as every 20 minutes. A rule of thumb is that a child 10 years of age or younger should drink until he or she does not feel thirsty and then should drink an additional half a glass (3 to 4 oz or $\frac{1}{3}$ to $\frac{1}{2}$ cup) of fluid.

Older children and adolescents should follow the same guidelines; however, they should consume an additional cup of fluid (8 oz). When relevant, regulations for competition should be modified to allow children to leave the playing field periodically to drink. One of the hurdles to getting children to consume fluids is to provide fluids they like. Providing a sports drink or slushy ice drink as described in the previous section that will maintain the drive to drink may be the key to keeping child athletes hydrated.

Older Athletes

Older, mature, or masters-level athletes are also at extra risk for dehydration and need to take precautions when exercising. Hypohydration (water loss exceeding water intake with a body water deficit) in older individuals can affect circulatory and thermoregulatory function to a greater extent and may be caused by the lower skin blood flow, causing core temperature to rise. Because the thirst drive is reduced in older adults, they need to drink adequately before exercise, well before they become thirsty (McArdle et al, 2013).

Hydration at High Altitudes

Unacclimated individuals undergo a plasma volume contraction when acutely exposed to moderately high altitude. This is the result of increased renal sodium and water excretion and decreased voluntary sodium and water intake. Respiratory losses are increased by high ventilatory rates and typically dry air. The result is an increase in serum hematocrit and hemoglobin, which increases the oxygen-carrying capacity of the blood, but at the cost of reduced blood volume, stroke volume, and cardiac output. Fluid requirements increase as a result. With acclimation, red blood cell production increases and plasma and blood volumes return to pre–high altitude levels.

OTHER CONSIDERATIONS

Carbohydrates
Chocolate Milk

Postexercise carbohydrate intake has been shown to augment recovery from heavy aerobic exercise. The effects of carbohydrate and protein coingestion have been investigated more recently, including the potential influences of chocolate milk.

The efficacy of carbohydrates and protein together could be due to influences on glycogen resynthesis, protein turnover, rehydration, attenuations in muscle disruption, or perhaps a combination of these factors. However, there are inconsistencies in the literature regarding the effects of carbohydrates and protein on these factors, and the mechanisms explaining potential influences after endurance exercise are not defined clearly.

Some studies report that carbohydrate and protein beverages such as chocolate milk can enhance subsequent exercise performance better than carbohydrate-only beverages, although others have reported no positive effects (Lunn et al, 2012; Peschek et al, 2013). Compared with placebo of an isocaloric carbohydrate–only beverage, chocolate milk has been shown to improve recovery from high intensity and endurance training in runners and cyclists. Postexercise chocolate milk supplementation also has been shown to improve subsequent exercise performance and muscle glycogen synthesis and provide a greater intracellular signaling stimulus for protein synthesis (Lunn et al, 2012). Chocolate milk can be an affordable recovery beverage for some athletes.

VITAMINS AND MINERALS

Micronutrients enable the use of macronutrients for all physiologic processes and are key regulators in health and work performance. Athletes who fail to consume a diet with adequate vitamins and minerals can become deficient, which can lead to impairments in training and performance. High training volume, exercise performed in stressful conditions including hot conditions, altitude, or training with substandard diets may promote excessive losses of micronutrients because of increased catabolism or excretion (Rodriquez et al, 2009).

Training and work schedules, low-nutrient snacks, infrequent nutrient-dense meals, and overall low calorie intakes may cause inadequate intakes of vitamins and minerals. Athletes who adopt popular diets that eliminate whole food groups such as meat, dairy, grains, or fruits, as in the case of vegetarians or Paleo enthusiasts, run the risk of poor micronutrient intake. Micronutrients such as calcium, zinc, iron, vitamin B_{12}, and others will be of concern.

Description of vitamin metabolism and resulting physical performance is very limited. Assessments of vitamin intake, biochemical measures of vitamin status, and determination of resulting physical performance are required; however, very few studies have provided this information.

A 2010 report reported numerous dietary vitamin and mineral deficiencies in elite female athletes including folate (48%), calcium (24%), magnesium (19%), and iron (4%) (Heaney et al, 2010). A 2014 report also highlighted the risk of injury in female athletes with iron, vitamin D, and calcium deficiencies (McClung et al, 2014).

A 2013 study of male athletes showed significant deficiencies in vitamin A (44% of group), vitamin C (80% of group), vitamin D (92% of group), folate (84% of group), calcium (52% of group), and magnesium, (60% of group) (Wierniuk and Włodarek, 2013).

Without a doubt, impaired micronutrient status affects exercise and work performance. Some of the deficiency signs and symptoms associated with exercise have been summarized in this section (see Table 23-4).

B Vitamins

Increased energy metabolism creates a need for more of the B vitamins, including thiamin, riboflavin, niacin, pyridoxine, folate, biotin, pantothenic acid, and choline, which serve as part of coenzymes involved in regulating energy metabolism by modulating the synthesis and degradation of carbohydrates, protein, fat, and bioactive compounds.

Some athletes who have poor diets and athletes such as wrestlers, jockeys, figure skaters, gymnasts, or rowers who consume low-calorie diets for long periods of time may be prone to deficiencies. A B-complex vitamin supplement to meet the RDA may be appropriate. However, there is no evidence that supplementing the well-nourished athlete with more B vitamins increases performance.

The intake of folic acid could potentially be low in athletes whose consumption of whole grains, whole fruits, and vegetables

TABLE 23-4 Vitamin and Mineral Deficiency Signs and Symptoms Associated with Exercise

Vitamin/ Mineral	Function	Deficiency Sign or Symptom	Evidence for Supplementation to Improve Performance
B_1 Thiamin	Carbohydrate and protein metabolism	Weakness, decreased endurance, muscle wasting, weight loss, pyruvate accumulation, increased circulating lactate, fatigue, reduced performance	To correct deficiency
B_2 Riboflavin	Oxidative metabolism, electron transport system	Altered skin and mucous membrane, and nervous system function limited	In athletes whose food availability may be at initiation of increased physical activity
B_3 Niacin	Oxidative metabolism, electron transport system	Irritability, diarrhea	Adequate in athletes, no impact on performance
B_6 Pyridoxine	Gluconeogenesis	Dermatitis, convulsions	Not shown effective
Folic Acid	Hemoglobin and nucleic acid formation	Anemia, fatigue	In deficiency
B_{12} Cyancobalamin	Hemoglobin formation	Anemia, neurological symptoms	In deficiency
Vitamin C	Antioxidant	Fatigue, loss of appetite	In depleted states, including environmental stress, infection altitude, high temperatures, cigarette smoking; 250 or 500 mg may reduce body heat, enhance immune function & facilitate recovery from intense training
Vitamin A	Antioxidant	Appetite loss, prone to infections	No evidence to suggest supplementation even in dietary deficient athletes
Vitamin E	Antioxidant	Nerve and muscle damage	Evidence lacking; results equivocal with regard to reducing exercised-induced damage
Magnesium	Energy metabolism, nerve and muscle contraction	Muscle weakness, nausea, irritability, impaired performance	May increase muscle strength, improve cellular function; lactate and oxygen update shown to decrease in exhaustive rowing; those with adequate status not shown to benefit
Iron	Hemoglobin synthesis	Anemia, cognitive impairment, immune abnormalities	Equivocal results in Fe-deficient nonanemic athletes; supplementation in women with depleted serum iron but not anemic enhanced muscle function
Zinc	Nucleic acid synthesis, glycolysis	Growth retardation, appetite loss, immune abnormalities	May benefit when zinc intake suboptimal; diet intakes within 70% maintains serum levels
Chromium	Glucose metabolism	Glucose intolerance	High-intensity exercise may increase urinary loss, albeit small; supplements not shown to improve body comp or performance or strength

is low; however, folate supplementation in deficient athletes has not been shown to improve performance. A deficiency of vitamin B_{12} could develop in a vegetarian athlete after several years of a strict vegan intake; thus a vitamin B_{12} supplement may be warranted. However B_{12} supplementation has not been shown to improve performance in athletes consuming adequate amounts of B_{12}.

Choline

Choline is a water-soluble nutrient typically found in foods rich in B vitamins. Choline is synthesized in the body from other nutrients and therefore is not considered essential. Some evidence suggests that choline, found in fatty foods, peanuts, dairy products, and egg yolks, is low in men and women, and is shown to decrease after certain types of strenuous exercise and this may affect performance (Penry and Manore, 2008).

Choline has been promoted to athletes to improve physical endurance by increasing fat lipolysis and acetylcholine production to increase muscle contractions and delay fatigue, although evidence does not support these claims (Castell et al, 2010).

Choline supplements may cause gastrointestinal side effects, including breakdown to trimethylamine, which leads to a fishy body odor.

Antioxidants

Antioxidants have been studied individually and collectively for their potential to enhance exercise performance or to prevent exercise-induced muscle tissue damage. Cells continuously produce free radicals and reactive oxygen species (ROS) as a part of metabolic processes. The rate of oxygen consumption during exercise may increase 10- to 15-fold, or as much as 100-fold in active peripheral skeletal muscles. This oxidative stress increases the generation of lipid peroxides and free radicals, and the magnitude of stress depends on the ability of the body's tissues to detoxify ROS (see Chapter 3).

Free radicals are neutralized by antioxidant defense systems that protect cell membranes from oxidative damage. These systems include catalase; superoxide dismutase; glutathione peroxidase; antioxidant vitamins A, E, and C; selenium; and phytonutrients such as carotenoids (see Chapter 3). Susceptibility to oxidative stress varies from person to person and the effect is influenced by diet, lifestyle, environmental factors, and training. Antioxidant nutrients may enhance recovery from exercise by maintaining optimal immune response, and lowering lipid peroxidation.

Although large-dose antioxidant supplementation attenuates exercise-induced reaction oxygen species (ROS) production and consequential oxidative damage, studies suggest oversupplementation may block necessary cellular adaptations to exercise (Sureda et al, 2013). In a recent study of 14 trained male runners, 152 mg of vitamin C and 50 mg vitamin E supplementation daily reduced oxidation of neutrophil proteins without inhibiting cellular adaptation to exercise. Further research is needed to assess the response to supplementation with varying degrees of exercise duration and intensity (Sureda et al, 2013). Another 2012 study showed that, although vitamin C and E supplementation may attenuate the acute exercise-induced increase in the inflammatory cytokine plasma IL-6, it does not seem to further decrease IL-6 levels after 12 weeks of supplementation combined with endurance training (Yfanti et al, 2012).

A diet rich in fruits and vegetables can ensure an adequate intake of antioxidants, and prudent use of an antioxidant supplement may provide insurance against a suboptimal diet and the increased stress from exercise.

Recent research has shown the positive benefits of phytonutrients with anti-inflammatory and antioxidant effects, especially anthocyanins found in purple and red fruits, and vegetables may help with posttraining inflammation. One review study suggests the benefits of quercetin found in red onions, blueberries, tomatoes, apples, black tea, purple grapes, and red onions. These compounds found in tart cherry juice can help to reduce inflammation, muscle damage, and oxidative stress after marathon running (Howatson et al, 2010). An unexpected effect of tart cherry juice is that it also may have a beneficial effect on sleep, which has been attributed to the high melatonin content of tart cherries (Howatson et al, 2010).

Vitamin C

Vitamin C is involved in a number of important biochemical pathways that are important to exercise metabolism. For example vitamin C is involved in the synthesis of carnitine, which transports long-chain fatty acids into the mitochondria for energy production. The effect of vitamin C supplementation on performance has received considerable attention, mainly because athletes consume vitamin C in large quantities, generally because of the volume of food they consume. Athletes generally have normal plasma vitamin C levels.

In studies in which athletes were deficient in vitamin C, supplementation improved physical performance, but a thorough analysis of these studies supports the general conclusion that vitamin C supplementation does not increase physical performance capacity in subjects with normal body levels of vitamin C. On the other hand, because exercise is a stressor to the body, some nutritionists recommend that the active individual may need more vitamin C than the DRI.

Fat-Soluble Vitamins

Vitamins A, D, E, and K have no direct role in energy metabolism; rather they play supportive roles in energy use. Vitamin A acts as an antioxidant in reducing muscle damage from exercise, whereas vitamin K functions in coagulation and bone formation.

Vitamin D

Over the past few years, vitamin D has been shown to play an increasingly important role in sports performance beyond its role in calcium absorption and use in bone formation (Todd et al, 2014). As a secosteroid hormone, upon activation to 1,25 hydroxyvitamin D_3, vitamin D responsive gene expression is altered with more than 1000 responsive genes affecting muscle protein synthesis, muscle strength, muscle size, reaction time, balance coordination, endurance, inflammation, and immunity, all of which are important to athletic performance.

Vitamin D deficiency may be more common in athletes than previously thought, especially in specific groups (Shuler et al, 2012). The prevalence appears to vary by sport, training location, and time of year and skin color (Larson-Meyer and Willis, 2010). Research has shown that more than 75% of Caucasians and 90% of African Americans and Latinos are possibly vitamin D deficient according to set values. It is possible that up to 77% of athletes who live in northern climates with little winter sunlight and who are indoor athletes, (94% of basketball players, and 83% of gymnasts) may be affected by deficiencies

BOX 23-6 Vitamin D and Athletic Performance

2,313 athletes in 23 studies – 56% were deficient
Football Players: 19.1% had adequate vitamin D levels; 50.6% had insufficient levels; 30.3% had deficient levels.

Vitamin D Potential Impact on Athletic Performance

Positive effect on muscle strength, power, and mass
Increased force and power output of skeletal muscle tissue
May influence maximal oxygen uptake (VO$_2$ Max)
Improved skeletal muscle function & bone strength
Potentially increased size and number of type II muscle fibers
Decreased recovery time from training
Increase testosterone production

From:

Dahlquist DT et al: Plausible ergogenic effects of vitamin D on athletic performance and recovery, *J Int Soc Sports Nutr*, 12:33, 2015.
Farrokhyar F et al: Prevalence of vitamin D inadequacy in athletes: a systematic-review and meta-analysis, *Sports Med* 45:365, 2015.
Maroon JC et al: Vitamin D profile in National Football League players, *Am J Sports Med* 43:1241, 2015.

of vitamin D (Cannell et al, 2009). Outdoor athletes may not have an advantage over indoor athletes; in a National Football league study, 81% of Caucasian and African American players may be at risk for deficiency (see Box 23-6). Blood tests can better determine deficiency states. A measurement of 25-(OH) D levels of 50 ng/ml or less is a value used to determine those at risk.

Although the specific amount of vitamin D needed to reverse deficiency states has not been determined, partly because it depends on the extent of deficiency, athletes should be tested and guided by a health professional if diagnosed with a deficiency (see Chapter 7 and Appendices 22 and 45).

Recent research suggests supplemental vitamin D increased serum 25(OH) D concentrations and enhanced the recovery in peak isometric force after the damaging event, and attenuated the immediate and delayed increase in circulating biomarkers representative of muscle damage (ALT or AST) (Barker et al, 2013).

After a detailed assessment, recommendations for attaining and maintaining optimal vitamin D levels can be individualized to the athlete's current 25-(OH)D concentration, diet, lifestyle habits, belief system, and clinical symptoms. The recommendation for fair-skinned individuals is to obtain 5 minutes and for dark skin 30 minutes of sunlight exposure to arms, legs, and back several times a week without sunscreen (see Appendix 45). Short-term, high-dose "loading" regimens for rapid repletion under the care of a physician also may be beneficial (Todd et al, 2014).

Vitamin E

Vitamin E is used widely as a supplement by athletes who hope to improve performance. Vitamin E may protect against exercise-induced oxidative injury and acute immune response changes.

MINERALS

Although 12 minerals have been shown to be designated as essential nutrients, iron, calcium, magnesium, and copper have biochemical functions with the potential to affect performance.

Iron

Iron is critical for sport performance because, as a component of hemoglobin, it is instrumental in transporting oxygen from the lungs to the tissues. It performs a similar role in myoglobin, which acts within the muscle as an oxygen acceptor to hold a supply of oxygen readily available for use by the mitochondria. Iron is also a vital component of the cytochrome enzymes involved in the production of ATP. Iron adequacy can be a limiting factor in performance because deficiency limits aerobic endurance and the capacity for work. Even partial depletion of iron stores in the liver, spleen, and bone marrow, as evidenced by low serum ferritin levels, may have a detrimental effect on exercise performance, even when anemia is not present (see Chapter 32).

Sports anemia is a term applied to at least three different conditions: hemodilution, iron deficiency anemia, and foot-strike anemia. Athletes at risk are the rapidly growing male adolescent; the female athlete with heavy menstrual losses; the athlete with an energy-restricted diet; distance runners who may have increased GI iron loss, hematuria, hemolysis caused by foot impact, and myoglobin leakage; and those training with heavy sweating in hot climates. Recent research suggests that anemia may be common in female athletes, especially adolescent and premenopausal females, long-distance runners, and vegetarians, who should be screened periodically to assess their iron status.

Heavy endurance training also can cause a transient decrease in serum ferritin and hemoglobin. This condition, known as sports or pseudoanemia is characterized by reduced hemoglobin levels resulting from expanding blood volumes that are almost those of clinical anemia, but return to pretraining normal levels. Performance does not appear to deteriorate and the pseudoanemia may in fact improve aerobic capacity and performance (McArdle et al, 2013).

Some athletes, especially long-distance runners, experience GI bleeding that is related to the intensity and duration of the exercise, the athlete's ability to stay hydrated, how well the athlete is trained, and whether he or she has taken ibuprofen before the competition. Iron loss from GI bleeding can be detected by fecal hemoglobin assays. See *Clinical Insight:* GI Issues in Athletes.

It is possible that using serum hemoglobin as the determining factor for identifying anemic athletes who may benefit from iron supplementation with performance improvement is not the best biomarker. Nonanemic athletes (with normal serum hemoglobins) who are supplemented with iron have shown improved performance (DellaValle, 2013). Optimal levels of serum ferritin, which is the most common index of body iron status associated with performance, and thus a better marker, may also be inadequate, because athletes supplemented with iron to achieve higher than "normal" serum ferritin levels have also shown improved performance (DellaValle, 2013). Some athletes experience iron deficiency without anemia, and have normal hemoglobin levels but reduced levels of serum ferritin (20-30 ng/ml; see Chapter 7).

Athletes should be assessed for their iron status using serum hemoglobin and serum ferritin at the beginning of and during the training season. This is especially important in those suspected to have sickle cell trait (SCT), because their rate of sudden death is 10 to 30 times higher than in non-SCT athletes. Typically deaths have occurred early in the season, during exhaustive drills in hot weather without adequate warmup time (Harris et al, 2012). In 2010 the NCAA instituted a universal screening program to test for SCT in all Division I athletes; however, in athletes at the high school level, in the NBA, NFL, Navy, Marines, and Air Force, testing is not required (Jung et al, 2011).

Although male athletes have been reported to consume at least the RDA for iron, female athletes tend to consume somewhat less for a variety of reasons, including low energy intake, lower intake of animal products, or adherence to a vegetarian or vegan diet (Woolf et al, 2009). Increasing dietary intake of iron or supplementation is the only way to replace iron losses and improve status.

Who should be supplemented and with how much iron remains to be answered. Given the evidence suggesting iron's role in overall health and physical performance, there is no debate that athletes with clinical deficiency should be identified and treated. Whether those with subclinical deficiency should be treated with iron supplementation remains controversial. Individuals with normal status typically do not benefit from supplementation, and concerns regarding unregulated doses and overload should be considered.

Calcium

Suboptimal levels of dietary calcium intake are seen in athletes. Because low levels of calcium intake have been shown to be a contributing factor in osteoporosis, young female athletes, especially those who have had interrupted menstrual function, may be at risk for decreased bone mass.

The FAT in women's athletics is discussed earlier in the chapter. Strategies to promote the resumption of menses include estrogen replacement therapy, weight gain, and reduced training. Regardless of menstrual history, most female athletes need to increase their calcium, vitamin D_3, and magnesium intake. Low-fat and nonfat dairy products, calcium-fortified fruit juices, calcium-fortified soy milk, and tofu made with calcium sulfate are good sources (see Appendices 45 and 46).

Magnesium

Magnesium is an essential mineral that supports more than 300 enzymatic reactions including glycolysis, fat and protein metabolism, and adenosine triphosphate hydrolysis, and is a regulator of neuromuscular, immune, and hormonal functions. Although hypomagnesemia has been seen in athletes possibly caused by excessive sweating while training and transient redistribution of magnesium indicating a release from one storage area to an active site, levels return to normal within 24 hours after exercise (Malliaropoulos et al, 2013).

True magnesium deficiency has been shown to impair athletic performance, causing muscle spasms and increased heart rate and oxygen consumption during submaximal exercise. For deficient athletes, supplemental magnesium has been shown to improve performance by improving cellular function, although in athletes with adequate status, performance outcomes are mixed (Kass, 2013). In one recent study with female volleyball players, magnesium supplementation improved alactic (does not produce any lactic acid) anaerobic metabolism, even though the players were not magnesium deficient (Setaro et al, 2013). In another study with young men participating in a strength training program for 7 weeks, daily magnesium intake of 8 mg/kg of body weight resulted in increases in muscle strength and power, whereas marathon runners with adequate stores did not seem to benefit (Moslehi et al, 2013).

COPPER

Copper is a cofactor in numerous enzymes that potentially can affect sports performance, including antioxidant defense,

oxygen transport and utilization, immune function, and catecholamine and connective tissue synthesis. Athletes who report persistent fatigue, frequent infections, and stress fractures should have their copper status assessed. Copper supplementation should not be undertaken without clinical justification, because it can be toxic.

ERGOGENIC AIDS

Ergogenic aids include any training technique, mechanical device, nutrition practice, pharmacologic method, or physiologic technique that can improve exercise performance capacity and training adaptations. Many athletes devote substantial time and energy striving for optimal performance and training and turn to ergogenic aids, especially dietary supplements.

The Food and Drug Administration (FDA) regulates dietary supplement products and ingredients in addition to labeling, product claims, package inserts, and accompanying literature. The Federal Trade Commission (FTC) regulates dietary supplement advertising (http://www.fda.gov/food/dietarysupplements/). See Chapter 12 for a definition of a dietary supplement as defined by the Dietary Supplement Health and Education Act (DSHEA) of 1994.

DSHEA protects dietary supplements from being required to demonstrate proof of efficacy or safety. Manufacturers are allowed to publish limited information about the benefits of dietary supplements in the form of statements of support, as well as so-called structure and function claims. This results in a great deal of printed material that can be confusing to athletes at the point of sale of nutritional products. In addition athletes are bombarded with advertisements and testimonials from other athletes and coaches about the effects of dietary supplements on performance.

The use of ergogenic aids in the form of dietary supplements is widespread in all sports. Many athletes, whether recreational, elite, or professional, use some form of dietary supplementation (e.g., substances obtainable by prescription or by illegal means or others marked as supplements, vitamins, or minerals) to improve athletic performance or to assist with weight loss (Maughan et al, 2011).

According to a survey, 88% of collegiate athletes report using one or more nutritional supplements (Buell et al, 2013). A recent study found 25,000 supplement inquiries to the Resource Exchange Center (REC) of the National Center for Drug Free Sport. Among dietary supplements, inquiries for amino acids and their metabolites, vitamins and minerals, and herbal products occurred most frequently, with banned substances accounting for 30% of all inquiries submitted to the REC, and 18% of all medications searched in the database (Ambrose et al, 2013).

Surveys show reasons for supplement use are varied and differ between genders. Women athletes often take supplements for their health, or to overcome an inadequate diet, whereas men may take supplements to improve speed, agility, strength, and power and also use them to help build body mass and reduce weight or excess body fat.

A recent survey of track and field athletes competing in the world championships showed 89% of females and 83% of males reported using supplements for the following reasons: 71% to aid in recovery from training; 52% for health; 46% to improve performance; 40% to prevent or treat an illness; and 29% to compensate for a poor diet (Maughan et al, 2007).

See Table 23-5 for discussion of ergogenic aids commonly used by athletes.

TABLE 23-5 Ergogenic Aids

Ergogenic Aid	Reported Action/Claim	Research on Ergogenic Effects	Side Effects
α-Ketoglutarate	Intermediate in Krebs cycle	Some evidence as anti-catabolic after surgery; may impact mitochondrial functioning at altitude	None
ALA	Enzyme found in mitochondria involved in energy production	No studies of use in humans for sport; used in Europe with persons with diabetes to treat insulin resistance and neuropathy	None
Arginine	Protein synthesis; precursor to creatine and potential to increase GH; precursor to NO	Improves aerobic endurance performance; increases plasma nitrite, reduces O2 consumption during submax exercise	GI distress
Branched-chain amino acids	Decrease mental fatigue; Decrease exercise-induced protein degradation and muscle enzyme release	Some evidence that decreased fatigue may occur at higher altitudes	Mild GI distress for some
EAAs	Increase strength, endurance; accelerate recovery	Limited; suggests 3-6 g of EAAs before exercise; stimulate protein synthesis	Same as protein
Glutamine	Boosts immunity; stimulates protein and glycogen synthesis	May boost immunity with branched-chain amino acids and enriched whey	None reported
HMB	Metabolite of EAA leucine; anticatabolic; enhances recovery by stimulating protein and glycogen synthesis	3 gm in 2 divided doses shown to improve performance; may increase upper-body strength and lean body mass and minimize muscle damage; decreases muscle catabolism	None reported
Carnitine	In skeletal muscle oxidizes fat and CHO during exercise; bioavailability from food poor; vegetarians have lower stores	Studies weak, no effect on performance, energy metabolism; limited stores may impact performance, supplementation may improve stores marginally	None reported
Choline	Lipolysis, weight loss, increased time to fatigue, improved work performance	Low plasma levels shown in endurance athletes, may decrease fatigue; strenuous and prolonged physical activity appears to significantly decrease circulating levels; no performance benefits in those with adequate stores	GI upset; fishy odor
Chondroitin sulfate	Builds and grows cartilage	No studies that it is effective in treating arthritis or joint damage or helps torn ligaments or cartilage.	None
Glucosamine	Serves as non-steroidal anti-inflammatory drug alternative	Readily absorbed; benefit in reducing pain and need for medication	None reported
Glycerol	Decreases heat stress, increases body fluid volume, facilitates water absorption from intestines, lowers heat stress, heart rate, body temp; enhances endurance performance in heat	Mixed—reduces heart rate, thirst sensation, improved endurance output and peak power output reported	Bloating, nausea, dizziness, light headedness
Glutamine	Conditionally essential amino acid; improves muscle recovery	Mixed, no effect on performance	None reported
Green tea extract	Antioxidant; increases energy expenditure	Limited; may increase energy expenditure	Same as caffeine
Nitrates (beet juice)	Vasodilator, reduced BP, increased performance, time to exhaustion	Mechanism unclear, research shows it to be strong NO precursor which reduces O2 cost of submaximal exercise, increases mitochondrial efficiency, contractile function	None reported
COQ10	Cofactor for ATP production; electron transport in mitochondria; reduces fatigue	Mixed: double-blinded, placebo, cross-over trial, 100 mg/d for 2 mo., lift loads of 75 g/kg of body weight 5x/30 s improved mean power; may improve in those with mitochondrial disorders or CoQ deficiency	

Continued

TABLE 23-5 Ergogenic Aids—cont'd

Ergogenic Aid	Reported Action/Claim	Research on Ergogenic Effects	Side Effects
Beta-alanine	As precursor to carnosine, buffer and antioxidant potential	Mixed; 4-10 weeks of supplementation can increase carnosine by 50-80%; effects seen in 30s-7min sports; acidosis during 6 minute high intensity training bout blunted w/4 weeks supplements; effects start 3-4 weeks following start of supplementation and for 1 month after D/C supplement	Skin prickling (paresthesia) when exceeding recommended dose 10mg/kg body weight)
Pyruvate	Augments endurance exercise performance; promote fat loss	Double-blind studies showed increased upper/lower body endurance performance by 20%; increased cycle ergometer time to exhaustion when diet contains adequate CHO 55%, supplement to increase pre-exercise muscle glycogen levels	None reported
Quercetin	Anti-inflammatory, anticarcinogenic, cardioprotective, neuroprotective	Mixed reduced muscle damage and body fat; increase in total time to exhaustion in badminton; no improvements in other studies	None reported
Ribose	Replenishes high-energy compounds following intense exercise; increases power	Limited; can increase exercise capacity in heart patients; no significant difference in double-blind hot environment; greater improvement in 1 rep MAX bench press; no effects on greater sprint performances	None reported
Sodium bicarbonate/ sodium citrate	Buffers lactic acid production; delays fatigue	Increases body's ability to buffer lactic acid during sub max exercise for events lasting 1-7 min	Stomach distress: bloating, diarrhea; dangerous in high doses; alkalosis
Sodium phosphate	Buffer	Some; increases VO_2max and anaerobic threshold by 5%-10%; improves endurance	Stomach distress
Creatine	Improves strength, power and intermittent sprint performance; accelerate training recovery	Increases muscle free creatine, phosphocreatine; performance effect seen in sprint/power through endurance by enhancing muscle glycogen storage; stimulates muscle anabolism, muscle relaxation; effects may fade after 2 months supplementation; consume with CHO to increase levels to greater extent	Weight gain 0.8-2.9%; watch with weight sensitive sports; unknown long term

ALA, α-Lipoic acid; *CF*, cardiorespiratory fitness; *EAA*, essential amino acid; *EP*, endurance performance; *GH*, growth hormone; *HMB*, β-hydroxy-β-methylbutyrate; *NO*, nitric oxide.

Research suggests that all too often physically active individuals, including high-level athletes, obtain nutrition information from unreliable sources, including coaches, fellow athletes, trainers, advertisements, and the Internet rather than well-informed and educated sports dietitians, physicians, and accredited exercise professionals (Morente-Sánchez and Zabala, 2013). Information on the efficacy and safety of many of these products used by athletes is limited or completely lacking.

The biggest concern for athletes is the use of drugs prohibited in sport and the possibility that a supplement may contain something that will result in a positive drug test, which may also apply to supplemental sport food products such as drinks, shakes, and bars. In fact a wide range of stimulants, steroids, and other agents that are included in the World Anti-Doping Agency's (WADA) prohibited list have been identified in supplements. This may occur in the preparation of the raw ingredients or in the formulation of the finished product. In some cases, the amount of product may be exceptionally higher or lower than the therapeutic dose (see Table 23-6).

Sports nutritionists need to know how to evaluate the scientific merit of articles and advertisements about exercise and nutrition products so that they can separate marketing hype from scientifically based training and nutrition practices (see Chapter 12).

ERGOGENIC AIDS FOR HIGH INTENSITY EXERCISE

Beta-Alanine

Intermittent bouts of **high-intensity interval training (HIIT)** deplete energy substrates and allow for metabolite accumulation.

Studies suggest that supplementation with beta-alanine may improve endurance performance as well as lean body mass (Kern and Robinson, 2011). Because of its relationship with carnosine, beta-alanine appears to have ergogenic potential. Carnosine is believed to be one of the primary buffering substances in muscle. Although carnosine is synthesized from two amino acids, beta-alanine and histidine, its synthesis appears to be limited by the availability of beta-alanine, thus taking supplemental beta-alanine can increase carnosine levels (Danaher et al, 2014).

This proposed benefit would help increase an athlete's capacity for training and increase time to fatigue. Supplementing with beta-alanine has been associated with improved strength, anaerobic endurance, body composition, and performance on various measures of anaerobic power output.

In one study, football players participated in 5 days a week training that included repeated sprints with low work-rest ratios three times a week and Olympic power-lifting four times per week. Football players taking 1.5 g of beta-alanine plus 15 g sugar (about the amount of sugar in 8 oz of a sports drink) gained an average of 2.1 lb of lean mass compared with controls who gained 1.1 lb in the same 8-week training cycle (Kern and Robinson, 2011). Another study showed that beta-alanine can result in greater training adaptations in 3 weeks of high-intensity interval training (Harris and Stellingwerff, 2013). More research is needed to confirm the effectiveness in football players and look for any long-term consequences.

TABLE 23-6	**Commonly Used Banned and Recreational Drugs Used by Athletes**		
Ergogenic Drug	**Goals of Use**	**Athletic Effect**	**Adverse Effects**
Alcohol	Reduce stress and inhibition; most widespread used drug in sport 88% intercollegiate athletes	No benefits	Dependence producing; twofold higher risk of injury; cardiovascular/liver disease; worsens left ventricular dysfunction; decreases amino acid, glucose utilization; decreases energy, hypoglycemia; dehydration; decreases skeletal muscle capillary density, cross sectional area; inhibits sarcolemmal calcium channel actions, impairs excitation-contraction coupling and diminishes performance; decreases muscle oxidative capability; compromises blood coagulation/fibrinolysis/post exercise perturbations in clotting factors; positive energy balance, obesity; increases HR and VO_2, reductions in power output
Nicotine	CNS psychostimulant	Mixed: Enhances brain norepinephrine and dopamine; higher doses enhances serotonin and opiate exerting calming and depressing effect, increases pain tolerance; increases muscle blood flow, lipolysis; may improve cognitive function, learning memory and reaction time and fine motor abilities; delays central fatigue	Addictive; may lead to development of respiratory, cardio and skin diseases and tobacco-related cancers if smoked; increased heart rate and blood pressure, cardiac stroke volume and output, and coronary blood flow; increases skin temp
Tetrahydrocannabionol (marijuana, cannabis)	Diminish nerves/pre competition stress, and anxiety; relax/decrease inhibition; improve sleep	No positive effect	Increases HR and BP at rest; physical work capacity decreases by 25%; decrease in standing steadiness, reaction time, psychomotor performance
Anabolic androgenic steroids	Gain muscle mass and strength	Increase muscle mass and strength especially when combined with strength training and high protein diets	Multiple organ systems including infertility, gynecomastia, female virilization, hypertension, atherosclerosis, physeal closure, aggression, depression, suicidal ideation
Androstendione	Increases testosterone to gain muscle mass and strength	Increase muscle strength and size	Tendopathy, rhabdomyolysis; tendon rupture
DHEA	Increases testosterone to gain muscle mass and strength	No measureable effect	Increases estrogens in men; impurities in preparation
Human Growth Hormone	Increase muscle mass, strength, and definition	Decreases subcutaneous fat and increases lipolysis; increases muscle mass and strength; improves wound healing; stimulates testosterone production	Acromegaly, glucose intolerance, physeal closure, increased lipids, myopathy
Stimulants (ephedrine alkaloids, amphetamines, cocaine)	Increases weight loss; fatigue delay	Increases metabolism, no clear performance benefit although may benefit power, endurance, strength, or speed; reduces tiredness; increases alertness and aggression	Muscle and joint pain; misjudgment in time orientation; tremors; cerebral vascular accident, arrhythmia, myocardial infarction, seizure, psychosis, hypertension, death
Arimidex, (anastrozole); selective estrogen receptor modulators (SERMs) like tamoxifen	Cancer drug used to decrease estrogen levels associated with testosterone use	None; increase testosterone, luteinizing hormone secretion; increase muscle strength and size; prevent bone loss	Side effects associated with taking these agents; early fatigue; increased bone resorption and decreased BMD (hip, lumber spine)
Ghrelin mimetics, (GHRP6 and GHRP2)	Increase GH secretion	Increase muscle mass; stimulates glycogenesis; anabolic effects on muscle mass	GH-associated side effects (see above)
Glucocorticoids	Alleviate pain; reduce tiredness	No improvement	Growth suppression, osteoporosis, avascular necrosis of femoral head; tendon or facial rupture (by local injections) osteoarthritis

Refs: Pesta, D et al 2013; Nikolopoulios, D et al 2011, Rogol A 2010; Hoffman J et al 2009.

Caffeine

Research on the physiologic benefits of caffeine on performance is extensive in areas of strength, endurance, rates of perceived effort, hydration, and recovery. The ergogenic benefits include:

(1) affecting the central nervous system (CNS) and cognitive performance
(2) mobilizing fat and sparing glycogen during exercise
(3) increasing intestinal absorption and oxidation of carbohydrates

(4) speeding up resynthesis of muscle glycogen in recovery
(5) reducing perceived exertion and pain of training.

Caffeine is classified as an "A" level effective and safe supplement by the Australian Institute of Sports Nutrition (AIS) because a large number of studies now show that caffeine intake can enhance performance at a dose of 1 to 3 mg/kg. The plateau in dose to performance appears to occur at 3 mg/kg (AIS, 2014).

According to the AIS, there is sound evidence that caffeine may enhance the performance of endurance sports (more than

60 min), brief, sustained high-intensity sports (1 to 60 min), and the work rates and skills and concentration of teams in intermittent sports. The effect of caffeine is still unclear in skill sports involving low-intensity exercise and in single efforts involving strength or power, in which the effects appear to be small and limited to certain muscle groups.

Caffeine contributes to endurance performance, apparently because of its ability to enhance mobilization of fatty acids and thus conserve glycogen stores. Caffeine also may directly affect muscle contractility, possibly by facilitating calcium transport. It could reduce fatigue as well by reducing plasma potassium accumulation, which contributes to fatigue. An energy-enhancing effect is seen with up to 3 mg/kg body mass or about 200 mg caffeine for the 150-lb athlete (Spriet, 2014). Unwanted side effects of overconsuming caffeine that may limit performance are headaches, insomnia, GI irritation, reflux, shakiness, heart palpitations, and increased urination.

Consumer demand for caffeine has resulted in greater accessibility and acceptance of a variety of beverages beyond coffee and tea. An emerging trend in sports nutrition is the intake of caffeine-containing energy drinks and shots for performance.

The growing availability and consumption of energy drinks with caffeine among all age groups is of concern, especially among young athletes because excessive amounts of caffeine have been shown to disrupt adolescent sleep patterns, exacerbate psychiatric disease, cause physiologic dependence, increase the risk of subsequent addiction and risk-taking behaviors, raise blood pressure, and cause dehydration, vomiting, irregular and rapid heartbeat, convulsions, coma, and death. Altered sleep patterns from excessive caffeine use can lead to poor performance, delayed reaction times, and increased risk for injuries.

Energy drinks consumed with alcohol are another growing concern among health experts, and in 2010 the US Food and Drug Administration (FDA) declared caffeine an "unsafe food additive" to alcoholic beverages, effectively banning premixed alcoholic energy drinks.

HERBS

Athletes' use of herbal supplements is higher than that of the general public and may change throughout the year as athletes move through training cycles. Reasons for athletes' use of herbs range from performance enhancement to immune function improvement to prevention of illness or healing of injuries. Many studies examining the pharmacologic effects of herbs on performance have been poorly designed, conducted only in animals, or lack consistency in the herbal preparation.

Nitrates and Beet Juice

Several studies suggest that inorganic nitrates may alter the physiologic responses to exercise and enhance performance by increasing vasodilation and glucose uptake and reducing blood pressure and the O_2 cost of submaximal exercise (Cermak et al, 2012). Because the consumption of nitrate salts may result in the production of harmful nitrogenous compounds, researchers have explored using natural nitrate-rich foods such as beetroot juice and powders. A dose of dietary nitrate, approximately 0.5L of beetroot juice, has been shown to increase plasma nitrite, which peaks within 3 hours and remains elevated for 6 to 9 hours before returning to baseline (Wylie et al, 2013).

In one study, supplementing the diet with 0.5 L of beetroot juice per day for 4 to 6 days reduced the steady state cost of submaximal exercise by 5% and extended the time to exhaustion during high-intensity cycling by 16%, which has been confirmed in other exercise populations including rowers and team sports. Although the mechanistic bases for the effects are unclear, evidence suggests mitochondrial efficiency and contractile function may be enhanced (Wylie et al, 2013).

It has been recommended to consume nitrate immediately before, during, and after long duration endurance exercise because of peak and maintenance level times. A daily dose of supplement has been shown to keep plasma nitrite elevated (Jones, 2013). Although there is a possibility that uncontrolled high doses of nitrate salts may be harmful to health, natural sources found in beetroot, spinach, lettuce, and celery are likely to promote health.

Ergogenic Aids for Muscle Building, Recovery, Antiinflammation

Amino Acids

The use of amino acids and protein by athletes is as old as the Olympic Games of ancient Greece. Athletes generally meet daily protein dietary recommendations, therefore on a dietary basis, protein or amino acid supplementation in the form of powders or pills is not necessary and should be discouraged, especially for teens and young children.

Taking large amounts of protein or amino acid supplements may be contrary to good performance and health and may lead to dehydration, hypercalciuria, weight gain, and stress on the kidney and liver. Taking single amino acids or in combination, such as arginine and lysine, may interfere with the absorption of certain other essential amino acids. An additional concern is that substituting amino acid supplements for food may cause deficiencies of other nutrients found in protein-rich foods such as iron, zinc, niacin, and thiamin.

A recent review suggests no relationship between consuming protein supplements and muscle recovery, soreness, or damage when protein supplements are consumed before, during, or after an endurance or resistance exercise training session. However some potential ergogenic effects of protein supplementation were shown in athletes who were in negative energy balance (Pasiakos et al, 2014).

Glutamine

Considered by some to be a conditionally essential amino acid, glutamine has many functions in the human body, including protein synthesis and energy source for cells in the immune system. Glutamine supplementation increases glycogen synthesis and muscle protein levels and may improve glucose utilization postworkout and increase growth hormone levels (Phillips, 2014).

Branched-Chain Amino Acids (BCAAs)

The BCAAs include leucine, isoleucine, and valine, and they make up 35% to 40% of the essential amino acids (EAAs) in the body's protein and 14% of the total AAs in muscle. To get energy, the body can break down muscle to use the BCAAs. During times of stress, BCAAs are required more than any other EAA.

BCAAs consumed before and after training have been shown to increase protein synthesis and muscle gains beyond normal adaptation. They have been reported to decrease exercise-induced protein breakdown and muscle enzyme release, a sign of muscle damage.

A combination of 3.2 g BCAA and 2.0 g taurine, three times a day, for 2 weeks before and 3 days after exercise was a useful

TABLE 23-7	Foods High in Branched-Chain Amino Acids	
Branched-Chain Amino Acid	**Food Sources**
Leucine	Meat, dairy, nuts, beans, brown rice, soy, and whole wheat
Isoleucine	Meat, chicken eggs, fish, almonds, chickpeas, soy protein, and most seeds
Valine	Meat, dairy, soy protein, grains, peanuts, and mushrooms

strategy reducing delayed muscle soreness (DOMS) and muscle damage (Ra et al, 2013).

Dairy products and red meat contain the greatest amounts of BCAAs with whey protein from dairy being a very concentrated source. Egg protein is also a good source (see Table 23-7).

Leucine is the most readily oxidized BCAA and is most effective at causing insulin secretion from the pancreas. It lowers blood sugar levels and aids in growth hormone production. Leucine works in conjunction with isoleucine and valine to protect muscle and act as fuel for the body. Doses of 3 to 5 g postworkout have been suggested by some experts for accelerating muscle repair and recovery (Churchward-Venne et al, 2014; Stark et al, 2012).

Beta-Hydroxy-Beta-Methylbutyrate (HMB)

HMB is an important compound made in the body and a metabolite of the essential amino acid leucine. In human research, HMB has been found to reduce muscle damage associated with exercise and to shorten recovery time. Supplementation has been found to inhibit muscle proteolysis, enhance protein synthesis, and increase body mass in the young, elderly, untrained, trained, and clinically cachexic.

Regarding HMB supplementation and exercise recovery, several studies have found that subjects supplemented with HMB may have less stress-induced muscle protein breakdown. Recent research suggests that acute and chronic administration of HMB are associated with less exercise-induced muscle damage and soreness (Wilson et al, 2013).

Creatine

As an amino acid, creatine is produced normally in the body from arginine, glycine, and methionine. Most dietary creatine comes from meat, but half is manufactured in the liver and kidneys. For meat eaters, dietary intake of creatine is approximately 1 g daily. The body also synthesizes approximately 1 g of creatine per day, for a total production of approximately 2 g daily.

In normal, healthy persons approximately 40% of muscle creatine exists as free creatine; the remainder combines with phosphate to form CP. Approximately 2% of the body's creatine is broken down daily to creatinine before excretion by the kidneys. The normal daily excretion of creatinine is approximately 2 g for most persons. Those with lower levels of intramuscular creatine such as vegetarians may respond to creatine supplementation (McArdle et al, 2013).

Creatine monohydrate is one of the most popular supplements used by strength and power athletes. Supplementation elevates muscle creatine levels and facilitates the regeneration of CP, which helps to regenerate ATP. A variety of synthetic creatine supplements have been developed including creatine malate, pyruvate, citrate, and many more with marketing claims of greater performance enhancement and absorption, although no advantage of one over the other has been reported.

Classical loading consists of an initial loading phase of 15 to 20 g per day for 4 to 7 days, followed by a maintenance dose of 2 to 5 g per day. However, alternative dosing methods also have been shown to effectively increase creatine stores and result in strength gains. Regimens without the loading include a dose of 0.3 g/kg body weight for 5 to 7 days, followed by maintenance dose of 0.03 g/kg body weight for 4 to 6 weeks. However, with this regimen creatine stores increase more slowly, and it may take longer to see the strength training effects (Buford et al, 2007; Hall and Trojian, 2013).

As one of the most researched supplements, numerous studies support the use and effectiveness of creatine for short-term, maximum output exercise such as weight lifting, running a 100-m sprint, swinging a bat, or punting a football. When creatine stores in the muscles are depleted, ATP synthesis is prevented and energy can no longer be supplied at the rate required by the working muscle. Improved athletic performance has been attributed to this ATP resynthesis.

Creatine supplementation increases body mass or muscle mass during training. It may improve submaximal exercise performance for HIIT, which promotes fitness similar to endurance training. A recent 2013 study on swimmers showed creatine supplementation improved swimming performance and reduced blood lactate levels after intermittent sprint swimming bouts (Dabidi Roshan et al, 2013).

Studies are conflicting on creatinine's effect on aerobic performance. In a double-blind, placebo-controlled study 16 male amateur soccer players, consuming 20 g of creatine per day, or a placebo for 7 days, experienced no beneficial effect on physical measures obtained during a 90-minute soccer test (Williams et al, 2013). More research in this area has been suggested because indirectly creatine supplementation may affectsubstrate utilization changes and enhanced muscle glycogen storage, which potentially can improve longer distance and timed sports (Cooper et al, 2012).

Creatine absorption appears to be stimulated by insulin. Therefore ingesting creatine supplements in combination with carbohydrate, amino acids, or protein can increase muscle creatine concentrations. Once creatine is taken up by the muscles, it is trapped within the muscle tissue. It is estimated that muscle creatine stores decline slowly and will still be elevated 2 to 3 months after ingestion of 20 g of creatine for 5 days.

Few data exist on the long-term benefits and risks of creatine supplementation. Because of the long-term risks, the American Orthopedic Society for Sports Medicine, the ACSM, and the AAP advises children and adolescents younger than 18 years and pregnant or nursing women to never take creatine supplements. People with kidney problems also should never take creatine supplements.

Betaine

A derivative of the amino acid glycine, one of the main functions of betaine is to maintain water retention of body cells. Some studies have suggested that betaine supplementation may reduce inflammation and also may contribute the compounds necessary to synthesize creatine in muscles; improve metabolically demanding strength-based and endurance performance; and promote adiposity reductions and lean mass gains, although the mechanisms are not completely understood and more research is recommended (Cholewa et al, 2014).

Betaine is a component of many foods, including wheat, spinach, beets, and shellfish. Betaine is also synthesized in the body. The daily intake of betaine is estimated to be 1 g to 2.5 g a day for individuals who consume the foods mentioned. Although one 2014 research review suggests that 2.5 g a day may result in performance benefits, because betaine research study doses have ranged from 2 to 5 g a day, more research is suggested to determine whether there is a dose-related response (Cholewa et al, 2014).

Quercetin

Quercetin, a natural flavonoid in many foods, including apples, cranberries, blueberries, and onions, has many beneficial biologic benefits such as antiinflammatory, anticarcinogenic, cardioprotective, and neuroprotective properties (Mason and Lavallee, 2012). Quercetin may enhance performance through a caffeine-like psychostimulant effect, or it may enhance mitochondrial biogenesis. In a recent study of 60 male students with an athletic history of at least 3 years, lean body mass, total body water, basal metabolic rate, and total energy expenditure increased significantly in the group given quercetin compared with the group without quercetin supplementation (Askari et al, 2013). Another 2009 study showed 2 weeks of quercetin supplementation in cyclists was effective in countering inflammation after 3 days of heavy exertion (Nieman et al, 2009). More studies are needed to confirm positive effects on postexercise inflammation markers, work performed in heat, and race performance.

PERFORMANCE ENHANCEMENT SUBSTANCES AND DRUGS (PES/PED): DOPING IN SPORT

The use of performance enhancement substances (PES) is not a new phenomenon in sports. As early as 776 BC the Greek Olympians were reported to use substances such as dried figs, mushrooms, and strychnine to perform better. Its use is prevalent in amateur and professional athletes, receiving even greater attention with the use by high-profile accomplished athletes such as Lance Armstrong, Alex Rodriquez, and Ryan Braun, and disqualification of some professional athletes for failed drug tests, and the seizure of companies caught with tainted supplements (Pope et al, 2013).

Since 2004, the World Anti-Doping Agency (WADA) has a list of banned drugs for athletes who compete and a strategy to detect drugs such as anabolic steroids, erythropoietin, human growth hormone (HgH), and insulin-like growth factor (IGF-1). WADA annually updates their prohibited list of supplements suspected of 1) illegally enhancing athletic performance, 2) representing an actual or potential health risk to the athlete, or 3) violating the spirit of the sport.

As the number of individuals participating in different sports increases so does the variety of doping agents. According to WADA, the rate of use has been fairly consistent, suggesting a prevalence of approximately 2% of elite athletes. Rates derived from self-reports have ranged from 1.2% to 26%. Between 10% and 24% of male athletes have reported they would use doping if it would help them achieve better results without the risk of consequences, with an additional 5% to 10%, indicating potential doping behavior regardless of health hazards. One report noted that 25% of male and female dancers surveyed would use doping if it were to ensure successful dance performance (Zenic et al, 2010).

Reasons given for using banned substances include achievement of athletic success by improving performance, financial gain, improving recovery and prevention of nutritional deficiencies, and the idea that others use them or the "false consensus effect."

Steroids

Androgenic-anabolic steroids (AASs) categorize all male sex steroid hormones, their synthetic derivatives, and their active metabolites used to enhance athletic performance and appearance. AAS use was reported in the 1950 Olympics and was banned in 1976. Steroids may be used as oral or intramuscular preparations.

The legal and illegal use of these drugs is increasing as a result of society's preoccupation with increasing muscle strength, size, and libido. Originally designed for therapeutic uses to provide enhanced anabolic potency, nontherapeutic use of AAS is increasing among adolescents and females. Anecdotal evidence suggests widespread use of anabolic steroids among athletes (20% to 90%), especially at the professional and elite amateur levels. Use among high school boys is approximately 5% to 10%; rates among college athletes are slightly higher.

Anabolic effects of AAS include increased muscle mass; increased bone mineral density; increased blood cell production; decreased body fat; increased heart, liver, and kidney size; vocal cord changes; and increased libido. Anabolic steroids increase protein synthesis in skeletal muscles and reverse catabolic processes, however, increased muscle mass and strength are observed only in athletes who maintain a high-protein, high-calorie diet during steroid administration. Androgenic effects are the development of secondary sexual characteristics in men, changes in genital size and function, and growth of auxiliary pubic and facial hair. Some adverse effects associated with steroid use are irreversible, especially in women.

Although steroid use has some valid medical uses (e.g., the treatment of delayed puberty, or body wasting resulting from disease), it also has adverse physical and emotional consequences in adolescents, such as arrested bone growth, internal organ damage, feminization in males, and masculinization in females. It also is associated with other high-risk behaviors, such as the use of other illicit drugs, reduced involvement in school, poor academic performance, engaging in unprotected sex, aggressive and criminal behavior, and suicidal ideation and attempted suicide.

Erythropoietin

EPO is used commonly to promote the body's production of red blood cells in patients with bone marrow suppression such as patients with leukemia, those who are receiving chemotherapy, or those with renal failure (see Chapters 35 and 36). In athletes, injections increase the serum hematocrit and oxygen-carrying capacity of the blood, and thus enhance VO_2max and endurance. EPO use as an ergogenic aid is difficult to detect because it is a hormone produced by the kidneys, although newer blood tests can detect its use. Typically, athletes with elevated hematocrit have been banned from endurance sports for suspected EPO misuse; however, despite its ban by the IOC, it is still commonly abused. Drastically high hematocrit combined with exercise-induced dehydration can lead to thick or viscous blood, which can lead to coronary or cerebral vascular occlusions, heart attack, or stroke. EPO also can cause elevated blood pressure or elevated potassium levels.

Human growth hormone (HGH) has many functions in the body, and it is produced naturally throughout life. It stimulates protein synthesis, enhances carbohydrate and fat metabolism, helps to maintain sodium balance, and stimulates bone and connective tissue turnover. HGH production decreases with age after the peak growth years. The amount secreted is affected by diet, stress, exercise, nutrition, and medications. HGH is banned by the IOC; however, it continues to be used by athletes. Potential side effects include skin changes, darkening of moles, adverse effects on glucose and lipid metabolism and the growth of bones as evidenced by development of a protruding jaw and boxy forehead.

Prohormones and Steroids

Prohormones are popular among bodybuilders, many of whom believe that these prohormones are natural boosters of anabolic hormones. Androstenedione, 4-androstenediol, 19-nor-4-androstenedione, 19-nor-4-androstenediol, 7-keto dehydroepiandrosterone (DHEA), and 7-keto DHEA are naturally derived precursors to testosterone and other anabolic steroids.

Androstenedione

Androstenedione (andro) is a prohormone, an inactive precursor to female estrogen and male testosterone. It has about one seventh of the activity of testosterone and is a precursor that directly converts to testosterone by a single reaction. It is produced naturally in the body from either DHEA or 17-alpha-hydroxyprogesterone. Some researchers have found that taking andro elevates testosterone more than DHEA does; however, the induced increase lasts only several hours and remains at peak levels for just a few minutes. Acute or long-term administration of testosterone precursors does not effectively increase serum testosterone levels and fails to produce any significant changes in lean body mass, muscle strength, or performance improvement.

Adverse reactions occur in male and female athletes, including muscle tightness and cramps, increased body weight, acne, GI problems, changes in libido, amenorrhea, liver damage, and stunted growth in adolescents. Consumption of a prohormone supplement can alter a patient's hypothalamic-pituitary-gonadal axis. Andro-related hormones may elevate abnormally estrogen-related hormones and alter elevations of serum estrogen, which is thought to increase the risk for developing prostate or pancreatic cancers. A significant decline in HDLs occur, leading to an increased cardiovascular disease risk. Therefore taking androstenedione may be irresponsible because of the potential risks associated with long-term use. Until there is scientific support for its use, andro should not be sold under the assumption that it is either an effective or a safe athletic ergogenic aid. Clearly adolescents and women of childbearing age should not use it. In 1998 andro was added to the list of banned substances by the IOC and several amateur and professional organizations, including the NFL and the NCAA.

Dehydroepiandrosterone (DHEA) is a weak androgen and product of dehydroandrosterone-3-sulfate (DHEA-S) and is used to elevate testosterone levels. It is a precursor to more potent testosterone and dihydrotestosterone. Although DHEA-S is the most abundant circulating adrenal hormone in humans, its physiologic role is poorly understood. DHEA has been labeled the "fountain of youth" hormone because its levels peak during early adulthood. The decline with aging has been associated with increased fat accumulation and risk of heart disease. Several studies have suggested a positive correlation between increased plasma levels of DHEA and improved vigor, health, and well-being in persons who range in age from 40 to 80 years. By decreasing cortisol output from the liver by 50%, DHEA could have an anabolic effect.

DHEA supplementation does not increase testosterone levels or increase strength in men, but it may increase testosterone levels in women with a virilizing effect. Because DHEA can take several different hormonal pathways, the one that it follows depends on several factors, including existing levels of other hormones. It can take several routes in the body and interact with certain enzymes along the sex-steroid pathway. Thus it can turn into less desirable byproducts of testosterone, including dihydrotestosterone, which is associated with male-pattern baldness, prostate enlargement, and acne.

The benefits of taking DHEA for sports performance have not been clearly established, and the effects of chronic DHEA ingestion are not known. Long-term safety has not been established, and there are concerns that chronic use in men may worsen prostate hyperplasia or even promote prostate cancer. DHEA is not recommended for athletic use because it can alter the testosterone-epitestosterone ratio so that it exceeds the 6:1 limit set by the IOC, the U.S. Olympic Committee, the NFL, and the NCAA.

CLINICAL CASE STUDY

Guillermo is a 32-year-old former college athlete who has been competing in long-distance triathlon and marathon events for the past year. He complains of low energy as training and racing duration increases and is plagued by gut issues—gas and bloating after meals, nausea, and vomiting during races. He also suffers from sleep issues, waking up frequently during the night. He works full time at a stressful job as manager of an electrical contracting firm and trains in swimming, cycling, and running 10 to 12 hours/week.

Assessment

His height is 5ft 9 in and his weight is 174 lb. His body composition analysis as measured by the RD using the ISAK method was 6.8% (10.4 lb body fat, 164 lb [74kg] FFM). He is satisfied with his body fat percentage but would like to reduce his weight if possible to lighten up for the running portion of his events.

Urine specific gravity was assessed to determine hydration status on three visits: 1.035, 1.025, and 1.030
Cholesterol levels were 250, HDL 50, LDL 170, triglycerides 160; all other values were within normal limits.
Using the Cunningham method to calculate REE:

$$500 + (22 \times FFM\ [Kg])\ 500 + (22 \times 74) = \mathbf{2128\ REE}$$

Day off training: Activity factor 1.2, = approx. 2553 calories
1-2 hours steady state training: Activity factor 1.4 = approx. 2979 calories
3-4 hours steady state training: Using Activity factor 1.6 = approx. 3404 calories
4-6 hours training steady state: Using 1.73 Activity factor = approximately 4581 calories

Continued

CLINICAL CASE STUDY—cont'd

Current Diet

Breakfast 1 hour before workout

12 oz coffee with 1 oz coffee creamer

3 eggs fried with onions, 2 slices bacon, 2 slices ham

1 spiced apple bran muffin

Analysis: 570 calories, 30 grams fat (49%), 40 grams carbs (28%) 570 mg cholesterol

Workout: 2000-yard swim, 2-hour bicycle ride, 4-mile run

During swim portion of workout (less than 1 hour): nothing

During cycle portion of workout: 2 hours

2 electrolyte pills every 20 minutes on bike—total 12 pills

Each pill contains: 40 mg Na—480 mg sodium

3 16 oz bottles fluid:

- 1 ×170 cal, 32 g cho, 10 g pro
- 1 bottle high carbohydrate, hypertonic sports drink with maltodextrin- 270 cal, 54 g carb, 7 g sugar and protein, 220 mg Na, 25 mg caffeine
- Water

1 gel pack every 30 minutes= 6 packs

Double latte with caffeine 110 cal, 27g carbs, 200 mg Na

During run portion of workout (less than 1 hour): nothing

Total workout fuel: 1100 calories, 248 g carbohydrates (124 g/hr cycling, 900 mg Na)

Immediately after workout: nothing

Breakfast

Coffee with half-and-half

1 plain bagel, cream cheese, jelly

Banana

12 ounces milk

Snack: none

Lunch

2-6 oz chicken breasts grilled with skin, 2 cups white rice, 1 cup black beans, ½ cup fried plantains

Snack: high-protein sports bar

Dinner

1 onion soup with melted cheese

12 oz grilled steak

1 c yellow rice

Sautéed mushrooms

Dietary Analysis

3041 calories, 216 g protein (2.77 g/Kg) (28%), 249 g carbohydrates (3.15 g/kg)(33%), 13.5% saturated fat, 1172 mg cholesterol, 5634 mg Na

RDA: 64% potassium, 85% Ca and folate, 26% C, 30% E, 13% K, dietary fluid intake= 9 cups

Assessment

Gut/Energy Antagonists

Whole food portion of diet appears to be:

Low in calories: 3041 calories (4141 with sport fuel) vs. 4581 calories required

Carbohydrates: 249 g carbohydrates (3.15 g/kg) (33%) (497 g sport fuel), vs. a minimum of 5 to 7 g/kg = 395-553 g

High in fat (38% total cal), saturated fat and cholesterol 1172 mg and sodium 5634 mg

Low in antioxidants

Excessive in fat pre-workout breakfast

Excessive in sport fuel carbohydrates and sodium for 2-hour bike portion of ride

Excessive in mealtime calories and protein

Questionable whether athlete can tolerate FODMAPs foods, i.e., onions, beans, mushrooms, cream cheese, dairy (lactose), sport fuel sources of HFCS, and gluten

Intervention

Increase meal frequency and calories while modifying fat, sat fat, and cholesterol

Increase plant-based tolerable sources of protein and complex carbohydrates

Modify amounts of animal protein at mealtime to 4 to 5 oz (30 to 35 g

Improve leafy green vegetable intake via juicing if whole food veggies not desired or tolerate

Improve intake of antioxidant rich fruits and fruit juices without added sugar

Recommendations

Probiotic, EAA to heal and strengthen gut; enzymes before meals

Adjust sport fuel intake, decrease electrolyte pills, reduce and modify carbohydrate-containing liquids and source, switch to waxy maize if maltodextrin or HFCS contributing to issue

Meditation or yoga on day off from training and/or prayer or meditation 5 to 10 minutes a day for relaxation

Melatonin and/or theanine for sleep issues, restlessness

Further Biochemical Evaluation and Testing

Hydrogen/methane breath testing, gut dysbiosis

Spectracell to determine extent of vitamin or mineral deficiency, assimilation, and absorption

Upper/lower GI series if elimination diet, FODMAPs diet, and adjustments in eating/sport fuel do not resolve problems during training and racing

Follow-up lipid profile after 9 to 12 weeks on modified fat, saturated fat, and cholesterol diet

Nutrition Care Questions

1. Calculate calorie and macronutrient needs using Cunningham Formula and guidelines provided in chapter
2. Assess what eating/lifestyle behaviors may be affecting this athlete's energy levels, i.e., sleep, stress, portion sizes at meal time
3. Calculate training/race day/recovery fuel formulas for preworkout, workout calories, carbohydrates, and sodium
4. List issues that appear to be a valid reason to initiate FODMAPs and elimination diet.
5. Provide a list and justification for supplementation based on the dietary information and performance enhancement information from this chapter.

USEFUL WEBSITES

Academy of Dietetics and Nutrition (AND)
http://www.eatright.org
Australian Institute of Sport
www.ausport.gov.au
(CDR) Board Certification Specialists in Sports Dietetics (CSSD)
http://www.scandpg.org/sports-nutrition/be-a-board-certified-sports-dietitian-cssd/
Collegiate and Professional Sports Dietitians Association (CPSDA)
http://www.sportsrd.org/

International Society for Sports Nutrition (ISSN)
http://www.sportsnutritionsociety.org/
Sports Nutrition Care Manual
https://sports.nutritioncaremanual.org/vault/sports/WeightLossAthletes1.pdf
United States Olympic Committee Sports Dietitian Registry (USOC)
http://www.teamusa.org/About-the-USOC/Athlete-Development/Sport-Performance/Nutrition/Sport-Dietitian-Registry

Resources, Fact Sheets, Books, Programs and Guides

Academy of Nutrition and Dietetics. Sports Nutrition Care Manual. 2014
http://www.nutritioncaremanual.org/about-sncm

Australian Institute of Sport
www.ausport.gov.au

Banned Substances Control Group
http://www.bscg.org

Informed Choice
www.informed-choice.org/registered-products

International Society of Sports Nutrition
www.theissn.org

MySportsDietitian, Blog, Podcasts, webinars, courses
https://www.mysportsD.com
https://mysportsduniversity.com

National Science Foundation (NSF), Certified for Sport
www.nsfsport.com/listings/certified_products.asp

Sports Nutrition: A Practice Manual for Professionals, 5th Edition.
Rosenblum C, Coleman E: Sports, Cardiovascular and Wellness Nutrition Dietetic Practice Group, Academy of Nutrition and Dietetics, 2012.

United States Olympic Committee (USOC), Sports Nutrition Performance
http://www.teamusa.org/About-the-USOC/Athlete-Development/Sport-Performance/Nutrition/Resources-and-Fact-Sheets

Supplement Education/Certification Information

Drug-Free Sport
http://www.drugfreesport.com

Natural Medicines Comprehensive Database
http://naturaldatabase.therapeuticresearch.com/(S(hmxif045lvxdjrn2rpkbfv45))/home.aspx?cs5&s5ND

Natural Standard
www.NaturalStandard.com

Taylor Hooton Foundation
Education programs created to help raise awareness and inform students, coaches and parents about the dangers of appearance and performance enhancing drugs (APEDs).
http://taylorhooton.org/

Company-Sponsored Websites for Research/Handouts

EAS Academy
http://easacademy.org/

Gatorade Sports Science Institute
www.gssiweb.com

Sport Science
www.sportsci.org

Whey Protein Institute
http://www.wheyoflife.org/

REFERENCES

Academy of Nutrition and Dietetics: *Sports Nutrition Care Manual (SNCM)*, 2014. http://www.nutritioncaremanual.org/about-sncm.

Aguirre N, et al: The role of amino acids in skeletal muscle adaptation to exercise, *Nestle Nutr Inst Workshop Ser* 76:85, 2013.

Ambrose PJ, et al: Characteristics and trends of drug and dietary supplement inquiries by college athletes, *J Am Pharm Assoc* 53:297, 2013.

Askari G, et al: Quercetin and vitamin C supplementation: effects on lipid profile and muscle damage in male athletes, *Int J Prev Med* 4(Suppl 1):S58, 2013.

Australian Institute of Sport (AIS): *Supplements: Executive Summary* (website), 2014. http://www.ausport.gov.au/ais/nutrition/supplements. Accessed December 1, 2015.

Barker T, et al: Supplemental vitamin D enhances the recovery in peak isometric force shortly after intense exercise, *Nutr Metab (Lond)* 10:69, 2013.

Bennett CB, et al: Metabolism and performance during extended high-intensity intermittent exercise after consumption of low- and high-glycemic index pre-exercise meals, *Br J Nutr* 108(Suppl 1):S81, 2012.

Brisswalter J, Louis J: Vitamin supplementation benefits in master athletes, *Sports Med* 44:311, 2014.

Buell JL, et al: National Athletic Trainers' Association position statement: evaluation of dietary supplements for performance nutrition, *J Athl Train* 48:124, 2013.

Buford TW, et al: International Society of Sports Nutrition position stand: creatine supplementation and exercise, *J Int Soc Sports Nutr* 4:6, 2007.

Burdon CA, et al: The effect of ice slushy ingestion and mouthwash on thermoregulation and endurance performance in the heat, *Int J Sport Nutr Exerc Metab* 23:458, 2013.

Burke LM: Fueling strategies to optimize performance: training high or training low? *Scand J Med Sci Sports* 20(Suppl 2):S48, 2010.

Campos-Ferraz PL, et al: Distinct effects of leucine or a mixture of the branched-chain amino acids (leucine, isoleucine, and valine) supplementation on resistance to fatigue, and muscle and liver-glycogen degradation, in trained rats, *Nutrition* 29:1388, 2013.

Cannell JJ, et al: Athletic performance and vitamin D, *Med Sci Sports Exerc* 41:1102, 2009.

Castell LM, et al: A-Z of nutritional supplements: dietary supplements, sports nutrition foods and ergogenic aids for health and performance Part 9, *Br J Sports Med* 44:609, 2010.

Cermak NM, et al: Nitrate supplementation's improvement of 10-km time-trial performance in trained cyclists, *Int J Sport Nutr Exerc Metab* 22:64, 2012.

Cermak NM, van Loon LJ: The use of carbohydrates during exercise as an ergogenic aid, *Sports Med* 43:1139, 2013.

Cholewa JM, et al: Effects of betaine on performance and body composition: a review of recent findings and potential mechanisms, *Amino Acids* 46:1785, 2014.

Churchward-Venne TA, et al: Leucine supplementation of a low-protein mixed macronutrient beverage enhances myofibrillar protein synthesis in young men: a double-blind, randomized trial, *Am J Clin Nutr* 99:276, 2014.

Colombani PC, et al: Carbohydrates and exercise performance in non-fasted athletes: a systematic review of studies mimicking real-life, *Nutr J* 12:16, 2013.

Cooper R, et al: Creatine supplementation with specific view to exercise/sports performance: an update, *J Int Soc Sports Nutr* 9:33, 2012.

Dabidi Roshan V, et al: The effect of creatine supplementation on muscle fatigue and physiological indices following intermittent swimming bouts, *J Sports Med Phys Fitness* 53:232, 2013.

Danaher J, et al: The effect of β et al: The effect of essplementation on muscle fatigue and physiological indices following intermittent swimming boutse, *ung mEur J Appl Physiol* 114:1715, 2014.

Daneshvar P, et al: Effect of eight weeks of quercetin supplementation on exercise performance, muscle damage and body muscle in male badminton players, *Int J Prev Med* 4(Suppl 1):S53, 2013.

DellaValle DM: Iron supplementation for female athletes: effects on iron status and performance outcomes, *Curr Sports Med Rep* 12:234, 2013.

De Lorenzo A, et al: A new predictive equation to calculate resting metabolic rate in athletes, *J Sports Med Phys Fitness* 39:213, 1999.

De Souza, et al: 2014 Female Athlete Triad Coalition consensus statement on treatment and return to play of the female athlete triad: 1st International Conference held in San Francisco, CA, May 2012, and 2nd International Conference held in Indianapolis, IN, May 2013, *Clin J Sport Med* 24:96, 2014.

Driskell J, Wolinsky I: *Nutrition assessment of athletes*, ed 3, Boca Raton, Fla, 2011, CRC Press.

Dugas J: Ice slurry ingestion increases running time in the heat, *Clin J Sport Med* 21:541, 2011.

Eijsvogels TM, et al: Sex difference in fluid balance responses during prolonged exercise, *Scand J Med Sci Sports* 23:198, 2013.

Engeln R, et al: Body talk among college men: content, correlates, and effects, *Body Image* 10:300, 2013.

Gibbs JC, et al: Prevalence of individual and combined components of the female athlete triad, *Med Sci Sports Exerc* 45:985, 2013.

Hall M, Trojian TH: Creatine supplementation, *Curr Sports Med Rep* 12:240, 2013.

Harris KM, et al: Sickle cell trait associated with sudden death in competitive athletes, *Am J Cardiol* 110:1185, 2012.

Harris RC, Stellingwerff T: Effect of β: Effect Stellingwerff T: Effect of ith sudden death in compete, *Nestle Nutr Inst Workshop Ser* 76:61, 2013.

Heaney S, et al: Comparison of strategies for assessing nutritional adequacy in elite female athletes' dietary intake, *Int J Sport Nutr Exerc Metab* 20:245, 2010.

Hoon MW, et al: The effect of nitrate supplementation on exercise performance in healthy individuals: a systematic review and meta-analysis, *Int J Sport Nutr Exerc Metab* 23:522, 2013.

Hosseinlou A, et al: The effect of water temperature and voluntary drinking on the post rehydration sweating, *Int J Clin Exp Med* 6:683, 2013.

Howatson G, et al: Influence of tart cherry juice on indices of recovery following marathon running, *Scand J Med Sci Sports* 37:843, 2010.

Institute of Medicine (IOM): *Dietary reference intakes for water, potassium, sodium, chloride, and sulfate*. Washington, DC, 2005, The National Academies Press.

International Olympic Committee (IOC): IOC consensus statement on sports nutrition 2010, *J Sports Sci* 29(Suppl 1):S3, 2011.

Jones AM, et al: Influence of dietary nitrate supplementation on exercise tolerance and performance, *Nestle Nutr Inst Workshop Ser* 75:27, 2013.

Jouris KB, et al: The effect of omega-3 fatty acid supplementation on the inflammatory response to eccentric strength exercise, *J Sports Sci Med* 10:432, 2011.

Jung AP, et al: Survey of sickle cell trait screening in NCAA and NAIA institutions, *Phys Sportsmed* 39:158, 2011.

Kass LS, et al: A pilot study on the effects of magnesium supplementation with high and low habitual dietary magnesium intake on resting and recovery from aerobic and resistance exercise and systolic blood pressure, *J Sports Sci Med* 12:144, 2013.

Kenefick RW, Cheuvront SN: Hydration for recreational sport and physical activity, *Nutr Rev* 70(Suppl 2):S137, 2012.

Kern BD, Robinson TL: Effects of β-alanine supplementation on performance and body composition in collegiate wrestlers and football players, *J Strength Cond Res* 25:1804, 2011.

Koncic MZ, Tomczyk M: New insights into dietary supplements used in sport: active substances, pharmacological and side effects, *Curr Drug Targets* 14:1079, 2013.

Larson-Meyer DE, Willis KS: Vitamin D and athletes, *Curr Sports Med Rep* 9:220, 2010.

Little JP, et al: The effects of low- and high-glycemic index foods on high-intensity intermittent exercise, *Int J Sports Physiol Perform* 4:367, 2009.

Lunn WR, et al: Chocolate milk and endurance exercise recovery: protein balance, glycogen, and performance, *Med Sci Sports Exerc* 44:682, 2012.

Lynch S: The differential effects of a complex protein drink versus isocaloric carbohydrate drink on performance indices following high-intensity resistance training: a two arm crossover design, *J Int Soc Sports Nutr* 10:31, 2013.

Malliaropoulos N, et al: Blood phosphorus and magnesium levels in 130 elite track and field athletes, *Asian J Sports Med* 4:49, 2013.

Mason BC, Lavallee ME: Emerging supplements in sports, *Sports Health* 4:142, 2012.

Maughan RJ, et al: Dietary supplements for athletes: emerging trends and recurring themes, *J Sports Sci* 29(Suppl 1):S57, 2011.

Maughan RJ, et al: The use of dietary supplements by athletes, *J Sports Sci* 25(Suppl 1):S103, 2007.

McArdle WD, et al: *Sports and exercise nutrition*, ed 4, Philadelphia, 2013, Lippincott Williams & Wilkins.

McClung JP, et al: Female athletes: a population at risk of vitamin and mineral deficiencies affecting health and performance, *J Trace Elem Med Biol* 28:388, 2014.

Megna M, et al: Effects of herbal supplements on the immune system in relation to exercise, *Int J Immunopathol Pharmacol* 25(Suppl 1):43S, 2012.

Mettler S, et al: Development and validation of a food pyramid for Swiss athletes, *Int J Sport Nutr Exerc Metab* 19:504, 2009.

Mettler S, et al: Increased protein intake reduces lean body mass loss during weight loss in athletes, *Med Sci Sports Exerc* 42:326, 2010.

Michael-Titus AT, Priestley JV: Omega-3 fatty acids and traumatic neurological injury: from neuroprotection to neuroplasticity? *Trends Neurosci* 37:30, 2014.

Morente-Sánchez J, Zabala M: Doping in sport: a review of elite athletes' attitudes, beliefs, and knowledge, *Sports Med* 43:395, 2013.

Moslehi N, et al: Does magnesium supplementation improve body composition and muscle strength in middle-aged overweight women? A double-blind, placebo-controlled, randomized clinical trial, *Biol Trace Elem Res* 153:111, 2013.

Mountjoy M, et al: The IOC consensus statement: beyond the Female Athlete Triad—Relative Energy Deficiency in Sport (RED-S), *Br J Sports Med* 48:491, 2014.

Murray SB, et al: A comparison of eating, exercise, shape, and weight related symptomatology in males with muscle dysmorphia and anorexia nervosa, *Body Image* 9:193, 2012.

Nieman DC, et al: Effects of quercetin and EGCG on mitochondrial biogenesis and immunity, *Med Sci Sports Exerc* 41:1467, 2009.

Ogan D, Pritchett K: Vitamin D and the athlete: risks, recommendations, and benefits, *Nutrients* 5:1856, 2013.

Pasiakos SM, et al: Effects of protein supplements on muscle damage, soreness and recovery of muscle function and physical performance: a systematic review, *Sports Med* 44:655, 2014.

Penry JT, Manore MM: Choline: an important micronutrient for maximal endurance exercise performance? *Int J Sport Nutr Exerc Metab* 18:191, 2008.

Peschek K, et al: The effects of acute post exercise consumption of two cocoa-based beverages with varying flavanol content on indices of muscle recovery following downhill treadmill running, *Nutrients* 6:50, 2013.

Pesta, et al: The effects of caffeine, nicotine, ethanol, and tetrahydrocannabinol on exercise performance, *Nutr Metab (Lond)* 10:71, 2013.

Pettersson S, et al: Practices of weight regulation among elite athletes in combat sports: a matter of mental advantage? *J Athl Train* 48:99, 2013.

Pettersson S, et al: The food and weight combat. A problematic fight for the elite combat sports athlete, *Appetite* 59:234, 2012.

Phillips SM: A brief review of critical processes in exercise-induced muscular hypertrophy, *Sports Med* 44(Suppl 1):S71, 2014.

Phillips SM: Dietary protein requirements and adaptive advantages in athletes, *Br J Nutr* 108(Suppl 2):S158, 2012.

Pope HG Jr, et al: Adverse health consequences of performance-enhancing drugs: an Endocrine Society scientific statement, *Endocr Rev* 35:341, 2014.

Ra SG, et al: Combined effect of branched-chain amino acids and taurine supplementation on delayed onset muscle soreness and muscle damage in high-intensity eccentric exercise, *J Int Soc Sports Nutr* 10:51, 2013.

Reidy PT, et al: Protein blend ingestion following resistance exercise promotes human muscle protein synthesis, *J Nutr* 143:410, 2013.

Rodriguez NR, et al: Position of the American Dietetic Association, Dietitians of Canada, and the American College of Sports Medicine: nutrition and athletic performance, *J Am Diet Assoc* 109:509, 2009.

Rosenbloom CA, Coleman E, editors: *Sports nutrition: a practice manual for professionals*, ed 5, Chicago, 2012, American Dietetic Association.

Rosenkilde M, et al: Changes in peak fat oxidation in response to different doses of endurance training, *Scand J Med Sci Sports* 2013, (Epub ahead of print).

Setaro L, et al: Magnesium status and the physical performance of volleyball players: effects of magnesium supplementation, *J Sports Sci* 32:438, 2014.

Shuler FD, et al: Sports health benefits of vitamin d, *Sports Health* 4:496, 2012.

Siegel R, et al: Pre-cooling with ice slurry ingestion leads to similar run times to exhaustion in the heat as cold water immersion, *J Sports Sci* 30:155, 2012.

Sousa M, et al: Dietary strategies to recover from exercise-induced muscle damage, *Int J Food Sci Nutr* 65:151, 2014.

Spriet LL: Exercise and sport performance with low doses of caffeine, *Sports Med* 44(Suppl 2):175, 2014.

Stark M, et al: Protein timing and its effects on muscular hypertrophy and strength in individuals engaged in weight-training, *J Int Soc Sports Nutr* 9:54, 2012.

Sureda A, et al: Prevention of neutrophil protein oxidation with vitamins C and E diet supplementation without affecting the adaptive response to exercise, *Int J Sport Nutr Exerc Metab* 23:31, 2013.

Suzuki A, et al: Thermoregulatory responses are attenuated after fructose but not glucose intake, *Med Sci Sports Exerc* 46:1452, 2014.

Taylor NA, Machado-Moreira CA: Regional variations in transepidermal water loss, eccrine sweat gland density, sweat secretion rates and electrolyte composition in resting and exercising humans, *Extrem Physiol Med* 2:4, 2013.

ter Steege RW, et al: Abdominal symptoms during physical exercise and the role of gastrointestinal ischaemia: a study in 12 symptomatic athletes, *Br J Sports Med* 46:931, 2012.

Tipton KD: Dietary strategies to attenuate muscle loss during recovery from injury, *Nestle Nutr Inst Workshop Ser* 76:73, 2013.

Tipton KD, Phillips SM: Dietary protein for muscle hypertrophy, *Nestle Nutr Inst Workshop Ser* 76:73, 2013.

Todd JJ, et al: Vitamin D: recent advances and implications for athletes, *Sports Med* 2014, (Epub ahead of print).

Tomlin DL, et al: Sports drink consumption and diet of children involved in organized sport, *J Int Soc Sports Nutr* 10:38, 2013.

Turocy PS, et al: National Athletic Trainers' Association position statement: safe weight loss and maintenance practices in sport and exercise, *J Athl Train* 46:322, 2011.

Van Proeyen K, et al: High-fat diet overrules the effects of training on fiber-specific intramyocellular lipid utilization during exercise, *J Appl Physion (1985)* 111:108, 2011.

Volek JS, et al: Rethinking fat as a fuel for endurance exercise, *Eur J Sport Sci* 2014, (Epub ahead of print).

Volpe SL, et al: Estimation of prepractice hydration status of National Collegiate Athletic Association Division I athletes, *J Athl Train* 44:624, 2009.

Wall BA, et al: Current hydration guidelines are erroneous: dehydration does not impair exercise performance in the heat, *Br J Sports Med* Sep 20, 2013, (Epub ahead of print).

Wierniuk A, Włodarek D: Estimation of energy and nutritional intake of young men practicing aerobic sports, *Rccz Panstw Zakl Hig* 64:143, 2013.

Williams J, et al: Effects of creatine monohydrate supplementation on simulated soccer performance, *Int J Sports Physiol Perform* 9:503, 2014.

Wilson JM, et al: International Society of Sports Nutrition position stand: beta-hydroxy-beta-methylbutyrate (HMB), *J Int Soc Sports Nutr* 10:6, 2013.

Woolf K, et al: Iron status in highly active and sedentary young women, *Int J Sport Nutr Exerc Metab* 19:519, 2009.

Wylie LJ, et al: Dietary nitrate supplementation improves team sport-specific intense intermittent exercise performance, *Eur J Appl Physiol* 113:1673, 2013.

Yeo WK, et al: Fat adaptation in well-trained athletes: effects on cell metabolism, *Appl Physiol Nutr Metab* 36:12, 2011.

Yfanti C, et al: Role of vitamin C and E supplementation on IL-6 in response to training, *J Appl Physiol (1985)* 112:990, 2012.

Zenic N, et al: Comparative analysis of substance use in ballet, dance sport, and synchronized swimming: results of a longitudinal study, *Med Probl Perform Art* 25:75, 2010.

24

Nutrition and Bone Health

Karen Chapman-Novakofski, PhD, RDN, LDN

KEY TERMS

25-hydroxyvitamin D_3 (calcifediol)
1,25-dihydroxy vitamin D_3 (calcitriol)
age-related primary osteoporosis
bisphosphonates
bone densitometry
bone mineral content (BMC)
bone mineral density (BMD)
bone modeling
bone remodeling
calcium homeostasis
calcitonin
cancellous bone

cholecalciferol (vitamin D_3)
cortical bone
estrogen-androgen deficient osteoporosis
estrogen receptor (ER)
estrogen replacement therapy (ERT)
hydroxyapatite
intermittent parathyroid hormone (PTH) therapy
osteoid
osteoblast
osteocalcin
osteoclast

osteocyte
osteomalacia
osteopenia
osteoporosis
parathyroid hormone (PTH)
peak bone mass (PBM)
secondary osteoporosis
selective estrogen receptor modulator (SERM)
trabecular bone

Adequate nutrition is essential for the development and maintenance of the skeleton. Although diseases of the bone such as osteoporosis and osteomalacia (a condition of impaired mineralization caused by vitamin D and calcium deficiency) have complex causes, the development of these diseases can be minimized by providing adequate nutrients throughout the life cycle. Of these diseases, osteoporosis is the most common and destructive on productivity and quality of life. As is true of many chronic diseases, signs and symptoms of osteoporosis become more evident in older age.

The number of people older than 65 years continues to increase: almost 25% of the population by 2020. As a result of the increasing numbers of older adults, osteoporosis with resulting hip fractures has become more significant in cost, morbidity, and mortality in the United States. Prevention and treatment are equally important to the quality of life.

BONE STRUCTURE AND BONE PHYSIOLOGY

Bone is a term used to mean an organ, such as the femur, and a tissue, such as trabecular bone tissue. Each bone contains bone tissues of two major types, trabecular and cortical. These tissues undergo bone modeling during growth (height gain) and bone remodeling after growth ceases.

Bone mass is a generic term that refers to bone mineral content (BMC). Bone mineral density (BMD) describes the mineral content of bone per unit of bone (or BMC/bone area). Neither BMC nor BMD provides information on the microarchitectural (three-dimensional) structural quality of bone tissue (i.e., index of risk of fracture).

Composition of Bone

Bone consists of an organic matrix, or osteoid, primarily collagen fibers, in which salts of calcium and phosphate are deposited in combination with hydroxyl ions in crystals of hydroxyapatite. The cable-like tensile strength of collagen and the hardness of hydroxyapatite combine to give bone its great strength. Other components of the bone matrix include osteocalcin, osteopontin, and several other matrix proteins.

Types of Bone Tissue

Approximately 80% of the skeleton consists of compact or cortical bone tissue. Shafts of the long bones contain primarily cortical bone, which consists of osteons or Haversian systems that undergo continuous but slow remodeling. Both contain an outer periosteal layer of compact circumferential lamellae and an inner endosteal layer of trabecular tissue. The remaining 20% of the skeleton is trabecular or cancellous bone tissue, which exists in the knobby ends of the long bones, the iliac crest of the pelvis, the wrists, scapulas, vertebrae, and the regions of bones that line the marrow. Trabecular bone is less dense than cortical bone as a result of an open structure of interconnecting bony spicules that resemble a sponge in appearance.

The elaborate interconnecting components (columns and struts) of trabecular bone add support to the cortical bone shell of the long bones and provide a large surface area that is exposed to circulating fluids from the marrow, and is lined by a disproportionately larger number of cells than cortical bone tissue. Therefore trabecular bone tissue is much more responsive to estrogens or the lack of estrogens than cortical bone tissue (see Figure 24-1). The loss of trabecular bone tissue late in life is largely responsible for the occurrence of fractures, especially those of the spine.

Bone Cells

Osteoblasts are responsible for the formation or production of bone tissue, and osteoclasts govern the resorption or breakdown of bone (also see Bone Modeling and Bone Remodeling

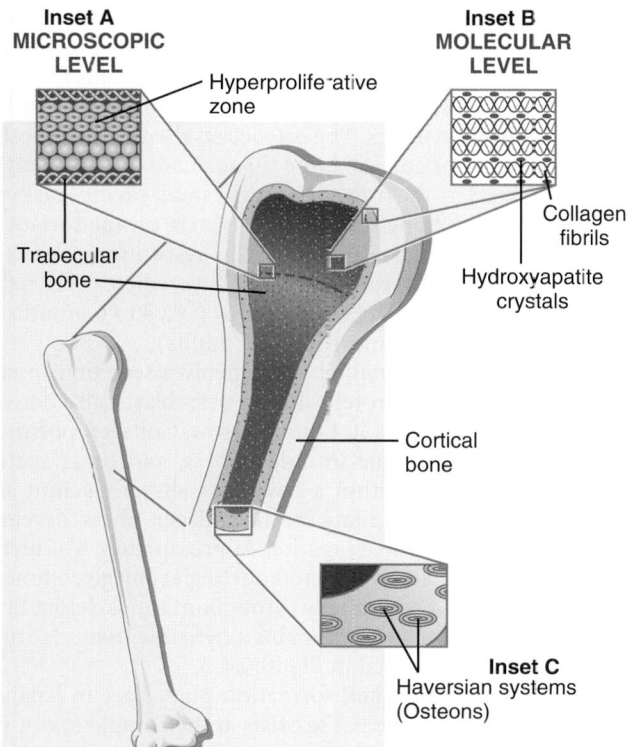

Inset A
MICROSCOPIC LEVEL

Hyperproliferative zone

Trabecular bone

Inset B
MOLECULAR LEVEL

Collagen fibrils

Hydroxyapatite crystals

Cortical bone

Inset C
Haversian systems (Osteons)

FIGURE 24-1 Schematic diagram of the structure of a long bone (hemisection of a long bone, such as the tibia). The ends of the long bones contain high percentages of trabecular (cancellous) bone tissue, whereas the shaft contains predominately cortical bone tissue. Inset A includes an enlarged section (approximately 100-fold) of the growth plate (epiphysis) and the subjacent hyperproliferative zone containing cartilage cells stacked like coins. Inset B includes a section of collagen molecules (triple helices) surrounded by mineralized deposits (dark spheroids) at a magnification of approximately 1,000,000-fold. These collagen-mineral complexes exist in trabecular and cortical bone tissues. Inset C shows the cross-section of half of the midshaft of a long bone (magnification 10-fold). This section of cortical bone tissue contains vertical Haversian systems (osteons) that run parallel with the shaft axis; many are required to extend this system from one end of the shaft to the other. At the center of each osteon is a canal that contains an artery that supplies bone tissues with nutrients and oxygen, a vein for removing wastes, and a nerve for returning afferent relays to the brain. (Copyright John J. B. Anderson and Sanford C. Garner.)

TABLE 24-1 **Functions of Osteoblasts and Osteoclasts**	
Osteoblasts	**Osteoclasts**
Bone Formation	**Bone Resorption**
Synthesis of matrix proteins: Collagen type 1 (90%) Osteocalcin and others (10%) Mineralization	Degradation of bone tissue via enzymes and acid (H+) secretion
Communication: Secretion of cytokines that act on osteoblasts	Communication: Secretion of enzymes that act on osteoclasts

later in this chapter). The functions of these two cell types are listed in Table 24-1.

Two other important cell types also exist in bone tissue, osteocytes and bone-lining cells (inactive osteoblasts), both of which are derived from osteoblasts. The origin of the osteoblasts is mesenchymal stem cells, whereas osteoclasts arise from hematopoietic stem cells (progenitors of macrophages) from the bone marrow, now known to be stimulated by hormones and growth factors as part of their differentiation to become mature, functional bone cells.

Cartilage

In the embryo, cartilage forms the first temporary skeleton, until it develops into a mature bone matrix. In the adult, cartilage is found as flexible supports in areas such as the nose and ear. Cartilage is not bone and is neither vascularized nor calcified.

Calcium Homeostasis

Bone tissue serves as a reservoir of calcium and other minerals. Calcium homeostasis refers to the process of maintaining a constant serum calcium concentration. The serum calcium is regulated by complex mechanisms that balance calcium intake and excretion with bodily needs. When calcium intake is not adequate, homeostasis is maintained by drawing on mineral from the bone to keep the serum calcium ion concentration at its set level (approximately 8.5-10 mg/dl). Homeostasis can be accomplished by drawing from two major skeletal sources: readily mobilizable calcium ions in the bone fluid, or through osteoclastic resorption from the bone tissue. The daily turnover of skeletal calcium ions (transfers in and out of bone) supports the dynamic activity of bone tissue in calcium homeostasis.

Serum calcium concentration is regulated by two calcium-regulating hormones: parathyroid hormone (PTH) and 1,25 dihydroxy vitamin D_3 (calcitriol). If serum calcium levels fall, PTH increases reabsorption from the kidney and bone, and calcitriol increases gut absorption and initiates osteoclastic activity for bone breakdown. Increased serum calcium or hypercalcemia, occurs primarily as a result of hyperparathyroidism. Serum calcium includes free calcium (formerly called ionized calcium) and albumin-bound calcium.

Bone Modeling

Bone modeling is the term applied to the growth of the skeleton until mature height is achieved. In long bones, growth occurs at terminal epiphyses (growth plates that undergo hyperproliferation) and circumferentially in lamellae; at each location cells undergo division and contribute to the formation of new bone tissue (see Figure 24-1). Bone modeling typically is completed in females by ages 16 to 18 and in males by ages 18 to 20.

During this growth period, formation exceeds the resorption of bone. Peak bone mass (PBM) is reached by 30 years of age or so (see Figure 24-2). The long bones stop growing in length by approximately age 18 in females and age 20 in males, but bone mass continues to accumulate for a few more years by a process known as consolidation (i.e., filling-in of osteons in the shafts of long bones). The age when BMD acquisition ceases varies, depending not only on diet but also on physical activity.

PBM is greater in men than in women because of men's larger frame size. BMC, but not necessarily BMD, is typically lower in women. The lean and fat components of body composition contribute to these differences in bone mass. BMD is also greater in blacks and Hispanics than in whites and Asians, related to larger muscle mass, differences in body weight, lifestyle

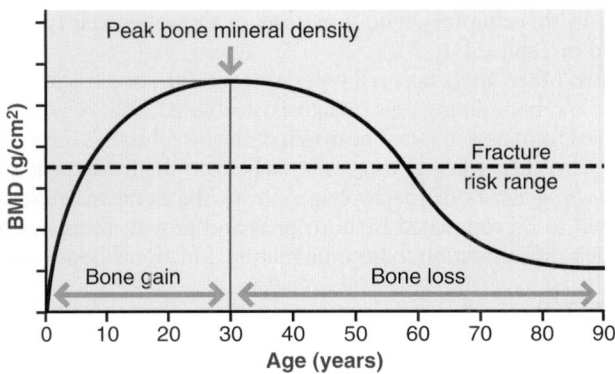

FIGURE 24-2 The early gain and later loss of bone in females. Peak bone mineral density (BMD) typically is achieved by age 30. Menopause occurs at approximately age 50 or within a few years. Postmenopausal women typically enter the fracture risk range after age 60. Men have a more gradual decline in BMD, which starts at 50 years. (Copyright John J. B. Anderson and Sanford C. Garner.)

factors, and dietary intake (Pothiwala et al, 2006; Reid, 2008). Heredity is a major factor contributing to BMD and may contribute as much as 50% to 80% of BMD.

PBM is related to appropriate nutrient intake, physical activity, and genetics. Because bone formation begins in the embryo, more attention is being focused on maternal nutrition and health as a predictor of the child's future PBM (Prentice et al, 2011). PBM is diminished in cases of anorexia nervosa (Misra and Klibanski, 2006), as well as in chronic and malabsorptive diseases.

Bone Remodeling

Bone is a dynamic organ both during growth and maintenance. Bone remodeling is a process in which bone is resorbed continuously through the action of the osteoclasts and reformed through the action of the osteoblasts. The remodeling process is initiated by the *activation* of preosteoclastic cells in the bone

marrow. Interleukin (IL)-1 and other cytokines released from bone-lining cells act as the triggers in the activation of precursor stem cells in bone marrow. The preosteoclast cells from the bone marrow migrate to the surfaces of bone while differentiating into mature osteoclasts. The osteoclasts then cover a specific area of trabecular or cortical bone tissue. Acids and proteolytic enzymes released by the osteoclasts form small cavities on bone surfaces and *resorb* bone mineral and matrix on the surface of trabecular bone or cortical bone. The resorptive process is rapid, and it is completed within a few days, whereas the refilling of these cavities by osteoblasts is slow (i.e., 3 to 6 months or even as long as a year or more in older adults).

The *rebuilding* or *formation* stage involves secretion of collagen and other matrix proteins by the osteoblasts, also derived from precursor stem cells in bone marrow. Collagen polymerizes to form mature triple-stranded fibers, and other matrix proteins are secreted. Within a few days salts of calcium and phosphate begin to precipitate on the collagen fibers, developing into crystals of hydroxyapatite. Approximately 4% of the total bone surface is involved in remodeling at any given time as new bone is renewed continually throughout the skeleton. Even in the mature skeleton, bone remains a dynamic tissue. Normal bone turnover is illustrated in Figure 24-3.

When the resorption and formation phases are in balance, the same amount of bone tissue exists at the completion of the formation phase as at the beginning of the resorption phase. The benefit to the skeleton of this remodeling is the renewal of bone without any microfractures. With aging, osteoclastic resorption becomes relatively greater than formation by osteoblasts (see Figure 24-4). This imbalance between formation and resorption is referred to as "uncoupling" of the osteoblastic and osteoclastic activity.

Because of this uncoupling of cell activity, age is an important determinant of BMD. At approximately age 40, BMD begins to diminish gradually in both sexes, but bone loss increases greatly in women after menopause because of the loss of estrogen's effects on bone. Men continue to have bone loss, but at a much lower rate than women of the same age until age 70, when the loss rates are about the same for both genders. Loss of

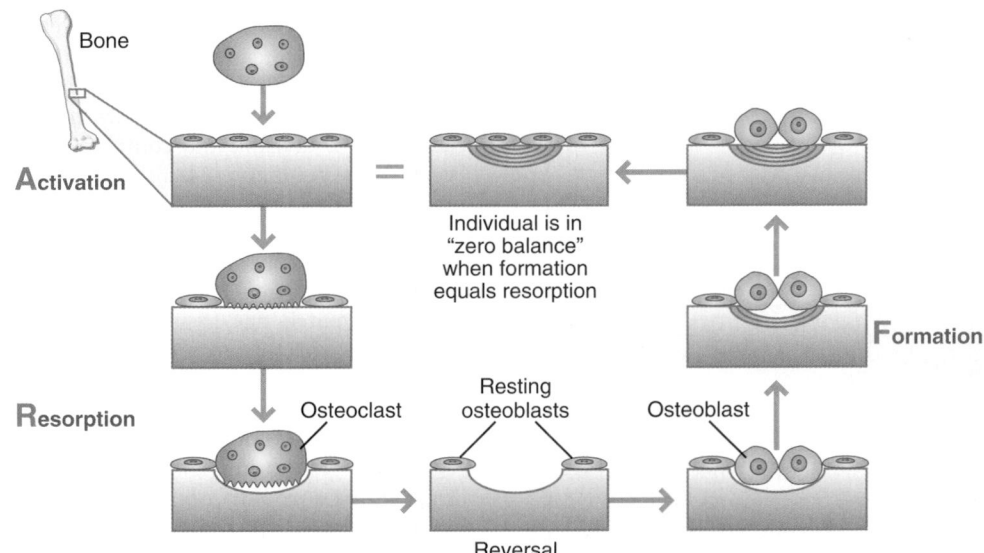

FIGURE 24-3 Normal bone turnover in healthy adults. (Copyright John J. B. Anderson and Sanford C. Garner.)

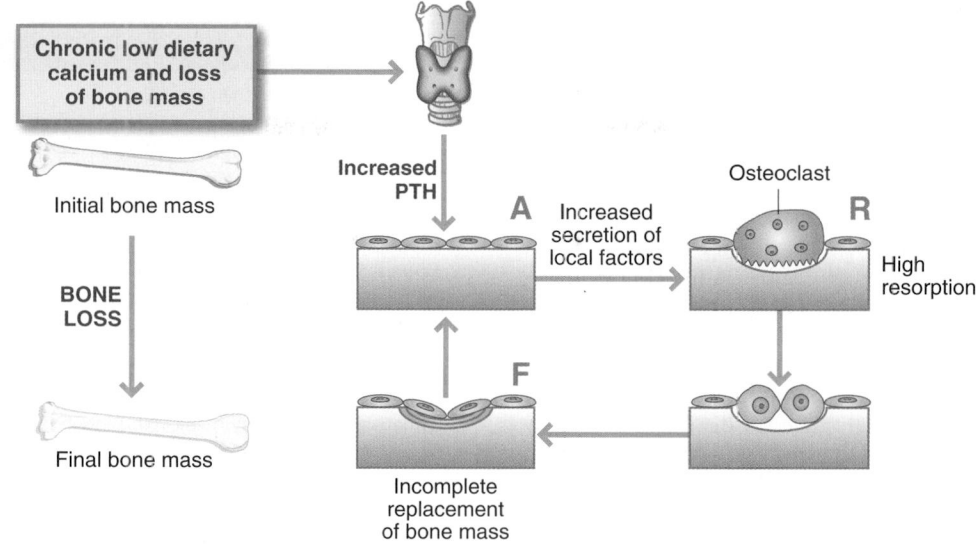

FIGURE 24-4 Effects of persistently elevated serum concentration of parathyroid hormone (PTH) on bone mass; this incorporates the effect of estradiol, counteracting the effect of PTH. (Copyright John J. B. Anderson and Sanford C. Garner.)

bone mass is the result of changes in the hormone-directed mechanisms that govern bone remodeling.

Cortical bone tissue and trabecular bone tissue undergo different patterns of aging. Loss of cortical bone eventually plateaus and may even cease late in life. Trabecular bone loss begins in both sexes as early as 40 years of age. Premenopausal loss of trabecular bone in women is much greater than that of cortical bone. Loss of both kinds of bone accelerates in women after menopause, although trabecular bone is lost at a much higher rate than cortical bone.

OSTEOPENIA AND OSTEOPOROSIS

This loss of bone can continue throughout aging, eventually leading to osteopenia or osteoporosis. However, not all older persons have poor bone health, and bone disease can occur in younger people, although rarely. Differences between normal and osteoporotic bone—both trabecular and cortical tissues—are shown in Figure 24-5.

Prevalence

It is estimated from the National Health and Nutrition Examination Survey of 2006 to 2008 that 9% of adults over age 50 have osteoporosis. Another 49% have low bone mass, or osteopenia, at the femur neck or spine, leaving about 49% with healthy bone. These results differ by age, gender, race and ethnicity, with the oldest having higher prevalence. Women more often have poor bone health than men, and for both genders, Hispanics are at higher risk than non-Hispanic whites, whereas African Americans are at lower risk (Looker et al, 2012).

Types of Osteoporosis

Osteoporosis is considered to have a broad spectrum of variant forms. There are two types of primary osteoporosis, distinguished in general by sex, the age at which fractures occur, and the kinds of bone involved. Secondary osteoporosis results when an identifiable drug or disease process causes loss of bone tissue (see Box 24-1).

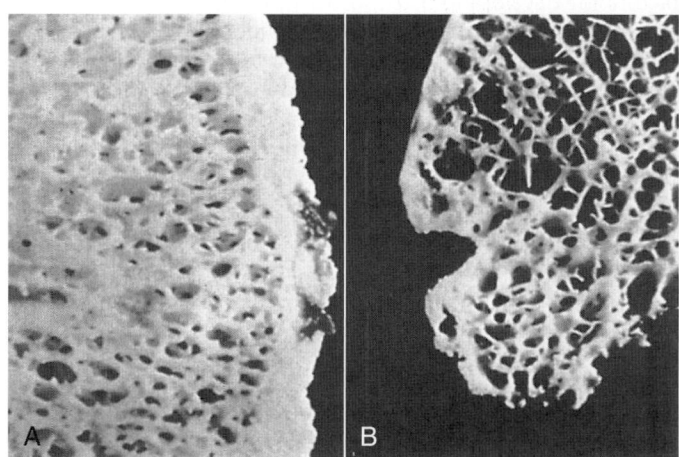

FIGURE 24-5 Difference between normal bone **(A)** and osteoporotic bone **(B).** (From Maher AB et al: Orthopaedic *nursing*, Philadelphia, 1994, Saunders.)

BOX 24-1   Medical Conditions that Increase the Risk of Osteoporosis

Chronic diarrhea or intestinal malabsorption (including celiac disease)
Chronic obstructive lung disease
Chronic renal disease
Diabetes
Hemiplegia
Hyperparathyroid disease
Hyperthyroidism
Subtotal gastrectomy

Estrogen-androgen deficient osteoporosis occurs in women within a few years of menopause from loss of trabecular bone tissue and cessation of ovarian production of estrogens. BMC and BMD measurements of the lumbar spine of women with postmenopausal osteoporosis may be as much as 25% to 40% lower than in age-matched nonosteoporotic control women of the same age range. Other bone sites with a preponderance of trabecular bone such as the pelvis, ribs, and proximal femur also display low BMD. Rarely, men may develop androgen-deficient osteoporosis if they have a significant decline in androgen production. This osteoporosis is characterized by fractures of the distal radius (Colles fractures) and "crush" fractures of the lumbar vertebrae that are often painful and deforming.

Age-related primary osteoporosis occurs at approximately age 70 and beyond. Many women lose several inches in height between 50 and 80 years of age (see Figure 24-6). Although age-associated osteoporosis affects both sexes, women are affected more severely because they have a smaller skeletal mass than men.

Causes and Risk Factors

Osteoporosis is a complex heterogeneous disorder, and many risk factors contribute during a lifetime. Low BMD is common to all types of osteoporosis, but an imbalance between bone resorption and formation results from an array of factors characteristic of each form of this disease. Risk factors for osteoporosis include age, race, gender, and factors noted in Box 24-2.

Alcohol and Cigarettes

Cigarette smoking and excessive alcohol consumption are risk factors for developing osteoporosis, probably because of toxic effects on osteoblasts. Moderate alcohol intake has no detrimental effect on bone, and some studies show a modest positive effect in postmenopausal women. Three or more drinks per day is associated with increased risk of falling and may pose other threats to bone health. The risk appears significant even after

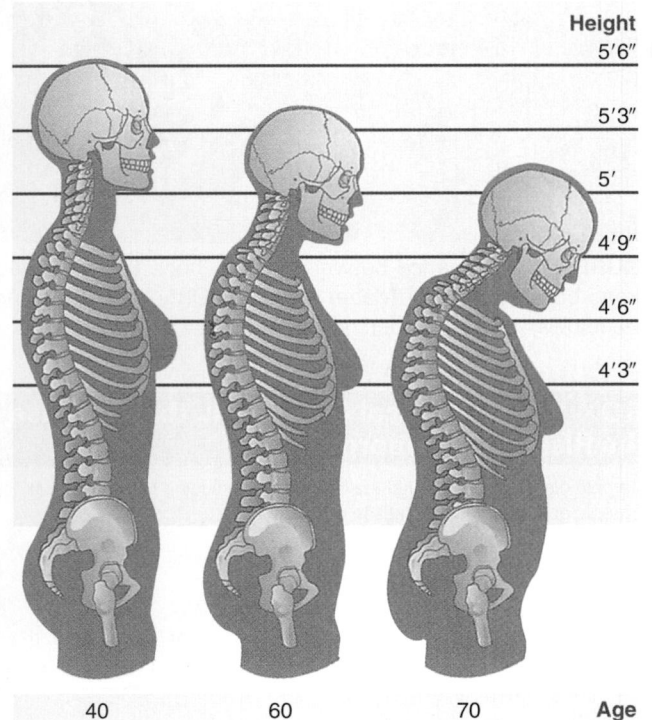

FIGURE 24-6 Normal spine at age 40 and osteoporotic changes at ages 60 and 70. These changes can cause a loss of as much as 6 to 9 inches in height and result in the dowager's hump *(far right)* in the upper thoracic vertebrae. (From Ignatavicius D, Workman M: *Medical-surgical nursing: critical thinking for collaborative care,* ed 5, Philadelphia, 2006, Saunders.)

> ### BOX 24-2 Risk Factors for Developing Osteoporosis
>
> Age, especially older than age 60
> Amenorrhea in women as a result of excessive exercise
> Androgen depletion with hypogonadism in men
> Cigarette smoking
> Estrogen depletion from menopause or early oophorectomy
> Ethnicity: white or Asian
> Excessive intake of alcohol, caffeine
> Female gender
> Family history of osteoporosis or parental history of hip fracture
> Inadequate calcium or vitamin D intake
> Lack of exercise
> Prolonged use of certain medications (see Box 24-3)
> Sarcopenia
> Underweight, low body mass index, low body fatness
>   Genetic diseases: Marfan syndrome, porphyria, homocystinuria, Gaucher disease, cystic fibrosis, glycogen storage disease, Ehlers-Danlos, hemochromatosis

adjusting for BMD when comparing smokers versus nonsmokers (North America Menopause Society, 2010). Excessive consumption (more than three drinks a day) for an extended period may result in bone loss. The combination of smoking and alcohol, common among young women and men, places them at increased risk for osteoporosis.

Low body weight is a principal determinant of bone density and fracture risk; adipose tissue mass is a major contributor (Reid, 2010). The greater the body mass, the greater the BMD. Fat and bone are linked by pathways involving adiponectin; insulin, amylin, and preptin; and leptin and adipocytic estrogens, which ultimately serve the function of providing a skeleton appropriate to the mass of adipose tissue it is carrying (Reid, 2010).

The lower the BMI, the lower the BMD is. Young girls who are typically premenarcheal may incur fractures with minimum trauma because of low BMC and BMD related to rapid growth in height that is not accompanied with a proportionate increase in weight. Young, overweight males with low bone mass also may suffer fractures (Goulding et al, 2005). Weight loss from dieting, bariatric surgery, or sarcopenia also are associated with bone loss. Thus being overweight is protective against osteoporosis and underweight is a risk factor for fractures (Reid, 2010).

Ethnicity

As previously noted, recent data suggest that Hispanics are at higher risk than non-Hispanic whites, whereas blacks are at lower risk for low bone density (Looker et al, 2012). However, non-Hispanic whites suffer more fractures than other racial or ethnic groups. Nevertheless, the incidence of fracture has declined in all racial and ethnic groups except Hispanics (Wright et al, 2012).

Limited Weight-Bearing Exercise

Maintenance of healthy bone requires exposure to weight-bearing pressures. A good diet plus exercise from roughly ages 10 to 20 years is particularly important for skeletal growth, accrual of bone mass, and increased femoral bone dimensions (Iuliano-Burns et al, 2005). Physical activity, especially upper body activities, is thought to contribute to an increase in bone mass or density (Chubak et al, 2006). Lack of exercise and a sedentary mode of living also may contribute to bone loss, although the most important influence is probably an inadequate accumulation of bone mass.

Exercise is beneficial for reducing skeletal inflammatory markers (see Chapters 3 and 7) in frail older individuals (Lambert et al, 2008). Stresses from muscle contraction and maintaining the body in an upright position against the pull of gravity stimulate osteoblast function. Bones not subjected to normal use rapidly lose mass.

Immobility in varying degrees is well recognized as a cause of bone loss. Invalids confined to bed or persons unable to move freely are commonly affected. Astronauts living in conditions of zero gravity for only a few days experience bone loss, especially in the lower extremities; appropriate exercise is a feature of their daily routines.

Loss of Menses

Loss of menses at any age is a major determinant of osteoporosis risk in women. Acceleration of bone loss coincides with menopause, either natural or surgical, at which time the ovaries stop producing estrogen. Estrogen replacement therapies have been shown to conserve BMD and reduce fracture risk within the first few years after menopause, at least in short-term studies.

Any interruption of menstruation for an extended period results in bone loss. The amenorrhea that accompanies excessive weight loss seen in patients with anorexia nervosa or in individuals who participate in high-intensity sports, dance, or other forms of exercise has the same adverse effect on bones as menopause. BMD in amenorrheic athletes has been measured at levels 25% to 40% below normal. Young women with the "female athlete triad" of disordered eating, amenorrhea, and low BMD are at increased risk for having fractures (see Chapter 23). These young women may benefit from the use of oral contraceptive agents plus calcium and vitamin D supplements.

Nutrients

Many nutrients and several nonnutrients have been implicated as causal risk factors for osteoporosis and have been discussed in previous paragraphs. Frank vitamin D deficiency has been widely reported at northern latitudes in North America and Europe. Vitamin D insufficiency also is now considered more common at latitudes closer to the equator than previously thought because of reduced exposure to sunlight. (Hypponen and Power, 2007). WHO recognizes that calcium, vitamin D, protein, phosphate, vitamin K, magnesium, and other trace elements and vitamins are related to bone health. Energy intake is related as well.

Medications

A number of medications contribute adversely to osteoporosis, either by interfering with calcium absorption or by actively promoting calcium loss from bone (see Box 24-3). For example, corticosteroids affect vitamin D metabolism and can lead to bone loss. Excessive amounts of exogenous thyroid hormone can promote loss of bone mass over time (see Chapter 8 and Appendix 23).

DIAGNOSIS AND MONITORING

Bone densitometry measures bone mass on the basis of tissue absorption of photons produced by x-ray tubes. DXA is available in most hospitals and many clinics for the measurement of the total body and regional skeletal sites, such as the lumbar

---

BOX 24-3 Medications that Increase the Risk of Osteoporosis

Aluminum-containing antacids
Corticosteroids
Cyclosporine
Heparin
Lasix and thiazide diuretics
Lithium
Methotrexate
Phenobarbital
Phenothiazine derivatives
Phenytoin (Dilantin)
Proton pump inhibitors (PPIs)
Thyroid hormone
Tetracycline

---

vertebrae and the proximal femur (hip). Results of DXA measurements are expressed commonly as T-scores and Z-scores. When the BMD T-score is 2.5 standard deviations (SD) below the mean, a diagnosis of osteoporosis is made; between 1 and 2.5 SD is considered low bone mass or osteopenia; and within 1 SD of the adult mean is considered normal. There are not separate standards for men yet, and so these standards for women are applied to men over the age of 50. For premenopausal women or men under the age of 50, Z-scores should be used. The diagnosis of osteoporosis should not be made in premenopausal women unless they experience a low trauma fracture or have Z-scores below 3 (National Osteoporosis Foundation (NOF), 2014). The International Society for Clinical Densitometry (ISCD) recommends separate diagnostic criteria to assess bone health in children and teens (http://www.iscd.org/official-positions/2013-iscd-official-positions-adult/).

Ultrasound Measurements of Bone

Ultrasound instruments measure the velocity of sound waves transmitted through bone and broadband ultrasound attenuation (BUA). Measurements at the calcaneus (heel) correlate fairly well with BMD measurements at this same skeletal site. However, ultrasound measurements are considered screening tools, whereas DEXA measurements are considered diagnostic.

Fracture Risk Assessment

The World Health Organization (WHO) developed an algorithm to predict fracture by using femoral head BMD and clinical indicators of low bone mass. This uses economic modeling to guide the most cost-effective instances to begin medications. Vertebral fractures that are confirmed by x-rays are a strong predictor of future vertebral fractures, as well as fractures at other sites (NOF, 2014).

Bone Markers

Enzymes or degradation products in serum or urine have been used for research and are beginning to be used more often to monitor drug treatment effectiveness. Serum procollagen type I N-terminal propeptide (P1NP), a bone formation marker, and serum collagen type I crosslinked C-telopeptide (sCTX), a bone resorption marker, are recommended by the International Osteoporosis Foundation and the International Federation of Clinical Chemistry and Laboratory Medicine, with caution because of the need for standardization of techniques and recognition of variation sources (Vasikaran et al, 2011).

Tools to Estimate Probability of Fracture

The World Health Organization developed a tool based on epidemiologic data to calculate the 10-year probability of fracture. The risk algorithm, known as FRAX, is a computer program that includes gender, age, body mass index, parental history of hip fracture, current tobacco smoking, long-term use of oral glucocorticoids, having rheumatoid arthritis or other secondary cause of osteoporosis, and alcohol intake of three or more servings daily. Bone mineral density data of the femoral neck also can be used in the FRAX assessment. The risk assessment does not include any diet or physical activity information, or information about the frequency of falling or likelihood of falling.

The FRAX is used by clinicians to help them decide when medications should be started. According to FRAX, a probability of more than a 20% risk of fracture indicates that some discussion should begin with the patient about whether medication should be started. However, the FRAX guidelines also should consider the patient's individual situation.

The tool has been adapted for use in many countries and is applicable for men and women between 40 and 90 years of age. However, the specificity of the tool for fracture risk is higher for women. One purpose of using the FRAX is to determine the point at which prescribing medications becomes cost effective. It is most valuable in determining risk of fracture in osteopenic individuals.

Used less in clinical practice are three other risk assessment tools: the Simple Calculated Osteoporosis Estimation (SCORE) survey, the Osteoporosis Risk Assessment Instrument (ARAI), and the Osteoporosis Index of Risk (OSIRIS). SCORE calculators are available online and include a person's race, existence of rheumatoid arthritis, estrogen therapy, number of previous fractures, age and weight. The ORAI includes age, weight and current estrogen use. The OSIRIS includes age, weight, estrogen use, and previous fractures.

NUTRITION AND BONE

Calcium, phosphate, and vitamin D are essential for normal bone structure and function. Protein, calories, and other micronutrients also help develop and maintain bone (Tucker, 2009).

Energy

Energy intake does not have a direct effect on bone; rather, inadequate energy intake leading to low body weight, or too many calories leading to overweight have effects on bone. Being underweight is considered a risk factor for osteoporosis, whereas being overweight may be protective.

Protein

Protein and calcium are important components of PBM, especially before puberty (Rizzoli, 2008). Adequate protein intake, with adequate calcium intake, is needed for optimal bone health. A meta-analysis of studies concerned with protein intake and indicators of bone health found a slight positive effect on BMD, but it did not influence the risk of fracture over the long term when total protein, animal protein, or vegetable protein intake were considered (Darling et al, 2009). Unfortunately, this analysis did not consider calcium intake.

The negative effects of either too high or too low an intake of protein is more pronounced with inadequate calcium intake, especially in seniors (Tucker, 2009). The theory that higher protein intakes produce a higher acidic load, which increases calcium urinary excretion, has not been verified (see *Clinical Insight:* Acid and Alkaline Diets in Chapter 35). Although dietary protein may increase acid load and thereby increase urinary calcium excretion, protein also may improve calcium absorption and increase growth factors, which also could improve bone health (Thorpe and Evans, 2011).

Very low protein intake may negatively affect bone turnover and development. In cases of negative nitrogen balance, such as with fracture or surgery, higher protein intake may be advised.

Minerals
Calcium

Calcium intake in the primary prevention of osteoporosis has received much attention. The Dietary Reference Intakes (DRIs) for calcium and vitamin D, are given as RDAs. The RDA for calcium from preadolescence (age 9 years) through adolescence (up to 19 years) was increased to 1300 mg/day for both genders

(IOM, 2011). The RDAs for calcium for adults, pregnant and lactating women, and children are listed on the inside front cover.

Most females older than age 8 do not meet the adequate intake level for calcium when all sources of calcium are considered; intake of males from birth until age 70 appears to be better, although many are still low. Calcium intake from all sources by males aged 70 and older is similar to females (Bailey et al, 2010).

Food sources are recommended first for supplying calcium needs because of the coingestion of other essential nutrients. In the United States the primary source of calcium is dairy foods, and this intake is higher in Caucasian than in African American women (Plawecki et al, 2009). However, calcium fortification of nondairy foods such as nondairy milks and other beverages, juices, breakfast cereals, bread, and some crackers is common.

Calcium bioavailability from foods is generally good, and the amount of calcium in the food is more important than its bioavailability. However, the order of concern relative to calcium absorption efficiency is first the individual's need for calcium, second the amount consumed because absorption efficiency is inversely related to amount consumed, and third the intake of absorption enhancers or inhibitors. For example, absorption from foods high in oxalic and phytic acid (certain vegetables and legumes) is lower than from dairy products.

The amount of calcium in foods varies with the brand, serving size, and whether it has been fortified. When reading the Nutrition Facts label to determine the amount of calcium per serving, multiply the daily value (DV) percentage by 10 to determine the milligrams of calcium per serving. For example, a 20% DV equals 200 mg of calcium (see Chapter 11). Labeling for "excellent" (more than 200 mg/serving) and "good" (100 to 200 mg/serving) sources of calcium are regulated by the Food and Drug Administration (FDA, 2013).

Reaching RDA levels for calcium from foods should be the first goal, but if insufficient amounts of calcium from foods are consumed, supplements of calcium should then be ingested to reach the age-specific RDA. Other sources of calcium include mineral water and medications, especially antacids. The amount of calcium in tap water across the U.S. and Canada is generally low, although ranges from 4 mg/L to 220 mg/L, with an average of about 50 mg/L, or the amount of calcium that could be found in a medium orange (Morr et al, 2006).

An increasing percentage of the population is taking calcium supplements. Persons who should take supplements include those not meeting the RDA on most days, those taking corticosteroids, those with low bone mass or osteoporosis, women who are perimenopausal or postmenopausal, and those who are lactose intolerant.

Calcium carbonate is the most common form of calcium supplement. It should be taken with food because an acidic environment enhances absorption. For those with achlorhydria, which often occurs in seniors, calcium citrate may be more appropriate because it does not require an acidic environment for absorption and does not further reduce the acidity of the stomach (Straub, 2007).

The absorption of calcium supplementation is optimal when taken as individual doses of 500 mg or less. Many formulations include vitamin D, because the likelihood of needing vitamin D is high if calcium supplementation is needed. Choosing a supplement that has the United States Pharmacopeia (USP) designation increases the likelihood that the supplement quantity is consistent with the label, and that good manufacturing practices are used. Calcium supplementation increases the risk of reaching the upper limit of safety (UL). The UL for calcium for each age group is listed in Table 24-2.

Phosphate

The body's reserve of phosphorus is found in the bone as hydroxyapatite. Phosphate salts are available in practically all foods either naturally or because of processing. In healthy adults, the urinary phosphorus excretion approximately equals intake.

Soft drinks are poor in nutrient value but often high in phosphate content. However, studies have found that the soft drink primarily displaces milk as a beverage, concluding that the negative effect is from lower calcium intake rather than higher phosphate intake. Another hypothesis about the negative affect of soft drink consumption on bones has to do with the rapid rate of phosphorus absorption and greater phosphorus bioavailability from processed foods such as cola drinks (Calvo and Tucker, 2013). Those at high risk and those who have osteoporosis may want to avoid these beverages (Tucker, 2009).

Trace Minerals

Few studies are available about the effects of trace minerals on bone. Iron, zinc, copper, manganese, and boron may function in bone cells, but their specific roles in preventing bone loss are not well established. In one study, 77 adults took a combination of nutrients most or all the time during a 12-month intervention period. The nutrients included docosahexaenoic acid, vitamin D, vitamin K, strontium, and magnesium along with a diet rich in calcium, and daily impact exercise. In the sample of 40 who completed the trial, about half demonstrated a >3%

change in bone mineral density at either the femoral neck, total hip, or spine (Genuis, Bouchard, 2012).

Fluoride ions enter the hydroxyapatite crystals of bone as substitutes for hydroxyl ions. Water containing 1 mg/liter has been determined to be optimal for dental health. The upper limits (UL) for fluoride vary by age, beginning with 0.7 mg/day for infants 0 through 6 months, and up to 10 mg/day for children over 8 years through adulthood (IOM, 1997) (see Chapter 25). Fluoride does not help bone in the same way that it helps tooth surfaces. Within narrow limits of safety (less than 2 ppm), fluoride ions have little effect on increasing the hardness of bone mineral.

Vitamins

Vitamin A

Vitamin A consumption consists of retinol (animal sources) and carotenoids (plant sources). Although the research is not definitive, a general guideline is that retinol intake should not be excessive, and carotenoids may have a beneficial role in bone health (Tanumihardjo, 2013). The window of safe consumption of retinol is fairly narrow, especially for older adults.

Vitamin D

In 2008, the Food and Drug Administration amended the label health claim regulations concerning calcium and osteoporosis so that they could also include vitamin D because of increasing recognition that vitamin D plays a pivotal role in calcium uptake and therefore bone homeostasis (FDA, 2008). Although the main function of vitamin D is to maintain serum calcium and phosphorus levels within a constant range, vitamin D is important in stimulating intestinal calcium transport. Vitamin D also stimulates activity of osteoclasts in bone. In both these areas the net desired effect is to increase calcium availability.

Vitamin D also may have a role in muscle tone and fall prevention. Although vitamin D supplementation for fall prevention has had positive and negative results (Theodoratou et al, 2014), older adults with vitamin D deficiency as measured by blood 25-hydroxyvitamin D_3 (calcifediol) levels had muscle weakness and poor balance (Hirani et al, 2014).

An individual's vitamin D status depends mostly on sunlight exposure, and secondarily on dietary intake of vitamin D. The synthesis of vitamin D by skin exposed to sunlight varies considerably as a result of many factors, including skin tone, sunscreen use, environmental latitude, and age (McCarty, 2008) (see Appendix 45). The skin of older individuals is less efficient at producing vitamin D after exposure to ultraviolet (UV) light because the skin is thinner and it contains fewer cells that can synthesize vitamin D. In addition, older adults living in nursing homes and similar institutions typically have little exposure to sunlight. Those who live at northern latitudes in the United States and Canada are at increased risk of osteoporosis because of limited UV light during winter months, although those at more southern latitudes also may be at risk if exposure to sunlight is limited (Hypponen and Power, 2007).

The few foods that naturally contain vitamin D are egg yolks, fatty fish such as salmon, mackerel, catfish, tuna, and sardines, cod liver oil, and some mushrooms (see Appendix 45). The vitamin D content of fish varies, as does the content in UV-exposed mushrooms. Fluid milk in the United States is fortified with vitamin D_2 at a standardized level of 400 IU vitamin D_2 per quart, whereas other foods, including juices, cereals, yogurt, and margarines, may be fortified in varying amounts. The RDAs for vitamin D across the life cycle are shown inside the

TABLE 24-2	Upper Limit for Calcium Intake
Age	**Amount, mg**
Birth to 6 months	1000
7 to 12 months	1500
1 to 8 years	2500
9 to 18 years	3000
19 to 50	2500
Over 50 years	2000

front cover. The upper limit is 100 µg (4000 IU) for everyone older than 8 years, and lower levels for younger children (see inside back cover). From any source, vitamin D must be hydroxylated in the kidney before becoming the physiologically active calcitriol (1,25-hydroxy vitamin D₃).

To prevent rickets, the American Academy of Pediatrics recommends that all infants who are exclusively breastfed be supplemented with 400 IU of vitamin D. Infants who are both formula and breastfed also should be supplemented until they are consistently taking 1 L (1 quart) of formula a day. They further recommend continuing the supplementation until 1 year of age, when children begin drinking vitamin D–fortified milk (Wagner and Greer, 2008).

The older adult is at increased risk for vitamin D deficiency because of the decreased synthesis of vitamin D by the skin secondary to age-related skin changes and decreased exposure to sunlight; increased body fat; decreased renal function that decreases the hydroxylation of vitamin D to its active form; and decreased levels of insulin-like growth factor 1, **calcitonin**, and estrogen, which affect hydroxylase activity. In general, seniors may benefit from daily vitamin D supplementation of 10 to 20 mcg (400 IU to 800 IU) to reach serum **25-hydroxy vitamin D (calcidiol)** levels of at least 30 ng/ml (75 nmol/L). Older adults who are frail or institutionalized may need up to 50 mcg (2000 IU)/day. Mobility, skin tone, body weight, and dietary habits may modify these recommendations (Oudshoorn et al, 2009). The most common blood test for vitamin D status is serum 25-(OH) D level, and the normal range is considered to be 30 to 75 ng/ml (Topiwala, 2013).

Vitamin K

Vitamin K is an essential micronutrient for bone health. Its role in post-translational modification of several matrix proteins, including **osteocalcin**, is well established. After bone resorption, osteocalcin is released and enters the blood. In this way, osteocalcin serves as a serum bone marker for predicting the risk of a fracture.

Most of the vitamin K intake by individuals in the United States is from green leafy vegetables, with about one third from fats and oils. Although menaquinones, a form of vitamin K, are formed in the gut by bacteria, the influence of this source on vitamin K status appears to be weak. Many older adults have inadequate intakes of vitamin K, primarily because their consumption of dark-green leafy vegetables is so low. It is important to consider the vitamin K intake in older persons who also may be taking blood-thinning medications (vitamin K antagonists) (see Chapter 8 and Appendix 23). Rather than having these patients avoid vitamin K in foods and thus jeopardize their bone status, it is better to have the vitamin K daily intake be consistent and regulate the vitamin K antagonist medication. In fact, it has been shown that therapeutic international normalized ratio (INR) ranges from blood thinning medication can be achieved with vitamin K in low-dose supplementation and when fluctuations are few (Ford and Moll, 2008).

Other Dietary Components

Several other dietary factors have been associated with bone health, but their relative quantitative importance is not clear.

Alcohol

Although previously mentioned as a risk factor, moderate consumption of wine and beer may be beneficial to bone in men and postmenopausal women. Nonalcoholic constituents, such as silicon in beer, need further investigation. In men, high liquor intakes (more than 2 drinks per day) are associated with significantly lower BMD (Kanis et al, 2005; Tucker et al, 2009). Heavy alcohol consumption also may be accompanied by poor dietary intake, cigarette smoking, poor balance, and an increased risk of falls.

Caffeine and Soft Drinks

The relationship of moderate consumption of caffeine to osteoporosis has not been clearly established. *Excessive* caffeine intake may have a deleterious effect on BMD (Ruffing et al, 2006). Intake of colas also is associated with lower BMD. Although the primary issue may be displacement of dairy beverages, there is also a potential direct effect (Tucker, 2009). Rapid metabolizers of caffeine may be a high risk group for bone loss (Hallström et al, 2010.)

Dietary Fiber

Excessive dietary fiber intake may interfere with calcium absorption, but any interference is considered extremely small in the typical low-fiber diet. Vegans who may consume as much as 50 g of fiber a day are most likely to have a significant depression in intestinal calcium absorption, but this is often offset by adequate calcium intake. Fiber includes a variety of different compounds, and so intake of "fiber" as a category can produce different effects on bone. The inulin-type fructans are a group of fiber compounds found in wheat, onion, bananas, garlic, and leeks that may enhance calcium and magnesium absorption (Roberfroid, 2007), whereas high-fiber foods that contain phytates or oxalates may lower calcium absorption. The calcium content of these foods, such as spinach or legumes, is also lower than in dairy foods (Dairy Research Institute, 2011).

Isoflavones

The isoflavones in soybeans function as estrogen agonists and antioxidants in bone cells. They inhibit bone resorption in female animal models without ovaries, but not in young adult females with normal estrogen status. Some, but not all, studies show modest skeletal benefits (Lagari, Levis, 2013).

High Acid or Alkaline Diets

Higher acid diets include those high in protein, dairy, and grains (see *Clinical Insight:* Acid and Alkaline Diets in Chapter 35). It is theorized that these higher acid diets may increase calcium excretion and have a detrimental effect on bone. The theory also supports a converse beneficial effect of an alkaline diet on bone. Several meta-analyses, experimental studies, and reviews have not supported either the negative effect of higher acid diets on bone or the positive effects of an alkaline diet on bone. Higher protein intake may, in fact, have a positive effect on bone (Cao and Nielsen, 2010; Fenton et al, 2010; Fenton et al, 2011; Frassetto et al, 2012; Hanley and Whiting, 2013).

Sodium

A high sodium intake may contribute to osteoporosis because of increased calcium excretion (Massey, 2005). Although the calciuric effect of sodium has been speculated, there seems to be no adverse effects when there is adequate calcium and vitamin D intake (Ilich et al, 2010).

Vegetarian Diets

Research is inconclusive concerning the effects of vegetarian diets on bone mass, bone density, and osteoporosis risk. Vegans and lactovegetarians differ in their intake of protein, calcium, and other nutrients, and often have lifestyle patterns that also differ from the general population. In addition, ethnicities with a traditional practice of vegetarianism may have differences in terms of genetics that influence body frame and size (Ho-Pham et al, 2009).

PREVENTION OF OSTEOPOROSIS AND FRACTURES

The increasing longevity of the population emphasizes the need for prevention of osteoporosis (see Box 24-4). Universal guidelines apply to everyone. Consuming adequate amounts of calcium, and vitamin D, along with lifelong muscle strengthening and weight-bearing exercise, avoidance of tobacco, moderate or no intake of alcohol, and steps to avoid falls are all part of the holistic approach to a lifestyle that promotes optimal bone health (NAMS, 2010).

Exercise

To preserve bone health through adulthood, the American Academy of Sports Medicine recommends weight-bearing activity three to five times per week and resistance exercise two to three times per week with moderate to high bone-loading force for a combination of 30 to 60 minutes per week. Regular walking and swimming appear to have minor benefits in older individuals. More active participation (such as weight-bearing exercises and intensive walking) have positive effects on BM (Guadalupe-Grau et al, 2009; Gomez-Cabello et al, 2012). For older adults, posture, balance, and flexibility are also important.

Diet

The National Osteoporosis Foundation recommends universal guidelines for all adults for the prevention of osteoporosis that includes adequate calcium and vitamin D, and a balanced diet of low-fat dairy, fruits, and vegetables. Although the NOF recommends the same amount of calcium intake as the IOM, the NOF recommends a higher intake of vitamin D than does the IM for those 50 years and older (800 to 1000 IU/day). If these intake goals are not reached by food, supplements should be considered (NOF, 2013). In addition, achieving and maintaining a healthy weight and consuming a lower sodium diet is recommended for optimal bone health for women (Cox et al, 2013).

FDA-Approved Drug Treatments

Raloxifene and tamoxiphen, which are **estrogen agonist/ antagonist agents**; alendronate sodium, risedronate sodium, and zoledronic acid, which are **bisphosphonates**; and **estrogen replacement therapy (ERT)** are all approved for the prevention of osteoporosis, especially for postmenopausal women (NOF, 2013). However, because of potential side effects, nonestrogen treatment for prevention is recommended, especially if menopausal symptom relief is not also a goal of the therapy (NOF, 2013). The **bisphosphonates** act as inhibitors on osteoclasts to reduce bone resorption. They have been shown to be effective in reducing the incidence of new fractures (Epstein, 2006). Side effects include gastrointestinal problems and rare cases of jaw necrosis. However, stopping the medication after 2 to 3 years is recommended. Estrogen agonists or antagonists, which used to be referred to as SERMS (**selective estrogen receptor modulators**), are able to stimulate **estrogen receptors (ER)** in bone tissue and yet have very little effect on the ERs of the breast or uterus. The most common side effect is hot flashes. Teriparatide, the only anabolic on the market, and Denosumab, a RANK (**Receptor Activator of Nuclear Factor κ B**) inhibitor are approved therapies. **Receptor Activator of Nuclear Factor κ B** is part of a signaling pathway that regulates osteoclast activation.

TREATMENT OF OSTEOPOROSIS

Medical Nutrition Therapy

Calcium (1000 mg/day) and vitamin D (800 to 1000 units/day) typically are recommended as supplements for patients being treated with one of the bone drugs, either antiresorptive or anabolic. These amounts are considered safe and sufficient for bone formation. Because of the range of nutrients involved in bone health, a healthy diet emphasizing the key nutrients seems most promising in achieving an intake for optimal bone health (Tucker, 2009). The dietitian nutritionist should evaluate the client's diet for all bone-related nutrients and tailor recommendations based on personal preferences, cultural differences, nutrient recommendations, and the need for supplements (McCabe-Sellers and Skipper, 2010).

Exercise

For those with osteoporosis, exercises that exert strong force against potentially weak bone are not recommended, such as sit-ups or twisting. Exercises should focus on posture, balance, gait, coordination, and hip and trunk stabilization (IOF, 2014). For those in need of rehabilitation, the client should be evaluated for capabilities and deficiencies, with attention to weight-bearing aerobic activities, posture, resistance training, stretching, and balance training (IOF, 2014).

FDA-Approved Drug Treatments

All the medications that are approved for prevention are also approved for treatment of osteoporosis, with the exception of estrogen replacement therapy. Another bisphosphonate, ibandronate sodium, is also approved only for treatment. In addition, **calcitonin**, the hormone, is used to inhibit osteoclastic bone resorption by blocking the stimulatory effects of PTH on these cells. Calcitonin can be administered by nasal spray. It improves BMD, especially of the lumbar spine, and it may reduce the recurrence of fractures in patients with osteoporosis. Calcitonin is approved by the FDA for postmenopausal treatment of osteoporosis, but it is recommended that the women be at least 5 years postmenopausal.

PTH therapy is approved by the FDA for the treatment of postmenopausal women and men at high risk for fracture and for those on long-term glucocorticoid therapy. Although the chronic, physiologic rise in PTH that can occur with aging or in

---

BOX 24-4 FDA-Approved Medications for Prevention or Treatment of Osteoporosis

Bisphosphonates
Calcitonin—treatment only
Estrogen—prevention only when menopausal symptoms are primarily being treated
Estrogen agonist/antagonist—treatment only
Tissue specific estrogen complex—treatment only
Parathyroid hormone (PTH)—treatment only
Receptor activator of nuclear factor k ligand (RANKL) inhibitor— treatment only

hyperparathyroidism resulting from other causes increases osteoclastic activity and decreases bone density, the **intermittent PTH therapy** has the opposite effect. The drug PTH works by increasing osteoblast number and function (Kousteni and Bilezikian, 2008). PTH increases spine, hip, and total body BMD. PTH is often prescribed first, followed by bisphosphonates, so that an increase in bone mass is followed by antiresorptive therapy (Cosman, 2008).

Denosumab, which works at the receptor level to inhibit RANKL, is approved by the FDA for men and women at high risk of fracture.

Drug Treatments Not Yet Approved by the FDA

There are many medications not approved by the FDA for prevention or treatment of osteoporosis. These include calcitriol (1,25-dihyroxy vitamin D_3); PTH 1-84, which is an intact human recombinant form of PTH; sodium fluoride; and strontium ranelate.

CLINICAL CASE STUDY

Liz B. is a 73-year-old white woman who is seeing her doctor for a regular physical. She is married and retired, but volunteers for several organizations and watches her grandchildren two mornings a week. She and her husband play golf about once a week during the spring, summer, and fall. She weighs 130 pounds and always thought she was 5'6". However, when she was measured at this physical, she was 5'4". Because of her age and height loss, she has a dual-energy x-ray absorptiometry (DEXA) measurement that shows that she has low bone mineral density (BMD) values of her proximal femur and lumbar vertebrae (both values are classified as osteoporotic according to World Health Organization definitions). A chest x-ray also revealed two vertebral fractures. However, she has no pain in her back or neck.

The RDN and Liz discuss her diet, concluding that her diet is low in calcium and vitamin D, but high in sodium. Along with suggestions to decrease her sodium intake and increase her fruit and vegetable intake, she is advised to start taking supplements of calcium (1000 mg/day) and vitamin D (800 units/day). They discuss avoiding high-impact exercise affecting the spine because of the low bone mass and existing vertebral fractures, but increasing flexibility, balance, and posture exercises. Because of the DXA results, she also begins on a bisphosphonate drug in addition to the calcium and vitamin D supplements. She receives baseline tests of bone turnover, to be rechecked in 6 months and an appointment for another DXA in 1 year.

After 1 year on the medication, supplements, diet and exercise changes, Liz has another DXA. Her BMD has improved to the osteopenia level, and she is taken off the bisphosphonate medication.

Nutrition Diagnostic Statement

Inadequate calcium and vitamin D intake related to avoidance of dairy products as evidenced by diet history revealing less than 20% of estimated requirements. NOTE: This may be resolved once she starts taking supplements.

Nutrition Care Questions

1. If Liz wants to increase her calcium through fortified foods rather than take a supplement, how would you counsel her?
2. Design a set (3 days minimum) of daily menus that provide approximately 800 mg of calcium from foods alone, which, coupled with a 500-mg supplement, would provide a total of 1300 mg daily, the current adequate intake for calcium. Similarly, design these same meals to include 400 units of vitamin D, with another 400 units coming from supplements.
3. If Liz's sodium intake is high, what foods would you advise her to eat less frequently?

USEFUL WEBSITES

Center for Disease Control and Prevention
http://www.cdc.gov/nutrition/everyone/basics/vitamins/calcium.html
International Osteoporosis Foundation
www.iofbonehealth.org/
Menopause
http://www.menopause.org/
National Institutes of Health—Bone Health
http://www.nichd.nih.gov/health/topics/bone_health.cfm
National Osteoporosis Foundation
http://www.nof.org/

REFERENCES

Bailey RL et al. Estimation of total usual calcium and vitamin D intakes in the United States. *J Nutr* 140:817, 2010.

Calvo MS, Tucker KL: Is phosphorus intake that exceeds dietary requirements a risk factor for bone health?, *Ann NY Acad Sci* 1301(29-35) 2013.

Cao JJ, Nielsen FH: Acid diet (high-meat protein) effects on calcium metabolism and bone health, *Curr Opin Clin Nutr Metab Care* 13(6):698-702, 2010.

Chubak J et al: Effect of exercise on bone mineral density and lean mass in postmenopausal women, *Med Sci Sports Exerc* 38:1236, 2006.

Cosman F: Parathyroid hormone treatment for osteoporosis, *Curr Opin Endocrin Diab Obes* 15:495, 2008.

Cox JT, Chapman-Novakofski K, Thompson C: Nutrition and women's health. Practice paper of the Academy of Nutrition and Dietetics. Available at http://www.eatright.org/Members/content.aspx?id=6442479072.

Dairy Research Institute: Calcium bioavailability. Scientific Status Report, 2011. Available at http://www.nationaldairycouncil.org/SiteCollection Documents/research/research-summaries/ScientificStatusReportCalcium Bioavailability.pdf. Accessed January, 2014.

Darling AL et al: Dietary protein and bone health: a systematic review and meta-analysis, *Am J Clin Nutr* 90:1674, 2009.

Epstein S: Update of current therapeutic options for the treatment of postmenopausal osteoporosis, *Clin Ther* 28:151, 2006.

FDA (Food and Drug Administration): *Title 21: Food and Drugs, Part 101 Food labeling. Subpart E. Specific Requirements for Health Claims. Health Claims: Calcium and Osteoporosis* (website): http://www.accessdata.fda.gov/scripts/cdrh/cfdocs/cfcfr/CFRSearch.cfm?fr=101.72, 2008. Accessed July, 2015,

FDA (Food and Drug Administration): *Guidance for Industry: A Food Labeling Guide (10. Appendix B: Additional Requirements for Nutrient Content Claims)* (website): http://www.fda.gov/Food/GuidanceRegulation/GuidanceDocumentsRegulatoryInformation/LabelingNutrition/ucm064916.htm, 2013. Accessed July, 2015.

Fenton TR et al: Low urine pH and acid excretion do not predict bone fractures or the loss of bone mineral density: a prospective cohort study, *BMC Musculoskelet Disord* 11:88, 2010.

Fenton TR: Causal assessment of dietary acid load and bone disease: a systematic review & meta-analysis applying Hill's epidemiologic criteria for causality, *Nutr J* 10:41, 2011.

Ford SK, Moll S: Vitamin K supplementation to decrease variability of international normalized ratio in patients on vitamin K antagonists: a literature review, *Curr Opin Hematol* 15:504, 2008.

Frassetto LA et al: No evidence that the skeletal non-response to potassium alkali supplements in healthy postmenopausal women depends on blood pressure or sodium chloride intake, *Eur J Clin Nutr* 66:1315, 2012.

Genuis SJ, Bouchard TP. Combination of micronutrients for bone (COMB) study: Bone density after micronutrient intervention, J Environ Pub Health Article ID 354151, 2012. Available at http://www.hindawi.com/journals/jeph/2012/354151/abs/

Gomez-Cabello et al. Effects of training on bone mass in older adults: a systematic review. *Sports Med* 42:301, 2012.

Goulding A et al: Bone and body composition of children and adolescents with repeated forearm fractures, *J Bone Miner Res* 20:2090, 2005.

Guadalupe-Grau et al. Exercise and bone mass in adults. *Sports Med* 39: 439, 2009.

Hallström H et al: Coffee consumption and CYP1A2 genotype in relation to bone mineral density of the proximal femur in elderly men and women: a cohort study, *Nutr Metab (Lond)* 7:12, 2010.

Hanley DA, Whiting SJ: Does a high dietary acid content cause bone loss, and can bone loss be prevented with an alkaline diet? *J Clin Densitom* 16:420, 2013.

Hirani V et al: Low levels of 25-hydroxy vitamin D and active 1,25-dihydroxyvitamin D independently associated with type 2 diabetes mellitus in older Australian men: the Concord Health and Ageing in Men Project. *J Am Geriatr Soc* 62:417, 2014.

Ho-Pham LT, Nguyen ND, Nguyen TV: Effect of vegetarian diets on bone mineral density: a Bayesian meta-analysis, *Am J Clin Nutr* 90:943, 2009.

Hypponen E, Power C: Hypovitaminosis D in British adults at age 45 y: nationwide cohort study of dietary and lifestyle predictors, *Am J Clin Nutr* 85:860, 2007.

Ilich JZ et al: Higher habitual sodium intake is not detrimental for bones in older women with adequate calcium intake, *Eur J Appl Physiol* 109:745, 2010.

International Osteoporosis Foundation (IOF): *Exercise Recommendations* (website): http://www.iofbonehealth.org/exercise-recommendations. Accessed January 2014.

Institute of Medicine (IOM): *Standing Committee on the Scientific Evaluation of Dietary Reference Intakes, Food and Nutrition Board: Dietary reference intakes for calcium and vitamin D* (website): www.nap.edu. http://www.nap.edu/openbook.php?record_id=5776 on Accessed July, 2015.

Institute of Medicine (IOM). Dietary Reference Intakes for Calcium, Phosphorus, Magnesium, Vitamin D, and Fluoride. (Website): www.nap.edu

Iuliano-Burns S et al: Diet and exercise during growth have site-specific skeletal effects: a co-twin study, *Osteoporos Int* 16:1225, 2005.

Kanis JA et al: Alcohol intake as a risk factor for fracture, *Osteoporos Int* 16:737, 2005.

Kousteni S, Bilezikian JP: The cell biology of parathyroid hormone in osteoblasts, *Curr Osteoporos Rep* 6:72, 2008.

Lagari VS, Levis S. Phytoestrogens in the prevention of postmenopausal bone. *J Clin Densitom* 16: 445, 2013.

Lambert CP et al: Exercise but not diet-induced weight loss decreases skeletal muscle inflammatory gene expression in frail obese elderly persons, *J Appl Physiol* 105:473, 2008.

Looker AC et al: *Osteoporosis or low bone mass at the femur neck or lumbar spine in older adults: United States, 2005–2008. NCHS data brief no 93*, Hyattsville, Md, 2012, National Center for Health Statistics.

McCabe-Sellers BJ, Skipper A, American Dietetic Association: Position of the American Dietetic Association: integration of medical nutrition therapy and pharmacotherapy, *J Am Diet Assoc* 110:950, 2010.

MacKinnon AS et al: Dietary restriction of lycopene for a period of one month resulted in significantly increased biomarkers of oxidative stress and bone resorption in postmenopausal women, *J Nutr Health Aging* 15:133, 2011.

Massey LK: Effect of dietary salt intake on circadian calcium metabolism, bone turnover, and calcium oxalate kidney stone risk in postmenopausal women, *Nutr Res* 25:891, 2005.

McCarty CA: Sunlight exposure assessment: can we accurately assess vitamin D exposure from sunlight questionnaires? *Am J Clin Nutr* 87:1097, 2008.

Misra M, Klibanski A: Anorexia nervosa and osteoporosis, *Rev Endocr Metab Disord* 7:91, 2006.

Morr S, et al:. How much calcium is in your drinking water? A survey of calcium concentrations in bottled and tap water and their significance for medical treatment and drug administration. *HHS* 2(2): 130, 2006.

National Osteoporosis Foundation (NOF) (website):http://www.nof.org/. Accessed January 2014.

Nieves JW: Osteoporosis: the role of micronutrients, *Am J Clin Nutr* 81:1232S, 2005.

North America Menopause Society (NAMS): Management of osteoporosis in post-menopausal women: 2010 position statement of the North America Menopause Society, *Menopause* 17:25, 2010.

Oudshoorn C et al: Ageing and vitamin D deficiency: effects on calcium homeostasis and considerations for vitamin D supplementation, *Br J Nutr* 101:1597, 2009.

Plawecki KL et al: Assessing calcium intake in postmenopausal women, *Prev Chronic Dis* 6:124, 2009.

Pothiwala P et al: Ethnic variation in risk for osteoporosis among women: a review of biological and behavioral factors, *J Womens Health* 15:709, 2006.

Prentice A: Milk intake, calcium and vitamin D in pregnancy and lactation: effects on maternal, fetal and infant bone in low- and high-income countries, *Nestle Nutr Workshop Ser Pediatr Progr* 67:1, 2011.

Reid IR: Fat and bone, *Arch Biochem Biophys* 503:20, 2010.

Reid IR: Relationships between fat and bone, *Osteoporos Int* 19:595, 2008.

Rizzoli R: Nutrition: its role in bone health, *Best Pract Res Clin Endocrinol Metab* 22:813, 2008.

Roberfroid MB: Inulin-type fructans: functional food ingredients, *J Nutr* 137(11 Suppl):2493S,, 2007.

Ruffing J et al: Determinants of bone mass and bone size in a large cohort of physically active young adult men, *Nutr Metabol* 3:14, 2006.

Straub DA: Calcium supplementation in clinical practice: a review of forms, doses, and indications, *Nutr Clin Pract* 22:286, 2007.

Tanumihardjo SA: Vitamin A and bone health: the balancing act, *J Clin Densitom* 16:414, 2013.

Theodoratou E, et al: Vitamin D and multiple health outcomes: umbrella review of systematic reviews and meta-analyses of observational studies and randomised trials. *BMJ* 1;348:g2035, 2014.

Thorpe MP, Evans EM: Dietary protein and bone health: harmonizing conflicting theories, *Nutr Rev* 69(4):215-230, 2011.

Topiwala S, for the US National Library of Medicine, US National Institute of Health and Human Services, NIH (website): http://www.nlm.nih.gov/medlineplus/ency/article/003569.htm, updated 2013. Accessed July, 2015.

Tucker KL: Osteoporosis prevention and nutrition, *Curr Osteoporos Rep* 7:111, 2009.

Tucker KL et al: Effects of beer, wine, and liquor intakes on bone mineral density in older men and women, *Am J Clin Nutr* 89:1188, 2009.

Vasikaran S et al: The International Osteoporosis Foundation and International Federation of Clinical Chemistry and Laboratory Medicine: Position on bone marker standards in osteoporosis, *Clin Chem Lab Med* 49:1271, 2011.

Wagner CL, Greer FR: American Academy of Pediatrics Section on Breastfeeding, American Academy of Pediatrics Committee on Nutrition: Prevention of rickets and vitamin D deficiency in infants, children, and adolescents, *Pediatrics* 122:1142, 2008.

Wright NC et al: Recent trends in hip fracture rates by race/ethnicity among older US adults, *J Bone Miner Res* 27:2325, 2012.

25

Nutrition for Oral and Dental Health

Diane Rigassio Radler, PhD, RDN

KEY TERMS

anticariogenic	dentin	lingual caries
calculus	early childhood caries (ECC)	periodontal disease
candidiasis	edentulism	plaque
cariogenic	enamel	remineralization
cariogenicity	fermentable carbohydrate	root caries
cariostatic	fluoroapatite	stomatitis
coronal caries	fluorosis	*Streptococcus mutans*
demineralization	gingiva	xerostomia
dental caries	gingival sulcus	xylitol
dental erosion	hydroxyapatite	

Diet and nutrition play key roles in tooth development, integrity of the gingiva (gums) and mucosa, bone strength, and the prevention and management of diseases of the oral cavity. Diet has a local effect on tooth integrity; the type, form, and frequency of foods and beverages consumed have a direct effect on the oral pH and microbial activity, which may promote dental decay. Nutrition systemically affects the development, maintenance, and repair of teeth and oral tissues.

Nutrition and diet affect the oral cavity, but the reverse is also true: that is, the status of the oral cavity may affect one's ability to consume an adequate diet and achieve nutritional balance. Indeed, there is a lifelong synergy between nutrition and the integrity of the oral cavity in health and disease related to the known roles of diet and nutrients in the growth, development, and maintenance of the oral cavity structure, bones, and tissues (Touger-Decker and Mobley, 2013).

NUTRITION FOR TOOTH DEVELOPMENT

Primary tooth development begins at 2 to 3 months' gestation. Mineralization begins at approximately 4 months' gestation and continues through the preteen years. Therefore maternal nutrition must supply the preeruptive teeth with the appropriate building materials. Inadequate maternal nutrition consequently affects tooth development.

Teeth are formed by the mineralization of a protein matrix. In dentin, protein is present as collagen, which depends on vitamin C for normal synthesis. Vitamin D is essential to the process by which calcium and phosphorus are deposited in crystals of hydroxyapatite, a naturally occurring form of calcium and phosphorus that is the mineral component of enamel and dentin. Fluoride added to the hydroxyapatite provides unique caries-resistant properties to teeth in prenatal and postnatal developmental periods.

Diet and nutrition are important in all phases of tooth development, eruption, and maintenance (see Figure 25-1). Posteruption diet and nutrient intake continue to affect tooth development and mineralization, enamel development and strength, and eruption patterns of the remaining teeth. The local effects of diet, particularly fermentable carbohydrates and eating frequency, affect the production of organic acids by oral bacteria and the rate of tooth decay as described later in this chapter.

DENTAL CARIES

Dental caries is one of the most common infectious diseases. According to a Surgeon General's report on oral health in 2000, dental caries is seven times more common than hay fever and five times more common than asthma. Unfortunately, differences are evident in caries prevalence; approximately 20% to 25% of U.S. children have 80% of the dental caries. Trends in dental caries have demonstrated that children who come from homes in which parents have a college education have fewer caries than children from homes in which parents have less than a college education (Centers for Disease Control and Prevention [CDC], 2010). These differences, or health disparities, may happen as a result of lack of access to care, cost of care not reimbursed by third-party payers (e.g., insurance, Medicaid), lack of knowledge of preventive dental care, or a combination of factors.

Pathophysiology

Dental caries is an oral infectious disease in which organic acid metabolites lead to gradual demineralization of tooth enamel, followed by rapid proteolytic destruction of the tooth structure. Caries can occur on any tooth surface. The cause of dental caries involves many factors. Four factors must be present simultaneously: (1) a susceptible host or tooth surface; (2) microorganisms such as *Streptococcus* or *Lactobacillus* in the dental plaque or oral

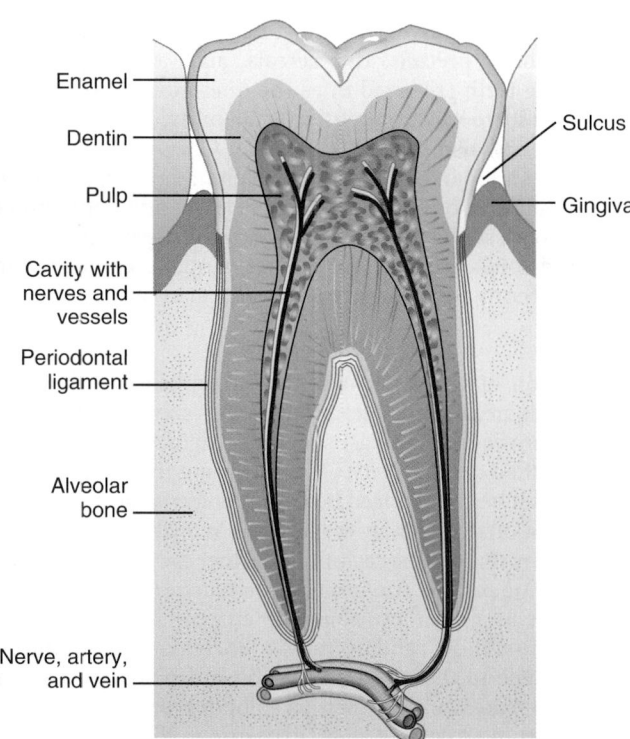

FIGURE 25-1 Anatomy of a tooth.

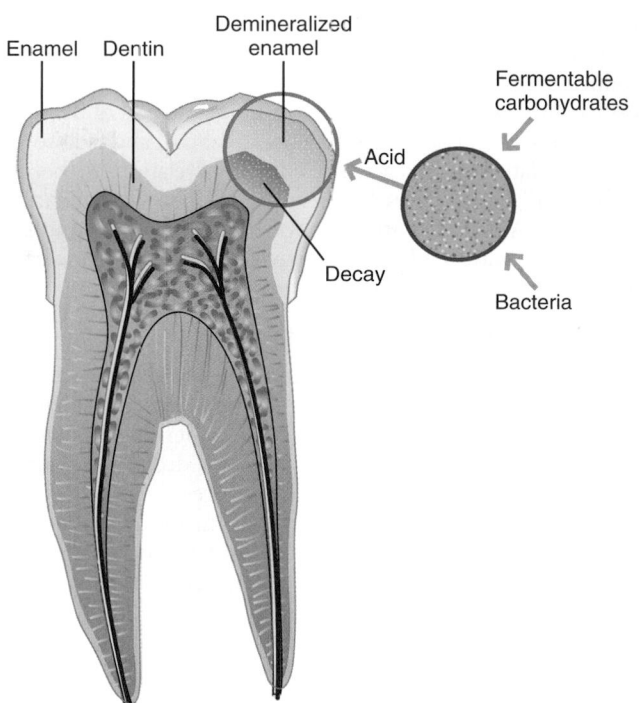

FIGURE 25-2 Formation of dental caries.

cavity; (3) fermentable carbohydrates in the diet, which serve as the substrate for bacteria; and (4) time (duration) in the mouth for bacteria to metabolize the fermentable carbohydrates, produce acids, and cause a drop in salivary pH to less than 5.5. Once the pH is acidic, which can occur within minutes, oral bacteria can initiate the demineralization process. Figure 25-2 shows the formation of dental caries.

Susceptible Tooth

The development of dental caries requires the presence of a tooth that is vulnerable to attack. The composition of enamel and dentin, the location of teeth, the quality and quantity of saliva, and the presence and extent of pits and fissures in the tooth crown are some of the factors that govern susceptibility. Alkaline saliva has a protective effect and acidic saliva increases susceptibility to decay.

Microorganisms

Bacteria are an essential part of the decay process. *Streptococcus mutans* is the most prevalent, followed by *Lactobacillus casein* and *Streptococcus sanguis*. All three contribute to the process because they metabolize carbohydrates in the mouth, producing acid as a byproduct, which is sufficient to cause decay. Genetic variations of the type and quantity of bacteria present in the oral cavity may put someone at an increased risk for caries and periodontal disease, but the quantity and quality of oral hygiene contributes directly to the risk of oral infectious disease.

Substrate

Fermentable carbohydrates, those carbohydrates susceptible to the actions of salivary amylase, are the ideal substrate for bacterial metabolism. The acids produced by their metabolism cause a drop in salivary pH to less than 5.5, creating the environment for decay. Bacteria are always present and begin to reduce pH when they have exposure to fermentable carbohydrates.

Although the Dietary Guidelines for Americans and the MyPlate Food Guidance system support a diet high in carbohydrates, it is important to be aware of the cariogenicity of foods. Cariogenicity refers to the caries-promoting properties of a diet or food. The cariogenicity of a food varies, depending on the form in which it occurs, its nutrient composition, when it is eaten in relation to other foods and fluids, the duration of its exposure to the tooth, and the frequency with which it is eaten (see Box 25-1). Individuals should be aware of the form of food consumed and the frequency of intake to integrate positive diet and oral hygiene habits to reduce risk of oral disease.

Fermentable carbohydrates are found in three of the five MyPlate food groups: (1) grains, (2) fruits, and (3) dairy. Although some vegetables may contain fermentable carbohydrates, little has been reported about the cariogenicity, or caries-promoting properties, of vegetables. Examples of grains and starches that are cariogenic by nature of their fermentable carbohydrate composition include crackers, chips, pretzels, hot and cold cereals, and breads.

All fruits (fresh, dried, and canned) and fruit juices may be cariogenic. Fruits with high water content, such as melons, have a lower cariogenicity than others such as bananas and dried fruits. Fruit drinks, sodas, ice teas, and other sugar-sweetened beverages; desserts; cookies; candies; and cake products may be cariogenic.

BOX 25-1 Factors Affecting Cariogenicity of Foods

Frequency of consumption
Food form (liquid or solid, slowly dissolving)
Sequence of eating certain foods and beverages
Combination of foods
Nutrient composition of foods and beverages
Duration of exposure of teeth

Dairy products sweetened with fructose, sucrose, or other sugars can also be cariogenic because of the added sugars; however, dairy products are rich in calcium, and their alkaline nature may have a positive influence, reducing the cariogenic potential of the food.

Like other sugars (glucose, fructose, maltose, and lactose), sucrose stimulates bacterial activity. The causal relationship between sucrose and dental caries has been established (Moynihan and Kelly, 2014). All dietary forms of sugar, including honey, molasses, brown sugar, agave, and corn syrup solids, have cariogenic potential and can be used by bacteria to produce organic acid.

Caries Promotion by Individual Foods

It is important to differentiate between cariogenic, cariostatic, and anticariogenic foods. Cariogenic foods are those that contain fermentable carbohydrates, which, when in contact with microorganisms in the mouth, can cause a drop in salivary pH to 5.5 or less and stimulate the caries process.

Cariostatic foods do not contribute to decay, are not metabolized by microorganisms, and do not cause a drop in salivary pH to 5.5 or less within 30 minutes. Examples of cariostatic foods are protein foods such as eggs, fish, meat, and poultry; most vegetables; fats; and sugarless gums. Sugarless gum may help to reduce decay potential because of its ability to increase saliva flow and because it uses noncarbohydrate sweeteners (Deshpande and Jadad, 2008; Splieth et al, 2009).

Anticariogenic foods are those that, when eaten before an acidogenic food, prevent plaque from recognizing the acidogenic food. Examples are aged cheddar, Monterey Jack, and Swiss because of the casein, calcium, and phosphate in the cheese. The five-carbon sugar alcohol, xylitol, is considered anticariogenic because bacteria cannot metabolize five-carbon sugars in the same way as six-carbon sugars such as glucose, sucrose, and fructose. It is not broken down by salivary amylase and is not subject to bacterial degradation. Salivary stimulation leads to increased buffering activity of the saliva and subsequent increased clearance of fermentable carbohydrates from tooth surfaces. Another anticariogenic mechanism of xylitol gum is that it replaces fermentable carbohydrates in the diet. *S. mutans* cannot metabolize xylitol and is inhibited by it. The antimicrobial activity against *S. mutans* and the effect of gum chewing on salivary stimulation are protective. Consumers should be advised to look for chewing gum in which xylitol is listed as the first ingredient.

Remineralization is mineral restoration of the hydroxyapatite in dental enamel. Casein phosphopeptide-amorphous calcium phosphate (CPP-ACP) is a substance that promotes remineralization of enamel surfaces (Cochrane et al, 2012). It is currently available as an ingredient trademarked as Recaldent (Cadbury Enterprises, Australia) in some brands of chewing gum (http://www.recaldent.com/c_faq.asp).

Factors Affecting Cariogenicity of Food

Cariogenicity also is influenced by the volume and quality of saliva; the sequence, consistency, and nutrient composition of the foods eaten; dental plaque buildup; and the genetic predisposition of the host to decay.

Form and Consistency

The form and consistency of a food have a significant effect on its cariogenic potential and pH-reducing or buffering capacity. Food form determines the duration of exposure or retention time of a food in the mouth, which, in turn, affects how long the decrease in pH or the acid-producing activity will last. Liquids are rapidly cleared from the mouth and have low adherence (or retentiveness) capabilities. Solid foods such as crackers, chips, pretzels, dry cereals, and cookies can stick between the teeth (referred to as the *interproximal spaces*) and have high adherence (or retention) capability.

Consistency also affects adherence. Chewy foods such as gum drops and marshmallows, although high in sugar content, stimulate saliva production and have a lower adherence potential than solid, sticky foods such as pretzels, bagels, or bananas. High-fiber foods with few or no fermentable carbohydrates, such as popcorn and raw vegetables, are cariostatic.

Exposure

The duration of exposure may be best explained with starchy foods, which are fermentable carbohydrates subject to the action of salivary amylase. The longer starches are retained in the mouth, the greater their cariogenicity. Given sufficient time, such as when food particles become lodged between the teeth, salivary amylase makes additional substrate available as it hydrolyzes starch to simple sugars. Processing techniques, either by partial hydrolysis or by reducing particle size, make some starches rapidly fermentable by increasing their availability for enzyme action.

Sugar-containing candies rapidly increase the amount of sugar available in the oral cavity to be hydrolyzed by bacteria. Sucking on hard candies such as lollipops or sugared breath mints results in prolonged sugar exposure in the mouth. Simple carbohydrate-based snacks and dessert foods (e.g., potato chips, pretzels, cookies, cakes, and doughnuts) provide gradually increasing oral sugar concentrations for a longer duration because these foods often adhere to the tooth surfaces and are retained for longer periods than candies. In school age children, more frequent snacking on carbohydrate-containing foods was associated with greater incidence of dental caries (Chankanka et al, 2011).

Nutrient Composition

Nutrient composition contributes to the ability of a substrate to produce acid and to the duration of acid exposure. Dairy products, by virtue of their calcium- and phosphorus-buffering potential, are considered to have low cariogenic potential. Evidence suggests that cheese and milk, when consumed with cariogenic foods, help to buffer the acid pH produced by the cariogenic foods. Because of the anticariogenic properties of cheese, eating cheese with a fermentable carbohydrate, such as dessert at the end of a meal, may decrease the cariogenicity of the meal and dessert (Ravishankar et al, 2012).

Nuts, which do not contain a significant amount of fermentable carbohydrates and are high in fat and dietary fiber, are cariostatic. Protein foods such as seafood, meats, eggs, and poultry, along with other fats such as oils, margarine, butter, and seeds, are also cariostatic.

Sequence and Frequency of Eating

Eating sequence and combination of foods also affect the caries potential of the substrate. Bananas, which are cariogenic because of their fermentable carbohydrate content and adherence capability, have less potential to contribute to decay when eaten with cereal and milk than when eaten alone as a snack. Milk, as a liquid, reduces the adherence capability of the fruit. Crackers eaten with cheese are less cariogenic than when eaten alone.

The frequency with which a cariogenic food or beverage is consumed determines the number of opportunities for acid production. Every time a fermentable carbohydrate is consumed, a decline in pH is initiated within 5 to 15 minutes, causing caries-promoting activity. Small, frequent meals and snacks, often high in fermentable carbohydrate, increase the cariogenicity of a diet more than a diet consisting of three meals and minimal snacks. Eating several cookies at once, followed by brushing the teeth or rinsing the mouth with water, is less cariogenic than eating a cookie several times throughout a day. Table 25-1 lists messages that can be given to children to reduce the risk of developing dental caries.

The Decay Process

The carious process begins with the production of acids as a byproduct of bacterial metabolism taking place in the dental plaque. Decalcification of the surface enamel continues until the buffering action of the saliva is able to raise the pH above the critical level. See Box 25-2 for prevention guidelines and the Practice Paper of the Academy of Nutrition and Dietetics on Oral Health and Nutrition (Mallonnee et al, 2014).

Plaque is a sticky, colorless mass of microorganisms and polysaccharides that forms around the tooth and adheres to teeth and gums. It harbors acid-forming bacteria and keeps the

---

BOX 25-2	Caries Prevention Guidelines

Brush at least twice daily, preferably after meals.
Rinse mouth after meals and snacks.
Chew sugarless gum for 15 to 20 min after meals and snacks.
Floss twice daily.
Use fluoridated toothpastes.
Pair cariogenic foods with cariostatic foods.
Snack on cariostatic and anticariogenic foods such as cheese, nuts, popcorn, and vegetables.
Limit between-meal eating and drinking of fermentable carbohydrates.

---

organic products of their metabolism in close contact with the enamel surface. As a cavity develops, the plaque blocks the tooth, to some extent, from the buffering and remineralization action of the saliva. In time the plaque combines with calcium and hardens to form **calculus**.

An acidic pH is also required for plaque formation. Soft drinks (diet and regular), sports beverages, citrus juices and "ades," and chewable vitamin C supplements have high acid content and may contribute to erosion (Tedesco et al, 2012). Research using National Health and Nutrition Examination Survey III data reported significantly more dental caries in children (ages 2-10 years) who consumed large amounts of carbonated soft drinks or juices compared with children who had high consumption of water or milk (Sohn et al, 2006). Other beverages and foods contribute to **dental erosion**, a loss of minerals from tooth surfaces by a chemical process in the presence of acid (Wongkhantee et al, 2006).

Roles of Saliva

Salivary flow clears food from around the teeth as a means to reduce the risk of caries. The bicarbonate-carbonic acid system, calcium, and phosphorus in saliva also provide buffering action to neutralize bacterial acid metabolism. Once buffering action has restored pH above the critical point, remineralization can occur. If fluoride is present in the saliva, the minerals are deposited in the form of **fluoroapatite**, which is resistant to erosion. Salivary production decreases as a result of diseases affecting salivary gland function (e.g., Sjögren syndrome); as a side effect of fasting; as a result of radiation therapy to the head and neck involving the parotid gland; normally during sleep and aging; with the use of medications associated with reduced salivary flow; or with **xerostomia**, dry mouth caused by inadequate saliva production. An estimated 400 to 500 medications currently available by prescription or over the counter may cause dry mouth. The degree of xerostomia may vary but may be caused by medications such as those to treat depression, hypertension, anxiety, human immunodeficiency virus (HIV), and allergies.

Caries Patterns

Caries patterns describe the location and surfaces of the teeth affected. **Coronal caries** affect the crown of the tooth, the part of the tooth visible above the gum line, and may occur on any tooth surface. Although the overall incidence of decay in the United States has declined, many states report 40% to 70% of children having some decay by age 8 (CDC, 2010).

Root caries, occurring on the root surfaces of teeth secondary to gingival recession, affect a large portion of the older population. Root caries is a dental infection that is increasing in older adults, partly because this population is retaining their natural teeth longer. The gums recede in

---

TABLE 25-1 Nutrition Messages Related to Oral Health for 3- to 10-Year-Old Children and Their Caregivers	
Message	**Rationale**
Starchy, sticky, or sugary foods should be eaten with nonsugary foods.	The pH will rise if a nonsugary item that stimulates saliva is eaten immediately before, during, or after a challenge.
Combine dairy products with a meal or snack.	Dairy products (nonfat milk, yogurt) enhance remineralization and contain calcium.
Combine chewy foods such as fresh fruits and vegetables with fermentable carbohydrates.	Chewy, fibrous foods induce saliva production and buffering capacity.
Space eating occasions at least 2 hours apart and limit snack time to 15 to 30 minutes. Limit bedtime snacks.	Fermentable carbohydrates eaten sequentially one after another promote demineralization. Saliva production declines during sleep.
Limit consumption of acidic foods such as sports drinks, juices, and sodas.	Acidic foods promote tooth erosion that increases risk for caries.
Combine proteins with carbohydrates in snacks. Examples: tuna and crackers, apples and cheese	Proteins act as buffers and are cariostatic.
Combine raw and cooked or processed foods in a snack.	Raw foods encourage mastication and saliva production, whereas cooked or processed foods may be more available for bacterial metabolism if eaten alone.
Encourage use of xylitol- or sorbitol-based chewing gum and candies immediately after a meal or snack.*	Five minutes of exposure is effective in increasing saliva production and dental plaque pH.
Recommend sugar-free chewable vitamin and mineral supplements and syrup-based medication.	Sugar-free varieties are available and should be suggested for high caries risk groups.
Encourage children with pediatric GERD to adhere to dietary guidelines.	GERD increases risk for dental erosion and thus increases risk for caries.

Modified from Mobley C: Frequent dietary intake and oral health in children 3 to 10 years of age, *Building Blocks* 25:17, 2001.
GERD, Gastroesophageal reflux disease.
*Gum is not recommended for children younger than 6 years old.

older age, exposing the root surface. Other factors related to the increased incidence of this decay pattern are lack of fluoridated water, poor oral hygiene practices, decreased saliva, frequent eating of fermentable carbohydrates, and dementia (Chalmers and Ettinger, 2008). Management of root caries includes dental restoration and nutrition counseling. Poor oral health from caries, pain, or edentulism often adversely affects dietary intake and nutritional status in older adults (Quandt et al, 2009).

Lingual caries, or caries on the lingual side (surface next to or toward the tongue) of the anterior teeth, are seen in persons with gastrointestinal reflux, bulimia, or anorexia-bulimia (see Chapter 22). Frequent intake of fermentable carbohydrates, combined with regurgitation or induced vomiting of acidic stomach contents, results in a constant influx of acid into the oral cavity. The acid contributes to erosion of tooth surfaces that can result in tooth sensitivity and dental caries. The pattern of erosion may be indicative of erosion from reflux versus from foods or beverages (Schlueter et al, 2012).

Fluoride

Fluoride is an important element in bones and teeth (Palmer and Gilbert, 2012). Used systemically and locally, it is a safe, effective public health measure to reduce the incidence and prevalence of dental caries (American Dental Association [ADA], 2014; CDC, 2013). Water fluoridation began in 1940; by 1999 the Centers for Disease Control and Prevention listed water fluoridation as one of the top 10 greatest public health achievements of the twentieth century because of its influence on decreasing the rate of dental caries (CDC, 2013). The effect of fluoride on caries prevention continues with water fluoridation, fluoridated toothpastes, oral rinses, and dentifrices, as well as beverages made with fluoridated water. Optimal water fluoridation concentrations (0.7-1.2 ppm) can provide protection against caries development without causing tooth staining (ADA, 2014). Despite the positions from the American Dental Association (ADA) and the Academy of Nutrition and Dietetics (AND), and the data from the CDC on fluoride for oral health, there is a controversy over the use of topical fluoride on teeth and systemic fluoridation in water supplies. Arguments against widespread fluoride use include claims that it can be carcinogenic and toxic; however, consumers should be urged to read the evidence (e.g., http://fluorideinfo.org/).

Mechanism of Action

There are four primary mechanisms of fluoride action on teeth: (1) when incorporated into enamel and dentin along with calcium and phosphorus, it forms fluoroapatite, a compound more resistant to acid challenge than hydroxyapatite; (2) it promotes repair and remineralization of tooth surfaces with early signs of decay (incipient carious lesions); (3) it helps to reverse the decay process while promoting the development of a tooth surface that has increased resistance to decay; and (4) helps to deter the harmful effects of bacteria in the oral cavity by interfering with the formation and function of microorganisms.

Food Sources

Most foods, unless prepared with fluoridated water, contain minimal amounts of fluoride, except for brewed tea, which has approximately 1.4 ppm (Morin, 2006). Fluoride may be added unintentionally to the diet in a number of ways, including through the use of fluoridated water in the processing of foods and beverages. Fruit juices and drinks, particularly white grape juice produced in cities with fluoridated water, may have increased fluoride content; however, because of the wide variation in fluoride content, it is difficult to estimate amounts consumed.

Supplementation

Health professionals should consider a child's fluid intake as well as food sources and the availability of fluoridated water in the community before prescribing fluoride supplements. Because bones are repositories of fluoride, bone meal, fish meal, and gelatin made from bones are potent sources of the mineral. In communities without fluoridated water, dietary fluoride supplements may be recommended for children ages 6 months to 16 years.

Fluoride can be used topically and systemically. When consumed in food and drink, it enters the systemic circulation and is deposited in bones and teeth. Systemic sources have a topical benefit as well by providing fluoride to the saliva. A small amount of fluoride enters the soft tissues; the remainder is excreted. The primary source of systemic fluoride is fluoridated water; food and beverages supply a smaller amount. Table 25-2 contains a schedule of fluoride supplementation.

Fluoride supplements are not recommended for formula-fed infants or for breast-fed infants living in fluoridated communities if these infants receive drinking water between feedings. If the infant does not drink water between feedings or drinks bottled water when on a diet of only breast milk, he or she should be supplemented according to the fluoride supplement guidelines. Fluoride supplements must be prescribed by the child's health care provider; they are not available as over-the-counter supplements (ADA, 2014).

Topical fluoride sources include toothpastes, gels, and rinses used by consumers daily, along with more concentrated forms applied by dental professionals in the form of gels, foams, and rinses. Frequent fluoride exposure via topical fluorides, fluoridated toothpastes, rinses, and fluoridated water is important in maintaining an optimal concentration of fluoride, but excess intake should be avoided.

Excess Fluoride

Fluorosis occurs when too much fluoride is provided during tooth development and can range from mild to severe and present on teeth from unnoticeable to very apparent dark spots on teeth (Bronckers, 2009). Causes of mild fluorosis from excessive fluoride intake include misuse of dietary fluoride supplements, ingestion of fluoridated toothpastes and rinses, or excessive fluoride intake secondary to fluoride in foods and beverages processed in fluoridated areas and transported to other areas. Topical fluorides, available as fluoridated toothpaste and mouthwashes, are effective

TABLE 25-2 Dietary Fluoride Supplement Schedule			
FLUORIDE ION LEVEL IN DRINKING WATER (ppm)*			
Age	**<0.3 ppm**	**0.3-0.6 ppm**	**>0.6 ppm**
Birth-6 mo	None	None	None
6 mo-3 yr	0.25 mg/day[†]	None	None
3-6 yr	0.50 mg/day	0.25 mg/day	None
6-16 yr	1.0 mg/day	0.50 mg/day	None

Approved by The American Dental Association, The American Academy of Pediatrics, and The American Academy of Pediatric Dentistry, 1994.
*1 ppm = 1 mg/L.
†2.2 mg of sodium fluoride contains 1 mg of fluoride ion.

sources of fluoride that can be used in the home, school, or dental office. Caries prevention efforts in preschool children include diet modification, water fluoridation or supplements in nonfluoridated areas, and supervised toothbrushing with fluoridated toothpaste (ADA, 2014).

Children younger than 6 years of age should not use fluoridated mouthwashes, and older children should be instructed to rinse, but not swallow, mouthwash. No more than a pea-size amount of toothpaste should be placed on a child's toothbrush to reduce the risk of accidental fluoride ingestion. Topical fluorides may be administered in the dental office.

Fluoride gels often are prescribed for adults and older adults. Such gels are effective in reducing the risk of coronal and root decay and tooth loss (Weintraub et al, 2006). Fluoride is most effective when given from birth through ages 12 to 13, the period when mineralization of unerupted permanent teeth occurs.

EARLY CHILDHOOD CARIES

Early childhood caries (ECC), often called "baby-bottle tooth decay," describes a caries pattern in the maxillary anterior teeth of infants and young children. Characteristics include rapidly developing carious lesions in the primary anterior teeth and the presence of lesions on tooth surfaces not usually associated with a high caries risk. Because tooth decay remains a common oral disease of childhood, caries are a primary marker for a child's oral health. Good behavioral habits and child nutrition patterns must be encouraged, beginning in infancy.

Pathophysiology and Incidence

Often ECC follows prolonged bottle-feeding, especially at night, of juice, milk, formula, or other sweetened beverages. The extended contact time with the fermentable carbohydrate–containing beverages, coupled with the position of the tongue against the nipple, which causes pooling of the liquid around the maxillary incisors, particularly during sleep, contributes to the decay process. The mandibular anterior teeth usually are spared (see Figure 25-3) because of the protective position of the lip and tongue and the presence of a salivary duct in the floor of the mouth. In general, children from low-income families and minority populations experience the greatest amount of oral disease, the most extensive disease, and the most frequent use of dental services for pain relief; yet these children have the fewest overall dental visits (CDC, 2010).

Nutrition Care

Management of ECC includes diet and oral hygiene education for parents, guardians, and caregivers. Messages should be

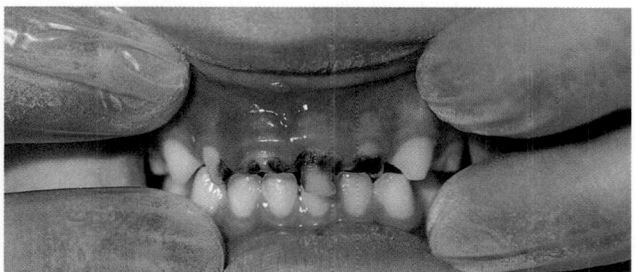

FIGURE 25-3 Early childhood caries. (From Swartz MH: *Textbook of physical diagnosis, history, and examination*, ed 5, Philadelphia, 2006, Saunders.)

targeted to counter the health habits that contribute to this problem: poor oral hygiene, failure to brush a child's teeth at least daily, frequent use of bottles filled with sweetened beverages, and lack of fluoridated water. Dietary guidelines include removal of the bedtime bottle and modification of the frequency and content of the daytime bottles. Bottle contents should be limited to water, formula, or milk. Infants and young children should not be put to bed with a bottle. Teeth and gums should be cleaned with a gauze pad or washcloth after all bottle feedings. All efforts should be made to wean children from a bottle by 1 year of age. Educational efforts should be positive and simple, focusing on oral hygiene habits and promotion of a balanced, healthy diet. Between-meal snacks should include cariostatic foods. When foods are cariogenic, they should be followed by tooth brushing or rinsing the mouth. Parents and caregivers need to understand the causes and consequences of ECC and how they can be avoided.

CARIES PREVENTION

Caries prevention programs focus on a balanced diet, modification of the sources and quantities of fermentable carbohydrates, and the integration of oral hygiene practices into individual lifestyles. Meals and snacks should be followed with brushing, rinsing the mouth vigorously with water, or chewing sugarless gum for 15 to 20 minutes, preferably gum that contains xylitol (Splieth et al, 2009). Positive habits should be encouraged, including snacking on anticariogenic or cariostatic foods, chewing sugarless gum after eating or drinking cariogenic items, and having sweets with meals rather than as snacks. Despite the potential for a diet that is based on the dietary guidelines to be cariogenic, with proper planning and good oral hygiene a balanced diet low in cariogenic risk can be planned (see Figure 25-4 for a sample diet).

Practices to avoid include sipping sugar-sweetened and low pH beverages for extended periods. Adding lemon and other fruits to water has become a common practice but this lowers the pH and in general should be avoided. Frequent snacking and harboring candy, sugared breath mints, or hard candies in the mouth for extended periods are discouraged. Over-the-counter chewable or liquid medications and vitamin preparations, such as chewable vitamin C or liquid cough syrup, may contain sugar and contribute to caries risk. Patients with dysphagia may use thickening agents in beverages or liquid foods (soups) to reduce the risk of aspiration. Good oral hygiene should be emphasized in these situations because the thickening agent may contain fermentable carbohydrate, and the type of dysphagia may contribute to inadequate clearing of food from the oral cavity.

Fermentable carbohydrates such as candy, crackers, cookies, pastries, pretzels, snack crackers, chips, and even fruits should be eaten with meals. Notably, "fat-free" snack and dessert items and "baked" chips and snack crackers tend to have a higher simple sugar concentration than their higher fat-containing counterparts.

TOOTH LOSS AND DENTURES

Tooth loss (edentulism) and removable prostheses (dentures) can have a significant effect on dietary habits, masticatory function, olfaction, and nutritional adequacy. As dentition status declines, masticatory performance is compromised and may have a negative effect on food choices, resulting in decreased intake of meat, whole grains, fruits, and vegetables (Tsakos et al, 2010). This

Breakfast:	1½ cups toasted oat cereal + 1 cup low-fat milk or 2 slices wheat toast with 1 oz melted cheese
	1 cup fresh berries
	coffee + low-fat milk
	BRUSH TEETH

Lunch:	2 slices of mushroom pizza
	small salad with 2 Tbs Italian dressing
	16 oz spring water
	banana
	FOLLOW WITH 2 PIECES XYLITOL GUM

| Afternoon snack: | 1 cup pretzels + 1 oz cheese |
| | **FOLLOW WITH 2 PIECES XYLITOL GUM** |

Dinner:	tossed salad with 2 Tbs grated cheese
	1½ cups spaghetti + 1 cup marinara sauce + ½ cup sauteed peppers
	1 cup fresh fruit salad
	1 slice Italian bread with 1 pat margarine
	½ cup ice cream
	1 cup low-fat milk

| Snack: | 4 cups popcorn |
| | **BRUSH TEETH BEFORE BED** |

FIGURE 25-4 A balanced diet plan with low cariogenic risk.

problem is more pronounced in older adults, whose appetite and intake may be compromised further by chronic disease, social isolation, and the use of multiple medications (see Chapter 8).

Dentures must be checked periodically by a dental professional for appropriate fit. Changes in body weight or changes in alveolar bone over time possibly may alter the fit of the dentures. This is a common problem in the elderly that interferes with eating. Counseling on appropriate food choices and textures is advocated.

Nutrition Care

Full dentures replace missing teeth but are not a perfect substitute for natural dentition. Before and after denture placement, many individuals may experience difficulty biting and chewing. The foods found to cause the greatest difficulty for persons with complete dentures include fresh whole fruits and vegetables (e.g., apples and carrots), hard-crusted breads, and whole muscle meats. Therefore dietary assessment and counseling related to oral health should be provided to the denture wearer. Simple guidelines should be provided for cutting and preparing fruits and vegetables to minimize the need for biting and reduce the amount of chewing. The importance of positive eating habits must be stressed as a component of total health. Overall, guidelines that reinforce the importance of a balanced diet should be part of the routine counseling given to all patients.

OTHER ORAL DISORDERS

Oral diseases extend beyond dental caries. Deficiencies of several vitamins (riboflavin, folate, B_{12}, and C) and minerals (iron and zinc) may be detected first in the oral cavity because of the rapid tissue turnover of the oral mucosa. Periodontal disease is a local and systemic disease. Select nutrients play a role, including vitamins A, C, E; folate; beta-carotene; and the minerals calcium, phosphorus, and zinc.

Oral cancer, often a result of tobacco and alcohol use, can have a significant effect on eating ability and nutritional status. This problem is compounded by the increased caloric and nutrient needs of persons with oral carcinomas. In addition, surgery, radiation therapy, and chemotherapy are modalities used to treat oral cancer that also can affect dietary intake, appetite, and the integrity of the oral cavity. Some but not all problems affecting the oral cavity are discussed here with relevant nutrition care. Patients may try over-the-counter natural products to prevent or treat oral disease or conditions (see *Clinical Insight:* Natural Products in Oral Health).

CLINICAL INSIGHT

Natural Products in Oral Health

Natural products include herbal and dietary supplements and probiotics (National Center for Complementary and Integrative Health [NCCIH], 2015). The following lists some herbal and dietary supplements that may be used to prevent or treat oral health issues. Other resources should be consulted to evaluate the efficacy and safety of natural products before choosing to use them in addition to or in place of conventional therapy.

Oral Use(s)	Natural Product	Use	Considerations
Mucositis	Hyaluronic acid	Topically (oral gel)	
	German chamomile	Oral rinse	May cause allergic reaction in sensitive individuals
	Glutamine	Oral rinse	
	Iodine	Oral rinse (in chemotherapy treatment)	
	Kaolin	Oral rinse (in radiation treatment)	
	Aloe	Oral rinse	Should not be ingested
Mucosal lesions	Slippery elm	Topically (lozenges)	
Periodontal disease	Coenzyme Q10	Systemically	
	Chitosan	Topically	
	Pomegranate extract and gotu kola extract	Topically	
Dental Caries	Fluoride	Topically	
	Xylitol	In chewing gum or in place of fermentable carbohydrate	

Natural Medicines Comprehensive Database (www.naturaldatabase.com).

PERIODONTAL DISEASE

Pathophysiology

Periodontal disease is an inflammation of the gingiva with infection caused by oral bacteria and subsequent destruction of the tooth attachment apparatus. Untreated disease results in a gradual loss of tooth attachment to the bone. Progression is influenced by the overall health of the host and the integrity of the immune system. The primary causal factor in the development of periodontal disease is plaque. Plaque in the gingival sulcus, a shallow, V-shaped space around the tooth, produces toxins that destroy tissue and permit loosening of the teeth. Important factors in the defense of the gingiva to bacterial invasion are (1) oral hygiene, (2) integrity of the immune system, and (3) optimal nutrition. The defense mechanisms of the gingival tissue, epithelial barrier, and saliva are affected by nutritional intake and status. Healthy epithelial tissue prevents the penetration of bacterial endotoxins into subgingival tissue.

Nutritional Care

Deficiencies of vitamin C, folate, and zinc increase the permeability of the gingival barrier at the gingival sulcus, increasing susceptibility to periodontal disease. Severe deterioration of the gingiva is seen in individuals with scurvy or vitamin C deficiency. Although other nutrients, including vitamins A, E, beta-carotene, and protein, have a role in maintaining gingival and immune system integrity, no scientific data support supplemental uses of any of these nutrients to treat periodontal disease. However when periodontal disease causes pain and avoidance of foods, nutrient intake may be limited and should be monitored (Staudte et al, 2012). The dietetics professional can make recommendations for modified food consistency to minimize nutrient deficits.

In societies in which malnutrition and periodontal disease are prevalent, poor oral hygiene is also usually evident. In such instances it is difficult to determine whether malnutrition is the cause of the disease or one of many contributing factors, including poor oral hygiene, heavy plaque buildup, insufficient saliva, or coexisting illness.

The roles of calcium and vitamin D relate to the link between osteoporosis and periodontal disease, in which bone loss may be the common denominator. Although causal relationships have not been determined, the association of calcium and dairy foods with periodontal disease warrants advocating a sufficient intake of dairy foods in those who tolerate them. Management strategies for the patient or client with periodontal disease follow many of the same guidelines as for caries prevention listed in Box 25-2.

Severe periodontal disease may be treated surgically. Diet adequacy is particularly important before and after periodontal surgery, when adequate nutrients are needed to regenerate tissue and support immunity to prevent infection. Adequacy of calories, protein, and micronutrients should be part of the postoperative care plan.

ORAL MANIFESTATIONS OF SYSTEMIC DISEASE

Acute systemic diseases such as cancer and infections, as well as chronic diseases such as diabetes mellitus, autoimmune diseases, and chronic kidney disease, are characterized by oral manifestations that may alter the diet and nutritional status. Cancer therapies, including irradiation of the head and neck region, chemotherapy, and surgeries to the oral cavity, have a significant effect on the integrity of the oral cavity and on an individual's eating ability, which may consequently affect nutrition status (see Chapter 36).

If the condition of the mouth adversely affects one's food choices, the person with chronic disease may not be able to follow the optimal diet for medical nutrition therapy. For example, poorly controlled diabetes may manifest in xerostomia or candidiasis, which may then affect the ability to consume a diet to appropriately control blood sugar, further deteriorating glucose control.

In addition, many medications alter the integrity of the oral mucosa, taste sensation, or salivary production (see Chapter 8). Phenytoin (Dilantin) may cause severe gingivitis. Many of the protease inhibitor drugs used to treat HIV and acquired immune deficiency syndrome (AIDS) are associated with altered taste and dry mouth. Reduced saliva may contribute to increased caries risk and also may alter the ability to form a bolus and swallow foods, especially dry foods that may crumble with mastication. Care should be taken to assess the effects of medication on the oral cavity and minimize these effects using alterations in diet or drug therapy.

Diabetes Mellitus

Diabetes is associated with several oral manifestations, many of which occur only in periods of poor glucose control. These include burning mouth syndrome, periodontal disease, candidiasis, dental caries, and xerostomia. The microangiopathic conditions seen in diabetes, along with altered responses to infection, contribute to risk of periodontal disease in affected persons. Tooth infection, more common in those with diabetes, leads to deterioration of diabetes control (Al-Khabbaz, 2014). In addition to blood glucose control, dietary management for people with diabetes after any oral surgery procedures or placement of dentures should include modifications in the consistency, temperature, and texture of food to increase eating comfort, reduce oral pain, and prevent infections or decay (see Chapter 30).

Fungal Infections

Oropharyngeal fungal infections may cause a burning, painful mouth and dysphagia. The ulcers that accompany viral infections such as herpes simplex and cytomegalovirus cause pain and can lead to reduced oral intake. Very hot and cold foods or beverages, spices, and sour or tart foods may cause pain and should be avoided. Consumption of temperate, moist foods without added spices should be encouraged. Small, frequent meals followed by rinsing with lukewarm water or brushing to reduce the risk of dental caries are helpful. Once the type and extent of oral manifestations are identified, a nutrition care plan can be developed. Oral high calorie–high protein supplements in liquid or pudding form may be needed to meet nutrient needs and optimize healing.

Head and Neck Cancers

Head, neck, and oral cancers can alter eating ability and nutrition status because of the surgeries and therapies used to treat these cancers. Surgery, depending on the location and extent, may alter eating or swallowing ability, as well as the capacity to produce saliva. Radiation therapy of the head and neck area and chemotherapeutic agents can affect the quantity and quality of saliva and the integrity of the oral mucosa. Thick, ropey saliva is often the result of radiation therapy to the head and neck

TABLE 25-3   Effects of Oral Infections

Location	Problem	Effect	Diet Management
Oral cavity	Candidiasis, KS, herpes, stomatitis	Pain, infection, lesions, altered ability to eat, dysgeusia	Increase kilocalorie and protein intake; administer oral supplements; provide caries risk reduction education
	Xerostomia	Increased caries risk, pain, difficulty with mastication, lack of saliva to form bolus, tendency of food to stick, dysgeusia	Moist, soft, nonspicy foods; "smooth" cool or warm foods and fluids; caries risk reduction education
Esophagus	Candidiasis, herpes, KS, cryptosporidiosis	Dysphagia, odynophagia	Try oral supplementation first; if that is unsuccessful, initiate NG feedings using silastic feeding tube or PEG
	CMV, with or without ulceration	Dysphagia, food accumulation	PEG

CMV, Cytomegalovirus; *KS,* Kaposi sarcoma; *NG,* nasogastric; *PEG,* percutaneous endoscopic gastrostomy.

area, causing xerostomia. Dietary management focuses on the recommendations described earlier for xerostomia, along with modifications in food consistency after surgery (see Chapters 36 and 40).

HIV Infection and AIDS

Viral and fungal infections, stomatitis, xerostomia, periodontal disease, and Kaposi sarcoma are oral manifestations of HIV that can cause limitations in nutrient intake and result in weight loss and compromised nutrition status. These infections often are compounded by a compromised immune response, preexisting malnutrition, and gastrointestinal consequences of HIV infection (see Chapter 37). Viral diseases, including herpes simplex and cytomegalovirus, result in painful ulcerations of the mucosa.

Stomatitis, or inflammation of the oral mucosa, causes severe pain and ulceration of the gingiva, oral mucosa, and palate, which makes eating painful. Candidiasis on the tongue, palate, or esophagus can make chewing, sucking, and swallowing painful (odynophagia), thus compromising intake. Table 25-3 outlines the effects of associated oral infections.

Xerostomia

Xerostomia (dry mouth) is seen in poorly controlled diabetes mellitus, Sjögren syndrome, other autoimmune diseases, and as a consequence of radiation therapy and certain medications (see Box 25-3). Xerostomia from radiation therapy may be more permanent than that from other causes (Kielbassa et al, 2006). Radiation therapy procedures to spare the parotid gland should be implemented when possible to reduce the damage to the salivary gland. Efforts to stimulate saliva production using pilocarpine and citrus-flavored, sugar-free candies may ease eating difficulty.

Individuals without any saliva at all have the most difficulty eating; artificial salivary agents may not offer sufficient relief. Lack of saliva impedes all aspects of eating, including chewing, forming a bolus, swallowing, and sensing taste; causes pain; and

increases the risk of dental caries and infections. Dietary guidelines focus on the use of moist foods without added spices, increased fluid consumption with and between all meals and snacks, and judicious food choices.

Problems with chewy (steak), crumbly (cake, crackers, rice), dry (chips, crackers), and sticky (peanut butter) foods are common in persons with severe xerostomia. Alternatives should be suggested, or the foods should be avoided to avert dysphagia risk. Drinking water with a lemon or lime twist or citrus-flavored seltzers or sucking on frozen tart grapes, berries, or sugar-free candies may help. Because these foods or beverages may contain fermentable carbohydrate or contribute to reduced pH, good oral hygiene habits are important in reducing the risk of tooth decay and should be practiced after all meals and snacks.

BOX 25-3   Medications that May Cause Xerostomia

Antianxiety agents	Diuretics
Anticonvulsants	Narcotics
Antidepressants	Sedatives
Antihistamines	Serotonin reuptake inhibitors
Antihypertensives	Tranquilizers

CLINICAL CASE STUDY

Gina is a 74-year-old woman with a history of type 2 diabetes, hypertension, and arthritis. She states that her dentist told her she has xerostomia and periodontal disease and will need multiple tooth extractions and a full maxillary (upper) and partial mandibular (lower) denture. Because of the condition of her teeth she consumes soft foods and lots of diet soda because her mouth always feels dry. She takes glyburide for glucose control, amlodipine (Norvasc) for blood pressure control, and glucosamine and chondroitin to alleviate her arthritis. She is 5'1" and weighs 176 lb. She lives alone, but receives assistance with food shopping and cooking from her family and friends. She occasionally conducts self-monitoring fasting glucose via fingerstick and states that her usual reading is 150 mg/dl.

Nutrition Diagnostic Statements

1. Chewing difficulty secondary to poor dentition and xerostomia as evidenced by patient report and choice of soft foods.
2. Altered nutrition-related laboratory value (glucose) secondary to diabetes and possibly food choices as evidenced by inadequate blood glucose control.

Nutrition Care Questions

1. What are the cultural, educational, and environmental influences affecting dental and nutritional health?
2. What are the diet counseling recommendations for the dental conditions (anticipated extractions, dry mouth, full and partial dentures)?
3. List an appropriate intervention for each of the diagnostic statements. How would you evaluate the impact of your intervention?
4. What would you assess at your follow-up (monitoring) appointment with Gina?

USEFUL WEBSITES

American Academy of Pediatric Dentistry
http://www.aapd.org/

American Dental Association
http://www.ada.org/

American Dental Hygienists Association
http://www.adha.org/

American Academy of Periodontology
http://www.perio.org/

Diabetes and Oral health
http://www.nidcr.nih.gov/OralHealth/Topics/Diabetes/
http://www.diabetes.org/living-with-diabetes/treatment-and-care/oral-health-and-hygiene/

HIV Dent
http://www.hivdent.org/

National Institute of Dental and Craniofacial Research
http://www.nidcr.nih.gov/

Oral Health America
http://oralhealthamerica.org/

Surgeon General Report on Oral Health
http://www.surgeongeneral.gov/library/reports/oralhealth/

World Health Organization on Oral Health
http://www.who.int/oral_health/en/

REFERENCES

Al-Khabbaz AK: Type 3 diabetes mellitus and periodontal disease severity, *Oral Health Prev Dent* 12:77, 2014.

American Dental Association: *ADA Fluoridation Policy & Statements* (website): http://www.ada.org/4045.aspx, 2014. Accessed December 20, 2014.

Bronckers A, Lyaruu D, DenBesten P: The impact of fluoride on ameloblasts and the mechanisms of enamel fluorosis, *J Dent Res* 88:877, 2009.

Centers for Disease Control and Prevention (CDC): Division of Oral Health. http://www.cdc.gov/oralhealth/, 2014. Accessed December 20, 2014.

Centers for Disease Control and Prevention (CDC): *National Oral Health Surveillance System* (website): http://www.cdc.gov/nohss/, 2010. Accessed December 20, 2014.

Chalmers JM, Ettinger RL: Public health issues in geriatric dentistry in the United States, *Dent Clin North Am* 52:423, 2008.

Chankanka O et al: Mixed dentition cavitated caries incidence and dietary intake frequencies, *Pediatric Dentistry* 33:233, 2011.

Cochrane NJ et al: Remineralization by chewing sugar-free gums in a randomized controlled in situ trial including dietary intake and gauze to promote plaque formation, *Caries Research* 46:147, 2012.

Deshpande A, Jadad AR: The impact of polyol-containing chewing gums on dental caries: a systematic review of original randomized trials and observational studies, *J Am Dent Assoc* 139 1602, 2008.

Kielbassa AM et al: Radiation-related damage to dentition, *Lancet Oncol* 7:326, 2006.

Mallonee LFH et al: Position Paper of the Academy of Nutrition and Dietetics on Oral Health and Nutrition, JAND 114:958, 2014.

Morin K: Fluoride: action and use, *MCN Am J Matern Child Nurs* 31:127, 2006.

Moynihan PJ, Kelly SA: Effect on caries of restricting sugars intake: Systematic review to inform WHO guidelines, *J Dent Res* 93:8, 2014.

National Center for Complementary and Integrative Health: Complementary, Alternative, or Integrative Health: What's in a Name? (website): https://nccih.nih.gov/health/integrative-health#types, 2015. Accessed September 13, 2015

Palmer CA, Gilbert JA: Position of the Academy of Nutrition and Dietetics: The impact of fluoride on health, *J Acad Nutr Diet* 112:1443, 2012.

Ravishankar TL et al: Effect of consuming different dairy products on calcium, phosphorus and pH levels of human dental plaque: a comparative study, *Eur Arch Paediatr Dent* 13:144, 2012.

Quandt SA et al: Food avoidance and food modification practices of older rural adults: association with oral health status and implications for service provision, *Gerontologist* 50:100, 2009.

Schlueter N et al: Is dental erosion really a problem? *Adv Dent Res* 24:68, 2012.

Sohn WB et al: Carbonated soft drinks and dental caries in the primary dentition, *J Dent Res* 85:262, 2006.

Splieth CH et al: Effect of xylitol and sorbitol on plaque acidogenesis, *Quintessence Int* 40:279, 2009.

Staudte H et al: Comparison of nutrient intake between patients with periodontitis and healthy subjects, *Quintessence Int* 43:907, 2012.

Tedesco TK et al: Erosive effects of beverages in the presence or absence of caries simulation by acidogenic challenge in human primary enamel: an in-vitro study, *Eur Arch Paediatr Dent* 13:36, 2012.

Touger-Decker R, Mobley C: Position of the Academy of Nutrition and Dietetics: oral health and nutrition, *J Acad Nutr Diet* 113:693, 2013.

Tsakos GK et al: Edentulism and fruit and vegetable intake in low-income adults, *J Dent Res* 89:462, 2010.

Weintraub JA et al: Fluoride varnish efficacy in preventing early childhood caries, *J Dent Res* 85:172, 2006.

Wongkhantee SV et al: Effect of acidic food and drinks on surface hardness of enamel, dentine, and tooth-coloured filling materials, *J Dent* 34:214, 2006.

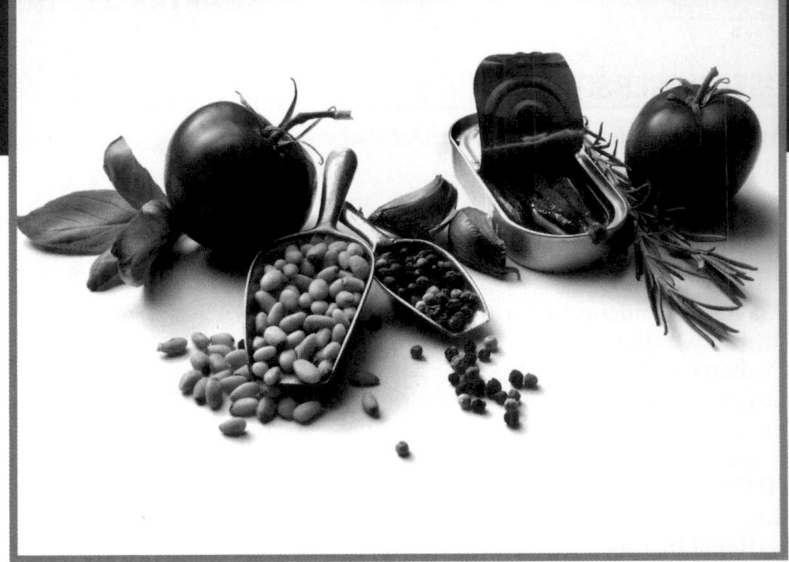

PART V

Medical Nutrition Therapy

This section contains chapters that reflect the evolution of nutritional science, from the identification of nutrient requirements and the practical application of this knowledge, to the concepts that relate nutrition to the prevention of chronic and degenerative diseases and optimization of health. The role of nutrition in reducing inflammation, a contributor to the state chronic disease, supports the awareness of diet in disease prevention and management.

Medical nutrition therapy (MNT) includes the assessment, nutrition diagnosis, interventions, monitoring, and evaluation of established disease. In some cases, medical nutrition therapy is a powerful preventive measure. The list of diseases amenable to nutrition intervention continues to increase, especially because hundreds of conditions are now known to have a genetic component and a connection with the nutrient-gene expression pathway.

Sophisticated feeding and nourishment procedures place an increased responsibility on those who provide nutrition care. The nutrition-related disorders included here can be managed by changes in dietary practices based on current knowledge. The goal in all cases is to move the individual along the continuum of disease and health management toward better nutritional health and overall well-being.

26

Medical Nutrition Therapy for Adverse Reactions to Food: Allergies and Intolerances

L. Kathleen Mahan, MS, RDN, CD
Kathie Madonna Swift, MS, RDN, LDN, FAND

Consultant Reviewer: Janice M. Joneja, PhD, RD

KEY TERMS

adverse reactions to food (ARF)
allergen
anaphylaxis
antibodies
antigen
antigen-presenting cell (APC)
atopic dermatitis (eczema)
atopy
basophils
B-cells
CAP–fluorescein-enzyme immunoassay (FEIA)
conformational epitopes
cow's milk protein allergy (CMPA)
cross-reactivity
cytokines
dendritic cells (DCs)
double-blind, placebo-controlled food challenge (DBPCFC)
dysbiosis
elimination diet
eosinophils
eosinophilic esophagitis (EoE)
eosinophilic gastroenteritis (EGE)
epigenetics
epitope

Food Allergen Labeling and Consumer Protection Act (FALCPA)
food allergen–specific serum IgE testing
food allergy
food and symptom record
food autoimmune or immune reactivity
food challenge
food dependent exercise-induced anaphylaxis (FDEIA)
food immunotherapy vaccine
food intolerance
food protein-induced enterocolitis syndrome (FPIES)
food protein-induced proctocolitis (FPIP)
food sensitivity
granulocyte
gut-associated lymphoid tissue (GALT)
hapten
histamine
increased intestinal permeability or "leaky gut"
IgE-mediated food allergy
immunoglobulin (Ig)
inflammatory mediators

latex-fruit syndrome or latex-food syndrome
"leaky gut"
lymphocyte
macrophage
mast cells
microbiome
microbiota
monocytes
natural rubber latex (NRL)
neutrophils
oral allergy syndrome (OAS)
oral tolerance
pollen-food syndrome (PFS)
prebiotics
probiotics
radioallergosorbent test (RAST)
sensitivity-related illness (SRI)
sensitization
skin-prick test
specific oral tolerance induction (SOTI)
T-cells
Th cells
Th1 cells
Th2 cells

There is growing evidence that adverse reactions to food (ARFs) are more prevalent than in the past, with a defined increase in severity and scope (Skypala, 2011). Changes in the modern diet and environmental influences interacting with genetic predisposition have been implicated in the escalation of ARFs and the parallel rise in other chronic disorders such as asthma and autoimmune diseases. Estimates suggest that 20% of the population alter their diet because of perceived ARFs (Sicherer and Sampson, 2010; Turnbull et al, 2015). Currently the prevalence of food allergy in the U.S. population, when documented objectively with serologic assessment and food challenges, is 2.5% to 3%. The prevalence is higher in children and is estimated to be about 4% to 7%, and in adults it is estimated to be 1% to 2% (Turnbull et al, 2015).

ARFs are implicated in many conditions as a result of the involvement of major organ systems, including the dermatologic, respiratory, gastrointestinal, and neurologic systems. The management of ARFs is complex because of the diverse response by which the body reacts to food constituents and the multifaceted nature of the mechanisms involved. The clinical relevance of ARFs should be carefully assessed and evaluated in the nutrition care process, because they can greatly affect a person's quality of life.

DEFINITIONS

It is important to comprehend the language of ARFs; it can be a source of confusion and misunderstanding (see Box 26-1).

BOX 26-1   Adverse Reactions to Foods: Definitions

- **Adverse reactions to food (ARFs)**: encompass food allergies and food intolerances, both of which can result in distressing symptoms and adversely affect health
- **Atopy**: a condition of genetic predisposition to produce excessive IgE antibodies in response to an allergen that results in the development of typical symptoms such as asthma, rhinoconjunctivitis, or eczema
- **Food allergy**: an adverse immune-mediated reaction to a food, usually a food protein, glycoprotein, or hapten that the person has been sensitized to, and which, when eaten, causes the release of inflammatory mediators or chemicals that act on body tissues and result in symptoms
- **Food autoimmune or immune reactivity**: the concept that when the body's normal tolerance of friendly antigenic substances (autoantigens produced by an individual's body) is disrupted because of disease, injury, shock, trauma, surgery, drugs, blood transfusion, or environmental triggers, the ingestion of foods containing antigenic substances with a composition similar to those of the body's autoantigens can result in the production of antibodies that react to the food antigens and the body's own tissues (Vojdani, 2015)

- **Food intolerance**: an adverse reaction to a food or food additive that does not involve the immune system and results from the body's inability to digest, absorb, or metabolize a food or component of the food
- **Food sensitivity**: a term often used to describe a reaction when it is unclear whether it is immunologically mediated or due to a biochemical or physiologic defect
- **Oral tolerance**: the process that allows an individual to eat food (which is "foreign") without any ill effects or reactions to it
- **Sensitivity-related illness**: the concept that an individual who is exposed to some type of toxicant or insult may then, by as yet unclear mechanisms, become sensitive to a food, inhalant, or chemical (Genuis, 2010)

Adverse reactions to food (ARF) encompass food allergies and food intolerances, both of which can result in distressing symptoms and adversely affect health. **Food allergy** is an immune system response that is triggered when a food is eaten by a person who has been sensitized to it. An **antigen** is any molecule that will elicit an immune response in the body. When it elicits a hypersensitivity reaction as in allergy, it is called an **allergen**. The key event in food allergy is the recognition of the food by components of the immune system, which then cause the release of chemicals (inflammatory mediators) that act on body tissues and result in a specific set of symptoms. The allergen is usually a food protein or a glycoprotein (protein to which a carbohydrate chain is attached) or a **hapten** (a small inorganic compound that can elicit an immune response when attached to a large carrier protein). An **epitope** is the actual section of the allergen that connects with the immune molecule. Some carbohydrates can act as allergens on their own and are referred to as carbohydrate epitopes (Soh et al, 2015). These carbohydrate epitopes are responsible for much of the cross-reactivity between allergens (Soh et al, 2015). There is also the possible contribution of genetically modified or engineered (GM or GE) molecules in food crops to act as epitopes and allergens and result in sensitization and food allergy. This remains an area of ongoing investigation (Ladics et al, 2014) (see *Focus On*: GMO or Genetically Engineered (GE) Foods).

The adverse reactions that occur are caused by the individual's unique response to the food, not by the food itself. Furthermore, the symptoms of the allergy in one individual can differ greatly from those in another in response to the same food. Symptoms of food allergy are noted in Box 26-2.

The definition of allergy has been broadened to encompass any immunologic reaction to a component of food resulting in adverse symptoms and now includes reactions to foods that include the following:

- Reactions that elicit production of specific IgE
- Reactions that result from release of inflammatory mediators in response to IgE produced against nonfood materials such as inhaled pollens or latex
- Reactions that result from inflammatory mediators released from granulocytes such as eosinophils in the digestive tract
- Food protein enteropathies due to proteins in milk or soy
- Food-associated disease such as gluten-sensitive enteropathy (celiac disease), which has an immune component

---

BOX 26-2   Symptoms of Food Allergy

Gastrointestinal

Abdominal pain
Abdominal bloating and distention
Indigestion
Belching
Nausea
Vomiting
Constipation
Diarrhea
Gastrointestinal bleeding
Oral and pharyngeal pruritus

Skin and Mucous Membranes

Urticaria (hives)
Angioedema (swelling of deeper tissues)
Eczema (atopic dermatitis)
Contact dermatitis
Erythema (skin inflammation)
Pruritus (itching)
Redness (erythema)
Oral allergy syndrome

Respiratory

Rhinitis
Rhinorrhea (runny nose)
Asthma
Bronchospasm
Cough
Laryngeal edema (throat tightening due to swelling of tissues)
Airway tightening
Hoarseness

Eyes, Ears, Nose, and Throat

Dark circles around eyes
Spots before eyes
Serous otitis media (earache with effusion)
Conjunctivitis (itchy, watery reddened eyes)

Systemic

Anaphylaxis
Hypotension
Dysrhythmias

Nervous System

Migraine headaches
Other headaches
Listlessness
Hyperactivity
Lack of concentration
Tension-fatigue syndrome
Fibromyalgia
Irritability
Chilliness
Dizziness

Other

Frequent urination
Bed-wetting
Excessive sweating
Pallor
Muscle aches
Low-grade fever

The umbrella generic term **food sensitivity** is used when it is unclear whether the reaction is immunologically related or due to a biochemical or physiologic defect (Joneja, 2013).

Food intolerance is an adverse reaction to a food or food additive that does not involve the immune system and results from the body's inability to digest, absorb, or metabolize a food or component of the food (Joneja, 2013; Turnbull et al, 2015). It may be caused by a toxic, gastrointestinal, pharmacologic, genetic/metabolic, psychogenic, or an idiopathic reaction to a food or chemical substances in that food. For example, an individual can be intolerant to milk not because of an allergy to milk protein, but because of an inability to digest the carbohydrate lactose (see Figure 26-1).

An emerging hypothesis called **sensitivity-related illness** proposes that an individual who is exposed to some type of toxicant or insult, usually in the GI tract, may subsequently become sensitive to food, inhalants, or chemicals (Genuis, 2010).

ETIOLOGY

ARFs illustrate the critical importance of appreciating "biochemical uniqueness" as a core clinical concept in nutrition assessment. Numerous factors, including genetics and epigenetics, intestinal barrier integrity, microbiota, and loss of biodiversity, maternal and early fetal and early life factors such as cesarean delivery and lack of breastfeeding, stress, psychologic factors, exercise, and environmental and physiologic influences such as changes in hormone levels, affect an individual's unique response to food or food component and its ultimate interpretation by the body as either "friend" or "foe."

Genetics and Epigenetics

Food allergy has a hereditary component that is not yet clearly defined. **Atopy** is a condition of genetic predisposition to produce IgE antibodies in response to an **allergen** and to develop typical symptoms. Atopic individuals, usually identified in infancy and confirmed by positive skin-prick test, are characterized

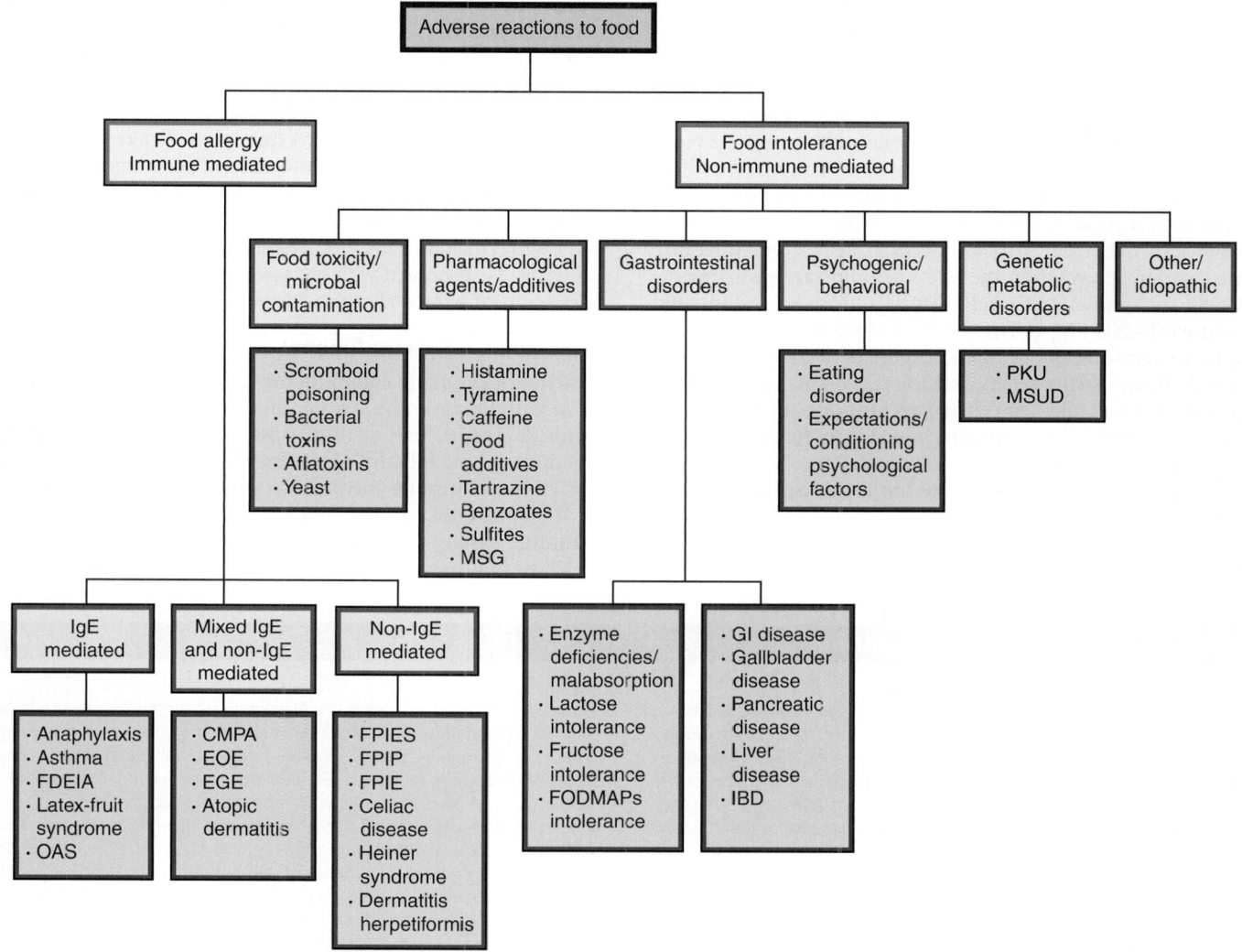

FIGURE 26-1 Adverse reactions to food. *CMPA,* cow's milk protein allergy; *EOE,* eosinophilic esophagitis; *EGE,* eosinophilic gastroenteritis; *FDEIA,* food dependent exercise-induced anaphylaxis; *FODMAPs,* fructose, oligo-, di-, monosaccharides, and polyols syndrome; *FPIE,* food protein-induced enteropathy; *FPIES,* food protein-induced enterocolitis syndrome; *FPIP,* food protein-induced proctocolitis; *IBD,* inflammatory bowel disease; *MSUD,* maple syrup urine disease; *OAS,* oral allergy syndrome; *PKU,* phenylketonuria.

by severe IgE-mediated reactions to dander, pollens, food, or other environmental factors, which present as food allergy, **atopic dermatitis (eczema)**, atopic conjunctivitis, atopic rhinitis, asthma, and symptoms in all organ systems, with the most severe being life-threatening anaphylaxis (see Box 26-2). A study of Finnish children showed that up to the age of 4 years, children with two parents reporting any type of allergic reaction were three times as likely to have a food allergy as children with allergy-free parents. Children with one allergic parent were twice as likely to have a food allergy (Pyrhönen et al, 2011).

However, genetic susceptibility alone does not completely explain the prevalence of food allergy. **Epigenetic** factors may alter the genetic expression of food allergy and atopy (see Chapter 5). Environmental exposures in early childhood such as diet, maternal or family smoking, air pollution, and microbial contact may, through epigenetic mechanisms, induce a long-lasting propensity that then influences the development of allergic symptoms (Tezza et al, 2013). Most likely it is multiple environmental changes or exposures over a lifetime at specific intervals (including pregnancy) that interact to predispose an individual to allergic sensitization and expression of allergic disease (Haahtela et al, 2013).

Antigen Exposure and Oral Tolerance

Humans are exposed to thousands of foreign molecules daily from food and the environment. Exposure to these foreign molecules in the digestive tract is usually followed by immune regulation or suppression, such that the food is recognized as "foreign but safe," which is a prerequisite for the development of tolerance to a food or food molecule. This is known as **oral tolerance** (Brandtzaeg, 2010; Weiner et al, 2011). Oral tolerance is mediated by several immune cells, including antigen-presenting cells, such as **dendritic cells (DCs)** and **macrophages**, and regulatory T-cells (T_{reg} cells), which are important suppressors of cellular and humoral immune responses (Bauer et al, 2015).

Food allergy occurs when oral tolerance fails and the food ingested acts as an allergen causing an immune-mediated reaction as discussed below. Ongoing research is focused on how oral tolerance develops and is maintained.

The amount of antigen presented to the sensitized immune cell also influences whether allergy symptoms develop. The effects of food antigens and other antigens may be additive. For example, clinical symptoms of food allergy may increase when inhalant allergies are exacerbated by seasonal or environmental changes. Similarly, the effects of environmental factors, toxins, tobacco smoke, stress, and exercise may exacerbate the clinical symptoms of food allergy.

The Gastrointestinal Function and the Microbiome

Gastrointestinal (GI) function and the ability to prevent the inappropriate passage of molecules through the intestinal wall is key to maintenance of oral tolerance and avoidance of the allergic response. Essential to this function of the GI tract is the presence of the **microbiota**, the population of bacteria that live in the human gut—about 10 trillion of them, with most of them residing in the lower GI tract. The **microbiome** is the collection of genes belonging to hundreds of different types of bacteria that live on the skin and in the gut. **Dysbiosis** exists when there is an imbalance in the microbiota, which can impair digestion and affect overall health.

Dysbiosis contributes to **increased intestinal permeability**, also referred to as "leaky gut," and the increased likelihood that inappropriate molecules will pass through and reach the lymphoid tissue, leading to allergy development. Disruptions in the microbiota and the intestinal wall barrier are the result of various factors, including cesarean delivery, lack of breastfeeding, antibiotics, chronic stress, infections, and alterations in the microbiota (see Chapters 1 and 28 for further discussion of the microbiota).

The **gut-associated lymphoid tissue (GALT)** is the largest mass of lymphoid tissue in the body. A leaky gut with altered GI permeability and possible dysbiosis allows antigen penetration and presentation to the GALT lymphocytes and sensitization (Fritscher-Ravens et al, 2014; Groschwitz and Hogan, 2009). Other conditions such as GI disease, malnutrition, fetal prematurity, and immunodeficiency also may be associated with increased gut permeability and risk of development of food allergy (see Figure 38-4).

The Immune System Arsenal

Antibodies contain a globulin protein; because of their association with the immune system, they are referred to as **immunoglobulins (Ig)**. Five distinct classes of antibodies have been identified: IgA, IgD, IgE, IgG, and IgM. Each Ig has a specific function in immune-mediated reactions (see Box 26-3).

Lymphocytes are the "command and control" cells of the immune system and include two important groups: **B-cells**, arising from stem cells in the bone marrow, and T-cells. **T-cells**

BOX 26-3   The Immunoglobulins

IgA

Found in two forms—serum IgA and secretory IgA (sIgA). The latter is present in mucus secretions in the mouth, respiratory and gastrointestinal tracts, vagina, and colostrum in mammalian milk. It includes a "secretory piece" in its structure that protects it from protein-destroying enzymes in the digestive tract so that it survives in an active form as a "first-line" defense against antigens entering from the external environment. Serum IgA, which does not have the secretory piece, is in the second highest amount in circulation, exceeded only by IgG.

IgD

Found in small amounts in the tissues that line the belly and chest; involved in immunoglobulin class switching; its role in allergy is probably minimal.

IgE

The classic allergy antibody of hay fever, asthma, eczema, and food-induced anaphylaxis, oral allergy syndrome, and immediate gastrointestinal hypersensitivity reactions. Immediate allergic reactions usually involve IgE and are the most clearly understood mechanisms.

IgG

The only antibody that crosses the placenta from mother to baby. Defends against pathogens and persists long after the threat is over; it may be responsible for some non–IgE-mediated hypersensitivity reactions. Four subtypes include IgG1, IgG2, IgG3, and IgG4. IgG4 has been implicated in some types of adverse reactions to food. Food protein–specific IgG antibodies tend to rise in the first few months after the introduction of a food and then decrease even though the food may continue to be consumed. It appears to be part of the process of development of tolerance to a food. A rise in antigen-specific IgG4 accompanied by a drop in IgE often indicates recovery (tolerance) from a food allergy. People with inflammatory bowel disorders such as celiac disease or ulcerative colitis often have high levels of IgG and IgM (Stapel et al, 2008), possibly indicating the passage of food molecules as "foreign invaders" into circulation.

IgM

The largest antibody; a first-line defender that can mop up many antigens at one time. It is produced by the fetus in utero and its level rises in the presence of an in utero infection.

also originate from stem cells but are later transported to the thymus gland, where they mature. Monocytes and macrophages are primarily phagocytes that engulf foreign material, break it apart, and display specific molecules of the material on their surfaces, making them antigen-presenting cells (APC). The antigenic component displayed on the surface is an epitope and is recognized by T-cells. T-cells respond by generating a cytokine message that stimulates their differentiation.

T-cells are a diverse group of lymphocytes with several different roles in the immune response under different circumstances, and they secrete different sets of cytokines. Th cells are helper cells that moderate and adjust the system. Th1 cells regulate the activities of the B-cells to produce antibodies and direct damage to target cells, resulting in the destruction of antigens. This function is useful in defending against bacteria, viruses, and other pathogenic cells. Th2 cells mediate the allergic response by regulating the production by B-cells of IgE sensitized to food or other allergens. Other T cells are T-regulatory cells (T-reg cells) and T- suppressor cells that regulate the immune response so that there is tolerance of the foreign but safe molecule.

In the process of making antibodies, the B-cells convert to plasma cells and the antibodies, or IgE, is generated from the plasma cells (see Figure 26-2). These allergen-specific antibodies attach themselves to mast cells (in the lungs, skin, tongue, and linings of the nose and intestinal tract) or basophils (in circulation).

Mast cells and basophils are granulocytes. Granulocytes contain intracellular granules, or small vessels that are storage depots for defense chemicals or inflammatory mediators that protect the body from invading pathogens but also cause allergic symptoms. Allergen-specific IgE antibodies attach to the surface of a mast cell by coupling with specific receptors on the cell's surface. When the eliciting allergens enter on a subsequent occasion, they attach to their matching (homologous) IgE antibodies on the mast cell's surface. The allergen attaches to two adjacent IgE molecules, forming a "bridge" between them. This bridging activates the mast cell by a series of energy-requiring processes, resulting in calcium channeling into the cell. This triggers degranulation of the intracellular granules, releasing the inflammatory mediators, such as histamine (in greatest amount), prostaglandins, leukotrienes, and cytokines.

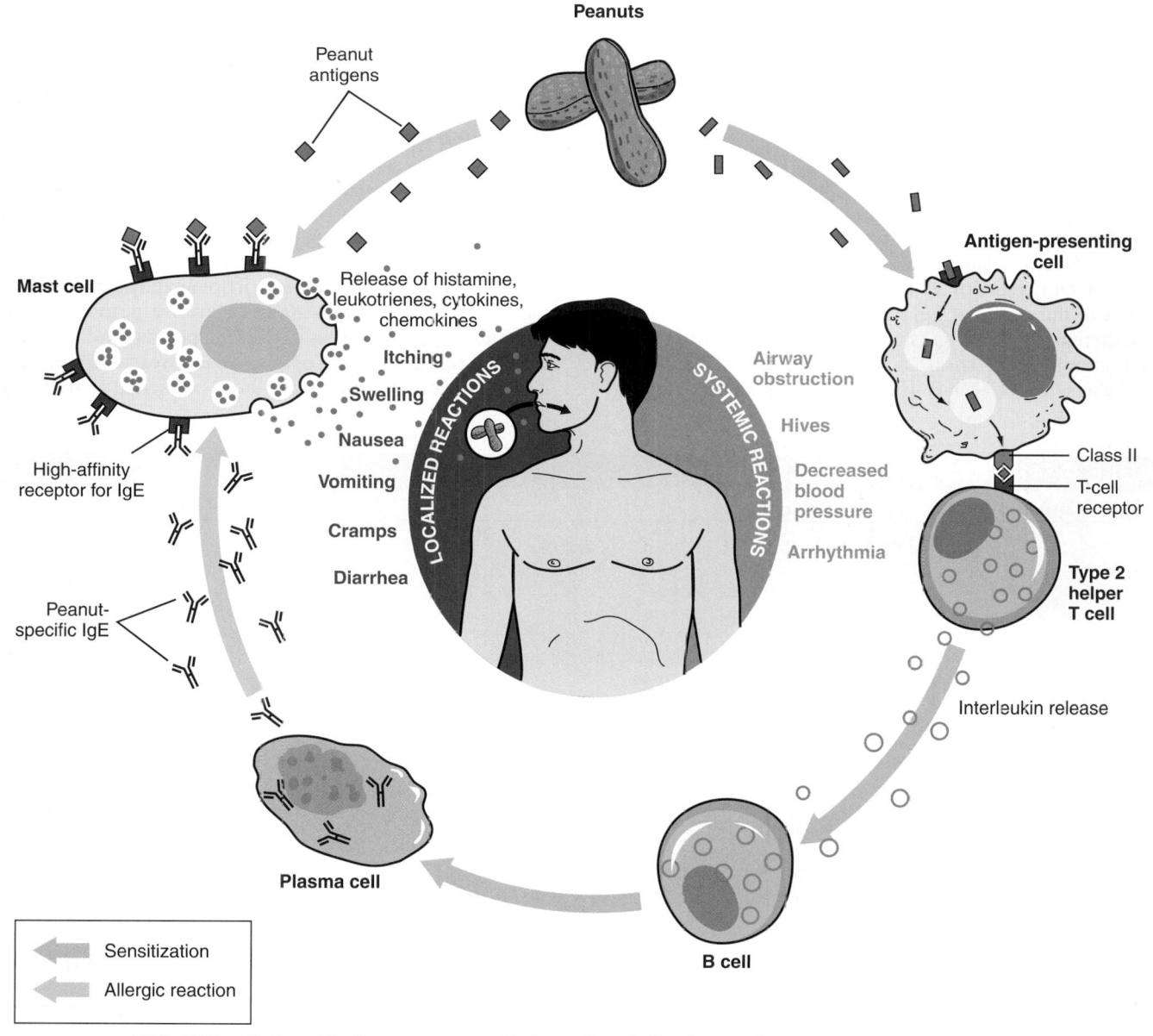

FIGURE 26-2 Sensitization process and IgE-mediated allergic reaction.

Each of the mediators has a specific effect on local tissues and at distant sites, resulting in the symptoms of allergy (Joneja, 2013). Other granulocytes such as neutrophils and eosinophils are attracted to the reaction site by mediators such as chemokines. These arise from degranulation of mast cells and release additional inflammatory chemicals, which further enhance the allergic response, resulting in increased symptom severity. This is also evidenced in a later biphasic reaction or reccurence of symptoms after the intial response has waned.

PATHOPHYSIOLOGY

The basic pathophysiology of the allergic response can be described in three phases: the breakdown of oral tolerance, allergen sensitization, and reactivity to allergens leading to allergy symptoms (Bauer et al, 2015). Other mechanisms still under investigation are increases in gastric pH, direct action of bioactive chemicals, neuroenteric hypersensitivity, and osmotic effects with luminal distention (Swift and Lisker, 2012).

Oral tolerance, as already discussed, is the norm in most individuals. It is the breakdown or loss of oral tolerance that promotes allergen sensitization. Loss of oral tolerance is associated with a lowered T_{reg} cell response and increased levels of APCs reaching the epithelial cells of the intestinal mucosa. With loss of oral tolerance, the immune system mistakenly recognizes a food or molecule as foreign.

When a food or molecule is no longer seen as safe, the second phase, sensitization, takes place, in which immune cells respond at this first exposure to the allergen. This is characterized by a Th-2 response and involves dendritic and epithelial cells.

The third phase is reactivity to allergens such that whenever that same foreign material or allergen enters the body, the immune system responds with an immune-mediated reaction, usually with the release of inflammatory mediators or defensive chemicals, resulting in allergic symptoms. Because individuals can develop immunologic sensitization, as evidenced by the production of allergen-specific IgE without having clinical symptoms upon subsequent exposure to those foods, an IgE-mediated food allergy requires the presence of sensitization and the development of specific signs and symptoms on exposure to the food. Sensitization alone is not sufficient to define food allergy (Boyce et al, 2011; NIH, NIAID, 2010; Vickery et al, 2011) (see Figure 26-2).

IgE-Mediated Reactions

IgE-mediated food allergic reactions are rapid in onset, occurring within minutes to a few hours of exposure. The methods of exposure include inhalation, skin contact, and ingestion. A wide range of symptoms has been attributed to this type of food allergy and frequently involve the GI, dermatologic, or respiratory systems and can range from mild hives to life-threatening multiple organ anaphylaxis.

A few foods account for the vast majority of IgE-mediated allergic reactions: milk, eggs, peanuts, tree nuts, soy, wheat, fish, shellfish, and sesame (see http://foodallergysupport.olicentral.com/index.php/topic,319.45.html for more information on sesame allergies). However, any food is capable of eliciting an IgE-mediated reaction after a person has been sensitized to it. Food-induced anaphylaxis, asthma, urticaria (hives), eczema, oral allergy syndrome (OAS), latex-fruit allergy, and food dependent exercise-induced anaphylaxis (FDEIA) are IgE-mediated immune reactions (see Table 26-1).

Food-Induced Anaphylaxis

Food-induced anaphylaxis is an acute, often severe, and sometimes fatal immune response that usually occurs within a limited period following exposure to an antigen. Multiple organ systems are affected. Symptoms can include respiratory distress, abdominal pain, nausea, vomiting, cyanosis, arrhythmia, hypotension, angioedema, urticaria, diarrhea, shock, cardiac arrest, and death. The vast majority of anaphylactic reactions to foods in adults in North America involve peanuts, tree nuts, fish, and shellfish, whereas in children peanuts and tree nuts are the most common causes of anaphylactic reactions but anaphylactic reactions to milk have been reported (Joneja, 2013).

TABLE 26-1 **Types of Allergic Reactions**		
Reaction/Classification	**IgE-Mediated**	**Mixed IgE- and Non-IgE-Mediated**
Mechanism	Th2 activation stimulates production of IgE antibodies by activated B-cell lymphocytes. The allergen binds with sensitized IgE antibodies on mast cells or basophils. Upon binding, chemical inflammatory mediators are released from the cell.	Antibodies and T-cells are associated with triggering inflammatory mediators and the development of symptoms.
Timing	First phase: Immediate hypersensitivity, minutes to 1 hour Late phase: May occur several hours after initial response, usually 4-6 hours after first phase	Delayed onset >2 hr; chronic, relapsing
Systemic	Anaphylaxis	
Skin and mucous membranes	Atopic dermatitis (eczema), angioedema, contact dermatitis, flushing, pruritus, urticarial (hives)	Atopic dermatitis, contact dermatitis, dermatitis herpetiformis
Gastrointestinal	Abdominal pain and bloating, belching, constipation, diarrhea, indigestion, nausea and vomiting	Eosinophilic esophagitis (EOE), eosinophilic gastroenteritis (EGE), food-protein-induced enteropathies (FPIES), celiac disease
Respiratory	Acute rhinitis (stuffy nose, hay fever), rhinorrhea (runny nose), allergic conjunctivitis (itchy, reddened, watery eyes) asthma, bronchospasm, laryngeal edema (throat tightening because of swelling of tissues)	Asthma, pulmonary hemosiderosis (Heiner syndrome)
Nervous system	Dizziness, headaches, hyperactivity, listlessness, irritability, migraine headaches, spots before eyes, tension-fatigue syndrome	Diverse symptoms similar to those listed for IgE mediated
Other	Bed-wetting, dark circles under eyes, excessive sweating, low-grade fever, hoarseness, myalgias, pallor	Diverse symptoms similar to those for IgE mediated

FPIES, Food protein–induced enterocolitis syndrome; Ig, immunoglobulin.
From Joneja JV: *The health professional's guide to food allergies and intolerances,* Chicago, 2013, Academy of Nutrition and Dietetics, p 44.

Peanuts are the most common food allergen in fatal anaphylactic reactions (Turnbull et al, 2015).

People with known anaphylactic reactions to food allergens should carry and be prepared to use, epinephrine via an injectable adrenaline at all times. Epinephrine is the drug of choice to reverse an allergic reaction, even with asthma (Franchini et al, 2010). Delayed use of epinephrine has been associated with an increased risk of biphasic reactions, in which a recurrence of symptoms 4 to 12 hours after the initial anaphylactic reaction may be fatal.

Oral Allergy or Pollen-Food Allergy Syndrome

The oral allergy syndrome (OAS), or pollen-food syndrome (PFS), results from direct contact with food allergens in a person primarily sensitized to a specific pollen. Symptoms of OAS are confined almost exclusively to the oropharynx and include itchy mouth, scratchy throat, or swelling of the lips, mouth, uvula, tongue, and throat tightness. Itchy ears are sometimes reported. Rarely, other target organs are involved. However, there may be a reaction later (biphasic) because of histamine release in the gastrointestinal tract. OAS may be severe and present as hives, wheezing, vomiting, diarrhea, and low blood pressure or even anaphylaxis, but this is rare (American College of Allergy, Asthma and Immunology [ACAAI], 2015; http://acaai.org/allergies/types/food-allergies/types-food-allergy/oral-allergy-syndrome, accessed March 20, 2015).

Sensitization to the pollen occurs through the respiratory system (Fernandez-Rivas et al, 2006). The reaction to foods occurs as a result of the presence of an antigen within the food that has a structure similar to that of the pollen; it is a situation of cross-reactivity between inhaled and ingested proteins. The primary sensitization is to the pollen, not the food. Symptoms are rapid and appear within 5 to 30 minutes upon ingestion of the allergen-containing food, and most often subside within 30 minutes. In severe cases, throat tightening can occur as a result of swelling of tissues within the area; asphyxiation has been reported in rare instances.

OAS is most commonly seen in individuals with coexisting seasonal allergic rhinitis to trees, in particular alder and birch, ragweed, other weeds (e.g., mugwort), or grass pollens, following ingestion of specific fruits, vegetables, and some nuts (Geroldinger-Simic et al, 2011). The cooked fruit or vegetable is often tolerated because the reactions are caused by predominately heat-labile proteins, which are changed during cooking. However, this is not always the case, and a careful history and questioning about the food is important (Kondo and Urisu, 2009). Box 26-4 lists the foods and pollens most commonly linked with OAS.

Because reactions are immediate after ingestion of the raw food, most individuals can identify the food culprit. However, if it is not obvious, an OAS elimination diet may be useful followed by careful challenge with a small amount of the food applied to the lip with observation for any reaction. Only those foods that cause an adverse reaction must be avoided.

Latex-Fruit or Latex-Food Syndrome

Natural rubber latex (NRL), used in latex rubber gloves, clothing, bottle nipples, children's rubber toys, elastic bands, and many other articles in the environment contain many proteins that can be highly allergenic. The allergic reaction is IgE-mediated and is often seen in health care workers (8% to 17%), other workers using latex rubber gloves such as hairdressers or house cleaners, those working in the latex industry, and in those undergoing multiple surgical procedures in which they have been exposed to latex rubber surgical gloves and appliances (68% of children with spina bifida) (American Latex Allergy Association, 2015, http://

BOX 26-4	**Foods and Pollens Involved in Oral Allergy Syndrome**			
Almonds	B	Melon	R, G
Apple	B	Nectarine	B
Apricot	B	Parsley	B
Banana	R	Parsnip	B
Carrot	B	Peanut	G
Celery	B	Peach	B
Chamomile	R	Pear	B
Cherry	B	Plum	B
Cucumber	R	Potato	B
Echinacea	R	Prune	B
Fennel	B	Pumpkin seed	B
Fig	B, G	Tomato	G
Green pepper	B	Walnut	B
Hazelnut	B	Zucchini	R
Kiwi	B		

B, Birch pollen; *G*, grass pollen; *R*, ragweed pollen.
From: Joneja JV: *The health professional's guide to food allergies and intolerances,* Chicago, 2013, Academy of Nutrition and Dietetics, p 311.

latexallergyresources.org/statistics). Symptoms of NRL allergy include contact dermatitis, eczema, angioedema, rhinoconjunctivitis, asthma, and, in severe cases, anaphylaxis.

It is estimated that 50% to 70% of people with latex allergies have IgE antibodies that can cross-react with antigens from foods, mostly fruits, and cause allergic symptoms of the latex-fruit syndrome or latex-food syndrome. Symptoms of latex-food allergy vary, with many being similar to those with NRL allergy, including anaphylaxis. The reaction is to the latex protein found in the food (Joneja, 2013) (see *Focus On:* Cross-Reactivity: How Does It Happen?)

Assessment of the problematic foods in latex-food allergy is difficult, because even though it is an IgE-mediated reaction, there usually is no food-specific IgE in the serum, so IgE tests are not useful. For those with NRL documented allergy, but with no symptoms after consumption of associated foods, it is important to keep in mind that every NRL-allergic individual reacts differently to foods with latex cross-reacting allergens. The most frequently reported foods in latex-food allergic reactions are listed in Box 26-5. Many clinicians advise NRL allergic individuals to avoid these foods in the interest of safety. However, it cannot be assumed that the NRL allergic person will react to these foods or that there will not be other NRL allergen-containing foods that may cause a reaction. Management is based on an exclusion diet that begins with avoidance of foods known to be reactive for that individual (Joneja, 2013).

◎ FOCUS ON

Cross-Reactivity: How Does it Happen?

Profilins are pathogenesis-related (PR) proteins found in fruits and vegetables that are produced in a plant when it is "under stress" and act as defensive chemicals. They are present in all eukaryotic cells, are similar in a wide range of plants, and can function as allergens. They may account for cross-reactivity between plant allergens. They occur in pollen, latex rubber, and other plants. They are often modified by processing or cooking, thus accounting for the observation that the raw food causes a reaction in an individual and when the cooked form does not.

Carbohydrate moieties are also now recognized as being able to function as allergens.

BOX 26-5   Foods Frequently Reported in Latex-Food Allergy

Avocado	Passion fruit
Banana	Tomato
Cassava	Turnip
Cherimoya	Zucchini
Chestnut	Bell pepper
Kiwi fruit	Celery
Mango	Potato
Papaya	Custard apple

Adapted from Joneja, JV: *The health professional's guide to food allergies and intolerances*, Academy of Nutrition and Dietetics, 2013, Chicago, p 321.

Food-Dependent, Exercise-Induced Anaphylaxis (FDEIA)

Food-dependent, exercise-induced anaphylaxis (FDEIA) is a distinct form of allergy in which an offending food triggers an IgE-mediated anaphylactic reaction only when the individual exercises within 2 to 4 hours after eating (DuToit, 2007). Signs of developing anaphylaxis are urticaria, pruritus (itching), and erythema (reddening) followed by breathing difficulty and GI symptoms. The food is not problematic in the absence of exercise. Usually a specific food causes FDEIA, but exercise-induced anaphylaxis (EIA) can happen following consumption of a meal, regardless of the foods in the meal.

FDEIA appears to be more common in adolescents and young adults and in those with known food allergy or a history of anaphylaxis (Joneja, 2013). Shellfish, seafood, certain fruits, milk, celery, a gliadin component in wheat, and other foods have been reported as offending agents (Morita et al, 2009). In FDEIA, the combination of a sensitizing food and exercise precipitates symptoms, possibly related to increased GI permeability and absorption, blood-flow redistribution, and increased osmolality (Robson-Ansley and Toit, 2010). Additional factors such as ingestion of aspirin may contribute to the reaction. The prevalence and causative agents and effective methods of diagnosis in FDEIA continue to be explored.

Mixed IgE-Mediated and Non–IgE-Mediated Reactions

Disorders involving IgE- and non-IgE mediated reactions are referred to as *mixed* and include cow's milk protein allergy (CMPA), eosinophilic esophagitis (EoE), eosinophilic gastroenteritis (EGE), and atopic dermatitis. They involve well-studied IgE-meditated reactions along with less well–understood non–IgE-mediated reactions.

Cow's Milk Protein Allergy (CMPA)

Cow's milk protein allergy (CMPA) is common in childhood; it is reported in 2% to 7% of babies under 1 year of age (Ludman et al, 2013). The IgE-mediated reactions are usually recognized because the urticaria, angioedema, eczema, GI symptoms, and respiratory symptoms appear within 2 hours of cow's milk protein (CMP) consumption. Non–IgE-mediated reactions are more difficult to identify because of the longer time between their appearance and the CMP consumption, sometimes as long as 20 hours. Symptoms may include gastroesophageal reflux disease (GERD), eczema, persistent crying, diarrhea, and constipation (Turnbull et al, 2015).

Exposure to CMP is through either formula or breastmilk if the mother is consuming cow's milk in her diet. Most children with CMPA outgrow it by 5 years for the IgE-mediated reactions and by 3 years for uncomplicated non–IgE-mediated reactions (Turnbull et al, 2015).

Eosinophilic Gastrointestinal Diseases (EGID)

The eosinophilic gastrointestinal diseases (EGID) are a group of GI disorders in which the accumulation of eosinophils (granulocytes capable of releasing inflammatory mediators) is diagnostic. Eosinophilic esophagitis (EoE) and eosinophilic gastroenteritis (EGE) are inflammatory disorders characterized by infiltration of the esophagus, stomach, or intestines with eosinophils. It is now thought that both conditions have an IgE and non-IgE component, although they are not clearly defined. Identification of specific offending allergens is not always possible (Merves et al, 2014).

Almost half of the patients who present with EGE have atopic features (Eroglu et al, 2009; Roy-Ghanta et al, 2008). EGE can occur at any age, and symptoms can easily be mistaken for functional GI disorders. EOE occurs most often in white men, usually starting some time between school age and midlife (Furuta and Katzka, 2015). Tests for food-specific IgE are invariably of no value in identification of the offending foods, calling into question the involvement of IgE reactions in their cause. Implementation of an elimination diet aimed at identifying and excluding food antagonists can be most helpful in the nutrition assessment and management of EGID. Heartburn with the ingestion of alcohol occurs in 30% of adult patients suggesting that the elimination of alcohol may also be useful (Straumann et al, 2012).

Non–IgE-Mediated Reactions

The contribution of non–IgE-mediated immune reactions to food intolerance continues to be investigated. These are associated with delayed or chronic reactions and typically appear before 6 months of age in formula-fed infants, but a few cases have been reported in breast-fed infants. It has been postulated that these reactions may play a role in atopic dermatitis, food protein–induced enterocolitis syndrome (FPIES), food protein–induced proctocolitis (FPIP), cow's milk–induced pulmonary hemosiderosis (Heiner syndrome), and food protein–induced enteropathies (Bone et al, 2009).

Multiple components of the immune system are likely to be involved with different underlying mechanisms. The reaction seems to involve Th cells that release TNF-alpha, which is a Th1 response. This is in contrast to the allergy Th2 response, which releases cytokines that result in the production of IgE. In the Th1 response, where there is release of TNF-alpha, there is also an abnormally low level of TGF-B, which is the cytokine involved in developing tolerance to foods. This suggests that the resulting lack of immunologic tolerance results in the immune system treating the food as if it were a foreign "threat" to the body's survival and becomes sensitized to it. Thus the next time the food is eaten, there is a release of mediators reflective of a Th1 response and the defensive reaction of vomiting and diarrhea. Not unexpectedly, tests for allergen-sensitized IgE are not useful in diagnosing these disorders.

Food Protein–Induced Enterocolitis Syndrome (FPIES)

An example of a non–IgE-meditated immune reaction to food is food protein–induced enterocolitis syndrome (FPIES). Although rare, it is seen in formula-fed infants and begins to appear around 6 months of age. It is typically provoked by cow's milk or soy protein–based formula (Mehr et al, 2009; Nowak-Wegrzyn and Muraro, 2009). A response to sheep or goat's milk or other solid foods is less common but also can occur (Järvinen and Chatchatee, 2009). The reaction is dramatic with immediate vomiting, often followed by diarrhea and abdominal pain. In chronic cases there may also be failure to thrive.

Occasionally FPIES is seen in breast-fed infants, presumably caused by milk proteins from the mother's diet crossing into her milk. Food-specific IgE antibodies have no value in this diagnosis; confirmation of FPIES is challenging because it mimics other GI inflammatory disorders.

Formula-fed infants should be switched to an extensively hydrolyzed casein formula (EHF) (see Box 26-9). If they do not tolerate this formula, they may require an elemental formula. Breast-fed infants should remain on the breast, and the mother should eliminate cow's milk and soy or other suspicious foods from her diet. FPIES usually resolves by 2 years of age.

Food Protein–Induced Proctitis or Proctocolitis (FPIP)

In food protein–induced proctitis or proctocolitis (FPIP), bloody and mucus-laden stools are seen in an otherwise apparently healthy baby, often at about 2 months of age. Parents are concerned when they see flecks of blood in their baby's stool, but it is usually slight and further development of anemia is rare. Common trigger foods are cow's milk protein or soy protein from infant formula, and their removal from the infant's diet usually solves the problem. In the case of the breast-fed infant, the mother should remove these foods from her diet and continue to breast-feed. For the formula-fed infant, it becomes necessary to switch to an extensively hydrolyzed formula (EHF), such as any of those listed in Box 26-9. However, sometimes the infant requires an elemental formula, examples of which are also listed in Box 26-9. The bleeding usually disappears within 3 days of implementing a formula change or change in the breastfeeding mother's diet. In most cases the FPIP resolves itself by the time the baby is 1 to 2 years old, and offending foods can be introduced with monitoring of the baby's stool for blood (Joneja, 2013).

FOOD INTOLERANCES

Food intolerances are ARFs that result in clinical symptoms but are not caused by an immune system reaction. They are caused by nonimmunologic mechanisms including toxic, pharmacologic, gastrointestinal, genetic, metabolic, psychogenic, or idiosyncratic reactions (see Table 26-2). Food intolerances are much more common than food allergies and are usually triggered by small-molecular weight chemical substances and biologically active components of food (Joneja, 2013). Symptoms caused by food intolerances are often similar to food allergy and include GI symptoms, cutaneous, respiratory, and neurologic manifestations such as headaches (see Table 26-2). Clinically, it is important to distinguish food intolerance from immune-mediated food allergy because food allergies can cause life-threatening anaphylactic reactions, whereas food intolerances do not.

Carbohydrate Intolerance

Carbohydrates—sugars, starches, and polysaccharides—are complex in structure and must be broken down by enzymes for optimal digestion, absorption, and assimilation. Adverse reactions can occur if there is a deficiency of enzymes responsible for carbohydrate digestion, especially of disaccharides, such as lactose or sucrose, or if there is malabsorption of the breakdown products.

Lactose Intolerance

Intolerance to the disaccharide lactose is the most common ARF, and most cases result from a genetically influenced reduction of intestinal lactase. It is estimated that up to 75% of the world's population has hypolactasia (Bulhoes et al, 2007; Jarvela et al, 2009). Abdominal bloating and cramping, flatulence, and diarrhea occur usually up to several hours following lactose ingestion. Because some of the GI symptoms are similar, lactose intolerance is often confused with allergy to cow's milk; however, most individuals who are allergic to cow's milk also have symptoms in other organ systems, including the respiratory tract, skin, and, in severe cases, systemic anaphylactic reactions. Deficiencies of lactase and other carbohydrate-digesting enzymes and their management are discussed further in Chapter 28.

Fructose Intolerance and the Inability to Digest Fructose Polymers (FODMAPs)

Fructose intolerance is evidenced by an inability to digest and absorb the monosaccharide fructose, either from a food containing fructose directly or the disaccharide sucrose (glucose + fructose) (see Chapter 28 for discussion of fructose intolerance and its management).

Maldigestion and malabsorption of the fructo-, oligo-, di-, and monosaccharides and polyols (FODMAPs) may also occur. Humans lack the hydrolase enzymes necessary to break down the bonds in the fructose polymer chains, so most individuals will develop symptoms if too much of these carbohydrates are consumed (Joneja, 2013). Intake of large quantities of FODMAPs will lead to bloating, diarrhea, cramping, and flatulence. The symptoms appear to be more common in individuals who have an underlying functional GI disorder, such as irritable bowel syndrome (see Chapter 28 for discussion of FODMAPs and the diet management, which eliminates excess fructose, fructose polymers, and the sugar alcohols).

Pharmacologic Reactions

An adverse reaction to a food may be the result of a response to a pharmacologically active component in that food. A wide range of allergy-like symptoms can result from ingestion of biogenic amines such as histamine and tyramine.

Histamine

Histamine is a biogenic amine produced endogenously with very important functions. It is released as the first inflammatory mediator in an allergic reaction or in a physical defense reaction. When released, it causes vasodilation, erythema, increased permeability of cell membranes, digestive tract upset, pruritus (itching), urticaria, angioedema (tissue swelling), hypotension, tachycardia (heart racing), chest pain, nasal congestion (rhinitis), runny nose (rhinorrhea), conjunctivitis (watery, reddened, irritated eyes), headache, panic, fatigue, confusion, and irritability.

Everyone has a level of histamine that is tolerated, and when that level is exceeded in the body, the symptoms of excessive histamine develop. Basal levels of 0.3 to 1 ng/ml are considered normal (Joneja, 2013). Some people are more sensitive to histamine than others, usually because of a genetically determined inability to catabolize or breakdown histamine fast enough to keep the levels manageable so that histamine-induced symptoms are not triggered.

Foods with a high histamine content include fermented foods, tomatoes, strawberries, sauerkraut, aged cheeses, processed meats and fish, alcoholic beverages (champagne and red wine), and leftovers. Symptoms of excessive histamine may be indistinguishable from those of food allergy because of histamine's mediator function in allergic reactions.

TABLE 26-2   Examples of Food Intolerances

Cause	Associated Food(s)	Symptoms
Gastrointestinal Disorders		
Enzyme Deficiencies and Malabsorptive Disorders		
Lactose intolerance (lactase deficiency)	Foods containing lactose and mammalian milk	Bloating, flatulence, diarrhea, abdominal pain
Glucose-6 phosphate dehydrogenase deficiency	Fava or broad beans	Hemolytic anemia
Fructose intolerance	Foods containing sucrose or fructose	Bloating, flatulence, diarrhea, abdominal pain
Diseases		
Cystic fibrosis	Symptoms may be precipitated by many foods, especially high-fat foods	Bloating, loose stools, abdominal pain, malabsorption
Gallbladder disease	Symptoms may be precipitated by high-fat foods	Abdominal pain after eating
Pancreatic disease Inflammatory bowel disease	Symptoms may be precipitated by eating	Anorexia, nausea, dysgeusia, and other gastrointestinal symptoms
Inborn Errors Of Metabolism		
Phenylketonuria	Foods containing phenylalanine	Elevated serum phenylalanine levels, mental retardation
Galactosemia	Foods containing lactose or galactose	Vomiting, lethargy, failure to thrive
Psychologic Or Neurologic Reactions		
	Symptoms may be precipitated by any food	Wide variety of symptoms involving any system
Reactions To Pharmacologic Agents In Foods		
Phenylethylamine	Chocolate, aged cheeses, red wine	Migraine headaches
Tyramine	Aged cheeses, brewer's yeast, Chianti wine, canned fish, chicken liver, bananas, eggplant, tomatoes, raspberries, plums	Migraine headaches, cutaneous erythema, urticaria and hypertensive crisis in patients taking monoamine oxidase inhibitors
Histamine	Aged cheeses, fermented foods (e.g., sauerkraut, yogurt, kefir), processed meats (e.g., sausage, bologna, salami), canned and smoked fish, red beans, soybeans, citrus, avocado, eggplant, olives, tomato products, chocolate, cocoa, tea, yeast, alcohol, many spices, food additives and preservatives	Dizziness, flushing, hives, erythema, runny nose, headaches, decreased blood pressure, nausea, vomiting, shortness of breath, edema
Histamine-releasing agents	Shellfish, egg whites, chocolate, avocado, strawberries, citrus, pineapple, tomatoes, spinach, nuts, peanuts, alcohol	Urticaria, eczema, pruritus
Reactions To Food Additives		
Artificial colors: tartrazine or FD&C yellow no. 5 and other azo dyes	Artificially colored yellow or yellow-orange foods, soft drinks, some medicines	Hives, rash, asthma, nausea, headaches
Benzoates: benzoic acid or sodium benzoate	Processed foods as antimicrobial preservatives; color preservatives; bleaching agents Naturally occurring in berries, cinnamon and other spices, tea, prunes	Hives, rash, asthma, angioedema, nasal congestion, headache, contact dermatitis, diverse digestive tract symptoms
Butylated hydroxyanisole (BHA); butylated hydroxytoluene (BHT)	Processed foods as antioxidants and used in food packaging materials	Skin reactions such as hives
Monosodium glutamate (MSG)	Processed foods: added as a flavor enhancer; often used in Asian cuisine	Facial numbness, tingling and numbness in hands and feet, dizziness, balance problems, visual disturbances, headaches, asthma, flushing, diverse digestive tract symptoms
Nitrates and nitrites	Processed foods containing sodium nitrite, sodium nitrate, potassium nitrite and potassium nitrate commonly found in cured meats, canned meats, smoked fish, pate, pickled meats	Flushing, hives, migraine, other headaches, digestive tract symptoms
Salicylates	Naturally occurring in a variety of fruits, vegetables and some spices	Angioedema, asthma, hives; people sensitive to aspirin higher risk for developing intolerance
Sulfites		
Sodium sulfite, potassium sulfite, sodium metabisulfite, potassium metabisulfite, sodium bisulfite, potassium bisulfite, sulfur dioxide	Shrimp, avocado, instant potatoes, dried fruits and vegetables, and fresh fruits and vegetables treated with sulfites to prevent browning, acidic juices, wine, beer, and many processed foods	Acute asthma and anaphylaxis in people with asthma, reactions in skin and mucous membranes
Reactions To Microbial Contamination Or Toxins In Foods		
Proteus, Klebsiella, or *Escherichia coli* bacteria cause histidine to break down to a histamine	Unrefrigerated scombroid fish (tuna, bonita, mackerel); heat-stable toxin produced	Scombroid fish poisoning (itching, rash, vomiting, diarrhea); anaphylactic-type reaction

BHA, Butylated hydroxyanisole; *BHT,* butylated hydroxytoluene.

However, histamine intolerance does not have an IgE-based mechanism for the release of histamine. One percent of the U.S. population suffers from histamine intolerance, and 80% of those sufferers are middle aged (Maintz and Novak, 2007). In histamine intolerance there is an excessive reaction to histamine for the following reasons: (1) certain foods naturally contain large amounts of histamine, or its precursor histidine, that cause a reaction in the histamine sensitive individual, (2) some individuals are not able to deactivate or metabolize histamine in a timely manner because of a deficiency of the enzymes diamine oxidase (DAO) or histamine-N-methyltransferase (HNMT), or (3) there is the presence of other amines that also influence the histamine reaction.

Foods such as strawberries, egg whites, shellfish, and some food additives (e.g., tartrazine) and preservatives (e.g., benzoates) stimulate histamine release from mast cells. The mechanisms for this reaction are not clear. Histamine intolerance or sensitivity may be suspected when an allergic cause has been ruled out (Maintz and Novak, 2007) (see Box 26-6 for histamine content of foods and a histamine-restricted diet).

BOX 26-6   Histamine Restricted Diet

Lists of histamine content of foods differ widely between testing laboratories. It is difficult to determine the accurate histamine content of food, especially of fruits and vegetables, because of variations in the foods, such as degree of ripeness, time and method of harvesting, storage conditions, degree of contamination, and differences in analytical techniques used by the testing lab.

1. Peeled, packaged fruits, salads, and vegetables often have a higher histamine content than fresh. Fresh, whole fruits and vegetables are protected from microbial invasion (and therefore histamine production) by their peels or skins. Products with cut surfaces (e.g., shredded or sliced packaged salads) are more susceptible to bacterial invasion and are therefore more likely to contain histamine. For example, packaged mung bean, lentil, and radish sprouts contain double the histamine content compared to homegrown sprouts. **Fresh is best!**

2. The restricted foods in this management program also include foods that release histamine by unkown mechanisms, such as egg white; some plant foods; and additives, such as azo dyes, sulfites, and benzoates whose adverse effects include an increase in histamine.

3. Therefore, these lists are not limited to foods reported as containing a high level of histamine when measured in the laboratory. Not all people will react to the additives, so judicious challenge after the initial trial will determine whether these need to be avoided in the long term.

The lists provided here have been compiled from a variety of resources and reflect the foods and additives that are most consistently associated with higher levels of histamine.

Histamine-Restricted Diet Guidelines
The following foods and additives are *avoided* during the 4-week elimination trial.

Fish, Eggs, Meat
- Fish and shellfish whether fresh, frozen, smoked, or canned, if processing is unkown. Note: If the fish is freshly caught, gutted, and cooked within 1/2 hour, it may be eaten.
- Eggs. Note: A small quantity of cooked egg in a baked product such as pancakes, muffins, cakes is usually tolerated.
- Processed, smoked, and fermented meats of all types such as luncheon meat, sausage, wiener, bologna, salami, pepperoni, smoked ham, cured bacon.
- Leftovers. Note: freeze any uneaten protein-based food. Bacteria will quickly act on protein at room and refrigerator temperatures, resulting in histamine production.

Milk and Milk Products
- All fermented milk products and those containing bacterial culture, including:
  - Cheese: any kind of fermented cheese such as cheddar, Colby, blue cheese, Brie, Camembert, feta, Romano, and so on
  - Cheese products such as processed cheese, cheese slices, cheese spreads
  - Cottage cheese
  - Ricotta cheese
  - Yogurt
  - Buttermilk
  - Kefir

Fruits
- Apricots
- Cherries
- Citrus fruits: Orange, grapefruit, lemon, lime
- Cranberries
- Currants (fresh or dried)
- Dates
- Grapes
- Loganberries
- Pineapple
- Prunes
- Raisins
- Raspberries
- Strawberries

Vegetables
- Avocado
- Eggplant
- Olives
- Pickles, relishes, and other foods containing vinegar
- Pumpkin
- Spinach
- Tomatoes, tomato sauces, ketchup

Legumes
- Red beans
- Soy and soy products

Food Additives
- Tartrazine and other artificial food colors
- Preservatives, especially benzoates and sulfites
- Medications and vitamin pills that contain artificial food colors, benzoates, or sufites (a pharmacist will be able to recommend additive-free supplements and medications)

Seasonings
- Chili powder
- Cinnamon
- Cloves
- Curry powder
- Nutmeg
- Thyme
- Vinegar

Miscellaneous
- Fermented soy products (such as soy sauce, miso)
- Fermented foods (such as sauerkraut)
- Tea (regular or green)
- Chocolate, cocoa, and cola drinks
- Alcoholic beverages of all types
- Nonalcoholic versions of alcoholic beverages (e.g., nonalcoholic beer, ale, wine, etc.)

(From: Joneja, JV: The Health Professional's Guide to Food Allergies and Intolerances, Academy of Nutrition and Dietetics, 2013, Chicago. p. 301-303-permission is needed.

Tyramine

Tyramine is formed from the amino acid tyrosine and can cause adverse reactions in individuals who are taking monoamine oxidase inhibitors (MAOIs), which interfere with the breakdown of tyramine. This is an example of a potentially serious ARF caused by a drug-food interaction. Fortunately, the MAOIs are not prescribed as frequently today as in the past. Tyramine sensitivity in those not taking MAOIs is probably due to a deficiency of monoamine oxidase, but this is not well understood. Ingestion of tyramine containing foods also may cause migraine headaches or chronic hives in tyramine-sensitive individuals, with the response being dose dependent (Joneja, 2013). Tyramine is found in some fermented foods such as aged cheeses, wines, vinegars, and naturally in chicken liver, bananas, eggplant, raspberries, plums, and tomatoes (see Box 8-4 in Chapter 8 and Chapter 41).

Reactions to Food Additives

At the present time, many of the reaction mechanisms to food additives are poorly understood. Food additives such as salicylates, carmine (cochineal extracts), artificial food dyes and colorings such as FD & C yellow #5, and preservatives such as benzoic acid, sodium benzoate, butylated hydroxyanisole (BHA), butylated hydroxytoluene (BHT), nitrates, sulfites, and monosodium glutamate (MSG) can cause adverse reactions in certain individuals (Vojdani et al, 2015).

Sulfites

Reactions to sulfites are most common in asthmatics and result in a range of symptoms in sulfite-sensitive individuals. These can include dermatitis, urticaria, hypotension, abdominal pain, diarrhea, and life-threatening asthmatic and anaphylactic reactions (Vally and Misso, 2012). The mechanisms remain unclear.

Monosodium Glutamate (MSG)

Adverse reactions to MSG were originally reported as the "Chinese restaurant syndrome" because of its use in Chinese cooking. Complaints of headache, nausea, flushing, abdominal pain, and asthma occurred after ingestion. MSG is widely distributed in the food supply (e.g., bouillon, meat tenderizers, canned food, frozen food, condiments) and occurs naturally in tomatoes, Parmesan cheese, mushrooms, and other foods. Results from double-blind, placebo-controlled food challenges (DBPCFC) found symptoms from MSG to not be persistent, clear, consistent, or serious (Geha et al, 2000; Williams and Woessner, 2009). However, more recent data in animals and humans have indicated that MSG consumption may be a contributing factor to increased risk of overweight independent of physical activity and total energy intake (He et al, 2011). Considering the ongoing debate about this common flavoring agent as an obesogenic agent, dietetic practitioners should be aware of MSG sensitivity (Savcheniuk et al, 2014).

Food Toxins and Microbial Contaminants

Food toxicity or food poisoning results from microbial contamination of food and causes a myriad of symptoms, including nausea, vomiting, diarrhea, abdominal pain, headache, and fever, many of which can be confused with an allergic reaction. It is estimated that in the United States 76 million people per year are affected by foodborne illness, and that 30% of all infections over the last 60 years worldwide were foodborne (Bold and Rastami, 2011). Fortunately, most episodes are self-limiting and should be distinguished from food allergy through a thorough history. If the cause of the symptoms cannot be determined to be a food toxin or microbial contamination, then a single food elimination diet followed by a challenge of that food may be necessary (see Table 26-3).

Psychogenic and Behavioral Factors

Evidence for the role of food allergy or intolerance in various disorders such as anxiety, depression, migraine headache, attention deficit hyperactivity disorder, and mood disorders is emerging. Increased intestinal permeability, dysbiosis, neurotransmitter production, and gut immune

---

TABLE 26-3 Protocol for Elimination and Challenge: Plan, Avoid, Challenge, and Evaluate (PACE)

Begin with the 4R Program:

1. **Remove** offending agents (already known adverse reacting foods, toxins, infections, chronic stress)
2. **Replace** digestive factors (enzymes or HCl)
3. **Repopulate** with pre- and probiotics
4. **Repair** with healing nutrients and botanicals

PLAN: Develop a tailored eating plan and timeline for the elimination diet based on review of the patient's medical and clinical history, findings from a thorough nutrition assessment, including a diet and symptom record kept for minimum of 1 week, and other patient information such as patient readiness.

AVOID: The elimination diet will be of either low, moderate, or high intensity and of duration of 2 to 4 weeks or longer if necessary, until the client's symptoms clear.

Level 1: a low-intensity diet will exclude those foods suspected by the individual to be problematic; it usually means avoidance of a few selected foods

Level 2: a medium-intensity elimination diet excludes many foods or food groups, and substitute food selections are based on the patient's preferences. The gluten- and casein-restricted diet or the Eight Food Elimination Diet are examples

Level 3: the highest intensity oligoantigenic diet, which excludes most foods and is based on just a few (maybe as few as 10), usually hypoallergenic foods. Medical foods or elemental formulas containing hypoallergenic, easily digested nutrients can be used to supplement the diet.

CHALLENGE: Reintroduction of the suspected and avoided foods is done one at a time. The diet should remain the same except for the introduction of the suspected food. A common method for reintroducing is to have the client eat a small amount of the food in the purest form at least 2 to 3 times per day on Day 1 with no test food on Day 2 and Day 3. The client will observe and document any food reactions during this 3 day period. The process is repeated with the next test food on Day 4, with no test food on Day 5 and Day 6. Again the patient observes and records for the period Day 4 to 6. Given that adverse food reactions (AFRs) can be delayed as much as 72 hours (3 days) it is important to not test another food sooner than 3 days. Foods being tested are rated as either safe, unsafe, or unsure. If the patient is unsure, he or she will wait a week and test the food again in the same manner as before.

EVALUATE: After the challenge phase is completed the clinician and client evaluate the responses and devise a long-term eating plan that prevents AFRs and maintains optimal health.

From: Swift KM, Lisker I: *Current concepts in nutrition: the science and art of the elimination diet*, Alternative and Complementary Therapies 18:5,251, 2012.

system response are currently being investigated as contributing factors (see Chapters 41 and 44). Even if a food-symptom relationship is not proven, but food avoidance is perceived as helpful because of personal experience, appropriate therapy can optimize nutritional status.

ASSESSMENT

Diagnosis of ARFs requires identification of the suspected food or food ingredient, proof that the food causes an adverse response, and verification of an immune or non–immune-mediated response. The first diagnostic tool is the detailed clinical history, and this is followed with appropriate testing (Skypala et al, 2015). Biochemical tests can rule out nonallergenic causes of symptoms. Tests that may be useful include a comprehensive metabolic profile with complete blood count and differential; stool tests for inflammatory markers, ova, parasites, or occult blood; breath hydrogen tests; intestinal permeability tests; genetic tests for celiac disease and gluten sensitivity profiles, or for histamine intolerance; tests for small intestinal bacterial

overgrowth (SIBO); and a sweat chloride test for cystic fibrosis (see Chapters 7, 27, 28, and 34). Tests for food reactivity remain controversial and should be used only in conjunction with a comprehensive history, physical, and nutrition assessment (see Table 26-4 for a complete description of tests).

Immunologic Testing
Skin-Prick Test

In skin-prick tests drops of standard food extracts are placed on the skin of the arm or back. The skin is then scratched or pricked with a lancet with each drop of extract. The areas of application are then observed for the development of the classic "wheal and flare" reaction. In theory, if the underlying mast cells have attached allergen-specific IgE, inflammatory mediators are released. The wheal and flare reaction results from the action of the mediators, especially histamine, on the surrounding tissue. These tests are the most economic immunologic tests of an Ig-E mediated reaction, providing results within 15 to 30 minutes. Comparison with the positive control (histamine) and the negative control (usually the solute used

TABLE 26-4 Tests Used in the Assessment of Adverse Reactions to Foods

Skin Tests

Skin testing (scratch, prick, or puncture)	A drop of antigen is placed on the skin, and the skin is then scratched or punctured to allow penetration of the antigen to reach sensitized IgE; assesses IgE-mediated sensitization.	Screening test; cannot be relied on as sole diagnostic tool; a history of food-symptom relationship also important; more reliable for negative findings than positive; negative results confirm absence of IgE-mediated allergic response.
Atopy patch test	Small pads soaked with allergen are applied to unbroken skin for 48 hours and read at 72 hours.	Variable sensitivity and specificity; used to assess delayed or non-IgE reactions; no clinical value in diagnosis of food allergy.
Intradermal testing also called skin endpoint titration (SET)	In a clinical setting, a small amount of allergen is injected directly into subcutaneous layer of skin; presence of wheal indicates reaction.	More sensitive than skin-prick testing, but with a greater risk of adverse reactions; not recommended as sole diagnostic tool.

Blood Tests

CAP-FEIA	Serum is mixed with food on a paper disk and then washed with radioactively labeled IgE. Compared with RAST, this test binds more allergen; best for assessing IgE-mediated reactions.	Reliable for six foods: milk, eggs, wheat, cow's milk, peanuts, and soy.
RAST	Being replaced with CAP-FEIA test; assesses IgE-mediated sensitization.	More sensitive assays now replace RAST; cannot be relied on as sole diagnostic tool. High sIgE values may not guarantee allergic reactivity, whereas low sIgE values may not eliminate the potential for allergic reactivity.
ELISA	Much like RAST, except that no radioactive material is used; being replaced with CAP-FEIA; assesses IgE-mediated sensitization.	Same as for RAST. Cannot be relied on as sole diagnostic tool. High sIgE values may not guarantee allergic reactivity, whereas low sIgE values may not eliminate the potential for allergic reactivity.
Specific IgG, IgM, IgA antibody assays	Techniques of precipitation hemagglutination complement fixation; requires special expertise.	Specific IgG not validated for diagnostic use; but still used clinically; reliability still questionable. Positive results may simply indicate previous exposure to the food.
Serum IgG4	Blood testing for food-specific IgG4.	Not validated for diagnostic use; tends to indicate previous exposure to the food, but still used clinically; reliability still questionable.
Basophil activation test (BAT)	Using whole blood, measures basophil response to allergenic cross-linking IgE on basophil granulocytes.	Not yet standardized for clinical diagnostic use. (Hoffman et al, 2015)
Cytotoxic testing *Antigen leukocyte cellular antibody test (ALCAT) *Mediator release test—(MRT)	Allergen is mixed with whole blood serum leukocyte suspension. Lysed leukocytes, primarily neutrophils, are measured against the food allergen. Changes in cell size and volume indicate response.	Nonstandardized; may result in false-positive or false-negative results; not widely validated for diagnostic use. (Pietschmann, 2015)

Continued

TABLE 26-4	Tests Used in the Assessment of Adverse Reactions to Foods—cont'd	
Other Tests		
Applied kinesiology, also called muscle strength testing	Subject's arm is extended and vial with test food is placed in the hand; test is considered a positive reaction if the muscle strength weakens and arm moves more easily after the food has been placed in hand.	Nonstandardized; may result in false-positive or false-negative results; not validated for diagnostic use.
Sublingual testing	Drops of allergen extract are placed under the tongue and symptoms are recorded.	May result in false-positive results; not validated for diagnostic use.
Provocation testing and neutralization	Subcutaneous injection of allergen extract elicits symptoms; this is then followed by injection of a weaker or stronger preparation to neutralize symptom.	May result in false-positive results; not validated for diagnostic use.

BAT, basophil activation test; *CAP-FEIA,* CAP-fluorescein-enzyme immunoassay; *CRD,* component-resolved diagnostics; *DBPCFC,* double-blind, placebo-controlled food challenge; *ELISA,* enzyme-linked immunosorbent assay; *Ig,* immunoglobulin; *MD,* medical doctor; *RAST,* radioallergosorbent test; *sIg,* secretory immunoglobulin.

for the antigen or saline) provide parameters necessary for accurate readings (see Figure 26-3). All skin-prick tests are compared with the control wheal. Test wheals that are 3 mm greater than the negative control usually indicate a positive result. Negative skin-prick tests have good negative predictive accuracy and suggest the absence of an IgE-mediated reaction. Positive skin-prick test results, however, indicate only IgE sensitization and the possibility of a food allergy reaction. In the patient with a suspected food allergy, the skin-prick test is useful in supporting the diagnosis. For children younger than 2 years of age, the skin test is reserved to confirm immunologic mechanisms after symptoms have been confirmed by a positive test result from a food challenge or when the history of the reaction is impressive.

In children with atopic dermatitis, skin-prick testing for food allergens is contraindicated because of the high reactivity of the skin, leading to false-positive reactions and the real danger of sensitization to the allergen through inflamed skin (see Figure 26-4).

All foods that test positive must correlate with a strong exposure history or be proven to cause allergic reactions through food challenges before they can be considered allergenic. The most common food allergens (milk, egg, peanut, soy, wheat, shellfish, fish, and tree nuts) account for most of the positive food skin-prick tests (Nowak-Wegrzyn and Sampson, 2006).

Serum Antibody Tests

Food allergen–specific serum IgE testing is used to identify foods that may be causing the allergic response. The **radioallergosorbent test (RAST),** an IgE test, and the enzyme-linked immunosorbent assay (ELISA), most often an Ig-G test, are

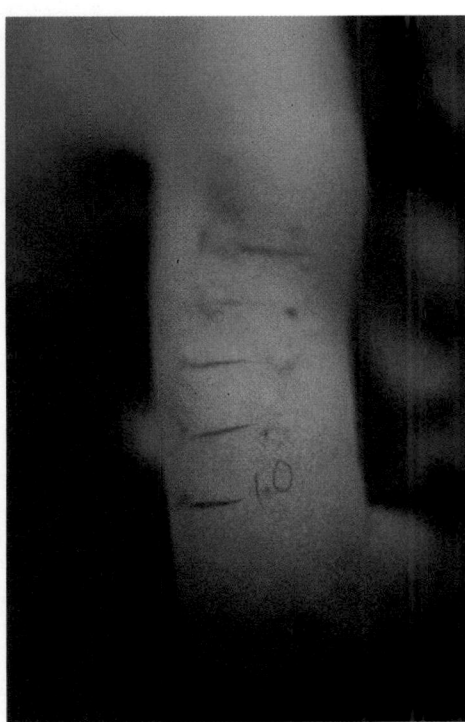

FIGURE 26-3 A skin-prick test showing the wheal and flare of the reaction to the allergen as compared with the reaction to the histamine control at the bottom.

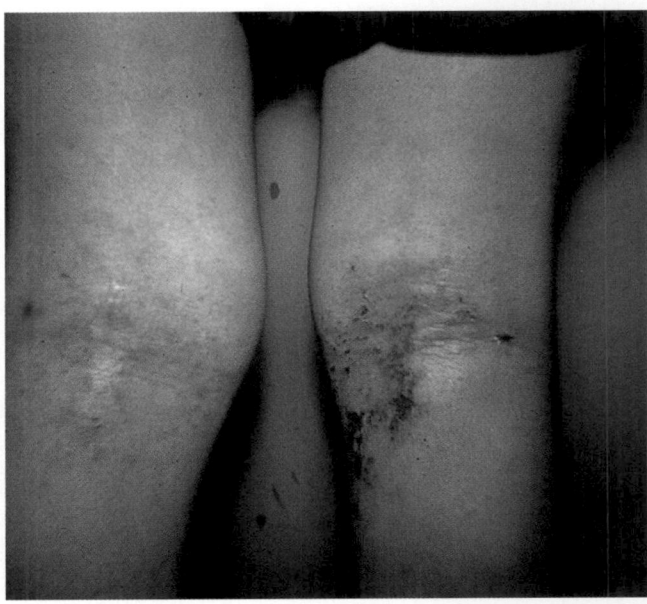

FIGURE 26-4 Atopic eczema: An IgE–mediated skin reaction to a food allergen, commonly seen on the back of knees and the inside of elbows.

TABLE 26-5 Food Challenges

DBPCFC	Allergen is disguised and given orally and patient monitored for reaction; patient and physician blinded; also tested with placebo.	"Gold standard" for food allergy testing.
Single-blind food challenge	Suspect food is disguised from patient and orally given by physician in a clinical setting.	Less time-consuming than DBPCFC; may be used in instances in which patient experiences çsymptoms secondary to fear or aversion to suspect food.
Open oral food challenge	Suspect food is orally given to patient in undisguised, natural form in gradual doses under medical supervision.	Less time-consuming than DBPCFC; should not be used in instances in which patient experiences symptoms secondary to fear or aversion to suspect food.
Food elimination diets	Suspect foods are eliminated from the diet for a set period to identify foods responsible for ARF. During gradual reintroduction symptoms are carefully observed.	May help identify foods responsible for ARF; strict, long-term elimination diets may require monitoring to ensure nutritional adequacy.

being replaced by the CAP–fluorescein-enzyme immunoassay (FEIA). The CAP-FEIA is a blood test that provides a quantitative assessment of allergen-specific IgE antibodies; higher levels of antibodies are often, but not always, predictors of clinical symptoms. The CAP-FEIA test has been approved for only six foods: egg, milk, peanut, fish, wheat, and soy (soy is still not as predictive) (Sampson, 2004). It is fairly effective as shown by testing known food-allergic children whose food allergies had been previously proven with DBPCFCs. Test results should be followed with either food elimination and challenge, or DBPCFCs to complete the diagnostic process. It should be noted that CAP-FEIA or skin testing results for IgE sensitization may remain positive even after the child has resolved the allergy, and the food can be eaten without symptoms (Sampson, 2004).

Other Tests

A number of laboratory tests are now available that attempt to identify an individual's specific ARFs. Some of these tests measure IgA, IgG, and IgG4 levels, whereas others measure the amount of cytokines released by lymphocytes and granulocytes upon degranulation in response to food antigen exposure. Continued scientific investigation into the evidence-based and validity of various types of food reactivity testing is warranted (Vojdani, 2015a; see Table 26-5).

MEDICAL NUTRITION THERAPY

A thorough history including prenatal history, method of birth (e.g., vaginal or C-section), early feeding practices (breastfed versus formula), current medical conditions, medications, dietary supplements, exercise patterns, lifestyle factors, and a nutrition-focused physical examination are important in assessing the patient with ARFs (see Chapters 4 and 7, and Appendices 21 and 22).

Anthropometric measurements for infants and children should be plotted on a growth chart and evaluated in relationship to earlier measurements (see Appendices 4 through 10). Because decreased weight-for-height measurements may be related to malabsorption or food allergy or intolerance, patterns of growth and their relationship to the onset of symptoms should be explored. Clinical signs of malnutrition should be assessed as part of the nutrition-focused physical exam.

Food and Symptom Record

A 7- to 14-day food and symptom record is extremely useful for uncovering ARFs (see Figure 26-4). This record also may be used to identify possible nutrient insufficiencies and deficiencies. The food and symptom record should include the time the food is eaten, the quantity and type of food, all food ingredients if possible, the time symptoms appear relative to the time of food ingestion, and any supplements or medications taken before or after the onset of symptoms. Other influences such as stress, physical exercise, and elimination and sleep patterns can provide valuable information in piecing together the factors that affect ARFs. The more thorough the information obtained about the adverse reaction, the more useful the record. For example, a reaction that appears to be caused by a food actually may be caused by a pet or a chemical or other environmental factor. The 1- to 2-week food and symptom record also can serve as a baseline for future interventions (see Chapter 4).

Food-Elimination Diets

The elimination diet followed by food challenges is the most useful tool in the diagnosis and management of ARFs when used in conjunction with a thorough history and nutrition assessment. With the elimination diet, suspect foods are eliminated from the diet for a specified period, usually 4 to 12 weeks, followed by a reintroduction and food-challenge phase. All forms (i.e., cooked, raw, frozen) of a suspected food are removed from the diet, and a food and symptom record (see Figure 26-5) is kept during the elimination phase. This record is used to ensure that all forms of suspected foods have been eliminated from the diet and to evaluate the nutritional adequacy of the diet.

Elimination diets should be personalized and may entail excluding only one or two suspect foods at a time to see if there is improvement in symptoms, or it may mean eliminating several foods if multiple foods are suspected. This would entail a more limited diet as shown in Table 26-6, but again the diet should be individualized as much as possible.

Elemental formulas, medical foods, or hypoallergenic formulas also may be used for additional nutrition support in adults on an elimination diet. An elemental formula provides high-quality calories in an easily digestible, hypoallergenic form and helps to optimize nutritional status. Because of low palatability and high cost, this should be reserved for the most restrictive cases. Hydrolyzed infant formulas or extensively hydrolyzed infant formulas may be required for the allergic infant who is not being completely breastfed and who needs to avoid several foods.

After the designated elimination phase, foods are systematically reintroduced into the diet one at a time to determine any adverse reactions while the person is carefully monitored. If

	DAY 1 DATE		DAY 2 DATE		DAY 3 DATE	
	FOOD	SYMPTOMS	FOOD	SYMPTOMS	FOOD	SYMPTOMS
Time: BREAKFAST						
Medications						
SUPPLEMENTS						
Snack Time:						
Time: LUNCH						
Medications						
SUPPLEMENTS						
Snack Time:						
Time: DINNER						
Medications						
SUPPLEMENTS						
Snack Time:						
MEDICATIONS						

Name _____

FIGURE 26-5 Food and symptom diary.

symptoms persist with careful avoidance of suspect foods, other causes for the symptoms should be considered. If a positive result has been obtained on a skin prick test or allergen-specific IgE blood test and symptoms improve unequivocally with the elimination of the food, that food should be excluded from the diet until an oral food challenge is appropriate. The oral food challenge will further prove or disprove a food-symptom relationship. If symptoms improve with the elimination of multiple foods, then multiple food challenges will be necessary.

An oral food challenge is conducted in a supervised medical setting once symptoms have resolved, and when the person is not taking any medications such as antihistamines. Foods are challenged one at a time on different days while the person is carefully observed in a medical setting for the recurrence of symptoms (see Box 26-7 for Food Challenge Protocols).

The form of the food ingested is an important consideration in the nutritional assessment of ARFs. For example, recent studies suggest that 70% to 80% of young children allergic to milk or eggs can tolerate baked (heat-denatured) forms of these proteins, but not the unbaked form. It is suggested that these children make IgE antibodies primarily to conformational epitopes (antigenic determinants on the surface of the food proteins that are recognized by the immune system) and represent those children who will naturally outgrow their food allergies (Sicherer and Sampson, 2010).

Allergic individuals and their families need guidelines and suggestions for avoiding allergenic foods and ingredients,

substituting permissible foods for restricted foods in meal planning and preparation, and selecting nutritionally adequate replacement foods.. Care providers and school personnel working with the food-allergic child must be trained to read labels carefully before purchasing or serving food. The Food Allergy and Anaphylaxis Network (www.foodallergy.org), a nonprofit organization created to support the child with food allergies, has worked with board-certified allergists and dietitians to develop an excellent education program for day-care or school programs.

To help identify and avoid offending foods, allergy-specific lists that describe foods to avoid, state key words for ingredient identification, and present acceptable substitutes, are useful and necessary in counseling (see Boxes 26-8 through 26-12).

Food ingredients to be avoided may be hidden in the diet in unfamiliar forms. When a food-sensitive person ingests a hidden allergen, the most common reason is that the "safe" food was contaminated. This may happen as a result of using common serving utensils such as at an ice cream stand, salad bar, or deli (where the meat slicer may be used to slice meat and cheese). Manufacturing plants or restaurants may use the same equipment to produce two different products (e.g., peanut butter and almond butter); despite cleaning, traces of an allergen may remain on the equipment between uses. Alternatively, a restaurant may use the same oil to fry potatoes and fish (see Box 26-13).

In addition, the food may have been genetically modified, changing its allergenicity. Here again, label reading is essential (see *Focus On:* GMO or Genetically Engineered (GE) Foods).

Text Continued on page 502

TABLE 26-6 Guidelines for Elimination Diets

These guidelines emphasize foods that are naturally nutrient rich.
Guidelines should be personalized according to the patient's history and should eliminate other foods that are already known allergens or foods that aggravate symptoms.
Refer to label reading guidelines to avoid ingredients to be eliminated (see Boxes 26-8 through 26-12).
Amounts should be individually tailored to energy needs.

	Foods Allowed	Foods to Avoid
Elimination Diet: Milk-, Egg-, and Wheat-Free		
Animal proteins	Fish, shellfish, turkey, chicken, beef, pork	Eggs, egg substitutes containing egg whites and all products containing eggs (see Box 26-8)
Plant proteins	Beans, lentils, split peas, organic soybeans, and soy products	Nonorganic soy (GMO containing)
Dairy alternatives	Nondairy beverage alternatives including organic soy beverages	Milk (cow, goat, sheep) and all products containing mammalian milk ingredients (see Box 26-9)
Grains	Amaranth, barley, buckwheat, corn, millet, oats, quinoa, rice, rye	Wheat, all forms of wheat (see Box 26-10)
Vegetables	All vegetables and starchy vegetables	Vegetable dishes containing milk, egg, or wheat (e.g., tempura, breaded)
Fruits	All fruits and 100% fruit juices	Fruit pies, pastries, cookies, etc., that contain milk, egg, or wheat
Fats and oils	Coconut oil, organic canola oil, grapeseed oil, olive oil, flaxseed oil, sesame oil, safflower oil, milk-free organic (nonhydrogenated) margarines	Butter, margarine, hydrogenated oils, shortening
Peanuts, nuts, and seeds	Peanuts, nuts, and natural nut butters, seeds and natural seed butters	Any peanut, nut, or seed product containing milk, egg, wheat (e.g., chocolate candy with nuts)
Beverages	Tea, herbal tea, coffee, decaffeinated tea, and coffee	Beverages containing milk (cow, goat, sheep)
Sweeteners	Cane or beet sugar, honey, maple syrup, black-strap molasses	Artificial sweeteners
Other	Salt, pepper, herbs, and spices	Egg-, milk-, or wheat-containing condiments; all artificial ingredients, salad dressing, mayonnaise, spreads containing milk, egg, wheat
Elimination Diet: Most Common 8 Allergens Elimination Diet: Milk, Egg, Wheat, Fish, Shellfish, Soy, Peanut and Tree Nut Free		
Animal proteins	Turkey, chicken, lean cuts of beef, lamb, pork	Fish, shellfish, eggs, processed meats such as sausages, deli meats, etc.
Plant protein sources	Beans, lentils, split peas	Soybeans and soy products, peanuts, tree nuts
Dairy alternatives	Nondairy, soy-free, nut-free beverage alternatives (i.e., rice, hemp beverages)	Milk and all dairy alternative beverages containing soy, oats or tree nuts
Grains	Amaranth, barley, buckwheat, millet, oats, quinoa, rice, teff, tapioca, wild rice	Wheat, spelt, kamut, triticale, and all wheat-containing products
Vegetables	Most vegetables and starchy vegetables	Vegetable dishes containing ingredients to avoid such as breaded, creamed, etc.
Fruits	Most fruits and 100% fruit juices	Fruit pies, pastries, cookies, etc., containing ingredients to avoid
Fats and oils	Olive oil, coconut oil, flaxseed oil, grapeseed oil, organic canola oil, safflower oil, sunflower oil	Butter, margarine, soy oil, peanut oil
Peanuts, nuts, and seeds	Seeds and seed butters, such as pumpkin seed, sunflower seed, flax seed, chia seed	Peanuts and peanut-containing products, tree nuts and tree nut–containing products
Beverages	Herbal tea, 100% unsweetened fruit or vegetable juice, water, nondairy soy-free beverages	Coffee, caffeinated tea, other caffeinated beverages, alcoholic beverages, soft drinks
Sweeteners	Honey, maple syrup, blackstrap molasses, agave, raw cane sugar	Artificial sweeteners
Other	Salt, pepper, all spices	Any food product containing any ingredient to avoid and all artificial ingredients
Elimination Diet: Few Foods/Limited Ingredients–		
Intended to be used in the short-term only		
Animal proteins	Chicken, turkey, lamb	
Grains	Brown rice	
Vegetables	Sautéed or steamed leafy green vegetables including spinach, green beans, summer squash	
Fruits	Banana	
Oils	Extra virgin olive oil	
Beverages	Water, herbal tea	
Sweeteners	Maple syrup	

BOX 26-7 Food Challenge Protocols

The three methods used to determine which foods when reintroduced into the diet are responsible for adverse reactions include the following:

1. Double-blind, placebo-controlled food challenge (DBPCFC): a food challenge in which neither the patient nor physician knows the identity of the test food component, which is usually disguised as a powder in a food known to be tolerated (such as applesauce) or in a gelatin capsule. The patient's reaction is compared to his or her reaction to the placebo, and the patient is monitored in a clinical setting.

2. Single-blind food challenge: a food challenge in which the patient is blinded to the challenge food's identity, but the clinician is not. The food or a powder of it is disguised in another food and reactions are observed and recorded.

3. Open food challenge: a food challenge in which the patient is knowingly given a serving of the suspect food and observed for several hours for a reaction

BOX 26-8 Eliminating Eggs: Label Reading and Strategies

People with an allergy to chicken eggs may also be allergic to other types of eggs, such as goose, duck, turkey, or quail.

Ingredients and Single-Ingredient Foods to Avoid*

- Albumin
- α-livetin
- Apovitellin
- Avidin
- Catalase
- Conalbumin
- Dried eggs
- Duck eggs
- Egg solids
- Egg substitutes
- Egg white
- Egg yolk
- Ficin inhibitor
- Flavoprotein

- Frozen eggs
- Globulin
- Goose eggs
- G2 and G3 globulins
- Imitation egg product
- Lecithin
- Lipovitellin
- Livetin
- Low-density lipoproteins
- Lysozyme
- Ovalbumin
- Ovoflavoprotein
- Ovoglobulin
- Ovoglycoprotein

- Ovoinhibitor
- Ovomacroglobulin
- Ovomucin
- Ovomucoid
- Ovomuxoid
- Ovotransferrin
- Ovovitellin
- Phosvitin
- Powdered egg
- Quail eggs
- Simplesse
- Turkey eggs
- Vitellin

Other Foods That Often Contain Eggs as an Ingredient

- Béarnaise sauce
- Eggnog
- Hollandaise sauce

- Mayonnaise
- Meringue
- Surimi

Note: Egg whites and shells may be used as a clarifying agent in soup stocks, consommés, wine, alcoholic beverages, and coffee drinks.

Egg Substitutes (Equivalent to 1 Egg) in Recipes

- 1 packet plain gelatin + 1 c boiling water; use 3 Tbsp of this mixture
- ½ tsp baking powder + 1 Tbsp liquid + 1 Tbsp vinegar
- 2 Tbsp fruit puree (use in baking for binding, but not leavening); apples, plums, peaches, or prunes
- To achieve an emulsifying effect in baking: 2 Tbsp whole wheat flour + ½ tsp oil + ½ tsp baking powder + 2 Tbsp milk, water, or fruit juice
- 1 Tbsp ground flax + 3 Tbsp water; blend and allow to sit for 10-15 minutes
- 1 tsp yeast dissolved in ¼ c warm water
- 1½ Tbsp water + 1½ Tbsp oil + 1 tsp baking powder
- ¼ c soft tofu, beaten
- 1 Tbsp chia seed + ⅓ cup water; blend and allow to sit for 10-15 minutes
- 1 Tbsp agar agar + 1 Tbsp water

- ½ mashed banana
- ¼ cup unsweetened applesauce

Always use caution and work closely with physicians or pharmacists to ensure that there are no egg ingredients in any of the following:
- Cosmetics
- Medications
- Vaccines
  - Albumin or chicken serum can be used in any vaccine
  - Influenza vaccines
  - MMR: measles, mumps, rubella vaccine
  - Rabies vaccine may contain small amounts
  - Typhus vaccine may contain small amounts
  - Yellow fever vaccine

*Eliminate these foods, as well as any foods containing any of these ingredients.
FARE Food Allergy Research & Education: *Tips for Avoiding Your Allergen* (website): www.foodallergy.org. Accessed Feb, 2014; Joneja JV: *The health professional's guide to food allergies and intolerances*, Chicago, 2013, Academy of Nutrition and Dietetics.

BOX 26-9 Eliminating Cow's Milk: Label Reading and Strategies

Ingredients and Single Ingredient Foods to Avoid*

- Acidophilus milk
- Ammonium caseinate
- Artifical butter flavor
- Butter
- Butter fat
- Butter oil
- Calcium caseinate
- Caramel
- Casein
- Casein hydrolysate
- Cheese and cheese flavor (e.g., cheddar, Colby, cream, Edam, Gouda, Monterey Jack, mozzarella, Muenster, Neufchâtel,, parmesan, provolone, ricotta, Romano, Swiss, etc)
- Chocolate milk
- Chocolate Sauce
- Condensed milk
- Cottage cheese
- Cultured buttermilk
- Curds
- Custard
- Delactosed whey
- Evaporated milk
- Ghee
- Goat milk‡
- Greek yogurt
- Half and half cream
- Hydrolysates (casein, milk protein, protein, whey, whey protein)
- Lactalbumin
- Lactalbumin phosphate
- Lactoferrin
- Lactoglobulin
- Lactose
- Lactulose
- Magnesium caseinate
- Milk (whole, 2%, 1½%, 1%, ½%, skim, evaporated, condensed)
- Milk powder (whole, low-fat, nonfat)
- Milk protein
- Potassium caseinate
- Rennet casein
- Semisweet chocolate
- Sheep milk‡
- Sodium caseinate
- Sour cream
- Sour cream solids
- Sour milk solids
- Sweet whey
- Sweetened condensed milk
- Whey
- Whey protein concentrate
- Whipping cream
- Yogurt, regular

Other Foods That Often Contain Cow's Milk as an Ingredient

- Alfredo sauce
- Bavarian cream flavoring
- Brown sugar flavoring
- Butter flavoring
- Caramel candy
- Caramel flavoring
- Carob candies
- Chocolate products
- Creamed candies such as caramel, fudge, taffy
- Cream dressings
- Cream sauces
- Cream soups
- Coconut cream flavoring
- Eggnog
- Gelato
- Hot cocoa mix
- Ice cream (low-fat, regular, fat free)
- Malted milk
- Milk chocolate
- Natural flavoring
- Nougat
- Protein powders
- Pudding
- Recaldent, used in tooth-whitening chewing gums
- Sherbet, most types
- Simplesse
- Sour cream dressings
- Yogurt, frozen

Milk Substitutes (Equivalent to 1 Cup Cow's Milk) in Recipes

- 1 c almond, coconut, hazelnut, or other nut milk beverage
- 1 c light colored fruit juice (e.g., apple, orange, white grape)
- 1 c flax, hemp, sunflower, or other seed beverages
- 1 c milk-free infant formula, mixed
- 1 c herbal tea
- 1 c oat, rice, quinoa, or other grain beverage
- 1 c soy milk
- 1 c water

Buttermilk Substitute (Equivalent to 1 Cup Cow's Milk) in Recipes

- Add 1 tablespoon vinegar to 1 cup alternative milk (soy, rice, oat, almond, coconut, etc.), stir and let sit for 5 minutes before using in recipe.

Intact Milk Protein–Free Formulas

Partially hydrolyzed (cow's milk protein) infant formula§
- Enfamil Gentlease (Mead Johnson) whey/casein protein blend
- Gerber Good Start Gentle (Nestle) 100% whey protein
- Gerber Good Start Protect (Nestle) 100% whey protein
- Some store brands (Perrigo Nutritionals) - check with manufacturer

Extensively hydrolyzed infant formula
- Nutramigen with Enflora LGG (Mead Johnson)
- Pregestimil (Mead Johnson)
- Similac Expert Care Alimentum (Abbott)

Free Amino-Acid Base Infant Formulas¶
- EleCare for Infants (Abbott)
- PurAmino (Mead Johnson)
- Neocate products (Nutrica)

Soy Infant Formula**
- Enfamil ProSobee (Mead Johnson)
- Gerber Good Start Soy (Nestle)
- Similac Soy Isomil (Abbott)
- Some store brands (Perrigo Nutritionals) - check with manufacturer

Organic Soy Infant Formula**
- Earth's Best Organic Soy (Hain Celestial Group)
- Soy Organic Infant Formula (Vermont Organics)

Individuals who must avoid all cow's milk sources frequently need a calcium supplement.

*Please also note that non-food products such as cosmetics, supplements, and medications can contain dairy ingredients and may cause an adverse reaction.

‡Goat and sheep milk proteins are similar to cow milk protein, and those with a cow milk allergy could experience similar symptoms with ingestion of these alternatives. Although occasionally this does not occur, they are not advised as cow milk substitutes when determining allergens (Ah-Leung et al, 2006). Goat's milk is not recommended as a cow's milk substitute, especially in infants, because it has a high renal solute load and is very low in folic acid compared with cow's milk.

§Partially hydrolyzed: Nonhypoallergenic; contains partially digested proteins that have a molecular weight greater than extensively hydrolyzed formula protein chains. May cause a reaction in one third to one half of individuals with a cow's milk protein allergy.

BOX 26-9 Eliminating Cow's Milk: Label Reading and Strategies—cont'd

¶Free amino acid-based infant formula: hypoallergenic; peptide-free formula that contains essential and nonessential amino acids. Usually tolerated by those allergic to extensively hydrolyzed formulas.

**Soy formula: Should not be used in infants younger than 6 months old with food allergies.

Ah-Leung S et al: Allergy to goat and sheep milk without allergy to cow's milk, *Allergy* 61(11):1358-1365, 2006; Bahna SL: Hypoallergenic formulas: optimal choices for treatment versus prevention, *Ann Allergy Asthma Immunol* 101:5, 2008; Greer FR et al: Effects of early nutritional interventions on the development of atopic disease in infants and children: the role dietary restriction, breastfeeding, timing of introduction of complementary foods, and hydrolyzed formulas, *Pediatrics* 121:183, 2008; Joneja JV: *The health professional's guide to food allergies and intolerances*, Chicago, 2013, Academy of Nutrition and Dietetics; Kneepkens CM, Meijer Y: Clinical practice: diagnosis and treatment of cow's milk allergy, *Eur J Pediatr* 168:891, 2009.

BOX 26-10 Eliminating Wheat: Label Reading and Strategies

Ingredients and Single Ingredient Foods to Avoid

- All-purpose flour
- Bran
- Bread crumbs
- Bread flour
- Bulgar
- Cake flour
- Cereal extract
- Couscous
- Cracked wheat
- Durum flour
- Durum wheat
- Einkorn
- Emmer
- Enriched flour
- Farina
- Farro
- Flour
- Gluten
- Graham flour
- High-gluten flour
- High-protein flour
- Kamut
- Kamut flour
- Laubina
- Leche alim
- Minchin
- Pastry flour
- Puffed wheat
- Red wheat flakes
- Rolled wheat
- Seitan
- Semolina flour
- Soft wheat flour
- Spelt
- Sprouted wheat
- Triticale
- Vegetable gums
- Vital gluten
- Wheat
- Wheat bran
- Wheat flakes
- Wheat flour
- Wheat germ
- Wheat gluten
- Wheat malt
- Wheat meal
- Wheat starch
- Wheat tempeh
- White flour
- Whole wheat berries
- Whole wheat flour
- Winter wheat flour

Other Foods That Often Contain Wheat as an Ingredient

- Ale and beer
- Baking mixes and baked products
- Bread
- Breaded or floured goods including batter-fried foods
- Cake
- Cookies
- Crackers
- Cracker crumbs
- Cream sauces
- Cream soups
- Gelatinized starch
- Hydrolyzed vegetable protein
- Licorice
- Malted cereals
- Meats containing fillers including processed meats
- Meatloaf
- Modified food starch
- Modified starch
- Multi-grain breads
- Multi-grain chips
- Multi-grain crackers
- Multi-grain flours
- Pastries
- Roux
- Shredded wheat
- Starch
- Soy sauce
- Tempura
- Tortillas
- Vegetable gums (guar, xanthan)
- Vegetable starch
- Wheat bread
- Wheat bread crumbs
- Wheat pasta
- Wheat protein beverage
- Wheat protein powder
- White bread

Wheat Substitutes (Equivalent to 1 Cup Wheat Flour) in Recipes

With any substitution, always read labels carefully and look for gluten-free labels to ensure that no cross-contamination with other grains and wheat has occurred, which can be common.

- All Purpose Blends:
  - ¾ cup brown rice flour, 3 tablespoons potato starch, 1 tablespoon tapioca flour, and ½ teaspoon xanthan gum

BOX 26-10 Eliminating Wheat: Label Reading and Strategies—cont'd

- ½ cup rice flour, ¼ cup tapioca flour, ¼ cup corn or potato starch
- High-Fiber Blend: Best for breads, pancakes, and snack bars
  - 1 cup brown rice or sorghum flour, ½ cup light teff flour, ½ cup millet flour, ⅔ cup tapioca flour, ⅓ cup corn or potato starch
- High-Protein Blend: Best for wraps and pie crusts
  - 1¼ cup bean flour, 1 cup arrowroot, corn, or potato starch, 1 cup tapioca flour, 1 cup brown rice flour
- Self-Rising Blend: Best for muffins, scones, cakes, or cupcakes
  - 1¼ cups white sorghum flour, 1¼ cups white rice flour, ½ cup tapioca flour, 2 teaspoons xanthan or guar gum, 4 teaspoons baking powder, ½ teaspoon salt
- Xanthan and guar gum can serve chemically as gluten substitutes in non-gluten flour blends, which can improve the texture of baked goods. Although usually made from corn, they can be made using wheat, dairy, or soy, so it is important to check the source.
  - Add ½ teaspoon per cup of flour for bars, cakes, cookies, muffins, and quick breads.
  - Add 1 teaspoon per cup of flour for baked items that call for yeast, such as pizza dough and yeasted bread.
- Pre-mixed wheat and gluten-free flour products are available commercially as well.

Wheat-Free Alternative Options

- Amaranth
- Barley (if no gluten intolerance)
- Buckwheat, raw groats
- Buckwheat, toasted kasha
- Chickpea/garbanzo
- Corn
- Job's tears (Hato Mugi)
- Lentil
- Millet
- Montina (Indian Rice Grass)
- Oats (if certified gluten free)
- Potato
- Quinoa
- Rice
- Rye (if no gluten intolerance)
- Sorghum
- Tapioca
- Teff
- Wild rice

*Please also note that non-food products such as cosmetics, supplements, and medications can contain wheat ingredients and may cause an adverse reaction.

Fenster, C, Case S. Gluten Free Whole Grains: *Whole Grains Council* (website): http://wholegrainscouncil.org/whole-grains-101/gluten-free-whole-grains, Accessed January 2014; Joneja JV: The Health Professional's Guide to Food Allergies and Intolerances, Chicago, 2013, Academy of Nutrition and Dietetics; Lair C: *Feeding the whole family,* ed 3, Seattle, 2008, Sasquatch Books; Living Without Magazine: *Gluten Free Flour Substitutions* (website): www.livingwithout.com/resources/substitutions.html. Accessed Feb., 2014.

BOX 26-11 Eliminating Peanuts: Label Reading and Strategies

Ingredients and Single Ingredient Foods to Avoid*

- Arachis oil
- Artificial tree nuts
- Beer nuts
- Cold pressed peanut oil
- Defattened peanuts
- Expelled or expressed peanut oil
- Extruded peanut oil
- Granulated peanuts
- Ground nuts
- Hydrolyzed plant protein
- Hydrolyzed vegetable protein
- Mandelonas

- Mixed nuts
- Monkey nuts
- Nut meat
- Nut pieces
- Nuts with artificial flavoring
- Peanuts, all varieties
- Peanut butter
- Peanut flakes
- Peanut flour
- Peanut meal
- Peanut oil
- Peanut protein hydrolysate

Other Foods That Often Contain Peanuts as an Ingredient†

- All candy (check ingredients)
- Baked goods
- Breading
- Cashew butter
- Cheesecake crusts
- Chili
- Chili sauce
- Chocolate candy
- Dog food and treats
- Egg rolls
- Enchilada sauce
- Foods fried in peanut sauce
- Frozen desserts
- Gravy
- Hamster feed

- High protein food
- Ice cream
- Livestock feed
- Marzipan
- Mole sauce
- Nougat
- Pancakes
- Pie crusts
- Rice Krispie treats
- Salad dressing
- Sauces
- Soups
- Stews
- Sunflower seeds

*Eliminate all sources of peanuts from diet including cross-contaminated food or utensils. There is a high risk of cross-contamination when eating out, especially at Asian, Chinese, Mexican, Thai, Mediterranean, and Indian restaurants.

*Please also note that non-food products such as cosmetics, supplements, and medications can contain peanut ingredients and may cause an adverse reaction.

†*Peanut powder, peanut butter, and peanuts may be used as an ingredient or garnish for many dishes*.

Joneja JV: *The health professional's guide to food allergies and intolerances,* Chicago, 2013, Academy of Nutrition and Dietetics; Peanut Allergy: *Food Allergy and Research Education* (website): https://www.foodallergy.org/allergens/peanut-allergy, Accessed February 2014.

BOX 26-12 Eliminating Soy: Label Reading and Strategies

Ingredients and Single Ingredient Foods to Avoid*

- Asian cuisine
- Chee-fan
- Deep-fried mature soy seed
- Edamame
- Fermented soybean paste
- Fermented soybeans
- Hamanatto
- Immature green soy seed
- Ketjap
- Miso
- Natto
- Shoyu sauce
- Soy albumin
- Soy cheese
- Soy fiber
- Soy ice cream
- Soy lecithin‡
- Soy milk
- Soy nuts
- Soy protein (concentrate, hydrolyzed, isolate)
- Soy protein powders
- Soy protein shakes
- Soy sauce
- Soybean curd
- Soybean flour
- Soybean granules
- Soybean grits
- Soybean oil‡
- Soybean sprouts
- Sufu
- Tamari
- Tao-cho
- Tao-si
- Taotjo
- Tempeh
- Textured soy protein
- Textured vegetable protein (TVP)
- Tofu
- Whey-soy drink

Other Foods That Often Contain Soy as an Ingredient

- Baked goods
- Canned broths and soups
- Canned tuna and meat
- Cereals
- Cold-pressed oils
- Cookies
- Crackers
- High-protein energy bars
- Hydrolyzed plant protein
- Hydrolyzed vegetable protein
- Low-fat peanut butter
- Natural flavoring
- Processed meats
- Sauces
- Vegetable broth
- Vegetable gum
- Vegetable starch

Soy Substitutes (Cup for Cup) in Recipes

- Light-colored fruit juice (e.g., apple, orange, white grape)
- Flax, hemp, sunflower, or other seed beverages
- Oat, rice, quinoa, or other grain beverages
- Almond, cashew, coconut, hazelnut, or other nut beverages

Soy Protein–Free Infant formulas
Standard Infant Formula

- Enfamil Premium Infant (Mead Johnson)
- Similac Advance (Abbott)
- Some store brands (Perrigo Nutritionals) - check with manufacturer

Partially Hydrolyzed (Cow's Milk Protein) Infant Formula§

- Gerber Good Start Gentle (Nestle) 100% whey protein
- Gerber Good Start Protect (Nestle) 100% whey protein
- Similac Total Comfort (Abbott) 100% whey protein
- Some store brands (Perrigo Nutritionals) - check with manufacturer

Extensively Hydrolyzed Infant Formula¶

- Nutramigen with Enflora LGG (Mead Johnson)
- Pregestimil (Mead Johnson)
- Similac Expert Care Alimentum (Abbott)

Free Amino-Acid Base Infant Formulas¶

- EleCare for Infants (Abbott)
- PurAmino (Mead Johnson)
- Neocate products (Nutricia)

There is a high risk of cross-contamination when eating out, especially dining at Asian restaurants.

*Please also note that non-food products such as cosmetics, supplements, and medications can contain soy ingredients and may cause an adverse reaction.

‡Several studies indicate that individuals who are soy allergic frequently tolerate soy lecithin and soy oil.

§Partially hydrolyzed: Nonhypoallergenic; contains partially digested cow's milk proteins that have a molecular weight greater than extensively hydrolyzed formula protein chains.

¶Free amino-acid based infant formula: Hypoallergenic; peptide-free formula that contains essential and nonessential amino acids. Usually tolerated by those allergic to extensively hydrolyzed formulas.

Joneja JV: *The health professional's guide to food allergies and intolerances,* Chicago, 2013, Academy of Nutrition and Dietetics; Kneepens CM, Meijer Y: Clinical practice. Diagnosis and treatment of cow's milk allergy, *Eur J Pediatr* 168: 891, 2009; *Soy Allergy, Food Allergy and Research Education* (website): https://www.foodallergy.org/allergens/soy-allergy. Accessed February 2014.

BOX 26-13   Reasons for Accidental Exposure to Allergens

- Common serving utensils used to serve different foods when some may contain the allergen
- Grocery store bulk bins contaminated with an allergen from another product bin
- Manufacture of two different food products using the same equipment without proper cleaning in between
- Misleading or inaccurate labels (e.g., nondairy creamers that contain sodium caseinate)
- Ingredients added for a specific purpose are listed on the label only in general terms of their purpose rather than as a specific ingredient (e.g., egg white that is simply listed as an "emulsifier")

- Addition of an allergenic product to a second product that bears a label listing only the ingredients of the second product (e.g., mayonnaise, without noting eggs)
- Switching of ingredients by food manufacturers (e.g., a shortage of one vegetable oil prompting substitution with another)
- A child being offered a food by an individual who is uneducated about the allergy

---

FOCUS ON: GMO or Genetically Engineered (GE) Foods

Christine McCullum-Gómez, PhD, RD, Food and Nutrition Consultant, Houston, TX

Genetic engineering is one type of genetic modification (GM) that involves the intentional introduction of a targeted change in a plant, an animal, or microbial gene sequence to achieve a specific result. Genetically engineered (GE) foods, also known as GMO (genetically modified organism) foods have been in the U.S. food supply for approximately 20 years. Plants that are GE can be made to tolerate herbicides and be insect resistant. GE or GMO crops are widely grown and consumed in a number of countries, including the United States (Agapito-Tenfen et al, 2013; Bohn et al, 2014). Some of the most commonly grown GE or GMO crops include soybeans, corn, cotton, canola, and sugar beets. Despite the widespread use of GE crops by various countries, the need for biosafety remains a concern as lack of stringent standards, international harmonization, and transparency, as well as remaining claims of confidentiality on biosafety-relevant data places additional burdens on regulatory agencies (Agapito-Tenfen, 2013; Nielson, 2013).

To date, risk assessment of GE plants has focused on potential allergenicity and toxicity. As part of a safety evaluation for GE crops, an allergenicity assessment is performed to: (1) ensure that an existing allergen or cross-reactive protein(s) is not transferred to a new GE crop; (2) demonstrate that a novel protein is unlikely to become a food allergen *de novo*; and (3) evaluate existing endogenous allergen levels for potential increases in the new GE crop (i.e., soybeans) versus its non-GE control (Ladics, 2008; Ladics et al, 2014).

With this information in mind, the lack of evidence that GE food is unsafe cannot be interpreted as proof that it is safe. As observed by Ladics and colleagues (2014), "the assessment of the allergy risk of a novel protein mainly focuses on its potential to elicit an allergic reaction in consumers already sensitized to a cross-reacting protein. However, reliable tests are missing to definitely predict on their own the potential of novel proteins to sensitize *de novo* atopic individuals. Such potential depends not only on the intrinsic characteristics of the protein (e.g., structure, function, and physiochemical properties) but also on complex interactions between the genetic background and physiology of the consumers and environmental conditions . . ." [Hence], "[a] sensitive and specific validated animal model would help in the identification of proteins that might present an increased risk of sensitizing consumers if introduced in a GE crop. While some progress has been reported with a limited number of proteins, none of the animal models that have been reviewed . . . have been thoroughly tested and validated with a wide range of allergens and non-allergens" (Ladics et al, 2014).

There are also long-term concerns beyond those related to the presence of unknown allergens. A long-term study of weaning and old mice consuming either GE corn or non-GE corn found that the mice consuming the GE corn had increased presence of several cytokines that are specifically involved in inflammatory and allergic responses, and alterations in the number of B-cells and T-cells, indicating an abnormal response to GE corn (Finamore et al, 2008). Histopathologic changes have been found in some organs (liver, kidney, and small intestine) of male rats fed GE corn (El-Shamei et al, 2012).

A published review concluded that there is an incomplete picture regarding the toxicity and safety of GE products consumed by humans and animals (Zdziarski et al, 2014). In addition, evaluations of possible unintended effects derived from GE crops by the use of proteomics and transcriptomics have been reported (Barros et al, 2010; Coll et al, 2011). Based on these results, further investigation of the long-term effects of GE food consumption is needed. Profiling techniques, such as proteomics, which studies the structure and functions of proteins, allow the simultaneous measurement and comparison of thousands of plant components without prior knowledge of their identity (Heinemann et al, 2011). "As global databases on outputs from 'omics' analysis become available, these [databases] could provide a highly desirable benchmark for safety assessments [of GE foods]" (Agapito-Tienfen et al, 2013).

To date, less attention has been given to the residues of herbicides and their degradation products that can accumulate in GE herbicide-tolerant plants, such as GE herbicide-tolerant soybeans (Bøhn et al, 2014). Bøhn and colleagues (2014) reported that GE herbicide-tolerant soybeans contained high residues of glyphosate and its main breakdown product aminomethylphosphonic acid (AMPA), whereas conventional and organic soybeans contained none of these same agrichemicals. In addition, the organic soybeans contained significantly more total protein and zinc and less saturated fat and total omega-6 fatty acids than conventional and GE soybeans (Bøhn et al, 2014). The increased use of glyphosate on GE herbicide-tolerant soybeans in the United States (Benbrook, 2012) may explain the observed plant tissue accumulation of glyphosate in GE herbicide-tolerant soybeans (Brohn et al, 2014). Some scientists have reported that although glyphosate and its degradation product AMPA showed little to no observable toxic effects in isolation, a glyphosate-based formulation containing adjuvants (Roundup)—which is used with GE herbicide-tolerant crops—induced cytotoxicity, oxidative effects, and apoptosis on human cells (Chaufan et al, 2014).

More recently, the International Agency for Research on Cancer (IARC) has classified glyphosate, the herbicide that is most widely used on GE crops, as a "probable human carcinogen (2A)" (Landrigan and Benbrook, 2015). The mechanistic evidence (genotoxicity and oxidative stress) provided independent support of the IARC's 2A classification (probably carcinogenic to humans) based on evidence of carcinogenicity in humans and experimental animals (Mesnage et al., 2015a). Results from DNA damage assays were considered to present solid mechanistic evidence supporting the 2A classification of glyphosate (Guyton et al., 2015; Mesnage et al., 2015a). In addition, chronic exposure to very low levels of glyphosate-based herbicides, which people are exposed to through drinking water, has been linked to liver and kidney damage in an established laboratory animal toxicity model system (Mesnage et al., 2015b). Finally, research indicates that xenobiotics (i.e., chemical compounds not produced by the body such as drugs and pesticides), are able to exert their toxic effects across several generations through epigenetic alterations (Nilsson and Skinner, 2015). Because the effects of reproductive toxicity of pesticides are not limited to a single generation, they have to be studied across several generations in multigenerational or transgenerational studies. However, no multigenerational or epigenetic study has been performed with the glyphosate-herbicide Roundup or its adjuvants (Mesnage et al., 2015a). As a result, some scientists are encouraging regulators "to ask for complete reassessment of glyphosate formulations, rather than glyphosate alone, in particular with a full life-span test on mammals at environmentally-relevant doses, with detailed blood and urine analyses, taking into account principles from endocrinology and epigenetics" (Mesagne et al., 2015a).

The first systems biology analysis conducted to assess the safety of GE organisms observed differences in two biomarkers, formaldehyde (a known toxin) and glutathione, which predict metabolic disruptions in

Continued

⊚ FOCUS ON: GMO or Genetically Engineered (GE) Foods—cont'd

Christine McCullum-Gómez, PhD, RD, Food and Nutrition Consultant, Houston, TX

one-carbon (C1) metabolism (Ayyadurai and Deonikar, 2015). In non-GE plants, formaldehyde remains at near zero levels, being naturally cleared through a process of formaldehyde detoxification. Concomitantly, glutathione, a known anti-oxidizing agent, in non-GE plants, is naturally replenished and remains at non-zero steady state levels to support systemic detoxification of formaldehyde (Kothandaram et al., 2015). However, in the case of GE herbicide-tolerant soybeans, accumulation of formaldehyde and a concomitant depletion of glutathione, suggests how a 'small' and single genetic modification can create 'large' and systemic perturbations to molecular systems equilibria. These authors note that given the potentially far-reaching effects of a single genetic modification, as this research suggests for the GE soybean, "at least a process, similar to the FDA clinical trials for single compound drugs, seems rational for GE safety assessment and approval" (Ayyadurai and Deonikar, 2015).

Adopting a computational systems biology approach (which aims to understand the complexity of the whole organism, as a system, rather than studying its parts in a reductionist manner) using biomarkers - such as

formaldehyde and glutathione – that predict metabolic disruptions, may be useful for modernizing the safety assessment of GE foods, while fostering a much-needed transparent, collaborative and scientific discourse. The substantial and material difference in the levels of biomarkers of formaldehyde and glutathione, across non-GE and GE soybeans, predicted from this systems biology analysis, however, demands *in vitro* and *in vivo* testing, including the development of objective standards on how such testing is to be performed (Ayyadurai and Deonikar, 2015). In the interim, some scientists have recommended labeling GE foods and long-term post-marketing surveillance to track any possible adverse effects (e.g., the emergence of novel food allergies and assessing the potential effects of synthetic herbicides applied to GE crops) (Landrigan and Benbrook, 2015).

Because using GE foods may complicate the elimination diet, or as already mentioned, aggravate an immune-mediated response, it may be prudent to advise those with documented food allergies to eat organic soybeans, corn, canola, cottonseed, beet sugar, and other foods for which there are GE versions in the food supply.

Another situation that may lead to the unknowing ingestion of an allergenic food occurs when one product is used to make a second product, and only the ingredients of the second product are listed on the food label. An example is the listing of mayonnaise as an ingredient in a salad dressing without specifically listing egg as an ingredient of the mayonnaise. Labels must be read often to ensure that ingredients have not changed in the processing of the food (see Box 26-14).

When foods are removed from the diet, alternative nutrient sources must be provided. Table 26-7 defines the levels of nutritional risk based on the types of food removed from the

---

BOX 26-14 Allergen Labeling of Foods

Since January 1, 2006, the updated US **Food Allergen Labeling and Consumer Protection Act (FALCPA)** requires the top allergens to be clearly listed by manufacturers as an ingredient or following the ingredient list on food labels. This includes ingredients in any amount and also mandates specific ingredients to be listed such as the type of nut or seafood.

Requirements of the Law

- **Top eight allergens must be clearly listed** by manufacturers as an ingredient or following the ingredient list on food labels of any food product containing allergens
- Applies to all packaged foods sold in the United States
- Does not apply to USDA-regulated products, including meat, poultry products, and some egg products
- Does not list sources of possible contamination
- Does not apply to prescription medication or alcoholic beverages
- Does not apply to foods packaged or wrapped after being ordered by the consumer

Top Allergens

- Any ingredient containing or derived from the top eight allergens—milk, eggs, fish, shellfish, tree nuts, peanuts, wheat, or soybeans
- For tree nuts, fish, and shellfish the specific type must be listed (e.g., walnut, pecan, shrimp, tuna)

Reading the Food Label

- Ingredients may be included within the food's ingredient list directly or in parentheses following the name, if an ingredient does not clearly identify the allergen
- Following the list of ingredients all food allergens may be listed in a "Contains" statement
- Manufacturers may voluntarily list potential unintended allergens that may be present due to cross contamination in a clear way that does not interfere with the required food ingredient list

Note: In 2013 the FDA issued a final rule defining "gluten-free" for food labeling. This final rule requires that items labeled "gluten-free" meet a defined standard for gluten content (see Chapter 28).

Note: It is being proposed that sesame be added to the list of top allergens required on labels.

TABLE 26-7 Risk of Nutritional Deficiency

Level of Risk	Food Characteristics/Examples
Low risk	Any food that can easily be eliminated with minimum or no nutritional risk to the patient; substitutes are easily incorporated into the diet; protein, fat, calorie and nutrient consumption is optimal. *Example:* Avoidance of a specific fruit or vegetable or tree nuts
Moderate risk	Any food that may be encountered frequently throughout the food supply, yet the elimination of which does not significantly limit food choices or vital nutrient sources; adequacy of protein, fat, calorie, and nutrient consumption need monitoring. *Example:* Avoidance of soy, fish, or eggs
High risk	Any food or usually group of foods that permeates the food supply, providing a significant source of specific nutrients that are not readily available through other foods that are a part of the normal diet; the elimination of which results in a significant lifestyle and dietary change because of the difficulty of avoiding that food and products containing that food; adequate protein, fat, calorie, and nutrient consumption unlikely; nutrient supplementation often necessary. *Example:* Avoidance of wheat, soy, egg, cow's milk, fish, or multiple foods

Rotation Diets—Where's the Science? Are They Clinically Useful?

Janice M Joneja, PhD, CDR

The Theory

Rotation diets, or the protocol of eating foods in the same food families no more often than every 4 to 10 days, were developed as a theoretical way to give the body a rest from each food family in an effort to prevent the development of food intolerances. In addition, it was claimed that rotation diets assisted in the identification of adverse food reactions and that by rotating the intake of the foods there could be freedom from allergic symptoms for a longer period.

The Data

- Evidence-based research studies to support these claims are lacking.
- Recent research has demonstrated that members of the same botanical food family are not necessarily related allergenically.
- There is often a closer antigenic association between unrelated foods than those within the same family. Examples that demonstrate this concept include oral allergy syndrome and latex-fruit syndrome.
- Diets based on the avoidance of entire food families is illogical.

Important Considerations

When an adverse reaction to foods is due to a non-immune-mediated reaction such as an enzyme deficiency (e.g., lactase), a diet that restricts the intake of all lactose-containing foods will ensure the tolerance level is not exceeded and thus symptoms are avoided. A "rotation type diet" that restricts the number and quantity of foods known to contain the culprit component is necessary to ensure that the dose of the reactive component is reduced.

Non-IgE-mediated food allergy may be dose related. A rotation diet that restricts the number and quantity of foods known to contain the culprit component is often beneficial (Joneja, 2013). However, when the food allergy is IgE mediated, there is no logic for a rotation diet. The problem food must be continually avoided until a food challenge shows that there is no longer a reaction. Then the food can be consumed on any schedule.

When the rotation diet is used, there is no scientific basis for a 4-, 5-, 7-, or even 30-day rotation of foods. All protocols have been used clinically. Such diets must be formulated on an individual basis to ensure that the dose of the reactive component is reduced to a minimum, whereas nutrients equivalent to those eliminated are supplied by alternative foods.

diet. For example, when eggs are omitted, other foods must provide choline, vitamin D, protein, and energy.

Healing the Gut and Restoring Immune Balance

Because approximately 70% of immune cells are located in the gut-associated lymphatic tissue (GALT), efforts to restore gut health should improve immune function and modulate allergic responses. Besides eliminating problematic foods, other measures include optimizing stomach acidity and enzyme function; identifying and treating pathogens such as bacteria, yeasts, and parasites; restoring intestinal barrier function; repleting nutritional status and restoring gut microbiota balance (see Chapters 27 and 28).

EMERGING THERAPIES

Food immunotherapy vaccines is a possible future treatment meant to complement food allergen avoidance, but these vaccines are still experimental. Recent research has produced encouraging evidence that specific oral tolerance induction (SOTI) can be achieved by introducing the culprit food via the digestive tract in minute then increasing quantities for

an extended period (Clark et al, 2009; Joneja, 2013; Zapatero et al, 2008).

Several potential treatments are under active investigation in animal and human studies. Some of these approaches include oral, sublingual, and epicutaneous immunotherapy, immunotherapy combined with anti-IgE, and Chinese herbal medicine. Also being studied are modified protein immunotherapy, adjuvants, DNA vaccines, and helminth administration (Keet and Wood, 2014).

Nutritional Adequacy

The nutritional adequacy of the diet should be monitored on a regular basis by conducting an ongoing evaluation of the patient's nutritional status and food and symptom records. The omission of foods from the diet on the basis of proper or improper diagnosis can and has impaired the nutritional status of the allergic individual. Malnutrition and poor growth may occur in children who consume improperly planned and nutritionally inadequate elimination diets (Keller et al, 2012). Vitamin and mineral supplementation may be needed to prevent this, especially when multiple foods are omitted. Nutrition assessment must be conducted on a regular basis.

Because food is an important part of a person's culture, the social aspects of eating can make adherence to an elimination diet challenging. Continued support from health care providers is needed to minimize the effect of dietary changes on family and social life. The strategies listed in Box 26-15 can help families and individuals cope with ARFs.

It was previously thought that most children would achieve tolerance and "outgrow" their food allergies by 3 years of age; however, it is becoming apparent that this is not the case. Only 11% of egg-allergic and 19% of milk-allergic children resolve their allergies by 4 years of age. However, almost 80% resolve these allergies by age 16 (Savage et al, 2007; Skripak et al, 2007). Peanut allergy tends to be lifelong for most children, with only about 20% of children able to resolve it (Sicherer and Sampson, 2010; NIH, NIAID, 2010). New therapies for peanut allergy are on the horizon, so this may change (DuToit et al, 2015, Fleischer et al, 2015).

PREVENTING FOOD ALLERGY

Intensive research is being focused on the pathogenesis and prevention of allergic disease, including the role of genetics, epigenetics, and environmental factors such as early dietary exposures and feeding practices. Allergy prevention guidelines have gradually shifted away from allergen avoidance to examination of the role of specific dietary and lifestyle factors in the development and prevention of allergic disease (Jennings and Prescott, 2010; Joneja, 2012). For prevention, focus is turning to lifestyle factors that promote oral tolerance (see Box 26-16).

Allergen Exposure

The traditional approach for dietary allergy prevention has been avoidance of food allergens in the maternal diet and early postnatal period. However, there is a lack of evidence that maternal dietary restrictions during pregnancy help prevent atopic disease in infants. Food restriction to avoid antigen exposure while breastfeeding does not appear to prevent atopic disease, with the possible exception of atopic eczema (Greer et al, 2008). However, recent research indicates that exposure to food antigens in the "safe" environment of pregnancy and in breast milk is more likely to lead to tolerance rather than sensitization to those foods in the infant. Current trials on infant feeding are

---

BOX 26-15 **Strategies for Coping with Food Allergy**

Food Substitutions

Try to substitute item-for-item at meals. For example, if the family is eating pasta for dinner, substitution of a gluten-free pasta may be better accepted for the gluten-sensitive or wheat-allergic person than a dissimilar item.

Dining Out and Eating Away from Home

Eating meals away from home can be risky for individuals with food allergies. Whether at a fancy restaurant or a fast-food establishment, inadvertent exposure to an allergen can occur, even among the most knowledgeable individuals. Here are some precautions to take:

- Bring "safe" foods along to make eating out easier. For breakfast, bring along an appropriate milk if others will be having cereal with milk.
- Alert the wait staff to the potential severity of the food allergy or allergies.
- Question the wait staff carefully about ingredients.
- Always carry medications.

Special Occasions

Call the host family in advance to determine what foods will be served. Offer to provide an acceptable dish that all can enjoy.

Grocery Shopping

Be informed about what foods are acceptable, and read labels carefully. Product ingredients change over time; continue to read the labels on foods, even if they were previously determined to be "safe" foods. Allow for the fact that shopping will take extra time.

Label Reading

Labeling legislation makes it easier for individuals with food allergies to identify certain potential allergens from the ingredient list on food labels. For example, when food manufacturers use protein hydrolysates or hydrolyzed vegetable protein, they must now specify the source of protein used (e.g., hydrolyzed soy or hydrolyzed corn). Although reactions to food colors or food dyes are rare, individuals who suspect an intolerance will find them listed separately on the food label, rather than categorized simply as "food color."

BOX 26-16 **Recommendations to Promote Oral Tolerance and Prevent Allergy**

- Support breastfeeding and delay introduction of solid foods until 4 to 6 months.
- Strengthen immunity by increasing connection to natural environments, pets, and farms.
- Strengthen immunity by regular physical exercise.
- Use antibiotics only when necessary; the majority of microbes are useful and help build healthy immune function.
- Consume fermented food or other probiotic preparations to strengthen immune system.
- Do not smoke: parental and family smoking around infants and children can increase risk of asthma.

From Haahtela T et al: The biodiversity hypothesis and allergic disease: world allergy organization position statement, *World Allergy Organ J* 6:3, 2013.

---

attempting to elucidate the concept of oral tolerance and define the effect that the timing of introduction of solids and allergenic foods has on development of allergic disease.

Breastfeeding

Breast milk contains a host of immunologically active compounds, such as transforming growth factor–beta, lactoferrin, lysozymes, long-chain fatty acids, antioxidants, and secretory IgA (sIgA), all of which have an effect on immune development, including oral tolerance, and help to reinforce the gut-epithelial barrier (Brandtzaeg, 2009; Jennings and Prescott, 2010). Breastfeeding without any maternal dietary restrictions is strongly encouraged, although the exact role of breastfeeding in allergy prevention is unclear. There is evidence that exclusive breastfeeding for at least 3 months protects against wheezing in early life (Greer et al, 2008). For infants at high risk of developing atopic disease (infants with a first-degree relative with allergy) exclusive breastfeeding for at least 4 months is recommended (Host et al, 2008). Continuation of breastfeeding through the time when solid foods are introduced is believed to further help prevent the development of food allergy.

Sensitivity to breast milk is rare but has been reported. Allergens such as cow's milk, eggs, and peanuts in the mother's diet can pass into the breast milk and cause an allergic reaction in the "exclusively" breast-fed infant, but cannot cause sensitization.

The infant may have been sensitized from an external source such as from small amounts of infant formula given to him or her.

Infant formulas should be given in the first 4 to 6 months only if exclusive breastfeeding is not possible for some reason. Soy-based infant formulas offer no advantage for the purpose of allergy prevention, and some infants may react adversely to these formulas. Extensively hydrolyzed formulas may be more protective than partially hydrolyzed formulas in prevention of atopic disease (Greer et al, 2008). Amino acid–based formulas may be used in managing an established food allergy but have not been adequately studied for atopy prevention (see Boxes 26-9 and 26-12).

Solid Food Introduction

Exclusive breastfeeding for 6 months is highly recommended. Complementary solid foods other than breast milk should not be introduced until 4 to 6 months of age. There is no convincing evidence that delaying introduction beyond this time prevents the development of atopic disease, and this even pertains to the introduction of foods that are considered to be highly allergenic, such as peanuts, eggs, and fish (Jennings and Prescott, 2010). In fact a recent study found that the early introduction of peanut in a powdered form as early as 4 to 11 months with a 3 times per week consumption, resulted in a significant and substantial decrease in the development of peanut allergy in high-risk infants. Peanut avoidance was associated with a greater frequency of peanut allergy by age 5 years than was peanut consumption (Du Toit et al, 2015).

Early Diet and Immunomodulatory Factors

A number of regulatory factors in early life may influence the development of asthma and other allergic diseases. The immunoregulatory network in newborns is orchestrated by a variety of events and agents, many incompletely understood. Nutrients such as vitamin A, vitamin D, omega-3 fatty acids, folate, and other micronutrients have been cited as potential influences (Brandtzaeg, 2010). The intestinal microbiota are important. For example parental sucking of their infant's pacifier has been shown to reduce the risk of allergy development, possibly by stimulation of the immune system by microbes transferred to the infant in the parent's saliva (Hesselmar et al, 2013).

Antioxidants

Diets high in antioxidants such as carotenoids and other phytonutrients, vitamin C, vitamin E, zinc, and selenium may prevent the development of food allergies. There have been positive associations found between maternal antioxidant status in pregnancy and cord blood immune responses (West et al, 2010). Higher maternal intake of green and yellow vegetables, citrus fruit, and beta-carotene during pregnancy was significantly associated with a reduced risk of eczema, but not wheezing, in the infants. Maternal vitamin E consumption was inversely related to the risk of infantile wheeze, but not eczema (Miyake et al, 2010). Thus, optimizing food sources of antioxidants from fruit and vegetable intake during pregnancy may be an effective effort for allergy risk reduction.

Vitamin D

It has been proposed that the increase in the development of food allergy in children may be due to an increased prevalence of vitamin D deficiency. Suboptimal vitamin D status in a developmentally critical period increases susceptibility to colonization of the gut with abnormal intestinal microbial flora and GI infections, contributing to an abnormally porous gut and inappropriate exposure of the immune system to dietary allergens. Vitamin D helps promote immunoregulation through T-cell differentiation. Cord blood levels of 25-OH vitamin D at birth have been found to be inversely correlated with reduced eczema at 6 months (Jones et al, 2015). It is suggested that early correction of vitamin D deficiency may promote mucosal immunity, healthy microbial ecology, and allergen tolerance and may prevent food allergy development (Jones et al, 2012; Rueter et al, 2014).

Folate

Folate deficiency has been associated with several disorders characterized by enhanced activation of the cellular, Th1-type immune response. An intriguing development has been the recognition of epigenetic effects of dietary folate in the development of asthma (Jennings and Prescott, 2010). DNA methylation and inflammation appear to be the two main pathways through which folate may influence the development of childhood asthma and allergy (Brown et al, 2014). The small increase in risk that has been reported was associated only with maternal folate exposure during late pregnancy (Brown et al, 2014). Impaired folate metabolism may be related to the development of atopy, but the relationship and the significance warrants further investigation (Binkley et al, 2011; Brown et al, 2014).

Polyunsaturated Fatty Acids (PUFAs)

The role of polyunsaturated fatty acids (omega-3 and omega-6 PUFAs) in allergy development has been the subject of investigation, because PUFAs have effects on inflammation and immune function. Some studies have suggested that maternal consumption of fish oil (a source of omega-3 fatty acids) in pregnancy protects against the development of asthma, eczema, and allergic sensitization, whereas others have not shown these results (Palmer et al, 2013). A recent systematic review indicates that it is not clear that supplementation with omega-3 and omega-6 oils will play a role in the prevention of sensitization or allergic disease (Miles and Calder, 2014). Further studies are needed to elucidate the role of fatty acids in allergy prevention and their role in the inflammatory cascade (see Chapter 3).

Pre- and Probiotics

Probiotics are defined as live microorganisms that, when administered in adequate amounts, impart health benefits to the host. Prebiotics are non-digestible, fermentable oligosaccharides that stimulate the growth and activity of the gastrointestinal microbiota, thus conferring benefits upon host health (International Scientific Association for Probiotics and Prebiotics [IASPP], 2015). The combination of pro- and prebiotics is sometimes referred to as a synbiotics (see Chapter 28).

The role of probiotics in allergy prevention continues to be investigated. The administration of probiotics during pregnancy and early infancy has been shown to reduce the risk of eczema (Fiocchi et al, 2015; West, 2014). The results of some studies support the use of probiotics during the first 6 months of life in infants at high risk of developing allergy, but more data are needed to recommend routine use of probiotics (Doege et al, 2011). The effect of the individual strain, timing of administration (pre-or postnatal), dosage, and environmental factors that affect colonization have yet to be determined (Esposito et al, 2014; Haahtela et al, 2015). It has been reported that low gut microbiota richness and an elevated ratio of the Enterobacteriaceae/Bacteroidaceae microbiota in early infancy are associated with subsequent food sensitization, and this may contribute to development of allergic disease, including food allergy (Azad et al, 2015). Interestingly, the Bacteroidaceae are one of the families of bacteria known to stimulate the production and degradation of mucin, so important in the maintenance of an intact microbiota-mucin barrier. Early deficiency of Bacteroidetes has been reported in infants with atopic dermatitis and food allergy (Ling et al, 2014).

CLINICAL CASE STUDY

Clara is 17 months old. At birth she was breastfed, but 2 weeks later cow's milk-based formula was introduced, which she did not appear to tolerate. Each feeding resulted in diarrhea and vomiting. The pediatrician recommended that her mother switch to a partially hydrolyzed casein infant formula, which Clara seemed to tolerate. However, at age 4 months she developed eczema that was treated with steroid creams. Cow's milk was introduced when Clara was 12 months of age. Her skin symptoms increased remarkably. When eggs and later peanut butter were introduced, she experienced immediate wheezing; watery, swelling eyes; hives; increased itchiness; and diarrhea. Clara's parents are unaware of how to look for egg or peanut sources; thus Clara has experienced several trips to the emergency room. The last reaction was much more intense. Her family physician suspects egg and peanut allergies and has sent her to see a board-certified allergist and a registered dietitian.

Nutrition Diagnostic Statements

- Food and nutrition-related knowledge deficit by parents related to food sources of eggs and peanuts as evidenced by serious reactions in their daughter following ingestion.
- Intake of unsafe foods related to ingestion of egg- and peanut-containing foods as evidenced by serious reactions to foods.

Nutrition Care Questions

- How many food allergen suspects are there, and what are they? Why?
- What measures will her parents need to take if Clara is to lose sensitivity to any of the food allergens?
- What other circumstances may arise that may warrant special instructions to caregivers?
- How often should Clara be checked for sensitivity changes?
- What would you tell Clara's parents to look for on food labels?
- What nutrient substitutions must be considered?

USEFUL WEBSITES AND APPS

Allergy Asthma Information Association—Canada
http://www.aaia.ca

American Academy of Allergy, Asthma, and Immunology
www.aaaai.org

The American Latex Allergy Association
http://www.latexallergyresources.org/

Anaphylaxis Canada
www.anaphylaxis.org

The Asthma and Allergy Foundation of America
www.aafa.org

Food Allergy and Anaphylaxis Network
www.foodallergy.org

Food Allergy Research Education (FARE)
http://blog.foodallergy.org/

Food Allergy Apps
http://www.healthline.com/health-slideshow/top-allergy-iphone-android-apps

Food and Symptom Record APPS
https://itunes.apple.com/us/app/mysymptoms-food-symptom-tracker/id405231632?mt=8.

International Network for Diet and Nutrition in Allergy (INDANA)
http://www.indana-allergynetwork.org/.

REFERENCES

Agapito-Tenfen SZ, Guerra MP, Wikmark OG, et al: Comparative proteomic analysis of genetically modified maize grown under different agroecosystems conditions in Brazil, *Proteome Sci* 11:46, 2013. http://www.proteomesci.com/content/11/1/46.

Ayyadurai VAS, Deonikar P: Do GMOs accumulate formaldehyde and disrupt molecular systems equilibria? Systems biology may provide answers, *Agric Sci* 6: 630, 2015. http://dx.doi.org/10.4236/as.2015.67062.

Azad MB, Konya T, Guttman DS, et al: Infantile gut microbiota and food sensitization: associations in the first year of life, *Clin Exp Allergy* 45:632, 2015.

Barros E, Lezar S, Anttonen MJ, et al: Comparison of two GM maize varieties with a near-isogenic non-GM variety using transcriptomics, proteomics and metabolomics, *Plant Biotechnol J* 8:436, 2010.

Bauer RN, Manohar M, Singh AM, et al: The future of biologics: applications for food allergy, *J Allergy Clin Immunol* 135:312, 2015.

Benbrook CM: Impacts of genetically engineered crops on pesticide use in the U.S.—the first sixteen years, *Environmental Science Europe* 24:24, 2012. doi:10.1186/2190-4715-24-24.

Binkley KE, et al: Antenatal risk factors for peanut allergy in children, *Allergy, Asthma & Clin Immunol*, 7:17, 2011.

Bøhn T, Cuhra M, Traavik T, et al: Compositional differences in soybeans on the market: glyphosate accumulates in Roundup Ready GM soybeans, *Food Chem* 153:207, 2014.

Brown SB, et al: Maternal folate exposure in pregnancy and childhood allergy: a systematic review, *Nutr Rev*, 72:55, 2014.

Chaufan G, Coalova I, Ríos de Molina Mdel C: Glyphosate commercial formulation causes cytotoxicity, oxidative effects, and apoptosis on human cells: differences with its active ingredients, *Int J Toxicol* 33:29, 2014.

Coll A, Nadal A, Rossignol M, et al: Proteomic analysis of MON810 and comparable non-GM maize varieties grown in agricultural fields, *Transgenic Res* 4:939, 2011.

Doege K, Grajecki D, Zyriax BC, et al: Impact of maternal supplementation with probiotics during pregnancy on atopic eczema in childhood – a meta-analysis, *Br J Nutr* 107:1, 2012.

DuToit G: Food-dependent exercise-induced anaphylaxis in childhood, *Pediatr Allergy Immunol* 18:455, 2007.

DuToit G, Roberts G, Sayre PH, et al: Randomized trial of peanut consumption in infants at risk for peanut allergy, *NEJM* 372:803, 2015.

El-Shamei ZS, Gab-Alla AA, Shatta AA, et al: Histopathological changes in some organs of male rats fed on genetically modified corn (Ajeeb YG), *J Am Sci* 8:684, 2012.

Eroglu Y, Lu H, Terry A, et al: Pediatric eosinophilic esophagitis: single-center experience in northwestern USA, *Pediatr Int* 51:612, 2009.

Esposito S, Castellazzi L, Garbarino F: Can probiotic administration during pregnancy and the first year of life effectively reduce the risk of infections and allergic diseases in childhood? *J Biol Regul Homeost Agents* 28:565, 2014.

Feuille EJ, Nowak-Węgrzyn A: Food protein-induced enterocolitis syndrome. In Sampson HA, editor: *Allergy and clinical immunology*, Chichester, UK, 2015, John Wiley & Sons, Ltd. doi: 10.1002/9781118609125.ch18.

Finamore A, Roselli M, Britti S, et al: Intestinal and peripheral immune response to MON810 maize ingestion in weaning and old mice, *J Agric Food Chem* 56:11533, 2008.

Fleischer DM, et al: Consensus communication on early peanut introduction and the prevention of peanut allergy in high-risk infants. *J Allergy Clin Immunol* 2015; 136:258-61.

Fiocchi A, Pawankar R, Cuello-Garcia C, et al: World Allergy Organization-McMaster University guidelines for allergic disease prevention (GLAD-P): Probiotics, *World Allergy Organ J* 8:4, 2015.

Food *Allergy Research and Education (FARE): About anaphylaxis* (website). https://www.foodallergy.org/anaphylaxis. Accessed July 31, 2015.

Food Allergy Research and Education (FARE): Who is likely to outgrow a food allergy? (website), 2013. http://blog.foodallergy.org/2013/09/13/who-is-likely-to-outgrow-a-food-allergy. Accessed July 30, 2015.

FPIES Foundation: *About food protein-induced enterocolitis syndrome* (website), 2011. http://fpiesfoundation.org/about-fpies-3. Accessed July 30, 2015.

Franchini S, Marinosci A, Cicenia G: Emergency treatment of asthma, *N Engl J Med* 363:2567, 2010.

Fritscher-Ravens A et al: Confocal endomicroscopy shows food-associated changes in the intestinal mucosa of patients with irritable bowel syndrome, *Gastroenterol* 147:1012, 2014.

Furuta GT, Katzka DA: Eosinophilic esophagitis, *N Engl J Med* 373:1640, 2015.

Geha RS, Beiser A, Ren C, et al: Multicenter, double-blind, placebo-controlled, multiple-challenge evaluation of reported reactions to monosodium glutamate, *J Allergy Clin Immunol* 106:973, 2000.

Genuis SJ: Sensitivity related illness: the escalating pandemic of allergy, intolerance and chemical sensitivity, *Sci Total Environ* 408:6047, 2010.

Geroldinger-Simic M, Zelniker T, Aberer W, et al: Birch pollen-related food allergy: clinical aspects and the role of allergen-specific IgE and IgG(4) antibodies, *J Allergy Clin Immunol* 127:616, 2011.

Greer FR, Sicherer SH, Burks AW, et al: Effects of early nutritional interventions on the development of atopic disease in infants and children: the role of maternal dietary restriction, breastfeeding, timing of introduction of complementary foods, and hydrolyzed formulas, *Pediatrics* 121:183, 2008.

Groschwitz KR, Hogan SP: Intestinal barrier function: molecular regulation and disease pathogenesis, *J Allergy Clin Immunol* 124:3, 2009.

Gruchalla RS, Sampson HA: Preventing peanut allergy through early consumption – Ready for prime time? *NEJM* 372:875, 2015.

Gupta RS, Lau CH, Sita EE, et al: Factors associated with reported food allergy tolerance among US children, *Ann Allerg Asthma Immunol* 111:194, 2013.

Guyton KZ, Loomis D, Grosse Y, et al: Carcinogenicity of tetrachlorvinphos, parathion, malathion, diazinon, and glyphosate, *Lancet Oncol* 16:490, 2015.

Haahtela T, Holgate S, Pawankar R, et al: The biodiversity hypothesis and allergic disease: world allergy organization position statement, *World Allergy Org J* 6:3, 2013.

He K, Du S, Xun P, et al: Consumption of monosodium glutamate in relation to incidence of overweight in Chinese adults: China Health and Nutrition Survey (CHNS), *Am J Clin Nutr* 93:1328, 2011.

Heimemann JA, Kurenbach B, Quist D: Molecular profiling: a tool for addressing emerging gaps in comparative risk assessment of GMOs, *Environ Int* 37:1285, 2011.

Hesselmar B, Sjöberg F, Saalman R, et al: Pacifier cleaning practices and risk of allergy development, *Pediatrics* 131:1, 2013.

Hoffmann HJ, Santos AF, Mayorga C, et al: The clinical utility of basophil activation testing in diagnosis and monitoring of allergic disease, *Allergy* 70:1393, 2015.

Host A, Halken S, Muraro A, et al: Dietary prevention of allergic diseases in infants and small children. Amendment to previous published articles in

Pediatric Allergy and Immunology 2004, by an expert group set up by the Section on Pediatrics, Europ Acad Allergology Clin Immunology, *Pediatr Allergy Immunol* 19:1, 2008.

International Scientific Association for Probiotics and Prebiotics: *Probiotic/Prebiotic Science* (website). http://www.isapp.net/Probiotics-and-Prebiotics/The-Science. Accessed April 26, 2015.

Järvinen KM, Chatchatee P: Mammalian milk allergy: clinical suspicion, cross-reactivities and diagnosis, *Curr Opin Allergy Clin Immunol* 9:251, 2009.

Jarvela I, Torniainen S, Kolho KL: Molecular genetics of human lactase deficiencies, *Ann Med* 41:568, 2009.

Jennings S, Prescott SL: Early dietary exposures and feeding practices: role in pathogenesis and prevention of allergic disease? *Postgrad Med J* 86:94, 2010.

Joneja JV: Infant nutrition – where are we now? *J Parenter Enteral Nutr* 36(Suppl 1):49S, 2012.

Joneja JV: *The health professional's guide to food allergies and intolerances*, Chicago, IL, 2013, Academy of Nutrition and Dietetics.

Jones AP, D'Vaz N, Meldrum S, et al: 25-hyroxyvitamin D3 status is associated with developing adaptive and innate immune responses in the first 6 months of life, *Clin Exp Allergy* 45:220, 2015.

Jones AP, Palmer D, Zhang G, et al: Cord blood 25-hydroxyvitamin D3 and allergic disease during infancy, *Pediatrics* 130: e1128, 2012.

Keet CA, Wood RA: Emerging therapies for food allergy, *J Clin Invest* 124:1880, 2014.

Keller MD, Shuker M, Heimall J, et al: Severe malnutrition resulting from use of rice milk in food elimination diets for atopic dermatitis, *Isr Med Assoc J* 14:40, 2012.

Kneepkens CM, Brand PL: Clinical practice: breastfeeding and the prevention of allergy, *Eur J Pediatr* 169:911, 2010.

Kondo Y, Urisu A: Oral allergy syndrome, *Allergol Int* 58:485, 2009.

Kothandaram S, Deonikar P, Mohan M, et al: In Silico Modeling of C1 Metabolism, *Am J Plant Sci* 6:1444, 2015. http://dx.doi.org/10.4236/ajps.2015.69144.

Lack G: The concept of oral tolerance induction to foods, *Clin Biochem* 47:715, 2014.

Lack G: Update on risk factors for food allergy, *J Allergy Clin Immmunol* 129:1187, 2012.

Ladics GS: Current Codex guidelines for assessment of potential protein allergenicity, *Food Chem Toxicol* 46:S20, 2008.

Ladics GS, Fry J, Goodman R, et al: Allergic sensitization: screening methods, *Clin Translational Allergy* 4:13, 2014.

Landrigan PJ, Benbrook C: GMOs, herbicides, and public health, *N Engl J Med* 373(8):693–695, 2015.

Ling Z, Li Z, Liu X, et al: Altered fecal microbiota composition for food allergy in infants, *Appl Environ Microbiol* 80:2546, 2014.

Ludman S, Shah N, Fox AT: Managing cow's milk protein allergy in children, *BMJ* 347:f5425, 2013.

Maintz L, Novak N: Histamine and histamine intolerance, *Am J Clin Nutr* 85:1185, 2007.

Merves J, Muir A, Modayur Chandramouleeswaran P, et al: Eosinophilic esophagitis, *Ann Allergy Asthma Immunol* 112:397, 2014.

Mesnage R, Arno M, Costanzo M, et al: Transcriptome profile analysis reflects rat liver and kidney damage following chronic ultra-low dose Roundup exposure, *Environ Health* 14:70, 2015. doi 10.1186/s12940-015-0056-1.

Mesnage R, Defarge N, Spiroux de Vendômois J, et al: Potential toxic effects of glyphosate and its commercial formulations below regulatory limits, *Food Chem Toxicol* 84:133–153, 2015.

Miles EA, Calder PC: Omega-6 and omega-3 polyunsaturated fatty acids and allergy diseases in infancy and childhood, *Curr Pharm Des* 20:946, 2014.

Miyake Y, Sasaki S, Tanaka K, et al: Consumption of vegetables, fruit, and antioxidants during pregnancy and wheeze and eczema in infants, *Allergy* 65:758, 2010.

Morita E, Matsuo H, Chinuki Y, et al: Food-dependent exercise-induced anaphylaxis-importance of omega-5 gliadin and HMW-glutenin as causative antigens for wheat-dependent exercise-induced anaphylaxis, *Allergol Int* 58:493, 2009.

National Institute of Health (NIH), National Institute of Allergy and Infectious Disease (NIAID), Boyce JA, et al: Guidelines for the diagnosis and management of food allergy in the United States: Report of the NIAID-sponsored Expert Panel, *J Allerg Clin Immunol* 126(6 Suppl):S1, 2010. www.niaid.nih.gov/topics/foodallergy/clinical/pages/default.aspx.

Nielsen KM: Biosafety data as confidential business information, *PLoS Biol* 11:e1001499, 2013.

Nilsson EE, Skinner MK: Environmentally induced epigenetic transgenerational inheritance of disease susceptibility, *Transl Res* 165(1):12–17, 2015.

Nowak-Wegrzyn A, Muraro A: Food protein-induced enterocolitis syndrome, *Curr Opin Allergy Clin Immunol* 9:371, 2009.

Palmer DJ, Sullivan T, Gold MS, et al: Randomized controlled trial of fish oil supplementation in pregnancy on childhood allergies, *Allergy* 68:1370, 2013.

Pietschmann N: Food intolerance: Immune activation through diet-associated stimuli in chronic disease, *Altern Ther Health Med* 21:42, 2015.

Pyrhönen K, Hiltunen L, Kaila M, et al: Heredity of food allergies in an unselected child population: an epidemiological survey from Finland, *Pediatr Allergy Immunol* 22(1pt2):e124, 2011.

Robson-Ansley P, Toit GD: Pathophysiology, diagnosis and management of exercise-induced anaphylaxis, *Curr Opin Allergy Clin Immunol* 10:312, 2010.

Roy-Ghanta S, Larosa DF, Katzka DA: Atopic characteristics of adult patients with eosinophilic esophagitis, *Clin Gastroenterol Hepatol* 6:531, 2008.

Rueter K, Siafarikas A, Prescott SL, et al: In utero and postnatal vitamin D exposure and allergy risk, *Expert Opin Drug Saf* 13:1601, 2014.

Sampson H: Update on food allergy, *J Allergy Clin Immunol* 113:5, 2004.

Savcheniuk OA, Virchenko OV, Falalyeyeva TM, et al: The efficacy of probiotics for monosodium glutamate-induced obesity: dietology concerns and opportunities for prevention, *EPMA J* 5:2, 2014.

Sicherer SH, Sampson HA: Food allergy, *J Allergy Clin Immunol* 125:S116, 2010.

Skypala IJ, Venter C, Meyer R, et al: The development of a standardized diet history tool to support diagnosis of food allergy, *Clin Transl Allergy* 5:7, 2015.

Soh JY, Huang CH, Lee BW: Carbohydrates as food allergens, *Asia Pac Allergy* 5:17, 2015.

Stapel SO, Asero R, Ballmer-Weber BK, et al: Testing for IgG4 against foods is not recommended as a diagnostic tool: EAACI Task Force Report, *Allergy* 63:793, 2008.

Straumanm A, Aceves SS, Blanchard C, et al: Pediatric and adult eosinophilic esophagitis: similarities and differences, *Allergy* 67:477, 2012.

Swift KM, Lisker I: Current concepts in nutrition: the science and art of the elimination diet, *Alternative and Complementary Therapies* 18:251, 2012.

Tezza G, Mazzei F, Boner A: Epigenetics of allergy, *Early Hum Dev* 89(Suppl 1):S20, 2013.

Turnbull JL, Adams HN, Gorard DA: Review article: the diagnosis and management of food allergy and food intolerances, *Aliment Pharmacol Ther* 41:3, 2015.

Vally H, Misso NL: Adverse reactions to the sulphite additives, *Gastroenterol Hepatol Bed Bench* 5:16, 2012.

Vickery BP, Chin S, Burks AW: Pathophysiology of food allergy, *Pediatr Clin North Am* 58:363, 2011.

Vojdani A: The evolution of reactivity testing: Why immunoglobulin G or immunoglobulin A antibody for food may not be reproducible from one lab to another, *Altern Ther Health Med* 21(Suppl 1):8S, 2015a.

Vojdani, A: Molecular mimicry as a mechanism for food immune reactivities and autoimmunity, *Altern Ther Health Med* 21(1):34S, 2015b.

Vojdani A, Vojdani C: Immune reactivity to food coloring, *Altern Ther Health Med* 21(Suppl 1): 52S, 2015.

Weiner HL, da Cunha AP, Quintana F, et al: Oral tolerance, *Immunol Rev* 241:241, 2011.

Werfel, Schwerk N, Hansen G, et al: The diagnosis and graded therapy of atopic dermatitis, *Dtsch Arztebl Int* 111:509, 2014.

West CE: Gut microbiota and allergic disease: new findings, *Curr Opin Clin Nutr Metab Care* 17:261, 2014.

West CE, Videky DJ, Prescott SL: Role of diet in the development of immune tolerance in the context of allergic disease, *Curr Opinion Pediatr* 22:635, 2010.

Williams AN, Woessner KM: Monosodium glutamate 'allergy': menace or myth? *Clin Exp Allergy* 39:640, 2009.

Zapatero L, Alonso E, Fuentes V, et al: Oral desensitization in children with cow's milk allergy, *J Invest Allergol Clin Immunol* 18:389, 2008.

Zdziarski IM, Edwards JW, Carman JA, et al: GM crops and the rat digestive tract: a critical review, *Environ Int* 73:423, 2014.

27

Medical Nutrition Therapy for Upper Gastrointestinal Tract Disorders

Gail Cresci, PhD, RDN, LD, CNSC; Arlene Escuro, MS, RDN, CNSC

KEY TERMS

achalasia
achlorhydria
achylia gastrica
atrophic gastritis
Barrett's esophagus (BE)
bezoar
Billroth I
Billroth II
dumping syndrome
duodenal ulcer
dyspepsia
dysphagia
endoscopy
esophagectomy
esophagitis
esophagogastroduodenoscopy (EGD)

functional dyspepsia
gastrectomy
gastric pull-up
gastric ulcer
gastritis
gastroesophageal reflux (GER)
gastroesophageal reflux disease (GERD)
gastroparesis
heartburn
Helicobacter pylori
hematemesis
hiatal hernia
lower esophageal sphincter (LES)
melena
mucosa-associated lymphoid tissue (MALT)

Nissen fundoplication
odynophagia
parietal cells
parietal cell vagotomy
peptic ulcer
pyloroplasty
Roux-en-Y
Rome III criteria
stress ulcer
upper esophageal sphincter (UES)
vagotomy
vagotomy, truncal
vagus nerve

Digestive disorders are among the most common problems in health care. Between 60 and 70 million people are affected by all digestive diseases, with more than 50 million ambulatory care visits made annually in the United States alone. More than 20 million diagnostic and surgical procedures involving the gastrointestinal (GI) tract are performed each year (CDC, 2014). Dietary habits and specific food types can play an important role in the onset, treatment, and prevention of many GI disorders. Nutrition therapy is integral in the prevention and treatment of malnutrition and deficiencies that can develop from a GI tract disorder. Diet and lifestyle modifications can improve a patient's quality of life by alleviating GI symptoms and decreasing the number of health care visits and costs associated with GI disease.

ASSESSMENT PARAMETERS

Components of a comprehensive nutrition assessment of patients with GI disorders include the clinical examination and evaluation of anthropometrics, biochemical markers, and the patient's nutrition history. A detailed nutrition history includes the typical dietary intake, changes in appetite, food allergies and intolerances, mastication and swallowing ability, and GI symptoms such as nausea, vomiting, diarrhea, constipation, and the use of dietary supplements (see Chapter 4). Assessment of body weight changes and evaluation of lean body mass (LBM) guide nutrition assessment, estimation of nutritional requirements, and the development of a nutrition care plan. Patients should

be evaluated for unexplained weight loss changes, particularly focusing on percent weight loss over a specified period of time (e.g., at least 5% in 1 month; at least 10% in 6 months). Patients with severe weight loss benefit from initiation of nutrition support early. In fact, "tuning up" a malnourished patient nutritionally before medical or surgical interventions is associated with improved patient outcomes.

Laboratory assessment can be useful to detect a subclinical nutrient deficiency or excess before physical signs manifest. Laboratory assessment should be guided by information obtained in the nutrition history for suspicion of deficiencies (see Chapter 7 and Appendix 22). Although an inadequate diet can result in suboptimal status of several nutrients, isolated vitamin, mineral, or trace element deficiencies also can be the result of disease state, medical interventions, or medication interactions (see Chapter 8 and Appendix 23).

THE ESOPHAGUS

The esophagus is a muscular tube that has an average length of 25 cm in adults (see Figure 27-1). It serves a single but very important function: conveying solids and liquids from the mouth to the stomach. It is lined with nonkeratinized stratified squamous epithelium, and submucosal glands secrete mucin, bicarbonate, epidermal growth factor, and prostaglandin E2, which protect the mucosa from gastric acid.

The top of the esophagus is connected to the pharynx and the bottom of the esophagus is connected to the stomach at the

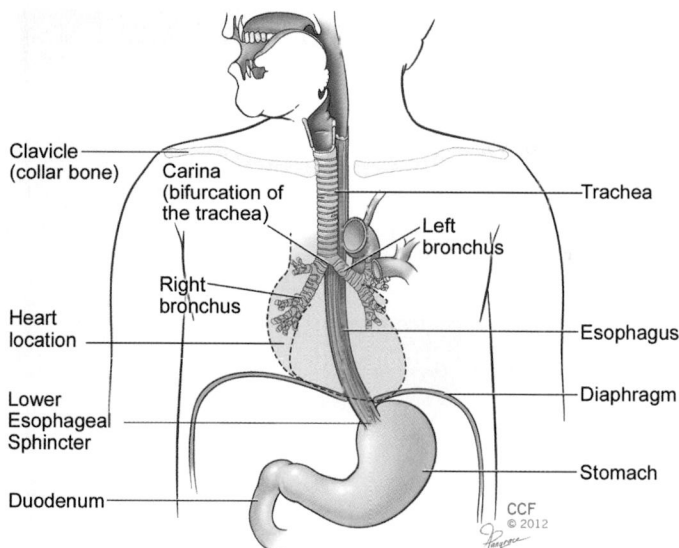

Clavicle (collar bone)
Carina (bifurcation of the trachea)
Trachea
Left bronchus
Right bronchus
Heart location
Esophagus
Lower Esophageal Sphincter
Diaphragm
Stomach
Duodenum
CCF © 2012

FIGURE 27-1 Normal esophagus. (Cleveland Clinic, Cleveland, Ohio.)

cardia. It is highly muscular, with muscles arranged in a way to facilitate the passage of food. As a bolus of food is moved voluntarily from the mouth to the pharynx, the **upper esophageal sphincter (UES)** relaxes, the food moves into the esophagus, and peristaltic waves move the bolus down the esophagus; the **lower esophageal sphincter (LES)** relaxes to allow the food bolus to pass into the stomach. The esophageal transit time takes an average of 5 seconds when in an upright position, and up to 30 seconds when in a supine position (la Roca-Chiapas and Cordova-Fraga, 2011).

The normal esophagus has a multitiered defense system that prevents tissue damage from exposure to gastric contents, including LES contraction, normal gastric motility, esophageal mucus, tight cellular junctions, and cellular pH regulators. Musculoskeletal disorders and motility disorders may result in dysphagia. For example, **achalasia** is characterized by a failure of esophageal neurons, resulting in a loss of ability to relax the LES and have normal peristalsis.

Gastroesophageal Reflux Disease (GERD) and Esophagitis
Etiology

Gastroesophageal reflux (GER) is considered a normal physiologic process that occurs several times a day in healthy infants, children and adults. GER generally is associated with transient relaxation of the LES independent of swallowing, which permits gastric contents to enter the esophagus. Limited information is known about the normal physiology of GER in infants, but regurgitation and spitting up, as the most visible symptom, is reported to occur daily in 50% of all infants (Lightdale et al, 2013).

Gastroesophageal reflux disease (GERD) is a more serious, chronic or long-lasting form of GER and is defined as symptoms or complications resulting from the reflux of gastric contents into the esophagus or beyond, and even into the oral cavity (including larynx) or lung.

In developed countries, the prevalence of GERD (defined by symptoms of **heartburn** [painful, burning sensation that radiates up behind the sternum of fairly short duration] and regurgitation, or both, at least once a week) is 10% to 20%, with a slightly lower prevalence in Asia (Jung, 2011). The types of GERD can be distinguished by **esophagogastroduodenoscopy (EGD)**, which uses a fiberoptic endoscope to directly visualize the esophagus, stomach, and duodenum. GERD can be classified as the presence of symptoms without abnormalities or erosions on endoscopic examination (nonerosive disease or NERD), or GERD with symptoms and erosions present (ERD). ERD generally is associated with more severe and prolonged symptoms compared with NERD (Katz et al, 2013).

Some patients experience GERD symptoms primarily in the evening (nocturnal GERD), which has a greater impact on quality of life compared with daytime symptoms. Nocturnal GERD is associated significantly with severe **esophagitis** (inflammation of the esophagus) and intestinal metaplasia (Barrett's esophagus) and can lead to sleep disturbance. Patients with ERD are more likely to be men, and women are more likely to have NERD. There is a definite relationship between GERD and obesity. Several meta-analyses suggest an association between body mass index (BMI), waist circumference, weight gain, and the presence of symptoms and complications of GERD. GERD is frequent during pregnancy, usually manifesting as heartburn, and may begin in any trimester. Significant predictors of heartburn during pregnancy are increasing gestational age, heartburn before pregnancy, and parity (Katz et al, 2013) (see Chapter 15).

Chest pain may be a symptom of GERD, and distinguishing cardiac from noncardiac chest pain is required before considering GERD as a cause of chest pain. Although the symptoms of dysphagia can be associated with uncomplicated GERD, its presence warrants investigation for a potential complication including an underlying motility disorder, stricture, or malignancy. Patients with disruptive GERD (daily or more than weekly symptoms) have an increase in time off work and decrease in work productivity, and a decrease in physical functioning (Katz et al, 2013).

Pathophysiology

The pathophysiology of GERD is complex. Box 27-1 describes possible mechanisms involved in GERD. Three components make up the esophagogastric junction: the lower esophageal sphincter (LES), the crural diaphragm, and the anatomic flap valve. This esophagogastric junction functions as an antireflux

---

BOX 27-1 Possible Mechanisms Involved in Gastroesophageal Reflux Disease (GERD)

- Decreased salivation
- Transient lower esophageal sphincter (LES) relaxation
- Reduced lower esophageal sphincter (LES) pressure
- Impaired esophageal acid clearance
- Increased esophageal sensitivity
- Acid pocket
- Increased intraabdominal pressure
- Delayed gastric emptying

Data from Beaumont H et al: The position of the acid pocket as a major risk factor for acidic reflux in healthy subjects and patients with GORD, *Gut* 59:441, 2010; Bredenoord AJ et al: Gastroesophageal reflux disease, *Lancet* 381:1933, 2013; Penagini R, Bravi I: The role of delayed gastric emptying and impaired esophageal motility, *Best Pract Res Clin Gastroenterol* 24:831, 2010.

PATHOPHYSIOLOGY AND CARE MANAGEMENT ALGORITHM

Esophagitis

ETIOLOGY

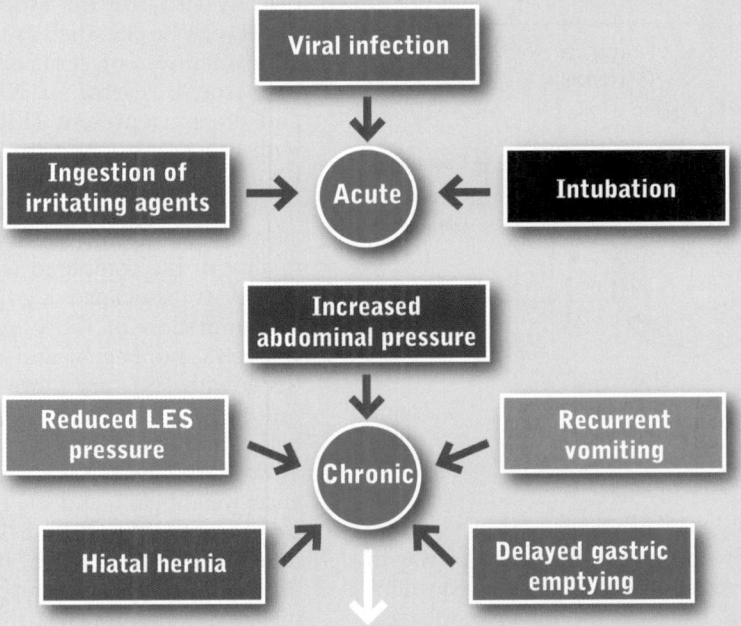

Viral infection

Ingestion of irritating agents → **Acute** ← Intubation

Increased abdominal pressure

Reduced LES pressure → **Chronic** ← Recurrent vomiting

Hiatal hernia → **Chronic** ← Delayed gastric emptying

PATHOPHYSIOLOGY

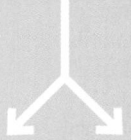

Reflux of gastric acid and/or intestinal contents through the lower esophageal sphincter (LES) and into the esophagus

MANAGEMENT

Behavioral Modification

Avoid:
- Eating within 3-4 hours of retiring
- Lying down after meals
- Tight-fitting garments
- Cigarette smoking

Medical/Surgical Management

- Proton pump inhibitors
- Histamine-2 receptor antagonists
- Antacids
- Prokinetic agents
- Fundoplication

Nutrition Management

Goal:
Decrease exposure of esophagus to gastric contents
Avoid:
- Large meals
- Dietary fat
- Alcohol

Goal:
Decrease acidity of gastric secretions
Avoid:
- Coffee
- Fermented alcoholic beverages

Goal:
Prevent pain and irritation
Avoid:
- Any food that the patient feels exacerbates his/her symptoms

barrier. The lower esophageal sphincter is a 3- to 4-cm segment of circular smooth muscle at the distal end of the esophagus. The resting tone of this muscle can vary among healthy individuals, ranging from 10 mm Hg to 35 mm Hg relative to the intragastric pressure. The most common mechanism for reflux is transient LES relaxations, which are triggered by gastric distention and serve to enable gas venting from the stomach. On average, transient LES relaxations persist for about 20 seconds, which is significantly longer than the typical swallow-induced relaxation (Bredenoord et al, 2013).

For reflux to take place, pressure in the proximal stomach must be greater than the pressure in the esophagus. Patients with chronic respiratory disorders, such as chronic obstructive pulmonary disease (COPD), are at risk for GERD because of frequent increases in intraabdominal pressure. A chronically increased pressure also is seen during pregnancy and in overweight and obese people.

Hypersensitivity to acid can occur in people with erosive esophagitis and in those with normal mucosa. A factor contributing to increased esophageal sensitivity to acid is impaired mucosal barrier function. In a systematic review, the overall rate of gastric emptying was delayed in patients with GERD (Penagini and Bravi, 2010). However, a relationship between delayed gastric emptying and increased reflux could not be seen in this study, suggesting that impaired emptying of the stomach as a whole is not an important determinant of GER.

Good peristaltic function is an important defense mechanism against GERD as prolonged acid clearance correlates with the severity of esophagitis and the presence of complication such as Barrett's esophagus. Acid pocket is an occurrence during the postprandial period when a layer of acidic gastric juice is ready to reflux resulting from absence of peristaltic contraction in the proximal stomach (Beaumont et al, 2010).

Prolonged acid exposure can result in esophagitis, esophageal erosions, ulceration, scarring, stricture, and in some cases dysphagia (see *Pathophysiology and Care Management Algorithm:* Esophagitis). Acute esophagitis may be caused by reflux, ingestion of a corrosive agent, viral or bacterial infection, intubation, radiation, or eosinophilic infiltration. Eosinophilic esophagitis (EOE) is characterized by an isolated, severe eosinophilic infiltration of the esophagus manifested by GERD-like symptoms that may be caused by an immune response (see Chapter 26).

The severity of the esophagitis resulting from the gastroesophageal reflux is influenced by the composition, frequency, and volume of the gastric reflux; the health of the mucosal barrier; length of exposure of the esophagus to the gastric reflux; and the rate of gastric emptying. Symptoms of esophagitis and GERD may impair the ability to consume an adequate diet and interfere with sleep, work, social events, and the overall quality of life (see Table 27-1).

Abnormalities in the body such as hiatal hernia also may contribute to gastroesophageal reflux and esophagitis. The esophagus passes through the diaphragm by way of the esophageal hiatus or ring. The attachment of the esophagus to the hiatal ring may become compromised, allowing a portion of the upper stomach to move above the diaphragm. Table 27-2 describes the four types of hiatal hernia. The most common symptom of hiatal hernia is heartburn. When acid reflux occurs with a hiatal hernia, the gastric contents remain above the hiatus longer than normal. The prolonged acid exposure

TABLE 27-1	Clinical symptoms associated with GERD
Dental corrosion	Slow, progressive tooth surface loss associated with acid regurgitation
Dysphagia	Difficulty initiating a swallow (oropharyngeal dysphagia) or sensation of food being hindered or "sticks" after swallowed (esophageal dysphagia)
Heartburn (pyrosis)	Painful, burning sensation that radiates up behind the sternum of fairly short duration
Odynophagia	Painful swallow
Regurgitation	Backflow of gastric content into the mouth not associated with nausea or retching
Noncardiac chest pain	Unexplained substernal chest pain resembling a myocardial infarction without evidence of coronary artery disease
Extraesophageal symptoms	Chronic cough, hoarseness, reflux-induced laryngitis, or asthma

Data from Bredenoord AJ et al: Gastro-esophageal reflux disease, *Lancet* 381:1933, 2013; Katz PO et al: Guidelines for the diagnosis and management of gastroesophageal reflux disease, *Am J Gastroenterol* 108:308, 2013.

TABLE 27-2	Types of Hiatal Hernia
Type 1 (sliding hiatal hernia)	Most common type; gastroesophageal junction is pushed above the diaphragm, causing a symmetric herniation of the proximal stomach.
Type 2 (true paraesophageal hernia)	Fundus slides upward and moves above the gastroesophageal junction
Type 3 (mixed paraesophageal hernia)	Combined sliding and paraesophageal herniation
Type 4 (complex paraesophageal hernia)	Less common form; intrathoracic herniation of other organs, such as the colon, and small bowel into the hernia sac

increases the risk of developing more serious esophagitis. Figure 27-2 illustrates a hiatal hernia *(A)*, and postsurgical reduction *(B)*. As the hiatal hernia enlarges, regurgitation may be more prominent, especially when lying down or when bending over. Epigastric pain occurs in the upper middle region of the abdomen after large, energy-dense meals. Weight reduction and decreasing meal size reduce the negative consequences of hiatal hernia.

Patients with type 3 hiatal hernia may present with severe chest pain, retching, vomiting, and hematemesis (vomiting of blood), because these hernias can twist and cause strangulation in the chest, which would be considered a surgical emergency (Hyun and Bak, 2011). Some patients can present with iron deficiency anemia without acute bleeding, because the diaphragm becomes so irritated that the patient may develop chronic blood loss.

Barrett's esophagus (BE) is a precancerous condition in which the normal squamous epithelium of the esophagus is replaced by an abnormal columnar-lined epithelium known as specialized intestinal metaplasia (tissue that is similar to the intestinal lining). The exact cause of BE is unknown, but GERD is a risk factor for the condition. The true prevalence of BE is unknown but is estimated to affect 1.6% to 6.8% of the general population (Gilbert et al, 2011). People with BE are at increased risk for a cancer called esophageal adenocarcinoma with

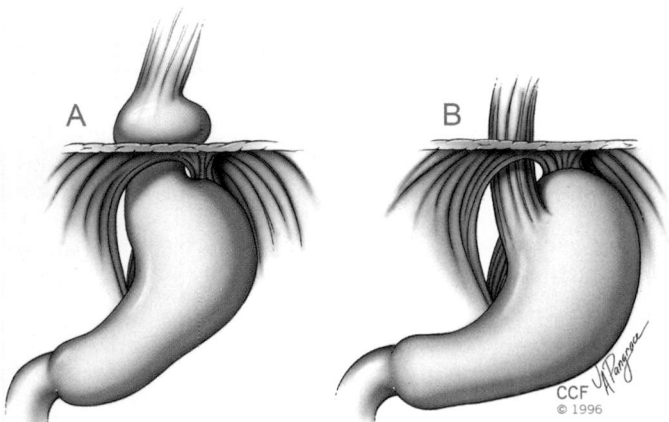

FIGURE 27-2 A, Hiatal hernia. **B,** Postsurgical reduction of hiatal hernia. (Cleveland Clinic, Cleveland, Ohio.)

Type of Medication	Common Names	Medication Function
Antacids	Magnesium, calcium, or aluminum bound to carbonate or phosphate	Buffers gastric acid
Antigas	Simethicone	Lowers surface tension of gas bubbles
Antidumping	Acarbose	Delays carbohydrate digestion by inhibiting alpha-glycoside hydrolase, which interferes with conversion of starch to monosaccharides
Antisecretory	Octreotide (somatostatin analog) Somatostatin	Inhibits release of insulin and other gut hormones; slows rate of gastric emptying and small intestine transit time; and increases intestinal water and sodium absorption
H_2 blocker	Cimetidine Ranitidine Famotidine Nizatidine	Blocks the action of histamine on parietal cells, decreasing the production of acid
Prokinetic	Metoclopramide Erythromycin Domperidone	Increases contractility of the stomach and shortens gastric emptying time
Proton pump inhibitor (PPI)	Omeprazole Lansoprazole Esomeprazole Pantoprazole Dexlansoprazole Rabeprazole	Inhibits acid secretion

TABLE 27-3 Common Medications Used in the Treatment of Upper Gastrointestinal Tract Disorders

incidence rising dramatically over the past 40 years and speculated to continue to rise during coming decades (Thrift and Whiteman, 2012). Risk factors for BE include prolonged history of GERD-related symptoms (more than 5 years), middle age, white male, obesity, smoking, and family history of BE or adenocarcinoma of the esophagus. Estrogen may be protective and account for the lower incidence of BE in females (Asanuma et al, 2016).

Medical and Surgical Management

The primary medical treatment of esophageal reflux is suppression of acid secretion. The aim in acid-suppression therapy is to raise the gastric pH above 4 during periods when reflux is most likely to occur. Proton pump inhibitors (PPIs), which decrease acid production by the gastric parietal cell, have been associated with superior healing rates and decreased relapses (Katz et al, 2013). Milder forms of reflux are managed by H_2 receptor (a type of histamine receptor on the gastric parietal cell) antagonists, and antacids, which buffer gastric acid in the esophagus or stomach to reduce heartburn. Prokinetic agents, which increase propulsive contractions of the stomach, may be used in persons with delayed gastric emptying. A trial of baclofen, a gamma-amino butyric acid (GABA) agonist, can be considered in patients with objective documentation of continued symptomatic reflux despite optimal PPI therapy (Katz et al, 2013). However, there have not been long-term data published regarding efficacy of baclofen in GERD. Refer to Table 27-3 for medications commonly used in upper GI disorders.

Of patients with severe GERD, 5% to 10% do not respond to medical therapy. The Nissen fundoplication was first described as a treatment for severe reflux esophagitis in 1956 and is still the most commonly performed antireflux surgery (see Figure 27-3). During this procedure, which can be done using either open or a laparoscopic technique, the fundus or top portion of the stomach is wrapped 360 degrees around the lower esophagus and sutured in place to limit reflux (see Figure 27-3). Surgical therapy is considered for individuals who have failed medical management, those who opt for surgery despite successful medical management (e.g., because of quality-of-life considerations, lifelong need for medication intake, expense of medications), those who experience complications of GERD

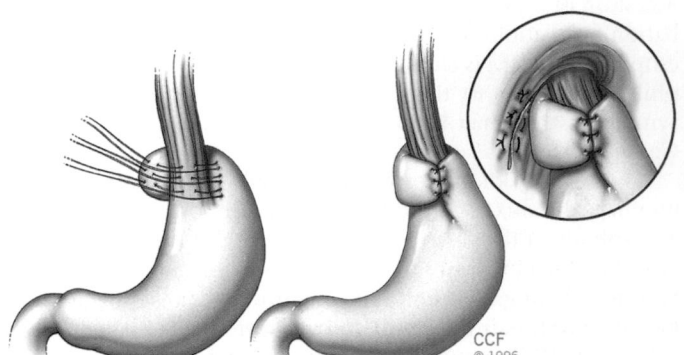

FIGURE 27-3 Nissen fundoplication. (Cleveland Clinic, Cleveland, Ohio.)

(Barrett's esophagus, peptic stricture), and those who have extraesophageal manifestations (asthma, hoarseness, cough, chest pain, aspiration) (Stefanidis et al, 2010). Surgical approaches are reserved for children who have intractable symptom unresponsive to medical therapy or who are at risk for life-threatening complications of GERD (Lightdale et al, 2013).

BOX 27-2 Dietary Guidelines After a Nissen Fundoplication

1. Start clear liquid diet after surgery.
2. Advance oral diet to soft, moist, solid foods. This could be ordered before hospital discharge or written in hospital discharge instructions when to start solids.
3. Follow soft, moist foods diet for about 2 months. Foods must be soft to pass through the esophagus.
4. Consume small, frequent meals.
5. Swallow small bites of food and chew thoroughly to allow an easy passage through the esophagus and avoid use of straw to consume liquids. Drink slowly.
6. Avoid foods and beverages that may cause backflow of stomach contents. This consists of citrus fruits and juices, tomato, pineapple, alcohol, caffeine, chocolate, carbonated beverages, peppermint or spearmint, fatty or fried foods, spicy foods, vinegar or vinegar-containing foods.
7. Avoid dry foods that are hard to pass through the esophagus, such as bread, steak, raw vegetables, rolls, dry chicken, raw fruits, peanut butter, other dry meats, or anything with skin, seeds, or nuts.
8. Avoid any food that may cause discomfort.
9. After 2 months, start to incorporate new foods into the diet. Try one new food item or beverage at a time. By 3 to 6 months, patient should be able to tolerate most foods.
10. Consult doctor or dietitian if having difficulty eating or losing weight.

Refer to Box 27-2 for dietary guidelines after Nissen fundoplication.

Lifestyle Modifications and Medical Nutrition Therapy

The first step in symptom management of GERD should consist of changes in lifestyle, including diet. The main factors that trigger reflux symptoms are caffeine, alcohol, tobacco, and stress. Initial recommendations should focus on meal size and content. Eating small rather than large meals reduces the probability that gastric contents will reflux into the esophagus.

Obesity is a contributing factor to GERD and hiatal hernia because it increases intragastric pressure, and weight reduction may reduce acid contact time in the esophagus leading to decreased reflux symptoms. The frequent advice to elevate the head of the bed by 6 to 8 inches would be rational for patients who have reflux episodes at night. Frequent bending over should be avoided. Use of loose-fitting garments in the waist area also is thought to decrease the risk of reflux.

Foods such as carminatives (such as peppermint and spearmint) and coffee have been reported to lower LES pressure, but little research has been done to establish their clinical significance in GERD when used in normal or small amounts. Fermented alcoholic beverages (such as beer and wine) stimulate the secretion of gastric acid and should be limited. Carbonated beverages enhance gastric distention, which increases transient LES relaxations. Highly acidic foods such as citrus juices and tomatoes should be avoided because they cause pain when the esophagus is already inflamed.

The role of spices in the pathologic conditions related to upper GI disorders is not clear. In patients with GI lesions, the use of foods highly seasoned with chili powder and pepper can cause discomfort. The type of chili and amount of capsaicin consumed make a difference (Milke et al, 2006). Chewing gum has been shown to increase salivary secretions, which help raise esophageal pH, but no studies have demonstrated its efficacy compared with other lifestyle measures. Limiting or avoiding

aggravating foods may improve symptoms in some individuals. Thus recommendations are to have a generally healthy diet and to avoid food items that, in the experience of the patient, trigger symptoms.

Lifestyle changes to treat GERD in infants may involve a combination of feeding changes and positioning therapy. Modifying the maternal diet if infants are breastfed, changing formulas, and reducing the feeding volume while increasing the frequency of feedings may be effective strategies to address GERD in many infants.. Thickened feedings appear to decrease observed regurgitation rather than the actual number of reflux episodes. Little is known about the effect of thickening formula on the natural history of infantile reflux or the potential allergenicity of commercial thickening agents (Lightdale et al, 2013).

Use of tobacco products is contraindicated with reflux. Cigarette smoking should be stopped because it is associated with decreased LES pressure and decreased salivation, thus causing prolonged acid clearance. Smoking tobacco products also compromises GI integrity and increases the risk of esophageal and other cancers.

Identification and treatment of the mechanism underlying the GERD is the first line of therapy. Box 27-3 lists lifestyle and dietary modifications that are aimed at minimizing the occurrence of reflux and optimizing esophageal acid clearance.

Head and Neck Cancer
Pathophysiology

Cancers of the upper aerodigestive tract, collectively referred to as head and neck cancers, comprise malignancies of the oral cavity (lips and inside of the mouth, including the front portion of the tongue, and the roof and floor of the mouth), the oropharynx (back portion of the tongue and the part of the throat behind the oral cavity), the larynx, and the esophagus. The patient diagnosed with head and neck cancer faces unique challenges in maintaining adequate nutrition. The disease and the treatments, especially surgery, chemo- and radiation therapy, have significant impact on upper digestive tract function, and oral intake is often insufficient during and after therapy. Almost all patients with head and neck cancer are malnourished at the time of diagnosis. Dysphagia is a hallmark of head and neck

---

BOX 27-3 Nutrition Care Guidelines for Reducing Gastroesophageal Reflux and Esophagitis

1. Avoid large, high-fat meals.
2. Avoid eating 2 to 3 hours before lying down.
3. Elevate the head of bed by 6 to 8 inches for individuals who have reflux episodes at night.
4. Avoid smoking.
5. Avoid alcoholic beverages.
6. Avoid caffeine-containing foods and beverages.
7. Remain upright for a while after eating.
8. Wear loose-fitting clothing around the stomach area; tight clothing can constrict the area and increase reflux.
9. Avoid acidic and highly spiced foods when inflammation exists.
10. Consume a healthy, nutritionally complete diet with adequate fiber.
11. Lose weight if overweight.

Data from National Digestive Diseases Information Clearinghouse: *Gastroesophageal Reflux (GER) and Gastroesophageal Reflux Disease (GERD) in Adults* (website): http://digestive.niddk.nih.gov/, 2014. Accessed February 1, 2015.

cancer; it occurs as a result of mechanical obstruction, sensory impairment, or odynophagia (painful swallowing). In these patients there is a high prevalence of alcohol abuse and long-term tobacco use, which are also associated with chronic malnutrition (Schoeff at al, 2013).

Medical Nutrition Therapy

Depending on the tumor site, the surgical procedure may significantly alter the anatomy and lead to scarring that can negatively affect swallowing. The patient is likely to be restricted from oral intake while healing from the surgery. Placement of a gastrostomy tube is the most common approach to ensure safe delivery of adequate nutrition, but the optimal timing is not defined. Although the goal is eventual transition to oral feeding, some patients will require additional enteral nutrition (EN) because of structural and sensory deficits.

Aggressive prophylactic swallowing therapy is a recent development in the treatment of dysphagia in patients with head and neck cancer. This approach focuses on maintaining or regaining function rather than simply accommodating dysfunction (reliance on feeding tube) and empowers patients to progress carefully with oral intake despite imperfect swallowing (Schoeff et al, 2013).

Surgery of the Esophagus

The primary indication for an esophagectomy is esophageal cancer or Barrett's esophagus with high-grade dysplasia. A patient undergoing esophagectomy often presents with dysphagia, decreased appetite, side effects from chemotherapy, and weight loss. Esophagectomy requires that there be another conduit in place to transport food from the oropharynx to the rest of the GI tract for digestion and absorption. Placement of an enteral feeding tube preoperatively, or at the time of surgery provides enteral access for patients who will experience eating challenges and a slow transition back to a normal diet. The enteral route of nutrition is preferred; however, if the GI tract is not functional, parenteral nutrition (PN) must be provided (see Chapter 13).

Medical Nutrition Therapy

Nutrition assessment of an esophagectomy candidate includes evaluation of treatment plans, history of weight loss, and the ability to swallow solid foods and liquids. Generally, the only esophagectomy patients screened at low nutrition risk preoperatively are those with Barrett's esophagus with high-grade dysplasia, or those who are asymptomatic.

Preoperative Phase. Swallowing difficulty (dysphagia) is the commonly identified problem in patients awaiting an esophagectomy. The dietary modifications may range from regular food with adequate chewing and slow eating, to soft foods, or to pureed or blenderized foods (see Chapter 13). Patients also benefit from calorically dense oral nutrition supplements to maximize energy and protein intake. Nutrition support from a nasoenteric feeding tube inserted in the preoperative patient may be necessary if the oral dietary modifications do not prevent further weight loss.

Postoperative Phase. A gastric pull-up procedure (see Figure 27-4) involves removal of a segment of or the entire esophageal tract and replacing it with the stomach tissue. Complications after this procedure include increased risk of aspiration, dysphagia, anastomosis leak, wound infection, and stricture at the anastomosis site. A jejunostomy feeding tube may be placed at surgery to provide postoperative nutrition until adequate oral intake is achieved. The tube feeding schedule is changed eventually from continuous to cyclical

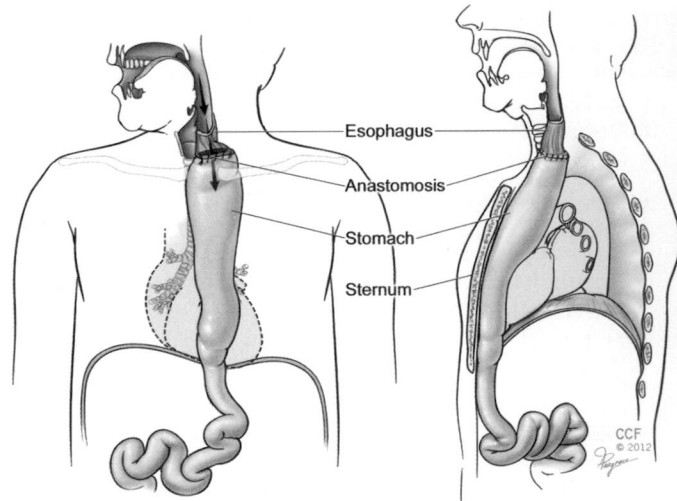

FIGURE 27-4 Gastric pull-up. (Cleveland Clinic, Cleveland, Ohio.)

BOX 27-4   Nutrition Guidelines After Esophagectomy

1. Nutrition support is provided through a jejunostomy feeding tube after esophagectomy.
   A patient cannot eat or drink anything by mouth until instructed by the doctor.
2. Once an oral diet can be started, patient is provided with specific guidelines on how to taper the tube feedings and how to advance the oral diet (from sips of clear liquids to very moist, tender foods).
3. It may take several weeks to taper the tube feedings and adjust to oral diet. When tube feeding is discontinued, the patient should continue to flush the jejunostomy tube daily. A patient will continue to adjust to oral feedings for about 3 months.
4. During the 3-month transition:
   • Eat 6 small meals per day and include sources of protein and fat at every small meal.
   • Choose very tender, moist foods that can be easily cut with the side of fork or spoon and use sauces or gravies to moisten food.
   • Gradually increase the volume and variety of foods at each meal.
   • Avoid skins, seeds, nuts, tough or dry meats, breads and rolls, peanut butter, fried and greasy foods, raw vegetables, cooked corn and peas, and raw fruits.
   • Avoid items that can cause heartburn and stomach reflux such as caffeine, citrus fruits, pineapples, tomatoes, carbonated beverages, mints, and alcohol.
   • Drink no more than 4 fluid ounces of water or other liquids with meals. Drink fluids about 30 minutes before or after the meal and sip slowly.
   • Avoid concentrated sweets and sugars.
   • Eat slowly and chew foods thoroughly.
5. After 3 months, more food should be added back into the diet. Try one new food or beverage at a time.
6. After 6 months, a patient should be eating normally. It is still advised to eat frequent small meals.

---

feedings at night as the patient is transitioned to an oral diet during the day.

Transition to oral intake postoperatively proceeds from clear liquids to a soft, moist foods diet. The patient is advised to eat small frequent meals with limited fluids at mealtimes. Some patients may experience dumping syndrome if food passes into the small intestine too quickly. The symptoms of dumping syndrome include abdominal pain, nausea, diarrhea, weakness, and dizziness. Box 27-4 lists dietary guidelines after esophageal surgery to prevent dumping syndrome (see Dumping Syndrome later in this chapter for more details).

THE STOMACH

The stomach accommodates and stores meals, mixes food with gastric secretions, and controls emptying into the duodenum. Gastric volume is approximately 50 ml when empty, but can expand to approximately 4 L. Gastric **parietal cells** (acid-producing cells) produce 1.5 to 2 L of acid daily resulting in a pH between 1 and 2 (see Chapter 1 for a detailed discussion of healthy stomach function).

The mucosa of the stomach and duodenum is protected from proteolytic actions of gastric acid and pepsin by a coating of mucus secreted by glands in the epithelial walls from the lower esophagus to the upper duodenum. The mucosa also is protected from bacterial invasion by the digestive actions of pepsin and hydrochloric acid (HCl). Prostaglandins play an important role in protecting the gastroduodenal mucosa by stimulating the secretion of mucus and bicarbonate and maintaining blood flow during periods of potential injury.

Dyspepsia and Functional Dyspepsia
Pathophysiology

Dyspepsia (indigestion) refers to nonspecific, persistent upper abdominal discomfort or pain. It affects an estimated 20% to 40% of the general population and significantly reduces quality of life (Ford and Moayyedi, 2013). The underlying causes of dyspepsia may include GERD, **peptic ulcer** disease, gastritis, gallbladder disease or other identifiable pathologic conditions.

Functional dyspepsia (FD) is defined by the **Rome III criteria** as the presence of symptoms thought to originate in the gastroduodenal region in the absence of any organic, systemic, or metabolic disease likely to explain the symptoms. Symptoms of FD do not consistently predict the underlying pathologic condition. Epigastric pain or discomfort is the hallmark symptom in patients with FD. The word discomfort is important to emphasize, because many patients will not complain of pain, but rather complain of burning, pressure, or fullness in the epigastric area, or that they cannot finish a normal-sized meal (early satiety). Other symptoms include postprandial nausea, belching, and abdominal bloating (Talley and Ford, 2015).

Medical Nutrition Therapy

Current treatments for FD have generally ignored the potential role of diet. The possible effect of specific foods and macronutrients and other dietary habits to induce or exacerbate FD symptoms has been poorly studied, and often there are conflicting results (Lacy et al, 2012). Using a food and symptom diary during a clinical evaluation of a patient with FD and assessing symptoms associated with eating patterns is useful. Dietary modifications such as consuming smaller meals with a reduction in dietary fat may be promising in FD therapy. Helping the client identify problematic foods also can be helpful.

Gastritis and Peptic Ulcers
Pathophysiology

Gastritis is a nonspecific term literally meaning inflammation of the stomach. It can be used to describe symptoms relating to the stomach, an endoscopic appearance of the gastric mucosa, or a histologic change characterized by infiltration of the epithelium with inflammatory cells such as polymorphonuclear cells

⊚ **FOCUS ON**

Changing Face of H. pylori and Gastric Cancer

Traditionally, gastric cancer was considered a single disease. However, scientists now classify gastric cancer by its location in either the top inch of the stomach near the esophagus (gastric cardia) or the rest of the stomach (noncardia).

This new classification of gastric cancers was adopted in part because of the role of *Helicobacter pylori*. *H. pylori* appears to be a strong risk factor for noncardia gastric cancer; however, the role of *H. pylori* in the development of gastric cardia cancer remains controversial.

A study of patients in Finland investigated *H. pylori* infection from blood obtained at the time of enrollment, before the patients actually developed cancer (Kamangar et al, 2006). When patients who developed cancer were compared with age-matched controls who did not develop cancer, *H. pylori* infection resulted in an eightfold increase in the incidence of noncardia gastric cancer but a 60% decrease in the incidence of cardia gastric cancer. The decrease in gastric cardia cancer with *H. pylori* infection was an unexpected finding because previous studies had not shown this. One reason that older studies may have had misleading results was that researchers did not check for the presence of *H. pylori* until after the diagnosis of gastric cancer, and *H. pylori* does not flourish on precancerous or malignant cells. Population studies support the protective effect of *H. pylori* on gastric cardia cancer (Whiteman et al, 2010).

Developed countries have seen a decrease in this infection in recent years because of increased information, testing, and effective treatment. Concomitantly, there has been a decreased incidence of noncardia gastric cancer, but an increase in the incidence of gastric cardia and esophageal cancers in these countries. The revelation that treating *H. pylori* infection decreases the risk for some cancers but may increase the risk of other cancers is prompting more research.

(PMNs). Acute gastritis refers to rapid onset of inflammation and symptoms. Chronic gastritis may occur over a period of months to decades, with reoccurring symptoms. Symptoms include nausea, vomiting, malaise, anorexia, hemorrhage, and epigastric pain. Prolonged gastritis may result in atrophy and loss of stomach parietal cells, with a loss of HCL secretion (achlorhydria) and intrinsic factor, resulting in pernicious anemia (see Chapter 32).

Helicobacter pylori Gastritis

Helicobacter pylori is a gram-negative bacteria that is somewhat resistant to the acidic environment in the stomach. *H. pylori* infection is responsible for most cases of chronic inflammation of the gastric mucosa and peptic ulcer, gastric cancer, and **atrophic gastritis** (chronic inflammation with deterioration of the mucous membrane and glands), resulting in achlorhydria and loss of intrinsic factor (Dos Santos and Carvalho, 2014; see *Focus On: Changing Face of H. pylori and Gastric Cancer*).

H. pylori infection prevalence generally correlates with geography and the socioeconomic status of the population and begins during childhood, but generally is not diagnosed until adulthood. *H. pylori* is believed to be spread through contaminated food and water. Its prevalence ranges from approximately 10% in developed countries to 80% to 90% in developing countries. Although gastritis is a characteristic observation, most people infected with *H. pylori* never develop ulcers. *H. pylori* infection does not resolve spontaneously, and risks of complications increase with the duration of the infection. Other risk factors contributing to pathology and disease severity include patient age at onset, specific strain and concentration of the organism, genetic factors related to the host, and the patient's lifestyle and overall health.

In the first week after *H. pylori* infection, many PMNs and a few eosinophils infiltrate the gastric mucosa. These are replaced gradually with the mononuclear cells. The presence of lymphoid follicles is called mucosa-associated lymphoid tissue (MALT). MALT may become autonomous to form a low-grade, B-cell lymphoma called MALT lymphoma. *H. pylori* can cause duodenitis if it colonizes gastric tissue that may be present in the duodenum.

Treating *H. pylori* with antibiotics can cause PMNs to disappear within a week or two, but a mild gastritis can persist for several years as the reduction in mononuclear cells is slow. In countries where *H. pylori* is common, so is gastric cancer. Because *H. pylori* can cause peptic ulcer and gastric cancer, antibiotic treatment is favored when it is diagnosed.

Non-*Helicobacter pylori* Gastritis

Aspirin and non-steroidal antiinflammatory drugs (NSAIDs) are corrosive; both inhibit prostaglandin synthesis, which is essential for maintaining the mucus and bicarbonate barrier in the stomach. Thus chronic use of aspirin or other NSAIDs, steroids, alcohol, erosive substances, tobacco, or any combination of these factors may compromise mucosal integrity and increase the chance for acquiring acute or chronic gastritis. Eosinophilic gastroenteritis (EGE) also may contribute to some cases of gastritis (see Chapter 26). Poor nutrition and general poor health may contribute to the onset and severity of the symptoms and can delay the healing process.

Medical Treatment

Treatment for gastritis involves removing the inciting agent (e.g., pathogenic organism, NSAIDs). Noninvasive methods for diagnosing *H. pylori* include a blood test for *H. pylori* antibodies, a urea breath test, or a stool antigen test. Endoscopy is a common invasive diagnostic tool (see *Focus On:* Endoscopy and Capsules). Antibiotics and proton pump inhibitors (PPIs) are the primary medical treatments. Side effects of chronic acid suppression either from disease or chronic use of PPIs should be considered (Katz, 2010). These include reduction of gastric secretion of HCL, which can reduce absorption of nutrients (e.g., vitamin B_{12}, calcium, and nonheme iron) that require intragastric proteolysis to make them bioavailable (McColl, 2009) (see Chapter 8 and Appendix 23.) Acid suppression may increase incidence of some bone fractures (Yang, 2012), as well as increase the risk for intestinal infection because gastric acidity is a primary defense against ingested pathogens (Linsky et al, 2010).

Peptic Ulcers
Etiology

Normal gastric and duodenal mucosa is protected from the digestive actions of acid and pepsin by the secretion of mucus, the production of bicarbonate, the removal of excess acid by normal blood flow, and the rapid renewal and repair of epithelial cell injury. Peptic ulcer refers to an ulcer that occurs as a result of the breakdown of these normal defense and repair mechanisms. Typically more than one of the mechanisms must be malfunctioning for symptomatic peptic ulcers to develop. Peptic ulcers typically show evidence of chronic inflammation and repair processes surrounding the lesion.

The primary causes of peptic ulcers are *H. pylori* infection, gastritis, use of aspirin, other NSAIDs and corticosteroids, and severe illness (see Stress Ulcers later in this chapter and *Pathophysiology and Care Management Algorithm:* Peptic Ulcer). Life stress may

FOCUS ON
Endoscopy and Capsules

The mucosa of the upper gastrointestinal (GI) tract can be viewed, photographed, and biopsied by means of endoscopy. a procedure that involves passing a flexible tube into the esophagus that has a light and camera on the distal end. It can be passed through the esophagus and into the stomach or upper small bowel. This procedure is called **esophagogastro-duodenoscopy (EGD)**. Inflammation, erosions, ulcerations, changes in the blood vessels, and destruction of surface cells can be identified. These changes can then be correlated with chemical, histologic, and clinical findings to formulate a diagnosis. This may be useful when physicians suspect certain conditions, such as complicated GERD strictures, BE, esophageal varices, or gastroduodenal ulcers or celiac disease.

EGD also can be used for a number of therapeutic purposes such as cauterization at ulcer sites, dilation or deployment of stents in areas of stricture, and placement of percutaneous feeding tubes. Endoscopy may be used in long-term monitoring of patients with chronic esophagitis and gastritis because of the possibility that they will develop premalignant lesions or carcinoma (Wong et al, 2010).

Capsules containing a miniaturized video camera, light, and radio transmitter that can be swallowed and the signal transmitted to a receiver worn on the waist of the patient, allowing wireless capsule endoscopy. Capsule endoscopy can be used to view segments of the GIT that are not accessible by standard EGD, to screen for abnormalities or bleeding, check pH, and measure the time it takes to pass through different segments of the GIT. The procedure is less invasive than normal endoscopy and provides the advantage of being able to observe, record, and measure GI function as the patient is ambulatory.

However, the images from capsule endoscopy can be blurred by rapid intestinal transit or limited in number after battery failure in cases of slow transit. In addition, reviewing the thousands of images obtained after each capsule endoscopy can be very time consuming. Prototypes of the newest generation of capsule endoscopy allow the physician to magnetically guide the capsule to a specific location by having the patient lie on a special table. Future generations of capsule endoscopy are on the drawing boards to hopefully allow therapeutic measures to be accomplished in the small bowel via capsule endoscopy.

lead to behaviors that increase peptic ulcer risk. Although excessive use of concentrated forms of ethanol can damage gastric mucosa, worsen symptoms of peptic ulcers, and interfere with ulcer healing, alcohol consumption in moderation does not cause peptic ulcers in healthy people. Use of tobacco products also is linked with peptic ulcer risk, because tobacco decreases bicarbonate secretion and mucosal blood flow, exacerbates inflammation, and is associated with additional complications of *H. pylori* infection. Other risk factors include gastrinoma and Zollinger-Ellison syndrome (see Chapter 29).

The incidence and number of surgical procedures related to peptic ulcers has decreased markedly in the past 3 decades because of recognition of symptoms and risk factors, and earlier screening for *H. pylori*. Peptic ulcers normally involve two major regions: gastric and duodenal. Uncomplicated peptic ulcers in either region may present with signs similar to those associated with dyspepsia and gastritis.

Abdominal discomfort is the most common symptom of duodenal and gastric ulcers. Felt anywhere between the navel and the breastbone, this discomfort usually is a dull or burning pain, occurs when the stomach is empty—between meals or during the night, may be briefly relieved by eating food, in the case of duodenal ulcers, or by taking antacids. In both types of peptic ulcers the symptoms last for minutes to hours and come and go for several days or weeks. Other symptoms include

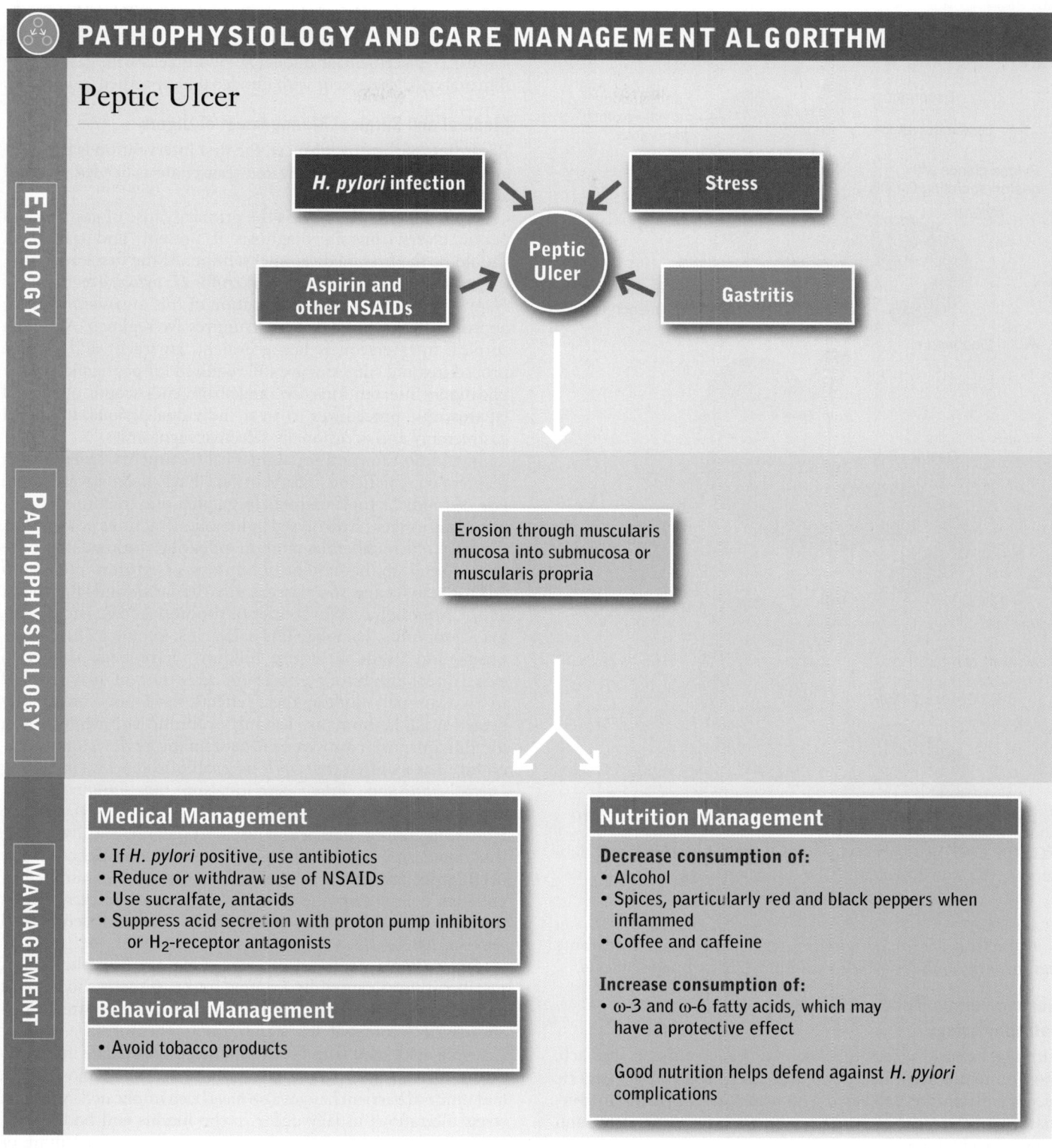

PATHOPHYSIOLOGY AND CARE MANAGEMENT ALGORITHM

Peptic Ulcer

ETIOLOGY

H. pylori infection → Peptic Ulcer ← Stress

Aspirin and other NSAIDs → Peptic Ulcer ← Gastritis

PATHOPHYSIOLOGY

Erosion through muscularis mucosa into submucosa or muscularis propria

MANAGEMENT

Medical Management

- If *H. pylori* positive, use antibiotics
- Reduce or withdraw use of NSAIDs
- Use sucralfate, antacids
- Suppress acid secretion with proton pump inhibitors or H$_2$-receptor antagonists

Behavioral Management

- Avoid tobacco products

Nutrition Management

Decrease consumption of:
- Alcohol
- Spices, particularly red and black peppers when inflammed
- Coffee and caffeine

Increase consumption of:
- ω-3 and ω-6 fatty acids, which may have a protective effect

Good nutrition helps defend against *H. pylori* complications

bloating, burping, nausea, vomiting, poor appetite, and weight loss. Some people experience only mild symptoms or none at all.

Peptic ulcers also may have "emergency symptoms," in which medical assistance should be sought immediately. These include sharp, sudden, persistent, and severe stomach pain, bloody or black stools (melena), bloody vomit (hematemesis), or vomit that looks like coffee grounds. These symptoms could be signs of a serious problem, such as acute or chronic GI bleeding—when acid or the peptic ulcer breaks a blood vessel; perforation—when the peptic ulcer burrows completely through the stomach or duodenal wall potentially penetrating an adjacent organ (e.g., pancreas); or obstruction—when the peptic ulcer blocks the path of food trying to leave the stomach.

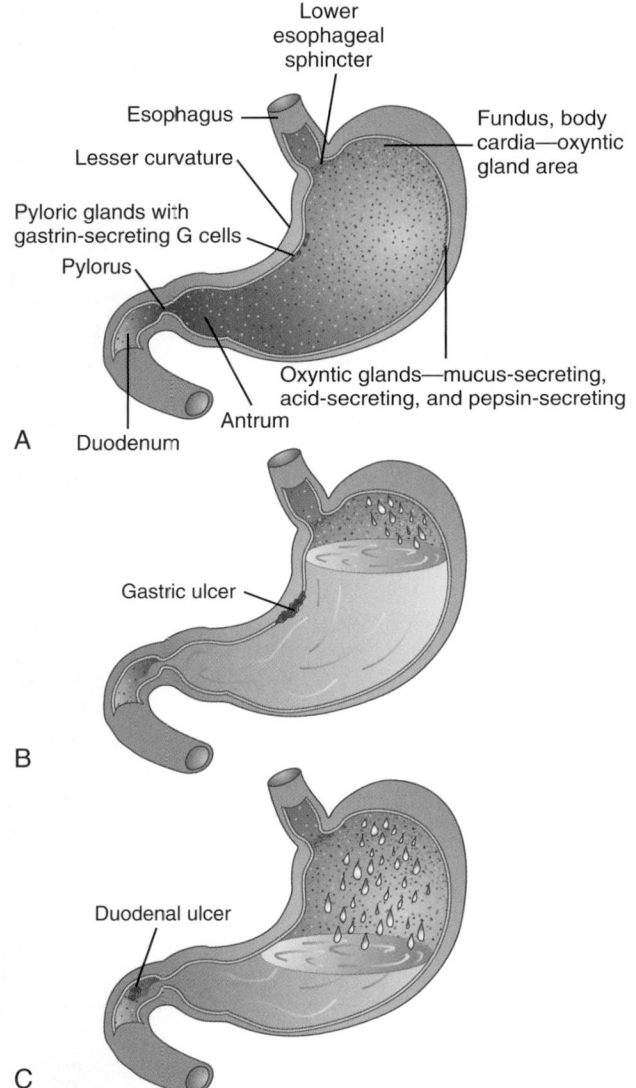

FIGURE 27-5 Diagram showing **(A)** normal stomach and duodenum; **(B)** a gastric ulcer; **(C)** a duodenal ulcer.

Complications of hemorrhage and perforation contribute significantly to the morbidity and mortality of peptic ulcers.

Gastric versus Duodenal Ulcers
Pathophysiology

Although gastric ulcers can occur anywhere in the stomach, most occur along the lesser curvature (see Figure 27-5). Gastric ulcers typically are associated with widespread gastritis, inflammatory involvement of parietal cells, and atrophy of acid- and pepsin-producing cells occurring with advancing age. In some cases gastric ulceration develops despite relatively low acid output. Antral hypomotility, gastric stasis, and increased duodenal reflux are associated commonly with gastric ulcers, and when present, may increase the severity of the gastric injury. The incidence of hemorrhage and overall mortality is higher with a gastric ulcer than a duodenal ulcer.

A duodenal ulcer is characterized by increased acid secretion throughout the entire day accompanied with decreased bicarbonate secretion. Most duodenal ulcers occur within the first few centimeters of the duodenal bulb, in an area immediately below

the pylorus. Gastric outlet obstruction occurs more commonly with duodenal ulcers than with gastric ulcers, and gastric metaplasia (e.g., replacement of duodenal villous cells with gastric-type mucosal cells) may occur with duodenal ulcer related to *H. pylori*.

Medical and Surgical Management of Ulcers

Regardless of the type of ulcer, the first intervention is to evaluate the patient endocopically and resuscitate as needed. Control acute bleeding if present.

Peptic Ulcers. *H. pylori* is the primary cause of gastritis and peptic ulcers, thus its diagnosis if present, and treatment, should be the first medical intervention. At the first endoscopy, diagnostic biopsies should be taken for *H. pylori*. Treatment of *H. pylori* infection entails eradication of this organism with the appropriate antibiotic and acid suppressive regimen. Although surgical intervention is less prevalent, emergent and elective procedures and surgeries are still required for peptic ulcer complications. Interventions can range from endoscopic, open, and laparoscopic procedures to treat individual lesions, to partial gastrectomy and occasionally selective vagotomies.

In addition to traditional medical treatments, several complementary medicine interventions have been investigated. Use of foods or their extracts (e.g., phenolic fractions of ginger and ginger hydrolysed phenolic fractions of ginger, *Zingiber officinale*) that contain phenolic antioxidants have been found to be potent inhibitors of proton potassium ATPase activity and *H. pylori* growth (Siddaraju and Dharmesh, 2007). Although certain species of probiotics (e.g., Lactobacillus acidophilus, Lactobacillus salivarius, Lactobacillus rhamnosus, and Bifidobacterium bifidum) have been shown to exert direct inhibitory effects on *H. pylori* in in-vitro and in-vivo animal models, these effects have not consistently been found in humans, leaving probiotic supplementation for this purpose controversial. Systematic reviews of the literature have shown that various probiotic species (including *Lactobacillus* spp., *Bifidobacterium* spp., *Saccharomyces* spp., and *Bacillus* spp.) can help diminish eradication-related side effects, including diarrhea, nausea, dyspepsia, and dysgeusia, thus increasing tolerability and therefore compliance. It has been postulated that it is this increase in the number of patients completing the therapy as prescribed that could, in turn, lead to higher eradication rates (Medeiros and Pereira, 2013).

Stress Ulcers. Stress ulcers may occur as a complication of metabolic stress caused by trauma, burns, surgery, shock, renal failure, or radiation therapy. A primary concern with stress ulceration is the potential for significant GI hemorrhage. Gastric ischemia associated with GI hypoperfusion, oxidative injury, reflux of bile salts and pancreatic enzymes, microbial colonization, and mucosal barrier changes also have been implicated. Although stress ulcerations usually occur in the fundus and body of the stomach, they also may develop in the antrum, duodenum, or distal esophagus. Typically shallow and causing oozing of blood from superficial capillary beds, stress ulcer lesions also may occur deeper, eroding into the submucosa, causing massive hemorrhage or perforation.

Stress ulcers that bleed can be a significant cause of morbidity in the critically ill patient (see Chapter 38). Although current prevention and treatment include sucralfate, acid suppressives, and antibiotics as needed, high-quality evidence to guide clinical practice in effective treatments is limited. Efforts to prevent gastric ulcers in stressed patients have focused on preventing or limiting conditions leading to hypotension and ischemia and coagulopathies. Avoiding NSAIDs and large doses of corticosteroids is also beneficial.

Providing oral or enteral feeding, when possible, increases GI vascular perfusion and stimulates secretion and motility. A meta-analysis of studies in critically ill patients that received an H2-receptor antagonist for stress ulcer prevention found this therapy to be preventative only in patients who did not receive enteral feeding. In fact, for patients receiving enteral feeding, H2-receptor antagonist therapy may increase the risk of pneumonia and death (Chanpura and Yende, 2012). Further research is needed to prospectively test the effect of enteral feeding on the risk of stress ulcer prophylaxis.

Medical Nutrition Therapy

In persons with atrophic gastritis, vitamin B_{12} status should be evaluated because of lack of intrinsic factor and gastric acid results in malabsorption of this vitamin (see Chapter 32). Low acid states may influence absorption of iron, calcium, and other nutrients because gastric acid enhances bioavailability. In the case of iron deficiency anemia, other causes may be the presence of H. pylori and gastritis. Eradication of H. pylori has resulted in improved absorption of iron and increased ferritin levels (Hershko and Ronson, 2009).

For several decades dietary factors have gained or lost favor as a significant component in the cause and treatment of dyspepsia, gastritis, and peptic ulcer disease. There is little evidence that specific dietary factors cause or exacerbate gastritis or peptic ulcer disease. Protein foods temporarily buffer gastric secretions, but they also stimulate secretion of gastrin, acid, and pepsin. Milk or cream, which in the early days of peptic ulcer management was considered important in coating the stomach, is no longer considered medicinal.

The pH of a food has little therapeutic importance, except for patients with existing lesions of the mouth or the esophagus. Most foods are considerably less acidic than the normal gastric pH of 1 to 3. The pH of orange juice and grapefruit is 3.2 to 3.6, and the pH of commonly used soft drinks ranges from approximately 2.8 to 3.5. On the basis of their intrinsic acidity and the amount consumed, fruit juices and soft drinks are not likely to cause peptic ulcers or appreciably interfere with healing. Some patients express discomfort with ingestion of acidic foods, but the response is not consistent among patients, and in some, symptoms may be related to heartburn. The dietary inclusion of "acidic foods" should be individualized based on the patient's perception of their effect.

Consumption of large amounts of alcohol may cause at least superficial mucosal damage and may worsen existing disease or interfere with treatment of the peptic ulcer. Modest consumption of alcohol does not appear to be pathogenic for peptic ulcers unless coexisting risk factors are also present. On the other hand, beers and wines significantly increase gastric secretions and should be avoided in symptomatic disease.

Coffee and caffeine stimulate acid secretion and also may decrease LES pressure; however, neither has been strongly implicated as a cause of peptic ulcers outside of the increased acid secretion and discomfort associated with their consumption.

When very large doses of certain spices are fed orally or placed intragastrically without other foods, they increase acid secretion and cause small, transient superficial erosions, inflammation of the mucosal lining, and altered GI permeability or motility. Most often incriminated are chili, cayenne, and black peppers. Small amounts of chili pepper or its pungent ingredient, capsicum, may increase mucosal protection by increasing production of mucus. However, large amounts may cause superficial mucosal damage, especially when consumed with alcohol. Another spice, curcumin, through its antiinflammatory activity that inhibits the NF-KB pathway activation may be a chemopreventative candidate against H. pylori–related cancer (Zaidi et al, 2009) (see Chapter 12).

The synergy of food combinations may inhibit the growth of H. pylori. Food provides an interesting alternative to therapies that include antibiotics, PPIs and bismuth salts (Kennan et al, 2010). Studies suggest that green tea, broccoli sprouts, black currant oil, and kimchi (fermented cabbage) help with H. pylori eradication. Probiotics species (Lactobacillus, Bifidobacterium) also have been studied for prevention, management, and eradication of H. pylori (Zhu et al, 2014).

Although these dietary supplements have some interesting results, they are not consistent, and therefore this therapy has not made it into general medical nutrition intervention. More controlled studies are needed.

Omega-3 and omega-6 fatty acids are involved in inflammatory, immune, and cytoprotective physiologic conditions of the GI mucosa, but they have not yet been found to be effective for treatment. Long-term clinical trials have not been performed.

Overall, a high-quality diet without nutrient deficiencies may offer some protection and may promote healing. Persons being treated for gastritis and peptic ulcer disease should be advised to avoid foods that exacerbate their symptoms and to consume a nutritionally complete diet with adequate dietary fiber from fruits and vegetables.

Carcinoma of the Stomach

Although the incidence and mortality have fallen dramatically over the last 50 years in many regions, gastric cancer is still the second most common cause of cancer death worldwide, with varying incidence in different parts of the world and among various ethnic groups (Nagini, 2012). Despite advances in diagnosis and treatment, the 5-year survival rate of stomach cancer is only 20%.

Etiology

The cause of gastric cancer is multifactorial, but more than 80% of cases have been attributed to H. pylori infection. In addition, diet, lifestyle, genetic, socioeconomic, and other factors contribute to gastric carcinogenesis. A Western diet, high in processed meats, fat, starches, and simple sugars, is associated with an increased risk of gastric cancer compared with a diet high in fruits and vegetables (Bertuccio et al, 2013). Other factors that may increase the risk of gastric cancer include alcohol consumption, excess body weight, smoking, intake of highly salted or pickled foods, or inadequate amounts of micronutrients. Certain cooking practices also are associated with increased risk of gastric cancer including broiling of meats, roasting, grilling, baking, and deep frying in open furnaces, sun drying, salting, curing, and pickling, all of which increase the formation of carcinogenic N-nitroso compounds. Polycyclic aromatic hydrocarbons such as benzo[a]pyrene formed in smoked food have been incriminated in many areas of the world (Nagini, 2012).

Pathophysiology

Stomach cancer refers to any malignant neoplasm that arises from the region extending between the gastroesophageal junction and the pylorus. Because symptoms are slow to manifest themselves and the growth of the tumor is rapid, carcinoma of the stomach frequently is overlooked until it is too late for a cure. Loss of appetite, strength, and weight frequently precede other symptoms. In some cases achylia gastrica (absence of HCl and pepsin) or achlorhydria (absence of HCl in gastric secretions) may exist for years before the onset of gastric carcinoma. Malignant gastric neoplasms can lead to malnutrition as a result of excessive blood and protein losses or, more commonly, because of obstruction and mechanical interference with food intake.

Medical and Surgical Management

Most cancers of the stomach are treated by surgical resection; thus part of the nutritional considerations includes partial or total resection of the stomach, a gastrectomy. Some patients may experience difficulties with nutrition after surgery.

Medical Nutrition Therapy

The dietary regimen for carcinoma of the stomach is determined by the location of the cancer, the nature of the functional disturbance, and the stage of the disease. The patient with advanced, inoperable cancer should receive a diet that is adjusted to his or her tolerances, preferences, and comfort. Anorexia is almost always present from the early stages of disease. In the later stages of the disease, the patient may tolerate only a liquid diet. If a patient is unable to tolerate oral feeding, consideration should be given to using an alternate route, such as a gastric or intestinal enteral tube feeding, or if this is not tolerated or feasible, parenteral feeding. The nutritional support for the patient should be in accordance with the patient's goals of care (see Chapter 13).

Gastric Surgeries

Because of increased recognition and treatment for *H. pylori* and acid secretion, gastric surgeries are performed less frequently. However, partial or total gastrectomy may still be necessary for patients with ulcer disease that does not respond to therapy, or for those with malignancy. Gastric surgeries performed for weight loss or bariatric surgeries are more common. These surgeries, such as Roux-en-Y gastric bypass, gastric banding, sleeve gastrectomy, vertical banding gastroplasty, and jejunoileal bypass are designed to induce weight loss though volume restriction, malabsorption, or both (see Chapter 21).

Types of Surgeries

A total gastrectomy involves removal of the entire stomach, whereas only a portion of the stomach is removed with a subtotal gastrectomy. A gastrectomy is accompanied by a reconstructive procedure. A total gastrectomy is performed for malignancies that affect the middle or upper stomach. The total stomach is removed and a Roux-en-Y reconstruction is performed to maintain GI tract continuity. With a Roux-en-Y, the jejunum is pulled up and anastomosed to the esophagus. The duodenum is then connected to the small bowel so that bile and pancreatic secretions can flow into the intestine. Billroth I (gastroduodenostomy) involves removal of the pylorus and/or antrum, and an anastomosis of the proximal end of the duodenum to the distal end of the remnant stomach. A Billroth II (gastrojejunostomy) involves removal of the stomach antrum and an anastomosis of the remnant stomach to the side of the jejunum, which creates a blind duodenal loop (see Figure 27-6).

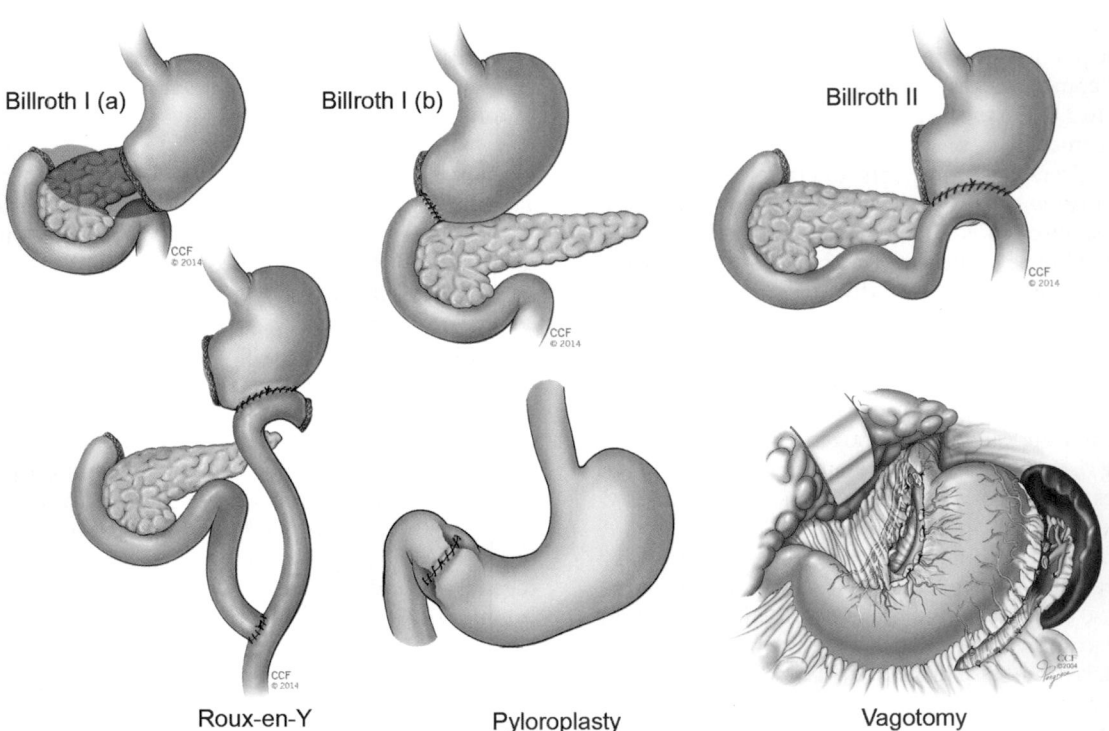

Billroth I (a)   Billroth I (b)   Billroth II

Roux-en-Y   Pyloroplasty   Vagotomy

FIGURE 27-6 Gastric surgical procedures [Bilroth I (A: preoperative and B: postoperative), Billroth II, Roux en Y, pylorplasty, vagotomy].

TABLE 27-4   Gastric Surgery–Related Nutrition Complications

Surgical Procedure	Potential Complications
Vagotomy	Impairs motor function of stomach
Total gastric and truncal vagotomy	Gastric stasis and poor gastric emptying
Total gastrectomy	Early satiety, nausea, vomiting Weight loss Inadequate bile acids and pancreatic enzymes available because of anastomotic changes Malabsorption Protein-energy malnutrition Anemia Dumping syndrome Bezoar formation Vitamin B_{12} deficiency Metabolic bone disease
Subtotal gastrectomy with vagotomy	Early satiety Delayed gastric emptying Rapid emptying of hypertonic fluids

Cresci G et al: *Nutrition essentials of general surgery*, ed 5, Lippincott Williams & Wilkins, 2013, Table 3-13, p 72.

The **vagus nerve** is responsible for not only motility, but also stimulation of parietal cells in the proximal stomach, therefore a **vagotomy** often is performed to eliminate gastric acid secretion. **Truncal vagotomy**, complete severing of the vagus nerve on the distal esophagus, decreases acid secretion by parietal cells in the stomach and decreases their response to the hormone gastrin. A **parietal cell vagotomy** (partial or selective) divides and severs only the vagus nerve branches that affect the proximal stomach where gastric acid secretion occurs, whereas the antrum and pylorus remain innervated. Vagotomy at certain levels can alter the normal physiologic function of the stomach, small intestine, pancreas, and biliary system. Vagotomy procedures commonly are accompanied by a drainage procedure (antrectomy or **pyloroplasty**) that aids with gastric emptying.

Postoperative Medical Nutrition Therapy

Oral intake of fluids and foods is initiated as soon as GI tract function returns (typically 24 to 72 hours postoperatively). Small frequent feedings of ice or water are normally initiated, followed by liquids and easily digested solid foods, after which the patient can progress to a regular diet. Although this is the common postoperative diet intervention, there is limited evidence supporting this practice. In fact, some studies suggest beginning a regular diet of tolerated foods as the first diet to improve patient tolerance (Warren et al, 2011). If the patient is unable to tolerate an oral diet for an extended period of time (e.g., 5 to 7 days), then enteral feeding should be considered if appropriate feeding access is available, and if not, parenteral nutrition should be considered.

Understanding the surgery performed and patient's resulting anatomy is paramount to providing proper nutritional care. Nutritional complications after gastric surgeries are varied (see Table 27-4). Complications such as obstruction, dumping, abdominal discomfort, diarrhea, and weight loss may occur, depending on the nature and extent of the disease and surgical interventions (see Figure 27-6). Patients may have difficulty regaining normal preoperative weight because of inadequate food intake related to (1) early satiety, (2) symptoms of dumping syndrome (see later in this chapter), or (3) nutrient malabsorption.

Patients with certain gastric surgeries, such as Billroth II, result in a mismatch in timing of food entry into the small intestine and the release and interaction with bile and pancreatic enzymes, contributing to impaired nutrient digestion and absorption. Patients who are lactose tolerant before gastric surgery may experience relative lactase deficiency, either because food enters the small intestine further downstream from adequate lactase presence, or because the rate of transit through the proximal small intestine is increased. Because of the complications of reflux or dumping syndrome associated with traditional gastrectomies, other procedures are used, including truncal, selective, or parietal cell vagotomy, pyloromyotomy, antrectomy, Roux-en-Y esophagojejunostomy, loop esophagojejunostomy, and pouches or reservoirs made from jejunal or ileocecal segments.

Some chronic nutritional complications that can occur after gastric surgery include anemia, osteoporosis, and select vitamin and mineral deficiencies resulting from inadequate intake and or malabsorption. Iron deficiency may be attributed to loss of acid secretion because gastric acid normally facilitates the reduction of iron compounds, allowing their absorption. Rapid transit and diminished contact of dietary iron with sites of iron absorption can also lead to iron deficiency.

Vitamin B_{12} deficiency may cause a megaloblastic anemia (see Chapter 32). If the amount of gastric mucosa is reduced, intrinsic factor may not be produced in quantities adequate to allow for complete vitamin B_{12} absorption, and pernicious anemia may result. Bacterial overgrowth in the proximal small bowel or the afferent loop contributes to vitamin B_{12} depletion because bacteria compete with the host for use of the vitamin. Therefore after gastrectomy patients should receive prophylactic vitamin B_{12} supplementation (injections) or take synthetic oral supplementation.

Dumping Syndrome
Etiology

The **dumping syndrome** is a complex GI and vasomotor response to the presence of large quantities of hypertonic foods and liquids in the proximal small intestine. Dumping syndrome usually occurs as a result of surgical procedures that allow excessive amounts of liquid or solid foods to enter the small intestine in a concentrated form. Milder forms of dumping may occur to varying degrees in persons without surgical procedures, and most of the symptoms can be reproduced in normal individuals by infusing a loading dose of glucose into the jejunum. Dumping may occur as a result of total or partial gastrectomy, manipulation of the pylorus, fundoplication, vagotomy, and some gastric bypass procedures for obesity. As a result of better medical management of peptic ulcers, use of selective vagotomies, and newer surgical procedures to avoid complications, classic dumping is encountered less frequently in clinical practice.

Pathophysiology

Symptoms can be divided into two stages of dumping of solids and liquids into the small intestine: early (within 10 to 30 minutes postprandially) and late (1-3 hrs postprandially). Characteristics and severity of symptoms vary between patients.

Early dumping is characterized by GI and vasomotor symptoms, which include abdominal pain, bloating, nausea, vomiting, diarrhea, headache, flushing, fatigue, and hypotension.

These early symptoms likely occur because of the rapid influx of hyperosmolar contents into the duodenum or small intestine. A subsequent fluid shift from the intravascular compartment to the intestinal lumen occurs resulting in small intestine distention potentially causing cramps and bloating.

Late symptoms are predominantly vasomotor and include perspiration, weakness, confusion, shakiness, hunger, and hypoglycemia (Tack et al, 2009). Late dumping is likely the result of reactive hypoglycemia. Rapid delivery, as well as hydrolysis and absorption of carbohydrates, produces an exaggerated rise in insulin level and a subsequent decline in blood glucose. The rapid changes in blood glucose and the secretion of gut peptides, glucose insulinotropic polypeptide, and glucagon-like polypeptide-1 appear to be at least partly responsible for the late symptoms (Deloose et al, 2014) (see Chapter 30).

Medical Management

Medical intervention typically involves dietary changes as the initial treatment, and they are usually effective. However, in 3% to 5% of patients, severe dumping persists despite dietary change. In these patients, medications may be used to slow gastric emptying and delay transit of food through the GI tract. Some, such as acarbose, inhibit alpha glycoside hydrolase and interfere with carbohydrate absorption, and octreotide, a somatostatin analog, inhibits insulin release (see Table 27-3 for common medications). Rarely, surgical intervention is used to treat dumping syndrome.

Medical Nutrition Therapy

Patients with dumping syndrome may experience weight loss and malnutrition caused by inadequate intake, malabsorption, or a combination of both. The prime objective of nutrition therapy is to restore nutrition status and quality of life. Because they are digested more slowly, proteins and fats are better tolerated than carbohydrates, particularly simple carbohydrates. Simple carbohydrates such as lactose, sucrose, fructose, glucose and dextrose are hydrolyzed rapidly and should be limited, but complex carbohydrates (starches) can be included in the diet.

Liquids leave the stomach and enter the jejunum rapidly; thus some patients have trouble tolerating liquids with meals. Patients with severe dumping may benefit from limiting the amount of liquids taken with meals and drinking liquids between meals without solid food. Reclining (approximately 30 degrees) after meals may also minimize severity of symptoms.

The use of fiber supplements, particularly pectin or gums (e.g., guar) can be beneficial in managing dumping syndrome because of fiber's ability to form gels with carbohydrates and fluids and delay GI transit. Patients may need to be taught about portion sizes of foods, especially of carbohydrate foods such as juices, soft drinks, desserts, and milk. The exchange list given in Appendix 27 can be used to calculate carbohydrate intake and teach about carbohydrate control.

Postgastrectomy patients often do not tolerate lactose, but small amounts (e.g., 6 g or less per meal) may be tolerated at one time. Patients typically do better with cheeses or unsweetened yogurt than with fluid milk. Nondairy milks are also useful. Vitamin D and calcium supplements may be needed when intake is inadequate. Commercial lactase-containing products are available for those with significant lactose malabsorption (see Chapter 28 for further discussion of lactose intolerance and its management).

When steatorrhea (greater than 7% of dietary fat in the stool) exists, reduced fat formulas or pancreatic enzymes may

---

BOX 27-5 Basic Guidelines for Dumping Syndrome

1. Eat small, frequent "meals" per day.
2. Limit fluids to 4 ounces (½ cup) at a meal, just enough to "wash" food down.
3. Drink remaining fluids at least 30 to 40 minutes before and after meals.
4. Eat slowly and chew foods thoroughly.
5. Avoid extreme temperatures of foods.
6. Use seasonings and spices as tolerated (may want to avoid pepper, hot sauce).
7. Remain reclined at least 30 minutes after eating.
8. Sugar-containing foods and liquids are limited. Examples: fruit juice, Gatorade, PowerAde, Kool Aid, sweet tea, sucrose, honey, jelly, corn syrup, cookies, pie, doughnuts
9. Complex carbohydrates are unlimited (e.g., bread, pasta, rice, potatoes, vegetables).
10. Include a protein-containing food at each meal.
11. Limit fats (less than 30% of total calories).
    Avoid fried foods, gravies, fat containing sauces, mayonnaise, fatty meats (sausage, hot dogs, ribs), chips, biscuits, pancakes.
12. Milk and dairy products may not be tolerated because of lactose. Introduce these slowly in the diet if they were tolerated preoperatively. Lactose-free milk or soy milk is suggested.

---

be beneficial. Box 27-5 provides general nutrition guidelines for patients with dumping syndrome after gastric surgery; however, each diet must be adjusted based on a careful dietary and social history from the patient.

GASTROPARESIS

Etiology

Gastroparesis, or delayed gastric emptying, is a complex and potentially debilitating condition. The nature of gastroparesis is complex in part because gastric motility is orchestrated by a variety of chemical and neurologic factors. Viral infection, diabetes, and surgeries are the most common causes for gastroparesis; however, more than 30% of cases are idiopathic. Numerous classes of clinical conditions are associated with gastroparesis, including acid-peptic diseases, gastritis, postgastric surgery, disorder of gastric smooth muscle, psychogenic disorders, long-term uncontrolled diabetes, and neuropathic disorders.

Pathophysiology

Clinical symptoms may include abdominal bloating, decreased appetite and anorexia, nausea and vomiting, fullness, early satiety, halitosis, and postprandial hypoglycemia. The gold-standard measure of gastric emptying rate is scintigraphy, a nuclear test of gastric emptying. This consists of the patient ingesting a radionucleotide-labeled meal (such as an egg labeled ^{90m}technetium), and scintigraphic images are taken over time (generally 4 hours) to assess the rate of gastric emptying. Gastric emptying is abnormal when greater than 50% of the meal is retained after 2 hours of study or when greater than 10% of the meal is retained after 4 hours (Maurer and Parkman, 2006).

Medical Management

Numerous symptoms of gastroparesis can affect oral intake, and the management of these symptoms generally improves nutrition status. Treatment of nausea and vomiting is perhaps the most vital, and prokinetics and antiemetics are the primary medical therapies (see Table 27-3). Metoclopramide and erythromycin are medications that may be used to promote gastric motility. Small intestinal bacterial overgrowth, appetite, ileal brake (the slowing effect of intestinal transit of undigested food, often fat, reaching the ileum), or formation of a bezoar (concentration of undigested material in the stomach) are other factors that may affect nutritional status. In a select patient population, implantation of gastric pacemakers may be advantageous to improve gastric emptying (Ross et al, 2014).

Bezoar formation may be related to undigested food such as cellulose, hemicellulose, lignin and fruit tannins (phytobezoars), or medications (pharmacobezoars) such as cholestyramine, sucralfate, enteric-coated aspirin, aluminum-containing antacids, and bulk-forming laxatives. Treatment of bezoars includes enzyme therapy (such as papain, bromelain, or cellulase), lavage, and sometimes endoscopic therapy to mechanically break up the bezoar. Most patients respond to some combination of medication and dietary intervention; however, unresponsive and more severe cases may benefit from placement of an enteral tube into the small intestine, such as a nasoenteric small bowel feeding tube (for less than 4-week need) or percutaneous endoscopic gastrostomy with jejunal extension (PEG/J) (for more than 4 week need). The latter allows for nutrition to bypass the stomach while providing an alternative route for venting of gastric secretions, which may relieve nausea and vomiting.

Medical Nutrition Therapy

The primary dietary factors that affect gastric emptying (in order of clinical importance) are volume, liquids versus solids, hyperglycemia, fiber, fat, and osmolality. Larger volumes of food that create stomach distension (approximately 600 ml) have been shown to delay gastric emptying and increase satiety (Oesch et al, 2006). Generally, patients benefit from smaller, more frequent meals. Patients with gastroparesis often continue to empty liquids, as they empty, in part, by gravity and do not require antral contraction.

Shifting the diet to more pureed and liquefied foods is often useful. A number of medications (such as narcotics and anticholinergics) slow gastric emptying and should be avoided if possible. Moderate to severe hyperglycemia (serum blood glucose more than 200 mg/dl) may acutely slow gastric motility, with long-term detrimental effects on gastric nerves and motility. Laboratory data considered in initial assessment include glycosylated hemoglobin A1C (if diabetes is present), ferritin, vitamin B_{12}, and 25-OH vitamin D (see Chapter 30).

Fiber, particularly pectin, can slow gastric emptying and increase risk of bezoar formation in patients who are susceptible. It is prudent to advise patients to avoid high-fiber foods and fiber supplements. The size of the fibrous particles, not the amount of fiber, is more important in bezoar risk (e.g., potato skins versus bran). This and the resistance to chewing are factors in bezoar formation. Examination of the patient's dentition is very important because patients who have missing teeth, a poor bite, or are edentulous are at greater risk. Even people with good dentition have swallowed and passed food particles up to 5 to 6 cm in diameter (potato skins, seeds, tomato skins, peanuts).

Fat is a powerful inhibitor of stomach emptying primarily mediated by cholecystokinin (Goetze et al, 2007); however, many patients tolerate fat well in liquid form. Fat should not be restricted in patients who are struggling to meet their daily caloric needs.

CLINICAL CASE STUDY

Jane is a 42-year-old female who presents with acute onset of epigastric abdominal pain associated with nausea and bilious vomiting, poor appetite, and 20-pound (9-kg) unintentional weight loss over the past 3 months. A nutrition consult is requested for assessment of nutritional status and strategies for treating nutritional issues associated with gastroparesis.

Nutrition Assessment

- Past medical history is significant for type I DM, GERD, gastroparesis, hypertension, chronic low back pain, and recent back surgery 3 months ago. Jane was discharged on narcotics, and then was recently hospitalized for similar symptoms that were attributed to diabetic gastroparesis exacerbated by narcotics use.
- Her medications on admission include insulin, Zofran, Prilosec, Reglan, lisinopril, Ultram.
- Oral intake has gradually decreased over the last 3 months to sips of liquids (water, soup, tea), and toast or crackers for the past 2 weeks. Upon further questioning, Jane reports frequent hypoglycemia after meals, early satiety, chronic constipation, and often wakes up in the morning feeling full. She has persistent epigastric abdominal pain accompanied by vomiting.
- Anthropometrics: Ht: 162.5 cm (64 inches); Wt: 72.7 kg (160 lb); BMI: 27.5 kg/m²
- Usual body weight: 81.8 kg (180 lbs); weight change: 11% change in 3 months (significant weight loss).
- Jane's nutrition-focused physical examination (NFPE) reveals the following: No evidence of muscle loss; stomach is smaller per patient report but otherwise no visible evidence of fat loss; no upper or lower extremity edema. Tongue is beefy red and swollen for the past few weeks (glossitis resulting from possible iron, folate, and vitamin B_{12} deficiency).

- Functional capacity: Little energy or motivation to do anything for past 3 months. Dizzy and lightheaded for past 1 week.
- Laboratory data: Hb A1C (glycosylated hemoglobin) level: 9.5% (high), blood pressure: 178/95 (high), blood glucose: 293 mg/dl (high)

Nutrition Diagnostic Statements (PES Statements)

- Suboptimal oral intake (P) related to inability to consume sufficient calories (E) as evidenced by report of nausea, vomiting, and persistent abdominal pain (S).
- Unintended weight loss (P) related to altered GI function (E) as evidenced by 11% weight loss over past 3 months (S).

Nutrition Interventions

1) What would you estimate to be Jane's daily energy and protein requirements?
2) What would you work out with Jane for timing and size of her meals?
3) Would you recommend a trial of oral nutrition supplements?
4) In educating Jane on dietary guidelines for DM and gastroparesis, what would you discuss with her?
5) What concerns would you have related to her use of antiemetics or prokinetic agents.
6) Would you recommend any nutritional supplements for Jane? Which nutrients would concern you?

Nutrition Monitoring and Evaluation

1) What would you monitor during your followup visits with Jane to ensure that her nutrition goals are being met?

USEFUL WEBSITES

American College of Gastroenterology
http://www.acg.gi.org/
American Gastroenterological Association
http://www.gastro.org/
International Foundation for Functional Gastrointestinal Disorders
http://www.aboutgimotility.org
The Gastroparesis and Dysmotilities Association
http://www.digestivedistress.com/
National Digestive Diseases Information Clearinghouse
http://www.digestive.niddk.nih.gov/

REFERENCES

Asanuma K, et al: Gender difference in gastro-esophageal reflux diseases, *World J Gastroenterol* 22:1800, 2016.

Beaumont H, Bennink RJ, de Jong J, et al: The position of the acid pocket as a major risk factor for acidic reflux in healthy subjects and patients with GORD, *Gut* 59:441, 2010.

Bertuccio P, Rosato V, Andreano A, et al: Dietary patterns and gastric cancer risk: a systematic review and meta-analysis, *Ann Oncol* 24:1450, 2013.

Bertuccio P, Rosato V, Andreano A, et al: Dietary patterns and gastric cancer risk: a systematic review and meta-analysis, *Ann Oncol* 24:1450, 2013.

Centers for Disease Control (CDC): *NAMCS and NHAMCS web tables* (website), 2014. http://www.cdc.gov/nchs/ahcd/web_tables.htm. Accessed February 1, 2015.

Chanpura T, Yende S: Weighing risks and benefits of stress ulcer prophylaxis in critically ill patients, *Critical Care* 16:322, 2012.

Deloose E, Bisschops R, Holvoet L, et al: A pilot study of the effects of the somatostatin analog pasireotide in postoperative dumping syndrome, *Neurogastroenterol Motil* 26:803, 2014.

Dos Santos AA, Carvalho AA: Pharmacological therapy used in the elimination of Helicobacter pylori infection: a review, *World J Gastroenterol* 21:139, 2015.

Ford AC, Moayyedi P: Dyspepsia, *Curr Opin Gastroenterol* 29:662, 2013.

Gilbert EW, Luna RA, Harrison VL, et al: Barrett's esophagus: a review of the literature, *J Gastrointest Surg* 15:708, 2011.

Goetze O, Steingoetter A, Menne D, et al: The effect of macronutrients on gastric volume responses and gastric emptying in humans: a magnetic resonance imaging study, *Am J Physiol Gastrointest Liver Physiol* 292:G11, 2007.

Hershko C, Ronson A: Iron deficiency, Helicobacter infection and gastritis, *Acta Haematol* 122:97, 2009.

Hyun JJ, Bak YT: Clinical significance of hiatal hernia, *Gut Liver* 5:267, 2011.

Jung HK: Epidemiology of gastroesophageal reflux disease in Asia: a systematic review, *J Neurogastroenterol Motil* 17:14, 2011.

Katz MH: Failing the acid test: benefits of proton pump inhibitors may not justify the risks for many users, *Arch Intern Med* 170:747, 2010.

Katz PO, Gerson LB, Vela MF: Guidelines for the diagnosis and management of gastroesophageal reflux disease, *Am J Gastrotenterol* 108:308, 2013.

Kennan JI, Salm N, Hampton MB, et al: Individual and combined effects of foods on Helicobacter pylori growth, *Phytother Res* 24:1229, 2010.

Lacy BE, Talley NJ, Locke GR 3rd, et al: Review article: current treatment options and management of functional dyspepsia, *Aliment Pharmacol Ther* 36:3, 2012.

la Roca-Chiapas JM, Cordova-Fraga T: Biomagnetic techniques for evaluating gastric emptying, peristaltic contraction and transit time, *World J Gastrointest Pathophysiol* 15:65, 2011.

Lightdale JR, Gremse DA, Section on Gastroenterology, Hepatology, and Nutrition: Gastroesophageal reflux: management guidance for the pediatrician, *Pediatrics* 131:e1684, 2013.

Linsky A, Gupta K, Lawler EV, et al: Proton pump inhibitors and risk for recurrent Clostridium difficile infection, *Arch Intern Med* 170:772, 2010.

McColl KE: Effect of proton pump inhibitors on vitamins and iron, *Am J Gastroenterol* 104(Suppl 2):S5, 2009.

Medeiros JA, Pereira MI: The use of probiotics in Helicobacter pylori eradication therapy, *J Clin Gastroenterol* 47:1, 2013.

Milke P, Diaz A, Valdovinos MA, et al: Gastroesophageal reflux in healthy subjects induced by two different species of chilli (Capsicum annum), *Dig Dis* 24:184, 2006.

Nagini S: Carcinoma of the stomach: a review of epidemiology, pathogenesis, molecular genetics and chemoprevention, *World J Gastrointest Oncol* 4:156, 2012.

Oesch S, Rüegg C, Fischer B, et al: Effect of gastric distension prior to eating on food intake and feelings of satiety in humans, *Physiol Behav* 87:903, 2006.

Penagini R, Bravi I: The role of delayed gastric emptying and impaired esophageal body motility, *Best Pract Res Clin Gastroenterol* 24:831, 2010.

Ross J, Masrur M, Gonzalez-Heredia R, et al: Effectiveness of gastric neurostimulation in patients with gastroparesis, *JSLS* 18:pii:e2014.00400, 2014.

Schoeff SS, Barrett DM, Gress CD, et al: Nutritional management of head and neck cancer patients, *Pract Gastroenterol* 121:43, 2013.

Siddaraju MN, Dharmesh SM: Inhibition of gastric H+, K+-ATPase and Helicobacter pylori growth by phenolic antioxidants of Zingiber officinale, *Mol Nutr Food Res* 51:324, 2007.

Stefanidis D, Hope WW, Kohn GP, et al: Guidelines for surgical treatment of gastroesophageal reflux disease, *Surg Endosc* 24:2647, 2010.

Tack J, Arts J, Caenepeel P, et al: Pathophysiology, diagnosis and management of postoperative dumping syndrome, *Nat Rev Gastroenterol Hepatol* 6:583, 2009.

Talley NJ, Ford AC: Functional dyspepsia, *N Engl J Med* 373:1853, 2015.

Thrift AP, Whiteman DC: The incidence of esophageal adenocarcinoma continues to rise: analysis of period and birth cohort effects on recent trends, *Ann Oncol* 23:3155, 2012.

Warren J, Bhalla V, Cresci G: Postoperative diet advancement: surgical dogma vs evidence-based medicine, *Nutr Clin Pract* 26:115, 2011.

Yang YX: Chronic proton pump inhibitor therapy and calcium metabolism, *Curr Gastroenterol Rep* 14:473, 2012.

Zaidi SF, Yamamoto T, Refaat A, et al: Modulation of activation-induced cytidine deaminase by curcumin in Helicobacter pylori-infected gastric epithelial cells, *Helicobacter* 14:588, 2009.

Zhu R, Chen K, Zheng YY, et al: Meta-analysis of the efficacy of probiotics in Helicobacter pylori eradication therapy, *World J Gastroenterol* 20:18013, 2014.

28

Medical Nutrition Therapy for Lower Gastrointestinal Tract Disorders

Gail Cresci, PhD, RD, LD, CNSC and Arlene Escuro, MS, RDN, CNSC

KEY TERMS

aerophagia
antibiotic-associated diarrhea (AAD)
Clostridium difficile infection (CDI)
celiac disease (CD)
colitis, collagenous
colitis, lymphocytic
colitis, microscopic
colostomy
constipation
Crohn's disease
dermatitis herpetiformis
diarrhea
dietary fiber
diverticulitis
diverticulosis
enterocutaneous fistula (ECF)
eructation
fecal microbiota transplant (FMT)
fistula
flatulence
flatus

FODMAPs
fructose malabsorption
functional constipation
glutamine
gluten
gluten intolerance
gluten-sensitive enteropathy
gluten sensitivity
high-fiber diet
high-output stoma (HOS)
hypolactasia
ileal J-pouch
ileal pouch anal anastomosis (IPAA)
ileostomy
inflammatory bowel disease (IBD)
intestinal ostomy
irritable bowel syndrome (IBS)
Koch pouch
lactose intolerance
medium-chain triglycerides (MCTs)
microbiota

osmotic agents
ostomy
polyp
pouchitis
prebiotics
probiotics
proctocolectomy
refractory celiac disease
Rome III criteria
short-bowel syndrome (SBS)
small intestine bacterial overgrowth (SIBO)
soluble fiber
S-pouch
steatorrhea
stimulant laxatives
stool softeners
synbiotics
tropical sprue
ulcerative colitis (UC)
W-pouch

Nutrition status and the digestive tract are inextricably linked. Dietary interventions for many diseases of the intestinal tract are designed primarily to alleviate symptoms and to correct nutrient deficiencies. A comprehensive nutritional assessment should be performed to determine the nature and severity of the gastrointestinal (GI) problem. Information to be obtained should include a history of weight change, medications used (including supplements), presence of GI and other symptoms that may affect oral intake or fluid loss, and potential signs and symptoms of micronutrient deficiencies.

COMMON INTESTINAL PROBLEMS

It is important to understand some of the common GI processes that occur in healthy people before discussing diseases relating to lower GI tract. Dietary ramifications of intestinal gas, flatulence, constipation, and diarrhea often are considered in the management of more serious GI disorders.

Sections of this chapter were written by Nora Decher, MS, RD, CNSD and Joseph S. Krenitsky, MS, RD for the previous edition of this text.

Intestinal Gas and Flatulence
Pathophysiology

The daily volume of human intestinal gas is about 200 ml, and it is derived from complex physiologic processes, including swallowed air (aerophagia) and bacterial fermentation by the intestinal tract. These gases are either expelled through belching (eructation) or passed rectally (flatus). Intestinal gases include carbon dioxide (CO_2), oxygen (O_2), nitrogen (N_2), hydrogen (H_2), and sometimes methane (CH_4). Studies have detected CH_4 production in about one third of healthy adult individuals (Sahakian et al, 2010). Intestinal CH_4 production is a complex mechanism involving metabolism of other gases, particularly H_2, and from specific bacteria in the colon. Abnormal CH_4 production has been considered in the pathogenesis of several intestinal disorders, such as colon cancer, inflammatory bowel disease (IBD), irritable bowel syndrome, and diverticulosis (Triantafyllou et al, 2014).

When patients complain about "excessive gas" or flatulence, they may be referring to increased volume or frequency of belching or passage of rectal gas. They also may complain of abdominal distention or cramping associated with the accumulation of gases in the upper or lower GI tract. The amount of air swallowed increases with eating or drinking too fast, smoking, chewing gum, sucking on hard candy, using a straw, drinking carbonated drinks, and wearing loose-fitting dentures. Foods that produce gas in one person may not cause gas in someone else, depending on the mix of microorganisms in the individual's colon. Inactivity, decreased motility, aerophagia, dietary components, and certain GI disorders can alter the amount of intestinal gas and individual symptoms.

Normally, the concentration of bacteria in the small intestine is significantly lower than that found in the colon. Various conditions can lead to overgrowth of bacteria in the small intestine causing bloating, distention, nausea, diarrhea, or other symptoms. Factors such as gastric acid, intestinal peristalsis, the ileocecal valve, bile acids, the enteric immune system, and pancreatic enzyme secretion prevent the overgrowth of bacteria within the small intestine.

Medical Nutrition Therapy

When evaluating a patient, clinicians must investigate and differentiate between increased production of gas and gas that is not being passed. It is also important to consider why a patient may have new or increased symptoms or if gas is accompanied by other symptoms such as constipation, diarrhea, or weight loss. Keeping a food diary to track eating habits and symptoms may help identify specific foods that cause gas. Careful review of the diet and the amount of burping or gas passed may help relate specific foods to symptoms and determine the severity of the problem.

If milk or milk products are causing gas, a patient is evaluated for lactose intolerance and advised to avoid milk products for a short time to see if symptoms improve. Recent viral or GI infection may induce temporary or even permanent impairment in the ability to digest lactose. Lactase tablets, drops, and lactose-free milk products are available to help digest lactose and reduce gas.

A sudden change in diet, such as a drastic increase in fiber intake, also can alter gas production. Specific foods that contain raffinose (a complex sugar resistant to digestion) such as beans, cabbage, broccoli, Brussels sprouts, asparagus, and some whole grains can increase gas production. Box 28-1 outlines foods that may cause increase in gas production.

BOX 28-1   Foods that may Increase Gas Production

1. Beans
2. Vegetables such as broccoli, cauliflower, cabbage, Brussels sprouts, onions, mushrooms, artichokes, and asparagus
3. Fruits such as pears, apples, and peaches
4. Whole grains such as whole wheat and bran
5. Sodas: fruit drinks especially apple juice and pear juice; and other drinks that contain high-fructose corn syrup, a sweetener made from corn
6. Milk and milk products such as cheese, ice cream, and yogurt
7. Packaged foods such as bread, cereal, and salad dressing that contain small amounts of lactose, a sugar found in milk and foods made with milk
8. Sugar-free candies and gums that contain sugar alcohols such as sorbitol, mannitol, and xylitol

From National Institute of Diabetes and Digestive and Kidney Diseases: *Digestive Diseases A-Z* (website): http://digestive.niddk.nih.gov/. Accessed January 4, 2014.

Changes in the intestinal flora occur over time after an increase in dietary fiber. A gradual introduction of fiber with adequate fluid consumption appears to reduce complaints of gas. Inactivity, constipation, intestinal dysmotility, or partial bowel obstruction may contribute to the inability to move normal amounts of gas produced.

Constipation

Constipation is a major problem worldwide. In the US, chronic constipation leads to 8 million visits to medical providers per year (Wald, 2016). Its exact prevalence is difficult to ascertain because only a minority of patients suffering from constipation seek health care. Reports of its prevalence have varied widely, ranging from 0.7% to 29.6% in children and from 2.5% to 79% in adults (Mugie et al, 2011). This worldwide variation in prevalence rates arises from factors such as cultural diversity, genetic, environmental and socioeconomic conditions, and different health care systems. Constipation has a significant impact on quality of life and it contributes to health care financial burden. Female gender in adults, elderly age, high body mass index, and low socioeconomic status seem to be associated with a higher prevalence of constipation (Mugie et al, 2011).

Etiology

Constipation is defined as difficulty with defecation characterized by frequency or dyschezia (painful, hard, or incomplete evacuations). Normal bowel movement frequency can range from three times per day to three times per week. Stool weight is used most frequently in medical practice and clinical descriptions as an objective measure of the amount or volume of stool. A volume of as little as 200 g daily is considered normal in healthy children and adults.

The causes of constipation are varied and may be multifactorial. Inadequate fiber intake has been cited as the primary culprit since the early 1970s. Box 28-2 outlines factors and conditions known to cause constipation. Treatment of the underlying disorder always should be the primary course of action. It is important to understand the symptom patterns and classification of constipation to tailor therapy based on the underlying pathophysiology.

Pathophysiology

Constipation is classified as primary or secondary. The primary causes of chronic constipation are classified further as normal transit constipation, slow transit constipation, and anorectal dysfunction (Andrews and Storr, 2011). The most common form of chronic constipation seen by clinicians is normal transit constipation (also known as functional constipation). Stool passes through the colon at a rate of about 5 days in persons with normal transit constipation. Box 28-3 outlines the Rome III diagnostic criteria for functional constipation. In **functional constipation**, patients report symptoms they believe to be consistent with constipation such as the presence of hard stools or a perceived difficulty with defecation. However, on testing, stool transit is not delayed and the stool frequency is often within the normal range. Patients may experience bloating and abdominal pain or discomfort. Symptoms of functional constipation typically respond with dietary fiber alone or with the addition of an osmotic agent.

Slow transit constipation causes infrequent bowel movements (typically less than once per week). Often patients do not feel the urge to defecate and may complain of associated

BOX 28-2 Causes of Constipation

Lifestyle and Diet
Lack of fiber in diet
Low total calorie and fluid intake
Iron and calcium supplements
Lack of exercise
Immobility
Laxative abuse
Postponing urge to defecate

Dysmotility Disorders
Chronic intestinal pseudoobstruction
Hypothyroidism
Colonic inertia
Gastroparesis
Hirschprung disease
Chagas disease
Metabolic and endocrine abnormalities such as diabetes

Neurologic Diseases
Amyotrophic lateral sclerosis
Multiple sclerosis
Muscular dystrophy
Parkinson's disease
Friedrich ataxia
Cerebral palsy

Para- or quadriplegia
Spinal cord injury
Cerebrovascular disease
Brain trauma

Pelvic Floor Disorders
Pregnancy
Dyssynergic defecation

Chronic Use of Opiates
Oncology patients
Chronic pain patients
Narcotic bowel syndrome

Other Gastrointestinal Disorders
Diseases of the upper gastrointestinal tract
Diseases of the large bowel resulting in:
Failure of propulsion along the colon (colonic inertia)
Anorectal malformations or outlet obstruction
Irritable bowel syndrome (IBS)
Anal fissure

Data from Andrews CN, Storr M: The pathophysiology of chronic constipation, *Can J Gastroenterol* 25(Suppl B):16B, 2011; Longstreth GF et al: Functional bowel disorders, *Gastroenterology* 130:1480, 2006; Schiller LR: Nutrients and constipation: cause or cure? *Pract Gastroenterol* 32:4, 2008.

BOX 28-3 Rome III Diagnostic Criteria for Functional Constipation

Criteria fulfilled for the last 3 months, with symptom onset at least 6 months before diagnosis
1. Must include two or more of the following:
   a. Straining during at least 25% of defecations
   b. Lumpy or hard stools in at least 25% of defecations
   c. Sensation of incomplete evacuation for at least 25% of defecations
   d. Sensation of anorectal obstruction/blockade for at least 25% of defecations
   e. Manual maneuvers to facilitate at least 25% of defecations (i.e., digital evacuation, support of the pelvic floor)
   f. Fewer than three defecations per week
2. Loose stools are rarely present without the use of laxatives.
3. There are insufficient criteria for irritable bowel syndrome (i.e., pain is not the predominant symptom).

Data from Longstreth GF et al: Functional bowel disorders, *Gastroenterology* 130:1480, 2006.

bloating and abdominal discomfort. Slowing of intestinal contents occurs more commonly in the rectosigmoid colon and results in decreased water content in the stool and reduced propulsive action. Treatment typically uses an aggressive laxative regimen. Select patients with slow transit constipation may respond well to surgical procedures such as subtotal colectomy and ileorectal anastomosis.

Anorectal dysfunction is a result of the pelvic floor muscle laxity, impaired rectal sensation, and decreased luminal pressure in the anal canal. Frequently, laxatives are highly ineffective in anorectal dysfunction. The use of biofeedback therapy to retrain the muscles can be used by patients with constipation caused by problems in the anorectal muscles. It uses a combination of diaphragmatic muscle training, simulated defecation, and manometric or EMG (electromyogram) guided anal sphincter and pelvic muscle relaxation, with a goal of improving recto-anal coordination and sensory awareness (Lee et al, 2014). The measurements are displayed on a video screen as line graphs and sounds indicate when the patient is using the correct muscles.

Medical Management for Adults

A thorough and meticulous history is most helpful in ruling out constipation secondary to medications or other underlying medical illness. After this is done, the first approach to treat mild and functional constipation is to ensure adequate dietary fiber and fluid intake, exercise, and heeding the urge to defecate. Patients who depend on laxatives are encouraged to use milder products, reducing the dose until withdrawal is complete.

When constipation persists despite lifestyle and dietary modifications, medications that promote regular bowel movements may be prescribed. Agents used in the treatment of constipation are categorized broadly as either stool softeners or stimulants. Stool softeners (i.e., docusate sodium) are anionic surfactants with an emulsifying detergent-like property that increases the water content in stool to make bowel movements easier to pass. Osmotic agents such as magnesium hydroxide, sorbitol, lactulose, and polyethylene glycol contain poorly absorbed or nonabsorbable sugars and work by pulling fluid into the intestinal lumen. Stimulant laxatives such as bisacodyl and senna increase peristaltic contraction and bowel motility and act to prevent water absorption. Chronic use of laxatives is associated with abdominal cramping and fluid imbalance.

Lubiprostone (Amitiza) was recently approved by the Food and Drug Administration for idiopathic constipation and to treat irritable bowel syndrome with constipation in adults. Lubiprostone is a chloride channel activator that increases intestinal fluid secretion and mobility; however, it does not alter sodium or potassium electrolytes (Bailes and Reeve, 2013). It increases spontaneous bowel movements and is contraindicated in patients with suspected or known mechanical GI obstruction.

Medical Management for Infants and Children

Constipation is often especially troubling in infants and young children. Approximately 3% to 5% of all pediatric visits are related to chronic constipation. Some patients have symptoms that persist for 6 months or more. Constipation may be related to inadequate intake of fiber or fluid, side effects of medication, inactivity, or disordered bowel motility. Historically, a high-fiber diet has been recommended for children with constipation. However, few studies document benefit (Kranz et al, 2012). A careful history and physical examination followed by parent and child education, behavioral intervention, and appropriate use of laxatives often lead to dramatic improvement.

Medical Nutrition Therapy

Primary nutrition therapy for constipation in otherwise healthy people is consumption of adequate amounts of fluids and dietary fiber, soluble and insoluble. Fiber increases colonic fecal fluid, microbial mass (which accounts for 60% to 70% of stool weight), stool weight and frequency, and the rate of colonic transit. With adequate intake of fluid, fiber may soften stools and make them easier to pass. Dietary Reference Intakes (DRI) recommend consumption of 14 g dietary fiber per 1000 kcal, or 25 g for adult women and 38 g for adult men. Appropriate kinds and amounts of dietary fiber for children, the critically ill, and the very old are unknown. Usual intake of dietary fiber in the United States is only about 16.2 g/day (Grooms et al, 2013).

Dietary fiber refers to edible plant materials not digested by the enzymes in the GI tract. It consists of cellulose, hemicellulose, pectins, gums, lignins, starchy materials, and oligosaccharides that are partially resistant to digestive enzymes. Fiber can be provided in the form of whole grains, fruits, vegetables, legumes, seeds, and nuts.

A high-fiber therapeutic diet may have to exceed 25 to 38 g/day. The high-fiber diet in Box 28-4 provides more than the amount of fiber recommended. It is important to assess dietary fiber intake before making recommendations for fiber supplementation. If a patient is already taking 25 to 30 g of dietary fiber daily, fiber supplementation is unlikely to be helpful. If less than this amount is being consumed, fiber should be added slowly in graduated doses to eventually reach 25 to 30 g per day. Amounts greater than 50 g/day are not necessary and may increase abdominal distention and excessive flatulence due to fermentation by the colonic flora.

Bran and fiber supplements may be helpful in persons who cannot or will not eat sufficient amounts of fiber-containing foods. Several of these commercial fiber supplements are palatable and can be added to cereals, yogurts, fruit sauces, juices, or soups. Cooking does not destroy fiber, but the structure may change. Consumption of at least eight 8-oz glasses (approximately 2 L) of fluids daily is recommended to facilitate the effectiveness of a high-fiber intake. Gastric obstruction and fecal impaction may occur when boluses of fibrous gels or bran are not consumed with sufficient fluid to disperse the fiber.

Increasing dietary fiber for laxation is unlikely to help patients who have serious dysmotility syndromes, neuromuscular disorders, chronic opioid use, pelvic floor disorders, or other serious GI disease. In some conditions, such as neuromuscular disorders, a specific laxative medication regimen is a necessary part of disease management.

Diarrhea

Diarrhea is defined by the World Health Organization as the passage of three or more loose or liquid stools per day. Diarrhea occurs when there is accelerated transit of intestinal contents through the small intestine, decreased enzymatic digestion of foodstuffs, decreased absorption of fluids and nutrients, increased secretion of fluids into the GIT, or exudative losses.

Pathophysiology

Diarrhea may be related to inflammatory disease; infections with fungal, bacterial, or viral agents; medications; overconsumption of sugars or other osmotic substances; an allergic response to a food, or insufficient or damaged mucosal absorptive surface.

Exudative diarrheas always are associated with mucosal damage, which leads to an outpouring of mucus, fluid, blood, and plasma proteins, with a net accumulation of electrolytes and water in the gut. Prostaglandin and cytokine release may be involved. Diarrhea associated with Crohn's disease, ulcerative colitis (UC), and radiation enteritis is often exudative.

Osmotic diarrheas occur when osmotically active solutes are present in the intestinal tract and are poorly absorbed. An example is the diarrhea that accompanies dumping syndrome in someone that consumes a beverage containing simple sugars after having a Billroth II procedure (gastrojejunostomy).

Secretory diarrheas are the result of active intestinal secretion of electrolytes and water by the intestinal epithelium, resulting from bacterial exotoxins, viruses, and increased intestinal hormone secretion. Unlike osmotic diarrhea, fasting does not relieve secretory diarrhea.

Malabsorptive diarrheas result when a disease process impairs digestion or absorption to the point that nutrients, such as fat, appear in the stool in increased amounts. Excess fat in the stool is called steatorrhea. Diarrhea occurs because of the osmotic action of these nutrients and the action of the bacteria on the nutrients that pass into the colon. Malabsorptive diarrhea occurs when there is not enough healthy absorptive area or inadequate production or interrupted flow of bile and pancreatic enzymes, or there is rapid transit, such as in inflammatory bowel disease (IBD) or after extensive bowel resection. Box 28-5 lists diseases and conditions associated with malabsorption and diarrhea.

Medication-induced diarrheas are frequent in hospitalized and long-term care patients. Medications that cause diarrhea do so by different mechanisms. For example, medications such as lactulose (used in the management of hepatic encephalopathy) and sodium polystyrene sulfonate with sorbitol (used to treat hyperkalemia) create increased bowel movements as part of their mechanism of action. Some antibiotics have direct effects on GI function (see Chapter 8). For example, as a motilin agonist, erythromycin increases lower GI motility; clarithromycin and clindamycin also increase GI secretions.

The human intestinal tract is home for trillions of bacteria microbiota (see Figure 28-1). In the normal GI tract, commensal gut microbiota ferment sloughed intestinal cells and undigested foodstuffs to gases and short-chain fatty acids (SCFAs). Absorption of SCFAs facilitates absorption of electrolytes and water from the colon. Broad-spectrum antibiotics decrease the number of commensal bacteria in the bowel and may result in decreased fermentation byproducts reducing the absorption of electrolytes and water, and causing diarrhea.

Some antibiotics allow proliferation of opportunistic pathogenic microorganisms normally suppressed by competitive

---

BOX 28-4 Guidelines for High-Fiber Diets

1. Increase consumption of whole-grain breads cereals, and other products to 6 to 11 servings daily.
2. Increase consumption of vegetables, legumes, fruits, nuts, and edible seeds to 5 to 8 servings daily.
3. Consume high-fiber cereals, granolas, and legumes to bring fiber intake to 25 g in women or 38 g in men or more daily.
4. Increase consumption of fluids to at least 2 L (or approximately 2 qt) daily.

Note: Following these guidelines may cause an increase in stool weight, fecal water, and gas. The amount that causes clinical symptoms varies among individuals, depending on age and presence of gastrointestinal (GI) disease, malnutrition, or resection of the GI tract.

BOX 28-5 Diseases and Conditions Associated with Malabsorption

Inadequate Digestion
Pancreatic insufficiency
Gastric acid hypersecretion
Gastric resection

Altered Bile Salt Metabolism with Impaired Micelle Formation
Hepatobiliary disease
Interrupted enterohepatic circulation of bile salts
Bacterial overgrowth
Drugs that precipitate bile salts

Genetic Abnormalities of Mucosal Cell Transport
Disaccharidase deficiency
Monosaccharide malabsorption
Specific disorders of amino acid malabsorption
Abetalipoproteinemia
Vitamin B_{12} malabsorption
Celiac disease

Inflammatory or Infiltrative Disorders
Crohn's disease
Amyloidosis
Scleroderma
Tropical sprue
Gastrointestinal allergy
Infectious enteritis
Whipple disease
Intestinal lymphoma
Radiation enteritis
Drug-induced enteritis
Endocrine and metabolic disorders
Short-bowel syndrome (SBS)

Abnormalities of Intestinal Lymphatics and Vascular System
Intestinal lymphangiectasia
Mesenteric vascular insufficiency
Chronic congestive heart failure

Data from Beyer PL: Short bowel syndrome. In Coulston AM et al, editors: *Nutrition in the prevention and treatment of disease,* ed 1, San Diego, 2001, Academic Press; Branski D et al: Chronic diarrhea and malabsorption, *Pediatr Clin North Am* 43:307, 1996; Fine KD: Diarrhea. In Feldman M et al, editors: *Gastrointestinal and liver disease,* ed 6, Philadelphia, 1998, Saunders; Mitra AD et al: Management of diarrhea in HIV-infected patients, *Int J STD AIDS* 12:630, 2001; Podolsky DK: Inflammatory bowel disease, *N Engl J Med* 347:417, 2002; Sundarum A et al: Nutritional management of short bowel syndrome in adults, *J Clin Gastroenterol* 34:207, 2002.

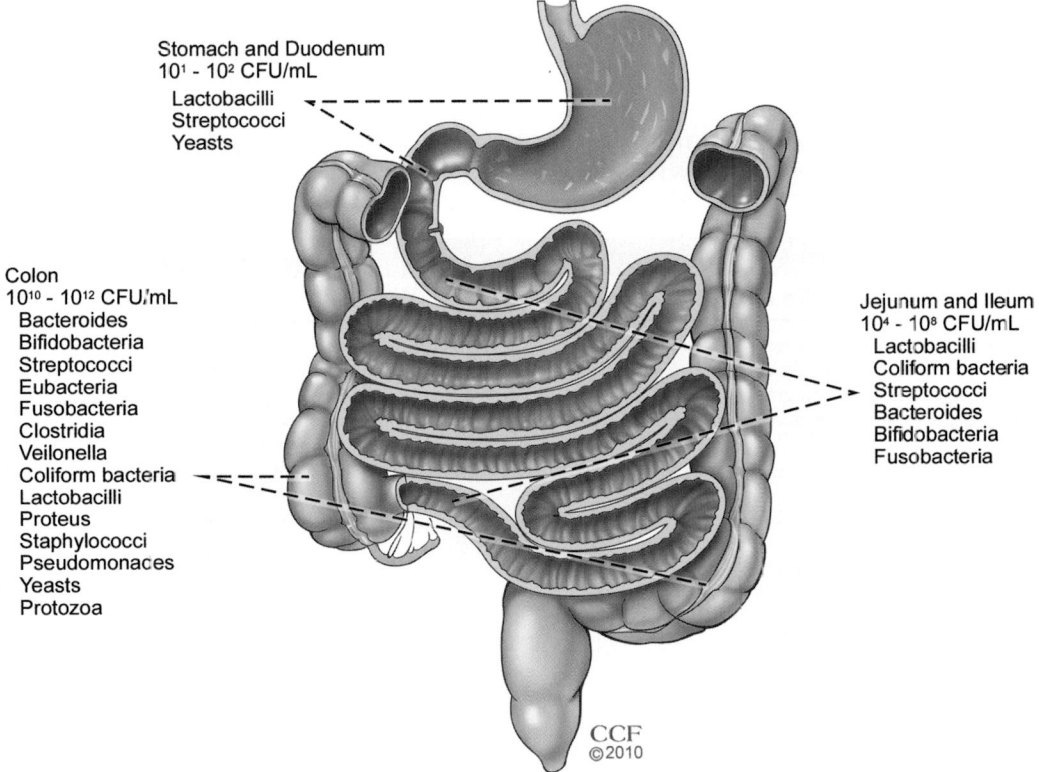

Stomach and Duodenum
$10^1 - 10^2$ CFU/mL
Lactobacilli
Streptococci
Yeasts

Colon
$10^{10} - 10^{12}$ CFU/mL
Bacteroides
Bifidobacteria
Streptococci
Eubacteria
Fusobacteria
Clostridia
Veilonella
Coliform bacteria
Lactobacilli
Proteus
Staphylococci
Pseudomonaces
Yeasts
Protozoa

Jejunum and Ileum
$10^4 - 10^8$ CFU/mL
Lactobacilli
Coliform bacteria
Streptococci
Bacteroides
Bifidobacteria
Fusobacteria

CCF
©2010

FIGURE 28-1 Gut microbiota.

microorganisms in the GI tract. The toxins produced by some opportunistic microorganisms can cause colitis and increased secretion of fluid and electrolytes. A rise in antibiotic use has led to an increase in antibiotic-associated diarrhea (AAD) and overgrowth of *Clostridium difficile* with resultant *C. difficile* infection (CDI). *C. difficile* is the leading cause of nosocomial (hospital-acquired) diarrhea in the United States (O'Keefe, 2010). This infection may cause colitis, secretory diarrhea, severe dilation of the colon (toxic megacolon), perforation of the bowel wall, peritonitis, or even death (Pattani et al, 2013).

In 2009 a survey of 12.5% of U.S. acute care facilities found a CDI prevalence rate among inpatients of 13.1 per 1000 patients (Borody and Khoruts, 2011). Resistant strains of *C. difficile* are less susceptible to treatment with antimicrobials and cause a more severe form of the disease with increased health care costs, and higher mortality (O'Keefe, 2010).

C. difficile is a spore-forming organism, and the spores are resistant to common disinfectant agents. The spore-forming ability of *C. difficile* allows the organism to be spread inadvertently to other patients by health care providers (iatrogenic infection) if strict infection control procedures are not followed. The presence of this infection is detected by analysis of a stool sample for the presence of the toxin produced by the organisms. Clindamycin, penicillins, and cephalosporins are associated most often with the development of *C. difficile* infection. Its occurrence depends on the number of antibiotics used, the duration of exposure to antibiotics, and the patient's overall health. Chronic suppression of stomach acid with proton pump inhibitor medications during broad-spectrum antibiotic therapy also may increase susceptibility to *C. difficile* infection (Howell et al, 2010; Linsky et al, 2010).

With human immunodeficiency virus (HIV) and other immune deficiency states, several factors contribute to the diarrhea, including the toxic effects of medications, proliferation of opportunistic organisms, and the GI manifestations of the disease itself (Kulkarni et al, 2009) (see Chapter 37). Increased risk of opportunistic infection also is associated with use of antineoplastic agents (such as chemotherapy) or with malnutrition.

Medical Management

Because diarrhea is a symptom, not a disease, the first step in medical treatment is to identify and treat the underlying problem. The next goal is to manage fluid and electrolyte replacement. In cases of severe diarrhea, restoring fluid and electrolyte is first priority. Electrolyte losses, especially potassium and sodium, should be corrected early by using oral glucose electrolyte solutions with added potassium. Oral rehydration solutions (ORS) work because they contain concentrations of sodium and glucose that are optimal for interaction with the sodium-glucose transport (SGLT) proteins in the intestinal epithelial cells (see Chapter 1).

With intractable diarrhea, especially in an infant or young child, parenteral feeding may be required. Parenteral nutrition (PN) may even be necessary if exploratory surgery is anticipated, or if the patient is not expected to resume full oral intake within 5 to 7 days (see Chapter 13).

Supplementation with **probiotics** shows some promise to prevent AAD and CDI, but there are inadequate data to recommend probiotics as a primary treatment for *C. difficile* infections (Pattani et al, 2013) (see *New Directions*: Probiotics and Prebiotics and the Gut Microbiota).

The best treatment currently is to employ **fecal microbiota transplant (FMT)** for refractory CDI. With the concept of the human gut microbiota as an organ, FMT may be considered an organ transplant. Basically the gut microbiota of the person infected with *C. difficile* is replaced with healthy donor stool, typically from a family member with similar dietary and living habits. The reported cumulative success rate of FMT in eradicating the infection is approximately 90% (Borody and Khoruts, 2011).

Products that combine probiotic microorganisms and a prebiotic fiber source have been described as **synbiotics** for their synergistic effects. However, no randomized controlled studies have systematically investigated the effectiveness of probiotics alone compared with synbiotics for the treatment of diarrhea. Controlled studies are needed to understand which strains of

---

✴ NEW DIRECTIONS

Probiotics and Prebiotics and the Gut Microbiota

Some gastrointestinal conditions such as *Clostridium difficile* infection, SIBO, antibiotic-associated diarrhea, and perhaps even inflammatory bowel disease may result or have exacerbated symptoms when there are alterations to the colonies of microorganisms that exist in the small or large intestines. Exposure to broad-spectrum antibiotics causes dramatic alterations to commensal gut microbiota, placing the patient at risk for overgrowth of potentially pathogenic microbes and opportunistic GI infections.

A **probiotic** is defined by the World Health Organization as "a live microbial feed that when consumed in adequate amounts confers a health benefit on the host." To be a probiotic, meaning "for life," a live microbial strain must meet very stringent criteria. These include, being of human origin, resistant to acid and bile, being able to survive the upper intestinal tract environment and reach the distal gut (ileum and colon) and attach to the intestinal epithelium, and being able to colonize the distal intestine, confer health benefit to the host, and have scientifically proven health benefits (Cresci, 2012). Because of this strict criteria, most supplements termed "probiotics" are not truly probiotics and their use may be misleading to clinicians and consumers.

Certain strains of bacteria have been identified as probiotics. These may be available in supplement form (e.g., capsules, powders) or included in fermented food products (e.g., yogurts, kefir). The exact dose, means for delivery, or the duration of viability are uncertain, probably vary for different probiotic strains, and may depend on the condition to be treated. It has been suggested that probiotics may restore the balance of intestinal microbes and improve symptoms and prevent or treat conditions in which a gut dysbiosis has occurred, such as antibiotic-associated diarrhea (Pattani et al, 2013). Certain types of probiotics may be effective in reducing the duration of enterovirus-induced acute infectious diarrhea in pediatric and adult patients and in those with IBD.

Like probiotics, prebiotics have strict criteria for their classification. Prebiotics, undigested polysaccharides, and sloughed proteins are the food source for the commensal gut microbiota.

A **prebiotic** is defined as "a selectively fermented ingredient that allows specific changes, both in the composition and activity in the gut microbiota, that confer benefits upon host well-being and health" (Cresci, 2012). Importantly, prebiotics must be resistant to gastric acidity, to hydrolysis by mammalian enzymes, and to GI absorption; must be fermented in the GI tract by the gut microbiota; and must be selective in the stimulation of the gut microbiota growth and activity that contribute to health and well-being. Prebiotics are naturally occurring or synthetic sugars and are not available to all gut microbial species. Upon reaching the distal gut, prebiotics are fermented by the gut microbiota to yield gases (carbon dioxide, hydrogen, and methane) and short-chain fatty acids. Short-chain fatty acids (acetate, propionate, butyrate) serve many biologic roles including aiding with water and electrolyte absorption, decreasing intraluminal pH, altering cell proliferation and differentiation, and modifying intestinal immune and inflammatory processes (Cresci, 2012). Although probiotics have reported safety issues with select clinical conditions, prebiotics carry little safety concerns but like probiotics, may contribute to GI discomfort (bloating, gas) if introduced too rapidly into the diet.

Because there is promise in theory and in select studies for correcting gut dysbiosis with supplements, further studies evaluating the optimal dose, timing, duration and indications for probiotics, prebiotics and their combinations are warranted.

probiotics should be provided, as well as type and amount of prebiotic fibers.

There is a long history of safe use of many strains of "live active cultures" in foods in healthy humans. However, the body of evidence is limited on the use of large doses of concentrated probiotic supplements, especially of specific strains that exhibit greater resistance to gastric acid or have increased ability to proliferate in the GI tract. Limited safety data support the use of concentrated probiotic supplements in patients with immunocompromised states, critical illness, or when probiotics are administered directly into the small intestine, as with jejunal feeding tubes, but research in this area continues (Stavrou et al, 2015). A number of case reports exist of hospitalized patients receiving concentrated strains of probiotics that have become septic because of infection in the bloodstream with the very same strain of probiotic being administered (Whelan and Myers, 2010). In a review of cases of adverse events related to probiotic administration in hospitalized patients, 25% of those adverse events resulted in the death of the patient (Whelan and Myers, 2010). Many of these case reports indicate the culprit probiotic was a nonpathogenic yeast, and since then product label warnings against providing this supplement to critically ill patients have been instated. In a large double-blind, randomized study of a high-dose multispecies probiotic administered via jejunal feeding tube in patients with severe acute pancreatitis, there were significantly more deaths in the patients who received probiotics compared with those receiving the inactive placebo (Besselink et al, 2008). Although this study is concerning and provides warning before administering live cultures to critically ill patients, study flaws lead to questions whether the increased mortality was solely the result of probiotic supplementation.

Probiotic preparations hold promise as an adjunctive or primary treatment in several gastrointestinal conditions, but additional studies are needed before routine use of these preparations is adopted, especially for hospitalized or immunocompromised patients. There remains much to be learned about true effectiveness, differences between probiotic strains, possible benefits of coadministration with prebiotics, best doses, safety, and cost-benefit of using probiotics.

Medical Nutrition Therapy

All nutrition interventions related to diarrhea must be viewed within the context of the underlying pathologic condition responsible for the diarrhea. Replacement of necessary fluids and electrolytes is the first step, using oral rehydration solutions (ORS), soups and broths, vegetable juices, and isotonic liquids. Restrictive diets, such as the BRAT diet made up of bananas, rice, applesauce, and toast, are nutrient poor; no evidence indicates that they are necessary during acute diarrheal illness. However, some clinicians recommend a progression of starchy carbohydrates such as cereals, breads, and low-fat meats, followed by small amounts of vegetables and fruits, followed by fats. The goal with this progression is to limit large amounts of hyperosmotic carbohydrates that may be maldigested or malabsorbed, foods that stimulate secretion of fluids, and foods that speed the rate of GI transit.

Sugar alcohols, lactose, fructose, and large amounts of sucrose may worsen osmotic diarrheas. Because the activity of the disaccharidases and transport mechanisms decrease during inflammatory and infectious intestinal disease, sugars may have to be limited, especially in children. Malabsorption is only one potential cause of diarrhea, and diarrhea may occur without

TABLE 28-1 Food to Limit in a Low-Fiber (Minimal Residue) Diet	
Food	**Comments**
Lactose (in lactose malabsorbers)	6 to 12 g is normally tolerated in healthy lactase-deficient individuals, but may not be in some individuals.
Insoluble fiber (quantities >20 g)	Modest amounts (10 to 15 g) may help maintain normal consistency of gastrointestinal (GI) contents and normal colonic mucosa in healthy states and GI disease.
Sorbitol, mannitol, and xylitol (excess, >10 g/day) Fructose (excess, 20-25 g/meal) Sucrose (excess, >25-50 g/meal)	Well tolerated in moderate amounts; large amounts may cause hyperosmolar diarrhea
Caffeine	Increases GI secretions, colonic motility
Alcoholic beverages (especially wine and beer)	Increase GI secretions

significant malabsorption of macronutrients (carbohydrate, fat, and protein). Absorption of most nutrients occurs in the small intestine; diarrhea related to colonic inflammation or disease preserves the absorption of most ingested nutrients.

Minimal fiber and low-residue diets are rarely indicated (see Table 28-1). Patients are encouraged to resume a regular diet as tolerated that contains moderate amounts of soluble fiber. The metabolism of soluble fiber and resistant starches by colonic bacteria leads to production of SCFAs, which in physiologic quantities serve as a substrate for colonocytes, facilitate the absorption of fluid and salts, and may help to regulate GI motility.

Fibrous material tends to slow gastric emptying, moderate overall GI transit, and pull water into the intestinal lumen. Providing fiber to patients with diarrhea does increase the volume of stool, and in some cases (such as small intestine bacterial overgrowth [SIBO]) initially can increase gas and bloating. Modest intake of prebiotic components and soluble fibers such as pectin or gum slows transit through the GI tract.

Several probiotics have been studied for preventing AAD. Currently, of those tested, *Saccharomyces boulardii* and *Lactobacillus*-based formulations appear to be most effective in reducing AAD (Pattani et al, 2013). Studies are still needed to find the optimal combination of probiotics and/or prebiotics, testing for dosing schedules, and concentrations.

Severe and chronic diarrhea is accompanied by dehydration and electrolyte depletion. If also accompanied by prolonged infectious, immunodeficiency, or inflammatory disease, malabsorption of vitamins, minerals, and protein or fat also may occur, and nutrients may have to be replaced parenterally or enterally. In some forms of infectious diarrhea, loss of iron from GI bleeding may be severe enough to cause anemia. Nutrient deficiencies themselves cause mucosal changes such as decreased villi height and reduced enzyme secretion, further contributing to malabsorption. As the diarrhea begins to resolve, the addition of more normal amounts of fiber to the diet may help to restore normal mucosal function, increase electrolyte and water absorption, and increase the firmness of the stool.

Food in the lumen is needed to restore the compromised GI tract after disease and periods of fasting. Early refeeding after rehydration reduces stool output and shortens the duration of illness. Micronutrient replacement or supplementation also may be useful for acute diarrhea, probably because it accelerates the normal regeneration of damaged mucosal epithelial cells.

Treating Diarrhea in Infants and Children

Acute diarrhea is most dangerous in infants and small children, who are easily dehydrated by large fluid losses. In these cases replacement of fluid and electrolytes must be aggressive and immediate. Standard ORS recommended by the World Health Organization and the American Academy of Pediatrics contain a 2% concentration of glucose (20 g/L), 45 to 90 mEq/L of sodium, 20 mEq/L of potassium, and a citrate base (see Table 28-2).

Newer reduced-osmolarity solutions (200 to 250 mOsm/L) have advantages over the traditional WHO-recommended ORS in treating acute diarrhea in children. The use of reduced-osmolarity ORS in children with acute diarrhea resulted in decreased need for intravenous therapy, significant reduction in stool output, and decreased vomiting compared with standard WHO-recommended ORS (Atia and Buchman, 2009). Commercial solutions such as Pedialyte, Infalyte, Lytren, Equalyte, and Rehydralyte typically contain less glucose and slightly less salt and are available in pharmacies, often without prescription. Oral rehydration therapy is less invasive and less expensive than intravenous rehydration and, when used with children, allows parents to assist with their children's recovery.

A substantial proportion of children 9 to 20 months of age can maintain adequate intake when offered either a liquid or a semisolid diet continuously during bouts of acute diarrhea. Even during acute diarrhea, the intestine can absorb up to 60% of the food eaten. Some practitioners have been slow to adopt the practice of early refeeding after severe diarrhea in infants despite evidence that "resting the gut" is actually more damaging.

Gastrointestinal Strictures and Obstruction
Pathophysiology

Patients with gastroparesis, adhesions, hernias, metastatic cancers, dysmotility, or volvulus are prone to obstruction, which can result in partial or complete blockage of movement of food or stool through the intestines. Obstructions may be partial or complete and may occur in the stomach (gastric outlet obstruction), small intestine, or large intestine. Symptoms include bloating, abdominal distention and pain, nausea, and vomiting.

Obstructions are not usually caused by foods in an otherwise healthy individual, however, when sections of the GI tract are partially obstructed or not moving appropriately, foods may contribute to obstruction. Researchers have not found that eating, diet, and nutrition play a role in causing or preventing the frequency of obstructive symptoms. It is believed that fibrous plant foods can contribute to obstruction because the fiber in the foods may not be completely chewed to pass through narrowed segments of the GI tract.

Medical Nutrition Therapy

Most clinicians would recommend patients prone to obstructions to chew food thoroughly and avoid excessive fiber intake. A patient with a partial bowel obstruction may be able to tolerate a restricted-fiber diet and liquids, depending on the location of stricture or obstruction in the GI tract. A more proximal (closer to the mouth) blockage may require a semisolid or liquid diet. However, the more distal (closer to the anus) the blockage, the less likely altering the consistency of the diet will help. Symptoms are more severe during complete obstruction. Patients may be intolerant of oral intake and of their own secretions leading to progressive dehydration, electrolyte imbalance, and systemic toxicity. Initial treatment consists of aggressive fluid resuscitation, nasogastric decompression, and administration of analgesics and antiemetics.

Patients with complete bowel obstruction may require surgical intervention. In some cases, enteral feeding beyond the point of obstruction may be feasible, but if enteral feeding is not possible for a prolonged period, parenteral nutrition may be needed. Working with the patient and physician is necessary to determine the nature, site, and duration of the obstruction so that nutrition therapy can be individualized.

DISEASES OF THE SMALL INTESTINE

Celiac Disease (Gluten-Sensitive Enteropathy)

The prevalence of celiac disease (CD) has been underestimated in the past and now is considered to affect at least 1 in 141 persons in the United States and varies by race and ethnicity, with a marked predominance among non-Hispanic whites (Rubio-Tapia et al, 2012). The onset and first occurrence of symptoms may appear any time from infancy to adulthood, but the peak in diagnosis occurs between the fourth and sixth decade. The disease may become apparent when an infant begins eating gluten-containing cereals. In some, it may not appear until adulthood, when it may be triggered or unmasked during GI surgery, stress, pregnancy, or viral infection. It may be discovered as a result of evaluation for another suspected problem. Approximately 20% of cases are diagnosed after the age of 60 years.

Etiology

The presentation in young children is likely to include the more "classic" GI symptoms of diarrhea, steatorrhea, malodorous stools, abdominal bloating, apathy, fatigue, and poor weight gain. Although GI-related symptoms often are thought to be most common, an increasing number of patients present without GI

TABLE 28-2	**Oral Rehydration Solution (ORS): Composition and Recipes**
Element	**Composition**
Glucose (g/100 ml)	20
Sodium (mEq/L)	90
Potassium (mEq/L)	20
Chloride (mEq/L)	80
Bicarbonate (mEq/L)	30
Osmolarity (mOsm/L)	330
Recipes* (each makes 1 liter)	
2 cups Gatorade, 2 cups water, ¾ tsp salt	28 g glucose, 82 mEq Na, 1.5 eEq K
or	
1 quart water, ¾ tsp salt, 6 teaspoons sugar	24 g glucose, 76 mEq Na, 0 mEq K

Data from Krenitsky J, McCray S: *University of Virginia Health System Nutrition Support Traineeship Syllabus*, Charlottesville, Va, 2010, University of Virginia Health System; *World Health Organization*: Guidelines for cholera control. http://whqlibdoc.who.int/publications/1993/924154449X.pdf, 1993, Geneva, Accessed January 31, 2015. Recipes from Parrish CR: The clinician's guide to short bowel syndrome, *Pract Gastroenterol* 29:67, 2005.
K, Potassium; *Na*, sodium.
*The solution should be made fresh every 24 hr.

BOX 28-6   Symptoms and Conditions Associated with Celiac Disease

Nutritional

Anemia (iron or folate, rarely B$_{12}$)
Osteomalacia, osteopenia, fractures (vitamin D deficiency, inadequate calcium absorption)
Coagulopathies (vitamin K deficiency)
Dental enamel hypoplasia
Delayed growth, delayed puberty, underweight
Lactase deficiency

Extraintestinal

Lassitude, malaise (sometimes despite lack of anemia)
Arthritis, arthralgia

Dermatitis herpetiformis
Infertility, increased risk of miscarriage
Hepatic steatosis, hepatitis
Neurologic symptoms (ataxia, polyneuropathy, seizures); may be partly nutrition related
Psychiatric syndromes

Associated Disorders

Autoimmune diseases: type 1 diabetes, thyroiditis, hepatitis, collagen vascular disease
Gastrointestinal malignancy
IgA deficiency

IgA, Immunoglobulin A.
Kupfer SS, Jabri B: Pathophysiology of celiac disease, *Gastrointest Endosc Clin N Am* 22:639, 2012.

symptoms. Fifty percent of celiac patients have few or no obvious symptoms, and some are overweight at presentation (Phatak and Pashankar, 2015). CD frequently is misdiagnosed as irritable bowel syndrome (IBS), lactase deficiency, gallbladder disease, or other disorders not necessarily involving the GI tract, because the presentation and onset of symptoms vary so greatly.

Patients may present with one or more of a host of conditions associated with CD: anemias, generalized fatigue, weight loss or failure to thrive, osteoporosis, vitamin or mineral deficiencies, and (although rare) GI malignancy. **Dermatitis herpetiformis**, yet another manifestation of CD, presents as an itchy skin rash; its presence is diagnostic of CD. Box 28-6 lists conditions associated with CD. Persons who are diagnosed late in life, who cannot or will not comply with the diet, or who were diagnosed as children, but told they would grow out of it, are at a higher risk for experiencing long-term complications from CD (Nachman et al, 2010).

Pathophysiology

CD, or **gluten-sensitive enteropathy**, is characterized by a combination of four factors: (1) genetic susceptibility, (2) exposure to gluten, (3) an environmental "trigger," and (4) an autoimmune response. Gluten refers to specific peptide fractions of proteins (prolamines) found in wheat (glutenin and gliadin), rye (secalin), and barley (hordein). These peptides are generally more resistant to complete digestion by GI enzymes and may reach the small intestine intact. In a normal, healthy intestine, these peptides are harmless as the intestinal barrier is intact and prevents translocation from the intestine. However, in persons with CD these peptides travel from the intestinal lumen, across the intestinal epithelium, and into the lamina propria, where they can trigger an inflammatory response that results in flattening of intestinal villi and elongation of the crypt cells (secretory cells), along with a more general systemic immune response (Sams and Hawks, 2014) (see Figure 28-2).

The term **gluten sensitivity** is used commonly to describe persons with nonspecific symptoms, without the immune response characteristic of CD or the consequential intestinal damage. **Gluten intolerance** describes individuals who have symptoms and who may or may not have CD. These two terms are used to describe symptoms such as nausea, abdominal cramps, or diarrhea after ingesting gluten. Patients who experience these symptoms generally should be advised against

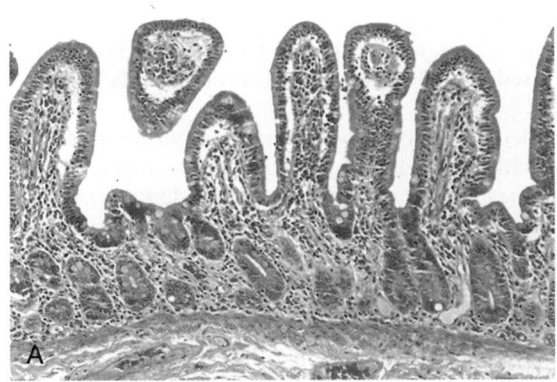
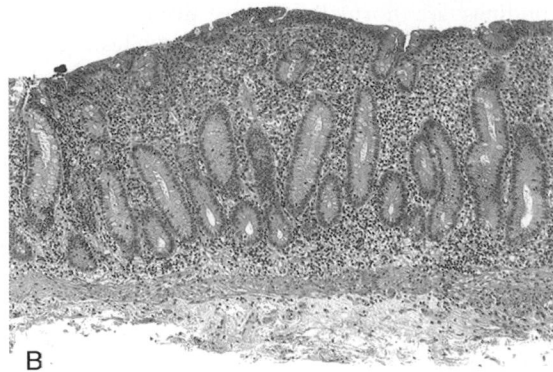

FIGURE 28-2 CD (gluten-sensitive enteropathy). **A,** Peroral jejunal biopsy specimen of diseased mucosa shows severe atrophy and blunting of villi, with a chronic inflammatory infiltrate of the lamina propria. **B,** Normal mucosal biopsy. (From Kumar V et al: *Robbins and Cotran pathologic basis of disease*, ed 7, Philadelphia, 2005, Saunders.)

following a gluten-free (GF) diet without having a workup to exclude or confirm a diagnosis of CD because (1) there may be an underlying medical condition for which a GF diet is not the treatment; (2) after following a GF diet for months or years, it is difficult to diagnose CD; and (3) although generally a healthy way to eat, a GF diet can be expensive and restrictive.

The "triggers" of CD are not well understood, but stressors (e.g., illness, inflammation) are thought to play a role. When CD remains untreated, the immune and inflammatory response eventually results in atrophy and flattening of villi. Over time, the process can cause enough damage to the intestinal mucosa to compromise normal secretory, digestive, and absorptive functions, leading to impaired micronutrient and macronutrient absorption (Kupfer and Jabri, 2012). Cells of the villi become deficient in the disaccharidases and peptidases needed for digestion and also in the carriers needed to transport nutrients into the bloodstream. The disease primarily affects the proximal and middle sections of the small bowel, although the more distal segments also may be involved (Sams and Hawks, 2014).

Assessment

The diagnosis of CD is made from a combination of clinical, laboratory, and histologic evaluations. Persons suspected of having CD should be evaluated for the overall pattern of symptoms and family history. Biopsy of the small intestine is the gold standard for diagnosis. An intestinal biopsy positive for CD generally shows villous atrophy, increased intraepithelial lymphocytes, and crypt cell hyperplasia. However, biopsy is not used for initial screening because of its cost and invasiveness.

Elevated blood levels of certain autoantibodies are found in people with celiac disease. To screen for celiac disease several serologic tests are evaluated. These tests identify the presence of antibodies in the blood, such as anti-tissue transglutaminase (anti-TTG), and antiendomysial antibodies, and deaminated gliadin peptide. The sensitivity and specificity of these tests are 90% to 99% (Schyum and Rumessen, 2013). There is a higher incidence of immunoglobulin A (IgA) deficiency in patients with CD; thus physicians often measure IgA levels when serologic findings are normal, but the overall clinical picture suggests CD (see *Clinical Insight:* Antibody Testing for Celiac Disease and Gluten Sensitivity). Using video capsule endoscopy to image the entire intestinal mucosa can show inflammation related to CD but is not currently used in the initial diagnosis (Bouchard et al, 2014). Because dietary change alters diagnostic results, initial evaluation should be done *before* the person has eliminated gluten-containing foods from his or her diet. Serologic tests also may be used to monitor the response of a newly diagnosed patient treated with a GF diet.

Lifelong, strict adherence to a GF diet is the only known treatment for CD (see Box 28-7 for a list of safe, questionable, and unsafe choices on the GF diet). The GF diet greatly diminishes the autoimmune process, and the intestinal mucosa usually reverts to normal or near normal. Within 2 to 8 weeks of starting the GF diet, most patients report that their clinical symptoms have abated. Histologic, immunologic, and functional improvements may take months to years, depending on the duration of the disease, age of the subject, and degree of dietary compliance. With strict dietary control, levels of the specific antibodies usually become undetectable within 3 to 6 months in most persons. In some individuals, recovery may be slow or incomplete.

A small percentage of patients are "nonresponders" to diet therapy. Inadvertent gluten intake is the most common offender, but another coexisting disorder may be present (such as pancreatic insufficiency, IBS, bacterial overgrowth, fructose intolerance, other GI maladies, or unknown causes). For nonresponders, intensive interviewing to identify a source of gluten contamination or treatment of another underlying disease may resolve the symptoms. Diagnosis of refractory celiac disease is made when patients do not respond or respond only temporarily to a GF diet, and all external causes have been ruled out, including inadvertent gluten ingestion. Patients with refractory disease may respond to steroids, azathioprine, cyclosporine, or other medications classically used to suppress inflammatory or immunologic reactions.

Several novel treatments for CD are being studied for their potential as alternative therapies. Researchers seek to treat CD by reducing gluten exposure (by digestion with added enzymes), decreasing uptake of gluten (by tightening junctions between intestinal epithelial cells), altering the immune response to gluten, or repairing intestinal injury.

Medical Nutrition Therapy

Elimination of gluten peptides from the diet is the only treatment for CD presently. The diet omits all dietary wheat, rye, and barley, which are the major sources of the prolamin fractions.

In general, patients should be assessed for nutrient deficiencies before supplementation is initiated. In all newly diagnosed patients, the clinician should consider checking levels of ferritin, red blood cell folate, and 25-OH vitamin D. If patients present with more severe symptoms, such as diarrhea, weight loss, malabsorption, or signs of nutrient deficiencies (e.g., nightblindness, neuropathy, prolonged prothrombin time), other vitamins such as fat-soluble vitamins (A, E, K) and minerals (zinc) should be checked.

CLINICAL INSIGHT

Antibody testing for Celiac Disease and Gluten Sensitivity by Ruth Leyse-Wallace, PhD, RDN

There are two different types of antibodies considered in celiac disease diagnosis: those which are "anti-gluten", and those which are "anti-self" (auto-immune). "Anti-gluten" antibodies are the anti-gliadin IgG and IgA. Ig stands for "immunoglobulin" or "antibody". "Anti-self" antibodies are anti-endomysial IgA and anti-tissue transglutaminase IgA (tTg IgA).

Antigliadin antibodies IgG and IgA recognize a small piece of the gluten protein called gliadin. Antigliadin IgG has good sensitivity, while antigliadin IgA has good specificity. Their combined use provides a screening test for celiac disease. Many normal individuals without celiac disease will have an elevated antigliadin IgG. It is estimated that 0.2-0.4% of the general population has selective IgA deficiency, while 2 to 3% or more of celiacs are IgA deficient.

If a celiac panel is only positive for antigliadin IgG, this is not highly suggestive for celiac disease if the patient has a normal total IgA level. An antigliadin IgG level 3 to 4 times the upper limit of normal for that lab is highly suggestive of a condition where the gut is abnormally permeable ("leaky") to gluten. This can happen with food allergies, cystic fibrosis, parasitic infections, Crohn's disease, and other types of autoimmune GI diseases. These antibodies may also be slightly elevated in individuals with no obvious disease.

The tTG IgA test is highly sensitive and specific. It correlates well with biopsy, is inexpensive, not subjective, and can be performed on a single drop of blood. However, it can be falsely positive in a patient who has other autoimmune conditions, such as type 1 diabetes. For those with a negative tTG IgA test, IgA deficiency should be considered. http://americanceliac.org/celiac-disease/diagnosis/)

BOX 28-7 The Basic Gluten-Free Diet

Foods	Safe Choices	Questionable	Avoid
Grains and flours	Amaranth, arrowroot, bean flours (such as garbanzo or fava bean), buckwheat, corn (maize) or cornstarch, flax, Job's tears, millet, potato, quinoa, ragi, rice, sorghum, soybean (soya), tapioca, teff	Carob-soy flour, buckwheat pancake mixes (often contain wheat flour), pure uncontaminated oats (note: a small percentage of people with celiac disease react to pure oats; discuss with health care provider first)	Wheat (bulghur, couscous, durum, farina, graham, kamut, semolina, spelt, triticale, wheat germ), rye, barley, oats (except pure, uncontaminated oats), low gluten flour. Caution: "wheat free" does not necessarily mean "gluten free"
Cereals—hot or dry	Cream of rice, cream of buckwheat, hominy, gluten-free dry cereals, grits	Puffed rice or corn cereals (possible contamination); pure uncontaminated oats (small percentage of people with CD react to oats)	Those with wheat, rye, oats (except pure, uncontaminated), barley, barley malt, malt favoring, wheat germ, bran
Potatoes, rice, starch	Any plain potatoes, sweet potatoes and yams, all types of plain rice, rice noodles, 100% buckwheat soba noodles, gluten-free pasta, polenta, hominy, corn tortillas, parsnips, yucca, turnips	Check labels for commercial potato or rice products with seasoning packets	Battered or deep-fried French fries (unless no other foods have been fried in the same oil), pasta, noodles, wheat starch, stuffing, flour tortillas, croutons
Crackers, chips, popcorn	Rice wafers or other gluten-free crackers, rice cakes; plain corn chips, corn tortilla chips, potato chips, and other root (taro, beet, sweet potato, or vegetable etc.) or grain (amaranth, quinoa) chips, plain popcorn	Flavored chips	On gluten-free crackers, graham crackers, rye crisps, matzo, croutons, pretzels
Desserts	Sorbet, popsicles, Italian ice	Check labels on ice cream and pudding	Ice cream with bits of cookies, "crispies," pretzels, etc; pie crust, cookies, cakes, ice cream cones, and pastries made from gluten-containing flours
Milk and yogurt	Any plain, unflavored milk or yogurt, buttermilk, cream, half and half	Flavored milks or yogurts (check labels)	Malted milk, yogurts with added "crunchies" or toppings
Cheese	Cheese (all styles including blue cheese and gorgonzola), processed cheese (i.e., American), cottage cheese	Cheese spreads or sauces (check labels)	
Eggs	All types of plain, cooked eggs	Eggs Benedict (sauce usually made with wheat flour)	
Meat, fish, shellfish, poultry	Any fresh, plain untreated meat, fish, shellfish, or poultry; fish canned in brine, vegetable broth, or water	Commercially treated, preserved, or marinated meats, luncheon meats, fish, shellfish; self-basting or cured poultry (check labels)	Breaded or battered meats
Beans and legumes	Any plain frozen, fresh, dried, or canned (no flavorings or sauces added) beans: garbanzo beans, kidney beans, lentils, pinto beans, edamame, lima, black beans, etc	Check labels for added ingredients—sauces may have gluten	
Soy products and meat analogs or alternatives	Plain tempeh, tofu, edamame	Check labels on miso, soy sauce, seasoned tofu and tempeh and hydrolyzed vegetable protein; meat analogs (imitation meat substitutes), imitation seafood and soy protein powdered drinks	Seitan; 3-Grain Tempeh
Nuts and seeds	Any plain (salted or unsalted) nuts, seeds or nut butters, coconut	Dry-roasted nuts (check with manufacturer—may dust with flour during processing)	Nut butters with gluten-containing ingredients
Fruits and juices	Any plain fresh, canned, frozen fruits or juices, plain dried fruit	Pie fillings (often thickened with gluten-containing flour)	Dried fruit dusted with flour
Vegetables	Any plain, fresh, canned or frozen vegetables including corn, peas, lima beans, etc.		Vegetables in gluten-containing sauce or gravy
Soups	Homemade soups with known allowed ingredients	Check labels on all commercial soups	
Condiments, jams, and syrups	Ketchup, mustard, salsa, wheat-free soy sauce, mayonnaise, vinegar (except malt vinegar), jam, jelly, honey, pure maple syrup, molasses	Check labels on soy sauce, salad dressings, commercial sauces, soup base, marinades, and coating mixes for gluten-free designation	Malt vinegar
Seasonings and flavorings	Any *plain* herb or spice; salt; pepper; brown or white sugar; or artificial sweetener (i.e., Equal, Sweet-N-Low, Splenda)	Seasoning mixes, bouillon; check labels for gluten-free designation	

Continued

BOX 28-7	The Basic Gluten-Free Diet—cont'd		
Foods	Safe Choices	Questionable	Avoid
Fats	Butter, margarine, all pure vegetable oils (including canola), mayonnaise, cream	Check labels on salad dressings, sandwich spreads	
Baking ingredients	Yeast, baking soda, baking powder, cream of tartar, regular chocolate baking chips		See grains and flours; Check label on grain sweetened, carob or vegan chocolate chips
Beverages	Coffee, tea, pure cocoa powder, sodas, Silk soymilk, Rice Dream beverage	Check labels on flavored instant coffee mixes (such as Swiss mocha, cappuccino); herbal teas, soy or rice drinks (may contain barley malt or rice syrup)	Malted beverages
Alcohol	Wine, all distilled liquor including vodka, tequila, gin, rum, whiskey and pure liqueurs, gluten-free beers (Redbridge, Bard's Tale beer, ciders)	Drink mixes	Beer, ale, lager
Candies	Check labels—many are gluten-free		Candy from bulk food bins Licorice

Adapted from Parrish CR et al: *University of Virginia Health System Nutrition Support Traineeship Syllabus,* Charlottesville, Va, 2010, University of Virginia Health System.
CD, Celiac disease.

The healing of the intestinal mucosa that occurs after initiation of a GF diet improves nutrient absorption, and many patients who eat well-balanced GF diets do not need nutritional supplementation. However, most specialty GF products are not fortified with iron, folate, and other B vitamins like other grain products, so the diet may not be as complete without at least partial supplementation. Anemia should be treated with iron, folate, or vitamin B_{12}, depending on the nature of the anemia. Patients with malabsorption may benefit from a bone density scan to assess for osteopenia or osteoporosis. Calcium and vitamin D supplementation are likely to be beneficial in these patients. Electrolyte and fluid replacement is essential for those dehydrated from severe diarrhea.

Those who continue to have malabsorption should take a general vitamin-mineral supplement to at least meet DRI recommendations. Lactose and fructose intolerance sometimes occur secondary to CD, and sugar alcohols are not well absorbed, even in a healthy gut. A low-lactose or low-fructose diet may be useful in controlling symptoms, at least initially. Once the GI tract returns to more normal function, lactase activity also may return, and the person can incorporate lactose and dairy products back into the diet.

In general, many fruits, vegetables, non–gluten containing grains, meats, and dairy products that are plain and unseasoned are safe to eat. Oats were once thought to be questionable for persons with CD; however, extensive studies have shown that they are safe in the GF diet as long as they are pure, uncontaminated oats (Garsed and Scott, 2007). However, a very small population of patients with CD may not tolerate even pure oats. In general, patients do not need to be advised against including GF oats in their diet unless they have demonstrated intolerance to GF oats.

Flours made from corn, potatoes, rice, soybean, tapioca, arrowroot, sorghum, garbanzo beans, nuts (such as almond flour), amaranth, quinoa, millet, teff, and buckwheat can be substituted in recipes. Patients can expect differences in textures and flavors of common foods using the substitute flours, but new recipes can be palatable once the adjustment is made. In GF baked goods, gums such as xanthan, guar, and cellulose (from nongluten grains) can be used to provide the elasticity needed to trap leavening gases in baked goods.

A truly GF diet requires careful scrutiny of the labels of all bakery products and packaged foods. Gluten-containing grains are not only used as primary ingredients in many products but also may be added during processing or preparation of foods. For example, hydrolyzed vegetable protein can be made from wheat, soy, corn, or mixtures of these grains.

In the US there is now a gluten-free labeling law that went into effect in September, 2014. (https://www.federalregister.gov/articles/2013/08/05/2013-18813/food-labeling-gluten-free-labeling-of-foods). This law states that all food carrying a gluten-free claim also must contain less that 20 ppm gluten (i.e., below 20 mg gluten per kg of food), including from cross-contact. Thompson discusses the law in detail (Thompson, 2015). Recent studies on the gluten content of labeled gluten-free food in the US showed that 95 – 99% of the products tested contained less than 20 ppm gluten (Sharma et al, 2015).

The diet for the person with CD requires a major lifestyle change because of the change from traditional grains in the diet. A tremendous number of foods made with wheat (in particular breads, cereals, pastas, and baked goods) are a common part of a Western diet. However, there is increasing awareness among food companies and restaurants of the expanding demand for GF foods, and food businesses are responding. The individual and family members should be taught about label reading, safe food additives, food preparation, sources of cross-contamination (such as toasters, condiment jars, bulk bins, and buffets), and hidden sources of gluten (such as medications and communion wafers) to be compliant with the diet. Box 28-8 provides sources of hidden gluten and cross-contamination. Eating in cafeterias, restaurants, vending outlets, street markets, at friends' homes, and at social events can be challenging, especially initially.

To avoid misinterpretation of information, newly diagnosed patients should be started with an in-depth instruction from a registered dietitian nutritionist (RDN) on the GF diet, along with reliable resources for further guidance and support. Persons with CD generally need several educational or counseling sessions and often benefit from a support group (American Gastroenterological Association [AGA], 2015) (see Box 28-9 for CD resources).

Marked gut improvement and a return to normal histologic findings occurs in the majority of patients after an average of 2 years (Hutchinson et al, 2010). Patients who are able to follow the GF diet closely have a better overall response (see *Pathophysiology and Care Management Algorithm: Celiac Disease*).

BOX 28-8   Hidden Gluten Exposure and Cross-Contamination

Hidden Gluten Exposure

Unfortunately, gluten is not always obvious. Review the list below for some "unsuspected" products that may contain gluten.

- Over-the-counter and prescription medications

The labeling requirements of the Food Allergen and Consumer Protection Act of 2004 (FALCPA) **do not** apply to medications (see Box 26-10 in Chapter 26). Check with your pharmacist or call the manufacturer to determine whether there is any gluten in your medications.

Note: Dietary supplements are covered under FALCPA regulations, so wheat must be clearly listed if it is an ingredient in a vitamin, mineral, or herbal supplement.

- Communion wafers

Gluten-free recipes are available.

- Uncommon sources

If laboratory values stay elevated and symptoms remain and, possible sources of gluten cannot be found in the diet, it may be worth checking into other sources such as toothpaste, mouthwash, or lipstick.

Cross-Contamination

Below are some of the most common sources of gluten contamination. A few crumbs that may not even be seen can cause damage to the intestine, so it is best to avoid these situations:

- Toasters used for gluten-containing foods

Keep two toasters at home and designate one as gluten free. Alternatively, there are now bags available that are designed to hold a piece of bread in the toaster.
- Bulk bins

Prepackaged food is a safer bet.
- Condiment jars (peanut butter, jam, mayonnaise, etc.)

It is best to keep a separate gluten-free jar for commonly used items and be sure to label it clearly. At the very least, make sure everyone in the house knows not to "double-dip."
- Buffet lines

Other customers may use one serving utensil for multiple items. Food from one area may be spilled into another food container. It may be safer to order from the menu.
- Deep-fried foods

Oil is typically used over and over to fry foods. It is highly likely that French fries (or other GF foods) are fried in the same oil as battered and breaded foods like fried chicken.

Adapted from Parrish CR et al: *University of Virginia Health System Nutrition Support Traineeship Syllabus*, Charlottesville, Va, 2010, University of Virginia Health System.
GF, Gluten free.

BOX 28-9   Celiac Disease Resources

Support Groups

Gluten Intolerance Group
Phone: 206-246-6652
E-mail: info@gluten.net
Website: www.gluten.net

Canadian Celiac Association
Phone: 800-363-7296
E-mail: customerservice@celiacs.ca
Website: www.celiac.ca

Celiac Disease Foundation
Phone: 818-990-2354
E-mail: cdf@celiac.org
Website: www.celiac.org

Celiac Sprue Association
Phone: 877-272-4272
E-mail: celiacs@csaceliacs.org
Website: www.csaceliacs.org

Medical Centers

Beth Israel Deaconess Celiac Center
Boston, Massachusetts
www.bidmc.harvard.edu/celiaccenter

University of Maryland Center for Celiac Research
Baltimore, Maryland
www.celiaccenter.org

Celiac Disease Center at Columbia University
New York, New York
www.celiacdiseasecenter.columbia.edu

University of Chicago Celiac Disease Program
Chicago, Illinois
www.celiacdisease.net

Other Celiac Organizations/Resources

National Foundation for Celiac Awareness
www.celiacawareness.org

Celiac listserv
www.enabling.org/ia/celiac

Gluten-free Restaurant Awareness Program
www.glutenfreerestaurants.org

Celiac Disease and Gluten-free Support Center
www.celiac.com

Clan Thompson Celiac Site (free newsletter)
http://finecooks.com/2009/01/clan-thompsons-gluten-free-list.html

PATHOPHYSIOLOGY AND CARE MANAGEMENT ALGORITHM

Celiac Disease (Gluten-Sensitive Enteropathy or Nontropical Sprue)

ETIOLOGY

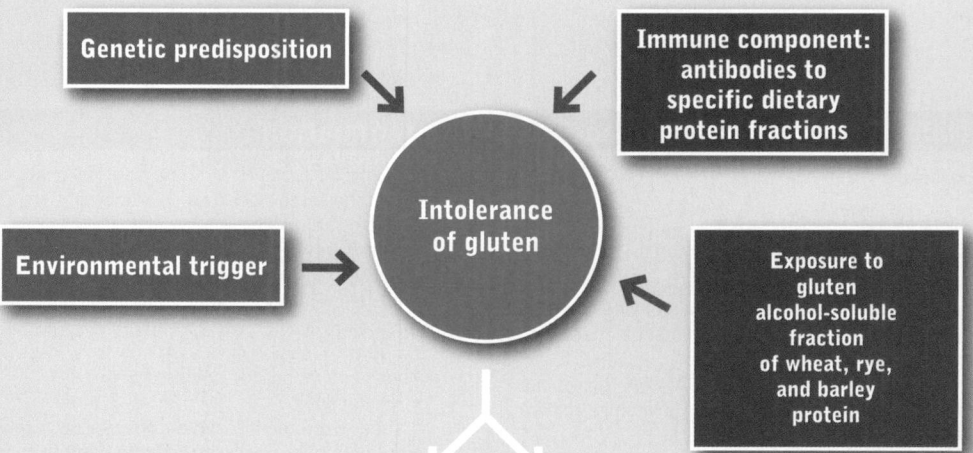

Genetic predisposition →

Immune component: antibodies to specific dietary protein fractions ↙

Environmental trigger → **Intolerance of gluten**

Exposure to gluten alcohol-soluble fraction of wheat, rye, and barley protein ↖

PATHOPHYSIOLOGY

Damage To Small Bowel
- Atrophy and flattening of villi
- Reduced area for absorption
- Cellular deficiency of disaccharidases and peptidases
- Reduced nutrient transport carriers

Extraintestinal Manifestations
- Anemia
- Bone loss
- Muscle weakness
- Polyneuropathy
- Endocrine disorders (e.g., infertility)
- Follicular hyperkeratosis
- Dermatitis herpetiformis

Intestinal Manifestations
- Chronic diarrhea
- Chronic constipation
- Malabsorption of vitamins and minerals

MANAGEMENT

Medical Management
- Electrolyte and fluid replacement
- Management of other co-morbid conditions

Nutrition Management
- Delete gluten sources (wheat, rye, barley) from diet
- Vitamin and mineral supplementation
- Substitute with corn, potato, rice, soybean, tapioca, arrowroot, and other non-gluten flours
- Calcium and vitamin D administration
- Read food labels carefully for hidden gluten-containing ingredients
- Supplementation with ω-3 fatty acids
- Guidance to support groups and reliable internet resources

Tropical Sprue

Tropical sprue is an acquired diarrheal syndrome with malabsorption that occurs in many tropical areas. In addition to diarrhea and malabsorption, anorexia, abdominal distention, and nutritional deficiency as evidenced by night blindness, glossitis, stomatitis, cheilosis, pallor, and edema can occur. Anemia may result from iron, folic acid, and vitamin B_{12} deficiencies.

Pathophysiology

Diarrhea appears to be an infectious type, although the precise cause and the sequence of pathogenic events remain unknown. The syndrome may include bacterial overgrowth, changes in GI motility, and cellular changes in the GI tract. Identified intestinal organisms may differ from one region of the tropics to the next. As in CD, the intestinal villi may be abnormal, but the surface cell alterations are much less severe. The gastric mucosa is atrophied and inflamed, with diminished secretion of hydrochloric acid and intrinsic factor (Langenberg et al, 2014).

Medical Treatment

Treatment of tropical sprue typically includes use of broad-spectrum antibiotics, folic acid, fluid, and electrolytes.

Medical Nutrition Therapy

Nutrition management includes restoration and maintenance of fluids, electrolytes, macronutrients, and micronutrients, and introduction of a diet that is appropriate for the extent of malabsorption (see Diarrhea earlier in this chapter). Along with other nutrients, B_{12} and folate supplementation may be needed if deficiency is identified. Nutritional deficiency increases susceptibility to infectious agents, further aggravating the condition.

INTESTINAL BRUSH-BORDER ENZYME DEFICIENCIES

Intestinal enzyme deficiency states involve deficiencies of the brush-border disaccharidases that hydrolyze disaccharides at the mucosal cell membrane. Disaccharidase deficiencies may occur as (1) rare congenital defects such as the sucrase, isomaltase, or lactase deficiencies seen in the newborn; (2) generalized forms secondary to diseases that damage the intestinal epithelium (e.g., Crohn's disease or CD); or, most commonly, (3) a genetically acquired form (e.g., lactase deficiency) that usually appears after childhood but can appear as early as 2 years of age. For this chapter, only lactose malabsorption is described in detail (see Chapter 43 for a discussion of inborn metabolic disorders).

Lactose Intolerance

Lactose intolerance is the syndrome of diarrhea, abdominal pain, flatulence, or bloating occurring after lactose consumption. Secondary lactose intolerance can develop as a consequence of infection of the small intestine, inflammatory disorders, HIV, or malnutrition. In children it is typically secondary to viral or bacterial infections. Lactose malabsorption commonly is associated with other GI disorders, such as IBS.

Etiology

High concentrations of the brush border enzyme, lactase, is present in the small bowel of all newborn mammals. After weaning, about 75% of the world's population dramatically decreases the synthesis of this enzyme despite continued exposure to lactose (Levitt et al, 2013). These people are termed to be lactase nonpersistent. The majority of adults of Asian, African, Latino, and Native American descent are lactase nonpersistent, whereas the majority of Caucasians are lactase persistent. Lactose malabsorption or intolerance has been reported to be low in children younger than age six but increases throughout childhood, peaking at age 10 to 16 years.

Little evidence indicates that lactose intolerance increases with increasing adult age (Suchy et al, 2010). Even in adults who retain a high level of lactase levels (75% to 85% of white adults of Western European heritage), the quantity of lactase is approximately half that of other saccharidases such as sucrase, alpha-dextrinase, or glucoamylase. The decline of lactase is commonly known as hypolactasia (see *Focus On:* Lactose Intolerance – NOT an Uncommon Anomaly).

Pathophysiology

When large amounts of lactose are consumed, especially by persons who have little remaining lactase enzyme or with concurrent GI problems, loose stools or diarrhea can occur. As is the case with any malabsorbed sugar, lactose may act osmotically and increase fecal water, as well as provide a substrate for rapid fermentation by intestinal bacteria, which may result in bloating, flatulence, and cramps. Malabsorption of lactose is due to a deficiency of lactase, the enzyme that digests the sugar

---

⊚ FOCUS ON

Lactose Intolerance: NOT an Uncommon Anomaly

When lactose intolerance was first described in 1963, it appeared to be an infrequent occurrence, arising only occasionally in the white population. Because the capacity to digest lactose was measured in people from a wide variety of ethnic and racial backgrounds, it soon became apparent that disappearance of the lactase enzyme shortly after weaning, or at least during early childhood, was actually the predominant (normal) condition in most of the world's population. With a few exceptions, the intestinal tracts of adult mammals produce little, if any, lactase after weaning (the milks of pinnipeds—seals, walruses, and sea lions—do not contain lactose).

The exception of lactose tolerance has attracted the interest of geographers and others concerned with the evolution of the world's population. A genetic mutation favoring lactose tolerance appears to have arisen approximately 10,000 years ago, when dairying was first introduced. Presumably, it would have occurred in places where milk consumption was encouraged because of some degree of dietary deprivation and in groups in which milk was not fermented before consumption (fermentation breaks down much of the lactose into monosaccharides). The mutation would have selectively endured, because it would promote greater health, survival, and reproduction of those who carried the gene.

It is proposed that the mutation occurred in more than one location and then accompanied migrations of populations throughout the world. It continues primarily among whites from northern Europe and in ethnic groups in India, Africa, and Mongolia. The highest frequency (97%) of lactose tolerance occurs in Sweden and Denmark, suggesting an increased selective advantage in those able to tolerate lactose related to the limited exposure to ultraviolet light typical of northern latitudes. Lactose favors calcium absorption, which is limited in the absence of vitamin D produced by skin exposure to sunlight.

Dairying was unknown in North America until the arrival of Europeans. Thus Native Americans and all of the non-European immigrants are among the 90% of the world's population who tolerate milk poorly, if at all. This has practical implications with respect to group feeding programs such as school breakfasts and lunches. However, many lactose-intolerant people are able to digest milk in small to moderate amounts (Shaukat et al, 2010).

in milk. Lactose that is not hydrolyzed into galactose and glucose in the upper small intestine passes into the colon, where bacteria ferment it to SCFAs, carbon dioxide, and hydrogen gas.

Medical Treatment

Lactose malabsorption is diagnosed by (1) an abnormal hydrogen breath test or (2) an abnormal lactose tolerance test. During a hydrogen breath test, the patient is given a standard dose of lactose after fasting, and breath hydrogen is measured. If lactose is not digested in the small intestine, it passes into the colon, where it is fermented by the gut microbiota to SCFAs, CO_2, and hydrogen. Hydrogen is absorbed into the bloodstream and is exhaled through the lungs. The breath hydrogen test shows increased levels 60 to 90 minutes after lactose ingestion.

During a lactose tolerance test, a dose of lactose is given, and if the individual has sufficient lactase enzyme, blood sugar rises, reflecting the digestion of lactose to galactose and glucose. If the individual is lactose intolerant (lactase deficient), blood sugar will not rise because the lactose is not absorbed; it passes into the colon and GI symptoms may appear. The lactose tolerance test was based originally on an oral dose of lactose equivalent to the amount in 1 quart of milk (50 g). Recently doses lower than 50 g of lactose have been used to approximate more closely the usual consumption of lactose from milk products.

Demonstrated lactose malabsorption does not always indicate a person will be symptomatic. Many factors play a role, including the amount of lactose ingested, the residual lactase activity, the ingestion of food in addition to lactose, the ability of the gut microbiota to ferment lactose, and the sensitivity of the individual to the lactose fermentation products (Misselwitz et al, 2013). Consumption of small amounts should be of little consequence because the SCFAs are readily absorbed and the gases can be absorbed or passed. Larger amounts, usually greater than 12 g/day, consumed in a single food (the amount typically found in a cup or 240 ml of milk) may result in more substrate entering the colon than can be disposed of by normal processes. Because serving sizes of milk drinks are increasing and more than one source of lactose may be consumed in the same meal, the amounts of lactose consumed may be more important than in years past (Misselwitz et al, 2013).

Medical Nutrition Therapy

Management of lactose intolerance requires dietary change. The symptoms are alleviated by reduced consumption of lactose-containing foods (see Table 28-3 for common foods containing lactose). Persons who avoid dairy products may need calcium and vitamin D supplementation or must be careful to get nondairy sources of these nutrients. A completely lactose-free diet is not necessary in lactase-deficient persons. Most lactose maldigesters can consume some lactose (up to 12 g/day) without major symptoms, especially when taken with meals or in the form of cheeses or fermented dairy products (Misselwitz et al, 2013).

Many adults with intolerance to moderate amounts of milk can ultimately adapt to and tolerate 12 g or more of lactose in milk (equivalent to one cup of full-lactose milk) when introduced gradually, in increments, over several weeks. Incremental or continuous exposure to increasing quantities of fermentable sugar can lead to improved tolerance, not as a consequence of increased lactase enzyme production but perhaps by altered gut microbiota composition. This has been shown with lactulose, a nonabsorbed carbohydrate that is biochemically similar to lactose (Lomer, 2014). Individual differences in tolerance may relate to the state of

TABLE 28-3 Lactose Content of Common Foods

Product	Serving Size	Approximate Lactose Content (grams)
Milk (nonfat, 1%, 2%, whole), chocolate milk, acidophilis milk, buttermilk	1 cup	10-12
Butter, margarine	1 tsp	trace
Cheese	1 ounce	0-2
Cheddar, sharp	1 ounce	0
American, Swiss, parmesan	1 ounce	1
Bleu cheese	1 ounce	2
Cottage cheese	½ cup	2-3
Cream (heavy), whipped cream	½ cup	3-4
Cream cheese	1 ounce	1
Evaporated milk	1 cup	24
Half-and-half	½ cup	5
Ice cream	½ cup	6
Ice milk	½ cup	9
Nonfat dry milk powder (unreconstituted)	1 cup	62
Sherbet, orange	½ cup	2
Sour cream	½ cup	4
Sweetened condensed milk, undiluted	1 cup	40
Yogurt, cultured, low-fat*	1 cup	5-10

*Note: Although yogurt does contain lactose, cultured yogurt is generally well tolerated by those with lactose intolerance.

colonic adaptation. Regular consumption of milk by lactase-deficient persons may increase the threshold at which diarrhea occurs.

Lactase enzyme in tablets or liquid or in milk products treated with lactase enzyme (e.g., Lactaid) are available for lactose maldigesters who have discomfort with milk ingestion. Commercial lactase preparations may differ in their effectiveness. Fermented milk products, such as aged cheeses and yogurts, are well tolerated because their lactose content is low. Tolerance of yogurt may be the result of a microbial galactosidase in the bacterial culture that facilitates lactose digestion in the intestine. The presence of galactosidase depends on the brand and processing method. Because this microbial enzyme is sensitive to freezing, frozen yogurt may not be as well tolerated. Although the addition of probiotics may change this, evidence is lacking (Morelli, 2014).

Fructose Malabsorption

Dietary fructose exists mainly in three forms: (1) the monosaccharide, (2) sucrose, a disaccharide of fructose and glucose, and (3) in chains as fructans. Consumption of fructose in the United States, especially from fruit juices, fruit drinks, and high fructose corn syrup (HFCS) in soft drinks and confections, has increased significantly in recent years. The human small intestine has a limited ability to absorb fructose, compared with the ability to absorb glucose rapidly and completely.

Etiology

Although fructose malabsorption is common in healthy people, its appearance depends on the amount of fructose ingested.

Absorption of fructose is improved when it is ingested with glucose (such as in sucrose) because glucose absorption stimulates pathways for fructose absorption. Although some degree of fructose malabsorption may be normal, those with coexisting GI disorders may be more likely to experience GI symptoms after fructose ingestion. Patients with IBS and visceral hypersensitivity may be more sensitive to gas, distension, or pain from fructose malabsorption, whereas those with small bowel bacterial overgrowth (SIBO) may experience symptoms from normal amounts of fructose.

Pathophysiology

Breath hydrogen testing has revealed that up to 75% of healthy people will incompletely absorb a large quantity of fructose (50 g) taken alone (Putkonen et al, 2013).

Fructose coexists in food with other poorly absorbed carbohydrates, which have been given the umbrella term of fermentable, oligosaccharides, disaccharides, monosaccharide, and polyols (**FODMAPs**). The efficacy of restricting all FODMAPs (see later in this chapter) compared with fructose alone for managing GI symptoms of fructose malabsorption has not been compared, but it may be a promising intervention (Staudacher et al, 2012).

Medical Nutrition Therapy

People with fructose malabsorption and those patients with GI conditions that experience symptoms of fructose malabsorption may not have problems with foods containing balanced amounts of glucose and fructose but may need to limit or avoid foods containing large amounts of free fructose. Pear, apple, mango, and Asian pear are notable in that they have substantially more "free fructose" (more fructose than glucose). In addition, most dried fruits and fruit juices may pose a problem in larger amounts because of the amount of fructose provided per serving. Foods sweetened with HFCS (as opposed to sucrose) are also more likely to cause symptoms. Hepatic fructose metabolism is similar to ethanol, in that they both serve as substrates for de novo lipogenesis, thus promoting hepatic insulin resistance, dyslipidemia, and hepatic steatosis (Lustig, 2010). The degree of fructose intolerance and tolerance to the symptoms of fructose malabsorption are so variable that intake of these foods must generally be individualized with each patient (see Table 28-7 for a list of foods high in fructose content).

INFLAMMATORY BOWEL DISEASES

The two major forms of IBD are Crohn's disease and UC. Crohn's disease and UC are relatively rare disorders, but they result in frequent use of health care resources. The prevalence and incidence is increasing as it emerges as a global disease. It is also becoming more prevalent in the elderly (Ye et al, 2015).

Etiology

The onset of IBD occurs most often in patients 15 to 30 years of age, but for some it occurs later in adulthood. Both sexes are equally affected. IBD occurs more commonly in developed areas of the world, in urban compared with rural environments, and in northern compared with southern climates. The reasons for the increased risk are not clear but are likely related to the increased inflammatory and proliferative state and nutritional factors affecting this.

Crohn's disease and UC share some clinical characteristics, including diarrhea, fever, weight loss, anemia, food intolerances, malnutrition, growth failure, and extraintestinal manifestations (arthritic, dermatologic, and hepatic). In both forms of IBD, the risk

of malignancy increases with the duration of the disease. Although malnutrition can occur in both forms of IBD, it is more of a lifelong concern in patients with Crohn's disease. The features that distinguish the forms of the disease in terms of genetic characteristics, clinical presentation, and treatment are discussed in Table 28-4.

Etiology

The cause of IBD is not completely understood, but it involves the interaction of the GI immunologic system and genetic and environmental factors. The genetic susceptibility is now recognized to be diverse, with a number of possible gene mutations that affect risk and characteristics of the disease. The diversity in the genetic alterations among individuals may help explain differences in the onset, aggressiveness, complications, location, and responsiveness to different therapies as seen in the clinical setting. The major environmental factors include resident and transient microorganisms in the GI tract and dietary components.

The genes affected (e.g., C677T mutation related to methylene-tetrahydrofolate reductase) normally play a role in the reactivity of the host GI immune system to luminal antigens such as those provided by intestinal flora and the diet. In animal models inflammatory disease does not occur in the absence of gut microbiota. Normally, when an antigenic challenge or trauma occurs, the immune response is initiated; it is then turned off and continues to be held in check after the challenge resolves. In IBD however, increased antigen exposure, decreased host defense mechanisms, and/or decreased tolerance to some components of the gut microbiota occurs. Inappropriate inflammatory response and an inability to suppress it play primary roles in the disease. For example, two genes, $NOD_2/CARD_{15}$ and the autophagy gene ATG16L1 have been linked to one functional pathway of bacterial sensing, invasion, and elimination. Failure of these genes to come

	Ulcerative Colitis	Crohn's Disease
TABLE 28-4	**Ulcerative Colitis versus Crohn's Disease**	
Presentation	Bloody diarrhea	Perianal disease, abdominal pain (65%), mass in abdomen
Gross Pathology	Rectum always involved	Rectum may not be involved
	Moves continuously proximally from rectum	Can occur anywhere along gastrointestinal tract
		Not continuous: "skip lesions"
	Thin wall	Thick wall
	Few strictures	Strictures common
	Diffuse ulceration	Cobblestone appearance
Histopathology	No granulomas	Granulomas
	Low inflammation	More inflammation
	Deeper ulcers (hence named ulcerative)	Shallow ulcers
	Pseudopolyps	Fibrosis
	Abscesses in crypts	
Extraintestinal manifestations	Sclerosing cholangitis	Erythema nodosum
	Pyoderma gangrenosum	Migratory polyarthritis Gallstones
Complications	Toxic megacolon	Malabsorption
	Cancer	Cancer
	Strictures and fistulas are very rare	Strictures or fistulas Perianal disease

together can lead to impaired autophagy and persistence of bacteria resulting in abnormal immune responses (Bossuyt and Vermeire, 2016).

Pathophysiology

Crohn's Disease and Ulcerative Colitis Crohn's disease may involve any part of the GIT, but approximately 50% to 60% of cases involve the distal ileum and the colon. Only the small intestine or only the colon is involved in 15% to 25% of cases. Disease activity in UC is limited to the large intestine and rectum. In Crohn's disease, segments of inflamed bowel may be separated by healthy segments, whereas in UC the disease process is continuous (see Figure 28-3). Mucosal involvement in Crohn's disease is transmural in that it affects all layers of the mucosa; in UC the disease normally is limited to the mucosa. Crohn's disease is characterized by abscesses, fistulas, fibrosis, submucosal thickening, localized strictures, narrowed segments of bowel, and partial or complete obstruction of the intestinal lumen. Bleeding is more common in UC (see Table 28-4).

The inflammatory response (e.g., increased cytokines and acute-phase proteins, increased GI permeability, increased proteases, and increased oxygen radicals and leukotrienes) results in GI tissue damage. In IBD either the regulatory mechanisms are defective or the factors perpetuating the immune and acute-phase responses are enhanced, leading to tissue fibrosis and destruction. The clinical course of the disease may be mild and episodic or severe and unremitting (see *Pathophysiology and Care Management Algorithm:* Inflammatory Bowel Disease).

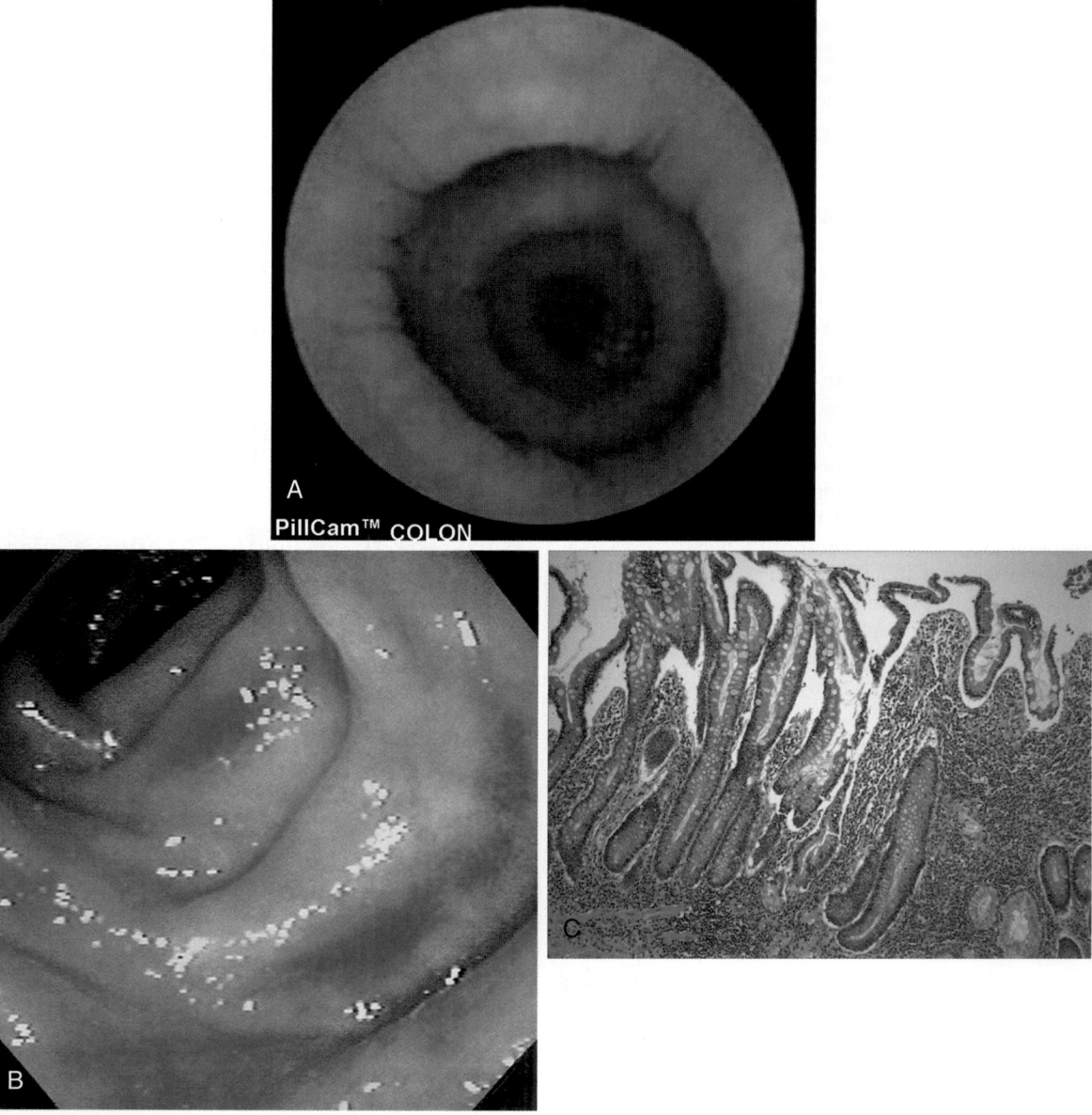

FIGURE 28-3 A, Normal colon. **B,** Ulcerative colitis. **C,** Crohn's disease. (*A,* From Fireman Z, Kopelman Y: The colon—the latest terrain for capsule endoscopy. *Dig Liver Dis* 39[10]:895-899, 2007. *B,* From Black JM, Hawks JH: Medical surgical nursing: clinical management for positive outcomes, ed 8, St Louis, 2009, Saunders. *C,* From McGowan, CE, Lagares-Garcia JA, Bhattacharya B: Retained capsule endoscope leading to the identification of small bowel adenocarcinoma in a patient with undiagnosed Crohn's disease, *Ann Diagn Pathol* 13[6]:390-393, 2009.)

PATHOPHYSIOLOGY AND CARE MANAGEMENT ALGORITHM

Inflammatory Bowel Disease

ETIOLOGY

Genetic predisposition →

Unknown "irritant" Viral? Bacterial? Autoimmune? →

Abnormal activation of the mucosal immune response. Secondary systemic response

← Vitamin D insufficiency

PATHOPHYSIOLOGY

Inflammatory Response

↓

Damage to the cells of the small and/or large intestine with malabsorption, ulceration, or stricture

↓

- Diarrhea
- Weight loss
- Poor growth
- Hyperhomocysteinemia
- Partial GI obstructions

MANAGEMENT

Medical Management

- Corticosteroids
- Anti-inflammatory agents
- Immunosuppressants
- Antibiotics
- Anticytokine medications

Surgical Management

- Bowel resection that can result in short bowel syndrome (SBS)

Nutrition Management

- Oral enteral formula (tube-feed if necessary)
- Use of foods that are well tolerated
- Parenteral nutrition in patients with severe disease or obstruction
- Multivitamin supplement containing folic acid, B_{12}, and B_6
- ω-3 fatty acid supplementation
- Consider use of prebiotics and probiotics
- Modify fiber intake as necessary
- Test for food intolerances

Diet is an environmental factor that may trigger relapses of IBD. Foods, microbes, individual nutrients, and incidental contaminants provide a huge number of potential antigens, especially considering the complexity and diversity of the modern diet. Malnutrition can affect the function and effectiveness of the mucosal, cellular, and immune barriers; diet also can affect the type and relative composition of the resident microflora. Several nutrients, such as dietary fats or vitamin D, can affect the intensity of the inflammatory response (Hlavaty et al, 2015; Sadeghian et al, 2015).

Food allergies and other immunologic reactions to specific foods have been considered in the pathogenesis of IBD and its symptoms; however, the incidence of documented food allergies, compared with food intolerances, is relatively small. The permeability of the intestinal wall to molecules of food and cell fragments is likely increased in inflammatory states, allowing the potential for increased interaction of antigens with host immune systems (Vermeire et al, 2011).

Food intolerances occur more often in persons with IBD than in the population at large, but the patterns are not consistent among individuals or even between exposures from one time to the next. Reasons for specific and nonspecific food intolerances are abundant and are related to the severity, location, and complications associated with the disease process. Partial GI obstructions, malabsorption, diarrhea, altered GI transit, increased secretions, food aversions, and associations are but a few of the problems experienced by persons with IBD. However, neither food allergies nor intolerances fully explain the onset or manifestations in all patients (see Chapter 26).

Medical Management

The goals of treatment in IBD are to induce and maintain remission and to improve nutrition status. Treatment of the primary GI manifestations appears to correct most of the extraintestinal features of the disease as well. The most effective medical agents include corticosteroids, antiinflammatory agents (aminosalicylates), immunosuppressive agents (cyclosporine, azathioprine, mercaptopurine), antibiotics (ciprofloxacin and metronidazole), and monoclonal tumor necrosis factor antagonists (anti-TNF), and infliximab, adalimumab, certolizumab, and natalizumab, agents that inactivate one of the primary inflammatory cytokines. Anti-TNF is normally used in severe cases of Crohn's disease and fistulas, but it has not been shown to be effective in UC.

Investigations of various treatment modalities for the acute and chronic stages of IBD are ongoing and include new forms of existing drugs as well as new agents targeted to regulate production and activity of cytokines, eicosanoids, or other mediators of the inflammatory and acute-phase response (Monteleone et al, 2014).

Surgical Management

In Crohn's disease, surgery may be necessary to repair strictures or remove portions of the bowel when medical management fails. Approximately 50% to 70% of persons with Crohn's disease undergo surgery related to the disease. Surgery does not cure Crohn's disease, and recurrence often occurs within 1 to 3 years of surgery. The chance of needing subsequent surgery in the patient's life is approximately 30% to 70%, depending on the type of surgery and the age at the first operation. Major resections of the intestine may result in varying degrees of malabsorption of fluid and nutrients. In

extreme cases patients may have extensive or multiple resections, resulting in short-bowel syndrome (SBS) and dependence on PN to maintain adequate nutrient intake and hydration (see Chapter 13).

With UC, approximately 20% of patients have a colectomy and removal of the colon, and this resolves the disease. Inflammation does not occur in the remaining GI tract. Whether a colectomy is necessary depends on the severity of the disease and indicators of increased cancer risk. After a colectomy for UC, surgeons may create an ileostomy with an external collection pouch and an internal abdominal reservoir fashioned with a segment of ileum or an ileoanal pouch, which spares the rectum, to serve as a reservoir for stool. The internal Koch pouch also may be used.

Medical Nutrition Therapy

Persons with IBD are at increased risk of nutrition problems for a host of reasons related to the disease and its treatment. Thus the primary goal is to restore and maintain the nutrition status of the individual. Foods, dietary and micronutrient supplements, and enteral and parenteral nutrition may be used to accomplish that mission. Oral diet and the other means of nutrition support may change during remissions and exacerbations of the disease.

Persons with IBD often have fears and misconceptions regarding GI symptoms and the role of food. Patients also often are confused by dietary advice from associates, various media, and health care providers. Education is a key form of nutrition intervention. There is no single dietary regimen for reducing symptoms or decreasing the flares in IBD. Diet and specific nutrients play a supportive role in maintaining nutrition status, limiting symptom exacerbations, and supporting growth in pediatric patients.

The ability of parenteral or enteral nutrition to induce remission of IBD has been debated for several years. Evaluation is confounded by the natural course of IBD with exacerbations and remissions and by the genetic diversity of the patients. Studies have concluded that (1) nutrition support may bring about some clinical remission when used as a sole source of treatment; (2) "complete bowel rest" using PN is not necessarily required; (3) enteral nutrition has the potential to feed the intestinal epithelium and alter GI flora and is the preferred route of nutrition support; (4) enteral nutrition may temper some elements of the inflammatory process, serve as a valuable source of nutrients needed for restoration of GI defects, and be steroid sparing; (5) children benefit from the use of enteral nutrition, either as sole source of nutrition or supplemental to an oral diet, to maintain growth and reduce the dependence on steroids that may affect growth and bone disease (Richmond and Rhodes, 2013). Patients and caretakers must be very committed when using enteral nutrition formulas or tube feeding because it takes 4 to 8 weeks before one sees the clinical effects.

Timely nutritional support is a vital component of therapy to restore and maintain nutritional health. Malnutrition compromises digestive and absorptive function by increasing the permeability of the GI tract to potential inflammatory agents. PN is not as nutritionally complete, has increased risk of infectious complications, and is more expensive than enteral nutrition. However, PN may be required in patients with persistent bowel obstruction, fistulas, and major GI resections that result in SBS where enteral nutrition is not possible.

Energy needs of patients with IBD are not greatly increased (unless weight gain is desired). Generally when disease activity increases basal metabolic rate, physical activity is greatly curtailed and overall energy needs are not substantially changed.

Protein requirements may be increased, depending on the severity and stage of the disease and the restoration requirements. Inflammation and treatment with corticosteroids induce a negative nitrogen balance and cause a loss of lean muscle mass. Protein losses also occur in areas of inflamed and ulcerated intestinal mucosa via defects in epithelial tight junctions (see Chapter 38). To maintain positive nitrogen balance, 1.3 to 1.5 g/kg/day of protein is recommended.

Supplemental vitamins, especially folate, B_6, and B_{12}, may be needed as well as minerals such as iron and trace elements to replace stores or for maintenance because of maldigestion, malabsorption, drug-nutrient interactions, or inadequate intake (Owczarek et al, 2016). Diarrhea can aggravate losses of zinc, potassium, and selenium. Patients who receive intermittent corticosteroids may need supplemental calcium and vitamin D. Patients with IBD are at increased risk of osteopenia and osteoporosis; 25-OH vitamin D levels and bone density should be monitored routinely and vitamin D supplemented appropriately (Hlavaty et al, 2015). Omega-3 fatty acid supplements in Crohn's disease significantly reduce disease activity. Use of omega-3 fatty acids or fish oil supplements in UC appears to result in a significant medication-sparing effect, with reductions in disease activity and increased time in remission reported (Farrukh and Mayberry, 2014). Use of foods and supplements containing prebiotics and probiotic supplements continues to be investigated for their potential to alter the gut microbiota; however, the benefit of either remains unproven (Sinegra et al, 2013).

In daily life people with IBD may have intermittent "flares" of the disease characterized by partial obstructions, nausea, abdominal pain, bloating, or diarrhea. Many patients report specific, individualized food intolerances (Hou et al, 2014). Patients sometimes are advised to eliminate the foods they suspect are responsible for the intolerance. Often, the patient becomes increasingly frustrated as the diet becomes progressively limited and symptoms still do not resolve. Malnutrition is a significant risk in patients with IBD, and an overly restricted diet only increases the likelihood of malnutrition and weight loss.

During acute and severe exacerbations of the disease, the diet is tailored to the individual. In people with rapid intestinal transit, extensive bowel resections, or extensive small bowel disease, absorption may be compromised. Here, excessive intake of lactose, fructose, or sorbitol may contribute to abdominal cramping, gas, and diarrhea; and high fat intake may result in steatorrhea. However, the incidence of lactose intolerance is no greater in patients with IBD than in the general population. Patients with IBD who tolerate lactose should not restrict lactose-containing foods because they can be a valuable source of high-quality protein, calcium, and vitamin D.

Patients with strictures or partial bowel obstruction benefit from a reduction in dietary fiber or limited food particle size. Small, frequent feedings may be tolerated better than large meals. Small amounts of isotonic, liquid oral supplements may be valuable in restoring intake without provoking symptoms. In cases in which fat malabsorption is likely, supplementation with foods made with **medium-chain triglycerides (MCTs)** may be useful in adding calories and serving as a vehicle for fat-soluble nutrients. However, these products are expensive and may be less effective than more basic treatments.

Factors associated with of the development of IBD in epidemiologic studies include increased sucrose intake, lack of fruits and vegetables, a low intake of dietary fiber, use of red meat and alcohol, and altered omega-6/omega-3 fatty acid ratios and insufficient vitamin D intake (Hlavaty, 2015). Yet dietary interventions to modify these factors during IBD flares are still under investigation (Owczarek et al, 2016).

The same foods that are responsible for GI symptoms (gas, bloating, and diarrhea) in a normal, healthy population are likely to be the triggers for the same symptoms in patients with mild stages of IBD or those in remission.

Patients receive nutritional information from a variety of sources, including support groups, Internet news groups, the audio and printed media, well-meaning friends, and food supplement salespersons. The information is sometimes inaccurate or exaggerated, or it may pertain only to one individual's situation and not to another's. The nutrition care provider can help patients sort out the role of foods in IBD management and teach them how to evaluate valid nutrition information from unproven or exaggerated claims. Patients' participation in the management of their disease may help to reduce not only the symptoms of the disease but also the associated anxiety level.

Microbiota. Probiotic foods and supplements have been investigated as potential therapeutic agents for IBD because of their ability to modify the gut microbiota and potentially modulate gut inflammatory response. Multistrain probiotic supplements (e.g., VSL#3) have been shown to be beneficial in maintaining disease remission in patients with UC who had **pouchitis**, inflammation in the ileal pouch surgically formed after colectomy. However, a different probiotic supplement at a lower dose did not significantly reduce symptoms (Holubar et al, 2010). Specific probiotic supplements also appear to be useful for induction and extension of remissions in pediatric and adult UC (Ghouri et al, 2014).

Although probiotics appear useful in UC, probiotic studies have not demonstrated significant improvement in Crohn's disease activity in adults or pediatric patients, nor do probiotic supplements appear to prolong remission in Crohn's disease (Ghouri et al, 2014).

Regular intake of prebiotic foods such as oligosaccharides, fermentable fibers, and resistant starches can beneficially affect the gut microbiota, feeding *Lactobacillus* and *Bifidobacteria* thus providing competition to and theoretically suppression of pathogenic or opportunistic microbiota. In addition, fermentation of prebiotics leads to increased production of SCFAs, theoretically creating a more acidic and less favorable environment for opportunistic bacteria.

Use of probiotics and prebiotics may prevent SIBO in predisposed individuals and may be used to treat diarrhea. Additional study is needed to identify the dose, the most effective prebiotic and probiotic foods, the form in which they can be used for therapeutic and maintenance purposes, and their relative value compared with other therapies (Ghouri et al, 2014).

Microscopic Colitis

Injury of the colon caused by UC, Crohn's disease, infections, radiation injury, and ischemic insult to the colon presents with abnormalities such as edema, redness, bleeding, or ulcerations that are visible on colonoscopy examination. Unlike the colitis of IBD, **microscopic colitis** is characterized by inflammation that is not visible by inspection of the colon during colonoscopy and is apparent only when the colon's lining is biopsied and then examined under a microscope. Patients with microscopic colitis can have diarrhea for months or years before the diagnosis is made. The cause of microscopic colitis is unknown.

Pathophysiology

There are two types of microscopic colitis. In **lymphocytic colitis**, there is an accumulation of lymphocytes within the lining of the colon. In **collagenous colitis**, there is also a layer of collagen (like scar tissue) just below the lining. Some experts believe that lymphocytic colitis and collagenous colitis represent different stages of the same disease. Symptoms include chronic, watery diarrhea, mild abdominal cramps, and pain. More than 30% of patients report weight loss. Microscopic colitis appears more frequently in patients aged 60 to 70 years, and collagenous colitis occurs more frequently in females (Ohlsson, 2015).

Medical Nutrition Therapy

Research is underway to determine possible effective treatments for microscopic colitis, including corticosteroids and immunosuppressive agents. Medical nutrition therapy is supportive with efforts to maintain weight and nutrition status, avoid symptom exacerbation, and maintain hydration, similar to that for IBD.

Irritable Bowel Syndrome

Irritable bowel syndrome (IBS) is a condition characterized by unexplained abdominal discomfort or pain that is associated with changes in bowel habits. Other common symptoms include gas, bloating, diarrhea and constipation, and increased GI distress associated with psychosocial distress. These symptoms may be vague and transient, making IBS a diagnosis of exclusion. It is classified as a functional disorder because tests show no diagnostic abnormalities and, therefore, diagnosis depends on symptoms. An estimated 10% to 20% of the United States population has IBS, with twice as many women as men being affected, although this may be a factor of reporting (Koff and Mullin, 2012). There are between 2.4 and 3.5 million annual physician visits for IBS in the United States alone. IBS is the most common disorder diagnosed by gastroenterologists and accounts for 20% to 40% of visits (International Foundation for Functional Gastrointestinal Disorders [IFFGD], 2013). Patients with IBS often have increased missed school and work days, decreased productivity, increased health care costs, and decreased quality of life as a result of their symptoms.

Etiology

No specific marker or test is diagnostic for IBS. When assessing a patient for IBS, the clinician must carefully review medication records because numerous over-the-counter and prescribed medications can cause abdominal symptoms such as pain and changes in bowel habits. In addition, the symptoms of IBS overlap with or are similar to, other GI diseases such as celiac disease, inflammatory bowel disease, functional dyspepsia, and functional constipation.

The **Rome III criteria** for IBS and its subtypes are used to define the diagnosis based on the presence of GI symptoms and exclusion of other disease processes (Longstreth et al, 2006). These diagnostic criteria are used in clinical research and to a lesser extent in clinical practice and are listed in Box 28-10. The diagnostic criteria also include a refining of subtypes of IBS based on predominant stool patterns (see Table 28-5).

BOX 28-10 Rome III Criteria for IBS

Criteria consists of recurrent abdominal pain or discomfort for at least 3 days per month in the last 3 months with onset at least 6 months before diagnosis and with 2 or more of the following:
1. Pain improvement with defecation
2. Change in stool frequency at onset
3. Change in stool form or appearance at onset

Data from Longstreth GF et al: Functional bowel disorders, *Gastroenterology* 130:1480, 2006.

TABLE 28-5 Subtypes of IBS Based on Stool Patterns

Type	Symptoms
IBS with constipation (IBS-C)	<3 bowel movements per week Hard or lumpy stools Straining during bowel movements
IBS with diarrhea (IBS-D)	≥3 bowel movements per day Fecal urgency Loose watery stools
Mixed IBS (IBS-M)	A mix of hard and loose stools over periods of hours to days
Unsubtyped IBS	Insufficient abnormality of stool patterns to meet criteria for IBS-C, D, or M

Data from Longstreth GF et al: Functional bowel disorders, *Gastroenterology* 130:1480, 2006.

Pathophysiology

The pathophysiology of IBS is not completely understood. A number of factors are presumed to play a role in the etiology of IBS, including nervous system alterations (abnormal GI motility and visceral hypersensitivity), gut flora alterations, genetics, and psychosocial stress. Research traditionally has focused on intestinal motility, however, studies of small bowel and colonic motility show inconsistent results and have not determined a predominant pattern of motor activity as a marker that would diagnose IBS.

Sensation in the GI tract results from stimulation of various receptors and sensory nerves in the gut wall, which transmit signals to the spinal cord and brain. Alterations in areas of the brain involved in pain modulation, autonomic nervous system dysregulation, and impaired brain-gut communication result in hyperalgesia (increased sensation to pain in the gut), visceral hypersensitivity, and altered motility (Anastasi et al, 2013). Dysregulation of serotonin concentrations in the GI tract has been correlated with the type of IBS a patient experiences; low serotonin concentrations are associated with constipation or a sluggish gut and higher serotonin concentrations are associated with diarrhea or increased peristalsis in the intestine (Kanazawa et al, 2011; Stasi et al, 2014).

Researchers believe that SIBO may contribute to IBS; however, many of these studies did not have the same results when repeated. Additional studies are needed to understand whether SIBO is directly connected to IBS or is a separate entity.

Psychologic conditions, such as depression and anxiety, often are observed in patients with IBS. Although it is unclear whether stress initiates IBS, it is accepted that stress can trigger or exacerbate symptoms in IBS. It is not unusual for patients with IBS to link their symptoms with lifetime or daily stress (Fadgyas-Stanculete et al, 2014).

Medical Management

The first step in the management of IBS and other functional GI disorders includes validating the reality of the patient's complaints and establishing an effective clinician-patient relationship. Patients with IBS should be educated that although their condition is not life threatening, it may be a lifelong struggle for them. Care should be tailored to help the patient deal with the symptoms and the factors that may trigger them. Clinician and patient should understand that no single therapy is proven to provide relief for all patients. Treatment options include medications focused mostly on symptom treatment or reduction, stress reduction and relaxation, and nutrition through diet modification. Drug therapy is aimed at management of symptoms associated with GI motility, visceral hypersensitivity, or psychologic issues. Generally, the treatment option is determined by the predominant bowel pattern and the symptoms that most disrupt the patient's quality of life (see Table 28-6).

Medical Nutrition Therapy

The goals of nutrition therapy for IBS are to ensure adequate nutrient intake, tailor the diet for the specific GI pattern of IBS, and explain the potential roles of foods in the management of symptoms. Implementation of nutrition interventions for IBS should take a stepwise approach from simple to complex. Initial steps during nutrition counseling should include (1) review of current medications for IBS and other medications; (2) review of GI symptoms (duration, severity, frequency); (3) assessment of nutritional status and food intake; (4) review of supplement intake (vitamins, minerals, fats, pre- and probiotics, herbals); and (5) review of use of mind-body therapies and the results achieved (Caldwell and Ireton-Jones, 2012).

TABLE 28-6 Treatment Options for IBS Symptoms

Symptom	Treatment
Abdominal pain and discomfort	Antispasmodic agents
	Tricyclic antidepressants
	Serotonin-directed agents (selective serotonin reuptake inhibitors, serotonin-3 receptor antagonists, or serotonin-4 receptor agonists)
Constipation	Fiber supplements
	Stool softeners
	Laxatives (osmotic, stimulant)
	Chloride channel activator (lubiprostone)
Diarrhea	Antidiarrheal agents (loperamide, diphenoxylate with atropine)
Small intestinal bacterial overgrowth (SIBO)	Antibiotics
Global symptoms and/or overall well-being	Psychotherapy (cognitive behavioral therapy, relaxation therapy, gut-directed hypnotherapy)
	Complementary and alternative medicine (acupuncture, meditation)
	Peppermint oil
	Probiotics
	Prebiotics

Data from Anastasi JK et al: Managing irritable bowel syndrome, *Am J Nurs* 113:42, 2013; Caldwell ME, Ireton-Jones C: Irritable bowel syndrome: new frontiers in treatment, *Support Line* 34(6):8, 2012; Clark C, DeLegge M: Irritable bowel syndrome: a practical approach, *Nutr Clin Pract* 23:263, 2008.

A review of foods to avoid that may aggravate IBS symptoms should be covered during the initial nutrition consultation. Little evidence exists for restricting particular foods. Large meals and certain foods may be poorly tolerated, such as excess quantities of dietary fat, caffeine, lactose, fructose, sorbitol, and alcohol. This is especially true in patients with diarrhea-predominant IBS or mixed IBS.

Most fiber or bulking agent studies in the IBS population have shown significant shortcomings (El-Salhy and Gundersen, 2015). A combination of soluble and insoluble fiber is targeted for constipation management. However, increasing the amount of insoluble fiber in the diet, especially in patients without constipation, actually may worsen IBS symptoms. Consumption of adequate fluid is recommended, especially when powdered fiber supplements are used. Although increasing fiber intake is a usual component of initial therapy for IBS, patients may have continuing symptoms possibly related to the type of fiber consumed. Recent studies show that certain carbohydrate containing foods that include highly fermentable carbohydrates in the presence of gut bacteria actually exacerbate IBS symptoms (Mullins et al, 2014).

FODMAPs Eating Plan

There is emerging research that a diet low in FODMAPs may be an effective therapy in the management of GI symptoms in patients with IBS (Halmos et al, 2014). The term FODMAPs was coined by a group of Australian researchers who theorize that foods containing these forms of carbohydrates worsen the symptoms of some digestive disorders such as IBS and IBD.

The low **FODMAPs** diet limits foods that contain lactose, fructose, fructo-oligosaccharides (fructans), galacto-oligosaccharides (galactans), and polyols or sugar alcohols (sorbitol, xylitol, mannitol, isomaltase, and maltitol). These short-chain carbohydrates are poorly absorbed in the small intestine, are highly osmotic, and are rapidly fermented by bacteria in the large intestine, resulting in gas, pain, and diarrhea in sensitive individuals. FODMAPs have a cumulative impact on GI symptoms. A cutoff value for acceptable amounts of FODMAPs has not been well defined and is likely patient specific. Patients may tolerate small amounts, but symptoms can develop if they consume quantities that surpass their threshold. Hydrogen breath testing, if readily available, can be useful to demonstrate which foods are problematic for the individual and help to tailor the diet. Examination of the patient's current diet to determine potential triggers and diet instructions regarding malabsorption and portion control of fructose containing foods are completed before the elimination phase.

Nutrition intervention begins with elimination of all high FODMAPs foods from the diet for a trial period of 6 to 8 weeks (Gibson, 2011). The challenge phase begins with a slow, controlled reintroduction of one FODMAPs diet category at a time to observe for symptoms and identify the most challenging foods (see Table 28-7).

Nutritional deficiencies that can arise with the low FODMAPs diet include folate, thiamin, and vitamin B_6 (from limiting cereals and breads), as well as calcium and vitamin D (from avoidance of dairy). The goal is to eventually reduce or eliminate GI symptoms, by creating a diet that includes FODMAPs at the most tolerable intake level, and with use of alternative foods. It does not present a cure but a dietary approach to

TABLE 28-7 **Foods Containing High FODMAPs, and Low FODMAP Diet Instructions**

FODMAP	High FODMAP Food
Excess free fructose	Fruits: apples, pears, mango, watermelon, boysenberries, cherries, figs, tamarillo
	Vegetables: asparagus, artichokes, sugar snap peas
	Sweeteners and condiments: honey, high fructose corn syrup, agave nectar, fructose, fruit juice concentrate
Lactose	Milk (cow, goat and sheep), ice cream, soft cheeses (e.g., ricotta, cottage cheese, cream cheese, mascarpone)
Oligosaccharides (fructans and galacto-oligosaccharides)	Fruits: nectarines, persimmon, watermelon, peaches, tamarillo
	Vegetables: artichokes (globe and Jerusalem), garlic, leeks, onions (yellow, red, white, onion powder), shallots, scallions (white part)
	Cereals: wheat, barley, and rye-based products (in large amounts)
	Legumes: chickpeas, lentils, beans (e.g., kidney, black, cannellini, great northern, pinto, navy, lima, butter, adzuki, soy, mung, and fava beans)
	Nuts: pistachios, cashews
Polyols	Fruits: apples, apricots, pear, nectarine, peaches, plums, prunes, watermelon, blackberries
	Vegetables: cauliflower, mushrooms, snow peas
	Sweeteners: sorbitol, mannitol, maltitol, xylitol, polydextrose, isomalt

Low FODMAP Diet Instructions

- Consider and look over the list of all high FODMAPs foods. If any of these foods are taken in too much, try cutting them out first.
- If symptoms do not improve, avoid all high FODMAPs foods for 6 to 8 weeks.
- Fructose containing foods with a 1:1 ratio of fructose to glucose are usually well tolerated as opposed to foods with excess fructose compared to glucose.
- Avoid foods that contain significant free fructose in excess of glucose (unless fructose malabsorption is not demonstrated).
- Foods containing excess fructose are those that contain 0.2 g or more of fructose compared with glucose per serving. Fructose and glucose content of foods can be found in the USDA database: http://ndb.nal.usda.gov/ndb/nutrients/index.
- Try ingesting a source of glucose with fructose-containing foods (i.e., sucrose contains equal amounts of glucose and fructose).
- Avoid foods that contain significant amounts of fructans and galacto-oligosaccharides (GOS) when first implementing the low FODMAPs diet because no one absorbs them well.
- Restrict lactose-containing foods (unless lactose malabsorption is not demonstrated).
- Avoid polyol-containing foods.
- Some FODMAPs cause more trouble in some people than others. This depends on the proportions of each FODMAPs in the diet, how well or poorly fructose or lactose is absorbed, and how sensitive one is to each FODMAPs.
- If symptoms have improved after 6 to 8 weeks, it is recommended to gradually reintroduce one FODMAPs group at a time.

Adapted from Shepherd SJ, Gibson PR: *The Complete Low FODMAP Diet*, New York, 2013, The Experiment Publishing.

FODMAPs, Fermentable oligo-, di-, monosaccharides and polyols.

improve symptoms and quality of life (Marcason, 2012) (see Table 28-7). An increasing number of resources facilitate adherence to the diet, including a mobile device app from the creators of the diet at Monash University in Australia, several cookbooks, and websites (Monash University, 2014).

Diverticular Disease

Diverticular disease is one of the most common medical conditions among industrialized societies. Diverticulosis is characterized by the formation of sac-like outpouchings or pockets (diverticula) within the colon that form when colonic mucosa and submucosa herniate through weakened areas in the muscle. The prevalence of diverticulosis is difficult to determine given that most individuals remain asymptomatic. This condition becomes more common as people age, particularly in people older than age 50 (Peery et al, 2012). Diverticulitis is a complication of diverticulosis that indicates inflammation of one or more diverticulum. It often represents a flare-up of diverticulosis, and after it subsides into a period of remission, it reverts to the state of diverticulosis. In Western populations, diverticulosis is found most often on the left side typically in the sigmoid colon; this is in contrast to right-sided colonic involvement found in the African and Asian populations (Feingold and Whelan, 2008).

Etiology

The cause of diverticulosis has not been elucidated clearly. Epidemiologic studies have implicated low-fiber diets in the development of diverticular disease. Low-fiber diets reduce stool volume, predisposing individuals to constipation and increased intracolonic pressures, which suggests that diverticulosis occurs as a consequence of pressure-induced damage to the colon. However, a study found that a low-fiber diet was not associated with diverticulosis and that a high-fiber diet and more frequent bowel movements may be linked to an increased rather than decreased chance of diverticula (Peery et al, 2012). Other studies have focused on the role of decreased levels of the neurotransmitter serotonin in causing decreased relaxation and increased spasms of the colon muscle. Studies also have found links between diverticular disease and obesity, vitamin D insufficiency, lack of exercise, smoking, and certain medications, including nonsteroidal antiinflammatory drugs such as aspirin and steroids (McGuire et al, 2015; Peery et al, 2012).

Pathophysiology

Evolving pathophysiologic mechanisms in diverticulosis and diverticulitis suggest chronic inflammation, alterations in colonic microbiota, disturbed colonic sensorimotor function, and abnormal colon motility have likely interrelated roles in the development of diverticular disease (Strate et al, 2012). Complications of diverticular disease range from painless, mild bleeding and altered bowel habits to diverticulitis. Acute diverticulitis includes a spectrum of inflammation, abscess formation, bleeding, obstruction, fistula, and sepsis from perforation (rupture).

Medical and Surgical Treatment

Treatment typically includes antibiotics and adjustment of oral intake as tolerated. Patients with severe cases of diverticulitis with acute pain and complications likely will require a hospital stay and treatment with intravenous (IV) antibiotics and a few days of bowel rest. Surgery is reserved for patients with recurrent episodes of diverticulitis and complications when there is little or no response to medication. Surgical treatment for diverticulitis removes the diseased part of the colon, most commonly, the left or sigmoid colon.

Medical Nutrition Therapy

Historically, it has been common in clinical practice to recommend avoidance of nuts, seeds, hulls, corn, and popcorn to prevent symptoms or complications of diverticular disease. However, an 18-year study found no association between nut, corn, or popcorn consumption and diverticular bleeding (Strate et al, 2008). In fact, an inverse relationship between nut and popcorn consumption and the risk of diverticulitis was demonstrated, suggesting a protective effect.

During an acute episode of diverticulitis or diverticular bleeding, oral intake is generally reduced until symptoms subside. Complicated cases may necessitate bowel rest and require parenteral nutrition (PN) support. Once oral intake has been resumed, or in mild to moderate cases, it is prudent to begin a low-fiber diet (10 to 15 g/day) as the diet is being advanced, followed by a gradual return to a high-fiber diet.

Although no convincing evidence exists that a high-fiber diet can reverse the pathophysiology of diverticular disease, there is reasonable evidence that this type of diet can improve diverticular symptoms (Tarleton and DiBaise, 2011). A high-fiber diet in combination with adequate hydration promotes soft, bulky stools that pass more swiftly and require less straining with defecation. Recommended intakes of dietary fiber, preferably from foods, are 25 g/day for adult women and 38 g/day for men.

Fiber intake should be increased gradually because it may cause bloating or gas. If a patient cannot or will not consume the necessary amount of fiber, methylcellulose or psyllium fiber supplements have been used with good results. A high-fiber diet possibly with fiber supplementation is advocated in asymptomatic diverticulosis to reduce the likelihood of disease progression, prevent the recurrence of symptom episodes, and prevent acute diverticulitis. Adequate fluid intake should accompany the high fiber intake. The potential role of altered bacterial flora in diverticular inflammation suggests that combining probiotic therapy with other therapies may prove effective in the management of this disorder (Maconi et al, 2013).

Intestinal Polyps and Colorectal Cancer

In the United States and worldwide, colorectal cancer (CRC) is the third most common cancer in adults and is also the second most common cause of cancer death. There are approximately 142,820 new cases of CRC per year, and the incidence is more common in men than women and among those of African American descent (National Cancer Institute, 2014).

Etiology

About 85% of CRCs are considered to be sporadic, whereas approximately 15% are familial. Familial adenomatous polyposis (FAP) accounts for less than 1% of CRCs. It is a hereditary syndrome characterized by the development of hundreds to thousands of polyps in the colon and rectum during the second decade of life. Almost all patients with FAP will develop CRC if they are not identified and treated at an early stage.

An evaluation of the association of major known risk factors for CRC with colorectal polyp risk by histology type, quantified the impact of lifestyle modifications on the prevention of polyps (Fu et al, 2012). Several lifestyle factors, including cigarette smoking, obesity, no regular use of nonsteroidal antiinflammatory drugs, high intake of red meat, low intake of fiber, low intake of calcium, and low vitamin D levels were found to be independently associated with the risk of polyps. The risk of polyps increased progressively with an increasing number of these adverse lifestyle factors (Bostick, 2015; Fu et al, 2012).

Pathophysiology

Polyps are established precursors of CRCs and defined as a mass that arises from the surface of the intestinal epithelium and projects into the intestinal lumen. Factors that increase the risk of CRC include family history, chronic IBD, FAP, adenomatous polyps, and several dietary components. Patterns of dietary practices rather than specific nutrients may be more predictive of the risk of developing CRC.

Medical Management

The treatment of a colorectal polyp is removal, usually by colonoscopy. Large polyps often require surgery for complete removal, even if the presence of cancer is not confirmed before resection. In a recent prospective analysis, it showed that compared with no endoscopy, colonoscopy and sigmoidoscopy are associated with a lower incidence of distal CRC, whereas only colonoscopy is associated with a reduced incidence of proximal colon cancer, and that reduction was modest. Furthermore, compared with no screening, screening colonoscopy and sigmoidoscopy are associated with lower mortality from CRC, whereas only colonoscopy is associated with lower mortality from proximal colon cancer (Nishihara et al, 2013). Patients diagnosed with CRC may require moderate to significant interventions, including, medications, radiation therapy, chemotherapy, surgery, enteral and/or PN support.

Medical Nutrition Therapy

Recommendations from national cancer organizations include sufficient exercise; weight maintenance or reduction; modest and balanced intake of lipids; adequate intake of micronutrients from fruits, vegetables, legumes, whole grains, and dairy products; and limited use of alcohol. Supplements are normally encouraged if the diet is not adequate. The diet for cancer survivors typically follows these prevention guidelines.

NUTRITIONAL CONSEQUENCES OF INTESTINAL SURGERY

Small Bowel Resections and Short-Bowel Syndrome

Short-bowel syndrome (SBS) can be defined as inadequate absorptive capacity resulting from reduced length or decreased functional bowel after resection. A loss of 70% to 75% of small bowel usually results in SBS, defined as 100 to 120 cm of small bowel without a colon, or 50 cm of small bowel with the colon remaining. A more practical definition of SBS is the inability to maintain nutrition and hydration needs with normal fluid and food intake, regardless of bowel length.

Patients with SBS often have complex fluid, electrolyte, and nutritional management issues. Consequences of SBS include malabsorption of micronutrients and macronutrients, frequent diarrhea, steatorrhea, dehydration, electrolyte imbalances, weight loss, and growth failure in children. Other complications include gastric hypersecretion, oxalate renal stones, and cholesterol gallstones. Individuals who eventually need long-term PN have increased risk of catheter infection, sepsis, cholestasis, and liver disease, and reduced quality of life associated with chronic intravenous nutrition support (DiBaise, 2014).

Etiology

The most common reasons for major resections of the intestine in adults include Crohn's disease, radiation enteritis, mesenteric infarct, malignant disease, and volvulus (Shatnawei et al, 2010). In the pediatric population most cases of SBS result from congenital anomalies of the GI tract, atresia, volvulus, or necrotizing enterocolitis.

Pathophysiology

Duodenal Resection. Resections of the duodenum (approximately 10 in) are rare, which is fortunate because it is the preferred site for absorption of key nutrients such as iron, zinc, copper, and folate. The duodenum is a key player in the digestion and absorption of nutrients, because it is the portal of entry for pancreatic enzymes and bile salts (see Chapter 1).

Jejunal Resections. The jejunum (6 to 10 ft) is responsible for a large portion of nutrient absorption. Normally most digestion and absorption of food and nutrients occurs in the first 100 cm of small intestine, which also includes the duodenum. Jejunal enterohormones play key roles in digestion and absorption. Cholecystokinin (CCK) stimulates pancreatic secretion and gallbladder contraction, and secretin stimulates secretion of bicarbonate from the pancreas. Gastric inhibitory peptide slows gastric secretion and gastric motility, whereas vasoactive inhibitory peptide inhibits gastric and bicarbonate secretion (see Table 1-3). What remains to be digested or fermented and absorbed are small amounts of sugars, resistant starch, lipids, dietary fiber, and fluids. After jejunal resections, the ileum typically adapts to perform the functions of the jejunum. The motility of the ileum is comparatively slow, and hormones secreted in the ileum and colon help to slow gastric emptying and secretions. Because jejunal resections result in reduced surface area and faster intestinal transit, the functional reserve for absorption of micronutrients, excess amounts of sugars (especially lactose), and lipids is reduced.

Ileal Resections. Significant resections of the ileum, especially the distal ileum, produce major nutritional and medical complications. The distal ileum is the only site for absorption of bile salts and the vitamin B12-intrinsic factor complex. The ileum also absorbs a major portion of the 7 to 10 L of fluid ingested and secreted into the GI tract daily (see Chapter 1). The ileocecal valve, at the junction of the ileum and cecum, maximizes nutrient absorption by controlling the rate of passage of ileal contents into the colon and

preventing reflux of colonic bacteria, which may decrease risk for SIBO.

Although malabsorption of bile salts may appear to be benign, it creates a cascade of consequences. If the ileum cannot "recycle" bile salts secreted into the GI tract, hepatic production cannot maintain a sufficient bile salt pool or the secretions to emulsify lipids. The gastric and pancreatic lipases are capable of digesting some triglycerides to fatty acids and monoglycerides, but, without adequate micelle formation facilitated by bile salts, lipids are poorly absorbed. This can lead to malabsorption of fats and fat-soluble vitamins A, D, E, and K. In addition, malabsorption of fatty acids results in their combination with calcium, zinc, and magnesium to form fatty acid–mineral soaps, thus leading to their malabsorption as well. To compound matters, colonic absorption of oxalate is increased, leading to hyperoxaluria and increased frequency of renal oxalate stones. Relative dehydration and concentrated urine, which are common with ileal resections, further increase the risk of stone formation (see Chapter 35).

Colon Resections

The colon (approximately 5 ft long) is responsible for reabsorbing 1 to 1.5 L of electrolyte-rich (particularly sodium and chloride) fluid each day but is capable of adapting to increase this capacity to 5 to 6 L daily. Preservation of colon is key to maintaining hydration status. However, if the patient has any colon left, malabsorption of bile salts can act as a mucosal irritant, increasing colonic motility with fluid and electrolyte losses. Consumption of high-fat diets with ileal resections and retained colon also may result in the formation of hydroxy fatty acids, which also increase fluid loss. Cholesterol gallstones occur because the ratio of bile acid, phospholipid, and cholesterol in biliary secretions is altered. Dependence on PN increases the risk of biliary "sludge," secondary to decreased stimulus for evacuation of the biliary tract (see Chapters 13 and 29).

Medical and Surgical Management of Resections

The first step in management is assessment of the remaining bowel length from patient surgical and health records or interview. Assessment should quantify dietary intake, as well as stool and urine output, over 24 hours. Medications and hydration status should be assessed. Medications may be prescribed to slow GI motility, decrease secretions, or treat bacterial overgrowth. The primary "gut slowing" medications include loperamide, and, if needed, narcotic medications. Somatostatin and somatostatin analogs; glucagon-like polypeptide 2; growth hormone; and other hormones with antisecretory, antimotility, or trophic actions have been studied for use to slow motility and secretions. Surgical procedures such as creation of reservoirs ("pouches") to serve as a form of colon, intestinal lengthening, and intestinal transplant have been performed to help patients with major GI resections. Intestinal transplant is very complex and is reserved for gut failure, or when patients develop significant complications from PN.

Medical Nutrition Therapy

Most patients who have significant bowel resections require PN initially to restore and maintain nutrition status. The duration of PN and subsequent nutrition therapy will be based on the extent of the bowel resection, the health of the patient, and the condition of the remaining GI tract. In general, older patients with major ileal resections, patients who have lost the ileocecal valve, and patients with residual disease in the remaining GI tract do not do as well. Enteral feeding provides a trophic stimulus to the GI tract; PN is used to restore and maintain nutrient status.

The more extreme and severe the problem, the slower the progression to a normal diet. Small, frequent mini meals (6 to 10 per day) are likely to be better tolerated than larger feedings. Tube feeding may be useful to maximize intake when a patient would not typically eat, such as during the night (see Chapter 13). Because of malnutrition and disuse of the GI tract, the digestive and absorptive functions of the remaining GI tract may be compromised, and malnutrition will delay postsurgical adaptation. The transition to more normal foods may take weeks to months, and some patients may never tolerate normal concentrations or volumes of foods and always require supplemental PN to maintain adequate fluid and nutritional status.

Maximum adaptation of the GI tract may take 1 to 2 years after surgery. Adaptation improves function, but it does not restore the intestine to normal length or capacity. Whole nutrients are the most important stimuli of the GI tract; other nutritional measures also have been studied as a means of hastening the adaptive process and decreasing malabsorption, but their evidence for use is limited. For example, **glutamine** is the preferred fuel for small intestinal enterocytes and thus may be valuable in enhancing adaptation. Nucleotides (in the form of purines, pyrimidine, ribonucleic acid) also may enhance mucosal adaptation, but unfortunately they are often lacking in parenteral and enteral nutritional products. SCFAs (e.g., butyrate, propionate, acetate), carbohydrate fermentation byproducts of commensal gut microbiota, are major fuels for the colonic epithelium (see *Clinical Insight*: Intestinal Adaptation: What Enhances It?).

Patients with jejunal resections and an intact ileum and colon will likely adapt quickly to normal diets. A normal balance of protein, fat, and carbohydrate sources is satisfactory. Six small feedings with avoidance of lactose, large amounts of concentrated sweets, and caffeine may help to reduce the risk of bloating, abdominal pain, and diarrhea. Because the typical American diet may be nutritionally lacking and the intake of some micronutrients may be marginal, patients should be advised that the quality of the diet is of utmost importance. A multivitamin and mineral supplement may be required to meet nutritional needs.

Patients with ileal resections require increased time and patience in the advancement from parenteral to enteral nutrition. Because of losses, fat-soluble vitamins, calcium, magnesium, and zinc may have to be supplemented. Dietary fat may have to be limited, especially in those with little remaining colon. Small amounts at each feeding are more likely to be tolerated and absorbed.

MCT products add to the caloric intake and serve as a vehicle for lipid-soluble nutrients. Because boluses of MCT oil (e.g., taken as a medication in tablespoon amounts) may add to the patient's diarrhea, it is best to divide the doses equally in feedings throughout the day. Fluid and electrolytes, especially sodium, should be provided in small amounts and frequently.

In patients with SBS an oral diet or enteral nutrition plus the use of gut-slowing medications should be maximized to prevent dependence on PN. Frequent meals, removal of osmotic medications and foods, use of oral hydration therapies, and other interventions should be pursued. In some cases, overfeeding in an attempt to compensate for malabsorption results in further malabsorption, not only of ingested foods and liquids but also of the significant amounts of GI fluids secreted in response to food ingestion. Patients with an extremely short bowel may depend on parenteral solutions for at least part of their nutrient and fluid supply. Small, frequent snacks provide some oral gratification for these patients, but typically they can supply only a portion of their fluid and nutrient needs (see Chapter 13 for discussion of home PN).

CLINICAL INSIGHT

Intestinal Adaptation: What Enhances It?

By Laura Matarese, PhD, RD

Short bowel syndrome (SBS) occurs after surgical resection, congenital defect, or disease of the bowel. The severity of SBS depends on the length and anatomy of the bowel resected, the health of the remaining mucosa, as well as the presence of an intact stomach, pancreas and liver (Jeejeebhoy, 2002). During the 2 years after resection, the remnant bowel undergoes an adaptation process that increases its absorptive capacity (Buchman et al, 2003). This intestinal adaptation is evidenced by hyperplasia of intestinal cells, an increase of villus height, deepening of intestinal crypts, and upregulation of transporter proteins.

Proper dietary management of SBS can augment this naturally occurring intestinal adaptation. Compared with parenteral nutrition (PN) and intravenous fluids (IV), enteral nutrition (EN) results in greater adaptation and should be instituted to the extent possible (Feldman et al, 1976; Ford et al, 1984; Johnson et al, 1975). The type of nutrition consumed has important effects. Complex luminal nutrients in the form of whole foods are potent stimuli to intestinal adaptation (Tappenden, 2006).

Hormonal therapy may facilitate intestinal adaptation in patients with SBS. Recombinant human growth hormone (rGH) and glucagon-like peptide 2 (GLP-2) have each been shown to enhance intestinal adaptation and nutrient absorption (Drucker et al, 1996; Jeppesen et al, 2001; Seguy et al, 2003). In a phase III trial conducted in PN-dependent patients with SBS,

administration of rGH (Zorbtive; EMD Serono, Rockland, MD) with modified diet and oral glutamine resulted in a significant decrease in necessary PN volume, calories, and infusion frequency compared with glutamine treatment with a modified diet (Byrne et al, 2005). In another recently published phase III trial, patients with SBS who received teduglutide (GATTEX; NPS Pharmaceuticals, Bedminster, NJ), a degradation-resistant analog of GLP-2, showed significant reductions in PN/IV volume and number of infusion days compared with patients who received placebo (Jeppesen et al, 2012).

Long-term PN/IV has been associated with complications such as catheter sepsis, vascular thrombosis, cholelithiasis, and metabolic bone disease. In addition, it is associated with high costs and diminished quality of life (Compher et al, 2008; Winkler, 2005). A reduction in PN days and volumes will allow the patient to sleep uninterrupted by excessive urination and have the freedom of a night without PN infusion.

The goal of SBS therapy should be to decrease PN/IV dependence to the extent possible. Even in the absence of complete weaning, reductions in the number of PN/IV days or session volumes can be beneficial to patients.

Introducing appropriate EN and hydration as soon as possible after resection facilitates intestinal adaptation and may promote eventual full weaning.

Small Intestine Bacterial Overgrowth

Small intestine bacterial overgrowth (SIBO) is a syndrome characterized by overproliferation of bacteria normally found in the large intestine within the small intestine. A number of physiologic processes normally limit the amount of bacteria in the small intestine. Gastric acid, bile, and pancreatic enzymes have bacteriostatic and bactericidal action within the small bowel. Normal propulsive action of bowel motility "sweeps" bacteria into the distal bowel. The ileocecal valve prevents retrograde migration of the large numbers of colonic bacteria into the small intestine. SIBO also has been referred to as "blind loop syndrome" because one cause of bacterial overgrowth can result from stasis of the intestinal tract as a result of obstructive disease, strictures, radiation enteritis, or surgical procedures that leave a portion of bowel without normal flow (a blind loop or Roux limb).

Etiology

Frequently, more than one of the normal homeostatic defenses must be impaired before small intestine bacteria overproliferate to the point that symptoms develop. Chronic use of medications that suppress gastric acid allow more ingested bacteria to survive and pass into the small bowel. Liver diseases or chronic pancreatitis can decrease the production or flow of bile and pancreatic enzymes that control bacterial growth, into the bowel. Gastroparesis, narcotic medications, or bowel dysmotility disorders decrease peristalsis and can impair the ability to propel bacteria to the distal bowel. Surgical resection of the distal ileum and ileocecal valve can result in retrograde proliferation of colonic bacteria.

Pathophysiology

Although symptoms vary depending on the amount and type of bacteria present in the small intestine, one of the most common symptoms of SIBO is chronic diarrhea from fat maldigestion. Bacteria within the small bowel deconjugate bile salts resulting in impaired formation of micelles and thus impaired fat digestion and steatorrhea. Carbohydrate malabsorption occurs because of injury to the brush border secondary to the toxic effects of bacterial products and consequent enzyme loss. The expanding numbers of bacteria use the available vitamin B_{12} and other nutrients for their own growth, and the host becomes deficient. Bacteria within the small bowel produce folic acid as a byproduct of their metabolism, and vitamin B_{12} deficiency with normal or elevated serum folic acid is common. Bloating and distention also are reported frequently in SIBO, resulting from the action of bacteria on carbohydrates with production of hydrogen and methane within the small bowel.

D-lactic acidosis is a rare neurologic complication of SIBO in SBS patients caused by malabsorption of a large carbohydrate load. A lower colonic pH, induced by a large production of lactate and short-chain fatty acids, promotes growth of acid-resistant bacteria that go on to produce D-lactate. Because of the lack of D-lactate dehydrogenase, humans cannot metabolize D-lactate and symptoms of D-lactic acidosis develop: from lethargy, altered mental status, ataxia, and slurred speech to aggression and coma (Htyte et al, 2011).

Medical Treatment

Treatment is directed toward control of the bacterial growth. Because of the difficulty of testing for SIBO in patients with SBS, prescribing a therapeutic trial of antibiotics when suspicion is high is considered acceptable. Generally a broad-spectrum antibiotic that covers aerobic and anaerobic bacteria is used. Treatment may involve cycling of several antibiotics until improvement of symptoms is observed. Typically a 7- to 10-day course of antibiotics is successful, but some patients may require 1 to 2 months of treatment (Bohm et al, 2013). The antibiotic should be rotated to prevent bacterial resistance. The addition of probiotics to the antibiotic treatment has not been well studied and the benefits are inconclusive. If probiotics are used, then strains that produce D-lactate (e.g., *Lactobacillus acidophilus, Lactobacillus fermenti*) should be avoided because this may increase the risk of developing D-lactic acidosis, which can be life threatening.

Medical Nutrition Therapy

Dietary modification should target alleviation of symptoms and correction of nutrient deficiencies. Part of the problem with bacterial overgrowth in the small intestine is that carbohydrates reaching the site where microbes are harbored serve as fuel for their proliferation, with subsequent increased production of gases and organic acids. At least theoretically then, a diet that limits refined carbohydrates that are readily fermented, such as refined starches and sugars (e.g., lactose, fructose, alcohol sugars), and substitutes whole grains, and vegetables, can limit the proliferation of bacteria and increase gut motility (see Table 28-7).

An assessment of the medical problem and the patient's dietary intake is necessary as vitamin B_{12} may be lost in fermentation, the diet may lack key dietary nutrients, or the absence or removal of greater than 60 cm of the terminal ileum has occurred, putting the patient at risk for deficiencies. A routine intramuscular vitamin B_{12} may be required. If bile salts are being degraded, as in the case of blind loop syndrome, MCTs may be helpful if they provide a source of lipid and energy. Deficiencies of fat soluble vitamins A, D, and E are of concern if fat malabsorption is present.

Fistula

A fistula is an abnormal passage of an organ to another organ, skin, or wound. An enterocutaneous fistula (ECF) is an abnormal passage from a portion of the intestinal tract to the skin or to a wound (e.g., colocutaneous fistula between the large intestine and the skin).

Etiology

Fistulas may occur in any part of the GI tract but frequently develop in the small and large intestine. ECF can be classified several ways: by volume of output per day, cause (surgical versus spontaneous), site of origin, and number of fistula tracts. Surgery accounts for the majority of ECF development and usually manifests 7 to 10 days postoperatively. Fistulas of the intestinal tract can be serious threats to nutrition status because large amounts of fluids and electrolytes are lost and malabsorption and sepsis can occur. Box 28-11 lists conditions associated with fistula development.

Medical Treatment

Definitive assessment of fistula source, fistula route, and presence of obstructions or abscesses is essential in determining the appropriate medical intervention (Frantz et al, 2012). A fistulogram is considered the gold standard for identifying

BOX 28-11 Conditions Associated with Fistula Development

Bowel resection for cancer
Bowel resection for inflammatory bowel disease
Surgery for pancreatitis
Surgery on radiated bowel
Emergent surgery
Surgical wound dehiscence
Inflammatory bowel disease (Crohn's disease or ulcerative colitis)
Radiation enteritis
Bowel ischemia
Diverticular disease

Data from Frantz D et al: Gastrointestinal disease. In Mueller CM et al, editors: *The A.S.P.EN. Adult Nutrition Support Core Curriculum*, ed 2, Silver Spring, Md, 2012, American Society for Parenteral and Enteral Nutrition.

TABLE 28-8 Potential Indications for Creation of Intestinal Ostomy

Ileostomy	Colostomy
Crohn's disease	Colon cancer
Ulcerative colitis	Rectal cancer
FAP	Diverticulitis
Colon cancer	Rectal trauma
Rectal cancer	Radiation proctitis
Bowel perforation	Distal obstruction
Bowel ischemia	Fecal incontinence
Rectal trauma	Complex fistula
Fecal incontinence	
Fecal diversion	
Colonic dysmotility	
Toxic colitis	
Anastomotic leak	
Distal obstruction	
Enterocutaneous fistula	

FAP, Familial adenomatous polyposis.

the location and route of the fistulous tract. Fluid and electrolyte balance must be restored, infection must be brought under control, and aggressive nutrition support may be necessary to permit spontaneous closure or to maintain optimal nutritional status before surgical closure.

Medical Nutrition Therapy

Nutrition management of patients with ECF can be very challenging. Initial management may include keeping the patient NPO (*nil per os*) as fistula output is quantified and administering nutritional support during the initial workup phase. PN, tube feeding, oral diet, or a combination is used in patients with ECF. The decision regarding which route to feed patients with ECF depends on several factors, including the origin of the fistula, the presence of obstructions or abscesses, the length of functional bowel, the likelihood of fistula closure, the ability to manage fistula output, and the patient's overall medical condition (see Chapter 13).

Intestinal Ostomies

The word ostomy, derived from the Latin word *ostium*, refers to mouth or opening. An **intestinal ostomy** is a surgically created opening between the intestinal tract and the skin, and is specifically named according to the site of origin along the intestinal tract. Approximately 100,000 people in the United States undergo operations that result in a colostomy or ileostomy each year (Sheetz et al, 2014). The high incidence of ostomy is due in part to the increasing prevalence of CRC and diverticular surgeries in the United States. Ostomies are created for many reasons; Table 28-8 lists indications for the creation of ostomies.

Colostomies and ileostomies can be categorized as either loop or end ostomies. A **loop ostomy** is formed when a loop of bowel is brought up to the skin, and an incision is made on one side. The distal end is sutured to the skin, whereas the proximal side of the loop is everted back on itself (Martin and Vogel, 2012). The result is a stoma with two openings: the proximal (functional) limb from which the effluent or stool is discharged, and the distal limb, which may connect to the anus and secrete mucus. A loop ostomy is used most often when a temporary ostomy is formed. **End ostomies** are created when the bowel is cut and the end is brought through the skin to create the stoma. End and loop ostomies are potentially reversible. The output from an ileostomy is termed effluent, whereas output from a colostomy is stool (Willcutts et al, 2005).

Colostomy

A **colostomy** is a surgically created opening from the colon to the skin when a portion of the large intestine is removed or bypassed (see Figure 28-4). It can originate from any part of the colon: ascending, transverse, descending, or sigmoid. It typically starts functioning 2 to 5 days after surgery and the amount and type of output varies slightly, depending on the amount of remaining colon. Stool from a colostomy on the left side of the colon is firmer than that from a colostomy on the right side, with stool output ranging from 200 to 600 ml/day. Patients with sigmoid colostomies have elimination patterns similar to their preoperative states, usually one to two soft stools daily.

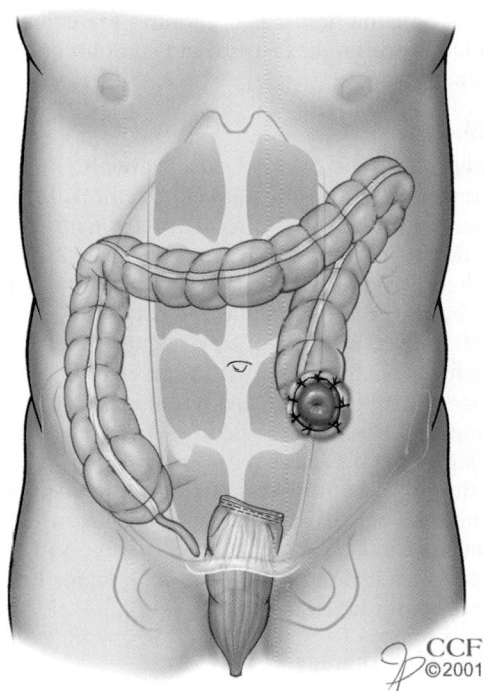

FIGURE 28-4 Colostomy. (Cleveland Clinic, Cleveland, Ohio, USA.)

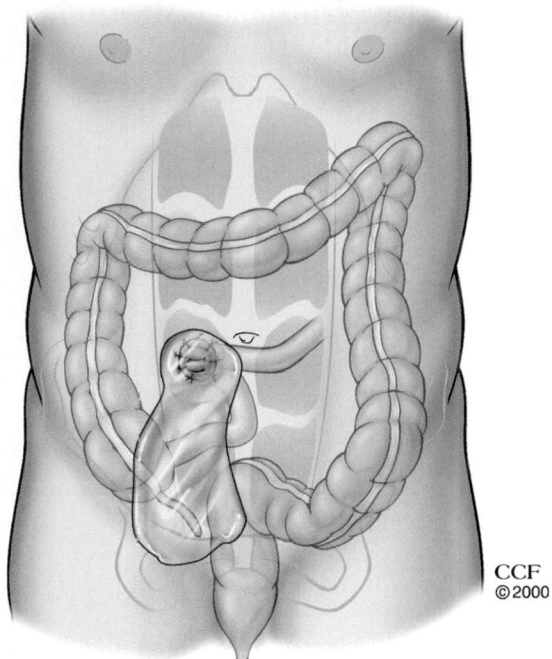

FIGURE 28-5 Ileostomy. (Cleveland Clinic, Cleveland, Ohio, USA.)

Ileostomy

An ileostomy is a surgically created opening from the distal small bowel (most often the terminal ileum) to the skin when the entire colon, rectum, and anus are removed or bypassed (see Figure 28-5). Typically, a new ileostomy will start functioning within 24 hours after surgery, and the effluent is initially bilious in color and watery (Willcutts and Touger-Decker, 2013). Stoma output increases initially to about 1200 ml per 24 hours for the first 1 to 2 weeks. As the bowel adapts over the next 2 to 3 months, the effluent thickens (semiliquid to porridge-like consistency) and output drops to less than a liter per day.

Medical Management

Management of a new ostomy patient involves maintenance of nutritional and hydration status, meticulous skin care, and adequate containment of the fecal stream using a pouching system in the hospital and as the patient transitions to home (McDonough, 2013). It is very helpful when a patient is evaluated by an enterostomal therapist (who specializes in the care of stomas) before surgery to mark the most appropriate site for an ostomy. This minimizes potential skin and pouch system problems. A poorly constructed ostomy can cause skin excoriation and difficulty with pouch application, and may significantly affect patient quality of life (QoL). A well-functioning ostomy is associated with a superior QoL. In those patients who express concerns regarding suboptimal QoL, social restrictions, psychosexual issues, and fear of the ostomy appliance leaking, seem to be the major limiting factors (Charua-Guindic et al, 2011).

Medical Nutrition Therapy

Traditional recommendations for postoperative feeding of patients with either a colostomy or ileostomy are to hold feeding until the bowel has started to "function" or put out stool or effluent. However, there is evidence that an oral diet or tube feeding can start early after surgery for any type of fecal diversion stoma that was created during an elective surgery. The Academy of Nutrition and Dietetics (AND) and the United Ostomy Association of America recommend a low fiber diet for approximately 6 to 8 weeks after surgery (AND, 2014; United Ostomy Associations of America, 2014). This advice is based on the premise that the bowel is edematous and therefore at risk for being damaged and or becoming obstructed after surgery. Most patients transition to a normal diet with a gradual increase in dietary fiber intake after approximately 6 weeks.

Vitamin B_{12} and bile salts or fat malabsorption are normally not a concern with a distal ileostomy. Greater than 100 cm of ileum must be resected before steatorrhea or fat-soluble vitamin deficiency occurs, and greater than 60 cm must be resected before vitamin B_{12} absorption is compromised (Parrish and DiBaise, 2014).

Controlling flatus and odor is a common concern for the colostomy patient rather than for a patient with an ileostomy. Many patients elect to limit foods that have the potential to increase flatus or cause increased odor of stool output. A patient must experiment with how different foods affect output. Deodorants are available, and ostomy appliances are made with odor-barrier material and can include charcoal filters that vent and deodorize gas.

Another concern for an ileostomy is the potential for intestinal blockage or obstruction at the stoma site resulting from narrowing of the intestinal lumen at the point where the ileum is brought through the abdominal wall. Patients are instructed to chew their food very well to reduce the chance of blockage. Ileostomy patients with higher volumes of watery effluent are encouraged to incorporate thickening foods to help thicken stoma output. The patient may have to experiment because thickened output may be desirable at times but can cause discomfort if output is thickened too much. Refer to Table 28-9 for the effects of various foods on ostomy output.

Maintenance of adequate fluid and electrolyte status is an important nutrition-related issue in managing a patient with colostomy or ileostomy. Patients with an ileostomy must recognize the symptoms of dehydration and understand the importance of maintaining adequate fluid intake throughout the day. In addition, patients may have to increase their salt, potassium, and magnesium intake resulting from losses in ileostomy output.

Ostomy output may become acutely or chronically elevated, and this is much more common with an ileostomy. The generally accepted definition of a high-output stoma (HOS) is output that exceeds 2000 ml/day over 3 consecutive days, at which point water, sodium, and magnesium depletion are expected (Baker et al, 2011). There are multiple potential causes of HOS, including inflammatory bowel disease, *Clostridium difficile*, intraabdominal sepsis, partial or intermittent obstruction, medication-related causes, drinking too much fluid (especially hypertonic fluids), or surgery that results in less than 200 cm of residual small bowel and no colon (Parrish and DiBaise, 2014).

Management of HOS includes assessment and correction of depleted electrolytes and minerals; initiation of an oral rehydration solution (ORS) sipped throughout the day; avoidance of hypertonic, simple sugar containing liquids and foods; restriction of foods high in insoluble fiber; separation of solids and liquids at meals; and consumption of smaller meals, more often (up to 6 to 8 per day) (McDonough, 2013; Parrish and

TABLE 28-9   Foods that may Alter Ostomy Output

Gas-Forming Foods	Odor-Producing Foods	Foods that May Control Odor
Broccoli	Asparagus	Buttermilk
Brussels sprouts	Beans	Cranberry juice
Cabbage	Broccoli	Orange juice
Cauliflower	Brussels sprouts	Yogurt
Garlic	Cabbage	Parsley
Onions	Cauliflower	Spinach
Fish	Garlic	Tomato juice
Eggs	Onions	
Carbonated beverages	Fish	
Alcoholic beverages	Eggs	
Dairy products	Some vitamins	
Legumes (dried beans)	Strong cheese	
Chewing gum		

Foods that may Thicken Stool	Foods that may Cause Obstruction	Foods that may Cause Diarrhea
Pasta	Apple peel	Alcoholic beverages
White bread	Orange	Caffeinated fluids
White rice	Pineapple	Chocolate
Potatoes	Grapes	Whole grains
Cheese	Dried fruits	Bran cereals
Pretzels	Raw cabbage	Fresh fruits
Creamy peanut butter	Raw celery	Grape juice
Applesauce	Chinese vegetables	Prune juice
Banana	Corn	Raw vegetables
Marshmallow	Mushrooms	Spicy foods
Tapioca	Coconut	Fried foods
	Popcorn	High-fat foods
	Nuts	Foods high in refined sugar or sorbitol

Data from Academy of Nutrition and Dietetics (AND): *Nutrition Care Manual, Ileostomy* (website): http://nutritioncaremanual.org/, 2014. Accessed March 16, 2014. McDonough MR: A dietitian's guide to colostomies and ileostomies, *Support Line* 35(3):3, 2013; United Ostomy Associations of America: *Diet and Nutrition Guide* (website): http://www.ostomy.org/ ostomy_info/pubs/OstomyNutritionGuide.pdf>, 2011 (Accessed 03.16.14); Willcutts K et al: Ostomies and fistulas: a collaborative approach, *Pract Gastroenterol* 29:63, 2005.

DiBaise, 2014). Malnutrition can occur in cases of persistent HOS, and many patients must increase their intake to maintain their nutritional status. Meeting the increased nutritional demand may not be possible via oral means for some patients, and nutrition support via enteral tube feeding may become necessary. Antidiarrheal and antisecretory medications are the two major classes of medications recommended to reduce output in HOS.

Restorative Proctocolectomy with Ileal Pouch Anal Anastomosis

Restorative proctocolectomy with ileal pouch anal anastomosis (IPAA) has evolved as the surgical treatment of choice for patients with medically refractory ulcerative colitis and familial adenomatous polyposis. About 30% of patients with ulcerative colitis eventually require colectomy, and the majority of these patients elect to have an IPAA. This procedure involves removal of the entire colon and rectum (proctocolectomy), while preserving the anal sphincter followed by creation of a reservoir using a portion of the distal ileum (ileal pouch). This pouch is then reconnected (pouch-anal anastomosis) to the preserved anal canal, thus maintaining continence and voluntary function. This offers a cure for the disease processes and avoids a permanent ileostomy.

Construction usually requires use of the distal-most 30 to 40 cm of ileum, with pouch configuration determined by the number of bowel limbs used. The most common pouch is the ileal J-pouch, which uses two limbs of bowel (see Figure 28-6).

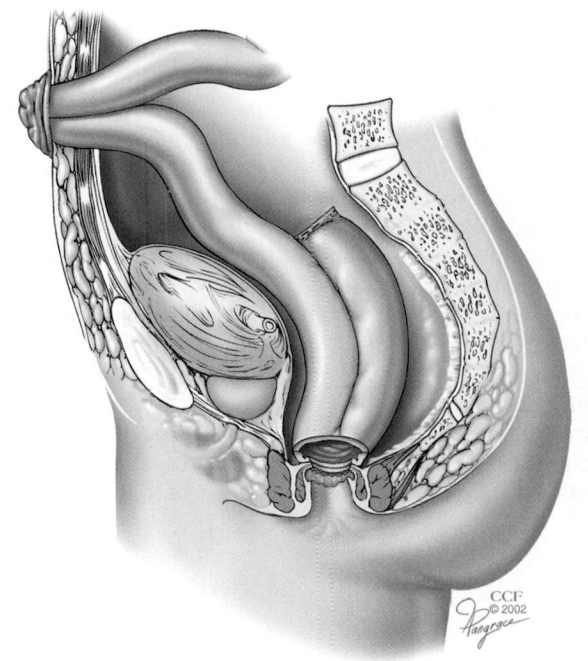

FIGURE 28-6 J-pouch. (Cleveland Clinic, Cleveland, Ohio, USA.)

It is the preferred ileal pouch because of the efficiency of construction and optimal functional results. Alternatives to the J-pouch configuration include three- and four-limbed pouches, such as an S-pouch or W-pouch. These alternative configurations are rarely performed because of the complexity of construction. The final decision as to which type is used remains at the discretion of the surgeon.

With any pouch surgery the recovery is longer than in those who have a conventional ileostomy because of the two-stage procedure. There will be a period of adaptation of the new reservoir after the ileostomy is closed. Initially, there could be up to 15 bowel movements a day with some problems of control and the need to get up several times at night. Eventually, most patients experience 4 to 6 bowel movements daily, have good control, and are not troubled by nighttime incontinence. This improves over time as the pouch capacity gradually increases.

A Koch pouch is a type of applianceless ileostomy that uses an internal reservoir with a one-way valve, constructed from a loop of intestine that is attached to the abdominal wall with a skin-level stoma. Patients must insert a tube or catheter into the stoma to open the valve and allow drainage of the ileostomy contents. The technical difficulties of surgical construction and the potential for complications has led to decreased use of the Koch pouch in favor of the ileal J-pouch.

Medical Management

Acute and chronic complications can necessitate removal of the ileal pouch and eventual construction of a permanent ileostomy. Pouchitis is a nonspecific inflammation of the mucosal tissue forming the ileal pouch and is the most frequent long-term complication of IPAA in patients with UC. The cause of pouchitis is not entirely clear, but it may be related to bacterial overgrowth, unrecognized Crohn's disease, immunologic changes, bile salt malabsorption, or insufficient short-chain fatty acid (SCFA) production. The usual presenting symptoms include increased stool frequency, urgency, incontinence, nocturnal seepage, abdominal cramps, and pelvic discomfort. Pouchitis may be classified based on the cause, disease duration and activity, and response to medical therapy. In the majority of patients, the etiology of pouchitis is not clear and thus termed as idiopathic pouchitis (Zezos and Saibil, 2015).

Pouch endoscopy is the main modality in the diagnosis and differential diagnosis in patients with pouch dysfunction. Antibiotic therapy is the mainstay of treatment for active pouchitis. Some patients may develop dependency on antibiotics, requiring long-term maintenance therapy. The evidence for the use of probiotics in maintenance treatment of pouchitis is controversial. There may be roles for postoperative probiotic supplementation to prevent pouchitis and in maintaining remission in antibiotic-dependent pouchitis (Shen et al, 2014). Clinical expert-generated guidelines concur that probiotics (VSL #3) can be effective for preventing recurrence of pouchitis (Ciorba, 2012).

Medical Nutrition Therapy

Patients who have undergone an IPAA procedure usually require supplemental vitamin B_{12} injections. The cause of vitamin B_{12} deficiency may be multifactorial: (1) there is reduced absorptive capacity because of distal ileal resection (main site of vitamin B_{12} absorption); (2) bacterial overgrowth is a well-known phenomenon in patients with an ileal pouch, and anaerobic bacteria can bind vitamin B_{12} in its free and intrinsic forms, leading to a decreased concentration available for absorption; and (3) there may be insufficient B_{12} intake. The anemia experienced by patients after IPAA can also be due to iron deficiency, because of impaired absorption, decreased oral intake, increased requirements, and blood loss.

Patients with a pouch often describe specific food sensitivities that may require diet alteration, even more so than do patients with permanent ileostomy (United Ostomy Associations of America, 2014). Problems commonly reported include obstructive symptoms and increased stool output, frequency, and gas. The incidence of obstruction may be avoided by limiting insoluble fibers, chewing thoroughly, and consuming small meals frequently throughout the day. Patients may try to experiment with timing of meals by eating larger meals earlier in the day and limiting the amount of food and fluid intake toward the end of the day to minimize sleep interruptions. The same dietary measures that are used to reduce excessive stool output (reduced caffeine, lactose avoidance if lactase-deficient, limitation of foods high in simple sugars, fructose and sorbitol) will likely reduce stool volume and frequency in patients with IPAA.

USEFUL WEBSITES

American Celiac Alliance
http://americanceliac.org/
Celiac Disease Awareness
http://celiac.nih.gov/
Gluten Intolerance Group
http://www.gluten.net/
Celiac Disease Foundation
http://www.celiac.org/
Celiac Sprue Association
http://www.csaceliacs.org/
Crohn's and Colitis Foundation of America
http://www.ccfa.org/
Fructose and Glucose Content of Foods
http://ndb.nal.usda.gov/ndb/nutrients/index/
Ileostomy, Colostomy, Pouches
National Digestive Diseases Information Clearinghouse
http://digestive.niddk.nih.gov/diseases/pubs/ileostomy/index.htm
United Ostomy Associations of America, Inc.
http://www.ostomy.org/
Wound, Ostomy and Continence Nurses Society
http://www.wocn.org

CLINICAL CASE STUDY

Lisa is a 35-year-old female with underlying diagnosis of fistulizing Crohn's colitis who underwent total abdominal colectomy (TAC) with end ileostomy. She had a difficult postoperative course complicated by ileus, high ostomy output, and slow introduction to oral diet. A nutrition consult was received for management of high ostomy output and malabsorption. Her ileostomy effluent was described as thin and watery.

Nutrition Assessment

- Anatomy: Patient has entire small bowel to ileostomy and no colon remaining, no ileocecal valve (ICV), no rectum, and no anus. The patient has no further potential for bowel reconnective surgery.
- Oral intake history: Decline in appetite and oral intake over past 3 months due to abdominal pain, nausea, and diarrhea. Before admission she was eating ½ of her usual meals. Unable to tolerate commercial nutrition supplements. Fluids: drinks "lots of fluids" (coffee, iced tea, water) , 8 to 10 glasses per day
- Current intake: taking 50% of meals provided, tolerating snacks, and sipping up to 500 mL of oral rehydration solution (ORS) daily. She feels that her appetite is slowly improving.
- Weight history: Ht: 152.4 cm (60 inches) Wt: 43.2 kg (95 lb), dosing weight BMI: 18.6 kg/m²
- Usual body weight: 51 kg (112 lb); weight change: 15% change × 3 months (significant weight loss)
- Physical examination: sunken, dark eye sockets, slight depression at temples, scapula protrudes, thin quadriceps and calves, fat loss at the ribs, no edema
- Functional capacity: low energy level over past 3 months, unable to go to her son's soccer games, fatigued and tired all the time
- Medications: started loperamide 2 mg before meals and bedtime, chewable multivitamin, KCl sustained release tablet, IV fluids to replace stoma losses
- 24 hour urine and ostomy output: 650 ml and 2200 ml
- Pertinent labs: serum sodium (130) low, serum potassium (3.4) low, serum magnesium (2.0) low normal, CRP: not available, stool toxin analysis for *Clostridium difficile* negative
- Current diet: GI Soft Fiber-controlled diet, Low Simple Sugars Diet

Nutrition Diagnoses (Pes Statement)

- Malnutrition (P) related to chronic illness (E) as evidenced by inadequate energy intake, weight loss, subcutaneous fat loss, muscle loss, and decline in functional capacity (S)
- Suboptimal protein-energy intake (P) related to altered GI function (E) as evidenced by high output stoma and weight loss (7.8 kg loss over 3 months representing 15% weight change × 3 months) (S)

Nutrition Interventions

- Estimated energy needs: 1300 to 1700 calories/day (30 to 40 kcal/kg/day)
- Estimated protein needs: 65 to 86 g protein/day (1.5 to 2.0 g protein/kg/day)
- Nutrition goal(s): Oral intake to meet estimated needs, and stabilize ostomy output to the point where patient's hydration is maintained.
- Replace electrolyte and fluid losses. Monitor fluid balance.
- Continue GI soft fiber-controlled, low simple sugars diet. Patient to make high-salt, high-starch, low simple sugar food choices from the menu. Encourage separation of beverages at mealtimes.
- Provide salty/starchy snacks between meals. Encourage "thickening foods," such as boiled white rice, pasta, noodles, bread, potatoes, banana, oatmeal, applesauce, peanut butter, cheese, and tapioca pudding.
- Sip 1 L of oral rehydration solution (ORS) between meals.
- Avoid caffeinated and hypertonic fluids.
- Consider trial of soluble fiber supplement to slow down transit time and thicken stoma output.
- Continue escalation of antidiarrheal medications depending on volume and consistency of ileostomy effluent.
- Diet education: discuss with patient and family nutrition management of high output stoma and maintaining hydration with ileostomy.
- Monitor ostomy output and assess need for home intravenous fluids (HIVF) versus home parenteral nutrition (HPN).

Nutrition Monitoring And Evaluation

- Monitor oral intake via calorie counts with a goal of meeting 75% to 100% of estimated energy and protein needs.
- Monitor ostomy output via intake/output records (I/Os) and stabilize to less than 1500 ml per day before hospital discharge.

REFERENCES

Academy of Nutrition and Dietetics (AND): *Ileostomy nutrition therapy* (website), 2014. http://nutritioncaremanual.org/index.cfm. Accessed March 16, 2001.

American Gastroenterological Association (AGA): *Understanding celiac disease* (website). http://www.gastro.org/patient-center/digestive-conditions/celiac-disease. Accessed January 22, 2015.

Anastasi JK, Capili B, Chang M: Managing irritable bowel syndrome, *Am J Nurs* 113:42, 2013.

Atia AN, Buchman AL: Oral rehydration solutions in non-cholera diarrhea: a review, *Am J Gastroenterol* 104:2596, 2009.

Bailes BK, Reeve K: Constipation in older adults, *The Nurse Practitioner* 38:21, 2013.

Baker ML, Williams RN, Nightingale JM: Causes and management of a high-output stoma, *Colorectal Dis* 3:191, 2011.

Besselink MG, van Santvoort HC, Buskens E: Probiotic prophylaxis in predicted severe acute pancreatitis: a randomised, double-blind, placebo-controlled trial, *Lancet* 371:651, 2008.

Bohm M, Siwiec RM, Wo JM: Diagnosis and management of small intestinal bacterial overgrowth, *Nutr Clin Pract* 28:289, 2013.

Borody TJ, Khoruts A: Fecal microbiota transplantation and emerging applications, *Nat Rev Gastroenterol Hepatol* 9:88, 2011.

Bostick RM: Effects of supplemental vitamin D and calcium on normal colon tissue and circulating biomarkers of risk for colorectal neoplasms, *J Steroid Biochem Mol Biol* 2015 148:86, 2015.

Bossuyt P, Vermeire S: Treat to target in inflammatory bowel disease, *Curr Treat Options Gastroenterol* Feb 11, 2016. Ahead of print.

Bouchard S, Ibrahim M, Van Gossum A: Video capsule endoscopy: perspectives of a revolutionary technique, *World J Gastroenterol* 20:17330, 2014.

Buchman AL, Scolapio J, Fryer J: AGA technical review on short bowel syndrome and intestinal transplantation, *Gastroenterology* 124:1111, 2003.

Byrne TA, Wilmore DW, Iyer K: Growth hormone, glutamine, and an optimal diet reduces parenteral nutrition in patients with short bowel syndrome: a prospective, randomized, placebo-controlled, double-blind clinical trial, *Ann Surg* 242:655, 2005.

Caldwell ME, Ireton-Jones C: Irritable bowel syndrome: new frontiers in treatment, *Support Line* 34(6):8, 2012.

Charua-Guindic L, Benavides-León CJ, Villanueva-Herrero JA: Quality of life in ostomized patients, *Cir Cir* 79:149, 2011.

Ciorba MA: A gastroenterologist's guide to probiotics, *Clin Gastroenterol Hepatol* 10:960, 2012.

Compher C, et al: Nutritional management of short bowel syndrome. In Marian M, et al, editors: *Clinical nutrition for surgical patients*, Sudbury, Mass, 2008, Jones and Bartlett.

Cresci G: Probiotics and prebiotics. In Mueller CG, editor: *ASPEN Adult Nutrition Support Core Curriculum*, ed 2, Silver Spring, Md, 2012, American Society for Parenteral Enteral Nutrition.

DiBaise JK: Short bowel syndrome and small bowel transplantation, *Curr Opin Gastroenterol* 30:128, 2014.

Drucker DJ, Erlich P, Asa SL, et al: Induction of intestinal epithelial proliferation by glucagon-like peptide 2, *Proc Natl Acad Sci U S A* 93:7911, 1996.

El-Salhy M, Gundersen D: Diet in irritable bowel syndrome, Nutr J 14:36, 2015.

Fadgyas-Stanculete M, Buga AM, Popa-Wagner A, et al: The relationship between irritable bowel syndrome and psychiatric disorders: from molecular changes to clinical manifestations, J Mol Psychiatry 2(1):4, 2014.

Farrukh A, Mayberry JF: Is there a role for fish oil in inflammatory bowel disease? *World J Clin Cases* 2:250, 2014.

Feingold DL, Whelan RL: Diverticulitis. In Bland KI, et al, editors: *General surgery: principles and international practice,* ed 2, London, 2008, Springer (pp 751–758).

Feldman EJ, Dowling RH, McNaughton J, et al: Effects of oral versus intravenous nutrition on intestinal adaptation after small bowel resection in the dog, *Gastroenterology* 70:712, 1976.

Ford WD, Boelhouwer RU, King WW, et al: Total parenteral nutrition inhibits intestinal adaptive hyperplasia in young rats: reversal by feeding, *Surgery* 96:527, 1984.

Frantz D, et al: Gastrointestinal disease. In Mueller CM, et al, editors: *The A.S.P.E.N. adult nutrition support core curriculum,* ed 2, Silver Spring, Md, 2012, American Society for Parenteral and Enteral Nutrition.

Fu Z, Shrubsole MJ, Smalley WE, et al: Lifestyle factors and their combined impact on the risk of colorectal polyps, *Am J Epidemiol* 176:766, 2012.

Garsed K, Scott BB: Can oats be taken in a gluten-free diet? A systematic review, *Scand J Gastroenterol* 42:171, 2007.

Ghouri YA, Richards DM, Rahimi EF, et al: Systematic review of randomized controlled trials of probiotics, prebiotics, and synbiotics in inflammatory bowel disease, *Clin Exp Gastroenterol* 7:473, 2014.

Gibson PR: Food intolerance and functional bowel disorders, *J Gastroenterol Hepatol* 26(suppl 3):128, 2011.

Grooms KN, Ommerborn MJ, Pham DQ, et al: Dietary fiber intake and cardiometabolic risk among US adults, NHANES 1999-2010, *Am J Med* 126:1059, 2013.

Halmos EP, Power VA, Shepherd SJ, et al: A diet low in FODMAPs reduces symptoms of irritable bowel syndrome, *Gastroenterology* 146:67, 2014.

Heizer WD, Southern S, McGovern S: The role of diet in symptoms of irritable bowel syndrome in adults: a narrative review, *J Am Diet Assoc,* 109:1204, 2009.

Hlavaty T, et al: Vitamin D therapy in inflammatory bowel diseases: who, in what form, and how much? *J Crohns Colitis.* 9:198, 2015.

Holubar SD, Cima RR, Sandborn WJ, et al: Treatment and prevention of pouchitis after ileal pouch-anal anastomosis for chronic ulcerative colitis, *Cochrane Database Syst Rev* 6:CD001176, 2010.

Hou JK, Lee D, Lewis J: Diet and Inflammatory Bowel Disease: Review of patient-targeted recommendations, *Clin Gastroenterol Hepatol* 12:1592, 2014.

Howell MD, Novack V, Grgurich P, et al: Iatrogenic gastric acid suppression and the risk of nosocomial Clostridium difficile infection, *Arch Int Med* 170:784, 2010.

Htyte N White L, Sandhu G, et al: An extreme and life-threatening case of recurrent D-lactate encephalopathy, *Nephrol Dial Transplant* 26:1432, 2011.

Hutchinson JM, West NP, Robins GG, et al: Long-term histological follow-up of people with coeliac disease in a UK teaching, *QJM* 103:511, 2010.

International Foundation for Functional Gastrointestinal Disorders (IFFGD): *About irritable bowel syndrome (IBS)* (website), 2014. http://www.aboutIBS.org. Accessed January 15, 2015.

Jeejeebhoy KN: Short bowel syndrome: a nutritional and medical approach, *CMAJ* 166:1297, 2002.

Jeppesen PB, Hartmann B, Thulesen J, et al: Glucagon-like peptide 2 improves nutrient absorption and nutritional status in short-bowel patients with no colon, *Gastroenterology* 120:806, 2001.

Jeppesen PB, Pertkiewicz M, Messing B, et al: Teduglutide reduces need for parenteral support among patients with short bowel syndrome with intestinal failure, *Gastroenterology* 143:1473, 2012.

Johnson LR, Copeland EM, Dudrick SJ, et al: Structural and hormonal alterations in the gastrointestinal tract of parenterally fed rats, *Gastroenterology* 68:1177, 1975.

Kanazawa M, Hongo M, Fukudo S: Visceral hypersensitivity in irritable bowel syndrome, *J Gastroenterol Hepatol* 26(Suppl 3):119, 2011.

Koff A, Mullin GE: Nutrition in irritable bowel syndrome. In Mullin GE, et al, editors: *Gastrointestinal and liver disease nutrition desk reference,* Boca Raton, Fla, 2012, CRC Press.

Kranz S, Brauchla M, Slavin JL, et al: What do we know about dietary fiber intake in children and health? The effects of fiber on constipation, obesity, and diabetes in children, *Adv Nutr* 3:47, 2012.

Kulkarni SV, Kairon R, Sane SS, et al: Opportunistic parasitic infections in HIV/AIDS patients presenting with diarrhea by the level of immunosuppression, *Indian J Med Res* 130:63, 2009.

Kupfer SS, Jabri B: Pathophysiology of celiac disease, *Gastrointest Endosc Clin N Am* 22:639, 2012.

Langenberg MC et al: Distinguishing tropical sprue from celiac disease in returning travellers with chronic diarrhoea: a diagnostic challenge? *Travel Med Infect Dis* 12:401, 2014.

Lee, YY et al: How to perform and assess colonic manometry and barostat study in chronic constipation, *J Neurogastroenterol Motil* 20:547, 2014.

Levitt M, Wilt T, Shaukat A: Clinical implications of lactose malabsorption versus lactose intolerance, *J Clin Gastroenterol* 47:471, 2013.

Linsky A, Gupta K, Lawler EV, et al: Proton pump inhibitors and risk for recurrent Clostridium difficile infection, *Arch Int Med* 170:772, 2010.

Liu LWC: Chronic constipation: current treatment options, *Can J Gastroenterol* 25(Suppl B):22B, 2011.

Lomer MC: Review article: the aetiology, diagnosis, mechanisms and clinical evidence for food intolerance, *Aliment Pharmacol Ther* 41:262–275, 2015.

Longstreth GF, Thompson WG, Chey WD, et al: Functional bowel disorders, *Gastroenterology* 130:1480, 2006.

Lustig RH: Fructose: metabolic, hedonic, and societal parallels with ethanol, *J Am Diet Assoc* 110:1307, 2010.

Maconi G et al: Diverticular disease of the colon: antibiotics or probiotics? *Int J Probiotics Prebiotics* 8(1):33, 2013.

Maguire LH et al. Association of geographic and seasonal variation with diverticulitis admissions. *JAMA Surg* 150:74, 2015.

Marcason W: What is the FODMAP diet? *J Acad Nutr Diet* 112:1696, 2012.

Martin ST, Vogel JD: Intestinal stomas: indications, management, and complications, *Adv Surg* 46:19, 2012.

McDonough MR: A dietitian's guide to colostomies and ileostomies, *Support Line* 35(3):3, 2013.

Misselwitz B, Pohl D, Frühauf H, et al: Lactose malabsorption and intolerance: pathogenesis, diagnosis and treatment, *United European Gastroenterol J* 1:151, 2013.

Monash University: *Low FODMAP diet for irritable bowel syndrome* (website), 2015. http://www.med.monash.edu/cecs/gastro/fodmap/. Accessed December 29, 2015.

Monteleone G, Caruso R, Pallone F, et al: Targets for new immunomodulation strategies in inflammatory bowel disease, *Autoimmun Rev* 13:11, 2014.

Morelli L: Yogurt, living cultures, and gut health, *Am J Clin Nutr* 99(Suppl 5):1248S, 2014.

Mugie SM, Benninga MA, Di Lorenzo C: Epidemiology of constipation in children and adults: a systematic review, *Best Pract Res Clin Gastroenterol* 25:3, 2011.

Mullins GE, Shepherd SJ, Chander Roland B, et al: Irritable bowel syndrome: contemporary nutrition management strategies, *J Parenter Enteral Nutr* 38:781, 2014.

Nachman F, del Campo MP, González A, et al: Long-term deterioration of quality of life in adult patients with celiac disease is associated with treatment noncompliance, *Dig Liver Dis* 42:685, 2010.

National Cancer Institute: *SEER stat fact sheets: colon and rectum cancer* (website), 2014). http://seer.cancer.gov/. Accessed March 8, 2014.

Navaneethan U, Shen B: Diagnosis and management of pouchitis and ileoanal pouch dysfunction, *Curr Gastroenterol Rep* 12:485, 2010.

Nishihara R, Wu K, Lochhead P, et al: Long-term colorectal cancer incidence and mortality after lower endoscopy, *N Engl J Med* 369:1095, 2013.

Ohlsson B: New insights and challenges in microscopic colitis, *Therap Adv Gastroenterol* 8:37, 2015.

O'Keefe SJ: Tube feeding, the microbiota, and Clostridium difficile infection, *World J Gastroenterol* 16:139, 2010.

Owczarek D et al: Diet and nutritional factors in inflammatory bowel diseases, *World J Gastroenterol* 22:895, 2016.

Parrish CR, DiBaise JK: Short bowel syndrome in adults- Part 2: nutrition therapy for short bowel syndrome in the adult patient, *Pract Gastroenterol* 138(10):40, 2014.

Pattani R, Palda VA, Hwang SW, et al: Probiotics for the prevention of antibiotic-associated diarrhea and Clostridium difficile infection among hospitalized patients: systematic review and meta-analysis, *Open Med* 7(2):e56, 2013.

Peery AF, Barrett PR, Park D, et al: A high fiber diet does not protect against asymptomatic diverticulosis, *Gastroenterology* 142:266, 2012.

Phatak UP and Pashankar DS: Obesity and gastrointestinal disorders in children, *J Pediatr Gastroenterol Nutr* 60:441, 2015.

Putkonen L, Yao CK, Gibson PR, et al: Fructose malabsorption syndrome, *Curr Opin Clin Nutr Metab Care* 16:473, 2013.

Richman E, Rhodes JM: Review article: evidence-based dietary advice for patients with inflammatory bowel disease, *Aliment Pharmacol Ther* 38:1156, 2013.

Rubio-Tapia A, Ludvigsson JF, Brantner TL, et al: The prevalence of celiac disease in the United States, *Am J Gastroenterol* 107:1538, 2012.

Sadeghian M et al: Vitamin D status in relation to Crohn's disease: A meta-analysis of observational studies, Nutrition Dec 22, 2015. Ahead of print.

Sams A, Hawks J: Celiac disease as a model for the evolution of multifactorial disease in humans, *Hum Biol* 86:19, 2014.

Schyum AC, Rumessen JJ: Serological testing for celiac disease in adults, *United European Gastroenterol J* 1:319, 2013.

Seguy D, Vahedi K, Kapel N, et al: Low-dose growth hormone in adult home parenteral nutrition-dependent short bowel syndrome patients: a positive study, *Gastroenterology* 124:293, 2003.

Sharma GM, Pereira M, Williams KM: Gluten detection in foods available in the United States – A market survey, *Food Chem* 169:120, 2015.

Shatnawei A, Parekh NR, Rhoda KM, et al: Intestinal failure management at the Cleveland Clinic, *Arch Surg* 145:521, 2010.

Shaukat A: Systematic review: effective management strategies for lactose intolerance, *Ann Intern Med* 152:797, 2010. http://www.ncbi.nlm.nih.gov/pubmed/20404262.

Sheetz KH, Waits SA, Krell RW, et al: Complication rates of ostomy surgery are high and vary significantly between hospitals, *Dis Colon Rectum* 57:632, 2014.

Shen J, Zuo ZX, Mao AP: Effect of probiotics on inducing remission and maintaining therapy in ulcerative colitis, Crohn's disease, and pouchitis: meta-analysis of randomized controlled trials, *Inflamm Bowel Dis* 20:21, 2014.

Sinagra E, Tomasello G, Cappello F, et al: Probiotics, prebiotics and symbiotics in inflammatory bowel diseases: state-of-the-art and new insights, *J Biol Regul Homeost Agents* 27:919, 2013.

Stasi C, Bellini M, Bassotti G, et al: Serotonin receptors and their role in the pathophysiology and therapy of irritable bowel syndrome, *Tech Coloproctol* 18:613, 2014.

Staudacher H, Lomer MC, Anderson JL, et al: Fermentable carbohydrate restriction reduces luminal bifidobacteria and gastrointestinal symptoms in patients with irritable bowel syndrome, *J Nutr* 142:1510, 2012.

Stavrou G, et al: The role of probiotics in the prevention of severe infections following abdominal surgery, *Int J Antimicrob Agents* 46(Suppl 1):S2, 2015.

Strate LL, Modi R, Cohen E, et al: Diverticular disease as a chronic illness: evolving epidemiologic and clinical insights, *Am J Gastroenterol* 107:1486, 2012.

Suchy FJ, Brannon PM, Carpenter TO, et al: National Institutes of Health Consensus Development Conference: lactose intolerance and health, *Ann Int Med* 152:792, 2010.

Tappenden KA: Mechanisms of enteral nutrient-enhanced intestinal adaptation, *Gastroenterology* 130(2 Suppl 1):S93, 2006.

Tarleton S, DiBaise JK: Low residue diet in diverticular disease: putting an end to a myth, *Nutr Clin Pract* 26:137, 2011.

Thompson T: The gluten-free labeling rule: what registered dietitian nutritionists need to know to help clients with gluten-related disorders, *J Acad Nutr Diet* 115:13, 2015.

Triantafyllou K et al: Methanogens, methane and gastrointestinal motility, *J Neurogastroenterol Motil* 20:31, 2014.

United Ostomy Associations of America: Diet and nutrition guide (website), 2011. http://www.ostomy.org/ostomy_info/pubs/OstomyNutritionGuide.pdf. Accessed March 16, 2014.

Vermeire S, Van Assche G, Rutgeerts P: Inflammatory bowel disease and colitis: new concepts from the bench and the clinic, *Curr Opin Gastroenterol* 27:32, 2011.

Wald A: Constipation: Advances in Diagnosis and Treatment, *JAMA* 315:185, 2016.

Whelan K, Myers CE: Safety of probiotics in patients receiving nutritional support: a systematic review of case reports, randomized controlled trials, and nonrandomized trials, *Am J Clin Nutr* 91:687, 2010.

Willcutts K, et al: Ostomies and fistulas: a collaborative approach, *Pract Gastroenterol* 29:63, 2005.

Willcutts K, Touger-Decker R: Nutritional management for ostomates, *Top Clin Nutr* 28:373, 2013.

Winkler MF: Quality of life in adult home parenteral nutrition patients, *J Parenter Enteral Nutr* 29:162, 2005.

Ye Y, et al: The epidemiology and risk factors of inflammatory bowel disease, *Int J Clin Exp Med* 8:22529, 2015.

Zezos P, Saibil F: Inflammatory pouch disease: The spectrum of pouchitis, World J Gastroenterol 21:8739, 2015.

29

Medical Nutrition Therapy for Hepatobiliary and Pancreatic Disorders

Jeanette M. Hasse, PhD, RDN , LD, CNSC, FADA,
Laura E. Matarese, PhD, RDN , LDN, CNSC, FADA, FASPEN, FAND

KEY TERMS

alcoholic liver disease
aromatic amino acids (AAAs)
ascites
bile
branched-chain amino acids (BCAAs)
calculi
cholangitis
cholecystectomy
cholecystitis
choledocholithiasis
cholelithiasis
cholestasis
cirrhosis
detoxification
fasting hypoglycemia
fatty liver

fulminant liver disease
hemochromatosis
hepatic encephalopathy
hepatic failure
hepatic osteodystrophy
hepatic steatosis
hepatitis
hepatorenal syndrome
jaundice
Kayser-Fleischer ring
Kupffer cells
nonalcoholic fatty liver disease (NAFLD)
nonalcoholic steatohepatitis (NASH)
oxidative deamination
pancreaticoduodenectomy (Whipple procedure)

pancreatic islet auto-transplantation
pancreatitis
paracentesis
portal hypertension
portal systemic encephalopathy
postcholecystectomy syndrome
primary biliary cirrhosis (PBC)
primary sclerosing cholangitis (PSC)
secondary biliary cirrhosis
steatorrhea
transamination
varices
Wernicke encephalopathy
Wilson's disease

The liver is of primary importance; one cannot survive without a liver. The liver and pancreas are essential to digestion and metabolism. Although it is important, the gallbladder can be removed, and the body will adapt comfortably to its absence. Knowledge of the structure and functions of these organs is vital. When they are diseased, the necessary medical nutrition therapy (MNT) is complex.

PHYSIOLOGY AND FUNCTIONS OF THE LIVER

Structure

The liver is the largest gland in the body, weighing approximately 1500 g. The liver has two main lobes: the right and left. The right lobe is further divided into the anterior and posterior segments; the right segmental fissure, which cannot be seen externally, separates the segments. The externally visible falciform ligament divides the left lobe into the medial and lateral segments. The liver is supplied with blood from two sources: the hepatic artery, which supplies approximately one third of the blood from the aorta; and the portal vein, which supplies the other two thirds and collects blood drained from the digestive tract.

Approximately 1500 mL of blood per minute circulates through the liver and exits via the right and left hepatic veins into the inferior vena cava. The liver has a system of blood vessels and a series of bile ducts. Bile, which is formed in the liver cells, exits the liver through a series of bile ducts that increase in size as they approach the common bile duct. Bile is a thick, viscous fluid secreted from the liver, stored in the gallbladder, and released into the duodenum when fatty foods enter the duodenum. It emulsifies fats in the intestine and forms compounds with fatty acids to facilitate their absorption.

Functions

The liver has the ability to regenerate itself. Only 10% to 20% of functioning liver is required to sustain life, although removal of the liver results in death, usually within 24 hours. The liver is integral to most metabolic functions of the body and performs more than 500 tasks. The main functions of the liver include (1) metabolism of carbohydrate, protein, and fat; (2) storage and activation of vitamins and minerals; (3) formation and excretion of bile; (4) conversion of ammonia to urea; (5) metabolism of steroids; (6) detoxification of substances such as drugs, alcohol, and organic compounds; and (7) function as a filter and flood chamber.

The liver plays a major role in carbohydrate metabolism. Galactose and fructose, products of carbohydrate digestion, are converted into glucose in the hepatocyte or liver cell. The liver stores glucose as glycogen (glycogenesis) and then returns it to the blood when glucose levels become low (glycogenolysis). The liver also produces "new" glucose (gluconeogenesis) from precursors such as lactic acid, glycogenic amino acids, and intermediates of the tricarboxylic acid cycle.

Important protein metabolic pathways occur in the liver. Transamination (transfer of an amino group from one compound to another) and oxidative deamination (removal of an amino group from an amino acid or other compound) are two such pathways that convert amino acids to substrates that are used in energy and glucose production as well as in the synthesis of nonessential amino acids. Blood-clotting factors such as fibrinogen and prothrombin as well as serum proteins including albumin, alpha-globulin, beta-globulin, transferrin, ceruloplasmin, and lipoproteins are formed by the liver.

Fatty acids from the diet and adipose tissue are converted in the liver to acetyl-coenzyme A by the process of beta-oxidation to produce energy. Ketones also are produced. The liver synthesizes and hydrolyzes triglycerides, phospholipids, cholesterol, and lipoproteins as well.

The liver is involved in the storage, activation, and transport of many vitamins and minerals. It stores all the fat-soluble vitamins in addition to vitamin B_{12} and the minerals zinc, iron, copper, and manganese. Hepatically synthesized proteins transport vitamin A, iron, zinc, and copper in the bloodstream. Carotene is converted to vitamin A, folate to 5-methyl tetrahydrofolic acid, and vitamin D to an active form (25-hydroxycholecalciferol) by the liver.

In addition to functions of nutrient metabolism and storage, the liver forms and excretes bile. Bile salts are metabolized and used for the digestion and absorption of fats and fat-soluble vitamins. Bilirubin is a metabolic end product from red blood cell destruction; it is conjugated and excreted in the bile.

Hepatocytes detoxify ammonia by converting it to urea, 75% of which is excreted by the kidneys. The remaining urea finds its way back to the gastrointestinal tract (GIT). The liver also metabolizes steroids. It inactivates and excretes aldosterone, glucocorticoids, estrogen, progesterone, and testosterone. It is responsible for the detoxification of substances, including drugs and alcohol as well as toxins such as pollutants, pesticides and herbicides, herbal products, and toxic mushrooms (*A. phalloides*). Finally, the liver acts as a filter and flood chamber by removing bacteria and debris from blood through the phagocytic action of Kupffer cells located in the sinusoids and by storing blood backed up from the vena cava as in right heart failure.

Laboratory Assessment of Liver Function

Biochemical markers are used to evaluate and monitor patients having or suspected of having liver disease. Enzyme assays measure the release of liver enzymes, and other tests measure liver function. Screening tests for hepatobiliary disease include serum levels of bilirubin, alkaline phosphatase, aspartate amino transferase, and alanine aminotransferase. Table 29-1 elaborates common laboratory tests for liver disorders (see also Appendix 22).

TABLE 29-1	**Common Laboratory Tests Used to Test Liver Function**
Laboratory Test	**Comment**
Hepatic Excretion	
Total serum bilirubin	When increased, may indicate bilirubin overproduction or impaired hepatic uptake, conjugation, or excretion
Indirect serum bilirubin	Unconjugated bilirubin; increased with excessive bilirubin production (hemolysis), immaturity of enzyme systems, inherited defects, drug effects
Direct serum bilirubin	Conjugated bilirubin; increased with depressed bilirubin excretion, hepatobiliary disease, intrahepatic or benign postoperative jaundice and sepsis, and congenital conjugated hyperbilirubinemia
Cholestasis	
Serum alkaline phosphatase	Enzyme widely distributed in liver, bone, placenta, intestine, kidney, leukocytes; mainly bound to canalicular membranes in liver; increased levels suggest cholestasis but can be increased with bone disorders, pregnancy, normal growth, and some malignancies
γ-Glutamyl transpeptidase (GGT)	Enzyme found in high concentrations in epithelial cells lining bile ductules in the liver; also present in kidney, pancreas, heart, brain; increased with liver disease, but also after myocardial infarction, in neuromuscular disease, pancreatic disease, pulmonary disease, diabetes mellitus, and during alcohol ingestion
Hepatic Serum Enzymes	
Alanine aminotransferase (ALT, formerly SGPT, serum glutamic pyruvic transaminase)	Located in cytosol of hepatocyte; found in several other body tissues but highest in liver; increased with liver cell damage
Aspartate aminotransferase (AST, formerly SGOT, serum glutamic oxaloacetic transaminase)	Located in cytosol and mitochondria of hepatocyte; also in cardiac and skeletal muscle, heart, brain, pancreas, kidney; increased with liver cell damage
Serum lactic dehydrogenase	Located in liver, red blood cells, cardiac muscle, kidney; increased with liver disease but lacks sensitivity and specificity because it is found in most other body tissues
Serum Proteins	
Prothrombin time (PT)	Most blood coagulation factors are synthesized in the liver; vitamin K deficiency and decreased synthesis of clotting factors increase prothrombin time and risk of bleeding.
International Normalized Ratio (INR)	A standardized way to report PT levels so that levels from different laboratories can be compared

Continued

TABLE 29-1	**Common Laboratory Tests Used to Test Liver Function—cont'd**	

Laboratory Test	Comment
Serum albumin	Main export protein synthesized in the liver and most important factor in maintaining plasma oncotic pressure; hypoalbuminemia can result from expanded plasma volume or reduced synthesis as well as increased losses as occurs with protein-losing enteropathy, nephrotic syndrome, burns, gastrointestinal bleeding, exfoliative dermatitis.
Serum globulin	Alpha₁ and alpha₂-globulins are synthesized in the liver; levels increase with chronic liver disease; limited diagnostic use in hepatobiliary disease although the pattern may suggest underlying cause of liver disease (e.g., elevated immunoglobulin [Ig]G suggests autoimmune hepatitis, elevated IgM suggests primary biliary cirrhosis, elevated IgA suggests alcoholic liver disease)
Markers of Specific Liver Diseases	
Serum ferritin	Major iron storage protein; increased level sensitive indicator of genetic hemochromatosis
Ceruloplasmin	Major copper-binding protein synthesized by liver; decreased in Wilson's disease
Alpha-fetoprotein	Major circulating plasma protein; increased with hepatocellular carcinoma
Alpha₁-antitrypsin	Main function is to inhibit serum trypsin activity; decreased levels indicate alpha₁-antitrypsin deficiency, which can cause liver and lung damage.
Markers for Viral Hepatitis	
Anti-HAV IgM (antibody to hepatitis A virus)	Marker for hepatitis A; indicates current or recent infection or convalescence
HBsAg (hepatitis B surface antigen)	Marker for hepatitis B; positive in most cases of acute or chronic infection
Anti-HBc (antibody to hepatitis B core antigen)	Antibody to hepatitis B core antigen; marker for hepatitis B; Recent or past hepatitis infection
Anti-HBs (antibody to hepatitis B surface antigen)	Antibody to HBsAg; marker for hepatitis B; denotes prior hepatitis B infection or hepatitis B vaccine; protective
HBeAg (hepatitis Be antigen)	Marker for hepatitis B; transiently positive during active virus replication; reflects concentration and infectivity of virus
Anti-HBe (antibody to hepatitis Be antigen)	Marker for hepatitis B; positive in all acute and chronic cases; positive in carriers; not protective
HBV-DNA (hepatitis B deoxyribonucleic acid)	Measures hepatitis B viral load
Anti-HCV (antibody to hepatitis C virus)	Marker for hepatitis C; positive 5-6 weeks after onset of hepatitis C virus; not protective; reflects infectious state and is detectable during and after treatment
HCV-RNA (hepatitis C virus ribonucleic acid)	Measures hepatitis C viral load
Anti-HDV	Marker for hepatitis D; indicates infection; not protective
Miscellaneous	
Ammonia	Liver converts ammonia to urea; may increase with hepatic failure and portal-systemic shunts

Data from Wedemeyer H, Pawlotsky JM: Acute viral hepatitis. In Goldman L et al, editors: *Goldman's Cecil medicine*, ed 24, Philadelphia, 2012, Elsevier Saunders. Pawlotsky JM, Mchuthinson J: Chronic viral and autoimmune hepatitis. In Goldman L et al, editors: *Goldman's Cecil medicine*, ed 24, Philadelphia, 2012, Elsevier Saunders. Woreta TA, Alqahtani SA: Evaluation of abnormal liver tests, *Med Clin North Am* 98:1, 2014. Martin P, Friedman LS: Assessment of liver function and diagnostic studies. In Friedman LS, Keeffe B, editors: *Handbook of liver disease*, ed 3, Philadephia, 2012, Elsevier Saunders; 2012. Khalili H et al: Assessment of liver function in clinical practice. In Gines P et al, editors: *Clinical gastroenterology: chronic liver failure*, New York, 2011, Springer.

Physical examination as well as diagnostic procedures (e.g., endoscopy) or abdominal imaging tests (e.g., abdominal ultrasound, magnetic resonance imaging, or computed tomography scan) can be used to diagnose or evaluate patients for liver disease. A liver biopsy is considered the gold standard to assess the severity of hepatic inflammation and fibrosis.

DISEASES OF THE LIVER

Diseases of the liver can be acute or chronic, inherited or acquired. The following section provides a brief overview of viral hepatitis, nonalcoholic fatty liver disease (NAFLD), alcoholic liver disease, cholestatic liver diseases, inherited disorders, and other liver diseases.

Viral Hepatitis

Viral **hepatitis** is a widespread inflammation of the liver and is caused by various hepatitis viruses including A, B, C, D, and E (see Figure 29-1 and Table 29-2). Hepatitis A and E are the infectious forms, mainly spread by fecal-oral route. Hepatitis B, C, and D are the serum forms that are spread by blood and body fluids (Wedemeyer and Pawlotsky, 2012). Minor agents such as Epstein-Barr virus, cytomegalovirus, and herpes simplex also can cause an acute hepatitis.

The clinical manifestations of acute viral hepatitis are divided into four phases. The first phase, the incubation phase, often is characterized by nonspecific symptoms such as malaise, loss of appetite, nausea, and right upper quadrant pain (Wedemeyer and Pawlotsky, 2012). This is followed by the preicteric phase, in which the nonspecific symptoms continue. In addition, about 10% to 20% of patients can have immune-mediated symptoms such as fever, arthralgia, arthritis, rash, and angioedema in the preicteric phase. The third phase is the icteric phase, in which **jaundice** (a yellowing of the skin, mucous membranes, and the eyes) appears and the nonspecific symptoms worsen. Finally, during the convalescent or recovery phase, jaundice and other symptoms begin to subside.

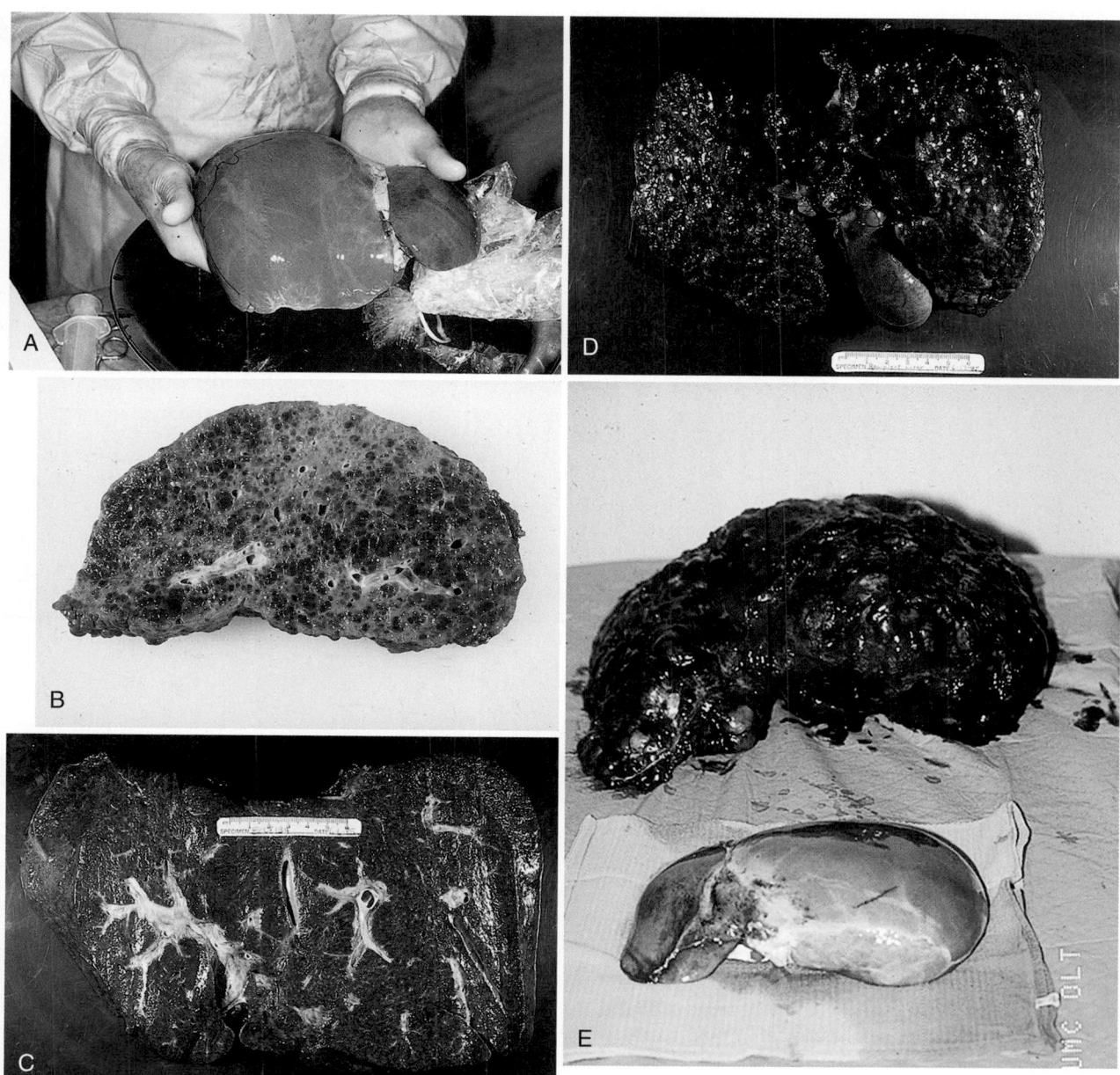

FIGURE 29-1 A, Normal liver. **B,** Liver with damage from chronic active hepatitis. **C,** Liver with damage from sclerosing cholangitis. **D,** Liver with damage from primary biliary cirrhosis. **E,** Liver with damage from polycystic liver disease *(background)* and normal liver *(foreground)*. (Courtesy Baylor Simmons Transplant Institute, Baylor University Medical Center, Dallas, TX.)

Complete spontaneous recovery is expected in all of hepatitis A cases, in nearly 90% of acute hepatitis B cases acquired as an adult, but in only 20% to 50% of acute hepatitis C cases. Chronic hepatitis usually does not develop with hepatitis E (Wedemeyer and Pawlotsky, 2012). There are vaccines only for hepatitis A and B; however, recent advances have resulted in effective antiviral drugs to treat chronic hepatitis B and C.

Nonalcoholic Fatty Liver Disease

Nonalcoholic fatty liver disease (NAFLD) is a spectrum of liver disease ranging from steatosis to steatohepatitis and cirrhosis. It involves the accumulation of fat droplets in the hepatocytes and can lead to fibrosis, cirrhosis, and even hepatocellular carcinoma. Causes of NAFLD can include drugs, inborn errors of metabolism, and acquired metabolic disorders (type 2 diabetes mellitus, lipodystrophy, jejunal ileal bypass, obesity, and malnutrition). However, NAFLD is associated most commonly with obesity, type 2 diabetes mellitus, dyslipidemia, and metabolic syndrome (Chalasani et al, 2012).

The initial stage of NAFLD is nonalcoholic fatty liver (NAFL) which is characterized by the simple accumulation of fat within the liver. Nonalcoholic steatohepatitis (NASH) is

TABLE 29-2	Types of Viral Hepatitis	
Virus	Transmission	Comments
Hepatitis A	Fecal-oral route; is contracted through contaminated drinking water, food, and sewage	Anorexia is the most frequent symptom, and it can be severe. Other common symptoms include nausea, vomiting, right upper quadrant abdominal pain, dark urine, and jaundice (icterus). Recovery is usually complete, and long-term consequences are rare. Serious complications may occur in high-risk patients; subsequently, great attention must be given to adequate nutritional intake.
Hepatitis B and C	HBV and HCV are transmitted via blood, blood products, semen, and saliva. For example, they can be spread from contaminated needles, blood transfusions, open cuts or wounds, splashes of blood into the mouth or eyes, or sexual contact.	HBV and HCV can lead to chronic and carrier states. Chronic active hepatitis also can develop, leading to cirrhosis and liver failure.
Hepatitis D	HDV is rare in the United States and depends on the HBV for survival and propagation in humans.	HDV may be a coinfection (occurring at the same time as HBV) or a superinfection (superimposing itself on the HBV carrier state). This form of hepatitis usually becomes chronic.
Hepatitis E	HEV is transmitted via the oral-fecal route.	HEV is rare in the United States (typically only occurs when imported), but it is reported more frequently in many countries of southern, eastern, and central Asia; northern, eastern, and western Africa; and Mexico. Contaminated water appears to be the source of infection, which usually afflicts people living in crowded and unsanitary conditions. HEV is generally acute rather than chronic.
Hepatitis G/GB	HGV and a virus labeled GBV-C appear to be variants of the same virus.	Although HGV infection is present in a significant proportion of blood donors and is transmitted through blood transfusions, it does not appear to cause liver disease.

HBV, Hepatitis B virus; *HCV,* hepatitis C virus; *HDV,* hepatitis D virus; *HEV,* hepatitis E virus; *HGV,* hepatitis G virus.

associated with hepatocyte injury with or without fibrous tissue in the liver. NASH can develop into chronic liver disease and NASH cirrhosis. The progression to cirrhosis is variable depending on age and the presence of obesity and type 2 diabetes, which contribute to a worsening prognosis (Chalasani, 2012).

The treatment recommendations for NAFLD from the American Association for the Study of Liver Diseases (AASLD) include weight loss, insulin-sensitizing drugs such as thiazolidinediones, and vitamin E (Chalasani et al, 2012). Based on the AASLD Guidelines, a 3% to 5% weight loss can improve steatosis, but up to 10% weight loss may be needed to improve necroinflammation. The AASLD Guidelines state that pioglitazone (an oral antihyperglycemia medication used to treat diabetes mellitus) may be considered for NASH treatment, although long-term safety and efficacy is not known. Vitamin E (800 IU/day of alpha-tocopherol) is considered first-line treatment for NASH in patients without diabetes (Chalasani et al, 2012; Lavine et al, 2011; Sanyal et al, 2010). Emerging data suggest drinking coffee is protective against NAFLD (Chen et al, 2013; Yesil and Yilmaz, 2013).

Alcoholic Liver Disease

Alcoholic liver disease is one of the most common liver diseases in the United States. In 2009, 48% of deaths from cirrhosis were related to alcohol (Yoon and Yi, 2012). Acetaldehyde is a toxic byproduct of alcohol metabolism that causes damage to mitochondrial membrane structure and function. Acetaldehyde is produced by multiple metabolic pathways, one of which involves alcohol dehydrogenase (see *Focus On: Metabolic Consequences of Alcohol Consumption*).

FOCUS ON

Metabolic Consequences of Alcohol Consumption

Ethanol is metabolized primarily in the liver by alcohol dehydrogenase. This results in acetaldehyde production with the transfer of hydrogen to nicotinamide adenine dinucleotide (NAD), reducing it to NADH. The acetaldehyde then loses hydrogen and is converted to acetate, most of which is released into the blood.

Many metabolic disturbances occur because of the excess of NADH, which overrides the ability of the cell to maintain a normal redox state. These include hyperlacticacidemia, acidosis, hyperuricemia, ketonemia, and hyperlipemia. The tricarboxylic acid (TCA) cycle is depressed because it requires NAD. The mitochondria, in turn, use hydrogen from ethanol rather than from the oxidation of fatty acids to produce energy via the TCA cycle, which leads to a decreased fatty acid oxidation and accumulation of triglycerides. In addition, NADH may actually promote fatty acid synthesis. Hypoglycemia also can occur in early alcoholic liver disease secondary to the suppression of the TCA cycle, coupled with decreased gluconeogenesis resulting from ethanol.

Several variables predispose some people to alcoholic liver disease. These include genetic polymorphisms of alcohol-metabolizing enzymes, gender (women more than men), simultaneous exposure to other drugs, infections with hepatotropic viruses, immunologic factors, obesity, and poor nutrition status. The pathogenesis of alcoholic liver disease progresses in three stages (see Figure 29-2): hepatic steatosis (see Figure 29-3), alcoholic hepatitis, and finally cirrhosis.

Fatty infiltration, known as hepatic steatosis or fatty liver, is caused by a culmination of these metabolic disturbances: (1) an increase in the mobilization of fatty acids from adipose tissue; (2) an increase in hepatic synthesis of

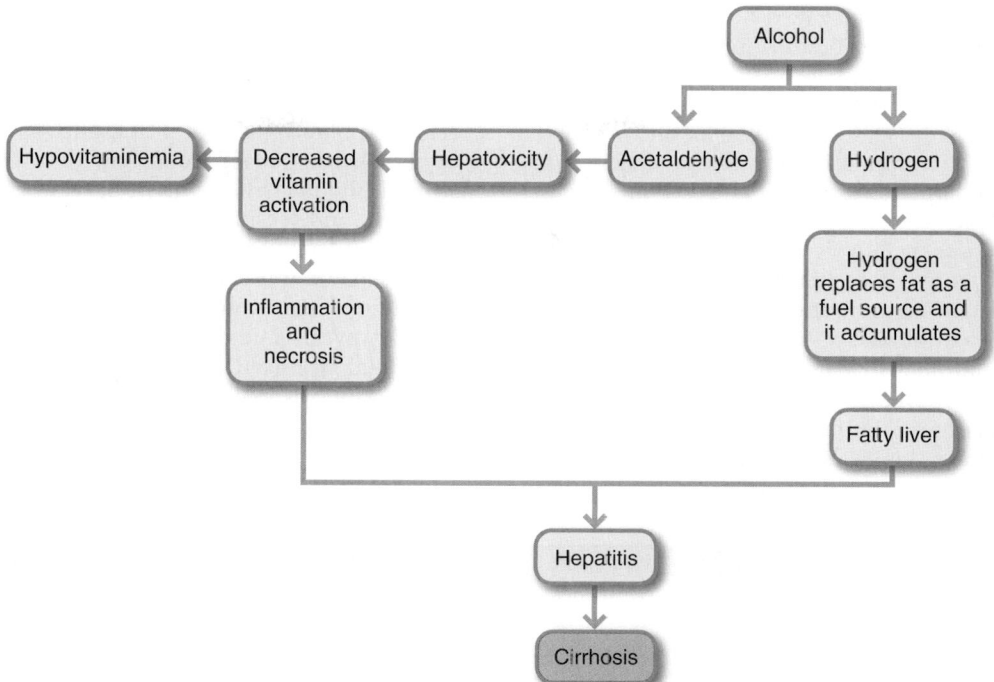

FIGURE 29-2 Complications of excessive alcohol consumption stem largely from excess hydrogen and from acetaldehyde. Hydrogen produces fatty liver and hyperlipemia, high blood lactic acid, and low blood sugar. The accumulation of fat, the effect of acetaldehyde on liver cells, and other factors as yet unknown lead to alcoholic hepatitis. The next step is cirrhosis. The consequent impairment of liver function disturbs blood chemistry, notably causing a high ammonia level that can lead to coma and death. Cirrhosis also distorts liver structure, inhibiting blood flow. High pressure in vessels supplying the liver may cause ruptured varices and accumulation of fluid in the abdominal cavity. Response to alcohol differs among individuals; in particular, not all heavy drinkers develop hepatitis and cirrhosis.

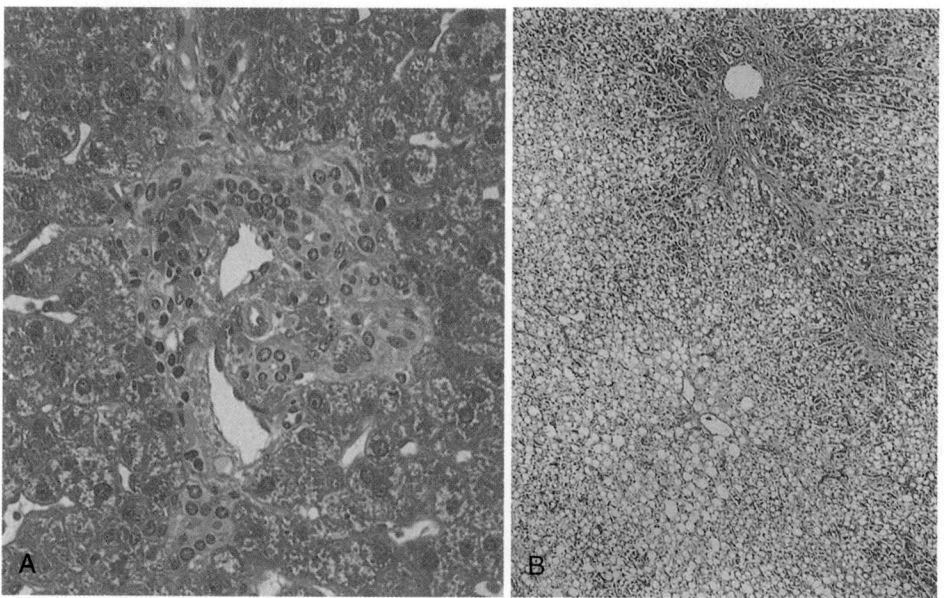

FIGURE 29-3 A, Microscopic appearance of a normal liver. A normal portal tract consists of the portal vein, hepatic arteriole, one to two interlobular bile ducts, and occasional peripherally located ductules. **B,** Acute fatty liver. This photomicrograph on low power exhibits fatty change involving virtually all the hepatocytes, with slight sparing of the liver cells immediately adjacent to the portal tract *(top)*. (From Kanel G, Korula J, editors: *Atlas of liver pathology,* Philadelphia, 1992, Saunders.)

fatty acids; (3) a decrease in fatty acid oxidation; (4) an increase in triglyceride production; and (5) a trapping of triglycerides in the liver. Hepatic steatosis is reversible with abstinence from alcohol. Conversely, if alcohol abuse continues, cirrhosis can develop. Patients with alcoholic fatty liver disease usually are asymptomatic but can have symptoms such as fatigue, poor appetite, right upper quadrant discomfort, or hepatomegaly.

Alcoholic hepatitis generally is characterized by hepatomegaly, modest elevation of serum transaminase levels, increased serum bilirubin concentrations, normal or depressed serum albumin concentrations, or anemia. Patients also may have abdominal pain, anorexia, nausea, vomiting, weakness, diarrhea, weight loss, or fever. Some patients can develop jaundice, coagulopathy, ascites, or encephalopathy. If patients discontinue alcohol intake, hepatitis may resolve; however, the condition often progresses to the third stage.

Clinical features of alcoholic cirrhosis, the third stage, vary. Symptoms can mimic those of alcoholic hepatitis; or patients can develop complications of cirrhosis such as gastrointestinal bleeding, hepatic encephalopathy, or portal hypertension (elevated blood pressure in the portal venous system caused by the obstruction of blood flow through the liver). Patients with alcoholic cirrhosis often develop ascites, the accumulation of fluid, serum protein, and electrolytes within the peritoneal cavity caused by increased pressure from portal hypertension and decreased production of albumin (which maintains serum colloidal osmotic pressure). A liver biopsy usually reveals micronodular cirrhosis, but it can be macronodular or mixed. Prognosis depends on abstinence from alcohol and the degree of complications already developed. Ethanol ingestion creates specific and severe nutritional abnormalities (see *Clinical Insight:* Malnutrition in the Alcoholic).

CLINICAL INSIGHT

Malnutrition in the Alcoholic

Several factors contribute to the malnutrition common in individuals with chronic alcoholic liver disease:

1. Alcohol can replace food in the diet of moderate and heavy drinkers, displacing the intake of adequate calories and nutrients. In light drinkers, it is usually an additional energy source, or empty calories. Although alcohol yields 7.1 kcal/g, when it is consumed in large amounts it is not used efficiently as a fuel source. When individuals consume alcohol on a regular basis but do not fulfill criteria for alcohol abuse, they are often overweight because of the increased calories (alcohol addition). This is different from the heavy drinker who replaces energy-rich nutrients with alcohol (alcohol substitution).

2. In the alcoholic, impaired digestion and absorption are related to pancreatic insufficiency, as well as morphologic and functional alterations of the intestinal mucosa. Acute and chronic alcohol intake impairs hepatic amino acid uptake and synthesis into proteins, reduces protein synthesis and secretion from the liver, and increases catabolism in the gut.

3. Use of lipids and carbohydrates is compromised. An excess of reduction equivalents (e.g., nicotinamide adenine dinucleotide phosphate [NADH])

and impaired oxidation of triglycerides result in fat deposition in the hepatocytes and an increase in circulating triglycerides. Insulin resistance is also common.

4. Vitamin and mineral deficiencies occur in alcoholic liver disease as a result of reduced intake and alterations in absorption, storage, and ability to convert the nutrients to their active forms. Steatorrhea resulting from bile acid deficiency is also common in alcoholic liver disease and affects fat-soluble vitamin absorption. Vitamin A deficiency can lead to night blindness. Thiamin deficiency is the most common vitamin deficiency in alcoholics and is responsible for Wernicke encephalopathy (Leevy et al, 2005). Folate deficiency can occur as a result of poor intake, impaired absorption, accelerated excretion, and altered storage and metabolism. Inadequate dietary intake and interactions between pyridoxal-5-phosphate (active coenzyme of vitamin B_6) and alcohol reduce vitamin B_6 status. Deficiency of all B vitamins and vitamins C, D, E, and K is also common. Hypocalcemia, hypomagnesemia, and hypophosphatemia are not uncommon among alcoholics; furthermore, zinc deficiency and alterations in other micronutrients can accompany chronic alcohol intake.

Cholestatic Liver Diseases

Cholestatic liver diseases refer to conditions affecting the bile ducts.

Primary Biliary Cirrhosis

Primary biliary cirrhosis (PBC) is a chronic cholestatic disease caused by progressive destruction of small and intermediate-size intrahepatic bile ducts. The extrahepatic biliary tree and larger intrahepatic ducts are normal. Ninety-five percent of patients with PBC are women. The disease progresses slowly, eventually resulting in cirrhosis, portal hypertension, liver transplantation, or death (Afdhal, 2012).

PBC is an autoimmune disorder. PBC typically presents with a mild elevation of liver enzymes with physical symptoms of pruritus and fatigue. Several nutritional complications from cholestasis can occur with PBC, including osteopenia, hypercholesterolemia, and fat-soluble vitamin deficiencies.

Primary Sclerosing Cholangitis

Primary sclerosing cholangitis (PSC) is characterized by fibrosing inflammation of segments of extrahepatic bile ducts, with or without involvement of intrahepatic ducts. The progressive disease can be characterized by three syndromes. The first is cholestasis with biliary cirrhosis followed by recurrent cholangitis with large bile duct strictures, and finally cholangiocarcinoma (Afdhal, 2012). Like PBC, PSC is considered an immune disorder. Of patients with PSC, 70% to 90% also have inflammatory bowel disease (especially ulcerative colitis), and men are more likely than women (2.3:1) to have PSC (Afdhal, 2012). Patients with PSC are also at increased risk of fat-soluble vitamin deficiencies resulting from steatorrhea associated with this disease. Hepatic osteodystrophy may occur from vitamin D and calcium malabsorption, resulting in secondary hyperparathyroidism, osteomalacia, or rickets. No treatment slows progression of the disease or improves survival. Ursodeoxycholic acid may improve laboratory values (serum bilirubin, alkaline phosphatase, and albumin), but has no effect on survival (Afdhal, 2012).

Inherited Disorders

Inherited disorders of the liver include hemochromatosis, Wilson's disease, alpha$_1$-antitrypsin deficiency, and cystic fibrosis.

Porphyria, glycogen storage disease, and amyloidosis are metabolic diseases with a genetic component.

Hemochromatosis

Hemochromatosis is an inherited disease of iron overload usually associated with the gene HFE (Bacon, 2012). Patients with hereditary hemochromatosis absorb excessive iron from the gut and may store 20 to 40 g of iron compared with 0.3 to 0.8 g in normal persons (see Chapter 32). Increased transferrin saturation (at least 45%) and ferritin (more than two times normal) suggest hemochromatosis. Hepatomegaly, esophageal bleeding, ascites, impaired hepatic synthetic function, abnormal skin pigmentation, glucose intolerance, cardiac involvement, hypogonadism, arthropathy, and hepatocellular carcinoma may develop. Early diagnosis includes clinical, laboratory, and pathologic testing, including elevated serum transferrin levels. Life expectancy is normal if phlebotomy is initiated before the development of cirrhosis or diabetes mellitus.

Wilson's Disease

Wilson's disease is an autosomal-recessive disorder associated with impaired biliary copper excretion. Copper accumulates in various tissues, including the liver, brain, cornea, and kidneys. Kayser-Fleischer rings are greenish-yellow pigmented rings encircling the cornea just within the corneoscleral margin, formed by copper deposits. Patients can present with acute, fulminant (occurring suddenly great severity), or chronic active hepatitis and neuropsychiatric symptoms. Low serum ceruloplasmin levels, elevated copper concentration in a liver biopsy, and high urinary copper excretion confirm the diagnosis.

Copper-chelating agents (such as D-penicillamine or trientine) and zinc supplementation (to inhibit intestinal copper absorption and binding in the liver) are used to treat Wilson's disease once it is diagnosed. Ongoing copper chelation is required to prevent relapses and liver failure; transplantation corrects the metabolic defect. A low-copper diet is no longer required but may be helpful in the initial phase of treatment. High-copper foods include organ meats, shellfish, chocolate, nuts, and mushrooms. For a comprehensive list of copper content of food, refer to the US Department of Agriculture National Nutrient Database (http://ndb.nal.usda.gov/). If this disease is not diagnosed until onset of fulminant failure, survival is not possible without transplantation.

Alpha₁-Antitrypsin Deficiency

Alpha$_1$-antitrypsin deficiency is an inherited disorder that can cause liver and lung disease. Alpha$_1$-antitrypsin is a glycoprotein found in serum and body fluids; it inhibits serine proteinases. Cholestasis or cirrhosis is caused by this deficiency, and there is no treatment except liver transplantation.

Other Liver Diseases

Liver disease can be caused by several conditions other than those already discussed. Liver tumors can be primary or metastatic, benign or malignant. Hepatocellular carcinoma (HCC) usually develops in cirrhotic livers. Although the incidence of HCC is rising worldwide, the majority of cases occur in Asia and Africa resulting from the high prevalence of hepatitis B and C in those continents (Dhanasekaran et al, 2012). The liver also can be affected by systemic diseases such as rheumatoid arthritis, systemic lupus erythematosus, polymyalgia, temporal arteritis, polyarteritis nodosa, systemic sclerosis, and Sjögren syndrome. When hepatic blood flow is altered, as in acute ischemic and chronic congestive hepatopathy, Budd-Chiari syndrome, and hepatic venoocclusive disease, dysfunction occurs. Individuals with hepatic or portal vein thromboses should be evaluated for a myeloproliferative disorder. Parasitic, bacterial, fungal, and granulomatous liver diseases also occur. Finally, cryptogenic cirrhosis is any cirrhosis for which the cause is unknown.

Classifying Liver Disease According to Duration

Liver disease can be classified according to the time of onset and duration of the disease. Liver disease can be fulminant, acute, and chronic.

Fulminant hepatitis is a syndrome in which severe liver dysfunction is accompanied by hepatic encephalopathy, a clinical syndrome characterized by impaired mentation, neuromuscular disturbances, and altered consciousness. Fulminant liver disease is defined by the absence of preexisting liver disease and the development of hepatic encephalopathy within 2 to 8 weeks of the onset of illness. The causes of fulminant hepatitis include viral hepatitis in approximately 75% of cases, chemical toxicity (e.g., acetaminophen, drug reactions, poisonous mushrooms, industrial poisons), and other causes (e.g., Wilson's disease, fatty liver of pregnancy, Reye syndrome, hepatic ischemia, hepatic vein obstruction, and disseminated malignancies). Extrahepatic complications of fulminant hepatitis are cerebral edema, coagulopathy and bleeding, cardiovascular abnormalities, renal failure, pulmonary complications, acid-base disturbances, electrolyte imbalances, sepsis, and pancreatitis (inflammation of the pancreas).

Acute liver disease is identified typically as liver dysfunction that has been present for less than 6 months. Recovery is expected in a majority of patients who develop acute liver disease.

To be diagnosed with chronic hepatitis, a patient must have at least a 6-month course of hepatitis or biochemical and clinical evidence of liver disease with confirmatory biopsy findings of unresolving hepatic inflammation. Chronic hepatitis can have autoimmune, viral, metabolic, drug, or toxin causes. The most common causes of chronic hepatitis are hepatitis B, hepatitis C, and autoimmune hepatitis. Other causes are drug-induced liver disease, metabolic diseases, and NASH. Cryptogenic cirrhosis is cirrhosis of an unknown cause.

Clinical symptoms of chronic hepatitis are usually nonspecific, occur intermittently, and are mild. Common symptoms include fatigue, sleep disorders, difficulty concentrating, and mild right upper quadrant pain. Severe advanced disease can lead to jaundice, muscle wasting, tea-colored urine, ascites, edema, hepatic encephalopathy, gastrointestinal varices (abnormal enlarged veins often caused by portal hypertension) with resultant gastrointestinal bleeding, splenomegaly, palmar erythema, and spider angiomata.

In some instances, chronic hepatitis leads to cirrhosis and end-stage liver disease. Cirrhosis has many clinical manifestations, as illustrated in Figure 29-4. Several major complications of cirrhosis and end-stage liver disease (ESLD), including malnutrition, ascites, hyponatremia, hepatic encephalopathy, glucose alterations, fat malabsorption, hepatorenal syndrome, and osteopenia, have nutrition implications.

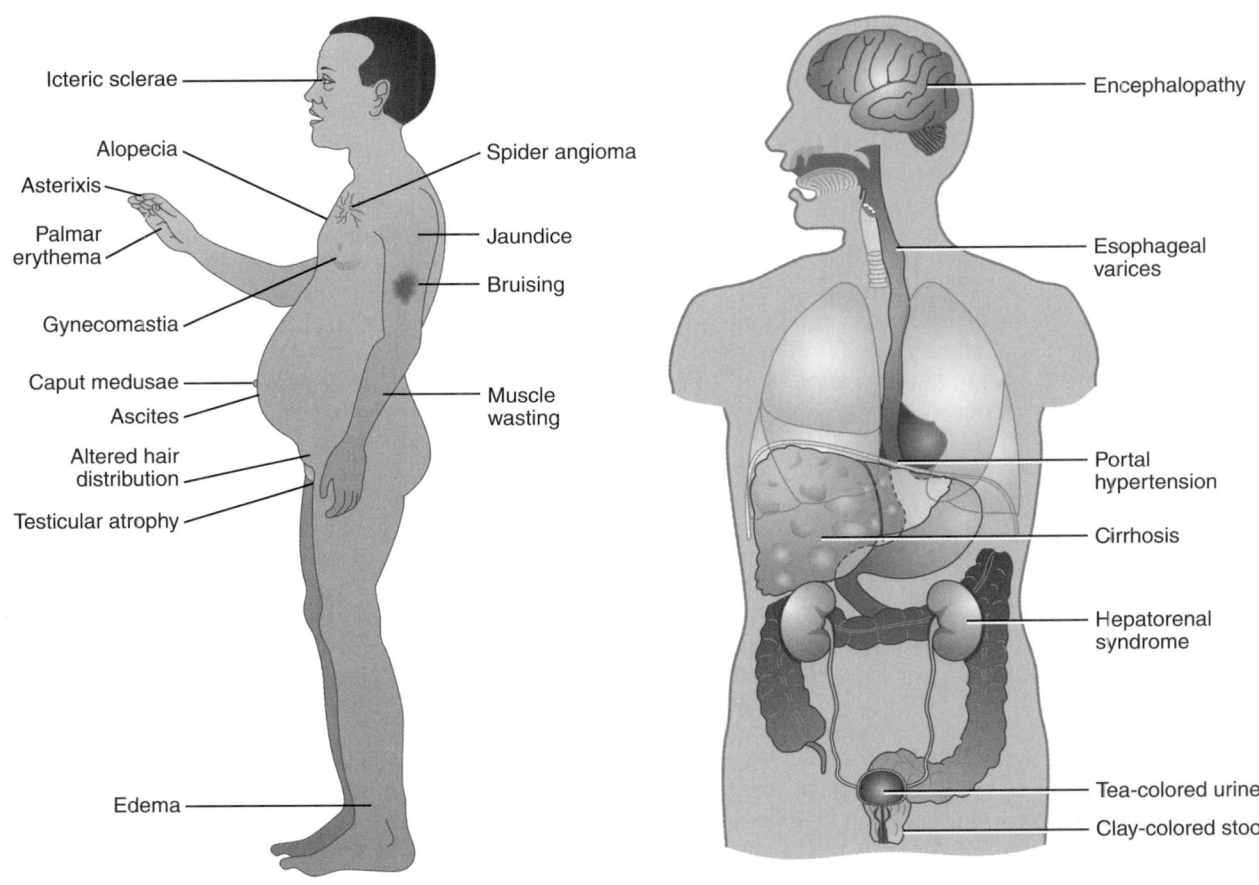

FIGURE 29-4 Clinical manifestations of cirrhosis.

Image labels (External Symptoms): Icteric sclerae, Alopecia, Asterixis, Palmar erythema, Gynecomastia, Caput medusae, Ascites, Altered hair distribution, Testicular atrophy, Edema, Spider angioma, Jaundice, Bruising, Muscle wasting

Image labels (Internal Symptoms): Encephalopathy, Esophageal varices, Portal hypertension, Cirrhosis, Hepatorenal syndrome, Tea-colored urine, Clay-colored stool

EXTERNAL SYMPTOMS

INTERNAL SYMPTOMS

COMPLICATIONS OF ESLD: CAUSE AND NUTRITION TREATMENT

End-stage liver disease can have several physical manifestations including portal hypertension, ascites and edema, hyponatremia, and hepatic encephalopathy. It is important to understand the underlying cause of these complications as well as the medical and nutrition treatment options.

Portal Hypertension
Pathophysiology and Medical Treatment

Portal hypertension increases collateral blood flow and can result in swollen veins (varices) in the GIT. These varices often bleed, causing a medical emergency. Treatment includes administration of alpha-adrenergic blockers to decrease heart rate, endoscopic variceal ligation, and radiologic placement of shunts. During an acute bleeding episode, somatostatin or its analog may be administered to decrease bleeding, or a nasogastric tube equipped with an inflatable balloon is placed to alleviate bleeding from vessels.

Medical Nutrition Therapy

During acute bleeding episodes, nutrition cannot be administered enterally; parenteral nutrition (PN) is indicated if a patient will be taking nothing enterally for at least 5 to 7 days (see Chapter 13). Repeated endoscopic therapies may cause esophageal strictures or impair a patient's swallowing. Finally, placement of shunts may

increase the incidence of encephalopathy and reduce nutrient metabolism because blood is shunted past the liver cells.

Ascites
Pathophysiology and Medical Treatment

Fluid retention is common, and ascites (accumulation of fluid in the abdominal cavity) is a serious consequence of liver disease. Portal hypertension, hypoalbuminemia, lymphatic obstruction, and renal retention of sodium and fluid contribute to fluid retention. Increased release of catecholamines, renin, angiotensin, aldosterone, and antidiuretic hormone secondary to peripheral arterial vasodilation causes renal retention of sodium and water.

Large-volume paracentesis may be used to relieve ascites. Diuretic therapy often is used and frequently includes spironolactone and furosemide. These drugs often are used in combination for best effect. Major side effects of loop diuretics such as furosemide include hyponatremia, hypokalemia, hypomagnesemia, hypocalcemia, and hypochloremic acidosis.

Conversely, spironolactone is potassium sparing. Therefore serum potassium levels must be monitored carefully and supplemented or restricted if necessary because deficiency or excess can contribute to metabolic abnormalities. Weight, abdominal girth, urinary sodium concentration, and serum levels of urea nitrogen, creatinine, albumin, uric acid, and electrolytes should be monitored during diuretic therapy.

Medical Nutrition Therapy

Dietary treatment for ascites includes sodium restriction. Sodium commonly is restricted to 2 g/day (see Chapter 33 and Appendix 30 for discussions of low-sodium diets). More severe limitations may be imposed; however, caution is warranted because of limited palatability and the risk of overrestricting sodium. Adequate protein intake is also important to replace losses from frequent paracentesis.

Hyponatremia
Pathophysiology

Hyponatremia often occurs because of decreased ability to excrete water resulting from the persistent release of antidiuretic hormone, sodium losses via paracentesis, excessive diuretic use, or overly aggressive sodium restriction.

Medical Nutrition Therapy

Fluid intake is often restricted to 1 to 1.5 L/day, depending on the severity of the edema and ascites although recent recommendations call for fluid restriction only if the sodium level is less than 125 mg/dl (Runyon, 2013). A moderate sodium intake of about 2000 mg/day should be continued because excessive sodium intake results in worsened fluid retention and the further dilution of serum sodium levels (hyponatremia).

Hepatic Encephalopathy
Pathophysiology and Medical Treatment

Hepatic encephalopathy is a syndrome characterized by impaired mentation, neuromuscular disturbances, and altered consciousness. Gastrointestinal bleeding, fluid and electrolyte abnormalities, uremia, infection, use of sedatives, hyperglycemia or hypoglycemia, alcohol withdrawal, constipation, azotemia, dehydration, portosystemic shunts, and acidosis can precipitate hepatic encephalopathy. Subclinical or minimal hepatic encephalopathy also affects patients with chronic hepatic failure. Hepatic or portal systemic encephalopathy results in neuromuscular and behavioral alterations. Box 29-1 describes the four stages of hepatic encephalopathy.

Different theories exist regarding the mechanism by which hepatic encephalopathy occurs. However, one of the most common theories involves ammonia accumulation because it is considered to be an important causal factor in the development of encephalopathy. When the liver fails, it is unable to detoxify ammonia to urea. Ammonia levels are elevated in the brain and bloodstream, leading to impaired neural function through a complex system. The main source of ammonia is its endogenous production by the GIT from the metabolism of protein and from the degradation of bacteria and blood from gastrointestinal bleeding. Exogenous protein is also a source of ammonia. Some clinicians suggest that dietary protein causes an increase in ammonia levels and subsequently hepatic encephalopathy, but this has not been proven in studies.

Drugs such as lactulose and rifaximin are given to treat hepatic encephalopathy. Lactulose is a nonabsorbable disaccharide. It acidifies the colonic contents, retaining ammonia as the ammonium ion. It also acts as an osmotic laxative to remove the ammonia. Rifaximin is a nonabsorbable antibiotic that helps decrease colonic ammonia production.

One nutrition-related hypothesis is the "altered neurotransmitter theory," which involves amino acid imbalance. A plasma amino acid imbalance exists in ESLD in which the branched-chain amino acids (BCAAs) valine, leucine, and isoleucine are decreased. The BCAAs furnish as much as 30% of energy requirements for skeletal muscle, heart, and brain when gluconeogenesis and ketogenesis are depressed causing serum BCAA levels to fall. Aromatic amino acids (AAAs) tryptophan, phenylalanine, and tyrosine, plus methionine, glutamine, asparagine, and histidine are increased. Plasma AAAs and methionine are released into circulation by muscle proteolysis, but the synthesis into protein and liver clearance of AAAs is depressed. This changes the plasma molar ratio of BCAAs to AAAs and has been theorized to contribute to the development of hepatic encephalopathy. Conversely, high levels of AAAs have been theorized to limit the cerebral uptake of BCAAs because they compete for carrier-mediated transport at the blood-brain barrier.

Medical Nutrition Therapy

The outdated practice of protein restriction in patients with low-grade hepatic encephalopathy is based on the premise that protein intolerance causes hepatic encephalopathy, but it has never been proven in a study. True dietary protein intolerance is rare except in fulminant hepatic failure, or in a rare patient with chronic endogenous hepatic encephalopathy. Unnecessary protein restriction may worsen body protein losses and must be avoided. In fact, patients with encephalopathy often do not receive adequate protein. More than 95% of patients with cirrhosis can tolerate mixed-protein diets up to 1.5 g/kg of body weight.

Studies evaluating the benefit of supplements enriched with BCAAs and restricted in AAAs have varied in study design, sample size, composition of formulas, level of encephalopathy, type of liver disease, duration of therapy, and control groups. When high methodological quality studies are evaluated, no significant improvements or survival benefits are associated with giving extra BCAAs to patients.

Other theories postulate that vegetable proteins and casein may improve mental status compared with meat protein. Casein-based diets are lower in AAAs and higher in BCAAs than meat-based diets. Vegetable protein is low in methionine and ammoniagenic amino acids but BCAA rich. The high-fiber content of a vegetable-protein diet also may play a role in the excretion of nitrogenous compounds.

Finally, it has been proposed that probiotics and synbiotics (sources of gut-friendly bacteria and fermentable fibers) can be used to treat hepatic encephalopathy. Probiotics may improve hepatic encephalopathy by reducing ammonia (Pereg et al, 2011) or by preventing production or uptake of lipopolysaccharides in the gut (Gratz et al, 2010). Thus they decrease inflammation and oxidative stress in the hepatocyte (thus increasing hepatic clearance of toxins including ammonia), and minimizing uptake of other toxins.

BOX 29-1 Four Stages of Hepatic Encephalopathy

Stage	Symptoms
I	Mild confusion, agitation, irritability, sleep disturbance, decreased attention
II	Lethargy, disorientation, inappropriate behavior, drowsiness
III	Somnolent but arousable, incomprehensible speech, confused, aggressive behavior when awake
IV	Coma

Glucose Alterations
Pathophysiology

Glucose intolerance occurs in almost two thirds of patients with cirrhosis, and as many as one third of patients develop overt diabetes. Glucose intolerance in patients with liver disease occurs because of insulin resistance in peripheral tissues. Hyperinsulinism also occurs in patients with cirrhosis, possibly because insulin production is increased, hepatic clearance is decreased, portal systemic shunting occurs, there is a defect in the insulin-binding action at the receptor site, or there is a postreceptor defect.

Fasting hypoglycemia, or low blood glucose, can occur because of the decreased availability of glucose from glycogen in addition to the failing gluconeogenic capacity of the liver when the patient has ESLD. Hypoglycemia occurs more often in acute or fulminant liver failure than in chronic liver disease. Hypoglycemia also may occur after alcohol consumption in patients whose glycogen stores are depleted by starvation because of the block of hepatic gluconeogenesis by ethanol.

Medical Nutrition Therapy

Patients with diabetes should receive standard medical and nutrition therapy to achieve normoglycemia (see Chapter 30). Patients with hypoglycemia should eat frequently to prevent this condition (see *Clinical Insight:* Fasting Hypoglycemia). Evening snacks may help prevent morning hypoglycemia.

CLINICAL INSIGHT

Fasting Hypoglycemia

Two thirds of the glucose requirement in an adult is used by the central nervous system. During fasting, plasma glucose concentrations are maintained for use by the nervous system and the brain because liver glycogen is broken down, or new glucose is made from nonglucose precursors such as alanine. Fasting hypoglycemia occurs when there is reduced synthesis of new glucose or reduced liver glycogen breakdown (see Chapter 30).

Causes of fasting hypoglycemia include cirrhosis, consumption of alcohol, extensive intrahepatic cancer, deficiency of cortisol and growth hormone, or non–beta-cell tumors of the pancreas (insulinomas). The method for detecting fasting hypoglycemia involves measuring plasma insulin when plasma glucose is low. The diagnostic hallmark of an insulinoma is altered insulin secretion in the presence of hypoglycemia. Fasting hypoglycemia also may be caused by spontaneously produced antibodies to insulin. All patients with liver or pancreatic disease should be monitored for fasting hypoglycemia. Nutrition therapy involves balanced meals with small, frequent snacks to avoid periods of fasting. Monitoring of blood glucose and insulin levels is required.

Fat Malabsorption
Pathophysiology

Fat absorption may be impaired in liver disease. Possible causes include decreased bile salt secretion (as in PBC, sclerosing cholangitis, and biliary strictures), administration of medications such as cholestyramine, and pancreatic enzyme insufficiency. Stools may be greasy, floating, or light- or clay-colored, signifying malabsorption, which can be verified by a 72-hour fecal fat study (see Chapter 28).

Medical Nutrition Therapy

If significant steatorrhea is present, replacement of some of the long-chain triglycerides or dietary fat with medium-chain triglycerides (MCTs) may be useful. Because MCTs do not require bile salts and micelle formation for absorption, they are readily taken up via the portal route (see Chapter 28). Some nutrition supplements contain MCTs, which can be used in addition to liquid MCT oil (see Chapter 13).

Significant stool fat losses may warrant a trial of a low-fat diet. If diarrhea does not resolve, fat restriction should be discontinued because it decreases the palatability of the diet and severely hampers adequate calorie intake. Because of the degree of malabsorption and steatorrhea, it is important to be suspicious that the patient may have deficiencies of multiple micronutrients especially fat-soluble vitamins.

Renal Insufficiency and Hepatorenal Syndrome
Pathophysiology, Medical, and Nutrition Therapies

Hepatorenal syndrome is renal failure associated with severe liver disease without intrinsic kidney abnormalities. Hepatorenal syndrome is diagnosed when the urine sodium level is less than 10 mEq/L and oliguria persists in the absence of intravascular volume depletion. If conservative therapies, including discontinuation of nephrotoxic drugs, optimization of intravascular volume status, treatment of underlying infection, and monitoring of fluid intake and output fail, dialysis may be required. In any case, renal insufficiency and failure may necessitate alteration in fluid, sodium, potassium, and phosphorus intake (see Chapter 35).

Osteopenia
Pathophysiology

Osteopenia often exists in patients with PBC, sclerosing cholangitis, and alcoholic liver disease. Depressed osteoblastic function and osteoporosis also can occur in patients with hemochromatosis, and osteoporosis is prevalent in patients who have had long-term treatment with corticosteroids. Corticosteroids increase bone resorption; suppress osteoblastic function; and affect sex hormone secretion, intestinal absorption of dietary calcium, renal excretion of calcium and phosphorus, and the vitamin D system.

Medical Nutrition Therapy

Prevention or treatment options for osteopenia include weight maintenance, ingestion of a well-balanced diet, adequate protein to maintain muscle mass, 1500 mg of calcium per day, adequate vitamin D from the diet or supplements, avoidance of alcohol, and monitoring for steatorrhea, with diet adjustments as needed to minimize nutrient losses (see Chapter 24).

NUTRITION ISSUES RELATED TO END-STAGE LIVER DISEASE

Nutrition Assessment

Nutrition assessment must be performed to determine the extent and cause of malnutrition in patients with liver disease. However, many traditional markers of nutrition status are affected by liver disease and its sequelae, making traditional assessment difficult. Table 29-3 summarizes the factors that affect interpretation of nutrition assessment parameters in patients with liver dysfunction.

Objective nutrition assessment parameters that are helpful when monitored serially include anthropometric measurements and dietary intake evaluation (see Chapters 4 and 7). Caution should be taken when assessing biochemical markers

TABLE 29-3 Factors That Affect Interpretation of Objective Nutrition Assessment Parameter in Patients with End-Stage Liver Disease

Parameter	Factors Affecting Interpretation
Body weight	Affected by edema, ascites, and diuretic use
Anthropometric measurements	Questionable sensitivity, specificity, and reliability
	Multiple sources of error
	Unknown if skinfold measurements reflect total body fat
	References do not account for variation in hydration status and skin compressibility
Nitrogen balance studies	Nitrogen is retained in the body in the form of ammonia
	Hepatorenal syndrome can affect the excretion of nitrogen
Single-frequency bioelectrical impedance	Invalid with ascites and edema

Modified from Hasse J: Nutritional aspects of adult liver transplantation. In Busuttil RW, Klintmalm GB, editors: *Transplantation of the liver,* ed 2, Philadelphia, 2005, Elsevier Saunders.

in the advanced liver disease patient because the typical nutrition criteria will be affected due to the liver disease itself. The best way to perform a nutrition assessment may be to combine these parameters with the subjective global assessment (SGA) approach, which has demonstrated an acceptable level of reliability and validity. The SGA gives a broad perspective, but it is not sensitive to changes in nutrition status. Other available parameters should also be reviewed. The SGA approach is summarized in Box 29-2.

BOX 29-2 Subjective Global Assessment Parameters for Nutrition Evaluation of Liver Disease Patients

History

Weight change (consider fluctuations resulting from ascites and edema)
Appetite
Taste changes and early satiety
Dietary intake (calories, protein, sodium)
Persistent gastrointestinal problems (nausea, vomiting, diarrhea, constipation, difficulty chewing or swallowing)

Physical Findings

Muscle wasting
Fat stores
Ascites or edema

Existing Conditions

Disease state and other problems that could influence nutrition status such as hepatic encephalopathy, gastrointestinal bleeding, renal insufficiency, infection

Nutritional Rating Based on Results

Well nourished
Moderately (or suspected of being) malnourished
Severely malnourished

From Hasse J: Nutritional aspects of adult liver transplantation. In: Busuttil RW, Klintmalm GB, editors: *Transplantation of the liver,* ed 2, Philadelphia, 2005, Elsevier Saunders.

Malnutrition

Moderate to severe malnutrition is a common finding in patients with advanced liver disease (see Figure 29-5). This is extremely significant, considering that malnutrition plays a major role in the pathogenesis of liver injury and has a profound negative effect on prognosis. The prevalence of malnutrition depends on nutrition assessment parameters used, type and degree of liver disease, and socioeconomic status (see Appendix 21).

Numerous coexisting factors are involved in the development of malnutrition in liver disease (see *Pathophysiology and Care Management Algorithm:* Malnutrition in Liver Disease). Inadequate oral intake, a major contributor, is caused by anorexia, dysgeusia, early satiety, nausea, or vomiting associated with liver disease and the drugs used to treat it. Another cause of inadequate intake is dietary restriction.

Maldigestion and malabsorption also play a role. **Steatorrhea,** presence of fat in the stool, is common in cirrhosis, especially if there is disease involving bile duct injury and obstruction. Medications also may cause specific malabsorptive losses. In addition, altered metabolism secondary to liver dysfunction causes malnutrition in various ways. Micronutrient function is affected by altered storage in the liver, decreased transport by liver-synthesized proteins, and renal losses associated with alcoholic and advanced liver disease. Abnormal macronutrient metabolism and increased energy expenditure also can contribute to malnutrition. Finally, protein losses can occur from large-volume **paracentesis** when several liters of fluid from the abdomen (ascites) are removed through a needle.

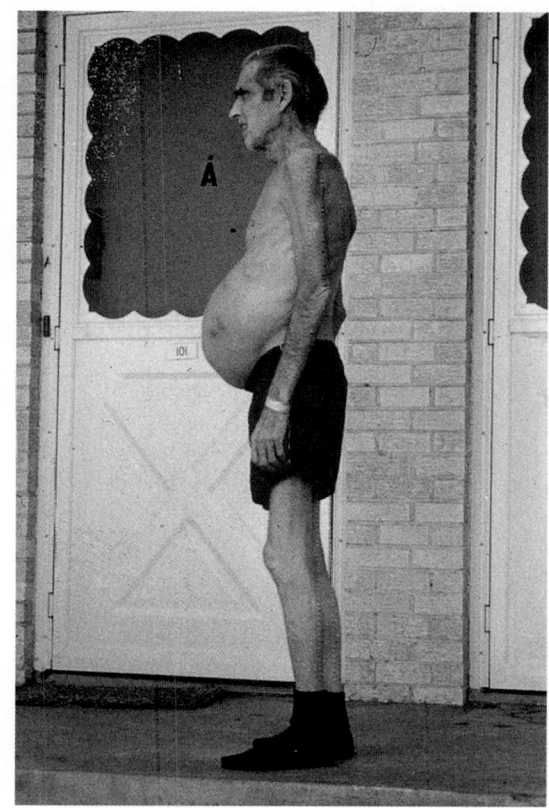

FIGURE 29-5 Severe malnutrition and ascites in a man with end-stage liver disease.

PATHOPHYSIOLOGY AND CARE MANAGEMENT ALGORITHM

Malnutrition in Liver Disease

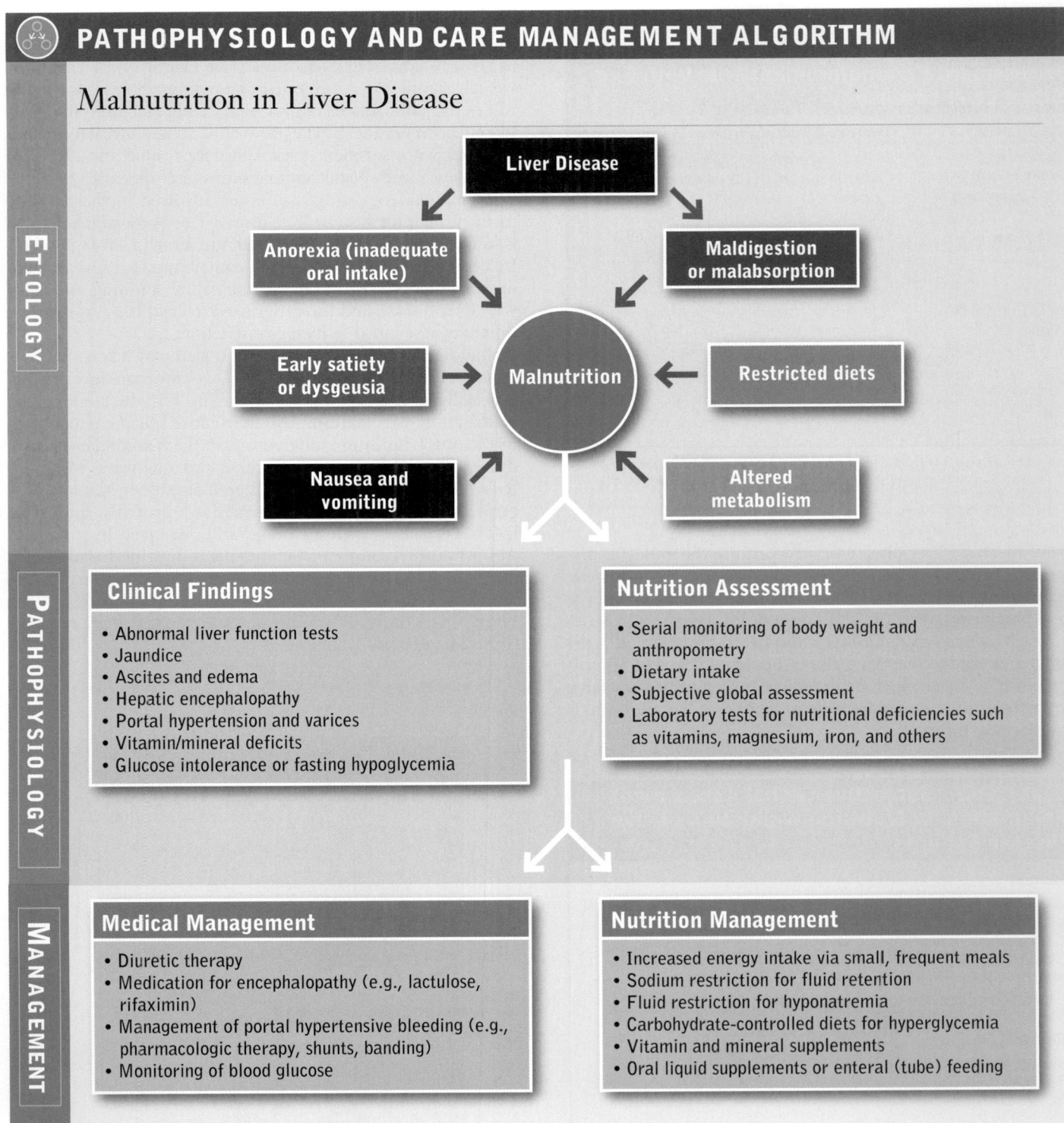

ETIOLOGY

Liver Disease

Anorexia (inadequate oral intake)

Maldigestion or malabsorption

Early satiety or dysgeusia → Malnutrition ← Restricted diets

Nausea and vomiting

Altered metabolism

PATHOPHYSIOLOGY

Clinical Findings

- Abnormal liver function tests
- Jaundice
- Ascites and edema
- Hepatic encephalopathy
- Portal hypertension and varices
- Vitamin/mineral deficits
- Glucose intolerance or fasting hypoglycemia

Nutrition Assessment

- Serial monitoring of body weight and anthropometry
- Dietary intake
- Subjective global assessment
- Laboratory tests for nutritional deficiencies such as vitamins, magnesium, iron, and others

MANAGEMENT

Medical Management

- Diuretic therapy
- Medication for encephalopathy (e.g., lactulose, rifaximin)
- Management of portal hypertensive bleeding (e.g., pharmacologic therapy, shunts, banding)
- Monitoring of blood glucose

Nutrition Management

- Increased energy intake via small, frequent meals
- Sodium restriction for fluid retention
- Fluid restriction for hyponatremia
- Carbohydrate-controlled diets for hyperglycemia
- Vitamin and mineral supplements
- Oral liquid supplements or enteral (tube) feeding

Route of Nutrition

Although oral diet is the preferred route of nutrition for patients with ESLD, anorexia, nausea, dysgeusia, and other gastrointestinal symptoms can make adequate nutrition intake difficult to achieve. Early satiety is also a frequent complaint such that smaller, more frequent meals are better tolerated than three large meals. In addition, frequent feedings may also improve nitrogen balance and prevent hypoglycemia. Oral liquid supplements should be encouraged, and, when necessary, enteral tube feedings used. Adjunctive nutrition support should be given to malnourished patients with liver disease if their intake is suboptimal and if they are at risk for fatal complications from the disease. Tube feeding is preferred over parenteral nutrition and history of varices are usually not a contraindication for tube feeding, provided there is no active bleeding (see *Portal Hypertension Pathophysiology and Medical Treatment*).

Treatment.

Although oral or enteral nutrition support may be necessary in malnourished patients or patients with inadequate nutrient intake, it is important to note that a recent trial and meta-analysis did not find survival benefits with oral or enteral nutrition in patients with cirrhosis (Dupont et al, 2012; Ney et al, 2013). However, study limitations and lack of statistical power preclude any firm conclusions on other benefits of oral or enteral nutrition support in these patients (Ney et al, 2013).

NUTRIENT REQUIREMENTS FOR CIRRHOSIS

Energy

Energy requirements vary among patients with cirrhosis. Several studies have measured resting energy expenditure (REE) in patients with liver disease to determine energy requirements. Some studies found that patients with ESLD had normal metabolism and that others had hypometabolism or hypermetabolism. Ascites or shunt placement may increase energy expenditure slightly.

In general, energy requirements for patients with ESLD and without ascites are approximately 120% to 140% of the REE. Requirements increase to 150% to 175% of REE if ascites, infection, and malabsorption are present, or if nutritional repletion is necessary. This equates to approximately 25 to 35 calories per kilogram body weight, although needs could be as low as 20 calories per kilogram for obese patients and as high as 40 calories per kilogram for underweight patients (Amodio et al, 2013). Estimated dry body weight or ideal weight should be used in calculations to prevent overfeeding.

Carbohydrate

Determining carbohydrate needs is challenging in liver failure because of the primary role of the liver in carbohydrate metabolism. Liver failure reduces glucose production and peripheral glucose use. The rate of gluconeogenesis is decreased, with preference for lipids and amino acids for energy. Alterations in the hormones insulin, glucagon, cortisol, and epinephrine are responsible in part for the preference for alternative fuels. In addition, insulin resistance can be present with liver dysfunction.

Lipid

In cirrhosis, plasma-free fatty acids, glycerol, and ketone bodies are increased in the fasting state. The body prefers lipids as an energy substrate. Lipolysis is increased with active mobilization of lipid deposits, but the net capacity to store exogenous lipid is not impaired. An average of 30% of calories as fat is sufficient, but additional fat can be given as a concentrated source of calories for those who need additional calories.

Protein

Protein is by far the most controversial nutrient in liver failure, and its management is also the most complex. Cirrhosis has long been thought of as a catabolic disease with increased protein breakdown, inadequate synthesis, depleted status, and muscle wasting. However, protein kinetic studies demonstrate increased nitrogen losses only in patients with fulminant hepatic failure or decompensated disease, but not in stable cirrhosis.

Patients with cirrhosis also have increased protein utilization. Studies suggest that 0.8 g of protein/kg/day is the mean protein requirement to achieve nitrogen balance in stable cirrhosis. Therefore in uncomplicated hepatitis or cirrhosis with or without encephalopathy, protein requirements range from 1 to 1.5 g/kg of ideal weight per day (Amodio et al, 2013).

To promote nitrogen accumulation or positive balance, at least 1.2 to 1.3 g/kg daily is needed. In situations of stress such as alcoholic hepatitis or decompensated disease (sepsis, infection, gastrointestinal bleeding, or severe ascites), at least 1.5 g of protein per kg per day should be provided.

Vitamins and Minerals

Vitamin and mineral supplementation is needed in all patients with ESLD because of the intimate role of the liver in nutrient transport, storage, and metabolism, in addition to the side effects of drugs (see Table 29-4). Vitamin deficiencies can contribute to complications. For example, folate and vitamin B_{12} deficiencies can lead to macrocytic anemia. Deficiency of pyridoxine, thiamin, or vitamin B_{12} can result in neuropathy. Confusion, ataxia, and ocular disturbances can result from a thiamin deficiency (Wernicke encephalopathy).

TABLE 29-4 Vitamin and Mineral Deficits in Severe Hepatic Failure

Vitamin or Mineral	Predisposing Factors	Signs of Deficiency (see Appendix 21)
Vitamin A	Steatorrhea, neomycin, cholestyramine, alcoholism	Night blindness, increased infection risk
Vitamin B_1 (thiamine)	Alcoholism, high-carbohydrate diet	Neuropathy, ascites, edema, central nervous system (CNS) dysfunction
Vitamin B_3 (niacin)	Alcoholism	Dermatitis, dementia, diarrhea, inflammation of mucous membranes
Vitamin B_6 (pyridoxine)	Alcoholism	Mucous membrane lesions, seborrheic dermatitis, glossitis, angular stomatitis, blepharitis, peripheral neuropathy, microcytic anemia, depression
Vitamin B_{12} (cyanocobalamin)	Alcoholism, cholestyramine	Megaloblastic anemia, glossitis, CNS dysfunction
Folate	Alcoholism	Megaloblastic anemia, glossitis, irritability
Vitamin D	Steatorrhea, glucocorticoids, cholestyramine	Osteomalacia, rickets (in children), possible link to cancer or autoimmune disorders
Vitamin E	Steatorrhea, cholestyramine	Peripheral neuropathy, ataxia, skeletal myopathy, retinopathy, immune system impairment
Vitamin K	Steatorrhea, antibiotics, cholestyramine	Excessive bleeding, bruising
Iron	Chronic bleeding	Stomatitis, microcytic anemia, malaise
Magnesium	Alcoholism, diuretics	Neuromuscular irritability, hypokalemia, hypocalcemia
Phosphorus	Anabolism, alcoholism	Anorexia, weakness, cardiac failure, glucose intolerance
Zinc	Diarrhea, diuretics, alcoholism	Immunodeficiency, impaired taste acuity, delayed wound healing, impaired protein synthesis

Deficiencies of fat-soluble vitamins have been found in all types of liver failure, especially in cholestatic diseases in which malabsorption and steatorrhea occur. Impaired dark adaptation can occur from vitamin A deficiency. Hepatic osteodystrophy or osteopenia can develop from vitamin D deficiency. Therefore supplementation is necessary, and may require using water-miscible forms. Intravenous or intramuscular vitamin K often is given for 3 days to rule out vitamin K deficiency as the cause of a prolonged prothrombin times. Water-soluble vitamin deficiencies associated with liver disease include thiamin (which can lead to Wernicke encephalopathy), pyridoxine (B$_6$), cyanocobalamin (B$_{12}$), folate, and niacin (B$_3$). Large doses (100 mg) of thiamin are given daily for a limited time if deficiency is suspected (see Appendix 22).

Mineral nutriture also is altered in liver disease. Iron stores may be depleted in patients experiencing gastrointestinal bleeding; however, iron supplementation should be avoided by persons with hemochromatosis or hemosiderosis (see Chapter 32). Manganese deposition has been noted to accumulate in brains of patients with cirrhosis leading to impaired motor function and parkinsonism (Butterworth, 2013). Elevated serum copper levels are found in cholestatic liver diseases (i.e., PBC and PSC).

In Wilson's disease, excess copper in various organs causes severe damage. Treatment typically includes administration of oral chelating agents such as D-penicillamine or trientine that release copper from organs where it can be filtered out of the blood and excreted in urine. Zinc acetate can block absorption of copper from food but typically is used with one of the chelating drugs. Dietary copper restriction can be useful during initial therapy. Copper also can be present in water where copper pipes are used. Running tap water for several seconds before using the water can reduce copper concentrations.

Zinc and magnesium levels are low in liver disease related to alcoholism, in part because of diuretic therapy. Calcium, as well as magnesium and zinc, may be malabsorbed with steatorrhea. Therefore the patient should take supplements of these minerals at least at the level of the DRI.

HERBAL SUPPLEMENTS AND LIVER DISEASE

Hepatotoxicity from herbal and dietary supplementation is one of the greatest concerns associated with herbal and dietary supplementation. There are many case reports of different herbal supplements resulting in liver failure. Some of the more commonly known hepatotoxic herbs are included in Box 29-3. However, one recent review lists more than 150 herbal products that have been reported to have caused hepatotoxicity (Teschke et al, 2013). This extensive list emphasizes the gravity of the potential for harm to the liver from herbal products and practitioners should be vigilant in asking patients about supplement usage.

Other dietary products also have been implicated in hepatotoxicity. Among the most common products are some Herbalife products, Hydroxycut, and OxyElite Pro (CDC, 2013; Fong et al, 2010; Jóhannsson et al, 2010; Schoepfer, 2007; Sharma et al, 2010). The most recent event was in 2013 when 56 individuals (43 in Hawaii) taking OxyElite Pro developed acute or fulminant liver failure. Several patients required liver transplantation and at least one patient died (CDC, 2013; Food and Drug Administration [FDA], 2013).

Despite reports of hepatotoxicity with numerous herbal supplements, some herbal supplements have been investigated

---

BOX 29-3 Selected Herbal Supplements Associated with Hepatotoxicity

Baikal skullcap (*Scutellaria*)
Chaparral (*Larrea tridentate*)
Pyrrolizidine alkaloids
Comfrey (*Symphytum*)
Heliotropium
Crotalaria
Germander (*Teucrium chamaedrys*)
Greater celandine (*Chelidonium majus*)
Saw palmetto (*Serrenoa repens*)
Noni juice (*Morinda citrifolia*)
Margosa oil (*Antelaea azadirachta*)
Aloe vera
Black cohosh (*Actea racemosa* or *Actea cimicifuga*)
LipoKinetix (usnic acid)
Astractylis gummifera
Impila (*Callilepis laureola*)
Mistletoe (*Viscum album*)
Valerian (*Valerian officinalis*)
Senna (*Cassia angustifolia*)
Pennyroyal (squawmint oil)
Kava (*Piper methysticum*)
Liatris callilepis
Green tea extract (*Camellia sinensis*)
Cascara sagrada
OxyElite Pro
Chinese herbal medicines
Jin Bu Huan (*Lycopodium serratum*)
Ma Huang (*Ephedra sinica*)
Dai-saiko-to (*Sho-saiko-to*)
Hydroxycut
Herbalife supplements
Ayurvedic herbal products

LipoKinetix (Syntrax Innovations, Inc, Cape Girardeau, MO), OxyElite Pro (USP Labs, LLC, Dallas, TX), Hydroxycut (Iovate Health Sciences USA, Inc, Blasdell, NY), Herbalife supplements (Herbalife International of America, Inc, Los Angeles, CA).
Reprinted with permission from: Corey RL, Rakela J: Complementary and alternative medicine: risks and special considerations in pre- and post-transplant patients, *Nutr Clin Pract* 29:322, 2014.

---

for benefits on liver disease. *S*-adenosyl-*L*-methionine (SAMe) is a complementary medicine product sometimes suggested for use with liver disease. It is purported to act as a methyl donor for methylation reactions and participates in glutathione (an antioxidant) synthesis. A Cochrane review did not find beneficial effects for SAMe in patients with alcoholic liver disease (Rambaldi and Gluud, 2006). Betaine has been evaluated for treatment of NASH. Although there is theoretical promise, there is a lack of strong evidence for benefit (Abdelmalek et al, 2009; Mukherjee, 2011).

Milk thistle appears to be the most popular and extensively studied herbal supplement for liver disease. The active component in milk thistle is silymarin with silybin (constituting 50% to 70% of silymarin) believed to have the most biologic activity. Milk thistle is proposed to reduce free radical production and lipid peroxidation associated with hepatotoxicity as well as block the binding of toxins to hepatocytes (Abenavoli, 2010). Milk thistle has been evaluated for viral hepatitis, alcoholic liver disease, and toxin-induced liver disease; its use also is being explored for treatment of NAFLD. Despite its popularity and widespread use, a clear consensus is lacking as to a beneficial effect of milk thistle on liver disease. However, data are not sufficient to suggest that it is unsafe or toxic for patients with liver disease.

LIVER RESECTION AND TRANSPLANTATION

As with any major surgery, protein and energy needs increase after liver resection. Needs also are increased for liver cell regeneration. Enteral tube feeding (EN) can be beneficial by providing portal hepatotropic factors necessary for liver cell proliferation. Optimal nutrition is most important for patients with poor nutrition status before hepatectomy (e.g., patients with hepatocellular carcinoma or cholangiocarcinoma).

Liver transplantation has become an established treatment for ESLD. Malnutrition is common in liver transplant candidates. Dietary intake often can be enhanced if patients eat small, frequent, nutrient-dense meals, and oral nutritional supplements also may be well tolerated. EN is indicated when oral intake is inadequate or contraindicated. Varices are not an absolute contraindication for placement of a feeding tube. Because PN can affect liver function adversely, EN is preferred. PN is reserved for patients without adequate gut function (see Chapter 13).

In the acute posttransplant phase, nutrient needs are increased to promote healing, deter infection, provide energy for recovery, and replenish depleted body stores. Nitrogen requirements are elevated in the acute posttransplant phase and can be met with early postoperative tube feeding. Early postoperative tube feeding has been associated with reduced infections in liver transplant recipients (Hasse et al, 1995; Ikegami et al, 2012). Administration of probiotics and fiber with tube feeding may reduce postoperative infection rate better than tube feeding or fiber alone (Rayes et al, 2005).

Multiple medications used after transplant have nutritional side effects such as anorexia, gastrointestinal upset, hypercatabolism, diarrhea, hyperglycemia, hyperlipidemia, sodium retention, hypertension, hyperkalemia, and hypercalciuria. Therefore dietary modification is based on the specific side effects of drug therapy (see Table 29-5). During the posttransplant phase, nutrient requirements are adjusted to prevent or treat problems of obesity, hyperlipidemia, hypertension, diabetes mellitus, and osteopenia. Table 29-6 summarizes nutrient needs after liver transplantation.

PHYSIOLOGY AND FUNCTIONS OF THE GALLBLADDER

The gallbladder lies on the undersurface of the right lobe of the liver (see Figure 29-6). The main function of the gallbladder is to concentrate, store, and excrete bile, which is produced by the liver. During the concentration process, water and electrolytes are resorbed by the gallbladder mucosa. Bile is composed of bile salts and excretory endogenous and exogenous compounds. Other components include fatty acids, cholesterol, phospholipids, bilirubin, protein and other compounds. Bile salts are made by liver cells from cholesterol and are essential for the digestion and absorption of fats, fat-soluble vitamins, and some minerals (see Chapter 1). Bilirubin, the main bile pigment, is derived from the release of hemoglobin from red blood cell destruction. It is transported to the liver, where it is conjugated and excreted via bile.

The primary transporter responsible for bile salt secretion is the bile salt export pump (BSEP). Overall, bile salts play a key role in a wide range of physiologic and pathophysiologic processes (Lam et al, 2010). Excreted into the small intestine via bile, bile salts are later resorbed into the portal system (enterohepatic circulation). This is the primary excretory pathway for the minerals copper and manganese.

TABLE 29-5	Drugs Commonly Used After Liver Transplantation	
Immunosuppressant Drug	**Possible Nutritional Side Effects**	**Proposed Nutrition Therapy**
Azathioprine	Macrocytic anemia	Give folate supplements.
	Mouth sores	Adjust food and meals as needed; monitor intake.
	Nausea, vomiting, diarrhea, anorexia, sore throat, stomach pain, decreased taste acuity	
Antithymocyte globulin (ATG), lymphocyte immune globulin	Nausea, vomiting	Adjust food and meals as needed; monitor intake.
Cyclosporine	Sodium retention	Decrease sodium intake
	Hyperkalemia	Decrease potassium intake.
	Hyperlipidemia	Limit fat and simple carbohydrate intake.
	Hyperglycemia	Decrease simple carbohydrate intake.
	Decreased serum magnesium level	Increase magnesium intake; give supplements.
	Hypertension	Limit sodium intake.
	Nausea, vomiting	Adjust food and meals as needed; monitor intake.
Glucocorticoids	Sodium retention	Decrease sodium intake.
	Hyperglycemia	Decrease simple carbohydrate intake.
	Hyperlipidemia	Limit fat and simple carbohydrate intake.
	False hunger	Avoid overeating.
	Protein wasting with high doses	Increase protein intake.
	Decreased absorption of calcium and phosphorus	Increase calcium and phosphorus intake; give supplements as needed.
Mycophenolate mofetil, mycophenolic acid	Nausea, vomiting, diarrhea	Adjust food and meals as needed; monitor intake.
Sirolimus	Possible GI symptoms	Adjust food and meals as needed; monitor intake.
	Hyperlipidemia	Limit fat and simple carbohydrate intake.
Tacrolimus	Hyperglycemia	Decrease simple carbohydrate intake.
	Hyperkalemia	Decrease potassium intake.
	Nausea, vomiting	Adjust food and meals as needed; monitor intake.

GI, Gastrointestinal.

TABLE 29-6	**General Nutrient Requirements for Liver Transplant Patients**		
	Pretransplantation	**Immediate Posttransplantation (First 2 Posttransplant Months)**	**Long-Term Posttransplantation**
Protein	Dependent on nutrition status and medical condition but usually 1-1.5 g/kg	Dependent on nutrition status, medical condition, and dialysis requirement but usually 1.2-1.75 g/kg	Maintenance – about 1 g/kg
Calories	Dependent on nutrition status and losses; usually 20%-50% above basal	Dependent on nutrition status and metabolic stress but usually 20%-30% above basal	Dependent on activity and weight goals; usually 20% above basal for sedentary activity if at goal weight
Fat	As needed	Approximately 30% of calories	Moderate fat (30% of calories)
Carbohydrate	Reduced carbohydrate if diabetes or obesity present	Reduced carbohydrate if diabetes present	Reduced simple carbohydrate, especially if diabetes or obesity present
Sodium	2 g/day	2 g/day (as indicated)	2 g/day (as indicated)
Fluid	Restrict to 1000-1500 mL/day (if hyponatremic)	As needed	As needed
Calcium	800-1200 mg/day	800-1200 mg/day	1200-1500 mg/day
Vitamins	Multivitamin/mineral supplementation to DRI levels; additional water- and fat-soluble vitamins as indicated	Multivitamin/mineral supplementation to DRI levels; additional water- and fat-soluble vitamins as indicated	Multivitamin/mineral supplementation to DRI levels

DRI, Dietary reference intake.
*Use estimated dry or ideal weight.

Bile contains immunoglobulins that support the integrity of the intestinal mucosa. Fibroblast growth factor receptor (FGFR4) controls bile acid metabolism and protects the liver from fibrosis; FGFR1 and FGFR2 assist in regeneration of the liver (Böhm et al, 2010). Molecular crosstalk between bile acid–activated nuclear receptors and proinflammatory nuclear mediators provides new understanding of inflammation-induced cholestasis (Kosters and Karpen, 2010; Lam et al, 2010).

Bile is removed by the liver via bile canaliculi that drain into intrahepatic bile ducts. The ducts lead to the left and right hepatic ducts, which leave the liver and join to become the common hepatic duct. The bile is directed to the gallbladder via the cystic duct for concentration and storage. The cystic duct joins the common hepatic duct to form the common bile duct. The bile duct then joins the pancreatic duct, which carries digestive enzymes.

During the course of digestion, food reaches the duodenum, causing the release of intestinal hormones such as cholecystokinin (CCK) and secretin. This stimulates the gallbladder and pancreas and causes the sphincter of Oddi to relax, allowing pancreatic juice and bile to flow into the duodenum at the ampulla of Vater to assist in fat digestion. For this reason diseases of the gallbladder, liver, and pancreas often are interrelated.

DISEASES OF THE GALLBLADDER

Disorders of the biliary tract affect millions of people each year, causing significant suffering and even death by precipitating pancreatitis and sepsis. A diverse spectrum of disease affects the biliary system, often presenting with similar clinical signs and symptoms. Treatment may involve diet, medication, or surgery.

Cholestasis
Pathophysiology and Medical Management

Cholestasis is a condition in which little or no bile is secreted or the flow of bile into the digestive tract is obstructed. This can occur in patients without oral or enteral feeding for a prolonged period, such as those requiring PN, and can predispose to acalculous cholecystitis. BSEP deficiency results in several different genetic forms of cholestasis and acquired forms of cholestasis such as drug-induced cholestasis and intrahepatic cholestasis of pregnancy (Lam et al, 2010). Prevention of cholestasis requires stimulation of biliary motility and secretions by at least minimum enteral feedings. If this is not possible, drug therapy is used.

Cholelithiasis
Pathophysiology

The formation of gallstones (calculi) is cholelithiasis. Virtually all gallstones form within the gallbladder. Gallstone disease affects millions of Americans each year and causes significant morbidity. In most cases gallstones are asymptomatic. Gallstones that pass from the gallbladder into the common bile duct

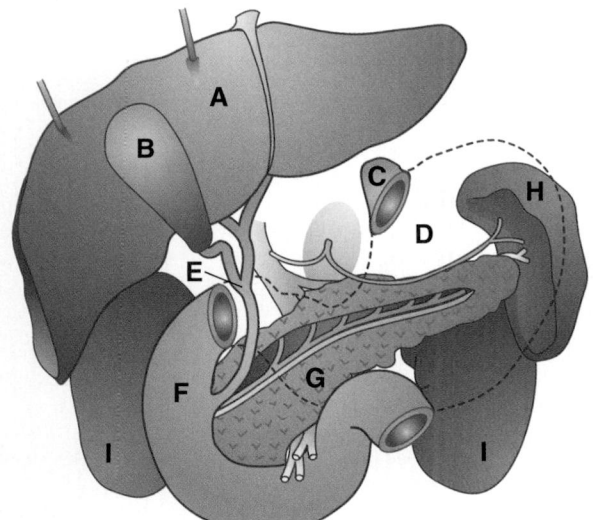

FIGURE 29-6 Schematic drawing showing relationship of organs of the upper abdomen. **A,** Liver (retracted upward); **B,** gallbladder; **C,** esophageal opening of stomach; **D,** stomach *(shown in dotted outline);* **E,** common bile duct; **F,** duodenum; **G,** pancreas and pancreatic duct; **H,** spleen; **I,** kidneys. (Courtesy Cleveland Clinic, Cleveland, Ohio, 2002.)

may remain there indefinitely without causing symptoms, or they may pass into the duodenum with or without symptoms.

Choledocholithiasis develops when stones slip into the bile ducts, producing obstruction, pain, and cramps. If passage of bile into the duodenum is interrupted, cholecystitis can develop. In the absence of bile in the intestine, lipid absorption is impaired, and without bile pigments, stools become light in color (acholic). If uncorrected, bile backup can result in jaundice and liver damage (secondary biliary cirrhosis). Obstruction of the distal common bile duct can lead to pancreatitis if the pancreatic duct is blocked.

Most gallstones are unpigmented cholesterol stones composed primarily of cholesterol, bilirubin, and calcium salts. Bacteria also play a role in gallstone formation. Low-grade chronic infections produce changes in the gallbladder mucosa, which affect its absorptive capabilities. Excess water or bile acid may be absorbed as a result. Cholesterol may then precipitate out and cause gallstones (Völzke et al, 2005).

High dietary fat intake over a prolonged period may predispose a person to gallstone formation because of the constant stimulus to produce more cholesterol for bile synthesis required in fat digestion. Rapid weight loss (as with jejunoileal and gastric bypass and fasting or severe calorie restriction) is associated with a high incidence of biliary sludge and gallstone formation. Indeed, cholelithiasis and fatty liver disease share risk factors, including central obesity, insulin resistance, and diabetes (Koller et al, 2012; Weikert et al, 2010).

Risk factors for cholesterol stone formation include female gender, pregnancy, older age, family history, obesity and truncal body fat distribution, diabetes mellitus, inflammatory bowel disease, and drugs (lipid-lowering medications, oral contraceptives, and estrogens). Certain ethnic groups are at greater risk of stone formation, including Pima Indians, Scandinavians, and Mexican Americans. In addition, approximately 30% of individuals with cirrhosis have gallstones (Acalovschi, 2014).

Pigmented stones typically consist of bilirubin polymers or calcium salts. They are associated with chronic hemolysis. Risk factors associated with these stones are age, sickle cell anemia and thalassemia, biliary tract infection, cirrhosis, alcoholism, and long-term PN.

Medical and Surgical Management

Cholecystectomy is surgical removal of the gallbladder, especially if the stones are numerous, large, or calcified. The cholecystectomy may be performed as a traditional open laparotomy or as a less invasive laparoscopic procedure.

Chemical dissolution with the administration of bile salts, chenodeoxycholic acid, and ursodeoxycholic acid (litholytic therapy) or dissolution by extracorporeal shockwave lithotripsy may also be used less often than surgical techniques. Patients with gallstones that have migrated into the bile ducts may be candidates for endoscopic retrograde cholangiopancreatography techniques.

Medical Nutrition Therapy

Gallstones are more prevalent in low-fiber, high-fat, westernized diets. Consumption of large amounts of animal protein and animal fat, especially saturated fat, and a lack of dietary fiber, promote gallstone development.

There also may be some benefit in replacing simple sugars and refined starches with high-fiber carbohydrates. Individuals consuming refined carbohydrates have a 60% greater risk for

developing gallstones, compared with those who consumed the most fiber, in particular insoluble fiber (Mendez-Sanchez et al, 2007). Thus plant-based diets may reduce the risk of cholelithiasis. Vegetarian diets are high in fiber and low in fat, consisting primarily of unsaturated fat. Vitamin C, which is generally high in vegetarian diets, affects the rate-limiting step in the catabolism of cholesterol to bile acids and inversely is related to the risk of gallstones in women.

Weight cycling (repeatedly losing and regaining weight), fasting, and very-low-calorie diets increase the likelihood of cholelithiasis. Along with weight reduction, some evidence indicates that physical activity reduces the risk of cholecystitis. In cholecystitis, MNT includes a high-fiber, low-fat, plant-based diet to prevent gallbladder contractions. Data are conflicting as to whether intravenous lipids stimulate gallbladder contraction.

After surgical removal of the gallbladder, oral feedings can be advanced to a regular diet as tolerated. In the absence of the gallbladder, bile is secreted directly by the liver into the intestine. The biliary tract dilates, forming a "simulated pouch" over time to allow bile to be held in a manner similar to the original gallbladder.

Cholecystitis
Pathophysiology

Inflammation of the gallbladder is known as cholecystitis, and it may be chronic or acute. It usually is caused by gallstones obstructing the bile ducts (calculous cholecystitis), leading to the backup of bile. Bilirubin, the main bile pigment, gives bile its greenish color. When biliary tract obstruction prevents bile from reaching the intestine, it backs up and returns to the circulation. Bilirubin has an affinity for elastic tissues (such as the eye and the skin); therefore when it overflows into the general circulation, it causes the yellow skin pigmentation and eye discoloration typical of jaundice.

Acute cholecystitis without stones (acalculous cholecystitis) may occur in critically ill patients or when the gallbladder and its bile are stagnant. Impaired gallbladder emptying in chronic acalculous cholecystitis appears to be due to diminished spontaneous contractile activity and decreased contractile responsiveness to cholecystokinin (CCK). The walls of the gallbladder become inflamed and distended, and infection can occur. During such episodes, the patient experiences upper-quadrant abdominal pain accompanied by nausea, vomiting, and flatulence.

Chronic cholecystitis is longstanding inflammation of the gallbladder. It is caused by repeated, mild attacks of acute cholecystitis. This leads to thickening of the walls of the gallbladder. The gallbladder begins to shrink and eventually loses the ability to perform its function: concentrating and storing bile. Eating foods that are high in fat may aggravate the symptoms of cholecystitis, because bile is needed to digest such foods. Chronic cholecystitis occurs more often in women than in men, and the incidence increases after the age of 40. Risk factors include the presence of gallstones and a history of acute cholecystitis.

Surgical Management

Acute cholecystitis requires surgical intervention unless medically contraindicated. Without surgery, the condition may either subside or progress to gangrene.

Medical Nutrition Therapy

Acute Cholecystitis In an acute attack, oral feedings are discontinued. PN may be indicated if the patient is malnourished and it is anticipated that he or she will not be taking anything orally for a prolonged period. When feedings are resumed, a low-fat diet is recommended to decrease gallbladder stimulation. A hydrolyzed low-fat formula or an oral low-fat diet consisting of 30 to 45 g of fat per day can be given. Table 29-7 shows a fat-restricted diet.

After cholecystectomy, patients may experience symptoms of gastritis secondary to duodenogastric reflux of bile acids. The reflux also may be responsible for symptoms in this postcholecystectomy syndrome. At present, there are no well-established pharmacologic approaches in the management of postcholecystectomy gastritis. The symptoms are not caused, but exacerbated, by the cholecystectomy. The addition of soluble fiber to the diet may act as a sequestering agent and bind the bile in the stomach between meals to avoid gastritis.

TABLE 29-7 Fat-Restricted Diet*

Food Allowed	Food Excluded
Beverages	
Skim milk or buttermilk made with skim milk; coffee, tea, Postum, fruit juice, soft drinks, cocoa made with cocoa powder and skim milk	Whole milk, buttermilk made with whole milk, chocolate milk, cream in excess of amounts allowed under fats
Bread and Cereal Products	
Plain, nonfat cereals, spaghetti, noodles, rice, macaroni; plain whole grain or enriched breads, air-popped popcorn, bagels, English muffins	Biscuits, breads, egg or cheese bread, sweet rolls made with fat; pancakes, doughnuts, waffles, fritters, popcorn prepared with fat; muffins, natural cereals and breads to which extra fat is added
Cheese	
Fat-free or low-fat cottage cheese, ¼ c to be used as substitute for 1 oz of cheese, or low-fat cheeses containing less than 5% butterfat	Whole-milk cheeses
Desserts	
Sherbet made with skim milk; nonfat frozen yogurt; nonfat frozen nondairy desserts; fruit ice; sorbet; gelatin; rice, bread, cornstarch, tapioca, or pudding made with skim milk; fruit whips with gelatin, sugar, and egg white; fruit; angel food cake; graham crackers; vanilla wafers; meringues	Cake, pie, pastry, ice cream, or any dessert containing shortening, chocolate, or fats of any kind, unless especially prepared using part of fat allowance
Eggs	
Three per week prepared only with fat from fat allowance; egg whites as desired; low-fat egg substitutes	More than one/day unless substituted for part of the meat allowed
Fats	
Choose up to the limit allowed among the following (1 serving in the amount listed equals 1 fat choice):	Any in excess of amount prescribed on diet; all others
1 tsp butter or margarine	
1 Tbsp reduced-fat margarine	
1 tsp shortening or oil	
1 tsp mayonnaise	
2 tsp Italian or French dressing	
1 Tbsp reduced-fat salad dressing	
1 strip crisp bacon	
⅛ avocado (4-inch diameter)	
2 Tbsp light cream	
1 Tbsp heavy cream	
6 small nuts	
5 small olives	
Fruits	
As desired	Avocado in excess of amount allowed on fat list
Lean Meat, Fish, Poultry, and Meat Substitutes	
Choose up to the limit allowed among the following: poultry without skin, fish, veal (all cuts), liver, lean beef, pork, and lamb, all with visible fat removed—1 oz cooked weight equals 1 equivalent; ¼ c water packed tuna or salmon equals 1 equivalent; tofu or tempeh—3 oz equals 1 equivalent	Fried or fatty meats, sausage, scrapple, frankfurters, poultry skins, stewing hens, spareribs, salt pork, beef unless lean, duck, goose, ham hocks, pig's feet, luncheon meats (unless reduced fat), gravies unless fat-free, tuna and salmon packed in oil, peanut butter
Milk	
Skim, buttermilk, or yogurt made from skim milk	Whole, 2%, 1%, chocolate, buttermilk made with whole milk
Seasonings	
As desired	None

TABLE 29-7 Fat-Restricted Diet—cont'd

Food Allowed	Food Excluded
Soups	
Bouillon, clear broth, fat-free vegetable soup, cream soup made with skim milk, packaged dehydrated soups	All others
Sweets	
Jelly, jam, marmalade, honey, syrup, molasses, sugar, hard sugar candies, fondant, gumdrops, jelly beans, marshmallows, cocoa powder, fat-free chocolate sauce, red and black licorice	Any candy made with chocolate, nuts, butter, cream, or fat of any kind
Vegetables	
All plainly prepared vegetables	Potato chips; buttered, au gratin, creamed, or fried potatoes and other vegetables unless made with allowed fat; casseroles or frozen vegetables in butter sauce

Daily Food Allowances for 40-g–Fat Diet

Food	Amount	Approximate Fat Content (g)
Skim milk	2 c or more	0
Lean meat, fish, poultry	6 oz or 6 equivalents	18
Whole egg or egg yolks	3 per week	2
Vegetables	3 servings or more, at least 1 or more dark green or deep yellow	0
Fruits	3 or more servings, at least 1 citrus	0
Breads, cereals	As desired, fat-free	0
Fat exchanges*	4-5 exchanges daily	20-25
Desserts and sweets	As desired from permitted list	0
	Total Fat	38-43

*Fat content can be reduced further by reducing the fat exchanges. 1 Fat exchange = 5 g of fat.

Chronic Cholecystitis. Patients with chronic conditions may require a long-term, low-fat diet that contains 25% to 30% of total kilocalories as fat (see Table 29-7). Stricter limitation is undesirable because fat in the intestine is important for some stimulation and drainage of the biliary tract. The degree of food intolerance varies widely among persons with gallbladder disorders; many complain of foods that cause flatulence and bloating. For this reason it is best to determine with the patient which foods should be eliminated (see Chapter 28 for a discussion of potential gas-forming foods). Administration of water-soluble forms of fat-soluble vitamins may be of benefit in patients with chronic gallbladder conditions or in those in whom fat malabsorption is suspected.

Cholangitis

Pathophysiology and Medical Management

Inflammation of the bile ducts is known as cholangitis. Patients with acute cholangitis need resuscitation with fluids and broad-spectrum antibiotics. If the patient does not improve with conservative treatment, placement of a percutaneous biliary stent or cholecystectomy may be needed.

Sclerosing cholangitis can result in sepsis and liver failure. Most patients have multiple intrahepatic strictures, which makes surgical intervention difficult, if not impossible. Patients are generally on broad-spectrum antibiotics. Percutaneous ductal dilation may provide short-term bile duct patency in some patients. When sepsis is recurrent, patients may require chronic antibiotic therapy (see Primary Sclerosing Cholangitis).

COMPLEMENTARY AND INTEGRATIVE MEDICINE

Patients often seek complementary and integrative approaches to disease of the gallbladder, including various nutritional supplements, herbal medications, and gallbladder flushes. Vitamin C deficiency has been linked to gallstone formation in animals models (Jenkins, 1978). The data in humans are limited but vitamin C supplementation has been associated with a decreased risk of gallstones in postmenopausal women who consume alcohol (Simon et al, 1998). Vitamin E has been shown to limit gallstone formation in hamsters provided with a high-fat diet (Christensen et al, 1953).

Choleretic herbs such as milk thistle, dandelion root, artichoke, turmeric, greater celandine, and Oregon grape stimulate bile flow and reduce the amount of cholesterol in bile. However, no trials in humans show benefit. Some integrative practitioners may prescribe gallbladder flushes that typically include olive oil, herbs, and fruit juice. The belief is that the monosaturated fat in olive oil may stimulate gallbladder contraction and improve bile flow. However, this has not been validated clinically and actually may trigger attacks of gallbladder pain.

PHYSIOLOGY AND FUNCTIONS OF THE EXOCRINE PANCREAS

The pancreas is an elongated, flattened gland that lies in the upper abdomen behind the stomach. The head of the pancreas is in the right upper quadrant below the liver within the curvature of the duodenum, and the tapering tail slants upward to the hilum of the spleen (see Figure 29-6). This glandular organ has an endocrine and exocrine function. Pancreatic cells manufacture glucagon, insulin, and somatostatin for absorption into the bloodstream (endocrine function) for regulation of glucose homeostasis (see Chapter 30). Other cells secrete enzymes and other substances directly into the intestinal lumen, where they aid in digesting proteins, fats, and carbohydrates (exocrine function).

In most people the pancreatic duct, which carries the exocrine pancreatic secretions, merges with the common bile duct into a unified opening through which bile and pancreatic juices drain into the duodenum at the ampulla of Vater. Many factors regulate exocrine secretion from the pancreas. Neural and hormonal responses play a role, with the presence and composition of ingested foods being a large contributor. The two primary hormonal stimuli for pancreatic secretion are secretin and CCK (see Chapter 1).

Factors that influence pancreatic secretions during a meal can be divided into three phases: (1) the cephalic phase, mediated through the vagus nerve and initiated by the sight, smell, taste, and anticipation of food that leads to the secretion of bicarbonate and pancreatic enzymes; (2) gastric distention with food initiates the gastric phase of pancreatic secretion, which stimulates enzyme secretion; and (3) the intestinal phase, mediated by the release of CCK, with the most potent effect.

DISEASES OF THE EXOCRINE PANCREAS

Pancreatitis

Pathophysiology and Medical Management

Pancreatitis is an inflammation of the pancreas and is characterized by edema, cellular exudate, and fat necrosis. The disease can range from mild and self-limiting to severe, with autodigestion, necrosis, and hemorrhage of pancreatic tissue. Ranson and colleagues (1974) identified 11 signs that could be measured during the first 48 hours of admission and that have prognostic significance (see Box 29-4). By using these observations, one can determine the likely outcome of hospitalization. Surgical intervention may be necessary. Pancreatitis is classified as either acute or chronic, the latter with pancreatic destruction so extensive that exocrine and endocrine function are severely diminished, and maldigestion and diabetes may result.

The symptoms of pancreatitis can range from continuous or intermittent pain of varying intensity to severe upper abdominal pain, which may radiate to the back. Symptoms may worsen with the ingestion of food. Clinical presentation also may include nausea, vomiting, abdominal distention, and steatorrhea. Severe cases are complicated by hypotension, oliguria, and dyspnea. There is extensive destruction of pancreatic tissue with subsequent fibrosis, enzyme production is diminished, and serum amylase and lipase may appear normal. However, absence of enzymes to aid in the digestion of food leads to steatorrhea and malabsorption. Table 29-8 describes several tests used to determine the extent of pancreatic destruction.

Medical Nutrition Therapy

Alcohol use, smoking, body weight, diet, genetic factors, and medications affect the risk of developing pancreatitis. Thus diet modification has an important role after diagnosis. Dietary recommendations differ, depending on whether the condition is acute or chronic. Obesity appears to be a risk factor for the development of pancreatitis and for increased severity (Martinez J et al, 2004).

Depressed serum calcium levels are common. Hypoalbuminemia occurs, with subsequent third spacing of fluid. The calcium, which is bound to albumin, is thus affected and may appear artificially low. Another occurrence is "soap" formation in the gut by calcium and fatty acids, created by the fat necrosis that results in less calcium absorption. Checking an ionized calcium level is a method of determining available calcium.

Acute Pancreatitis. Pain associated with acute pancreatitis (AP) is partially related to the secretory mechanisms of pancreatic enzymes and bile. Therefore nutrition therapy is adjusted to provide minimum stimulation of these systems (see *Pathophysiology and Care Management Algorithm: Pancreatitis*). The basis for nutrition therapy is to put the pancreas "at rest." In less severe attacks, a clear liquid diet with negligible fat may be given once abdominal pain is decreasing and inflammatory markers are improving, generally within a few days (International Association of Pancreatology [IAP], American Pancreatic Association [APA], 2013). Several recent randomized controlled trials demonstrated that starting these patients on a low-fat diet is as safe as a clear liquid diet, with varying effect on length of hospital stay (Jacobson BC et al, 2007; Moraes et al, 2010; Rajkumar et al, 2013; Sathiaraj et al, 2008; Teich N et al, 2010). The patient should be monitored for any symptoms of pain, nausea, or vomiting. The diet should be progressed as tolerated to easily digested foods with a low fat content with more fat added as tolerated. Foods may be better tolerated if they are divided into six small meals (see Table 29-7).

BOX 29-4 Ranson's Criteria to Classify the Severity of Pancreatitis

At Admission or Diagnosis

Age >55 yr
White blood cell count >16,000 m³
Blood glucose level >200 mg/100 mL
Lactic dehydrogenase >350 units/L
Aspartate transaminase >250 units/L

During the Initial 48 Hours

Hematocrit decrease of >10%
Blood urea nitrogen increase of >5 mg/dL
Arterial PO_2 <60 mm Hg
Base deficit >4 mEq/L
Fluid sequestration >6000 mL
Serum calcium level <8 mg/mL

Modified from Ranson JH et al: Prognostic signs and the role of operative management in acute pancreatitis, *Surg Gynecol Obstet* 139:69, 1974.

TABLE 29-8 Some Tests of Pancreatic Function

Test	Significance
Secretin stimulation test	Measures pancreatic secretion, particularly bicarbonate, in response to secretin stimulation
Glucose tolerance test	Assesses endocrine function of the pancreas by measuring insulin response to a glucose load
72-hr stool fat test	Assesses exocrine function of the pancreas by measuring fat absorption that reflects pancreatic lipase secretion
Fecal elastase	Enzyme most commonly used to determine pancreatic function; indirect test. Levels >200 mcg/g are considered normal; concentration <15 mcg/g of feces consistent with pancreatic exocrine insufficiency

PATHOPHYSIOLOGY AND CARE MANAGEMENT ALGORITHM

Pancreatitis

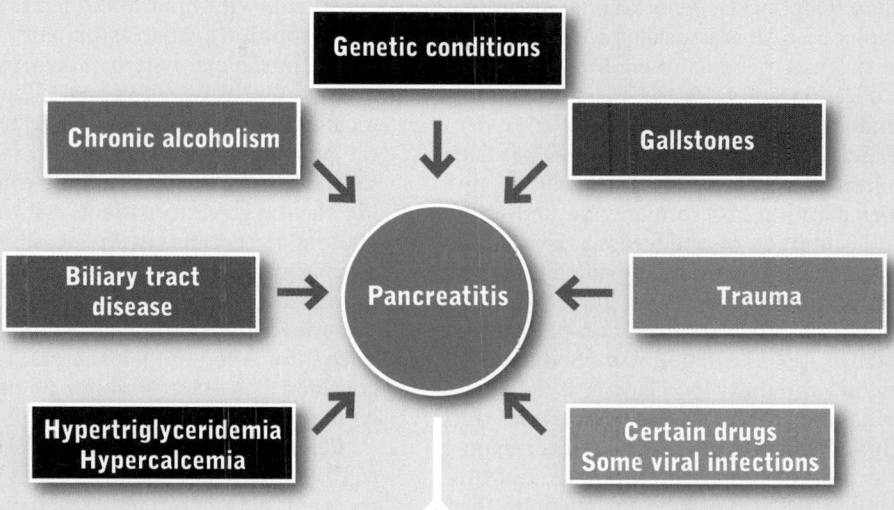

ETIOLOGY

- Genetic conditions
- Chronic alcoholism
- Gallstones
- Biliary tract disease
- Pancreatitis
- Trauma
- Hypertriglyceridemia Hypercalcemia
- Certain drugs Some viral infections

PATHOPHYSIOLOGY

Diagnosis

  I: Apply Ranson's criteria
 II: Tests of pancreatic function
    Secretin stimulation test
    Glucose tolerance test
    72-hour stool fat test
    Fecal elastase

Clinical Findings

Symptoms:
- Abdominal pain and distention
- Nausea
- Vomiting
- Steatorrhea

In severe form:
- Hypotension
- Oliguria
- Dyspnea

MANAGEMENT

Medical Management

Acute:
- Withhold oral feeding
- Give IV fluids
- Administer H_2-receptor antagonists, somatostatin

Chronic:
- Manage intestinal pH with:
  - Antacids
  - H_2-receptor antagonists
  - Proton pump inhibitors
- Administer insulin for glucose intolerance

Nutrition Management

Acute:
- Withhold oral and enteral feeding
- Support with IV fluids
- If oral nutrition cannot be initiated in 5 to 7 days, start tube feeding
- Once oral nutrition is started, provide
  - Easily digestible foods
  - Low-fat diet
  - 6 small meals
  - Adequate protein intake
  - Increased calories

Chronic:
- Provide oral diet as in acute phase
- TF can be used when oral diet is inadequate or as a treatment to reduce pain
- Supplement pancreatic enzymes
- Supplement fat-soluble vitamins and vitamin B_{12}

Severe acute pancreatitis (SAP) results in a hypermetabolic, catabolic state with immediate metabolic alterations in the pancreas and also in remote organs. Metabolic demands are similar to those of sepsis. Amino acids are released from muscle and used for gluconeogenesis. These patients often exhibit signs of stress-induced malnutrition such as decreased serum levels of albumin, transferrin, and lymphocytes reflecting the inflammatory response (see Chapter 3). SAP is associated with significant morbidity and mortality. These patients often develop complications such as fluid collections, pseudocysts, pancreatic necrosis, and infection or multisystem organ failure.

The optimal route and timing of nutrition in SAP has been the subject of much controversy. PN and EN are equally effective in terms of days to normalization of serum amylase and serum albumin levels, days to resumption of oral feeding, days to clear nosocomial infections, and the clinical outcome in patients with mild to moderate pancreatitis (Petrov et al, 2009; Wu et al, 2014). The favorable effect of either EN or PN on patient outcome may be enhanced by supplementation with modulators of inflammation and systemic immunity (McClave et al, 2006) (see Chapter 3). However, failure to use the gastrointestinal tract (GIT) in patients with SAP may exacerbate the stress response and disease severity, leading to more complications and prolonged hospitalization; thus EN is preferred for nutrition therapy (Al-Omran et al, 2010; McClave, 2013; Mirtallo et al, 2012). Some data support the use of early EN in acute pancreatitis. In a meta-analysis of observational data from individuals with acute pancreatitis, starting EN within 24 hours after hospital admission, compared with after 24 hours, was associated with a reduction in complications (Bakker et al, 2014).

Nasogastric EN has been shown to be efficacious in SAP (Nally et al, 2014). However, to minimize pancreatic stimulation it is best to place jejunal feeding tubes endoscopically as far down the intestine as possible, generally more than 40 cm past the ligament of Treitz (O'Keefe et al, 2001).

EN results in a substantial cost savings with fewer septic complications and overall reduction of morbidity and mortality (Petrov et al, 2008; Sun et al, 2013). The location of the feeding and the composition of the formula is thought to determine the degree of pancreatic stimulation. Infusion into the jejunum eliminates the cephalic and gastric phases of exocrine pancreatic stimulation. The use of jejunal feedings may be better tolerated and allow for an increase in the amount of nutrition that is delivered in the face of AP. However, not any controlled trial has clearly demonstrated a significant improvement of feeding tolerance, mortality, or length of ICU stay with the use of jejunal feeding compared with gastric feedings (Zhang et al, 2013). Because the placement of a nasogastric feeding tube is easier than a jejunal tube, it is reasonable to consider gastric feedings for AP and reserve jejunal feedings for those who are intolerant to gastric feeding (Petrov, 2014). For those patients with severe AP complicated by organ failure, pancreatic necrosis, or fluid collections, nasojejunal feeding is the preferred method of delivery (Seminerio et al, 2014) to minimize pancreatic stimulation (see Chapter 13 for jejunal feeding details).

Although various formulations have been used in pancreatitis, no studies have determined the relative merits of standard, partially digested, elemental, or "immune-enhanced" formulations. Polymeric formulas infused at various sections of the gut stimulate the pancreas more than elemental and hydrolyzed formulas. Peptide-based formula can be used safely and standard formulas can be tried if the patient is tolerant (Mirtallo et al, 2012). Close observation for patient tolerance is important. Tolerance may be enhanced with the use of supplemental pancreatic enzymes during enteral feeding (Berry, 2014). These can be provided by mouth, mixed with water and delivered via the feeding tube, or added directly to the enteral formula. When the patient is allowed to eat, supplemental pancreatic enzymes may also be required to treat steatorrhea. In severe, prolonged cases, PN may be necessary.

Patients with mild to moderate stress can tolerate dextrose-based solutions, whereas patients with more severe stress require a mixed fuel system of dextrose and lipid to avoid complications of glucose intolerance. Lipid emulsion should not be included in a PN regimen if hypertriglyceridemia is the cause of the pancreatitis (Patel et al, 2014). A serum triglyceride level should be obtained before lipid-containing PN is initiated. Lipids may be given to patients with triglyceride values less than 400 mg/dL. Because of the possibility of pancreatic endocrine abnormalities and a relative insulin resistance, close glucose monitoring also is warranted. H_2-receptor antagonists may be prescribed to decrease hydrochloric acid production, which reduce stimulation of the pancreas. The hormone somatostatin is considered the best inhibitor of pancreatic secretion and may be used in conjunction with PN.

Chronic Pancreatitis. In contrast to AP, chronic pancreatitis (CP) evolves insidiously over many years. CP is characterized by recurrent attacks of epigastric pain of long duration that may radiate into the back. The pain can be precipitated by meals. Associated nausea, vomiting, or diarrhea make it difficult to maintain adequate nutrition status (Verhaeqh et al, 2013).

Patients with CP are at increased risk of developing protein-calorie malnutrition because of pancreatic insufficiency and inadequate oral intake. Patients with CP admitted to a tertiary care center usually have malnutrition, increased energy requirements, weight loss, deficits of lean muscle and adipose tissue, visceral protein depletion, impaired immune function, and vitamin deficiencies (Duggan et al, 2014) (see Appendix 21).

The objective of therapy for patients is to prevent further damage to the pancreas, decrease the number of attacks of acute inflammation, alleviate pain, decrease steatorrhea, and correct malnutrition. Dietary intake should be as liberal as possible, but modifications may be necessary to minimize symptoms.

The first goal of MNT is to provide optimal nutrition support, and the second is to decrease pain by minimizing stimulation of the exocrine pancreas. Because CCK stimulates secretion from the exocrine pancreas, one approach is to decrease CCK levels. If postprandial pain is a limiting factor, alternative enteral therapies that minimally stimulate the pancreas are warranted. Nutrition counseling, antioxidants, and pancreatic enzymes may play a role in effective management of CP as well (Afghani et al, 2014).

When pancreatic function is diminished by approximately 90%, enzyme production and secretion are insufficient; maldigestion and malabsorption of protein and fat thus become a problem. Large meals with high-fat foods and alcohol should be avoided.

The patient may present with weight loss despite adequate energy intake and will complain of bulky, greasy stools. This is definitely the case with idiopathic CP associated with a cystic fibrosis gene mutation; therapies directed toward cystic fibrosis may benefit these patients (see Chapter 34). Of these therapies, pancreatic enzyme replacement is mandatory at this time. Pancreatic enzyme replacements are given orally with meals; the dosage should be at least 30,000 units of lipase with each meal. To promote weight gain, the level of fat in the diet should be the maximum a patient can tolerate without increased steatorrhea or pain.

Additional therapies that may be tried to maintain nutrition status and minimize symptoms in patients with maximum enzyme supplementation include a lower-fat diet (40 to 60 g/day) (see Table 29-7) or substitution of some dietary fat with MCT oil to improve fat absorption and weight gain (see Chapter 13). The diet should be low fat, primarily from vegetable-based oils such as olive oil. Trans fatty acids, found in commercially baked goods and other processed foods should be eliminated. Meals should be small and frequent.

Malabsorption of the fat-soluble vitamins may occur in patients with significant steatorrhea. Also, deficiency of pancreatic protease, necessary to cleave vitamin B_{12} from its carrier protein, potentially could lead to vitamin B_{12} deficiency. With appropriate supplemental enzyme therapy, vitamin absorption should be improved; however, the patient should still be monitored periodically for vitamin deficiencies. Water-miscible forms of the fat-soluble vitamins or parenteral administration of vitamin B_{12} may be necessary. Some evidence indicates that increasing intake of antioxidants (found in fruits and vegetables) may help protect against pancreatitis or alleviate symptoms of the condition (Ahmed et al, 2014).

Because pancreatic bicarbonate secretion is frequently defective, medical management also may include maintenance of an optimal intestinal pH to facilitate enzyme activation. Antacids, H_2-receptor antagonists, or proton pump inhibitors that reduce gastric acid secretion may be used to achieve this effect.

In chronic pancreatitis with extensive pancreatic destruction, the insulin-secreting capacity of the pancreas decreases, and glucose intolerance develops. Treatment with insulin and nutrition therapy is then required (see Chapter 30). Management is delicate and should focus on control of symptoms rather than normoglycemia.

Effort should be made to cater to the patient's tolerances and preferences for nutritional management; however, alcohol is prohibited because of the possibility of exacerbating the pancreatic disease. There is evidence that the progressive destruction of the pancreas will be slowed in the alcoholic patient who abstains from alcohol (Nordback et al, 2008).

COMPLEMENTARY AND INTEGRATIVE MEDICINE

The role of complementary and integrative medicine in the treatment of pancreatic disorders remains unclear (Saxena et al, 2014). Certainly, non–FDA-approved proteolytic enzymes can be purchased without a prescription. No data support their use, especially in those individuals with pancreatic disease. Several supplements such as oral calcium, saw palmetto, and other herbs have been suggested for treatment in pancreatitis. However, many of these supplements cause pancreatitis (Kim et al, 2013; Lesser and Hillesheim, 2007; Proniseva et al, 2014; Wargo et al, 2010). Melatonin may have a protective effect and may alter the disease progression (Belyaev et al, 2011; Jaworek et al, 2012; Jin et al, 2013).

PANCREATIC SURGERY

A surgical procedure often used for pancreatic carcinoma is a **pancreaticoduodenectomy (Whipple procedure)**, in which distal segment (antrum) of the stomach, the first and second portions of the duodenum, the head of the pancreas, the common bile duct, and the gallbladder are removed. The basic concept behind the pancreaticoduodenectomy is that the head of the pancreas and the duodenum share the same arterial blood supply (the gastroduodenal artery). These arteries run through the head of the pancreas, so both organs must be removed if the single

blood supply is severed. If only the head of the pancreas were removed, it would compromise blood flow to the duodenum, resulting in tissue necrosis. A cholecystectomy, vagotomy, or a partial gastrectomy also may be performed during the surgery. The pancreatic duct is reanastomosed to the jejunum. Partial or complete pancreatic insufficiency can result, depending on the extent of the pancreatic resection. Most patients who have undergone pancreatic resection are at risk for vitamin and mineral deficiencies and will benefit from vitamin and mineral supplementation. Nutrition care is similar to that for CP.

Pancreatic and Islet Cell Transplantation

There have been significant improvements in the outcomes of patients undergoing pancreatic transplants or pancreatic transplants combined with a kidney transplant. In patients with brittle diabetes who suffer from bouts of hyper- and hypoglycemia, transplantation can restore normal glucose homeostasis and prevent, halt, or reverse the progression of secondary complications (Dunn, 2014; Gruessner et al, 2013).

Pancreatic islet allo-transplantation is a procedure in which islets from the pancreas of a deceased organ donor are purified, processed, and transferred into a recipient. It is performed in certain patients with type 1 diabetes mellitus whose blood glucose levels are extremely labile and difficult to control. **Pancreatic islet autotransplantation** is performed after total pancreatectomy in patients with severe and chronic, or long-lasting, pancreatitis that cannot be managed by other treatments. After pancreatectomy, islets are extracted and purified from the pancreas. The islets then are infused through a catheter into the liver. The goal is to give the body enough healthy islets to make insulin. A person who receives a pancreatic islet cell transplant should follow a meal plan designed for a person with diabetes (see Chapter 30). Immunosuppressive medications are required for allo- but not auto-transplantation; these medications can contribute to weight gain, hypertension, dyslipidemia, and labile blood glucose levels (Chhabra et al, 2014).

CLINICAL CASE STUDY 1

A 62-year-old man is admitted to the hospital from the doctor's office with altered mental status. Past medical history reveals cirrhosis resulting from hepatitis C, esophageal varices, hepatic encephalopathy, and ascites. The patient reports missing his doses of lactulose the two previous days. Muscle wasting is noted in the form of squared shoulders, prominent clavicle, temporal wasting, and thin extremities. He has 3+ edema in his lower extremities and a protuberant abdomen from ascites. His abnormal laboratory values on admission included elevated liver function enzymes and total bilirubin, sodium 127 mEq/L, glucose 68 mg/dL. Nutritional data include height, 177.8 cm; weight, 71.8 kg; ideal body weight, 75 kg; recent body weight range due to fluid fluctuations, 63.6 kg to 90.9 kg.

Nutrition Diagnostic Statements

1. Involuntary weight loss related to cirrhosis as evidenced by loss of dry body weight and physical signs of malnutrition.
2. Altered laboratory values related to cirrhosis as evidenced by hyponatremia and hypoglycemia.

Interventions

Initiate 2 g sodium diet with small, frequent meals.
Initiate commercial beverage twice daily.

Monitoring and Evaluation

Monitor food and beverage intake.
Assess food and nutrition knowledge.
Assess adherence to prescribed diet.

CLINICAL CASE STUDY 2

A 42-year-old female presents with a history of chronic pancreatitis resulting from pancreatic divisum (a congenital abnormality in which there are two pancreatic ducts instead of one). The patient has had multiple hospitalizations for acute pancreatitis. Despite placement of pancreatic stents, she has developed chronic pancreatitis (confirmed by abnormal endoscopic ultrasound and low fecal elastase) and depends on chronic pain medications. She presents for evaluation of total pancreatectomy with islet-autotransplantation. The patient is thin with apparent muscle wasting and reports that she is very fatigued and no longer able to work because of chronic pain. She describes chronic abdominal pain that worsens with eating so that she is only drinking clear soft drinks throughout the day and eating only one small meal per day. She often is constipated, but this can alternate with diarrhea with greasy, foul-smelling loose stools. Her nutritional data include height, 160 cm; weight, 40.5 kg; ideal body weight, 52.3 kg; usual body weight, 54.5 kg (1 year ago). Her 25-hydroxy-vitamin D level is <10 ng/mL.

Nutrition Diagnostic Statements

1. Involuntary weight loss due to pain with eating as evidenced by 31-lb weight loss.
2. Altered nutrition-related laboratory values due to malabsorption as evidenced by vitamin D level <10 ng/mL.

Interventions

Insert feeding tube (for supplemental nocturnal nutrition)
Nutrition-related medication management (start pancreatic enzymes with meals)
Initiate vitamin D supplement.

Monitoring and Evaluation

Monitor total energy intake.
Monitor enteral intake – formula/solution (for tolerance and adequacy).
Monitor vitamin A, D, E levels.

USEFUL WEBSITES

American Liver Foundation
http://www.liverfoundation.org
National Institute on Alcohol Abuse and Alcoholism
http://www.niaaa.nih.gov
Transplant Living
http://www.transplantliving.org/

REFERENCES

Abdelmalek MF, Sanderson SO, Angulo P, et al: Betaine for nonalcoholic fatty liver disease: results of a randomized placebo-controlled trial, *Hepatology* 50:1818, 2009.

Abenavoli L, Capasso R, Milic N, et al: Milk thistle in liver diseases: past, present, future, *Phytother Res* 24:1423, 2010.

Acalovschi M: Gallstones in patients with liver cirrhosis: incidence, etiology, clinical and therapeutical aspects, *World J Gastroenterol* 20:7277, 2014.

Afdhal NH: Diseases of the gallbladder and bile ducts. In Goldman L, et al, editors: *Goldman's Cecil medicine,* ed 24, Philadelphia, 2012, Elsevier Saunders.

Afghani E, Sinha A, Singh VK, et al: An overview of the diagnosis and management of nutrition in chronic pancreatitis, *Nutr Clin Pract* 29:295, 2014.

Ahmed AU, Jens S, Busch OR, et al: Antioxidants for pain in chronic pancreatitis, *Cochrane Database Syst Rev* 8:CD008945, 2014. doi: 10.1002/14651858.CD008945.pub2.

Al-Omran M, Albalawi ZH, Tashkandi MF, et al: Enteral versus parenteral nutrition for acute pancreatitis, *Cochrane Database Syst Rev* CD002837, 2010.

Amodio P, Bemeur C, Butterworth R, et al: The nutritional management of hepatic encephalopathy in patients with cirrhosis: International Society for Hepatic Encephalopathy and Nitrogen Metabolism Consensus, *Hepatology* 58:325, 2013.

Bacon BR: Inherited and metabolic disorders of the liver. In Goldman L, et al, editors: *Goldman's Cecil medicine,* ed 24, Philadelphia, 2012, Elsevier Saunders.

Bakker OJ, van Brunschot S, Farre A, et al: Timing of enteral nutrition in acute pancreatitis: meta-analysis of individuals using a single-arm of randomized trials, *Pancreatology* 14:340, 2014.

Belyaev O, Herzog T, Munding J, et al: Protective role of endogenous melatonin in the early course of human acute pancreatitis, *J Pineal Res* 50:71, 2011.

Berry AJ: Pancreatic enzyme replacement therapy during pancreatic insufficiency, *Nutr Clin Pract* 29:312, 2014.

Böhm F, Speicher T, Hellerbrand C, et al: FGF receptors 1 and 2 control chemically-induced injury and compound detoxification in regenerating livers of mice, *Gastroenterology* 139:1385, 2010.

Butterworth RF: Parkinsonism in cirrhosis: pathogenesis and current therapeutic options, *Metab Brain Dis* 28:261, 2013.

Centers for Disease Control and Prevention (CDC): Notes from the field: acute hepatitis and liver failure following the use of a dietary supplement intended for weight loss or muscle building—May-October 2013, *MMWR Morb Mortal Wkly Rep* 62:817, 2013.

Chalasani N, Younossi Z, Lavine JE, et al: The diagnosis and management of non-alcoholic fatty liver disease: practice guideline by the American Association for the Study of Liver Diseases, American College of Gastroenterology, and the American Gastroenterological Association, *Hepatology* 55:2005, 2012.

Chalasani NP: Alcoholic and nonalcoholic steatohepatitis. In Goldman L, et al, editors: *Goldman's Cecil medicine,* ed 24, Philadelphia, 2012, Elsevier Saunders.

Chen S, Teoh NC, Chitturi S, et al: Coffee and non-alcoholic fatty liver disease: brewing evidence for hepatoprotection? *J Gastroenterol Hepatol* 29:435, 2014.

Chhabra P, Brayman KL: Overcoming barriers in clinical islet transplantation: current limitations and future prospects, *Curr Prob Surg* 51:49, 2014.

Christensen F, Dam H, Prange I: Alimentary production of gallstones in hamsters. II, *Acta Physiol Scand* 27:315, 1953.

Dhanasekaran R, Limaye A, Cabrera R: Hepatocellular carcinoma: current trends in worldwide epidemiology, risk factors, diagnosis, and therapeutics, *Hepat Med* 4:19, 2012.

Duggan SN, Smyth ND, O'Sullivan M, et al: The prevalence of malnutrition and fat-soluble vitamin deficiencies in chronic pancreatitis, *Nutr Clin Pract* 29:348, 2014.

Dunn TB: Life after pancreas transplantation: reversal of diabetic lesions, *Curr Opin Organ Transplant* 19:73, 2014.

Dupont B, Dao T, Joubert C, et al: Randomised clinical trial: enteral nutrition does not improve the long-term outcome of alcoholic cirrhotic patients with jaundice, *Aliment Pharmacol Ther* 35:1166, 2012.

Food and Drug Administration (FDA): *OxyElite Pro supplements recalled* (website), 2013. http://www.fda.gov/ForConsumers/ConsumerUpdates/ucm374742.htm. Accessed April 24, 2014.

Fong TL, Klontz KC, Canas-Coto A, et al: Hepatotoxicity due to Hydroxycut: a case series, *Am J Gastroenterol* 105:1561, 2010.

Gratz SW, Mykkanen H, El-Nezami HS: Probiotics and gut health: a special focus on liver diseases, *World J Gastroenterol* 16:403, 2010.

Gruessner RW, Gruessner AC: Pancreas transplant alone: a procedure coming of age, *Diabetes Care* 36: 2440, 2013.

Hasse JM, Blue LS, Liepa GU, et al: Early enteral nutrition support in patients undergoing liver transplantation, *J Parenter Enteral Nutr* 19:437, 1995.

Ikegami T, Shirabe K, Yoshiya S, et al: Bacterial sepsis after living donor liver transplantation: the impact of early enteral nutrition, *J Am Coll Surg* 214:288, 2012.

International Association of Pancreatology (IAP), American Pancreatic Association (APA): IAP/APA evidence-based guidelines for the management of acute pancreatitis, *Pancreatology* 13(4 Suppl 2):e1, 2013. doi: 10.1016/j.pan.2013.07.063.

Jacobson BC, Vander Vliet MB, Hughes MD, et al: A prospective, randomized trial of clear liquids versus low-fat solid diet as the initial meal in mild acute pancreatitis, *Clin Gastroenterol Hepatol* 5:946, 2007.

Jaworek J, Szklarczyk J, Jaworek AK, et al: Protective effect of melatonin on acute pancreatitis, *Int J Inflam* 2012:173675, 2012.

Jenkins SA: Biliary lipids, bile acids and gallstone formation in the hypovitaminotic C guinea-pigs, *Br J Nutr* 40:317, 1978.

Jin Y, Lin CJ, Dong LM, et al: Clinical significance of melatonin concentrations in predicting the severity of acute pancreatitis, *World J Gastroeterol* 19:4066, 2013.

Jóhannsson M, Ormarsdóttir S, Olafsson S: Hepatotoxicity associated with the use of Herbalife, *Laeknabladid* 96:167, 2010.

Kim DB, Cho YK, Song HJ, et al: A case of acute pancreatitis and acute hepatitis caused by ingestion of Ceramium kondoi, *Korean J Gastroenterol* 62:306, 2013.

Koller T, Kollerova J, Hlavaty T, et al: Cholelithiasis and markers of non-alcoholic fatty liver disease in patients with metabolic risk factors, *Scand J Gastroenterol* 47:197, 2012.

Kosters A, Karpen SJ: The role of inflammation in cholestasis: clinical and basic aspects, *Semin Liver Dis* 30:186, 2010.

Lam P, Soroka CJ, Boyer JL: The bile salt export pump: clinical and experimental aspects of genetic and acquired cholestatic liver disease, *Semin Liver Dis* 30:125, 2010.

Lavine JE, Schwimmer JB, Van Natta ML, et al: Effect of vitamin E or metformin for treatment of nonalcoholic fatty liver disease in children and adolescents: the TONIC randomized controlled trial, *JAMA* 305:1659, 2011.

Leevy CM, Moroianu SA: Nutritional aspects of alcoholic liver disease. *Clin Liver Dis.* 9:67, 2005.

Lesser D, Hillesheim P: Pancreatitis in a woman taking an herbal supplement, *South Med J* 100:59, 2007.

Martinez J, Sánchez-Payá J, Palazón JM, et al: Is obesity a risk factor in acute pancreatitis? A meta-analysis, *Pancreatology* 4:42, 2004.

McClave SA, Chang WK, Dhaliwal R, et al: Nutrition support in acute pancreatitis: a systematic review of the literature, *J Parenter Enteral Nutr* 30:143, 2006.

McClave SA: Nutrition in pancreatitis, *World Rev Nutr Diet* 105:160, 2013.

Mendez-Sanchez N, Zamora-Valdés D, Chávez-Tapia NC, et al: Role of diet in cholesterol gallstone formation, *Clin Chim Acta* 376:1, 2007.

Mirtallo JM, Forbes A, McClave SA, et al: International consensus guidelines for nutrition therapy in pancreatitis, *JPEN J Parenter Enteral Nutr* 36:284, 2012.

Moraes JM, Felga GE, Chebli LA, et al: A full solid diet as the initial meal in mild acute pancreatitis is safe and result in a shorter length of hospitalization: results from a prospective, randomized, controlled, double-blind clinical trial, *J Clin Gastroenterol* 44:517, 2010.

Mukherjee S: Betaine and nonalcoholic steatohepatitis: back to the future? *World J Gastroenterol* 17:3663, 2011.

Nally DM, Kelly EG, Clarke M, et al: Nasogastric nutrition is efficacious in severe acute pancreatitis: a systematic review and meta-analysis, *Br J Nutr* 112:1769, 2014.

Ney M, Vandermeer B, van Zanten SJ, et al: Meta-analysis: Oral or enteral nutritional supplementation in cirrhosis, *Aliment Pharmacol Ther* 37:672, 2013.

Nordback I, Pelli H, Lappalainen-Lehto R, et al: The recurrence of acute alcohol-associated pancreatitis can be reduced: a randomized controlled trial, *Gastroenterology* 136:848, 2008.

O'Keefe SJ, Cariem AK, Levy M: The exacerbation of pancreatic endocrine dysfunction by potent pancreatic exocrine supplements in patients with chronic pancreatitis, *J Clin Gastroenterol* 32:319, 2001.

Patel KS, Noel P, Singh VP: Potential influence of intravenous lipids on the outcomes of acute pancreatitis, *Nutr Clin Pract* 29:291, 2014.

Pereg D, Kotliroff A, Gadoth N, et al: Probiotics for patients with compensated liver cirrhosis: a double-blind placebo-controlled study, *Nutrition* 27:177, 2011.

Petrov MS: Gastric feeding and gut rousing in acute pancreatitis, *Nutr Clin Pract* 29:287, 2014.

Petrov MS, Pylypchuk RD, Emelyanov NV: Systematic review: nutrition support in acute pancreatitis, *Aliment Pharmacol Ther* 28:704, 2008.

Petrov MS, Pylypchuk RD, Uchugina AF: A systematic review on the timing of artificial nutrition in acute pancreatitis, *Br J Nutr* 101:787, 2009.

Pronisceva V, Sebastian J, Joseph S, et al: A case report on over-replacement of oral calcium supplements causing acute pancreatitis, *Ann R Coll Surg Engl* 96:94E, 2014.

Rajkumar N, Karthikeyan VS, Ali SM, et al: Clear liquid diet vs soft diet as the initial meal in patients with mild acute pancreatitis: a randomized interventional trial, *Nutr Clin Pract* 28:365, 2013.

Rambaldi A, Gluud C: S-adenosyl-L-methionine for alcoholic liver diseases, *Cochrane Database Syst Rev* 19(2): CD002235, 2006.

Ranson JH, Rifkind KM, Roses DF, et al: Prognostic signs and the role of operative management in acute pancreatitis, *Surg Gynecol Obstet* 139:69, 1974.

Rayes N, Seehofer D, Theruvath T, et al: Supply of pre- and probiotics reduces bacterial infection rates after liver transplantation—a randomized, double-blind trial, *Am J Transplant* 5:125, 2005.

Runyon BA: Management of adult patients with ascites due to cirrhosis: update 2012, *Hepatology* 49:2087, 2013.

Sanyal AJ, Chalasani N, Kowdley KV, et al: Pioglitazone, vitamin E, or placebo for nonalcoholic steatohepatitis, *N Engl J Med* 362:1675, 2010.

Sathiaraj E, Murthy S, Mansard MJ, et al: Clinical trial: oral feeding with a soft diet compared with clear liquid diet as initial meal in mild acute pancreatitis, *Aliment Pharmacol Ther* 28:777, 2008.

Saxena P, Chen JA, Mullin GE: The role of complementary and alternative medicine for pancreatic disorders, *Nutr Clin Pract* 29:409, 2014.

Schoepfer AM, Engel A, Fattinger K, et al: Herbal does not mean innocuous: ten cases of severe hepatotoxicity associated with dietary supplements from Herbalife products, *J Hepatol* 47:521, 2007.

Seminerio J, O'Keefe SJ: Jejunal feeding in patients with pancreatitis, *Nutr Clin Pract* 29:283, 2014.

Sharma T, Wong L, Tsai N, et al: Hydroxycut (herbal weight loss supplement) induced hepatotoxicity: a case report and review of literature, *Hawaii Med J* 69:188, 2010.

Simon JA, Grady D, Snabes MC, et al: Ascorbic acid supplement use and the prevalence of gallbladder disease. Heart & Estrogen-Progestin Replacement Study (HERS) Research Group, *J Clin Epidemiol* 51: 257, 1998.

Sun JK, Mu XW, Li WQ, et al: Effects of early enteral nutrition on immune function of severe acute pancreatitis patients, *World J Gastroenterol* 19:917, 2013.

Teich N, Aghdassi A, Fischer J, et al: Optimal timing of oral refeeding in mild acute pancreatitis: results of an open randomized multicenter trial, *Pancreas* 39:1088, 2010.

Teschke R, Schwarzenboeck A, Eickhoff A, et al: Clinical and causality assessment in herbal hepatotoxicity, *Expert Opin Drug Saf* 12:339, 2013.

Verhaegh BP, Reijven PL, Prins MH, et al: Nutritional status in patients with chronic pancreatitis, *Eur J Clin Nutr* 67:1271, 2013.

Völzke H, Baumeister SE, Alte D, et al: Independent risk factors for gallstone formation in a region with high cholelithiasis prevalence, *Digestion* 71:97, 2005.

Wargo KA, Allman E, Ibrahim F, et al: A possible case of saw palmetto-induced pancreatitis, *South Med J* 103:683, 2010.

Wedemeyer H, Pawlotsky JM: Acute viral hepatitis. In: Goldman L et al, editors: *Goldman's Cecil medicine*, ed 24, Philadelphia, 2012, Elsevier Saunders.

Weikert C, Weikert S, Schulze MB, et al: Presence of gallstones or kidney stones and risk of type 2 diabetes, *Am J Epidemiol* 171:447, 2010.

Wu LM, Sankaran SJ, Plank LD, et al: Meta-analysis of gut barrier dysfunction in patients with acute pancreatitis, *Br J Surg* 101:1644, 2014

Yesil A, Yilmaz Y: Review article: coffee consumption, the metabolic syndrome and non-alcoholic fatty liver disease, *Aliment Pharmacol Ther* 38:1038, 2013.

Yoon YH, Yi HY: *Surveillance Report #93: Liver Cirrhosis Mortality in the United States, 1970–2009.* Bethesda, MD: National Institute on Alcohol Abuse and Alcoholism (website), 2012. Accessed November 7, 2014. http://pubs.niaaa.nih.gov/publications/Surveillance93/Cirr09.htm.

Zhang Z, Xu X, Ding J, et al: Comparison of postpyloric tube feeding and gastric tube feeding in intensive care unit patients: a meta-analysis, *Nutr Clin Pract* 28:371, 2013.

Zou L, Ke L, Li W, et al: Enteral nutrition within 72 h after onset of acute pancreatitis vs delayed initiation, *Eur J Clin Nutr* 68:1288, 2014.

30

Medical Nutrition Therapy for Diabetes Mellitus and Hypoglycemia of Nondiabetic Origin

Marion J. Franz, MS, RDN, LD, CDE, Alison B. Evert, MS, RDN, CDE

KEY TERMS

acanthosis nigricans
amylin
autonomic symptoms
carbohydrate counting
continuous glucose monitoring (CGM)
correction factor (CF)
counterregulatory (stress) hormones
dawn phenomenon
diabetic ketoacidosis (DKA)
fasting hypoglycemia
gastroparesis
gestational diabetes mellitus (GDM)
glucagon
glucose-lowering medications
glucotoxicity
glycemic index (GI)
glycemic load (GL)
glycosylated hemoglobin (A1C)

honeymoon phase
hyperglycemia
hyperglycemic hyperosmolar state (HHS)
hypoglycemia (or insulin reaction)
hypoglycemia of nondiabetic origin
immune-mediated diabetes mellitus
impaired fasting glucose (IFG)
impaired glucose tolerance (IGT)
incretins
insulin
insulin deficiency
insulin resistance
insulin secretagogues
latent autoimmune diabetes of aging (LADA)
lipotoxicity
macrosomia

macrovascular diseases
metabolic syndrome
microvascular diseases
neuroglycopenic symptoms
polydipsia
polyphagia
polyuria
postprandial (after a meal) blood glucose
postprandial (reactive) hypoglycemia
prediabetes
preprandial (fasting/premeal) blood glucose
self-monitoring of blood glucose (SMBG)
Somogyi effect
type 1 diabetes (T1DM)
type 2 diabetes (T2DM)
Whipple's triad

Diabetes mellitus is a group of diseases characterized by high blood glucose concentrations resulting from defects in insulin secretion, insulin action, or both. **Insulin** is a hormone produced by the beta-cells of the pancreas that is necessary for the use or storage of body fuels (carbohydrate, protein, and fat). Persons with diabetes do not produce adequate insulin; with **insulin deficiency**, **hyperglycemia** (elevated blood glucose) occurs.

Diabetes mellitus contributes to a considerable increase in morbidity and mortality rates, which can be reduced by early diagnosis and treatment. Direct medical expenditures such as inpatient care, outpatient services, and nursing home care are astronomical and indirect costs such as disability, work loss, and premature mortality are equally high. Average medical expenditures among people with diabetes are double that of people who do not have diabetes. Thus providing medical nutrition therapy (MNT) for prevention and treatment of diabetes has tremendous potential to reduce these costs. Fortunately, people with diabetes can take steps to control the disease and lower the risk of complications or premature death.

INCIDENCE AND PREVALENCE

In 2014 total prevalence of diabetes in the United States in all ages was 29.1 million people (15.5 million adult men and 13.4 adult women), or 9.3% of the population. Of these, 21.0 million are diagnosed, and 8.1 million undiagnosed. In 2012 1.7 million new cases of diabetes were diagnosed in people age 20 years or older (CDC, 2014). Diabetes prevalence also increases with age, affecting 11.2 million people age 65 years and older, or 25.9% of all people in this age group.

Much of the increase in prevalence is because the prevalence of type 2 diabetes is increasing dramatically in younger age groups in the last decade, especially in minority populations. Among youth with newly diagnosed diabetes, approximately 20% have type 2 diabetes. The prevalence of type 2 diabetes is highest in ethnic groups in the United States. Data indicate in people aged 20 years or older, 15.9% of American Indians and Alaska Natives, 13.2% of non-Hispanic blacks, 12.8% of Hispanics, and 9.0% of Asian Americans had diagnosed diabetes. Among Hispanics, rates were 14.8% for Puerto Ricans, 13.9% for Mexican Americans, and 9.3% for Cubans (CDC, 2014). Of great concern, are the 86 million people (37% of adults 20 years or older and 51% of adults 60 years or older) with **prediabetes**, which includes **impaired glucose tolerance (IGT)** and **impaired fasting glucose (IFG)** (ADA, 2014b). All are a high risk for conversion to type 2 diabetes and cardiovascular disease (CVD) if lifestyle prevention strategies are not implemented.

CATEGORIES OF GLUCOSE INTOLERANCE

Assigning a type of diabetes to an individual often depends on the circumstances present at the time of diagnosis, and many individuals do not easily fit into a single category. Thus it is less important to label the particular type of diabetes than it is to understand the pathogenesis of the hyperglycemia and to treat it effectively (ADA, 2014a). What is essential is the need to intervene early with lifestyle interventions, beginning with prediabetes and continuing through the disease process.

Prediabetes

Individuals with a stage of impaired glucose homeostasis that includes IFG and IGT are referred to as having prediabetes, indicating their relatively high risk for the development of diabetes and CVD. People at risk may have IFG (fasting plasma glucose 100-125 mg/dL), IGT (2-hour postchallenge glucose of 140 to 199 mg/dl), both, or a hemoglobin A1c (A1C) of 5.7% to 6.4% and should be counseled about strategies, such as reduced energy intake, weight loss, and physical activity, to lower their risks.

Type 1 Diabetes

At diagnosis, people with **type 1 diabetes (T1DM)** often experience excessive thirst, frequent urination, and significant weight loss. The primary defect is pancreatic beta-cell destruction, usually leading to absolute insulin deficiency and resulting in hyperglycemia, **polyuria** (excessive urination), **polydipsia** (excessive thirst), **polyphagia** (excessive hunger), weight loss, dehydration, electrolyte disturbance, and ketoacidosis. The rate of beta-cell destruction is variable, proceeding rapidly in infants and children and slowly in others (mainly adults.) The capacity of a healthy pancreas to secrete insulin is far in excess of what is needed normally. Therefore the clinical onset of diabetes may be preceded by an extensive asymptomatic period of months to years, during which beta-cells are undergoing gradual destruction.

T1DM accounts for 5% to 10% of all diagnosed cases of diabetes. Persons with T1DM are dependent on exogenous insulin to prevent ketoacidosis and death. T1DM can develop at any age. Although more cases are diagnosed in people before the age of 30 years, it also occurs in older individuals. Most individuals are lean but some are diagnosed without any or with more subtle symptoms and may be overweight, reflecting the trend of increasing obesity among children and adults.

T1DM has two forms: immune-mediated and idiopathic. **Immune-mediated diabetes mellitus** results from an autoimmune destruction of the beta-cells of the pancreas, the only cells in the body that make the hormone insulin. Idiopathic T1DM refers to forms of the disease that have no known etiology. Although only a minority of individuals with T1DM fall into this category, of those who do, most are of African or Asian ancestry (ADA, 2014b). At this time there are no known means to prevent T1DM.

Autoimmune thyroid disease and celiac disease are two immune-mediated diseases that occur with increased frequency in persons with type 1 diabetes. Autoimmune thyroid disease occurs in 17% to 30% of persons with type 1 diabetes, and celiac disease occurs in 1% to 16% of individuals compared with 0.3% to 1% in the general population (ADA, 2014b). Children with type 1 diabetes should be screened for celiac disease soon after diagnosis. If celiac disease is biopsy-confirmed, children should be placed on a gluten-free diet by a RDN experienced in managing diabetes and celiac disease (Chiang et al, 2014).

Pathophysiology

Markers of the immune destruction of the beta-cells include islet cells autoantibodies, autoantibodies to insulin, autoantibodies to glutamic acid decarboxylase (GAD65) (a protein on the surface of the beta-cells), and autoantibodies to the tyrosine phosphatases IA-2 and IA-2beta. One and usually more of these autoantibodies are present in 85% to 90% of individuals when fasting hyperglycemia is detected initially. The disease also has strong genetic factors, which involve the association between T1DM and histocompatibility locus antigen (HLA) with linkage to the DQA and DQB genes, and is influenced by the DRB genes. These HLA-DR/DQ alleles can be either predisposing or protective (ADA, 2014a).

The rate of clinical beta-cell destruction is quite variable, being rapid in some individuals (mainly infants and children) and slow in others (mainly adults). Hyperglycemia and symptoms develop only after greater than 90% of the secretory capacity of the beta-cell mass has been destroyed.

Frequently, after diagnosis and the correction of hyperglycemia, metabolic acidosis, and ketoacidosis, endogenous insulin secretion recovers. During this **honeymoon phase** exogenous insulin requirements decrease dramatically for up to 1 year or longer, and good metabolic control may be easily achieved. However, the need for increasing exogenous insulin replacement is inevitable and always should be anticipated. Intensive insulin therapy along with attention to MNT and self-monitoring of glucose from early diagnosis has been shown to prolong insulin secretion. Within 5 to 10 years after clinical onset, beta-cell loss is complete, and circulating islet cell antibodies can no longer be detected.

Amylin, a glucoregulatory hormone also is produced in the pancreatic beta-cell and cosecreted with insulin. Amylin complements the effects of insulin by regulating postprandial glucose levels and suppressing glucagon secretion. T1DM is also an amylin-deficient state. Individuals with T1DM are also prone to other autoimmune disorders such as Graves' disease, Hashimoto's thyroiditis, Addison's disease, vitiligo, celiac disease, autoimmune hepatitis, myasthenia gravis, and pernicious anemia.

Latent autoimmune diabetes of aging (LADA) may account for as many as 10% of cases of insulin-requiring diabetes in older individuals and represents a slowly progressive form of autoimmune diabetes that frequently is confused with T2DM. Adults with LADA have HLA genetic susceptibility as well as autoantibodies. Their diabetes may be controlled initially with nutrition therapy but within a relatively short period of time glucose-lowering medication and progression to insulin treatment are required (Naik et al, 2009).

Type 2 Diabetes

Type 2 diabetes (T2DM) accounts for 90% to 95% of all diagnosed cases of diabetes and is a progressive disease that, in many cases, is present long before it is diagnosed. Hyperglycemia develops gradually and is often not severe enough in the early stages for the person to notice any of the classic symptoms of diabetes. Although undiagnosed, these individuals are at increased risk of developing macrovascular and microvascular complications.

Most persons with T2DM are obese, and obesity itself causes some degree of **insulin resistance**. Persons who are not obese

PATHOPHYSIOLOGY AND CARE MANAGEMENT ALGORITHM

Type 1 Diabetes Mellitus

ETIOLOGY

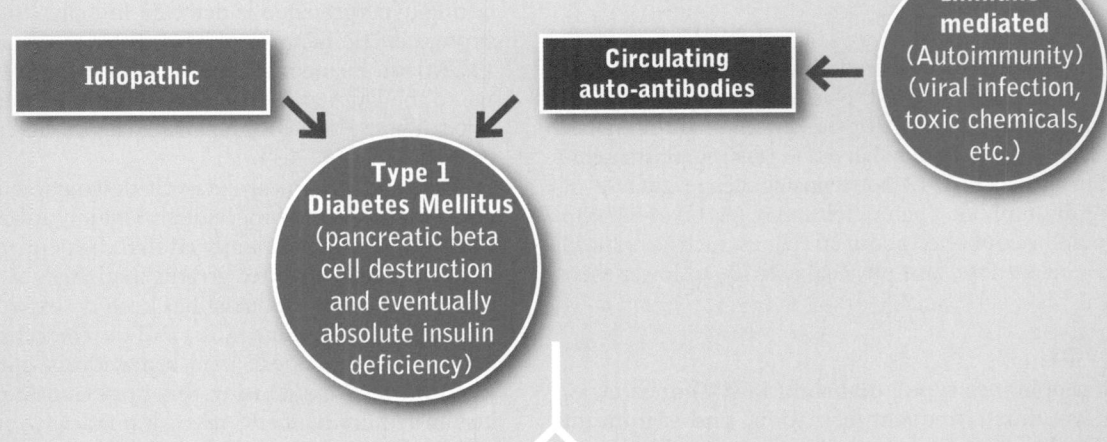

Idiopathic

Circulating auto-antibodies

Immune-mediated (Autoimmunity) (viral infection, toxic chemicals, etc.)

Type 1 Diabetes Mellitus (pancreatic beta cell destruction and eventually absolute insulin deficiency)

PATHOPHYSIOLOGY

Symptoms

- Hyperglycemia
- Excessive thirst
- Frequent urination
- Significant weight loss
- Electrolyte disturbances

Complications

Ketoacidosis
Macrovascular diseases
- Coronary heart disease
- Peripheral vascular disease
- Cerebrovascular disease

Microvascular diseases
- Retinopathy
- Nephropathy

Neuropathy

MANAGEMENT

Medical Management

Medical nutrition therapy
Medications
- Insulin by injection or insulin infusion pumps

Monitoring
- Self-monitoring of blood glucose
- A1C testing
- Lipids
- Blood pressure
- Ketones
- Weight and growth in children

Self-management education

Medical Nutrition Therapy (MNT)

- Integrate insulin regimen into preferred eating and physical activity schedule; consistency in timing and amount of carbohydrate eaten if on fixed insulin doses
- Adjust premeal insulin dose based on insulin-to-carbohydrate ratios
- Energy intake to prevent weight gain in adults
- Adequate energy and nutrient intake to promote growth and development in children
- Cardioprotective nutrition interventions

by traditional weight criteria may have an increased percentage of body fat distributed predominately in the abdominal region. However, many obese persons never develop T2DM. Therefore obesity combined with a genetic predisposition may be necessary for T2DM to occur. Other risk factors include genetic and environmental factors, including a family history of diabetes, older age, physical inactivity, a prior history of gestational diabetes, prediabetes, hypertension or dyslipidemia, and race or ethnicity.

Pathophysiology

T2DM is characterized by a combination of insulin resistance and beta-cell failure. Endogenous insulin levels may be normal, depressed, or elevated, but they are inadequate to overcome concomitant insulin resistance (decreased tissue sensitivity or responsiveness to insulin.) As a result, hyperglycemia ensues. The inflammatory response to excess weight, insulin resistance, and beta-cell failure occurs approximately 5 to 10 years before the elevation of glucose above normal. When T2DM is diagnosed, it is estimated that people already have lost approximately 50% of their beta-cell function. There is disagreement among researchers whether this is loss of beta-cell mass or function. Persons in the upper tertile of IGT before the diagnosis of T2DM are reported to have lost more than 80% of their beta-cell function.

Insulin resistance is demonstrated first in target tissues, mainly muscle, liver, and adipose cells. Initially there is a compensatory increase in insulin secretion (hyperinsulinemia), which maintains glucose concentrations in the normal or prediabetic range. In many persons the pancreas is unable to continue to produce adequate insulin, hyperglycemia occurs, and the diagnosis of diabetes is made. Therefore insulin levels are always deficient relative to elevated glucose levels before hyperglycemia develops.

Hyperglycemia is first exhibited as an elevation of postprandial (after a meal) blood glucose caused by insulin resistance at the cellular level and is followed by an elevation in fasting glucose concentrations. As insulin secretion decreases, hepatic glucose production increases, causing the increase in preprandial (fasting) blood glucose levels. The insulin response is also inadequate in suppressing alpha-cell glucagon secretion, resulting in glucagon hypersecretion and increased hepatic glucose production. Compounding the problem is glucotoxicity, the deleterious effect of hyperglycemia on insulin sensitivity and insulin secretion; hence the importance of achieving near-euglycemia in persons with T2DM.

Insulin resistance also is demonstrated at the adipocyte level, leading to lipolysis and an elevation in circulating free fatty acids. In particular, excess intraabdominal obesity, characterized by an excess accumulation of visceral fat around and inside abdominal organs, results in an increased flux of free fatty acids to the liver, leading to an increase in insulin resistance. Increased fatty acids also cause a further decrease in insulin sensitivity at the cellular level, impair pancreatic insulin secretion, and augment hepatic glucose production (lipotoxicity). The above defects contribute to the development and progression of T2DM and are also primary targets for pharmacologic therapy.

Persons with T2DM may or may not experience the classic symptoms of uncontrolled diabetes (polydipsia, polyuria, polyphagia, weight loss) and they are not prone to develop ketoacidosis except during times of severe stress. The progressive loss of beta-cell secretory function means that persons with T2DM require more medication(s) over time to maintain the same level of glycemic control; eventually exogenous insulin will be required. Insulin is also required sooner for control during periods of stress-induced hyperglycemia, such as during illness or surgery.

If at diagnosis it is not clear whether T1DM or T2DM is present, C-peptide may be measured. When the pancreas produces insulin, it begins as a large molecule—proinsulin. This molecule splits into two equal-sized pieces: insulin and C-peptide. A person with T1DM has a low level of C-peptide, whereas as a person with T2DM can have a normal or high level of C-peptide. As T2DM progresses, C-peptide also may be measured to see if endogenous insulin is still being produced by the pancreas. If it is not, exogenous insulin is needed.

Gestational Diabetes Mellitus

Gestational diabetes mellitus (GDM) occurs in about 7% of all pregnancies (ranging from 1% to 14% depending on the population studied), resulting in more than 200,000 cases annually (ADA, 2014a). After delivery, about 90% of all women with GDM become normoglycemic but are at increased risk of developing GDM earlier in subsequent pregnancies. Immediately after pregnancy, 5% to 10% of women with GDM are diagnosed with T2DM. Women who have had GDM have a 35% to 60% chance of developing diabetes in the next 5 to 10 years (CDC, 2014). Lifestyle modifications aimed at reducing or preventing weight gain and increasing physical activity after pregnancy may reduce the risk of subsequent diabetes.

Previously GDM was defined as any degree of glucose intolerance with onset or first recognition during pregnancy. However, the number of pregnant women with undiagnosed diabetes has increased and therefore it has now been recommended that women with risk factors for diabetes should be screened for undiagnosed T2DM at the first prenatal visit, using standard diagnostic criteria. Women found to have diabetes in the first trimester should receive a diagnosis of overt, not gestational, diabetes (ADA, 2014b).

All women not previously known to have diabetes should be screened for GDM at 24 to 28 weeks of gestation. GDM is diagnosed most often during the second or third trimester of pregnancy because of the increase in insulin-antagonist hormone levels and insulin resistance that normally occurs at this time. GDM screening can be accomplished with either of two strategies:

1. "One-step" 3-hr 75-g OGTT. A fasting glucose >92 mg/dl (5.1 mmol/L), a 1-hour >180 mg/dL (10 mmol/L), or a 2-hr >153 mg/dl (8.4 mmol/L) is diagnostic of GDM
2. "Two-step" approach with a 1-hr 50-g (nonfasting) screen followed by a 3-hr 100-g OGTT for those with plasma glucose ≥140 mg/dl (10.0 mmol/L). The diagnosis of GDM is made when the plasma glucose level measured 2 hr after the test is ≥140 mg/dl (7.8 mmol/L).

During pregnancy, treatment to normalize maternal blood glucose levels reduces the risk of adverse maternal, fetal, and neonatal outcomes. Extra glucose from the mother crosses the fetal placenta and the fetus' pancreas responds by releasing extra insulin to cope with the excess glucose. The excess glucose is converted to fat, which results in macrosomia. The fetus may become too large for a normal birth resulting in the need for cesarean delivery. Neonatal hypoglycemia at birth is another common problem. The above normal levels of maternal glucose have caused the fetus to produce extra insulin. However, after

PATHOPHYSIOLOGY AND CARE MANAGEMENT ALGORITHM

Type 2 Diabetes Mellitus

ETIOLOGY

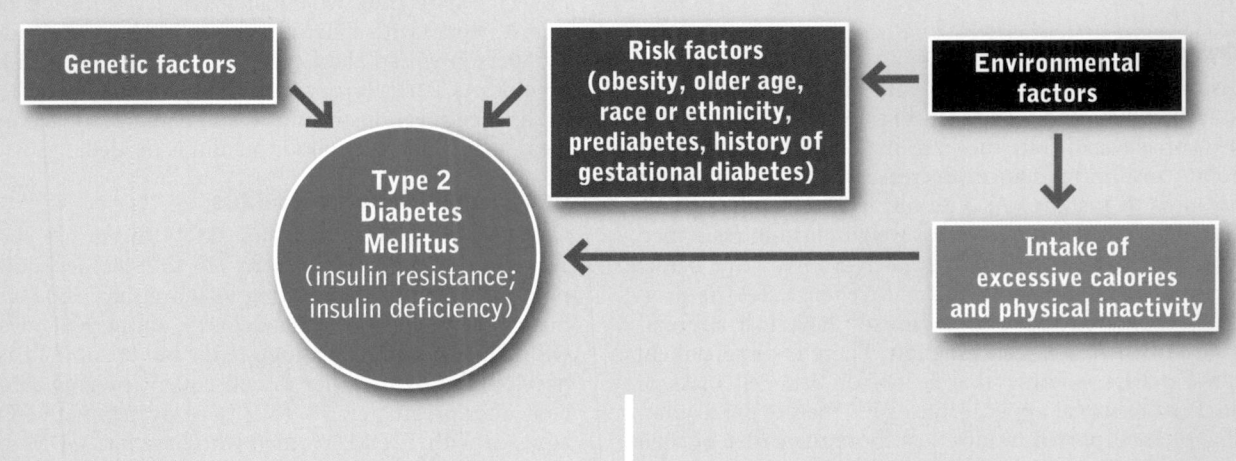

Genetic factors

Risk factors (obesity, older age, race or ethnicity, prediabetes, history of gestational diabetes)

Environmental factors

Type 2 Diabetes Mellitus (insulin resistance; insulin deficiency)

Intake of excessive calories and physical inactivity

PATHOPHYSIOLOGY

Symptoms (variable)

- Hyperglycemia
- Fatigue
- Excessive thirst
- Frequent urination

Clinical Findings

- Abnormal patterns of insulin secretion and action
- Decreased cellular uptake of glucose and increased postprandial glucose
- Increased release of glucose by liver (gluconeogenesis) resulting in fasting hyperglycemia
- Central obesity
- Hypertension
- Dyslipidemia

MANAGEMENT

Medical Management

Medical nutrition therapy
Physical activity
Medications
- Glucose-lowering medications
- Insulin
Monitoring
- Self-monitoring of blood glucose
- A1C testing
- Lipids
- Blood pressure
- Weight
Self-management education

Medical Nutrition Therapy (MNT)

- Lifestyle strategies (food/eating and physical activity) that improve glycemia, dyslipidemia, and blood pressure
- Nutrition education (carbohydrate counting and fat modification) and counseling
- Energy restriction
- Blood glucose monitoring to determine adjustments in food or medications
- Cardioprotective nutrition interventions

birth the extra glucose is no longer available to the fetus, but until his or her pancreas can adjust, the neonate may require extra glucose through intravenous feedings for a day or two to keep blood glucose levels normal.

GDM does not cause congenital anomalies. Such malformations occur in women with diabetes before pregnancy who have uncontrolled blood glucose levels during the first 6 to 8 weeks of pregnancy when fetal organs are being formed. Because GDM does not appear until later in pregnancy, the fetal organs were formed before hyperglycemia became a problem.

When optimal blood glucose levels are not being maintained with MNT or the rate of fetal growth is excessive, pharmacologic therapy is needed (AND, 2008b). Research supports the use of insulin, insulin analogs, metformin, and glyburide during pregnancy. Women with GDM should be screened for diabetes 6 to 12 weeks postpartum and should have lifelong screening for the development of diabetes or prediabetes at least every 3 years (ADA, 2014b).

Other Types of Diabetes

This category includes diabetes associated with specific genetic syndromes (such as maturity-onset diabetes of youth), genetic defects in insulin action, diseases of the exocrine pancreas (such as cystic fibrosis), endocrinopathies, (such as acromegly or Cushing's syndrome), drug or chemical induced (such as in the treatment of HIV/AIDS or after organ transplantation), infections, and other illnesses. Such types of diabetes may account for 1% to 5% of all diagnosed cases of diabetes (ADA, 2014a).

SCREENING AND DIAGNOSTIC CRITERIA

Screening for Diabetes

Screening for diabetes should be considered in all adults who are overweight (body mass index [BMI] $\geq$25 kg/m2) and who have one or more additional risk factors for T2DM listed below. In those without these risk factors, testing should begin at age 45 years. If tests are normal, testing should be done at 3-year intervals; A1C, FPG, or 2-h OGTT, can be used to test for either prediabetes or diabetes (ADA, 2014b). Additional risk factors for diabetes are the following:

- Physical inactivity
- First-degree relative with diabetes
- Members of a high-risk population (African Americans, Latino, Native American, Asian American, and Pacific Islander)
- Women who have delivered a baby weighing more than 9 lb or have been diagnosed with GDM
- Hypertensive (blood pressure $\geq$140/90 mm Hg or taking medication for hypertension)
- High-density lipoprotein (HDL) cholesterol level <35 mg/dl (0.9 mmol/L) and/or a triglyceride level >250 mg/dl (2.82 mmol/L)
- Women with polycystic ovary syndrome (PCOS)
- A1C $\geq$5.7%, IGT, or IFG on previous testing
- Other clinical condition associated with insulin resistance (e.g., severe obesity, acanthosis nigricans [gray-brown skin pigmentations])
- History of CVD

Consistent with screening recommendations for adults, children and youth at increased risk for T2DM should be tested. The age of initiation of screening is age 10 years or at onset of puberty, and the frequency is every 3 years (ADA, 2014b). Youth who are overweight (BMI >85th percentile for age and sex, weight for height above the 85th percentile, or weight more than 120% of ideal for height) and have any two of the following risk factors should be screened:

- Family history of T2DM in first- or second-degree relative
- Race/ethnicity (Native American, African American, Latino, Asian American, Pacific Islander)
- Signs of insulin resistance (acanthosis nigricans, hypertension, dyslipidemia, PCOS, or small-for-gestational-age birth weight)
- Maternal history of diabetes or GDM during the child's gestation

Diagnostic Criteria

Four diagnostic methods may be used to diagnose diabetes and each, in the absence of unequivocal hyperglycemia, must be confirmed, on a subsequent day, by repeat testing. It is preferable that the same test be repeated for confirmation (ADA, 2014b). Diagnostic criteria for diabetes and prediabetes are summarized in Table 30-1.

Plasma glucose criteria, either the fasting plasma glucose (FPG) or the 2-hr plasma glucose after a 75-g OGTT, was the method usually used to diagnosis diabetes. However, the A1C assay now is highly standardized and is a reliable measure of chronic glucose levels. The A1C test reflects longer-term glucose concentrations and is assessed from the results of glycosylated hemoglobin (simplified as A1C) tests. When hemoglobin and other proteins are exposed to glucose, the glucose becomes attached to the protein in a slow, nonenzymatic, and concentration-dependent fashion. Measurements of A1C therefore reflect a weighted average of plasma glucose concentration over the preceding weeks. In nondiabetic persons A1C values are 4% to 6%; these values correspond to mean blood glucose levels of

TABLE 30-1	Criteria for the Diagnosis of Diabetes Mellitus and Increased Risk for Diabetes (Prediabetes)
Diagnosis	**Criteria**
Diabetes	A1C $\geq$6.5%*
	OR
	FPG $\geq$126 mg/dl ($\geq$7.0 mmol/L)*
	OR
	2-h PG $\geq$200 mg/dl ($\geq$11.1 mmol/L) during an OGTT*
	OR
	In patients with classic symptoms of hyperglycemia or hyperglycemic crisis, a random PG $\geq$200 mg/dL ($\geq$11.1 mmol/L)
Prediabetes	FPG 100-125 mg/dL (5.6-6.9 mmol/L) [Impaired fasting glucose]
	OR
	2-hPG in the 75-g OGTT 140-199 mg/dl (7.8-11.0 mmol/L) (Impaired glucose tolerance)
	OR
	A1C 5.7-6.4%
Normal	FPG <100 mg/dL (<5.6 mmol/L)
	2-hPG <140 mg/dL (<7.8 mmol/L)
	A1C 4 to 5.6%

Data from American Diabetes Association: Diagnosis and classification of diabetes mellitus, *Diabetes Care* 37(S1):S5, 2014.

*In the absence of unequivocal hyperglycemia, criteria 1 to 3 should be confirmed by repeat testing.

FPG, fasting plasma glucose; *2-hPG*, 2-hour plasma glucose level (measured 2 hours after an oral glucose tolerance test [OGTT] with administration of 75 g of glucose).

about 70 to 126 mg/dL (3.9 to 7.0 mmol/L). A1C values vary less than FPG, and testing is more convenient because patients are not required to be fasting or to undergo an OGTT. However, A1C levels may vary with person's race/ethnicity as glycation rates may differ by race (ADA, 2014b). It is also unclear if the same A1C cutoff point should be used to diagnose children or adolescents with diabetes, because studies used to recommend A1C to diagnose diabetes have all been performed in adult populations. For conditions with abnormal red cell turnover, such as hemolysis (blood loss), pregnancy, or iron deficiency, the diagnosis of diabetes must use glucose criteria exclusively (ADA, 2014b). The A1C test should be performed using a method certified by the National Glycohemoglobin Standardization Program.

MANAGEMENT OF PREDIABETES

In no other disease does lifestyle—healthy and appropriate food choices and physical activity—play a more important role in prevention and treatment than in diabetes. Studies comparing lifestyle modifications to medication have provided support for the benefit of weight loss (reduced energy intake) and physical activity as the first choice to prevent or delay diabetes. Clinical trials comparing lifestyle interventions to a control group have reported risk reduction for T2DM from lifestyle interventions ranging from 29% to 67% (Youssef, 2012). Two frequently cited studies are the Finnish Diabetes Prevention Study and the Diabetes Prevention Program (DPP), in which lifestyle interventions focused on a weight loss of 5% to 10%, physical activity of at least 150 min/week of moderate activity, and ongoing counseling and support. Both reported a 58% reduction in the incidence of T2DM in the intervention group compared with the control group and persistent reduction in the rate of conversion to T2DM within 3 to 14 years postintervention follow-up (DPP Research Group, 2009; Li et al, 2008; Lindström et al, 2006).

Medical Management

Use of the pharmacologic agents metformin, alpha-glucosidase inhibitors, orlistat, and thiazolidinediones has been shown to decrease incidence of diabetes by various degrees (Youssef, 2012). At this time, metformin is the only drug that should be considered for use in diabetes prevention. It is the most effective in those with a BMI of at least 35 kg/m2 and who are under age 30. For other drugs, issues of cost, side effects, and lack of persistence of effect are of concern.

Medical management must include lifestyle changes. Physical activity is important to prevent weight gain and maintain weight loss. For cardiovascular fitness and to reduce risk of T2DM, recommendations include moderate-intensity aerobic physical activity a minimum of 30 minutes 5 days per week (150 min/week) (i.e., walking 3 to 4 miles/hr) or vigorous-intensity aerobic physical activity a minimum of 20 minutes 3 days per week (90 min/week). Muscle-strengthening activities involving all major muscle groups two or more days per week are also recommended (US Department of Health and Human Services [USDHHS], 2008). Physical activity independent of weight loss improves insulin sensitivity.

Medical Nutrition Therapy for Prediabetes

Goals of MNT for prediabetes emphasize the importance of food choices that facilitate moderate weight loss. Structured programs that emphasize lifestyle changes that include moderate weight loss (7% of body weight) with strategies including reduced calories and reduced intake of fat are effective. More recently, moderate to high adherence to a Mediterranean-style eating pattern characterized by high levels of monounsaturated fatty acids such as olive oil, high intake of plant-based foods (vegetables, legumes, fruits, and nuts), moderate amounts of fish and wine, and a low intake of red and processed meat and whole-fat dairy products versus low adherence has been associated with a lower incidence of diabetes (Youssef, 2012).

In addition, whole grains and dietary fiber are associated with reduced risk of diabetes. Increased intake of whole grain–containing foods improves insulin sensitivity independent of body weight, and increased intake of dietary fiber has been associated with improved insulin sensitivity and improved ability to secrete insulin adequately to overcome insulin resistance. Moderate consumption of alcohol (1 to 3 drinks per day [15 to 45 g alcohol]) is linked with decreased risk of T2DM, coronary heart disease, and stroke. But the data do not support recommending alcohol consumption to persons at risk for diabetes who do not already drink alcoholic beverages.

High consumption of sugar-sweetened beverages, which includes soft drinks, fruit drinks, and energy and vitamin water-type drinks containing sucrose, high-fructose corn syrup, and/or fruit juice concentrates is associated with the development of T2DM (Malik et al, 2010). Studies also have reported that an eating pattern high in saturated fatty acids and trans fatty acids is associated with increased markers of insulin resistance and risk for type 2 diabetes, whereas unsaturated fatty acid intake is associated inversely with risk of diabetes (Youssef, 2012). Therefore individuals at increased risk for T2DM should be encouraged to limit their intake of sugar-sweetened beverages and decrease saturated fat intake.

Adhering to a combination of healthy lifestyle habits (a healthy eating pattern, participating in regular physical activity, maintaining a normal body weight, moderate alcohol intake, and being a nonsmoker) was shown to reduce the risk of developing T2DM by as much as 84% for women and 72% for men (Reis et al, 2011).

Bariatric Surgery and Prediabetes

Observational studies have demonstrated that bariatric surgery reduces the incidence of T2DM, but there are no randomized controlled trials (RCTs) on the role of bariatric surgery in the prevention of diabetes (Reis et al, 2011). Possible mechanisms for this weight-independent impact of bariatric surgery on glucose include enterohormonal changes and neurohormonal events resulting from the anatomic changes of the surgery (Lautz et al, 2011).

MANAGEMENT OF DIABETES

Two classic clinical trials have demonstrated beyond a doubt the clear link between glycemic control and the development of complications in persons with T1DM and T2DM, as well as the importance of nutrition therapy in achieving control. The Diabetes Control and Complications Trial (DCCT) studied approximately 1400 persons with T1DM treated with either intensive (multiple injections of insulin or use of insulin infusion pumps guided by blood glucose monitoring results) or conventional (one or two insulin injections per day) regimens. Epidemiology of Diabetes Interventions (EDIC) is an observational study following the DCCT cohort. A 30-year follow-up of the DCCT/EDIC cohort convincingly demonstrated that an intervention that aimed to achieve glycemia as close to the nondiabetic range as safely possible reduced all of the microvascular and cardiovascular complications of diabetes and should be implemented as early as possible after diagnosis (Nathan, 2014). Another study, the United Kingdom Prospective Diabetes Study (UKPDS), demonstrated conclusively that glucose and blood pressure control decreased the risk of long-term complications in T2DM (Holman et al, 2008). A reduction in energy intake was at least as important, if not more important, than the actual weight lost.

Medical Management

The management of all types of diabetes includes MNT, physical activity, monitoring, medications, and self-management education and support. An important goal of medical treatment is to provide the individual with diabetes with the necessary tools to achieve the best possible control of glucose, lipids, and blood pressure to prevent, delay, or manage the microvascular and macrovascular complications while minimizing hypoglycemia and excess weight gain. Insulin, the primary hormone in glucose control is also anticatabolic and anabolic and facilitates cellular transport (see Table 30-2). In general, the counterregulatory (stress) hormones (glucagon, growth hormone, cortisol, epinephrine, and norepinephrine) have the opposite effect of insulin.

The ADA's glycemic treatment goals for persons with diabetes are listed in Table 30-3. Achieving goals requires open communication between the health care provider and the persons with diabetes and appropriate self-management education. Patients can assess day-to-day glycemic control by self-monitoring of blood glucose (SMBG) and measurement of urine or blood ketones. Longer-term glycemic control is assessed by A1C testing. Lipid levels and blood pressure also must be monitored (see Table 30-4). In most adults, lipids should be measured at least annually and blood pressure at every routine visit (ADA, 2014b). Optimal control of diabetes also requires the restoration of normal carbohydrate, protein, and fat metabolism.

It is important that people with diabetes receive medical care from a team that may include physicians, dietitians, nurses, pharmacists, and mental health professionals with expertise in diabetes. Individuals with diabetes also must assume an active role in their care. For T1DM a flexible, individualized management program using the principles of intensive insulin therapy is essential. T2DM is a progressive disease. The "diet" doesn't fail; the pancreas fails to secrete enough insulin to maintain adequate glucose control. As the disease progresses, MNT alone is not enough to keep A1C level at 7% or less. Therapy must intensify over time. Medications, and eventually insulin, have to be combined with nutrition therapy. Through the collaborative development of individualized nutrition interventions and ongoing support of behavior changes, health care professionals can facilitate the achievement of the person with diabetes health goals.

Medical Nutrition Therapy for Diabetes

MNT is integral to total diabetes care and management. To integrate MNT effectively into the overall management of diabetes requires a registered dietitian nutritionist (RDN) who is knowledgeable and skilled in implementing current nutrition therapy recommendations into the medical management of diabetes. MNT requires an individualized approach and effective nutrition self-management education, counseling, and

TABLE 30-2	Action of Insulin on Carbohydrate, Protein, and Fat Metabolism		
Effect	**Carbohydrates**	**Protein**	**Fat**
Anticatabolic (prevents breakdown)	Decreases breakdown and release of glucose from glycogen in the liver	Inhibits protein degradation, diminishes gluconeogenesis	Inhibits lipolysis, prevents excessive production of ketones and ketoacidosis
Anabolic (promotes storage)	Facilitates conversion of glucose to glycogen for storage in liver and muscle	Stimulates protein synthesis	Facilitates conversion of pyruvate to free fatty acids, stimulating lipogenesis
Transport	Activates the transport system of glucose into muscle and adipose cells	Lowers blood amino acids in parallel with blood glucose levels	Activates lipoprotein lipase, facilitating transport of triglycerides into adipose tissue

TABLE 30-3	Recommendations for Glycemic Control for Adults with Diabetes	
Glycemic Control	**Criteria**	
A1C	<7.0%*	
Preprandial capillary plasma glucose	80-130 mg/dL* (4.4-7.2 mmol/L)	
Peak postprandial capillary plasma glucose†	<180 mg/dL* (<10.0 mmol/L)	

Modified from American Diabetes Association: Standards of medical care in diabetes—2014, *Diabetes Care* 37(S1):S14, 2014.

*Goals should be individualized, such as for the elderly, individuals with a history of cardiovascular disease, or hypoglycemia unawareness

†Postprandial glucose measurements should be made 1 to 2 hr after the beginning of the meal, generally peak levels in patients with diabetes.

TABLE 30-4	Recommendations for Lipid and Blood Pressure for Most Adults with Diabetes	
Lipids/Blood Pressure	**Criteria**	
LDL cholesterol	<100 mg/dl (<2.6 mmol/l)*	
HDL cholesterol		
Men	>40 mg/dl (>1.1 mmol/l)	
Women	>50 mg/dl (>1.4 mmol/l)	
Triglycerides	<150 mg/dl (<1.7 mmol/l)	
Blood pressure	<140/90 mm Hg	

Modified from American Diabetes Association: Standards of medical care in diabetes—2014, *Diabetes Care* 37(S1):S14, 2014.

*In individuals with overt CVD, a lower LDL cholesterol goal of <70 mg/dl (1.8 mmol/l), using a high dose of a statin, is an option.

support. Monitoring glucose, A1C and lipid levels, blood pressure, weight, and quality-of-life issues is essential in evaluating the success of nutrition-related recommendations. If desired outcomes from MNT are not met, changes in overall diabetes care and management should be recommended (Evert et al, 2013). Effective nutrition therapy interventions may be implemented in individualized sessions or in a comprehensive diabetes education program.

The Academy of Nutrition and Dietetics (AND) published evidence-based nutrition practice guidelines (EBNPG) for T1DM and T2DM in adults in their Evidence Analysis Library and in print (AND, 2008a; Franz et al, 2010). The ADA nutrition recommendations are published in a position statement and are summarized in their annual standards of care (Evert et al, 2013; ADA, 2014b).

Goals and Desired Outcomes

The goals for MNT for diabetes emphasize the role of lifestyle in improving glucose control, lipid and lipoprotein profiles, and blood pressure. Goals of MNT are summarized in Box 30-1. Medicare reimburses qualified RDN providers for providing evidence-based MNT for diabetes management to eligible participants. Improving health through food choices and physical activity is the basis of all nutrition recommendations for the treatment of diabetes.

Besides being skilled and knowledgeable in assessing and implementing MNT, RDNs also must be aware of expected outcomes from MNT, when to assess outcomes, and what feedback, including recommendations, should be given to referral sources. Furthermore, the effect of MNT on A1C will be known by 6 weeks to 3 months, at which time the RDN must assess whether the goals of therapy have been met by changes in lifestyle or whether changes or additional medications are needed (Evert et al, 2013; AND, 2008a).

Multiple research studies support MNT as an effective therapy in reaching diabetes treatment goals. MNT implemented by RDNs reduced A1C levels by an average of 1% to 2% depending on the type and duration of diabetes and the A1C level at implementation (Pastors and Franz, 2012). These outcomes are similar or greater to those from glucose-lowering medications. MNT also is reported to improve lipid profiles, decrease blood

pressure, promote weight loss, decreased need for medications, and decrease risk of onset and progression to diabetes-related comorbidities. A variety of nutrition therapy interventions such as reduced energy/fat intake, carbohydrate counting, simplified meal plans, healthy food or exchange choices, use of insulin-to-carbohydrate ratios, physical activity, and/or behavioral strategies can be implemented. A unified focus of MNT for T2DM is a reduced energy intake and for T1DM carbohydrate counting is used to adjust bolus (premeal) insulin doses (insulin-to-carbohydrate ratios).

Energy Balance and Weight Management

Facilitating the achieving and maintaining of body weight goals is another important focus of MNT for diabetes. Provision of adequate calories for normal growth and development for children and adolescents with T1DM is a key component of MNT. Therefore it is important to monitor growth by measuring height and weight every 3 months and recording it on growth charts (Chiang et al, 2014). Although caloric requirements based on age, sex, and activity level are available, assessing usual calorie and nutrient intake is recommended. Usual caloric intake then can be adjusted to accommodate growth or to prevent excessive weight gain. For youth with T2DM, nutrition therapy goals include ceasing of excessive weight gain with normal linear growth. For adults with T1DM, attention to weight goals is also important.

Overweight and obesity are, however, common health problems in persons at risk for and with T2DM. Weight loss frequently is recommended as the solution to improve glycemic control (Evert et al, 2013). Weight loss interventions implemented in persons with prediabetes and newly diagnosed with T2DM have been shown to be effective in improving glycemic control, but the benefit of weight loss interventions in T2DM of longer duration is controversial (Franz, 2013). The AND EBNPG reported that approximately half of the weight loss intervention studies in persons with T2DM improved A1C at 1 year and one-half did not (AND, 2008a). In the weight loss studies lasting 1 year or longer reviewed by the ADA only 2 study groups achieved weight losses of 5% or greater: a Mediterranean-style eating pattern (−6.2 kg) in persons with newly diagnosed diabetes and the intensive lifestyle intervention in the Look AHEAD (Action for Health in Diabetes) (−8.4 kg) (Esposito et al, 2009; Look AHEAD Research Group, 2010). The other weight loss interventions resulted in weight losses of less than 5% (4.8 kg or less) at 1 year (Evert et al, 2013). The weight losses greater than 5% resulted in consistent improvements in A1C, lipids, and blood pressure; however, weight losses less than 5% did not result in consistent 1 year improvements in A1C, lipids, or blood pressure (AND, 2008a; Franz, 2013). Furthermore, it appears to be more difficult for persons with diabetes to lose weight. In a systematic review of 80 studies with 26,455 participants primarily without diabetes, the average weight loss was 7.5 kg (8% of baseline weight) (Franz et al, 2007). Therefore the RDN should collaborate with individuals who have diabetes to integrate nutrient-dense eating patterns that focus on a reduced energy intake (which may or may not lead to weight loss) and regular physical activity. Support for lifestyle changes is also essential.

Bariatric Surgery

Bariatric surgery can be an effective weight loss treatment for severely obese patients with T2DM and can result in marked

---

BOX 30-1   Goals of Medical Nutrition Therapy that Apply to Adults with Diabetes

1. To promote and support healthful eating patterns, emphasizing a variety of nutrient-dense foods in appropriate portion sizes, to improve overall diet and specifically to:
   - Attain individualized glucose, blood pressure, and lipids goals
   - Achieve and maintain body weight goals
   - Delay or prevent complications of diabetes
2. To address individual nutrition needs based on personal and cultural preferences, health literacy and numeracy, access to healthful food choices, willingness and ability to make behavioral changes.
3. To maintain the pleasure of eating by providing positive messages about food choices while limiting food choices only when indicated by scientific evidence.
4. To provide the individual with diabetes with practical tools for day-to-day meal planning rather than focusing on individual macronutrients, micronutrients, or single foods.

Adapted from Evert AB et al: Nutrition therapy recommendations for the management of adults with diabetes, *Diabetes Care* 36:3821, 2013.

improvements in glycemia (Schauer et al, 2014). The ADA states it may be considered for adults with BMI of at least 35 kg/m2 and T2DM, especially if the diabetes or associated comorbidities are difficult to control with lifestyle and pharmacologic therapy (ADA, 2014b). In 4434 adults with T2DM, gastric bypass surgery resulted in 68.2% initial complete diabetes remission within 5 years after surgery (Arterburn et al, 2013). However, 35.1% had redeveloped diabetes within the next 5 years and the median duration of remission was 8.3 years. Predictors of relapse were poor preoperative glycemic control, insulin use, and longer diabetes duration.

Macronutrient Percentages and Eating Patterns

Although numerous studies have attempted to identify the optimal percentages of macronutrients for the Eating Plan of persons with diabetes, review of the evidence shows clearly that there is not an ideal percentage of calories from carbohydrate, protein, and fat for all persons with diabetes (Evert et al, 2013). Total energy intake rather than the source of the energy is the priority. However, even total energy intake is determined by changes that the individual with diabetes is willing and able to make.

The ADA also reviewed research on eating patterns (Mediterranean-style, vegetarian and vegan, low-fat, low-carbohydrate, and DASH) implemented for diabetes management and concluded that a variety of eating patterns are acceptable (Evert et al, 2013). The RDN must take into consideration personal preferences and metabolic goals when recommending one eating pattern over another.

Because macronutrients require insulin for metabolism and influence healthy eating, they still, however, must be reviewed. Although numerous factors influence glycemic response to foods, monitoring total grams of carbohydrates, whether by use of carbohydrate counting or experienced based estimation remains a key strategy in achieving glycemic control (Evert et al, 2013). Evidence exists that the quantity and type of carbohydrate eaten influence blood glucose levels; however, the total amount of carbohydrate eaten is the primary predictor of glycemic response. Day-to-day consistency in the amount of carbohydrate eaten at meals and snacks is reported to improve glycemic control, especially in persons on either MNT alone, glucose-lowering medications, or fixed insulin regimens. Whereas in persons with T1DM or T2DM who adjust their mealtime insulin doses or who are on insulin pump therapy, insulin doses should be adjusted to match carbohydrate intake (Evert et al, 2013).

Carbohydrate counting is an Eating Plan method based on the principle that all types of carbohydrate (except fiber) are digested with the majority being absorbed into the bloodstream as molecules of glucose and that the total amount of carbohydrate consumed has a greater effect on blood glucose elevations than the specific type. Carbohydrate foods include starches, such as breads, cereals, pasta, rice, beans and lentils, starchy vegetables, crackers, and snack chips; fruits and fruit juices; milk, milk substitutes and yogurt; and sweets and desserts. One carbohydrate choice or serving is a portion of food containing 15 grams of carbohydrate. A RDN and the person with diabetes collaboratively create an eating plan that lists the number of carbohydrate choices to be selected for meals and, if desired, for snacks. Individuals are encouraged to keep protein and fat food sources as consistent as possible because they do not greatly affect blood glucose levels even though they require insulin for

metabolism. Energy needs determine daily total servings of macronutrients.

There are two main Eating Plans using carbohydrate counting; using insulin-to-carbohydrate ratios to adjust premeal insulin doses for variable carbohydrate intake (physiologic insulin regimens), or following a consistent carbohydrate Eating Plan when using fixed insulin regimens. Testing premeal and postmeal glucose levels is important for making adjustments in either food intake or medication to achieve glucose goals.

Carbohydrate Intake

Sugars, *starch*, and *fiber* are the preferred carbohydrate terms. As noted earlier, blood glucose levels after eating are determined primarily by the rate of appearance of glucose from carbohydrate digestion and absorption into the bloodstream, and the ability of insulin to clear glucose from the circulation. Low-carbohydrate diets may seem to be a logical approach to lowering postprandial glucose. However, foods that contain carbohydrates (whole grains, legumes, fruits, vegetables, and low-fat milk) are excellent sources of vitamins, minerals, dietary fiber, and energy and are encouraged over other sources of carbohydrates, or sources with added fats, sugars, or sodium to improve overall nutrient intake (Evert et al, 2013).

The long-held belief that sucrose must be restricted based on the assumption that sugars are more rapidly digested and absorbed than starches is not justified. The total amount of carbohydrate eaten at a meal, regardless if the source is starch or sucrose, is the primary determinant of postprandial glucose levels. The glycemic effect of carbohydrate foods cannot be predicted based on their structure (i.e., starch versus sugar) owing to the efficiency of the human digestive tract in reducing starch polymers to glucose. Starches are rapidly metabolized into 100% glucose during digestion, in contrast to sucrose, which is metabolized into only approximately 50% glucose and approximately 50% fructose. Fructose has a lower glycemic response, which has been attributed to its slow rate of absorption and its storage in the liver as glycogen. Sucrose-containing foods can be substituted for isocaloric amounts of other carbohydrate foods. However, as for the general population, care should be taken to avoid excess energy intake and to avoid displacing nutrient-dense food choices. The ADA advises that people with or at risk for diabetes avoid sugar-sweetened beverages (soft drinks, fruit drinks, energy and vitamin-type water drinks containing sucrose, high-fructose corn syrup, and/or fruit juice concentrates) to reduce the risk of worsening the cardiometabolic risk profile and to prevent weight gain.

Glycemic Index and Glycemic Load

The glycemic index (GI) of food was developed to compare the physiologic effects of carbohydrates on glucose. The GI measures the relative area under the postprandial glucose curve of 50 g of digestible carbohydrates compared with 50 g of a standard food, either glucose or white bread. When bread is the reference food, the GI value for the food is multiplied by 0.7 to obtain the GI value that is comparable to glucose being used as the reference food (GI of glucose = 100; GI of white bread = 70.) The GI does not measure how rapidly blood glucose levels increase. The peak glucose response for individual foods and meals, either high or low GI, occurs at approximately the same time (Brand-Miller et al, 2009).

The estimated glycemic load (GL) of foods, meals, and dietary patterns is calculated by multiplying the GI by the amount of available carbohydrate (divided by 100) in each food and then totaling the values for all foods in a meal or dietary pattern. For example, two slices of white bread with a GI of 75 and 30 g of carbohydrate has a GL of 22.5 (75 × 30/100 = 22.5) (see Appendix 37 for GI and GL of foods).

In studies comparing low- and high-GI diets, total carbohydrate first is kept consistent. The ADA systematic review of macronutrients concluded that, in general, there is little difference between low-GI and high-GI or other diets in terms of glycemic control and cardiovascular risk (Wheeler et al, 2012). The review notes that a slight improvement in glycemia may result from a lower-GI diet; however, confounding by higher fiber is not accounted for in some of the studies. A major problem with the GI is the variability of response to a specific carbohydrate food. For example, the mean glycemic response and standard deviation of 50 grams of carbohydrate from white bread tested in 23 subjects was 78 ± 73 with an individual coefficient of variation (CV) of 94%. Although the average GI of bread from three tests was 71%, the range of GI values was broad, ranging from 44 to 132 and the CV was 34% (Vega-López et al, 2007).

Studies are complicated further by differing definitions of "high GI" or "low GI" diets or quartiles. GIs in the low GI diets range from 38% to 77% and in the high GI diets from 63% to 98%. More recently, two trials, each 1 year in duration, reported no significant differences in A1C levels from a low GI versus high GI diet or a more usual diet (Ma et al, 2008; Wolever et al, 2008). Furthermore, most people appear to consume a moderate GI diet. It is unknown if reducing the usual GI by a few percentage points will result in improved glycemic control.

Fiber and Whole Grains

Evidence is lacking to recommend a higher fiber intake for people with diabetes than for the population as a whole. Thus recommendations for fiber intake for people with diabetes are similar to the recommendations for the general public. Although diets containing 44 to 50 g of fiber daily improve glycemia, more usual fiber intakes (up to 24 g daily) have not shown beneficial effects. It is unknown if free-living individuals can daily consume the amount of fiber needed to improve glycemia. However, consuming foods containing 25 g fiber per day for adult women and 38 g per day for adult men is encouraged (Evert et al, 2013). As with the general population, individuals with diabetes should consume at least half of all grains as whole grains.

Grams of fiber (and sugar alcohols) are included on food labels and are calculated as having about half the energy (2 kcal/g) of most other carbohydrates (4 kcal/g.) However, for most people, it is not necessary to subtract the amount of dietary fiber (or sugar alcohols) when carbohydrate counting (Evert et al, 2013). Adjustments in carbohydrate intake values is practical only if the amount per serving is more than 5 g. In that case, counting half of the carbohydrate grams from fiber (and sugar alcohols) would be useful in calculating food choices for food labels or recipes.

Non-nutritive and Hypocaloric Sweeteners

Reduced calorie sweeteners approved by the Food and Drug Administration (FDA) include sugar alcohols (erythritol, sorbitol, mannitol, xylitol, isomalt, lactitol, and hydrogenated starch hydrolysates) and tagatose. They produce a lower glycemic response and contain, on average, 2 calories per gram. There is no evidence that the amounts of sugar alcohols likely to be consumed will reduce glycemia or energy intake. Although their use appears to be safe, some people report gastric discomfort after eating foods sweetened with these products, and consuming large quantities may cause diarrhea, especially in children.

Saccharin, aspartame, neotame, acesulfame potassium, and sucralose are non-nutritive sweeteners currently approved for use by the FDA. All such products must undergo rigorous testing by the manufacturer and scrutiny from the FDA for effectiveness and safety before they are approved and marketed to the public. For all food additives, including non-nutritive sweeteners, the FDA determines an *acceptable daily intake* (ADI), defined as the amount of a food additive that can be consumed safely on a daily basis over a person's lifetime without risk. The ADI generally includes a 100-fold safety factor and greatly exceeds average consumption levels. For example, aspartame actual daily intake in persons with diabetes is 2 to 4 mg/kg of body weight daily, well below the ADI of 50 mg/kg daily. The stevia-derived sweetener, Rebaudioside A, and monk fruit are generally recognized as safe (GRAS) and are currently being marketed. However, as new so-called "natural" and other sweeteners (such as agave nectar) appear in the market, people with diabetes should be aware that many do contain energy and carbohydrate as do foods sweetened with them.

All FDA-approved non-nutritive sweeteners, when consumed within the established daily intake levels, can be used by persons with diabetes, including pregnant women. Furthermore, nonnutritive sweeteners could facilitate reductions in added sugars intake; thereby resulting in decreased total energy and promoting beneficial effects on related metabolic parameters (Gardner et al, 2012).

Protein Intake

The amount of protein usually consumed by persons with diabetes (15% to 20% of energy intake) has minimal acute effects on glycemic response, lipids, and hormones, and no long-term effect on insulin requirements. For people with diabetes, evidence is inconclusive to recommend an ideal amount of protein intake for optimizing glycemic control or improving CVD risk factors; therefore goals should be individualized (Evert et al, 2013).

Although nonessential amino acids undergo gluconeogenesis, in well-controlled diabetes, the glucose produced does not appear in the general circulation; the glucose produced is likely stored in the liver as glycogen. When glycolysis occurs, it is unknown if the original source of glucose was carbohydrate or protein. Although protein is just as potent a stimulant of acute insulin release as carbohydrate, it has no long-term effect on insulin needs. Adding protein to the treatment of hypoglycemia does not prevent subsequent hypoglycemia and the addition of protein only adds unnecessary and usually unwanted calories. Furthermore, protein does not slow the absorption of carbohydrates and should not be added to snacks (or meals) to prevent hypoglycemia.

Fat Intake

Evidence is also inconclusive for an ideal amount of total fat for people with diabetes and therefore goals should be individualized (Evert et al, 2013). The type of fat consumed is more important than total fat in terms of metabolic goals and influencing CVD risk. Individuals should be encouraged, however, to moderate their fat intakes to be consistent with their goals to lose or maintain weight.

Monounsaturated fatty acid (MUFA)-rich foods as a component of the Mediterranean-style eating pattern are associated with improved glycemic control and improved CVD risk factors in persons with type 2 diabetes. Controversy exists on the best ratio of omega-6 to omega-3 fatty acids; however, polyunsaturated fatty acids (PUFAs) and MUFAs are recommended as substitutes for saturated fatty acids (SFAs) or trans fatty acids. The amount of SFAs, cholesterol, and trans fat recommended for people with diabetes is the same as for the general population.

There is evidence from the general population that foods containing omega-3 fatty acids have beneficial effects on lipoproteins and prevention of heart disease. Therefore the recommendations for the general public to eat fish (particularly fatty fish) at least two times (two servings) per week is also appropriate for people with diabetes. However, evidence from RCT does not support recommending omega-3 supplements for people with diabetes for the prevention or treatment of CVD despite evidence from observational and preclinical studies (Evert et al, 2013).

Alcohol

Moderate amounts of alcohol ingested with food have minimum, if any, acute effect on glucose and insulin levels. If individuals choose to drink alcohol, daily intake should be limited to one drink or less for adult women and two drinks or less for adult men (1 drink = 12 oz beer, 5 oz of wine, or 1.5 oz of distilled spirits.) Each drink contains =15 g alcohol. The type of alcoholic beverage consumed does not make a difference. The same precautions that apply to alcohol consumption for the general population apply to persons with diabetes. Abstention from alcohol should be advised for people with a history of alcohol abuse or dependence; for women during pregnancy; and for people with medical problems such as liver disease, pancreatitis, advanced neuropathy, or severe hypertriglyceridemia.

Alcohol consumption may place people with diabetes who take insulin or insulin secretagogues at increased risk for delayed hypoglycemia. Consuming alcohol with food can minimize the risk of nocturnal hypoglycemia. Education and awareness of delayed hypoglycemia after consuming alcoholic beverages is important. Alcoholic beverages should be considered an addition to the regular food and meal plan for all persons with diabetes. No food should be omitted, given the possibility of alcohol-induced hypoglycemia and because alcohol does not require insulin to be metabolized. Excessive amounts of alcohol (three or more drinks per day) on a consistent basis, contribute to hyperglycemia which improves as soon as alcohol use is discontinued.

In persons with diabetes, light-to-moderate amounts of alcohol (1 to -2 drinks per day; 15- to 30 g of alcohol) are associated with a decreased risk of coronary heart disease, likely because of improved insulin sensitivity associated with alcohol consumption. Ingestion of light-to-moderate amounts of alcohol does not raise blood pressure or triglycerides; whereas excessive, chronic ingestion of alcohol does raise blood pressure and may be a risk factor for stroke.

Micronutrients and Herbal Supplements

No clear evidence has been established for benefits from vitamin or mineral supplements in persons with diabetes (compared with the general population) who do not have underlying deficiencies (Evert et al, 2013). Because diabetes may be a state of increased oxidative stress, there has been interest in prescribing antioxidant vitamins in people with diabetes. Clinical trial data not only indicate the lack of benefit from antioxidants on glycemic control and progression of complications but also provide evidence of the potential harm. Therefore routine supplementation is not advised. At this time there is also insufficient evidence to support the routine use of micronutrients such as chromium, magnesium, and vitamin D as well as use of cinnamon or other herbs/supplements for the treatment of diabetes.

In addition, herbal products are not standardized and vary in their content of active ingredients and have the potential to interact with and potentiate the effect of other medications. Therefore it is important that people with diabetes report the use of supplements and herbal products to their health care provider/RDN. Without well-designed clinical trials to prove efficacy, the benefit of pharmacologic doses of supplements is unknown, and findings from small clinical and animal studies frequently are extrapolated to clinical practice.

Physical Activity/Exercise

Physical activity involves bodily movement produced by the contraction of skeletal muscles that requires energy expenditure in excess of resting energy expenditure. Exercise is a subset of physical activity: planned, structured, and repetitive bodily movement performed to improve or maintain one or more components of physical fitness. Aerobic exercise consists of rhythmic, repeated, and continuous movements of the same large muscle groups for at least 10 minutes at a time. Examples include walking, bicycling, jogging, swimming, and many sports. Resistance exercise consists of activities that use muscular strength to move a weight or work against a resistive load. Examples include weight lifting and exercises using resistance-providing machines.

Physical activity should be an integral part of the treatment plan for persons with diabetes. Exercise helps all persons with diabetes improve insulin sensitivity, reduce cardiovascular risk factors, control weight, and improve well-being. Given appropriate guidelines, the majority of people with diabetes can exercise safely. The activity plan will vary, depending on interest, age, general health, and level of physical fitness.

Despite the increase in glucose uptake by muscles during exercise, glucose levels change little in individuals without diabetes. Muscular work causes insulin levels to decline, while counterregulatory hormones (primarily glucagon) rise. As a result, the increased glucose use by the exercising muscles is matched with increased glucose production by the liver. This balance between insulin and counterregulatory hormones is the major determinant of hepatic glucose production, underscoring the need for insulin adjustments in addition to adequate carbohydrate intake during exercise for people with diabetes.

In persons with T1DM, the glycemic response to exercise varies, depending on overall diabetes control, plasma glucose and insulin levels at the start of exercise; timing, intensity, and duration of the exercise; previous food intake; and previous conditioning. An important variable is the level of plasma insulin during and after exercise. Hypoglycemia can occur because of insulin-enhanced muscle glucose uptake by the exercising muscle.

In persons with T2DM, blood glucose control can improve with physical activity, largely because of decreased insulin resistance and increased insulin sensitivity, which results in increased peripheral use of glucose not only during but also after the activity. This exercise-induced enhanced insulin sensitivity occurs independent of any effect on body weight. Structured exercise interventions of at least 8 weeks' duration are reported to lower A1C. Exercise also decreases the effects of counterregulatory hormones; this, in turn, reduces the hepatic glucose output, contributing to improved glucose control.

Potential Problems with Exercise

Hypoglycemia is a potential problem associated with exercise in persons taking insulin or insulin secretagogues. Hypoglycemia can occur during, immediately after, or many hours after exercise. Hypoglycemia has been reported to be more common after exercise—especially exercise of long duration—strenuous activity or play, or sporadic exercise, than it is during exercise. This is because of increased insulin sensitivity after exercise and the need to replete liver and muscle glycogen, which can take up to 24 to 30 hours (see Chapter 23).

Blood glucose levels before exercise reflect only the value at that time, and it is unknown if this is a stable blood glucose level or a blood glucose level that is dropping. If blood glucose levels are dropping before exercise, adding exercise can contribute to hypoglycemia during exercise. Furthermore, hypoglycemia on the day before exercise may increase the risk of hypoglycemia on the day of exercise as well.

Hyperglycemia also can result from exercise of high intensity, likely because the effects of counterregulatory hormones. When a person exercises at what for him or her is a high level of exercise intensity, there is a greater-than-normal increase in counterregulatory hormones. As a result, hepatic glucose release exceeds the rise in glucose use. The elevated glucose levels also may extend into the postexercise state. Hyperglycemia and worsening ketosis also can result in persons with T1DM who are deprived of insulin for 12 to 48 hours and are ketotic. Vigorous activity should be avoided in the presence of ketosis (ADA, 2014b). It is not, however, necessary to postpone exercise based simply on hyperglycemia, provided the individual feels well and urine and/or blood ketones are negative. High-intensity exercise is more likely to be the cause of hyperglycemia than insulin deficiency.

Exercise Guidelines

The variability of glucose responses to exercise contributes to the difficulty in giving precise guidelines for exercising safely. Frequent blood glucose monitoring before, during, and after exercise helps individuals identify their response to physical activities. To meet their individual needs, individuals must modify general guidelines to reduce insulin doses before (or after) or ingest carbohydrates after (or before) exercise. Similar to the general population without diabetes, it is also important for individuals with diabetes to stay hydrated when performing physical activities.

Carbohydrate for Insulin or Insulin Secretagogue Users. During moderate-intensity exercise, glucose uptake is increased by 8 to 13 g/hr; this is the basis for the recommendation to add 15 g carbohydrate for every 30 to 60 minutes of activity (depending on the intensity) over and above normal routines. Moderate exercise for less than 30 minutes usually does not require any additional carbohydrate or insulin adjustment, unless the individual is hypoglycemic before the start of exercise. Added carbohydrates should be ingested if pre-exercise glucose levels are less than 100 mg/dl (5.6 mmol/L). Supplementary carbohydrate is generally not needed in individuals

with T2DM who are not treated with insulin or insulin secretagogues; it simply adds unnecessary calories (ADA, 2014b).

In all persons, blood glucose levels decline gradually during exercise, and ingesting a carbohydrate feeding during prolonged exercise can improve performance by maintaining the availability and oxidation of blood glucose. For the exerciser with diabetes whose blood glucose levels may drop sooner and lower than the exerciser without diabetes, ingesting carbohydrate after 40 to 60 minutes of exercise is important and also may assist in preventing hypoglycemia. Drinks containing 6% or less of carbohydrates empty from the stomach as quickly as water and have the advantage of providing both needed fluids and carbohydrates. Consuming carbohydrates immediately after exercise optimizes repletion of muscle and liver glycogen stores. For the exerciser with diabetes, this takes on added importance because of increased risk for late-onset hypoglycemia.

Insulin Guidelines. It is often necessary to adjust the insulin dosage to prevent hypoglycemia. This occurs most often with moderate to strenuous activity lasting more than 45 to 60 minutes. For most persons a modest decrease (of about 1 to 2 units) in the rapid- (or short-) acting insulin during the period of exercise is a good starting point. For prolonged vigorous exercise, a larger decrease in the total daily insulin dosage may be necessary. After exercise, insulin dosing also may have to be decreased.

Precautions for Persons with Type 2 Diabetes. Persons with T2DM may have a lower VO_{2max} and therefore need a more gradual training program. Rest periods may be needed, but this does not impair the training effect from physical activity. Autonomic neuropathy or medications, such as for blood pressure, may not allow for increased heart rate, and individuals must learn to use perceived exertion as a means of determining exercise intensity. Blood pressure also may increase more in persons with diabetes than in those who do not have diabetes, and exercise should not be undertaken if systolic blood pressure is greater than 180 to 200 mm Hg (ADA, 2014b).

Exercise Recommendations

Adults with diabetes should be advised to perform at least 150 min/week of moderate-intensity aerobic physical activity (50% to 70% of maximum heart rate), or at least 90 min/week of vigorous aerobic exercise (more than 70% of maximum heart rate), spread over at least 3 days/week with no more than 2 consecutive days without physical activity. In the absence of contraindications, adults with T2DM should be encouraged to perform resistance exercise at least twice per week with each session consisting of at least one set of five or more different resistance exercises involving large muscle groups. There is an additive benefit of combined aerobic and resistance training in adults with T2DM. Children with diabetes or prediabetes should be encouraged to engage in at least 60 min/day of physical activity (ADA, 2014b).

Routine screening pre-exercise is not recommended. Providers should use clinical judgment in this area. High-risk patients should be encouraged to start with short periods of low-intensity exercise and increase the intensity and duration slowly (ADA, 2014b).

Medications

A consensus statement on the approach to management of hyperglycemia in T2DM has been published by the ADA and the European Association for the Study of Diabetes (Inzucchi et al, 2015). Interventions at the time of diagnosis include healthy eating, weight control, physical activity, and diabetes education. Metformin is the preferred initial pharmacologic agent for type 2 diabetes, either in addition to lifestyle counseling and support for weight loss and physical activity, or when lifestyle efforts alone have not achieved or maintained glycemic goals. If A1C target goals are not reached after approximately 3 months, a second oral agent, a glucagon-like peptide 1 (GLP-1) receptor agent, or basal insulin is added. If A1C goals are not reached after another approximately 3 months, a three-drug intervention is implemented. If this combination therapy that includes a long-acting insulin does not achieve A1C goals, a more complex insulin therapy involving multiple daily doses, usually in combination with one or more noninsulin agents, is implemented. A patient-centered approach is stressed, including patient preferences, cost and potential side effects (ADA, 2014b). The overall objective is to achieve and maintain glycemic control and to change interventions, including the use of insulin, when therapeutic goals are not being met.

All persons with T1DM and many persons with T2DM who no longer produce adequate endogenous insulin need replacement of insulin. Circumstances that require the use of insulin in T2DM include the failure to achieve adequate control with administration of glucose-lowering medications; periods of acute injury, infection, extreme heat exposure, surgery, or pregnancy.

Glucose-Lowering Medications for Type 2 Diabetes

Understanding that T2DM is a progressive disease is important for the understanding of treatment choices. Assisting individuals with diabetes to understand the disease process also helps them to understand and accept changes in medications that occur over time. Diabetes is first diagnosed when there is insufficient insulin available to maintain euglycemia, and as insulin deficiency progresses, medications and eventually insulin will be required to achieve glycemic goals. This is not a "diet failure" or a "medication failure" but rather a failure of the insulin secreting capacity of the beta-cells.

Glucose-lowering medications target different aspects of the pathogenesis of T2DM—insulin resistance at the cellular level, incretin system defects, endogenous insulin deficiency, elevated levels of glucagon, and excessive hepatic glucose release. Because the mechanisms of action differ, the medications can be used alone or in combination. Table 30-5 lists the generic and brand names of glucose-lowering medications and their principal sites of action for persons with T2DM.

Biguanides. Metformin is the most widely used first-line type 2 medication. It suppresses hepatic glucose production, is not associated with hypoglycemia, may cause small weight losses when therapy begins, and is relatively inexpensive. The most common side effects are gastrointestinal, which often

	TABLE 30-5	Glucose-Lowering Medications for Type 2 Diabetes		
Class	**Brand Name**	**Site and Mechanism of Action**	**Adverse Effects/Nutrition Considerations**	
Biguanide	Metformin (Glucophage) Metformin Extended Release (Glucophage XR)	Liver Decrease hepatic glucose production and may help reduce insulin resistance	Nausea, vomiting, diarrhea, and gas May be able to reduce side effects by slowly increasing dose and taking with a meal	
Sulfonylureas (second-generation)	Glipizide (Glucotrol) Glipizide (Glucotrol XL) Glyburide (Glynase Prestabs) Glimepiride (Amaryl)	Pancreas Stimulate insulin secretion from the beta-cells	Hypoglycemia	
Meglitinides (Glinides)	Repaglinide (Prandin) Nateglinide (Starlix)	Pancreas Stimulate insulin secretion from beta-cells	Hypoglycemia	
Thiazolidinediones	Pioglitazone (Actos) Rosiglitazone (Avandia)	Muscle Improve peripheral insulin sensitivity	Weight gain, fluid retention	
Glucagon-like peptide-1 (GLP-1) Receptor Agonists	Exenatide (Byetta) Exenatide Extended Release (Bydureon) Liraglutide (Victoza) Albiglutide (Tanzeum) Dulaglutide (Trulicity)	Pancreas, liver, and gastrointestinal tract Enhances glucose-dependent insulin secretion Suppresses postprandial glucagon secretion Slows gastric emptying Increases satiety	Nausea, vomiting, and hypoglycemia if taken with a sulfonylurea or insulin Exenatide can be injected up to 60 minutes before meal. If nausea and/or vomiting occur, try moving injection closer to meal: 10-20 minutes or immediately before eating	
Dipeptidyl peptidase-4 (DPP-4) inhibitors	Sitaglipton (Januvia) Saxagliptin (Onglyza) Linagliptin (Tradjenta) Alogliptin (Nesina)	Pancreas and liver Enhance the effects of GLP-1 and GIP by preventing degradation	No major side effects Possible cold symptoms	
Alpha glucosidase inhibitors	Acarbose (Precose) Miglitol (Glyset)	Small intestine Delay carbohydrate absorption	Diarrhea, gas, and nausea (can lessen effects by slowly increasing dose) If mild to moderate hypoglycemia occurs in combination with another antidiabetic drug such as a sulfonylurea or insulin, the hypoglycemia should be treated with oral glucose (dextrose) instead of sucrose (table sugar) because the drug blocks the digestion of sucrose to glucose.	

Continued

Class	Brand Name	Site and Mechanism of Action	Adverse Effects/Nutrition Considerations
Amylin agonists	Pramlintide (Symlin)	Liver, gastrointestinal tract, brain Decreases glucagon production, which decreases mealtime hepatic glucose release and prevents postprandial hyperglycemia	Bladder infections
Sodium-glucose transport protein inhibitors (SGLT)	Canagliflozin (Invokana) Dapagliflozin (Farxiga) Empagligloxin (Jardiance)	Kidney Reduces the reabsorption of glucose in the kidneys via sodium glucose cotransporter-2 (SGLT2) inhibition	Constipation, diarrhea, nausea, urinary frequency and genitourinary infections
Insulins	See Table 30-6	Supplements endogenous insulin	Hypoglycemia

TABLE 30-5   Glucose-Lowering Medications for Type 2 Diabetes—cont'd

Adapted from Inzucchi SE et al: Management of hyperglycemia in type 2 diabetes: a patient-centered approach, *Diabetes Care* 35:1364, 2012.

disappear with time. To minimize these effects, the medication should be taken with food consumption and the smallest dose (500 mg) given twice a day for a week and gradually increased to maximum doses. A rare side effect is severe lactic acidosis, which can be fatal. The acidosis usually occurs in patients who use alcohol excessively, have renal dysfunction, or have liver impairments.

Sulfonylureas. The sulfonylureas are insulin secretagogues and promote insulin secretion by the beta-cells of the pancreas. First- and second-generation sulfonylurea drugs differ from one another in their potency, pharmacokinetics, and metabolism. Disadvantages of their use include weight gain and the potential to cause hypoglycemia. They have the advantage of being inexpensive.

Thiazolidinediones (TZDs). Thiazolidinediones (TZDs) or glitazones (pioglitazone [Actos] and rosiglitazone [Avandia]) decrease insulin resistance in peripheral tissues and thus enhance the ability of muscle and fat cells to take up glucose. TZDs also have a favorable effect on lipids and do not independently cause hypoglycemia. Adverse effects include weight gain, fluid retention leading to edema and/or heart failure, and increased risk of bone fractures.

Glucagon-like Peptide-1 (GLP-1) Receptor Agonist. Incretins are hormones made by the gastrointestinal tract and includes GLP-1. GLP-1 is released during nutrient absorption, which increases glucose-dependent insulin secretion, slows gastric emptying, decreases glucagon production, and enhances satiety. Exenatide (Byetta) and liraglutide (Victoza) are synthetic drugs that have many of the same glucose lowering effects as the body's naturally occurring incretin, GLP-1. A primary benefit is weight loss (liraglutide has also been approved as a weight-loss drug). Typically exenatide is injected twice a day, at breakfast and at the evening meal and liraglutide is injected once a day, at any time, independent of meals. There are two once-weekly injection GLP-1s: exenatide extended (Bydureon) and dulaglutide (Trulicity).

Dipeptidyl Peptidase 4 Inhibitors (DPP-4). GLP-1 and glucose-dependent insulinotropic peptide (GIP), the main intestinal stimulants of insulin are rapidly degraded by DPP-4. As a result, incretins have very short half-lives of 2 to 3 minutes. DPP-4 inhibitors prolong their half-lives. Oral DPP-4 inhibitors are sitagliptin (Januvia), saxagliptin (Onglyza), linagliptin (Tradjenta), and alogliptin (Nesina). They have a modest effect on A1C; however, advantages include being weight neutral and relatively well tolerated. Furthermore, they do not cause hypoglycemia when used as monotherapy.

Alpha Glucosidase Inhibitors. Acarbose (Precose) and miglitol (Glyset) are alpha-glucosidase inhibitors that work in the small intestine to inhibit enzymes that digest carbohydrates, thereby delaying carbohydrate absorption and lowering postprandial glycemia. They do not cause hypoglycemia or weight gain when used alone, but they can frequently cause flatulence, diarrhea, cramping, or abdominal pain. Symptoms may be alleviated by initiating therapy at a low dose and gradually increasing the dose to therapeutic levels.

Glinides. The meglitinides repaglinide (Prandin) and nateglinide (Starlix) differ from the sulfonylureas in that they have short metabolic half-lives, which result in brief episodic stimulation of insulin secretion. They are given before meals decreasing postprandial glucose excursions and less risk of hypoglycemia. Nateglinide only works in the presence of glucose and is a somewhat less potent secretagogue. Risk of weight gain is similar to sulfonylureas.

Sodium-Glucose Transporter 2 (SGLT-2) Inhibitors. Canagliflozin (Invokana), dapagliflozin (Farxiga) and empaglifloxin (Jardiance) are drugs in a new class that target blood glucose lowering action in the kidneys. SGLT-2 inhibitors block a transporter protein that returns glucose to the bloodstream after it is filtered through the kidneys. Blocking this protein causes more glucose to be flushed out in the urine. Used independently it does not cause hypoglycemia or weight gain.

Amylin Agonists (Pramlintide). Pramlintide (Symlin) is a synthetic analog of the hormone amylin, a hormone normally cosecreted with insulin by the beta-cell in response to food that is deficient in people with T1DM and T2DM. It is injected before meals slowing gastric emptying and inhibiting glucagon production, resulting in a decrease in postprandial glucose excursions, which is related to a decrease in glucagon production from the pancreatic alpha cells. It must be injected separately from insulin.

Insulin. Insulin strategies for persons with T2DM may begin with basal insulin at bedtime to suppress nocturnal hepatic glucose production and to normalize fasting glucose levels. Glucose-lowering medications usually are continued during the day. The next step is to add one mealtime rapid-acting insulin with the basal insulin or use of premixed insulin twice daily. If

A1C goals are not achieved, mealtime rapid-acting insulin is used before each meal. Insulin secretagogues usually are stopped but other glucose lowering agents may be continued.

Insulin

Insulin has three characteristics: onset, peak, and duration (see Table 30-6). U-100 is the concentration of insulin used in the United States. This means it has 100 units of insulin per milliliter of fluid (100 units/ml). U-100 syringes deliver U-100 insulin; however, insulin pens are now being used more frequently as an alternative to the traditional syringe-needle units. Humulin R U-500 (500 units/ml) is useful in the treatment of insulin-resistant patients who require daily doses more than 200 units.

Rapid-Acting Insulins. Included are insulin lispro (Humalog), insulin aspart (Novolog), and insulin glulisine (Apidra) and are used as bolus (premeal or prandial) insulins. They are insulin analogs that differ from human insulin in amino acid sequence but bind to insulin receptors and thus function in a manner similar to human insulin. To determine the accuracy of the dose, blood glucose checking is done before meals and 2 hours after the start of the meals.

Regular Insulin. A short-acting insulin with a slower onset of action and later activity peak. For best results the slow onset of regular insulin requires it to be taken 30 to 60 minutes before meals.

Intermediate-Acting Insulin. NPH is the only available intermediate-acting insulin and is cloudy in appearance.

Long-Acting Insulins. Insulin glargine (Lantus) and insulin determir (Levemir) are long-acting insulins. Insulin glargine is an insulin analog that, because of its slow dissolution at the injection site, results in a relatively constant and peakless delivery over 24 hours. Because of its acidic pH, it cannot be mixed with any other insulin in the same syringe before injection and

usually is given at bedtime. However, glargine can be given before any meal, but, whichever time is chosen, it must be given consistently at that time. Insulin determir is absorbed from the subcutaneous tissue relatively quickly but then binds to albumin in the bloodstream, resulting in a prolonged action time of approximately 17 hours. Therefore it may have to be given twice a day. Basal insulin analogs decrease the chances of hypoglycemia, especially nocturnal hypoglycemia.

Premixed Insulins. Included are 70% NPH/30% regular, 75% lispro protamine (NPL [addition of neutral protamine to lispro to create an intermediate-acting insulin])/25% lispro, 50% lispro protamine and 50% lispro, and 70% protamine (addition of neutral protamine to aspart to create an immediate-acting insulin)/30% aspart. Persons using premixed insulins must eat at specific times and be consistent in carbohydrate intake to prevent hypoglycemia.

Insulin Regimens. All persons with T1DM and those with T2DM who no longer produce adequate endogenous insulin need replacement of insulin that mimics normal insulin action. After individuals without diabetes eat, their plasma glucose and insulin concentrations increase rapidly, peak in 30 to 60 minutes, and return to basal concentrations within 2 to 3 hours. To mimic this, rapid-acting (or short-acting) insulin is given before meals, and this is referred to as bolus or mealtime insulin.

Mealtime insulin doses are adjusted based on the amount of carbohydrate in the meal. An insulin-to-carbohydrate ratio can be established for an individual that will guide decisions on the amount of mealtime insulin to inject. Basal or background insulin dose is that amount of insulin required in the postabsorptive state to restrain endogenous glucose output primarily from the liver. Basal insulin also limits lipolysis and excess flux of free fatty acids to the liver. Long-acting insulins are used for basal insulin (see Figure 30-1).

TABLE 30-6 Action Times of Human Insulin Preparations

Type of Insulin	Onset of Action	Peak Action	Usual Effective Duration	Monitor Effect In
Rapid-Acting				
Insulin lispro (Humalog)	<0.25-0.5 hr	0.5-2.5 hr	3-6.5 hr	1-2 hr
Insulin aspart (NovoLog)	<0.25 hr	0.5-1.0 hr	3-5 hr	1-2 hr
Insulin glulisine (Apidra)	<0.25 hr	1-1.5 hr	3-5 hr	1-2 hr
Short-Acting				
Regular (Humulin R and Novolin R)	0.5-1 hr	2-3 hr	3-6 hr	4 hr (next meal)
Intermediate-Acting				
NPH	2-4 hr	4-10 hr	10-16 hr	8-12 hr
Long-Acting				
Insulin glargine (Lantus)	2-4 hr	Peakless	20-24 hr	10-12 hr
Insulin determir (Levemir)	0.8-2 hr (dose dependent)	Peakless	12-24 hr (dose dependent)	10-12 hr
Mixtures				
70/30 (70% NPH, 30% regular)	0.5-1 hr	Dual	10-16 hr	
Humalog Mix 75/25 (75% neutral protamine lispro [NPL], 25% lispro)	<0.25 hr	Dual	10-16 hr	
Humalog Mix 50/50 (50% protamine lispro, 50% lispro)	<0.25 hr	Dual	10-16 hr	
NovoLog Mix 70/30 (70% neutral protamine aspart [NPA], 30% aspart)	<0.25 hr	Dual	15-18 hr	

Adapted from Kaufman FR editor: *Medical management of type 1 diabetes,* ed 6, Alexandria, Va, 2012, American Diabetes Association.

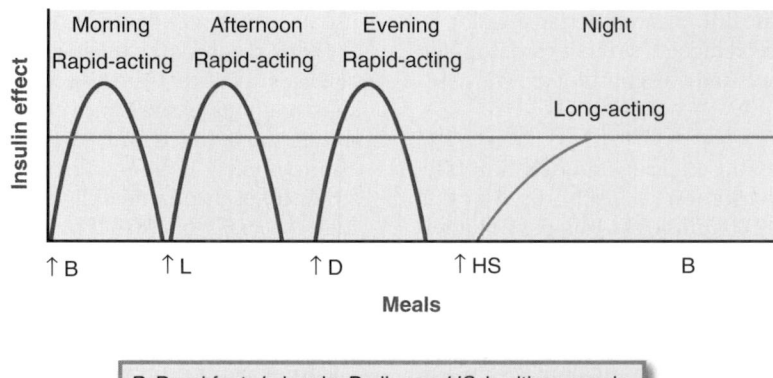

FIGURE 30-1 Time actions of flexible insulin regimens.(Modified from Kaufman FR, *editor: Medical management of type 1 diabetes, ed 6, Alexandria, Va, 2012, American Diabetes Association.*)

These physiologic insulin regimens allow increased flexibility in the type and timing of meals. For normal-weight persons with T1DM, the required insulin dosage is about 0.5 to 1 unit/kg of body weight per day. About 50% of the total daily insulin dose is used to provide for basal or background insulin needs. The remainder (rapid-acting insulin) is divided among the meals either proportionately to the carbohydrate content or by giving about 1 to 1.5 units of insulin per 10 to 15 g of carbohydrates consumed. As a result of the presence in the morning of higher levels of counterregulatory hormones many individuals may require larger doses of mealtime insulin for carbohydrates consumed at breakfast than meals later in the day. Persons with T2DM may require insulin doses in the range of 0.5 to 1.2 units/kg of body weight daily. Large doses, even more than 1.5 units/kg of body weight daily, may be required at least initially to overcome prevailing insulin resistance. The type and timing of insulin regimens should be individualized, based on eating and exercise habits and blood glucose concentrations.

Insulin Regimens: Continuous Sustained Insulin Infusion (CSII) or Insulin Pump Therapy. The insulin (usually a rapid-acting insulin) is pumped continuously by a mechanical device in micro amounts through a subcutaneous catheter. The pump delivers insulin in two ways: in a steady, measured, and continuous dose (basal insulin) and as a surge (bolus) dose before meals. Pump therapy requires a committed and motivated person who is willing to do a minimum of four blood glucose tests per day, understand increased risk of **diabetic ketoacidosis,** and learn the technical features of pump use such as the bolus calculator and "insulin-on-board" features. The individual also should be educated on MNT, including carbohydrate counting/estimation. Prandial boluses are dependent on carbohydrate intake as well as circadian variation in insulin sensitivity, current blood glucose levels, and planned physical activity. Regularly scheduled outpatient follow-up with diabetes care providers knowledgeable in the use of CSII is recommended to optimize glycemic control long term.

Self-Management Education

Diabetes management is a team effort. Persons with diabetes must be at the center of the team because they have the responsibility for day-to-day management. RDNs, nurses, physicians, and other health care providers contribute their expertise to developing therapeutic regimens that help the person with diabetes achieve the best metabolic control possible. The goal is to provide patients with the knowledge, skills, and motivation to incorporate self-management into their daily lifestyles. The Academy of Nutrition and Dietetics (AND) Evidence-Based Nutrition Practice Guidelines (EBNPG) recommends that individuals with diabetes be referred for MNT early after the diagnosis of diabetes. MNT is to be provided by a RDN in an initial series of three to four encounters each lasting 45 to 90 minutes. This series should be completed within 3 to 6 months, and the RDN should determine whether additional encounters are needed after the initial series based on the nutrition assessment of learning needs and progress toward desired outcomes. At least one follow-up encounter is recommended annually to reinforce lifestyle changes and to evaluate and monitor outcomes that affect the need for changes in MNT or medication(s). The RDN should again determine whether additional MNT encounters are needed. Although glycemic control is the primary focus for diabetes management, cardioprotective nutrition interventions for the prevention and treatment of CVD also should be implemented in the initial series of encounters (AND, 2008a; Franz et al, 2010).

Dietitians can demonstrate their specialized diabetes knowledge by obtaining certification beyond the RDN credential. Two diabetes care certifications available to RDs are the Certified Diabetes Educator (CDE), a specialty certification, and Board Certified-Advanced Diabetes Management (BC-ADM), an advanced practice certification.

Monitoring

The health care team, including the individual with diabetes, should work together to implement blood glucose monitoring and establish individual target blood glucose goals (see Table 30-3). Several methods are available to assess the effectiveness of the diabetes management plan on glycemic control: SMBG or **continuous glucose monitoring (CGM)** of interstitial glucose and A1C. SMBG is used on a day-to-day basis to manage diabetes effectively and safely; however, measurement of A1C levels provides the best available index of overall diabetes control.

Self-Monitoring of Blood Glucose (SMBG)

The ADA recommendations state that persons on multiple-dose insulin (MDI) or insulin pump therapy should do SMBG before meals and snacks, occasionally postprandially at bedtime, before exercise, when they suspect low blood glucose, after treating low blood glucose until they are normoglycemic, and before critical tasks such as driving. For persons using less frequent insulin injections or noninsulin therapies, SMBG results may be helpful to guide treatment decisions (ADA, 2014b).

The AND EBNPG for diabetes reviewed the evidence on glucose monitoring and recommended that for persons with T1DM or T2DM on insulin therapy, at least three to four glucose tests per days are needed to determine the accuracy of the insulin dose(s) and to guide adjustments in insulin dose(s), food intake, and physical activity. Once established some insulin regimens require less frequent SMBG. For persons on MNT alone or MNT in combination with glucose-lowering medications, frequency and timing are dependent on diabetes management goals and therapies.

Self-management education and training is necessary to use SMBG devices and data correctly (ADA, 2014b). Individuals must be taught how to adjust their management program based on the results of SMBG. The first step in using such records is to learn how to identify patterns in blood glucose levels taken at the same time each day that are outside the target range—generally high readings for three or more days in a row or low readings 2 days in a row. The next step is to determine whether a lifestyle factor (meal times, carbohydrate intake, quantity and time of physical activity) or medication dose adjustment is needed.

If changes in medication doses such as insulin are needed, adjustments are made in the insulin (or mediations) acting at the time of the problem glucose readings. After pattern management is mastered, algorithms for insulin dose changes to compensate for an elevated or low glucose value can be used. A commonly used formula determines the insulin sensitivity, or **correction factor (CF)**, which defines how many milligrams per deciliter a unit of rapid- (or short-acting) insulin will lower blood glucose levels over a 2- to 4-hr period (Kaufman, 2012). The CF is determined by using the "1700 rule," in which 1700 is divided by the total daily dose (TDD) of insulin the individual typically takes. For example, if the TDD is 50 units of insulin, the CF = 1700/50 = 35. In this case 1 unit of rapid-acting insulin should lower the individual's blood glucose level by 35 mg/dl (2 mmol/L).

In using blood glucose monitoring records, remember that factors other than food affect blood glucose concentrations. An increase in blood glucose can be the result of insufficient insulin or insulin secretagogue; too much food; or increases in glucagon and other counterregulatory hormones as a result of stress, illness, or infection. Factors that contribute to hypoglycemia include too much insulin or insulin secretagogue, not enough food, unusual amounts of exercise, and skipped or delayed meals. Urine glucose testing, used in the past, has so many limitations that it should not be used.

Continuous Glucose Monitoring (CGM)

CGM systems include a tiny glucose-sensing device called a sensor that is inserted under the skin in the subcutaneous fat tissue for several days at a time. The sensor measures glucose in interstitial fluid and transmits readings every 5 minutes to a monitor that is worn or carried externally. CGM devices also provide information not just on current glucose level, but also on the trend and rate of change in glucose levels (i.e., whether the glucose level is rising or falling and how quickly). Other features include alerts for glucose highs and lows and the ability to download data and track trends over time. The ADA recommends that CGM in conjunction with intensive insulin regimens can be a useful tool to lower A1C in selected adults (age of more than 25 years) with T1DM. Evidence is less strong for A1C lowering in children, teens, and younger adults; however, CGM may be also helpful in these groups (ADA, 2014b).

A1C Monitoring

A1C tests should be done at least twice a year in persons who are meeting treatment goals and have stable glycemic control. They should be done quarterly in persons whose therapy has changed or who are not meeting glycemic goals. In persons without diabetes A1C values are 4% to 6%. These values correspond to mean plasma glucose levels of approximately 70 to 126 mg/dl (3.9 to 7.0 mmol/L). Correlation between A1C levels and average glucose levels recently have been verified. An A1C of 6% reflects an average glucose level of 126 mg/dL (7.0 mmol/L). Lowering A1C to below or around 7% is a reasonable goal for many nonpregnant adults with diabetes. An A1C less than 7% has been shown to reduce cardiovascular complications of diabetes and is associated with long-term reduction of macrovascular disease (ADA, 2014b). Less stringent goals, such as less than 8% may be appropriate for individuals with advanced macrovascular and microvascular complications, history of severe hypoglycemia, or other extensive comorbid conditions.

Ketone, Lipid, and Blood Pressure Monitoring

Urine or blood testing can be used to detect ketones. Testing for ketonuria or ketonemia should be performed regularly during periods of illness and when blood glucose levels consistently exceed 240 mg/dl (13.3 mmol/L). The presence of persistent, moderate, or large amounts of ketones, along with elevated blood glucose levels, requires insulin adjustments. Persons with T2DM rarely have ketosis; however, ketone testing should be done when the person is seriously ill.

For most adults, lipids should be measured at least annually; however, in adults with low-risk lipid values, assessments may be repeated every 2 years. Blood pressure should be measured at every routine diabetes visit (ADA, 2014b).

IMPLEMENTING THE NUTRITION CARE PROCESS

The nutrition care process (NCP) articulates the consistent and specific steps used to deliver MNT (AND, 2012). For some individuals with diabetes MNT will be implemented in individual sessions and for others in group sessions. Providing nutrition interventions in groups is becoming increasingly important; however, group interventions must also allow for individualization of MNT and evaluation of outcomes. The following sections review implementation of individual MNT.

Nutrition Assessment

The nutrition assessment involves obtaining information before and during the encounter needed to identify nutrition-related problems. Assessment data can be obtained from the referral source or the patient's medical records and from the patient/client. Patient/client data can be collected from forms the patient completes before the first encounter or directly from the patient. By collecting as much data as possible before the first session, completion of the assessment and implementation of interventions can begin more efficiently. Nutrition assessment is an ongoing process that involves not only initial data collection but also reassessment and analysis of patient data and needs. Box 30-2 provides a summary of assessment categories (Franz et al, 2012).

The AND EBNPG for diabetes highlights three specific assessment recommendations. First, the RDN should assess food intake (focusing on carbohydrates) medication, metabolic control (glycemia, lipids, and blood pressure), anthropometric measurements, and physical activity as the basis for the implementation of the nutrition prescription, goals, and interventions (see Chapters 4 and 7). Second, the RDN should assess glycemic control and focus MNT to achieve and maintain blood glucose levels in the target range. However, the need for cardioprotective nutrition interventions also should be assessed. Third, the RDN should assess the relative importance of weight management for persons with diabetes who are overweight or obese. Although modest weight loss has been shown to improve insulin resistance in overweight and obese insulin-resistant individuals, research on sustained weight loss interventions lasting 1 year or longer report inconsistent effects on A1C (AND, 2008a).

Nutrition Diagnosis

The nutrition diagnosis identifies and describes a specific nutrition problem that can be resolved or improved through treatment/intervention by an RDN. Patients may have more than one nutrition diagnoses, in which case the RDN will need to prioritize them in the nutrition intervention step. The nutrition diagnostic language includes three domains: (1) intake problems related to the quantity of intake versus requirements, (2) clinical findings/problems related to medical (or physical) condition, and (3) behavioral-environmental findings/problems related to knowledge, attitudes/beliefs,

physical environment, and access to food. A nutrition diagnosis is written in the PES format that states the *problem* (P), the *etiology* (E), and *signs and symptoms* (S). Examples of diabetes-related nutrition diagnoses are listed in Box 30-3 (Franz et al, 2012).

Nutrition Interventions

Nutrition interventions include two distinct steps: planning the nutrition goals and implementing the actual interventions. Planning involves prioritizing the nutrition diagnoses, conferring with the persons with diabetes and others, reviewing current nutrition practice guidelines for diabetes, setting goals, determining the nutrition prescription, and choosing specific intervention strategies.

Implementation is the action phase. In the food and nutrient delivery phase, an individualized eating plan is developed and specific nutrient recommendations are included. Nutrition

---

BOX 30-2 Nutrition Assessment

Nutrition Assessment Categories

- Biochemical data, medical tests, and procedures, which include laboratory data such as for A1C, glucose, lipids, kidney function, and blood pressure measurements
- Anthropometric measurements, which include height, weight, body mass index (BMI), waist circumference, growth rate, and rate of weight change
- Client history, which includes:
  - General patient information, such as age, gender, race/ethnicity, language, literacy, and education
  - Medical/health history and medical treatment, including goals of medical therapy and prescribed medications related to medical condition for which MNT is being implemented
  - Readiness to change nutrition-related behaviors
  - Weight management goals
  - Physical activity history and goals
  - Social history, such as social and medical support, cultural and religious beliefs, and socioeconomic status
  - Other medical or surgical treatments, therapy, and alternative medicine
- Food/nutrition history
  - Food intake, nutrition and health knowledge and beliefs
  - Food availability
  - Supplement use

Modified from Franz MJ et al: *ADA pocket guide to lipid disorders, hypertension, diabetes, and weight management,* Chicago, 2012, Academy of Nutrition and Dietetics.

BOX 30-3 Examples of PES Statements Related to Diabetes Mellitus

Nutrition Diagnosis: Inconsistent carbohydrate intake

- Inconsistent carbohydrate intake (P) related to incorrect application of carbohydrate counting (E) as evidenced by food records revealing 2 additional carbohydrate servings for many meals and wide fluctuations in blood glucose levels, most days of the week (S).

Nutrition Diagnosis: Inconsistent carbohydrate intake

- Inconsistent carbohydrate intake (P) related to inconsistent timing of meals (E) as evidenced by wide fluctuations in blood glucose levels (S).

Nutrition Diagnosis: Excessive carbohydrate intake

- Excessive carbohydrate intake (P) compared with insulin dosing related to inaccurate carbohydrate counting (E) as evidenced by the number of carbohydrate servings per meal noted in food record and postmeal glucose levels consistently >200 mg/dl (S).

Nutrition Diagnosis: Inappropriate intake of food fats

- Excessive saturated fat intake (P) related to lack of knowledge of saturated fat content of foods (E) as evidenced by self-report of high saturated fat intake (S).

Nutrition Diagnosis: Altered laboratory values

- Altered blood glucose values (P) related to insufficient insulin (E) as evidenced by hyperglycemia despite very good eating habits (S).

Nutrition Diagnosis: Overweight/obesity

- Overweight (P) related to excessive energy intake with limited physical activity (E) as evidenced by a BMI of 30 and food history indicating consumption of 2800 kcal per day vs 2200 calories (estimated needs) and sedentary lifestyle (S).

Nutrition Diagnosis: Food- and nutrition-related knowledge deficit

- Food- and nutrition-related knowledge deficit (P) related to lack of exposure to information (E) as evidenced by new diagnosis of diabetes (or prediabetes, lipid disorder, hypertension) (S)

Nutrition Diagnosis: Not ready for lifestyle change

- Not ready for lifestyle change (P) related to denial of need to change in precontemplation (E) as evidenced by reluctance to begin participation in physical activity program (S)

Modified from Franz MJ et al: *ADA pocket guide to lipid disorders, hypertension, diabetes, and weight management,* Chicago, 2012, Academy of Nutrition and Dietetics.

education involves the transfer of knowledge to the specific deficits identified in the nutrition diagnosis statements. Nutrition counseling involves behavior and attitude change through the use of strategies that promote behavior changes and/or motivation and intention to change (see Chapter 14). Nutrition care also must be coordinated with other health care providers that can assist in the implementation of the nutrition prescription and nutrition therapy. If home care is needed, follow-up should take place.

Nutrition Therapy Interventions for All People with Diabetes

The first priority is to promote and support a healthful eating pattern, emphasizing a variety of nutrient dense foods in appropriate portion sizes. However, monitoring carbohydrate intake also can be important nutrition therapy strategy for persons with all types of diabetes. It is important that individuals with diabetes know what foods contain carbohydrates—starchy vegetables, grains, fruit, milk and milk products, vegetables, and sweets; portion sizes; and how many servings they should select for meals (and if they desire, snacks). When choosing carbohydrate foods, nutrient-dense, high-fiber foods are recommended whenever possible instead of processed foods with added sodium, fat, and sugars. Sugar-sweetened beverages also should be avoided.

Nutrition Therapy Interventions for Specific Populations

Persons with T1DM and Insulin-Requiring T2DM. The first priority is to integrate an insulin regimen into the usual eating habits and physical activity schedule. With the many insulin options now available (rapid- and long-acting insulins), an insulin regimen can be planned that will conform to an individual's preferred meal routines and food choices. It is no longer necessary to create unnatural or artificial divisions of meals and snacks.

Physiologic insulin regimens that mimic natural insulin secretion involve multiple injections (three or more insulin injections per day) or use of insulin pump therapy. These types of insulin regimens allow increased flexibility in choosing when and what to eat. Mealtime insulin doses are adjusted to match carbohydrate intake (insulin-to-carbohydrate ratios). Therefore, it is important that individuals learn how to count carbohydrates or use another meal planning approach to quantify carbohydrate intake. The insulin action times of the currently available rapid-acting insulin analogs are: onset 5 to 15 minutes, a peak between 30 to 90 minutes, and a duration of approximately 4 to 6 hours. "Lag time" is defined as the amount of time that elapses between the injection of rapid-acting insulin and the meal; it is critical in control of postprandial hyperglycemia and in later risk of hypoglycemia. Given the pharmacodynamics of insulin analogs, a sufficient lag time of approximately 10 to 15 minutes before start of meal helps to decrease postprandial hyperglycemia.

For persons who receive fixed insulin regimens such as with the use of premixed insulins or those who do not adjust their mealtime insulin doses, day-to-day consistency in the timing and amount of carbohydrates eaten is recommended. Insulin doses also must be taken at consistent times every day. The amount of carbohydrate is individualized to the person's nutritional needs. The amount of mealtime insulin (rapid- or short-acting) that the person takes only changes for the blood glucose level. Some people with T1DM or insulin-requiring T2DM still use this method for a variety of reasons, such as age, cost, fewer required injections, lack of access to insulin analogs, personal preference, or prescribing habits of the health care provider.

With so much attention focused on the carbohydrate component of the diabetes Eating Plan, consideration also must be paid to total energy intake. Weight gain may adversely affect glycemia, lipids, blood pressure, and general health; thus prevention of weight gain in adults is desirable. Furthermore, it is assumed that protein and fat content is kept fairly consistent. However, there may be occasions when fat and protein intake is significantly increased and small amounts of additional bolus insulin may be needed for their metabolism (Wolpert et al, 2013).

Persons with Type 2 Diabetes on MNT Alone or with Glucose-Lowering Medications. The first priority is to adopt lifestyle interventions that improve the metabolic abnormalities of glycemia, dyslipidemia, and hypertension. Lifestyle interventions independent of weight loss that can improve glycemia include reduced energy intake and increased energy expenditure through physical activity. Because many persons also have dyslipidemia and hypertension, a cardioprotective eating pattern also is recommended. These interventions should be implemented as soon as the diagnosis of diabetes is made.

MNT interventions for established T2DM differ from interventions for prevention. Because of the progressive nature of T2DM, MNT interventions progress from prevention of obesity, to the prevention or delay of T2DM, to strategies for improved metabolic control. Modest weight loss is beneficial in persons with insulin resistance; however, as the disease progresses to insulin deficiency, medications usually have to be combined with MNT. Emphasis should be on blood glucose control, improved food choices, increased physical activity, and moderate energy restriction rather than weight loss alone as it is unclear whether weight loss alone may or may not improve glycemic control (AND, 2008a).

The first step in food and meal planning is teaching which foods are sources of carbohydrate, appropriate portion sizes, and how many servings to select at meals (and snacks, if desired). Important components of successful MNT for T2DM include: teaching that unsaturated fats should be substituted for foods high in saturated and trans fats, encouraging physical activity, and using blood glucose monitoring to adjust food and eating patterns; medications are also important components of successful MNT for T2DM. Frequent follow-up with an RDN can provide the problem-solving techniques, encouragement, and support that lifestyle changes require.

Physical activity improves insulin sensitivity, acutely lowers blood glucose in persons with diabetes, and also may improve cardiovascular status. By itself it has only a modest effect on weight; however, it is essential for long-term weight maintenance.

Youth with Type 1 Diabetes. Involvement of a multidisciplinary team, including a physician, RDN, nurse, and behavioral specialist, all trained in pediatric diabetes, is the best means of achieving optimal diabetes management in youth. However, the most important team members are the child or adolescent and his or her family/caregiver.

A major nutrition goal for children and adolescents with T1DM is maintenance of normal growth and development. Possible causes of poor weight gain and linear growth include poor glycemic control, inadequate insulin, and overrestriction of calories. The last may be a consequence of the common erroneous belief that restricting food, rather than adjusting insulin, is the way to control blood glucose. Additional reasons for poor weight gain unrelated to diabetes management may include other autoimmune conditions such as thyroid abnormalities

(Hashimoto's thyroiditis) and malabsorption syndromes (celiac disease) or disordered eating behaviors or insulin omission. Excessive weight gain can be caused by excessive caloric intake, overtreatment of hypoglycemia, or overinsulinization. Other causes include low physical activity levels and hypothyroidism, accompanied by poor linear growth (Chiang et al, 2014).

The nutrition prescription is based on the nutrition assessment. Newly diagnosed children often present with weight loss and hunger; as a result, the initial meal plan must be based on adequate calories to restore and maintain appropriate body weight. In about 4 to 6 weeks the initial caloric level may need to be modified to meet more usual caloric requirements. Nutrient requirements for children and adolescents with diabetes appear to be similar to those of children and adolescents without diabetes. The DRIs can be used to determine energy requirements (IOM, 2002). However, it may be preferable to use a food and nutrition history of typical daily intake, providing that growth and development are normal, to determine an individual child's or adolescent's energy needs.

Consultation with an RDN to develop and discuss the eating plan is encouraged (Chiang et al, 2014). Because energy requirements change with age, physical activity, and growth rate, an evaluation of height, weight, BMI, and the eating plan must be updated at least every year. Height and weight should be recorded on a Centers for Disease Control and Prevention (CDC) pediatric growth charts every 3 months. Good metabolic control is essential for normal growth and development (for growth charts see Appendices 4 through 11). Linear growth can be affected by an insulin prescription that is not adjusted as the child grows. Chronic undertreatment with insulin along with longstanding poor diabetes control often leads to poor growth and weight loss. However, withholding food or having the child eat consistently without an appetite for food in an effort to control blood glucose should be discouraged. Calories should be adequate for growth and restricted if the child becomes overweight.

Individualized Eating Plans, insulin regimens using basal (background) and bolus (mealtime) insulins, and insulin algorithms or insulin pumps can provide flexibility for children with T1DM as well as their families. This approach accommodates irregular meal times and schedules and varying appetites and activity levels. Blood glucose records are essential to assist in making appropriate changes in insulin regimens. Daily eating patterns in young children generally include three meals and two or three snacks, depending on the length of time between meals and the child's physical activity level. Children often prefer smaller meals and snacks. Snacks can prevent hypoglycemia between meals and provide adequate calories. Older children and teens may prefer only three meals. Blood glucose monitoring data are then used to integrate an insulin regimen into the meal, snack, and exercise schedules.

After the appropriate nutrition prescription has been determined, the meal planning approach can be selected. A number of meal planning approaches can be used. Carbohydrate counting for food planning provides youth and their families with guidelines that facilitate glycemic control while still allowing the choice of many common foods that children and adolescents enjoy. However, whatever approach to food planning is used, the youth and family must find it understandable and applicable to their lifestyle.

Youth with Type 2 Diabetes. Childhood obesity has been accompanied by an increase in the prevalence of T2DM among children and adolescents. IGT has been shown to be highly prevalent in obese youth, irrespective of ethnic group, and is associated with insulin resistance. Once T2DM develops, beta-cell

failure is also a factor. Thus T2DM in youth follows a progressive pattern similar to T2DM in adults. However, because of the increase in overweight and obesity in children and adolescents, it can be difficult to determine immediately whether a youth has T1DM or T2DM. Testing for islet antibodies is performed, but it may take weeks to get the results of the test. Therefore guidelines for the management of type 2 diabetes in youth recommend starting the youth on insulin if it is unclear whether the youth has T1DM or T2DM (Springer et al, 2013). When the youth has been diagnosed with T2DM, metformin and lifestyle changes, including nutrition therapy and physical activity, are recommended (Copeland et al, 2013).

Successful lifestyle treatment of T2DM in children and adolescents involves cessation of excessive weight gain, promotion of normal growth and development, and the achievement of blood glucose and A1C goals. Nutrition guidelines also should address comorbidities such as hypertension and dyslipidemia. Offer behavior modification strategies to decrease intake of high-caloric, high-fat, and high-carbohydrate foods (extralarge desserts) and sugar-sweetened beverages while encouraging healthy eating habits and regular physical activity for the entire family. Youth with T2DM should be encouraged to exercise at least 60 minutes a day and to limit their nonacademic "screen time" (video games, television) to less than 2 hours a day (Springer et al, 2013). The guidelines also emphasize the importance of a team effort using not only the physician but also the skills of an RDN, diabetes educator, and a psychologist or social worker to deal with the emotional and/or behavioral problems that may accompany T2DM.

Women with Preexisting Diabetes and Pregnancy. Normalization of blood glucose levels during pregnancy is very important for women who have preexisting diabetes or who develop GDM. Table 30-7 lists glucose goals for pregnancy. The MNT goals are to assist in achieving and maintaining optimal blood glucose control and to provide adequate maternal and fetal nutrition throughout pregnancy, energy intake for appropriate maternal weight gain, and necessary vitamins and minerals (Reader, 2012). Nutrition recommendations during pregnancy and lactation appear to be similar for women with and without diabetes; therefore the DRIs can be used to determine energy and nutrient requirements during pregnancy and for lactation (IOM, 2002) (see Chapter 15).

TABLE 30-7	**Plasma Glucose Goals during Pregnancy**
Gestational diabetes	Preprandial: ≤95 mg/dl (5.3 mmol/L) and EITHER
	1-h postmeal: ≤140 mg/dl (7.8 mmol/L)
	OR
	2-h postmeal: ≤120 mg/dl (6.7 mmol/L)
Preexisting type 1 or type 2 diabetes*	Premeal, bedtime, and overnight glucose: 60-99 mg/dl (3.3-5.5 mmol/L)
	Peak postprandial glucose: 100-129 mg/dl (5.5-7.2 mmol/L)
	A1C: <6.0%
Normal	Preprandial: ~75 mg/dL (4.1mmol/L)
	1-h postmeal: 105 mg/dL (5.8 mmol/L)
	Peak postprandial glucose: 110 mg/dL (6.1 mmol/L)

*If goals can be achieved without excessive hypoglycemia
Modified from Reader, D: Nutrition therapy for pregnancy, lactation, and diabetes. In Franz MJ, Evert AB editors: *American Diabetes* Association Guide to nutrition therapy for diabetes, ed 2, Alexandria, Va, American Diabetes Association, 2012, p 188.

Preconception counseling and the ability to achieve near-normal blood glucose levels before pregnancy have been shown to be effective in reducing the incidence of anomalies in infants born to women with preexisting diabetes to nearly that of the general population. As a result of hormonal changes during the first trimester, blood glucose levels are often erratic. Although caloric needs do not differ from those preceding pregnancy, the Eating Plan may have to be adjusted to accommodate the metabolic changes. Women should be educated about the increased risk of hypoglycemia during pregnancy and cautioned against overtreatment.

The need for insulin increases during the second and third trimesters of pregnancy. At 38 to 40 weeks' postconception, insulin needs and levels peak at two to three times prepregnancy levels. Pregnancy-associated hormones that are antagonistic to the action of insulin lead to elevated blood glucose levels. For women with preexisting diabetes, this increased insulin need must be met with increased exogenous insulin.

Eating Plan adjustments are necessary to provide the additional calories required to support fetal growth, and weight should be monitored. During pregnancy the distribution of energy and carbohydrate intake should be based on the woman's food and eating habits and blood glucose responses. Insulin regimens can be matched to food intake, but maintaining consistency of times and amounts of food eaten are essential to avoid hypoglycemia caused by the continuous fetal draw of glucose from the mother. Smaller meals and more frequent snacks often are needed. A late-evening snack is often necessary to decrease the likelihood of overnight hypoglycemia and fasting ketosis. Records of food intake and blood glucose values are essential for determining whether glycemic goals are being met and for preventing and correcting ketosis.

Regular follow-up visits during pregnancy are needed to monitor caloric and nutrient intake, blood glucose control, and whether there is starvation ketosis. Urine or blood ketones during pregnancy may signal starvation ketosis that can be caused by inadequate energy or carbohydrate intake, omission of meals or snacks, or prolonged intervals between meals (e.g., more than 10 hours between the bedtime snack and breakfast). Ketonemia during pregnancy has been associated with reduced IQ scores in children, and women should be instructed to test for ketones periodically before breakfast.

Women with Gestational Diabetes Mellitus.

MNT for GDM involves primarily a carbohydrate-controlled meal plan that promotes optimal nutrition for maternal and fetal health with adequate energy for appropriate gestational weight gain, achievement and maintenance of normoglycemia, and absence of ketosis. Specific nutrition and food recommendations are determined and modified based on individual assessment and blood glucose records. Monitoring blood glucose, fasting ketones, appetite, and weight gain can aid in developing an appropriate, individualized meal plan and in adjusting the meal plan throughout pregnancy.

Nutrition practice guidelines for gestational diabetes have been developed and field-tested (AND, 2008b). All women with GDM should receive MNT at diagnosis of GDM. Monitoring records guide nutrition therapy and are used to determine whether additional therapy is needed. Insulin, metformin, or glyburide therapy is added if glucose goals exceed target range (see Table 30-7) on two or more occasions in a 1- to 2-week period without some obvious explanation. Lack of weight gain and ketone testing can be useful in determining whether women are undereating to keep glucose levels within target range in an effort to avoid insulin therapy.

Carbohydrates should be distributed throughout the day into three small-to-moderate size meals and two to four snacks. All pregnant women require a minimum of 175 g of carbohydrates daily (Reader, 2012). An evening snack usually is needed to prevent accelerated ketosis overnight. Carbohydrates are not as well tolerated at breakfast as they are at other meals because of increased levels of cortisol and growth hormones. To compensate for this, the initial Eating Plan may have approximately 30 g of carbohydrate at breakfast. To satisfy hunger, protein foods can be added because they do not affect blood glucose levels.

Although caloric restriction must be viewed with caution, a modest energy restriction to slow weight gain is recommended for overweight or obese women with GDM. A slight calorie restriction results in a slowing of maternal weight gain in obese women with GDM without causing maternal or fetal compromise and/or ketonuria (Reader, 2012). Energy intake below approximately 1700 to 1800 kcal/day is not advised. Weight gain during pregnancy for women with GDM should be similar to that of women without diabetes.

Exercise assists in overcoming peripheral resistance to insulin and in controlling fasting and postprandial hyperglycemia and may be used as an adjunct to nutrition therapy to improve maternal glycemia. The ideal form of exercise is unknown, but a brisk walk after meals is often recommended.

Women with GDM (and women with preexisting diabetes) should be encouraged to breastfeed because breastfeeding is associated with a reduced incidence of future T2DM (Stuebe et al, 2005) (see Chapter 15). For women with GDM who are overweight/obese or with above-recommended weight gain during pregnancy, weight loss is advised after delivery. Weight loss reduces the risks of recurrent GDM or future development of T2DM (Reader, 2012). It has been shown that diabetes can be prevented or its onset delayed with lifestyle interventions of weight reduction and physical activity as was shown in the Diabetes Prevention Program and other prevention trials (Youssef, 2012).

Older Adults.

The prevalence of diabetes and IGT increases dramatically as people age. Many factors predispose older adults to diabetes: age-related decreases in insulin production and increases in insulin resistance, adiposity, decreased physical activity, multiple prescription medications, genetics, and coexisting illnesses. A major factor appears to be insulin resistance. Controversy persists as to whether the insulin resistance is a primary change or whether it is attributable to reduced physical activity, decreased lean body mass (sarcopenia), and increased adipose tissue, which are common in older adults. Furthermore, medications used to treat coexisting diseases may complicate diabetes therapy in older persons.

Despite the increase in glucose intolerance with age, aging should not be a reason for suboptimal control of blood glucose. Even if it is incorrectly assumed that preventing long-term diabetic complications is not relevant to the care of older adults, persistent hyperglycemia has deleterious effects on the body's defense mechanisms against infection. It also increases the pain threshold by exacerbating neuropathic pain, and it has a detrimental effect on the outcome of cerebrovascular accidents.

Nutrition recommendations for older adults with diabetes should include meeting the DRI for age for nutrients, evaluating fluid intake, avoiding significant weight loss, and being sensitive to individual preferences and longstanding food habits while advocating good nutrition (Stanley, 2012) (see Chapter 20). Physical activity can reduce the decline in aerobic capacity significantly that occurs with age, improve risk factors for atherosclerosis, slow the decline in age-related lean body mass, decrease central adiposity, and improve insulin sensitivity; thus it should be encouraged.

Malnutrition, not obesity, is the more prevalent nutrition-related problem in older adults. It often remains subclinical or unrecognized because the result of malnutrition—excessive loss of lean body mass—resembles the signs and symptoms of the aging process. Malnutrition and diabetes adversely affect wound healing and defense against infection, and malnutrition is associated with depression and cognitive deficits. The most reliable indicator of poor nutrition status in older adults is a change in body weight; involuntary weight gain or loss of more than 10 pounds or 10% of body weight in less than 6 months indicates a need to evaluate the reason.

It is essential that older adults, especially those in long-term care settings, receive an eating plan that meets their nutritional needs, enables them to attain or maintain a reasonable body weight, helps control blood glucose, and is palatable. Dietary restriction is not warranted for older residents in long-term health facilities. Residents should be served the regular, unrestricted menu with consistency in the amount and timing of carbohydrates (Swift, 2012).

Hyperglycemia and dehydration can lead to a serious complication of diabetes in older adults: **hyperglycemic hyperosmolar state (HHS)**. Patients with HHS have a very high blood glucose level (ranging from 400-2800 mg/dl, [22.2 to 155.6 mmol/L] with an average of 1000 mg/dl [55.6 mmol/L]) without ketones. Patients are markedly dehydrated, and mental alterations range from mild confusion to hallucinations or coma. Patients who have HHS have sufficient insulin to prevent lipolysis and ketosis. Treatment consists of hydration and small doses of insulin to control hyperglycemia.

The Nutrition Prescription

To develop, educate, and counsel individuals regarding the nutrition prescription, it is essential to learn about their lifestyle and eating habits. Food and eating histories can be done several ways, with the objective being to determine a schedule and pattern of eating that will be the least disruptive to the lifestyle of the individual with diabetes and, at the same time, will facilitate improved metabolic control. With this objective in mind, asking the individual either to record or report what, how much, and when he or she typically eats during a 24-hour period may be the most useful. Another approach is to ask the individual to keep and bring a 3-day or 1-week food intake record (see Chapter 4 and Fig. 4-6). The request to complete a food record can be made when an appointment with the RDN is scheduled. It is also important to learn about daily routine and schedule. The following information is needed: (1) time of waking; (2) usual meal and eating times; (3) work schedule or school hours; (4) type, amount, and timing of exercise; (5) usual sleep habits; (6) type, dosage and timing of diabetes medication; and (7) SMBG data.

Using the assessment data and food and nutrition history information, a preliminary Eating Plan can then be designed, and, if the individual desires, sample menus provided. Developing an Eating Plan does not begin with a set calorie or macronutrient prescription; instead, it is determined by modifying the individual's usual food intake as necessary. The worksheet in Figure 30-2 can be used to record the usual foods eaten and

Food Group	Meal/Snack/Time						Total servings/day	CHO (g)	Protein (g)	Fat (g)	Calories
	Breakfast	Snack	Lunch	Snack	Dinner	Snack					
Starches								15	3	1	80
Fruit								15			60
Milk								12	8	1	100
Vegetables								5	2		25
Meats/Substitutes									7	5(3)	75(55)
Fats										5	45
CHO Choices								Total grams			
							Calories/gram	X4=	X4=	X9=	Total calories
							Percent calories				

Calculations are based on medium-fat meats and skim/very low-fat milk. If diet consists predominantly of low-fat meats, use the factor 3 g instead of 5 g fat; if predominantly high-fat meats, use 8 g fat. If low-fat (2%) milk is used, use 5 g fat; if whole milk is used, use 8 g fat.

FIGURE 30-2 Worksheet for assessment and design of a meal or food plan. *CHO,* Carbohydrate.

to modify the usual food and nutrient intake as necessary. The macronutrient and caloric values for the food lists are listed on the form and in Table 30-8; see Appendix 27 for portion sizes of the foods on the food lists. These tools are useful in evaluating nutrition assessments.

Using the form in Figure 30-2, the RDN begins by totaling the number of servings from each food list and multiplying this number by the grams of carbohydrate, protein, and fat contributed by each. Next the grams of carbohydrate, protein, and fat are totaled from each column; the grams of carbohydrates and protein are then multiplied by 4 (4 kcal/g of carbohydrates and protein), and the grams of fat are multiplied by 9 (9 kcal/g of fat.) Total calories and percentage of calories from each macronutrient can then be determined. Numbers derived from these calculations are then rounded off. Figure 30-3 provides an example of a preliminary Eating Plan. In this example the nutrition prescription would be the following: 1900 to 2000 calories, 230 g of carbohydrates (50%), 90 g of protein (20%), 65 g of fat (30%.) The number of carbohydrate choices for each meal and snack is the total of the starch, fruit, and milk servings. Vegetables, unless starchy or eaten in very large amounts (three or more servings per meal), generally are considered "free foods." The carbohydrate choices are circled under each meal and snack column.

The next step is to evaluate the preliminary Eating Plan. First and foremost, does the individual think it is feasible to implement the Eating Plan into his or her lifestyle? Second, is it appropriate for diabetes management? Third, does it encourage healthful eating? Fourth, if the individual is taking diabetes medicine is the Eating Plan coordinated with the medication plan to reduce risk of hypoglycemia and/or minimize postprandial hyperglycemia?

To discuss feasibility, the Eating Plan is reviewed with the individual in terms of general food intake. Timing of meals and snacks and approximate portion sizes and types of foods are discussed. Calorie levels are only approximate, and adjustments in calories can be made during follow-up visits. A meal-planning approach can be selected later that will assist the patient in making his or her own food choices. At this point it must be determined whether this Eating Plan is reasonable.

To determine the appropriateness of the Eating Plan for diabetes management, distribution of the meals or snacks must be assessed along with the types of medications prescribed and treatment goals. For patients with T2DM receiving MNT alone or MNT with glucose-lowering medications, often the Eating Plan begins with three or four carbohydrate servings per meal for adult women and four or five for adult men and, if desired, one or two for a snack. Eating snacks when not hungry simply provides unnecessary calories. There is also no research to support the need to add protein to a snack for an individual with diabetes. Results of blood glucose monitoring before the meal and 2 hours after the meal, plus feedback from the person with diabetes, are used to assess if these recommendations are feasible and realistic and to determine whether target glucose goals are being achieved.

For people who require insulin, the timing of eating is important as insulin must be synchronized with food consumption (see Medications earlier in the chapter.) If the Eating Plan is determined first, an insulin regimen can be selected that will fit with it. The best way to ensure that the eating plan encourages healthful eating is to encourage individuals to eat a variety of foods from all the food groups. The Dietary Guidelines for Americans, with its suggested number of servings from each food group, can be used to compare the individual's Eating Plan

TABLE 30-8 Macronutrient and Caloric Values for Food Lists*
The following chart shows the macronutrients and calories from each list.

Food List	Carbohydrate (grams)	Protein (grams)	Fat (grams)	Calories
Carbohydrates				
Starch: breads, cereals and grains, starchy vegetables, crackers, snacks, and beans, peas, and lentils	15	3	1	80
Fruits	15	—	—	60
Milk and milk substitutes	12	8	0-3	100
Fat-free, low-fat, 1%	12	8	5	120
Reduced-fat, 2%	12	8	8	160
Whole				
Sweets, desserts, and other carbohydrates	15	Varies	Varies	Varies
Nonstarchy vegetables	5	2	—	25
Proteins				
Lean	—	7	2	45
Medium-fat	—	7	5	75
High-fat	—	7	8	100
Plant-based protein	—	7	Varies	Varies
Fats	—	—	5	45
Alcohol (1 alcohol equivalent)	Varies	—	—	100

From American Diabetes Association and Academy of Nutrition and Dietetics: *Choose your foods: food lists for diabetes,* Alexandria, Va, Chicago, 2014 American Diabetes Association, Academy of Nutrition and Dietetics.
*See Appendix 34.

Food Group	Breakfast 7:30 AM	Snack 10:00	Lunch 12:00	Snack 3:00	Dinner 6:30	Snack 10:00	Total servings/day	CHO (g)	Protein (g)	Fat (g)	Calories
Starches	2	1	2–3	1	2–3	1–2	10	15 / 150	3 / 30	1 / 10	80
Fruit	1		1		1	0–1	3	15 / 45			60
Milk	1				1		2	12 / 24	8 / 16	1 / 2	100
Vegetables			✓		✓			5 / 10	2 / 4		25
Meats/Substitutes			2–3		3–4		6		7 / 42	5(3) / 30	75(55)
Fats	1	0–1	1–2	0–1	1–2	0–1	5			5 / 25	45
CHO Choices	3–4 CHO	1 CHO	3–4 CHO	1 CHO	4–5 CHO	1–2 CHO	Total grams	229	92	67	
	1900–2000 calories	230 g CHO–50%	90 g protein–20%	65 g fat–30%			Calories/gram	X4= 916	X4= 368	X9= 603	Total calories
							Percent calories	50	19	30	1900–2000

Calculations are based on medium-fat meats and skim/very low-fat milk. If diet consists predominantly of low-fat meats, use the factor 3 g, instead of 5 g fat; if predominantly high-fat meats, use 8 g fat. If low-fat (2%) milk is used, use 5 g fat; if whole milk is used, use 8 g fat.

FIGURE 30-3 An example of a completed worksheet from the assessment, the nutrition prescription, and a sample 1900- to 2000-calorie meal plan. *CHO*, Carbohydrate.

with the nutrition recommendations for all Americans (see Chapter 11).

Nutrition Education and Counseling

Implementation of MNT begins with the RDN selecting from a variety of interventions (reduced energy and fat intake, carbohydrate counting, simplified meal plans, healthy food choices, individualized meal planning strategies, insulin-to-carbohydrate ratios, physical activity and behavioral strategies) (Pastors and Franz, 2012). All of the above interventions have been shown to lead to improved metabolic outcomes. Furthermore, nutrition education and counseling must be sensitive to the personal needs, willingness to change, and ability to make changes, of the individual with diabetes (see Figure 30-3). Assessing the individual's health literacy and numeracy also may be beneficial. No single eating plan approach has been shown to be more effective than any other, and the eating plan approach selected should allow individuals with diabetes to select appropriate foods for meals and snacks.

A popular approach to eating planning is carbohydrate counting. It can be used as a basic meal-planning approach or for more intensive management. Carbohydrate-counting educational tools are based on the concept that, after eating it is the carbohydrate in foods that is the major predictor of postprandial blood glucose levels. One carbohydrate serving contributes 15 g of carbohydrates. Basic carbohydrate counting emphasizes the following topics: basic facts about carbohydrates, primary food sources of carbohydrate, average portion sizes and the importance of consistency and accurate portions, amount of carbohydrates that should be eaten, and label reading. Advanced

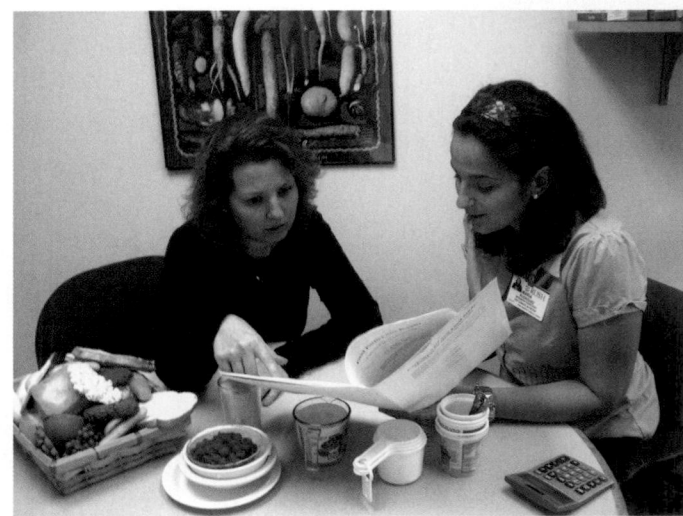

FIGURE 30-4 A woman with Type 1 DM is learning about carbohydrate counseling from her RDN counselor.

carbohydrate counting emphasizes the importance of record keeping, calculating insulin-to-carbohydrate ratios, and pattern management.

An important goal of nutrition counseling is to facilitate changes in existing food and nutrition-related behaviors and the adoption of new ones. The combined use of behavior change theories may potentially have a greater impact than any individual theory or technique used alone (Franz et al, 2012). The following "five As" can guide the education/counseling sessions: step 1: ask; step 2: assess; step 3: advise; step 4: agree; and step 5: arrange. The "ask" step emphasizes the importance of questions as the RDN aims to develop a relationship with the client. Motivational interviewing techniques are used initially and throughout all of the encounters. In the "assess" step, the RDN evaluated the client's readiness to change. Different intervention strategies may be needed for individuals at different stages of the change process (see Chapter 14). The "advise" step uses a client-centered framework that adapts nutrition interventions to meet the client's needs, wants, priorities, preferences and expectations. In the "agree" step the RDN facilitates the client's process of setting his or her own short-term goals related to nutrition, physical activity, or glucose monitoring (if appropriate) and helps outline the client's potential methods for accomplishing lifestyle changes. In the "arrange" step, plans for follow-up are identified to evaluate responses to nutrition interventions. The individual also is given information on how to call or email with questions and concerns. In making plans for the next encounter, the patient is asked to keep a 3-day or weekly food record with blood glucose–monitoring data.

Nutrition Monitoring and Evaluation

Food intake, medication, metabolic control (glycemia, lipids, and blood pressure), anthropometric measurements, and physical activity should be monitored and evaluated (AND, 2008a; Franz et al, 2010). Medical and clinical outcomes should be monitored after the second or third visit to determine whether the individual is making progress toward established goals. If no progress is evident, the individual and RDN must reassess and perhaps revise nutrition interventions. Blood glucose monitoring results can be used to determine whether adjustments in foods and meals will be sufficient to achieve blood glucose goals or if medication additions or adjustments have to be combined with MNT. Nutrition care must be coordinated with an interdisciplinary team.

Documentation in the individual's medical record serves as a communication tool for members of the health care team. The medical record also serves as a legal document of what was done and not done and supports reimbursement of nutrition services billed to insurance carriers. There are many different formats available for medical record documentation. The appropriate format depends on where the RDN practices and whether electronic health records are used. Regardless of the specific format, the RDN can document using the ADIME content; Box 30-4 lists key elements.

Follow-Up Encounters

Successful nutrition therapy involves a process of assessment, problem solving, adjustment, and readjustment. Food records can be compared with the eating plan, which will help to determine whether the initial eating plan needs changing, and can be integrated with the blood glucose–monitoring

---

BOX 30-4   Nutrition Care Documentation

Nutrition assessment
- Date and time of assessment
- Pertinent data collected and comparisons with standards (e.g., food and nutrition history, biochemical data, anthropometric measurements, client history, medical therapy, and supplement use
- Patient's readiness to learn, food and nutrition-related knowledge, and potential for change
- Physical activity history and goals
- Reason for discontinuation of nutrition therapy, if appropriate

Nutrition diagnoses
- Date and time
- Concise written statement of nutrition diagnosis (or nutrition diagnoses) written in the PES format (problem, etiology, signs and symptoms). If there is no existing or predicted nutrition problem that requires a nutrition intervention, state "no nutrition diagnosis at this time."

Nutrition interventions
- Date and time
- Specific treatment goals and expected outcomes
- Recommended nutrition prescription and nutrition interventions (individualized for the patient)
- Any adjustments to plan and justifications
- Patient's receptivity regarding recommendations
- Changes in patient's level of understanding and food-related behaviors
- Referrals made and resources used
- Any other information relevant to providing care and monitoring progress over time
- Plans for follow-up and frequency of care

Nutrition monitoring and evaluation
- Date and time
- Specific nutrition outcomes indicators and results relevant to the nutrition diagnosis (or diagnoses) and intervention plans and goals, compared with previous status or reference goals
- Progress toward nutrition intervention goals
- Factors facilitating or hindering progress
- Other positive or negative outcomes
- Future plans for nutrition care, monitoring, and follow-up or discharge

Adapted from Writing Group of the Nutrition Care Process/Standardized Language Committee: Nutrition Care Process Part II: Using the International Dietetics and Nutrition Terminology to Document the Nutrition Care Process, J Am Diet Assoc *108:1287, 2008.*

---

records to determine changes that can lead to improved glycemic control.

Nutrition follow-up visits should provide encouragement and ensure realistic expectations for the individual with diabetes. A change in eating habits is not easy for most people, and they become discouraged without appropriate recognition of their efforts. Individuals should be encouraged to speak freely about problems they are having with their eating plan. Furthermore, there may be major life changes that require changes in the eating plan. Job and schedule changes, travel, illness, and other factors all have an impact on the meal plan.

ACUTE COMPLICATIONS

Hypoglycemia and diabetic ketoacidosis are the two most common acute complications related to diabetes.

Hypoglycemia

A low blood glucose, or **hypoglycemia (or insulin reaction)**, is a common side effect of insulin therapy, although individuals taking insulin secretagogues also can be affected. **Autonomic symptoms** arise from the action of the autonomic nervous system and are often the first signs of mild hypoglycemia. Adrenergic symptoms include shakiness, sweating, palpitations, anxiety, and hunger. **Neuroglycopenic symptoms**, related to an insufficient supply of glucose to the brain, also can occur at similar glucose levels as autonomic symptoms but with different manifestations. The earliest signs of neuroglycopenia include a slowing down in performance and difficulty concentrating and reading. As blood glucose levels drop further, the following symptoms occur: frank mental confusion and disorientation, slurred or rambling speech, irrational or unusual behaviors, extreme fatigue and lethargy, seizures, and unconsciousness. Symptoms differ for different people but tend to be consistent from episode to episode for any one person. Several common causes of hypoglycemia are listed in Box 30-5.

In T1DM and T2DM it has been demonstrated that counterregulatory responses to hypoglycemia steadily decline with frequent and repetitive episodes. It can become a vicious cycle as hypoglycemic episodes impair defenses against a subsequent hypoglycemic episode and thus can result in recurrent hypoglycemia. Hypoglycemia causes increased morbidity in most people with T1DM and many with long-duration T2DM and is sometimes fatal.

In general, a blood glucose of 70 mg/dl (3.9 mmol/L) or lower should be treated immediately. Treatment of hypoglycemia requires ingestion of glucose or carbohydrate-containing food. Although any carbohydrate will raise glucose levels, glucose is the preferred treatment. The form of carbohydrates (i.e., liquid or solid) used to treat does not make a difference. Commercially available glucose tablets have the advantage of being premeasured to help prevent overtreatment. Ingestion of 15 to 20 g of glucose is an effective but temporary treatment. Initial response to treatment should be seen in about 10 to 20 minutes; however, blood glucose should be evaluated again in about 60 minutes as additional carbohydrate may be necessary (see Box 30-6).

BOX 30-6   Treatment of Hypoglycemia

- Immediate treatment with carbohydrates is essential.
  If the blood glucose level falls below 70 mg/dL (3.9 mmol/L), treat with 15 g of carbohydrates, which is equivalent to:
  15 g carbohydrate from glucose tablets (4) or glucose gel
  4-6 ounces of fruit juice or regular soft drinks
  6 ounces (1/2 can) of regular soda pop (not sugar free)
  8 ounces (1 cup) of sports drink (not sugar free)
  1 tablespoon of sugar, syrup or honey
- Retest in approximately 10-15 minutes. If the blood glucose level remains <70 mg/dl (<3.9 mmol/l), treat with an additional 15 g of carbohydrates.
- Repeat testing and treatment until the blood glucose level returns to within normal range.
- If it is more than 1 hour to the next meal, test again 60 minutes after treatment as additional carbohydrate may be needed.

Adapted from Kaufman F: *Medical management of Type 1 diabetes*, ed 6, Alexandria, Va, 2012, American Diabetes Association.

Severely low blood glucose can cause loss of consciousness or seizures. If individuals are unable to swallow, administration of subcutaneous or intramuscular glucagon may be needed. Parents, roommates, and spouses should be taught how to mix, draw up, and administer glucagon so that they are properly prepared for emergency situations. Kits that include a syringe prefilled with diluting fluid are available. After the injection, turn the patient on their side to prevent choking in case of vomiting. Nausea and vomiting are common side effects of glucagon. The patient should be given food or beverage containing carbohydrate as soon as they regain consciousness and can swallow.

Self-monitoring of blood glucose is essential for prevention and treatment of hypoglycemia. Changes in insulin injections, eating, exercise schedules, and travel routines warrant increased frequency of monitoring. Some patients experience hypoglycemia unawareness, which means that they do not experience the usual symptoms of hypoglycemia. Patients must be reminded of the need to treat hypoglycemia, even in the absence of symptoms. Short-term relaxation of glycemic targets generally assists in the correction of hypoglycemia unawareness (ADA, 2014b).

Hyperglycemia and Diabetic Ketoacidosis

Hyperglycemia can lead to **diabetic ketoacidosis (DKA)**, a life-threatening but reversible complication characterized by severe disturbances in carbohydrate, protein, and fat metabolism. DKA is always the result of inadequate insulin for glucose use. As a result, the body depends on fat for energy, and ketones are formed. Acidosis results from increased production and decreased use of acetoacetic acid and 3-beta-hydroxybutyric acid from fatty acids. Ketones spill into the urine; hence the reliance on testing for ketones.

DKA is characterized by elevated blood glucose levels (>250 mg/dl but generally <600 mg/dl) and the presence of ketones in the blood and urine. Symptoms include polyuria, polydipsia, hyperventilation, dehydration, the fruity odor of ketones, and fatigue. SMBG, testing for ketones, and medical intervention can help prevent DKA. If left untreated, DKA can lead to coma and death. Treatment includes supplemental insulin, fluid and electrolyte replacement, and medical monitoring. Acute illnesses such as flu, colds, vomiting, and diarrhea, if not managed appropriately, can lead to the development of DKA. Patients need to know the steps to take during acute illness to prevent

---

BOX 30-5   Common Causes of Hypoglycemia

Medication errors
- Inadvertent or deliberate errors in medication (generally insulin) dosages
- Excessive insulin or oral secretagogue dosages
- Reversal of morning or evening insulin doses
- Improper timing of insulin in relation to food intake

Nutrition therapy or exercise
- Omitted or inadequate food intake
- Timing errors; delayed meals or snacks
- Unplanned or increased physical activities or exercise
- Prolonged duration or increased intensity of exercise

Alcohol and drugs
- Alcohol intake without food
- Impaired mentation associated with alcohol, marijuana, or other illicit drugs

Adapted from Kaufman F: *Medical management of type 1 diabetes*, ed 6, Alexandria, Va, 2012, American Diabetes Association.

BOX 30-7 Sick-Day Guidelines for Persons with Diabetes

1. During acute illnesses, usual doses of insulin and other glucose-lowering medications are required. The need for insulin continues, or may even increase, during periods of illness. Fever, dehydration, infection, or the stress of illness can trigger the release of counterregulatory or "stress" hormones, causing blood glucose levels to become elevated.
2. Blood glucose levels and urine or blood testing for ketones should be monitored at least four times daily (before each meal and at bedtime). Blood glucose readings exceeding 250 mg/dl and the presence of ketones are danger signals indicating that additional insulin is needed.
3. Ample amounts of liquid need to be consumed every hour. If vomiting, diarrhea, or fever is present, small sips—1 or 2 tablespoons every 15 to 30 min—can usually be consumed. If vomiting continues and the individual is unable to take fluids for longer than 4 hr, the health care team should be notified.
4. If regular foods are not tolerated, liquid or soft carbohydrate-containing foods (such as regular soft drinks, soup, juices, and ice cream) should be eaten. Eating about 10 to 15 g of carbohydrate every 1 to 2 hr (or 50 g of carbohydrate every 3 to 4 hr) is usually sufficient.
5. The health care team should be called if illness continues for more than 1 day.

Adapted from Kaufman F: *Medical management of type 1 diabetes*, ed 6. Alexandria, Va, 2012, American Diabetes Association.

DKA (see Box 30-7). During acute illness, oral ingestion of about 150 to 200 g of carbohydrates per day (45-50 g every 3-4 hr) should be sufficient, along with medication adjustments, to keep glucose in the goal range and to prevent starvation ketosis.

Fasting hyperglycemia is a common finding in persons with diabetes. The amount of insulin required to normalize blood glucose levels during the night is less in the predawn period (from 1:00-3:00 AM) than at dawn (4:00-8:00 AM). The increased need for insulin at dawn causes a rise in fasting blood glucose levels referred to as the dawn phenomenon. It results if insulin levels decline between predawn and dawn or if overnight hepatic glucose output becomes excessive as is common in T2DM. To identify the dawn phenomenon, blood glucose levels are monitored at bedtime and at 2:00 to 3:00 AM. With the dawn phenomenon, predawn blood glucose levels will be in the low range of normal but not in the hypoglycemic range. For patients with T2DM, metformin often is used because it decreases hepatic glucose output. For persons with T1DM, administering insulin that does not peak at 1:00 to 3:00 AM such as a long-acting insulin should be considered.

Hypoglycemia followed by "rebound" hyperglycemia is called the Somogyi effect. This phenomenon originates during hypoglycemia with the secretion of counterregulatory hormones (glucagon, epinephrine, growth hormone, and cortisol) and usually is caused by excessive exogenous insulin doses. Hepatic glucose production is stimulated, thus raising blood glucose levels. If rebound hyperglycemia goes unrecognized and insulin doses are increased, a cycle of overinsulinization may result. Decreasing evening insulin doses or, as for the dawn phenomenon, taking a long-acting insulin should be considered.

LONG-TERM COMPLICATIONS

Long-term complications of diabetes include macrovascular diseases, microvascular diseases, and neuropathy. Macrovascular diseases involve diseases of large blood vessels; microvascular diseases associated with diabetes involve the small blood vessels and include nephropathy and retinopathy. In contrast, diabetic neuropathy is a condition characterized by damage to the nerves. MNT is important in managing several long-term complications of diabetes. Nutrition therapy is also a major component in reducing risk factors for chronic complications, especially those related to macrovascular disease.

Macrovascular Diseases

Insulin resistance, which may precede the development of T2DM and macrovascular disease by many years, induces numerous metabolic changes known as the metabolic syndrome (see Chapter 21). It is characterized by intraabdominal obesity or the android distribution of adipose tissue (waist circumference greater than 102 cm [40 in] in men and greater than 88 cm [35 in] in women) and is associated with dyslipidemia, hypertension, glucose intolerance, and increased prevalence of macrovascular complications. Other risk factors include genetics, smoking, sedentary lifestyle, high-fat diet, renal failure, and microalbuminuria.

Macrovascular diseases, including atherosclerotic cardiovascular disease (ASCVD), peripheral vascular disease (PVD), and cerebrovascular disease are more common, tend to occur at an earlier age, and are more extensive and severe in people with diabetes. Persons with diabetes have the CVD risk equivalent as persons with preexisting CVD and no diabetes (Buse et al, 2007). Furthermore, in women with diabetes the increased risk of mortality from heart disease is greater than in men, in contrast to the nondiabetic population, in which heart disease mortality is greater in men than in women.

Dyslipidemia

Patients with diabetes have an increased prevalence of lipid abnormalities that contribute to higher rates of CVD. In T2DM the prevalence of an elevated cholesterol level is about 28% to 34%. About 5% to 14% of patients with T2DM have high triglyceride levels; also, lower HDL cholesterol levels are common. Persons with T2DM typically have smaller, denser LDL particles, which increase atherogenicity even if the total LDL cholesterol level is not significantly elevated. Lifestyle intervention, including MNT, weight loss through reduced energy intake and increased physical activity, and smoking cessation always should be implemented. Evidence is inconclusive for ideal amount of total fat intake; fat quality may as important as quantity (Evert et al, 2013). Diet should be focused on reduction of saturated fat, trans fat and cholesterol and increased intake of omega-3 fat (in food, not as supplements), viscous fiber, and plant stanols/sterols (Diabetes Care 2015). In people with T2DM, a Mediterranean-style, MUFA-rich eating pattern may benefit glycemic control and CVD risk factors. Other CVD nutrition recommendations for people with diabetes are the same as for the general public. The most current AHA/ACC recommendations are for use of the DASH diet eating pattern (see Chapter 33). Statin therapy is added to nutrition therapy, regardless of lipid levels, for persons with diabetes (ADA, 2014b).

Hypertension

Hypertension is a common comorbidity of diabetes, with about 67% of adults with diabetes having blood pressure of 140/90 mm Hg or higher or using prescription medications for hypertension (CDC, 2014). Treatment of hypertension in persons with diabetes should be vigorous to reduce the risk of macrovascular and microvascular disease. Blood pressure should be measured at every routine visit with a goal for blood pressure control of less than 140/80 mm Hg. MNT interventions for persons with hypertension include weight loss, if overweight; DASH-style eating pattern (Appendix 26); reducing sodium intake and increasing potassium intake; moderation of alcohol intake; and increased physical activity (see Chapter 33). The recommendation for the general population to reduce sodium to less than 2300 mg/day is also appropriate for people with diabetes and hypertension (Evert et al, 2013). For individuals with both diabetes and hypertension, further reduction in sodium intake should be individualized. Consideration must be given to issues such as the availability, palatability, and additional cost of low sodium food products. Pharmacologic therapy for hypertension includes either an angiotensin-converting enzyme (ACE) inhibitor or an angiotensin receptor blocker (ARB); however, multiple drug therapy is generally required (ADA, 2014b).

Microvascular Diseases
Diabetic Kidney Disease

In the United States and Europe diabetic kidney disease (DKD) or diabetic nephropathy occurs in 20% to 40% of patients with diabetes and is the single leading cause of end-stage renal disease (ESRD). Because of the much greater prevalence of T2DM, such patients constitute over half of the patients with diabetes currently starting on dialysis (see Chapter 36).

An annual screening to quantitate urine albumin excretion rate should be performed in patients who have had T1DM for more than 5 years, and in all patients with T2DM starting at diagnosis (ADA, 2014b). The serum creatinine is used to estimate glomerular filtration rate (GFR) and stage the level of chronic kidney disease (CKD), if present.

To reduce the risk and slow the progression of DKD, glucose and blood pressure control should be optimized. Although low protein diets have been shown to lower albuminuria, they do not alter the course of GFR decline or improve glycemic or CVD risk measures, and therefore are not recommended (Evert et al, 2013).

Retinopathy

Diabetic retinopathy is estimated to be the most frequent cause of new cases of blindness among adults 20 to 74 years of age. Glaucoma, cataracts, and other disorders of the eye also occur earlier and more frequently with diabetes (ADA, 2014b). Laser photocoagulation surgery can reduce the risk of further vision loss but usually does not restore lost vision—thus the importance for a screening program to detect diabetic retinopathy.

Neuropathy

Chronic high levels of blood glucose also are associated with nerve damage, and 60% to 70% of people with diabetes have mild to severe forms of nervous system damage (CDC, 2014). Intensive treatment of hyperglycemia reduces the risk and slows progression of diabetic neuropathy but does not reverse neuronal loss. Peripheral neuropathy usually affects the nerves that control sensation in the feet and hands. Autonomic neuropathy affects nerve function controlling various organ systems. Cardiovascular effects include postural hypotension and decreased responsiveness to cardiac nerve impulses, leading to painless or silent ischemic heart disease. Sexual function may be affected, with impotence the most common manifestation.

Damage to nerves innervating the gastrointestinal tract can cause a variety of problems. Neuropathy can be manifested in the esophagus as nausea and esophagitis, in the stomach as

unpredictable emptying, in the small bowel as loss of nutrients, and in the large bowel as diarrhea or constipation.

Gastroparesis is characterized by delayed gastric emptying in the absence of mechanical obstruction of the stomach (Camilleri, 2007). Symptoms are reported by 5% to 12% of persons with diabetes. It results in delayed or irregular contractions of the stomach, leading to various gastrointestinal symptoms such as feelings of fullness, bloating, nausea, vomiting, diarrhea, or constipation. Gastroparesis should be suspected in individuals with erratic glucose control.

The first step in management of patients with neuropathy should be to aim for stable and optimal glycemic control. MNT involves minimizing abdominal stress. Small, frequent meals may be better tolerated than three full meals a day; and these meals should be low in fiber and fat. If solid foods are not well tolerated, liquid meals may have to be recommended. For patients using insulin, as much as possible, the timing of insulin administration should be adjusted to match the usually delayed nutrient absorption. Insulin injections may even be required after eating. Frequent blood glucose monitoring is important to determine appropriate insulin therapy.

A prokinetic agent such as erythromycin, is used most commonly to treat gastroparesis. Antiemetic agents may be helpful for the relief of symptoms. In very severe cases, generally with unintentional weight loss, a feeding tube is placed in the small intestine to avoid the stomach. Gastric electric stimulation with electrodes surgically implanted in the stomach may be used when medications fail to control nausea and vomiting.

HYPOGLYCEMIA OF NONDIABETIC ORIGIN

Hypoglycemia of nondiabetic origin has been defined as a clinical syndrome with diverse causes in which low levels of plasma glucose eventually lead to neuroglycopenia. Hypoglycemia means low (hypo-) blood glucose (glycemia). Normally the body is remarkably adept at maintaining fairly steady blood glucose levels—usually between 60 and 100 mg/dl (3.3-5.6 mmol/L), despite the intermittent ingestion of food. Maintaining normal levels of glucose is important because body cells, especially the brain and central nervous system, must have a steady and consistent supply of glucose to function properly. Under physiologic conditions the brain depends almost exclusively on glucose for its energy needs. Even with hunger, either because it has been many hours since food was eaten or because the last meal was small, blood glucose levels remain fairly consistent.

Pathophysiology

In a small number of people, blood glucose levels drop too low. Symptoms are often felt when blood glucose is below 65 mg/dl (3.6 mmol/l.) If the brain and nervous system are deprived of the glucose they need to function, symptoms such as sweating, shaking, weakness, hunger, headaches, and irritability can develop. Symptoms of hypoglycemia have been recognized at plasma glucose levels of about 60 mg/dl, and impaired brain function has occurred at levels of about 50 mg/dl.

Hypoglycemia can be difficult to diagnose because these typical symptoms can be caused by many different health problems. For example, adrenaline (epinephrine) released as a result of anxiety and stress can trigger the symptoms similar to those of hypoglycemia. The only way to determine whether hypoglycemia is causing these symptoms is to measure blood glucose levels while an individual is experiencing the symptoms. Hypoglycemia can best be defined by the presence of three features known as **Whipple's triad**: (1) a low plasma or blood glucose level; (2) symptoms of hypoglycemia at the same time; and (3) amelioration of the symptoms by correction of the hypoglycemia.

A fairly steady blood glucose level is maintained by the interaction of several mechanisms. After eating, carbohydrates are broken down into glucose and enters the bloodstream. As blood glucose levels rise, the pancreas responds by releasing the hormone insulin, which allows glucose to leave the bloodstream and enter various body cells, where it fuels the body's activities. Glucose is also taken up by the liver and stored as glycogen for later use.

When glucose concentrations from the last meal decline, the body goes from a "fed" to a "fasting" state. Insulin levels decrease, which keeps the blood glucose levels from falling too low. Stored glucose is released from the liver back into the bloodstream with the help of **glucagon** from the pancreas. Normally the body's ability to balance glucose, insulin, and glucagon (and other counterregulatory hormones) keeps glucose levels within the normal range. Glucagon provides the primary defense against hypoglycemia; without it full recovery does not occur. Epinephrine is not necessary for counterregulation when glucagon is present. However, in the absence of glucagon, epinephrine has an important role.

Types of Hypoglycemia

Two types of hypoglycemia can occur in people who do not have diabetes. If blood glucose levels fall below normal limits within 2 to 5 hours after eating, this is postprandial (reactive) hypoglycemia. It can be caused by an exaggerated or late insulin response caused by either insulin resistance or elevated GLP-1; alimentary hyperinsulinism; renal glycosuria; defects in glucagon response; high insulin sensitivity; rare syndromes such as hereditary fructose intolerance, galactosemia, leucine sensitivity; or a rare beta-cell pancreatic tumor (insulinoma), causing blood glucose levels to drop too low. Alimentary hyperinsulinism is common after gastric surgery, associated with rapid delivery of food to the small intestine, rapid absorption of glucose, and exaggerated insulin response. These patients respond best to multiple, frequent feedings.

The ingestion of alcohol after a prolonged fast or the ingestion of large amounts of alcohol and carbohydrates on an empty stomach ("gin-and-tonic" syndrome) also may cause hypoglycemia within 3 to 4 hours in some healthy persons.

Idiopathic reactive hypoglycemia is characterized by normal insulin secretion but increased insulin sensitivity and, to some extent, reduced response of glucagon to acute hypoglycemia symptoms. The increase in insulin sensitivity associated with a deficiency of glucagon secretion leads to hypoglycemia late postprandially. Idiopathic reactive hypoglycemia has been inappropriately overdiagnosed by physicians and patients, to the point that some physicians doubt its existence. Although rare, it does exist but can be documented only in persons with hypoglycemia that occurs spontaneously and who meet the criteria of Whipple's triad.

Fasting hypoglycemia, or postabsorptive hypoglycemia, often is related to an underlying disease. This food-deprived hypoglycemia may occur in response to having gone without food for 8 hours or longer and can be caused by conditions that upset the body's ability to balance blood glucose. These include eating disorders and other serious underlying medical conditions, including hormone deficiency states (e.g., hypopituitarism, adrenal insufficiency, catecholamine or glucagon deficiency), acquired liver disease, renal disease, certain drugs (e.g., alcohol, propranolol, salicylate), insulinoma (of which most are benign, but 6%-10% can be malignant), and other nonpancreatic tumors. Taking high doses of aspirin also may lead to fasting hypoglycemia. Factitious hypoglycemia, or self-administration of insulin or sulfonylurea in persons who do not have diabetes, is a cause as well. Symptoms related to fasting hypoglycemia tend to be particularly severe and can include a loss of mental acuity, seizures, and unconsciousness. If the underlying problem can be resolved, hypoglycemia is no longer a problem.

Diagnostic Criteria

One of the criteria used to confirm the presence of hypoglycemia is a blood glucose level of less than 50 mg/dl (2.8 mmol/L). Previously the OGT test was the standard test for this condition; however, this test is no longer used. Recording finger stick blood glucose measurements during spontaneous, symptomatic episodes at home is used to establish the diagnosis. An alternative method is to perform a glucose test in a medical office setting, in which case the patient is given a typical meal that has been documented in the past to lead to symptomatic episodes; Whipple's triad can be confirmed if symptoms occur. If blood glucose levels are low during the symptomatic period and if the symptoms disappear on eating, hypoglycemia is probably responsible. It is essential to make a correct diagnosis in patients with fasting hypoglycemia because the implications are serious.

Management of Hypoglycemia

The management of hypoglycemic disorders involves two distinct components: (1) relief of neuroglycopenic symptoms by restoring blood glucose concentrations to the normal range and (2) correction of the underlying cause. The immediate treatment is to eat foods or beverages containing carbohydrates. As the glucose from the breakdown of carbohydrates is absorbed into the bloodstream, it increases the level of glucose in the blood and relieves the symptoms. If an underlying problem is causing hypoglycemia, appropriate treatment of this disease or disorder is essential.

Almost no research has been done to determine what type of food-related treatment is best for the prevention of hypoglycemia. Traditional advice has been to avoid foods containing sugars and to eat protein- and fat-containing foods. Recent research on the GI and sugars has raised questions about the appropriateness of restricting only sugars because these foods have been reported to have a lower GI than many of the starches that were encouraged in the past. Restriction of sugars may contribute to a decreased intake in total carbohydrates, which may be more important than the source of the carbohydrates.

The goal of treatment is to adopt eating habits that will keep blood glucose levels as stable as possible (International Diabetes Center, 2013). To stay symptom free, it is important for individuals to eat five to six small meals or snacks per day. Doing this provides manageable amounts of glucose to the body. Recommended guidelines are listed in Box 30-8.

Patients with hypoglycemia also may benefit from learning carbohydrate counting and, to prevent hypoglycemia, eating three to four carbohydrate servings (15 g of carbohydrate per serving) at meals and one to two for snacks (see Appendix 27). Foods containing protein that are also low in saturated fat can be eaten at meals or with snacks. These foods would be expected to have minimum effect on blood glucose levels and can add extra food for satiety and calories. However, because protein and carbohydrate stimulate insulin release, a moderate intake may be advisable.

BOX 30-8   Guidelines for Preventing Hypoglycemic Symptoms in People Who Do Not Have Diabetes

1. Eat small meals, with snacks interspersed between meals and at bedtime. This means eating five to six small meals rather than two to three large meals to steady the release of glucose into the bloodstream.
2. Spread the intake of carbohydrate foods throughout the day. Most individuals can eat two to four servings of carbohydrate foods at each meal and one to two servings at each snack. If carbohydrates are removed from the diet completely, the body loses its ability to handle carbohydrates properly, so this is not recommended. Carbohydrate foods include starches, fruits and fruit juices, milk and yogurt, and foods containing sugar.
3. Avoid or limit foods high in sugar and carbohydrate, especially on an empty stomach. Examples of these foods are regular soft drinks, syrups, candy, fruit juices, regular fruited yogurts, pies, and cakes.
4. Avoid beverages and foods containing caffeine. Caffeine can cause the same symptoms as hypoglycemia and make the individual feel worse.
5. Limit or avoid alcoholic beverages. Drinking alcohol on an empty stomach and without food can lower blood glucose levels by interfering with the liver's ability to release stored glucose (gluconeogenesis). If an individual chooses to drink alcohol, it should be done in moderation (one or two drinks no more than twice a week), and food always should be eaten along with the alcoholic beverage.

Modified from International Diabetes Center: *Reactive and fasting hypoglycemia*, Minneapolis, 2013, International Diabetes Center.

CLINICAL CASE STUDY

Maria P is a 65 year old, non-smoker Hispanic female who is coming to see you for management of her Type 2 diabetes. Her blood glucose levels are uncontrolled as evidenced by an A1C >10, and she complains of increasing numbness in her feet and occasionally in her fingers, and frequent urination during the day and overnight. From interviewing her and reviewing her health record, you learn the following about her:

Education: Did not complete high school, attended through middle school.
Occupation: Not employed outside the home, babysits infant grandchild on a daily basis
Household Members: Lives with her husband and with one of her four adult children.
Ethnic Background: Latin American, born in Mexico, emigrated to US in 1980
Religious Affiliation: Catholic
Language: Native Spanish, speaks English – has difficulty reading English
Patient History: Weighed more than 9 lb at birth.
Maria was diagnosed with T2DM, 10 or 15 years ago and her diabetes management history is as follows:
Type of Treatment: Nutrition therapy plus oral diabetes medication and long-acting insulin at bedtime (HS)
Medications: Meds: glargine 80 units at HS, metformin XR 1000 mg BID, enalapril 10 mg daily, simvastatin 40 mg daily, levothyroxine 75 mcg daily
Family history: Mother had type 2 diabetes, 12 year old grandson recently diagnosed with prediabetes
Medical History: type 2 diabetes, hypertension, hyperlipidemia, hypothyroidism, episodic migraines (last occurrence 2012)
Physical exam shows the following: Weight: 201 lbs.
    Height: 5'2" inches,
    Temp: 98.6 F
    BP: 143/88 mm Hg
    Heart rate; 80 bpm
Labs: A1C 9.8%, TSH 8, FT4 0.3; Total cholesterol 144 mg/dL, LDL 116 mg/dL, HDL 54 mg/dL; Triglycerides 545 mg/dL, BUN 14
Self-monitoring of blood glucose record shows:
Aggregate mean: 218 mg/dL, Standard deviation: 48 (n = 68) over last 30 days
Frequency – 2 x/day
Fasting (6 AM): 173 mg/dL, Standard deviation: 35 (n = 21)
Prebreakfast (9 AM): 248 mg/dL, Standard deviation: 30 (n = 6)
Prelunch: (1 PM): 193 mg/dL, Standard deviation: 47 (n = 17)
Predinner (6 PM): 195 mg/dL, Standard deviation: 33 (n = 11)
Bedtime (n = 9): 260 mg/dL, Standard deviation 34 (n = 13)
Range: 69 mg/dL to 304 mg/dL
Nutrition History:
General: Good appetite, with wide consumption of foods and beverages native to the region in Mexico where she was born. She plans and prepares meals for the household.
Performed a 24-hour diet recall.
    Breakfast: coffee with milk and sugar (several spoons) + sweet bread 3 to 4 pieces
    Lunch: chicken and vegetable soup + corn tortillas (4-6), home-prepared fruit juice (1-2 x 16 ounce glass)

    Dinner: Largest meal – chicken/beef, rice (~2 cups) and beans (1½ - 2 cups), + corn tortillas (4-6), home-prepared fruit juice (1-2 x 16 ounce glass)
    Afternoon snack: 1 can "natural" cola + 3 to 4 sugar-free cookies
    HS snack: cereal + milk
Food allergies/intolerances/aversions: None
Previous nutrition therapy: Several years ago when diagnosed
Vitamin/supplement intake: Vitamin D3 – 2000 IU per day, One A Day vitamin supplement

Tx Plan:

1. Referral to RDN, CDE for instruction on carbohydrate counting for use with a basal-bolus insulin plan.
2. Physician prescribed:
    a. rapid-acting insulin analog lispro.
Premeal dose
breakfast 10 units,
lunch 15 units,
dinner 20 units
Correction insulin (insulin sensitivity factor) 1 unit to drop blood glucose level 50 mg/dL when premeal blood glucose > 150 mg/dL
    b. Increased self-monitoring of blood glucose premeal (breakfast, lunch and dinner) and 2 hour postprandial blood glucose after dinner.

Nutrition Care Questions

1) Why did Maria's physician prescribe mealtime insulin? Would another medication have been more effective at this stage of her disease?
2) What is a potential problem of the current mealtime insulin plan using "set" or "fixed" doses of premeal insulin?
3) Will the long-acting insulin need to be adjusted? If so, why?
4) What is the proposed mechanism of action of metformin? Why did her physician leave Maria on this medication after the insulin was initiated?
5) Identify at least two reasons why regular physical activity such as walking would be beneficial for Maria?
6) What is causing the numbness and tingling in Maria's feet and occasionally in her fingers?

Nutrition Assessment

7) Determine Maria's nutrition requirements
    a) Identify two methods for determination of Maria's energy requirements.
    b) Calculate body mass index, percent usual body weight (UBW), percent ideal body weight?
8) Intake Domain:
    a) Dietary factors associated with increase of overweight/obesity and hyperglycemia are large portions of food, no regular physical activity, and increased consumption of sugar-sweetened beverages. Identify foods in Maria's diet history that fit these criteria.
    b) Increased vegetable and fruit intake is associated with a reduced risk of overweight. Using Maria's usual intake, is her vegetable and fruit intake adequate?

CLINICAL CASE STUDY—cont'd

c) Using the carbohydrate counting Eating Plan approach with 3 to 4 carbohydrate choices per meal (Breakfast/Lunch and Dinner) and 1 carbohydrate choice at HS, plan a 1 day menu for Maria.

9) Clinical Domain:
   a) Why does Maria's physician order pre- and 2 hour postmeal blood glucose monitoring?
   b) What are the pre/postmeal glucose targets?

10) Behavioral-Environmental Domain:
   a) What behaviors might be contributing to Maria's overweight and obesity?
   b) Identify one specific physical activity recommendation for Maria that she could do during the day when she is caring for her grandchild.

Nutrition Diagnostic Statements

Select two of Maria's nutrition problems and complete PES statements for each one.

PES Statements:

1) Food and nutrition-related knowledge deficit related to lack of previous diabetes nutrition education as evidenced by patient's nutrition history.

2) Limited adherence to nutrition-related recommendations related to poor understanding as evidenced by elevated hemoglobin A1C and food records that indicate that patient is consuming excessive amounts of carbohydrate and calories.

3) Altered blood glucose levels related to inability to match insulin to carbohydrate intake as evidenced by patient's nutrition history and glucose monitoring download data report.

Nutrition Intervention

4) For each of the two PES statements, write a goal, based on signs and symptoms.

5) For the two goals, write 2 to 3 nutrition interventions, based on the etiology that would be appropriate for Maria.

NOTE: In a real face-to-face appointment between an RDN/CDE and Maria, they would collaboratively develop Maria's goals together.

Nutrition Evaluation and Monitoring

a) When should the next nutrition counseling session be scheduled for Maria?

b) What would you assess at the follow-up visit based on the nutrition goals and interventions developed at the initial appointment?

USEFUL WEBSITES

American Association of Diabetes Educators (AADE)
http://www.diabeteseducator.org

American Diabetes Association (ADA)
http://www.diabetes.org

Academy of Nutrition and Dietetics (AND)
AND Evidence Analysis Library
http://www.adaevidencelibrary.com

Diabetes Care and Education Practice Group (DCE)
http://www.dce.org

DCE Patient Education Handouts
http://www.dce.org/pub_publications/education.asp

International Diabetes Center (IDC), Minneapolis, Minnesota
http://www.idcdiabetes.org

IDC Publishing
http://www.idcpublishing.com

Joslin Diabetes Center
Resources for Healthcare Professionals
http://www.joslin.org

National Diabetes Education Program (NDEP)
http://www.ndep.nih.gov

National Institute of Diabetes and Digestive Kidney Diseases (NIDDK)
http://www.niddk.nih.gov

REFERENCES

Academy of Nutrition and Academy of Nutrition and Dietetics: *Diabetes Type 1 and Type 2 for Adults Evidence-Based Nutrition Practice Guidelines* (website), http://www.adaevidencelibrary.com/topic.cfm?=3251, 2008a. Accessed February 2, 2014.

Academy of Nutrition and Dietetics: *Gestational Diabetes Mellitus (GDM): Executive Summary of Recommendations* (website), 2008b. http://www.adaevidencelibrary.com/topic.cfm?format_tables=0&cat=3731. Accessed February 3, 2014.

Academy of Nutrition and Dietetics: *International Dietetics & Nutrition Terminology (IDNT) reference manual. Standardized language for the nutrition care process*, ed 4, Chicago, 2012, American Dietetic Association.

American Diabetes Association: Diagnosis and classification of diabetes mellitus, *Diabetes Care* 37(S1):S5, 2014a.

American Diabetes Association: Standards of medical care in diabetes—2014, *Diabetes Care* 37(S1):S14, 2014b.

American Diabetes Association: Standards of medical care in diabetes – 2015, Cardiovascular disease and risk management, *Diabetes Care* 38:S49, 2015.

Arterburn DE, et al: A multisite study of long-term remission and relapse of type 2 diabetes mellitus following gastric bypass, *Obes Surg* 23:93, 2013.

Brand-Miller JC, et al: Glycemic index, postprandial glycemia, and the shape of the curve in healthy subjects: analysis of a database of more than 1000 foods, *Am J Clin Nutr* 89:97, 2009.

Buse JB, et al: Primary prevention of cardiovascular diseases in people with diabetes mellitus: A scientific statement from the American Heart Association and the American Diabetes Association, *Diabetes Care* 30:162, 2007.

Camilleri M: Diabetic gastroparesis, *N Engl J Med* 356:820, 2007.

Centers for Disease Control and Prevention: *National diabetes statistics report: estimates of diabetes and its burden in the United States, 2014.* Atlanta, 2014, U.S. Department of Health and Human Services.

Chiang JL, et al: Type 1 diabetes through the life span: a position statement of the American Diabetes Association, *Diabetes Care* 37:2034, 2014.

Copeland KC, et al: Clinical practice guidelines management of newly diagnosed type 2 diabetes mellitus (T2DM) in children and adolescents, *Pediatrics* 131:364, 2013.

Diabetes Prevention Program Research Group: 10-year follow-up of diabetes incidence and weight loss in the Diabetes Prevention Program Outcome Study, *Lancet* 374:1677, 2009.

Esposito K, et al: Effects of a Mediterranean-style diet on the need for antihyperglycemic drug therapy in patients with newly diagnosed type 2 diabetes: a randomized trial, *Ann Intern Med* 151:306, 2009.

Evert AB, et al: Nutrition therapy recommendations for the management of adults with diabetes, *Diabetes Care* 36:3821, 2013.

Franz MJ: The obesity paradox and diabetes, *Diabetes Spectrum* 26:145, 2013.

Franz MJ, et al: *ADA pocket guide to lipid disorders, hypertension, diabetes, and weight management,* Chicago, 2012, Academy of Nutrition and Dietetics.

Franz MJ, et al: The evidence for medical nutrition therapy for type 1 and type 2 diabetes in adults, *J Am Diet Assoc* 110:1852, 2010.

Franz MJ, et al: Weight loss outcomes: a systematic review and meta-analysis of weight-loss clinical trials with a minimum 1-year follow-up, *J Am Diet Assoc* 107:1755, 2007.

Gardner C, et al: Nonnutritive sweeteners: current use and health perspectives: a scientific statement from the American Heart Association and the American Diabetes Association, *Diabetes Care* 35:1798, 2012.

Holman RR, et al: 10-year follow-up of intensive glucose control in type 2 diabetes, *N Eng J Med* 359:1577, 2008.

Institute of Medicine: *Dietary reference intakes: energy, carbohydrate, fiber, fat, fatty acids, cholesterol, protein, and amino acids*, Washington, DC, 2002, National Academies Press.

International Diabetes Center: *Reactive and fasting hypoglycemia*, ed 4, Minneapolis, 2013, International Diabetes Center.

Inzucchi SE, et al: Management of hyperglycemia in type 2 diabetes, 2015: a patient-centered approach. Update to a position statement of the American Diabetes Association (ADA) and the European Association for the Study of Diabetes (EASD), *Diabetes Care* 38:140, 2015.

Kaufman FR, editor: *Medical management of type 1 diabetes*, ed 6, Alexandria, Va, 2012, American Diabetes Association.

Li G, et al: The long-term effect of lifestyle interventions to prevent diabetes in the China Da Qing Diabetes Prevention Study: a 20-year follow-up study, *Lancet* 371:1783, 2008.

Lindström J, et al: Sustained reduction in the incidence of type 2 by lifestyle intervention: follow-up of the Finnish Diabetes Prevention Study, *Lancet* 368:1673, 2006.

Lautz D, et al: The great debate: medicine or surgery: what is best for the patient with type 2 diabetes? *Diabetes Care* 34:763, 2011.

Look AHEAD Research Group: Long-term effects of a lifestyle intervention on weight and cardiovascular risk factors in individuals with type 2 diabetes mellitus: four year results of the Look AHEAD trial, *Arch Intern Med* 170:1566, 2010.

Ma Y, et al: A randomized clinical trial comparing low-glycemic index versus ADA dietary education among individuals with type 2 diabetes, *Nutrition* 24:45, 2008.

Malik VS, et al: Sugar-sweetened beverages and risk of metabolic syndrome and type 2 diabetes, *Diabetes Care* 33:2477, 2010.

Naik RG, et al: Latent autoimmune diabetes in adults. *J Clin Endocrinol Practice* 94:4635, 2009.

Nathan DM: The Diabetes Control and Complications Trial/Epidemiology of Diabetes Interventions and Complications Study at 30 Years: Overview, *Diabetes Care* 37:9, 2014.

Pastors JG, Franz MJ: Effectiveness of medical nutrition therapy in diabetes. In Franz MJ, Evert AB editors: *American Diabetes Association Guide to Nutrition Therapy for Diabetes*, ed 2, Alexandria, Va, 2012, American Diabetes Association, p 1.

Reader D: Nutrition therapy for pregnancy, lactation, and diabetes. In Franz MJ, Evert AB editors: *American Diabetes Association Guide to Nutrition Therapy for Diabetes*, ed 2, Alexandria, Va, 2012, American Diabetes Association, p 181.

Reis JP, et al: Lifestyle factors and risk of new-onset diabetes: a population-based cohort study, *Ann Intern Med* 155:292, 2011.

Schauer PR, et al: Bariatric surgery versus intensive medical therapy for diabetes—3-year outcomes, *N Engl J Med* 370:2002, 2014.

Springer SC, et al: Management of type 2 diabetes mellitus in children and adolescents, *Pediatrics* 131:e648, 2013.

Stanley K: Nutrition therapy for older adults with diabetes. In Franz MJ, Evert AB editors: *American Diabetes Association Guide to Nutrition Therapy for Diabetes*, ed 2, Alexandria, Va, 2012, American Diabetes Association, p 169.

Stuebe AM, et al: Duration of lactation and incidence of type 2 diabetes, *JAMA* 294:2601, 2005.

Swift CS: Nutrition therapy for the hospitalized and long-term care patient with diabetes. In Franz MJ, Evert AB editors: *American Diabetes Association Guide to Nutrition Therapy for Diabetes*, ed 2, Alexandria, Va, 2012, American Diabetes Association, pp 229.

U.S. Department of Health and Human Services: *2008 Physical Activity Guidelines for Americans*, 2008. http://www.health.gov/paguidelines. Accessed December 19, 2014.

Vega-López S, et al: Interindividual variability and intra-individual reproducibility of glycemic index values for commercial white bread, *J Am Diet Assoc* 30:1412, 2007.

Wheeler ML, et al: Macronutrients, food groups, and eating patterns in the management of diabetes: a systematic review of the literature, 2010, *Diabetes Care* 35:434, 2012.

Wolever TMS, et al: The Canadian Trial of Carbohydrates in Diabetes, a 1-y controlled trial of low-glycemic index dietary carbohydrate in type 2 diabetes: no effect on glycated hemoglobin but reduction in C-reactive protein, *Am J Clin Nutr* 87:114, 2008.

Wolpert HA, et al: Dietary fat acutely increases glucose concentrations and insulin requirements in patients with type 1 diabetes, *Diabetes Care* 36:810, 2013.

Writing Group of the Nutrition Care Process/Standardized Language Committee: Nutrition Care Process Part II: Using the International Dietetics and Nutrition Terminology to Document the Nutrition Care Process, *J Am Diet Assoc* 108:1287, 2008.

Youssef G: Nutrition therapy and prediabetes. In Franz MJ, Evert AB editors: *American Diabetes Association Guide to Nutrition Therapy for Diabetes*, ed 2, Alexandria, Va, 2012, American Diabetes Association, pp 469–500.

31

Medical Nutrition Therapy for Thyroid, Adrenal, and Other Endocrine Disorders

Sheila Dean, DSc, RDN, LD, CCN, CDE

KEY TERMS

5-deiodinase
Addison's disease
adrenal fatigue
autoimmune thyroid disorders
(AITDs)
calcitonin
cortisol
cretinism
euthyroid sick syndrome
free T$_4$
goitrin

Graves' disease
Hashimoto's thyroiditis
hyperthyroidism
hypothalamus
hypothalamic-pituitary-thyroid
(HPT) axis
hypothyroidism
pituitary gland
polycystic ovary syndrome (PCOS)
reverse T$_3$ (rT$_3$)
Schmidt syndrome

thyroid-binding globulin (TBG)
thyroglobulin antibodies (TGB Ab)
thyroid peroxidase (TPO)
thyroid peroxidase antibodies (TPO Ab)
thyroid-stimulating hormone (TSH)
thyrotropin-releasing hormone
(TRH)
thyrotoxicosis
thyroxine (T$_4$)
triiodothyronine (T$_3$)
tyrosine

Diabetes mellitus appears to be the most common endocrine-related chronic disease (CDC, 2014; NIH, MedlinePlus, 2014). However, according to a comprehensive review of the prevalence and incidence of endocrine and metabolic disorders in the United States (2009), about 5% of the U.S. population age 12 and older has hypothyroidism, and more than half remain undiagnosed. Furthermore, individuals with diabetes tend to have a higher prevalence of thyroid disorders.

Thyroid-related diseases often are poorly diagnosed, and much about their treatment requires greater clarification and study. For example, radiation exposure of the thyroid at a young age is a risk factor for the development of thyroid cancer, lasting for a lifetime after exposure (Sinnott et al, 2010). Efforts to reduce exposure from medical x-ray examinations can protect the thyroid gland.

Genetic factors promote the endocrine autoimmune diseases. Recent genome-wide association studies (GWAS) have enabled identification of relevant immune response pathways; the same allele that predisposes to a certain autoimmune disease can be protective in another (Wiebolt et al, 2010). Thus endocrine GWAS are needed, especially for Graves' disease, Hashimoto's thyroiditis, and Addison's disease. Each of these disorders has stages beginning with genetic susceptibility, environmental triggers, and active autoimmunity, followed by metabolic derangements with overt symptoms of disease (Michels and Eisenbarth, 2010). Research is needed to clarify how nutrients interact with genetics, especially in these **autoimmune thyroid disorders (AITDs)**.

THYROID PHYSIOLOGY

The thyroid gland is a small, butterfly-shaped gland found just below the Adam's apple. Although it weighs less than an ounce, it produces hormones that influence essentially every organ, tissue, and cell in the body, thus having an enormous effect on health. The thyroid gland responds to stimulation by **thyroid-stimulating hormone (TSH)**, a hormone secreted by the pituitary gland. When stimulated, the thyroid gland produces two main hormones: **thyroxine (T$_4$)**, a thyroid hormone named for its four molecules of iodine, and **triiodothyronine (T$_3$)**, a thyroid hormone named for its three molecules of iodine. T$_3$ is the most predominant and active form of thyroid hormone that the body can use. The thyroid gland regulates many processes in the body, including fat and carbohydrate metabolism, body temperature, and heart rate. The thyroid also produces **calcitonin**, a hormone that helps regulate the amount of blood calcium. Last, **reverse T$_3$ (rT$_3$)**, an isomer of T$_3$, is derived from T$_4$ through the action of deiodinase. The body cannot use rT$_3$.

The synthesis of these hormones requires **tyrosine**, a key amino acid involved in the production of thyroid hormone, and the trace mineral iodine. Within the cells of the thyroid gland, iodide is oxidized to iodine by hydrogen peroxide, a reaction termed the *organification* of iodide. Two additional molecules of iodine bind to the tyrosyl ring in a reaction that involves **thyroid peroxidase (TPO)**, an enzyme in the thyroid responsible for thyroid hormone production. Completed thyroid hormones are released into the circulation; however, metabolic effects of thyroid hormones result when the hormones ultimately occupy specific thyroid receptors. It is estimated that a cell needs five to seven times more T_4 to bind to the nuclear receptors to have a physiologic effect compared with T_3.

The biosynthetic processes resulting in generation of thyroid hormones within the thyroid gland are controlled by feedback mechanisms within the **hypothalamic-pituitary-thyroid axis (HPT axis)**. The HPT axis is part of the endocrine system responsible for the regulation of metabolism. As its name suggests, it depends on the **hypothalamus** (a tiny, cone-shaped structure located in the lower center of the brain that communicates between the nervous and endocrine systems), the **pituitary gland** (the master gland of the endocrine system located at the base of the brain), and the thyroid gland (see Figure 31-1).

The hypothalamus produces and secretes **thyrotropin-releasing hormone (TRH)**, which travels to the pituitary gland, stimulating it to release TSH, which signals the thyroid gland to upregulate its synthetic machinery. Although T_4, T_3, and rT_3 are generated within the thyroid gland, T_4 is quantitatively the major secretory product. All T_4 found in circulation is generated in the thyroid unless exogenously administered. Production of T_3 and rT_3 within the thyroid is relegated to very small quantities and is not considered significant compared with their peripheral production (see Figure 31-2).

When T_4 is released from the thyroid, it is primarily in a bound form with **thyroid-binding globulin (TBG)**, a protein that transports thyroid hormones through the bloodstream, with lesser amounts bound to T_4-binding prealbumin. It is estimated that only 0.03% to 0.05% of T_4 within the circulatory system is in a free or unbound form; this unbound T_4 is called **free T_4**. In peripheral tissues, approximately 70% of T_4 produced is either deiodinated and converted to T_3 or rT_3, or eliminated. As mentioned, T_3 is considered to be the most metabolically active thyroid hormone. Although some T_3 is

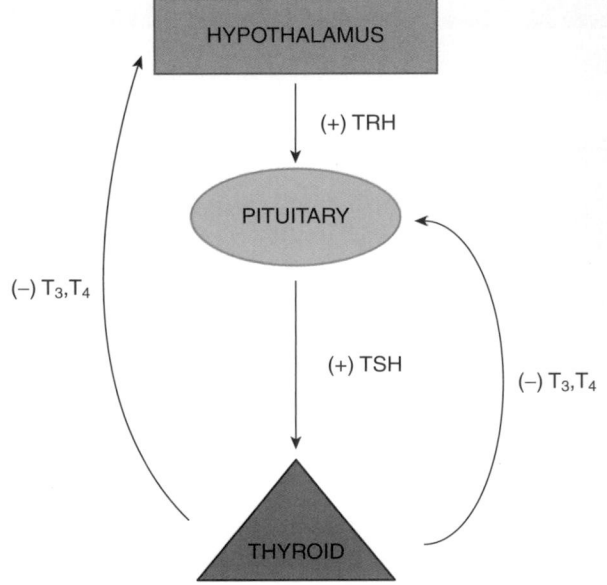

$(+)$ = positive feedback or stimulation
$(-)$ = negative feedback or inhibition

FIGURE 31-1 The hypothalamus-pituitary-thyroid axis.

produced in the thyroid, approximately 80% to 85% is generated outside the thyroid gland, primarily by conversion of T_4 in the liver and kidneys. The pituitary and nervous system are also capable of converting T_4 to T_3 so are not reliant on T_3 produced in the liver or kidney. Within the liver and kidney, the enzyme responsible for production of T_3 is a selenium-dependent

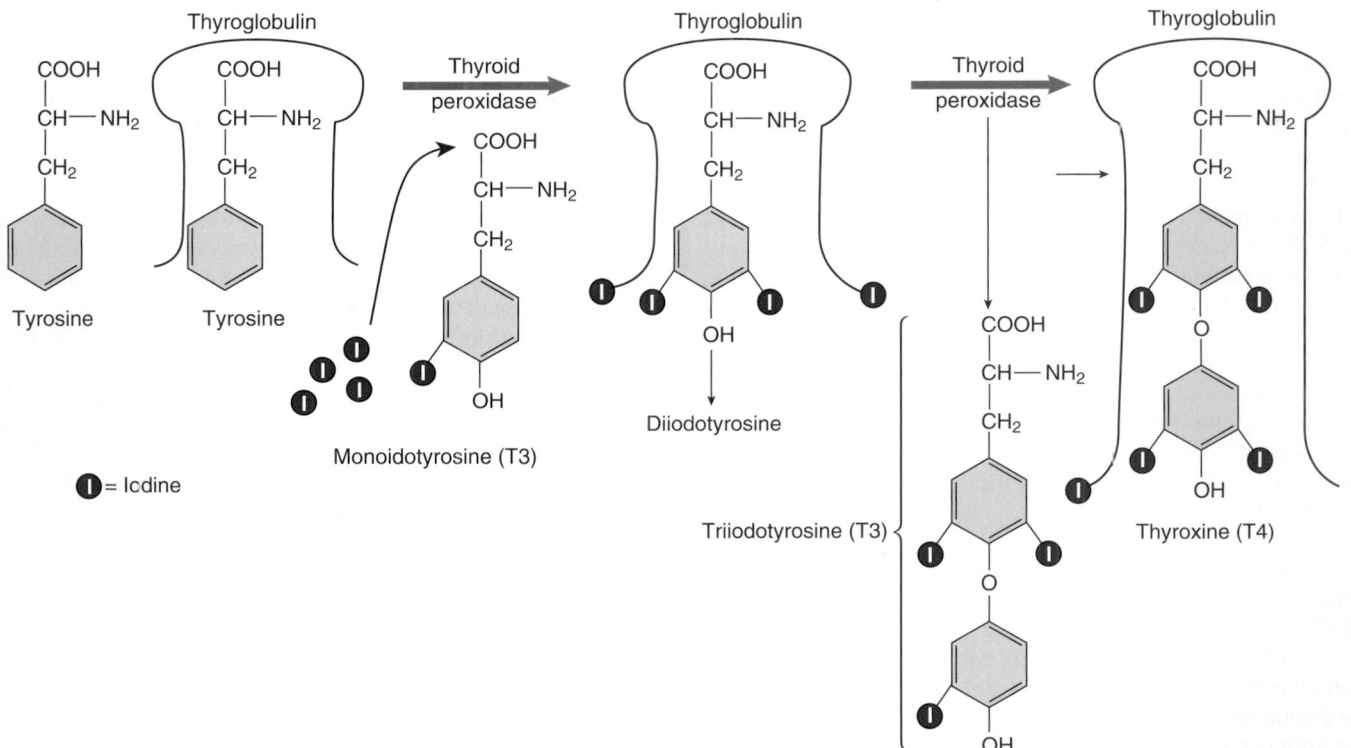

FIGURE 31-2 Constructing thyroid hormones. (1) Accumulation of the raw materials tyrosine and iodide (I-), (2) fabrication or synthesis of the hormone, and (3) secretion of hormone into the blood either bound or as free T_4.

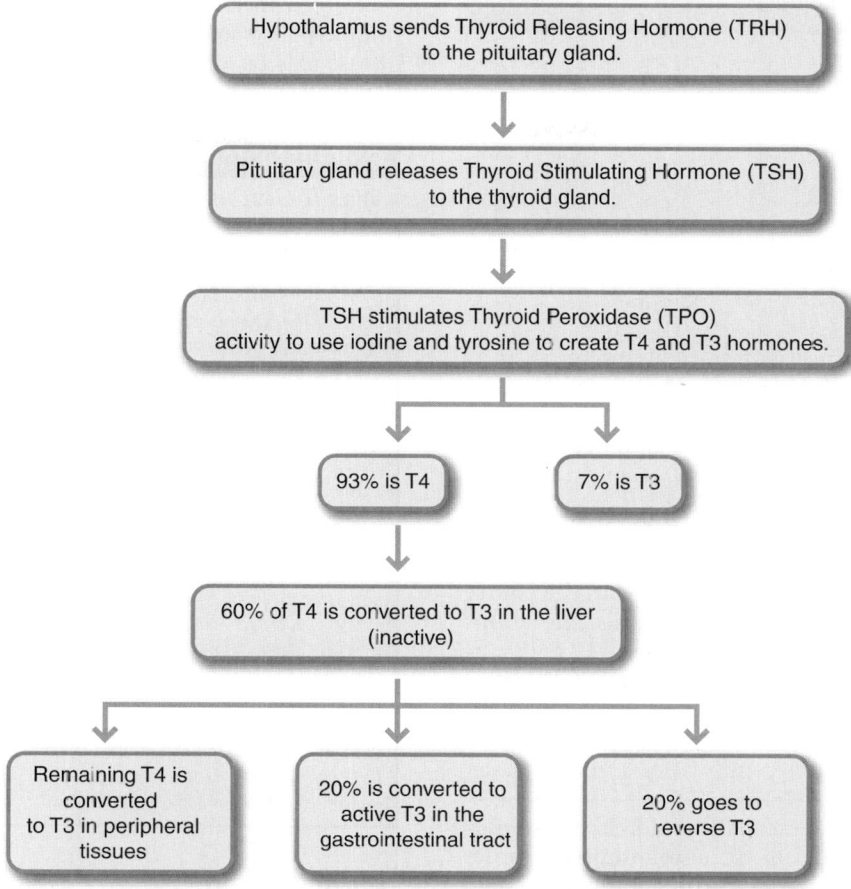

FIGURE 31-3 Thyroid metabolism.

enzyme called 5-deiodinase, an enzyme that removes one molecule of iodine from T_4 to form either T_3 or rT_3 (see Figure 31-3).

ASSESSMENT IN THYROID DISORDERS

Assessment begins with an evaluation of thyroid status based on laboratory data such as a full thyroid panel. In the absence of a full thyroid panel, a serum thyrotropin (also known as TSH) is the single best screening test for primary thyroid dysfunction, (when it does not include thyroid associated autoimmune conditions), for the vast majority of outpatient clinical situations (Garber et al, 2012). Assessments also may include a diet history to evaluate micronutrients pertaining to thyroid health along with an evaluation of calorie and carbohydrate intake. In addition, an assessment of dietary intake of goitrogenic foods may be warranted.

Laboratory Norms: Functional versus Pathologic Ranges

A typical (statistical) reference range for TSH in many laboratories is approximately 0.2 to 5.5 mIU/L. Individuals with TSH values greater than 2 mIU/L have an increased risk of developing overt hypothyroidism during the next 20 years. Subclinical autoimmune thyroid disease is so common in the population that laboratory reference ranges derived from testing apparently healthy subjects easily could be misconstrued for those with disease. Importantly, several studies have detected an increase in TPO antibody positivity with TSH

concentrations outside the narrow range of 0.2 to 1.9 mIU/L (Downs et al, 2008; Fjaellagaard et al, 2014). This fact provides evidence that TSH in the upper reference range often is associated with abnormal pathologic findings (Hak et al, 2000; Khandelwal and Tandon, 2012; Saravanan et al, 2002), mitochondrial dysfunction and morphologic skeletal muscle alterations including myalgia, muscle cramps, and weakness (Dunn et al, 2009). Additional evidence that thyroid function within the laboratory reference ranges can be associated with adverse outcomes is shown in Table 31-1. Conversely,

TABLE 31-1	Variation In Thyroid Function Within Reference Range and Adverse Outcomes
TSH >2 mIU/L*	Increased 20-year risk of hypothyroidism
TSH >2 mIU/L*	Increased frequency of thyroid autoantibodies
TSH >4 mIU/L*	Increased risk of heart disease
TSH 2-4 mIU/L*	Cholesterol values respond to thyroxine replacement
Free T_4 <10.4 pmol/L†	Impaired psychomotor development of infant if occurs in first trimester of pregnancy

T_3, Triiodothyronine; T_4, thyroxine; *TSH*, thyroid-stimulating hormone.
*Typical reference ranges: TSH 0.2-5.5 mIU/L
†Typical reference ranges: free T4 9.8-25 pml/L

decreased TSH levels combined with normal to high T_4 or T_3 levels may be suggestive of hyperthyroidism (see Thyroid Function Tests in Appendix 22).

Changes in 5-deiodination occur in a number of situations, such as stress, poor nutrition, illness, selenium deficiency, and drug therapy. Toxic metals such as cadmium, mercury, and lead have been associated with impaired hepatic 5-deiodination in animal models. Free radicals are also involved in inhibition of 5-deiodinase activity. In the course of chronic liver disease such as hepatic cirrhosis, alterations in hepatic deiodination resulting in increased rT_3 and a simultaneous decrease in T_3 levels also have been observed (see Box 31-1 and Chapter 29).

HYPOTHYROIDISM

Of the detected cases of underactive thyroid (hypothyroidism), more than half are due to an autoimmune disorder called Hashimoto's thyroiditis, in which the immune system attacks and destroys thyroid gland tissue. A common clinical presentation of patients with functional changes of the endocrine system is altered thyroid function. Indeed *subclinical* hypothyroidism represents the first signs of thyroid hormone dysfunction for many individuals. Typical symptoms include low energy, cold hands and feet, fatigue, hypercholesterolemia, muscle pain, depression, and cognitive deficits (see Box 31-2). Evaluation of thyroid hormone metabolism is needed before thyroid hormone replacement therapy.

BOX 31-2	Common Symptoms of Hypothyroidism and Hyperthyroidism

Hypothyroidism	Hyperthyroidism
Fatigue	Heat intolerance, sweating
Forgetfulness	Weight loss
Depression	Alterations in appetite
Heavy menses	Frequent bowel movements
Dry, coarse hair	Changes in vision
Mood swings	Fatigue and muscle weakness
Weight gain	Menstrual disturbance
Hoarse voice	Impaired fertility
Dry, coarse skin	Mental disturbances
Constipation	Sleep disturbances
	Tremors
	Thyroid enlargement

From Shomon M: Thyroid *Disease Symptoms—Hypothyroidism and Hyperthyroidism* (website): http://thyroid.about.com/cs/basics_starthere/a/symptoms.htm, 2008. Accessed December 8, 2014.

Women are five to eight times more likely than men to suffer from hypothyroidism. In addition, individuals who have celiac disease may be at risk (see *Clinical Insight:* Was It Gluten That Caused Her Hypothyroidism?)

CLINICAL INSIGHT
Was It Gluten That Caused Her Hypothyroidism?

A case report described a 23-year-old woman with a diagnosis of hypothyroidism caused by Hashimoto's thyroiditis and autoimmune Addison's disease who was found in evaluation to have elevated antiendomysial antibody levels. During a 3-month period on a gluten-free diet, the patient demonstrated remarkable clinical improvement in her GI related symptoms and, more importantly, in her thyroid function. She required progressively less thyroid and adrenal replacement therapy. After 6 months her endomysial antibody level became negative, her antithyroidal antibody titer decreased significantly, and thyroid medication was discontinued. This case report points out the important effect of a hypoallergenic diet on thyroid function in relation to the potential reduction of antithyroid antibodies.

A number of studies show the importance of gluten in the induction of endocrine autoantibodies and organ system dysfunction in adolescent celiac patients (Cassio et al, 2010; Meloni et al., 2009). Furthermore, the genetic risk for celiac disease is largely related to human leukocyte antigen genotypes, which in turn is largely accountable for its link to autoimmune thyroid disease (Barker and Liu, 2008). It has been reported that gluten-dependent diabetes and thyroidal-related antibodies were found in patients with celiac disease, but were abolished after a gluten-free diet was followed (Duntas, 2009). Similarly, there is a high prevalence of thyroid disorders in untreated adult patients with celiac disease; gluten withdrawal through dietary avoidance may reverse this abnormality. This is another important dietary variable that can modify thyroid hormone activity.

Pathophysiology

Hashimoto's thyroiditis is an autoimmune disorder in which the immune system attacks and destroys the thyroid gland. It is the most common form of hypothyroidism. The enlarged, chronically inflamed thyroid gland becomes nonfunctional, with reactive parts of the gland deteriorating after several years. Thyroid autoantibodies indicate the body's immune system is attacking itself and whether an autoimmune thyroid condition is present, be it hypothyroidism or hyperthyroidism. Epstein-Barr virus (EBV) has been implicated as a critical etiopathogenic factor in autoimmune thyroid disease. Janegova et al demonstrated a high prevalence of EBV infection in cases of Hashimito's thyroiditis (80.7%) as well as in samples of Graves' disease (62.5%).

Specific antibody tests identify Hashimoto's thyroiditis. Thyroid peroxidase antibodies (TPO Ab) are immune cells that indicate the immune system is attacking TPO in the thyroid gland. The TPO Ab test is the most important, because TPO is the enzyme responsible for the production of thyroid hormones, and the most frequent target of attack in Hashimoto's. Thyroglobulin antibodies (TGB Ab) are immune cells that indicate the immune system is attacking thyroglobulin in the thyroid gland. Sometimes this test is necessary as well because it is the second most common target for Hashimoto's disease.

Schmidt syndrome refers to hypothyroidism with other endocrine disorders, including Addison's disease (adrenal insufficiency), hypoparathyroidism, and diabetes mellitus, all of which may be autoimmune in nature. Euthyroid sick syndrome is hypothyroidism, associated with a severe systemic illness that causes decreased peripheral conversion of T_4 to T_3, an increased conversion of T_3 to the inactive rT_3, and decreased binding of thyroid hormones. Conditions commonly associated with this syndrome include protein-calorie malnutrition, surgical trauma, myocardial infarction, chronic renal failure, diabetic ketoacidosis, anorexia nervosa, cirrhosis, thermal injury, and sepsis. Once the underlying cause is treated, the condition usually is resolved (see *Pathophysiology and Care Management Algorithm: Thyroid Dysfunction*).

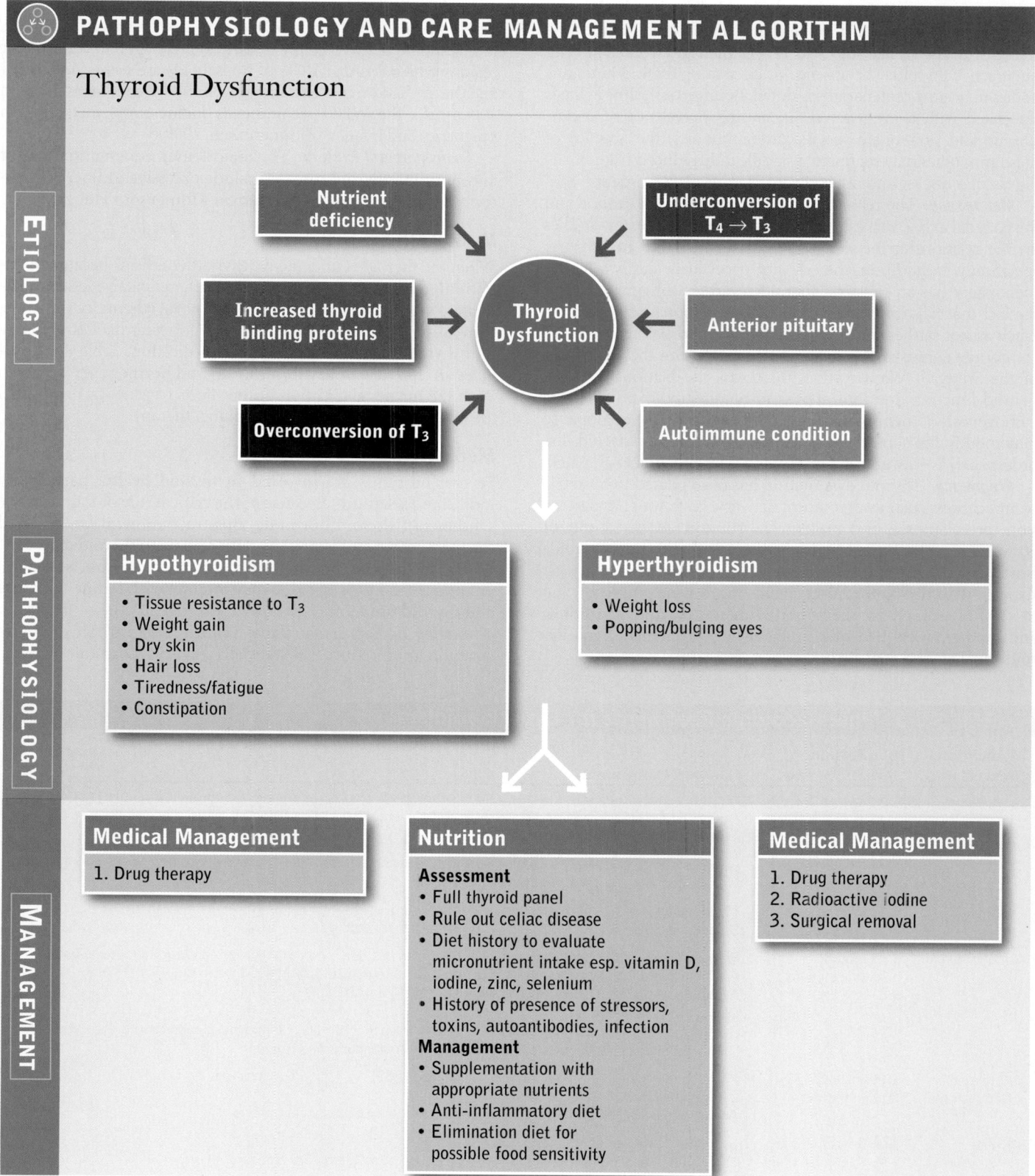

PATHOPHYSIOLOGY AND CARE MANAGEMENT ALGORITHM

Thyroid Dysfunction

ETIOLOGY

- Nutrient deficiency
- Underconversion of $T_4 \rightarrow T_3$
- Increased thyroid binding proteins
- Anterior pituitary
- Overconversion of T_3
- Autoimmune condition

→ Thyroid Dysfunction

PATHOPHYSIOLOGY

Hypothyroidism

- Tissue resistance to T_3
- Weight gain
- Dry skin
- Hair loss
- Tiredness/fatigue
- Constipation

Hyperthyroidism

- Weight loss
- Popping/bulging eyes

MANAGEMENT

Medical Management

1. Drug therapy

Nutrition

Assessment
- Full thyroid panel
- Rule out celiac disease
- Diet history to evaluate micronutrient intake esp. vitamin D, iodine, zinc, selenium
- History of presence of stressors, toxins, autoantibodies, infection

Management
- Supplementation with appropriate nutrients
- Anti-inflammatory diet
- Elimination diet for possible food sensitivity

Medical Management

1. Drug therapy
2. Radioactive iodine
3. Surgical removal

Triggers

Adrenal Stress and Oxidative Stress. Low thyroid function is almost always secondary to some other condition, often adrenal fatigue (Kaltsas et al, 2010) (see Adrenal Disorders later in this chapter).

Aging. Maintaining thyroid hormone function throughout the aging process appears to be an important hallmark of healthy aging. The incidence of hypothyroidism (underactive thyroid) increases with age. By age 60, 9% to 17% of men and women have an underactive thyroid. The absence of circulating thyroid autoantibodies in healthy centenarians is noted. Because unhealthy aging is associated with a progressively increasing prevalence of organ-specific and non–organ-specific autoantibodies, the absence of these antibodies may represent a significantly reduced risk for cardiovascular disease and other chronic age-related disorders.

Menopause. The relationship between thyroid hormone and the gonadal axis is well established; however, there are few studies on the relationship between thyroid function and menopause specifically. In addition, they do not necessarily clarify whether menopause has an effect on thyroid regardless of aging, despite the fact that hypothyroid symptoms and menopause symptoms (such as hot flashes, insomnia, irritability, and palpitations) are commonly confused. According to a report from the evaluation of the Study of Women's Health Across the Nation (SWAN), thyroid function does not appear to be directly involved in the pathogenesis of menopausal complications; however, menopause may modify the clinical expression of autoimmune thyroid disorders such as Hashimoto's thyroiditis (Del Ghianda et al, 2013).

Pregnancy. Thyroid dysfunction has been related to obstetric complications such as premature delivery, gestational hypertension, preeclampsia, and placental abruption. Nearly 1 out of 50 women in the United States is diagnosed with hypothyroidism during pregnancy. Out of every 100 miscarriages, 6 are associated with thyroid hormone deficiency during pregnancy; up to 18% of women are diagnosed with postpartum thyroiditis; and approximately 25% of women develop permanent hypothyroidism (De Vivo et al, 2010; Yassa et al, 2010).

The World Health Organization (WHO) recently increased the recommended iodine intake during pregnancy from 200 to 250 mcg/day and suggested that a median urinary iodine (UI) concentration of 150 to 249 mcg/L indicates adequate iodine intake in pregnant women. In areas of severe iodine deficiency, maternal and fetal hypothyroxinemia can cause cretinism (condition of stunted physical and mental growth) and adversely affect cognitive development in children (see Chapter 15). To prevent fetal damage, iodine should be given before or early in pregnancy. In countries or regions where less than 90% of households are using iodized salt and the median UI concentration in school-age children is less than 100 mcg/L, the WHO recommends iodine supplementation in pregnancy and infancy (Zimmermann, 2009).

Environmental Factors. The major environmental triggers of autoimmune thyroid disease include excessive iodine, medications, infection, smoking, and stress (Tomer and Huber, 2009).

Medical Management

When the thyroid is underactive (hypothyroidism) because of autoimmune disease (Hashimoto's disease), radioactive iodine treatment, congenital defects, or surgical removal (thyroidectomy), the conventional pharmacologic approach for treatment is prescription thyroid hormone replacement medication. Table 31-2 provides an overview of key forms of thyroid hormone replacement. With the further elucidation of the effects of genetics, new agents are likely to become available as adjunct therapy.

Medical Nutrition Therapy

Several nutrients are involved in thyroid health, particularly iodine and selenium. Because of the critical role of iodine in the synthesis of thyroid hormone, this trace mineral has received the most attention historically with respect to thyroid disorders. Other deficiencies of micronutrients such as iron, selenium, vitamin A, and possibly zinc may interact with iodine nutriture and thyroid function (Hess, 2010; Köhrle, 2013).

Fasting or Restrictive Diets. Calorie and carbohydrate restriction may reduce substantially thyroid hormone activity.

TABLE 31-2 Pharmacologic Treatments for Hypothyroidism

Medication Brand Name	Medication Generic Name	Use and Comments
Synthroid, Levoxyl	Levothyroxine— (synthetic T_4)	Most commonly prescribed synthetic form of thyroid hormone replacement drug (thyroxine) that provides a steady dose of T_4 for the body to convert to T_3. Available in a wide range of doses. Inactive ingredients include lactose and cornstarch.
Tirosint	Levothyroxine	A synthetic form of replacement hormone that includes only three inactive ingredients - gelatin, glycerin and water. Is produced in a dedicated facility to eliminate the risk of cross-exposure.
Cytomel	Liothyronine— (synthetic T_3)	Synthetic form of T_3, which can also be compounded. Sometimes prescribed in addition to T_4. Only effective for approximately 10 hours and must be taken twice daily.
Armour Thyroid	Desiccated natural thyroid	Prepared from dried or powdered porcine (pig) or mixed beef and pork thyroid gland for therapeutic use. Available by prescription and frequently used as an alternative to synthetic thyroid drugs. All brands contain a mixture of approximately 80% T_4 and 20% T_3. Difficult to standardize Compounded T_3 medication is available as a time-released formula. Compounded medications are frequently not insurance covered but are less expensive than standard medications.
WP Thyroid, Nature-Throid	Dessicated natural thyroid	Provides the full range of thyroid hormones, including T_4, T_3, T_2 and T_1 which may be beneficial for those who have difficulty with T_4-T_3 conversion. Available in 8-13 different strengths, ranging from low to high concentrations.
Thyrolar	Liotrix—(synthetic T_4-T_3 combination)	Synthetic combination of T_4 and T_3 Sometimes used in lieu of Armour Thyroid because of problem with standardization.

From Shomon M: *What is the best thyroid drug?* (website): http://thyroid.about.com/cs/thyroiddrugs/a/bestdrug.htm, 2014. Accessed December 8, 2014.
T_3, Triiodothyronine; T_4, thyroxine.

This varies widely between individuals. Genetics, obesity, gender, and the macronutrient content of the hypocaloric diet influence the response. Nutritional status and energy expenditure influence thyroid function centrally at the level of TSH secretion, deiodination, and possibly elsewhere. Because an increase of rT_3 is found at the expense of T_3 during caloric restriction, it is possible that the hepatic pathways play a substantial role in metabolic control during energy balance. However, when caloric restriction is longer than 3 weeks, T_4 and rT_3 levels return to normal values (DeVries et al, 2015).

Fasting also exerts a powerful influence on the metabolism of thyroid hormones to save energy and limit catabolism. Mild elevations in endogenous cortisol levels may be partly responsible. Fasting decreases serum T_3 and T_4 concentrations, whereas intrahepatic thyroid hormone concentrations remain unchanged. However, ketones generated from calorie deprivation do not appear to suppress T_3 generation and hepatic 5-deiodinase activity. It appears that fasting-induced changes in liver thyroid hormone metabolism are not regulated via the hepatic autonomic input in a major way and more likely reflect a direct effect of humoral factors on the hepatocyte. Overall during fasting, there is a down regulation of the hypothalamus-pituitary-thyroid axis, which is assumed to represent an energy-saving mechanism, instrumental in times of food shortage (DeVries et al, 2015).

Goitrogens. Cyanogenic plant foods (cauliflower, broccoli, cabbage, Brussels sprouts, mustard seed, turnip, radish, bamboo shoot, and cassava) exert antithyroid activity through inhibition of TPO. The hydrolysis of some glucosinolates found in cruciferous vegetables (e.g., progoitrin) may yield **goitrin**, a compound known to interfere with thyroid hormone synthesis. The hydrolysis of indole glucosinolates results in the release of thiocyanate ions, which can compete with iodine for uptake by the thyroid gland. Increased exposure to thiocyanate ions from cruciferous vegetable consumption, however, does not increase the risk of hypothyroidism unless accompanied by iodine deficiency.

Soybean, an important source of protein in many developing countries, also has goitrogenic properties when iodine intake is limited. The isoflavones, genistein and daidzein, inhibit the activity of TPO and can lower thyroid hormone synthesis. Furthermore, soybean interrupts the enterohepatic cycle of thyroid hormone metabolism. However, high intakes of soy isoflavones do not appear to increase the risk of hypothyroidism when iodine consumption is adequate.

Since the addition of iodine to soy-based formulas in the 1960s, there have been no further reports of hypothyroidism developing in soy formula-fed infants. Soybeans are by far the most concentrated source of isoflavones in the human diet. Small amounts are found in a number of legumes, grains, and vegetables. Average dietary isoflavone intakes in Asian countries, in particular in Japan and China, range from 11 to 47 mg/day because of intake of the traditional foods made from soybeans, including tofu, tempeh, miso, and matte, whereas intakes are considerably lower in Western countries (2 mg/day). Soy products (meat substitutes, soy milk, soy cheese, and soy yogurt), however, are gaining popularity in Western countries. Although research has not determined the exact effect of soy on the metabolic fate of thyroid hormones, excessive soy consumption is best approached cautiously in those with suspected impairment of thyroid metabolic pathways.

Iodine. As a trace element, iodine is present in the human body in amounts of 10 to 15 mg, and 70% to 80% of it is located in the thyroid gland. Ninety percent of it is organically bound to thyroglobulin (Tg). Iodide is actively absorbed in the thyroid gland to help produce the biochemically active thyroid hormones T_4 and T_3 (see Figure 31-2). The thyroid gland must capture an estimated minimum of 60 mcg of iodide (the ionic form of iodine) daily to ensure an adequate supply for the production of thyroid hormone (Gropper et al, 2012). Inadequate intake of iodine impairs thyroid function and results in a spectrum of disorders. Randomized controlled intervention trials in iodine deficient populations have shown that providing iron along with iodine results in greater improvements in thyroid function and volume than providing iodine alone (Hess, 2010). It is also vital to thyroid function, as it is a major cofactor and stimulator for the enzyme TPO.

In autoimmune Hashimoto's, supplementing with iodine may exacerbate the condition. Because iodine stimulates production of TPO, this in turn increases the levels of TPO antibodies (TPO Abs) dramatically, indicating an autoimmune flare-up. Some people develop symptoms of an overactive thyroid, whereas others have no symptoms despite tests showing an elevated level of TPO Abs. Therefore one must be cautious regarding the use of iodine. Furthermore, although iodine deficiency is the most common cause of hypothyroidism for most of the world's population (Melse-Boonstra and Jaiswal, 2010), in the United States and other westernized countries, Hashimoto's accounts for the majority of cases (Ebert, 2010).

Although the risk of iodine deficiency for populations living in iodine-deficient areas without adequate iodine fortification programs is well recognized, concerns have been raised that certain subpopulations may not consume adequate iodine in countries considered iodine-sufficient. Vegetarian and nonvegetarian diets that exclude iodized salt, fish, and seaweed have been found to contain very little iodine. Furthermore, UI excretion studies suggest that iodine intakes are declining in Switzerland, New Zealand, and the United States, possibly because of increased adherence to dietary recommendations to restrict salt intake for reducing the incidence of hypertension.

Severe iodine deficiency during pregnancy has been shown to increase the risk of stillbirths, spontaneous abortions, and congenital abnormalities. The most severe is **cretinism**, which is a state of mental retardation mostly in combination with dwarfism, deaf-mutism, and spasticity (Chen and Hetzel, 2010). These conditions are largely irreversible. The consequences of severe iodine deficiency during pregnancy on pregnancy outcome and early infant development have been described extensively (Zimmermann, 2009); other details can be found in Chapter 15.

Iron. Historically, it has been thought that low thyroid function may cause anemia. Recent studies suggest that low thyroid function may be secondary to low iron status or anemia. The reason for this is because TPO is a glycosylated heme enzyme that is iron-dependent. The insertion of heme iron into TPO is necessary for the enzyme to translocate to the apical cell surface of thyrocytes (or thyroid epithelial cells), thus assisting TPO to catalyze the two initial steps of thyroid hormone synthesis. A full assessment of iron status could likely help to identify the cause of many cases of thyroid malfunction (Dobbs and Titchenal, 2009).

Selenium. Selenium, as selenocysteine, is a cofactor for 5-deiodinase. If selenium is deficient, the deiodinase activity is impaired, resulting in a decreased ability to deiodinate T_4 to T_3. In animals, deficiencies of selenium are associated with impaired 5-deiodinase activity in the liver and kidney, as well as reduced T3 levels. Evidence suggests a strong linear association between lower T_3/T_4 ratios and reduced selenium status, even among individuals considered to be euthyroid based on standard laboratory parameters. This association is particularly strong in older adults, possibly as the result of impaired peripheral conversion. An inverse relationship between T3 and breast cancer is associated with decreased selenium status, even when plasma T_4 and TSH concentrations may be similar. This combination of factors strongly suggests that low T_3 may be due to faulty conversion of T_4 to T_3 expected in selenium deficiency.

Selenium participates in the antioxidant network. It assists in detoxification as part of glutathione peroxidase, an enzyme whose main biologic role is to protect the organism from oxidative damage. Several studies reported on the benefit of selenium treatment in Hashimoto's thyroiditis and Graves' disease.

Evidence also suggests that high intakes of selenium may exert a detrimental influence on thyroid hormone metabolism. Although individuals exposed to high dietary levels of selenium typically have normal levels of T_4, T_3, and TSH, a significant inverse correlation has been found between T_3 and selenium. Some researchers have hypothesized the activity of 5-deiodinase may become depressed after a high dietary intake of selenium, suggesting a safe level of dietary selenium at or below 500 mcg daily (Köhrle and Gärtner, 2009).

POLYCYSTIC OVARY SYNDROME

Polycystic ovary syndrome (PCOS) is a common endocrine disorder of unknown cause that affects an estimated 3% to 12% of women of reproductive age in Western societies (Moran et al, 2010; Velez and Motta, 2014). The condition is characterized by reproductive issues such as amenorrhea or other menstrual irregularities, anovulation, enlarged ovaries with multiple cysts, and infertility. More generalized symptoms include acne, hirsutism (excessive or abnormal distribution of hair growth), male-pattern baldness, obesity, and sleep apnea (see Table 31-3).

Pathophysiology

Biochemical and endocrine abnormalities in women with PCOS include a hyperandrogenic state in which there is a higher concentration of free androgens (dehydroepiandrosterone, testosterone, and androstenedione) and decreased hepatic production of sex hormone binding globulin (Sirmans and Pate, 2013). In addition to the elevated levels of androgens, hyperinsulinemia (which results from insulin resistance), impaired glucose tolerance, and hyperlipidemia are seen. Hyperandrogenism is responsible for many of the symptoms of PCOS, such as reproductive

and menstrual abnormalities, hirsutism, and acne. Elevated androgen levels, in turn, appear to be due in part to hyperinsulinemia, which triggers the increase in androgen production. Thus interventions that improve insulin resistance and hyperinsulinemia may reverse some of the manifestations of PCOS.

The insulin resistance seen in 50% to 70% of women with PCOS is unique in that it occurs independent of body weight to some extent and is not always corrected by weight loss. It appears to result from insulin receptor phosphorylation abnormalities in an insulin-mediated signaling pathway (Sirmans and Pate, 2013). Conventional treatment of PCOS includes diet and exercise to promote weight loss. In women who are obese, weight loss may improve insulin resistance, decrease androgen levels and hirsutism, and restore ovulation in some cases. Low–glycemic index diets historically have been recommended without evidence of their clinical effectiveness. However, the capacity of dietary carbohydrates to increase postprandial blood sugar response may be an important consideration for optimizing metabolic and clinical outcomes in PCOS. Furthermore, independent of weight loss, a low–glycemic index diet appears to result in greater improvements in health, including improved insulin sensitivity, improved menstrual regularity, better emotion scores (on a questionnaire designed to detect changes in quality of life), and decreased markers of inflammation compared with a conventional low-fat diet when matched closely for macronutrient and fiber content (Marsh et al, 2010).

Medical Management

Hypothyroidism occurs in some cases of PCOS. Laboratory tests for thyroid function are frequently normal in patients with clinical evidence of hypothyroidism, and treatment with thyroid hormone results in clinical improvement in many patients. Therefore an empirical trial of thyroid hormone should be considered for patients with PCOS who have clinical evidence of hypothyroidism.

Thyroid antibody status should be taken into account when considering empirical treatment with thyroid hormone in women with PCOS. Metformin frequently is prescribed to improve insulin resistance, and treatment with this drug may lead to resumption of ovulation. Other therapies include the drugs clomiphene citrate (to induce ovulation) and spironolactone (an antiandrogen), as well as oral contraceptives (to treat menstrual irregularities and hirsutism).

Medical Nutrition Therapy

Nutritional interventions that may be beneficial for women with PCOS include dietary modifications designed to enhance insulin sensitivity. This includes restricting refined carbohydrates and total calories; consuming high-fiber foods; and eating small, frequent meals. Some patients with insulin resistance fare better on a diet high in complex carbohydrates (approximately 60% of total calories), whereas others respond better to a low-carbohydrate diet (≤40% of total calories). In addition, supplementation with vitamin D_3 (up to 10,000 IU/day), (Nazarian et al, 2011) and chromium picolinate (200 to 1000 mcg/day) has been reported to improve glucose tolerance, insulin secretion, and insulin sensitivity in human subjects (Lydic et al, 2006) and laboratory animals (Abdourahman and Edwards, 2008). Short-term treatment with N-acetylcysteine (600 mg twice a day) may be useful as an adjunct to clomiphene citrate in women with clomiphene citrate-resistant infertility (Rizk et al, 2005). In addition, treatment with thyroid hormone may be beneficial for women who have laboratory or clinical evidence of hypothyroidism (see Table 31-3).

TABLE 31-3 Nutrition Treatment For Polycystic Ovary Syndrome

Obesity	Institute weight management program of diet and exercise.
Insulin resistance	Restrict refined carbohydrates (low glycemic index diet) and total calories. Increase high-fiber foods. Recommend small, frequent meals. Monitor carefully to ascertain benefit from high- versus low-carbohydrate diet. Consider supplementation with chromium picolinate.
Low serum 25 hydroxy vitamin D	Administer vitamin D_3 (cholecalciferol).
Clomiphene-citrate resistant infertility	Use short-term NAC as adjunct.
Laboratory or clinical evidence of hypothyroidism	Institute thyroid hormone replacement. Use foods or supplements with selenium and iodine.

NAC, N-acetylcysteine.

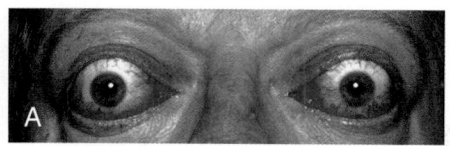

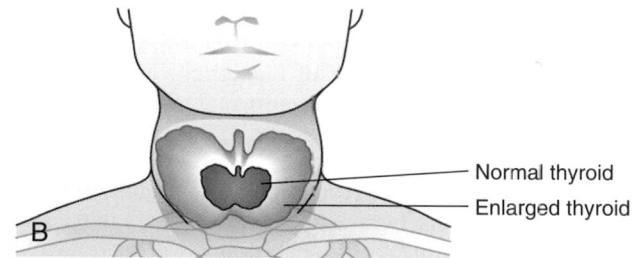

Normal thyroid

Enlarged thyroid

FIGURE 31-4 A, Exophthalmos. (From SPL/Photo Researchers, Inc.) **B,** Thyroid enlargement. (From Buck C: *2011 ICD-9-CM, for Hospitals,* vols 1-3, St Louis, 2011, WB Saunders.)

HYPERTHYROIDISM

Graves' disease is an autoimmune disease in which the thyroid is diffusely enlarged (goiter) and overactive, producing an excessive amount of thyroid hormones. It is the most common cause of hyperthyroidism (overactive thyroid) in the United States. Physical symptoms frequently include red, dry, swollen, puffy, and bulging eyes (exophthalmos), heat intolerance, difficulty sleeping, and anxiety (see Box 31-2). However, the most common sign of Graves' disease is goiter or thyroid enlargement (see Figure 31-4). The excessive thyroid hormones may cause a serious metabolic imbalance, thyrotoxicosis. The prevalence of maternal thyrotoxicosis is approximately 1 case per 1500 persons, with maternal Graves' disease being the most common cause (80% to 85%) (American Thyroid Association, 2012).

Pathophysiology

Commonly, patients have a family history involving a wide spectrum of autoimmune thyroid diseases, such as Graves' disease, Hashimoto's thyroiditis, or postpartum thyroiditis. In Graves' disease, the TRH receptor itself is the primary autoantigen and is responsible for the manifestation of hyperthyroidism. The thyroid gland is under continuous stimulation by circulating autoantibodies against the TRH receptor, and pituitary TSH secretion is suppressed because of the increased production of thyroid hormones. These thyroid-stimulating antibodies cause release of thyroid hormone and thyroglobulin (Tg) and they also stimulate iodine uptake, protein synthesis, and thyroid gland growth.

The Tg and TPO Abs appear to have little role in Graves' disease. However, as mentioned earlier, they are markers of Hashimoto's autoimmune disease against the thyroid. A TSH antibody—typically referred to as thyroid-stimulating immunoglobulin—test is used to identify hyperthyroidism, or Graves' disease.

Triggers

Graves' disease is an autoimmune disorder, influenced by a combination of environmental and genetic factors. Genetic factors contribute to approximately 20% to 30% of overall susceptibility. Other factors include infection, excessive iodide intake, stress, female gender, steroids, and toxins. Smoking has been implicated in the worsening of Graves' ophthalmopathy. Graves' disease also has been associated with infectious agents such as *Yersinia enterocolitica* and *Borrelia burgdorferi.*

Genetics. Several autoimmune thyroid disease susceptibility genes have been identified and appear to be specific to either Graves' disease or Hashimoto's thyroiditis, whereas others confer susceptibility to both conditions. The genetic predisposition to thyroid autoimmunity may interact with environmental factors or events to precipitate the onset of Graves' disease. HLA-DRB1 and HLA-DQB1 appear to be associated with Graves' disease susceptibility.

Stress. Stress can be a factor for thyroid autoimmunity. Acute stress-induced immunosuppression may be followed by immune system hyperactivity, which could precipitate autoimmune thyroid disease. This may occur during the postpartum period, in which Graves' disease may occur 3 to 9 months after delivery. Estrogen may influence the immune system, particularly the beta-cells. Trauma to the thyroid also has been reported to be associated with Graves' disease. This may include surgery of the thyroid gland, percutaneous injection of ethanol, and infarction of a thyroid adenoma.

Medical Management

For patients with sustained forms of hyperthyroidism, such as Graves' disease or toxic nodular goiter, antithyroid medications can be used. The goal with this form of drug therapy is to prevent the thyroid from producing hormones (see Table 31-4).

The effects of immunotherapy are also being evaluated (Salvi, 2014) (see *Pathophysiology and Care Management Algorithm:* Thyroid Dysfunction).

TABLE 31-4   Treatments for Hyperthyroidism

Medication Brand Name	Medication Generic Name	Use and Comments
Tapazole	Methimazole (MMI)	Both drugs interfere with the thyroid gland's production of hormones. Both have side effects, which include rash, itching, joint pain, and fever.
Northyx	Propylthiuracil (PTU)	Liver inflammation or reduction in white blood cells may occur. Underlying hyperthyroidism can return when patient is no longer taking the medication.
Radioactive iodine		This is the most widely recommended permanent treatment of hyperthyroidism. Thyroid cells absorb radioactive iodine, which damages or kills them. If too many of the thyroid cells are damaged, remaining thyroid does not produce enough hormone, resulting in hypothyroidism, and supplemental thyroid hormone may be necessary.

Surgical Treatment
- Partial or complete removal of the thyroid
- Not as common as pharmacologic modes of treatment

MANAGING IMBALANCES OF THE HYPOTHALAMUS-PITUITARY-THYROID AXIS

The thyroid has a relationship to hypothalamic, pituitary, immune, adrenal, and cardiovascular functions that affect clinical, cellular, and molecular outcomes. A checklist of considerations is found in Box 31-3 and is discussed here.

Provide adequate precursors for the formation of T_4. Iodide is a limiting nutrient in many individuals for the production of T_4. Adequate levels of organic iodide, which can come from sea vegetables, iodized salt, and seafood, are important in T_4 production. Adequate dietary protein intake is important in establishing proper protein calorie nutrition. Supplementation with tyrosine does not appear to have a beneficial effect on elevating thyroid hormones.

Reduce antithyroidal antibodies. A variety of food antigens could induce antibodies that crossreact with the thyroid gland. A food elimination diet using gluten-free grains and possible elimination of casein, the predominant milk protein, may be considered for hypothyroidism of unexplained origin. It also has been suggested that environmental toxins may play a role in inducing autoimmune thyroiditis and thyroid dysfunction. Implementing nutritional support and providing adequate levels of vitamin D to support the immune system may be beneficial.

Improve the conversion of T_4 to T_3. Nutritional agents that help support proper deiodination by the type 1 5-deiodinase enzyme include selenium (as L-selenomethionine) and zinc (as zinc glycinate or zinc citrate). Human studies repeatedly have demonstrated consequent reduced concentrations of thyroid hormones when a zinc deficiency is present (Blazewicz et al, 2010). In children with Down syndrome, zinc sulfate may reduce thyroidal antibodies, improve thyroid function, and reduce the incidence of subclinical hypothyroidism.

Enhance T_3 influence on mitochondrial bioenergetics. A number of important nutritional relationships improve thyroid hormones' effects on the mitochondria. Selenium supplementation in animals can improve the production of T_3 and lower autoantibodies to thyroid hormones, while improving energy production. Supplementation with selenomethionine results in improved deiodination of T_4, which may improve adenosine triphosphate formation by supporting improved mitochondrial activity. Food sources of selenium include the Brazil nut, snapper, cod, halibut, yellow fin tuna, salmon, sardines, shrimp, mushrooms, and barley.

BOX 31-3 Factors Promoting Thyroid Health in Adults

Consider
  Protein: 0.8 g/kg/day
  Iodine (once autoimmune disease has been ruled out): 150 mcg/day
  Selenium (as L-selenomethionine): 75 to 200 mcg/day
  Zinc (as zinc citrate): 10 mg/day
  Vitamin D (as D_3 or cholecalciferol): 1000 IU/day
  Vitamin E (as D-alpha tocopherol succinate): 100 IU/day
  Vitamin C (as ascorbic acid): 100 to 500 mg/day
  Guggulsterones (from guggul extract):100 mg/day
  Ashwaganda: 100 mg/day
Reduce or eliminate
  Gluten (found in wheat, rye, oats, and barley)
  Processed soy
  Excessive uncooked goitrogenic foods
  Stress

Monitor use of botanical products. Based on animal studies, it appears that certain botanical preparations influence thyroid activity. The most significant products include *Commiphora mukul* (guggulsterones, from guggul extract) and *Withania somnifera* (ashwagandha). *C. mukul* demonstrates strong thyroid stimulatory action. Its administration (1 mg/100 g body weight) increases iodine uptake by the thyroid, increases TPO activity, and decreases lipid peroxidation, suggesting that increased peripheral generation of T_3 might be mediated by this plant's antioxidant effects. *W. somnifera* (ashwagandha) root extract (1.4 g/kg) may increase T_3 and T_4 concentrations without changing 5-deiodinase activity.

Avoid disruption of thyroid hormone metabolism from flavonoids. Flavonoids, natural and synthetic, have the potential to disrupt thyroid hormone metabolism. Synthetic flavonoid derivatives can decrease serum T_4 concentrations and inhibit the conversion of T_4 to T_3 and the metabolic clearance of rT_3 by the selenium-dependent 5-deiodinase. Naturally occurring flavonoids appear to have a similar inhibitory effect. Of the naturally occurring flavonoids, luteolin (most often found in leaves, but also seen in celery, thyme, dandelion, green pepper, thyme, perilla, chamomile tea, carrots, olive oil, peppermint, rosemary, and oregano) is the most active inhibitor of 5-deiodinase activity. Because isolated or concentrated flavonoids are increasingly used as therapeutic interventions, more research on the potential influence of these substances on thyroid hormone metabolism is desirable (Goncalves et al, 2013).

Use caution with supplements. Lipoic acid reduces the conversion of T_4 to T_3. Because it is usually not a therapeutic advantage to decrease peripheral activation of T_3 subsequent to T_4 therapy, use of lipoic acid supplements in hypothyroid patients receiving exogenous hormone therapy should be approached with caution.

Maintain vitamin sufficiency. One nutrient that is critically important for establishing immune balance and preventing the production of autoantibodies is vitamin D. Vitamin D is considered a prohormone with antiproliferative, differentiating, and immunosuppressive activities. Vitamin D is an effective immune modulator and may suppress the development of autoimmune diseases, such as arthritis and multiple sclerosis (Baeke et al, 2010). Conversely, a vitamin D deficiency is associated with numerous autoimmune conditions, including Hashimoto's. More than 90% of people with autoimmune thyroid disease have a genetic defect affecting their ability to metabolize vitamin D (Feng et al, 2013; Kivity et al, 2011). Vitamin D also appears to work with other nutritional factors to help regulate immune sensitivity and may protect against development of autoantibodies. After exposure to heavy metals, decreases in a variety of hepatic antioxidant lipid peroxidation (the oxidative degradation of lipids) systems have been observed. Ascorbic acid has been shown to be effective in preventing cadmium-induced decreases in T_3 and hepatic 5-deiodination.

ADRENAL DISORDERS

Cushing's Syndrome

In Cushing's syndrome, too much cortisol remains in the bloodstream over a long period. The exogenous form occurs when individuals take steroids or other similar medications and ceases when the medication is stopped. Endogenous Cushing's syndrome is rare and occurs as the result of a tumor on the adrenal or pituitary gland. Weight gain, easy bruising, depression, muscle loss, and weakness are common symptoms. A weight management protocol may be needed.

Addison's Disease

Primary adrenal insufficiency, also known as Addison's disease, is rare. In this condition, insufficient steroid hormones are produced in spite of adequate levels of the hormone ACTH. Regulation of blood glucose levels and stress management are affected. Loss of appetite, fatigue, low blood pressure, nausea and vomiting, and darkening of skin on the face and neck may occur. Patients with Addison's disease should not restrict their salt intake unless they have concurrent hypertension. Those patients who live in warm climates and therefore have increased losses through perspiration may need to increase salt intake.

Adrenal Fatigue

Adrenal fatigue has been identified as a collection of signs and symptoms caused by the decreased ability of the adrenal glands to respond adequately to stress. A variety of terms are found in the scientific literature that address adrenal fatigue, including subclinical adrenal insufficiency, adrenal stress, adrenal exhaustion, adrenal burnout, and adrenal imbalance (Allen, 2013). The adrenals are the two triangular-shaped glands located at the top of each kidney and are responsible primarily for governing the body's adaptations to stress of any kind. However, adrenal fatigue can occur whether the source of stress, physical, emotional or psychologic, is chronic and continues to persist causing a cumulative effect, or is a very intense single event stressor. In other words, the adrenal glands are unable to keep pace with the demands of perpetual fight-or-flight arousal, resulting in subclinical adrenal dysfunction. The most common symptoms of adrenal fatigue include, but are not limited to, excessive fatigue and exhaustion, hair loss, hormone imbalance, poor digestion, low immune function, slow recovery from illness, inability to concentrate, and inability to cope with stressors.

Chronic adrenal stress causes the following:
- Affects communication between the brain and hormone-secreting glands. The hypothalamus and pituitary gland direct hormone production, including that of the thyroid. When the hypothalamus and pituitary weaken because of chronic adrenal stress, they are not able to communicate well with the thyroid gland
- Increases thyroid-binding protein activity, so that thyroid hormones cannot get into cells to do their job
- Hampers the conversion of T_4 to active forms of T_3 that the body can use
- Interferes with the detoxification pathways through which unnecessary thyroid hormones exit the body, leading to thyroid hormone resistance
- Causes cells to lose sensitivity to thyroid hormones
- Weakens the immune barriers of the digestive tract, lungs, and brain; promotes poor immune regulation

These factors increase the risk for triggering Hashimoto's or exacerbating it. These are some of the ways adrenal stress directly affect thyroid function.

Chronic adrenal stress affects other systems of the body, which in turn, decrease thyroid function. For example, the adrenal hormone **cortisol** plays a large role in thyroid health. Cortisol is a life-sustaining hormone essential to the maintenance of homeostasis. If often is called the "stress hormone" because it influences, regulates, or modulates many of the changes that occur in the body in response to stress, including but not limited to the following:
- Antiinflammatory actions
- Blood glucose levels
- Blood pressure
- Central nervous system activation
- Fat, protein, and carbohydrate metabolism to maintain blood glucose
- Heart and blood vessel tone and contraction
- Immune responses

Cortisol levels follow a circadian rhythm and normally fluctuate throughout the day and night, peaking at about 8:00 AM and reaching a low at about 4:00 PM (Allen, 2013). It is very important that bodily functions and cortisol levels return to normal after a stressful event. Adrenal fatigue appears to occur when the amount of stress or combined stresses overextend the capacity of the body to compensate for and recover from that stress. When this happens repeatedly, it exhausts the adrenal and thyroid glands, as well as the hypothalamus and the pituitary gland. Over time, this exhaustion leads to functional hypothyroidism. In addition, constant cortisol production weakens the gastrointestinal (GI) tract, making one more susceptible to inflammation, dysbiosis (poor gut health), and infection. Thus a vicious cycle weakens the thyroid.

With proper care, most people who experience adrenal fatigue can expect to regain their normal quality of life. Some of the conventional approaches in the treatment of adrenal fatigue may include the following (Allolio, 2007):
- B-complex vitamins
- Exercise in moderation
- DHEA (dehydroepiandosterone)
- Proper diet
- Relaxation
- Sleep
- Stress relief and management

CLINICAL CASE STUDY

Frank is a 72-year-old man from Jamaica who moved to the United States 2 years ago. He has been diagnosed with hypothyroidism this past year. He comes to your clinic with his medicine and traditional folk remedies, including Synthroid, garlic, and chamomile. His diet history indicates daily use of chicken, rice, celery, dandelion, green pepper, mango, and papaya. He states that he has been very tired lately, has little energy, and has constipation. His hormone levels on his last medical report were thyroxine (T_4): 1.7, triiodothyronine (T_3): 75, and thyroid-stimulating hormone (TSH): 15, indicative that his hypothyroidism is still not well controlled.

Nutrition Diagnostic Statement

Food-drug interaction related to mixing Synthroid with foods and herbs that aggravate thyroid function as evidenced by fatigue, constipation, high TSH, and low serum T_3 and T_4.

Nutrition Care Questions

1. What other information do you need for a more thorough assessment?
2. What advice would you offer Frank about his diet?
3. What foods and herbs conflict with Synthroid?
4. Because traditional folk remedies are commonly used, how do you plan to discuss these issues with Frank?

USEFUL WEBSITES

American Association of Clinical Endocrinologists
http://www.aace.com/
American Thyroid Association
http://www.thyroid.org/
Endocrine Web
http://www.endocrineweb.com/
Thyroid Disease Information
http://thyroid.about.com/

REFERENCES

Abdourahman A, Edwards JG: Chromium supplementation improves glucose tolerance in diabetic Goto-Kakizaki rats, *IUBMB Life* 60:541, 2008.

Abdullatif H, Ashraf A: Reversible subclinical hypothyroidism in the presence of adrenal insufficiency, *Endocr Pract* 12:572, 2006.

Allen LV: Adrenal fatigue, *Int J Pharm Compd* 17:39, 2013.

Allolio B, et al: Why, when and how much-DHEA replacement in adrenal insufficiency, *Ann Endocrinol* 68:268, 2007.

American Thyroid Association: *Thyroid Disease and Pregnancy* (website), 2012. http://www.thyroid.org/thyroid-disease-and-pregnancy/. Accessed January 13, 2014.

Baeke F, et al: Vitamin D: modulator of the immune system, *Curr Opin Pharmacol* 10:482, 2010.

Barker J, Liu E: Celiac disease: pathophysiology, clinical manifestations, and associated autoimmune conditions, *Adv Pediatr* 55:349, 2008.

Blazewicz A, et al: Determination of cadmium, cobalt, copper, iron, manganese, and zinc in thyroid glands of patients with diagnosed nodular goitre using ion chromatography, *J Chromatogr B Analyt Technol Biomed Life Sci* 878:34, 2010.

Cassio A, et al: Long-term clinical significance of thyroid autoimmunity in children with celiac disease, *J Pediatr* 156:292, 2010.

Centers for Disease Control: National Diabetes Statistics Report, 2014 (website), 2014. http://www.cdc.gov/diabetes/pubs/statsreport14/national-diabetes-report-web.pdf. Accessed December 8, 2014.

Chen ZP, Hetzel BS: Cretinism revisited, *Best Pract Res Clin Endocrinol Metab* 24:39, 2010.

De Vivo A, et al: Thyroid function in women found to have early pregnancy loss, *Thyroid* 20:633, 2010.

Del Ghianda S, et al: Thyroid and menopause, *Climacteric* 17:225, 2014.

De Vries EM, et al: Differential effects of fasting vs food restriction on liver thyroid hormone metabolism in male rats, *J Endocrinol* 224:25, 2015.

Dobbs J, Titchenal A: *Iron Plays an Important Role for the Thyroid* (website), 2009. http://www.nutritionatc.hawaii.edu/HO/2009/415.htm. Accessed July 10, 2010.

Downs H, et al: Clinical inquiries: How useful are autoantibodies in diagnosing thyroid disorders? *J Fam Pract* 57:615, 2008.

Dunn M, et al: Clinical Case Report: Ultrastructural evidence of skeletal muscle mitochondrial dysfunction in patients with subclinical hypothyroidism, *Thyroid Science* 4:1, 2009.

Duntas LH: Does celiac disease trigger autoimmune thyroiditis? *Nat Rev Endocrinol* 5:190, 2009.

Ebert E: The thyroid and the gut, *J Clin Gastroenterol* 44:402, 2010.

Feng M, et al: Polymorphisms in the vitamin D receptor gene and risk of autoimmune thyroid diseases: a meta-analysis, *Endocrine* 43:318, 2013.

Fjaellagaard K, et al: Well-being and depression in individuals with subclinical hypothyroidism and thyroid autoimmunity – a general population study, *Nord J Psychiatry* 1:1, 2014. Epub ahead of print.

Garber JR, et al: Clinical practice guidelines for hypothyroidism in adults: co-sponsored by the American Association of Clinical Endocrinologists and the American Thyroid Association, *Endocrine Pract* 18:988, 2012.

Golden SH, et al: Prevalence and incidence of endocrine and metabolic disorders in the United States: a comprehensive review, *J Clin Endocrinol Metab* 94:1853, 2009.

Goncalves CF, et al: Flavonoid rutin increases thyroid iodide uptake in rats, *PLoS One* 8:e73908, 2013, doi: 10.1371/journal.pone.0073908. eCollection 2013.

Gropper S, Smith JL: *Advanced nutrition and human metabolism*, ed 6, Belmont, Calif, 2012, Wadsworth Cengage Learning.

Hak AE, et al: Subclinical hypothyroidism is an independent risk factor for atherosclerosis and myocardial infarction in elderly women: the Rotterdam study, *Ann Intern Med* 132:270, 2000.

Hess SY: The impact of common micronutrient deficiencies on iodine and thyroid metabolism: the evidence from human studies, *Best Pract Res Clin Endocrinol Metab* 24:117, 2010.

Janegova A, Jenega P, Rychly B, Kuracinova K, Babal P: The role of Epstein-Barr virus infection in the development of autoimmune thyroid disease, *Endokrynol Pol* 66(2):132, 2015.

Kaltsas G, et al: Fatigue, endocrinopathies and metabolic disorders, *PMR* 2:393, 2010.

Khandelwal D, Tandon N: Overt and subclinical hypothyroidism: who to treat and how, *Drugs* 72:17, 2012.

Kivity S, et al: Vitamin D and autoimmune thyroid diseases, *Cell Mol Immunol* 8:243, 2011.

Köhrle J: Selenium and the thyroid, *Curr Opin Endocrinol Diabetes Obes* 20:441, 2013.

Kohrle J, Gärtner R: Selenium and thyroid, *Best Pract Res Clin Endocrinol Metab* 23:815, 2009.

Lydic M, et al: Chromium picolinate improves insulin sensitivity in obese subjects with polycystic ovary syndrome, *Fertil Steril* 86:243, 2006.

Marsh KA, et al: Effect of a low glycemic index compared with a conventional healthy diet on polycystic ovary syndrome, *Am J Clin Nutr* 92:83, 2010.

Meloni A, et al: Prevalence of autoimmune thyroiditis in children with celiac disease and effect of gluten withdrawal, *J Pediatr* 155:51, 2009.

Melse-Boonstra A, Jaiswal N: Iodine deficiency in pregnancy, infancy and childhood and its consequences for brain development, *Best Pract Res Clin Endocrinol Metab* 24:29, 2010.

Michels AW, Eisenbarth GS: Immunologic endocrine disorders, *J Allergy Clin Immunol* 125:S226, 2010.

Moran LJ, et al: Polycystic ovary syndrome and weight management, *Women's Health* 6:271, 2010.

National Institutes of Health, MedlinePlus: *Endocrine Diseases* (website), 2014. http://www.nlm.nih.gov/medlineplus/endocrinediseases.html. Accessed December 8, 2014.

Nazarian S, et al: Vitamin D3 supplementation improves insulin sensitivity in subjects with impaired fasting glucose, *Transl Res* 158:276, 2011.

Rizk AY, et al: N-acetyl-cysteine is a novel adjuvant to clomiphene citrate in clomiphene citrate-resistant patients with polycystic ovary syndrome, *Fertil Steril* 83:367, 2005.

Salvi M: Immunotherapy for Graves' ophthalmopathy, *Curr Opin Endocrinol Diabetes Obes* 21:409, 2014.

Saravanan P, et al: Psychological well-being in patients on "adequate" doses of L-thyroxine: results of a large controlled community based questionnaire study, *Clin Endocrinol* 57:577, 2002.

Sinnott B, et al: Exposing the thyroid to radiation: a review of its current extent, risks, and implications, *Endocr Rev* 31:756, 2010.

Sirmans SM, Pate KA: Epidemiology, diagnosis, and management of polycystic ovary syndrome, *Clin Epidemiol* 18(6):1, 2013.

Tomer Y, Huber A: The etiology of autoimmune thyroid disease: A story of genes and environment, *J Autoimmun* 32:231, 2009.

Velez LM, Motta AB: Association between polycystic ovary syndrome and metabolic syndrome, *Curr Med Chem* 21:3999, 2014.

Wiebolt J, et al: Endocrine autoimmune disease: genetics become complex, *Eur J Clin Invest* 40:1144, 2010.

Yassa L, et al: Thyroid hormone early adjustment in pregnancy (the THERAPY) trial, *J Clin Endocrinol Metab* 95:3234, 2010.

Zimmermann MB: Iodine deficiency in pregnancy and the effects of maternal iodine supplementation on the offspring: a review, *Am J Clin Nutr* 89(2):668S, 2009.

32

Medical Nutrition Therapy for Anemia

Tracy Stopler, MS, RDN
Susan Weiner, MS, RDN, CDE

KEY TERMS

anemia	iron deficiency anemia	restless legs syndrome (RLS)
aplastic anemia	koilonychia	serum
ceruloplasmin	macrocytic anemia	sickle cell anemia (SCA)
ferritin	meat-fish-poultry (MFP) factor	sideroblastic (pyridoxine-responsive)
ferroprotein	megaloblastic anemia	anemia
hematocrit	microcytic anemia	soluble serum transferrin receptors
heme iron	nonheme iron	(STFRs)
hemochromatosis	nutritional anemias	sports anemia
hemoglobin	pagophagia	thalassemia
hemolytic anemia	pernicious anemia	total iron-binding capacity (TIBC)
hepcidin	plasma	transferrin
holotranscobalamin II (holo TCII)	polycythemia	transferrin receptor
hypochromic	protoporphyrin	transferrin saturation
intrinsic factor (IF)	reticulocytosis	

It is important for nutrition professionals to understand the myriad of terms related to blood disorders. Hemoglobin is a conjugated protein containing four heme groups and globin; it is the oxygen-carrying pigment of the erythrocytes. The hematocrit is the volume percentage of erythrocytes in the blood. Plasma is the liquid portion of whole blood containing coagulation factors; serum is the liquid portion of whole blood without coagulation factors.

Anemia is a deficiency in the size or number of red blood cells (RBCs) or the amount of hemoglobin they contain. This deficiency limits the exchange of oxygen and carbon dioxide between the blood and the tissue cells. Anemia classification is based on cell size—macrocytic (large), normocytic (normal), and microcytic (small)—and on hemoglobin content—hypochromic (pale color from deficiency of hemoglobin) and normochromic (normal color) (see Table 32-1).

Macrocytic anemia presents with larger-than-normal RBCs, plus increased mean corpuscular volume (MCV) and mean corpuscular hemoglobin concentration (MCHC). Microcytic anemia is characterized by smaller-than-normal erythrocytes and less circulating hemoglobin, as in iron deficiency anemia and thalassemia.

Most anemias are caused by a lack of nutrients required for normal erythrocyte synthesis, principally iron, vitamin B_{12}, and folic acid. These anemias that result from an inadequate intake of iron, protein, certain vitamins, copper, and other heavy metals are called nutritional anemias. Other anemias result from conditions such as hemorrhage, genetic abnormalities, chronic disease states, or drug toxicity, and have varying degrees of nutritional consequence.

IRON-RELATED BLOOD DISORDERS

Iron status can range from overload to deficiency and anemia. Routine measurement of iron status is necessary because approximately 6% of Americans have a negative iron balance, approximately 10% have a gene for positive balance, and approximately 1% have iron overload. As shown in Figure 32-1, stages of iron status range from iron overload to iron deficiency anemia and are summarized as follows:

a. Stage I and Stage II negative iron balance (i.e., iron depletion). In these stages iron stores are low and there is no dysfunction. In Stage I negative iron balance, reduced iron absorption produces moderately depleted iron stores. Stage II negative iron balance is characterized by severely depleted iron stores.

b. Stage III and IV negative iron balance (i.e., iron deficiency). Iron deficiency is characterized by inadequate body iron, possibly causing dysfunction and disease. In Stage III negative iron balance, dysfunction is not accompanied by anemia; anemia develops in Stage IV negative iron balance.

c. Stage I and II positive iron balance. Stage I positive balance usually lasts for several years with no dysfunction. Supplements of iron and/or vitamin C promote

*Thank you to Melissa Fraser RD, CDN, and Mollie Kurshan RD, CDN, for their help and research for this chapter.
In memory of Victor Herbert, MD, JD, for his inspiration in the writing of the chapter.

TABLE 32-1   Morphologic Classification of Anemia

Morphologic Type of Anemia	Underlying Abnormality	Clinical Syndromes	Treatment
Macrocytic (MCV > 94; MCHC > 31)			
Megaloblastic	Vitamin B_{12} deficiency	Pernicious anemia	Vitamin B_{12}
	Folic acid deficiency	Nutritional megaloblastic anemias, sprue, and other malabsorption syndromes	Folic acid
	Inherited disorders of DNA synthesis	Orotic aciduria	Treatment based on the nature of the disorder
		Sickle cell anemia	
	Drug-induced disorders of DNA synthesis	Side effects of chemotherapeutic agents, anticonvulsants, oral contraceptives,	Discontinue offending drug and administer folic acid
Nonmegaloblastic	Accelerated erythropoiesis	Hemolytic anemia	Treatment of underlying disease
Hypochromic Microcytic (MCV < 80; MCHC < 31)			
	Iron deficiency	Chronic loss of blood,	Ferrous sulfate and correction of underlying cause
	Disorders of globin synthesis	Thalassemia	Nonspecific
		Hemoglobin E	Mild – does not require treatment;
		Hemoglobin C	Severe –frequent blood transfusions to provide healthy RBCs with normal hgb
	Disorders of porphyrin and heme synthesis	Pyridoxine-responsive anemia	Pyridoxine
	Other disorders of iron metabolism	Copper deficiency	Copper
Normochromic Normocytic (MCV 82-92; MCHC > 30)			
	Recent blood loss	Various	Transfusion, iron, correction of underlying condition
	Overexpansion of plasma volume	Edema of pregnancy	Restore homeostasis
	Hemolytic diseases	Overhydration	Treatment based on the nature of the disorder
	Hypoplastic bone marrow	Aplastic anemia	Transfusion
		Pure red blood cell aplasia	Androgens
	Infiltrated bone marrow	Leukemia, multiple myeloma, myelofibrosis	Chemotherapy
	Endocrine abnormality	Hypothyroidism, adrenal insufficiency	Treatment of underlying disease
	Chronic disease		Treatment of underlying disease
	Renal disease	Renal disease	Treatment of underlying disease
	Liver disease	Cirrhosis	Treatment of underlying disease

Modified from Wintrobe MM et al: *Clinical hematology,* ed 8, Philadelphia, 1981, Lea & Febiger.
DNA, Deoxyribonucleic acid; *MCHC,* Mean corpuscular hemoglobin concentration: concentration of hemoglobin expressed in grams per deciliter (g/dl); *MCV,* mean corpuscular volume: volume of one red blood cell expressed in femtoliters (fl).

progression to dysfunction or disease, whereas iron removal prevents progression to disease. Iron overload disease develops in persons with stage II positive balance after years of iron overload have caused progressive damage to tissues and organs.

Iron status has a variety of indicators. Serum ferritin is an iron apoferritin complex, one of the chief storage forms of iron. Serum ferritin levels are in equilibrium with body iron stores. Very early (stage I) positive iron balance may best be recognized by measuring total iron-binding capacity (TIBC), the capacity of transferrin to take on or become saturated with iron. Conversely, measurement of serum or plasma ferritin levels may best reveal early (stage I or II) negative iron balance, although serum TIBC may be as good an indicator (see Chapter 7). Transferrin saturation is the measure of the amount of iron bound to transferrin and is a gauge of iron supply to the tissues; the percent saturation = serum iron/TIBC × 100.

Iron Deficiency Anemia
Pathophysiology

Iron deficiency anemia is characterized by the production of (microcytic) erythrocytes and a diminished level of circulating hemoglobin. This microcytic anemia is the last stage of iron deficiency, and it represents the end point of a long period of iron deprivation. There are many causes of iron deficiency anemia as discussed in Box 32-1.

With few exceptions, iron deficiency anemia in adult men is the result of blood loss. Large losses of menstrual blood can cause iron deficiency in women, many of whom are unaware that their menses are unusually heavy.

Because anemia is the last manifestation of chronic, long-term iron deficiency, the symptoms reflect a malfunction of a variety of body systems. Inadequate muscle function is reflected in decreased work performance and exercise tolerance. Neurologic

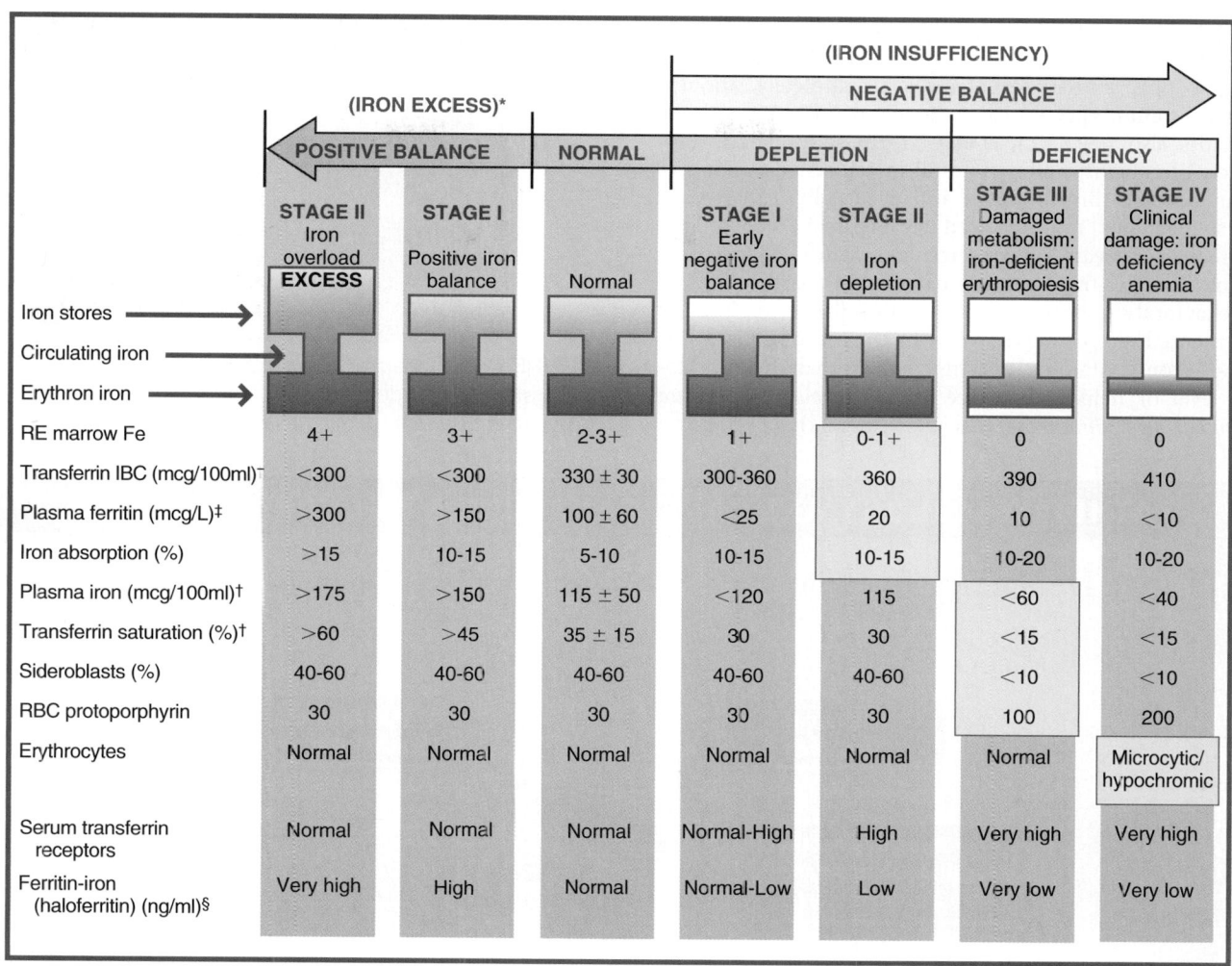

| | (IRON EXCESS)* | | | | (IRON INSUFFICIENCY) NEGATIVE BALANCE | |
| | POSITIVE BALANCE | | NORMAL | DEPLETION | | DEFICIENCY | |
	STAGE II Iron overload EXCESS	STAGE I Positive iron balance	Normal	STAGE I Early negative iron balance	STAGE II Iron depletion	STAGE III Damaged metabolism: iron-deficient erythropoiesis	STAGE IV Clinical damage: iron deficiency anemia
Iron stores							
Circulating iron							
Erythron iron							
RE marrow Fe	4+	3+	2-3+	1+	0-1+	0	0
Transferrin IBC (mcg/100ml)†	<300	<300	330 ± 30	300-360	360	390	410
Plasma ferritin (mcg/L)‡	>300	>150	100 ± 60	<25	20	10	<10
Iron absorption (%)	>15	10-15	5-10	10-15	10-15	10-20	10-20
Plasma iron (mcg/100ml)†	>175	>150	115 ± 50	<120	115	<60	<40
Transferrin saturation (%)†	>60	>45	35 ± 15	30	30	<15	<15
Sideroblasts (%)	40-60	40-60	40-60	40-60	40-60	<10	<10
RBC protoporphyrin	30	30	30	30	30	100	200
Erythrocytes	Normal	Normal	Normal	Normal	Normal	Normal	Microcytic/ hypochromic
Serum transferrin receptors	Normal	Normal	Normal	Normal-High	High	Very high	Very high
Ferritin-iron (haloferritin) (ng/ml)§	Very high	High	Normal	Normal-Low	Low	Very low	Very low

*Randall Lauffer of Harvard and Joe McCord of University of Colorado–Denver hold that *any* storage iron is excessive because of its potential to promote excessive free radical generation. (Herbert V et al: Most free radical injury is iron related, *Stem Cells* 12:289, 1994.)
†Inflammation reduces transferrin (and the plasma iron on it), because transferrin is a reverse acute-phase reactant.
‡Inflammation produces elevated ferritin, because ferritin protein is an acute-phase reactant.
§Ferritin-iron is unaffected by inflammation, so it is reliable when ferritin, transferrin, and plasma iron are not.
Dallman (pediatrician) definition of negative balance: less absorbed than *excreted.*
Herbert (internist) definition of negative balance: less absorbed than *needed.*

FIGURE 32-1 Sequential stages of iron status. *IBC,* Iron-binding capacity; *RBC,* red blood cell; *RE,* reticuloendothelial cells. (Copyright Victor Herbert, 1995.)

BOX 32-1 Causes of Iron Deficiency Anemia

1. Inadequate dietary intake secondary to a poor diet without supplementation
2. Inadequate absorption resulting from diarrhea, achlorhydria, intestinal disease such as celiac disease, atrophic gastritis, partial or total gastrectomy, or drug interference
3. Inadequate utilization secondary to chronic gastrointestinal disturbances
4. Increased iron requirement for growth of blood volume, which occurs during infancy, adolescence, pregnancy, and lactation and which is not being matched with intake
5. Increased excretion because of excessive menstrual blood (in females); hemorrhage from injury; or chronic blood loss from a bleeding ulcer, bleeding hemorrhoids, esophageal varices, regional enteritis, celiac disease, Crohn's disease, ulcerative colitis, parasitic or malignant disease
6. "Increased destruction" of iron from iron stores into the plasma and defective iron use caused by a chronic inflammation or other chronic disorder

involvement is manifested by behavioral changes such as fatigue, anorexia, and pica, especially pagophagia (ice eating). Abnormal cognitive development in children suggests iron deficiency before it has developed into overt anemia.

Growth abnormalities, epithelial disorders, and a reduction in gastric acidity are also common. A possible sign of early iron deficiency is reduced immunocompetence, particularly defects in cell-mediated immunity and the phagocytic activity of neutrophils, which may lead to frequent infections. Restless legs syndrome (RLS) with leg pain or discomfort may result from a lack of iron in the brain; this alters dopamine production and movement. Besides iron deficiency, kidney failure, Parkinson's disease, diabetes, rheumatoid arthritis, and pregnancy can aggravate RLS (Allen et al, 2013; National Institutes of Health [NIH], National Heart Blood and Lung Institute [NHBLI], 2010).

As iron deficiency anemia becomes more severe, defects arise in the structure and function of the epithelial tissues, especially of the tongue, nails, mouth, and stomach. The skin may appear pale, and the inside of the lower eyelid may be light pink instead of red. Mouth changes include atrophy of the lingual papillae, burning, redness, and in severe cases a completely smooth, waxy, and glistening appearance of the tongue (glossitis). Angular stomatitis also may occur, as may a form of dysphagia. Gastritis occurs frequently and may result in achlorhydria. Fingernails can become thin and flat, and eventually koilonychia (spoon-shaped nails) may be noted (see Figure 32-2).

Progressive, untreated anemia results in cardiovascular and respiratory changes that can eventually lead to cardiac failure. Some behavioral symptoms respond to iron therapy before the anemia is cured, suggesting they may be the result of tissue depletion of iron-containing enzymes rather than from a decreased level of hemoglobin (see *Pathophysiology and Care Management Algorithm:* Iron Deficiency Anemia).

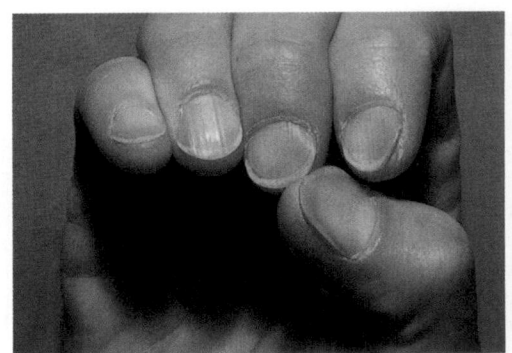

FIGURE 32-2 Fingernails with cuplike depressions (koilonychia) are a sign of iron deficiency in adults. (From Callen JP et al: *Color atlas of dermatology,* Philadelphia, 1993, Saunders.)

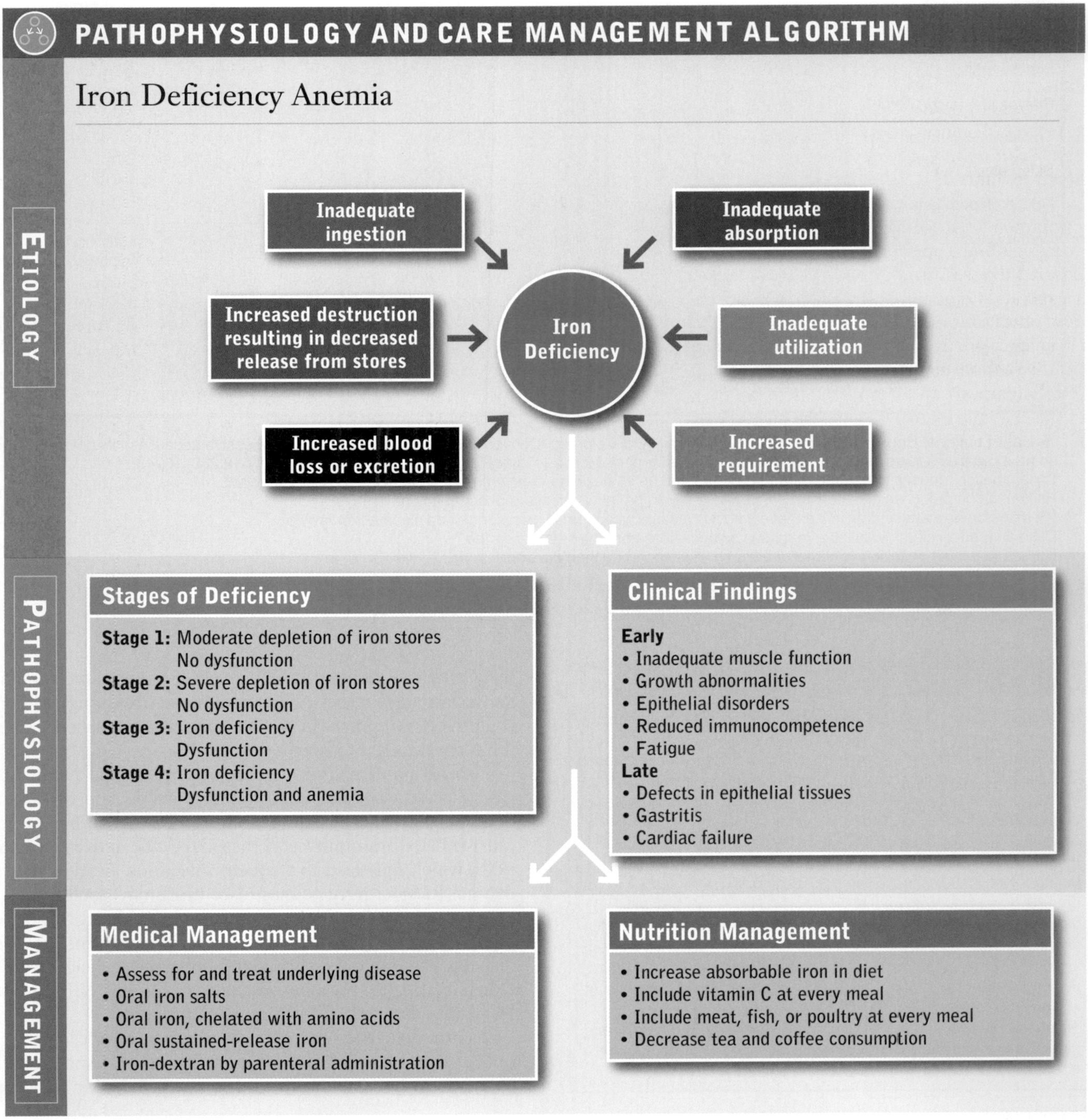

PATHOPHYSIOLOGY AND CARE MANAGEMENT ALGORITHM

Iron Deficiency Anemia

ETIOLOGY

- Inadequate ingestion
- Inadequate absorption
- Increased destruction resulting in decreased release from stores
- Inadequate utilization
- Increased blood loss or excretion
- Increased requirement

→ **Iron Deficiency**

PATHOPHYSIOLOGY

Stages of Deficiency

Stage 1: Moderate depletion of iron stores
No dysfunction
Stage 2: Severe depletion of iron stores
No dysfunction
Stage 3: Iron deficiency
Dysfunction
Stage 4: Iron deficiency
Dysfunction and anemia

Clinical Findings

Early
- Inadequate muscle function
- Growth abnormalities
- Epithelial disorders
- Reduced immunocompetence
- Fatigue

Late
- Defects in epithelial tissues
- Gastritis
- Cardiac failure

MANAGEMENT

Medical Management

- Assess for and treat underlying disease
- Oral iron salts
- Oral iron, chelated with amino acids
- Oral sustained-release iron
- Iron-dextran by parenteral administration

Nutrition Management

- Increase absorbable iron in diet
- Include vitamin C at every meal
- Include meat, fish, or poultry at every meal
- Decrease tea and coffee consumption

Assessment

A definitive diagnosis of iron deficiency anemia requires more than one method of iron evaluation; serum ferritin, iron and transferrin are the most useful. The evaluation also should include an assessment of cell morphology. By itself, hemoglobin concentration is unsuitable as a diagnostic tool in cases of suspected iron deficiency anemia for three reasons: (1) it is affected only late in the disease, (2) it cannot distinguish iron deficiency from other anemias, and (3) hemoglobin values in normal individuals vary widely.

After absorption, iron is transported by plasma transferrin— a beta-1 globulin (protein) that binds iron derived from the gastrointestinal tract, iron storage sites, or hemoglobin breakdown—to the bone marrow (hemoglobin synthesis), endothelial cells (storage), or placenta (fetal needs). Transferrin molecules are generated on the surface of RBCs in response to the need for iron. With iron deficiency, so many transferrin receptors are on the cell surface looking for iron that some of them break off and float in the serum. Their presence is an early measurement of developing iron deficiency; a higher quantity of soluble serum transferrin receptors (STFRs) means greater deficiency of iron. Progressive stages of iron deficiency can be evaluated by measurements, as shown in Table 32-2.

Protoporphyrin is the iron-containing portion of the respiratory pigments that combines with protein to form hemoglobin or myoglobin. The zinc protoporphyrin (ZnPP)/heme ratio is measured to assess iron deficiency. However, both this ZnPP/heme ratio and hemoglobin levels are affected by chronic infection and other factors that can produce a condition that mimics iron deficiency anemia when, in fact, iron is adequate.

With higher altitudes, where there is a lower availability of oxygen, hematocrit and hemoglobin levels increase to adapt. This must be considered in any anemia assessment strategies (Zubieta-Calleja et al, 2007). High altitude is 4900 to 11,500 feet; very high altitude is 11,500 to 18,000 feet; extreme altitude is above 18,000 feet.

Medical Management

Treatment of iron deficiency anemia should focus primarily on the underlying cause, although this is often difficult to determine. The goal is repletion of iron stores.

Oral Supplementation. The chief treatment for iron deficiency anemia involves oral administration of inorganic iron in the ferrous form. Although the body uses ferric and ferrous iron, the reduced ferrous is easier on the gut and better absorbed. At a dose of 30 mg, absorption of ferrous iron is three times greater than if the same amount were given in the ferric form.

Iron is best absorbed when the stomach is empty; however, under these conditions it tends to cause gastric irritation. Gastrointestinal side effects can include nausea, epigastric discomfort and distention, heartburn, diarrhea, or constipation. If these side effects occur, the patient is told to take the iron with meals instead of on an empty stomach; however, this sharply reduces the absorbability of the iron. Gastric irritation is a direct result of the high quantity of free ferrous iron in the stomach. Chelated forms of iron (combined with amino acids) are more bioavailable than nonchelated iron. Chelated iron is less affected by phytate, oxalate, phosphate, and calcium (all iron absorption inhibitors). Chelated iron causes less gastrointestinal disturbances than elemental iron because it is needed in lower doses when it is absorbed into mucosal cells (Ashmead, 2001).

Health professionals usually prescribe oral iron three times daily for 3 months to treat iron deficiency. Depending on the severity of the anemia and the patient's tolerance, the daily dose of elemental iron recommended is 50-100 mg three times daily for adults and 4-6 mg/kg of body weight divided into three doses per day for children. Vitamin C greatly increases iron absorption and gastric irritation somewhat through its capacity to maintain iron in the reduced state (Aditi and Graham, 2012).

Absorption of 10 to 20 mg of iron per day permits RBC production to increase to approximately three times the normal rate and, in the absence of blood loss, hemoglobin

TABLE 32-2 Biochemical Evaluation of Iron Deficiency

Measure	Reference Range	Deficiency
Serum or plasma ferritin	Newborn 25–200 ng/mL; 25–200 mcg/dL Neonate—5 mos 50–200 ng/mL; 50–200 mcg/dL 6 mos–15 yr 7–142 ng/mL; 7–142 mcg/dL F 15 yr + 10–150 ng/mL; 10–150 mcg/dL M 15 yr + 12–300 ng/mL; 12–300 mcg/dL	The most sensitive indicator of iron deficiency. Low levels of ferritin are also seen in severe protein depletion. Females — < 10 mcg/dL Males — < 12 mcg/dL
Serum or plasma iron	F 40–150 mcg/dL; 7.2–26.9 mmol/L M 50–160 mcg/dL; 8.9–28.7 mmol/L	A good measure of quantity of iron bound to transferrin Females — < 40 mcg/dL Males — <50 mcg
Total Iron Binding Capacity (TIBC) (Quantity of serum total circulating transferrin)	250–460 mcg/dL; 45–82 mmol/L	TIBC primarily reflects liver function and is an indirect measurement of transferrin. < 250 mcg/dL
Percent saturation of circulating transferrin	F 15–50% M 20–50%	Measures the iron supply to the tissues. It is calculated by dividing serum iron by the TIBC. Levels less than 16% are considered inadequate for erythropoiesis.
Soluble serum transferrin receptor (STFR)	F: 1.9–4.4 mg/L M: 2.2–5 mg/L	STFR reflects the rate of RBC production in bone marrow. Ordered to differentiate between anemia caused by iron deficiency and anemia caused by chronic and inflammatory diseases. It is more sensitive than serum ferritin because it is elevated with iron deficiency, is WNL in chronic disease or inflammation, and is low with iron overload.

Created with assistance by Mary Litchford, PhD, RDN, LDN

concentration to rise at a rate of 0.2 g/dl daily. Increased reticulocytosis (an increase in the number of young RBCs) is seen within 2 to 3 days after iron administration, but affected persons may report subjective improvements in mood and appetite sooner. The hemoglobin level will begin to increase by day 4. Iron therapy should be continued for 4 to 5 months, even after restoration of normal hemoglobin levels, to allow for repletion of body iron reserves.

Parenteral Iron-Dextran. If iron supplementation fails to correct the anemia, (1) the patient may not be taking the medication as prescribed due to gastric distress; (2) bleeding may be continuing at a rate faster than the erythroid marrow can replace blood cells; or (3) the supplemental iron is not being absorbed, possibly as a result of malabsorption secondary to steatorrhea, celiac disease, or hemodialysis. In these circumstances parenteral administration of iron in the form of iron dextran may be necessary. Although replenishment of iron stores by this route is faster, it is more expensive than, and not as safe as, oral administration.

Medical Nutrition Therapy

In addition to iron supplementation and its dosage adjustment depending on patient tolerance, attention should be given to the amount of absorbable dietary iron consumed. A good source of iron contains a substantial amount of iron in relation to its calorie content and contributes at least 10% of the recommended dietary allowance (RDA) for iron. Liver; kidney; beef; dried fruits; dried peas and beans; nuts; dark green leafy vegetables; and fortified whole-grain breads, muffins, cereals, and nutrition bars are among the foods that rank highest in iron content (see Appendix 49). It is estimated that 1.8 mg of iron must be absorbed daily to meet the needs of 80% to 90% of adult women and adolescent boys and girls.

Bioavailability of Dietary Iron. Because typical Western diets generally contain 6 mg/1000 kcal of iron, the bioavailability of iron in the diet is more important in correcting or preventing iron deficiency than the total amount of dietary iron consumed. The rate of absorption depends on the iron status of the individual, as reflected in the level of iron stores. The lower the iron stores, the greater the rate of iron absorption. Individuals with iron deficiency anemia absorb approximately 20% to 30% of dietary iron compared with the 5% to 10% absorbed by those without iron deficiency.

Form of Iron. Heme iron (approximately 15% of which is absorbable) is the organic form in meat, fish, and poultry, and is known as the **meat-fish-poultry (MFP) factor**. It is much better absorbed than nonheme iron. Nonheme iron can also be found in MFP, as well as in eggs, grains, vegetables, and fruits, but it is not part of the heme molecule. The absorption rate of nonheme iron varies between 3% and 8%, depending on the presence of dietary enhancing factors, specifically vitamin C and meat, fish, and poultry. Vitamin C not only is a powerful reducing agent, but also binds iron to form a readily absorbed complex. The mechanism by which the MFP factor potentiates the absorption of nonheme iron in other foodstuffs is unknown.

Inhibitors. Iron absorption can be inhibited to varying degrees by factors that chelate iron, including carbonates, oxalates, phosphates, and phytates (unleavened bread, unrefined cereals, and soybeans). Factors in vegetable fiber may inhibit nonheme iron absorption. If taken with meals, tea and coffee can reduce iron absorption by 50% through the formation of insoluble iron compounds with tannin. Iron in egg yolk is poorly absorbed because of the presence of phosvitin.

IRON OVERLOAD

Excess iron is stored as ferritin and hemosiderin in the macrophages of the liver, spleen, and bone marrow. The body has a limited capacity to excrete iron. Approximately 1 mg of iron is excreted daily through the gastrointestinal tract, urinary tract, and skin. To maintain a normal iron balance, the daily obligatory loss must be replaced by the absorption of heme and nonheme food iron. Persons with iron overload excrete increased amounts of iron, especially in the feces, to compensate partially for the increased absorption and higher stores.

Excessive iron intake usually stems from accidental incorporation of iron into the diet from environmental sources. In developing countries the iron overload can result from eating foods cooked in cast iron cooking vessels or contaminated by iron-containing soils. In developed countries it likely results from excessive intake of iron-supplemented foods or multivitamin and mineral supplementation containing iron.

Uncommon disorders associated with iron overload or toxicity include thalassemias, sideroblastic anemia, chronic hemolytic anemia, ineffective erythropoiesis, transfusional iron overload (secondary to multiple blood transfusions), porphyria cutanea tarda, aplastic anemia, and alcoholic cirrhosis. Aplastic anemia is a normochromic-normocytic anemia accompanied by a deficiency of all the formed elements in the blood; it can be caused by exposure to toxic chemicals, ionizing radiation, and medications, although the cause is often unknown.

Brain iron increases with age, is higher in men, and is abnormally elevated in neurodegenerative diseases, including Alzheimer's disease and Parkinson's disease (Bartzokis et al, 2010). Several gene variants affect iron metabolism and may contribute to early onset of these conditions.

Hemochromatosis

Hemochromatosis is the most common form of iron overload that causes progressive hepatic, pancreatic, cardiac, and other organ damage. People with this condition absorb three times more iron from their food than those without hemochromatosis. This disease, associated with the HFE gene, often is underdiagnosed. Persons who have two affected genes (homozygotes) will die of iron overload unless they donate blood frequently. Otherwise, the excessive iron absorption continues unabated.

Asians and Pacific Islanders have the highest levels of iron in their blood of all racial and ethnic groups, but they have the lowest prevalence of the gene mutation found with the typical form of hemochromatosis The Hemochromatosis and Iron Overload Screening Study notes that non-Hispanic whites have the highest prevalence of the C282Y mutation of the hereditary iron (HFE) gene and thus hemochromatosis, followed by Native Americans, Hispanics, African Americans, Pacific Islanders, and Asians (Moretti et al, 2013).

In women, monthly menses slow the associated organ damage until after menopause (Moretti et al, 2013). Men are particularly susceptible to hemochromatosis because they have no physiologic mechanisms for losing iron such as menstruation, pregnancy, or lactation.

Pathophysiology

Hepcidin is a peptide synthesized in the liver that functions as the principal regulator of systemic iron homeostasis. It regulates iron transport from iron-exporting tissues into plasma. Hepcidin deficiency underlies most known forms of hereditary hemochromatosis Hepcidin inhibits the cellular efflux of iron by binding to and inducing the degradation of ferroprotein, the sole iron exporter in iron-transporting cells. Hepcidin controls plasma iron concentration and tissue distribution of iron by inhibiting intestinal iron absorption, iron recycling by macrophages, and iron mobilization from hepatic stores (Ganz, 2011).

Hepcidin synthesis is increased by iron loading and decreased by anemia and hypoxia. Its synthesis is also greatly increased during inflammation, trapping iron in macrophages, decreasing plasma iron concentrations, and causing iron-restricted erythropoiesis that is characteristic of anemia of chronic disease. There is evidence that the mutation of the HFE gene leading to hemochromatosis is also associated with increased levels of gastrin in the stomach, leading to increased levels of gastric acid and thus increased absorption of iron (Ganz, 2011). In hemochromatosis iron absorption is enhanced, resulting in a gradual, progressive accumulation of iron. Most affected persons do not know they have it. In its early stages iron overload may result in symptoms similar to iron deficiency such as fatigue and weakness; later it can cause chronic abdominal pain, aching joints, impotence, and menstrual irregularities.

A progressive, positive iron balance may result in a variety of serious problems, including hepatomegaly, skin pigmentation, arthritis, heart disease, hypogonadism, diabetes mellitus, and cancer. Individuals with abnormally high iron levels are more likely to develop cancer of the colon. Iron is a prooxidant that can be used for tumor cell growth and proliferation. There also seems to be increased risk for age-related macular degeneration and Alzheimer's disease because of the oxidant effect of iron overload (Fleming and Ponka, 2012; Leskovjan et al, 2011).

Assessment

If an iron overload is suspected, the following screening tests should be performed: serum ferritin level (storage iron), serum iron concentration, TIBC, and percent of transferrin saturation ([serum iron/TIBC] $\times$ 100). Iron overload may be present if the percent of transferrin saturation is greater than 50 in women and 60 in men, and if the serum iron level is greater than 180 mg/dl. Deoxyribonucleic acid (DNA) testing, using blood or cheek cell samples, is also available for early detection of hemochromatosis. Liver biopsy is the gold standard for the diagnosis of iron overload.

Medical Management

The patient with iron overload may simultaneously be anemic as a result of damage to the bone marrow, an inflammatory disorder, cancer, internal bleeding, or chronic infection. Iron supplements should not be taken until the cause is known.

For patients with significant iron overload, weekly phlebotomy for 2 to 3 years may be required to eliminate all excess iron. Treatment for iron overload also may involve iron depletion with intravenous desferrioxamine-B, a chelating agent that is excreted by the kidneys, or with calcium disodium ethylenediaminetetraacetic acid (EDTA). Morbidity is reduced if excess body iron is removed by phlebotomy therapy before hepatic cirrhosis develops. Patients diagnosed as having hemochromatosis should inform all blood relatives so that they can be evaluated.

Medical Nutrition Therapy

Individuals with iron overload should ingest less heme iron from meat, fish, and poultry compared with nonheme iron from plant foods. Persons with iron overload also should avoid alcohol and vitamin C supplements because both enhance iron absorption. In addition, vitamin C supplements may cause release of harmful free radical–generating excess iron from body stores.

Affected persons should avoid foods that are fortified with iron (i.e., breakfast cereals, "energy" or sports bars, and meal-replacement drinks or shakes). They should also avoid iron supplements or multiple vitamin and mineral supplements that contain iron. The recommended dietary allowance (RDA) for iron should not be exceeded, and perhaps the intake of iron should be less than that in some persons. The dietary reference intakes (DRIs) for iron are RDAs and are summarized on the inside front cover. The RDA for women in their childbearing years is 18 mg; for pregnant women, 27 mg; and the RDA for adult men, and women 51 years of age and older is 8 mg.

MEGALOBLASTIC ANEMIAS

Megaloblastic anemia reflects a disturbed synthesis of DNA, which results in morphologic and functional changes in erythrocytes, leukocytes, platelets, and their precursors in the blood and bone marrow. This anemia is characterized by the presence of large, immature, abnormal, RBC progenitors in the bone marrow; 95% of cases are attributable to folic acid or vitamin B_{12} deficiency. Two disorders of cobalamin metabolism arise from mutations of the methionine synthase and methionine synthase reductase genes; these disorders feature megaloblastic anemia and neurologic manifestations (see Chapter 5).

Both vitamins are essential to the synthesis of nucleoproteins. Hematologic changes are the same for both; however, the folic acid deficiency is the first to appear. Normal body folate stores are depleted within 2 to 4 months in individuals consuming folate-deficient diets. By contrast, vitamin B_{12} stores are depleted only after several years of a vitamin B_{12}–deficient diet. In persons with vitamin B_{12} deficiency, folic acid supplementation can mask B_{12} deficiency (see Figure 32-3).

In correcting the anemia, the vitamin B_{12} deficiency may remain undetected, leading to the irreversible neuropsychiatric damage that is corrected **only** with B_{12} supplementation (see Chapter 41).

Folic Acid Deficiency Anemia
Etiology

Folic acid deficiency anemia is associated with tropical sprue, can affect pregnant women, and occurs in infants born to mothers with folic acid deficiency. Folic acid deficiency in early pregnancy also can result in an infant born with a neural tube defect (see Chapter 15). Prolonged inadequate diets, inadequate absorption, inadequate use of folic acid caused by genetic aberrations resulting in reduced methylation of folic acid, and increased requirements resulting from pregnancy or growth are believed to be the most frequent causes. Other causes are gluten-induced enteropathy (childhood and adult celiac disease), idiopathic steatorrhea, nontropical sprue, and use of certain drugs (anticonvulsants, barbiturates, cycloserine, sulfasalazine, cholestyramine, and metformin), amino acid excess (glycine and methionine), and alcohol.

Because alcohol interferes with the folate enterohepatic cycle, most alcoholics have a negative folate balance or a folate deficiency. Alcoholics constitute the only group that generally has all six causes of folic acid deficiency simultaneously: inadequate

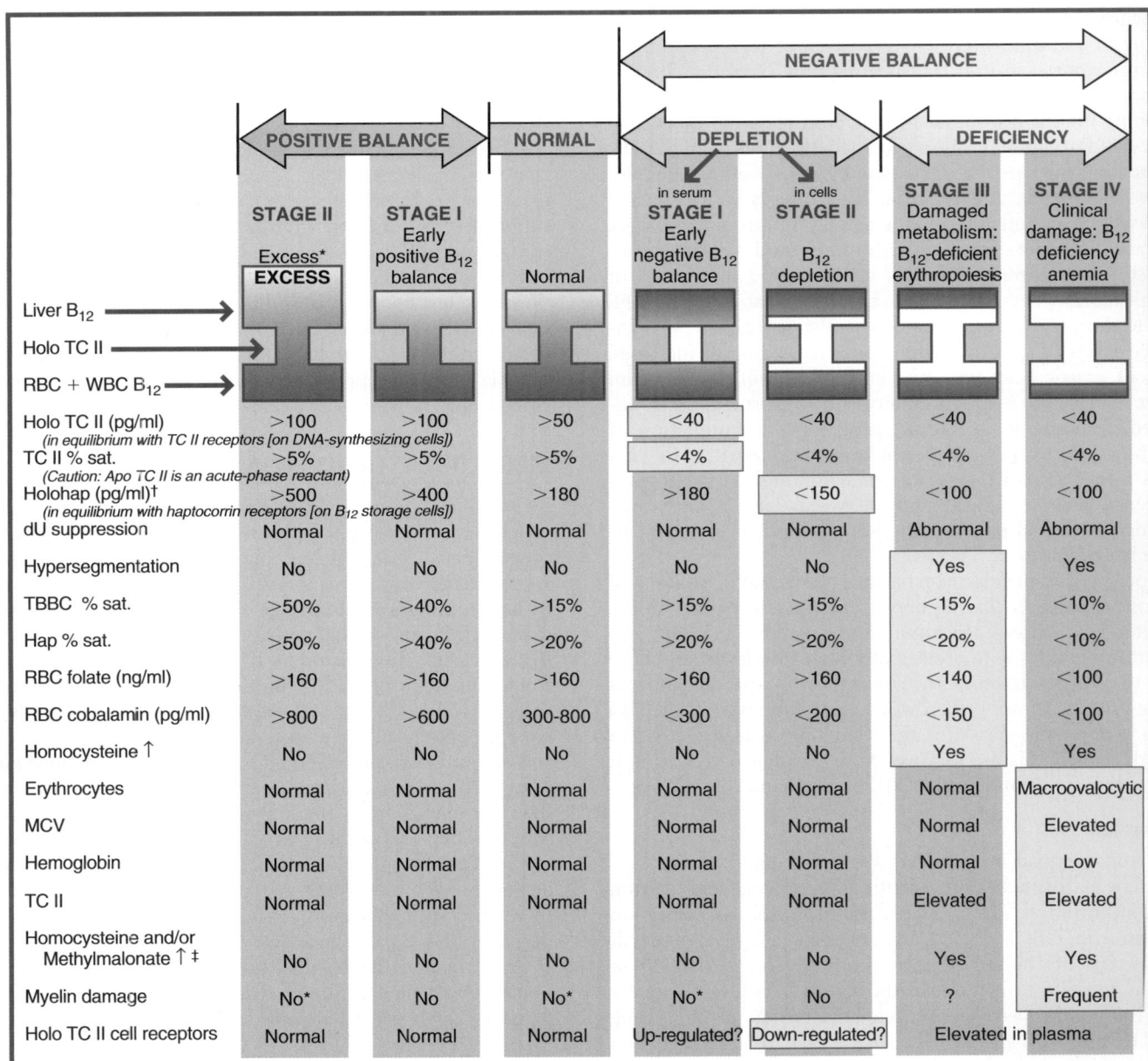

	POSITIVE BALANCE		NORMAL	DEPLETION		DEFICIENCY	
	STAGE II Excess* **EXCESS**	STAGE I Early positive B12 balance	Normal	STAGE I Early negative B12 balance (in serum)	STAGE II B12 depletion (in cells)	STAGE III Damaged metabolism: B12-deficient erythropoiesis	STAGE IV Clinical damage: B12 deficiency anemia
Liver B12							
Holo TC II							
RBC + WBC B12							
Holo TC II (pg/ml) *(in equilibrium with TC II receptors [on DNA-synthesizing cells])*	>100	>100	>50	<40	<40	<40	<40
TC II % sat. *(Caution: Apo TC II is an acute-phase reactant)*	>5%	>5%	>5%	<4%	<4%	<4%	<4%
Holohap (pg/ml)† *(in equilibrium with haptocorrin receptors [on B12 storage cells])*	>500	>400	>180	>180	<150	<100	<100
dU suppression	Normal	Normal	Normal	Normal	Normal	Abnormal	Abnormal
Hypersegmentation	No	No	No	No	No	Yes	Yes
TBBC % sat.	>50%	>40%	>15%	>15%	>15%	<15%	<10%
Hap % sat.	>50%	>40%	>20%	>20%	>20%	<20%	<10%
RBC folate (ng/ml)	>160	>160	>160	>160	>160	<140	<100
RBC cobalamin (pg/ml)	>800	>600	300-800	<300	<200	<150	<100
Homocysteine ↑	No	No	No	No	No	Yes	Yes
Erythrocytes	Normal	Normal	Normal	Normal	Normal	Normal	Macroovalocytic
MCV	Normal	Normal	Normal	Normal	Normal	Normal	Elevated
Hemoglobin	Normal	Normal	Normal	Normal	Normal	Normal	Low
TC II	Normal	Normal	Normal	Normal	Normal	Elevated	Elevated
Homocysteine and/or Methylmalonate ↑‡	No	No	No	No	No	Yes	Yes
Myelin damage	No*	No	No*	No*	No	?	Frequent
Holo TC II cell receptors	Normal	Normal	Normal	Up-regulated?	Down-regulated?	Elevated in plasma	

Holo TC II, Holotranscobalamin II; *MCV,* mean corpuscular volume; *% sat.,* percent saturation; *RBC,* red blood cell; *TBBC,* total B12 binding capacity.

* Cyanocobalamin excesses (injected or intranasal) produce transient increases in B12 delivery protein (TC II); the significance of such increases is unknown. Cyanocobalamin acts as an anti–B12 agent in a rare congenital defect in B12 metabolism.

† In serum and urine.

‡ Low holohaptocorrin correlates with **liver cell** B12 depletion, except in liver disease and myeloproliferative disorders, in which serum B12 and binding proteins are artificially elevated.

There may be hematopoietic cell and glial cell B12 depletion **prior to** liver cell depletion, and those cells may be in stage III or IV negative B12 balance, whereas liver cells are still in stage II.

FIGURE 32-3 Sequential stages of vitamin B12 status. (From Herbert V: Staging vitamin B12. In Ziegler EE, Filer LJ, editors: *Present knowledge in nutrition,* ed 7, Washington, DC, 1996, International Life Sciences Institute Press.)

ingestion, absorption, and use, increased excretion, requirement, and destruction of folic acid (see Chapter 29). Box 32-2 describes the causes of folate deficiency.

Folate absorption takes place in the small intestine. Enzyme conjugases (e.g., pteroylpolyglutamate hydrolase, the folate conjugase), found in the brush border of the small intestine, hydrolyze the polyglutamates to monoglutamates and reduce them to dihydrofolate and tetrahydrofolic acid (THFA) in the small intestinal epithelial cells (enterocytes). From the enterocytes these forms are transported to the circulation, where they are bound to protein and transported as methyl THFA into the cells of the body.

In the absence of vitamin B12, 5-methyl THFA, the major circulating and storage form of folic acid, is metabolically inactive.

BOX 32-2   Causes of Folate Deficiency

Inadequate Ingestion

Poor diet (lack of or overcooked fruits and vegetables), vitamin B_{12} or vitamin C deficiency, chronic alcoholism

Inadequate Absorption

Gluten-induced enteropathy or celiac disease, tropical sprue, drug interactions, congenital defects

Inadequate Utilization

Antagonists, anticonvulsants, enzyme deficiency, vitamin B_{12} and vitamin C deficiency, chronic alcoholism, excess glycine and methionine

Increased Requirement

Extra tissue demand, infancy, increased hematopoiesis, increased metabolic activity, Lesch-Nyhan syndrome, drugs

Increased Excretion

Vitamin B_{12} deficiency, liver disease, kidney dialysis, chronic exfoliative dermatitis

Increased Destruction

Dietary oxidants

Modified from Herbert V, Das KC: Folic acid and vitamin B_{12}. In Shils ME et al, editors: *Modern nutrition in health and disease*, ed 3, vol 1, Philadelphia, 1994, Lea & Febiger.

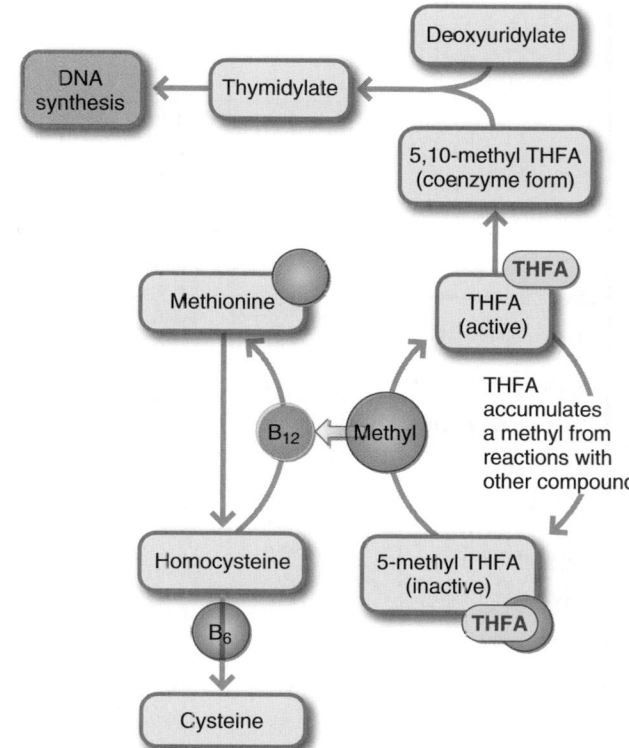

FIGURE 32-4 Methylfolate trap. A deficiency of vitamin B_{12} can result in a deficiency of folic acid because folate is trapped in the form of 5-methyltetrahydrofolate (5-methyl THFA), which cannot be converted to THFA and methyl groups donated by the vitamin B_{12}–dependent pathway. *DNA,* Deoxyribonucleic acid.

To be activated the 5-methyl group is removed, and THFA is cycled back into the folate pool, where it functions as the main 1-carbon-unit acceptor in mammalian biochemical reactions. THFA may then be converted to the coenzyme form of folate required to convert deoxyuridylate to thymidylate, which is necessary for DNA synthesis.

MTHFR Allele. A genetic defect found in 10% of whites is the methylenetetrahydrofolate reductase (MTHFR) deficiency (see Chapter 5). The allele is problematic in pregnancy and may contribute to miscarriages, anencephaly, or neural defects (see Chapter 15). Because MTHFR irreversibly reduces 5,10-methylenetetrahydrofolate to 5-methyltetrahydrofolate, its deficiency may result in developmental delay, motor and gait dysfunction, seizures, neurologic impairment, extremely high levels of homocysteine, clotting disorders, and other conditions.

Methylfolate Trap. Vitamin B_{12} deficiency can result in a folic acid deficiency by causing folate entrapment in the metabolically useless form of 5-methyl THFA (see Figure 32-4). The lack of vitamin B_{12} to remove the 5-methyl unit means that metabolically inactive methyl THFA is trapped. It cannot release its 1-carbon methyl group to become THFA, the basic 1-carbon carrier that picks up 1-carbon units from one molecule and delivers them to another. Hence a functional folic acid deficiency results.

Pathophysiology

Folate deficiency develops in four stages: two that involve depletion, followed by two marked by deficiency (see Figure 32-5):

Stage 1: Characterized by early negative folate balance (serum depletion to less than 3 ng/ml)

Stage 2: Characterized by negative folate balance (cell depletion), with a decrease in erythrocyte folate levels to less than 160 ng/ml

Stage 3: Characterized by damaged folate metabolism, with folate-deficient erythropoiesis. This stage is characterized by slowed DNA synthesis, manifested by an abnormal diagnostic deoxyuridine (dU) suppression test correctable in vitro by folates, granulocyte nuclear hypersegmentation, and macro-ovalocytic red cells.

Stage 4: Characterized by clinical folate-deficiency anemia, with an elevated MCV and anemia.

Because of their interrelated roles in the synthesis of thymidylate in DNA formation, a deficiency of either vitamin B_{12} or folic acid results in a megaloblastic anemia. The immature nuclei do not mature properly in the deficient state; and large (macrocytic), immature (megaloblastic) RBCs are the result. The common clinical signs of folic acid deficiency include fatigue, dyspnea, sore tongue, diarrhea, irritability, forgetfulness, anorexia, glossitis, and weight loss.

Normal body folate stores are depleted within 2 to 4 months on a folate-deficient diet, resulting in a macrocytic, megaloblastic anemia with a decreased number of erythrocytes, leukocytes, and platelets. Folate-deficiency anemia is manifested by very low serum folate (<3 ng/ml) and RBC folate levels of less than 140 to 160 ng/ml. Whereas a low serum folate level merely diagnoses a negative balance at the time the blood is drawn, a red cell folate (RCF) level measures actual body folate stores, and thus is the superior measurement for determining folate nutriture. To differentiate folate deficiency from vitamin B_{12} deficiency, levels of serum folate, RCF, serum vitamin B_{12}, and vitamin B_{12} bound to transcobalamin II (TCII) can be measured simultaneously using a radioassay kit. Also diagnostic for folate deficiency is an elevated level of formiminoglutamic acid in the urine, as well as

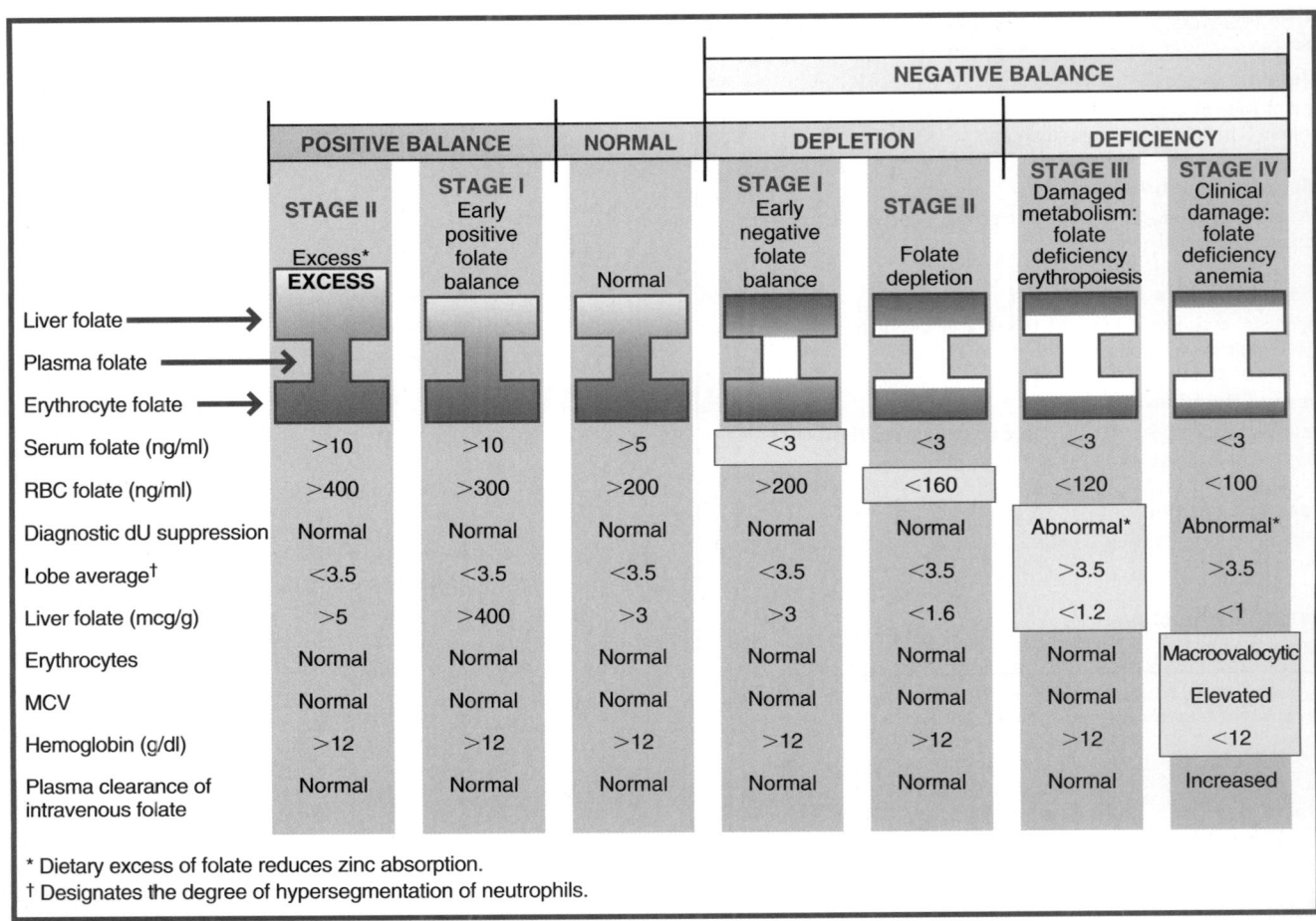

	POSITIVE BALANCE		NORMAL	DEPLETION		NEGATIVE BALANCE — DEFICIENCY	
	STAGE II Excess* **EXCESS**	STAGE I Early positive folate balance	Normal	STAGE I Early negative folate balance	STAGE II Folate depletion	STAGE III Damaged metabolism: folate deficiency erythropoiesis	STAGE IV Clinical damage: folate deficiency anemia
Serum folate (ng/ml)	>10	>10	>5	<3	<3	<3	<3
RBC folate (ng/ml)	>400	>300	>200	>200	<160	<120	<100
Diagnostic dU suppression	Normal	Normal	Normal	Normal	Normal	Abnormal*	Abnormal*
Lobe average†	<3.5	<3.5	<3.5	<3.5	<3.5	>3.5	>3.5
Liver folate (mcg/g)	>5	>400	>3	>3	<1.6	<1.2	<1
Erythrocytes	Normal	Normal	Normal	Normal	Normal	Normal	Macroovalocytic
MCV	Normal	Normal	Normal	Normal	Normal	Normal	Elevated
Hemoglobin (g/dl)	>12	>12	>12	>12	>12	>12	<12
Plasma clearance of intravenous folate	Normal	Normal	Normal	Normal	Normal	Normal	Increased

* Dietary excess of folate reduces zinc absorption.
† Designates the degree of hypersegmentation of neutrophils.

FIGURE 32-5 Sequential stages of folate status. *dU*, Deoxyuridine; *MCV*, mean corpuscular volume; *RBC*, red blood cell. (From Herbert V: Folic acid. In Shils ME et al, editors: *Modern nutrition in health and disease*, ed 9, Philadelphia 1998, Lea & Febiger.)

the dU suppression test in bone marrow cells or peripheral blood lymphocytes (see Chapter 7 and Appendix 22).

Medical Management

Before treatment is initiated, it is important to diagnose the cause of the megaloblastosis correctly. Administration of folate corrects megaloblastosis from either folate or vitamin B_{12} deficiency, but it can mask the neurologic damage of vitamin B_{12} deficiency, allowing the nerve damage to progress to the point of irreversibility.

A dosage of 1 mg of folate taken orally every day for 2 to 3 weeks replenishes folate stores. Maintaining repleted stores requires an absolute minimum oral intake of 50 to 100 mcg of folic acid daily. When folate deficiency is complicated by alcoholism, genetic aberrations, or other conditions that suppress hematopoiesis, increase folate requirements, or reduce folate absorption, therapy should remain at 500 to 1000 mcg daily. Symptomatic improvement, as evidenced by increased alertness, cooperation, and appetite, may be apparent within 24 to 48 hours, long before hematologic values revert to normal, a gradual process that takes approximately a month.

Medical Nutrition Therapy

After the anemia is corrected, the patient should be instructed to eat at least one fresh, uncooked fruit, or dark green vegetable or to drink a glass of vegetable or fruit and vegetable juice daily (see

Appendix 40 for a list of folate-containing foods). Fresh, uncooked fruits and vegetables are good sources of folate because folate can easily be destroyed by heat. In 1998 the Food and Drug Administration required that grains be fortified with folic acid. The DRIs for folate are RDAs and are summarized on the inside front cover of this text. The RDA for adults is 400 mcg daily. The Dietary Guidelines for Americans recommend that women of childbearing age who may become pregnant and those in their first trimester of pregnancy consume adequate synthetic folic acid (600 mcg/day) from fortified foods and supplements in addition to consuming a variety of foods containing folate.

Vitamin B_{12} Deficiency and Pernicious Anemias

Intrinsic factor (IF) is a glycoprotein in the gastric juice that is necessary for the absorption of dietary vitamin B_{12}. Secreted by parietal cells of the gastric mucosa, IF is necessary for the absorption of exogenous vitamin B_{12}. Ingested vitamin B_{12} is freed from protein by gastric acid and gastric and intestinal enzymes. The free vitamin B_{12} attaches to salivary R-binder, which has a higher affinity for the vitamin than does IF. An acid pH (2.3) is needed, such as that found in the healthy stomach.

Etiology

The release of pancreatic trypsin into the proximal small intestine destroys R-binder and releases vitamin B_{12} from its complex with R-protein. With an alkaline pH (6.8) in the intestine, IF binds the vitamin B_{12}. The vitamin B_{12}–IF complex is then carried to the ileum. In the ileum, with the presence of ionic calcium (Ca^{2+}) and a pH (>6), the complex attaches to the surface vitamin B_{12}–IF receptors on the ileal cell brush border. Here, the vitamin B_{12} is released and attaches to holotranscobalamin II (holo TCII). Holo TCII is vitamin B_{12} attached to the beta-globulin, the major circulating vitamin B_{12} delivery protein. Like IF, holo TCII plays an active role in binding and transporting vitamin B_{12}. The TCII–vitamin B_{12} complex then enters the portal venous blood.

Other binding proteins in the blood include haptocorrin, also known as transcobalamin I (TCI) and transcobalamin III (TCIII). These are alpha-globulins, larger macromolecular-weight glycoproteins that make up the R-binder component of the blood. Unlike IF, the R-proteins are capable of binding not only vitamin B_{12} but also many of its biologically inactive analogs. Although approximately 75% of the vitamin B_{12} in human serum is bound to haptocorrin and roughly 25% is bound to TCII, only TCII is important in delivering vitamin B_{12} to all the cells that need it. After transport through the bloodstream, TCII is recognized by receptors on cell surfaces. Patients with haptocorrin abnormalities have no symptoms of vitamin B_{12} deficiency. Those lacking TCII rapidly develop megaloblastic anemia. Vitamin B_{12} is excreted in urine.

Pathophysiology

Pernicious anemia is a megaloblastic, macrocytic anemia caused by a deficiency of vitamin B_{12}, most commonly from a lack of IF. Rarely, vitamin B_{12} deficiency anemia occurs in strict vegetarians whose diet contains no vitamin B_{12} except for traces found in plants contaminated by microorganisms capable of synthesizing vitamin B_{12}. Other causes include antibody to IF in saliva or gastric juice; small intestinal disorders affecting the ileum such as celiac disease, idiopathic steatorrhea, tropical sprue, cancers involving the small intestine; drugs (paraamino-salicylic acid, colchicine, neomycin, metformin, antiretrovirals); and long-term ingestion of alcohol or calcium-chelating agents (see Box 32-3).

Aging is associated with B_{12} deficiency for various reasons as discussed in Chapter 20. Approximately 1% to 2% of the U.S. population over the age of 51 years has clinical B_{12} deficiency, and it is thought that 10% to 20% have subclinical deficiency (Carmel, 2011).

BOX 32-3 Causes of Vitamin B_{12} Deficiency

Inadequate ingestion	Poor diet resulting from a vegan diet and lack of supplementation, chronic alcoholism, poverty
Inadequate absorption	Gastric disorders, small intestinal disorders, competition for absorption sites, pancreatic disease, HIV, or AIDS
Inadequate use	Vitamin B_{12} antagonists, congenital or acquired enzyme deficiency, abnormal binding proteins
Increased requirement	Hyperthyroidism, increased hematopoiesis
Increased excretion	Inadequate vitamin B_{12} binding protein, liver disease, renal disease
Increased destruction	Pharmacologic doses of ascorbic acid when it functions as a prooxidant

AIDS, Acquired immune deficiency syndrome; *HIV,* human immunodeficiency virus.

Stages of Deficiency

As a result of normal enterohepatic circulation (i.e., excretion of vitamin B_{12} and analogs in bile and resorption of vitamin B_{12} in the ileum), it generally takes decades for strict vegetarians who are not receiving vitamin B_{12} supplementation to develop a vitamin B_{12} deficiency. Serum B_{12}, homocysteine, and methylmalonic acid levels are not as effective as predictors of B_{12}-responsive neurologic disorders; patients with unexplained leukoencephalopathy should be treated proactively because even long-standing deficits may be reversible (Graber et al, 2010).

Stage 1: Early negative vitamin B_{12} balance begins when vitamin B_{12} intake is low or absorption is poor, depleting the primary delivery protein, TCII. A low TCII (<40 pg/ml) may be the earliest detectable sign of a vitamin B_{12} deficiency (Serefhanoglu et al, 2008). This is a vitamin B_{12} pre-deficiency stage.

Stage 2: Vitamin B_{12} depletion shows a low B_{12} on TCII and a gradual lowering of B_{12} in haptocorrin (holohap <50 pg/ml), the storage protein.

Stage 3: Damaged metabolism and vitamin B_{12}–deficient erythropoiesis includes an abnormal dU suppression, hypersegmentation, a decreased TIBC and holohap percent saturation, a low RCF level (<140 ng/ml), and subtle neuropsychiatric damage (impaired short-term and recent memory).

Stage 4: Clinical damage occurs, including vitamin B_{12} deficiency anemia; includes all preceding parameters, including macroovalocytic erythrocytes, elevated MCV, elevated TCII levels, increased homocysteine, methylmalonic acid levels, and myelin damage. Leukoencephalopathy and autonomic dysfunction occur with very low serum B_{12} levels (<200 pg/ml); psychiatric changes, neuropathy, and dementia also may occur (Graber et al, 2010) (see Figure 32-3).

Clinical Findings

Pernicious anemia affects not only the blood but also the gastrointestinal tract and the peripheral and central nervous systems. This distinguishes it from folic acid deficiency anemia. The overt symptoms, which are caused by inadequate myelinization of the nerves, include paresthesia (especially numbness and tingling in the hands and feet), diminution of the senses of vibration and position, poor muscular coordination, poor memory, and hallucinations. If the deficiency is prolonged, the nervous system damage may be irreversible, even with initiation of vitamin B_{12} treatment.

Helicobacter pylori causes peptic ulcer disease and chronic gastritis (see Chapter 27). Both conditions are associated with hypochlorhydria, reduced production of IF by epithelial cells in the stomach, vitamin B_{12} malabsorption, and pernicious anemia. There is also a correlation between autoimmune gastritis and pernicious anemia. More than 90% of patients with pernicious anemia have parietal cell antibodies (PCAs), and 50% to 70% have elevated IF antibodies. Serum vitamin B_{12} levels of the *H. pylori*–infected patients are significantly lower than that of uninfected patients (Sato et al, 2013).

A study on *H. pylori* infection and autoimmune type atrophic gastritis examined serum markers for gastric atrophy (pepsinogen I, pepsinogen I/II, and gastrin) and autoimmunity. Positive serum autoimmune markers (IF antibodies and PCA) suggest that *H. pylori* contributes to autoimmune gastritis and pernicious anemia (Aditi and Graham, 2012).

Vitamin B_{12} deficiency is an important modifiable risk factor for osteoporosis in men and women. Adults with vitamin B_{12}

levels below 148 pg/ml have a lower average bone mineral density and greater risk for osteoporosis (Tucker et al, 2005).

Reduced vitamin B_{12} status and elevated homocysteine concentrations are common. These alterations are problematic among vegans (Sato et al, 2013). B_{12}-folate-homocysteine interactions aggravate heart disease and may lead to adverse pregnancy outcomes (Moreiras et al, 2009) (see Chapters 15 and 33).

Assessment

Vitamin B_{12} stores are depleted after several years without vitamin B_{12} intake. A low holo-TCII value (<40 pg/ml) is a sign of early B_{12} deficiency. Radioassays measure more than one component within the same biologic medium. The Becton-Dickinson SimulTRAC Radioassay Kit measures the levels of serum vitamin B_{12} and serum folate simultaneously in a single test tube.

Other laboratory tests that may be helpful in diagnosing a vitamin B_{12} deficiency and determining its cause include measurements of unsaturated B_{12} binding capacity, IF antibody (IFAB), the Schilling test, and tests to determine serum homocysteine and serum methionine levels (see Chapter 7 and Appendix 22). The IFAB and Schilling urinary excretion tests can determine whether the deficiency is caused by a lack of IF. The IFAB assay is performed on a patient's serum, whereas the Schilling test requires that the patient first swallow radioactive B_{12} alone and then a second time with IF (http://www.nlm.nih.gov/medlineplus/ency/article/003572.htm).

Patients with pernicious anemia excrete very little vitamin B_{12} during the first step because little or no vitamin B_{12} is absorbed. However, during the second step the urinary excretion becomes almost normal because more vitamin B_{12} is absorbed with the addition of the IF. Vitamin B_{12} deficiency secondary to malabsorption syndrome and not IF deficiency is manifested by a decrease in urinary excretion of B_{12} that remains unchanged with IF administration. The Schilling test is ordered less often today because it uses a radioactive B_{12} molecule which is not as available, and because the treatment, a large injection of B_{12}, is the same whether or not the malabsorption is due to inadequate IF.

Medical Management

Treatment usually consists of an intramuscular or subcutaneous injection of 100 mcg or more of vitamin B_{12} once per week. After an initial response is elicited, the frequency of administration is reduced until remission can be maintained indefinitely with monthly injections of 100 mcg. Very large oral doses of vitamin B_{12} (1000 mcg daily) are also effective, even in the absence of IF, because approximately 1% of vitamin B_{12} is absorbed by diffusion. Initial doses should be increased when vitamin B_{12} deficiency is complicated by debilitating illness such as infection, hepatic disease, uremia, coma, severe disorientation, or marked neurologic damage. A response to treatment is evidenced by improved appetite, alertness, and cooperation, followed by improved hematologic results, as manifested by marked reticulocytosis within hours of an injection.

Medical Nutrition Therapy

A high-protein diet (1.5 g/kg of body weight) is desirable for liver function and for blood regeneration. Because green leafy vegetables contain iron and folic acid, the diet should contain increased amounts of these foods. Meats (especially beef and pork), eggs, milk, and milk products are particularly rich in vitamin B_{12} (see Appendix 40).

For those individuals prescribed metformin for treatment of diabetes, 10% to 30% have reduced vitamin B_{12} absorption. Metformin negatively affects the calcium-dependent membrane and the B_{12}-IF complex by decreasing the absorbability by the ileal cell surface receptors. Increased intake of calcium reverses the vitamin B_{12} malabsorption.

The Dietary Guidelines for Americans recommend that people older than age 50 consume vitamin B_{12} in its crystalline form (i.e., in fortified cereals or supplements) to overcome the effects of atrophic gastritis. The DRIs for B_{12} are RDAs and are summarized on the inside front cover. The RDA for adult men and women is 2.4 mcg daily.

OTHER NUTRITIONAL ANEMIAS

Anemia of Protein-Energy Malnutrition

Protein is essential for the proper production of hemoglobin and RBCs. Because of the reduction in cell mass and thus oxygen requirements in protein-energy malnutrition (PEM), fewer RBCs are required to oxygenate the tissue. Because blood volume remains the same, this reduced number of RBCs with a low hemoglobin level (hypochromic, normocytic anemia), which can mimic an iron deficiency anemia, is actually a physiologic (nonharmful) rather than harmful anemia. In acute PEM, the loss of active tissue mass may be greater than the reduction in the number of RBCs, leading to polycythemia (an increase in RBCs where they make up a larger proportion of the blood volume). The body responds to this RBC production, which is not a reflection of protein and amino acid deficiency but of an oversupply of RBCs. Iron released from normal RBC destruction is not reused in RBC production, but is stored so that iron stores are often adequate. Iron deficiency anemia can reappear with rehabilitation when RBC mass expands rapidly.

The anemia of PEM may be complicated by deficiencies of iron and other nutrients and by associated infections, parasitic infestation, and malabsorption. A diet lacking in protein is usually deficient in iron, folic acid, and, less frequently, vitamin B_{12}. The nutrition counselor plays an important role in assessing recent and typical dietary intake of these nutrients.

Copper Deficiency Anemia

Copper and other heavy metals are essential for the proper formation of hemoglobin. Ceruloplasmin, a copper-containing protein, is required for normal mobilization of iron from its storage sites to the plasma. In a copper-deficient state, iron cannot be released; this leads to low serum iron and hemoglobin levels, even in the presence of normal iron stores. Other consequences of copper deficiency suggest that copper proteins are needed for use of iron by the developing erythrocyte and for optimal functions of the erythrocyte membrane. The amounts of copper needed for normal hemoglobin synthesis are so minute that they are usually amply supplied by an adequate diet; however, copper deficiency may occur in infants who are fed cow's milk or a copper-deficient infant formula. It also may be seen in children or adults who have a malabsorption syndrome or who are receiving long-term total parenteral nutrition that does not supply copper.

Sideroblastic (B₆-Responsive) Anemia

Sideroblastic (pyridoxine-responsive) anemia is characterized by a derangement in the final pathway of heme synthesis, leading to a buildup of immature RBCs. It has four primary characteristics: (1) microcytic and hypochromic RBCs; (2) high serum and tissue iron levels (causing increased transferrin saturation); (3) the presence of an inherited defect in the formation of δ-aminolevulinic acid synthetase, an enzyme involved in heme synthesis (pyridoxal-5-phosphate is necessary in this reaction); and (4) a buildup of iron-containing immature RBCs (sideroblasts, for which the anemia is named). The iron that cannot be used for heme synthesis is stored in the mitochondria of immature RBCs. These iron-laden mitochondria do not function normally, and the development and production of RBCs become ineffective. The symptoms are those of anemia and iron overload. Even though the anemia responds to the administration of pharmacologic doses of pyridoxine and thus is referred to as *pyridoxine–responsive anemia,* the neurologic and cutaneous manifestations of vitamin B_6 deficiency are not observed. This distinguishes it from anemia caused by a dietary vitamin B_6 deficiency.

Treatment consists of a therapeutic trial dose of 50 to 200 mg daily of pyridoxine or pyridoxal phosphate (PLP or pyridoxal-5-phosphate) which is 25 to 100 times the RDA. If the anemia responds to one or the other, pyridoxine therapy is continued for life. However, if the anemia is only partially corrected; a normal hematocrit value is never regained. Patients respond to this treatment to varying degrees, and some may only achieve near-normal hemoglobin levels.

Acquired sideroblastic anemias such as those attributable to drug therapy (isoniazid, chloramphenicol), copper deficiency, hypothermia, and alcoholism are not responsive to B_6 administration.

Vitamin E–Responsive Hemolytic Anemia

Hemolytic anemia occurs when defects in RBC membranes lead to oxidative damage and eventually to cell lysis.

This anemia is caused by shortened survival of mature RBCs. Vitamin E, an antioxidant, is involved in protecting the membrane against oxidative damage, and one of the few signs noted in vitamin E deficiency is early hemolysis of RBCs. Vitamin E–responsive hemolytic anemia in neonates is discussed in Chapter 42.

NONNUTRITIONAL ANEMIAS

Anemia of Pregnancy

A physiologic anemia is the anemia of pregnancy, which is related to increased blood volume and usually resolves with the end of the pregnancy. However, demands for iron during pregnancy also are increased so that inadequate iron intake may also play a role in whether it develops (see Chapter 15 for further discussion).

Anemia of Chronic Disease

Anemia of chronic disease occurs from inflammation, infection, or malignancy because there is decreased RBC production, possibly as a result of disordered iron metabolism. Ferritin levels are normal or increased, but serum iron levels and TIBC are low (see Chapter 7). It is important that this form of anemia, which is mild and normocytic, not be mistaken for iron deficiency anemia; iron supplements should not be given. Recombinant erythropoietin therapy usually corrects this anemia.

Sickle Cell Anemia
Pathophysiology

Sickle cell anemia (SCA), a chronic hemolytic anemia also known as *hemoglobin S disease,* affects about 1 of 500 African Americans in the United States as a result of homozygous inheritance of hemoglobin S. It also affects Hispanic Americans, but at a much lower rate. This results in defective hemoglobin synthesis, which produces sickle-shaped RBCs that get caught in capillaries and do not carry oxygen well (see Figure 32-6). The sickle-shaped RBCs die in 10 to 20 days. The bone marrow cannot make new cells fast enough to replace them; they are dying much faster than normal RBCs. The disease usually is diagnosed toward the end of the first year of life and is thought to affect 70,000 to 100,000 in the United States, although 2 million Americans have the sickle cell trait (NIH, NHLBI, 2012).

In addition to the usual symptoms of anemia, SCA is characterized by episodes of pain resulting from the occlusion of small blood vessels by the abnormally shaped erythrocytes. The occlusions frequently occur in the abdomen, causing acute, severe abdominal pain. The hemolytic anemia and vasoocclusive disease result in impaired liver function, jaundice, gallstones, and deteriorating renal function. The constant hemolysis of erythrocytes increases iron stores in the liver; however, iron deficiency anemia and SCA can coexist. Iron overload is less common and is usually a problem only in those who have received multiple blood transfusions.

Typically serum homocysteine levels are elevated, which may be due to low concentrations of vitamin B_6. Children with SCA were found to have these lower vitamin B_6 levels despite B_6 intakes comparable to those of unaffected children.

Medical Management

A new set of guidelines for managing sickle cell disease recommends using monthly blood transfusions and the drug

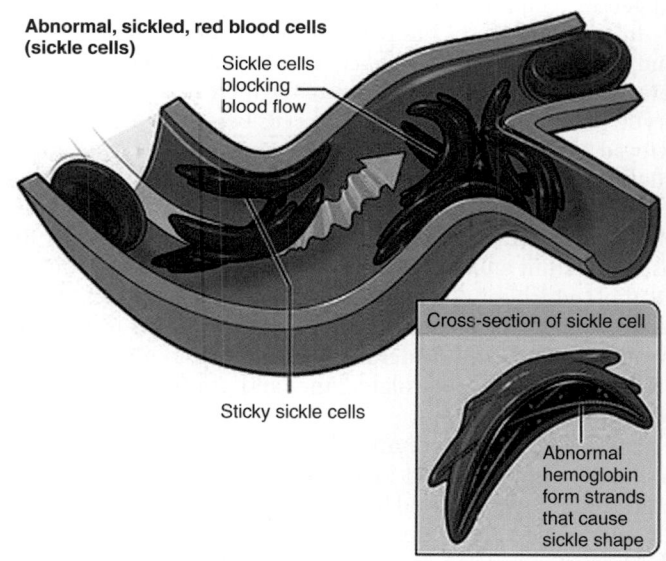

Abnormal, sickled, red blood cells (sickle cells)

Sickle cells blocking blood flow

Cross-section of sickle cell

Sticky sickle cells

Abnormal hemoglobin form strands that cause sickle shape

FIGURE 32-6 Sickled red blood cells. (From National Institutes of Health (NIH), National Heart, Lung and Blood Institute (NHLBI): What is sickle cell anemia? (website): http://www.nhlbi.nih.gov/health/health-topics/topics/sca/, 2012. Accessed January 8, 2015.)

hydroxyurea (Yawn et al, 2014). Consistent blood transfusions stop the body from producing sickle cells and attempts to normalize red blood cell count. Hydroxyurea increases the production of healthy fetal hemoglobin, reducing hospitalizations. Because hydroxyurea also lowers the number of white blood cells, patients must be monitored regularly with blood tests.

Other treatment for SCA focuses on relieving pain during a crisis, keeping the body oxygenated (using oxygen therapy if needed), and possibly administering an exchange transfusion. It is important that SCA not be mistaken for iron deficiency anemia, which can be treated with iron supplements, because iron stores in the patient with SCA secondary to transfusions are frequently excessive.

Zinc can increase the oxygen affinity of normal and sickle-shaped erythrocytes. Thus zinc supplements may be beneficial in managing sickle cell disease, especially because decreased plasma zinc is common in children with the SS genotype sickle cell disease and is associated with decreased linear and skeletal growth, muscle mass, and sexual maturation. Zinc supplementation (as little as 10 mg daily) also may prevent the deficit in growth that appears in these children (Zemel et al, 2007). Because zinc competes with copper for binding sites on proteins, the use of high doses of zinc may precipitate copper deficiency.

Medical Nutrition Therapy

Children with SCA and their families should receive instruction about how they can develop a well-balanced food plan providing enough calories and protein for growth and development. Their dietary intake may be low because of the abdominal pain characteristic of the disease. They also have increased metabolic rates, leading to a need for a higher caloric intake. This hypermetabolism probably is due to a constant inflammation and oxidative stress (Yawn et al, 2014). Therefore their diets must be high enough in calories to meet these needs and must provide foods high in folate and the trace minerals zinc and copper (see Appendix 53 for sources of zinc).

In addition, these children may be low in vitamins A, C, D, and E, folate, calcium, and fiber. The diet should be high in folate (400 to 600 mcg daily) because the increased production of erythrocytes needed to replace the cells being continuously destroyed also increases folic acid requirements (see Appendices 40 through 43).

When assessing the nutrition status of patients with SCA, clinicians must pay attention to the questions related to the use of vitamin and mineral supplements, the consumption of alcohol (which increases iron absorption), and sources of protein (animal sources being high in zinc and iron) in the diet. A multivitamin and mineral supplement containing 50% to 150% of the RDA for folate, zinc, and copper (not iron) is recommended.

Dietary fluid and sodium intake influence the risk for vaso-occlusive events in SCA; increasing fluid intake and limiting high-sodium foods should be discussed (Fowler et al, 2010) (see Chapter 33 and Appendix 30). Intake of 2 to 3 quarts of water daily is recommended. Finally, it is important to remember that patients with sickle cell disease may require higher than RDA amounts of protein.

If it is necessary for the diet to be low in absorbable iron, the diet should emphasize vegetable proteins. Iron-rich foods, such as liver, iron-fortified formula, iron-fortified cereals, and iron-fortified energy bars and iron-fortified sport drinks should be excluded. Substances such as alcohol and vitamin C supplements, both of which enhance iron absorption, should be avoided. However, iron deficiency may be present in some patients with SCA owing to repeated phlebotomies, excessive transfusions, or hematuria secondary to renal papillary necrosis. This should be assessed and the diet adjusted appropriately.

Hypochromic Microcytic Transient Anemia (Sports Anemia)

Increased RBC destruction, along with decreased hemoglobin, serum iron, and ferritin concentrations, may occur at the initiation and early stages of a vigorous training program. Once called *march hemoglobinuria* (an unusual appearance of hemoglobin in the urine), this anemia was believed to arise in soldiers as a result of mechanical trauma incurred by erythrocytes (RBCs) during long marches. The RBCs in the capillaries are compressed every time the foot lands until they burst, releasing hemoglobin. It was thought that a similar situation existed in runners, especially long-distance runners; however, it is now thought that sports anemia is a physiologic anemia (i.e., a transient problem of blood volume and dilution) (see Chapter 23 for further discussion).

Athletes who have hemoglobin concentrations below those needed for optimal oxygen delivery may benefit from consuming nutrient and iron-rich foods; ensuring that their diets contain adequate protein; and avoiding tea, coffee, antacids, H_2-blockers, and tetracycline, all of which inhibit iron absorption. No athlete should take iron supplements unless true iron deficiency is diagnosed based on a complete blood cell count with differential, serum ferritin level, serum iron level, TIBC, and percent saturation of iron-binding capacity. Athletes who are female, vegetarian, involved in endurance sports, or entering a growth spurt are at risk for iron deficiency anemia and therefore should undergo periodic monitoring (see Chapter 23).

Thalassemias

Thalassemias (alpha and beta) are severe inherited anemias characterized by microcytic, hypochromic, and short-lived RBCs resulting from defective hemoglobin synthesis, which affects primarily persons in the Mediterranean region. The ineffective erythropoiesis leads to an increase in plasma volume, progressive splenomegaly, and bone marrow expansion with the result of facial deformities, osteomalacia, and bone changes. Ultimately there is increased iron absorption and progressive iron deposition in tissues, resulting in oxidative damage. The accumulation of iron causes dysfunction of the heart, liver, and endocrine glands. Because these patients require transfusions to stay alive, they also must have regular chelation therapy to prevent the damaging buildup of iron that can occur. Impaired growth in children accompanying thalassemia major can be partially corrected by increasing caloric intake.

Medical Nutrition Therapy

The diet should be high in protein, B vitamins, especially folic acid, and zinc. Multivitamin and mineral supplements that contain amounts of iron and vitamin C above the RDA should be avoided. Increased calcium intake may be required in some patients because of bone formation issues (NIH, National Library of Medicine [NLM], 2014; NIH, 2012). Patients should stay well hydrated.

CLINICAL CASE STUDY

Marisa, a 27-year-old female, reports increased symptoms of restless leg syndrome, fatigue, and painful abdominal bloating and heavy menses for the past year. A physical examination reveals inflammation and tenderness around her knee and ankle joints.

MEDICATIONS: None

HT: 5'5"

WT: 215 lb

LABORATORY VALUES:

	Client	Normal Range	
WBC	8.3	3.8 – 10.5	K/uL
RBC	4.86	3.8 – 5.20	M/uL
HGB	10.8 L	12.0 – 16.0	g/dL
HCT	32.7 L	34.5 -45.0	%
MCV	74.1 L	80.0 – 100.0	fl
MCH	24.3 L	27.0 – 34.0	pg
MCHC	30.4 L	32.0 – 36.0	gm/dL
IRON	28 L	40 – 160	ug/dL
UIBC	429 H	110 – 370	ug/dL
TIBC	508 H	220 – 430	ug/dL
% Saturation, Iron	12 L	14-50	%
Transferrin	435 H	200 – 400	mg/dL
Ferritin	12 L	15-150	ng/mL
C-Reactive Protein	0.96 H	0.00 – 0.40	mg/dL
Vitamin D	14.6 L	30.0 – 100.0	ng/mL

Nutrition Diagnostic Statements

Increased nutrient needs (iron) related to heavy menses and suboptimal intake of dietary iron as evidenced by multiple low iron status labs including HCT, HGB and ferritin.

Altered nutrition related laboratory value related to predicted pro-inflammatory diet pattern as evidenced by low intake of omega-3 fatty acids and bioactive compounds, elevated c-reactive protein (CRP) and painful joints.

Nutrition Care Questions:

1) How should Marisa be further evaluated?
2) What vitamin/mineral supplements, if any, should be part of her treatment plan?
3) What factors play a role in her nutritional plan?
4) Evaluate her laboratory test results. Do you recommend further blood tests?
5) With her input devise an nutrition action plan that she can follow.
6) What lab tests or questions would you include in your followup with her?

USEFUL WEBSITES

Anemia Institute for Research and Education
http://www.anemiainstitute.org
Anemia Lifeline
http://www.anemia.com
CDC Centers for Disease Control and Prevention
http://www.cdc.gov/nutrition/everyone/basics/vitamins/iron.html
Iron Disorders Institute
http://www.irondisorders.org/
National Heart Lung and Blood Institute
http://www.nhlbi.nih.gov/health/health-topics/topics/anemia/

REFERENCES

Aditi A, Graham D: Vitamin C, gastritis, and gastric disease: a historical review and update, *Dig Dis Sci* 57:2504, 2012.

Allen R, et al: The prevalence and impact of restless legs syndrome on patients with iron deficiency anemia, *Am J Hematol* 88:261, 2013.

Ashmead HD: The absorption and metabolism of iron amino acid chelate, *Arch Latinoam Nutr* 51(Suppl 1):13, 2001.

Bartzokis G, et al: Prevalent iron metabolism gene variants associated with increased brain ferritin iron in healthy older men, *J Alzheimers Dis* 20:333, 2010.

Carmel R: Biomarkers of cobalamin (vitamin B12) status in the epidemiologic setting: a critical overview of context, applications, and performance characteristics of cobalamin, methylmalonic acid, and holotranscobalamin II, *Am J Clin Nutr* 94(Suppl 1):348S, 2011.

Fleming R, Ponka P: Iron overload in human disease, *N Engl J Med* 366:348, 2012.

Fowler KT, et al. Dietary water and sodium intake of children and adolescents with sickle cell anemia, *J Pediatr Hematol Oncol* 32:350, 2010.

Ganz T: Hepcidin and iron regulation, 10 years later, *Blood* 117:4425, 2011.

Graber JJ, et al. Vitamin B12-responsive severe leukoencephalopathy and autonomic dysfunction in a patient with "normal" serum B12 levels, *J Neurol Neurosurg Psychiatry* 81:1369, 2010.

Leskovjan AC, et al. Increased brain iron coincides with early plaque formation in a mouse model of Alzheimer's disease, *Neuroimage* 55(1):32, 2011.

Moreiras GV, et al. Cobalamin, folic acid, and homocysteine, *Nutr Rev* 67(Suppl 1): S69, 2009.

Moretti D, et al. Relevance of dietary iron intake and bioavailalitiy in the management of HFE hemochromatosis: a systematic review, *Am J Clin Nutr* 98:468, 2013.

National Institutes of Health (NIH), National Heart, Blood and Lung Institute (NHBLI): *What is restless leg syndrome?* (website), 2010. http://www.nhlbi.nih.gov/health/dci/Diseases/rls/rls_WhatIs.html. Accessed January 8, 2015.

National Institutes of Health (NIH), National Heart, Blood and Lung Institute (NHBLI): *What is sickle cell anemia?* (website), 2012. http://www.nhlbi.nih.gov/health/health-topics/topics/sca. Accessed December 17, 2014.

National Institutes of Health (NIH), National Library of Medicine (NLM): *Thalassemia* (website), 2014. http://www.nlm.nih.gov/medlineplus/thalassemia.html. Accessed January 6, 2015.

Sato Y, et al: Relationship between metformin use, vitamin B12 deficiency, hyperhomocysteinemia and vascular complications in patients with type 2 diabetes, *Endocr J* 60:1275, 2013.

Serefhanoglu S, et al: Measuring holotranscobalamin II, an early indicator of negative B12 balance, by radioimmunoassay in patients with ischemic cerebrovascular disease, *Ann Hematol* 87:391, 2008.

Tucker K, et al: Low plasma vitamin B12 is associated with lower bone mineral density: the Framingham Osteoporosis Study, *J Bone Miner Res* 20:152, 2005.

Yawn BP, et al: Management of sickle cell disease: summary of the 2014 evidence-based report by expert panel members, *JAMA* 312:1033, 2014, doi:10.1001/jama.2014.10517.

Zemel BS, et al: Effects of delayed pubertal development, nutritional status, and disease severity on longitudinal patterns of growth failure in children with sickle cell disease, *Pediatr Res* 61:607, 2007.

Zubieta-Calleja GR, et al: Altitude adaptation through hematocrit changes, *J Physiol Pharmacol* 58(Suppl 5):811, 2007.

33

Medical Nutrition Therapy for Cardiovascular Disease

Janice L. Raymond, MS, RDN, CD, CSG
Sarah C. Couch, PhD, RDN

KEY TERMS

3-hydroxy-3-methylglutaryl–
  coenzyme A (HMG-CoA)
angina
angiography
apolipoproteins
atherosclerotic cardiovascular disease
  (ASCVD)
atheroma
bile acid sequestrant
blood pressure
B-natriuretic peptide
cardiac cachexia
cardiac catheterization
cardiovascular disease (CVD)
C-reactive protein (CRP)
chylomicron
coronary artery bypass graft (CABG)
diastolic blood pressure (DBP)
Dietary Approaches to Stop Hypertension (DASH)

dyslipidemia
dyspnea
edema
endothelial cell
essential hypertension
familial combined hyperlipidemia
  (FCHL)
familial dysbetalipoproteinemia
familial hypercholesterolemia
fatty streak
foam cells
heart failure (HF)
high-density lipoprotein (HDL)
homocysteine
hypertension
hypertriglyceridemia
intermediate-density lipoprotein (IDL)
ischemia
left ventricular hypertrophy (LVH)
lipoprotein

low-density lipoprotein (LDL)
Mediterranean Diet (MeD)
metabolic syndrome
myocardial infarction (MI)
nitric oxide (NO)
orthopnea
plaque
prehypertension
renin-angiotensin system (RAS)
secondary hypertension
statins
stroke
syncope
systolic blood pressure (SBP)
thrombus
trans fatty acids
trimethylamine-N-oxide (TMAO)
very-low-density lipoprotein (VLDL)
xanthoma

Cardiovascular disease (CVD) is a group of interrelated diseases that include atherosclerosis, hypertension, ischemic heart disease, peripheral vascular disease, and heart failure (HF). These diseases are interrelated and often coexist. An estimated 81,100,000 adult Americans (one in three) have one or more types of CVD (see Box 33-1).

CVD remains the number one killer of men and women in the United States; one of every 2.9 deaths is attributed to CVD. In 2010 it is estimated that 1.26 million Americans had a new or recurrent coronary attack. Every 25 seconds an American suffers a coronary event and about every minute someone will die of one (American Heart Association [AHA], 2015). The lifetime risk for CVD in American men is two in three and for women is one in two (AHA, 2015). Worldwide, 18 million deaths per year are attributed to CVD (Yusuf, 2014).

Of all causes of death, CVD, cancer, and stroke are the leaders (AHA, 2015). Atherosclerotic cardiovascular disease (ASCVD) involves the narrowing of small blood vessels that oxygenate the heart muscle by the build-up of plaque (the lesion in the blood vessels). The plaque, known as atherosclerosis, can rupture, causing a blood clot to form that blocks the artery or travels somewhere else in the body, causing blockage at that

site. The result can be a myocardial infarction (MI), which is also called a heart attack or stroke. Heart disease and stroke cause the most deaths in both sexes of all ethnic groups, increasing with age. Until the age of 65 years, black men have the highest rates of ASCVD deaths; thereafter, white men have the highest rates. Black women have higher rates than white women at all ages. Among Caucasians older than age 18, 12.1% have CVD. In the same age group, 10.2% of African Americans have heart disease, and in Hispanics the incidence is 8.1%. The incidence in adult Native Americans is 12.1%, in Native Hawaiians or other Pacific Islanders it is 19.7 %, and in Asians it is 5.2% (AHA 2015). This chapter discusses the incidence, pathophysiologic findings, prevention, and treatment of each of the CVDs.

ATHEROSCLEROSIS AND CORONARY HEART DISEASE

Anatomy and Physiology

Blood vessels are composed of three layers. The outer layer is mainly connective tissue that gives structure to the vessels. The middle layer is smooth muscle that contracts and dilates to control blood flow and blood pressure. The inner lining is a thin layer of **endothelial cells** (the endothelium) that in a healthy state is smooth and responsive. The endothelium functions as a protective barrier between tissues and circulating blood. It facilitates bidirectional passage of macromolecules and blood gases to and from tissues and blood. **Endothelial cells** sense changes in blood flow and respond with the release of bioactive substances that maintain vascular homeostasis. One such substance is **nitric oxide (NO)**. NO is a soluble gas continually synthesized from the amino acid L-arginine in endothelial cells. NO has a wide range of biologic properties that maintain vascular homeostasis. It appears to be involved in protection from injurious substances and plays a key role in vasodilation (Tousoulis et al, 2012). Decreased NO is a factor in the endothelial cell dysfunction that disrupts vascular balance and can result in vasoconstriction, platelet activation, leukocyte adherence, and vascular inflammation.

Pathophysiology

ASCVD involves the accumulation of plaque within the walls of the arteries. It starts with injury to the endothelial cells with an associated inflammatory response involving phagocytes and monocytes. Once in the tissue, monocytes evolve into macrophages that ingest oxidized cholesterol and become **foam cells** and then **fatty streaks** in these vessels. Intracellular microcalcification occurs, forming deposits within the vascular smooth muscle cells of the surrounding muscular layer (see Figure 33-1).

A protective fibrin layer (**atheroma**) forms between the fatty deposits and the artery lining. Atheromas produce enzymes that cause the artery to enlarge over time, thus compensating for the narrowing caused by the plaque. This "remodeling" of the shape and size of the blood vessel may result in an aneurysm.

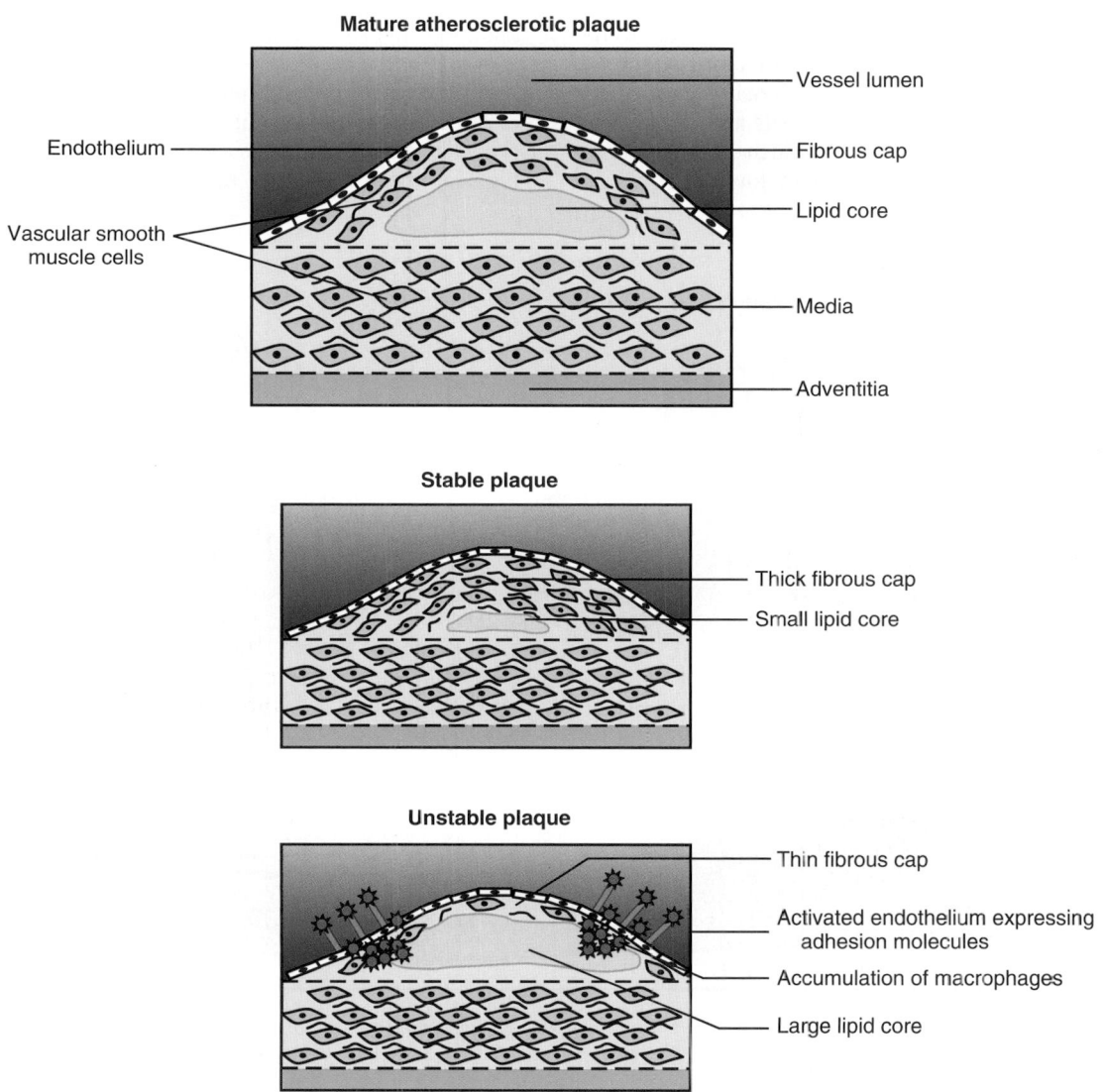

FIGURE 33-1 The structure of mature, stable, and unstable plaque. (From Rudd JHF et al: Imaging of atherosclerosis—can we predict plaque rupture? *Trends Cardiovasc Med* 15:17, 2005.)

Atheromas can rupture or break off, forming a thrombus (blood clot), where they attract blood platelets and activate the clotting system in the body. This response can result in a blockage and restricted blood flow.

Only high-risk or vulnerable plaque forms thrombi. Vulnerable plaque are lesions with a thin fibrous cap, few smooth muscle cells, many macrophages (inflammatory cells), and a large lipid core (see Figure 33-2). Arterial changes begin in infancy and progress asymptomatically throughout adulthood (see Figure 33-3).

The clinical outcome of impaired arterial function arising from atherosclerosis depends on the location of the impairment. In the coronary arteries atherosclerosis can cause angina (chest pain), MI, and sudden death; in the cerebral arteries it causes strokes and transient ischemic attacks; and in the peripheral circulation it causes intermittent claudication, limb ischemia (inadequate blood supply), and gangrene (see Figure 33-4). Thus atherosclerosis is the underlying cause of many forms of CVD.

Dyslipidemia refers to a blood lipid profile that increases the risk of developing atherosclerosis. Three important biochemical measurements in ASCVD include lipoproteins, total cholesterol, and triglycerides. Cholesterol is delivered into cell walls by low-density lipoprotein (LDL), especially smaller particles. To attract and stimulate the macrophages, the cholesterol must be released from the LDL particles and oxidized, a key step in the ongoing inflammatory process. Additionally, macrophages must move excess cholesterol quickly into high-density lipoprotein (HDL) particles to avoid becoming foam cells and dying. The typical dyslipidemic condition is one in which LDL levels are elevated (hyperlipidemia) and HDL levels are low.

Lipoproteins

Lipids are not water soluble, so they are carried in the blood bound to protein. These complex particles, called lipoproteins, vary in composition, size, and density. Lipoproteins measured in clinical practice—chylomicrons, very-low-density lipoprotein (VLDL), low-density lipoproteins (LDL), and high-density lipoproteins (HDL)—consist of varying amounts of triglyceride, cholesterol, phospholipid, and protein. Each class of lipoprotein actually represents a continuum of particles. The ratio of protein to fat determines the density; thus particles with higher levels of protein are the most dense (e.g., HDLs have more protein than LDLs). The physiologic role of lipoprotein includes transporting lipid to cells for energy, storage, or use as substrate for synthesis of other compounds such as prostaglandins, thromboxanes, and leukotrienes.

The largest particles, chylomicrons, transport dietary fat and cholesterol from the small intestine to the liver and periphery. Once in the bloodstream, the triglycerides within the chylomicrons are hydrolyzed by lipoprotein lipase (LPL), located on the endothelial cell surface in muscle and adipose tissue. Apolipoproteins carry lipids in the blood and also control the metabolism of the lipoprotein molecule. Apo C-II, one of the apolipoproteins, is a cofactor for LPL. When approximately 90% of the triglyceride is hydrolyzed, the particle is released back into the blood as a remnant. The liver metabolizes these chylomicron remnants, but some deliver cholesterol to the arterial wall and thus are considered atherogenic. Consumption of high-fat meals produces more chylomicrons and remnants.

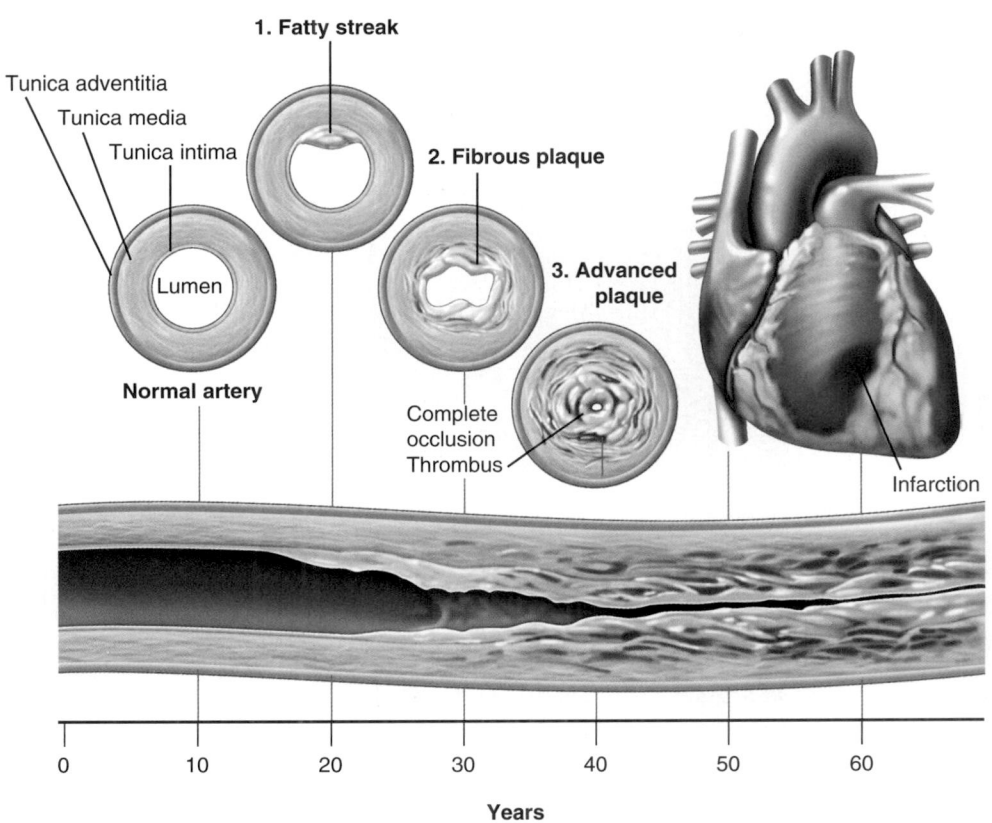

FIGURE 33-2 Natural progression of atherosclerosis. (From Harkreader H: *Fundamentals of nursing: caring and clinical judgment,* Philadelphia, 2007, Saunders.)

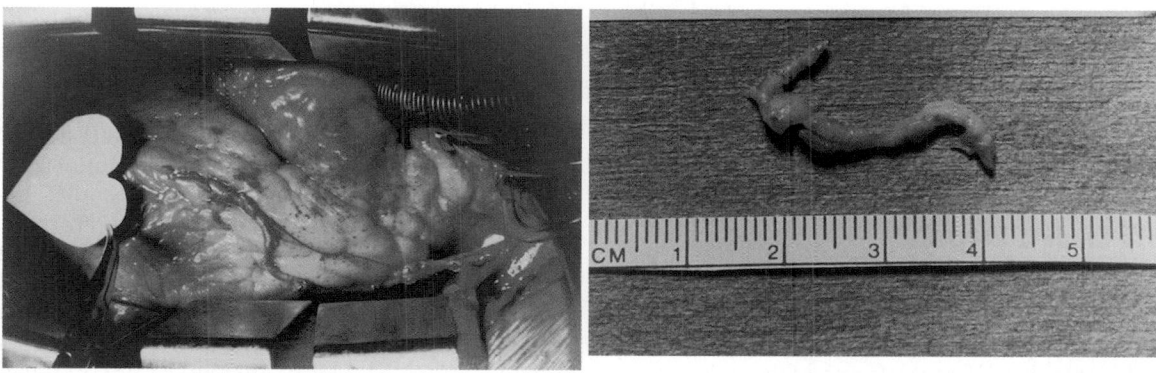

FIGURE 33-3 Plaque that can be surgically removed from the coronary artery. (Photographs courtesy Ronald D. Gregory and John Riley, MD.)

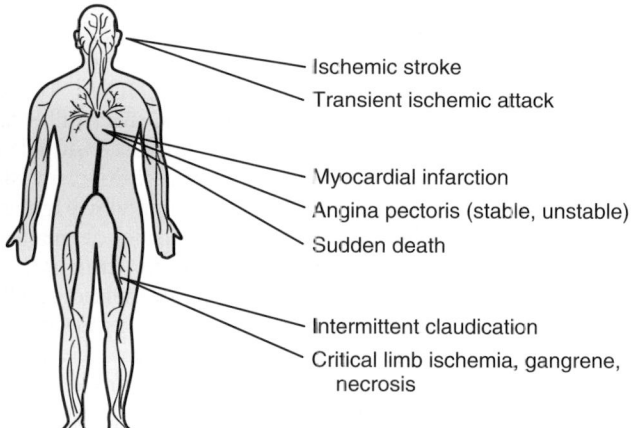

- Ischemic stroke
- Transient ischemic attack

- Myocardial infarction
- Angina pectoris (stable, unstable)
- Sudden death

- Intermittent claudication
- Critical limb ischemia, gangrene, necrosis

FIGURE 33-4 Major clinical manifestations of atherothrombotic disease. (From Viles-Gonzalez JF et al: Atherothrombosis: a widespread disease with unpredictable and life-threatening consequences, *Eur Heart J* 25:1197, 2004.)

Plasma studies are done when fasting; chylomicrons are normally absent.

VLDL particles are synthesized in the liver to transport endogenous triglyceride and cholesterol. Triglyceride accounts for 60% of the VLDL particle. The large, buoyant VLDL particle is believed to be nonatherogenic. Vegetarian and low-fat diets increase the formation of large VLDL particles. Smaller VLDL particles (i.e., remnants) are formed from triglyceride hydrolysis by LPL. Normally these remnants, called intermediate-density lipoproteins (IDLs), are atherogenic and are taken up by receptors on the liver or converted to LDLs. Some of the smaller LDL particles stay in the blood, are oxidized, and are then taken into the arterial wall. Clinically, a total triglyceride level is a measurement of the triglycerides carried on the VLDL and the IDL remnants.

LDL is the primary cholesterol carrier in blood, formed by the breakdown of VLDL. High LDL cholesterol is associated specifically with atherosclerosis (Stone et al, 2013). A recent change in recommendations from AHA/ACC was to drop the actual serum LDL ASCVD prevention target. LDL levels are used for dosing medication but are otherwise only considered part of a bigger picture of risk and should not be assessed in isolation. After LDL formation, 60% is taken up by LDL receptors on the liver, adrenals, and other tissues. The remainder is metabolized via nonreceptor pathways. The number and activity of these LDL receptors are major determinants of the LDL level in the blood. Apolipoprotein B is the structural protein for all of the atherogenic lipoproteins (VLDL, IDL, LDL) and modulates the transport of lipids from the gut and liver to the tissues. The two forms, apo B and apoB-100 are synthesized in the liver. ApoB-100 constitutes 95% of the apolipoproteins in LDL. ApoB-48 is synthesized in the intestines and is the structural component of chylomicrons.

HDL particles contain more protein than any of the other lipoproteins, which accounts for their metabolic role as a reservoir of the apolipoproteins that direct lipid metabolism. Apo A-I, the main apolipoprotein in HDL, is an antiinflammatory, antioxidant protein that also helps to remove cholesterol from the arterial wall to the liver for excretion or repackaging. This process prevents the build-up and oxidation of cholesterol in the arteries. Evaluation of apo A-I or the ratio of apo B to apo A-I has been proposed to assess risk and determine treatment (Navab et al, 2011). The lower the ratio, the lower the ASCVD risk. Both apo C and apo E on HDL are transferred to chylomicrons. Apo E helps receptors metabolize chylomicron remnants and also inhibits appetite. Therefore high HDL levels are associated with low levels of chylomicrons; VLDL remnants; and small, dense LDLs. Epidemiologic studies have shown an inverse correlation between HDL levels and risk of cardiovascular events. Subsequently, high HDL implies lower atherosclerotic risk, except in patients with specific genetic causes of hypercholesterolemia who can have a triglyceride-enriched HDL$_3$ fraction that is proatherogenic (Ottestad et al, 2006).

Total Cholesterol

A total cholesterol measurement captures cholesterol contained in all lipoprotein fractions: 60% to 70% is carried on LDL, 20% to 30% on HDL, and 10% to 15% on VLDL.

Triglycerides

The triglyceride-rich lipoproteins include chylomicrons, VLDLs, and any remnants or intermediary products formed in metabolism. Of these triglyceride-rich lipoproteins, chylomicrons and VLDL remnants are known to be atherogenic because they activate platelets, the coagulation cascade, and clot formation. All contain the apo B lipoprotein. Fasting triglyceride levels are classified as normal (<150 mg/dl), borderline high (150 to 199 mg/dl), high (200 to 499 mg/dl), and very high (<500 mg/dl) (Stone et al, 2013).

Patients with familial dyslipidemias have high triglyceride levels (hypertriglyceridemia). Triglycerides in the very high range place the patient at risk for pancreatitis. Triglyceride measurements are now considered along with glucose intolerance, hypertension, low HDL cholesterol, and high LDL cholesterol as part of the metabolic syndrome.

GENETIC HYPERLIPIDEMIAS

The study and identification of the genes responsible for the familial forms of hyperlipidemia have provided insight into the roles of enzymes, apolipoproteins, and receptors on cells involved in lipid metabolism. Several forms of hyperlipidemia have strong genetic components and are described here.

Familial Hypercholesterolemia

Familial hypercholesterolemia (FH) (type IIa hyperlipidemia) is a monogenetic disorder that is seen around the world, with an estimated 14 to 34 million people being affected (Nordestgaard et al, 2013). In FH elevated cholesterol is already present at birth and results in early atherosclerotic disease. The optimal age range for screening is between 2 and 10 years. Currently, it is considered unreasonable to start a restricted diet before age 2, and there are no safety data on the use of statins before age 8 to 10 (Nordestgaard et al, 2013). Men with FH seem to develop CVD before women. Hypertension, smoking, diabetes, and high triglycerides and low HDL cholesterol are all well-established additional risk factors in FH.

Defects in the LDL receptor gene cause FH; 800 mutations have been identified. Treatment with statin drugs improves arterial function and structure (Masoura et al, 2011). Ultrasound of the Achilles tendon for xanthomas (cholesterol deposits from LDL) correctly identifies the majority of FH patients.

Polygenic Familial Hypercholesterolemia

Polygenic FH is the result of multiple gene defects. The apo E-4 allele is common in this form. The diagnosis is based on two or more family members having LDL cholesterol levels above the 90th percentile without any tendon xanthomas. Usually these patients have lower LDL cholesterol levels than patients with the nonpolygenic form, but they remain at high risk for premature disease. The treatment is lifestyle change in conjunction with cholesterol-lowering drugs.

Familial Combined Hyperlipidemia

Familial combined hyperlipidemia (FCHL) is a disorder in which two or more family members have serum LDL cholesterol or triglyceride levels above the 90th percentile. Several lipoprotein patterns may be seen in patients with FCHL. These patients can have (1) elevated LDL levels with normal triglyceride levels (type IIa), (2) elevated LDL levels with elevated triglyceride levels (type IIb), or (3) elevated VLDL levels (type IV). Often these patients have the small, dense LDL associated with ASCVD. Consequently all forms of FCHL cause premature disease; approximately 15% of patients who have an MI before the age of 60 have FCHL. The defect in FCHL is hepatic overproduction of apo B-100 (VLDL) or a defect in the gene that produces hepatic lipase, the liver enzyme involved in triglyceride removal from the bloodstream. Patients with FCHL usually have other risk factors such as obesity, hypertension, diabetes, or metabolic syndrome. If lifestyle measures are ineffective, treatment includes medication. Patients with elevated triglyceride levels also need to avoid alcohol.

Familial Dysbetalipoproteinemia

Familial dysbetalipoproteinemia (type III hyperlipoproteinemia) is relatively uncommon. Catabolism of VLDL and chylomicron remnants is delayed because apo E-2 replaces apo E-3 and apo E-4. For dysbetalipoproteinemia to be seen, other risk factors such as older age, hypothyroidism, obesity, diabetes, or other dyslipidemias such as FCHL must be present. Total cholesterol levels range from 300 to 600 mg/dl, and triglyceride levels range from 400 to 800 mg/dl. This condition creates increased risk of premature ASCVD and peripheral vascular disease. Diagnosis is based on determining the isoforms of apo E. Treatment involves weight reduction, control of hyperglycemia and diabetes, and dietary restriction of saturated fat and cholesterol. If the dietary regimen is not effective, drug therapy is recommended.

Medical Diagnosis

Noninvasive tests such as electrocardiograms, treadmill stress tests, thallium scans, and echocardiography are used initially to establish a cardiovascular diagnosis. A more definitive, invasive test is angiography (cardiac catheterization), in which a dye is injected into the arteries, and radiographic images of the heart are obtained. Most narrowing and blockages from atherosclerosis are readily apparent on angiograms; however, neither smaller lesions nor lesions that have undergone remodeling are visible.

Magnetic resonance imaging (MRI) scans show the smaller lesions and can be used to follow atherosclerosis progression or regression after treatments. To predict MI or stroke, measuring the intimal thickness of the carotid artery may be used. Intracoronary thermography helps to determine the presence of vulnerable plaque.

Finally, the calcium in atherosclerotic lesions can be assessed. Electron beam computed tomography (ECT) measures calcium in the coronary arteries; persons with a positive scan are far more likely to have a future coronary event than those with a negative scan.

Approximately two thirds of cases of acute coronary syndromes (unstable angina and acute MI) happen in arteries that are minimally or mildly obstructed. This illustrates the role of thrombosis in clinical events. In the ischemia of an infarction, the myocardium or other tissue is deprived of oxygen and nourishment. Whether the heart is able to continue beating depends on the extent of the musculature involved, the presence of collateral circulation, and the oxygen requirement.

Prevention and Management of Risk Factors

The identification of risk factors for ASCVD and stroke has been a landmark achievement. The primary prevention of these disorders involves the assessment and management of the risk factors in the asymptomatic person. Persons with multiple risk factors are the target population, especially those with modifiable factors (see Box 33-2).

Risk factor reduction has been shown to reduce CVD in persons of all ages. Many coronary events could be prevented with adoption of a healthy lifestyle (eating a heart-healthy diet, exercising regularly, managing weight, and not using tobacco) and adherence to lipid and hypertension drug therapy (Stone et al, 2013). The Framingham Study, conducted over several decades, has provided a plethora of useful information to researchers (see *Focus On*: Framingham Heart Study).

BOX 33-2 Cardiovascular Disease Risk Factors

Major Risk Factors

Hypertension
Age (older than 45 years for men, 55 years for women)
Diabetes mellitus
Estimated glomerular filtration rate <60 ml/min
Microalbuminuria
Family history of premature cardiovascular disease (men <55 years of age, or women <65 years of age)

Modifiable Cardiovascular Risk Factors

Lipoprotein profile
Low-density lipoprotein cholesterol, elevated
Total triglycerides, elevated
Elevated TMAO (Trimethylamine N-oxide)
High-density lipoprotein (HDL) cholesterol, low
Inflammatory markers

Fibrinogen
C-reactive protein

Lifestyle Risk Factors

Tobacco use, particularly cigarettes
Physical inactivity
Poor diet
Stress
Insufficient sleep
Excessive alcohol consumption

Related Conditions

Hypertension
Obesity (body mass index >30)
Metabolic syndrome (including reduced HDL, elevated triglycerides, abdominal obesity)

Modified from National Institutes of Health, National Heart, Lung, and Blood Institute National High Blood Pressure Education Program: The Seventh Report of the Joint National Committee on Prevention, Detection, Evaluation, and Treatment of High Blood Pressure, NIH Publication No. 04-5230, August 2004.

FOCUS ON

Framingham Heart Study

Since 1948 various leading investigators (Dr. Joseph Mountain, Dr. Thomas Dawber, Dr. William Kannel, and Dr. William Castelli) have been studying the population (28,000) of Framingham, Massachusetts, to determine the prevalence and incidence of cardiovascular disease and factors related to its development. This is the largest epidemiologic study of cardiovascular disease in the world. Initial study participants (*n* = 5209) were healthy adults between 30 and 62 years of age. The study continues today, looking at the children and grandchildren of the original cohort. Through this cohort study, the concept of risk factors and thus prevention was born. Modifiable risk factors not only predict disease in healthy adults but also contribute to the disease process in those who have atherosclerotic disease. The seven major risk factors identified by the Framingham study are age, sex, blood pressure, total and high-density lipoprotein cholesterol, smoking, glucose intolerance, and left-ventricular hypertrophy (Opie et al, 2006).

Milestones of the Framingham Study

1960 Cigarette smoking found to increase the risk of heart disease.
1961 Cholesterol level, blood pressure, and electrocardiogram abnormalities found to increase the risk of heart disease.
1967 Physical activity found to reduce the risk of heart disease, and obesity found to increase the risk of heart disease.
1970 High blood pressure found to increase the risk of stroke.

1976 Menopause found to increase the risk of heart disease.
1978 Psychosocial factors found to affect heart disease.
1988 High levels of high-density lipoprotein cholesterol found to reduce risk of death.
1994 Enlarged left ventricle (one of two lower chambers of the heart) found to increase the risk of stroke.
1996 Progression from hypertension to heart failure described.
2006 Genetic Research Study begins to identify genes underlying cardiovascular diseases in 9000 participants from three generations.
2008 Discovery and publication of four risk factors that raise probability of developing precursor of heart failure; new 30-year risk estimates developed for serious cardiac events.
2009 Researchers find parental dementia may be linked to poor memory in middle-aged adults.
2011 Blood lipids and the incidence of atrial fibrillation: The multiethnic study of atherosclerosis and the Framingham Heart Study.

In 1971 the offspring study was begun to measure the influence of heredity and environment on the offspring of the original cohort. The younger group appears to be more health conscious because they have lower rates of smoking, lower blood pressures, and lower cholesterol levels than their parents at the same age. The Generation III Cohort Study of the grandchildren is presently underway.

Data from Framingham Heart Study: *A Timeline of Milestones from The Framingham Heart Study* (website): http://www.framingham.com/heart/timeline.htm, 2015. Accessed May 2, 2015.

In the medical model, primary prevention of ASCVD and stroke involves altering similar risk factors toward a healthy patient profile. For ischemic stroke, atherosclerosis is the underlying disease. Therefore optimal lipid levels, as determined by the National Cholesterol Education Program (NCEP) for hypercholesterolemia, are also the target levels to prevent stroke.

Although the National Heart, Lung and Blood Institute created the NCEP, the American Heart Association (AHA) has endorsed it. AHA suggests that primary prevention of CVD should begin in children older than age 2 (Gidding et al, 2009). Dietary recommendations for children are a bit more liberal than those for adults. Activity is emphasized in maintaining ideal body weight. Early screening for dyslipidemia is recommended for children with a family history of hypercholesterolemia or ASCVD.

For adults, a total cholesterol level of 170 mg/dl or less is now considered optimal, including an HDL of at least 50 mg/dl. The new 2013 guidelines no longer rely strictly on cholesterol levels for advising patients or dosing medications. Instead the patient's overall health is evaluated for treatment decisions. The guidelines advise assessing factors such as age, gender, race, whether a patient smokes, blood pressure and whether it is being treated, whether a person has diabetes, as well as blood cholesterol levels in determining their risk. They also suggest that health care providers should consider other factors, including family history. Only after that very personalized assessment is a decision made on what treatment would work best. The Risk Calculator developed by the ACC/AHA expert panel is available at http://tools.acc.org/ASCVD-Risk-Estimator/

Inflammatory Markers

Fifty percent of heart attacks occur in individuals with normal serum cholesterol, which has led to research on other risk markers. Increasing knowledge about the role of inflammation in ASCVD gives credence to the use of inflammatory markers to indicate the presence of atherosclerosis in asymptomatic individuals or the extent of atherosclerosis in patients with symptoms. Several markers have been suggested (see Box 33-3), and research continues to look at the effects of diet on these biomarkers. Plasma levels of omega-3 fatty acids are inversely associated with the inflammatory markers CRP, IL-6, fibrinogen, and homocysteine (Kalogeropoulos et al, 2010). An inflammatory marker specific to vascular inflammation has recently become available. The PLAC™ test measures Lp-PLA2 (Jellinger et al, 2012). Lp-PLA2 levels indicate ASCVD risk independent from other markers and provides information on the relationship between inflammation and atherosclerosis (see Chapters 3 and 7).

Fibrinogen. Most MIs are the result of an intracoronary thrombosis. Prospective studies have shown that plasma fibrinogen is an independent predictor of ASCVD risk. Factors associated with an elevated fibrinogen are smoking, diabetes, hypertension, obesity, sedentary lifestyle, elevated triglycerides, and genetic factors. More clinical trials are needed to determine whether fibrinogen is involved in atherogenesis or is just a marker of vascular damage. Blood thrombogenicity increases with high LDL cholesterol and in diabetes.

C-Reactive Protein. C-reactive protein is synthesized in the liver as the acute-phase response to inflammation. In a normal individual without infection or inflammation, CRP levels are very low, less than 0.6 mg/dl. Because atherogenesis is an inflammatory process, CRP has been shown to be elevated (>3 mg/dl) in people with angina, MI, stroke, and peripheral vascular disease; the elevated levels are independent of other risk factors (see Chapter 7). Despite a lack of specificity for the cause of the inflammation, data from more than 30 epidemiologic studies have shown significant association between elevated blood levels of CRP and the prevalence of atherosclerosis (Morrow, 2014).

CRP levels are categorized for risk as low (<1 mg/L), average (2 to 3 mg/L), and high (>3 mg/L) after the average of two measurements are taken at least 2 weeks apart. CRP levels have been shown to be inversely correlated with a vegetable-based diet (Bloomer et al, 2010; Lee et al, 2014).

Homocysteine. Homocysteine, an amino acid metabolite of methionine, is a risk factor for CVD. It was first observed that children who were deficient in cystathionine B synthase, the essential enzyme for the breakdown of homocysteine, had premature atherosclerosis in some blood vessels. Elevated total homocysteine (tHcy) independently increases the odds of stroke, especially in younger individuals (Towfighi et al, 2010). Although evidence suggests that homocysteine may promote atherosclerosis, no causal link has been established. Homocysteine levels are influenced strongly by genetic factors and diet. Giving supplemental vitamins B_6 and B_{12}, which lower homocysteine levels, is being investigated actively as a treatment for CVD but as of now is not widely recommended.

Trimethylamine-N-oxide. Trimethylamine-N-oxide (TMAO) is a gut biota-dependent metabolite that contributes to heart disease (Tang et al, 2013). It is produced by the liver after intestinal bacteria have digested animal protein. TMAO has been shown to predict cardiac risk in individuals not identified by traditional risk factors and blood tests.

Lifestyle Guidelines

Lifestyle modification remains the backbone of CVD prevention and treatment. Adhering to a heart-healthy diet, regular exercising, avoidance of tobacco products, and maintenance of a healthy weight are known lifestyle factors that, along with genetics, determine CVD risk. Three critical questions (CQs) were addressed in the 2013 ACC/AHA Lifestyle modification guidelines. CQ1 presents evidence on dietary patterns and macronutrients and their effect on blood pressure and lipids, CQ2 presents evidence on the effect of dietary sodium and potassium intake on blood pressure and CVD outcomes, and CQ3 presents the evidence on the effect of physical activity on lipids and blood pressure. The recommendations are summarized in Box 33-4.

Diet

The importance of diet and nutrition in modifying the risk of CVD has been known for some time. However, in general, individual dietary components have been the predominant focus. Because foods are consumed typically in combinations rather than individually and because of the possibility of synergist relationships between nutrients, there has been increasing attention to dietary patterns and their relationship to health outcomes such as CVD.

The Mediterranean Diet

There is no uniform definition of the Mediterranean Diet (MeD) in the published studies. Common features of the diet are greater number of servings of fruits and vegetables (mostly fresh) with an emphasis on root vegetables and greens, whole grains, fatty fish (rich in omega-3 fatty acids), lower amounts of red meat and with an emphasis on lean meats, lower fat dairy products, abundant nuts and legumes, and use of olive oil, canola oil, nut oil, or margarine blended with rapeseed oil or flaxseed oil. The MeD dietary patterns that have been studied were moderate in total fat (32% to 35%), relatively low in saturated fat (9% to 10%), high in polyunsaturated fatty acids (especially omega-3), and high in fiber (27 to 37 g per day).

BOX 33-3 Inflammatory Markers for Cardiovascular Risk

Genetic markers: angiotensin II receptor type-1 polymorphism	Interleukin-6
	Tumor necrosis factor-alpha
Oxidized low-density lipoprotein cholesterol	Acute-phase reactants
	Fibrinogen
Adhesion molecules	C-reactive protein
Selectins	Serum amyloid A
Free fatty acids	White blood cell count
Cytokines	Erythrocyte sedimentation rate
Interleukin-1	TMAO

Derived from Fung MM et al: Early inflammatory and metabolic changes in association with AGTR1 polymorphisms in prehypertensive subjects, *Am J Hypertens* 24:225, 2011; Pearson TA et al: Markers of inflammation and cardiovascular disease: application to clinical and public health practice: a statement for healthcare professionals from the Centers for Disease Control and Prevention and the American Heart Association, *Circulation* 107:499, 2003.

BOX 33-4 Summary of ACC/AHA
Recommendations for Lifestyle Management

BOX 33-4 Summary of ACC/AHA Recommendations for Lifestyle Management

DIET

LDL-C

Advise adults who would benefit from LDL-C lowering to

1. Consume a dietary pattern that emphasizes intake of vegetables, fruits, and whole grains; includes low-fat dairy products, poultry, fish, legumes, nontropical vegetable oils and nuts; and limits intake of sweets, sugar-sweetened beverages and red meats.
   a. Adapt this dietary pattern to appropriate calorie requirements, personal and cultural food preferences, and nutrition therapy for other medical conditions (including diabetes mellitus).
   b. Achieve this pattern by following plans such as the DASH dietary pattern, the USDA Food Pattern, or the AHA Diet.
2. Aim for a dietary pattern that achieves 5% to 6% of calories from saturated fat.
3. Reduce percent of calories from saturated fat.
4. Reduce percent of calories from trans fat.

Blood Pressure (BP)

Advise adults who would benefit from BP lowering to

1. Consume a dietary pattern that emphasizes intake of vegetables, fruits, and whole grains; includes low-fat dairy products, poultry, fish, legumes, nontropical vegetable oils and nuts; and limits intake of sweets, sugar-sweetened beverages, and red meats.
   a. Adapt this dietary pattern to appropriate calorie requirements, personal and cultural food preferences, and nutrition therapy for other medical conditions (including diabetes mellitus).
   b. Achieve this pattern by following plans such as the DASH dietary pattern, the USDA Food Pattern, or the AHA Diet.
2. Lower sodium intake.
3. a. Consume no more than 2400 mg of sodium/day.
   b. Further reduction of sodium intake to 1500 mg/day is desirable because it is associated with even greater reduction in BP.
   c. Reduce intake by at least 1000 mg/day because that will lower BP, even if the desired daily sodium.
4. Combine the DASH dietary pattern with lower sodium intake.

PHYSICAL ACTIVITY

Lipids

In general, advise adults to engage in aerobic physical activity to reduce LDL–C and non-HDL–C: 3 to 4 sessions a week, lasting on average 40 minutes per session, and involving moderate-to-vigorous intensity physical activity.

Blood Pressure

In general, advise adults to engage in aerobic physical activity to lower BP: 3 to 4 sessions a week, lasting on average 40 minutes per session, and involving moderate to-vigorous intensity physical activity.

The Dietary Approaches to Stop Hypertension (DASH) Diet

The **DASH** dietary pattern is high in fruits and vegetables, low-fat dairy products, whole grains, fish, and nuts and low in animal protein and sugar. Two DASH variations were studied in the OmniHeart (Optimal Macronutrient Intake Trial for Heart Health) trial, one that replaced 10% of total daily energy from carbohydrate with protein; the other that replaced the same amount of carbohydrate with unsaturated fat. The former had showed better results than the latter in lowering CVD risk (Swain et al, 2008). See Appendix 26.

Vegan Diet

A vegan diet is a strict vegetarian diet that includes no dietary sources from animal origins (see Appendix 39). There is ongoing research to suggest only this type of very restricted diet can actually reverse ASCVD (Esselstyn and Goulubic, 2014).

Physical Inactivity

Physical inactivity and a low level of fitness are independent risk factors for ASCVD. Physical activity is associated with ASCVD, independent of the common cardiometabolic risk factors of obesity, serum lipids, serum glucose and hypertension, in men and women (McGuire et al, 2009). With the high prevalence of obesity, physical activity is a high priority. Physical activity lessens ASCVD risk by retarding atherogenesis, increasing vascularity of the myocardium, increasing fibrinolysis, increasing HDL cholesterol, improving glucose tolerance and insulin sensitivity, aiding in weight management, and reducing blood pressure.

The 2013 ACC/AHA recommendations for exercise are based on studies on the role of exercise in preventing and treating CVD alone, not in combination with other interventions. Their recommendation based on the evidence is for three to four sessions of aerobic exercise per week for an average of 40 minutes duration.

Stress

Stress activates a neurohormonal response in the body that results in increased heart rate, blood pressure, and cardiac excitability. The stress hormone angiotensin II is released after stimulation of the sympathetic nervous system (SNS); exogenous infusion of angiotensin II accelerates the formation of plaque. The INTERHEART study found that the effect of stress on CVD risk is comparable to that of hypertension. Stress management was not part of the 2013 ACC/AHA lifestyle modification guidelines.

Diabetes

Diabetes is a disease that is an independent risk factor. The prevalence of diabetes mirrors that of obesity in the United States. Type 2 diabetes has continued to increase in incidence (see Chapter 30). Any form of diabetes increases the risk for ASCVD, with occurrence at younger ages. Most people with diabetes die of CVD. Similarly, 75% of people with diabetes have more than two risk factors for ASCVD (McCollum et al, 2006). Some of the increased risk seen in patients with diabetes is attributable to the concurrent presence of other risk factors, such as dyslipidemia, hypertension, and obesity. Thus diabetes is now considered an ASCVD risk factor (see Chapter 30).

Metabolic Syndrome

Since the early findings of the Framingham study, it has been known that a clustering of risk factors markedly increases the risk of CVD (see Chapter 21 for an in-depth discussion of metabolic syndrome).

Obesity

Obesity has now reached epidemic levels in children and adults in many developed countries. Body mass index (BMI) and CVD are positively related; as BMI goes up, the risk of CVD also increases. The prevalence of overweight and obesity is the highest that it has ever been in the United States; 65% of adults are overweight, and 31% are obese (Blumenthal et al, 2010). Obesity rates vary by race and ethnicity in women. Non-Hispanic black women have the highest prevalence, followed by Mexican American women, American Indians, Alaskan natives, and non-Hispanic whites. In men the rates of obesity vary from 25% to 28% of the population.

An obese-years metric was developed using more than 5000 participants of the Framingham Heart Study that captures the cumulative damage of obesity over years. The obese-years metric is calculated by multiplying the number of BMI units above 29 kg/m2 by the number of years lived at that BMI. Higher obese-years were associated with higher CVD risk in the study. The metric was found to provide a slightly more accurate measure of CVD risk than obesity alone (Abdullah et al, 2014).

Carrying excess adipose tissue greatly affects the heart through the many risk factors that are often present: hypertension, glucose intolerance, inflammatory markers (IL-6, TNF-α, CRP), obstructive sleep apnea, prothrombotic state, endothelial dysfunction, and dyslipidemia (small dense LDL, increased apo B, low HDL, high triglyceride levels). Many inflammatory proteins are now known to come from the adipocyte (see Chapters 3 and 21). These concurrent risk factors may help to explain the high morbidity and mortality rates observed in people who are obese.

Weight distribution (abdominal versus gynoid) is also predictive of CVD risk, glucose tolerance, and serum lipid levels. Central or abdominal length of adiposity also has been strongly related to markers of inflammation, especially CRP. Therefore a waist circumference of less than 35 inches for women and 40 inches for men is recommended (see Chapter 21).

Small weight losses (10 to 20 lb) can improve LDL cholesterol, HDL cholesterol, triglycerides, high blood pressure, glucose tolerance, and CRP levels, even if an ideal BMI is not achieved. Weight loss also has been correlated with lower CRP levels. However, to restore vascular function, the amount of weight that must be lost, the time of weight maintenance, or the amount of improvement in endothelial function that lessens cardiovascular events is still unknown.

Nonmodifiable Risk Factors
Age and Sex
With increasing age, higher mortality rates from CVD are seen in both genders. However, gender is a factor for the assessment of risk. The incidence of premature disease in men 35 to 44 years of age is three times as high as the incidence in women of the same age. Therefore being older than 45 years of age is considered a risk factor for men. For women the increased risk comes after the age of 55 years, which is after menopause for most women. Overall the increased risk for CVD parallels age.

Family History and Genetics
A family history of premature disease is a strong risk factor, even when other risk factors are considered. A family history is considered to be positive when MI or sudden death occurs before the age of 55 years in a male first-degree relative or the age of 65 in a female first-degree relative (parents, siblings, or children). The presence of a positive family history, although not modifiable, influences the intensity of risk factor management.

Menopausal Status
Endogenous estrogen confers protection against ASCVD in premenopausal women, probably by preventing vascular injury. Loss of estrogen after natural or surgical menopause is associated with increased ASCVD risk. Rates of ASCVD in premenopausal women are low except in women with multiple risk factors. During the menopausal period total cholesterol, LDL cholesterol, and triglyceride levels increase; HDL cholesterol level decreases, especially in women who gain weight.

Medical Nutrition Therapy
Medical nutrition therapy (MNT), which includes discussion of physical activity, is the primary intervention for patients with elevated LDL cholesterol (see Box 33-4). Physicians are encouraged to refer patients to registered dietitian nutritionists (RDNs) to help patients meet goals for therapy based on LDL cholesterol levels.

With diet, exercise, and weight reduction, patients can decrease LDL cholesterol and reduce body inflammation. The complexity of changes, number of changes, and motivation of the patient will dictate how many patient visits it will take for the adherent client to be successful. An initial visit of 45 to 90 minutes followed by two to six visits of 30 to 60 minutes each with the RDN is recommended (American Dietetic Association [ADA] Evidence Library, 2006). Consequently these interventions are tried before drug therapy and also continue during pharmacologic treatment to enhance effectiveness of the medication (see *Pathophysiology and Care Management Algorithm: Atherosclerosis*).

Lifestyle Recommendations
The ACC/AHA recommends diet and lifestyle changes to reduce ASCVD risk in all people older than the age of 2 (Eckel et al, 2013). The ACC/AHA recommendations are for a diet high in vegetables, fruits, whole grains, low-fat poultry, fish, nontropical vegetable oils, nuts, and low-fat dairy and low in sweets, sugar-sweetened beverages, and red meat. The DASH diet pattern or USDA food pattern (MyPlate) is recommended to achieve this diet. The Mediterranean Diet was not specifically recommended because in the evidence evaluated the diet was not specific or consistent enough to draw conclusions. In general, the Mediterranean diet pattern (see Figure 33-5) fits the recommendations. A study recently presented at the American College of Cardiology supports the Mediterranean diet pattern for CVD risk reduction (American College of Cardiology, 2015). The study included more than 2500 Greek adults over more than 10 years. Nearly 20% of men and 12% of women in the study developed or died from heart disease. People who closely followed the Mediterranean diet were 47% less likely to develop heart disease than those who did not follow the diet. The Mediterranean Diet Score Tool was used (see Figure 33-5) to validate the dietary pattern. A Mediterranean diet may also reduce recurrent CVD by 50% to 70% and has been shown to affect lipoprotein levels positively in high-risk populations (Carter et al, 2010).

Saturated Fatty Acids. Currently in the United States the average intake of saturated fat is 11% of calories. The recommendation for decreasing LDL cholesterol is 5% to 6%. The guidelines have no specific recommendation for trans fatty acid intake but recommend it be decreased with the saturated fat. Saturated fat is generally found in animal proteins. It is recommended that intake of animal protein, especially red meat and high fat dairy be decreased.

Trans Fatty Acids. Trans fatty acids (stereoisomers of the naturally occurring cis-linoleic acid) are produced in the hydrogenation process used in the food industry to increase shelf life of foods and to make margarines, made from oil, firmer. Most trans fatty acids intake comes from these partially hydrogenated oils (PHOs). In 2013 the FDA made a decision to remove PHOs from the "generally recognized as safe" list. This was based on the mounting evidence that trans fats contributed to ASCVD and was associated with increased LDL cholesterol

PATHOPHYSIOLOGY AND CARE MANAGEMENT ALGORITHM

Atherosclerosis

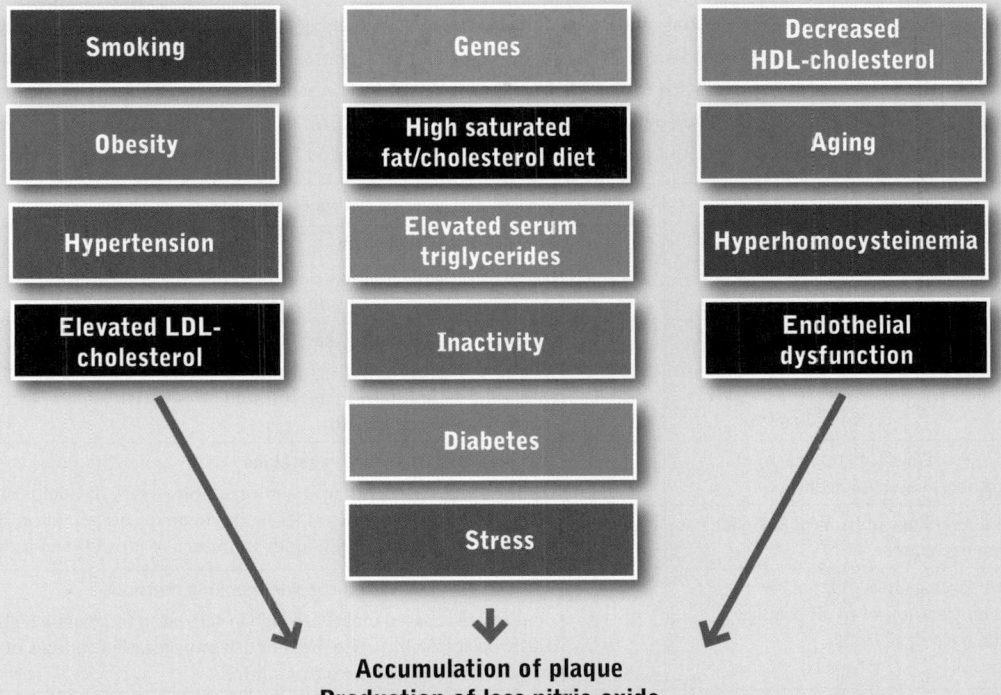

ETIOLOGY

Smoking

Obesity

Hypertension

Elevated LDL-cholesterol

Genes

High saturated fat/cholesterol diet

Elevated serum triglycerides

Inactivity

Diabetes

Stress

Decreased HDL-cholesterol

Aging

Hyperhomocysteinemia

Endothelial dysfunction

Accumulation of plaque
Production of less nitric oxide
Oxidized LDL cholesterol taken up by macrophages
Formation of foam cells and fatty streaks

PATHOPHYSIOLOGY

Clinical Findings

- Elevated LDL cholesterol
- Elevated serum triglycerides
- Elevated C-reactive protein
- Low HDL-cholesterol

Nutrition Assessment

- BMI evaluation
- Waist circumference; waist to hip ratio (WHR)
- Dietary assessment for:
  SFA, *trans*-fatty acids, ω-3 fatty acids, fiber, sodium, alcohol, sugar and phytonutrients

MANAGEMENT

Medical Management

- Lifestyle change
- HMG CoA reductase inhibitors (statins)
- Triglyceride-lowering medication
- Blood pressure—lowering medication
- Medication for glucose management
- Percutaneous coronary intervention (PCI)
  - Balloon
  - Stent
- Coronary artery bypass graft (CABG)
- Antiplatelet Therapy

Nutrition Management

- DASH dietary pattern
- Mediterranean diet pattern
- Weight reduction if needed
- Increase dietary fiber to 25–30 g/day or more
- Add ω-3 fats from food sources
- Add fruits and vegetables
- CoQ$_{10}$ for those on statin drugs

MEDITERRANEAN DIET SCORE TOOL

A Mediterranean dietary pattern ('Med diet') is typically one based on whole or minimally processed foods. It's rich in protective foods (fruits, vegetables, legumes, wholegrains, fish and olive oil) and low in adverse dietary factors (fast food, sugar-sweetened beverages, refined grain products and processed or energy-dense foods) with moderate red meat and alcohol intake.

Evidence shows **overall dietary pattern** (reflected in TOTAL SCORE) as well as **individual components** reflect risk; a higher score is associated with lower risk of CVD and all-cause mortality (BMJ 2008;337:a1344). During rehabilitation patient scores should ideally rise in response to dietary advice and support.

This tool can be used by health professionals with appropriate nutritional knowledge and competencies, such as Registered Dietitians (NICE, 2007, 2013). It can be used as both an *audit tool* and *as part of a dietary assessment* at baseline, end of programme and 1 year follow-up, along with assessment and advice for weight management, salt intake and eating behaviours. For information on complete requirements for dietary assessments and advice, please refer to the latest NICE/Joint British Societies guidelines (BACPR, 2012. The BACPR Standards and Core Components for Cardiovascular Disease Prevention and Rehabilitation, 2nd Ed.).

	Question	Yes	No	Nutritional issue to discuss in response
1.	Is olive oil the main culinary fat used?			**Choosing Healthier Fats** Olive oil is high in monounsaturated fat. Using unsaturated fats instead of saturated fats in cooking and preparing food is advisable.
2.	Are ≥ 4 tablespoons of olive oil used each day?			**Healthy fats are better than very low fat** Med diet is more beneficial than a very low fat diet in prevention of CVD. So replacing saturated with unsaturated fat is better than replacing it with carbohydrates or protein.
3.	Are ≥ 2 servings (of 200g each) of vegetables eaten each day?			**Eat plenty of fruits and vegetables** Eating a wide variety of fruit and vegetables every day helps ensure adequate intake of many vitamins, minerals, phytochemicals and fibre. Studies have shown that eating plenty of these foods is protective for CVD and cancer.
4.	Are ≥ 3 servings of fruit (of 80g each) eaten each day?			
5.	Is < 1 serving (100-150g) of red meat/ hamburgers/ other meat products eaten each day?			**Choose lean meats and consider cooking methods** Red and processed meats are high in saturated fat, can be high in salt and are best replaced with white meat or fish or vegetarian sources of protein. Grill or roast without fat, casserole or stir fry.
6.	Is < 1 serving (12g) of butter, margarine or cream eaten each day?			**Keep saturated fat low** These foods are high in saturated fat which can increase your blood cholesterol level. Choose plant-based or reduced-fat alternatives.
7.	Is < 1 serving (330ml) of sweet or sugar sweetened carbonated beverages consumed each day?			Excessive consumption of sugar-sweetened beverages can worsen many risk factors for CVD: keep consumption to < 1/day.
8.	Are ≥ 3 glasses (of 125ml) of wine consumed each week?			**Moderate alcohol intake with meals** While this does have some protective effect but **there is no evidence that non-drinkers should take up drinking alcohol.**
9.	Are ≥ 3 servings (of 150g) of legumes consumed each week?			**Include soluble fibre** These foods are high in soluble fibre and other useful nutrients. Regular consumption is advisable for raised cholesterol.
10.	Are ≥ 3 servings of fish (100-150g) or seafood (200g) eaten each week?			**Eat more oily and white fish** Oily fish is an excellent source of essential omega-3 fats. White fish is very low in saturated fat.
11.	Is < 3 servings of commercial sweets/pastries eaten each week?			**Eat less processed food** These foods are usually high in saturated fat, salt or sugar and often contain trans fats. Replacing these with healthy snacks such as fruit or unsalted nuts is beneficial.
12.	Is ≥ 1 serving (of 30g) of nuts consumed each week?			**Snack on modest servings of unsalted nuts** Nuts are rich in unsaturated fat, phytosterols, fibre, vitamin E and iron, **e.g. walnuts, almonds, hazelnuts**
13.	Is chicken, turkey or rabbit routinely eaten instead of veal, pork, hamburger or sausage?			'White meat' choices are lower in saturated fat. Remove the skin and consider your cooking method.
14.	Are pasta, vegetable or rice dishes flavoured with garlic, tomato, leek or onion eaten ≥ twice a week?			Using a tomato and garlic or onion or leek-based sauce regularly is a key feature of the Med diet.
TOTAL SCORE (total no. of 'yes' answers)				

26.09.13
Version 1

Alison Hornby, Katherine Paterson

FIGURE 33-5 Mediterranean Diet Score Tool. (Courtesy of Alison Hornby and Katherine Paterson.)

levels. Trans fat intake is inversely associated with HDL levels (Yanai et al, 2015).

Monounsaturated Fatty Acids. Oleic acid (C18:1) is the most prevalent MUFA in the American diet. Substituting oleic acid for carbohydrate has almost no appreciable effect on blood lipids. However, replacing SFAs with MUFAs (as would happen when substituting olive oil for butter) lowers serum cholesterol levels, LDL cholesterol levels, and triglyceride levels. Oleic acid as part of the Mediterranean diet (see Figure 33-6) has been shown to have antiinflammatory effects.

Polyunsaturated Fatty Acids. The essential fatty acid linoleic acid (LA) is the predominant PUFA consumed in the American diet; its effect depends on the total fatty acid profile of the diet. When added to study diets, large amounts of LA decrease HDL serum cholesterol levels. High intakes of omega-6 PUFAs may exert adverse effects on the function of vascular endothelium or stimulate production of proinflammatory cytokines (Harris et al, 2009). Replacing PUFAs for carbohydrate in the diet results in a decline in serum LDL cholesterol. When SFAs are replaced with PUFAs in a low-fat diet, LDL and HDL cholesterol levels are lowered. Overall, eliminating SFAs is twice as effective in lowering serum cholesterol levels as increasing PUFAs.

Omega-3 Fatty Acids. The main omega-3 fatty acids (eicosapentaenoic acid [EPA] and docosahexaenoic acid [DHA]) are high in fish oils, fish oil capsules, and ocean fish. Some studies have shown that eating fish is associated with a decreased ASCVD risk. The recommendation for the general population is to increase fish consumption specifically of fish high in omega-3 fatty acids (salmon, tuna, mackerel, sardines). Patients who have hypertriglyceridemia need 2 to 4 g of EPA and DHA per day for effective lowering. Omega-3 fatty acids lower triglyceride levels by inhibiting VLDL and apo B-100 synthesis, thereby decreasing postprandial lipemia. Fish oil consumption has been associated with high levels of HDL cholesterol (Yanai et al, 2015). See Appendix 34.

An omega-3 fatty acid from vegetables, alpha-linolenic acid (ALA), has antiinflammatory effects (see Chapter 3). CRP levels are reduced when patients consume 8 g of ALA daily (Basu et al, 2006). Omega-3 fatty acids are thought to be cardioprotective because they interfere with blood clotting and alter prostaglandin synthesis. Omega-3 fat stimulates production of nitric oxide, a substance that stimulates relaxation of the blood vessel wall (vasodilation). Unfortunately, high intakes prolong bleeding time, a common condition among Arctic Native populations

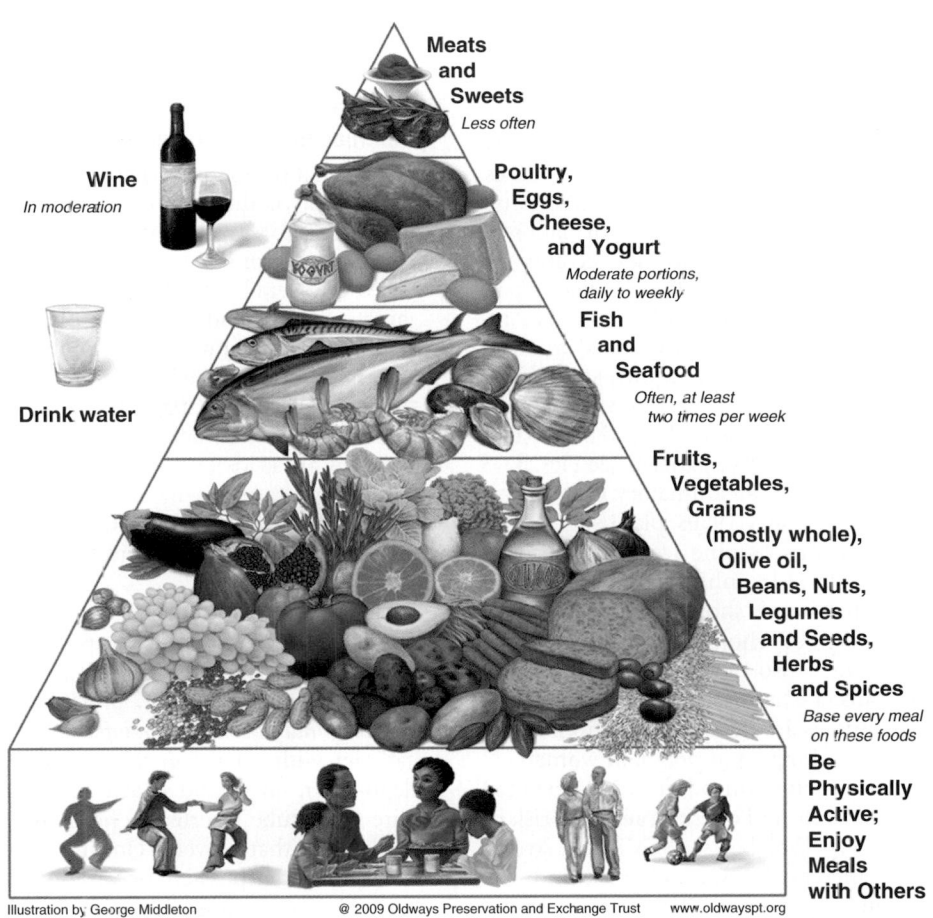

FIGURE 33-6 The Traditional Healthy Mediterranean Diet Pyramid. (Courtesy Oldways Preservation and Exchange Trust, www.oldwayspt.org.) (http://www.cardiacrehabilitation.org.uk/docs/Mediterranean-Diet-Score.pdf)

with high omega-3 fat dietary intakes and low incidence of ASCVD.

Dietary Cholesterol. Previous recommendations have been to decrease dietary cholesterol to decrease LDL cholesterol and reduce ASCVD risk. The ACC/AHA 2013 guidelines no longer make this recommendation, and they specifically state that dietary cholesterol does not raise LDLs. The 2015 US Dietary Guidelines also eliminate the recommendation to restrict cholesterol (see Chapter 11). However it is important to remember that most high cholesterol foods are also high in saturated fats that do raise LDL cholesterol.

Fiber. High intake levels of dietary fiber are associated with significantly lower prevalence of ASCVD and stroke (Anderson et al, 2009). The USDA MyPlate, the DASH diet, and the Mediterranean diet pattern emphasize fruits, vegetables, legumes, and whole grains, so they are innately high in fiber. This combination of foods provides a combination of soluble and insoluble fiber. Proposed mechanisms for the hypocholesterolemic effect of soluble fiber include the following: (1) the fiber binds bile acids, which lowers serum cholesterol and (2) bacteria in the colon ferment the fiber to produce acetate, propionate, and butyrate, which inhibit cholesterol synthesis. The role of fiber, if any, on inflammatory pathways is not well established. Minerals, vitamins, and antioxidants that are components of a high-fiber diet further enrich the diet.

Insoluble fibers such as cellulose and lignin have no effect on serum cholesterol levels. For the purpose of heart disease prevention, most of the recommended 25 to 30 g of fiber a day should be soluble fiber.

Antioxidants. Two dietary components that affect the oxidation potential of LDL cholesterol are the level of LA in the particle and the availability of antioxidants. Vitamins C, E, and beta-carotene at physiologic levels have antioxidant roles in the body. Vitamin E is the most concentrated antioxidant carried on LDLs, the amount being 20 to 300 times greater than any other antioxidant. A major function of vitamin E is to prevent oxidation of PUFAs in the cell membrane. The AHA does not recommend vitamin E supplementation for CVD prevention. A dietary pattern that includes increased amounts of whole grains has increased amounts of vitamin E. Foods with concentrated amounts of antioxidants are found in phytochemicals known as catechins and have been found to improve vascular reactivity. Red grapes, red wine, tea (especially green tea), berries, and broad beans (fava beans) are part of the Mediterranean diet pattern. See Figs. 33-5 and 33-6 and Appendix 31, The Anti-inflammatory Diet.

Stanols and Sterols. Since the early 1950s, plant stanols and sterols isolated from soybean oils or pine tree oil have been known to lower blood cholesterol by inhibiting absorption of dietary cholesterol. Stanols and sterols should be part of dietary recommendations for lowering LDL cholesterol in adults (Yanai et al, 2015). Because these esters also can affect the absorption of and cause lower beta-carotene, alpha-tocopherol, and lycopene levels, further safety studies are needed for use in normocholesterolemic individuals, children, and pregnant women.

Weight Loss. More than 78 million adults in the United States were obese in 2009 to 2010, and obesity raises the risk of hypertension, dyslipidemia, type 2 diabetes, ASCVD, and stroke. Obesity is associated with increased risk in all-cause and cardiovascular disease mortality (Stone et al, 2014) (see Treatment Algorithm—The Chronic Disease Management Model for Primary Care of Patients with Overweight and Obesity). Recommendations of the panel are summarized in Box 33-5.

> ### BOX 33-5 Recommendations from the AHA/ACC/TOS Obesity Guideline
>
> 1. Patient/provider encounter for obesity prevention and management: a patient encounter is defined as an interaction with a primary care provider who assesses weight status to determine need for further assessment and treatment.
> 2. Measure weight and height and calculate BMI.
> 3. BMI 25 <30 (overweight) or BMI 30 <35 (class I obese) or BMI 35 <40 class II obese or BMI > 40 (class III obese): these BMI cutpoints define overweight and obese individuals who are at increased risk of CVD. Within these categories, additional personal risk assessment is needed.
> 4. Assess and treat CVD risk factors and obesity-related comorbidities: A waist circumference measurement is recommended for individuals with BMI 25 to 35 to provide additional information on risk. It is not necessary to measure waist circumference in patients with BMI >35 because the waist circumference will likely be elevated and it will add no additional information. Increased cardiometabolic risk is defined as >88 cm or >35 in for women and >102 cm or >40 in for men.
> 5. Assess weight and lifestyle histories: Ask questions about history of weight gain and loss over time, details of previous weight loss attempts, dietary habits, physical activity, family history of obesity and other medical conditions and medications that may affect weight.
> 6. Assess need to lose weight: Weight loss treatment is indicated for (1) obese (2) overweight with one or more indicators of increased CVD risk.
> 7. Advise to avoid weight gain and address other risk factors.

Jensen, et al, 2013 AHA/ACC/TOS Guideline for the Management of Overweight and Obesity in Adults. Circulation, 129:S102, 2014.

Medical Management
Pharmacologic Management

Determination of drug therapy depends on risk category and attainment of the LDL cholesterol goal. The 2013 ACC/AHA Guidelines for Treatment of Blood Cholesterol have updated recommendations for prescribing statin drugs to be more focused on overall patient risk than on specific serum cholesterol targets. See Appendix 22 for a discussion of the guidelines for treatment with statin drugs. The primary treatment for those at risk of ASCVD are the HGM-CoA reductase inhibitors, of which there are many (see Chapter 8). The classes of drugs include the following: (1) **bile acid sequestrants** such as cholestyramine (adsorbs bile acids); (2) nicotinic acid; (3) **statins**, or **3-hydroxy-3-methylglutaryl–coenzyme A (HMG-CoA)** reductase inhibitors, which inhibit the rate-limiting enzyme in cholesterol synthesis; (4) fibric acid derivatives; and (5) probucol.

Medical Intervention

Medical interventions such as percutaneous coronary intervention (PCI) are now performed in patients with asymptomatic ischemia or angina. PCI, previously known as *percutaneous transluminal coronary angioplasty,* is a procedure that uses a catheter with a balloon that, once inflated, breaks up plaque deposits in an occluded artery. Coronary stenting involves a wire mesh tube inserted to hold an artery open; it can release medication that prevents clotting (Thom et al, 2006).

PCI is often possible because of earlier detection of blockages. The most common problem with PCI is restenosis of the artery. A recent study examined more than 2200 patients, half of whom received intervention of medication and lifestyle changes such as quitting smoking, exercise, and nutrition, and half of whom received lifestyle changes as well as angioplasty. After 5 years it was observed that the number who had heart attacks, were hospitalized, or died because of their heart problems was virtually identical in both groups. Angioplasty did not appear to provide an additional benefit versus lifestyle changes combined with medication (Boden et al, 2007).

Because PCI is performed with the patient under local anesthesia in a cardiac catheterization laboratory, recovery is quicker than with coronary artery bypass graft (CABG) surgery. In CABG surgery, an artery from the chest is used to redirect blood flow around a diseased vessel. Candidates for CABG usually have more than two occluded arteries. CABG surgeries have decreased since 1995 because more PCI procedures are being done. These surgeries improve survival time, relieve symptoms, and markedly improve the quality of life for patients with ASCVD. However, CABG does not cure atherosclerosis; the new grafts are also susceptible to atherogenesis. Consequently, restenosis is common within 10 years of surgery.

HYPERTENSION

Hypertension is persistently high arterial blood pressure, the force exerted per unit area on the walls of arteries. The systolic blood pressure (SBP), the upper reading in a blood pressure measurement, is the force exerted on the walls of blood vessels as the heart contracts and pushes blood out of its chambers. The lower reading, known as diastolic blood pressure (DBP), measures the force as the heart relaxes between contractions. Blood pressure is measured in millimeters (mm) of mercury (Hg). Adult blood pressure is considered normal at 120/80 mm Hg.

The evidence-based guideline from the Joint National Committee (JNC) Eight Report (James et al., 2014) on the management of high blood pressure in adults indicates that adults aged 60 years or older should be treated with medication if their blood pressure exceeds 150/90, which sets a higher bar for treatment than the former guideline of 140/90 (see Table 33-1). The expert panel also recommends that individuals with diabetes and chronic kidney disease younger than 60 years be treated at the same point as everyone else that age, when their blood pressure exceeds 140/90. Until now, people with those chronic conditions have been prescribed medication when their blood pressure exceeded 130/80. The recommendations are based on clinical evidence showing that stricter guidelines for these patients provided no additional benefit. Importantly, the guidelines emphasize that people with high blood pressure should follow a healthy diet and lifestyle along with medication management. Diet and lifestyle modifications are important part of primary prevention of hypertension.

Hypertension is a common public health problem in developed countries. In the United States one in three adults has high blood pressure (AHA, 2013). Untreated hypertension leads to many degenerative diseases, including heart failure (HF), end-stage renal disease, and peripheral vascular disease. It is often called a "silent killer" because people with hypertension can be asymptomatic for years and then have a fatal stroke or heart attack. Although no cure is available, hypertension is easily detected and usually controllable. Some of the decline in CVD mortality during the last two decades has been attributed to the increased detection and control of hypertension. The emphasis on lifestyle modifications has given diet a prominent role in the primary prevention and management of hypertension.

Of those persons with high blood pressure, 90% to 95% have essential hypertension (hypertension of unknown cause) or primary hypertension. The cause involves a complex interaction between poor lifestyle choices and gene expression. Lifestyle factors that have been implicated include poor diet (i.e., high sodium, low fruit and vegetable intake), smoking, physical inactivity, stress, and obesity. Vascular inflammation has also been implicated (Hall et al, 2012). Many genes play a role in hypertension; most relate to the renal or neuroendocrine control of blood pressure. Evaluations of more than 2.5 million genotyped polymorphisms have identified more than 40 genetic loci associated with monogenic blood pressure syndromes (Padmanabhan et al, 2012). Hypertension that arises as the result of another disease, usually endocrine, is referred to as secondary hypertension. Depending on the extent of the underlying disease, secondary hypertension can be cured.

Prevalence and Incidence

Approximately 78 million American adults age 20 and older have hypertension or are taking antihypertensive medication (AHA, 2013). Projections show that by 2030, prevalence of hypertension will increase by 7.2% from 2013 estimates. Non-Hispanic black adults have a higher age-adjusted prevalence of hypertension (42.6% of men; 47% of women) than non-Hispanic whites (33.4% of men; 30.7% of women) and Mexican Americans (30.1% of men; 28.8% of women) (AHA, 2013). The prevalence of high blood pressure in blacks is one of the highest rates seen anywhere in the world. Because blacks develop hypertension earlier in life and maintain higher blood pressure levels, their risk of fatal stroke, heart disease, or end-stage kidney disease is higher than whites (AHA, 2013).

A person of any age can have hypertension. Approximately 16% of boys and 9% of girls have elevated blood pressure (Ostchega et al, 2009). With aging, the prevalence of high blood pressure increases (see Figure 33-7). Before the age of 45 more men than women have high blood pressure, and after age 65 the rates of high blood pressure among women in each racial group surpass those of the men in their group (Go et al, 2014). Because the prevalence of hypertension rises with increasing age, more than half the older adult population (more than 65 years of age) in any racial group has hypertension. Although lifestyle interventions targeted to older persons may reduce the prevalence of hypertension, early intervention programs provide the greatest long-term potential for reducing overall blood pressure-related complications (Lloyd-Jones, 2012).

The relationship between blood pressure and risk of CVD events is continuous and independent of other risk factors. The higher the blood pressure, the greater is the chance of target organ damage, including left ventricular hypertrophy (LVH),

TABLE 33-1 **Classification of Blood Pressure for Adults Ages 18 Years or Older**				
	Systolic BP (mm Hg)*		Diastolic BP (mm Hg)*	
Normal, <60yrs	140	and	90	
≥60yrs	150	or	<90	

James PA, et al : 2014 evidence-based guideline for the management of high blood pressure in adults: Report from the panel members appointed to the Eighth Joint National Committee (JNC 8), JAMA 311 : 5C7 , 2014.
*Definitions of hypertension and pre-hypertension not addressed, goals of treatment now specific to presence of diabetes and kidney disease

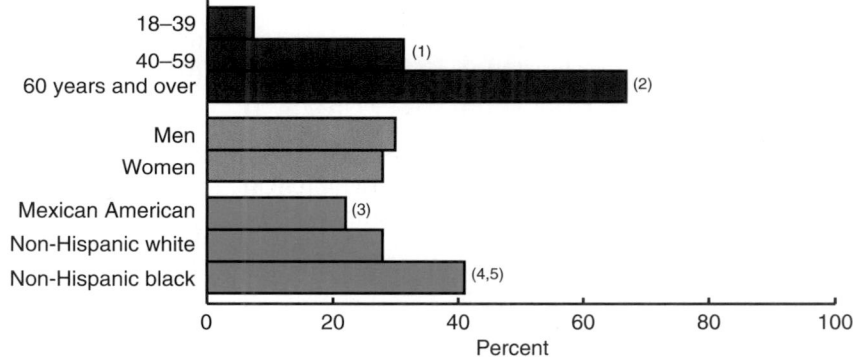

18–39

40–59 (1)

60 years and over (2)

Men

Women

Mexican American (3)

Non-Hispanic white

Non-Hispanic black (4,5)

0 20 40 60 80 100

Percent

[1]Statistically significant difference between ages 18–39 and 40–59 years.
[2]Statistically significant difference between ages 40–59 and 60 years and over.
[3]Statistically significant difference between the non-Hispanic white and Mexican-American populations.
[4]Statistically significant difference between the non-Hispanic white and non-Hispanic black populations.
[5]Statistically significant difference between the non-Hispanic black and Mexican-American populations.
SOURCE: CDC/NCHS, National Health and Nutrition Examination Survey.

FIGURE 33-7 Age-specific and age-adjusted prevalence of hypertension in adults: United States, 2005-2006. (Ostchega Y et al: *Hypertension awareness, treatment, and control—continued disparities in adults: United States, 2005-2006.* NCHS data brief no. 3, Hyattsville, Md, 2008, National Center for Health Statistics.)

HF, stroke, chronic kidney disease, and retinopathy (ADA, 2013). As many as 28% of adults with hypertension have treatment-resistant hypertension, which means that their blood pressure remains high despite the use of three or more antihypertensive drugs from different classes (Egan et al, 2010). Treatment-resistant hypertension puts an individual at greater risk of target organ damage. Older age and obesity are two of the strongest risk factors associated with the condition. Identification and reversal of lifestyle factors contributing to treatment resistance, along with diagnosis and appropriate treatment of secondary causes and use of effective multidrug regimens are essential treatment strategies.

Adults with diabetes have CVD death rates two to four times higher than adults without diabetes (AHA, 2013). Consequently, national health organizations, including the American Diabetes Association (ADA, 2013), have set the target blood pressure goal for antihypertensive therapy for individuals with diabetes lower than that recommended for the general population, which is 140/90 mm Hg. A recent update of the JNC 8 Report (James et al, 2014) recommends similar treatment goals for all hypertensive populations, including those with diabetes, citing insufficient evidence from randomized clinical trials (RCTs) of CVD benefits for lowered blood pressure targets. RCTs provide the highest quality of scientific evidence regarding the efficacy of treatment approaches to lower blood pressure.

Although hypertensive patients are often asymptomatic, hypertension is not a benign disease. Cardiac, cerebrovascular, and renal systems are affected by chronically elevated blood pressure. High blood pressure was the primary or a contributory cause in 348,000 of the 2.4 million U.S. deaths in 2009 (AHA, 2013). Between 1999 and 2009 the age-adjusted death rate from hypertension increased by 17.1%; overall deaths from hypertension increased by 43.6%. Death rates from hypertension are approximately three times higher in blacks than in whites (AHA, 2013). Hypertension is a major contributing factor to atherosclerosis, stroke, renal failure, and MI. Factors associated with a poor prognosis in hypertension are shown in Box 33-6.

BOX 33-6   Risk Factors and Adverse Prognosis in Hypertension

Risk Factors

Black race
Youth
Male gender
Persistent diastolic pressure >115 mm Hg
Smoking
Diabetes mellitus
Hypercholesterolemia
Obesity
Excessive alcohol intake
Evidence of end organ damage

Cardiac

Cardiac enlargement

Electrocardiographic signs of ischemia or left ventricular strain
Myocardial infarction
Heart failure

Eyes

Retinal exudates and hemorrhages
Papilledema

Renal

Impaired renal function

Nervous system

Cerebrovascular accident

From Fisher ND, Williams GH: Hypertensive vascular disease. In Kasper DL et al, editors: *Harrison's principles of internal medicine,* ed 16, New York, 2005, McGraw-Hill.

Pathophysiology

Blood pressure is a function of cardiac output multiplied by peripheral resistance (the resistance in the blood vessels to the flow of blood). Thus the diameter of the blood vessel markedly affects blood flow. When the diameter is decreased (as in atherosclerosis) resistance and blood pressure increase. Conversely, when the diameter is increased (as with vasodilator drug therapy), resistance decreases and blood pressure is lowered.

Many systems maintain homeostatic control of blood pressure. The major regulators are the sympathetic nervous system (SNS) for short-term control and the kidney for long-term control. In response to a fall in blood pressure, the SNS secretes norepinephrine, a vasoconstrictor, which acts on small arteries and arterioles to increase peripheral resistance and raise blood pressure. Conditions that result in overstimulation of the SNS (i.e., certain adrenal disorders or sleep apnea) result in increased blood pressure. The kidney regulates blood pressure by controlling the extracellular fluid volume and secreting renin,

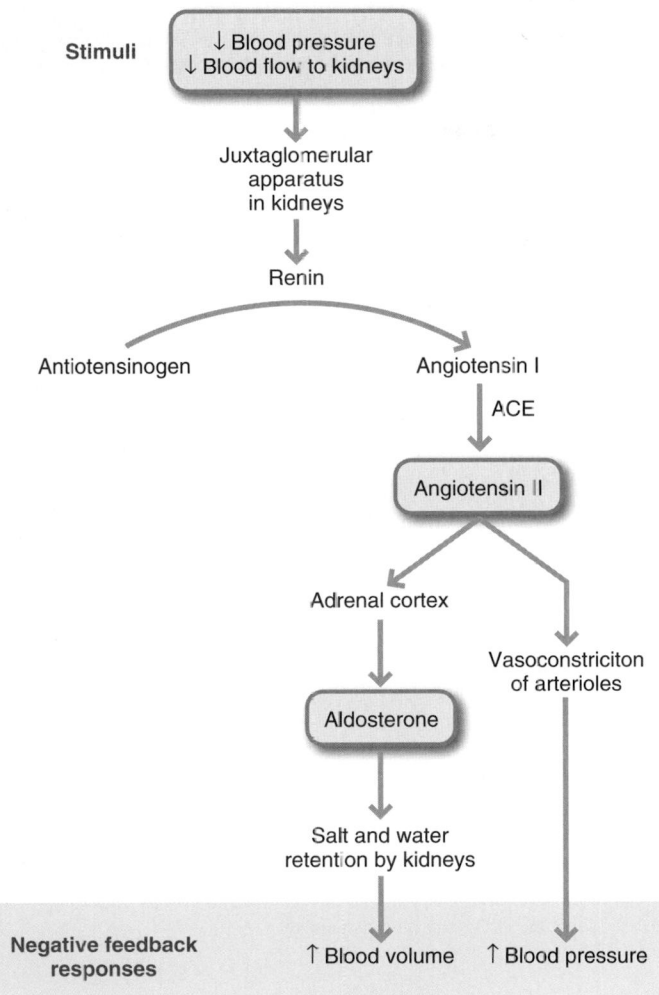

Stimuli

↓ Blood pressure
↓ Blood flow to kidneys

Juxtaglomerular
apparatus
in kidneys

Renin

Antiotensinogen   Angiotensin I

ACE

Angiotensin II

Adrenal cortex

Vasoconstriciton
of arterioles

Aldosterone

Salt and water
retention by kidneys

**Negative feedback
responses**

↑ Blood volume   ↑ Blood pressure

FIGURE 33-8 Renin-angiotensin cascade. *ACE,* Angiotensin-converting enzyme. (Reprinted with permission from Fox SI: Human physiology, ed 6, New York, 1999, McGraw-Hill.)

which activates the **renin-angiotensin system (RAS)** (see Figure 33-8). Abnormal blood pressure is usually multifactorial. In most cases of hypertension, peripheral resistance increases. This resistance forces the left ventricle of the heart to increase its effort in pumping blood through the system. With time, left ventricular hypertrophy (LVH) and eventually HF can develop.

Common genetic variants of the RAS gene, including angiotensin-converting enzyme (ACE) and angiotensinogen, have shown relationships with hypertension (Norton et al, 2010). An increased production of these proteins may increase production of angiotensin II, the primary mediator of the RAS, thus increasing blood pressure. Angiotensin II may also trigger low-grade inflammation within the blood vessel wall, a condition that predisposes to hypertension (Savoia et al, 2011).

Hypertension often occurs with other risk factors for CVD, including visceral (intraabdominal) obesity, insulin resistance, high triglycerides, and low HDL cholesterol levels. The coexistence of three or more of these risk factors leads to metabolic syndrome. It is unclear whether one or more of these risk factors precede the others or whether they occur simultaneously. Accumulation of visceral fat synthesizes increased amounts of angiotensinogen, which activates the RAS and

increases blood pressure (Zhou et al, 2012). Also, angiotensin II, the primary mediator of the RAS, promotes the development of large dysfunctional adipocytes, which produce increased amounts of leptin and reduced quantities of adiponectin. Higher levels of leptin and lower amounts of circulating adiponectin activate the SNS, a key component of the hypertensive response (DeMarco et al, 2014).

Primary Prevention

Positive changes in hypertension awareness, treatment, and control have occurred during the last several years. Based on analysis of National Health and Nutrition Examination Survey (NHANES) data from 2007 to 2010, 81.5% of people with hypertension are aware that they have it (Go et al, 2014), up from 72% in 1999 to 2004. Although current hypertension treatment and control rates have increased from 48.4% to 53.3%, respectively, during this same time period, additional efforts are needed to meet the *Healthy People 2020* objective of 61.2%. In 2010, women, younger adults (aged 18 to 39 years), and Hispanic individuals had lower rates of blood pressure control compared with men, younger individuals, and non-Hispanic whites. Improving hypertension treatment through targeted intervention programs should have a positive effect on CVD outcomes. Blood pressure treatment guidelines highlight the importance of evaluating patients for the presence of multiple CVD risk factors and individualizing lifestyle modification and drug therapies accordingly.

Changing lifestyle factors have documented efficacy in the primary prevention and control of hypertension. These factors were systematically reviewed and categorized by the Academy of Nutrition and Dietetics (AND) in 2009 and more recently by the ACC and AHA in 2013 (Eckel et al, 2013). These guidelines made a strong recommendation (i.e., high benefit/risk ratio with supporting evidence) for reducing intake of dietary sodium. A strong recommendation also was made for fruits and vegetables and dietary patterns emphasizing these foods, as well as weight management to lower blood pressure. Increasing physical activity was recommended, although the ACC/AHA felt that data showing that physical activity lowers blood pressure were limited in diverse populations. The ACC/AHA did not make a recommendation for potassium, citing insufficient evidence from RCTs to determine whether increasing dietary potassium intake without use of nutritional supplements lowers blood pressure. The AND provided a "fair" recommendation for this nutrient with consideration given to studies that included dietary and supplemental intake of potassium. A summary of recommendations and ratings from the ACC/AHA and the AND can be found in Table 33-2.

Fats

Although the total quantity of dietary fat, SFA, and omega-6 PUFAs do not seem to affect blood pressure (Cicero et al, 2009), evidence from short-term feeding trials documented that MUFA, when used as a replacement for SFAs, PUFA, or carbohydrate, lowered blood pressure in some individuals with hypertension (Appel et al, 2005). In a large population study spanning different continents and diverse dietary patterns, higher intake of dietary MUFA (~13 g/day), especially oleic acid from plant oils, was associated with significantly lower DBP (Miura et al, 2013). In a recent meta-analysis, including 9 RCTs, examining the effect of MUFA on blood pressure, SBP (net change: −2.26 mm Hg), and DBP (net change: −1.15 mm Hg)

TABLE 33-2 Recommendations on Blood Pressure in Hypertensive Adults from Evidence Analysis Library (2009) and American College of Cardiology/American Heart Association (2013)

Food or Nutrient	EAL Recommendation	Rating	ACC/AHA Recommendation	Rating
Sodium	Sodium intake should be limited to no more than 2300 mg/day; if adherent to this recommendation and BP target not achieved, a further reduction in dietary sodium to 1600 mg/day should be encouraged in combination with a DASH dietary pattern.	Strong	Lower sodium intake. Consume no more than 2400 mg of sodium/day; further reduction of sodium to 1500 mg/day is desirable because it is associated with even greater reduction in BP; reduce intake by at least 1000 mg/day because that will lower BP, even if the desired daily sodium intake is not achieved.	Strong Moderate
Dietary patterns emphasizing fruits and vegetables	Individuals should adopt the DASH dietary pattern, which is rich in fruits, vegetables, low-fat dairy, and nuts; low in sodium, total fat, and saturated fat; and adequate in calories for weight management.	Consensus	Consume a dietary pattern that emphasizes intake of vegetables, fruits, and whole grains; includes low-fat dairy products, poultry, fish, legumes, nontropical vegetable oils and nuts; and limits intake of sweets, sugar-sweetened beverages, and red meat; adapt the pattern to appropriate calorie requirements; achieve this pattern by following plans such as DASH, USDA food pattern or the AHA Diet; combine the DASH dietary pattern with lower sodium intake.	Strong
Fruits and vegetables	Fruits and vegetables should be recommended at a level of five to ten servings per day for significant BP reduction.	Strong		Not evaluated
Weight management	Optimal body weight should be achieved and maintained (BMI 18.5-24.9) to reduce BP.	Consensus	Counsel overweight and obese adults with high BP that lifestyle changes that produce even modest, sustained weight loss of 3% to 5% produce clinically meaningful benefits (e.g., reduce TG, blood sugar, HbA1C); >5% will reduce BP and reduce the need for medications to control BP.*	Strong
Physical activity	Individuals should be encouraged to engage in aerobic physical activity for at least 30 minutes per day on most days of the week, because it reduces SBP.	Consensus	Advise adults to engage in aerobic physical activity to lower BP: 3-4 sessions a week, lasting on average 40 minutes per session, and involving moderate-to-vigorous intensity physical activity.	Moderate
Alcohol	For individuals who can safely consume alcohol, consumption should be limited to no more than two drinks (24 oz beer, 10 oz wine, or 3 oz of 80-proof liquor) per day in most men and to no more than one drink per day in women.	Consensus		Not evaluated
Potassium	Studies support a modest relationship between increasing intake of potassium and a lower sodium-potassium ratio with lowered blood pressure.	Fair	Insufficient evidence	Low
Calcium	The effect of increasing calcium intake with lowered blood pressure is unclear; although some research indicates minimal benefit.	Fair		Not evaluated
Magnesium	The effect of increasing magnesium intake with lowered blood pressure is unknown; although some research indicates minimal benefit.	Fair		Not evaluated
Omega-3 fatty acids	Studies investigating increased consumption of omega-3 fatty acids have not demonstrated a beneficial effect on BP.	Fair		Not evaluated

BMI, Body mass index; *BP,* blood pressure; *DASH,* Dietary Approaches to Stop Hypertension; *SBP,* systolic blood pressure.

Recommendations listed are for those rated by the Academy of Nutrition and Dietetics and the American Academy of Cardiology (ACC) / American Heart Association (AHA) as strong, fair/moderate, and consensus; for those with weak ratings consult the American Dietetic Association Evidence Analysis Library for Hypertension (2009) http://www.adaevidencelibrary.com/topic.cfm?cat=3259 or the ACC/AHA data supplement at http://circ.ahajournals.org/lookup/suppl/doi:10.1161/01.cir.0000437740.48606.d1/-DC1

*Weight management guidelines are from Jensen MD et al: 2013 AHA/ACC/TOS guideline for the management of overweight and obesity in adults: a report of the American College of Cardiology/American Heart Association Task Force on Practice Guidelines, and the Obesity Society, *J Am Coll Cardiol* 63:2985, 2014.

TABLE 33-3 Manifestations of Target Organ Disease from Hypertension

Organ System	Manifestations
Cardiac	Clinical, electrocardiographic, or radiologic evidence of arterial wall thickening left ventricular hypertrophy; left ventricular malfunction or cardiac failure
Cerebrovascular	Transient ischemic attack or stroke
Peripheral	Absence of one or more pulses in extremities (except for dorsalis pedis) Ankle-Brachial Index < 0.9
Renal	Serum creatinine elevated: Men 1.3-1.5 mg/dL, Women 1.2-1.4 mg/dL
	Calculated GFR <60 mL/min/1.73 m2
	Elevated albumin excretion
Retinopathy	Hemorrhages or exudates, with or without papilledema

Adapted from: Schmieder R: End organ damage in hypertension, *Dtsch Arztebl* 107:866 2010.

reductions were significantly greater among participants assigned to high MUFA diets compared with those on control diets (Schwingshackl et al, 2011). Taken together, these findings suggest that diets high in MUFA may be a useful component of blood pressure–lowering diets.

Supplementation with n-3 PUFAs (EPA + DHA) in doses higher than 2 g/day also can give modest reductions in SBP and DBP, especially in untreated hypertensive persons (Miller et al, 2014).

Protein

Evidence from observational studies and RCTs suggests replacement of protein for fat or carbohydrate in an isocaloric diet results in lowered blood pressure (Bazzano et al, 2013). Protein supplementation in doses of 60 g/day reduced SBP by 4.9 mm Hg and DBP by 2.7 mm Hg as compared with 60 g/day of carbohydrate in overweight individuals with prehypertension and untreated stage 1 hypertension (Teunissen-Beekman and van Baak, 2013). Although soy protein may contribute to the lowering of blood pressure, the effect of increased soy food intake on blood pressure remains controversial (AND, 2009).

Dietary Patterns Emphasizing Fruits and Vegetables

Several dietary patterns have been shown to lower blood pressure. Plant-based dietary patterns have been associated with lower SBP in observational studies and clinical trials. Average SBP reductions of 5 to 6 mm Hg have been reported. Specifically, the Dietary Approaches to Stop Hypertension (DASH) controlled feeding study showed that a dietary pattern emphasizing fruits, vegetables, low-fat dairy products, whole grains, lean meats, and nuts significantly decreased SBP in hypertensive and normotensive adults. The DASH diet (Appendix 26) was found to be more effective than just adding fruits and vegetables to a low-fat dietary pattern and was equally effective in men and women of diverse racial and ethnic backgrounds (Appel et al, 2006). This dietary pattern serves as the core for the ACC/AHA dietary recommendations for lowering blood pressure (Eckel et al, 2013). Although the DASH diet is safe and currently advocated for preventing and treating hypertension, the diet is high in potassium, phosphorus, and protein, depending on how it is planned. For this reason the DASH diet is not advisable for individuals with end-stage renal disease (Appel et al, 2006).

Several versions of the DASH diet have been examined in regard to blood pressure–lowering potential. The OmniHeart trial compared the original DASH diet to a high-protein version of the DASH diet (25% of energy from protein, approximately half from plant sources), and a DASH diet high in unsaturated fat (31% of calories from unsaturated fat, mostly monounsaturated). Although each diet lowered SBP, substituting some of the carbohydrate (approximately 10% of total calories) in the DASH diet with either protein or monounsaturated fat achieved the best reduction in blood pressure and blood cholesterol (Appel et al, 2005; Miller et al, 2006). This could be achieved by substituting nuts for some of the fruit, bread, or cereal servings.

Because many hypertensive patients are overweight, hypocaloric versions of the DASH diet also have been tested for efficacy in promoting weight loss and blood pressure reduction. A hypocaloric DASH diet versus a low-calorie, low-fat diet produces a greater reduction in SBP and DBP. More recently, the ENCORE study showed that the addition of exercise and weight loss to the DASH diet resulted in greater blood pressure reductions, greater improvements in vascular function, and reduced left ventricular mass compared with the DASH diet alone (Hinderliter et al, 2014).

The MeD dietary pattern has many similarities to the DASH diet but is generally higher in fat, primarily MUFA from olive oil, nuts, and seeds. A traditional MeD diet also contains fatty fish rich in omega-3 fatty acids. A recent systematic review of the MeD diet and CVD risk factors, found that although limited, evidence from RCTs was suggestive of a blood-pressure lowering effect of this style dietary pattern in adults with hypertension (Rees et al, 2013). According to the ACC/AHA (Eckel et al, 2013), more studies on diverse populations are warranted before recommendations can be made related to the MeD diet for use in blood pressure management.

Weight Reduction

There is a strong association between BMI and hypertension among men and women in all race or ethnic groups and in most age groups. It is estimated that at least 75% of the incidence of hypertension is related directly to obesity (AHA, 2013). Weight gain during adult life is responsible for much of the rise in blood pressure seen with aging.

Some of the physiologic changes proposed to explain the relationship between excess body fat and blood pressure are overactivation of the SNS and RAS and vascular inflammation (Mathieu et al, 2009). Visceral fat in particular promotes vascular inflammation by inducing cytokine release, proinflammatory transcription factors, and adhesion molecules (Savoia et al, 2011). Low-grade inflammation occurs in the vasculature of individuals with elevated blood pressure; whether it precedes the onset of hypertension is unclear. Weight loss, exercise, and a MeD-style diet are beneficial. Also see Appendix 31.

Virtually all clinical trials on weight reduction and blood pressure support the efficacy of weight loss on lowering blood pressure. Reductions in blood pressure can occur without attainment of desirable body weight in most participants. Larger blood pressure reductions are achieved in participants who lost more weight and were also taking antihypertensive medications. This latter finding suggests a possible synergistic effect between weight loss and drug therapy. Although weight reduction and maintenance of a healthy body weight is a major effort, interventions to prevent weight gain are needed before midlife. In addition, BMI is recommended as a screening tool in adolescence for future health risk.

Sodium

Evidence from a variety of studies supports lowering blood pressure and CVD risk by reducing dietary sodium. For example, in the Trials of Hypertension Prevention more than 2400 individuals with moderately elevated blood pressure were assigned randomly to either cut their sodium by 750 to 1000 mg per day or to follow general guidelines for healthy eating for 18 months to 4 years. In 10 to 15 years after the studies ended, individuals who cut their sodium experienced a 25% to 30% lower risk of heart attacks, strokes, or other cardiovascular events compared with the group that did not (Cook et al, 2007). A recent meta-analysis of 37 RCTs confirmed these positive effects of sodium reduction on blood pressure and cardiovascular outcomes for normotensive and hypertensive individuals (Aburto et al, 2013).

The DASH sodium trials tested the effects of three different levels of sodium intake (1500 mg, 2400 mg, and 3300 mg/day) combined with either a typical U.S. diet or the DASH diet in persons with prehypertension or stage 1 hypertension (Appel et al, 2006). The lowest blood pressures were achieved by those eating the 1500-mg sodium level in the DASH diet. In the DASH diet and the typical American diet groups, the lower the sodium, the lower the blood pressure. Such data provide the basis for the 2013 ACC/AHA (Eckel et al, 2013) sodium guideline for adults with elevated blood pressure to consume no more than 2400mg/day. For those with normal blood pressure, the Dietary Guidelines for Americans recommend an intake of less than 2300 mg of sodium, the equivalent of 6 g of salt, each day (USDA, 2015). This goal is supported by the AND Practice Guidelines (AND, 2009) and other organizations.

Some experts, including the AHA, have suggested that all individuals should aim for the lower level of 1500 mg of sodium per day, the amount considered optimal for at-risk individuals but thought to be beneficial for all. In a recent report, *Sodium Intake in Populations: Assessment of Evidence,* the Institute of Medicine (IOM, 2013) systematically reviewed the effects of sodium on clinical events, rather than blood pressure as the end point. The IOM concluded that there was insufficient evidence of benefit in the general U.S. population and some evidence suggesting risk of adverse outcomes in specific populations (specifically those with mid-to-late stage heart failure receiving aggressive medical therapy) associated with sodium intake less than 2300 mg per day. Further research is needed, the IOM concluded, on associations between lower levels of sodium (between 1500 and 2300 mg/day range) and health outcomes. Nevertheless, the 2013 guidelines from the ACC/AHA advocate for sodium reduction to 1500 mg/day in at-risk adults based on evidence of improved blood pressure reduction (Eckel et al, 2013).

There is agreement that some persons with hypertension show a greater decrease in their blood pressures in response to reduced sodium intake than others. The term salt-sensitive hypertension has been used to identify these individuals. Salt-resistant hypertension refers to individuals with hypertension whose blood pressures do not change significantly with lowered salt intakes. Salt sensitivity varies, with individuals having greater or lesser degrees of blood pressure reduction. In general, individuals who are more sensitive to the effects of salt and sodium tend to be individuals who are black, obese, and middle-aged or older, especially if they have diabetes, chronic kidney disease, or hypertension. Currently, there are no clinical tests methods for identifying the salt-sensitive individual from the salt-resistant individual.

Calcium and Vitamin D

Higher dairy versus supplemental calcium is associated with lower risk of hypertension (van Mierlo et al, 2008). In particular, low-fat dairy intake reduced the risk of hypertension by 13%, whereas supplemental calcium intake and high fat dairy sources had no effect. At least 2.5 servings of low-fat dairy per day are necessary for blood pressure improvement (Rice et al, 2013). Mechanistically, dairy intake, a major source of dietary calcium, potentiates an increase in intracellular calcium concentration. This in turn increases 1, 25-vitamin D_3 and parathyroid hormone levels, causing calcium influx into vascular smooth muscle cells and greater vascular resistance (Kris-Etherton et al, 2009). Alternatively, peptides derived from milk proteins, especially fermented milk products, may function as ACEs, thereby lowering blood pressure (Qin et al, 2009). The DASH trial found that 8-week consumption of a diet high in fruits, vegetables, and fiber; three servings of low-fat dairy products/day; and lower total and saturated fat could lower SBP by 5.5 mm Hg and DBP by 3 mm Hg further than the control diet. The fruit and vegetable diet without dairy foods resulted in blood pressure reductions approximately half that of the DASH diet. The AND Practice Guidelines recommend a diet rich in fruits, vegetables, and low-fat dairy products (versus calcium supplements) for the prevention and management of elevated blood pressure (AND, 2009). An intake of dietary calcium to meet the DRI is recommended.

Cross-sectional studies suggests lower 25-hydroxy vitamin D (25(OH)D) levels are associated with higher blood pressure levels (Fraser et al, 2010) and higher rates of incident hypertension (Kunutsor et al, 2013). Mechanistically, vitamin D has been shown to improve endothelial function, reduce RAS activity, and lower PTH levels. However, recent evidence suggests that supplementation with vitamin D is not effective as a blood pressure lowering agent and therefore is not recommended as a antihypertension agent (Beveridge, 2015).

Magnesium

Magnesium is a potent inhibitor of vascular smooth-muscle contraction and may play a role in blood pressure regulation as a vasodilator. High dietary magnesium often is correlated with lower blood pressure (Sontia and Touyz, 2007). Trials of magnesium supplementation have shown decreases in SBP of 3 to 4 mm Hg and DBP of 2 to 3 mm Hg with greater dose-dependent effects at supplementation of at least 370 mg/day (Kupetsky-Rincon and Uitto, 2012). The DASH dietary pattern emphasizes foods rich in magnesium, including green leafy vegetables, nuts, and whole-grain breads and cereals. Overall food sources of magnesium rather than supplemental doses of the nutrient are encouraged to prevent or control hypertension (AND, 2009).

Potassium

Supplemental doses of potassium in the range of 1900 to 4700 mg/day lower blood pressure approximately 2 to 6 mm Hg DBP and 2 to 4 mm Hg SBP (Dickinson et al, 2006). The effects of potassium are greater in those with higher initial blood pressure, in blacks compared with whites, and in those with higher intakes of sodium. Higher potassium intake also is associated with a lower risk of stroke (Aburto et al, 2013). Although the mechanism by which potassium lowers blood pressure is uncertain, several potential explanations have been offered, including decreased vascular smooth muscle contraction by altering membrane potential or restoring endothelium-dependent vasodilation (Bazzano et al, 2013). Failure of the kidney to adapt to a diet lower in potassium has been linked to sodium-sensitive hypertension.

The large number of fruits and vegetables recommended in the DASH diet makes it easy to meet the dietary potassium recommendations—approximately 4.7 g/day (AND, 2009). In individuals with medical conditions that could impair potassium excretion (e.g., chronic renal failure, diabetes, and congestive HF), a lower potassium intake (less than 4.7 g/day) is appropriate to prevent hyperkalemia. See Appendix 51.

Physical Activity

Less active persons are 30% to 50% more likely to develop hypertension than their active counterparts. Despite the benefits of activity and exercise in reducing disease, many Americans remain inactive. Hispanics (33% men, 40% women), African Americans (27% men, 34% women), and Caucasians (18% men, 22% women) all have a high prevalence of sedentary lifestyles (AHA, 2013). Exercise is beneficial to blood pressure. Increasing the amount of moderate-intensity physical activity to a minimum of 40 minutes on 3 to 4 days per week is an important adjunct to other blood pressure–lowering strategies (Eckel et al, 2013).

Alcohol Consumption

Excessive alcohol consumption is responsible for 5% to 7% of the hypertension in the population (Appel and American Society of Hypertension Writing Group, 2009). A three drink per day amount (a total of 3 oz of alcohol) is the threshold for raising blood pressure and is associated with a 3-mm Hg rise in SBP. For preventing high blood pressure, alcohol intake should be limited to no more than two drinks per day (24 oz of beer, 10 oz of wine, or 2 oz of 80-proof whiskey) in men, and no more than one drink a day is recommended for lighter-weight men and for women.

Medical Management

The goal of hypertension management is to reduce morbidity and mortality from stroke, hypertension-associated heart disease, and renal disease. The three objectives for evaluating patients with hypertension are to (1) identify the possible causes, (2) assess the presence or absence of target organ disease and clinical CVD, and (3) identify other CVD risk factors that help guide treatment. The presence of risk factors and target organ damage determines treatment priority.

Lifestyle modifications are definitive therapy for some and adjunctive therapy for all persons with hypertension. Several months of compliant lifestyle modifications should be tried before drug therapy is initiated. An algorithm for treatment of hypertension is shown in Figure 33-9. Even if lifestyle modifications cannot completely correct blood pressure, these approaches help increase the efficacy of pharmacologic agents and improve other CVD risk factors. Management of hypertension requires a lifelong commitment.

Pharmacologic therapy is necessary for many individuals with hypertension, especially if blood pressure remains elevated after 6 to 12 months of lifestyle changes. The blood pressure target for initiating pharmacologic treatment is 140/90 mm Hg in adults with diabetes, kidney disease, and in the general population of 60 years of age or less to reduce risk of stroke, heart failure, and ASCVD. For individuals more than 60 years of age, the blood pressure target is 150/90 mm Hg because additional health benefits in lowering blood pressure further have not been demonstrated (James et al, 2014). Most patients with

hypertension more severe than stage 1 hypertension require drug treatment; however, lifestyle modifications remain a part of therapy in conjunction with medications. Recommended pharmacologic treatment includes thiazide-type diuretics, calcium channel blockers (CCB), angiotensin-converting enzyme inhibitors (ACEI), or angiotensin receptor blockers (ARB). Thiazide-type diuretics and CCBs are recommended in black populations, including those with diabetes, because they have been shown to be more effective in improving CVD outcomes compare to other classes of medications (James et al, 2014). All these drugs can affect nutrition status (see Chapter 8).

Diuretics lower blood pressure in some patients by promoting volume depletion and sodium loss. At high doses other water-soluble nutrients are also lost and may have to be supplemented. Thiazide diuretics increase urinary potassium excretion, especially in the presence of a high salt intake, thus leading to potassium loss and possible hypokalemia. Except in the case of a potassium-sparing diuretic such as spironolactone or triamterene, additional potassium usually is required. Grapefruits and grapefruit juice can affect the action of many of the calcium channel blockers and should not be consume while taking the medication.

A number of medications either raise blood pressure or interfere with the effectiveness of antihypertensive drugs. These include oral contraceptives, steroids, nonsteroidal anti-inflammatory drugs, nasal decongestants and other cold remedies, appetite suppressants, cyclosporine, tricyclic antidepressants, and monoamine-oxidase inhibitors (see Chapter 8 and Appendix 23).

In addition to standard, conventional medical care, more than 1/3 of Americans also use complementary approaches and this includes treatment of hypertension. Table 33-4 lists some that are most common.

Medical Nutrition Therapy

The appropriate course of nutrition therapy for managing hypertension should be guided by data from a detailed nutrition assessment. Weight history; leisure-time physical activity; and assessment of intake of sodium, alcohol, fat type (e.g., MUFA versus SFA), and other dietary patterns (e.g., intake of fruits, vegetables, and low-fat dairy products) are essential components of the medical and diet history. Nutrition assessment should include evaluation of the individual in the following specific domains to determine nutrition problems and diagnoses: food and nutrient intake; knowledge, beliefs, and attitudes; behavior; physical activity and function; and appropriate biochemical data. Following are the components of the current recommendations for managing elevated blood pressure.

Energy Intake

For each kilogram of weight lost, reductions in SBP and DBP of approximately 1 mm Hg are expected. Hypertensive patients who weigh more than 115% of ideal body weight should be placed on an individualized weight-reduction program that focuses on hypocaloric dietary intake and exercise (see Chapter 21). A modest caloric reduction is associated with a significant lowering of SBP and DBP, and LDL cholesterol levels. Hypocaloric diets that include a low-sodium DASH dietary pattern have produced more significant blood pressure reductions than low-calorie diets emphasizing only low-fat foods. Another benefit of weight loss on blood pressure is the synergistic effect with drug therapy. Weight loss should be an adjunct to drug therapy because it may decrease the dose or number of drugs necessary to control blood pressure.

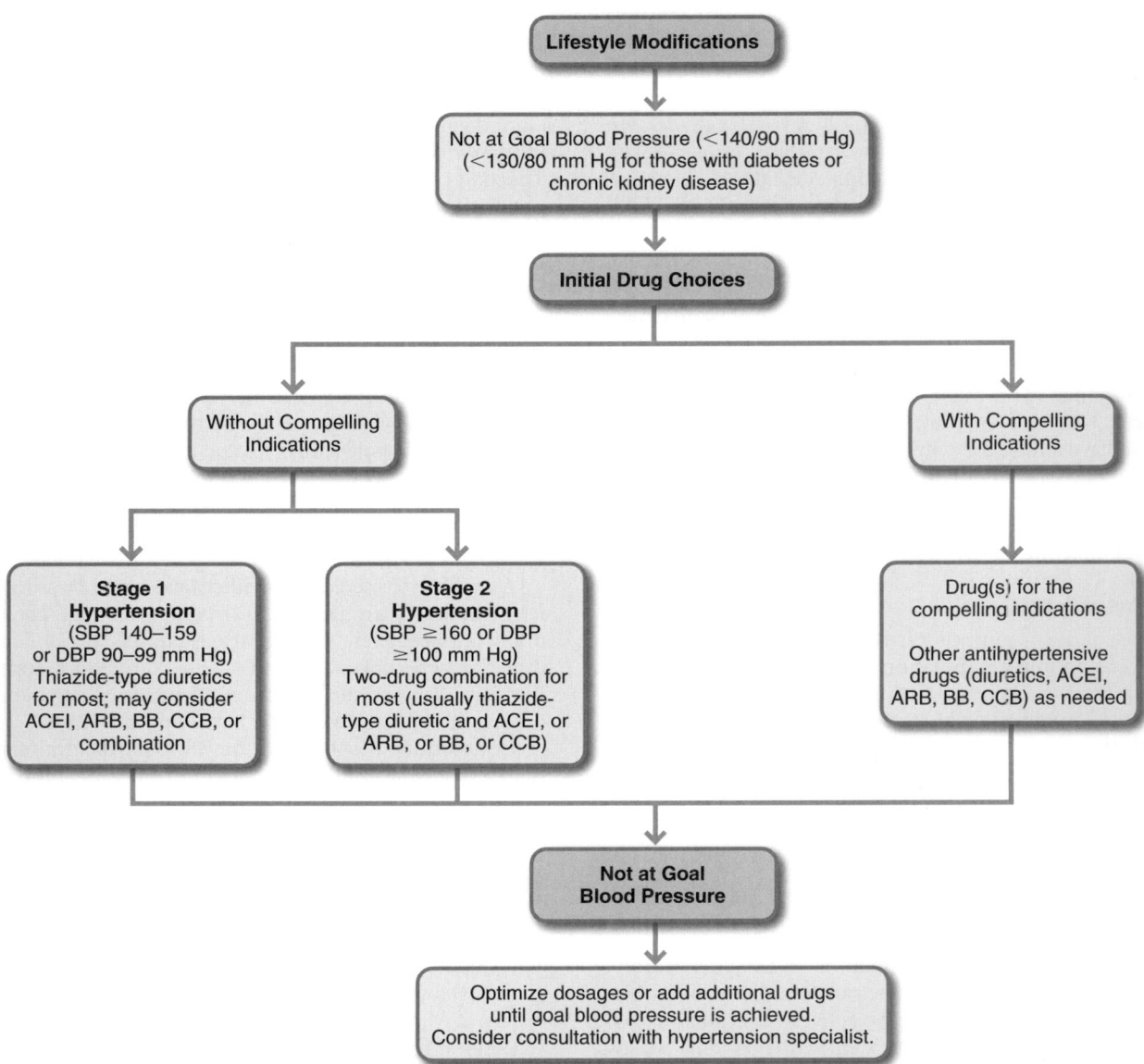

FIGURE 33-9 Algorithm for treatment of hypertension. *ACEI,* Angiotensin-converting enzyme inhibitor; *ARB,* angiotensin-receptor blocker; *BB,* beta-blocker; *CCB,* calcium channel blocker; *DBP,* diastolic blood pressure; *SBP,* systolic blood pressure. (From National Institutes of Health, National Heart, Lung and Blood Institute National High Blood Pressure Education Program: The Seventh Report of the Joint National Committee on Prevention, Detection, Evaluation, and Treatment of High Blood Pressure, NIH Publication No. 04-5230, August 2004.)

DASH Diet

The DASH diet is used for preventing and controlling high blood pressure (see Appendix 26). Successful adoption of this diet requires many behavioral changes: eating twice the average number of daily servings of fruits, vegetables, and dairy products; limiting by one third the usual intake of beef, pork, and ham; eating half the typical amounts of fats, oils, and salad dressings; and eating one quarter the number of snacks and sweets. Lactose-intolerant persons may need to incorporate lactase enzyme or use other strategies to replace milk. Assessing patients' readiness to change and engaging patients in problem solving, decision making, and goal setting are behavioral strategies that may improve adherence (Appel et al, 2006).

The high number of fruits and vegetables consumed on the DASH diet is a marked change from typical patterns of Americans. To achieve the 8 to 10 servings, two to three fruits and vegetables should be consumed at each meal. Importantly, because the DASH diet is high in fiber, gradual increases in fruit, vegetables, and whole-grain foods should be made over time. Eight to 10 cups of fluids daily should be encouraged. Slow changes can reduce potential short-term gastrointestinal disturbances associated with a high-fiber diet, such as bloating and diarrhea. The DASH pattern is advocated in the 2013 ACC/AHA nutrition guidelines on lifestyle management to reduce CVD risk (Eckel et al, 2013). Servings for different calorie levels are shown in Appendix 26.

TABLE 33-4	**Complementary and Alternative Approaches to Lowering Blood Pressure**		
Common Name	**Scientific Name**	**Effect on BP and Mechanism of Action**	**Side Effects and Risks**
Coenzyme Q_{10}	Ubiquinone	Decreases SBP and DBP via a direct effect on the vascular endothelium and smooth muscle	May cause gastrointestinal discomfort, nausea, flatulence, and headaches
Vitamin C and vitamin E taken in combination as supplement	Ascorbic acid α-tocopherol	Decreases SBP and DBP, decreases arterial stiffness, and improves endothelial function by improving antioxidant status	Vitamin E supplementation alone may increase BP
Vitamin D	1,25-dihydroxy vitamin D_3	Decreases SBP via suppression of renin expression and vascular smooth muscle cell proliferation	Hypercalcemia may occur depending on level of supplementation
Fish oil	Omega-3 polyunsaturated fatty acid	At very high doses in hypertensive individuals, SBP and DBP reductions may occur by increasing the endothelium-dependent vasodilatory response; it may also increase the bioavailability of NO in the vascular wall	May cause gastrointestinal discomfort, belching, bad breath, and altered taste
Garlic	Allium sativum	Reduces SBP and DBP in individuals with hypertension via vasodilation resulting from activation of potassium channels; may also be due to activation of NOS	May cause bad breath and body odor
Resveratrol	Trans-3,4′,5-trihydroxystilbene	Reduces systolic BP in animals via enhanced NOS expression in the aorta	Unknown
Mistletoe	Viscum album	Reduces systolic BP in animals via a sympathetic mechanism	Unknown
Hawthorn berry	Crataegus oxycantha, Crataegus monogyna	Exerts a mild, gradual BP lowering effect. The mechanism is unclear	Unknown
Mulberry	Morus alba	Reduces SBP and DBP in animals; the mechanism is unclear	Unknown
Roselle	Hibiscus sabdariffa	Lowers SBP in pre- and mildly hypertensive adults via calcium channel activation	None
Dogbane plant	Rauwolfia serpentine	Reduces SBP by depleting catecholamines and serotonin from central and peripheral synapses	None
Quercetin	3,3′,4′,5,7-pentahydroxyflavone	Reduced SBP via a direct vasodilator effect; also may cause an increase in the bioavailability and biologic activity of NO	May cause joint discomfort with long-term use and gastrointestinal upset unless taken with meals. May increase estradiol and reduce the effectiveness of other forms of estrogen

Data from Fragakis AS, Thomson C: *The health professional's guide to popular dietary supplements*, ed 3, Chicago, 2007, American Dietetic Association. © American Dietetic Association. Reprinted with permission.

BP, Blood pressure; *DBP*, diastolic blood pressure; *NO*, nitric oxide; *NOS*, nitric oxide synthase; *SBP*, systolic blood pressure.

Salt Restriction

The Dietary Guidelines for Americans recommend that young adults consume less than 2300 mg of sodium per day. To lower blood pressure, people with hypertension, African Americans, and middle-aged and elderly people—almost half the population—should heed this advice (Eckel, 2013). Although further blood pressure improvements may be achieved by reducing sodium to 1500 mg/day (Appel et al, 2006), patients with heart failure should be cautioned against use of this dietary approach because adverse health effects of very low sodium diets in these patients have been reported (IOM, 2013). Adherence to diets containing less than 2 g/day of sodium is very difficult to achieve.

In addition to advice to select minimally processed foods, dietary counseling should include instruction on reading food labels for sodium content, avoidance of discretionary salt in cooking or meal preparation (1 tsp salt = 2400 mg sodium), and use of alternative flavorings to satisfy individual taste. The DASH eating plan is rich in fruits and vegetables, which are naturally lower in sodium that many other foods.

Because most dietary salt comes from processed foods and eating out, changes in food preparation and processing can help patients reach the sodium goal. Sensory studies show that commercial processing could develop and revise recipes using lower sodium concentrations and reduce added sodium without affecting consumer acceptance. The food industry is embarking on efforts to reduce sodium in the American diet (see *Focus On: Sodium and the Food Industry*).

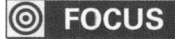 **FOCUS ON**

Sodium and the Food Industry

Most foods sold in supermarkets and restaurants are high in salt. The dramatic differences in sodium from brand to brand suggest that many companies could easily achieve significant reductions without sacrificing taste. According to the Center for Science in the Public Interest (Liebman, 2014), processed foods and restaurant foods contribute approximately 80% of the sodium in Americans' diets; 10% comes from salt added during cooking at home or at the table; the remaining 10% is naturally occurring. Americans now consume approximately 4000 mg of sodium per day—about twice the recommended amount. To help address this problem, the National Academy of Science and Institute of Medicine (2010) issued a report calling for urgent government action to reduce salt in packaged and restaurant foods. The report recommends five strategies to reduce sodium levels in America's food supply. The primary strategy is to set a mandatory national sodium level standard for foods. The interim strategy is voluntary reduction of sodium content in foods by food manufacturers. Supporting strategies are for government agencies, public health and consumer organizations, and the food industry to administer activities to support the reduction of sodium in the food supply and consumers' intake of sodium. An interim investigation of sodium changes made to a representative sample of foods in 2013 suggests an absence of any statistically significant changes in sodium content of the food supply over 6 years (Jacobson et al, 2013). The authors suggest that voluntary action by the food industry has not produced the results that were expected and that stronger action on the part of the FDA is required to reduce the sodium content of packaged and restaurant foods.

Potassium-Calcium-Magnesium

Consuming a diet rich in potassium may lower blood pressure and blunt the effects of salt on blood pressure in some individuals (Appel et al, 2006). The recommended intake of potassium for adults is 4.7 g/day (IOM, 2004). Potassium-rich fruits and vegetables include leafy green vegetables, fruits, and root vegetables. Examples of such foods include oranges, beet greens, white beans, spinach, bananas, and sweet potatoes. Although meat, milk, and cereal products contain potassium, the potassium from these sources is not as well absorbed as that from fruits and vegetables (USDA, 2010).

Increased intakes of calcium and magnesium may have blood pressure benefits, although there are not enough data to support a specific recommendation for increasing levels of intake (AND, 2009). Rather, recommendations suggest meeting the AI intake for calcium and the recommended dietary allowance for magnesium from food sources rather than supplements. The DASH diet plan encourages foods that would be good sources of both nutrients, including low-fat dairy products, dark green leafy vegetables, beans, and nuts.

Lipids

Current recommendations for lipid composition of the diet are recommended to help control weight and decrease the risk of CVD. Omega-3 fatty acids are not highlighted in blood pressure treatment guidelines (AND, 2009), although intakes of fish oils exceeding 2 g/day may have blood pressure benefits.

Alcohol

The diet history should contain information about alcohol consumption. Alcohol intake should be limited to no more than two drinks daily in men, which is equivalent to 2 oz of 80-proof whiskey, 10 oz of wine, or 24 oz of beer. Women or lighter-weight men should consume half this amount.

Exercise

Moderate to-vigorous aerobic activity such as brisk walking done at least three to four times per week, lasting on average 40 minutes per session, is recommended as an adjunct therapy in hypertension management (Eckel et al, 2013). Because exercise is associated strongly with success in weight-reduction and weight-maintenance programs, any increase in activity level should be encouraged for those trying to lose weight. For substantial health benefits, the dietary guidelines recommends at least 2 hours and 30 minutes a week of moderate-intensity physical activity as well as muscle-strengthening activities that include all major muscle groups on 2 or more days for all Americans (USDA, 2010).

Treatment of Hypertension in Children and Adolescents

The prevalence of primary hypertension among children in the United States is increasing in concert with rising obesity rates and increased intakes of high-calorie, high-salt foods (Flynn, 2013). Hypertension tracks into adulthood and has been linked with carotid intimal-medial thickness, LVH, and fibrotic plaque formation. Secondary hypertension is more common in preadolescent children, mostly from renal disease; primary hypertension caused by obesity or a family history of hypertension is more common in adolescents (Miller and Joye Woodward, 2014). In addition, intrauterine growth retardation leads to hypertension in childhood (Longo et al, 2013).

High blood pressure in youth is based on a normative distribution of blood pressure in healthy children. Hypertension is defined as an SBP or DBP of greater than the 95th percentile for age, sex, and height. The designation for prehypertension in children is SBP or DBP of greater than the 90th percentile. Therapeutic lifestyle changes are recommended as an initial treatment strategy for children and adolescents with prehypertension or hypertension. These lifestyle modifications include regular physical activity, avoiding excess weight gain, limiting sodium, and consuming a DASH-type diet.

Weight reduction is considered the primary therapy for obesity-related hypertension in children and adolescents. Unfortunately, sustained weight loss is difficult to achieve in this age group. The Framingham Children's Study showed that children with higher intakes of fruits, vegetables (a combination of four or more servings per day), and dairy products (two or more servings per day) had lower SBP compared with those with lower intakes of these foods. Couch and colleagues (2008) showed that adolescents with prehypertension and hypertension could achieve a significant reduction in SBP in response to a behaviorally oriented nutrition intervention emphasizing the DASH diet. Because adherence to dietary interventions may be particularly challenging among children and teenagers, innovative nutrition intervention approaches that address the unique needs and circumstances of this age group are important considerations in intervention design (see Chapters 17 and 18).

Treatment of Blood Pressure in Older Adults

More than half of the older population has hypertension; this is not a normal consequence of aging. The lifestyle modifications discussed previously are the first step in treatment of older adults, as with younger populations. The Trial of Nonpharmacologic Interventions in the Elderly study found that losing weight (8 to 10 lb) and reducing sodium intake (to 1.8 g/day) can lessen or eliminate the need for drugs in obese, hypertensive older adults. Although losing weight and decreasing sodium in older adults are very effective in lowering blood pressure, knowing how to facilitate these changes and promote adherence remains a challenge for health professionals.

Blood pressure should be controlled regardless of age, initial blood pressure level, or duration of hypertension. Severe sodium restrictions are not adopted because these could lead to volume depletion in older patients with renal damage. Drug treatment in the older adult is supported by very strong data. Additionally, the benefits of treating hypertensive persons age 60 years and older to reach a blood pressure goal of less than 150/90 mm Hg are well supported in the literature (James et al, 2014).

HEART FAILURE

Normally the heart pumps adequate blood to perfuse tissues and meet metabolic needs (see Figure 33-10). In **heart failure (HF)**, formerly called congestive heart failure, the heart cannot provide adequate blood flow to the rest of the body, causing symptoms of fatigue, shortness of breath (**dyspnea**), and fluid retention. Diseases of the heart (valves, muscle, blood

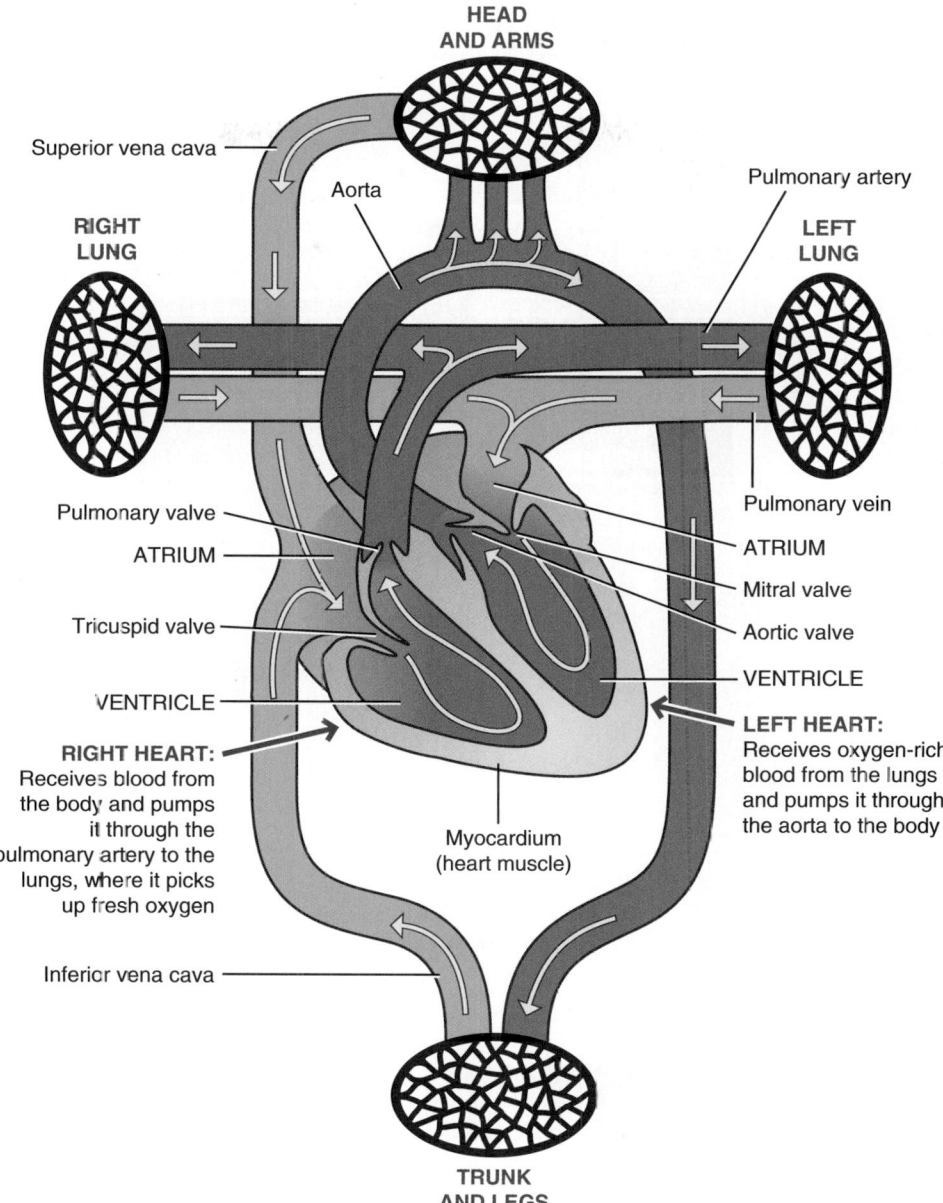

FIGURE 33-10 Structure of the heart pump.

vessels) and vasculature can lead to HF (see *Pathophysiology and Care Management Algorithm:* Heart Failure). HF can be right-sided or left-sided or can affect both sides of the heart. It is further categorized as systolic failure when the heart cannot pump, or eject, blood efficiently out of the heart or diastolic failure, meaning the heart cannot fill with blood as it should.

The lifetime risk of developing HF is 20% for Americans age 40 or older. Approximately 5.1 million in the United States have HF. The incidence increases with age, rising from approximately 20 per 1000 individuals 65 to 69 years to greater than 80 per 1000 in those individuals 85 and older (Stone et al, 2014). Black men have been shown to be at the highest risk of HF; white women have the lowest. HF in non-Hispanic black males and females has a prevalence of 4.5% and 3.8% respectively, versus 2.7% and 1.8% in non-Hispanic white males and females, respectively (Stone et al, 2014).

Pathophysiology

The progression of HF is similar to that of atherosclerosis because there is an asymptomatic phase when damage is silently occurring (stages A and B) (see Figure 33-11). HF is initiated by damage or stress to the heart muscle either of acute MI or insidious (hemodynamic pressure or volume overloading) onset (see Table 33-5 for classifications of HF).

The progressive insult alters the function and shape of the left ventricle such that it hypertrophies in an effort to sustain blood flow, a process known as cardiac remodeling. Symptoms do not usually arise until months or years after cardiac remodeling begins. Many compensatory mechanisms from the SNS, RAS, and cytokine system are activated to restore

PATHOPHYSIOLOGY AND CARE MANAGEMENT ALGORITHM

Heart Failure

ETIOLOGY

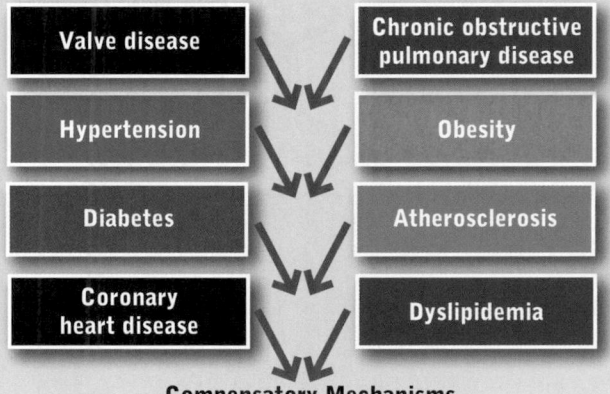

Valve disease	Chronic obstructive pulmonary disease
Hypertension	Obesity
Diabetes	Atherosclerosis
Coronary heart disease	Dyslipidemia

Compensatory Mechanisms
Sympathetic nervous system
Renin-angiotensin system
Cytokine system

Left Ventricular Hypertrophy or Hemodynamic Stress on a Diseased Heart

Dietary sodium excess
Medication noncompliance
Arrhythmias
Pulmonary embolism
Infection
Anemia

Heart Failure

PATHOPHYSIOLOGY

Clinical Findings

- Shortness of breath
- Fatigue
- Fluid retention
- Peripheral vasoconstriciton
- Elevated B-natriuretic peptide
- Mental confusion
- Memory loss
- Anxiety
- Insomnia
- Syncope and headache
- Dry cough

Nutrition Assessment

- Anorexia
- Nausea, abdominal pain and feeling of fullness
- Constipation
- Malabsorption
- Malnutrition
- Cardiac cachexia
- Hypomagnesemia
- Hyponatremia

MANAGEMENT

Medical Management

- ACE inhibitors
- Angiotensin receptor blockers
- Aldosterone blockers
- β-blockers
- Digoxin
- Vasodilators
- Implantable defibrillator
- Heart transplant

Nutrition Management

- Diet low in saturated fat, *trans* fat
- Restricted sodium diet—<3 gm/day
- Increased use of whole grains, fruits, vegetables
- Limit fluid to 2 L per day
- Lose to or maintain appropriate weight
- Magnesium supplementation
- Thiamin supplementation
- Increase physical activity as tolerated
- Avoid tobacco
- Avoid alcohol

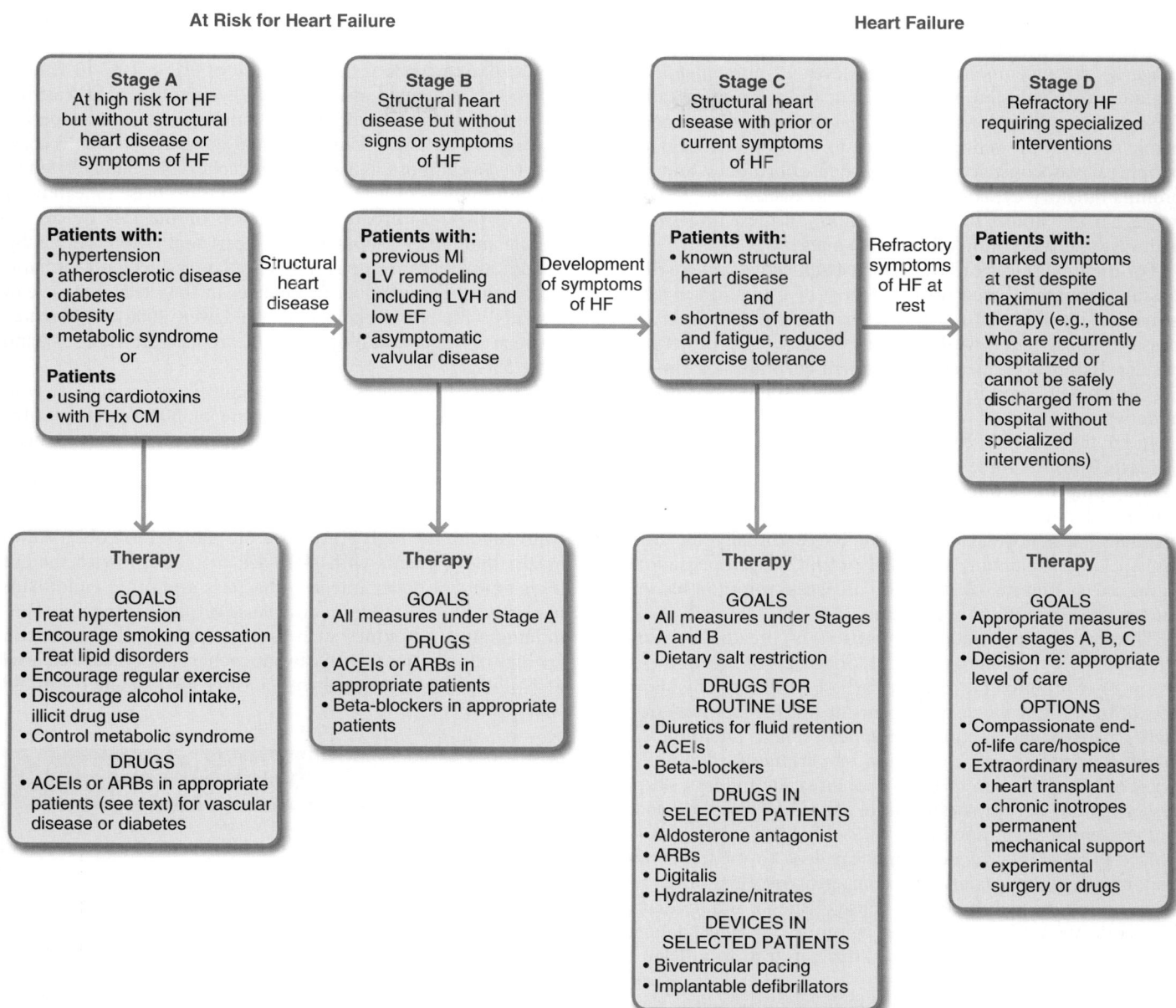

FIGURE 33-11 Stages of heart failure and recommended therapy by stage. *ACEI,* Angiotensin-converting enzyme inhibitor; *ARB,* angiotensin receptor blocker; *CM,* cardiomyopathy; *EF,* ejection fraction; *FHx,* family history; *HF,* heart failure; *IV,* intravenous; *MI,* myocardial infarction; *LV,* left ventricular; *LVH,* left ventricular hypertrophy. (From Hunt SA et al: ACC/AHA 2005 guideline update for the diagnosis and management of chronic heart failure in the adult: a report of the American College of Cardiology/American Heart Association Task Force, *J Am Coll Cardiol* 46:e1, 2005.)

TABLE 33-5	Classifications of Heart Failure
Class I	No undue symptoms associated with ordinary activity and no limitation of physical activity
Class II	Slight limitation of physical activity; patient comfortable at rest
Class III	Marked limitation of physical activity; patient comfortable at rest
Class IV	Inability to carry out physical activity without discomfort; symptoms of cardiac insufficiency or chest pain at rest

Modified from Hunt SA et al: ACC, AHA, 2005 guideline update for the diagnosis and management of chronic heart failure in the adult: a report of the American College of Cardiology/American Heart Association Task Force on practice guidelines, *J Am Coll Cardiol* 46:e1, 2005.

homeostatic function. Proinflammatory cytokines, such as TNF-alpha, IL-1, and IL-6, are increased in blood and the myocardium and have been found to regulate cardiac remodeling.

Another substance, **B-natriuretic peptide (BNP)**, is secreted by the ventricles in response to pressure and is predictive of the severity of HF and mortality at any level of BMI. BNP is often highly elevated in patients with HF (greater than 100 pg/ml is abnormal, and some patients have levels more than 3000 pg/ml). For every 100 pg/mL rise in BNP concentration, there is a corresponding 35% increase in the relative risk of death (Desai, 2013).

Eventually overuse of compensatory systems leads to further ventricle damage, remodeling, and worsening of symptoms (stage C). HF patients have elevated levels of norepinephrine, angiotensin II, aldosterone, endothelin, and vasopressin; all of these are neurohormonal factors that increase the hemodynamic stress on the ventricle by causing sodium retention and peripheral vasoconstriction. These neurohormones and the proinflammatory cytokines contribute to disease progression; hence, current studies focus on inhibition of these undesirable pathways and promotion of desirable ones.

For the final stages of HF, there is a subjective scale used to classify symptoms based on the degree of limitation in daily activities (see Table 33-6). The severity of symptoms in this classification system is weakly related to the severity of left ventricular dysfunction; therefore treatment encompasses improving functional capacity and lessening progression of the underlying disease.

In HF the heart can compensate for poor cardiac output by (1) increasing the force of contraction, (2) increasing in size, (3) pumping more often, and (4) stimulating the kidneys to conserve sodium and water. For a time this compensation maintains near-normal circulation, but eventually the heart can no longer maintain a normal output (decompensation). Advanced symptoms can develop in weeks or months, and sudden death can occur at any time.

Three symptoms—fatigue, shortness of breath, and fluid retention—are the hallmarks of HF. Shortness of breath on exertion, or effort intolerance, is the earliest symptom. This shortness of breath gets worse and occurs at rest (orthopnea) or at night (paroxysmal nocturnal dyspnea). Fluid retention can manifest as pulmonary congestion or peripheral edema. Evidence of hypoperfusion includes cool forearms and legs, sleepiness, declining serum sodium level caused by fluid overload, and worsening renal function.

Decreased cranial blood supply can lead to mental confusion, memory loss, anxiety, insomnia, syncope (loss of oxygen to the brain causing brief loss of consciousness), and headache. The latter symptoms are more common in older patients and often are the only symptoms; this can lead to a delay in diagnosis. Often the first symptom in older adults is a dry cough with generalized weakness and anorexia.

Cardiac cachexia is the end result of HF in 10% to 15% of patients. It is defined as involuntary weight loss of at least 6% of nonedematous body weight during a 6-month period (Springer et al, 2006). Unlike normal starvation, which is characterized by adipose tissue loss, this cachexia is characterized by a significant loss of lean body mass. This decrease in lean body mass further exacerbates HF because of the loss of cardiac muscle and the development of a heart that is soft and flabby. In addition, there are structural, circulatory, metabolic, inflammatory, and neuroendocrine changes in the skeletal muscle of patients with HF (Delano and Moldawer, 2006). Differences between younger and older patients are listed in Box 33-7 and Table 33-7.

Cardiac cachexia is a serious complication of HF with a poor prognosis and mortality rate of 50% in 18 months (Carlson and Dahlin, 2014). Symptoms that reflect inadequate blood supply to the abdominal organs include anorexia, nausea, a feeling of fullness, constipation, abdominal pain, malabsorption, hepatomegaly, and liver tenderness. All of these contribute to the high prevalence of malnutrition observed in hospitalized patients with HF. Lack of blood flow to the gut leads to loss of bowel integrity; bacteria and other endotoxins may enter the bloodstream and cause cytokine activation. Proinflammatory cytokines such as TNF-alpha and adiponectin are highest in patients with cardiac cachexia. An increased level of TNF-alpha is associated with a lower BMI, smaller skinfold

---

BOX 33-7 Principal Effects of Aging on Cardiovascular Structure and Function

Increased vascular stiffness
Increased myocardial stiffness
Decreased beta-adrenergic responsiveness
Impaired mitochondrial ATP production
Decreased baroreceptor responsiveness
Impaired sinus node function
Impaired endothelial function
Net effect: Marked reduction in cardiovascular reserve

From Rich MW: Office management of heart failure in the elderly, *Am Med* 118:342, 2005.
ATP, Adenosine triphosphate.

TABLE 33-6 Skeletal Muscle Changes in Heart Failure

Function loss	Weakness
	Fatigability
Structural	Loss of muscle mass
	Atrophy, fibrosis, no ≠ apoptosis
	Fiber type switch type I–type IIb
	Loss of mitochondria
	Endothelial damage
Blood flow	Capillary density ↓
	Vasodilation
	Peak leg blood flow ↓
Metabolism	Proteolysis
	Oxidative metabolism ↓ Acidosis glycolysis ≠
Inflammation	Cytokine and oxidative markers
Neuroendocrine	GH, IGF-1, epinephrine, norepinephrine, cortisol
Inactivity	TNF-α ≠ ≠
Genetic factors	Myostatin, IGF

From Strassburg S et al: Muscle wasting in cardiac cachexia, *Int J Biochem Cell Biol* 37:1938, 2005.
GH, Growth hormone; *IGF,* insulin-like growth factor; *TNF-α.* tumor necrosis factor-α.

TABLE 33-7 Heart Failure in Middle Age versus Older Adulthood

	Middle Age	Older Adulthood
Prevalence	<1%	≈10%
Sex	Men > women	Women > men
Cause	CAD	Hypertension
Clinical features	Typical	Atypical
LVEF	Reduced	Normal
Comorbidities	Few	Multiple
RCTs	Many	Few
Therapy	Evidence-based	Empiric
Physician treating HF	Cardiologist	Primary care

From Rich MW: Office management of heart failure in the elderly, *Am J Med* 118:342, 2005.
CAD, Coronary artery disease; *HF,* heart failure; *LVEF,* left ventricular ejection fraction; *RCT,* randomized clinical trial.

measurements, and decreased plasma total protein levels, indicative of a catabolic state.

Adiponectin levels are high in HF and are a marker for wasting and a predictor of mortality. As with TNF-alpha, adiponectin levels also are correlated inversely with BMI. Pharmacological treatments for muscle wasting are being explored.

Risk Factors

The Framingham Study (see *Focus On:* Framingham Heart Study) showed the risk factors for HF were hypertension, diabetes, ASCVD, and left ventricular hypertrophy (LVH) (enlargement of the left ventricle of the heart). Antecedent hypertension is present in about three fourths of HF patients. Individuals who have diabetes mellitus and ischemic heart disease more frequently develop HF compared with patients without diabetes (Rosano et al, 2006). Diabetes is an especially strong risk factor for HF in women. The prevalence of hypertension and diabetes increases with age, making the elderly particularly vulnerable to HF. Another large cohort study of older adults (70 to 79 years) showed that waist circumference and percentage of body fat were the strongest predictors of who would develop HF (Nicklas et al, 2006). Numerous changes in cardiovascular structure and function also place the elderly at high risk for developing HF (see Box 33-7).

Prevention

Because long-term survival rates for persons with HF are low, prevention is critical. HF is categorized into four stages ranging from persons with risk factors (stage A—primary prevention) to persons with advanced HF (stage D—severe disease). For stages A and B the aggressive treatment of underlying risk factors and diseases such as dyslipidemia, hypertension, and diabetes is critical to prevent structural damage to the myocardium and the appearance of HF symptoms. Such prevention has been very effective. Even patients who experience an MI can reduce the risk of HF with antihypertensive therapy. Patients are often asymptomatic during these two stages.

For stages C and D, secondary prevention strategies to prevent further cardiac dysfunction are warranted. These strategies include the use of ACE inhibitors (first line of therapy), angiotensin receptor blockers, aldosterone blockers, beta-blockers, and digoxin. Early detection, correction of asymptomatic left ventricular dysfunction, and aggressive management of risk factors are needed to lower the incidence and mortality of HF.

Medical Management

Therapy recommendations correspond to the stage of HF. For patients at high risk of developing HF (stage A), treatment of the underlying conditions (hypertension, dyslipidemia, thyroid disorders, arrhythmias), avoidance of high-risk behaviors (tobacco, excessive alcohol, illicit drug use), and lifestyle changes (weight reduction, exercise, reduction of sodium intake, heart-healthy diet) are recommended. All these recommendations are carried through the other stages. In addition, an implantable defibrillator, which shocks the heart when it stops, can be placed in patients at risk of sudden death. Pharmacologic treatment of HF is the hallmark of therapy with progressive stages.

The last stage also includes surgically implanted ventricular-assist devices, heart transplantation, and continual intravenous therapy.

The short-term goals for the treatment of HF are to relieve symptoms, improve the quality of life, and reduce depression if it is present. The long-term goal of treatment is to prolong life by lessening, stopping, or reversing left ventricular dysfunction. Medical management is tailored to clinical and hemodynamic profiles with evidence of hypoperfusion and congestion. In some cases, surgical procedures are needed to alleviate the HF caused by valvular disease; medical management is limited in these instances.

Standard fluid restrictions are to limit total fluid intake to 2 L (2000 ml) daily. When patients are severely decompensated, a more restrictive fluid intake (1000 to 1500 ml daily) may be warranted for adequate diuresis. A sodium-restricted diet should be maintained despite low-sodium blood levels because in this case the sodium has shifted from the blood to the tissues. Serum sodium appears low in a patient who is fluid overloaded because of dilution; diuresis improves the levels by decreasing the amount of water in the vascular space.

An ACE inhibitor is the first line of pharmacologic treatment for HF. As the stages progress, a beta-blocker or angiotensin receptor blocker may be added. In Stages C and D selected patients also may take a diuretic, aldosterone antagonists, digitalis, and vasodilators (e.g., hydralazine). Basically these medications reduce excess fluid, dilate blood vessels, and increase the strength of the heart's contraction. Several of these medications have neurohormonal benefits along with their primary mechanism of action. For example, ACE inhibitors (e.g., captopril, enalapril) not only inhibit the RAS but also improve symptoms, quality of life, exercise tolerance, and survival. Similarly, spironolactone has diuretic and aldosterone-blocking functions that result in reduced morbidity and mortality in patients. Most of these medications can affect nutrition status (see Chapter 8).

Medical Nutrition Therapy

The RDN provides MNT, which includes assessment, a nutrition diagnosis, and interventions (education, counseling). As part of a multidisciplinary team (physician, pharmacist, psychologist, nurse, and social worker), the RDN positively affects patient outcomes. Reduced readmission to the hospital, fewer days in the hospital, improved compliance with restricted sodium and fluid intakes, and improved quality of life scores are the goals in HF patients.

Nutrition screening for HF in older adults can help prevent disease progression and improve disease management, overall health, and quality-of-life outcomes. The first step in screening is determination of body weight. Altered fluid balance complicates assessment of body weight in the patient with HF. Weights should be taken before eating and after voiding at the same time each day. A dry weight (weight without edema) should be determined on the scale at home. Patients should record daily weights and advise their care providers if weight gain exceeds more than 1 lb a day for patients with severe HF, more than 2 lb a day for patients with moderate HF, and more than 3 to 5 lb with mild HF. Restricting sodium and fluids along with diuretic therapy may restore fluid balance and prevent full-blown HF.

TABLE 33-8 Dietary Sodium Intake in Heart Failure

Guideline	Year	Sodium/Fluid Restriction Recommendations	Level of Evidence
National Heart Foundation of Australia/ Cardiac Society of Australia and New Zealand	2006[7]	<3 g/d for NYHA class II without peripheral edema/<2 g/d for NYHA class III and IV	C
		<2 L/d for all patients and <1.5 L/d during fluid retention episodes	
Heart Failure Society, India	2007[5]	<2 g/d	Not stated
		<2 L/d	
European Society of Cardiology	2008[5]	Moderate restriction 1.5-2 L/d in patients with severe symptoms and especially with hyponatremia	C
Canadian Cardiovascular Society	2008[6]	<2 g/d	Not stated
		2 L/d	
American College of Cardiology/ American Heart Association	2009[2]	Moderate restriction (≤2 g/d, if volume overload, followed by fluid intake restriction to 2 L/d if fluid retention persists)	C
Royal College of Physicians	2010[3]	*Salt reduction Fluid restriction*	Limited; further research required
Heart Failure Society of America	2010[8]	2-3 g/d; <2 g/d may be considered in moderate to severe heart failure	C
		<2 L/d, if fluid retention persists and if severe hyponatremia (serum Na <130 mEq/L) is present	
Scottish Intercollegiate Guidelines Network	2010[9]	<2.4 g/d tailored fluid restriction	1+
American Dietetic Association	2011[10]	<2 g/d1.4-1.9 L/d depending on clinical symptoms	Fair

Level of Evidence: *C*, Limited populations evaluated. Only consensus opinion of experts, case studies, or standard of care; *Fair*, Benefits exceed the harms but quality of evidence is not as strong; *1+*, well-conducted meta-analysis, systemic reviews, or randomized controlled trials with low risk of bias.
NYHA, New York Heart Association.
From American Heart Association: *Contemporary Reviews in Cardiovascular Medicine* (website): http://circ.ahajournals.org/content/126/4/479/T1.expansion.html, 2015. Accessed May 2, 2015.

Dietary assessments in HF patients reveal that more than half have malnutrition, usually related to the cardiac cachexia mentioned earlier. Negative energy balance and negative nitrogen balances can be noted. In overweight patients, caloric reduction must be monitored carefully to avoid excessive and rapid body protein catabolism. Nutrition education to promote behavior change is a critical component of MNT. The benefits of MNT should be communicated to patients.

The total diet must be addressed in patients with HF because underlying risk factors are often present; dietary changes to modify these risk factors are an important component of MNT. For dyslipidemia or atherosclerosis, a heart-healthy diet low in SFAs, trans fatty acids, and cholesterol and high in fiber, whole grains, fruits, and vegetables is recommended. For persons with hypertension, the DASH diet is recommended. Both of these dietary patterns emphasize lower-sodium foods and higher intake of potassium. Total energy expenditure is higher in HF patients because of the catabolic state, adequate protein and energy should be provided.

Salt Restriction

Excessive sodium intake is associated with fluid retention and edema. A 2-g sodium restriction is regularly prescribed for patients with HF. The AND (2012) evidence analysis library recommends a 2-g sodium restriction but notes that the evidence for this recommendation is only "fair." The Heart Failure Society of America recommends 2 to 3 g of sodium daily unless severe symptoms are present, then the recommendation is for 2 g (Gupta et al, 2012). The updated AHA recommendation is for "moderate" sodium restriction. Table 33-8 summarizes the recommendations from multiple organizations. The inconsistencies in the different organizations are due to the weak database of studies. Many have small sample sizes and many were not randomized trials. Three of the larger studies that were randomized had consistent results but showed that sodium restriction was associated with worse outcome (Gupta et al, 2012). It is hypothesized that this effect may be related to neurohormones including aldosterone, norepinephrine, and angiotensin II, all of which increased with dietary restriction. These hormones act to conserve fluid, thus trying to restore blood flow. Aldosterone promotes sodium reabsorption, and vasopressin promotes water conservation in the distal tubules of the nephron. This complex balance is further complicated by the medications used for HF.

Patient compliance with sodium restriction of 2 g/day has been shown to be poor. This can lead to generally inadequate nutritional intake that may be a contributing factor to poor outcomes associated with sodium restriction. A one-size-fits-all sodium restriction is not possible. The HF stage, amount of edema present, overall nutritional status, and medications must be taken into consideration. There is consensus that high sodium intake (above 3 g/day) is contraindicated for HF.

The degree of restriction depends on the individual (see *Focus On*: Sodium and Salt Measurement Equivalents).

⊚ FOCUS ON

Sodium and Salt Measurement Equivalents

Sodium chloride is approximately 40% (39.3%) sodium and 60% chloride. To convert a specified weight of sodium chloride to its sodium equivalent, multiply the weight by 0.393. Sodium also is measured in milliequivalents (mEq). To convert milligrams of sodium to mEq, divide by the atomic weight of 23. To convert sodium to sodium chloride (salt), multiply by 2.54. Millimoles (mmol) and milliequivalents (mEq) of sodium are the same. For example:

1 tsp of salt = approximately 6 g NaCl = 6096 mg NaCl
6096 mg NaCl × 0.393 = 2396 mg Na (approximately 2400 mg)
2396 mg Na/23 = 104 mEq Na
1 g Na = 1000 mg/23 = 43 mEq or mmol
1 tsp of salt = 2400 mg or 104 mEq Na

Adherence to sodium restrictions can be problematic for many individuals, and individualized instruction is recommended. Ethnic differences in sodium consumption must be considered. Some cultures have traditional diets that are very high in sodium such as Kosher and Asian diets. In some cases regional cooking, like in some areas in the southern United States, depends heavily on salt.

Positive outcomes (i.e., decreased urinary sodium excretion, less fatigue, less frequent edema) have been observed in HF patients receiving MNT. The type of sodium restriction prescribed should be the least restrictive diet that will achieve the desired results. The first step is to minimize or eliminate the use of table salt and high-sodium foods (see Box 33-8) (see Appendix 30 for further explanation of the sodium-restricted diet).

Poor adherence to low-sodium diets occurs in part as a result of lack of knowledge about sodium and lower-sodium food choices by the patient, and perception that the diet interferes with the social aspects of eating. Lack of cooking skills or adequate cooking facilities is another obstacle because it leads patients to eat premade foods that tend to be high in salt. Memory loss, severe fatigue, and economic issues are all challenges to following a low-sodium diet. In addition, food labels, although informative, may be hard for many patients or their caregivers to comprehend (see Box 33-9).

Alcohol

In excess, alcohol contributes to fluid intake and raises blood pressure. Many cardiologists recommend avoiding alcohol. Chronic alcohol ingestion may lead to cardiomyopathy and HF (Li and Ren, 2006). Although heavy drinking should be discouraged, there is no evidence to support total abstinence from alcohol (AND, 2012). Quantity, drinking patterns, and genetic factors influence the relationship between alcohol consumption and HF (Djousse and Gaziano, 2008). If alcohol is consumed, intake should not exceed one drink per day for women and two drinks per day for men. A drink is equivalent to 1 oz of alcohol (1 oz of distilled liquor), 5 oz of wine, or 12 oz of beer.

BOX 33-8 Top Ten Categories of High-Sodium Foods

1. Smoked, processed, or cured meats and fish (e.g., ham, bacon, corned beef, cold cuts, hot dogs, sausage, salt pork, chipped beef, pickled herring, anchovies, tuna, and sardines)
2. Tomato juices and tomato sauce, unless labeled otherwise
3. Meat extracts, bouillon cubes, meat sauces, MSG,* and taco seasoning
4. Salted snacks (potato chips, tortilla chips, corn chips, pretzels, salted nuts, popcorn, and crackers)
5. Prepared salad dressings, condiments, relishes, ketchup, Worcestershire sauce, barbecue sauce, cocktail sauce, teriyaki sauce, soy sauce, commercial salad dressings, salsa, pickles, olives, and sauerkraut
6. Packaged mixes for sauces, gravies, casseroles, and noodle, rice, or potato dishes; macaroni and cheese; stuffing mix
7. Cheeses (processed and cheese spreads)
8. Frozen entrees and pot pies
9. Canned soup
10. Foods eaten away from home

*MSG, Monosodium glutamate.
Note: Reading labels is most important; some brands are lower in sodium than others.

BOX 33-9 Food Labeling Guide for Sodium

Sodium-free	Less than 5 mg per standard serving; cannot contain any sodium chloride
Very low sodium	35 mg or less per standard serving
Low sodium	140 mg or less per standard serving
Reduced sodium	At least 25% less sodium per standard serving than in the regular food
Light in sodium	50% less sodium per standard serving than in the regular food
Unsalted, without added salt, or no salt added	No salt added during processing; the product it resembles is normally processed with salt
Lightly salted	50% less added sodium than is normally added; product must state "not a low-sodium food" if that criterion is not met

http://www.fda.gov/Food/IngredientsPackagingLabeling/LabelingNutrition/ucm315393.htm. Accessed March 25, 2016.

Caffeine

Until now caffeine has been considered detrimental to patients with HF because it contributes to irregular heartbeats. However, a study in the Netherlands suggests that moderate intake of either tea or coffee reduces ASCVD risk; tea actually reduces ASCVD deaths (de Konig Gans et al, 2010). Researchers in the United States followed 130,054 men and women and found that those who reported drinking four or more cups of coffee each day had an 18% lower risk of hospitalization for heart rhythm disturbances. Those who reported drinking one to three cups each day had a 7% reduction in risk (Klatsky, 2010). The antioxidant effects of coffee and tea may be beneficial.

Calcium

Patients with HF are at increased risk of developing osteoporosis because of low activity levels, impaired renal function, and prescription drugs that alter calcium metabolism (Zittermann et al, 2006). Cachectic HF patients have lower bone mineral density and lower calcium levels than HF patients without cachexia (Anker et al, 2006). Caution must be used with calcium supplements because they may aggravate cardiac arrhythmias.

L-Arginine

In patients with HF, decreased exercise capacity may be in part due to reduced peripheral blood flow related to impairment of endothelium-dependent vasodilation. L-Arginine is converted to nitric oxide, an endothelium-derived relaxing factor. At least four studies have showed some benefit with supplementation. The studies were small, and more research is needed to establish clear recommendations.

Coenzyme Q10

Some studies on the use of coenzyme Q_{10} (CoQ_{10}) supplementation in HF patients showed positive outcome. Outcomes included significantly improved exercise tolerance, decreased symptoms, and improved quality of life. CoQ_{10} levels are generally low in HF patients; it is postulated that repletion can prevent oxidative stress and further myocardial damage. A systematic review of 7 studies and over 900 patients on the use of CoQ10 in HF patients concluded that the studies were too small and too diverse in study design to draw any useful conclusions (Madmani et al, 2014). Patients on statins (HMG-CoA reductase inhibitors) may have a different reason to consider supplementation. HMG-CoA reductase inhibitors are a class of cholesterol-lowering drugs that are known to interfere with synthesis of CoQ_{10} (see Chapter 8).

D-Ribose

D-ribose is a component of ATP for cellular metabolism and energy production. Myocardial ischemia lowers cellular energy levels, integrity, and function. The failing heart is energy starved. D-ribose is being tested to correct this deficient cellular energy as a naturally occurring carbohydrate (Shecterle et al, 2010).

Energy

The energy needs of patients with HF depend on their current dry weight, activity restrictions, and the severity of the HF. Overweight patients with limited activity should be encouraged to maintain an appropriate weight that will not stress the myocardium. However, the nutrition status of the obese patient must be assessed to ensure that the patient is not malnourished. In patients with HF, energy needs are unclear. At least two studies found that standard energy equations used to determine calorie needs underestimated the needs of HF patients. Another study found lower calorie needs when compared with healthy controls (AND, 2012). This area requires more research. Standard nutritional assessment should be employed with careful monitoring.

Fats

Fish consumption and fish oils rich in omega-3 fatty acids can lower elevated triglyceride levels and may prevent atrial fibrillation in HF patients (Roth and Harris, 2010). Intake of at least 1 g daily of omega-3 fatty acids from either oily fish or fish-oil supplements was used in the study. However, further studies are needed. Some evidence suggests that high saturated fat feeding in mild to moderate HF preserves contractile function and prevents the switch from fatty acid to glucose metabolism, thus serving a cardioprotective role (Chess et al, 2009; Christopher et al, 2010).

Meal Strategies

Patients with HF often tolerate small, frequent meals better than larger, infrequent meals because the latter are more tiring to consume, can contribute to abdominal distention, and markedly increase oxygen consumption. All these factors tax the already stressed heart. Caloric supplements can help to increase energy intake; however, this intervention may not reverse this form of malnutrition (Anker et al, 2006).

Folate, Vitamin B₆, and Vitamin B₁₂

High dietary intakes of folate and vitamin B_6 have been associated with reduced risk of mortality from HF and stroke in some populations (Cui et al, 2010). However, deficiencies of vitamin B12 and folate have been studied and found to be relatively rare in HF patients (van der Wall et al 2015).

Magnesium

Magnesium deficiency is common in patients with HF as a result of poor dietary intake and the use of diuretics, including furosemide. As with potassium, the diuretics used to treat HF increase magnesium excretion. Magnesium deficiency aggravates changes in electrolyte concentration by causing a positive sodium and negative potassium balance. Because deficient magnesium status is associated with poorer prognosis, blood magnesium levels should be measured in HF patients and treated accordingly. Magnesium supplementation (800 mg/day) produces small improvements in arterial compliance (Fuentes

et al, 2006). Poor dietary intake of magnesium has been associated with elevated CRP, a product of inflammation. Hypermagnesemia may be found in some cases of renal failure, HF, and high doses of furosemide.

Thiamin

Patients with HF are at risk for thiamin deficiency because of poor food intake; use of loop diuretics, which increases excretion; and advanced age. Thiamin is a required coenzyme in the energy-producing reactions that fuel myocardial contraction. Therefore, thiamin deficiency can cause decreased energy and weaker heart contractions. Studies have shown thiamin deficiency to be associated with HF, in great part due to the effect of commonly used medications. Loop diuretics (e.g. furosemide) can deplete body thiamin and cause metabolic acidosis. Supplementation with thiamin has been shown to improve cardiac function, urine output, weight loss and signs and symptoms of HF (DiNicolantonio et al, 2013). Thiamin deficiency is diagnosed using erythrocyte thiamin pyrophosphate. Thiamin status should be assessed in HF patients on loop diuretics and appropriate supplementation recommended if necessary. Thiamin supplementation (e.g., 100 mg/day) can improve left ventricular ejection fraction (fraction of blood pumped out of the ventricles with each heartbeat) and symptoms.

Vitamin D

Patients with a polymorphism of the vitamin D receptor gene have higher rates of bone loss than HF patients without this genotype. Vitamin D may improve inflammation in HF patients (Vieth and Kimball, 2006). In a double-blind, randomized, placebo-controlled trial, supplementation with vitamin D (50 mcg or 2000 international units of vitamin D_3 per day) for 9 months increased the anti-inflammatory cytokine IL-10 and decreased the proinflammatory factors in HF patients (Schleithoff et al, 2006). As a steroid hormone, vitamin D regulates gene expression and inversely regulates renin secretion (Meems et al, 2011). However, it remains unclear if vitamin D supplementation truly is needed in HF patients.

CARDIAC TRANSPLANTATION

Cardiomyopathies represent a heterogeneous group of diseases that often lead to progressive HF; types include dilated cardiomyopathy, hypertrophic cardiomyopathy, restrictive cardiomyopathy, and arrhythmogenic right ventricular cardiomyopathy (Wexler et al, 2009). Cardiac transplantation is the only cure for refractory, end-stage HF. Because the number of donor hearts is limited, careful selection of recipients with consideration of the likelihood for adherence to lifelong therapeutic regimen and their quality of life is imperative. Nutrition support before and after transplantation is crucial to decrease morbidity and mortality. Thus the nutrition care of the heart transplant patient can be divided into three phases: pretransplant, immediate posttransplant, and long-term posttransplant.

Pretransplant Medical Nutrition Therapy

A comprehensive nutrition assessment of the pretransplant patient should include a history, physical and anthropometric assessment, and biochemical testing. Recommended lifestyle changes before transplantation include restricting alcohol consumption, losing weight, exercising, quitting smoking, and eating a low-sodium diet (Wexler et al, 2009). Extremes in body weight (less than 80% or more than 140% of ideal body weight) increase the patient's risk for infection, diabetes, morbidity, and higher mortality. Pretransplant comorbidities such as hyperlipidemia and hypertension also reduce survival rates. If oral intake is inadequate, an enteral feeding should be tailored to the nutritional and comorbid conditions of the patient.

Immediate Posttransplant Nutrition Support

Nutrition guidelines are consistent for all types of organ transplants and not specific just to heart transplants (see Table 33-9). The nutritional goals in the acute posttransplant patient are to (1) provide adequate protein and calories to treat catabolism and promote healing, (2) monitor and correct electrolyte abnormalities, and (3) achieve optimal blood glucose control (Hasse, 2015). In the immediate posttransplant period nutrient needs are increased, as is the case after any major surgery. Protein needs are increased because of steroid-induced catabolism, surgical stress, anabolism, and wound healing.

Patients progress from clear liquids to a soft diet given in small, frequent feedings. Enteral feeding may be appropriate in the short term, especially if complications arise. Nutrient intake is often maintained by using liquid supplements and foods of high caloric density, especially in patients with poor appetite. Weight gain to an ideal weight is the nutritional goal for patients who were cachectic before transplant. The increase in cardiac function helps to halt the presurgical cachectic state. Hyperglycemia can be exacerbated by the stress of the surgery and the immunosuppressive drug regimen. Dietary adjustments can be made to aid in glucose control (see Table 33-9).

Long-Term Posttransplant Nutrition Support

Comorbid conditions that often occur after transplantation include hypertension, excessive weight gain, hyperlipidemia, osteoporosis, and infection. Hypertension is managed by diet, exercise, and medications. Minimizing excessive weight gain is important because patients who become obese after transplantation are at higher risk for rejection and lower rates of survival.

Increases in total LDL cholesterol and triglycerides are a consequence of immunosuppressive drug therapy and increase the risk of HF after transplantation. Along with a heart-healthy diet, patients also need a lipid-lowering drug regimen to normalize blood lipids. Statins are recommended in the early and long-term postoperative periods. Because of their LDL-lowering effect, stanols or sterols may be helpful to reduce statin dosages (Goldberg et al, 2006).

Before transplantation, patients are likely to have osteopenia because of their lack of activity and cardiac cachexia. After transplantation, patients are susceptible to steroid-induced osteoporosis. Patients require optimal calcium and vitamin D intake to slow bone loss; weight-bearing exercise and antiresorptive drug therapy are often necessary. Infection must be avoided because of the necessity of lifelong use of immunosuppressive drugs. Food safety should be discussed.

TABLE 33-9   Posttransplant Nutrient Recommendations

Nutrient	Short-Term Recommendations	Long-Term Recommendations
Calories	120%-140% of BEE (30-35 kcal/kg) or measure REE	Maintenance: 120%-130% BEE (20-30 kcal/kg) depending on activity level
Protein	1.3-2 g/kg/day	1 g/kg/day
Carbohydrate	~50% of calories Restrict simple sugars if glucose level elevated	~50% of calories Restrict simple sugars and encourage high-fiber complex carbohydrate choices
Fat	30% of calories (or higher with severe hyperglycemia)	≤30% of total calories <10% of calories as saturated fat
Calcium	1200 mg/day	1200-1500 mg/day (consider the need for estrogen or vitamin D supplements)
Sodium	2 g/day	2 g/day
Magnesium and phosphorus	Encourage intake of foods high in these nutrients Supplement as needed	Encourage intake of foods high in these nutrients Supplement as needed
Potassium	Supplement or restrict based on serum potassium levels	Supplement or restrict based on serum potassium levels
Other vitamins and minerals	Multivitamin/mineral– supplement to RDI levels May need additional supplements to replete suspected or confirmed deficiencies	Multivitamin/mineral– supplement to RDI levels May need additional supplements to replete suspected or confirmed deficiencies
Other	Avoid complementary or alternative products without proven safety and effectiveness in transplant patients	Avoid complementary or alternative products without proven safety and effectiveness in transplant patients

CLINICAL CASE STUDY

Tom is a 55-year-old single man with hypertension (blood pressure 145/92), high low-density lipoprotein cholesterol (241), and low high-density lipoprotein cholesterol (38) and a CRP of 4mg/L. He has a strong family history of heart disease. He reports that he often eats in his car, so he frequents fast-food restaurants. He works long hours and, other than gardening on the weekends, he does not exercise. He is 5'10" and 220 lb. His breakfast is usually a cheese-egg biscuit, bacon, and coffee without milk or cream. Lunch is often a bean and cheese burrito and ice cream. His favorite dinner is fried chicken, mashed potatoes with gravy, collards sautéed with bacon fat, and pie.

Using the following list, what are Tom's nutritional diagnoses? Which should be the top priority?

Nutrition Diagnostic Term

Excessive energy intake
Excessive intake of fats
Excessive alcohol intake
Inadequate fiber intake
Inadequate calcium intake
Inadequate magnesium intake
Inadequate potassium intake
Excessive sodium intake
Overweight or obesity
Food- and nutrition-related knowledge deficit
Undesirable food choices
Physical inactivity

Nutrition Care Questions

Which interventions would be most beneficial for Tom?
What signs and symptoms would you want to monitor and evaluate?

USEFUL WEBSITES

American Association of Cardiovascular and Pulmonary Rehabilitation
http://www.aacvpr.org/
American Dietetic Association, Evidence Analysis Library
http://www.eatright.org/
American Heart Association
http://www.heart.org/
Framingham Heart Study
http://www.framinghamheartstudy.org
NCEP Adult Treatment Panel Guidelines
http://www.nhlbi.nih.gov/guidelines/cholesterol/atp_iii.htm

REFERENCES

Abdullah A, et al: Estimating the risk of cardiovascular disease using an obese-years metric, *BMJ Open* 4:e005629, 2014.

Aburto NJ, et al: Effect of lower sodium intake on health: systematic review and meta-analyses, *BMJ* 346:f1326, 2013.

Academy of Nutrition and Dietetics (AND): *Hypertension, AND Evidence Analysis Library*, Chicago, IL, 2009, AND.

Academy of Nutrition and Dietetics (AND): *Evidence Analysis Library, Recommendations Summary: Heart Failure*, Updated 2012. Accessed April 10, 2015.

American College of Cardiology: Mediterranean diet cuts heart disease risk by nearly half, March 2, 2015. http://www.acc.org/about-acc/press-releases/2015/03/04/16/36/mediterranean-diet-cuts-heart-disease-risk-by-nearly-half. Accessed September 8, 2015.

American Diabetes Association: *National Diabetes Factsheet*, Alexandria. Va, 2013, American Diabetes Association.

American Diabetes Association: Standards of medical care in diabetes–2013, *Diabetes Care* 36(Suppl 1):S11, 2013.

American Heart Association: *Heart Disease and Stroke Statistics: 2013 Update At-A-Glance*, Dallas, Texas, 2013, American Heart Association.

American Heart Association: *Heart and Stroke Statistics*, 2015. http://www.heart.org/HEARTORG/General/Heart-and-Stroke-Association-Statistics_UCM_319064_SubHomePage.jsp. Accessed April 25, 2015.

American Heart Association (AHA) Nutrition Committee, et al: Diet and lifestyle recommendations revision 2006: a scientific statement from the American Heart Association Nutrition Committee, *Circulation* 114:82, 2006.

Anderson JW, et al: Health benefits of dietary fiber, *Nutr Rev* 67:188, 2009.

Anker SD, et al: ESPEN guidelines on enteral nutrition: cardiology and pulmonology, *Clin Nutr* 25:311, 2006.

Appel LJ, American Society of Hypertension Writing Group: ASH position paper: dietary approaches to lower blood pressure, *J Am Soc Hypertens* 3:321, 2009.

Appel LJ, et al: Dietary approaches to prevent and treat hypertension: a scientific statement from the American Heart Association, *Hypertension* 47:296, 2006.

Appel LJ, et al: Effects of protein, monounsaturated fat, and carbohydrate intake on blood pressure and serum lipids: results of the OmniHeart randomized trial, *JAMA* 294:2455, 2005.

Basu A, et al: Dietary factors that promote or retard inflammation, *Arterioscler Thromb Vasc Biol* 26:995, 2006.

Bazzano LA, et al: Dietary approaches to prevent hypertension, *Curr Hypertens Rep* 15:694, 2013.

Beveridge LA, et al: Effect of vitamin D supplementation on blood pressure: a systematic review and meta-analysis incorporating individual patient data, *JAMA Intern Med* March 16, 2015, (Epub ahead of print).

Bloomer RJ, et al: Effect of a 21 day Daniel Fast on metabolic and cardiovascular disease risk factors in men and women, *Lipids Health Dis* 9:94, 2010.

Blumenthal JA, et al: Effects of the DASH diet alone and in combination with exercise and weight loss on blood pressure and cardiovascular biomarkers in men and women with high blood pressure: the ENCORE study, *Arch Int Med* 170:126, 2010.

Boden WE, et al: Optimal medical therapy with or without PCI for stable coronary disease, *N Engl J Med* 356:1503, 2007.

Carlson H, Dahlin CM: Managing the effects of cardiac cachexia, *J Hosp Palliat Nurs* 16:15, 2014.

Carter SJ, et al: Relationship between Mediterranean diet score and atherothrombotic risk: findings from the Third National Health and Nutrition Examination Survey (NHANES-III), 1988-1994. *Atherosclerosis* 210:630, 2010.

Chess DJ, et al: A high-fat diet increases adiposity but maintains mitochondrial oxidative enzymes without affecting development of heart failure with pressure overload, *Am J Physiol Heart Circ Physiol* 297:1585, 2009.

Chobanian AV, et al: The Seventh Report of the Joint National Committee on the Prevention, Evaluation and Treatment of High Blood Pressure: the JNC 7 report, *JAMA* 289:2560, 2003.

Christopher BA, et al: Myocardial insulin resistance induced by high fat feeding in heart failure is associated with preserved contractile function, *Am J Physiol Heart Circ Physiol* 299:H1917, 2010.

Cicero AF, et al: Omega-3 polyunsaturated fatty acids: their potential role in blood pressure prevention and management, *Curr Vasc Pharmacol* 7:330, 2009.

Cook NR, et al: Long term effects of dietary sodium reduction on cardiovascular disease outcomes: observational follow-up of the trials of hypertension prevention (TOHP), *BMJ* 334:885, 2007.

Couch SC, et al: The efficacy of a clinic-based behavioral nutrition intervention emphasizing a DASH-type diet for adolescents with elevated blood pressure, *J Pediatr* 152:494, 2008.

Cui R, et al: Dietary folate and vitamin B6 and B12 intake in relation to mortality from cardiovascular diseases: Japan collaborative cohort study, *Stroke* 41:1285, 2010.

de Koning Gans JM, et al: Tea and coffee consumption and cardiovascular morbidity and mortality, *Arterioscler Thromb Vasc Biol* 30:1665, 2010.

Delano MJ, Moldawer LL: The origins of cachexia in acute and chronic inflammatory diseases, *Nutr Clin Pract* 21:68, 2006.

DeMarco VG, et al: The pathophysiology of hypertension in patients with obesity, *Nat Rev Endocrinol* 10:364, 2014.

Desai AS: Controversies in cardiovascular medicine. Are serial BNP measurements useful in heart failure management?, *Circulation* 127: 509, 2013.

Dickinson HO, et al: Lifestyle interventions to reduce raised blood pressure: a systematic review of randomized controlled trials, *J Hypertens* 24:215, 2006.

DiNicolantonio JJ, et al: Thiamine supplementation for the treatment of heart failure: a review of the literature, *Congest Heart Fail* 19:214, 2013.

Djousse L, Gaziano JM: Alcohol consumption and heart failure: a systematic review, *Curr Atheroscler Rep* 10:117, 2008.

Eckel RH, et al: 2013 AHA/ACC guideline on lifestyle management to reduce cardiovascular risk: a report of the American College of Cardiology/American Heart Association Task Force on Practice Guidelines, *Circulation* 129(Suppl 2):S76, 2013.

Egan BM, et al: US trends in prevalence, awareness, treatment, and control of hypertension, 1988-2008, *JAMA* 303:2043, 2010.

Esselstyn C, Golubic M: The nutritional reversal of cardiovascular disease – Fact or fiction? Three case reports, *Cardiology* 20:1901, 2014.

Flynn J: The changing face of pediatric hypertension in the era of the childhood obesity epidemic, *Pediatr Nephrol* 28:1059, 2013.

Fraser A, et al: Associations of serum 25-hydroxyvitamin D, parathyroid hormone and calcium with cardiovascular risk factors: analysis of 3 NHANES cycles (2001-2006), *PLoS One* 5:e13882, 2010.

Fuentes JC, et al: Acute and chronic oral magnesium supplementation: effects on endothelial function, exercise capacity, and quality of life in patients with symptomatic heart failure, *Congest Heart Fail* 12:9, 2006.

Gidding SS, et al: Implementing American Heart Association pediatric and adult nutrition guidelines: a scientific statement from the American Heart Association Nutrition Committee of the Council on Nutrition, Physical Activity and Metabolism, Council on Cardiovascular Disease in the Young, Council on Arteriosclerosis, Thrombosis and Vascular Biology, Council on Cardiovascular Nursing, Council on Epidemiology and Prevention, and Council for High Blood Pressure Research, *Circulation* 119:1161, 2009.

Go AS, et al: Heart disease and stroke statistics – 2014 update: a report from the American Heart Association, *Circulation* 129:e28, 2014.

Goldberg AC, et al: Effect of plant stanol tablets on low-density lipoprotein cholesterol lowering in patients on statin drugs, *Am J Cardiol* 97:376, 2006.

Gupta D, et al: Dietary sodium intake in heart failure, *Circulation* 126:479, 2012.

Hall JE, et al: Hypertension: physiology and pathophysiology, *Compr Physiol* 2:2393, 2012.

Harris WS, et al: Omega-6 fatty acids and risk for cardiovascular disease: a science advisory from the American Heart Association Nutrition Subcommittee of the Council on Nutrition, Physical Activity, and Metabolism; Council on Cardiovascular Nursing; and Council on Epidemiology and Prevention, *Circulation* 119:902, 2009.

Hasse JM: Nutritional aspects of transplantation in adults. In Busuttil RW, Klintmalm GB, editors: *Transplantation of the Liver*, ed 3, St Louis, 2015, Elsevier Saunders, pp 4994–4509.

Hinderliter AL, et al: The long-term effects of lifestyle change on blood pressure: 1-year follow-up of the ENCORE Study, *Am J Hypertens* 27:734, 2014.

Institute of Medicine (IOM): *Dietary reference intakes: water, potassium, sodium chloride and sulfate*, ed 1, Washington, DC, 2004, National Academies Press.

Institute of Medicine (IOM): *Sodium intake in populations: assessment of evidence*, Washington, DC, 2013, National Academies Press.

Jacobson MF, et al: Changes in sodium levels in processed and restaurant foods, 2005 to 2011, *JAMA Intern Med* 173:1285, 2013.

James PA, et al: 2014 evidence-based guideline for the management of high blood pressure in adults: Report from the panel members appointed to the Eighth Joint National Committee (JNC 8), *JAMA* 311:507, 2014.

Jellinger PS, et al: American Association of Clinical Endocrinologists' guidelines for management of dyslipidemia and prevention of atherosclerosis, *Endocr Pract* 18(Suppl 1):1, 2012.

Kalogeropoulos N, et al: Unsaturated fatty acids are inversely associated and ω-6/ω-3 ratios are positively related to inflammation and coagulation markers in plasma of apparently healthy adults, *Clin Chim Acta* 411:584, 2010.

Klatsky AL: *Coffee drinking and caffeine associated with reduced risk of hospitalization for heart rhythm disturbance.* AHA 50th Annual Conference on Cardiovascular Disease, Epidemiology and Prevention, San Francisco, Calif, 2010.

Kris-Etherton PM, et al: Milk products, dietary patterns and blood pressure management, *J Am Coll Nutr* 28:103S, 2009.

Kunutsor SK, et al: Vitamin D and risk of future hypertension: meta-analysis of 283,537 participants, *Eur J Epidemiol* 28:205, 2013.

Kupetsky-Rincon RA, Uitto J: Magnesium: novel applications in cardiovascular disease – a review of the literature, *Ann Nutr Metab* 61:102, 2012.

Lee Y, et al: Effect of dietary patterns on serum C-reactive protein level, *Nutr Metab Cardiovasc Dis* 24:1004, 2014.

Li Q, Ren J: Cardiac overexpression of metallothionein attenuates chronic alcohol intake-induced cardiomyocyte contractile dysfunction, *Cardiovasc Toxicol* 6:173, 2006.

Liebman B: *Salt, Shaving Salt, Saving Lives*, 2014. http://www.cspinet.org/nah/articles/salt.html. Accessed April 28, 2015.

Lloyd-Jones DM: Improving the cardiovascular health of the US population, *JAMA* 307:1314, 2012.

Longo S, et al: Short-term and long-term sequelae in intrauterine growth retardation (IUGR), *J Matern Fetal Neonatal Med* 26:222, 2013.

Madmani ME, et al: Coenzyme Q10 for heart failure, *Cochrane Database Syst Rev* 6:CD008684, Jun 2, 2014.

Masoura C, et al: Arterial endothelial function and wall thickness in familial hypercholesterolemia and familial combined hyperlipidemia and the effect of statins. A systemic review and meta-analysis, *Atherosclerosis* 214:129, 2011.

Mathieu P, et al: Visceral obesity: the link among inflammation, hypertension and cardiovascular disease, *Hypertension* 53:577, 2009.

McCollum M, et al: Prevalence of multiple cardiac risk factors in US adults with diabetes, *Curr Med Res Opin* 22:1031, 2006.

McGuire KA, et al: Ability of physical activity to predict cardiovascular disease beyond commonly evaluated cardiometabolic risk factors, *Am J Cardiol* 104:1522, 2009.

Meems LM, et al: Vitamin D biology in heart failure: molecular mechanisms and systematic review, *Curr Drug Targets* 12:29, 2011.

Mehta PK, Griendling KK: Angiotensin II cell signaling: physiological and pathological effects in the cardiovascular system, *Am J Physiol Cell Physiol* 292:C82, 2007.

Miller D, Joye Woodward N: Clinical inquiries. Whom should you test for secondary causes of hypertension? *J Fam Pract* 63:41, 2014.

Miller ER III, et al: The effects of macronutrients on blood pressure and lipids: an overview of the DASH and OmniHeart trials, *Curr Atheroscler Rep* 8:460, 2006.

Miller PE, et al: Long-chain omega-3 fatty acids eicosapentaenoic acid and docosahexanoic acid and blood pressure: a meta-analysis of randomized controlled trials, *Am J Hypertens* 27:885, 2014.

Miura K, et al: Relationship of dietary monounsaturated fatty acids to blood pressure: the International Study of Macro/Micronutrients and Blood Pressure, *J Hypertens* 31:1144, 2013.

Morrow DA: C-reactive protein in cardiovascular disease, *UpToDate*, http://www.uptodate.com/contents/c-reactive-protein-in-cardiovascular-disease. 2014, Wolters Kluwer, Accessed September 8, 2015.

Navab M, et al: HDL and cardiovascular disease: atherogenic and atheroprotective mechanisms, *Nat Rev Cardiol* 8:222, 2011.

Nicklas BJ, et al: Abdominal obesity is an independent risk factor for chronic heart failure in older people, *J Am Geriatr Soc* 54:413, 2006.

Nordestgaard M, et al: Familial hypercholesterolaemia is underdiagnosed and undertreated in the general population: guidance for clinicians to prevent coronary heart disease: consensus statement of the European Atherosclerosis Society, *Eur Heart J* 34:3478, 2013.

Norton GR, et al: Gene variants of the renin-angiotensin system and hypertension: from a trough of disillusionment to a welcome phase of enlightenment? *Clin Sci (Lond)* 118:487, 2010.

Opie LH, et al: Controversies in stable coronary artery disease, *Lancet* 367:69, 2006.

Ostchega Y, et al: Trends of elevated blood pressure among children and adolescents: data from the National Health and Nutrition Examination Survey 1988-2006. *Am J Hypertens* 22:59, 2009.

Ottestad IO, et al: Triglyceride-rich HDL3 from patients with familial hypercholesterolemia are less able to inhibit cytokine release or to promote cholesterol efflux, *J Nutr* 136:877, 2006.

Padmanabhan S, et al: Genetic basis of blood pressure and hypertension, *Trends Genet* 28:397, 2012.

Qin LQ, et al: Milk consumption and circulating insulin-like growth factor-I level: a systematic literature review, *Int J Food Sci Nutr* 60(Suppl 7):330, 2009.

Rees K, et al: Mediterranean dietary pattern for the primary prevention of cardiovascular disease, *Cochrane Database Syst Rev* 8:CD00985, 2013.

Rice BH, et al: Meeting and exceeding dairy recommendations: effect of dairy consumption on nutrient intakes and risk of chronic disease, *Nutr Rev* 71:209, 2013.

Rosano GM, et al: Metabolic therapy for patients with diabetes mellitus and coronary artery disease, *Am J Cardiol* 98:14, 2006.

Roth EM, Harris WS: Fish oil for primary and secondary prevention of coronary heart disease, *Curr Atheroscler Rep* 12:66, 2010.

Savoia C, et al: Angiotensin II and vascular phenotype in hypertension, *Exp Rev Mol Med* 13:e11, 2011.

Shecterle LM, et al: The patented uses of D-ribose in cardiovascular diseases, *Recent Pat Cardiovasc Drug Discov* 5:138, 2010.

Schleithoff SS, et al: Vitamin D supplementation improves cytokine profiles in patients with congestive heart failure: a double-blind, randomized, placebo-controlled trial, *Am J Clin Nutr* 83:754, 2006.

Schwingshackl L, et al: Effects of monounsaturated fatty acids on cardiovascular risk factors: a systematic review and meta-analysis, *Ann Nutr Metab* 59:176, 2011.

Sontia B, Touyz RM: Role of magnesium in hypertension, *Arch Bioch Biophys* 458:33, 2007.

Stone NJ, et al: 2013 ACC/AHA guideline on the treatment of blood cholesterol to reduce atherosclerotic cardiovascular risk in adults, *Circulation* 129(Suppl 2):S1, 2014.

Swain JF, et al: Characteristics of the diet patterns tested in the optimal macronutrient intake trial to prevent heart disease (OmniHeart): options for a heart-healthy diet, *J AmCiet Assoc* 108:257, 2008.

Tang WH, et al: Intestinal microbial metabolism of phosphatidylcholine and cardiovascular disease, *N Engl J Med* 368:1575, 2013.

Teunissen-Beekman KF, van Baak MA: The role of dietary protein in blood pressure regulation, *Curr Opin Lipidol* 24:65, 2013.

Thom T, et al: Heart disease and stroke statistics—2006 update from the American Heart Association Statistics Committee, *Circulation* 113:e85, 2006.

Tousoulis D, et al: The role of nitric oxide in endothelial function, *Curr Vasc Pharmacol* 10:4, 2012.

Towfighi A, et al: Pronounced association of elevated serum homocysteine with stroke in subgroups of individuals: a nationwide study, *J Neurol Sci* 298:153, 2010.

US Department of Agriculture (USDA), United States Department of Health and Human Services (USDHHS): *Dietary Guidelines for Americans 2010*, 2015. http://www.health.gov/dietaryguidelines/2010.asp. Accessed April 28, 2015.

Vieth R, Kimball S: Vitamin D in congestive heart failure, *Am J Clin Nutr* 83:731, 2006.

van der Wal HH, et al: Vitamin B12 and folate deficiency in chronic heart failure, *Heart* 101:302, 2015.

van Mierlo LA, et al: Blood pressure response to calcium supplementation: a meta-analysis of randomized controlled trials, *J Hum Hypertension* 20:571, 2006.

Wexler RK, et al: Cardiomyopathy: an overview, *Am Fam Physician* 79:778, 2009.

Yanai H, et al: Effects of dietary fat intake on HDL metabolism, *J Clin Med Res* 7:145, 2015.

Yusuf S, et al: Cardiovascular risk and events in 17 low-, middle-, and high-income countries, *N Engl J Med* 371:818, 2014.

Zhou MS, et al: Link between the renin-angiotensin system and insulin resistance: implications for cardiovascular disease, *Vasc Med* 17:330, 2012.

Zittermann A, et al: Markers of bone metabolism in congestive heart failure, *Clin Chim Acta* 366:27, 2006.

34

Medical Nutrition Therapy for Pulmonary Disease

Sameera H. Khan, RDN, PA-C, MBA
Ashok M. Karnik, MD, FACP, FCCP, FRCP

KEY TERMS

acinar
acinus
acute respiratory distress syndrome (ARDS)
adiponectin
asthma
aspiration pneumonia
bronchiectasis
bronchogenic carcinomas
bronchopulmonary dysplasia (BPD)
cancer cachexia syndrome
chronic bronchitis
chronic obstructive pulmonary disease (COPD)
cilia
chylothorax
clubbing

continuous positive airway pressure (CPAP)
cor pulmonale
cystic fibrosis (CF)
cystic fibrosis related diabetes (CFRD)
distal intestinal obstruction syndrome (DIOS)
dyspnea
elastase
emphysema
ghrelin
hypercapnia
hypopnea
kyphosis
leptin
obesity hypoventilation syndrome (OHS)
obstructive sleep apnea (OSA)

osteopenia
pancreatic enzyme replacement therapy (PERT)
pancreatic insufficiency (PI)
pneumonia
pulmonary cachexia
pulmonary function tests
pulse oximetry
resistin
resolvin
respiratory quotient (RQ)
spirometry
steatorrhea
surfactant
tachypnea
tuberculosis (TB)

During fetal life, from birth to maturity, and throughout adulthood, the pulmonary system is intertwined with nutrition. Optimal nutrition permits the proper growth and development of the respiratory organs, supporting structures of the skeleton and muscles, and related nervous, circulatory, and immunologic systems. A well-functioning pulmonary system enables the body to obtain the oxygen needed to meet its cellular demands for energy from macronutrients and to remove metabolic byproducts. Overall, a person's nutritional well-being and proper metabolism of nutrients are essential for the formation, development, growth, maturity, and protection of healthy lungs and associated processes throughout life.

THE PULMONARY SYSTEM

The respiratory structures include the nose, pharynx, larynx, trachea, bronchi, bronchioles, alveolar ducts, and alveoli. Supporting structures include the skeleton and the muscles (e.g., the intercostal, abdominal, and diaphragm muscles). Within a month after conception, pulmonary structures are recognizable. The pulmonary system grows and matures during gestation and childhood, and no new alveoli are produced after

approximately age 20 years. As aging occurs, there is a loss of lung capillaries and the lungs lose elasticity.

The primary function of the respiratory system is gas exchange, and the anatomy and physiology is geared to fulfill this function (see Figure 34-1). The lungs enable the body to obtain the oxygen needed to meet its cellular metabolic demands and to remove the carbon dioxide (CO_2) produced. Healthy nerves, blood, and lymph are needed to supply oxygen and nutrients to all tissues. The lungs also filter, warm, and humidify inspired air.

The respiratory center is the name for structures involved in the generation of rhythmic respiratory movements and reflexes, and is located in the medulla and pons (see Figure 41-1). The electrical impulses generated by the respiratory center are carried by the phrenic nerves to the diaphragm and other respiratory muscles. Contraction of diaphragm and other muscles increases the intrathoracic volume, which creates negative intrathoracic pressure and allows air to be sucked in. The air traverses through upper and lower airways (see Figure 34-1, *A*) and reaches alveoli (see Figure 34-1, *B*). The alveoli are surrounded by capillaries where gas exchange takes place (see Figure 34-1, *C*). The large pulmonary blood vessels and the conducting airways are located in a well-defined connective tissue compartment—the pleural cavity.

The lungs are an important part of the body's immune defense system, because inspired air is laden with particles and microorganisms. Mucus keeps the airways moist and traps the particles and microorganisms from inspired air. The airways

Portions of this chapter were written by Donna H. Mueller, PhD, RD, FADA, LDN, for the previous edition.

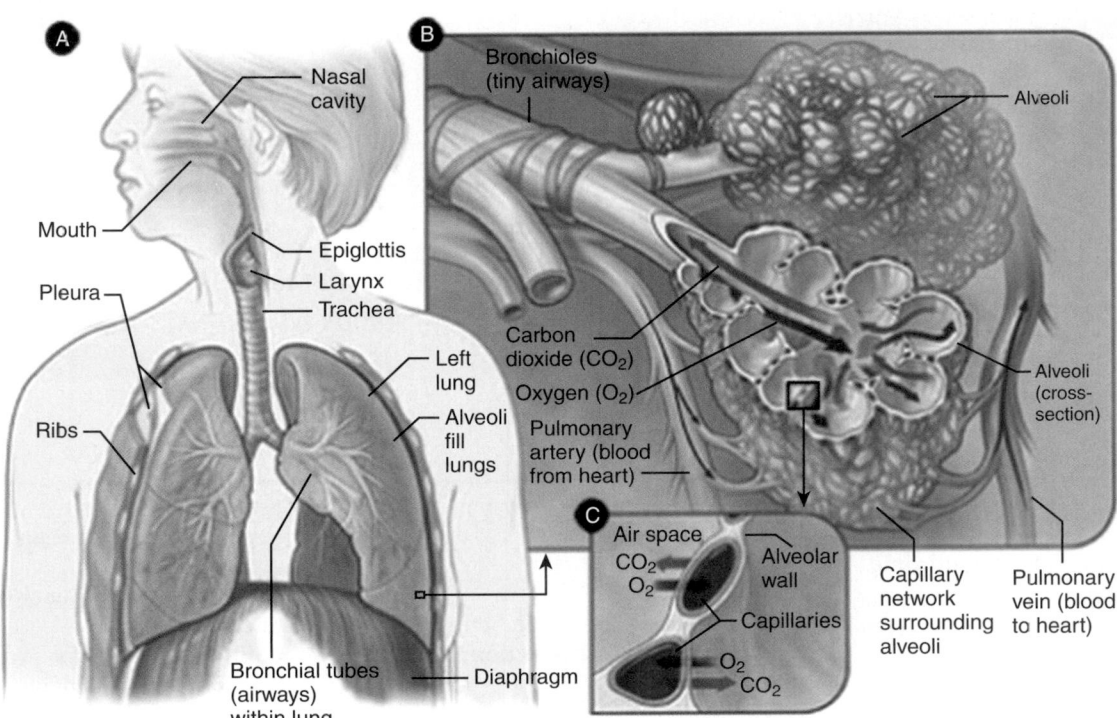

FIGURE 34-1 Functional anatomy and physiology of the respiratory system. **A,** Various parts of respiratory system. **B,** Gas exchange unit. **C,** Alveolar-capillary interface. *National Heart, Lung, and Blood Institute; National Institutes of Health; U.S. Department of Health and Human Services.*

have 12 types of epithelial cells, and most cells that line the trachea, bronchi, and bronchioles have **cilia.** The cilia are "hair-like" structures that move the superficial liquid lining layer from deep within the lungs, toward the pharynx to enter the gastrointestinal tract, thereby playing an important role as a lung defense mechanism by clearing bacteria and other foreign bodies. Each time a person swallows, the particle- and microorganism-containing mucus passes into the digestive tract. When bacteria inhaled by the patient are not cleared effectively, the patient is prone to develop recurrent chest infections that may eventually lead to bronchiectasis.

The epithelial surface of the alveoli contains macrophages. By the process of phagocytosis, these alveolar macrophages engulf inhaled inert materials and microorganisms and digest them. The alveolar cells also secrete surfactant, a compound synthesized from proteins and phospholipids that maintains the stability of pulmonary tissue by reducing the surface tension of fluids that coat the lung.

The lungs have several metabolic functions. For example, they help regulate the body's acid-base balance (see Chapter 6). The body's pH is maintained partially by the proper balance of CO_2 and O_2. The lungs also synthesize arachidonic acid that ultimately may be converted to prostaglandins or leukotrienes. These appear to play a role in bronchoconstriction seen in asthma. The lungs convert angiotension I to angiotensin II by the angiotension-converting enzyme (ACE) found mainly in the numerous capillary beds of the lungs. Angiotensin II increases blood pressure. Because of the ultrastructure and the fact that they receive the total cardiac output, lungs are well suited to function as a chemical filter. They protect the systemic circulation from exposure to high levels of circulating vasoactive substances. Although serotonin, 5-hydroxytryptamine (5 HT), and norepinephrine are totally or partially eliminated or inactivated in the pulmonary circulation, epinephrine and histamines pass through the lungs unchanged.

Effect of Malnutrition on the Pulmonary System

The relationship between malnutrition and respiratory disease has long been recognized. Malnutrition adversely affects lung structure, elasticity, and function; respiratory muscle mass, strength, and endurance; lung immune defense mechanisms; and control of breathing. For example, protein and iron deficiencies result in low hemoglobin levels that diminish the oxygen-carrying capacity of the blood. Low levels of calcium, magnesium, phosphorus, and potassium compromise respiratory muscle function at the cellular level. Hypoalbuminemia, as measured by serum albumen, contributes to the development of pulmonary edema by decreasing colloid osmotic pressure, allowing body fluids to move into the interstitial space. Decreased levels of surfactant contribute to the collapse of alveoli, thereby increasing the work of breathing. The supporting connective tissue of the lungs is composed of collagen, which requires ascorbic acid for its synthesis. Normal airway mucus is a substance consisting of water, glycoproteins, and electrolytes, and thus requires adequate nutritional intake.

Effect of Pulmonary Disease on Nutritional Status

Pulmonary disease substantially increases energy requirements. This factor explains the rationale for including body composition and weight parameters in nutrition assessment. Weight loss from inadequate energy intake is significantly correlated with a poor prognosis in persons with pulmonary diseases. Malnutrition leading to impaired immunity places any patient at high risk for developing respiratory infections. Malnourished patients with pulmonary disease who are hospitalized are likely to have lengthy stays and are susceptible to increased morbidity and mortality.

The complications of pulmonary diseases or their treatments can make adequate food intake and digestion difficult. Absorption and metabolism of most nutrients are affected. As pulmonary disease progresses, several conditions may interfere with food intake and overall nutrition status. For example, abnormal production of sputum, vomiting, tachypnea (rapid breathing), hemoptysis, thoracic pain, nasal polyps, anemia, depression, and altered taste secondary to medications are often present. Weight loss, low body mass index (BMI), and other adverse effects are listed in Box 34-1.

Medical Management

Pulmonary system disorders may be categorized as primary, such as tuberculosis (TB), bronchial asthma, and cancer of the lung; or secondary when associated with cardiovascular disease, obesity, human immunodeficiency virus (HIV) infection, sickle cell disease, or scoliosis. Conditions also may be acute or hronic. Examples of acute conditions include aspiration pneumonia, airway obstruction from foods such as peanuts, and allergic anaphylaxis from consumption of shellfish. Examples of chronic conditions include cystic fibrosis (CF) and chronic obstructive pulmonary disease (COPD).

The assessment of pulmonary status generally starts with physical examination using percussion and auscultation. These bedside techniques provide important information on the patient's breathing. Numerous diagnostic and monitoring tests such as imaging procedures, arterial blood gas determinations, sputum cultures, and biopsies also can be employed. Signs and symptoms of pulmonary disease include cough, dyspnea (shortness of breath), fatigue, early satiety, anorexia, and weight loss.

Pulmonary function tests are used to diagnose or monitor the status of lung disease; they are designed to measure the ability of the respiratory system to exchange oxygen and CO_2. Pulse

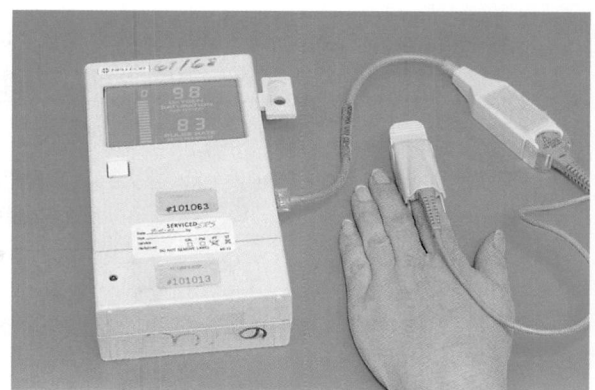

FIGURE 34-2 Pulse oximeter.

oximetry is one such test. A small device called a pulse oximeter, which uses light waves to measure the oxygen saturation of arterial blood, is placed on the end of the finger (see Figure 34-2). Normal for a young, healthy person is 95% to 99%. Spirometry is another common pulmonary function test. This involves breathing into a spirometer that gives information on lung volume and the rate at which air can be inhaled and exhaled.

CHRONIC PULMONARY DISEASE

Cystic Fibrosis

Cystic fibrosis (CF) is a life-threatening autosomal recessive inherited disorder that is most commonly seen in the Caucasian population with a CF incidence of 1 out of 3500 babies born in the United States (Culhane et al, 2013). It is caused by mutations in the cystic fibrosis transmembrane conductance regulator (CFTR) protein, a complex chloride channel and regulatory protein found in all exocrine tissues. This defect causes impaired transport of chloride, sodium and bicarbonate, which results in the production of thick, viscous secretions in the lungs, pancreas, liver, intestines and reproductive tract, and leads to increased salt content in the sweat gland secretions. Most of the clinical manifestations are related to the thick, viscid secretions (see Figure 34-3). Lung disease and malnutrition are predominant burdens of the disease.

In the past, most patients were diagnosed with CF because of symptoms related to various organ systems. During the past decade, newborn screening programs have been expanded and a large number of CF cases are diagnosed before development of symptoms. In 2001 less than 10% of CF cases were diagnosed during the newborn screening programs; by 2011, almost 60% were diagnosed during screening (Katkin, 2014). When a patient has clinical disease in one or more organs and has elevated sweat chloride (more than 60 mmol/L), it is called a "typical" or "classic" presentation. About 2% of patients present with the typical clinical picture, but have a normal or intermediate sweat chloride level; this is called nonclassic presentation (Katkin, 2014).

Pathophysiology
Pulmonary and Sinus Disease

CF patients present with chronic persistent cough, dyspnea, and wheezing. As the disease progresses, patients develop bronchiectasis, a chronic condition of dilatation of the bronchi that develops as a result of recurrent lung infections. Examination of

---

BOX 34-1 Adverse Effects of Lung Disease on Nutrition Status

Increased Energy Expenditure

Increased work of breathing
Chronic infection
Medical treatments (e.g., bronchodilators, chest physical therapy)

Reduced Intake

Fluid restriction
Shortness of breath
Decreased oxygen saturation while eating
Anorexia resulting from chronic disease
Gastrointestinal distress and vomiting

Additional Limitations

Difficulty preparing food because of fatigue
Lack of financial resources
Impaired feeding skills (for infants and children)
Altered metabolism
Food-drug interaction

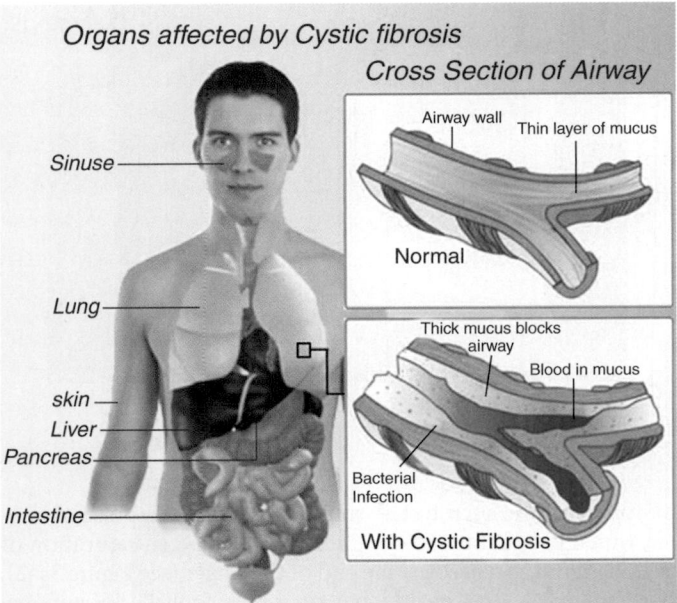

FIGURE 34-3 Illustration showing multi system involvement in CF and tenacious secretions.

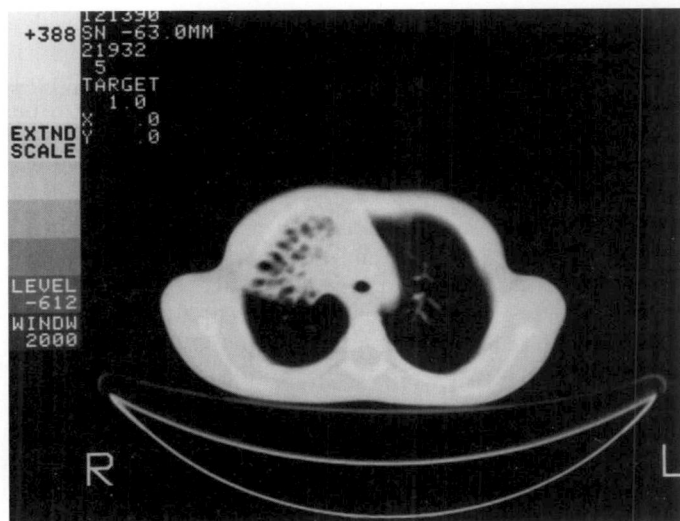

FIGURE 34-5 CT scan of a patient showing cystic changes of bronchiectasis in right upper lobe.

a patient with bronchiectasis may show presence of clubbing. Digital clubbing is characterized by increased digital tip mass and increased longitudinal and transverse nail plate curvature (see Figure 34-4), and lung auscultation reveals crackles in the lungs. Chest radiograph may show hyperinflation, and a CT scan may show the classical picture of cystic bronchiectasis (see Figure 34-5). Pulmonary function testing shows airways obstruction. The spirogram shows reduced forced vital capacity (FVC), known as "restrictive pattern." The reduced forced expiratory volume (FEV_1) and the reduced FEV_1/FVC ratio are suggestive of airways obstruction.

Early in life, the airways are colonized by bacteria. Although *Staphylococcus aureus, Haemophilus influenzae,* and *Pseudomonas aeruginosa* are common colonizers, recent research has shown that the lung may be colonized by multiple pathogens rather than one dominant organism. Many children with CF develop chronic rhinosinusitis with nasal polyposis. Some questions remain unanswered as to the origin of

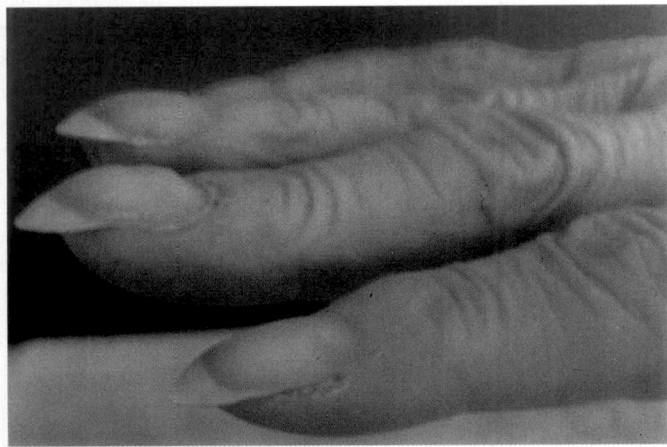

FIGURE 34-4 Illustration of clubbing in a patient of "yellow nail syndrome."

polyps in CF patients. Chronic colonization of *Pseudomonas aeruginosa* and CF genotypes are argued to play major roles (Vital et al, 2013).

Pancreatic Disease

Several different types of pancreatic disease occur in CF patients.

Pancreatic Insufficiency. Pancreatic insufficiency (PI), in which the pancreas fails to make adequate enzymes to digest food in the small intestine, is the most common gastrointestinal complication of CF, affecting approximately 90% of patients at some time in their lives (Rogers, 2013).

Up to 90% of patients exhibit fat malabsorption by 1 year of age. The production of pancreatic enzymes is decreased, which leads to the malabsorption of fats and steatorrhea. Steatorrhea, is characterized by foul smelling, bulky, oily stools and failure to thrive or poor weight gain. Such patients may also present with clinical features of deficiency of the fat-soluble vitamins A, D, E, and K. The CF population frequently presents with suboptimal vitamin D status. CF patients also suffer from vitamin K deficiencies and need routine supplementation.

Pancreatitis. The abnormal pancreatic secretions cause progressive pancreatic damage, so these patients can present with acute or recurrent pancreatitis.

CF-Related Diabetes. Patients with exocrine pancreatic insufficiency also may develop impaired function of the endocrine pancreas, leading to the development of cystic fibrosis related diabetes (CFRD). Twenty five percent of CF patients develop CFRD, which is associated with poor growth, clinical and nutritional deterioration, and early death. The American Diabetes Association (ADA) and the Cystic Fibrosis Foundation (CFF) recommend yearly CFRD screenings, starting at age 10 (see Chapter 30 for discussion of diabetes management).

Bone Disease

Bone disease is common in CF patients and is characterized by increased fracture rates, low bone density, and kyphosis, which is increased curvature of the upper back, causing a hunchback.

Multiple risk factors contribute to developing bone disease—chronic corticosteroid use, failure to thrive, malabsorption of calcium, vitamin D, vitamin K and magnesium, inadequate overall intake, and reduced weight-bearing activities.

Other Conditions

Meconium ileus, rectal prolapse, biliary disease, infertility, musculoskeletal disorders, and recurrent venous thrombosis are other conditions that occur in patients with CF. CF patients are susceptible to SIBO (small intestine bacterial overgrowth) secondary to decreased motility. This disorder interferes with fat absorption and appetite (Baker et al, 2013) (see Chapter 28).

Medical Management

Cystic fibrosis is a multisystem disease and its management requires a multidisciplinary approach. Involvement of respiratory and gastrointestinal systems is responsible for significant mortality and morbidity. Sinus infection, glucose control, nutritional status, and psychosocial issues must be assessed and managed at regular intervals (see Figure 34-6).

Ivacaftor (VX-770) is a small molecular weight oral drug that is designed specifically to treat patients who have a G551D mutation in at least one of their CFTR genes. Ivacaftor is the first approved CF therapy that restores the functioning of a mutant CF protein rather than trying to target one or more of its downstream consequences (Davis, 2011).

Cystic fibrosis patients are prone to recurrent chest infections, requiring treatment with antibiotics, bronchodilators, and chest physiotherapy. Inhalants help to clear purulent and tenacious secretions. Antiinflammatory agents such as macrolide antibiotics, ibuprofen, and systemic and inhaled steroids are used with the objective of controlling excessive and harmful inflammatory reaction in the lungs. Influenza and pneumococcal vaccines are used as preventive measures. Hypoxemic patients need supplemental oxygen. Some patients are considered for bilateral lung transplantation.

Because of the pancreatic insufficiency, pancreatic enzyme replacement therapy (PERT) is an important component of the management for CF patients to adequately absorb carbohydrates, protein, and fat. The pancreatic ducts are obstructed in approximately 85% to 90% of CF individuals, and this prevents pancreatic enzymes such as lipase, amylase, and protease from secreting into the small intestine. The build-up of these enzymes in the pancreas leads to auto digestion of the pancreas, and destruction of acinus. Pancreatic acinus is the secretory unit of exocrine pancreas, where pancreatic juice is produced. Destruction of pancreatic acinus, or acinar destruction, results in impaired secretion of pancreatic juice, which results in loose, oily, frequent stools and malabsorption. These individuals need PERT to combat the pancreatic insufficiency and maintain adequate absorption and digestion of nutrients (see Focus On: PERT).

Medical Nutrition Therapy

Medical nutrition therapy (MNT), critical to management of all the conditions described earlier, is vital in promoting longevity and positive outcomes. MNT begins with evaluation of the nutritional status of the patient (Baker et al, 2013) (see Chapters 4 and 7 and Appendix 22). CF patients frequently have growth failure, the cause of which is multifactorial: malabsorption, increased energy needs, and reduced appetite. There is a close correlation between pulmonary function tests (PFT) and nutritional status. All patients with CF should have regular

---

◎ FOCUS ON

PERT

Pancreatic enzyme replacement therapy (PERT) is the first step taken to correct maldigestion and malabsorption. The microspheres, designed to withstand the acidic environment of the stomach, release enzymes in the duodenum, where they digest protein, fat, and carbohydrate. Pharmaceutical advancements have improved the medications. The quantity of enzymes to be taken with food depends on the degree of pancreatic insufficiency; the quantity of food eaten; the fat, protein, and carbohydrate content of food consumed; and the type of enzymes used.

Enzyme dosage per meal or snack is adjusted empirically to control gastrointestinal symptoms, including steatorrhea, and to promote growth appropriate for age. Following the manufacturer's directions about storage and administration of a particular brand of enzyme is important to emphasize. If gastrointestinal symptoms cannot be controlled, enzyme dosage, patient adherence, and enzyme type should be reevaluated. Fecal elastase (protein-digesting enzyme secreted by the pancreas and involved in hydrolysis of peptide bonds), fecal fat, or nitrogen balance studies may help to evaluate the adequacy of enzyme supplementation.

The acidic environment of the stomach does not allow the enzymes of the enteric coated PERT to be degraded. This normally occurs once the pH is above 5.5, usually when the PERT reaches the duodenal jejunum. A common practice is placing CF patients on proton pump inhibitors in order to increase the duodenal pH by decreasing gastric acid secretion (Rogers, 2013).

Intestinal abnormalities such as gastroesophageal reflux disease (GERD), meconium ileus (MI), distal intestinal obstruction syndrome (DIOS), which is the blockage of intestines resulting from stool and intussusceptions, are some of the complications seen in patients (Katkin, 2014).

Hepatobiliary problems are seen more commonly now in this population because of an increased survival rate. In the liver, the CFTR is located in the biliary epithelium. Bile produced in patients with CF is thick and tenacious, causing blockage of the intrahepatic bile ducts. Blockage of these ducts eventually leads to cirrhosis. Use of ursodeoxycholic acid (UDCA) may delay the progression of liver disease (Kappler et al, 2012) (see Chapter 29).

---

nutritional assessments at 3-month intervals for early detection of nutritional status deterioration (see Pathophysiology and Care Management Algorithm: Cystic Fibrosis).

Children with CF should be monitored annually for parathyroid hormone (PTH) levels, 25 hydroxy-vitamin D levels, and serum calcium and phosphate levels. Older children should be evaluated for bone density using the dual energy x-ray absorptiometry (DXA) (see Chapter 24).

Major goals of nutritional therapy are increasing muscle strength, promoting optimal growth and weight maintenance and enhancing the quality of life. To achieve these goals, the objectives of treatment are to correct maldigestion and malabsorption and to provide nutrients that are commonly deficient.

Energy. Because body mass index (BMI) is more sensitive to lung function in CF patients than percentage ideal body weight (IBW), in 2011 the CF foundation discontinued using the %IBW as an assessment tool in CF patients. Instead recommendations are for maintaining a BMI at or above the 50th percentile between ages 2 to 19 and a median BMI of 22.1 kg/m2 for adults 20 to 40 years of age (Culhane et al, 2013).

A broad range of energy requirements are reported in patients with CF, ranging from 120% to 150% of recommendations for the general population, depending on the CF mutation, the patient's age, and the current state of health (Rogers, 2013). Although an energy-dense diet is important, achieving that

PATHOPHYSIOLOGY AND CARE MANAGEMENT ALGORITHM

Cystic Fibrosis

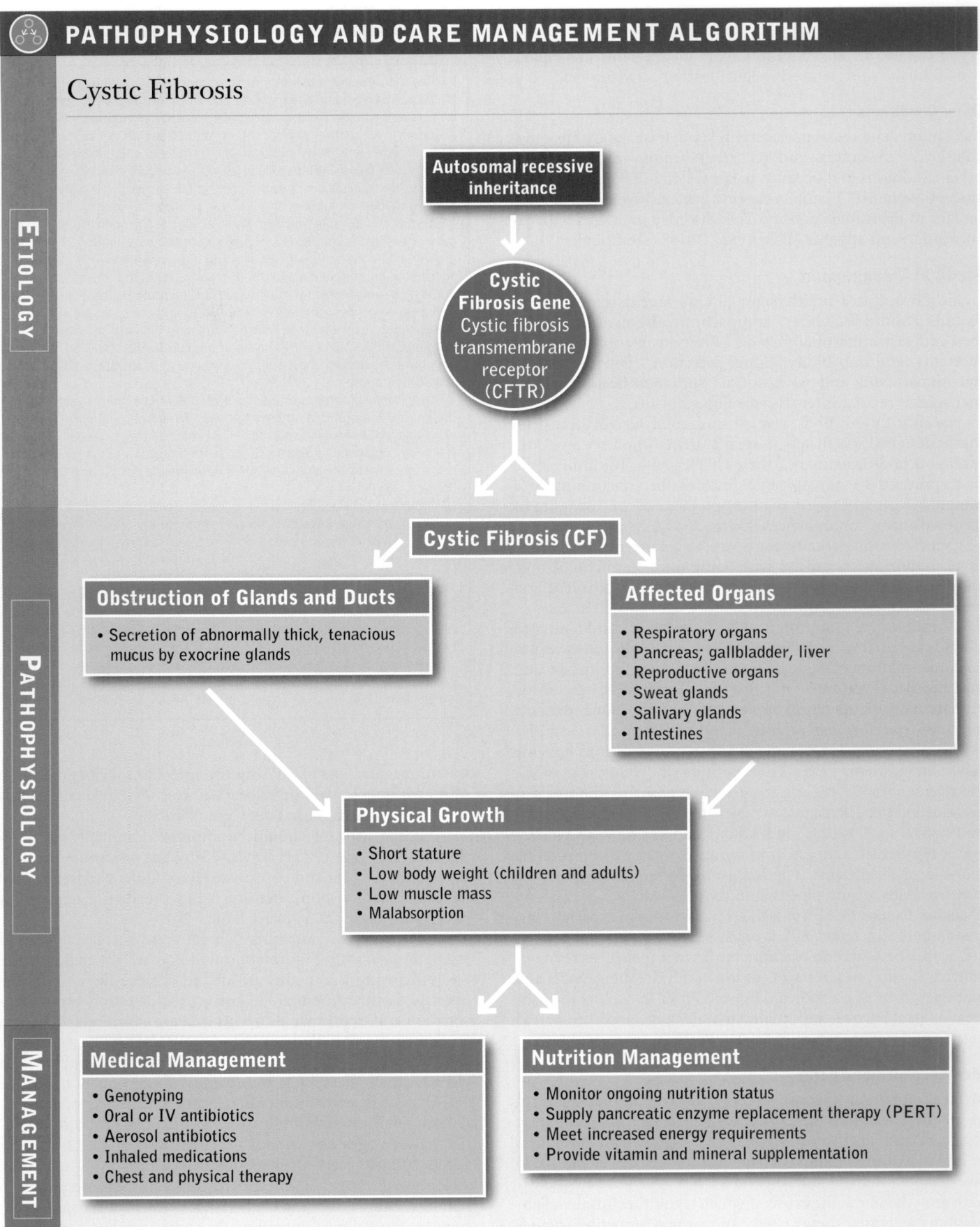

FIGURE 34-6 Algorithm for diagnosis and management of cystic fibrosis.

with high-glycemic index (GI) carbohydrates can be a problem, because a high GI diet can promote impaired glucose tolerance (CF-IGT) and CFRD by exceeding the capabilities of insulin production in CF (Balzer et al, 2012) (see Chapter 30).

Fat-soluble Vitamins. In CF patients, liver disease and pancreatic dysfunction lead to fat malabsorption, which predisposes these patients to deficiencies of fat-soluble vitamins A, D, E and K. The deficiency of vitamins A, D, E, and K, which significantly affects CF patients, reduces their response to pulmonary infections. Because bone disease is common in patients with CF and progresses with age (Rana et al, 2014), the CF foundation recommends patients be treated with cholecalciferol (D$_3$). A daily vitamin D dosage of 1500 to 2000 IU is suggested by the Endocrine Society with dosages increasing to 10,000 IU daily for CF patients 18 or older (Rogers, 2013).

It is also recommended that the CF patient be supplemented with vitamin K. Taking at least 1000 mcg/day was found to achieve an optimal status of vitamin K (Rogers, 2013).

Fat-soluble vitamin testing is important in the identification of deficiencies in CF patients with pancreatic insufficiency. Fat-soluble vitamins are supplemented routinely and annually monitored. Patients may be noncompliant with vitamin supplementation or require higher dosages (Rana et al, 2014).

Salt. Excessive sodium loss in perspiration in patients with CF predisposes them to hyponatremic dehydration under conditions of heat stress. Most patients need supplementation of sodium chloride. The amount of salt supplementation should be increased under circumstances such as high temperature and humidity; a dry, desert climate; strenuous exercise in hot weather; excessive sweating; fever; and presence of diarrhea or vomiting.

High levels of linoleic acid (LNA) (an omega-6 fatty acid) and low levels of alpha linoleic acid (ALA) (an omega-3 fatty acid) are seen in the development of fatty acid alterations in CF patients (Katrangi et al, 2013). Although nutrition therapy consisting of a high caloric and high fat intake counteracts the effect of malabsorption in CF, no recommendations exist regarding the best type of fat for the diet. However, data suggest that the increased LNA:ALA ratio may contribute to the increased metabolic abnormalities of CF and CF-related inflammation. More research is needed to determine the role of specific fat sources in treating CF patients (Katrangi et al, 2013).

A challenging issue while working with CF individuals is the gastrostomy tube feeds and administration of pancreatic enzymes. Overnight enteral pump feedings often are required for CF patients in order to supplement the daytime oral intake and provide an additional 6 to 8 hours of energy intake. Questions still remain on the optimal level of enzymes to be provided with overnight feeds (Matel, 2012).

Tube feeding options include gastrostomy tube, nasogastric tube, and jejunostomy tube. The most common delivery option is the percutaneous endoscopic gastrostomy (PEG) tube (see Chapter 13). When CF patients have trouble maintaining sufficient caloric intake because of recurrent infections, abdominal issues, and increased breathing, supplemental enteral feedings are of great benefit; PERT is still required (Rogers, 2013).

ASTHMA

Asthma is a chronic disorder that affects the airways and is characterized by bronchial hyper-reactivity, reversible airflow obstruction, and airway remodeling. Asthmatic symptoms include periodic episodes of chest tightness, breathlessness, and wheezing. Asthma has become more prevalent and has been increasing at the rate of 25% to 75% every decade since 1960 in westernized countries (Allan and Devereux, 2011).

Pathophysiology

Asthma is the result of a complex interaction between environmental exposures and genetics. When people are genetically susceptible, environmental factors exacerbate airway hyper-responsiveness, airway inflammation, and atopy (tendency to develop allergic reaction) that eventually leads to asthma.

Environmental factors that are linked to the development of asthma include indoor allergies (dust mites, animal allergies) and outdoor allergies (pollen and fungi). Increased risk of asthma development also has been linked to air pollution, tobacco smoke exposure, small size at birth, respiratory infection, and lower socioeconomic status (McCloud and Papoutsakis, 2011).

Clinicians identify three key areas when diagnosing asthma:
1. Airflow obstruction that is at least partially reversible
2. Airflow obstruction that recurs
3. Exclusion of other diagnoses

Symptoms such as wheezing, coughing, shortness of breath, and chest tightness occur in most patients, and symptoms that worsen at night is a common feature. Although allergic asthma or "extrinsic asthma" is due to chronic allergic inflammation of the airways, "intrinsic asthma" is triggered by nonallergic factors such as exercise, certain chemicals, and extreme emotions (Chih–Hung Guo et al, 2012).

A life-threatening situation with markedly narrow airways, known as status asthmaticus, can result when asthma has not been treated properly. Corticosteroid therapy is often prescribed, but chronic use may place the individual at risk for osteopenia (precursor to osteoporosis), bone fractures, or steroid-induced hyperglycemia (see Chapter 8 and Appendix 23.). Some evidence supports the effectiveness of sublingual immunotherapy in the treatment of asthma and rhinitis, but more studies are needed on optimal dosages (Lin et al, 2013).

Medical Management

The essential components of asthma therapy are routine monitoring of symptoms and lung function, patient education, control of environmental triggers, and pharmacotherapy.

Pharmacologic treatment must be tailored to the individual patient and is used in a stepwise manner. The medications and the regime chosen depend on the severity of the asthma, which can be classified as an acute attack, intermittent, mild persistent, moderate persistent, or severe persistent.

Quick relief and long-term controller medications are used as therapy for asthma. Although quick-relief medications include short-acting beta agonists (bronchodilators) and steroid pills, long-term controller medications include inhaled long-acting beta agonists and leukotriene modifiers.

Inhaled corticosteroids are the cornerstone of pharmacologic management with persistent asthma. Some younger patients with refractory asthma need maintenance doses of systemic steroids. Because steroids change bone metabolism and the development of osteoporosis, these children benefit from increased calcium intake (see Table 34-1). Two newer therapies are anti-IgE (anti-immunoglobulin E) therapy and

TABLE 34-1 Recommended Calcium Intakes for Children Receiving Steroids Compared with Those for Healthy Children

Age in Years	Recommendations for Healthy Children (mg/day)	Recommendations for Children Taking Steroids (mg/day)
1-3	700	1000
4-8	1000	1500
9-13	1300	1900
14-18	1300	1900

Adapted from McCloud E, Papoutsakis C: A medical nutrition therapy primer for childhood asthma: current and emerging perspectives, *J Am Diet Assoc* 111:1052, 2011. McEvoy GK, Snow EK: *AHFS drug information*, Bethesda, Md, American Society of Health System Pharmacists, 2015.

bronchial thermoplasty, which are used in selected cases of severe asthma. Immunomodulator therapies with anti-IL-5 (anti-interleukin-5) antibodies, anti-IL-4 alpha subunit antibodies, human necrosis factor TNF-alpha (tumor necrosis factor-alpha) inhibitors, and the use of macrolide antibiotics for their antiinflammatory actions are some of the experimental approaches (Wenzel, 2014).

Antibiotics for exacerbation of asthma are not recommended by current clinical practice guidelines, because respiratory infection triggering asthma attacks are more often viral rather than bacterial.

Medical Nutrition Therapy

When treating asthma, the dietitian nutritionist addresses the dietary triggers, corrects energy and nutrient deficiencies and excesses in the diet, educates the patient on a personalized diet that provides optimal levels of nutrients, monitors growth in children, and watches for food-drug interactions.

Modulation of antioxidant intake with nutritional supplementation has a beneficial effect on the severity and progression of asthma. Although a slight inverse association was seen between a low vitamin E intake and wheezing symptoms, no association was found between vitamin E and asthma. Further studies are required to understand the mechanism of vitamin E on the inflammation of the immune system (Fabian et al, 2013). Low blood carotenoid levels also have been linked with asthma. A diet rich in antioxidants and monounsaturated fats seems to have a protective effect on childhood asthma by counteracting oxidative stress (Garcia-Marcos L et al, 2013). Studies have also associated asthma with reduced selenium status (Allan and Devereux, 2011).

In the childhood asthma prevention study omega-3 polyunsaturated fatty acid (PUFA) fish oil was supplemented throughout childhood and wheezing was reduced. This effect did not continue into later childhood. Supplementation of vitamin C and zinc also have been reported to improve asthma symptoms and lung function (Allan and Devereux, 2011).

Conflicting results on the efficacy of vitamin D supplementation have been reported. In one study an insufficient serum level of less than 30 ng/dL of vitamin D was associated with an increase in asthma exacerbation in the form of ER visits and hospitalizations (Brehm et al, 2010). In another, high doses of vitamin D supplementation were not shown to have any protective effect (Litonjua et al, 2014).

A higher than desirable BMI during childhood is associated with a significant increase in the development of asthma.

Institution of diets that help with weight loss in asthmatic obese children seem to show improvements with the control of asthma, static lung function, and improved quality of life (Gibson et al, 2013).

Gastroesophageal reflux disease (GERD) and food allergens are the two most common dietary triggers for asthma. GERD is highly prevalent in asthmatic patients. A critical component of medical nutrition therapy for asthmatic patients is a diet free of known irritants such as spicy foods, caffeine, chocolate, and acidic foods (see Chapter 27). Limiting the intake of high fat foods and portion control can prevent gastric secretions, which exacerbate GERD.

Food allergens and food additives are other potential dietary triggers for asthma. An immunoglobulin E-mediated reaction to a food protein can lead to bronchoconstriction. Completely avoiding the allergenic food protein is the only dietary treatment currently available for food allergies. Some sulfites, such as potassium metasulfite and sodium sulfide, used in the processing of foods, have been found to be a trigger for asthmatics (Gaur et al, 2013) (see Chapter 26).

Some asthma patients need maintenance oral steroids, and these patients are prone to develop drug-nutrient interaction problems (see Chapter 8).

CHRONIC OBSTRUCTIVE PULMONARY DISEASE

COPD is now the third most common cause of death in the world and is predicted to be the fifth most common cause of disability by 2020 (Burney et al, 2014). Smoke from cigarettes is a major risk factor, along with that from biomass fuel used for cooking and heating in rural areas of developing countries. Occupational smoke or dust, air pollution, and genetic factors are also factors in the development of COPD (see Table 34-2). Patients with COPD suffer from decreased food intake and malnutrition that causes respiratory muscle weakness, increased disability, increased susceptibility to infections, and hormonal alterations.

Pathophysiology

COPD is a term that encompasses **chronic bronchitis** (a long-term condition of COPD in which inflamed bronchi lead to mucus, cough and difficulty breathing) and **emphysema** (a form of long-term lung disease characterized by the destruction of lung parenchyma with lack of elastic recoil). These conditions may coexist in varying degrees and are generally not reversible. Figure 34-7 shows the overlap between these three conditions, asthma, chronic bronchitis and emphysema.

Patients with primary emphysema suffer from greater dyspnea and cachexia. On the other hand patients with bronchitis have hypoxia, **hypercapnia** (increased amount of carbon dioxide), and complications such as pulmonary hypertension and right heart failure (Papaioannou et al, 2013).

TABLE 34-2 Risk Factors for COPD

Definite	Probable
Tobacco smoking	Pulmonary tuberculosis
Occupational exposure	Repeated lower respiratory infection during childhood
Exposure to biomass fuel smoke	Poorly treated asthma
Environmental tobacco smoke	

Adapted from Gupta D et al: Guidelines for diagnosis and management of chronic obstructive pulmonary disease: Joint ICS/NCCP (I) recommendations, *Lung India* 30:228, 2013.

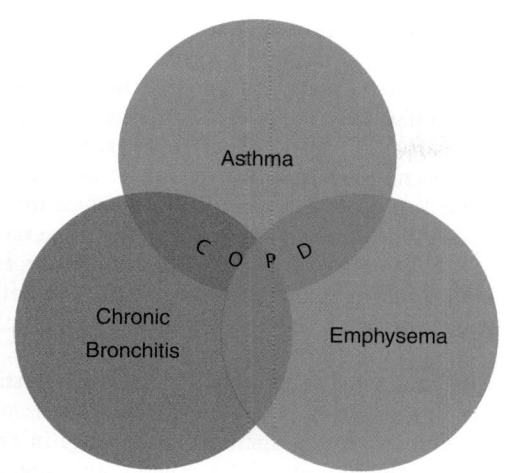

FIGURE 34-7 The overlap of asthma, chronic bronchitis, and emphysema making up COPD.

Alpha-1 antitrypsin deficiency is present in 1% to 2% of COPD patients and is likely underrecognized. COPD exacerbations can be caused by *Haemophilus influenzae*, Moraxella catarrhalis, *S. pneumonia*, rhinovirus, coronavirus, and to a lesser degree, organisms such as *P. aeruginosa*, *S. aureus*, *Mycoplasma* spp., and *Chlamydia pneumoniae*. Allergies, smoking, congestive heart failure, pulmonary embolism, pneumonia, and systemic infections are the reason for 20% to 40% of COPD exacerbations (Nakawah et al, 2013).

Although cigarette smoking is considered a major risk factor for developing COPD, only about 20% of smokers develop the disease (Hirayama et al, 2010). Osteoporosis in COPD patients not only predisposes patients to painful vertebral fractures but also affects lung function by altering the configuration of the chest wall. Frequent acute exacerbations in COPD patients increase the severity of chronic system inflammation. This leads to bone loss by inhibiting bone metabolism. Lack of sun exposure and physical activity with COPD leads to a lack of 25-hydroxy vitamin D (25-OHD), which regulates bone metabolism by promoting the absorption of calcium (Xiaomei et al, 2014).

Factors that influence the prognosis of COPD are the severity of disease, genetic predisposition, nutritional status, environmental exposures, and acute exacerbations.

Medical Management

In general, COPD therapies have a limited effect compared with therapies in asthma. No disease-modifying medications exist that can change the progression of airway obstruction in COPD.

Inhaled bronchodilators remain the mainstay of treatment for COPD patients. Usually these are given by metered dose inhalers (MDI), but for severe dyspnea, may be administered in a nebulized form. Anticholinergic medications such as ipratropium bromide or Spiriva (tiotropium bromide), a long-acting anticholinergic agent with specificity for muscarinic receptors, can be added to the treatment. Theophylline continues to be used in some cases. Inhaled steroids and a trial of oral steroids may be required for some patients. Antibiotics often are prescribed when an exacerbation is considered to be due to bacterial infection.

Pulmonary hypertension is a risk factor that shortens life expectancy and is common in advanced COPD. The first step in treating pulmonary hypertension in patients with COPD is appropriate management of their obstructive lung disease as mentioned earlier. The exact indication for pulmonary hypertension specific therapies in COPD patients is unclear. Current recommendations state that pulmonary hypertension specific therapies should be considered when pulmonary hypertension is persistent despite optimization of COPD management and when pulmonary hypertension is out of proportion to the degree of air flow obstruction (Minai et al, 2010).

Patients who are hypoxemic need supplemental oxygen. Pulmonary rehabilitation may be helpful in advanced COPD. Patients with severe COPD may suffer respiratory failure related to complications such as pneumothorax, pneumonia, and congestive heart failure, or due to uncontrolled administration of high-dose oxygen or narcotic sedatives. The patients in respiratory failure need mechanical ventilation (see Figure 34-8).

In addition to facing major physical impairment and chronic dyspnea, COPD patients are at an increased risk of developing depression that should be identified and treated.

Medical Nutrition Therapy

Malnutrition is a common problem associated with COPD, with prevalence rates of 30% to 60% due to the extra energy required by the work of breathing and frequent and recurrent respiratory infections. Breathing with normal lungs expends 36 to 72 kcal/day; it increases 10-fold in patients with COPD (Hill et al, 2013). Infection with fever increases metabolic rate even further (see Chapter 2). An independent predictor of increased mortality in COPD patients is low body weight. Weight loss in advanced COPD is considered an independent risk factor for mortality, whereas weight gain reverses the negative effect of decreased body weight (Berman, 2011).

Low body weight is due to poor nutritional intake, an increased metabolic rate, or both. Inadequate food intake and poor appetite are the primary targets for intervention in patients with COPD. These two issues mean COPD patients struggle to meet their nutritional needs. Depletion of protein and vital minerals such as calcium, magnesium, potassium, and phosphorus contribute to respiratory muscle function impairment. In severe malnutrition inadequate electrolyte repletion during aggressive nutrition repletion can lead to severe metabolic consequences related to refeeding syndrome (see Chapter 13).

There are two main goals in managing the hypermetabolism seen in stable COPD: 1) the prevention of weight loss, and

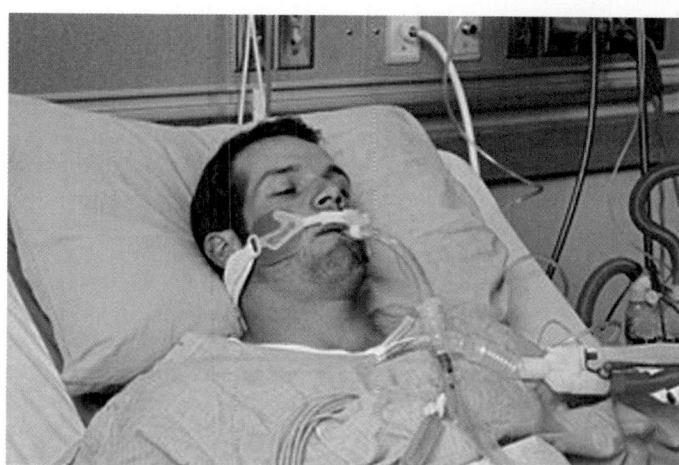

FIGURE 34-8 An ICU patient on ventilator.

2) the prevention of the loss of lean body mass (LBM). These goals can be achieved by ensuring the following:

- Small frequent meals that are nutritionally dense
- The patient eats the main meal when energy level is at its highest
- Adequate calories, protein, vitamins, and minerals to maintain a desirable weight - a BMI of 20 to 24 kg/m2
- Availability of foods that require less preparation and can be heated easily in a microwave oven
- Limitation of alcohol to fewer than 2 drinks/day (30 g alcohol)
- A period of rest before mealtimes

People with COPD suffer a poor prognosis when they have malnutrition that predisposes them to infections. The ability to produce lung surfactant, exercise tolerance, and respiratory muscle force are reduced in the presence of infection. Weight loss leads to an increased load on the respiratory muscles, contributing to the onset of acute respiratory failure (Hill et al, 2013).

Many factors affect nutritional status during the progression of COPD. Although body weight and BMI should be followed because they are easily obtained markers of nutritional status in patients, they can underestimate the extent of nutritional impairment (Hill et al, 2013).

Current evidence suggests that a prudent diet pattern helps in protecting smokers against malnutrition. A combination of nutritional counseling and nicotine replacement seems to optimize success (Hill et al, 2013).

Studies have shown an inverse relationship between dietary iron and calcium intake and COPD risk. Iron deficiency anemia is seen in 10% to 30% of patients with COPD. It has been seen that correcting the anemia and iron deficiency by either blood transfusions or intravenous iron therapy improves dyspnea in COPD patients (Silverberg et al, 2014). COPD patients are also at higher risk of developing osteoporosis resulting from steroid usage, smoking, and vitamin D depletion. Maintaining adequate levels of vitamin D (25-OHD) is a health-promoting strategy for COPD patients (Lee et al, 2013; see Appendix 45).

The primary goals of nutrition care for patients with COPD are to facilitate nutritional well-being, maintain an appropriate ratio of lean body mass to adipose tissue, correct fluid imbalance, manage drug-nutrient interactions (see Chapter 8 and Appendix 23), and prevent osteoporosis.

Nutritional depletion may be evidenced clinically by low body weight for height and decreased grip strength. Calculation of BMI may be insufficient to detect changes in fat and muscle mass. Instead, determination of body composition helps to differentiate lean muscle mass from adipose tissue and overhydration from dehydration. In patients with cor pulmonale (increased blood pressure which leads to enlargement and failure of the right ventricle of the heart) and the resultant fluid retention, weight maintenance, or gain from fluid may camouflage actual wasting of lean body mass. Thus for patients retaining fluids, careful interpretation of anthropometric measurements, biochemical indicators, and functional measures of nutrition status is necessary (see Chapter 7 and Appendices 21 and 22).

A combination of nutritional supplements and anabolic steroids can increase muscle mass and reverse any negative effects of weight loss. Exercise tolerance has been shown to improve with a dietary supplement that contains omega-3 PUFA, which has antiinflammatory effects (Berman, 2011) (see Chapter 3).

Adipokines is a generic term for the bioactive proteins that are secreted by adipocytes. They include adiponectin, leptin, IL-6, and TNF-alpha. They play a vital role in influencing the nutritional status and regulating the appetite. Leptin (satiety hormone) is secreted promptly in response to food intake, and plays a role in suppressing appetite and enhancing energy expenditure. It has been suggested that measuring levels of leptin in the sputum can be useful in determining the severity of lung disease because it has been shown to increase during acute exacerbations (Itoh et al, 2013). Adiponectin (a protein involved in fatty acid breakdown and glucose regulation), like leptin, is secreted from adipocytes, but has an opposite effect. Adiponectin enhances appetite, has an antiinflammatory, antidiabetic, and antiatherosclerotic effect and is considered beneficial. Resistin, another adipokine, induces inflammation and insulin resistance. In addition to being an appetite stimulant, ghrelin also stimulates growth hormone secretion, with antagonistic effects to leptin. Table 34-3 summarizes the functions and change in the blood levels of these adipokines in COPD patients, and how they can influence management and recovery (Itoh et al, 2013).

Macronutrients

In stable COPD, requirements for water, protein, fat, and carbohydrate are determined by the underlying lung disease, oxygen therapy, medications, weight status, and any acute fluid fluctuations. Attention to the metabolic side effects of malnutrition and the role of individual amino acids is necessary. Determination of a specific patient's macronutrient needs is made on an individual basis, with close monitoring of outcomes.

Energy

Meeting energy needs can be difficult. For patients participating in pulmonary rehabilitation programs, energy requirements depend on the intensity and frequency of exercise therapy and can be increased or decreased. It is crucial to remember that energy balance and nitrogen balance are intertwined. Consequently, maintaining optimal energy balance is essential to

TABLE 34-3   Blood Levels of Hormones and Adipokines in Patients with COPD

Hormone	Function	Changes in blood levels with COPD
Leptin	• Suppresses appetite • Promotes inflammation • Regulates hematopoiesis, angiogenesis, and wound healing	Decreased in patients with a low BMI compared with patients with a normal and high BMI
Ghrelin	Stimulates appetite and release of growth hormone	Increased in underweight patients compared with normal weight patients
Adiponectin	• Stimulates fatty acid oxidation • Increases insulin sensitivity, and inhibits inflammatory process	Increased during acute exacerbation Decreased levels in current smokers
Resistin	Promotes inflammation and insulin resistance by the production of IL-6 and TNF-alpha	Inversely correlated with predicted FEV_1 %
TNF-alpha	Antagonizes insulin signaling, and promotes inflammation.	Increased compared with healthy individuals
IL-6	• Loss of appetite • Promotes inflammation	Increased compared with healthy individuals

Adapted from Itoh M et al: Undernutrition in patients with COPD and its treatment, *Nutrients* 5:1316, 2013.

preserving visceral and somatic proteins. Preferably, indirect calorimetry should be used to determine energy needs and to prescribe and monitor the provision of sufficient, but not excessive calories. When energy equations are used for prediction of needs, increases for physiologic stress must be included. Caloric needs may vary significantly from one person to the next and even in the same individual over time (see Chapter 2).

Fat

Omega-3 and omega-6 are PUFAs that are essential fatty acids. The simplest forms of these fatty acids are the omega-6 linoleic acid (LA) and alpha-linolenic acid (ALA). The body is unable to synthesize them, and they must be consumed in the human diet. These fatty acids are desaturated to form long chain omega-3 PUFAs or omega-6 PUFAs. Docosahexaenoic acid (DHA) and eicosapentaenoic acid (EPA) and alpha-linolenic acid (ALA) are the major omega-3 PUFAs, and the major long-chain omega–6 fatty acids are linoleic acid (LA) and arachidonic acid (AA). See Appendix 34 for the sources of these fatty acids in the diet. In theory, intake of long-chain omega-3 PUFAs, which reduces inflammation, should improve the efficacy of COPD treatments. PUFA supplementation is beneficial in COPD, but various factors such as supplement adherence, comorbidities, and duration of the supplementation play vital roles(Fulton et al, 2012).

Dietary supplementation of DHA and AA has been shown to delay and reduce risk of upper respiratory infections and asthma, with lowering the incidence of bronchiolitis during the first year of life (Shek et al, 2012). Data from various studies have shown the positive impact of long-chain PUFAs in initiating and providing resolution of inflammation in respiratory diseases (Shek et al, 2012). It has been shown that aspirin helps to trigger resolvin, a molecule naturally made by the body from omega-3 fatty acids. Resolvin resolves or turns off the inflammation in underlying destructive conditions such as inflammatory lung diseases (Dalli et al, 2013).

Protein

Sufficient protein of 1.2 to 1.5 g/kg of dry body weight is necessary to maintain or restore lung and muscle strength, as well as to promote immune function. A balanced ratio of protein (15% to 20% of calories) with fat (30% to 45% of calories) and carbohydrate (40% to 55% of calories) is important to preserve a satisfactory respiratory quotient (RQ) from substrate metabolism use (see Chapter 2). Repletion but not overfeeding is particularly critical in patients with compromised ability to exchange gases as excess feeding of calories results in CO_2 that must be expelled. Other concurrent disease processes such as cardiovascular or renal disease, cancer, or diabetes affect the total amounts, ratios, and kinds of protein, fat, and carbohydrate prescribed.

Vitamins and Minerals

As with macronutrients, vitamin and mineral requirements for individuals with stable COPD depend on the underlying pathologic conditions of the lung, other concurrent diseases, medical treatments, weight status, and bone mineral density. For people continuing to smoke tobacco, additional vitamin C is necessary (see Appendix 42).

The role of minerals such as magnesium and calcium in muscle contraction and relaxation may be important for people with COPD. Intakes at least equivalent to the dietary reference intake (DRI) should be provided. Depending on bone mineral density test results, coupled with food intake

history and glucocorticoid medications use, additional vitamins D and K also may be necessary (see Chapter 24).

Patients with cor pulmonale and subsequent fluid retention require sodium and fluid restriction. Depending on the diuretics prescribed, increased potassium supplementation may be required (see Chapter 8 and Appendix 23). And other water soluble vitamins, particularly thiamin, may need to be supplemented.

Patients are recommended to drink adequate fluids and stay hydrated to help sputum consistency and easier expectoration. The Parenteral and Enteral Nutrition Group (PENG) recommends a fluid intake of 35 ml/kg body weight daily for adults 18 to 60 years and 30 ml of fluid/kg body daily for adults over 60 years (PENG, 2011).

COPD patients report difficulties with eating because of low appetite, increased breathlessness when eating, difficulty shopping and preparing meals, dry mouth, early satiety and bloating, anxiety and depression, and fatigue. In addition to the above, inefficient and overworking respiratory muscles lead to increased nutritional requirements (Evans, 2012).

Patients in the Advanced Stage of COPD

Patients with advanced COPD are undernourished and in a state of pulmonary cachexia. The cause of cachexia in advanced COPD is poorly understood. The role for myostatin has been suggested. Myostatin is a member of the transforming growth factor-beta superfamily that functions as a negative regulator of muscle growth. This has been suggested by the significantly high levels of myostatin in patients with stable COPD compared with healthy individuals (Benedik et al, 2011).

These cachectic patients have anorexia as a typical symptom. Pulmonary cachexia is an independent risk factor and is common in the advanced stage of COPD. Pharmacotherapy and nonpharmacotherapeutic treatments such as respiratory rehabilitation and nutrition counseling are the mainstays of COPD treatment in such patients (Itoh et al, 2013). Sarcopenia and cachexia result from the accelerated loss of lean tissue (Raguso and Luthy, 2011). This muscle wasting has a detrimental effect on the respiratory function (Collins et al, 2012).

Osteoporosis exists as a significant problem in 24% to 69% of patients with advanced COPD (Evans and Morgan, 2014). Any sudden drop in height is a mark of developing osteoporosis. As COPD progresses, osteoporosis results because of immobility, which also leads to deconditioning and dyspnea. Smoking, low BMI, low skeletal muscle mass, and corticosteroid usage can lead to bone loss along with low serum vitamin D levels (Evans and Morgan, 2014) (see Box 34-2).

BOX 34-2 Planning the Diet for the Patient with Pulmonary Cachexia

Energy requirements during healing = 30 kcal/kg of usual body weight or 13.7 cal/usual body weight (pounds)

Protein (gm)/day during healing = [(1.2 g – 1.4 g) × body weight (kg) or 0.55 × usual body weight (pounds)

Fluid requirements = body weight (lb)/2 = ounces per day **or** body wt (lb) × 9/16 = cups per day

Fluid requirements are increased because of fever, chemotherapy regimen, oxygen use, and presence of COPD. Lack of energy or dehydration increases fatigue and constipation. Fluid deficits of 1% body weight lower metabolic function by 5%.

Levin RM: *Nutrition in the Patient with Lung Cancer, Caring Ambassadors Lung Cancer Choices* (website): http://lungcancercap.org/wp-content/uploads/2014/10/Chapter_8_2014.pdf, 2012. Accessed December 31, 2014.

TUBERCULOSIS

Mycobacterium tuberculosis, the causative organism of **tuberculosis (TB)**, is an intracellular bacterial parasite, has a slow rate of growth, is an obligate aerobe, and induces a granulomatous response in the tissues of a normal host.

Even though TB is not as common in the United States as in some other countries, there has been a resurgence associated with human immunodeficiency virus (HIV) and drug-resistant forms of TB (see Chapter 37). The World Health Organization (WHO) estimates approximately 630,000 cases of TB worldwide. In 2013 TB remained a major health concern with resistance to multidrug-resistant TB on the rise. Increase in relocation of this population of patients, the HIV pandemic, and increase in multidrug-resistant TB poses global concerns in the management of TB (Abubakar et al, 2013).

Pathophysiology

When an infectious TB patient coughs, the cough droplets contain tuberculous bacilli. Small particles penetrate deep into the lungs. Each of these tiny droplets may carry 1 to 5 bacilli, which are enough to establish infection. This is the reason why cases of active TB must be isolated till they become noninfectious. In about 5% of cases, the infection progresses and produces active tuberculosis. In 95% of cases when a host has an effective cell-mediated immune response, the infection is contained. When patients with active TB, are left untreated, they can die as a result of progression and complications (Hood, 2013).

Although there may be minimal symptoms and the diagnosis is suspected because of an abnormal chest radiograph, most patients with pulmonary TB present with chronic cough, prolonged fever, night sweats, anorexia, and weight loss.

Management

An important component of management is to place these patients in respiratory isolation to prevent spread of infection, until the smear for sputum acid fast bacillus (AFB) comes back negative. As soon as the diagnosis is established, treatment with four anti-TB medications - INH, rifampin, pyrazinamide and ethambutol - is started. Each drug has food-nutrient interactions (see Chapter 8 and Appendix 23). These medications are continued for 2 months, and then only rifampin and INH are continued for 4 more months. Duration of treatment may be longer in some patients.

Medical Nutrition Therapy

Malnutrition is common in patients with pulmonary TB, and nutritional supplementation is necessary. Markers of protein nutritional status are low levels of the inflammatory proteins (see Table 7-4), anthropometric indices, and the micronutrient status of TB patients (Miyata et al, 2013).

TB leads to or worsens any preexisting condition of malnutrition and increases catabolism. The WHO guidelines suggest hospitalization of patients who are severely undernourished in view of their mortality risk. Dietary supplementation is recommended until the patient achieves a BMI of 18.5 (Bhargava et al, 2013).

Active TB is associated with weight loss, cachexia, and low serum concentration of leptin. There is a synergistic interaction between malnutrition and infection. Recurrent infection leads to worsening nutritional status and loss of body nitrogen. The resulting malnutrition, in turn, creates a higher susceptibility to infection (Miyata et al, 2013).

In the short term, malnutrition increases the risk of infection and early progression of infection to produce active TB. In the long term, malnutrition increases the risk of reactivation of the TB disease. Malnutrition also can lower the effectiveness of the anti-TB drug regime, which patients have to be on for several months. The efficacy of Bacillus Calmette-Guerin (BCG) vaccine can also be impaired by malnutrition.

Upon correction of nutritional deficiencies, malnutrition-induced loss of certain immune processes can be reversed rapidly. Nutritional intervention in combination with appropriate medications does improve the outcome of malnourished TB patients.

Energy

Current energy recommendations are those for undernourished and catabolic patients, 35 to 40 kcal/kg of ideal body weight. For patients with any concomitant infections such as HIV, energy requirements increase by 20% to 30% to maintain body weight.

Protein

Protein is vital in preventing muscle tissue wastage and an intake of 15% of energy needs or 1.2 to 1.5 g/kg ideal body weight, approximately 75 to 100 g per day, is recommended.

Vitamins and Minerals

A multivitamin and mineral supplement that provides 50% to 150% of the RDA is helpful, because TB patients have increased requirements that are impossible to meet with diet alone. Nutrients such as vitamin A, the B vitamins, vitamins C and E, zinc, and selenium are usually deficient in TB patients. These are vital for the integrity of the immune response. Vitamin D deficiencies are common with TB and result because of an insufficient vitamin D intake and limited exposure to sunlight (Desai et al, 2012; see Appendix 45).

Isoniazid is an antagonist of vitamin B_6 (pyridoxine) and is frequently used in TB treatment. It may cause rare instances of peripheral neuropathy resulting from the nutritional depletion of vitamin B_6. A standard procedure is to supplement adults with 25 mg of vitamin B_6 per day to overcome this drug-nutrient interaction. Vitamin B_6 supplementation is not routinely used with children, but if large dosages of isoniazid are used or the child has a low blood vitamin B_6 level, 25 mg of B_6 supplementation is recommended (Nutrition Information Center University of Stellenbosch [NICUS], 2009).

Studies have documented an increased prevalence of anemia with TB patients, which is associated with increased risk of death. To guide clinical decision making and provide treatment recommendations, factors that contribute to the TB-associated anemia have to be characterized. Although other causes do coexist, iron deficiency anemia is the most important contributor in the development of anemia in TB patients (Isanaka et al, 2012).

Evidence indicates that excess iron supplementation may be dangerous to TB patients, and the use of iron therapy is not universally recommended. However, if iron studies show iron deficiency, iron therapy is then initiated (see Chapter 32 for management of iron deficiency anemia).

LUNG CANCER

Lung cancer remains the leading cause of cancer deaths for males and females in the United States. In 2012 1.8 million patients worldwide were diagnosed with lung cancer (Mannino et al, 2014).

Neoplasms of the lower respiratory tract are a heterogeneous group of tumors. The group commonly called **bronchogenic carcinomas** comprises squamous cell carcinoma, adenocarcinoma, small cell undifferentiated carcinoma, and large cell undifferentiated carcinoma, and account for 90% of all the neoplasms of the lower respiratory tract. Mortality is more common in males than females, although this difference is diminishing. While the female incidence rate is stabilizing, the male incidence rate seems to be decreasing (Baldini et al, 2014).

Pathophysiology

Often lung cancer is detected on a routine chest radiograph in an asymptomatic smoker. Other patients may present with symptoms related to the tumor itself, symptoms related to the local extension of the tumor or widespread metastases, or systemic symptoms such as anorexia, weight loss, weakness, and paraneoplastic syndromes.

Dyspnea is the most burdensome cancer symptom, and occurs in 15% to 55% of lung cancer patients at diagnosis. In addition to the tumor, other factors contribute to the symptom of dyspnea – factors such as pericardial effusion, anemia, fatigue, depression, anxiety, metastatic involvement of other organs, aspiration, anorexia-cachexia syndrome, and pleural effusion.

Patients with lung cancer suffer from progressive *weight loss* with changes in body composition. Malnutrition impairs the contractility of the respiratory muscles, affecting endurance and respiratory mechanics.

Cough is present in 50% to 75% of lung cancer patients at presentation and occurs most frequently in squamous cell and small cell carcinoma because of their tendency to involve central airways (Huhmann and Camporeale, 2012).

Pain and fatigue are common symptoms associated with lung cancer. The tumor may produce pleuritic pain because of tumor extension into the pleura, or musculoskeletal type pain because of extension into the chest wall. Bone pain may occur as a result of metastases to the bones. Bone metastases in patients with lung cancer account for 30% to 40% of the pain. About 50% of early stage cancer and 75% to 100% of advanced stage cancer patients report fatigue (Huhmann and Camporeale, 2012).

Pulmonary cachexia syndrome affects patients with advanced lung disease and is defined by a BMI of less than 20 or a weight less than 90% of IBW (Bellini, 2013). In lung cancer, weight loss is associated with increasing mortality, and weight loss of even 5% indicates a poor prognosis. Although anorexia and cachexia are two different entities they often are used interchangeably (Huhmann and Camporeale, 2012) (see Chapter 36).

Medical Management

The choice of definitive management for a particular patient is determined by numerous factors, such as the tumor cell type, tumor stage, resectability of the tumor, and suitability of the patient for general anesthesia and surgery. Some patients need general palliative care in terms of psychologic support, control of distressing symptoms, and palliative radiation. Nutritional support plays a very important role in the management of advanced lung cancer.

Medical Nutrition Therapy

The National Comprehensive Cancer Network (NCCN) guidelines include nutritional assessments, medications, and nonpharmacologic approaches to achieve the following:

1. Treat the reversible causes of anorexia such as early satiety
2. Evaluate the rate and severity of weight loss
3. Treat the symptoms interfering with food intake: nausea and vomiting, dyspnea, mucositis, constipation, and pain
4. Assess the use of appetite stimulants like megestrol acetate and Decadron (corticosteroids)
5. Provide nutritional support (enteral or parenteral) (Del Ferraro et al, 2012)

Cancer cachexia syndrome (CCS) is the presence of a metabolic state that leads to energy and muscle store depletion in lung cancer patients. When patients experience CCS, they lose adipose and skeletal muscle mass. Changes in hormone and cytokine levels, along with tumor byproducts, cause CCS. Weight loss seen with CCS, unlike starvation, is irreversible and continues to worsen despite increased nutritional intake (Huhmann and Camporeale, 2012) (see Chapter 36).

However, despite these findings, reversible causes of anorexia should be sought and treated. Although nutritional support does not improve spirometric values and arterial blood gas and does not stop weight loss, it does modestly improve clinical outcomes such as the 6-minute walk test, quality of life, and inspiratory and expiratory muscle strength (Bellini, 2013).

Nutrition repletion is problematic in advanced lung disease because fatigue and dyspnea tend to interfere with the preparation and consumption of food. Alterations in the taste of food because of chronic sputum production, early satiety resulting from flattening of the diaphragm, nausea and indigestion resulting from side effects of medications, and lack of motivation to eat because of depression make it difficult for the patient to take adequate nutrition by the oral route. However, accepted components of oral nutrition therapy are the following:

1. Small frequent meals that are high in fat and protein and low in carbohydrate
2. Provision of adequate calories that meet or exceed the resting energy expenditure (REE)
3. Rest before meals
4. Meals that require minimal preparation
5. Oral supplements with the ratio of fat: carbohydrate of 3:1 that are better tolerated because the respiratory quotient for carbohydrates is 1.0 and for fats is only 0.7 and thus results in decreased work of breathing (Bellini, 2013)

With pulmonary cancer cachexia syndrome, patients are unable to gain weight with nutritional interventions alone. Prokinetic agents for delayed gastric emptying can be used with careful consideration of side effects. Megestrol acetate, an appetite stimulant, may result in increasing appetite and caloric intake. **Ghrelin** (a growth hormone releasing peptide) lowers fat use and stimulates feeding through growth hormone independent mechanisms, thereby inducing a positive energy balance. Studies have shown that repeated IV administration of ghrelin improves body composition, lowers muscle wasting, and increases functional capacity (Bellini, 2013).

One study suggests that whole body protein metabolism in pulmonary patients may benefit from branched-chain amino acid (BCAA) supplementation. This study was the first of its kind in assessing the clinical benefits of supplementing BCAA in a preoperative pulmonary rehabilitation center; 6.2 g of

BCAA supplementation was the recommended daily dosage. However, the effect of BCAA supplementation for lung cancer patients has not been clarified and requires further study before specific recommendations can be made. A comprehensive pulmonary rehabilitation protocol includes nutritional support and physical exercise (Harada et al, 2013).

OBESITY HYPOVENTILATION SYNDROME

Obesity hypoventilation syndrome (OHS) is defined as a BMI of more than 30 kg/m^2 and alveolar hypoventilation defined by arterial carbon dioxide (Paco$_2$) level of more than 45 mm Hg during wakefulness, which occurs in the absence of other conditions that cause hypoventilation (Piper and Grunstein, 2011).

Alveolar hypoventilation in OHS is related to the multiple physiologic abnormalities related to obesity: obstructive sleep apnea (OSA), increased work of breathing, respiratory muscle impairment, a depressed central ventilator drive, and reduced effects of neurohumoral modulators (e.g., leptin) (Koenig, 2011; Piper and Grunstein, 2007).

Obstructive sleep apnea (OSA) is a common chronic disorder, which is characterized by loud snoring, excessive daytime sleepiness, and witnessed breathing interruptions or awakenings because of gasping or choking. The presence or absence of OSA and its severity usually is confirmed by a "sleep study" (polysomnography, PSG) before initiating treatment. The PSG also serves as a baseline to establish the effectiveness of the subsequent treatment (Epstein et al, 2009).

Medical Management

Depending on the number of episodes of apnea or hypopnea (overly shallow breathing) per hour, OSA is graded as mild, moderate, or severe. The patients with OSA commonly are treated with continuous positive airway pressure (CPAP) provided by custom made oral appliances or with various surgical methods. These primary treatment modalities for OSA must be used in addition to weight loss because of the low success and low cure rates by dietary approach alone (Epstein et al, 2009).

Medical Nutrition Therapy

Weight reduction by medical nutrition therapy or, in morbid obesity, by bariatric surgery remains an important component of management of these cases (see Chapter 21).

A 13% weight reduction has been shown to decrease the upper airway collapsibility by modifying its anatomy and function. Even modest weight loss of 10% achieved by reduced caloric intake can lead to a reduction in the apnea-hypopnea index (AHI) from 55 to 29 per hour (Shah and Roux, 2009).

Chylothorax

Chylothorax is a rare cause of pleural effusion. It is caused by the disruption or obstruction of the thoracic duct, which results in the leakage of chyle (lymphatic fluid of intestinal origin) into the pleural space. The fluid typically has a milky appearance. A pleural fluid triglyceride concentration of more than 110 mg/dl strongly supports the diagnosis of a chylothorax (Heffner, 2013).

Chylothorax can result from nontraumatic causes such as sarcoidosis or benign idiopathic chylothorax. It can occur because of surgical trauma such as postoperative chylothorax or postpneumonectomy chylothorax. A unique case of recurrent bilateral chylothoraces resulting from push-ups has even been

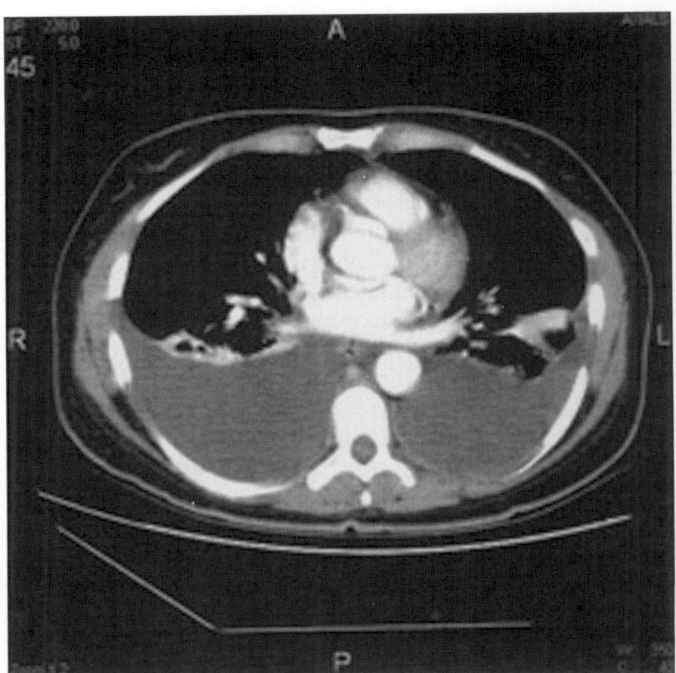

FIGURE 34-9 CT scan showing bilateral pleural effusions.

reported (Karnik and Patel, 2011). Figure 34-9 is a CT scan of the patient showing bilateral pleural effusion. It shows the milky white chylous fluid aspirated from the patient. The milky white color seen in chylothorax is because of very high triglyceride levels.

Medical Management

The principles of management of chylothorax are (1) treatment of the underlying condition such as sarcoidosis, infection, lymphoma, or metastatic carcinoma and (2) pleural drainage to relieve dyspnea. Those patients who do not improve by thoracentesis and dietary control measures may have to be treated by pleurodesis or thoracic duct ligation (Heffner, 2013).

Medical Nutrition Therapy

MNT is the primary therapy and includes manipulation of dietary contents aimed at decreasing the formation of chyle itself. For example, it has been shown that if a patient is placed on a long-chain fatty acid restricted diet, and medium-chain triglyceride (MCT) supplements are given, there can be resolution of pleural effusion as shown by serial chest radiographs over the course of as little as 4 days (Karnik and Patel, 2011). Because the MCTs are absorbed directly into the portal system rather than into the gastrointestinal lymphatics, using them for energy in the diet results in less lymphatic flow and thus faster healing of the thoracic duct.

ACUTE RESPIRATORY DISTRESS SYNDROME

Acute respiratory distress syndrome (ARDS) is a clinical state in which patients develop diffuse pulmonary infiltrates, severe hypoxia, and respiratory failure. Underlying clinical events such as sepsis or trauma that lead to the development of ARDS also result in a hypermetabolic state that markedly increases nutritional requirements.

Pathophysiology

For normal gas exchange, it is essential that dry, patent alveoli be in close proximity to capillaries. When an injury produces diffuse alveolar damage, proinflammatory cytokines are released. These cytokines recruit neutrophils to the lungs, where they become activated and release toxic mediators, which produce further damage to the alveolar epithelium and capillary endothelium. This damage allows protein to escape into the interstitium. Alveoli get filled with bloody, proteinaceous fluid which interferes with gas exchange and severe, refractory hypoxemia results. Various clinical conditions can lead to the development of ARDS (see Table 34-4).

Patients with ARDS present with acute onset of shortness of breath, tachypnea, and hypoxemia, which is refractory to oxygen supplementation.

Medical Management

The principles of ARDS management are the following:
- Treatment of underlying cause such as sepsis, aspiration, or bacterial pneumonia
- Mechanical ventilatory support
- Ensuring hemodynamic stability
- Prevention of complications such as stress ulcers, deep venous thrombosis, and aspiration pneumonia
- Nutritional support (Saguil and Fargo, 2012)

Therapies with corticosteroids, exogenous surfactant, antioxidants, and inhaled nitric oxide have been used but have not shown consistent benefit.

Medical Nutrition Therapy

Malnutrition is common in these patients who require mechanical ventilation. Patients with advanced respiratory disease have increased metabolic needs, and require prompt initiation of supplemental nutrition. It is important to consider issues related to protein use, and excess carbon dioxide production in these patients (Bellini, 2013).

Nutrition support in ARDS patients is necessary for preventing cumulative caloric deficits, loss of lean body mass, malnutrition and deterioration of respiratory muscle strength (Krzak et al, 2011).

Patients with ARDS are at high risk for complications as a result of underfeeding or overfeeding (see Table 34-5). Reduction in respiratory muscle strength is a deleterious effect of underfeeding, which leads to problems in weaning from mechanical ventilation. In addition, poor wound healing, immunosuppression, and risk of nosocomial infections increase related to inadequate calories and protein. Overfeeding leads to undesirable

TABLE 34-4 Common Clinical Conditions Associated with ARDS

Most Common	Less Common
Pneumonia	Drug toxicity
Sepsis	Aspiration
	Inhalation injury
	Near drowning
	Respiratory Syncytial virus
	Transfusion related acute lung injury
	Trauma

Adapted from Saguil A, Fargo M: Acute respiratory distress syndrome: diagnosis and management, *Am Fam Phys* 85:352, 2012.

TABLE 34-5 Complications Resulting from Overfeeding and Underfeeding in ARDS Patients

Overfeeding	Underfeeding
Nosocomial infections	Nosocomial infections
Hypercapnia	Immunosuppression
Immunosuppression	Depressed respiratory muscle strength
Failure in weaning from mechanical ventilator	Failure in weaning from mechanical ventilator
Poor wound healing	Low ventilatory drive
Electrolyte imbalance	
Azotemia	

Adapted from Krzak A et al: Nutrition therapy for ALI and ARDS, *Crit Care Clin* 27:647, 2011.

outcomes such as stress hyperglycemia, delayed weaning from mechanical ventilation and delayed wound healing (Krzak et al, 2011). Effective MNT requires careful assessment and monitoring. Indirect calorimetry is a useful tool for determining and monitoring energy needs (see Chapter 2). See Chapter 38 for further discussion on MNT for metabolically stressed patients.

PNEUMONIA

An inflammatory condition of the lungs that causes chest pain, fever, cough, and dyspnea is called **pneumonia**. In the clinical setting there are various kinds of pneumonias, such as community-acquired pneumonia, which may be viral or bacterial; hospital-acquired pneumonia; pneumonia in an immune compromised host; ventilator-associated pneumonia (VAP); and aspiration pneumonia, which will be discussed here. Aspiration is a common event even in healthy adults and usually causes no deleterious effects. At least one half of healthy adults aspirate during sleep. However, when this aspirate results in pulmonary consequences, it results in **aspiration pneumonia** (see Box 34-3).

Pathophysiology

Two conditions must exist for aspiration pneumonia to develop. First, there is a breach in the normal defense mechanisms, such as failure of glottis closure or impaired cough reflex, and second, a large enough inoculum enters the lungs. The aspirate contains

BOX 34-3 Conditions That Predispose a Patient to Aspiration Pneumonia

- Impaired level of consciousness, with compromised closure of glottis and impaired cough reflex
- Dysphagia from neurologic conditions
- Gastric reflux, disorders of or surgery on the upper gastrointestinal tract
- Mechanical disruption of the glottis closure because of endotracheal tube, tracheostomy, bronchoscopy, and interference with the cardiac sphincter by gastroduodenal endoscopy or placement of a nasogastric tube
- Miscellaneous conditions such as protracted vomiting, feeding via gastrostomy at less than a 45-degree angle and persistent recumbent position

Bartlett JG: Aspiration pneumonia in adults. In Baslow DS, editor: Wolters Kluwer: *UpToDate*, Waltham, Mass, 2012. Accessed October 26, 2013. Retrieved from http://www.uptodate.com/contents/aspiration-pneumonia-in-adults

gastric acid, which has a direct toxic effect on the lungs, particulate matter that may cause airway obstruction and atelectasis, and oral bacteria, which can result in infection and pneumonia. Pathogens such as *Streptococcus pneumonia*, *Haemophilus influenza*, gram-negative bacilli, and *Staphylococcus aureus* are virulent, and only a small inoculum is needed to cause pneumonia. By convention, aspiration pneumonia is caused by less-virulent organisms such as anaerobes, which are part of the normal oral flora, with predisposing situations (see Box 34-3).

Medical Management

Three clinical syndromes exist within the category of aspiration pneumonia: (1) chemical pneumonitis resulting from aspiration of acid, (2) bacterial infection, and (3) airway obstruction. The clinical features depend on which of these predominates, but often there is an overlap. The details of the management of these syndromes is beyond the scope of this chapter, but understanding of pathophysiology and predisposing conditions helps in the effective treatment and prevention of aspiration pneumonia.

Patients who are observed to have aspirated should be cleared of the fluids or food with immediate tracheal suction. However, this maneuver will not necessarily protect the lungs from chemical injury, which occurs instantly (Bartlett, 2012). The main treatment in this situation is to support the pulmonary function. Use of glucocorticoids in chemical pneumonitis is controversial.

Aspiration pneumonia usually presents with indolent symptoms. Many patients present with complications such as lung abscess, emphysema, and necrotizing pneumonia. Once a patient has been diagnosed with aspiration pneumonia, antibiotic therapy should include coverage for anaerobic pathogens because they may cause significant disease when present (Allen et al, 2013).

Medical Nutrition Therapy

As per the 2009 Society of Critical Care Medicine and American Society for Parenteral and Enteral Nutrition (SCCM/ASPEN) guidelines, nutritional interventions for preventing aspiration pneumonia and managing it when it exists in the patient in the acute care setting are the following:

- Direct tube feedings into the small bowel rather than the stomach
- Implement continuous feedings rather than bolus feedings recommended
- Elevate the head of the patient's bed to 45 degrees
- Use prokinetic agents
- Minimize use of sedatives
- Optimize oral hygiene
- Use naloxone to improve gut motility (Allen et al, 2013)

BRONCHOPULMONARY DYSPLASIA

Bronchopulmonary dysplasia (BPD) is a chronic neonatal lung disease that causes respiratory morbidity in preterm newborns. Bronchopulmonary dysplasia occurs in 25% to 42% of preterm neonates, who show impaired growth during early stages of infancy (Jain and Bancalari, 2014). BPD affects 20% of infants born prematurely and 60% of infants born before completing 26 weeks (Ghanta et al, 2013).

Common interventions have little impact on long-term outcomes, with respiratory care remaining supportive. Decreased lung compliance and increased need for respiratory support exists in these patients (Dani and Poggi, 2012).

Medical Management

Management should minimize any further injuries, while providing an optimal environment for growth and recovery (Adams and Stark, 2014).

Ongoing pulse oximetry is used to monitor oxygenation, whereas intermittent blood gas sampling monitors pH and $Paco_2$. Periodic attempts are made to progressively wean infants from ventilator support. Prolonged ventilation is associated with laryngeal injury and subglottic stenosis, especially with infants who require multiple intubations. Suctioning should be limited to only when needed because it is associated with tracheal and bronchial injury (Adams and Stark, 2014).

The use of supplemental oxygen is challenging in patients with BPD because of the need to treat hypoxemia on one hand and on other, to avoid exposure to excess oxygen. Increasing the inhaled oxygen concentrations could have a negative affect by increasing the risk of retinopathy, pulmonary edema, or inflammation.

Most infants are managed with a modest fluid restriction of 140 to 150 ml/kg per day. Although diuretic therapy may improve short-term pulmonary status, there is no evidence that it improves clinical outcomes. Use of diuretics leads to serum electrolyte abnormalities such as hyponatremia and hypokalemia (Adams and Stark, 2014).

Medical Nutrition Therapy

Using the criteria in Box 34-4, assessment of the infant with BPD begins MNT (see Box 34-4). Energy needs of infants with BPD are 15% to 20% higher than those of healthy infants, and they benefit from 140 to 150 kcal/kg/day during active stages of the disease (Dani and Poggi, 2012). Inadequate caloric

---

BOX 34-4 Components of Nutrition Assessment for Infants with Bronchopulmonary Dysplasia

History
Birthweight
Gestational age
Medical history
Nutrition history
Previous growth pattern

Medical Status
Respiratory status
Oxygen saturation
Use of medications
Emesis
Stool pattern
Urine output
Urine specific gravity
Ventilator dependency

Nutrition-Biochemical Measures
Anthropometrics
Weight
Length
Growth percentiles
Head circumference

Hemoglobin
Hematocrit
Serum electrolytes
C-reactive protein

Feeding History
Volume of intake
Frequency of feedings
Behavior during feedings
Formula composition
Use of solid foods
Developmental feeding milestones
Swallowing difficulty
Gastroesophageal reflux

Environmental Concerns
Parent-child interaction
Home facilities
Access to safe food supply
Community resources
Economic resources
Access to adequate food and nutrients

intake leads to a catabolic state and muscle fatigue of the diaphragm. Adequate nutrition is essential for lung growth, alveolar development, surfactant production, and protection against infections.

Infants with BPD have decreased lean body mass, indicating an inadequate protein intake. Treatment with corticosteroids also increases body fat and lowers protein, thereby altering the composition of weight gain. Protein intakes of 3.5 to 4.0 g/kg body weight in infants with BPD help in meeting the growth and anabolic needs (Dani and Poggi, 2012). Amino acids are administered within the first 26 hours of life because they are well tolerated, improve glucose tolerance, and create positive nitrogen balance. An amino acid requirement of 1.5 to 2 g/kg/day is suggested for term infants, 2 to 3 g/kg/day for infants at 30 to 36 weeks, and 3.6 to 4.8 g/kg/day for infants at 24 to 30 weeks (Dani and Poggi, 2012) (see Chapter 42).

Although lipids remain a vital component in providing essential fatty acids and meeting energy goals, the role of lipid administration remains controversial. Lipids are held or administered in small quantities because they can cause hyperbilirubinemia and increase the risk of kernicterus in these infants. Lipids result in less carbon dioxide production compared to carbohydrate and although high-fat formulas do not show a significant change in respiration in adults, infants who receive fat-free formulas exhibit decreased carbon dioxide production and improved respiration (Dani and Poggi, 2012). Further investigation is required to determine the optimal lipid intake for infants with BPD. The European Society of Pediatric Gastroenterology, Hepatology and Nutrition (ESPGHAN) recommends a reasonable range of 4.4 to 6.0 g of fat/100 kcal or 40% to 55% of caloric intake.

Sodium and potassium depletion are seen in infants with BPD who are treated with diuretics. Because sodium administration counteracts the action of diuretics, mild deficiencies in sodium and chloride are anticipated (Dani and Poggi, 2012).

Decreased bone mineralization is seen in infants with BPD. Urinary loss of calcium is increased with the administration of corticosteroids and diuretics. Osteopenia of prematurity is common in infants with BPD resulting from nutritional deficiencies of calcium and phosphorus. Enteral feeds are not useful in providing adequate amounts of calcium and phosphorus,

whereas parenteral feeds restrict the intake because of limited solubility of calcium and phosphorus.

Infants with BPD are monitored every 1 to 2 weeks for calcium, and phosphorus and it is recommended to supplement with vitamin D (Dani and Poggi, 2012) and milk fortifiers (see Chapter 42).

The use of vitamin A, corticosteroids, and caffeine have been shown to reduce BPD at 36 weeks of age. 5000 IU of vitamin A was administered intramuscularly three times a week for a month to show a significant reduction in BPD and death in those infants receiving the supplementation (Ehrenkranz, 2014).

Parenteral nutrition is continued along with enteral feeds till the feeding volume reaches 100 ml/kg/day. Starting enteral feeds earlier induces gastric motility and promotes progression to full enteral feedings. Better neurologic development in preterm infants with BPD can be accomplished with early nutrition support, appropriate enteral feeds, and parenteral feed selection (Dani and Poggi, 2012). See Chapter 42 for further discussion on feeding the low birthweight infant.

USEFUL WEBSITES

American Academy of Allergy, Asthma, and Immunology
http://www.aaaai.org/home.aspx
American Association for Respiratory Care
http://www.aarc.org
American Lung Association
http://www.lungusa.org
American Thoracic Society
http://www.thoracic.org
Cystic Fibrosis Foundation
http://www.cff.org
Cystic Fibrosis Genetic Analysis Consortium (Cystic Fibrosis Mutation Database)
http://www.genet.sickkids.on.ca/cftr
National Cancer Institute (Lung Cancer)
http://www.cancer.gov/cancertopics/types/lung
National Institute of Diabetes and Digestive and Kidney Diseases—Cystic Fibrosis Research
http://www.niddk.nih.gov

CLINICAL CASE STUDY

Esther is an 80-year-old widow who is a retired secretary. She started smoking when she was 15, and she smoked two packs per day until 7 years ago. She has been diagnosed with COPD and has been admitted to the rehabilitation center with a broken hip following a fall at home. Significant findings are weight 101 lb, height 5'3", blood pressure 127/65 mm Hg, heart rate 82/minute, respiratory rate 18/minute, temperature 98.6° F, oxygen saturation 95% on 3L of O_2. History and physical examination reveal severe dyspnea on exertion, including showering, carrying packages, making the bed, and pushing a vacuum cleaner; orthopnea (two or three pillows); and decreased breath sounds. Prescribed medications include theophylline (300 mg twice daily), prednisone (20 mg once daily in the morning), furosemide 20 mg twice daily, fluticasone (Flovent; 220 mcg, four puffs twice daily), albuterol and ipratropium (Atrovent; two puffs as needed). Over-the-counter medications include vitamin C (250 mg twice daily), and calcium (500 mg daily). She says she has no appetite and is eating very little. Her stated usual weight is 115 lbs and she admits to recent weight loss.

Nutrition Diagnosis Statement

Significant weight loss related to decreased food intake due to lung disease and surgery.

Nutrition Care Questions

1. What dietary interventions can you suggest to increase intake of calories and protein?
2. What are the interrelationships between chronic obstructive pulmonary disease, food intake, and nutrient metabolism?
3. Are there any food-drug interactions that are a concern for Esther?
4. What are the principles of medical nutrition therapy in this clinical situation? Explain the scientific rationale for each.
5. What do you think of Esther's nutrient supplementation program? Would you have her change it?
6. You are planning a session on nutrition for the clients and their families who participate in the Pulmonary Rehabilitation Program. What topics would you cover? What educational techniques would you use?

REFERENCES

Abubakar, et al: Drug resistant tuberculosis: time for visionary political leadership, *Lancet Infec Dis* 13:529, 2013.

Adams JM, Stark AR: Management of bronchopulmonary dysplasia. In Basow DS, editor: *UpToDate*, Waltham, 2014, Mass. http://www.uptodate.com/contents/management-of-bronchopulmonary-dysplasia. Accessed February 5, 2014.

Allan K, Devereux G: Diet and asthma: nutritional implications from prevention to treatment, *J Amer Diet Assoc* 111:258, 2011.

Allen KS, et al: When does nutrition impact respiratory function, *Curr Gastroenterol Rep* 15:327, 2013.

Baker RD, et al: Cystic fibrosis: nutritional issues. In Basow DS, editor: *UpToDate*, Waltham, 2013, Mass. Accessed February 7, 2014.

Baldini EH, et al: Women and lung cancer. In Basow DS, editor: *UpToDate*, Waltham, 2014, Mass. http://www.uptodate.com/contents/women-and-lung-cancer. Accessed November 16, 2014.

Balzer BWR, et al: Low glycemic index dietary interventions in youth with cystic fibrosis: a systemic review and discussion of the clinical implications, *Nutrients* 4:286, 2012.

Bartlett JG: Aspiration pneumonia in adults. In Baslow DS, editor: *Wolters Kluwer: UpToDate*, Waltham, 2012, Mass. http://www.uptodate.com/contents/aspiration-pneumonia-in-adults. Accessed October 26, 2013.

Bellini L: Nutritional support in advanced lung disease. In Baslow DS, editor: *UpToDate*, Waltham, 2013, Mass. http://www.uptodate.com/contents/nutritional-support-in-advanced-lung-disease. Accessed November 20, 2013.

Benedik B, et al: Mini nutritional assessment, body composition, and hospitalizations in patients with chronic obstructive pulmonary disease, *Respir Med* 105(Suppl 1):S38, 2011.

Berman AR: Management of patients with end stage chronic obstructive pulmonary disease, *Prim Care* 38:277, 2011.

Bhargava A, et al: Nutritional status of adult patients with pulmonary tuberculosis in rural central India and its association with mortality, *pLos One* 8:e77979, 2013.

Brehm JM, et al: Serum vitamin D levels and severe asthma exacerbations in the Childhood Asthma Management Program Study, *J Allergy Clin Immunol* 126:52, 2010.

Burney P, et al: Chronic obstructive pulmonary disease mortality and prevalence: the associations with smoking and poverty—a BOLD analysis, *Thorax* 69:465, 2014.

Chih–Hung Guo, et al: Nutritional supplement therapy improves oxidative stress, immune response, pulmonary function, and quality of life in allergic asthma patients: an open label pilot study, *Altern Med Rev* 17:42, 2012.

Collins PF, et al: Nutritional support in chronic obstructive pulmonary disease: a systemic review and meta analysis, *Am J Clin Nutr* 95:1385, 2012.

Culhane S, et al: Malnutrition in cystic fibrosis: a review, *Nutr Clin Pract* 28:676, 2013.

Dalli J, et al: Resolvin D3 and aspirin-triggered Resolvin D3 are potent immune resolvents, *Chem Biol* 20:188, 2013.

Dani C, Poggi C: Nutrition and bronchopulmonary dysplasia, *J Matern Fetal Neonatal Med* 25(Suppl 3):37, 2012.

Davis PB: Therapy for cystic fibrosis—the end of the beginning, *New Engl J Med* 365:1734, 2011.

Del Ferraro C, et al: Management of anorexia-cachexia in late-stage lung cancer patients, *J Hosp and Palliat Nurs* 14:1, 2012.

Desai NS, et al: Effects of sunlight and diet on vitamin D status of pulmonary tuberculosis patients in Tbilisi, Georgia, *Nutrition* 28:362, 2012.

Ehrenkranz RA: Ongoing issues in the intensive care for the periviable infant-nutritional management and prevention of bronchopulmonary dysplasia and nosocomial infections, *Semin Perinatol* 38:25, 2014.

Epstein LJ, et al: Clinical guidelines for the evaluation, management and long-term care of obstructive sleep apnea in adults, *J Clin Sleep Med* 5:263, 2009.

Evans A: Nutrition screening in patients with COPD, *Nurs Times* 108:12, 2012.

Evans RA, Morgan MD: The systemic nature of chronic lung disease, *Clin Chest Med* 35:283, 2014.

Fabian E, et al: Nutritional supplements and plasma antioxidants in childhood asthma, *Wien Klin Wochenschr* 125:309, 2013.

Fulton AS, et al: Feasibility of omega-3 fatty acid supplementation as an adjunct therapy for people with chronic obstructive pulmonary disease: study protocol for a randomized controlled trial, *Trials* 14:107, 2012.

Garcia-Marcos L, et al: Influence of Mediterranean diet on asthma in children: a systematic review and meta-analysis, *Pediatr Allergy Immunol* 24:330, 2013.

Gaur P, et al: Nutritional scenario in bronchial asthma, *Int J Curr Microbiol Appl Sci* 2:119, 2013.

Ghanta S, et al: An update on pharmacologic approaches to bronchopulmonary dysplasia, *Semin Perinatol* 37:115, 2013.

Gibson JME, et al: Diet induced weight loss in obese children with asthma: a randomized control trial, *Clin Exp Allergy* 43:775, 2013.

Harada H, et al: Multidisciplinary team–based approach for comprehensive preoperative pulmonary rehabilitation including intensive nutritional support for lung cancer patients, *PLoS One* 8:e59566, 2013.

Heffner JE: Management of chylothorax. In Basow DS, editor: UpToDate, Waltham, 2013, Mass. http://www.uptodate.com/contents/management-of-chylothorax. Accessed August 20, 2013.

Hill K, et al: The importance of components of pulmonary rehabilitation, other than exercise training in COPD, *Eur Respir Rev* 22:405, 2013.

Hirayama F, et al: Folate intake associated with lung function, breathlessness and the prevalence of chronic obstructive pulmonary disease, *Asia Pac J Clin Nutr* 19:103, 2010.

Hood MLH: A narrative review of recent progress in understanding the relationship between tuberculosis and protein energy malnutrition, *Eur J Clin Nutr* 67:1122, 2013.

Huhmann M, Camporeale J: Supportive care in lung cancer: clinical update, *Semin Oncol Nurs* 28(2):e1, 2012.

Isanaka S, et al: Iron deficiency and anemia predict mortality in patients with tuberculosis, *J Nutr* 142:350, 2012.

Itoh M, et al: Undernutrition in patients with COPD and its treatment, *Nutrients* 5:1316, 2013.

Jain D, Bancalari E: Bronchopulmonary dysplasia: clinical perspective, *Birth Defects Res A Clin Mol Teratol* 100:134, 2014.

Kappler M, et al: Ursodeoxycholic acid therapy in cystic fibrosis liver disease-a retrospective long-term follow-up case control study, *Aliment Pharmacol Ther* 36:266, 2012.

Karnik AA, Patel NP: A curious case of chylothorax, *J Postgrad Med* 57:259, 2011.

Katkin JP: Cystic fibrosis: clinical manifestations and diagnosis. In Baslow DS, editor: *UpToDate*, Waltham, 2014, Mass. http://www.uptodate.com/contents/cystic-fibrosis-clinical-manifestations-and-diagnosis?source=search_result&search=cystic+fibrosis&selectedTitle=1~150. Accessed January 25, 2014.

Katrangi W, et al: Interactions of linoleic and alpha-linolenic acids in the development of fatty acid alterations in cystic fibrosis, *Lipids* 48:333, 2013.

Koenig SM: Pulmonary complications of obesity, *Am J Med Sci* 321:249, 2011.

Krzak A, et al: Nutrition therapy for ALI and ARDS, *Crit Care Clin* 27:647, 2011.

Lee H, et al: Nutritional status and disease severity in patients with chronic obstructive pulmonary disease (COPD), *Arch Gerontol Geriatr* 56:518, 2013.

Lin SY, et al: Sublingual immunotherapy for the treatment of allergic rhino-conjunctivitis and asthma, a systematic review, *JAMA* 309:1278, 2013.

Litonjua AA, et al: The Vitamin D Antenatal Asthma Reduction Trial (VDAART): rationale, design, and methods of a randomized, controlled trial of vitamin D supplementation in pregnancy for the primary prevention of asthma and allergies in children, *Contemp Clin Trials* 38:37, 2014.

Mannino DM, et al: Cigarette smoking and other risk factors for lung cancer. In Baslow DS, editor: *UpToDate*, Waltham, 2014, Mass. http://www.uptodate.com/contents/cigarette-smoking-and-other-risk-factors-for-lung-cancer?source=search_result&search=cigarette+smoking+and+other+risks+for+lung+cancer&selected. Accessed October 25, 2014.

Matel JL: Nutritional management of cystic fibrosis, *JPEN J Parenter Enteral Nutr* 36(Suppl 1):S60, 2012.

McCloud E, Papoutsakis C: A medical nutrition therapy primer for childhood asthma: current and emerging perspectives, *J Am Diet Assoc* 111:1052, 2011.

McEvoy GK, Snow EK: *AHFS drug information*, Bethesda, Md, 2015, American Society of Health System Pharmacists.

Minai OA, et al: Pulmonary hypertension in COPD: epidemiology, significance and management: pulmonary vascular disease: the global perspective, *Chest* 137(Suppl 6):S39, 2010.

Miyata S, et al: The prognostic significance of nutritional status using malnutrition universal screening tool in patients with pulmonary tuberculosis, *Nutr J* 12:42, 2013.

Nakawah MO, et al: Asthma, chronic obstructive pulmonary disease (COPD) and the overlap syndrome, *J Am Board of Fam Med* 26:470, 2013.

Nutrition Information Center University of Stellenbosch (NICUS): *Tuberculosis and Nutrition*, 2009. http://www.health24.com/Medical/Tuberculosis/Living-with-TB/TB-and-nutrition-20120721. Accessed January 2, 2015.

Papaioannou I, et al: Global assessment of the COPD patient: time to look beyond FEV$_1$? *Respir Med* 103:650, 2013.

Parenteral and Enteral Nutrition Group (PENG): *A pocket guide to clinical nutrition*, ed 4, Birmingham, 2011, British Dietetic Association.

Piper AJ, Grunstein RR: Current perspectives on the obesity hypoventilation syndrome, *Curr Opin Pulm Med* 13:490, 2007.

Piper AJ, Grunstein RR: Obesity hypoventilation syndrome: mechanisms and management, *Am J Respir Crit Care Med* 183:292, 2011.

Raguso CA, Luthy C: Nutritional status in chronic obstructive pulmonary disease: role of hypoxia, *Nutrition* 27:138, 2011.

Rana M, et al: Fat soluble vitamin deficiency in children and adolescents with cystic fibrosis, *J Clin Pathol* 67:605, 2014.

Rogers CL: Nutritional management of the adult with cystic fibrosis – Part 1, *Practical Gastroenterology Series* 113:10, 2013.

Saguil A, Fargo M: Acute respiratory distress syndrome: diagnosis and management, *Am Fam Physician* 85:352, 2012.

Shah N, Roux F: The relationship of obesity and obstructive sleep apnea, *Clin Chest Med* 30:3, 2009.

Shek LP, et al: Role of dietary long-chain polyunsaturated fatty acids in infant allergies and respiratory diseases, *Clin Dev Immunol* 1:1, 2012.

Silverberg DS, et al: Anemia and iron deficiency in COPD patients: prevalence and the effects of correction of the anemia with erythropoiesis stimulating agents and intravenous iron, *BMC Pulm Med* 24:14, 2014.

Vital D, et al: Nasal polyposis in lung transplant recipients with cystic fibrosis, *Journal of Cyst Fibros* 12:266, 2013.

Wenzel S: Treatment of severe asthma in adolescents and adults. In Baslow DS, editor: *UpToDate*, Waltham, 2014, Mass. http://www.uptodate.com/contents/treatment-of-severe-asthma-in-adolescents-and-adults?source=search_result&search=treatment+of+severe+asthma+in+adolescents&selectedTitle=8~115. Accessed on November 20, 2014.

Xiaomei W, et al: Bone metabolism status and associated risk factors in elderly patients with chronic obstructive pulmonary disease (COPD), *Cell Biochem Biophys* 70:129, 2014.

35

Medical Nutrition Therapy for Renal Disorders

Katy G. Wilkens, MS, RDN, Veena Juneja, MScRD, RDN,
Elizabeth Shanaman, RDN

KEY TERMS

acute glomerulonephritides
acute kidney injury (AKI)
acute renal failure (ARF)
adynamic (low turnover) bone disease
antidiuretic hormone (ADH)
azotemia
blood urea nitrogen (BUN)
calciphylaxis
chronic interstitial nephritis
chronic kidney disease (CKD)
continuous renal replacement therapy (CRRT)
continuous venovenous hemodialysis (CVVHD)
continuous venovenous hemofiltration (CVVH)
creatinine
dialysate
end-stage renal disease (ESRD)
estimated glomerular filtration rate (eGFR)

erythropoietin (EPO)
Fanconi syndrome
fistula
glomerular filtration rate (GFR)
graft
hemodialysis (HD)
hypercalciuria
hyperoxaluria
idiopathic hypercalciuria (IH)
intradialytic parenteral nutrition (IDPN)
intraperitoneal nutrition (IPN)
Kidney Dialysis Outcome Quality Initiative (KDOQI)
kinetic modeling
Kt/V
metastatic calcification
nephritic syndrome
nephrolithiasis
nephrotic syndrome

oliguria
osteitis fibrosa cystica
osteomalacia
peritoneal dialysis (PD)
phosphate binders
protein-nitrogen appearance (PNA) rate
pyelonephritis
recombinant human EPO (rHuEPO)
renal failure
renal osteodystrophy
renal replacement therapy (RRT)
renal tubular acidosis (RTA)
renin-angiotensin mechanism
syndrome of inappropriate antidiuretic hormone (SIADH)
ultrafiltrate
urea reduction ratio (URR)
uremia
vasopressin

PHYSIOLOGY AND FUNCTION OF THE KIDNEYS

The main function of the kidney is to maintain the balance of fluids, electrolytes, and organic solutes. The normal kidney performs this function over a wide range of fluctuations in sodium, water, and solutes. This task is accomplished by the continuous filtration of blood with alterations in secretion and reabsorption of this filtered fluid. The kidney receives 20% of cardiac output, filtering approximately 1600 L/day of blood and producing 180 L of fluid called ultrafiltrate. Through active processes of reabsorbing certain components and secreting others, composition of this ultrafiltrate is changed into the 1.5 L of urine excreted in an average day.

Each kidney consists of approximately 1 million functioning nephrons (see Figure 35-1), consisting of a glomerulus connected to a series of tubules. Tubules consist of different segments: the proximal convoluted tubule, loop of Henle, distal tubule, and collecting duct. Each nephron functions independently and contributes to the final urine, although all are under similar control and coordination. If one segment of a nephron is destroyed, that complete nephron is no longer functional.

The glomerulus is a spheric mass of capillaries surrounded by a membrane, Bowman's capsule. The glomerulus produces the ultrafiltrate, which then is modified by the next segments of the nephron. Production of ultrafiltrate is mainly passive and relies on the perfusion pressure generated by the heart and supplied by the renal artery.

The tubules reabsorb the vast majority of components that compose the ultrafiltrate. Much of this process is active and requires a large expenditure of energy in the form of adenosine triphosphate (ATP). The tubule is a unique structure; differences in permeability between the various segments and hormonal responses allow the tubule to produce the final urine, which can vary widely in concentration of electrolytes, osmolality, pH, and volume. Ultimately, this urine is funneled into common collecting tubules and into the renal pelvis. The renal pelvis narrows into a single ureter per kidney, and each ureter carries urine into the bladder, where it accumulates before elimination.

The kidney has almost unlimited ability to regulate water homeostasis. Its ability to form a large concentration gradient between its inner medulla and outer cortex allows the kidney to excrete urine as dilute as 50 mOsm or as concentrated as 1200 mOsm. Given a daily fixed solute load of approximately

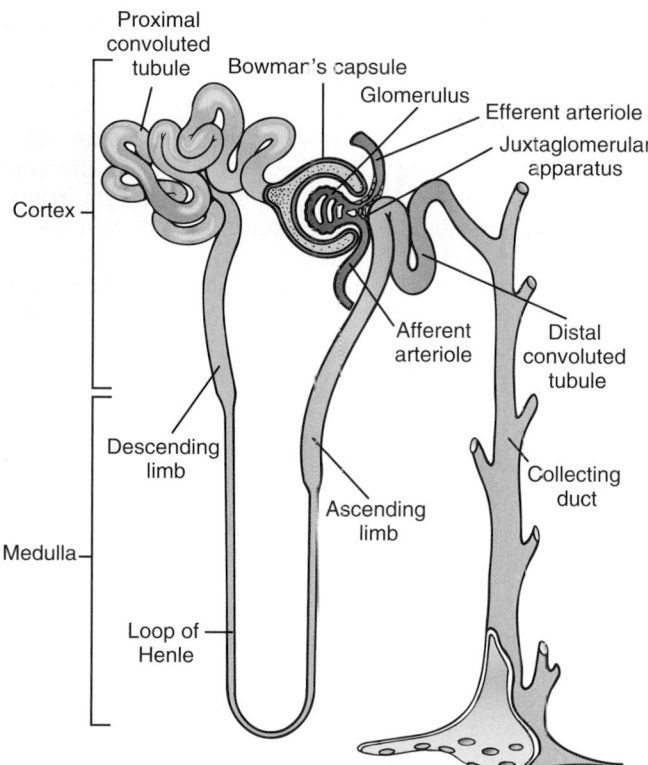

FIGURE 35-1 The nephron. (Modified from Patton KT, Thibodeau GA: *The human body in health and disease,* ed 6, Maryland Heights, Mo, 2013, Mosby.)

600 mOsm, the kidney can get rid of as little as 500 ml of concentrated urine or as much as 12 L of dilute urine. Control of water excretion is regulated by **vasopressin** (**antidiuretic hormone [ADH]**), a small peptide hormone secreted by the posterior pituitary. An excess of relative body water, indicated by a low osmolality, leads to prompt shut-off of all vasopressin secretion. Likewise, a small rise in osmolality brings about marked vasopressin secretion and water retention. However, the need to conserve sodium sometimes leads to a sacrifice of the homeostatic control of water for the sake of volume (see *Focus On:* Syndrome of Inappropriate Antidiuretic Hormone (SIADH)).

⊚ **FOCUS ON**

Syndrome of Inappropriate Antidiuretic Hormone

Syndrome of inappropriate antidiuretic hormone (SIADH) is seen when there is an excessive amount of antidiuretic hormone released from the pituitary gland. Common causes include head injury, meningitis, cancer, infection, and hypothyroidism. The result is hyponatremia caused by hemodilution. It is characterized by a serum sodium less than 135 mEq/L and a urine sodium concentration greater than 20 mEq/L. If left untreated it can result in seizures and coma. It is treated with fluid restriction, generally less than 1800 ml/day, and may require intravenous sodium administration. Oral sodium supplementation is contraindicated.

The minimum urinary volume capable of eliminating a relatively fixed 600 mOsm of solute is 500 ml, assuming that the kidney is capable of maximum concentration. Urinary volume of less than 500 ml/day is called **oliguria**; it is impossible for such a small urine volume to eliminate all of the daily waste.

The majority of the solute load consists of nitrogenous wastes, primarily the end products of protein metabolism. Urea predominates in amount, depending on the protein content of the diet. Uric acid, **creatinine** (Cr), and ammonia are present in small amounts. If normal waste products are not eliminated appropriately, they collect in abnormal quantities in the blood, known as **azotemia**. The ability of the kidney to adequately eliminate nitrogenous waste products is defined as renal function. Thus **renal failure** is the inability to excrete the daily load of wastes.

The kidney also performs functions unrelated to excretion. One of these involves the **renin-angiotensin mechanism**, a major control of blood pressure. Decreased blood volume causes cells of the glomerulus (the juxtaglomerular apparatus) to react by secreting renin, a proteolytic enzyme. Renin acts on angiotensinogen in the plasma to form angiotensin I, which is converted to angiotensin II, a powerful vasoconstrictor and a potent stimulus of aldosterone secretion by the adrenal gland. As a consequence, sodium and fluid are reabsorbed, and blood pressure is returned to normal.

The kidney also produces the hormone **erythropoietin (EPO)**, a critical determinant of erythroid activity in the bone marrow. Deficiency of EPO is the primary cause of the severe anemia present in chronic renal disease.

Maintenance of calcium-phosphorus homeostasis involves the complex interactions of parathyroid hormone (PTH); calcitonin; active vitamin D; and three effector organs: the gut, kidney, and bone. The role of the kidney includes production of the active form of vitamin D—1,25-dihydroxycholecalciferol $(1,25\text{-}[OH]_2D_3)$—as well as elimination of calcium and phosphorus. Active vitamin D promotes efficient absorption of calcium by the gut and is one of the substances necessary for bone remodeling and maintenance. Active vitamin D also suppresses PTH production, which is responsible for mobilization of calcium from bone (see Chapter 24).

RENAL DISEASES

The manifestations of renal disease are significant. They can be ordered by degree of severity: (1) kidney stones, (2) acute kidney injury (AKI), (3) chronic kidney disease (CKD), and (4) end-stage renal disease (ESRD) (National Kidney Foundation, 2002). Objectives of nutritional care depend on the abnormality being treated.

Kidney Stones (Nephrolithiasis)

Nephrolithiasis, the presence of kidney stones, is a significant health problem in the United States. The prevalence of kidney stones from the National Health and Nutrition Examination Survey (NHANES) 2007 to 2010 data is 8.8% (Scales et al, 2012). It is characterized by frequent occurrences during the fourth and fifth decades of life and a high recurrence rate. The risk doubles in those with a family history of kidney stones; stone formers often have first-degree relatives with kidney stones. Increased frequency of obesity, diabetes, and metabolic syndrome have resulted in increasing rates of nephrolithiasis. Thought to be a predominantly male disease, its prevalence is fast increasing in women (7.1%) and in men at 10.6%, changing the male/female ratio. Kidney stones affect people of all ethnic groups. NHANES reveals a lower occurrence rate in black non-Hispanic and Hispanic individuals compared with white non-Hispanic individuals (Scales et al, 2012).

Health care cost of evaluation, hospitalization, and treatment of kidney stone disease in the United States exceeds 4.5 billion dollars per year. Preventing recurrence can have a significant cost-saving potential as a result of reduced stone burden. Medical nutrition therapy can play an important role in prevention (Morgan, 2016). A low urine volume is the single most important risk factor for all types of nephrolithiasis.

Pathophysiology

Kidney stone formation is a complex process that consists of saturation; supersaturation; nucleation; crystal growth or aggregation; crystal retention; and stone formation in the presence of promoters, inhibitors, and complexors in urine. A typical metabolic evaluation is described in Table 35-1.

Calcium stones are the most common: 60% of stones are calcium oxalate, 10% calcium oxalate and calcium phosphate, and 10% calcium phosphate. Other stones are 5% to 10% uric acid, 5% to 10% struvite, and 1% cystine.

TABLE 35-1 Baseline Information and Metabolic Evaluation of Urolithiasis

Information	Description and Data
History of urolithiasis	History of onset, frequency
	Family history
	Spontaneous passage or removal
	Retrieval, analysis of stone
	Current status with radiologic examination
Medical history, investigation	Hyperparathyroidism
	Renal tubular acidosis
	Urinary tract infection
	Sarcoidosis
	Hypertension
	Osteoporosis
	Inflammatory bowel disease, malabsorption syndrome, intestinal bypass surgery for obesity (Roux-en Y or gastric banding/sleeve gastrectomy)
	Metabolic syndrome or insulin resistance
	Diabetes mellitus
	Obesity
Blood tests	Serum—calcium, phosphorus, creatinine, uric acid, CO_2, albumin, parathyroid hormone, Hgb A1C
Urinalysis	Urine analysis with pH
	Urine culture
24-hr urine collection	Volume, calcium, oxalate, uric acid, sodium, citrate, magnesium, phosphorus
	Urea
	Creatinine
	Qualitative cystine
Medications and vitamins	Thiazide, allopurinol, vitamin C, vitamin B_6, vitamin D, cod liver oil, calcium carbonate, glucocorticoid therapy, potassium citrate, antacids
Occupation history and strenuous exercise	Dermal water losses
	Dehydration
	Low urine volume
	Type of job and activity level
Environment	Hard water area
Dietary evaluation	Intake of calcium, oxalate, animal protein, salt, purines, fructose, potassium
	Fruits and vegetables (related to urine pH)
	Herbal products; fish oils
	Volume of fluid intake
	Type of fluids containing citrate, malate, caffeine, fructose, phosphoric acid; mineral water; sports drinks

CO_2, Carbon dioxide; *Hgb A1C,* hemoglobin A1C.

Obese stone formers excrete increased amounts of sodium, calcium, uric acid, and citrate, and have lower urine pH. Obesity is the strongest predictor of stone recurrence in first-time stone formers. As body weight increases, the excretion of calcium, oxalate, and uric acid also increases. Patients with a higher body mass index (BMI) have a decrease in ammonia excretion and impaired hydrogen ion buffering. With increasing BMI, uric acid stones become more dominant than calcium oxalate stones, especially in men. Based on urinary supersaturation index and urinary risk factors total body fat and truncal fat mass are associated more strongly with uric acid stones than total body weight and lean body mass (Pigna et al, 2014).

Uric acid stones are common in the presence of type 2 diabetes. Hyperinsulinemia also may contribute to the development of calcium stones by increasing urinary calcium excretion.

In postmenopausal women as the amount not the intensity of physical activity increases, the risk of incident stones declines (Sorensen et al, 2014).

Weight control may be considered one of the preventive modalities and in stone formers, a BMI of 18 to 25 kg/m^2 is recommended.

With malabsorptive bariatric procedures such as Roux-en-Y gastric bypass (RYGB), urolithiasis is higher than in obese controls, probably because of the increased prevalence of hyperoxaluria and hypocitraturia in RYGB patients. However, restrictive gastric surgery (i.e., gastric banding or sleeve gastrectomy) is not associated with increased risk of kidney stones (Semins et al, 2010).

Agents added intentionally or unintentionally to food or drug products have led to the appearance of new types of stones containing melamine and indinavir (Zilberman et al, 2010) (see Table 35-2).

Calcium Stones. One third to one half of patients with calcium stones are hypercalciuric. **Hypercalciuria** describes a value of calcium in excess of 300 mg (7.5 mmol) per day in men, 250 mg (6.25 mmol) per day in women, or 4 mg (0.1 mmol)/kg/day for either in random urine collections of outpatients on unrestricted diets. The classic definition of hypercalciuria of upper normal limit of 200 mg per day is based on a constant diet restricted in calcium, sodium, and animal protein (Pak et al, 2011).

Idiopathic hypercalciuria (IH) is a familial disorder characterized by abnormal serum calcium in the absence of known causes of hypercalciuria, such as primary hyperparathyroidism, sarcoidosis, excess vitamin D intake, hyperthyroidism, glucocorticoid use, or renal tubular acidosis (RTA). Ninety percent of patients with IH never form a kidney stone. However, they are more sensitive to forming stones, as relatively small increases in urine calcium increase calcium oxalate supersaturation.

TABLE 35-2 Causes and Composition of Renal Stones

Pathogenetic Causes	Composition of Stone
Hypercalciuria, hyperoxaluria, hyperuricosuria, or hypocitraturia	Calcium oxalate
Primary hyperparathyroidism	Calcium oxalate
Cystinuria	Cystine
Infection	Struvite
Acid urine pH	Uric acid
Hyperuricosuria	Uric acid
Renal tubular acidosis	Calcium phosphate
Alkaline urine pH	Calcium phosphate

Formation of a stone in a person with IH can be triggered by an excessive dietary calcium intake, increased intestinal absorption of calcium that may or may not be vitamin D–mediated, decreased renal tubular reabsorption of calcium, or prolonged bed rest. Increased gut absorption of calcium even when on a restricted calcium, sodium and animal protein diet is noted particularly in patients with absorptive hypercalciuria. Urinary calcium levels higher than normal at any level of net calcium absorption suggests that some of the urine calcium is derived from the bone. Negative calcium balance appears to be greater in stone formers than in non–stone formers.

When challenged with a very-low-calcium diet, the loss of more calcium in the urine than is in the diet indicates a net loss of total body calcium. The source of this additional calcium is the skeleton (Krieger and Bushinsky, 2013). Patients with IH tend toward negative phosphorus balance even on normal intakes. The defective phosphate metabolism may lead to increased $1,25(OH)_2D_3$ levels, and increased intestinal calcium absorption.

Bone loss can be high in patients with IH in whom low calcium intake exaggerates bone loss from increased net acid excretion (NAE). For decades low-calcium diets were recommended to reduce the hypercalciuria in these stone formers. However, chronic prolonged calcium restriction, deficient calcium intake, and increased losses from hypercalciuria decrease bone mineral density. The decreased BMD also correlates with an increase in markers of bone turnover as well as increased fractures (Krieger and Bushinsky, 2013). Vertebral fracture risk increases fourfold among urolithiasis patients in comparison with the general population.

Undesirable bone resorption may be enhanced by a high protein intake of nondairy origin. An inadequate calcium intake along with high protein intake induces metabolic acidosis, increases calcium excretion, and lowers urinary pH. This acid load inhibits the renal reabsorption of calcium. A reduction in nondairy animal protein may be recommended (see *Clinical Insight:* Urinary pH—How Does Diet Affect It?).

Calcium supplements do not have the same protective effect against stone formation as dietary calcium. Widespread use of calcium supplements to prevent osteoporosis corresponds to an increase in kidney stones in women. A trial of combined calcium–vitamin D supplementation to prevent bone loss and fractures led to a 17% increase in new stone formation in women who increased their calcium intake to 2000 mg a day by adding a 1000 mg calcium supplement to their baseline diet (Wallace et al, 2011).

If calcium is taken as a supplement, timing is important. Calcium supplements taken with meals increase urinary calcium and citrate, but decrease urinary oxalate; thus the increase in citrate and decrease in oxalate counterbalance the effects of elevated urinary calcium. Therefore, if used by patients who

CLINICAL INSIGHT

Acid and Alkaline Diets

by Sheila Dean, DSc, RDN, LD, CCN, CDE

Dietary intake can influence the acidity or alkalinity of the urine (Berardi et al, 2008). It has been shown that excessive dietary protein (particularly high in sulfur-containing amino acids such as methionine and cysteine), and chloride, phosphorous, and organic acids are the main sources of dietary acid load. When these animal proteins, such as meat and cheese, are eaten concomitantly with other acid-producing foods and not balanced with alkaline-producing foods, such as fruit and vegetables, there is an increased risk of chronic acidosis. Acidosis (which is not to be confused with acidemia) has been linked to inflammatory-related chronic diseases such as urolithiasis, hypertension, insulin resistance, low immune function, and osteoporosis (Adeva and Souto, 2011; Minich and Bland, 2007).

Consequently, when working with higher protein intakes it is important to provide a diet balanced in high alkaline foods. The most abundant alkaline foods are plant-based foods; particularly vegetables and fruit abundant in alkalinizing micronutrients such as magnesium, calcium, sodium, and potassium. A more alkaline diet consisting of a higher fruit and vegetable intake is associated with a low potential renal acid load (PRAL) (Remer and Manz, 1995). Lower consumption of meat, which is also associated with a lower PRAL, may thus ameliorate not only the elevated blood pressure of hypertension but also the concurrent excess of morbidity and mortality of the concurrent cardiac, vascular, and metabolic aspects of the hypertensive state. Although acute acid loading may only temporarily disrupt acid-base equilibrium, a chronic perturbation occurs when metabolism of the diet repeatedly releases acids into the systemic circulation in amounts that exceed the amount of base released at the same time. To overcome the imbalance, the skeleton, which serves as the major reservoir of base, provides the buffer needed to maintain blood pH and plasma bicarbonate concentrations. To some degree, skeletal muscle also acts as a buffer. Other compensatory mechanisms occur as well, all in response to the acidic load (Pizzorno et al, 2010).

Remer and Manz developed a physiologically based model to calculate the PRAL of selected, frequently consumed foods. By means of these PRAL data, the daily net acid excretion can be calculated, allowing for an accurate prediction of the effects of diet on acid load. This has been a reason to recommend animal protein limited diets, to control the dietary source of acids (Kiwull-Schone et al, 2008). The following food lists serve as a guide to influencing potential renal acid load (PRAL).

Potentially Acid Foods

Protein: meat, fish, fowl, shellfish, eggs, all types of cheese, peanut butter, peanuts
Fat: bacon, butternuts, walnuts, pumpkin seeds, sesame seeds, sunflower seeds, creamy salad dressings
Carbohydrate: all types of bread including cornbran, oats, macaroni, rice-bran, rye, wheat, and especially wheat gluten
Sweets: gelatin desserts (dry mix with and without aspartame), pudding (instant, dry mix)

Potentially Basic or Alkaline Foods

Fat: dried beechnuts, dried chestnuts, acorn
Vegetables: all types including legumes but especially beets, beet greens, Swiss chard, dandelion greens, kale, leeks, mustard greens, spinach, turnip greens
Fruit: all types, especially currants, dates, figs, bananas, dried apricots, apples, prunes, raisins
Spices/Herbs: all types, especially fresh dill weed and dried spices/herbs such as spearmint, basil, coriander, curry powder, oregano, parsley
Sweets: sorghum syrup, sugar (brown), molasses, cocoa (dry powder)
Beverages: coffee

Neutral Foods

Fats: butter, margarine, oils
Dairy: milk
Vegetables: corn
Sweets: sugar (white), most syrups, honey
Beverages: water, tea

cannot tolerate dairy products because of lactose intolerance, allergies, or preference, calcium supplements should be taken with meals. Urine calcium should be measured before starting the supplement and afterward to see the effect; if urine calcium increases, patients should increase fluid intake to dilute the urine concentration of calcium.

Higher dietary calcium from either nondairy or dairy foods is independently associated with a lower kidney stone risk (Taylor and Curhan, 2013). Therefore, based on DRI recommendations for age (see inside front cover), patients may select calcium from dairy or nondairy choices. Given recent concerns for increased risk for cardiovascular disease and kidney stones with increased use of calcium supplements, women should aim to meet DRI recommendations from a calcium-rich diet, taking calcium supplements only if needed to reach DRI goals (Manson and Bassuk, 2014). Calcium should be taken in divided doses, choosing a source with each meal to maximize oxalate binding. Low-fat dairy choices are good options for their lower saturated fat content.

Oxalate Stones. Hyperoxaluria (more than 40 mg of oxalate in urine per day) plays an important role in calcium stone formation and is observed in 10% to 50% of recurrent stone formers. Primary hyperoxaluria is a feature of an autosomal-recessive genetic defect of a hepatic enzyme that results in overproduction of oxalate and a urinary oxalate concentration three to eight times normal. Multiple stones occur in these children, causing renal failure and early death.

Patients with inflammatory bowel diseases or gastric bypass often develop hyperoxaluria related to fat malabsorption. The bile acids produced during the digestive process normally are reabsorbed in the proximal gastrointestinal (GI) tract, but when this fails to occur, bile salts and fatty acids increase colonic permeability to oxalate (see Chapter 28). The unabsorbed fatty acids also bind calcium to form soaps, decreasing availability of calcium in a soluble form. With less calcium available to bind oxalate in the gut and prevent its absorption, serum oxalate and thus urinary oxalate levels increase.

Urinary oxalate also comes from endogenous synthesis, proportional to lean body mass. Ascorbic acid accounts for 35% to 55%, and glyoxylic acid accounts for 50% to 70% of urinary oxalate. In patients with CKD, excessive vitamin C intake may lead to stone formation. Oxalate synthesis is not increased with a high protein diet (Knight et al, 2009). Because pyridoxine acts as a cofactor in the conversion of glyoxylate to glycine, its deficiency could increase endogenous oxalate production.

The bioavailability of food oxalate and urine oxalate are affected by salt forms of oxalate, food processing and cooking methods, meal composition, and the presence of *Oxalobacter formigenes (OF)* in the GI tract (Siener et al, 2013). Stone-forming patients who lack this bacteria have significantly higher urinary oxalate excretion and stone episodes compared with patients colonized with the bacteria. There is a 70% risk reduction in calcium-oxalate stone formers when there is OF colonization of their stool (Lange, 2014).

Administration of *O. formigenes* as enteric-coated capsules significantly reduces urine oxalate in patients with primary hyperoxaluria. Dietary advice for reducing urinary oxalate should include use of this probiotic and reduction of dietary oxalate, if needed, and simultaneous consumption of calcium-rich food or supplement to reduce oxalate absorption (Knight et al, 2009; see Box 35-1).

BOX 35-1 Foods to Avoid for a Low-Oxalate Diet

Rhubarb
Spinach
Strawberries
Chocolate
Wheat bran and whole-grain wheat products
Nuts (almonds, peanuts, or pecans)
Beets
Tea (green, black, iced, or instant)
High doses of turmeric

Data from Siener R et al: Oxalate content of cereals and cereal products, *J Agric Food Chem* 54:3008, 2006.

Uric Acid Stones. Uric acid is an end product of purine metabolism from food, de novo synthesis, and tissue catabolism. Approximately half of the purine load is from endogenous sources and is constant. Exogenous dietary sources provide the other half, accounting for the variation in urinary uric acid. The solubility of uric acid depends on urine volume, the amount excreted, and urine pH (see Table 35-3). Uric acid stones form when urine is supersaturated with undissociated uric acid, which occurs at urinary pH less than 5.5.

The most important feature in uric acid stone formers is low urine pH resulting from increased NAE and impaired buffering caused by reduced urinary ammonium excretion. The former can be a result of low intake of alkali-producing foods or increased consumption of acid-producing foods (see *Clinical Insight:* Urine pH—How Does Diet Affect It?).

Inflammatory bowel disease results in chronically acidic urine, usually from dehydration. GI bicarbonate loss from diarrhea may predispose these patients to uric acid stones. Uric acid stones also are associated with lymphoproliferative and myeloproliferative disorders, with increased cellular breakdown that releases purines and thus increases uric acid load. Diabetes, obesity, and hypertension appear to be associated with nephrolithiasis; diabetes is a common factor in uric acid stone development (Scales et al, 2012). Besides diabetes management for patients with uric acid lithiasis and hyperuricosuric calcium oxalate stones, dietary purines also should be restricted.

Meat, fish, and poultry are rich in purines and acid ash and thus should be used in moderation to meet DRI for protein. Purines and metabolism of sulfur-rich amino acids, cystine and methionine, in animal protein confer an acid load to the kidney, thus lowering urine pH. PRAL value is assigned to groups of foods in terms of their positive or negative effect on acidic load (Trinchieri, 2012, 2013). Foods specifically high in purines should be avoided, including organ meats, anchovies, herrings, sardines, meat-based broth, and gravy (see Box 39-3). Dietary noncompliance or persistence of hyperuricosuria warrants use of medication such as allopurinol. Uric acid stones are the only stones amenable to dissolution therapy by urine

TABLE 35-3 Effect of Urine pH on Stone Formation

pH	State of Urate	Likely Stone Development
<5.5	Undissociated urate	Uric acid stones
5.5-7.5	Dissociated urate	Calcium oxalate stones
>7.5	Dissociated urate	Calcium phosphate stones

alkalinization to a pH of 6 to 6.5. Potassium citrate has been used as the therapy of choice. Sodium bicarbonate increases urinary monosodium urate and calcium and should not be used as a supplement.

Cystine Stones. Cystine stones represent 1% to 2% of urinary calculi and are caused by homozygous cystinuria. Cystine stones affect approximately 1 in 15,000 persons in the United States. Whereas normal individuals daily excrete 20 mg or less of cystine in their urine, stone-forming cystinuric patients excrete more than 250 mg/day. Cystine solubility increases when urine pH exceeds 7; therefore an alkaline urine pH must be maintained 24 hours per day, even while the patient sleeps. This is achieved almost always with the use of medication. Fluid intake of more than 4 L daily is recommended to prevent cystine crystallization. Lower sodium intake may be useful in reducing cystine in the urine. Restriction of animal protein is associated with lower intake of cystine and methionine, a precursor of cystine. Ingestion of vegetables and fruit high in citrate and malate, such as melons, limes, oranges and fresh tomato juice, may help alkalinize the urine (Heilberg and Goldfarb, 2013).

Melamine and Indinavir Stones. Kidney stones, ARF, and death have been reported in young children who received melamine-contaminated infant formula. Melamine is an organic base synthesized from urea. When added to liquid milk or milk powder, it deceptively increases the protein content. Melamine precipitates in the distal renal tubules, forming crystals and sandlike stones. Hydration and urine alkalinization help with stone passage.

The treatment of human immunodeficiency virus infection with protease inhibitors has led to the appearance of another previously unknown urinary calculus: indinavir. Hypocitraturia is universal in all patients with indinavir stones as well as decreased solubility in a low urine volume with a low pH. These stones are soft, gelatinous, and radiolucent and are not amenable to basket removal or ureteroscopy. Intravenous (IV) hydration and temporary cessation of indinavir should be the first choice of treatment (Zilberman et al, 2010).

Struvite Stones. Struvite stones are composed of magnesium ammonium phosphate and carbonate apatite. They are also known as triple-phosphate or infection stones. Unlike most urinary stones, they occur more commonly in women than in men, at a ratio of 2:1. They form only in the presence of bacteria such as *Pseudomonas, Klebsiella, Proteus mirabilis*, and *Urealyticum*, which carry urease, a urea-splitting enzyme. Urea breakdown results in ammonia and carbon dioxide (CO_2) production, thus raising urine pH and the level of carbonate. Struvite stones grow rapidly to large staghorn calculi in the renal pelvic area. The mainstay of treatment is extracorporeal shockwave lithotripsy (ECSWL) with adjunctive culture-specific antimicrobial therapy that uses urease inhibitors. The goal is to eliminate or prevent urinary tract infections by regularly screening and monitoring urine cultures. Because of their infectious origin, diet has no definitive role except avoidance of urine alkalinization.

Medical Management

Uric acid stones are the only type amenable to dissolution therapy, or dissolving of the stone by alkalinization of the urine. This is done with consumption of a more vegetarian diet, that is also lower in purines, or use of medication. Shockwave lithotripsy and endourologic techniques almost have replaced the open surgical procedures of stone removal of 20 years ago.

Struvite stones also are treated with adjunctive culture-specific antimicrobial therapy that uses urease inhibitors. Management strategies are now aimed at kidney stone prevention.

Medical Nutrition Therapy

After corrective treatment, nutrition assessment is needed to determine risk factors for stone recurrence. The risk in men and women rises with increasing urine calcium and oxalate and decreases with increasing citrate and urine volume. There is a continuum of risk related to increasing urinary calcium and urinary oxalate. For patients with no metabolic abnormality there is a graded increase in stone risk that begins when the rate of urinary excretion of calcium, oxalate, and citrate is still within the normal range (Curhan and Taylor, 2008). Because urine chemistries change from day to day based on changes in the environment and diet, two 24-hour urine specimens are needed based on a usual diet, one during a weekday and one on the weekend. Specific medical nutrition therapy (MNT) is then based on comprehensive metabolic evaluations. Nutrition counseling and metabolic monitoring can be effective (see Table 35-4).

When a patient passes a stone, it should be determined whether it is a new stone or a preexisting one and advisement given accordingly. The effectiveness of any MNT should be monitored with evaluation of subsequent 24-hour urine collections. This gives the nutritionist and patient a measure of the effect of dietary changes. Once diet therapy is initiated, the goal is to prevent new stones from forming and preexisting stones from growing (see *Pathophysiology and Care Management Algorithm: Kidney Stones*).

TABLE 35-4	**Recommendations for Diet and 24-Hour Urine Monitoring in Kidney Stone Disease**	
Diet Component	**Intake Recommendation**	**24-Hour Urine**
Protein	Normal intake: avoid excess	Monitor urinary urea
Calcium	Normal intake: 1000 mg if age <50 years; 1200 mg if age >50 years Divide intake between three or more eating sessions. Choose from dairy or non-dairy sources	Calcium <150 mg/L (<3.75 mmol/L)
Oxalate	Avoid moderate- to high-oxalate foods if urinary oxalate is high	Oxalate <20 mg/L (<220 µmol/L)
Fluid	2.5 L or more; assess type of fluids consumed; provide guidelines	Volume > 2 L/day
Purines	Avoid excessive protein intake; avoid specific high-purine foods	Uric acid <2 mmol/L (<336 mg/L)
Vitamin C	Avoid supplementation	Monitor urinary oxalate
Vitamin D	Meet DRI for vitamin D intake. Use supplements to reach DRI	Serum 25(OH)D$_3$ in acceptable range
Vitamin B$_6$	40 mg or more per day reduces risk. No recommendation made	
Sodium	<100 mmol/day	Monitor urinary sodium

PATHOPHYSIOLOGY AND CARE MANAGEMENT ALGORITHM

Kidney Stones

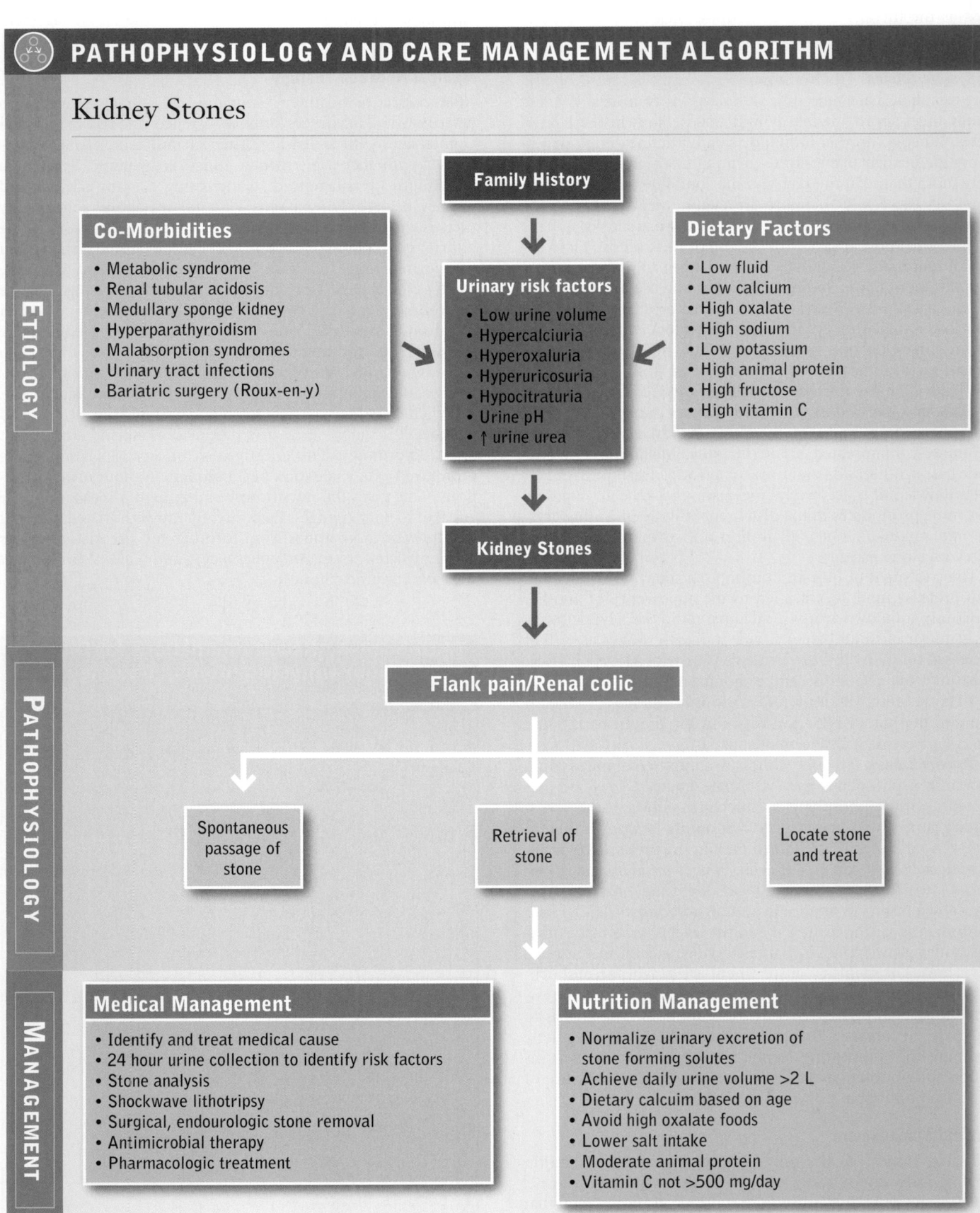

ETIOLOGY

Family History

Co-Morbidities
- Metabolic syndrome
- Renal tubular acidosis
- Medullary sponge kidney
- Hyperparathyroidism
- Malabsorption syndromes
- Urinary tract infections
- Bariatric surgery (Roux-en-y)

Urinary risk factors
- Low urine volume
- Hypercalciuria
- Hyperoxaluria
- Hyperuricosuria
- Hypocitraturia
- Urine pH
- ↑ urine urea

Dietary Factors
- Low fluid
- Low calcium
- High oxalate
- High sodium
- Low potassium
- High animal protein
- High fructose
- High vitamin C

Kidney Stones

PATHOPHYSIOLOGY

Flank pain/Renal colic

Spontaneous passage of stone

Retrieval of stone

Locate stone and treat

MANAGEMENT

Medical Management
- Identify and treat medical cause
- 24 hour urine collection to identify risk factors
- Stone analysis
- Shockwave lithotripsy
- Surgical, endourologic stone removal
- Antimicrobial therapy
- Pharmacologic treatment

Nutrition Management
- Normalize urinary excretion of stone forming solutes
- Achieve daily urine volume >2 L
- Dietary calcium based on age
- Avoid high oxalate foods
- Lower salt intake
- Moderate animal protein
- Vitamin C not >500 mg/day

Fluid and Urine Volume. A low urine volume is by far the most common abnormality noted in the metabolic evaluation of stone formers, and its correction with a high fluid intake should be the focus with all types of kidney stones. The objective is to maintain urinary solutes in the undersaturated zone to inhibit nucleation; this is accomplished by an increase in urine volume and reduction of solute load. The goal is the amount of urine flow rather than a specified fluid intake. High urine flow rate tends to wash out any formed crystals, and a urine volume of 2 to 2.5 L/day should prevent stone recurrence. Fluid intake should change based on different rates of extrarenal fluid loss that affect rate of urine flow. The concentration of urinary risk factors is important, not the absolute amount excreted, the former will be high when the urine volume is low. The goal should be to maintain appropriate concentration of solutes per liter of urine.

Achieving a urine volume of 2 to 2.5 L/day usually requires an intake of 250 ml of fluid at each meal, between meals, at bedtime, and when arising to void at night. Hydration during sleep hours is important to break the cycle of the "most-concentrated" morning urine. Half of this daily 2.5 L should be taken as water. Even higher fluid intake, perhaps as much as 3 L/day, may be necessary to compensate for any GI fluid loss, excessive sweating from strenuous exercise, or an excessively hot or dry environment. Barriers to fluid intake success include lack of knowledge about the benefits of fluid or not remembering to drink, disliking the taste of water, lack of thirst, lack of availability of water, needing to void frequently, and not wanting workplace disruptions. Fluid intake behavior can be improved by specifically addressing barriers relevant to the individual patient.

Not all fluids are equally beneficial for reducing the risk of kidney stones. Cranberry juice acidifies urine and is useful in the treatment of struvite stones. Black currant juice increases urinary citrate and oxalate and, because of its urine alkalinizing effect, may prevent the occurrence of uric acid stones.

Tea, coffee, decaffeinated coffee, orange juice, beer, and wine have been associated with reduced risk of stone formation. Coffee and tea induce moderate diuresis because of their caffeine content. Because decaffeinated coffee has no caffeine, it is suggested that other mechanisms may be involved, such as phytochemicals with antioxidant properties. Alcohol also helps because of diuresis. Orange juice has citrate that delivers an alkali load (Taylor and Curhan, 2008a).

The oxalate content of tea brewed from regular black or green tea is 300 to 1500 μmol/L. Because of this high oxalate content of black tea, it should be taken with generous amounts of added milk; milk appears to reduce oxalate absorption by binding it in the gut lumen as calcium oxalate, making it less absorbable. Herbal teas have much lower oxalate content of 31 to 75 μmol/L and are an acceptable alternative (Kaufman et al, 2008).

Animal Protein. Epidemiologic studies find a correlation between improved standard of living, high animal protein intake, and the rising incidence of kidney stones. Meat, fish, poultry, eggs, cheese, and grains are the primary contributors of acid; a LAKE (load of acid to kidney evaluation) score can be a simple and useful tool to evaluate dietary PRAL (potential renal acid load). Dietary modifications can be made to achieve LAKE reduction for the prevention of kidney stones. Fruits, juices, vegetables, potatoes, and legumes have negative PRAL values (Trinchieri, 2012) (see *Clinical Insight:* Urine pH—How Does Diet Affect It?). An adequate-calcium, low–animal protein, low-salt diet (less than 4 g) reduces oxalate excretion more than a traditional low oxalate diet.

Oxalate. Because much less oxalate than calcium exists in urine (the ratio is 1:5), changes in oxalate concentration have a greater effect than changes in urinary calcium. However, oxalate absorption, which is 3% to 8% of the amount in food, is affected by the amount of dietary calcium. Dietary calcium reduces oxalate absorption, and appears to have more impact on urinary oxalate than the amount of dietary oxalate. The impact of dietary oxalate on urinary oxalate appears to be small. For many stone formers, restricting dietary oxalate may be a relatively ineffective intervention to decrease urinary oxalate excretion (Agarwal et al, 2011). On very low calcium intakes of less than 200 mg/day, oxalate absorption rises; it falls when more calcium (1200 mg) is ingested. Age is associated independently and inversely with urinary oxalate.

Dietary counseling to reduce oxalate absorption is beneficial for stone-forming individuals who have large intakes of high-oxalate foods and who excrete more than 30 mg (350 μmol) of oxalate per day. Based on the available evidence, severe oxalate restriction is not necessary. The oxalate content of foods can be found at http://regepi.bwh.harvard.edu/health/oxalate/files/oxalate. However, avoidance of excessive dietary oxalate intake is reasonable, and should be coupled with advice for increasing calcium intake (Agarwal et al, 2011). The patient is advised to add calcium to each meal to bind oxalate. The total calcium intake for the day can be divided between at least three meals or as many eating occasions as possible. It takes 150 mg of calcium to bind 100 mg of oxalate. Patients should include approximately 150 mg calcium in each meal, such as that found in $^1/_2$ cup milk, ice cream, pudding, yogurt, or $^3/_4$ oz cheese (Kaufman et al, 2008).

Potassium. Stone formers often have a low to normal potassium intake and high sodium intake that results in an adversely raised Na:K ratio. Potassium intake is related inversely to the risk of kidney stones. Estimation of fruit and vegetable intake should be included in the metabolic evaluation. Stone formers should be encouraged to increase the potassium in their diets by choosing low-oxalate fruit and vegetables many times throughout the day (see Appendix 51 and Box 35-1). Foods high in potassium are replete with alkali, which stimulates urinary citrate excretion. Every 20 mEq/day increase in urinary potassium is associated with a 17 mg/day decrease in urinary calcium (Nouvenne et al, 2010).

Magnesium. Magnesium is a low-molecular-weight inhibitor that forms soluble complexes with oxalate. Like calcium, it inhibits oxalate absorption and may have a role to play in hyperoxaluric patients.

Phosphate. Excess urine phosphate contributes to calcium phosphate stone risk, but it is not as important a risk factor as urinary pH, which determines how much phosphate will be in the form of hydrogen phosphate (HPO_4). Calcium phosphate stones tend to occur in pregnant women in the second and third trimester of pregnancy.

Sodium. The daily amount of sodium chloride in modern diets reaches excessive levels of up to 10 g/day. The amount of sodium in the urine and hypercalciuria are correlated directly because sodium and calcium are reabsorbed at common sites in the renal tubule. The risk for nephrolithiasis is significantly higher in hypertensive individuals compared with normotensive individuals. A low-sodium diet and water therapy lowered urine sodium, calcium, and oxalate in idiopathic hypercalciuric stone formers compared with controls on water therapy alone

(Taylor et al, 2009). Urine sodium is associated positively with urine calcium and urine volume and negatively with urine calcium-oxalate supersaturation. Increased volume may confer a protective effect.

Sodium intake should be lowered to less than 2300 mg/day in patients with hypercalciuria. Consumption of a diet modeled on the Dietary Approaches to Stop Hypertension (DASH) diet reduces the risk for kidney stones (Baia et al, 2012; Trinchieri, 2013). Higher DASH scores are associated with higher intakes of calcium, potassium, magnesium, oxalate, and vitamin C and lower intakes of sodium as the diet is moderately high in low-fat dairy products, fruits and vegetables, and nuts and low in animal proteins (see Appendix 26).

Citrate. Citrate inhibits urinary stones by forming a complex with calcium in urine. Thus less calcium is available to bind urinary oxalate, which helps prevent the formation of calcium oxalate or calcium phosphate stones. Distal renal tubular acidosis (RTA) is an acidosis accompanied by hypokalemia. RTA, malabsorption syndrome with enteric hyperoxaluria, and excessive meat intake (lower urine pH) are associated with decreased urinary citrate levels.

Many citrate-containing beverages have been tested for their effect on urine. Several diet sodas contain moderate amounts of citrate and malate, bicarbonate precursors; malate increases the total alkali load delivered, which augments citraturia. One commercial sports drink tested in non–stone formers increased urine citrate as much as 170 mg/day, but many sports drinks contain too much fructose and do not increase urinary citrate. Melon juice has citrate and malate and a PRAL value more negative than orange juice (Kang et al, 2007). Fresh tomato juice has citrate and malate and is low in sodium and oxalate.

Hypocitraturia is most commonly idiopathic but also may be caused by acidosis accompanied by hypokalemia, malabsorption syndrome with enteric hyperoxaluria, excessive meat intake, and acid ash. Half of recurrent calcium stone formers have hypocitraturia (urinary citrate of less than 300 mg/day). Normal daily urinary citrate level should be more than 640 mg/day. Long-term lemonade or lime or lemon juice therapy in hypocitraturic stone formers results in increased urinary citrate levels and decreased stone formation rate (Taylor and Curhan, 2008b). Mineral water, with its magnesium and bicarbonate content, raises urine pH and stone inhibition.

Fructose. Fructose intake has increased approximately 2000% during the past 30 years from the widespread use of high-fructose corn syrup in foods. Fructose may increase urinary excretion of calcium and oxalate. It is the only carbohydrate known to increase the production of uric acid and its urinary excretion. Fructose also may increase insulin resistance, which is associated with low urine pH. Fructose intake has been positively associated with risk for all types of kidney stones (Tang et al, 2012). Increased fruit and vegetable consumption is recommended to increase potassium intake, but because of the fructose content of fruit, there should be more emphasis on vegetables.

Vitamins. Vitamin C supplementation at 1000 mg/day was associated with twofold increased risk of kidney stones in men. Compared with less than 90 mg/day vs. 1000 mg/day the latter results in 6.8 mg more oxalate in urine (Agarwal et al, 2011). In another study, which included women, total vitamin C intake and supplement vitamin C intake correlated with risk for stone formation in men, but not women. The same was observed for supplemental vitamin C intake, but not dietary vitamin C intake in both men and women (Ferraro et al, 2016). Thus individuals with

calcium oxalate stone disease and high levels of urine oxalate should avoid vitamin C supplementation greater than 90 mg/day.

Vitamin B_6 in the form of pyridoxal phosphate is a required cofactor in oxalate metabolism; marginal B_6 status should be avoided. Supplementing with 2 to 10 mg/day of vitamin B_6 may reduce urinary oxalate in some calcium oxalate stone formers.

The role of vitamin D in stone diease is controversial. From NHANES III data based on serum 25-OH vitamin D concentration, a high concentration was not associated with prevalent kidney stone disease in the participants (Tang et al, 2012). Vitamin D in doses producing desirable levels of 25(OH) D at 100 to 150 nmol/L or 40 to 60 ng/ml does not adversely affect components of kidney stones (Heany, 2013, http://www.grassrootshealth.net).

Omega-3 Fatty Acids. Elevated levels of arachidonic acid (AA) in cell membranes may promote hypercalciuria and hyperoxaluria. The intake of omega-3 fatty acids such as eicosapentaenoic acid (EPA) and docosahexaenoic acid (DHA) may decrease the AA content of cell membranes and reduce urinary excretion of calcium and oxalate. EPA is an inhibitor of AA metabolism resulting in decreased synthesis of prostaglandin 2 (E-2 (PGE2)), a substance known to potentiate urine calcium excretion. EPA and DHA through fish oil supplementation did not reduce the risk of incident kidney stones and fatty acid intake of AA, and linoleic acid did not increase the risk of developing kidney stones in observational studies (Taylor et al, 2005). The use of fish oil (omega-3 FA at 1200 mg/day) in the treatment of hypercalciuric stone formers combined with empiric diet counseling resulted in a measurable decrease in urine calcium (24% became normocalciuric) and oxalate excretion, and an increase in urinary citrate. Calcium-oxalate supersaturation decreased in 38% of subjects (29). EPA at 1800 mg/day showed significant reduction in stone episodes (Yasui et al, 2008).

ACUTE KIDNEY INJURY (ACUTE RENAL FAILURE)

Pathophysiology

Acute kidney injury (AKI), formerly acute renal failure (ARF), is characterized by a sudden reduction in glomerular filtration rate (GFR), the amount of filtrate per unit in the nephrons, and altered ability of the kidney to excrete the daily production of metabolic waste. AKI can occur in association with oliguria (decreased output of urine) or normal urine flow, but it typically occurs in previously healthy kidneys. Duration varies from a few days to several weeks. The causes of AKI are numerous and can occur simultaneously (see Table 35-5). These causes are generally classified into three categories: (1) inadequate renal perfusion (prerenal), (2) diseases within the renal parenchyma (intrinsic), and (3) urinary tract obstruction (postrenal).

A new form of classification to help clinicians assess the severity and progression of acute kidney injury, using the acronym RIFLE (Risk, Injury, Failure, Loss and ESRD), indicates the likelihood of a patient recovering or progressing to chronic renal failure. This, in turn, helps dietitians know whether to increase protein intake goals or be more moderate to preserve kidney function.

Medical Management

The ratio of blood urea nitrogen (BUN) to creatinine can be used diagnostically to assess the location of damage to the kidney. Depending on where the insult occurs, BUN is

TABLE 35-5 Some Causes of Acute Kidney Injury

Causes	Condition
Prerenal inadequate renal perfusion	Severe dehydration Circulatory collapse
Intrinsic diseases within the renal parenchyma	Acute tubular necrosis • Trauma, surgery • Septicemia Ischemic acute tubular necrosis Nephrotoxicity • Antibiotics, contrast agents, and other drugs Local reaction to drugs Vascular disorders • Bilateral renal infarction Acute glomerulonephritis of any cause • Poststreptococcal infection • Systemic lupus erythematosus
Postrenal urinary tract obstruction	Benign prostatic hypertrophy with urinary retention Carcinoma of the bladder or prostate Retroperitoneal or pelvic cancer Bilateral ureteral stones and obstruction Rhabdomyolysis

increased because of poor filtration and is more actively reabsorbed. In this situation, with a BUN/Cr ratio greater than 20:1, damage is prerenal (before the kidney). When damage is intrinsic (within the kidney), the BUN/Cr ratio decreases to less than 10:1. Generally, if careful attention is directed at diagnosing and correcting the prerenal or obstructive causes, AKI is short lived and requires no particular nutritional intervention.

Intrinsic AKI can result from causes listed in Table 35-5; of these, a prolonged episode of ischemia leading to ischemic acute tubular necrosis is the most devastating. Typically patients develop this illness as a complication of an overwhelming infection, severe trauma, surgical accident, or cardiogenic shock. The clinical course and outcome depends mainly on the underlying cause. Patients with AKI caused by drug toxicity generally recover fully after they stop taking the drug. On the other hand, the mortality rate associated with ischemic acute tubular necrosis caused by shock is approximately 70%. Typically these patients are highly catabolic, and extensive tissue destruction occurs in the early stages. Hemodialysis (HD) is used to reduce the acidosis, correct the uremia, and control hyperkalemia.

If recovery is to occur, it generally takes place within 2 to 3 weeks after the insult is corrected. The recovery (diuretic) phase is characterized first by an increase in urine output and later by a return of waste elimination. During this period dialysis may still be required, and careful attention must be paid to fluid and electrolyte balance and appropriate replacement.

Medical Nutrition Therapy

Nutritional care in AKI is particularly important because the patient not only has uremia, metabolic acidosis, and fluid and electrolyte imbalance but also usually suffers from physiologic stress (e.g., infection or tissue destruction) that increases protein needs. The problem of balancing protein and energy needs with treatment of acidosis and excessive nitrogenous waste is complicated and delicate. In the early stages of AKI the patient is often unable to eat. Mortality in AKI is high, especially among those who are

previously malnourished (Coca et al, 2009). Early attention to nutritional support and early dialysis improves patient survival.

At the onset of AKI, depending on severity, some patients can be treated with medical management, other patients require **renal replacement therapy (RRT)** with standard **hemodialysis (HD)** or **peritoneal dialysis (PD)** to remove wastes and fluids until kidney function returns. In significant AKI, a patient in the intensive care unit (ICU) may require continuous treatments, rather than periodic dialysis. **Continuous renal replacement therapy (CRRT)** is the broad category term that includes a whole host of modalities (see *Focus On:* Continuous Renal Replacement Therapy or CRRT). Most often used are **continuous venovenous hemofiltration (CVVH)** and **continuous venovenous hemodialysis (CVVHD)**, which use a small ultrafiltration membrane to produce an ultrafiltrate that can be replaced by parenteral nutrition (PN) fluids. This treatment allows parenteral feeding without fluid overload.

◎ FOCUS ON

Continuous Renal Replacement Therapy or CRRT

CRRT typically is used when patients develop anasarca (extreme generalized edema) or elevated blood pressure and are unable to excrete fluid or uremic wastes. It is the therapy chosen when periodic hemodialysis is to be avoided because rapid removal of fluid and wastes may put the kidney into a less active state causing decreased blood flow to the kidney and a delay in regaining of kidney function.

	CVVH-Diffusion	CVVH-Convection	CVVHD	SCUF
Definition	Continuous venovenus hemodialysis using diffusion	Continuous venovenus hemodialysis using convection	Continuous venovenus hemodiafiltration	Slow continuous ultrafiltration
Advantages	Good removal of small molecules. Do not need replacement fluids.	Better removal of middle weight molecules. Good fluid removal.	Best removal of fluid and middle weight solutes. Also used in treatment of severe sepsis.	Best treatment for fluid overload. Used primarily for fluid removal.
Contraindications	May add considerable calorie load, less effective removal of middle weight molecules.	10% to 15% protein losses in ultrafiltrate. Protein lost must be replaced, along with other fluid replacement.	Replacement fluids required. Considerable calorie load from dextrose solution possible.	Does not remove urea or other small or middle weight molecules well.

Protein. The amount of protein recommended is influenced by the underlying cause of AKI and the presence of other conditions. A range of recommended levels can be found in the literature, from 0.5 to 0.8 g/kg for nondialysis patients to 1 to 2 g/kg for patients receiving dialysis. With CRRT protein losses are high, and estimated protein needs increase to 1.5 to 2.5 g/kg. As the patient's overall medical status stabilizes and improves, metabolic requirements decrease. During this stable period before renal function returns, a minimum protein intake of 0.8 to 1 g/kg of body weight should be given. This remains dependent on the patient's overall status and comorbidities and should be evaluated individually.

Energy. Energy requirements are determined by the underlying cause of AKI and comorbidity. Energy needs can be measured at the bedside by indirect calorimetry in most ICUs (see Chapter 2). If this equipment is not available, calorie needs should be estimated at 25 to 40 cal/kg of upper end IBW or adjusted IBW per day. Excessive calorie intake can lead to excess CO_2 production, depressing respiration (see Chapter 34). With newer solutions available, glucose can be either absorbed or lost, depending on the concentration or type of solution used, and can be a source of calorie loss or gain. Large intakes of carbohydrate and fat are needed to prevent the use of protein for energy production. For patients who receive PN, high concentrations of carbohydrate and lipid can be administered to fulfill these needs as long as respiratory status is monitored.

A high-calorie, low-protein diet may be used in cases in which dialysis or hemofiltration is unavailable. In addition to the usual dietary sources of refined sweets and fats, special high-calorie, low-protein, and low-electrolyte formulas have been developed to augment the diet. However, care must be taken with these products because hyperglycemia is not uncommon as a result of glucose intolerance, and additional insulin often is needed.

Fluid and Sodium. During the early (often oliguric) phase of AKI, meticulous attention to fluid status is essential. Ideally fluid and electrolyte intake should balance the net output. With negligible urine output, significant contributions to total body water output include emesis and diarrhea, body cavity drains, and skin and respiratory losses. If fever is present, skin losses can be excessive; whereas if the patient is on humidified air, almost no losses occur. Because of the numerous IV drugs, blood, and blood products necessitated by the underlying disease, the challenge in managing patients at this point becomes how to cut fluid intake as much as possible while providing adequate protein and energy.

Sodium is restricted, based on decreased urinary production. In the oliguric phase when the sodium output is very low, intake should be low as well, perhaps as low as 20 to 40 mEq/day. However, limiting sodium is often impossible because of the requirement for many IV solutions (including IV antibiotics, medications for blood pressure, and PN). The administration of these solutions in electrolyte-free water in the face of oliguria quickly leads to water intoxication (hyponatremia). For this reason, all fluid above the daily calculated water loss should be given in a balanced salt solution.

Potassium. Most of the excretion of potassium and the control of potassium balance are normal functions of the kidney. When renal function is impaired, potassium balance should be scrutinized carefully. In addition to dietary sources, all body tissues contain large amounts of potassium; thus tissue destruction can lead to potassium overload. Potassium levels can shift abruptly and have to be monitored frequently. Potassium intake must be individualized according to serum levels (see Appendices 29 and 51). The primary mechanism of potassium removal during AKI is dialysis. Control of serum potassium levels between dialysis

TABLE 35-6 Summary of Medical Nutrition Therapy for Acute Kidney Injury

Nutrient	Amount
Protein	0.8-1 g/kg IBW increasing as GFR returns to normal; 60% should be HBV protein
Energy	30-40 kcal/kg of body weight
Potassium	30-50 mEq/day in oliguric phase (depending on urinary output, dialysis, and serum K⁺ level); replace losses in diuretic phase
Sodium	20-40 mEq/day in oliguric phase (depending on urinary output, edema, dialysis, and serum Na⁺ level); replace losses in diuretic phase
Fluid	Replace output from the previous day (vomitus, diarrhea, urine) plus 500 ml
Phosphorus	Limit as necessary

GFR, Glomerular filtration rate; *HBV,* high biologic value; *IBW,* ideal body weight; *K⁺,* potassium; *Na⁺,* sodium.

administrations relies mainly on IV infusions of glucose, insulin, and bicarbonate, all of which drive potassium into cells. Exchange resins, such as sodium polystyrene sulfonate (Kayexalate), which exchange potassium for sodium in the GI tract, can be used to treat high potassium concentrations; however, for many reasons these resins are less than ideal. Table 35-6 summarizes MNT for AKI.

DISEASES OF THE TUBULES AND INTERSTITIUM

To a great extent, the functions of the kidney tubules make them susceptible to injury. The enormous energy requirements and expenditures of the tubules for active secretion and reabsorption often leave this part of the kidney particularly vulnerable to ischemic injuries. Many toxic drugs can destroy or damage various segments of the tubules. The high-solute concentration generated in the medullary interstitium exposes it to damage from oxidants and precipitation of calcium-phosphate product (extraosseous calcification) and favors the sickling of red blood cells in sickle cell anemia. Indeed, a wide variety of diseases or disorders of the tubules and interstitium exists. They share common manifestations and can be considered together with respect to nutritional management.

Chronic interstitial nephritis can occur as a result of analgesic abuse, sickle cell disease, diabetes mellitus, or vesicoureteral reflux and manifests primarily as inability to concentrate the urine and as mild renal insufficiency. A hereditary disorder of the interstitium, medullary cystic disease, also presents with this picture. Dietary management consists of adequate fluid intake, which can require several liters of extra fluid. This is generally well tolerated by the patient, except when intercurrent illness occurs.

Fanconi syndrome is characterized by an inability to reabsorb the proper amount of glucose, amino acids, phosphate, and bicarbonate in the proximal tubule, thus causing urinary excretion of these substances. Adults with this syndrome present with acidosis, hypokalemia, polyuria, or osteomalacia, whereas children present with polyuria, growth retardation, rickets, and vomiting. No specific medical treatment is available to treat Fanconi syndrome; therefore dietary treatment is the main form of management. Replacement therapy usually consists of large volumes of water and dietary supplements of bicarbonate, potassium, phosphate, calcium, and vitamin D.

Renal tubular acidosis (RTA), a defect in tubular handling of bicarbonate, can be caused by either a defect in the distal tubule (type 1) or a proximal tubular defect (type 2). Distal RTA leads to severe osteomalacia, kidney stones, or even nephrocalcinosis (calcification of the kidney). Distal RTA is treated with small amounts of bicarbonate, 70 to 100 mEq/day, with complete resolution of disease manifestations. Isolated proximal RTA in the adult is a benign disease, which often is made worse with bicarbonate and therefore should not be treated.

Pyelonephritis, a bacterial infection of the kidney, does not require extensive dietary management. However, in chronic cases the use of cranberry juice to reduce bacteriuria may be useful (Wang et al, 2012). Concentrated tannins or proanthocyanidins in cranberry juice and blueberry juice may inhibit the adherence of *Escherichia coli* bacteria to the epithelial cells of the urinary tract (see *Clinical Insight:* Urinary Tract Infections and Cranberry Juice). However, a study that reviewed 24 studies did find substantial benefit (Freire, 2013).

CLINICAL INSIGHT

Urinary Tract Infections and Cranberry Juice

Urinary tract infections (UTIs) are much more common in women than men because of the shorter female urethra. Elderly women have the highest incidence of UTI, and it is thought to be related to the loss of estrogen after menopause. Patients who are catheterized are also at high risk. The bacteria most commonly involved are *E. coli* resulting from the close proximity of the anus to a woman's urethra. Treatment is usually antibiotics to resolve the infection and phenazopyridine is used as an anesthetic to decrease symptoms. It temporarily changes the color of a woman's urine to bright orange or red. It is contraindicated in renal failure.

Nutritionally, tannins or proanthocyanidins in cranberry juice and blueberry juice may inhibit the adherence of *E. coli* bacteria to the epithelial cells. Coffee, alcohol, and sodas should be avoided because they irritate the urinary tract and cause dehydration. In normal kidney function drinking 6 to 8 ounces of water daily is recommended.

GLOMERULAR DISEASES

The functions of the glomerulus that are important with respect to disease are production of an adequate ultrafiltrate and prevention of certain substances from entering this ultrafiltrate.

Nephritic Syndrome

Nephritic syndrome incorporates a group of diseases characterized by inflammation of the capillary loops of the glomerulus. These acute glomerulonephritides are sudden in onset and brief and may proceed to complete recovery, development of chronic nephrotic syndrome, or ESRD. The primary manifestation of these diseases is hematuria (blood in the urine), a consequence of the capillary inflammation that damages the glomerular barrier to blood cells. The syndrome also is characterized by hypertension and mild loss of renal function. The most common presentation follows a streptococcal infection and is usually, although not always, self-limiting. Other causes include primary kidney diseases such as immunoglobulin A nephropathy (IgA); hereditary nephritis; and secondary diseases such as systemic lupus erythematosus (SLE), vasculitis, and glomerulonephritis (GN) associated with endocarditis, abscesses, or infected ventriculoperitoneal shunts.

Pathophysiology

Nephrotic syndrome comprises a group of diseases that derive from a loss of the glomerular barrier for protein. Large urinary protein losses lead to hypoalbuminemia with consequent edema, hypercholesterolemia, hypercoagulability, and abnormal bone metabolism. More than 95% of the cases of nephrotic syndrome stem from three systemic diseases: (1) diabetes mellitus, (2) systemic lupus erythematosus (SLE), and (3) amyloidosis; and from four diseases that are primarily of the kidney: (1) minimum change disease (seen only with electron microscopy), (2) membranous nephropathy, (3) focal glomerulosclerosis, and (4) membranoproliferative glomerulonephritis. Although renal function can deteriorate during the course of these diseases, it is not a consistent feature.

CHRONIC KIDNEY DISEASE

Many forms of kidney disease, two of which are described earlier, are characterized by a slow, steady decline in renal function and lead to renal failure in some patients, whereas other patients have a benign course without loss of renal function. It is unclear why some patients remain stable with chronic kidney disease (CKD) for many months to years, whereas others progress rapidly to renal failure and dialysis. The nature of this progressive loss of function has been the subject of an enormous amount of basic and clinical research during the past several decades and the subject of several excellent reviews (National Kidney Foundation, 2000; Yang et al, 2014). Medical nutrition therapy begins when the patient is diagnosed with the goal of preventing the progression of the disease as well as mitigating symptoms.

Pathophysiology

Once approximately one half to two thirds of kidney function has been lost, regardless of the underlying disease, progressive further loss of kidney function ensues. This is true even in diseases in which the underlying cause has been eliminated completely, such as in vesicoureteral reflux, cortical necrosis of pregnancy, or analgesic abuse. It is thought that, in response to a decreasing GFR, the kidney undergoes a series of adaptations to prevent decline. Although in the short term this leads to improvement in filtration rate, in the long term it leads to an accelerated loss of nephrons and progressive renal insufficiency. The nature of these adaptations involves a change in the hemodynamic characteristics of the remaining glomeruli, specifically leading to increased glomerular pressure. Factors that increase glomerular pressure tend to accelerate this process, whereas factors that decrease glomerular pressure tend to alleviate it (Grams et al, 2013).

Diabetes is the leading risk factor for CKD followed by hypertension and glomerulonephritis. The National Kidney Foundation (NKF) divides CKD into five stages related to the estimated GFR (eGFR) the rate at which the kidneys are filtering wastes (see Table 35-7). Stages 1 and 2 are early stages with markers such as proteinuria, hematuria, or anatomic issues. Stages 3 and 4 are considered advanced stages. Stage 5 results in death unless dialysis or transplantation is initiated.

Medical Management

The prevalence of CKD is now estimated at approximately 10% of adults in the United States, or greater than 20 million Americans. This estimated prevalence of CKD shows that 1 in

TABLE 35-7 Stages of Chronic Kidney Disease

Stage	eGFR	Description
1	90-130 ml/min	Kidney damage, but normal to increased kidney function
2	60-89 ml/min	Mild decrease in kidney function
3	30-59 ml/min	Moderate decrease in kidney function
4	15-29 ml/min	Severe decrease in kidney function
5	Less than 15 ml/min	Kidney failure requires dialysis, transplantation, or medical management (death with dignity)

eGFR, Estimated glomerular filtration rate.

3 people with diabetes and 1 in 5 people with hypertension have CKD (CDC, 2014). Many states now urge clinical laboratories reporting serum creatinine also to report the patient's **eGFR**. Patients with a low calculated eGFR do not necessarily have CKD. They must have several blood samples drawn 3 months apart that are consistently low (showing eGFR of less than 60) (see Table 35-7). This testing alerts primary care physicians to monitor for possible presence of kidney disease. Further research using eGFR cystatin C followed by eGFR pairing cystatin C and creatinine is now recognized as the most precise measure (Inker et al, 2012).

An online eGFR calculator can be found at the NKF site at http://www.kidney.org/professionals/kdoqi/gfr_calculator.cfm. With screening tools such as the calculated eGFR and a greater awareness of the progressive nature of CKD, more attention has focused on its social, medical, and financial effects. For example, CKD is strongly linked with cardiovascular disease (see *Clinical Insight:* Chronic Kidney Disease and Heart Disease—A Deadly Union).

Medical Nutrition Therapy

With each level of CKD, a different nutritional therapy may be proposed. The primary objectives of MNT are to manage the symptoms associated with the syndrome (edema,

hypoalbuminemia, and hyperlipidemia), decrease the risk of progression to renal failure, decrease inflammation, and maintain nutritional stores. Patients are treated primarily with statins to correct hyperlipidemia, low-sodium diets, and diuretics (Turner et al, 2012). Patients with an established severe protein deficiency who continue to lose protein may require an extended time of carefully supervised nutritional care. The diet should attempt to provide sufficient protein and energy to maintain a positive nitrogen balance and to support tissue synthesis while not overtaxing the kidneys. In most cases, sufficient intake from carbohydrate and fats is needed to spare protein for anabolism.

Some of the more common nutrition diagnoses in the CKD population include the following:
- Inadequate mineral intake
- Excessive mineral intake
- Imbalance of nutrients
- Excessive fluid intake
- Impaired nutrient utilization
- Altered nutrition-related laboratory values
- Food-medication interaction
- Food- and nutrition-related knowledge deficit

Depending on the nutrition diagnosis, MNT interventions are adjusted for various intakes of minerals, protein, and fluids. Some benefit has been seen in CKD with dietary interventions to lower inflammation. Cooking techniques, a more plant-based diet, and a focus on foods that lower inflammation are being studied (Abboud and Henrich, 2010).

Protein. The recommended dietary protein level for CKD patients has changed over time. Historically, these patients received diets high in protein (up to 1.5 g/kg/day) in an attempt to increase serum albumin and prevent protein malnutrition. However, studies have shown that a reduction of protein intake to as low as 0.8 mg/kg/day may decrease proteinuria without adversely affecting serum albumin. Serum albumin is a marker of inflammation, not protein malnutrition. Dietary protein has been championed as a factor that increases glomerular pressure and thus leads to accelerated loss of renal function. Numerous studies in experimental models of moderate renal insufficiency demonstrate a significant decline in this process with protein restriction. Clinical studies demonstrate a role for protein restriction in the management of patients with mild to moderate renal insufficiency to preserve renal function. To allow for optimal protein use, 50% to 60% of the protein should be from sources of high biologic value (HBV), meaning that the body is easily able to digest and use the amino acids.

A large multicenter trial, Modification of Diet in Renal Disease (MDRD), attempted to determine the role of protein, phosphorus restriction, and blood pressure control in the progression of renal disease. Thus the National Institute of Diabetes and Digestive and Kidney Diseases (NIDDKD) developed recommendations for the management of patients with progressive renal disease or pre-ESRD. Those recommendations for dietary protein intake in progressive renal failure are 0.8 g/kg/day with 60% HBV for patients whose GFR is greater than 55 ml/min, and 0.6 g/kg/day with 60% HBV for patients whose GFR is 25 to 55 ml/min.

The NKF's **Kidney Dialysis Outcome Quality Initiative (KDOQI)** panel suggests that patients whose GFR is less than 25 ml/min and who have not yet begun dialysis should be maintained on 0.6 g/kg/day of protein and 35 kcal/kg/day. If patients cannot maintain an adequate caloric intake on this protein recommendation, their protein intake should be increased to 0.75 g/kg/day. In both cases approximately 50% of the protein should be of HBV.

The potential benefits of protein restriction in the patient with moderate renal insufficiency must be weighed against the potential hazards of such treatment (i.e., protein malnutrition). If protein is restricted, careful monitoring and anthropometric studies should be carried out periodically as directed by the KDOQI guidelines.

Systemic hypertension, which aggravates the progressive loss of renal function, must be well controlled to produce benefits from protein restriction. Also important in the control of the progression of renal failure in people with diabetes is good blood glucose control. In a national multicenter trial, the Diabetes Control and Complications Trial (DCCT) showed that blood glucose control was more important than protein restriction in delaying the onset of renal failure in individuals who have diabetes (see Chapter 30).

Research continues about the use of more plant-based proteins in CKD, including tofu and legumes. Some benefits can be assessed looking at inflammation and improvement in mortality rates, but it is not yet conclusive if this is related to the plant-based proteins, or the nutrition and lifestyle associated with a more plant-based diet (Chen et al, 2016).

Energy. Energy intake should be approximately 35 kcal/kg/day for adults to spare protein for tissue repair and maintenance. In patients who are significantly overweight, some adjustment should be made to normalize requirements (see Box 2-1).

Sodium. Edema, the most clinically apparent manifestation, indicates total body sodium overload. In addition, because of low oncotic pressure from hypoalbuminemia, the volume of circulating blood may be reduced because of migration of fluid to interstitial space. Attempts to severely limit sodium intake or to use diuretics may cause marked hypotension, exacerbation of coagulopathy, and deterioration of renal function. Therefore control of edema in this group of diseases should be with dietary intake of 1500 g of sodium daily (Whelton et al, 2012).

Potassium. Potassium management is possible through use of medications such as diuretics, individualized diet prescription,

and rate of progression of CKD. Many patients in early-stage CKD take potassium-wasting diuretics (e.g., furosemide) that require supplementation of potassium. When urine output drops below 1 L/day, these same patients may require a change to potassium restriction as the kidney is no longer able to excrete all the potassium ingested. This typically occurs rather late in stage 4 CKD.

Phosphorus. The importance of controlling phosphate in patients with early stage disease often is overlooked. Serum phosphorous levels elevate at the same rate as eGFR decreases. Early initiation of phosphate reduction therapies is advantageous for delaying hyperparathyroidism and bone disease. Unfortunately, patients are often asymptomatic during the early phase of hyperparathyroidism and hyperphosphatemia; they may not attend to their modified diets or understand the need to take **phosphate binders** with meals.

Those with an eGFR of less than 60 should be evaluated for renal bone disease and benefit from phosphorus restriction. Ongoing monitoring of patient's phosphorus and use of phosphate binders is recommended. The diet typically is modified to allow no more than 1000 mg of phosphates daily, a limit that allows approximately 1 to 2 dairy foods per day. Because of the decrease in protein intake, the control of phosphorus is somewhat easier to manage. Patients who are in later stages of CKD and intolerant of red meats because of uremic taste alterations often are able to substitute milk foods for meat and still maintain a limited phosphate intake.

Lipids. The important consequence of dyslipidemia is cardiovascular disease. Pediatric patients with frequently relapsing or resistant nephrotic syndrome are at particular risk for premature atherosclerosis. Certain lipid-lowering agents in combination with a cholesterol-lowering diet can reduce total cholesterol, low-density lipoprotein cholesterol, and triglycerides in these patients (see Chapter 33). Lowering protein intake in adult patients also may involve lowering fat and cholesterol intake from animal sources.

Vitamins. CKD patients routinely are recommended a water-soluble renal customized vitamin supplement, because restrictions on fruits, vegetables and dairy foods may cause the diet to be inadequate.

END-STAGE RENAL DISEASE

End-stage renal disease (ESRD) reflects the kidney's inability to excrete waste products, maintain fluid and electrolyte balance, and produce certain hormones. As renal failure slowly progresses, the level of circulating waste products eventually leads to symptoms of uremia (see *Pathophysiology and Care Management Algorithm:* Chronic Kidney Disease and End-Stage Renal Disease). **Uremia** is a clinical syndrome of malaise, weakness, nausea and vomiting, muscle cramps, itching, metallic taste in the mouth, and neurologic impairment that is brought about by an unacceptable level of nitrogenous wastes in the body.

Pathophysiology

ESRD can result from a wide variety of different kidney diseases. Currently 90% of patients reaching ESRD have chronic (1) diabetes mellitus, (2) hypertension, or (3) glomerulonephritis. The manifestations are somewhat nonspecific and vary by patient. No reliable laboratory parameter corresponds directly with the beginning of symptoms. However, as a rule of thumb, BUN of more than 100 mg/dl and creatinine of 10 to 12 mg/dl are usually close to this threshold.

PATHOPHYSIOLOGY AND CARE MANAGEMENT ALGORITHM

Chronic Kidney Disease and End-Stage Renal Disease

ETIOLOGY

Hypertension

Glomerulonephritis

Diabetes mellitus

Other Disorders
(i.e., polycystic kidney disease, congenital anomalies, etc.)

CKD Chronic Kidney Disease

CKD Medical Management

- Blood pressure control
- Blood sugar control
- Immunosuppressant therapy
- Erythropoietin
- Active vitamin D

CKD Nutrition Management

- Sodium restriction
- Possible protein restriction
- Monitor electrolytes and acid base balance
- Phosphate binders
- Decrease cardiac risk factors

PATHOPHYSIOLOGY

End-Stage Renal Disease
(renal failure)

Inability to

- Excrete waste products
- Maintain fluid and electroyte balance
- Produce hormones

Uremia

Unacceptable level of nitrogenous wastes

Symptoms

- Malaise
- Weakness
- Nausea and vomiting
- Muscle cramps and itching
- Metallic taste in mouth
- Neurologic impairment

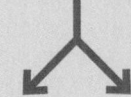

MANAGEMENT

ESRD Medical Management

- Dialysis
- Kidney transplantation
- Immunosuppressant therapy
- Psychologic support
- Conservative treatment and preparation for death
- Erythropoietin
- Active vitamin D

ESRD Nutrition Management

Goals
- Prevent nutrient deficiencies
- Control edema and serum electrolytes
  - Sodium and potassium restriction
- Prevent renal osteodystrophy
  - Use of phosphate binders, low phosphorus diet, and calcium supplementation
- Provide a palatable and attractive diet

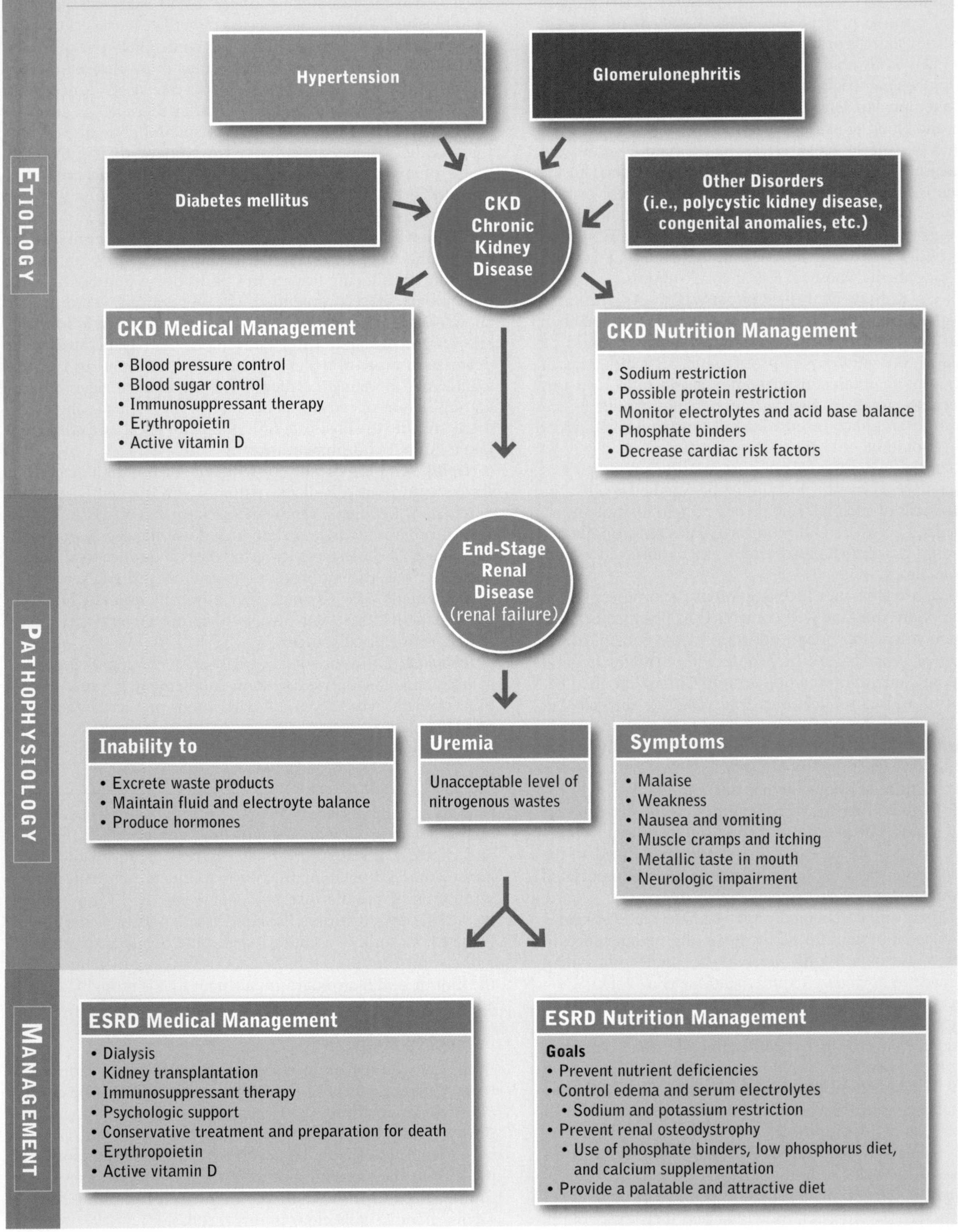

Medical Treatment

Once the patient progresses from stage 4 to stage 5 CKD, options for treatment for ESRD include dialysis, transplantation, or medical management progressing to death. Patients do best if they have some control and choice over their options (Wingard et al, 2007).

Dialysis

Patients may choose to dialyze in an outpatient dialysis facility or they may prefer hemodialysis (HD) at home using either conventional daily or nocturnal dialysis. They may choose peritoneal dialysis (PD) and have a choice of continuous ambulatory peritoneal dialysis (CAPD) or automated peritoneal dialysis (APD, formerly called continuous cyclic peritoneal dialysis, or CCPD), or combinations of the two. Patients, families, and their physicians together evaluate the therapy that best meets the patient's needs. Factors that come into account in this decision are availability of family or friends to assist with therapy, type of water supply to the home, capability of the patient or involved family (including eyesight and ability to perform sterile technique), previous abdominal surgeries, membrane characteristics of the individual's peritoneal membrane, body size, cardiac status, ability to create a vascular access, desire to travel, and a host of other considerations (see Table 35-9).

HD requires permanent access to the bloodstream through a fistula created by surgery to connect an artery and a vein (see Figure 35-2). If the patient's blood vessels are fragile, an artificial vessel called a graft may be implanted surgically. Large needles are inserted into the fistula or graft before each dialysis and removed when dialysis is complete. Temporary access through subclavian catheters is common until the patient's permanent access can be created or can mature; however, problems with infection make these catheters undesirable (Gomes et al, 2013).

The HD fluid and electrolyte content is similar to that of normal plasma. Waste products and electrolytes move by diffusion, ultrafiltration, and osmosis from the blood into the dialysate and are removed (see Figure 35-3) (Himmelfarb and Ikizler,

2010). Outpatient HD usually requires treatment of 3 to 5 hours three times per week in a dialysis unit (see Figure 35-4). Newer therapies can shorten the duration of treatment by increasing its frequency. Patients on these more frequent dialysis therapies have lower mortality rates, approaching that of transplantation. Patients on daily dialysis at home typically have treatments lasting from 2 to 3.5 hours 5 to 6 days a week, whereas some home dialysis patients receive nocturnal dialysis 3 to 6 times a week for 8 hours, while they sleep.

Peritoneal dialysis (PD) makes use of the body's own semipermeable membrane, the peritoneum. A catheter is implanted surgically through the abdomen and into the peritoneal cavity. Dialysate containing a high-dextrose concentration is instilled into the peritoneum, where diffusion carries waste products from the blood through the peritoneal membrane and into the dialysate; water moves by osmosis. This fluid then is withdrawn and discarded, and new solution is added multiple times each day.

Several types of PD exist. In CAPD, the dialysate is left in the peritoneum and exchanged manually, by gravity. Exchanges of dialysis fluid are done four to five times daily, making it a 24-hour treatment (see Figure 35-5). In APD, patient treatments are done at night by a machine that mechanically performs the exchanges. During the day these patients sometimes keep a single dialysate exchange in the peritoneal cavity for extended periods (called a long dwell), perhaps the entire day. Several combinations of CAPD and APD are possible and are referred to here as *PD*.

Advantages of PD are avoidance of large fluctuations in blood chemistry, longer residual renal function, and the ability of the patient to achieve a more normal lifestyle. Complications include peritonitis, hypotension that requires fluid and sodium replacement, and weight gain. Tissue weight gain is experienced by most patients as a result of absorbing 400 to 800 calories per day from the glucose in the dialysate. The amount depends on the concentration of the dialysate solution and how many exchanges are done daily. This may be desirable in patients who

TABLE 35-8 Nutrient Requirements of Adults with Renal Disease Based on Type of Therapy

Therapy	Energy	Protein	Fluid	Sodium	Potassium	Phosphorus
Impaired renal function	30-35 kcal/kg IBW	0.6-1.0 g/kg IBW	Ad libitum	Variable, 1.5-2 g/day	Variable, usually ad libitum or increased to cover losses from diuretics	0.8-1.2 g/day or 8-12 mg/kg IBW
Hemodialysis	35 kcal/kg IBW	1.2 g/kg IBW	750-1000 ml/day plus urine output	1.5-2 g/day	2-3 g/day or 40 mg/kg IBW	0.8-1.2 g/day or <17 mg/kg IBW
Peritoneal dialysis (CAPD)(CCPD)	30-35 kcal/kg IBW	1.2-1.5 g/kg BW	Ad libitum (minimum of 1000 ml/day from urine plus output)	1.5-4 g/day	3-4 g/day	0.8-1.2 g/day
Transplant, 4-6 weeks after transplant	30-35 kcal/kg IBW	1.3-2 g/kg IBW	Ad libitum	1.5-2 g/day	Variable; may require restriction with cyclosporine-induced hyperkalemia	Calcium 1.2 g/day No need to limit phosphorus
6 weeks or longer after transplant	Kcal/kg To achieve/maintain IBW Limit simple CHO Fat <35% cal Cholesterol < 400 mg/day PUFA/SFA ratio > 1	1 g/kg BW	Ad libitum	1.5-2 g/day	Variable	Calcium 1.2 g/day No need to limit phosphorus

Modified from National Kidney Foundation: KDOQI clinical practice guidelines for nutrition in chronic renal failure, *Am J Kidney Dis* 35(suppl 2):S1, 2000; Wiggins K: Guidelines for nutrition care of renal patients, ed 3, Chicago, 2002, American Dietetic Association.
CAPD, Continuous ambulatory peritoneal dialysis; *CCPD*, continuous cyclical peritoneal dialysis; *IBW*, ideal body weight; *PUFA*, polyunsaturated fat; *SFA*, saturated fat.

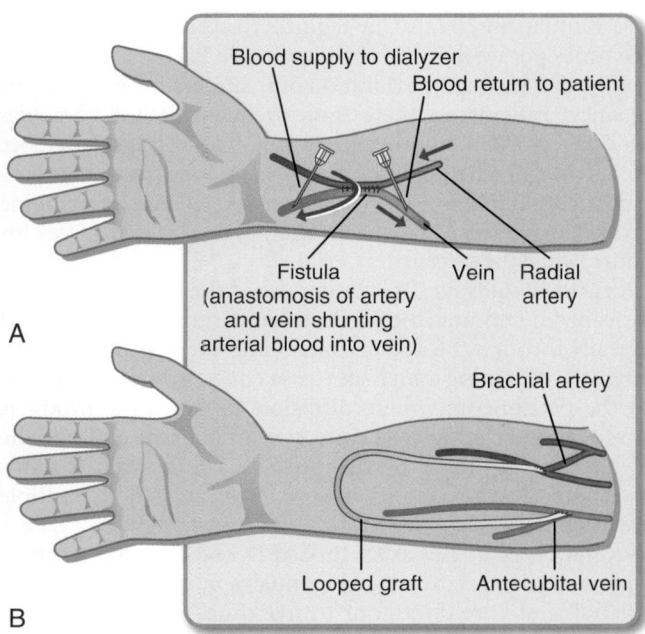

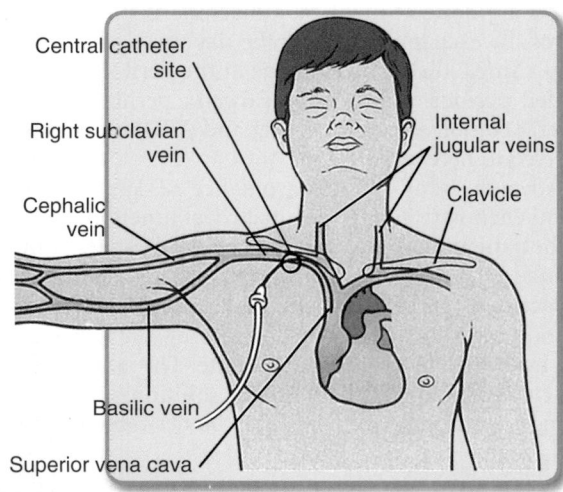

FIGURE 35-2 Types of access for hemodialysis. **A,** Arteriovenous fistula. **B,** Artificial loop graft. **C,** Subclavian catheter (usually temporary). (From Lewis SL, et al: *Medical-surgical nursing: assessment and management of clinical problems,* ed 9, St Louis, 2013, Elsevier Mosby.)

are underweight, but eventually dietary intake or activity must be modified to account for the energy absorbed from dialysate. Icodextrin (Extraneal, Baxter) is a long-chain, nonabsorbable sugar available for long dwell times. It offers superior fluid removal (ultrafiltration) without excess dextrose absorption. This can be useful for patients with diabetes and those with excessive tissue weight gain but can cause other complications.

Evaluation of Dialysis Efficacy

Kinetic modeling is a method for evaluating the efficacy of dialysis that measures the removal of urea from the patient's blood over a given period. This formula, often called **Kt/V** (where *K* is the urea clearance of the dialyzer, *t* is the length of time of dialysis, and *V* is the patient's total body water volume), should ideally produce a result higher than 1.4 per HD, or 3.2 per week. These calculations are somewhat complex and are

typically calculated using a computer program. A more accurate method for determining adequacy of HD is the eKt/V, in which *e* stands for equilibrated and takes into account the amount of time it takes for urea to equilibrate across cell membranes after dialysis has stopped. An acceptable eKt/V is 1.2 or greater.

Another method to determine effective dialysis treatment is the **urea reduction ratio (URR)**, which looks at the reduction in urea before and after dialysis. The patient is considered well dialyzed when a 65% or greater reduction in the serum urea occurs during dialysis. Unlike Kt/V, this calculation can be done quickly at the patient's bedside by the practitioner. The method for calculating the efficacy of PD is somewhat different, but a weekly Kt/V of 2 is the goal. The Kt/V can be altered by several patient- and dialysis-associated variables. The calculations for Kt/V can also be used to determine the patient's **protein-nitrogen appearance (PNA) rate**, which compares to a simplified nitrogen balance study in the dialysis patient. The PNA values should be between 0.8 and 1.4. Patients on short daily HD and nocturnal HD require different calculations to estimate their Kt/V.

Medical Nutrition Therapy

Goals of medical nutrition therapy in the management of ESRD are intended to do the following:
1. Prevent deficiency and maintain good nutrition status (and, in the case of children, growth) through adequate protein, energy, vitamin, and mineral intake (see Table 35-8)
2. Control edema and electrolyte imbalance by controlling sodium, potassium, and fluid intake
3. Prevent or slow the development of renal osteodystrophy by balancing calcium, phosphorus, vitamin D, and PTH
4. Enable the patient to eat a palatable, attractive diet that fits his or her lifestyle as much as possible
5. Coordinate patient care with families, dietitian nutritionists, nurses, and physicians in acute care, outpatient, or skilled nursing facilities
6. Provide initial nutrition education, periodic counseling and long-term monitoring of patients, with the goal of patients receiving enough education to direct their own care and diet.

Table 35-10 presents a guide for teaching patients about their blood values and control of their disease. Because dialysis is done at home or in an outpatient unit, most all patients with ESRD assume responsibility for their own diets. Most long-term patients know their diets very well (see Figure 35-6), having been instructed many times by renal dietitian nutritionists at their dialysis units.

Protein

Dialysis is a drain on body protein, so protein intake must be increased. In addition, exposure of patients' blood to an artificial membrane three or more times a week induces a state of chronic inflammation and distorts protein metabolism. Protein losses of 20 to 30 g can occur during a 24-hour PD, with an average of 1 g/hr. Those receiving PD need a daily protein intake of 1.2 to 1.5 g/kg of body weight. At least 50% should be HBV protein. Patients who receive HD three times per week require a daily protein intake of 1.2 g/kg of body weight. Serum BUN and serum Cr levels, uremic symptoms, and weight should be monitored, and the diet should be adjusted accordingly.

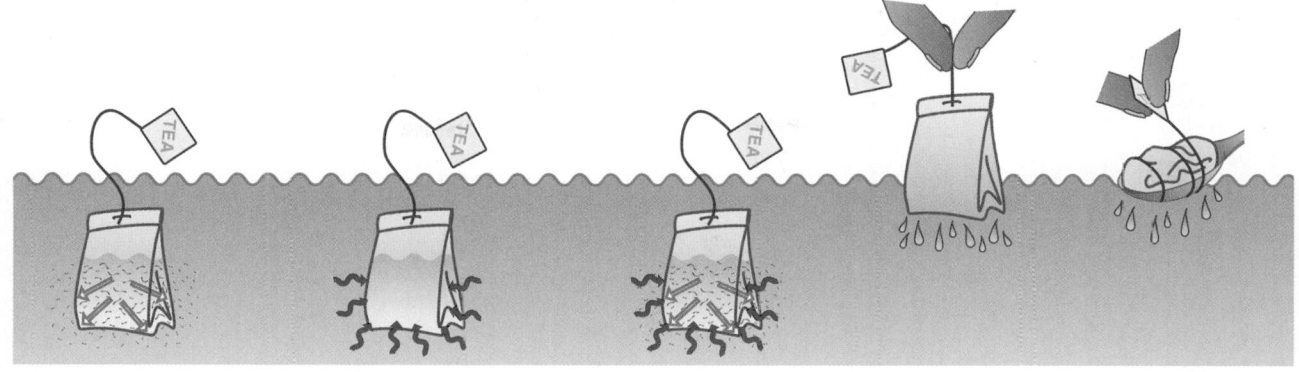

Diffusion is the passage of particles through a semipermeable membrane. Tea, for example, diffuses from a tea bag into the surrounding water.

Osmosis is the movement of fluid across a semipermeable membrane from a lower concentration of solutes to a higher concentration of solutes. (The water moves into the teabag.)

Diffusion and **Osmosis** can occur at the same time. (Particles move out and fluid moves in at the same time.)

Filtration is the passage of fluids through a membrane.

Ultrafiltration provides additional pressure to squeeze extra fluid through the membrane.

FIGURE 35-3 Dialysis: how it works. (Modified from Core curriculum for the dialysis technician: a comprehensive review of hemodialysis, 2001, AMGEN, Inc.)

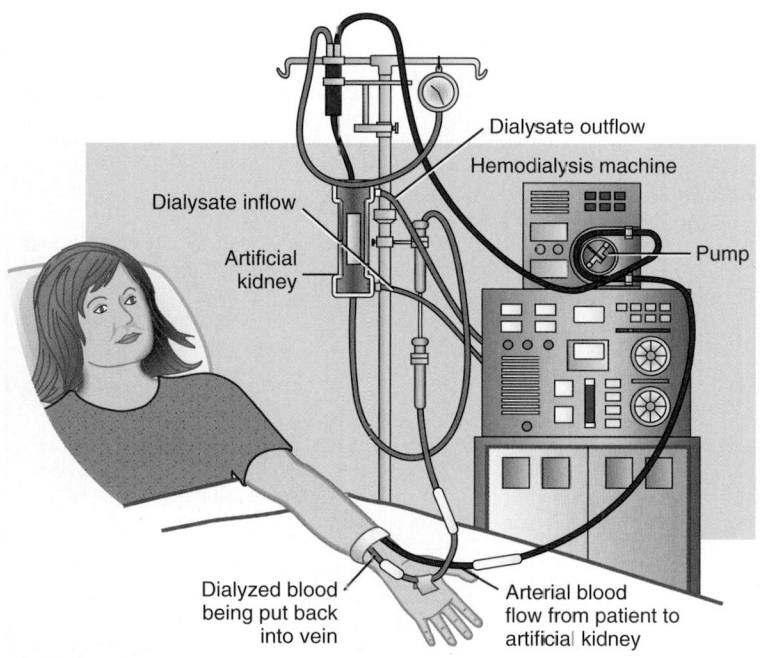

FIGURE 35-4 Hemodialysis. Treatment is usually for 3 to 5 hours, three times per week.

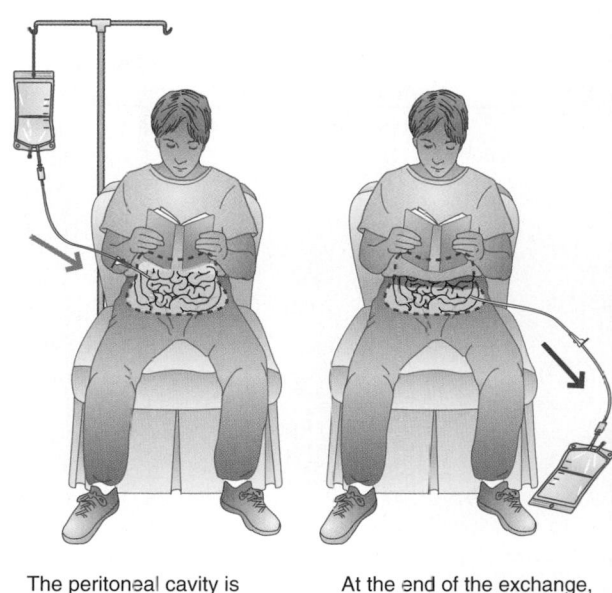

The peritoneal cavity is filled with dialysate, using gravity.

At the end of the exchange, the dialysate is drained into the bag, again using gravity.

FIGURE 35-5 Continuous ambulatory peritoneal dialysis; 20-minute exchanges are given four to five times daily every day.

In renal failure, prealbumin, which is metabolized by the kidney, is not a good nutritional marker, because values are routinely elevated. Albumin is not recommended by the Academy of Nutrition and Dietetics to be used as an indicator of protein nutriture but continues to be routinely used in evaluating ESRD patients (Friedman and Fadem, 2010; Gama-Axelsson et al, 2012). However, because of the complexity of either acute or chronic inflammation, albumin remains predictive more of poor survival in ESRD and less of nutritional status. Hypoalbuminemia is multifactorial and may be related to poor nutrition, inflammation, or comorbid disease. When interpreting albumin values, it is important to know the laboratory's methodology for measuring serum albumin, because different laboratory techniques give different results in renal failure (see Table 35-10). Federal mandates require some nutrition intervention at levels below 4 g/dl to attempt to improve albumin to this level despite the evidence that low albumin is not a function of nutritional intake.

Most patients find it challenging to consume adequate protein because uremia itself causes taste aberrations, notably to red meats. Some patients cannot even tolerate the smell of meat cooking. Often this protein aversion makes it difficult to achieve

TABLE 35-9 Options for Treatment in ESRD

	Hemodialysis	Peritoneal Dialysis	Short Daily Hemodialysis or Nocturnal Dialysis	Transplant
Primary treatment responsibility	Health care personnel	Patient and/or family member	Patient and/or family member	Patient
Diet	Low K, low PO$_4$, low Na, moderate protein, fluid restriction	High K, low PO$_4$, low Na, high protein, moderate fluid restriction	High K, low PO$_4$, low Na, high protein, moderate fluid restriction	High and moderate protein, no K or PO$_4$ restrictions, no fluid restriction.
Location	Clinical dialysis unit	Home, office, vacation	Home, vacation	No limitations
Risks	Bleeding, sepsis, infection	Peritonitis, hernia, constipation, exit site infections, poorly controlled diabetes, weight gain, early satiety	Unattended dialysis, rare user error bleeding	Immuno-compromised, diabetes, cancer
Contraindications	Poor cardiac status, poor blood vessels for access creation	Multiple abdominal surgeries, lack of a clean home, altered mental status	Dementia, illiteracy, inability to communicate, lack of a clean home	High BMI, noncompliance with medications, less than 5 year hx of cancer

TABLE 35-10 Guide to Blood Values in End-Stage Renal Disease Patients

This guide is to help in understanding laboratory reports. In the following table, the normal values are for people with good kidney function. Acceptable values for dialysis patients are also given. Many things affect blood values. Diet is only one of these. Underlying disease, adequacy of treatment, medications, and complications all may affect laboratory values.

Substance	Normal Values	Normal for People on Dialysis	Function	Diet Changes
Sodium	135-145 mEq/L	135-145 mEq/L	Found in salt and many preserved foods. A diet high in sodium causes thirst. When patients drink too much fluid, it may actually dilute their sodium, and serum levels will appear low. If patients eat too much sodium and do not drink water, sodium may be high. Too much sodium and water raise blood pressure and can cause fluid overload, pulmonary edema, and congestive heart failure.	High: Check fluid status. If high fluid gains, tell patient to eat fewer salty foods. If low fluid gains, make sure patient is gaining about 1.5 kg between dialyses (or <4% body weight) and is not dehydrated (this is rare). Low: If high fluid gains, tell patient to eat less salt and fluid. Check fluid status—patient is probably drinking too much fluid. Limit weight gains to less than 4% of body weight between runs, and ask patient to eat fewer salty foods and limit fluid to 3 C plus urine output.
Potassium	3.5-5.5 mEq/L	3.5-5.5 mEq/L	Found in most high-protein foods, milk, fruits, and vegetables. Affects muscle action, especially the heart. High levels can cause the heart to stop. Low levels can cause symptoms such as muscle weakness and atrial fibrillation.	High: Ascertain that no other causes, such as gastrointestinal bleeding, trauma, or medications are creating high potassium values. Tell patient to avoid foods with more than 250 mg/serving and limit daily intake to 2000 mg. Consider lowering potassium in dialysate bath. Recheck blood level next treatment. Low: Add one high-potassium food/day, and recheck blood level. Consider raising potassium in dialysate bath if diet changes not working.
Urea nitrogen (BUN)	7-23 mg/dl	50-100 mg/dl	Waste product of protein breakdown. Unlike creatinine, this is affected by the amount of protein in the diet. Dialysis removes urea nitrogen.	High: Patient is probably underdialyzed. Check eKt/V. Check nPNA. Low: Underdialysis is also a cause. BUN may decrease if patient is not eating because of uremic symptoms. Also decreases with loss of muscle.
Creatinine	0.6-1.5 mg/dl	Less than 15 mg/dl	A normal waste product of muscle breakdown. This value is controlled by dialysis. Patients have a higher amount because they are not dialyzing 24 hours a day, 7 days a week, as they would with normal kidney function.	Dialysis normally controls creatinine. Low creatinine may indicate good dialysis or low body muscle. Check the clearance of urea during dialysis (Kt/V) to assess dialysis adequacy. If patient losing weight, will break down more muscle, so creatinine may be higher. Patient may need to eat more protein and calories to stop weight loss.
URR	N/A	Above 65% (or 0.65)	A measure of reduction of urea that occurs during a dialysis treatment. Postdialysis BUN is subtracted and divided by predialysis BUN to give a percentage.	No diet changes, but catabolism or anabolism will affect values, as with Kt/V and equilibrated clearance of urea during dialysis (eKt/V).

TABLE 35-10 Guide to Blood Values in End-Stage Renal Disease Patients—cont'd

Substance	Normal Values	Normal for People on Dialysis	Function	Diet Changes
eKt/V	N/A	Above 1.2	A mathematic formula that attempts to quantify how well a patient is dialyzed. Represents the clearance of urea by the dialyzer, multiplied by the minutes of treatment, and divided by the volume of water the patient's body holds.	No diet changes. Low: Values below 1.2 are associated with increased morbidity and mortality. High: Higher values are associated with better outcomes.
Kt/V		Above 1.4 for hemodialysis Above 2 for peritoneal dialysis	Not adjusted for urea equilibration. See above.	No diet changes. See above.
nPNA	N/A	0.8-1.4	A calculation used to look at the rate of protein turnover in the body. Assumes patient is not catabolic because of infection, fever, surgery, or trauma. A good indicator of stable patient's protein intake, when combined with dietary history and albumin. The term *normalized* means that values have been adjusted to the patient's "normal" or ideal weight.	High: Patient may need to decrease protein intake. Have patient consult with nutritionist. Patient may be catabolic. Patient may be eating large amounts of protein. Low: Patient may need to increase protein intake. If patient is putting out urine, a small urine volume can make a big difference in results. Have patient keep a 48-hour urine collection.
Albumin	3.5-5 g/dl (bromcresol green) 3-4.5 g/dl (bromcresol purple)	3.5-5 g/dl Above 4 g/dl	Good measure of health in dialysis patients. Protein is lost with all dialysis. If albumin is below 2.9, fluid will "leak" from blood vessels into the tissue, thus causing edema. When fluid is in the tissue, it is more difficult to remove with dialysis. Low albumin is closely associated with increased risk of death in dialysis patients.	Low: Increase intake of protein-rich foods: meat, fish, chicken, eggs. A protein supplement may be needed. Intravenous albumin corrects short-term problems with oncotic pressure but does not change serum albumin levels.
Calcium	8.5-10.2 mg/dl	8.5-10.2 mg/dl	Found in dairy products. Dialysis patients' intakes are usually low. Active vitamin D is needed for absorption. The calcium value multiplied by the phosphorus value should not exceed 59, or patient will get calcium deposits in soft tissue. Because it is bound to albumin, calcium can be falsely lower if albumin is low. Ionized calcium is a more accurate test in this case.	High: Check with doctor if patient is taking calcium supplement or a form of active vitamin D. These should be temporarily stopped. Low: If albumin is low, suggest an ionized calcium be drawn. Patient may need a calcium supplement between meals and active vitamin D. Check with physician.
Phosphorus	2.5-4.8 mg/dl	3-6 mg/dl	Found in milk products, dried beans, nuts, and meats. Used to build bones and helps the body produce energy. Acceptable levels depend on variety of factors, including calcium, PTH levels, and the level of phosphorus in diet. If calcium and PTH levels are normal, a slightly higher-than-normal level of phosphorus is acceptable.	High: Limit milk and milk products to 1 serving/day. Remind patient to take phosphate binders as ordered with meals and snacks. Noncompliance with binders is the most common cause of high phosphorus. Low: Add 1 serving milk product or other high-phosphorus food per day or decrease phosphate binders.
PTH intact (I-PTH)	10-65 pg/ml	200-300 pg/ml	A high level of PTH indicates that calcium is being pulled out of bone to maintain serum calcium levels. This syndrome is called secondary hyperparathyroidism. Leads to osteodystrophy. Pulsed doses of oral or IV vitamin D usually lower PTH.	High: Check whether patient taking oral or IV active vitamin D. Contact patient's physician regarding therapy. If patient has no symptoms (high phosphorus, bone pain, fractures), treat less aggressively. Low: No treatment available.
Aluminum	0-10 mcg/L	Less than 40 mcg/L	Patients taking aluminum hydroxide phosphate binders may develop aluminum toxicity, which can cause bone disease and dementia. Value should be checked every 6 months.	High: Discontinue aluminum hydroxide treatment.

Continued

TABLE 35-10 Guide to Blood Values in End-Stage Renal Disease Patients—cont'd

Substance	Normal Values	Normal for People on Dialysis	Function	Diet Changes
Magnesium	1.5-2.4 mg/dl	1.5-2.4 mg/dl	Magnesium normally is excreted in the urine and can become toxic to dialysis patient. High levels may be caused by antacids or laxatives that contain magnesium such as Milk of Magnesia or Maalox.	No dietary changes, except to use nontoxic methods such as fiber to aid in relief of constipation. If magnesium is used as a phosphate binder, levels will have to be checked more often.
Ferritin	Male: 20-350 mcg/L Female: 6-350 mcg/L	300-800 mcg/L with EPO; 50 mcg/L without EPO	This is the way iron is stored in the liver. If iron stores are low, red blood cell production is decreased.	Low: Iron in food is not well absorbed. Most patients need an IV iron supplement. Patients should not take oral iron at same time as phosphate binders.
CO_2	22-25 mEq/L	22-25 mEq/L	Dialysis patients are often acidotic because they do not excrete metabolic acids in their urine. Acidosis may increase the rate of muscle and bone catabolism.	Low: Review eKt/V, BUN, nPNA. Oral sodium bicarbonate may be given to raise CO_2, but it presents a significant sodium load to patient.
Glucose	65-114 mg/dl	Same for nondiabetic patients Less than 300 mg/dl (patients with diabetes)	Because the kidney metabolizes insulin, low blood sugar levels caused by a longer half-life of insulin are possible. For patients with diabetes: a high blood sugar may increase thirst.	Most people need 6-11 servings of breads and starches or cereals per day and 2-4 servings of fruit per day to provide energy. Patients with diabetes should avoid concentrated sweets, unless blood sugar level is low.

BUN, Blood urea nitrogen; *CO₂,* carbon dioxide; *DHT,* dihydrotachysterol; *EPO,* erythropoietin; *IV,* intravenous; *N/A,* not applicable; *nPNA,* normalized protein nitrogen appearance; *PTH,* parathyroid hormone: *URR,* urea reduction ratio.
Developed by Katy G. Wilkens, MS, RD, Northwest Kidney Centers, Seattle, Washington.

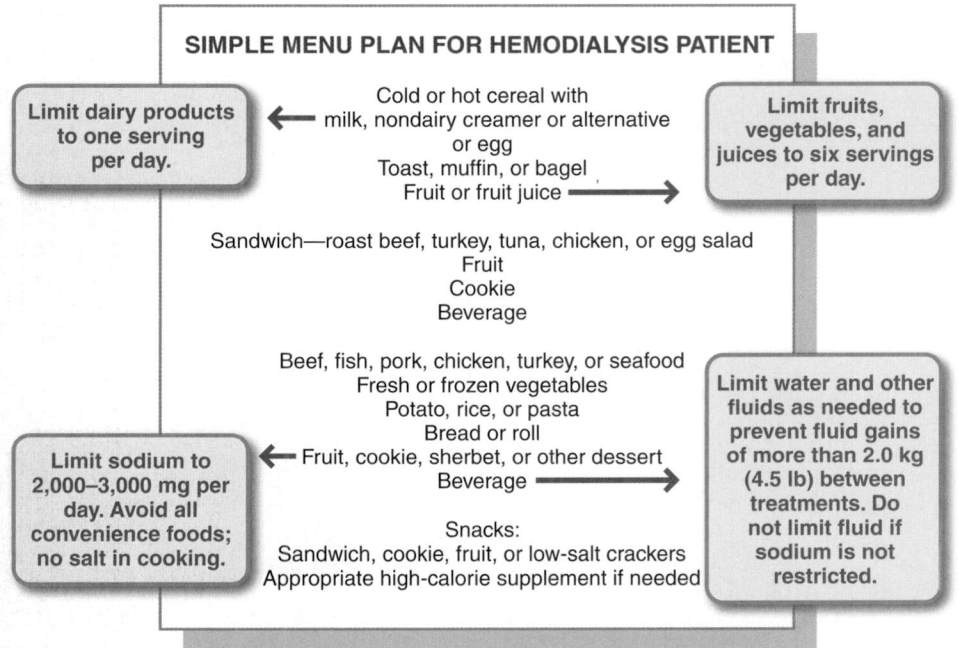

SIMPLE MENU PLAN FOR HEMODIALYSIS PATIENT

Cold or hot cereal with milk, nondairy creamer or alternative or egg
Toast, muffin, or bagel
Fruit or fruit juice

Limit dairy products to one serving per day.

Limit fruits, vegetables, and juices to six servings per day.

Sandwich—roast beef, turkey, tuna, chicken, or egg salad
Fruit
Cookie
Beverage

Beef, fish, pork, chicken, turkey, or seafood
Fresh or frozen vegetables
Potato, rice, or pasta
Bread or roll
Fruit, cookie, sherbet, or other dessert
Beverage

Limit sodium to 2,000–3,000 mg per day. Avoid all convenience foods; no salt in cooking.

Limit water and other fluids as needed to prevent fluid gains of more than 2.0 kg (4.5 lb) between treatments. Do not limit fluid if sodium is not restricted.

Snacks:
Sandwich, cookie, fruit, or low-salt crackers
Appropriate high-calorie supplement if needed

FIGURE 35-6 A simple menu plan for a patient on hemodialysis. The diet should allow for less than 4% fluid weight gain between dialyses.

recommended high biologic value protein intake. Patients may tolerate eggs, tofu, and "white" meats better. They also can use spices to hide the taste of meats, or serve animal proteins cold, to minimize the urea taste. Nutritional supplements may be helpful in some patients, and occasionally the phosphate restriction may have to be lifted to allow the consumption of dairy products to meet protein needs. As with all the nutritional parameters, meeting patient needs must be individualized.

Energy

Energy intake should be adequate to spare protein for tissue protein synthesis and to prevent its metabolism for energy (Therrien, 2015). Depending on the patient's nutrition status and degree of stress, between 25 and 40 kcal/kg of body weight should be provided, with the lower amount for transplantation and PD patients and the higher level for the nutritionally depleted patient (see *Clinical Insight:* Calculating BMI and

Determining Appropriate Body Weight in Chapter 7). Tools have been developed to allow the renal dietitian to assess the quality of the patient's nutrition status (see Chapter 7 and Appendices 21 and 22).

Fluid and Sodium Balance

The kidney's ability to handle sodium and water in ESRD must be assessed frequently through measurement of blood pressure, edema, fluid weight gain, serum sodium level, and dietary intake. The vast majority of dialysis patients need to restrict sodium and fluid intakes. Excessive sodium intake is responsible for increased thirst, increased fluid gain, and resultant hypertension. Even those patients who do not experience these symptoms but produce minimal amounts of urine benefit from a reduced sodium intake to limit their thirst and prevent large intradialytic fluid gains.

In the patient who is maintained on HD, sodium and fluid intake are regulated to allow for a weight gain of 4 to 5 lb (2 to 3 kg) from increased fluid in the vasculature between dialyses. The goal is a fluid gain of less than 4% of body weight. A sodium intake of 65 to 87 mEq (1500 to 2000 mg) daily and a limit on fluid intake (usually about 750 ml/day plus the amount equal to the urine output) is usually sufficient to meet these guidelines. Only fluids that are liquid at room temperature are included in this calculation. The fluid contained in solid foods is not included in the 750 ml limit. Solid foods in the average diet contribute approximately 500 to 800 ml/day of fluid. This fluid in solid food is calculated to approximately replace the 500 ml/day net insensible water loss.

A 65 to 87 mEq (1500 to 2000 mg) sodium diet requires no salt in cooking; no salt at the table; no salted, smoked, enhanced, or cured meat or fish; no cheese except swiss or cream cheese and no salted snack foods, canned soups, packaged bread products, or high-sodium convenience foods. In today's marketplace, increased intake of convenience foods is the norm and it is estimated that 75% to 90% of sodium intake is consumed in convenience foods, with only 10% to 25% added to foods in cooking or at the table.

The most effective way to reduce the renal patient's thirst and fluid intake is to decrease sodium intake. It is salt intake that drives fluid consumption. Appendix 30 gives the details of a low-sodium meal plan. Attempts to restrict fluid in patients who are not on a restricted sodium diet are futile, because feelings of thirst become overwhelming to the patient with a high sodium intake.

When educating about fluid balance, the health care provider must teach the patient how to deal with thirst without drinking. Sucking on a few ice chips, cold sliced fruit, or sour candies or using artificial saliva are good suggestions. In approximately 15% to 20% of patients, hypertension is not alleviated even after meticulous attention to fluid and water balance. In these patients hypertension usually is perpetuated by a high level of renin secretion and requires medication for control.

Although the majority of patients with ESRD retain sodium, a small number may lose it. Examples of conditions with a salt-losing tendency are polycystic disease of the kidney, medullary kidney disease, chronic obstructive uropathy, chronic pyelonephritis, ostomy losses, and analgesic nephropathy. To prevent hypotension, hypovolemia, cramps, and further deterioration of renal function, extra sodium may be required. A diet for these types of patients may contain 130 mEq (3 g) or more of sodium per day. Not limiting sodium in the diet can satisfy the need for extra sodium. The number of patients who require this level of sodium intake is small, but these patients exemplify the need for individual consideration of the diet prescription and a thorough understanding of the patient's underlying disease and present diet.

Potassium

Potassium usually requires restriction, depending on the serum potassium level, urine output, medications, and the frequency of HD. The daily intake of potassium for most Americans is 75 to 100 mEq (3 to 4 g). This usually is reduced in ESRD to 60 to 80 mEq (2.3 to 3.1 g) per day and is reduced for the anuric patient on dialysis to 51 mEq (2 g) per day. Some patients (i.e., those on high-flux dialysis or with increased dialysis times or frequencies such as PD, short daily or nocturnal) require higher intakes. Again, a close monitoring of the patient's laboratory values, potassium content of the dialysate, and dietary intake is essential.

The potassium content of foods is listed in Appendix 44. When counseling HD patients on a low-potassium diet, clinicians should take care to point out that some low-sodium foods contain potassium chloride as a salt substitute rather than sodium chloride. Nutrition labels for products such as salt substitutes, LiteSalt, and low-sodium herb mixtures must be checked carefully to be sure they do not contain dangerous levels of potassium. Low-sodium soy sauces, low-sodium soups, and other low-sodium products may require particular review by a trained professional (see Chapter 11 for labeling definitions). Reviewing food preparation techniques should include anyone who may be cooking for the patient, such as family members, a church group, or neighbors.

When a thorough diet history does not reveal the reason for elevated serum potassium, other nondietetic sources of potassium should be researched. Examples include poor dialysis adequacy or missed dialysis treatments, too high a concentration of potassium in the dialysate bath, very elevated blood sugar, acidosis, constipation, significant GI bleeding, some medications, blood transfusions, major trauma, chemotherapy, or radiation therapy. Occasionally, blood samples are handled improperly, resulting in hemolysis and falsely elevated potassium levels.

Phosphorus

More than 99% of excess phosphate is excreted in the urine. However, as GFR decreases, phosphorus is retained in the plasma. Because of the large molecular weight of the phosphate molecule, it is not easily removed by dialysis, and patients experience net "gain" of about one half of the phosphate they consume daily. Phosphate intake is lowered by restricting dietary sources to 1200 mg/day or less. The difficulty in implementing the phosphorus restriction comes from the necessity for a high-protein diet. High-protein foods, such as meats, contain high levels of phosphorus in the form of ATP. In addition, other sources of protein—dairy products, nuts, and legumes—are also high in phosphorus. Thus high-phosphorus foods cannot be eliminated without restricting protein, creating a challenge to balance intake with dietary intervention alone.

The American diet, which contains highly processed foods, has resulted in increases in the types and amounts of phosphorus available for absorption, making compliance with a phosphorus restriction more difficult. Naturally occurring phosphate in food is only approximately 60% absorbed. Commonly used phosphate additives such as trisodium phosphate, disodium phosphate, and dicalcium phosphate are nearly 100% absorbed, making the processed diet a contributor to elevated phosphorus levels (Leon et al, 2013). Dietary intervention should focus on a balance of limiting dairy, nuts, beans, and processed foods while still encouraging enough HBV proteins to meet dietary needs.

Because dietary restrictions alone are not adequate to control serum phosphorus, nearly all patients who undergo dialysis require phosphate-binding medications. Phosphate binders such as calcium carbonate, calcium acetate, sevelamer carbonate, sucroferric oxyhydroxide, ferric citrate, and lanthanum carbonate are used routinely with each meal or snack to bind to phosphorus in the gut. These medications bind excess dietary phosphate and transport it through the GI tract for elimination, thus preventing its absorption into the blood. Side effects of taking these medications over long periods are common. Some may cause GI distress, diarrhea, or gas. Severe constipation, leading to intestinal impaction, is a potential risk of excessive use of some types of phosphate binders; occasionally this may lead to perforation of the intestine resulting in peritonitis or death. Common medications are listed in Table 35-11 (see *Clinical Insight:* Why Don't Clients Take Their Phosphate Binders?).

CLINICAL INSIGHT

Why Don't Clients Take Their Phosphate Binders?

Phosphate binders are prescribed to be taken with all meals and snacks, whether the client eats at home, at work, or in a restaurant. Reasons clients give for not taking their phosphate binders are that they:
- cause gastrointestinal discomfort and acid reflux
- cause severe constipation and can lead to bowel impaction
- may be difficult to chew or swallow
- may need to take an average of 2 to 5 pills each meal
- forget to take them
- do not like to be reminded of being "sick"
- cannot feel a difference when taking them
- may be expensive and not always covered by insurance

Calcium and Parathyroid Hormone

In ESRD, the body's ability to maintain phosphorus-calcium balance is complicated by calcium and PTH controls. As GFR decreases, the serum calcium level declines for several reasons. First, decreased ability of the kidney to convert to inactive vitamin D to its active form, $1,25\text{-}(OH)_2D_3$ leads to poor GI absorption of calcium. Second, the need for serum calcium increases as serum phosphate levels increase. Both of these causes lead to hypertrophy of the parathyroid gland, which is responsible for calcium homeostasis. The resultant oversecretion of PTH increases resorption of bone to provide a calcium source.

The resulting metabolic bone disease, **renal osteodystrophy**, is essentially one of four types: (1) **osteomalacia**, (2) **osteitis fibrosa cystica**, (3) **metastatic calcification**, or (4) **adynamic bone disease**. With a deficit of calcium available from dietary absorption, the low calcium level triggers the release of PTH from the parathyroid glands. This acts to increase release of calcium from the bones by stimulating osteoclast activity. This can lead to osteomalacia or bone demineralization, as a result of lack of osteoblast stimulation to replace lost calcium in the bones.

TABLE 35-11 Common Medications and Nutritional Supplements for Patients with End-Stage Renal Disease

Phosphate Binders
Taken with meals and snacks to prevent dietary phosphorus absorption

Calcium carbonate	TUMS, Os-Cal, Calci-Chew, Calci-Mix
Calcium acetate	PhosLo
Mg/Ca++ carbonate	MagneBind
Sevelamer carbonate	Renvela
Lanthanum carbonate	Fosrenol
Aluminum hydroxide	AlternaGEL
Iron-based binders	Velphoro, Auryxia

Vitamins
Increased need for water-soluble vitamins because of losses during dialysis
Fat-soluble vitamins A, E, and K are not supplemented

Dialysis Recommendations

Vitamin C	60 mg (not to exceed 200 mg daily)
Folic acid	1 mg
Thiamin	1.5 mg
Riboflavin	1.7 mg
Niacin	20 mg
Vitamin B_6	10 mg
Vitamin B_{12}	6 mcg
Pantothenic acid	10 mg
Biotin	0.3 mg

Brand names include Nephrocap, Nephron FA, Nephplex, Nephrovites, and Dia-tx

Iron
Iron needs are increased because of EPO therapy

IV iron	Iron dextran (Infed), Iron gluconate (Ferrlecit), Iron sucrose (Venofer)

EPO
Stimulates bone marrow to produce red blood cells

IV or IM	Epogen

Activated Vitamin D
Used for the management of hyperparathyroicism

Oral	Calcitriol (Rocaltrol), doxercalciferol (Hectorol)
IV	Calcitriol (Calcijex), paricalcitol (Zemplar)

Biphosphonates
Inhibit bone resorption by blocking osteoclast activity

Oral	Alendronate (Fosamax)
IV	Pamidronate (Aredia)

Calcium Supplements
TUMS, Os-Cal, Calci-Chew

Phosphorus Supplements

	Kphos neutral, NutraPhos, NutraPhos K

Calcimimetics

Mimic calcium and bind to parathyroid gland	Cinacalcet (Sensipar)

Cation Exchange Resin
For the treatment of hyperkalemia

Oral or rectal	SPS (Kayexalate)

Developed by Fiona Wolf, RD, and Thomas Montemayor, RPh, Northwest Kidney Centers, Seattle, Washington, 2015.
Ca++, Calcium; *CHO,* cholesterol; *EPO,* epoetin; *ESRD,* end-stage renal disease; *IV,* intravenous; *IM,* intramuscular; *MVI;* Multiple vitamin injection; *SPS,* sodium polystyrene sulfonate.

Ongoing low calcium causes the parathyroid glands to continue producing PTH in an attempt to elevate serum calcium levels. In time this leads to secondary hyperparathyroidism, in which even the baseline production of PTH by these enlarged glands is enough to cause severe bone demineralization (osteitis fibrosis cystica), which is characterized by dull, aching bone pain.

Even though the serum calcium level is elevated in response to PTH, serum phosphate concentration remains high as the GFR falls lower. If the product of serum calcium multiplied by the serum phosphate level is greater than 70, metastatic calcification is imminent. Metastatic calcification occurs when calcium phosphate, removed from bones, is deposited in nonbone cells. This extraskeletal calcification may develop in joints, soft tissue, and vessels.

Calciphylaxis occurs when calcium phosphate is deposited in wound tissues with resultant vascular calcification, thrombosis, nonhealing wounds, and gangrene. It is frequently fatal. Clinical management aims to keep the product of serum calcium multiplied by serum phosphorus below 55 by preventing elevations in serum phosphate and calcium. Phosphorus intake must be controlled to as great a degree as possible to avoid aggravation of the delicate situation posed by hyperparathyroidism, phosphate retention, vitamin D deficiency, and hypocalcemia in renal failure. Newer treatments pair calcium and phosphorus control with increased dialysis, antibiotic therapy, sodium thiosulfate, and hyperbaric chamber treatments (Baldwin et al, 2011; Cohen and Vyas, 2013).

Many patients on dialysis suffer from hypocalcemia, despite calcium supplementation. Because of this, the routine drug of choice is active vitamin D, $1,25\text{-}(OH)_2D_3$, available as calcitriol (Rocaltrol and Calcijex). Analogs such as doxercalciferol (Hectorol) and paricalcitol (Zemplar) are also effective in lowering PTH and raising calcium levels, but with less enhancement of gut absorption of calcium than the 1,25 forms.

Other mechanisms for controlling PTH include the medication cinacalcet (Sensipar), a calcimimetic or calcium-imitating drug, which binds to sites on the parathyroid gland and gives the gland a false impression that calcium levels are elevated. The drug is effective in suppressing PTH production and also may lower calcium levels dramatically, with significant benefit. Overall, close monitoring is essential.

In more extreme cases of hyperparathyroidism, use of surgical excision of portions of the parathyroid glands can be used in an attempt to restore balance. This creates the risk of low PTH, and can lead to adynamic (low turnover) bone disease, characterized by decreased levels of bone turnover and suppression of both osteoclasts and osteoblasts. This condition is unique to ESRD, in which oversuppression of the parathyroid gland and too much active vitamin D lead to decreased bone formation and fragile bones with very little matrix. Usually diagnosed by a low PTH level, this disease results in a high risk of nonhealing fractures. Oversuppression of the parathyroid gland by use of vitamin D or its analogs can mimic this as well.

Overall the dietary balance of phosphorus, the use of phosphate binders and vitamin D analogs, the removal of phosphate by dialysis, and intense monitoring of laboratory values contribute to bone management in ESRD.

Lipid

Atherosclerotic cardiovascular disease is the most common cause of death among patients maintained on long-term dialysis (Iff et al, 2014). This appears to be a function of underlying disease (e.g., diabetes mellitus, hypertension, nephrotic syndrome) and a lipid abnormality common among patients with ESRD. The patient with ESRD typically has an elevated triglyceride level with or without an increase in cholesterol. The lipid abnormality likely represents increased synthesis of very-low-density lipoprotein and decreased clearance as well as increased reliance on animal-based proteins.

Treatment of hyperlipidemia with diet or pharmacologic agents remains controversial. Epidemiologic evidence demonstrating increased incidence of atherosclerotic coronary disease is balanced by studies that demonstrate that patients with clearly defined clinical evidence of atherosclerosis at the initiation of dialysis are at no increased risk for a cardiovascular event. Although routine treatment appears unwarranted, a good case can be made for dietary and pharmacologic treatment of patients with ESRD with underlying lipid disorders and evidence of atherosclerosis. Lipid-lowering drugs, including most statins, may have a significant effect on better management (see Chapter 33).

On the other hand, low cholesterol levels can be a significant predictor of mortality in ESRD. They can indicate poor oral intake and may be a useful tool in diagnosing malnutrition. Use of lipid-lowering drugs should be monitored and cut back if necessary in these patients, particularly if they are underweight or suffering from malnutrition.

Iron and Erythropoietin

The anemia of chronic renal disease is caused by an inability of the kidney to produce EPO, the hormone that stimulates the bone marrow to produce red blood cells, an increased destruction of red blood cells secondary to circulating uremic waste products; and blood loss with dialysis or blood sampling. A synthetic form of EPO, recombinant human EPO (rHuEPO), is used to treat this form of anemia. Clinical trials have demonstrated a dramatic improvement in correcting anemia and restoring a general sense of well being (Trkulja, 2012). Recent studies have indicated that higher dosages of EPO pose increased risk of stroke, adverse cardiac events, and death, so close monitoring and balancing the needs of the patient are essential in good management (Koulouridis et al, 2013).

Use of EPO increases red blood cell production 2.5-fold. Almost always accompanying the rise in hematocrit is an increased need for iron that requires IV supplementation. Oral iron alone is not effective in maintaining adequate iron stores in patients who take EPO. Unless a documented allergic reaction exists, almost all patients taking EPO require periodic IV or intramuscular iron. For patients who are allergic to IV iron, several better-tolerated forms are now available as iron dextran (Infed), iron gluconate (Ferrlecit), and iron sucrose (Venofer).

Serum ferritin is an accurate indicator of iron status in renal failure. Patients who have received several transfusions and who are storing extra iron may have high serum ferritin levels of 800 to 5000 ng/ml (a normal level is 68 ng/ml for women and 150 ng/ml for men; see Appendix 22). In patients who are receiving EPO, ferritin should be kept above 300 ng/ml but below 800 ng/ml. When ferritin values fall below 100 ng/ml, IV iron is usually given. The percent of transferrin saturation is another useful indicator of iron status in these patients and should be between 25% to 30%.

Vitamins

Water-soluble vitamins are rapidly lost during dialysis. In general, ascorbic acid and most B vitamins are lost through dialysate at approximately the same rate they would have been lost in the urine (depending on the type and duration of treatment), with the exception of folate, which is highly dialyzable. Patients who still produce urine may be at increased risk of loss of water-soluble vitamins. Folate is recommended to be supplemented at 1 mg/day based on extra losses. Because vitamin B_{12} is protein-bound, losses of this B vitamin during dialysis are minimal. Altered metabolism and excretory function, as well as drug administration, also may affect vitamin levels. Little is known about GI absorption of vitamins in uremia, but it may be significantly decreased. Uremic toxins may interfere with the activity of some vitamins, such as inhibition of phosphorylation of pyridoxine and its analogs.

Another cause of decreased vitamin intake in uremia is the restriction of dietary phosphorus and potassium. Water-soluble vitamins are usually abundant in high-potassium foods such as citrus fruits, vegetables, and high-phosphorus foods such as milk. Diets for patients on dialysis tend to be low in folate, niacin, riboflavin, and vitamin B_6. With frequent episodes of anorexia or illness, vitamin intake is decreased further. Whereas levels of water-soluble vitamins decrease as a result of dialysis, replacement of fat-soluble vitamins usually is not required in renal disease.

Several vitamin supplements that fit the needs of the uremic patient or the dialysis patient are now available by prescription: Nephrocaps, Renavite, Dialyvite, Folbee Plus, and Renal Caps. An over-the-counter supplement containing the vitamin B complex and vitamin C often is used and can be less expensive than a prescription, but additional supplements of folic acid and pyridoxine may be needed.

Niacin has been found to be helpful in lowering phosphate levels in ESRD patients. It interferes with the sodium-phosphate pump in the GI lumen, causing decreased transport of phosphate, and thus works with a different mechanism than phosphate binders (Cheng et al, 2006, 2008). It has shown benefit in improving outcomes in patients that struggle with a serum phosphorus of more than 6.0 when used in conjunction with phosphate binders as a once-daily pill. Potential side effects such as GI bleeding, liver disease, and flushing must be carefully considered.

Nutrition Support in End-Stage Renal Disease
Enteral Tube Feeding

Patients with ESRD who require enteral tube feeding generally can use standard formulas used for most tube-fed patients (see Chapter 13) and do not require a "specialty" or renal formula. Formulas marketed as renal products are more calorie-dense, higher in protein and lower in specific nutrients such as potassium and phosphorus. If patients are receiving renal products only, they may develop problems with low phosphorus or potassium levels as these products are designed to be used in conjunction with oral intake.

Oral Protein Supplementation During Dialysis

Recent research has focused on use of oral protein supplements while a patient is receiving dialysis treatments. The theory is that muscle protein will be replaced, offsetting catabolism, which occurs during dialysis. This is thought to be similar to what an athlete might experience using a protein supplement immediately after exercise. Study results show possible links to reduction in mortality from use during dialysis treatments, but no improvement in serum albumin levels (Lacson et al, 2012).

Parenteral Nutrition

Parenteral nutrition (PN) in ESRD is similar to PN used for other malnourished patients with respect to protein, carbohydrates, and fat, but differs in use of vitamins and minerals. Most researchers agree that vitamin needs for ESRD during PN differ from normal requirements; however, they do not agree on recommendations for individual nutrients. Folate, pyridoxine, and biotin should be supplemented. Vitamin A should not be provided parenterally unless retinol-binding protein is monitored during each HD treatment because it is elevated in patients with ESRD. Because there is currently no parenteral vitamin that is specifically designed for patients with renal failure, a standard vitamin preparation usually is administered. Little information related to parenteral trace mineral supplementation is available. Because most trace minerals, including zinc, chromium, and magnesium, are excreted in the urine, a close monitoring of these minerals in the serum seems to be appropriate.

Intradialytic Parenteral Nutrition

Malnourished patients with chronic renal failure who are on HD have easy access to PN because of the direct blood access required by the dialysis therapy itself. Intradialytic PN (IDPN) can be administered if necessary without additional invasive procedures or need for a separate port. It is administered typically through a connection to the venous side of the extracorporeal circuit during dialysis. Because of the high blood flow rate achieved through use of the surgically created fistula and the high blood pump speeds that are attained, hypertonic glucose and protein can be administered without danger of phlebitis. Lipids also may be administered. Reimbursement issues are complex because IDPN is a supplemental feeding that requires the patient to have at least a functioning GI tract and only supplies an average of 700 - 1000 calories during each HD treatment, depending on composition, dose, and administration time.

Complications are similar to those encountered in usual PN, with the exception of postdialysis hypoglycemia caused by the abrupt ending of the glucose supply. To avoid this problem, administration of IDPN containing glucose is tapered down during the last half hour of the 3- to 5-hour treatment. Insulin can be given, and may be administered in the bag of the dextrose–amino acid solution so that the patient does not become hypoglycemic if the infusion must be stopped. Blood sugar levels typically are monitored during the therapy. Some patients may benefit from a complex carbohydrate snack toward the end of the treatment or afterwards to avoid posttreatment rebound hypoglycemia. Amino acid losses through the dialysate only average approximately 10%.

Another method of nutrition support in PD patients is called intraperitoneal nutrition (IPN) using a peritoneal dialysate solution that contains amino acids instead of dextrose. Typically one bag of this solution is used per day. Some patients experience side effects from this treatment, which may include too much fluid removal. Reimbursement issues with this therapy are significant.

End-Stage Renal Disease in Patients with Diabetes

Because renal failure is a complication of diabetes, approximately 40% to 50% of all new patients starting dialysis have diabetes (MacIsaac et al, 2014). The need to control blood sugar in these patients requires specialized diet therapy. The diet for diabetes management (see Chapter 30) can be modified for the patient on dialysis. In addition, the diabetic patient on dialysis often has other complications such as retinopathy, neuropathy, gastroparesis, and amputation, all of which can place this patient at high nutritional risk. The National Kidney Foundation (NKF) has established guidelines for managing diabetes in the presence of CKD at the Kidney Disease Outcome Quality Initiative at www.kdoqi.org (National Kidney Foundation, 2012).

Increased osmolality caused by high serum levels of glucose may cause water and potassium to be pulled out of cells, with resultant hyperkalemia. Interpretation of commonly used laboratory values will change when a diabetic patient develops renal failure. Hemoglobin A1C (Hgb A1C) measures the glycosylation of hemoglobin. The shortened half-life of red blood cells from uremia and the losses in the dialysis process cause Hgb A1C values to appear lower than they really are (Vos et al, 2012).

Chronic Kidney Disease and End-Stage Renal Disease in Children

Although CKD may occur in children at any age, from the newborn infant to the adolescent, it is a relatively uncommon diagnosis. Causal factors in children include congenital defects, anatomic defects (urologic malformations or dysplastic kidneys), inherited disease (autosomal-recessive polycystic kidney disease), metabolic disorders that eventually result in renal failure (cystinosis or methylmalonic aciduria), or acquired conditions or illnesses (untreated kidney infections, physical trauma to kidneys, exposure to nephrotoxic chemicals or medications, hemolytic anemia resulting from *E. coli* 0157 ingestion, or glomerular nephritis).

As with all children, the major concern is to promote normal growth and development. Without aggressive monitoring and encouragement, the child with renal failure rarely meets his or her nutritional requirements. If the renal disease is present from birth, nutrition support needs to begin immediately to avoid losing the growth potential of the first few months of life. Growth in children with CKD usually is delayed. Although no specific therapy ensures normal growth, factors capable of responding to therapy include metabolic acidosis, electrolyte depletion, osteodystrophy, chronic infection, and protein-calorie malnutrition. Energy and protein needs for children with chronic renal disease are at least equivalent to the DRIs for normal children of the same height and age. If nutrition status is poor, energy needs may be even higher to promote weight gain and linear growth.

Feeding by tube is required in the presence of poor intake, particularly in the critical growth period of the first 2 years of life. Gastrostomy tubes almost always are placed in these children to enhance nutritional intake and facilitate growth. PN rarely is initiated unless the GI tract is nonfunctional. For the nutritional requirements of children with renal failure see www.kdoqi.org (National Kidney Foundation, 2008).

Control of calcium and phosphorus balance is especially important for maintaining good growth. The goal is to restrict phosphorus intake while promoting calcium absorption with the aid of $1,25\text{-}(OH)_2D_3$. This helps prevent renal osteodystrophy, which can cause severe growth retardation. Use of calcium carbonate formulations to supplement the dietary intake enhances calcium intake while binding excess phosphorus. Persistent metabolic acidosis is often associated with growth failure in infancy. In chronic acidosis the titration of acid by the bone causes calcium loss and contributes to bone demineralization. Bicarbonate may be added to the infant formula to counteract this effect.

Restriction of protein in pediatric diets is controversial. The so-called "protective" effect on kidney function must be weighed against the clearly negative effect of possible protein malnutrition on growth (Chaturvedi and Jones, 2007). The recommended dietary allowance for protein for age is usually the minimum amount given.

Each child's diet should be adjusted to his or her food preferences, family eating patterns, and biochemical needs. This is often not an easy task. In addition, care must be taken not to place too much emphasis on the diet to avoid food becoming a manipulative tool and an attention-getting device. Special encouragement, creativity, and attention are required to help the child with CKD consume the necessary energy. When possible, PD is given intermittently during the day and continuously at night because it allows liberalization of the diet. The child is more likely to meet nutritional requirements with fewer dietary restrictions and therefore experience better growth. See www.kidney.org for further tips on pediatric renal nutrition support.

Other treatments that help renal disease in children include the use of rHuEPO and recombinant deoxyribonucleic acid–produced human growth hormone. EPO usually is started when the child's serum hemoglobin falls below 10 g/dl, with a goal of maintaining hemoglobin between 11 and 12 g/dl. Correction of anemia with the use of rHuEPO may increase appetite, intake, and feeling of well-being, but it has not been found to affect growth, even with seemingly adequate nutrition support.

Medical Nutrition Therapy for Transplantation

The nutritional care of the adult patient who has received a transplanted kidney is based mainly on the metabolic effects of the required immunosuppressive therapy. Medications typically used for the long term include azathioprine (Imuran), corticosteroids (e.g., prednisone), calcineurin inhibitors (cyclosporine A, Gengraf, SangCya, Sandimmune, tacrolimus [Prograf, F506]), sirolimus (Rapamune), everolimus (Zortress), mycophenolate mofetil (CellCept), and mycophenolic acid (Myfortic). Corticosteroids are associated with accelerated protein catabolism, hyperlipidemia, sodium retention, weight gain, hyperglycemia, osteoporosis, and electrolyte disturbances. Calcineurin inhibitors are associated with hyperkalemia, hypertension, hyperglycemia, and hyperlipidemia. The doses of these medications used after transplantation are decreased over time until a "maintenance level" is reached.

During the first 6 weeks after surgery, a high-protein diet is often recommended (1.2 to 1.5 g/kg ideal body weight [IBW]) with an energy intake of 30 to 35 kcal/kg IBW, to prevent negative nitrogen balance. A moderate sodium restriction of 2 to 3 g/day during this period minimizes fluid retention and helps to control blood pressure. After recovery, protein intake should be decreased to 1 g/kg IBW, with calorie intake providing sufficient energy to maintain or achieve an appropriate weight for height. A balanced low-fat diet aids in lowering cardiac complications, whereas sodium intakes are individualized based on fluid retention and blood pressure (see Appendix 30).

Hyperkalemia warrants a temporary dietary potassium restriction. After transplantation, many patients exhibit hypophosphatemia and mild hypercalcemia caused by bone resorption; this is associated with persistent hyperparathyroidism and the effects of steroids on calcium, phosphorus, and vitamin D metabolism. The diet should contain adequate amounts of calcium and phosphorus (1200 mg of each daily) and cholecalciferol (vitamin D_3, 2000 IU daily). Supplemental phosphorus also may be necessary to correct hypophosphatemia.

Hydration must also be monitored closely after transplantation. Because most kidney recipients required a fluid restriction while on dialysis, they must be reminded of the importance of maintaining fluid intake after transplant. Typically, patients are encouraged to drink 2 L/day, but their overall needs depend on their urine output.

The majority of transplant recipients have elevated serum triglycerides or cholesterol for a variety of reasons. Intervention consists of medications, calorie restriction for those who are overweight, cholesterol intake limited to less than 300 mg/day, and limited total fat (see Chapter 33). In patients with glucose intolerance, limiting carbohydrates and a regular exercise regimen are appropriate. Tissue weight gain with resultant obesity is common after transplantation. Medication side effects, fewer dietary restrictions, and the lack of physical exercise can contribute to posttransplant weight gain.

Because of immunosuppression, care must be taken with food safety similar to other significantly at risk groups. Handwashing, food temperature monitoring, and avoidance of uncooked foods remain appropriate infection control behaviors.

Referral to bariatric surgery is being seen in patients needing weight loss to qualify for a transplant. Much coordination and collaboration is needed between the bariatric RDN and the renal RDN to be sure that the patient's very specific diet needs are met based on their treatment modality and progression of kidney disease (see Chapter 21).

Counseling and Education of Patients with End-Stage Renal Disease

For effective intervention, it is important to look at the long-range goals for educating the patient with ESRD about his or her nutritional needs. The average patient survives on dialysis 7 to 10 years, the average mortality is approximately 20% per year, equal to that of serious cancers such as ovarian cancer. However, some patients with a relatively benign diagnosis may look forward to life spans of 20 to 40 years, particularly if they receive kidney transplants as a part of their treatment. The challenge for the dietitian is educating the patient with a chronic disease who will be primarily responsible for implementing nutritional recommendations for the rest of his or her life. Thus intervention for ESRD and that for diabetes share many similarities.

It is incumbent on the renal dietitian nutritionist to develop a long-standing rapport with the patient and his or her family, and to serve as an ally to help them make the best nutritional choices over an extended period. Understanding the burdens of a complex, challenging, ever-changing diet suggests the transfer of information to the renal patient and family in a workable, flexible, and easily understood manner. Skills for this task are just as challenging, if not more so, than maintaining a patient's iron status or keeping the patient at a good body weight. Empathy and use of techniques such as motivational interviewing or cognitive behavioral therapy are essential tools (see Chapter 14).

Coordination of Care in End-Stage Renal Disease

The position of the RDN in the care of dialysis patients is unique because it is a federally mandated position. So, too, is the RDN's place on the mandated interdisciplinary health care team that exists within each dialysis unit. The team approach is an important aspect of all health care; however, its importance is magnified in the dialysis team, which consists of the patient, renal nurse, renal social worker, nephrologist, and renal dietitian nutritionist. Care of these complex, long-term ESRD patients requires the skill and compassion of each member of the health care team working together. Advanced levels of practice are available for dietitians who wish to be certified as renal RDNs; they can be certified through examination by the Academy of Nutrition and Dietetics, and become a Board Certified Specialist in Renal Nutrition.

Emergency Diets for Dialysis Patients

When power outages, flooding, storms, hurricanes, or earthquakes threaten a community, they threaten the most vulnerable people in that community. Patients on HD require power and water sources to do their own treatments at home. If they travel to a dialysis unit, they need access to transportation. Because of poor outcomes in recent natural disasters, the federal government's ESRD program has specified that patients and caregivers must be familiar with alternative nutritional therapies when dialysis is not available because of a natural or manmade emergency. Box 35-2 demonstrates the type of nutrient and practical information that must be considered when patients may be without dialysis for days, or because they must be evacuated to a site that cannot meet their urgent nutritional needs.

Medical Management (Conservative Treatment) or Palliative Care

The decision to forego or discontinue dialysis and opt for end-of-life care is a difficult and emotional one. Factors such as religious practices, age, quality of life, and comorbid disease play a role. Patients who are poor candidates for dialysis or transplantation may benefit from a low-protein, low-sodium diet to minimize physical symptoms, such as shortness of breath and uremia. Palliative care can be offered with the goal of balancing patient wishes for food choice with these complex side effects (Germain et al, 2011).

BOX 35-2 Emergency Dialysis Diet Plan

This plan will work for short periods (5 days or less) when patients cannot dialyze.

The Emergency Diet Plan does not replace dialysis; it should be used only in case of an emergency.

Guidelines

1. Limit meat to 3-4 oz/day.
2. Avoid all high-potassium fruits and vegetables.
3. Consume only one to two 8-oz cups of fluid per day.
4. Choose low-salt foods.
5. Do not use salt or salt substitute.
6. Use fats and sugars for extra calories.
7. If the power is off for a day, foods in refrigerator should be eaten first.
8. Patients should eat food from the freezer while they still have ice crystals in the center.

9. Patients should have a portable Emergency Kit they can take with them to a disaster relief center. Sample foods are listed in the following diet plan.

Emergency Diet Plan

If a food is not on this list, dialysis patients should not eat it.

Meat and Protein Foods (three to four 1-oz choices/day)

1 egg
1 ounce meat, fish, tofu or poultry
1/4 cup unsalted or rinsed canned fish or poultry
2 tablespoons unsalted peanut butter
1/4 cup cottage cheese
1/2 can commercial liquid nutritional supplement

BOX 35-2 Emergency Dialysis Diet Plan—cont'd

Starch (six to ten choices/day)
1 slice white bread
½ English muffin or bagel
5 unsalted crackers
2 graham crackers
6 shortbread cookies, vanilla wafers
1 cup unsalted rice, noodles, pasta
1 cup puffed wheat, rice, shredded wheat
1 cup of rice or pasta

Vegetables (one choice/day)
½-cup serving of green beans, summer squash, corn, beets, carrots, or peas
Should be fresh or frozen, not canned

Fruits (three to four choices/day)
1 small apple
15 grapes
½ cup serving of berries, cherries, applesauce, canned pears or canned pineapple

Fats and Oil (six or more choices/day)
1 tsp butter, margarine, oil or mayonnaise

Fluids (one to two choices/day)
1 cup water, coffee, tea, soda
½ cup Ensure Plus, Boost Plus or Nepro
½ cup serving of milk, half and half, soy, or rice milk
Cranberry, apple, or grape juice; or Kool-Aid

Emergency Kit
Have the following things stored in a box or bag easily accessible:
Foods listed in the Emergency Diet Plan
Can opener
Two gallon jugs of distilled water
Bleach, 1 Tbsp/gallon of water to sterilize
Flashlight and extra batteries
Sharp knife
Aluminum foil
Plastic mixing containers and lids
Measuring cup
Fork, knife, spoon
Battery-operated transistor radio
One-week supply of personal medicines kept in a handy place, including blood pressure medications and phosphate binders (insulin and some other medications must be kept refrigerated or cold)

Storage Tips
1. Store things in a clean, dry place such as a new garbage can or rubber tub.
2. Label and date when food is put in storage.
3. Change all food and water once a year. Eat unused food or donate to a food bank.

Dialysis Emergency Diet information from Katy Wilkens, MS, RD. Copyright Northwest Kidney Centers, 2011. For more emergency diet info see www.nwkidney.org or your local Network Coordinating Council website.

CLINICAL CASE STUDY

Fred, a 67-year-old Caucasian man, is seen by his primary care physician. Fred lives with a significant other and has an active lifestyle (golfing, biking, swimming) and a history of hemicolectomy, diverticulitis, and hypertension. His weight is 240 lb. His laboratory values show serum creatinine of 3.3 mg/dl, BUN of 72 mg/dl, albumin of 4.1 mg/dL, potassium of 5.5 mEq/L, phosphate of 6.7 mg/dl, calcium of 8.3 mg/dl, and his parathyroid hormone is 365 pg/ml. Blood pressure is 160/92.

Nutrition Diagnostic Statement
Altered laboratory values related to hypertension as evidenced by estimated glomerular filtration rate (eGFR) calculation.

Nutrition Care Questions
1. What is Fred's calculated eGFR?
2. What is his stage of chronic kidney disease (CKD)?
3. What is the first goal for your education of Fred?
4. What dietary factors would you address based on Fred's laboratory values?
5. What is the goal for his protein intake?
6. How would you assess Fred for improvement or stability of his CKD?
7. What would you expect for him during the next few years if no diet intervention is followed?

USEFUL WEBSITES

Academy of Nutrition and Dietetics and the National Renal Diet
www.eatright.org
Agency for Healthcare Research and Quality
www.effectivehealthcare.ahrq.gov/reports/final.cfm
American Society of Nephrology
www.asn.online.org/education/kidneyweek
American Urological Association
www.auanet.org

European Association of Urology
http://www.uroweb.org/gls/pdf/21_Urolithiasis_LR.pdf
Kidney Disease Outcome Quality Initiative
www.kdoqi.org
Life Options
www.lifeoptions.org
National Institute of Diabetes and Digestive and Kidney Diseases
http://www.niddk.nih.gov/Pages/default.aspx
National Kidney Foundation
www.kidney.org
Nationwide End-Stage Renal Network
www.esrdnetworks.org
Northwest Kidney Centers
www.nwkidney.org
Renal Support Network
www.rsnhope.org
United States Renal Data Systems
www.usrds.org

REFERENCES

Abboud H, Henrich WL: Clinical practice: stage IV chronic kidney disease, *N Engl J Med* 362:56, 2010.

Agarwal MM, et al: Preventive fluid and dietary therapy for urolithiasis: An appraisal of strength, controversies and lacunae of current literature, *Indian J Urol* 27:310, 2011.

Adeva MM, Souto G: Diet-induced metabolic acidosis, *Clin Nutr* 30:416, 2011.

Baia LC, et al: Non-citrus alkaline fruit: a dietary alternative for the treatment of hypocitraturic stone formers, *J Endourol* 26:1221, 2012.

Baldwin C, et al: Multi-intervention management of calciphylaxis: a report of 7 cases, *Am J Kidney Dis* 58:988, 2011.

Berardi JM, et al: Plant based dietary supplement increases urinary pH, *J Int Soc Sports Nutr* 5:20, 2008.

Centers for Disease Control (CDC): *National Chronic Kidney Disease Fact Sheet*, 2014. http://www.cdc.gov/diabetes/pubs/pdf/kidney_factsheet.pdf. Accessed February 7, 2015.

Chaturvedi S, Jones C: Protein restriction for children with chronic kidney disease, *Cochrane Database Syst Rev* 17:CD006863, 2007.

Chen X, et al: The associations of plant protein intake with all-cause mortality in CKD, *Am J Kidney Dis* 67:423, 2016.

Cheng SC, Coyne DW: Niacin and niacinamide for hyperphosphatemia in patients undergoing dialysis, *Int Urol Nephrol* 38:171, 2006.

Cheng S, et al: A randomized, double-blind, placebo-controlled trial of niacinamide for reduction of phosphorus in hemodialysis patients, *Clin J Am Soc Nephrol* 3:1131, 2008.

Coca SG, et al: Long term risk of mortality and other adverse outcomes after acute kidney injury: a systematic review and meta-analysis, *Am J Kidney Dis* 53:961, 2009.

Cohen G, Vyas NS: Sodium thiosulfate in the treatment of calciphlaxis, *J Clin Aesthet Dermatol* 6:41, 2013.

Curhan GC, Taylor EN: 24-h uric acid excretion and the risk of kidney stones, *Kidney Int* 73:489, 2008.

Ferraro JM et al: Total, dietary and supplemental vitamin C intake and risk of incident kidney stones, *Am J Kidney Dis* 67:400, 2016.

Freire GC: Cranberries for preventing urinary tract infections, *Sao Paulo Med J* 131:363, 2013.

Friedman AN, Fadem SZ: Reassessment of albumin as a nutritional marker in kidney disease, *J Am Soc Nephrol* 21:223, 2010.

Gama-Axelsson T, et al: Serum albumin as a predictor of nutritional status in patients in ESRD, *J Am Soc Nephrol* 7:1446, 2012.

Germain M, et al: When enough is enough: the nephrologists responsibility in ordering dialysis treatments, *Am J Kidney Dis* 58:135, 2011.

Gomes A, et al: Re-envisioning fistula first in a patient-centered culture, *Clin J Am Soc Nephrol* 8:1791, 2013.

Grams M, et al: Lifetime incidence of CKD stages 3-5 in the United States, *Am J Kidney Dis* 62:245, 2013.

Heaney RP: *GrassrootsHealth/Vitamin D action-kidney stones not caused by vitamin D*, 2013. http://www.grassrootshealth.net.

Heilberg IP, Goldfarb DS: Optimum nutrition for kidney stone disease, *Adv Chronic Kidney Dis* 20:165, 2013.

Himmelfarb J, Ikizler TA: Hemodialysis, *N Engl J Med* 363:1833, 2010.

Iff S, et al: Relative energy balance, CKD, and risk of cardiovascular and all-cause mortality, *Am J Kidney Dis* 63:437, 2014.

Inker LA, et al: Estimating glomerular filtration rate from serum creatinine and cystatin C, *N Engl J Med* 367:20, 2012.

Kang DE, et al. Long-term lemonade based dietary manipulation in patients with hypocitraturic nephrolithiasis, *J Urol* 177:1358, 2007.

Kiwull-Schone H, et al: Food composition and acid-base balance: alimentary alkali depletion and acid load in herbivores, *J Nutr* 138: S431, 2008.

Knight J, et al: Increased protein intake on controlled oxalate diets does not increase urinary oxalate excretion, *Urol Res* 37: 63, 2009.

Koulouridis I, et al: Dose of erythropoiesis-stimulating agents and adverse outcomes in CKD: a metaregression analysis, *Am J Kidney Dis* 61:44, 2013.

Krieger NS, Bushinsky DA: The relation between bone and stone formation, *Calcif Tissue Int* 93:374, 2013.

Lacson E, et al: Outcomes associated with intradialytic oral nutrition supplements in patients undergoing maintenance hemodialysis: a quality improvement report, *Am J Kidney Dis* 60:591, 2012.

Lange D: Dietary habits may influence oxalate degradation by intestinal bacteria commentary on: The role of oxalobacter formigenes colonization in calcium oxalate stone disease, *Urology* 84:1263, 2014.

Leon J, et al: The prevalence of phosphorus-containing food additives in top-selling foods in grocery stores, *J Ren Nutr* 23:265, 2013.

MacIsaac R, et al: Markers of and risk factors for the development and progress of diabetic kidney disease, *Am J Kidney Dis* 63(Suppl 2):S39, 2014.

Manson JE, Bassuk SS: Calcium supplements: do they help or harm? *Menopause* 21:106, 2014.

Minich DM, Bland JS: Acid-alkaline balance: role in chronic disease and detoxification, *Altern Ther Health Med* 13:62, 2007.

Morgan MSC, Pearle MS: Medical management of kidney stones. *BMJ* 352: 152, 2016.

National Kidney Foundation: *KDOQI Clinical Practice Guideline for Children with Chronic Kidney Disease*, 2008.

National Kidney Foundation: *KDOQI Clinical Practice Guideline for Chronic Kidney Disease*, 2000.

National Kidney Foundation: *KDOQI Clinical Practice Guideline for Chronic Kidney Disease and Diabetes*, 2012.

Nouvenne A, et al: Effects of a low salt diet on idiopathic hypercalciuria in calcium oxalate stone formers: a 3-month randomized controlled trial, *Am J Clin Nutr* 91:565, 2010.

Ortiz-Alvarado O, et al: Omega-3 fatty acids eicosapentaenoic acid and docosahexaenoic acid in the management of hypercalciuric stone formers, *Urology* 79:282, 2012.

Pak CY, et al: Defining hypercalciuria in nephrolithiasis, *Kidney Int* 80:777, 2011.

Pigna F, et al: Body fat content and distribution and urinary risk factors for nephrolithiasis, *Clin J Am Soc Nephrol* 9:159, 2014.

Pizzorno J, et al: Diet induced acidosis: is it real and clinically relevant? *Br J Nutr* 103:1185, 2010.

Remer T, Manz F: Potential renal acid load of foods and its influence on urine pH, *J Am Diet Assoc* 95:791, 1995.

Scales CD, et al: Prevalence of kidney stones in the United States, *Eur Urol* 62(1):160, 2012.

Semins MJ, et al: The effect of restrictive bariatric surgery on urinary stone risk factors, *Urology* 76:826, 2010.

Siener R, et al: The role of oxalobacter formigenes colonization in calcium oxalate stone disease, *Kidney Int,* 83:1144, 2013.

Sorensen MD, et al: Activity, energy intake, obesity and the risk of incident kidney stones in postmenopausal women: A report from the Women's Health Initiative, *J Am Soc Nephrol* 25:362, 2014.

Tang J, et al: Association between serum 25-hydroxyvitamin D and nephrolithiasis: the National Health and Nutrition Examination Survey III, 1988-94, *Nephrol Dial Transplant* 27:4385, 2012.

Taylor EN, Curhan GC: Determinants of 24-h urinary oxalate excretion, *Clin J Am Soc Nephrol* 3:1453, 2008a.

Taylor EN, Curhan GC: Dietary calcium from dairy and nondairy sources, and risk of symptomatic kidney stones, *J Urol* 190:1255, 2013.

Taylor EN, Curhan GC: Fructose consumption and the risk of kidney stones, *Kidney Int* 73:207, 2008b.

Taylor EN, et al: DASH-style diet associates with reduced risk of kidney stones, *J Am Soc Nephrology* 20:2253, 2009.

Taylor EN, et al: Fatty acid intake and incident nephrolithiasis, *Am J Kidney Dis* 45:267, 2005.

Therrien M, et al: A Review of Dietary Intake Studies in Maintenance Dialysis Patients, *J Ren Nutr* 25:4, 2015.

Trinchieri A: Development of a rapid food screener to assess the potential renal acid load of diet in renal stone formers (LAKE score), *Arch Ital Urol Adrol* 84:36, 2012.

Trinchieri A: Diet and renal stone formation, *Minerva Med* 104:41, 2013.

Trkulja V: Treating anemia associated with chronic renal failure with erythropoiesis stimulators: recombinant human erythropoietin might be the best among the available choices, *Med Hypotheses* 78:157, 2012.

Turner JM, et al: Treatment of chronic kidney disease, *Kidney Int* 81:351, 2012.

Vos FE, et al: Assessment of markers of glycaemic control in diabetic patients with chronic kidney disease using continuous glucose monitoring, *Nephrology* 17:182, 2012.

Wallace RB, et al: Urinary tract stone occurrence in the Women's Health Initiative randomized clinical trial of calcium and vitamin D supplements, *Am J Clin Nutr* 94:270, 2011.

Wang CH, et al: Cranberry-containing products for prevention of urinary tract infections in susceptible populations: a systemic review and meta-analysis of randomized controlled trials, *Arch Intern Med* 172:988, 2012.

Whelton PK, et al: Sodium, blood pressure, and cardiovascular disease: further evidence supporting the American Heart Association sodium reduction recommendations, *Circulation* 126:2880, 2012.

Wingard R, et al: Early intervention improves mortality and hospitalization rates in incident hemodialysis: RightStart program, *Clin J Am Soc Nephrol* 2:1170, 2007.

Yang W, et al: Association of Kidney Disease Outcomes with risk factors for CKD: Findings from the Chronic Renal Insufficiency cohort (CRIC) Study, *Am J Kidney Dis* 63:236, 2014.

Yasui T, et al: Eicosapentanoic acid has protective effect on the recurrence of nephrolithissis, *Urol Int* 81:135, 2008.

Zilberman DE, et al: The impact of societal changes on patterns of urolithiasis, *Curr Opin Urol* 20:148, 2010.

36

Medical Nutrition Therapy for Cancer Prevention, Treatment, and Survivorship

Kathryn K. Hamilton, MA, RDN, CSO, CDN, FAND
Barbara L. Grant, MS, RDN, CSO, LD, FAND

KEY TERMS

antiangiogenic agents
antineoplastic therapy
antioxidants
apoptosis
benign
biotherapy
bisphenol A (BPA)
cancer cachexia
carcinogen
carcinogenesis
certified specialist in oncology
    nutrition (CSO)
chemoprevention
chemotherapy
complementary therapies
cytokines
dumping syndrome
emetogenic
energy balance

graft-versus-host disease (GVHD)
hematopoietic cell transplantation
    (HCT)
hematopoietic growth factors
hormonal therapy
hospice
initiation
insulin-like growth factor-1 (IGF-1)
integrative medicine
malignant neoplasm
metastasis
mucositis
myelosuppression
neoplasm
neutropenia
nutrition impact symptoms
oncogenes
oncology
osteoradionecrosis

palliate (palliative care)
pancytopenia
phytochemicals
polycyclic aromatic hydrocarbons
    (PAHs)
progression
promotion
radiation enteritis
radiation therapy
sinusoidal obstructive syndrome
    (SOS)
tumor-node-metastasis (TNM) staging
    system
trismus
tumor
tumor angiogenesis
tumor necrosis factor-α (cachectin)
tumor suppressor genes
venoocclusive disease

Cancer involves the abnormal division and reproduction of cells that can spread throughout the body. Usually thought of as a single disease, cancer actually consists of more than 100 distinct types. The American Cancer Society (ACS) predicts the lifetime risk for developing cancer in the United States is slightly less than half of men and a little more than one third of women (ACS, 2014a). Annually in the United States, cancer is responsible for almost one in four deaths (ACS, 2014a). It is estimated that one third of the more than 580,000 anticipated cancer deaths can be attributed to nutrition and lifestyle behaviors such as poor diet, physical inactivity, alcohol use, and overweight and obesity. Tobacco use also contributes significantly to death from cancer with more than 15 million lives lost since the Surgeon General released the warning in 1964. Today, nearly one in five deaths from cancer and other diseases in the United States are caused by tobacco use (ACS, 2014a). Tobacco use has been shown to reduce life expectancy, on average, by approximately 14 years and is responsible for the loss of millions of dollars in health care costs and early loss of life.

The cost of cancer care in the United States is estimated to be more than $216.6 billion annually, $86.6 billion for direct medical costs, and $130 billion for loss of productivity resulting from premature death (ACS, 2014a) (see Figure 36-1).

The ACS established *2015 Challenge Goals* to improve cancer prevention and early detection efforts for lowering cancer incidence and mortality rates. These national recommendations outline specific measures to expand the use of established screening guidelines for the early detection of cancer and ways to influence individual health behaviors, such as protection from the sun, reducing tobacco use, maintaining a healthy body weight, improving diet, and increasing regular physical activity (ACS, 2013).

Overall, fewer Americans are dying from cancer, a trend that began more than 15 years ago. For many, cancer is now a chronic disease, like heart disease and diabetes. According to the American Cancer Society, there are 13.7 million American cancer survivors living with a history of cancer; this means they are cancer free, are living with evidence of disease, or are undergoing cancer treatment (ACS, 2014a). As a result of progress in early detection of cancer and the development of new anticancer therapies, survivorship for all cancers is now 67%, up from 47% in the 1970s (ACS, 2014a). The Annual Report to the Nation on the Status of Cancer, 1975-2010, released in December 2013, found rates of new diagnoses and rates of death from the major cancers continue to decline for men and women, as well as for the major racial and ethnic populations (Edwards et al,

Estimated New Cases

			Males	Females			
Prostate	220,800	20%		Breast	231,840	29%
Lung & bronchus	115,610	14%		Lung & bronchus	105,590	13%
Colon & rectum	69,090	8%		Colon & rectum	63,610	8%
Urinary bladder	56,320	7%		Uterine corpus	54,870	7%
Melanoma of the skin	42,670	5%		Thyroid	47,230	6%
Non-Hodgkin lymphoma	39,850	5%		Non-Hodgkin lymphoma	32,000	4%
Kidney & renal pelvis	38,270	5%		Melanoma of the skin	31,200	4%
Oral cavity & pharynx	32,670	4%		Pancreas	24,120	3%
Leukemia	30,900	4%		Leukemia	23,370	3%
Liver & intrahepatic bile duct	25,510	3%		Kidney & renal pelvis	23,290	3%
All Sites	**848,200**	**100%**		**All Sites**	**810,170**	**100%**

Estimated Deaths

			Males	Females			
Lung & bronchus	86,380	28%		Lung & bronchus	71,660	26%
Prostate	27,540	9%		Breast	40,290	15%
Colon & rectum	26,100	8%		Colon & rectum	23,500	9%
Pancreas	20,710	7%		Pancreas	19,850	7%
Liver & intrahepatic bile duct	17,030	5%		Ovary	14,180	5%
Leukemia	14,210	5%		Leukemia	10,240	4%
Esophagus	12,600	4%		Uterine corpus	10,170	4%
Urinary bladder	11,510	4%		Non-Hodgkin lymphoma	8,310	3%
Non-Hodgkin lymphoma	11,480	4%		Liver & intrahepatic bile duct	7,520	3%
Kidney & renal pelvis	9,070	3%		Brain & other nervous system	6,380	2%
All Sites	**312,150**	**100%**		**All Sites**	**277,280**	**100%**

FIGURE 36-1 New cases of cancer. (Printed with permission of the American Cancer Society, Cancer Facts & Figures 2015.)

2014). Although cancer rates continue to be higher for men than for women, combined rates of death from cancer decreased by 1.5% per year from 2001 through 2010; overall incidence rates decreased in men and stabilized in women (Edwards et al, 2014).

PATHOPHYSIOLOGY

Carcinogenesis is the origin or development of cancer. **Oncology** is the study of all forms of cancer. Researchers believe changes in gene function cause normal cells to transform into cancerous cells. Thus the study of genetic material and its function, genomics, is of great scientific interest in cancer and its treatment (see Chapter 5 and *Pathophysiology and Care Management Algorithm:* Cancer).

Oncogenes are altered genes that promote tumor growth and change programmed cell death (**apoptosis**). The inhibition of cell death pathways allows for survival of the genetically damaged cancer cells. **Tumor suppressor genes** are the opposite of oncogenes; these genes become deactivated in cancer cells. This loss in function can lead to unregulated cell growth and, ultimately, cancer. Examples of tumor suppressor

genes include adenomatosis polyposis coli (APC), breast cancer types BRCA1 and BCRA, and tumor suppressor p53, a protein that is involved in preventing cancer. Only approximately 5% to 10% of all cancers occur as result of inherited genetic alterations (ACS, 2014b). Factors observed in families with hereditary cancers include the following:

- Many cases of an uncommon or rare type of cancer
- A cancer diagnosis at an earlier age than normal for certain kinds of cancer
- Individuals with one type of cancer being diagnosed with a second type of cancer
- More than one childhood cancer diagnosed in a set of siblings
- Certain types of cancers observed in specific ethnic populations (e.g., individuals of Ashkenazi Jewish ancestry with breast and ovarian cancer)
- Recognized cancer syndromes, such as hereditary nonpolyposis colorectal cancer or Lynch syndrome, which cause individuals to be at greater risk for developing gastrointestinal (GI), ovarian, uterine, brain, or skin cancer (NIH)

Genetic counselors assist individuals and their families to evaluate their risk of hereditary predisposition, such as testing positive for gene mutations.

Phases of Carcinogenesis

A carcinogen is a physical, chemical, or viral agent that induces cancer. Carcinogenesis is a biologic, multistage process that proceeds on a continuum in three distinct phases: initiation, promotion, and progression. Initiation involves transformation of cells produced by the interaction of chemicals, radiation, or viruses with cellular deoxyribonucleic acid (DNA). This transformation occurs rapidly, but cells can remain dormant for a variable period until they are activated by a promoting agent. After the initial cellular damage has occurred, transformation from normal cells to a detectable cancer can take many years or even decades. During promotion, initiated cells multiply and escape the mechanisms set in place to protect the body from the growth and spread of such cells. A neoplasm, new and abnormal tissue with no useful function, is established. In the third phase, progression, tumor cells aggregate and grow into a fully malignant neoplasm or a tumor.

In the process known as metastasis, the neoplasm has the capacity for invasion that can spread to distant tissues and organs. For a cancer to metastasize, it must develop its own blood supply to sustain its growth of rapidly dividing abnormal cells. In normal cells, angiogenesis promotes the formation of new blood vessels, which are essential to supply the body's tissues with oxygen and nutrients. In cancer cells, tumor angiogenesis occurs when tumors release substances that aid in the development of new blood vessels needed for their growth and metastasis.

NUTRITION AND CARCINOGENESIS

Nutrition may modify the carcinogenic process at any stage, including carcinogen metabolism, cellular and host defense, cell differentiation, and tumor growth. Gene expression can be promoted or altered by nutrients during pregnancy, childhood, and throughout the lifecycle. Estimates produced by the World Cancer Research Fund indicate a quarter to a third of all of the cancers that occur in higher-income countries such as the United States are due to poor nutrition, physical inactivity, and excess weight (ACS, 2014a). The strong influence of diet and nutrients is seen readily in studies of migration between cultures. Patterns of cancer occurrence often change over time to resemble those of the new country. For example, in Japan mortality from breast and colon cancer is low and mortality from stomach cancer is high; the reverse is true among Japanese individuals living in the United States. After two or three generations, the cancer patterns in individuals become similar to those in the population in the new location.

Studies looking at the role of nutrition and diet as causal factors of cancer seek to identify relationships between the diets of population groups and categories of individuals and the incidence of specific cancers (Thomson et al, 2014). Sets of individuals are compared in case control, cohort, or cross-sectional studies. The strongest evidence comes from consistent findings of these different types of epidemiologic studies in diverse populations. In cancer research, epidemiologists look at human populations and evaluate how many people are diagnosed with cancer, what types of cancer occur in different populations and cultures, and what factors, such as diet and lifestyle, play a role in the development of the cancers.

The sheer complexity of diverse diet patterns presents a difficult challenge for study. Thousands of chemicals are found in a normal diet; some compounds are well studied and some less known and unmeasured. Some dietary carcinogens are naturally occurring pesticides or herbicides produced by plants for protection against fungi, insects, animal predators, or mycotoxins, which are secondary metabolites produced by molds present in foods (e.g., aflatoxins, fumonisins, or ochratoxin). Food preparation and preservation methods also may contribute to dietary carcinogen ingestion. Fortunately, diets contain both inhibitors, as well as enhancers of carcinogenesis. Dietary carcinogen inhibitors include antioxidants (e.g., vitamin C, vitamin A and the carotenoids, vitamin E, selenium, zinc) and phytochemicals (biologically active components of plants) (see Table 36-1).

Examples of dietary enhancers of carcinogenesis may be the saturated fat in red meat or the polycyclic aromatic hydrocarbons (PAHs) that form on the surface of meat when grilling at high temperatures. Complicating the study of nutrition, diet, and cancer is the fact that an alteration of one major component of the diet can precipitate a change in other facets of the diet. For example, decreasing animal protein also decreases animal fat. This cascade event makes the interpretation of research findings difficult because the effects cannot be associated clearly with one single factor.

Additional complications in interpretation can result from the fact that cancer cells can either be fast growing or have a long latent or dormant period. The slow-growing, latent, or dormant aspect of the disease progression makes pinpointing dietary patterns at the time of cancer cell initiation or promotion, and not at time of diagnosis, difficult. Select prospective epidemiologic studies attempt to deal with this challenge by measuring diet at one point in time and following the same subjects for several years. Studies done with laboratory animals test this effect, and since the early part of the last century, laboratory scientists have shown that various nutritional manipulations influence the development of cancerous tissue in animals. Epidemiologic research, together with animal studies, provides a viable method for discovering the links between nutrition and cancer in humans.

Alcohol

Alcohol consumption accounted for 3.5% of cancer-related deaths in 2009, representing more than 19,000 deaths and 18 years of potential life lost (Voelker, 2013). It is associated with increased cancer risk for cancers of the mouth, pharynx, larynx, esophagus,

TABLE 36-1 Phytochemicals in Vegetables and Fruits that may have Cancer Protective Properties		
Color	**Phytochemical**	**Vegetables and Fruits**
Red	Lycopene	Tomatoes and tomato products, pink grapefruit, watermelon
Red and purple	Anthocyanins, polyphenols	Berries, grapes, red wine, plums
Orange	Alpha- and beta-carotene	Carrots, mangos, pumpkin
Orange and yellow	Cryptoxanthin, flavonoids	French cantaloupe, peaches, oranges, papaya, nectarines
Yellow and green	Lutein, zeaxanthin	Spinach, avocado, honeydew, collard and turnip greens, asparagus
Green	Sulforaphanes, indoles	Cabbage, broccoli, Brussels sprouts, cauliflower
White and green	Allyl sulfides	Leeks, onion, garlic, chives

lung, colon, rectum, liver, and breast (pre- and postmenopausal women). For cancers of the mouth, pharynx, larynx, and esophagus, daily consumption of 1½ to 3 drinks increases risk significantly compared with nondrinkers (Voelker, 2013; WCRF and AICR, 2007).

Alcohol can also negatively affect health for cancer survivors. Although the research is inconsistent, alcohol consumption after breast cancer diagnosis has been shown in select studies to increase recurrence risk, especially among postmenopausal and overweight or obese women (Kwan et al, 2010; Rock et al, 2012). However, a clear association has been documented between continued alcohol consumption after treatment for head and neck cancers and its negative impact on survival (Rock et al, 2012). In the United States, alcohol results in 10 times as many deaths as it prevents, after the consideration of possible benefit from low-level consumption on cardiovascular and diabetes risk (Voelker, 2013).

Concurrent tobacco and alcohol use greatly increases cancer risk, particularly for cancers of the upper digestive area and respiratory tract (AICR C.U.P., 2015; WCRF and AICR, 2007). In addition, malnutrition associated with alcoholism is likely to be important in the increased risk for certain cancers. In the United States, if individuals choose to drink, men are recommended to limit alcohol intake to no more than two drinks per day and women to one drink per day. Serving sizes of popular alcoholic drinks include beer (12 oz), wine (5 oz), and liquors (1.5 oz of 80-proof liquors) (Kushi et al, 2012; WCRF and AICR, 2007).

Energy Intake and Body Weight

Obesity is a risk factor for cancer and may account for 14% to 20% of all cancer-related mortality (Kushi et al, 2012). Currently 69.2% of all American adults are overweight or obese (CDC, 2013). The relationship between body weight, body mass index (BMI), or relative body weight and site-specific cancer has been widely investigated; a positive association has been seen with cancers of the esophagus, pancreas, gallbladder, breast (postmenopausal), endometrium, kidney, colon, and rectum (Bender et al, 2013; WCRF and AICR, 2007). Metabolic operations (bariatric surgeries) seem to have a significant impact on cancer incidence and mortality, particularly with female obesity-related cancers (see Chapter 21). Researchers speculate the underlying mechanisms are weight dependent and weight independent with beneficial effects from dramatic weight loss, including improved insulin resistance, decreased oxidative stress and inflammation, modulation of sex steroids, gut hormones, cellular energetics, immune system, and adipokines (Ashrafian et al, 2011).

The optimal adult BMI should be between 21 and 23, depending on the normal range with different populations (WCRF and AICR, 2007). Body weight throughout childhood should be at the lower end of normal BMI, because excessive weight in adolescence has been correlated with increased risk of cancer development in adulthood (Kelsey et al, 2014).

Obesity, age, hyperglycemia, and the incidence of metabolic syndrome play a role in the circulating levels of insulin-like growth factor-1 (IGF-1), a potentially cancer-causing compound. IGF-1 is a polypeptide secreted primarily by the liver and plays a key role in normal growth and development. It can promote the development and progression of prostate, breast, lung, and colon cancer. It has been hypothesized to stimulate the growth of cancer cells and inhibit their death (Pollack, 2008; Zhou et al, 2007). IGF-1 secretion is increased when insulin levels are elevated. Obesity and high simple carbohydrate intakes

potentially increase insulin resistance and raise circulating insulin levels. This area of research connects several known risk factors between nutrition, diet, and cancer (Parekh et al, 2010).

Overweight and obese cancer survivors are at risk for recurrence and for developing additional problems after surgery, including impaired wound healing, lymphedema after lymph node dissections, second cancers, heart disease, and diabetes mellitus (Ligibel et al, 2014).

Physical activity is a critical component of weight management and energy balance. The ACS Nutrition and Physical Activity Guidelines for Cancer Prevention and the Guidelines for Cancer Survivors encourage individuals to strive for a minimum of 150 minutes per week of moderate activity or a minimum of 75 minutes per week of vigorous activity (Kushi et al, 2012; Rock et al, 2012) (see Table 36-2).

Achieving and maintaining energy balance and a reasonable weight should be a primary health goal for all individuals, including cancer survivors, because being overweight or obese appears to increase risk of developing cancer, cancer recurrence, and decreased survival (Kushi et al, 2012; Rock et al, 2012) (see the New Directions box Does Eating Less Reduce the Risk for Cancer?).

TABLE 36-2 American Cancer Society: Moderate and Vigorous Physical Activity

	Moderate Activities*	Vigorous Activities†
Exercise and leisure	Walking, dancing, leisurely bicycling, ice and roller skating, horseback riding, canoeing, yoga	Jogging or running, fast bicycling, circuit weight training, aerobic dance, martial arts, jumping rope, swimming
Sports	Volleyball, golfing, softball, baseball, badminton, doubles tennis, downhill skiing	Soccer, field or ice hockey, lacrosse, singles tennis, racquetball, basketball, cross-country skiing
Home activities	Mowing the lawn, general yard and garden maintenance	Digging, carrying and hauling, masonry, carpentry
Workplace activity	Walking and lifting as part of the job (custodial work, farming, auto or machine repair)	Heavy manual labor (forestry, construction, fire fighting)

American Cancer Society (ACS): www.cancer.org. Accessed February 20, 2015; Kushi LH et al: American Cancer Society guidelines on nutrition and physical activity for cancer prevention: reducing the risk of cancer with healthy food choices and physical activity, *CA Cancer J Clin* 62:30, 2012.
*Moving fast enough that you can speak but you cannot sing.
†Moving fast enough that you can speak a few words but not in complete sentences.

✳ NEW DIRECTIONS

Does Eating Less Reduce the Risk for Cancer?

Animal studies have demonstrated that chronic restriction of food inhibits the growth of most experimentally induced cancers and the occurrence of many spontaneous cancers. This effect is observed even when underfed animals ingested more dietary fat than control animals ingested. Caloric restriction, without malnutrition, appears to have a positive effect on cancer prevention in animals; it is unclear whether that effect translates to humans (Longo and Fontana, 2010).

Fat

Dietary fat has been studied in relationship to cancer risk and recurrence, and right now there appears to be an inconsistent link between certain types of cancer and the amount of fat in the diet. Of note, diets that contain a significant amount of fat often contain more meat and more calories, which can contribute to overweight and obese conditions and increased cancer risk.

To further complicate the picture, an additional link between fat, meat, and cancer risk results from meat preparation and processing, such as the presence of heterocyclic amines (HCAs) and or polycyclic aromatic hydrocarbons (PAHs) from cooking, formation of carcinogenic N-nitroso compounds (NOCs) from processing, and the potential cancer-promoting influence of heme-iron (WCRF and AICR, 2007).

Because dietary fat intake is correlated with the intake of other nutrients and dietary components, it is difficult to distinguish between the effects of dietary fat, protein, total calories, and carcinogenic compounds in cancer prevention. So, the current ACS recommendation is to limit consumption of processed meats and red meats (Kushi et al, 2012).

Two large prospective randomized studies examined dietary fat consumption as part of the diet composition, and breast cancer recurrence showed mixed results. The Women's Intervention Nutrition Study (WINS) found that interventions that reduced dietary fat intake to 20% of total calories and precipitated a modest reduction in body weight may favorably influence breast cancer prognosis. However, the Women's Healthy Eating and Living (WHEL) study, which included significant amounts of vegetables, fruit, and dietary fiber and was low in fat, demonstrated no significant survival benefit (Pierce et al, 2007).

What does seem to be important is eating more omega-3 fatty acids (foods such as fatty fish, flaxseed oil, walnuts, and certain algae) in relation to omega-6 fatty acids (polyunsaturated fats such as, safflower oil and sunflower oil) because this potentially reduces risk of cancer by acting to decrease inflammation, cell proliferation, and angiogenesis while increasing apoptosis (Bender et al, 2013).

A Plant-Based Diet

Plant foods may aid in cancer prevention by functioning as cancer inhibitors through antiinflammatory mechanisms and changes in gene expression and hormone activity (Bender et al, 2013). Fruits, vegetables, and whole grains contain biologically active phytochemicals, vitamins, minerals, and dietary fiber that have demonstrated functions in preventing and treating disease (see Table 36-3). In addition, the ACS Prevention Guidelines suggest that individuals who eat more vegetables and fruits further benefit by experiencing less weight gain, and greater satiety and are at a lower risk of developing obesity, thereby reducing overall cancer risk (Kushi et al, 2012).

Nonnutritive and Nutritive Sweeteners

The Food and Drug Administration (FDA) has approved eight nonnutritive sweeteners (acesulfame-K, aspartame, luo han guo fruit extract, neotame, saccharin, stevia, advantame, and sucralose) for use in the food supply and regulates them as food additives; they are generally recognized to be safe (GRAS) when used in moderation (www.fda.gov). Described as "high-intensity" sweeteners, nonnutritive sweeteners provide little or no energy because they sweeten in minute amounts. Nonnutritive sweeteners have been investigated primarily in relation to potential adverse health concerns, including long-term safety and carcinogenicity, but multiple studies during the past 20 or more years have indicated that

TABLE 36-3 Diet and Cancer-Site Risk Reduction	
Nutrition and Dietary Factors	**Cancer-Risk Correlation**
Obesity	Esophagus
	Colorectum
	Pancreas
	Stomach
	Breast (postmenopausal)
	Endometrium
	Limited and suggestive: renal
Dietary fat (specifically saturated fat), red and processed meats	Colorectum
	Endometrium
	Limited and suggestive: lymphoid, hematologic cancers, esophagus, stomach, lung, pancreas, breast, prostate, endometrium, renal, and ovarian
Omega 3 fatty acids—*protective*	Colon
Plant-based diet (low fruit, vegetable and complex carbohydrate intake)—*protective*	Prostate
	Mouth
	Pharynx
	Larynx
	Esophagus
	Stomach
	Lung
	Colorectum
	Prostate

Ferguson LR: Meat and Cancer, *Meat Sci* 84:308, 2010.
Kushi LH et al: American Cancer Society guidelines on nutrition and physical activity for cancer prevention: reducing the risk of cancer with healthy food choices and physical activity, *CA Cancer J Clin* 62:30, 2012.
World Cancer Research Fund (WCRF), American Institute for Cancer Research (AICR): *Food, nutrition, physical activity, and the prevention of cancer: a global perspective,* Washington, DC, 2007, AICR.

when consumed in reasonable amounts, they are safe. Additional sugar substitutes on the market include sugar alcohols (e.g., mannitol, sorbitol, xylitol) and blue agave. Sugar alcohols are not considered nonnutritive sweeteners even though they are used in a similar way. Blue agave is the juice from the *Agave tequiliana* plant and has no proven health benefits over sugar.

Protein

Most diets that contain significant amounts of protein also contain significant amounts of meat and fat and insignificant amounts of fiber. The effect of protein on carcinogenesis depends on the tissue of origin and the type of tumor as well as the type of protein and the calorie content of the diet. In general, tumor development is suppressed by diets that contain levels of protein below that required for optimal growth and development; whereas it is enhanced by protein levels two to three times the amount that is required. The effects may be attributable to specific amino acids, a general effect of protein, or, in the case of low-protein diets, depressed food intake. Epidemiologic studies have found limited and conflicting results. Recommendations for lowering cancer risk and improving overall health encourage intake of plant foods and limiting foods from animal sources, including red meat and processed meats and poultry (WCRF and AICR, 2007).

Smoked, Grilled, and Preserved Foods

Nitrates are added as preservatives to processed meats. Nitrates can be readily reduced to form nitrites, which in turn can interact with dietary substrates such as amines and amides to produce

N-nitroso compounds (NOCs): nitrosamines and nitrosamides, which are known mutagens and carcinogens. Nitrates or nitrites are used in smoked, salted, and pickled foods. Sodium and potassium nitrates are present in a variety of foods and give hot dogs and processed deli meats their pink color, but the main dietary sources are vegetables and drinking water.

NOCs are also produced endogenously in the stomach and colon of people who eat large amounts of red meat. Studies looking at the detrimental effects of smoked foods have not demonstrated a clear, consistent connection between these foods and stomach cancer (WCRF and AICR, 2007). Diets with high amounts of fruits and vegetables that contain vitamin C and phytochemicals that can retard the conversion of nitrites to NOCs should be encouraged (Kushi et al, 2012).

Charring or cooking meat at high temperatures over an open flame (400° F or more) can cause the formation of polycyclic aromatic hydrocarbons (PAHs) and heterocyclic amines (HCAs). PAHs have shown clear indications of mutagenicity and carcinogenicity. Normal roasting or frying food does not produce large amounts of PAHs compared with the amount produced when cooking over open flames. Animal proteins that produce the greatest dripping of fat on to the flames register the highest PAH formation. For example, grilled beef produces larger amounts of PAHs than grilled chicken, which produces higher amounts than oven-grilled chicken. The source of the flame can also influence PAH production; charcoal grilling promotes the most, followed by flame gas, and finally oven grilling (Farhadian et al, 2010).

Toxic Environments

The Environmental Protection Agency (EPA) was established in 1970 for the purpose of overseeing the acute and long-term health threats caused by substances in the environment. As part of this protection, the Toxic Substances Control Act passed in 1976 requires manufacturers to submit health and safety information on all new chemicals. However, many were grandfathered in with the passage of this law and are still untested. To date, 54 compounds have been identified by the National Institute of Health as carcinogenic (NIH, NIEHS, 2003).

Everyday activities expose people to a myriad of chemicals through air, water, food, and beverages. In fact, an estimated six percent of cancers diagnosed each year (2% from environmental exposures and 4% from occupational exposures) are likely caused by these very common exposures (Israel, 2010; NIH, NIEHS, 2003). Health care practitioners grapple with assessing exposure to so many different agents. A good environmental history can be performed at clinical visits and then quickly reviewed for outdoor air pollutants such as nitrogen dioxide, ozone, and carbon monoxide, which pose health risks. Exposure to heavy metals, pesticides, herbicides, and occupational exposures also may be noted. In addition to determining the patient's environmental exposure, practitioners must determine exposure of family members or others living in the same household. Oxidative stress caused by these environmental exposures can be alleviated by changes in lifestyle, including eliminating smoking and implementing dietary changes. Routine consumption of antioxidant-rich foods and a nutrient-rich diet (not supplementation) is suggested (Kushi et al, 2012).

Toxicity from Bisphenol A (BPA)

Bisphenol A (BPA) is an industrial chemical used since the 1960s in the manufacturing of many hard plastic bottles and the epoxy linings of metal-based food and beverage cans. It is also an ingredient in the production of epoxy resin used in

---

> ### BOX 36-1   Tips from FDA to Minimize Exposure to BPA
>
> - Check plastic container recycle codes on the bottom of container. Some, but not all, plastics that are marked with recycle codes 3 or 7 may be made with BPA.
> - Avoid putting very hot or boiling liquids in plastic containers made with BPA. BPA levels rise in food when containers and products made with the chemical are heated and come in contact with the food.
> - Do not use bottles with scratches, because these may harbor bacteria and, if the bottles are BPA-containing, the damage may lead to greater release of the BPA into the liquid.

FDA, 2014.

---

paints and adhesives. Studies done when the product was developed indicated it was safe to use in food and beverage containers. However, recent studies have demonstrated that BPA may disrupt the function of some hormones, including sex hormones, leptin, insulin, and thyroxin and it causes hepatotoxic, immunologic, and carcinogenic effects (Michalowicz, 2014).

Other findings from the combined efforts of the National Institute of Environmental Health Sciences, the National Toxicology Program, and FDA scientists at the National Center for Toxicological Research Program conclude that the health threat from BPA is less than previously estimated. Health damage from BPA may not be as likely because based on mathematical models, BPA rapidly metabolizes in the body, rather than accumulating (FDA, 2014).

Until more is known, the current goal is to reduce the use and exposure to BPA through several actions: restricting the use of BPA in baby bottles, using alternatives to the glue used in food containers, and increasing the oversight on the use of BPA in manufacturing and testing. The U.S. Department of Health and Human Services (USDHHS) supports eliminating it from all food-related product production. Originally it was thought to leach from the plastic only when exposed to heat; now it is believed to leach even at cold temperatures (FDA, 2014) (see Box 36-1).

CHEMOPREVENTION

Eating behaviors play a very important role in health promotion and disease prevention. Chemoprevention is defined as the use of drugs, vitamins, or other agents to reduce the risk of, or delay the development or recurrence of, cancer (NIH, NCI, 2015). Examples include nonsteroidal antiinflammatory drugs that may protect against colon cancer, and metformin, a commonly used medication to treat diabetes; these are currently being explored as cancer prevention and treatment agents (Guppy et al, 2011; Quinn et al, 2013). Other natural products or molecules currently being investigated include the hundreds of polyphenols in fruits and vegetables, green tea, curcumin (turmeric and curry), and resveratrol from red grapes and berries. Phenolic acid, flavonoids, stilbenes, and lignans are the most abundant polyphenols; the chemopreventive potential of these compounds comes from their ability to modulate epigenetic alterations in cancer cells (Choi and Friso, 2010).

The epigenetic modification step occurs early in the development of a cancer cell, at a time when it is potentially reversible. Scientists do not fully understand how this process works, yet it is reasonable to recommend a health-promoting and possibly cancer-preventing diet rich in fruits, vegetables, soy, therapeutic culinary herbs such as turmeric and cinnamon, green tea, and coffee (Link et al, 2010). The overall evidence of association between these and other dietary factors

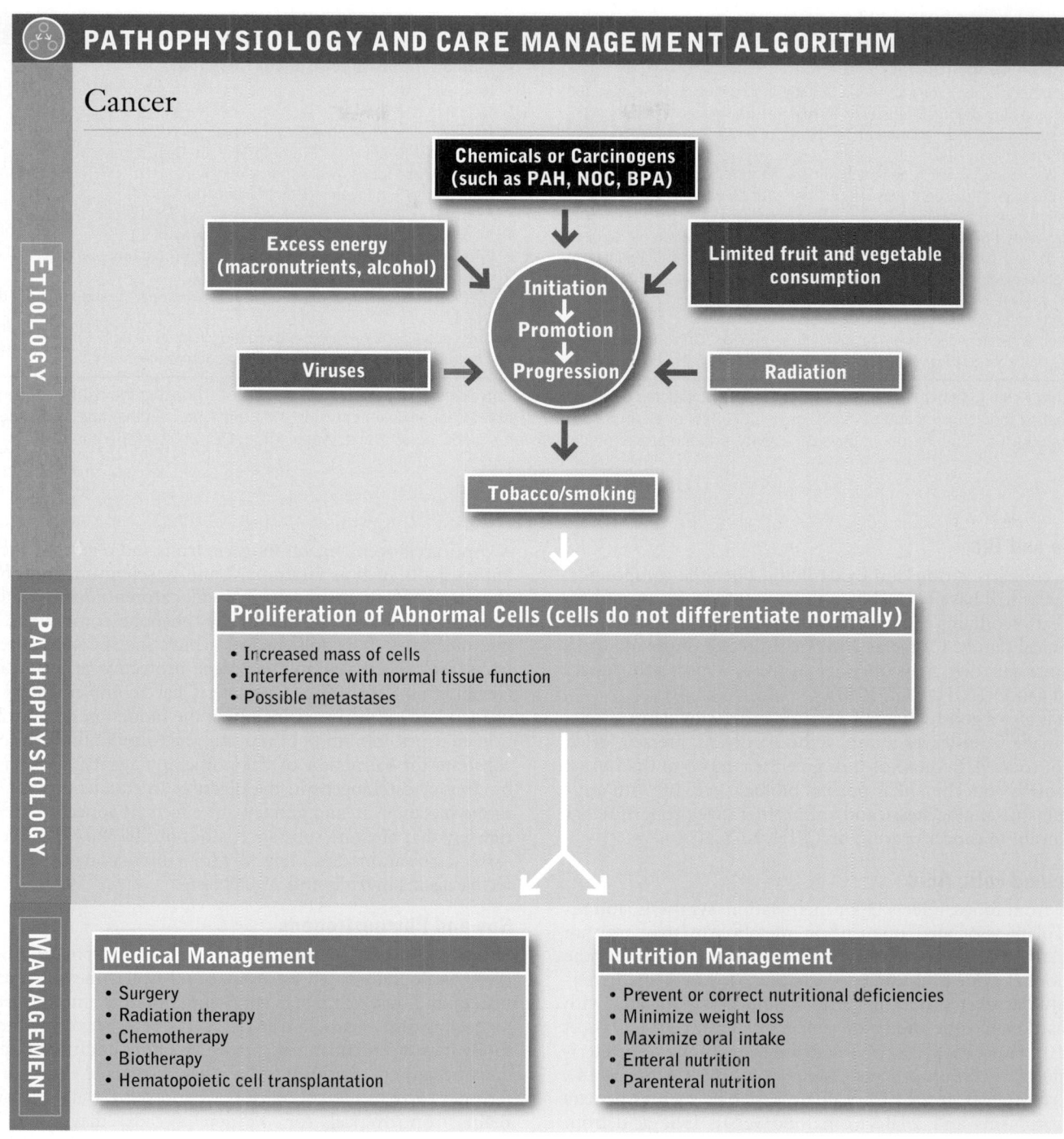

PATHOPHYSIOLOGY AND CARE MANAGEMENT ALGORITHM

Cancer

ETIOLOGY

Chemicals or Carcinogens (such as PAH, NOC, BPA)

Excess energy (macronutrients, alcohol)

Limited fruit and vegetable consumption

Initiation → Promotion → Progression

Viruses

Radiation

Tobacco/smoking

PATHOPHYSIOLOGY

Proliferation of Abnormal Cells (cells do not differentiate normally)

• Increased mass of cells
• Interference with normal tissue function
• Possible metastases

MANAGEMENT

Medical Management

• Surgery
• Radiation therapy
• Chemotherapy
• Biotherapy
• Hematopoietic cell transplantation

Nutrition Management

• Prevent or correct nutritional deficiencies
• Minimize weight loss
• Maximize oral intake
• Enteral nutrition
• Parenteral nutrition

enable health organizations to draft diet and lifestyle recommendations for the purpose of reducing cancer risk (see the American Cancer Society website (www.cancer.org) and Box 36-2).

Vitamin D and Calcium

Studies have reported an association of poor vitamin D status and greater incidence of cancer. For years, public health messages have encouraged use of sunscreens and less direct exposure to the sun. Because of these recommendations, there is reduced conversion of vitamin D on the skin surface, leading to the potential increase in deficiencies. Studies have reported that higher serum 25-hydroxyvitamin D (25[OH]D) levels are associated with lower incidence of some cancers, while some

studies report a higher risk for other cancers with high levels of vitamin D. More work must be done in this area to determine if supplementation with vitamin D can prevent cancer, or if low levels of the vitamin simply increases an individual's cancer risk (ACS, 2013b). Until more is learned about the interaction between vitamin D_3 and cancer prevention, taking 800 IU of vitamin D per day to maintain normal serum 25(OH)D levels is considered safe (ACS, 2013b). Individuals with abnormal serum levels should consult their medical team for supplement suggestions, monitoring, and evaluation. Correcting a deficiency in vitamin D may be important for its health promotion benefits as well as its effect on calcium absorption, as calcium supplementation and dairy, especially milk, may be associated with lower colorectal cancer risk (Kushi et al, 2012).

BOX 36-2   Cancer Prevention Recommendations

American Cancer Society

- Adopt a physically active lifestyle. Adults should engage in at least 150 minutes of moderate intensity or 75 minutes of vigorous intensity activity each week, or an equivalent combination, preferably spread throughout the week.
- Achieve and maintain a healthy body weight throughout life. Be as lean as possible throughout life without being underweight. Avoid excess weight gain at all ages.
- Consume a healthy diet, with an emphasis on plant sources. Choose foods and beverages in amounts that help achieve and maintain a healthy weight. Limit consumption of processed meat and red meat. Eat at least 2½ cups of vegetables and fruits each day. Choose whole grains instead of refined grain products.
- If you drink alcoholic beverages, limit consumption. Drink no more than one drink per day for women or two per day for men.

American Institute for Cancer Research

- Body Fatness: Be as lean as possible within the normal range of body weight.
- Physical Activity: Be physically active as part of everyday life.
- Foods and Drinks That Promote Weight Gain: Limit consumption of energy-dense foods. Avoid sugary drinks.
- Plant Foods: Eat foods mostly of plant origin.
- Animal Foods: Limit intake of red meat and avoid processed meat.
- Alcoholic Beverages: Limit alcoholic beverages.
- Preservation, Processing, Preparation: Limit consumption of salt. Avoid moldy cereals (grains) or pulses (legumes).
- Dietary Supplements: Aim to meet nutritional needs through diet alone.
- Breastfeeding: Mothers to breastfeed; children to be breastfed.
- Cancer Survivors: Follow the same recommendations.

Data from Kushi LH et al: American Cancer Society guidelines on nutrition and physical activity for cancer prevention: reducing the risk of cancer with healthy food choices and physical activity, CA Cancer J Clin 62:30, 2012; World Cancer Research Fund (WCRF), American Institute for Cancer Research (AIRC): Food, nutrition, physical activity, and the prevention of cancer: a global perspective, Washington, DC, 2007, WCRF and AIRC.

Coffee and Tea

Coffee contains various antioxidant and phenolic compounds, some of which have been shown to have anticancer properties. Coffee also contains caffeine, a compound in the alkaloid phytochemical family. Coffee as a major source of antioxidants in the American diet may offer its drinkers a protective effect against cancer (NIH, NCI, 2010).

Tea is also a good source of phenols and antioxidants. Green tea is made from leaves that have been cooked, pressed, dried and not roasted. Because of this, green tea, more so than black tea, contains catechins that possess biologic activity with antioxidant, anti-angiogenesis, and antiproliferative properties that are relevant to cancer prevention (NIH, NCI, 2010).

Folate and Folic Acid

Folate, from foods, affects DNA methylation, synthesis, and repair. Folate-associated one-carbon metabolism may play an important role in colorectal carcinogenesis because of gene variations (Levine et al, 2010; see Chapter 5). Several epidemiologic studies suggest that higher folate intake is associated with decreased pancreatic and colon cancer risk (ACS, 2011; Oaks et al, 2010). However, excessive folate may contribute to deleterious effects in certain cancers (Bailey et al, 2010; MNT, 2014). More research is needed to evaluate variables such as genetic polymorphisms and folate from food versus folic acid from supplements.

Fruits and Vegetables

Fruit intake is protective against cancers of the mouth, pharynx, larynx, esophagus, cervix, lung, and stomach (WCRF, AICR, 2007). Health benefits from vegetables are more difficult to quantify. Nonstarchy vegetables, such as spinach, tomatoes, and peppers, probably provide protection against mouth, pharynx, larynx, and esophageal cancers; all vegetables, but particularly green and yellow ones, probably protect against stomach cancer (WCRF, AICR, 2007). Most countries have recommendations for the consumption of vegetables and fruits that vary but generally are for three or more servings of vegetables and two or more servings of fruit daily with a serving being approximately 80 g or ½ cup (Norat, 2014).

Anticarcinogenic agents found in fruits and vegetables include antioxidants such as vitamins C and E, selenium, and phytochemicals. Phytochemicals include carotenoids, flavonoids, isoflavones, lignans, organosulfides, phenolic compounds, and monoterpenes. It is still unclear which specific substances of fruits and vegetables are the most protective against cancer (Kushi et al, 2012). These substances have complementary and overlapping mechanisms, including the induction of detoxification enzymes, inhibition of nitrosamine formation, provision of substrate for formation of chemotherapy agents, dilution and binding of carcinogens in the digestive tract, alteration of hormone metabolism, and antioxidant effects. It appears extremely unlikely that any one substance is responsible for all of the observed associations. See Table 36-1 for a discussion of chemoprotective agents in fruits and vegetables.

Soy and Phytoestrogens

Soy is a plant-based protein, and it contains phytoestrogens (very weak plant-based estrogens) and isoflavones such as genistein and daidzein. Diets containing modest amounts of soy protect against breast cancer (ACS, 2012), especially if the soy foods have been consumed before reaching adulthood apparently because of exposure to the weak estrogenic effects of isoflavones early in life (ACS, 2012). However, the use of soy remains controversial for women already diagnosed with hormone-sensitive cancers (e.g., breast, endometrium) and for postmenopausal women.

Commercially prepared soy supplement powders and foods made from soy products can but may not always contain isoflavones at much higher concentrations than traditional whole soy foods such as edamame beans, tofu, or soy milk (U.S. Department of Agriculture [USDA], 2014). The ACS advises breast cancer survivors to limit the consumption of soy foods to no more than three servings daily and to avoid using prepared soy supplement powders and products (Rock et al, 2012). Unlike the advice for women, men with hormone-sensitive cancer such as prostate cancer may benefit from regular consumption of soy foods. Prostate cancer is a testosterone-driven cancer and estrogens (or phytoestrogens) are antagonists.

MEDICAL DIAGNOSIS AND STAGING OF CANCER

Despite the progress made in understanding possible prevention strategies, cancer remains a significant health threat and, for most adults, is second to heart disease as a cause of death in the United States. Assessing symptoms of cancer at the earliest stage is critical for treatment effectiveness and survival. Table 36-4 summarizes constitutional or systemic symptoms of cancer and metastatic disease. Many symptoms of early or metastatic cancer affect an individual's ability to eat, digest, or absorb. According to the ACS, the following early warning signs and symptoms of cancer are described using the acronym "CAUTION":

Change in bowel or bladder habits

A sore that does not heal

Unusual bleeding or discharge

Thickening or lump in breast or elsewhere

Indigestion or difficulty in swallowing or chewing

Obvious change in a wart or mole

Nagging cough or hoarseness

When symptoms or screening tests suggest cancer, physicians use the following to establish a definitive diagnosis: evaluation of an individual's medical, social, and family histories; physical examination; laboratory tests; imaging procedures; and tissue biopsy. Laboratory evaluation is composed of analysis of blood, urine, and other body fluids. In particular, oncologists evaluate tumor markers (e.g., alpha-fetoprotein [AFP], cancer antigen [CA] 125, CA 19-9, carcinoembryonic antigen [CEA],

prostate-specific antigen [PSA]) and other substances in blood or body fluids that can be elevated in cancer. Imaging procedures and studies help determine a diagnosis (Table 36-5). Pathologists perform cytologic examinations by analyzing body fluids, sputum, urine, or tissue under a microscope. To detect malignant cells, they use a histopathologic examination to review specially stained tissue, flow cytometry to count and examine cells and chromosomes, immunohistochemistry to review antibodies for specific cell proteins, and cytogenetics to visualize genetic defects.

Oxidative damage to lipids in cellular membranes, proteins, and DNA is often permanent. Thus biomarkers may be used to estimate the DNA damage after exposure to cancer-causing agents, such as tobacco smoke, asbestos fibers, heavy metals, and PAHs. 8-hydroxy-2-deoxyguanosine (8-OHdG) is a new biomarker for the measurement of endogenous oxidative DNA damage and risk for cancer (Valavanidis et al, 2009).

Staging is used to identify how much a cancer has spread throughout the body. The stage of the cancer at the time of diagnosis is a strong predictor of survival, and it directs oncologists to the most effective treatment plan. Cancer staging is most frequently described as stage I, II, III, or IV—stage I being the least amount of disease and stage IV being the most advanced. The tumor-node-metastasis (TNM) staging system is also commonly used by oncologists. *T* stands for the size of the tumor, *N* stands for nodes or whether it has spread into lymph nodes, and *M* stands for metastasis, or whether the cancer has spread to distant organs.

For classification, tumors are often referred to as *solid* cancers, and hematologic-related cancers of the blood are frequently called *liquid* cancers. The classification of tumors is based on their tissue of origin, their growth properties, and their invasion of other tissues. Tumors that are not malignant typically are described as benign.

Because cancer occurs in cells that are replicating, the patterns of cancer are different in children and adults. In early life the brain, nervous system, bones, muscles, and connective tissues are still growing; therefore cancers involving these tissues are more prevalent in children than in adults. Common childhood cancers include neuroblastoma; medulloblastoma; osteosarcoma; and soft tissue sarcomas such as rhabdomyosarcoma, schwannoma, and germ cell tumors. Conversely, adult cancers

TABLE 36-4 Signs and Symptoms of Cancer

Constitutional Symptoms of Cancer	Signs and Symptoms of Metastatic Cancer
Anorexia	Pain
Fatigue	Enlarged lymph nodes or body organs
Weight loss	Cough with or without hemoptysis
Fever	Bone pain with or without fracture
Sweating	Neurologic symptoms
Anemia	

Data from National Institutes of Health (NIH), National Cancer Institute (NCI): *NCI Dictionary of Cancer Terms*, http://www.cancer.gov/dictionary. Accessed April 16, 2014.

TABLE 36-5 Imaging Studies for Cancer Diagnosis and Disease Monitoring

Type of Imaging	Description and Use in Cancer Diagnosis and Treatment
Computed tomography (CT) scan	**Description:** A CT scan is a radiographic procedure in which a series of detailed pictures of areas inside the body are taken from different angles. Images are created by a computer and are linked to an x-ray machine. **Use:** A CT scan is used to evaluate for abnormalities of possible cancer in a general anatomic area such as the head, chest, abdomen, or pelvis. Radiologists use CT scans to visualize suspicious lesions, internal organs, and lymph nodes.
Magnetic resonance imaging (MRI) scan	**Description:** An MRI scan is an imaging procedure that uses radio waves and a powerful magnet linked to a computer to create detailed pictures of areas inside the body. This type of scanning often creates better images of body organs and soft tissue than other type of scanning methods. **Use:** Images produced show differences between normal and cancerous tissue. In particular, an MRI scan is used to evaluate suspicious areas of the brain, spinal cord, and liver.
Positron emission tomography (PET) scan	**Description:** A PET scan is a procedure in which a small amount of radioactive glucose is injected into a vein and a scanner is used to make detailed, computerized pictures of areas where glucose is used in the body. **Use:** Cancerous cells have an enhanced rate of glycolysis (they use more glucose than normal cells). Areas of glucose metabolism with high activity or "hot spots" appearing on the PET scan generally correlate to findings of cancer.

Data from American Cancer Society (ACS): *Cancer Glossary* (website): http://www.cancer.org/cancer/cancerglossary/index. Accessed April 16, 2014. National Institutes of Health (NIH), National Cancer Institute (NCI): NCI Dictionary of Cancer Terms. http://www.cancer.gov/publications/dictionaries/cancer-terms?expand=.; Accessed September 18, 2015.
CT, Computed tomography; *MRI*, magnetic resonance imaging; *PET*, positron emission tomography.

frequently involve epithelial tissues that cover and line the body's internal and external surfaces. Cancers of the epithelial tissues include cancers of the skin, and circulatory, digestive, endocrine, reproductive, respiratory, and urinary systems. Cancers arising from these tissues are referred to as carcinomas, and common types are classified as adenocarcinomas, basal cell carcinomas, papillomas, and squamous cell carcinomas.

Leukemias, lymphomas, and myelomas are cancers of the immune system and can occur in children or adults. Leukemias arise most frequently from white blood cells of the bone marrow. Lymphomas are cancers that develop in the lymphatic system—its nodes, glands, and organs. Myeloma is cancer that originates in the plasma cells of the bone marrow and most frequently occurs in older adults.

Other types of cancer are related to infectious causes and cancer experts recommend antibiotics, vaccines, and changes in behavior for their prevention (ACS, 2014b). Examples include hepatocellular carcinoma linked to hepatitis B virus (HBV) exposure and alcoholic-related cirrhosis, oropharyngeal and cervical cancers linked to human papillomavirus infection (HPV), and stomach cancer caused by chronic inflammation by *Helicobacter pylori* (see Chapter 27).

MEDICAL TREATMENT

In the United States and in hundreds of countries across the world, cancer treatment is guided by oncologists, medical doctors specializing in the prevention, treatment, and palliation of cancer, and by evidence-based standards known as the National Comprehensive Cancer Network (NCCN) Clinical Practice Guidelines in Oncology (2015). The NCCN Guidelines encompass evidence-based care for 97% of all cancers treated in oncology practice. Also listed with these guidelines are evidence-based recommendations for providing supportive care (e.g., survivorship, palliative care, cancer-related pain, fatigue, distress, and antiemesis).

Conventional modalities include antineoplastic therapy (e.g., chemotherapy, biotherapy, or hormonal therapy), radiation therapy, and surgery used alone or in combination with other cancer therapies. Solid tumors and hematologic malignant diseases such as leukemias, lymphomas, and multiple myelomas may be treated with hematopoietic cell transplantation (HCT).

Chemotherapy is the use of chemical agents or medications to systematically treat cancer. These agents interfere with the steps or phases of the cell-cycle, specifically with the synthesis of DNA and replication of cancer cells. The basic five phases of cell reproduction in normal and malignant cells are the following (Polovich et al, 2014):

G0—resting phase
G1—postmitotic phase; RNA and protein are synthesized
S—DNA is synthesized
G2—premiotic phase; the second phase where RNA and protein synthesized
M—mitosis; cell division

Most chemotherapy agents are categorized by their biochemical activity and their mechanism of action such as alkylating agents (cell-cycle nonspecific), antimetabolites (cell-cycle specific, usually S-phase), and taxanes (m-phase specific). Biotherapy is the use of biologic agents to produce anticancer effects indirectly by inducing, enhancing, or suppressing an individual's own immune response. Antiangiogenic agents are used to inhibit the development of new blood vessels needed by cancers (tumor vasculature) and thus prevent their growth, invasion, and spread. Hormonal therapy is systemic therapy used for the treatment of hormone-sensitive cancers (e.g., breast, ovarian, prostate) by blocking or reducing the source of a hormone or its receptor site.

Radiation oncologists work in the area of therapeutic radiation therapy, which uses high-energy (ionizing radiation) in multiple fractionated doses, or radioactive chemicals to treat cancer. Surgery involves the surgical removal of cancerous tissue.

Response to cancer treatment is defined as complete or partial response (improvement), stable disease (same), or disease progression (worsening). Factors that affect an individual's response to treatment include tumor burden (the larger the tumor, the greater risk of metastatic disease), rate of tumor growth (rapidly growing tumors are usually more responsive to therapy), and drug resistance (tumors mutate as they grow, and with successive mutations new cancer cells become more likely to be resistant to therapy). Other factors contributing to an individual's response to cancer treatment include comorbid diseases (e.g., diabetes, renal disease, cardiopulmonary disease), age, performance status, psychosocial support systems, bone marrow reserve, and overall general health (NIH, NCI, 2014c; Polovich et al, 2014).

Goals of Treatment

The goal of cancer treatment may be to cure, control, or palliate. Cure is a complete response to treatment. Even if a treatment cannot cure a cancer, often there can be cancer control that extends life when a cure is not possible. *Control* measures may obscure microscopic metastases after tumors are surgically removed, reduce the size of tumors before surgery or radiation therapy, or alleviate symptoms and side effects of cancer. If a cancer cannot be cured or controlled, palliative care is offered. Palliative care helps individuals be as comfortable as possible. Palliation is designed to relieve pain and manage symptoms of illness; lessen isolation, anxiety and fear; and help maintain independence as long as possible (National Hospice and Palliative Care Organization [NHPCO], 2014). Hospice is care for individuals with a life expectancy of months and focuses on relieving symptoms, controlling pain, and providing support to patients and their families. Patients are made as comfortable as possible through the end of their lives.

MEDICAL NUTRITION THERAPY

The Commission on Dietetic Registration has developed a board certification in oncology nutrition: certified specialist in oncology nutrition (CSO). To further assist clinicians working in the cancer care setting the Academy of Nutrition and Dietetics (AND) has developed the Oncology Toolkit with MNT protocols for breast, colorectal, esophageal, gastric, head and neck, hematologic, lung, and pancreatic cancers (AND, 2010). Another Academy resource for clinicians when providing MNT in the cancer care setting is the Pocket Guide to the Nutrition Care Process in Cancer (Grant, 2015).

Nutrition Screening and Assessment

With the recent shift of cancer care from the hospital setting to outpatient settings, nutrition screening and assessment should continue throughout the continuum of care. Ideally, nutrition screening and assessment for risk of nutrition problems should be interdisciplinary, instituted at the time of diagnosis, and re-evaluated and monitored throughout treatment and recovery. See Chapter 4 for the following screening tools validated for use with individuals diagnosed with cancer (AND, 2013):

- Patient Generated-Subjective Global Assessment (PG-SGA) for inpatient and outpatient settings (http://www.ncbi.nlm.nih.gov/pubmed/12122555).
- Malnutrition Screening Tool (MST) for inpatient and outpatient settings (http://www.ncbi.nlm.nih.gov/pubmed/10378201.)
- Malnutrition Screening Tool for Cancer Patients (MSTC) for inpatient settings (http://www.ncbi.nlm.nih.gov/pubmed/21813215).
- Malnutrition Universal Screening Tool (MUST) for inpatient and outpatient settings (http://www.ncbi.nlm.nih.gov/pubmed/22142968).

Other assessment tools specific to patients with cancer are the Activities of Daily Living (ADLs) tool, the Common Toxicity Criteria for Adverse Events (CTCAE), and the Karnofsky Performance Scale (KPS) Index. CTCAE is an outcome measure used in anticancer therapy that compares acute toxicities of cancer treatment, and KPS is a scoring index that associates an individual's functional status with disease status and survival (Polovich et al, 2014).

In-depth assessment is undertaken to obtain more information and to identify nutrition problems (see Chapter 7 and Appendix 22). Careful review of the individual's appetite and oral intake is required, with an assessment of symptoms (e.g., nausea, vomiting, and diarrhea), weight status, comorbidities, and laboratory studies. A nutrition-focused physical examination is recommended to evaluate fully nutrition status and degree of risk (see Appendix 21). Components of this type of assessment include a general survey of the body, review of vital signs and anthropometrics, and an evaluation of subcutaneous fat stores, muscle mass, and fluid status (see Chapter 7).

Energy

Determining individualized energy needs is vital to helping people maintain an energy balance and achieve a healthy weight; it is also vital to preventing unintentional weight gain or loss associated with cancer and cancer treatment. Methods used to estimate energy requirements for adults include using standardized equations or measuring resting metabolic rate using indirect calorimetry (Hamilton, 2013; see Chapter 2 for methods for determining energy requirements). To ensure that adequate energy is being provided, the individual's diagnosis, presence of other diseases, intent of treatment (e.g., curative, control, or palliation), anticancer therapies (e.g., surgery, chemotherapy, biotherapy, or radiation therapy), presence of fever or infection, and other metabolic complications such as refeeding syndrome must be considered. Evidence-based guidelines from the American Society for Parenteral and Enteral Nutrition (ASPEN) for quickly estimating energy needs of people with cancer based on body weight are shown in Table 36-6.

Protein

An individual's need for protein is increased during times of illness and stress. Additional protein is required by the body to repair and rebuild tissues affected by cancer treatments and to maintain a healthy immune system (Hamilton, 2013). Adequate energy should be provided, or the body will burn its lean body mass as a fuel source. The degree of malnutrition, extent of disease, degree of stress, and ability to metabolize and use

TABLE 36-6 Estimating Energy Needs of People with Cancer

Condition	Energy Needs
Cancer, nutritional repletion, weight gain	30-35 kcal/kg/day
Cancer, inactive, non-stressed	25-30 kcal/kg/day
Cancer, hypermetabolic, stressed	35 kcal/kg/day
Hematopoietic cell transplant	30-35 kcal/kg/day
Sepsis	25-30 kcal/kg/day

Data from Gottschlich MM, editor: *The A.S.P.E.N. nutrition support core curriculum: a case-based approach—the adult patient*, Silver Spring, Md, 2007, American Society for Parenteral and Enteral Nutrition; Hamilton KK: Nutrition needs of the adult oncology patient. In Leser M et al, editors: *Oncology nutrition for clinical practice*, Chicago, 2013, Oncology Nutrition Dietetic Practice Group of the Academy of Nutrition and Dietetics.

protein are factors in determining protein requirements (Hamilton, 2013). For example, protein needs for a catabolic client may be 1.2 g/kg/day or more, and protein needs for an individual undergoing a hematopoietic cell transplant may be 1.5 g/kg/day. Daily protein requirements generally are calculated using actual body weight rather than ideal body weight.

Fluid

Fluid management in cancer care must ensure adequate hydration and electrolyte balance and prevent dehydration and hypovolemia. Altered fluid balance may occur with fever, ascites, edema, fistulas, profuse vomiting or diarrhea, multiple concurrent intravenous (IV) therapies, impaired renal function, or medications such as diuretics. Individuals need close monitoring for dehydration (e.g., intracellular fluid losses caused by inadequate intake of fluid because of mucositis or anorexia), hypovolemia (e.g., extracellular fluid losses from fever or GI fluids such as vomiting, diarrhea, or malabsorption), and nephrotoxic effects from anti-cancer treatments. Common nephrotoxic chemotherapy agents include the following (Polovich et al, 2014):

Alkylating agents: cisplatin, oxaliplatin, ifosfamide
Antimetabolites: methotrexate
Antitumor antibiotics: mitomycin-c
Cytokines: interleukin-2

Signs and symptoms of dehydration include fatigue, acute weight loss, hypernatremia, poor skin turgor, dry oral mucosa, dark or strong smelling urine, and decreased urine output. To carefully assess for hypovolemia, levels of serum electrolytes, blood urea nitrogen, and creatinine also should be evaluated.

A general guideline for estimating fluid needs for all adults without renal concerns is 20 to 40 ml/kg (Hamilton, 2013). Another method to assess fluid needs recommends 1 ml fluid per 1 kcal of estimated calorie needs (Hamilton, 2013). Intravenous hydration (IV) may be recommended for individuals struggling to achieve adequate hydration, but infusion frequency and volume must be determined on an individual basis, considering fluid intake and output.

Vitamins and Minerals

Individuals diagnosed with cancer are often interested in taking vitamin and mineral supplements because they believe these dietary supplements can improve their tolerance of treatment, enhance their immune system, or even reverse the course of their disease. Others may see dietary supplementation as a way to make up for presumed nutritional deficiencies at the time of diagnosis caused by poor diet and lifestyle choices. If individuals are experiencing difficulty with eating and treatment-related side effects, a standard multivitamin and mineral supplement that provides no more than 100% of the dietary reference intakes (DRIs) is considered safe (Rock et al, 2012). In contrast, the American Institute for Cancer Research (AICR) encourages all people (including cancer survivors) not to use dietary supplements for cancer prevention, citing evidence that high-dose dietary supplementation can have cancer-promoting effects (Martinez et al, 2012; Moyer, 2014; WCRF, AICR, 2007). According to the recommendations from leading national scientific groups, whether for primary or secondary prevention, individuals should attempt to meet vitamin and mineral needs though the foods they eat rather than use dietary supplements. In some instances during and after a cancer diagnosis, supplementation or restriction of specific micronutrients may be required above or below DRI levels, depending on medical diagnosis and laboratory analysis (e.g., iron supplementation for iron-deficiency anemia, B_{12} injections, and folic acid supplementation during treatment with the chemotherapy agent pemetrexed [Alimta]).

Supplement Use

Despite recommendations to the contrary, the majority of cancer survivors continue to use dietary supplements during all phases of anticancer treatment. Unless specifically instructed to do so, oncology practitioners ask that cancer survivors avoid use of dietary supplements during treatment, particularly the antioxidant dietary supplements such as vitamins A, C, E, beta-carotene, zinc, selenium, coenzyme Q10, and green tea extract, as the practice remains controversial. Studies have shown inhibition and enhancement of the antitumor effects of radiation therapy and chemotherapy (Rock et al, 2012). Well-designed studies evaluating larger numbers of individuals are still needed.

Nutrition Diagnosis

Nutrition diagnosis identifies the specific nutrition problems that can be resolved or improved through nutrition intervention (AND, 2012a; see the Clinical Insight box Common Nutrition Diagnoses for Patients with Cancer).

Nutrition Intervention

Nutrition intervention outlines specific actions to manage a nutrition diagnosis (see Chapter 10). It includes two distinct, interrelated components—planning and implementing nutrition interventions (AND, 2013). The Oncology Toolkit (www.eatright.org) recommends careful appraisal if the planned nutrition intervention will negatively affect patient safety or possibly interfere with the cancer treatment (AND, 2010). The Toolkit also advises evaluation of the nutrition intervention's likely effectiveness for improving nutrition status, possible financial burden, and patient acceptance.

Intervention goals should be specific, achievable, and individualized to encourage cooperation. Goals must be directed toward an objective measure such as body weight or some other meaningful index. Another goal is to minimize the effects of "nutrition impact symptoms" and to maximize the individual's nutritional parameters. Nutrition impact symptoms can be defined as symptoms and side effects of cancer and cancer treatment that directly affect the nutrition status. Consultation with the individual, caregivers, or family members regarding expected problems and their possible solutions should be initiated early in the course of cancer therapy and should continue in conjunction with follow-up nutrition assessment and care.

The adverse nutritional effects of cancer can be severe and may be compounded by the effects of the treatment regimens and the psychological effects of cancer. The result is often a profound depletion of nutrient stores and deterioration in nutrition status. Malnutrition, anorexia (loss of appetite), and weight loss are significant issues in cancer care and are often present in many individuals at the time of diagnosis, even in children. The incidence of malnutrition among individuals with cancer has been estimated to be between 15% and 80% (Santarpia et al, 2011). Studies consistently show that even small amounts of weight loss (less than 5% of body weight) before treatment is associated with a poorer prognosis and decreased quality of life, thus reinforcing the importance of early MNT (Fearon, 2008).

CLINICAL INSIGHT

Common Nutrition Diagnoses for Patients with Cancer
Using the Problem, Etiology, and Signs and Symptoms Format

Intake Domain
- Inadequate oral intake *related to* pelvic radiation therapy *as evidenced by* diarrhea and 2½ lb weight loss in the preceding week
- Inadequate enteral nutrition (EN) infusion *related to* intolerance of EN *as evidenced by* nausea, abdominal distention, and weight loss of 3 lb in the preceding 5 days
- Malnutrition *related to* cancer cachexia *as evidenced by* wasting of temporalis and interosseous muscles, and weight loss of more than 7.5% in 3 months

Clinical Domain
- Altered GI function *related to* recent ileostomy surgery *as evidenced by* 2 L/day ostomy diarrhea output, and the need for daily IV hydration during the preceding week
- Altered GI function *related to* biweekly chemotherapy *as evidenced by* nausea, vomiting, and anorexia in the preceding 4 days

- Swallowing difficulty *related to* an obstructing esophageal tumor *as evidenced by* dysphagia, odynophagia, and 10-pound weight loss in the preceding month

Behavioral-Environmental Domain
- Limited access to nutrition-related supplies *related to* lack of insurance and financial resources *as evidenced by* not using the prescribed amount of tube feeding formula and continued weight loss to 80% of usual weight during the preceding month
- Intake of unsafe food *related to* exposure to contaminated food while neutropenic *as evidenced by* hospitalization, diarrhea, and positive stool culture for salmonella
- Undesirable food choices *related to* an unwillingness to apply nutrition information *as evidenced by* ongoing diarrhea and diet history of continued high fiber food intake while undergoing pelvic radiation therapy

Oral Nutrition Management Strategies

Oral feeding is the goal, however individuals often experience symptoms that make it difficult. Strategies for modifying dietary intake may be necessary and depend on the specific eating problem and the individual's nutritional status. Food and its presentation may need modification. Liquid medical food supplements may be recommended for those unable to consume enough energy and protein to maintain weight and nutrition status, however real food is optimal (see Chapter 13). Education materials with suggestions for improving oral intake and managing treatment-related side effects are at the end of the chapter and include Eating Hints, Chemotherapy and You, and Radiation Therapy and You (NIH, NCI, 2011a, 2011b, 2012). Table 36-7 outlines examples of nutrition intervention strategies.

Managing Anorexia and Alterations in Taste and Smell

Sometimes even before diagnosis, and then throughout cancer treatment, individuals may report anorexia, early satiety, and decreased food intake. Alterations in taste and smell are common problems. Taste alterations can be associated with the disease itself, certain chemotherapy agents, radiation therapy, or surgery to the head and neck. Chemotherapy-induced, learned taste aversions have been reported in adults and children. Individuals also may develop a heightened sense of smell that results in sensitivity to food preparation odors and aversions to nonfood items such as soaps or perfumes. These sensation abnormalities do not consistently correlate with the tumor site, extent of tumor involvement, tumor response to therapy, or food preferences and intake. Nutrition interventions that decrease the aroma of foods, such as serving foods cold instead of hot, may be helpful.

Alterations in Energy Metabolism Resulting from Cancer

Energy metabolism is related intimately to carbohydrate, protein, and lipid metabolism, all of which are altered by tumor growth. Tumors exert a consistent demand for glucose, exhibit a

---

TABLE 36-7   Nutrition Intervention Strategies for Patients with Cancer

Side Effect or Symptom	Strategies
Anorexia, poor appetite	• Encourage small, more frequent nutrient dense meals and snacks. • Recommend adding protein and calories to favorite foods. • Recommend use of protein and calorie-containing supplements (e.g., whey or soy powder, nutritional supplements). • Keep nutrient dense foods close at hand and snack frequently. • Advise capitalizing on times when feeling best. • Recommend eating meals and snacks in a pleasant atmosphere. • Suggest viewing eating as part of treatment. • Encourage activities of daily living and physical activity as able.
Nausea and vomiting	• Recommend eating small, more frequent meals and snacks. • Suggest sipping on cool or room temperature clear liquids in small amounts. • Advise the avoidance of high-fat, greasy, spicy, or overly sweet foods. • Advise the avoidance of foods with strong odors. • Encourage the consumption of bland, soft, easy-to-digest foods on scheduled treatment days. • Encourage compliance with medications that are prescribed to control nausea.
Diarrhea	• Encourage the intake of hydrating liquids such as water, clear juices, broth, gelatin, popsicles, sports drinks. • Recommend a low-fiber diet and the avoidance of high-fiber foods, such as nuts, raw fruits and vegetables, and whole-grain breads and cereals. • Advise the avoidance of sugar alcohol–containing foods such as sugar-free candies and gums (e.g., mannitol, xylitol, sorbitol). • Encourage the intake of soluble fiber such as applesauce, bananas, canned peaches, white rice, or pasta. • Encourage compliance with medications prescribed to control diarrhea.
Constipation	• Recommend increasing the intake of high-fiber foods such as whole grains, fresh or cooked fruits and vegetables, especially those with skins and seeds, dried fruits, beans, and nuts. • Encourage the intake of 64 ounces of fluid each day. • Recommend the use of probiotic-containing foods or supplements. • Encourage activities of daily living and physical activity as able. • Encourage compliance with fiber supplements and/or medications that affect bowel function and are prescribed to manage constipation.
Sore throat, esophagitis	• Recommend the intake of softer, moister foods with extra sauces, dressings, or gravies. • Advise the avoidance of dry, coarse, or rough foods. • Avoid alcohol, citrus, caffeine, tomatoes, vinegar, and hot peppers. • Suggest experimenting with food temperatures (e.g. warm, cool, or icy) to find which temperature is the most soothing. • Encourage compliance with medications prescribed to manage esophagitis and/or painful swallowing.
Sore mouth, mucositis, or thrush	• Recommend good oral hygiene (e.g., rinse mouth frequently, keep mouth clean). • Recommend the intake of softer, moister foods with extra sauces, dressings, and gravies. • Suggest serving foods at cool or room temperatures. • Advise the avoidance of alcoholic beverages, citrus, caffeine, tomatoes, vinegar and hot peppers; and dry, coarse, or rough foods. • Suggest eating foods at room temperature or chilled. • Encourage compliance with medications prescribed to manage oral pain and/or infection.

Continued

TABLE 36-7	Nutrition Intervention Strategies for Patients with Cancer—cont'd
Side Effect or Symptom	**Strategies**
Fatigue	• Recommend the intake of small, frequent meals and snacks. • Recommend the intake of easy-to-prepare, easy-to-eat foods. • Advise keeping nutrient dense snacks close at hand and snack frequently. • Suggest eating when appetite is best. • Encourage activities of daily living and physical activity as able.
Neutropenia	• Advise frequent hand washing and keep kitchen surfaces and utensils clean. • Advise the avoidance of raw or undercooked animal products, including meat, pork, game, poultry, eggs, and fish. • Advise washing all fresh fruits and vegetables before eating. • "When in doubt, throw out" and "No oldy or moldy."
Altered taste or smell	• Recommend good oral hygiene practices (e.g., rinse mouth frequently, keep mouth clean). • Suggest trying marinades and spices to mask strange tastes. • Recommend using plastic utensils if metallic tastes are a problem. • Recommend eating cooler foods, rather than warmer foods.
Thickened saliva	• Suggest sipping on liquids throughout the day to keep the oral cavity moist. • Recommend thinning oral secretions with club soda, seltzer water, or papaya nectar. • Suggest trying guaifenesin to help thin oral secretions. • Recommend using a cool mist humidifier while sleeping.
Xerostomia	• Suggest sipping on liquids throughout the day to keep the oral cavity moist. • Suggest trying tart foods to stimulate saliva, if open sores are not present. • Recommend alternating bites of food with sips of liquids at meals. • Recommend eating soft, moist foods with extra sauces, dressings, or gravies. • Advise avoidance of alcoholic beverages and alcohol-containing mouthwash. • Recommend good oral hygiene (e.g., rinse mouth frequently, keep mouth clean). • Recommend a cool mist humidifier while resting or sleeping.

Data from Grant BL et al, editors: *American Cancer Society's complete guide to nutrition for cancer survivors*, ed 2, Atlanta, 2010, American Cancer Society; National Cancer Institute (NCI): *Eating Hints* (website): http://www.cancer.gov/publications/patient-education/eatinghints.pdf, 2011. Accessed March 29, 2014; Elliot L: Symptom management of cancer thera-pies. In Leser M et al, editors: *Oncology nutrition for clinical practice*, Chicago, 2013, Oncology Nutrition Dietetic Practice Group of the Academy of Nutrition and Dietetics.

characteristically high rate of anaerobic metabolism, and yield lactate as the end product. This expanded lactic acid pool requires an increased rate of host gluconeogenesis via Cori cycle activity, which is increased in some people with cancer but not in others. Protein breakdown and lipolysis take place at increasing rates to maintain high rates of glucose synthesis. There is glucose intolerance and insulin resistance, characterized by excess fatty acid oxidation and decreased uptake and use of glucose by muscle.

Alterations in protein metabolism appear to be directed toward providing adequate amino acids for tumor growth. Most notable is the loss of skeletal muscle protein caused by increased protein breakdown, as well as decreased protein synthesis.

Managing Cancer Cachexia

A common secondary diagnosis in people with advanced cancer is a variant of protein-energy malnutrition. This syndrome is termed cancer cachexia and is characterized by progressive weight loss, anorexia, generalized wasting and weakness, immunosuppression, altered basal metabolic rate, and abnormalities in fluid and energy metabolism. There is also increased loss of adipose tissue, which is related to an increased rate of lipolysis, rather than a decrease in lipogenesis. Increased levels of lipid-mobilizing factor and proteolysis-inducing factor secreted by tumor cells will lead to increased loss of fat and muscle mass. Individuals at the time of diagnosis with breast or hematologic cancers rarely present with significant weight loss, whereas individuals with lung, esophageal, or head and neck cancers often exhibit substantial weight loss. Cancer cachexia is caused in part by cytokines (immune-modulating agents), produced by the cancer itself or by the immune system in response to the cancer. Cytokines can cause metabolic changes and wasting that is similar to changes seen in inflammation (see Chapter 3.) Proinflammatory cytokines include tumor necrosis factor (TNF)-α (cachectin) and TNF-β, interleukin (IL)-1, IL-6, and interferon-α. These cytokines have overlapping physiologic activities, which makes it likely that no single substance is the sole cause. Resting energy expenditure (REE) is elevated, which is in contrast to the REE in chronic starvation, wherein the body adapts to conserve energy and preserve body tissue. Cancer cachexia and the associated wasting often increase closer to the time of death.

Pharmacotherapy

The pharmacologic management of cachexia and anorexia requires careful evaluation based on the individual's treatment goals and prognosis and on close monitoring of symptoms. Although cancer cachexia cannot be reversed by conventional nutrition support, anorexia, a common cancer-related condition, is amenable to treatment with nutrition counseling, diet modification, and pharmacotherapy. A number of pharmacologic agents are currently under investigation for their impact on anorexia, including antihistamines (Periactin), corticosteroids (Decadron, Solu-medrol), progestational agents (Provera, Megace), prokinetic agents (Reglan), and antidepressants (Remeron) (Elliot, 2013).

Medical marijuana, or cannabis, is a controlled substance in the United States, and it is illegal except in the few states that have enacted laws to legalize its use. According to the NCI PDQ, cannabinoids, which are the active chemicals in cannabis, can be useful in treating the side effects of nausea and vomiting and anorexia from cancer and cancer treatment (NIH, NCI, 2014b).

The FDA has not approved medical marijuana for cancer or cancer treatment application; however, it has approved two cannabinoids, Marinol and Cesamet, for individuals experiencing chemotherapy–related nausea and vomiting (NIH, NCI, 2014b).

Managing Other Cancer-Related Metabolic Abnormalities

Metabolic alterations vary by tumor type. An individual's immunologic function can be impaired, apparently as the result of the disease, cancer treatment, or progressive malnutrition. In addition to the cancer-induced metabolic effects, the mass of the tumor may anatomically alter the physiology of specific organ systems. The activity of several enzyme systems involved with digestion and absorption can be affected, as can certain endocrine functions.

Critical imbalances in fluid and electrolyte status can occur in people who have cancers or are undergoing cancer treatments that promote excessive diarrhea, vomiting, or malabsorption. Profuse and often severe diarrhea can result from partial bowel obstructions and endocrine-secreting tumors such as those secreting serotonin (carcinoid tumors), calcitonin, or gastrin (Zollinger-Ellison syndrome). The use of antimetabolites, alkylating agents, and antibiotics may also lead to the development of severe diarrhea. In some instances, people who are immunocompromised or have undergone GI surgery may experience profuse diarrhea that is caused by intestinal pathogens such as *Clostridium difficile.*

Persistent vomiting is associated with intestinal obstruction, radiation therapy to the stomach and abdomen or brain, highly emetogenic (nausea-causing) chemotherapy agents, intracranial tumors, and advanced cancer (Iwamoto et al, 2012). Careful assessment and evaluation of the cause of the diarrhea or vomiting is critical for effective management. Malabsorption may be caused by treatment-related pancreatic dysfunction, postsurgical short gut syndrome, acute or chronic radiation enteritis (inflammation of the GI tract tissues secondary to radiation), excess serotonin, steatorrhea, or chronic diarrhea.

Hypercalcemia may occur in individuals with bone metastases, caused by the osteolytic activity of tumor cells releasing calcium into the extracellular fluid. Hypercalcemia is potentially fatal and is associated most commonly with multiple myeloma, lung cancer, and advanced breast and prostate cancer. Nausea, weakness, fatigue, lethargy, and confusion occur. Medical management of hypercalcemia includes rehydration and use of antihypercalcemic agents. Calcium supplementation from dietary supplements and antacids should be avoided. Restricting the intake of foods containing calcium is not indicated because the consumption of these foods has little effect in the overall management of hypercalcemia.

NUTRITIONAL IMPACT OF CANCER TREATMENTS

Chemotherapy

Chemotherapy uses chemical agents or medications to treat cancer. Classifications of chemotherapy cytotoxic agents include alkylating agents, antimetabolites, antitumor antibiotics, miscellaneous agents, nitrosoureas, and plant alkaloids (Wilkes and Barton-Burke, 2013). Once in the bloodstream, these agents are carried through the body to reach as many cancer cells as possible. Routes of administration for chemotherapy include the following:
- Oral: capsule, pill, or liquid
- Intravenous (IV): delivery of medication via an injection or an indwelling catheter into a vein

- Intraperitoneal: delivery of medication via a catheter directly into the abdominal cavity
- Intravesicular: delivery of medication via a Foley catheter directly into the bladder
- Intrathecal: delivery of medication via an injection into the central nervous system using an Ommaya reservoir or a lumbar puncture (Polovich et al, 2014)

Whereas surgery and radiation therapy are used to treat localized tumors, chemotherapy is a systemic therapy that affects the malignant tissue and normal cells as well. Cells of the body with a rapid turnover such as bone marrow, hair follicles, and the mucosa of the alimentary tract are the most affected. As a result, nutrition intake and nutrition status can be adversely affected. Nutrition-related symptoms include myelosuppression (suppression of bone marrow production of neutrophils, platelets, and red blood cells), anemia, fatigue, nausea and vomiting, loss of appetite, mucositis, changes in taste and smell, xerostomia (mouth dryness), dysphagia, and altered bowel function such as diarrhea or constipation (Table 36-8).

The severity of the side effects depends on the specific agents used, dosage, duration of treatment, number of treatment cycles, accompanying drugs, individual response, and current health status. The timely and appropriate use of supportive therapies such as antiemetics, antidiarrheals, hematopoietic agents, and antibiotics, as well as dietary changes, is important. Many people experience significant side effects, especially in "dose-intensive" multiple-agent chemotherapy regimens; neutropenia (reduced white blood cells or neutrophils) and myelosuppression are the primary factors limiting chemotherapy administration. Commonly experienced chemotherapy induced toxicities affecting the GI system include mucositis, nausea, vomiting, diarrhea, and constipation. Chemotherapy related taste abnormalities can lead to anorexia and decreased oral intake. Symptoms of GI toxicity are usually temporary; however, some multiagent chemotherapy regimens may lead to lasting GI side effects.

Diarrhea

Diarrhea is a common side effect of certain chemotherapy agents. Left unmanaged, it can lead to depletion of fluids, electrolytes, malnutrition, and even hospitalization. The intestinal mucosa and digestive processes can be affected, thus altering digestion and absorption to some degree. Protein, energy, and vitamin metabolism may be impaired.

Nausea and Vomiting

Chemotherapy induced nausea and vomiting are commonly classified as anticipatory (occurs before receiving treatment), acute (occurs within the first 24 hours after receiving treatment), or delayed (occurs 1 to 4 days after treatment), each of which is characterized by distinct pathophysiologic events and requires different therapeutic interventions. Effective agents for treatment-related nausea and vomiting are the serotonin antagonists (e.g., ondansetron, granisetron, and dolasetron), neurokinin-1 (NK-1) receptor antagonists (e.g., aprepitant), dopamine antagonists (e.g., metoclopramide, prochlorperazine), and corticosteroids such as dexamethasone (Polovich et al, 2014). Other antiemetic agents include cannabinoids (e.g., dronabinol, nabilone) and benzodiazepines (e.g., lorazepam, diazepam).

Food-Drug Interactions

Nutrition professionals can gain valuable insights regarding possible drug-nutrient interactions and contraindications by reviewing product medication inserts, pharmacy resource books,

TABLE 36-8 Nutrition-Related Effects of Antineoplastic Agents: Chemotherapy, Biotherapy, and Hormone Therapy

Agent Classification	Common Nutrition Impact Symptom
CHEMOTHERAPY **Alkylating Agents** • Bendamustine (Treanda), cisplatin (Platinol), cyclophosphamide (Cytoxan), oxaliplatin (Eloxatin), temozolomide (Temodar)	• Myelosuppression, anorexia, nausea, vomiting, fatigue, renal toxicity
Antitumor Antibiotics • Bleomycin (Blenoxane), doxorubicin (Adriamycin), Mitomycin (Mutamycin)	• Myelosuppression, anorexia, nausea, vomiting, fatigue, diarrhea, mucositis
Antimetabolites • Capecitabine (Xeloda), cytarabine (ARA-C), 5-fluorouracil (5-FU), gemcitabine (Gemzar), methotrexate	• Myelosuppression, anorexia, nausea, vomiting, fatigue, diarrhea, mucositis
Plant Alkaloids • Camptosar (Irinotecan), etoposide (VP-16), docetaxel (Taxotere), paclitaxel (Taxol), vinorelbine (Navelbine)	• Myelosuppression, anorexia, nausea, vomiting, fatigue, peripheral neuropathy
Miscellaneous • Procarbazine (Matulane)	• Myelosuppression, nausea, vomiting, diarrhea, MAO inhibitor/avoid foods high in tyramine
BIOTHERAPY **Cytokines** • Interferon-alfa (Intron A), interleukin (IL-2)	• Myelosuppression, anorexia, fatigue, nausea, flu-like symptoms, chills
Monoclonal Antibodies • Cetuximab (Erbitux), Rituximab (Rituxan), Trastuzumab (Herceptin)	• Infusion reaction of chills, fever, headache, hypotension; myelosuppression; nausea; vomiting; rash
Protein-Targeted Therapies: Small Molecule Inhibitors • Tyrosine kinase inhibitors: erlotinib (Tarceva), imatinib mesylate (Gleevec) • mTOR inhibitors: everolimus (Affinitor), temsirolimus (Torisel) • Proteasome inhibitor: bortezomib (Velcade)	• Fever, chills, rash, diarrhea, fatigue, anorexia
Angiogenesis Inhibitors • Bevacizumab (Avastin), lenalidomide (Revlimid), thalidomide	• Hypertension, arterial thromboembolic events, gastrointestinal perforation, hemorrhage, proteinuria, hypothyroidism
Cancer Vaccines • Sipuleucel-T (Provenge)	• Fever, chills, back pain, loss of appetite, fatigue, nausea, flu-like symptoms
HORMONE THERAPY **Antiandrogens** • Bicalutamide (Casodex); flutamide (Eulexin)	• Hot flashes, weight gain, fatigue, bone pain
Luteinizing Hormone-Releasing Hormone (LHRH) Antagonist • Leuprolide (Lupron), goserelin (Zoladex)	• Hot flashes, fatigue, edema, nausea, bone pain, muscle weakness, headache
Selective Estrogen Receptor Modulators (SERMs) • Raloxifene (Evista), tamoxifen (Novadex), toremifene (Fareston)	• Thromboembolic events, fluid retention, hot flashes, nausea, joint discomfort, diarrhea, weight gain
Aromatase Inhibitors (AIs) • Anastrozole (Arimidex), letrozole (Femara), exemestane (Aromasin)	• Hot flashes, nausea, vomiting, thromboembolic events, fever, joint aches and pains
Progesterones • Megestrol acetate (Megace)	• Increased appetite, weight gain, fluid retention; thromboembolic events

Data from Polovich M et al: *Chemotherapy and biotherapy guidelines and recommendations for practice*, ed 4, Pittsburgh, 2014, Oncology Nursing Society; Wilkes GM, Barton-Burke M: *2014 Oncology nursing drug handbook*, Burlington, 2013, Jones and Bartlett; Chu E, Devita VT: *Physician's cancer chemotherapy drug manual*, Boston, 2014, Jones and Bartlet, http://www.chemocare com. Accessed on March 29, 2014.

and medication databases or by consulting with pharmacy personnel (see Chapter 8). Some chemotherapy agents can cause potentially severe adverse events (Grant, 2013), for example:

• Individuals with certain types of lung cancer who are being treated with pemetrexed (Alimta) require vitamin B_{12} (often by injection) and folic acid supplementation throughout the duration of their therapy to avoid significant anemia associated with this chemotherapy agent.

• A severe hypertensive event is possible when tyramine-rich foods and beverages are consumed while taking procarbazine (Matulane), a chemotherapy agent commonly used to treat brain cancer (see Box 8-4).

- Individuals with colon cancer receiving oxaliplatin (Eloxatin) should not drink, eat, or handle cold drinks or foods for up to 5 days because of treatment-related dysesthesias or transient paresthesias of the hands, feet, and throat.
- To prevent unnecessary gastric upset, individuals taking the medication capecitabine (Xeloda) must take the medication within 30 minutes of eating food or a meal. Conversely, medications such as erlotinib (Tarceva) should not be taken with food; it can cause a rash and profound diarrhea unless taken on an empty stomach.

Oral Changes

People with altered taste acuity (dysgeusia, hypogeusia, ageusia) may benefit from increased use of flavorings and seasonings during food preparation. Meat aversions may require the elimination of red meats, which tend to be strong in flavor, or the substitution of alternative protein sources. Herpes simplex virus and *Candida albicans* (thrush) account for most oral infections. In addition to causing oral infections, some agents, especially corticosteroids, can cause hyperglycemia and can lead to excessive losses of urinary protein, potassium, and calcium.

Mucositis

Oral **mucositis**, an inflammation of the mucous membranes lining the oropharynx and esophagus, is a common side effect of some types of chemotherapy (Figure 36-2). Although many interventions exist, most strategies lack scientific evidence (Brown, 2009). General care guidelines include recommending daily oral care (e.g., keeping the mouth clean, avoidance of tobacco, alcohol, and irritating foods) and the use of bland rinses (e.g., baking soda or saline rinses). Bland liquids and soft solids are usually better tolerated in individuals with oral or esophageal mucositis and strong-flavored, acidic, or spicy foods also should be avoided. Commercially prepared liquid medical food supplements can be useful.

Biotherapy

Biotherapy is immunotherapy, in which a group of cancer treatment drugs prescribed to stimulate the body's own immune system and natural defenses are used to treat cancer. Biotherapy is sometimes used by itself, but it is given most often in combination with chemotherapy drugs. Different kinds of biotherapy drugs used to help the immune system recognize cancer cells and strengthen its ability to destroy them include:

- Cytokines such as interferon and IL-2 for treatment of malignant melanoma and metastatic melanoma.
- Monoclonal antibodies such as trastuzumab (Herceptin) for treatment of specific types of breast cancer, and rituximab (Rituxan) for treatment of non-Hodgkin lymphoma.
- Antiangiogenesis inhibitors prevent and reduce the growth of new blood vessels and prevent tumor invasion. These agents are most frequently used in combination with other chemotherapy agents to maximize their effectiveness. An example of an antiangiogenic agent used to treat colon or brain cancer is bevacizumab (Avastin).
- Cancer vaccines such as sipuleucel-T (Provenge) made from an individual's own cancer or substances from tumor cells are currently under investigation in clinical cancer trials (Grant, 2013; Wilkes and Barton-Burke, 2013).

Other types of biotherapy drugs are groups of proteins that cause blood cells to grow and mature (NIH, NCI, 2015). These drugs are called **hematopoietic growth factors**. They include supportive care medications such as darbepoetin (Aranesp) or epoetin alfa (Procrit) to stimulate red blood cell production, and filgrastim (Neupogen) or pegfilgrastim (Neulasta) to stimulate the production of neutrophils in the bone marrow. Individuals receiving these agents may experience fatigue, chills, fever, and flu-like symptoms.

Hormone Therapy

Hormone therapy adds, blocks, or removes hormones to slow or stop the growth of hormone-sensitive breast or prostate cancer (NIH, NCI, 2015). Examples of these agents include tamoxifen (Nolvadex) and anastrozole (Arimidex) for breast cancer and leuprolide (Lupron) or bicalutamide (Casodex) for prostate cancer. Side effects commonly include hot flashes, decreased libido, and bone pain (Wilkes and Barton-Burke, 2013).

Radiation Therapy

Radiation therapy, ionizing radiation used in multiple fractionated doses, is used to cure, control, or palliate cancer. Radiation therapy can be delivered externally into the body from a megavoltage machine or with brachytherapy by placing a radioactive source (implant) in or near the tumor to deliver a highly localized dose. Advances in technology to deliver radiation therapy with precise accuracy include radiation surgery (e.g., stereotactic radiosurgery) and intensity-modulated radiation therapy (IMRT). Whereas chemotherapy is a systemic therapy, radiation therapy affects only the tumor and the surrounding area. The side effects of radiation therapy are usually limited to the specific site being irradiated. Chemotherapy agents may also be given in combination with radiation therapy to produce a radiation-enhancing effect. People receiving

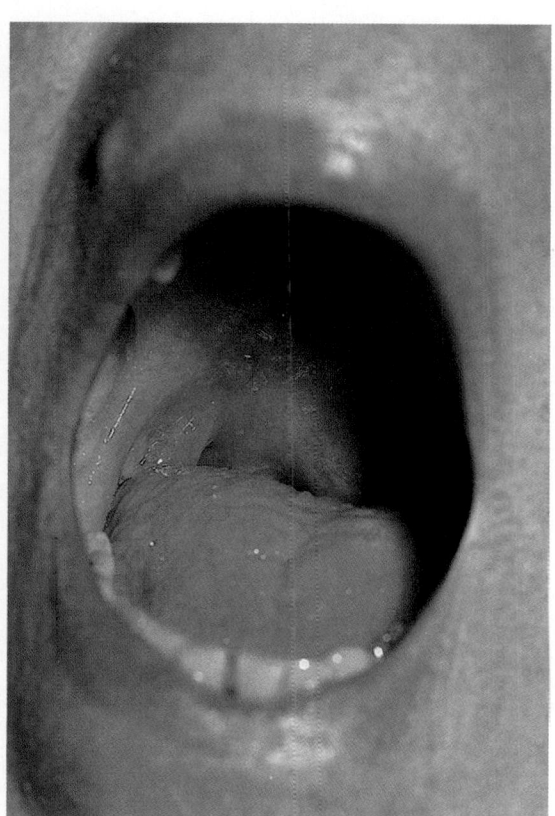

FIGURE 36-2 Oral mucositis. (From Kanski JL: *Clinical diagnosis in ophthalmology,* ed 1, 2006, Elsevier.)

multimodality therapy often experience side effects sooner and with greater intensity.

The acute side effects of radiation therapy when used alone generally occur around the second or third week of treatment and usually resolve within 2 to 4 weeks after the radiation therapy has been completed. Late effects of radiation therapy may happen several weeks, months, or even years after treatment. Commonly experienced nutrition-related symptoms include fatigue, loss of appetite, skin changes, and hair loss in the area being treated (Table 36-9).

Radiation to the Head and Neck

Treatment for head and neck cancer usually includes a multimodality approach with aggressive chemotherapy, radiation therapy, and often surgery. Radiation therapy to the head and neck can cause acute nutrition-related symptoms: sore mouth, altered taste and smell, dysphagia and odynophagia, mucositis, xerostomia, anorexia, fatigue, and weight loss (Havrila et al, 2010). Prophylactic placement of percutaneous endoscopic gastrostomy (PEG) feeding tubes can help to reduce treatment-associated weight loss and malnutrition (NCCN, 2013).

Salivary stimulants and substitutes or oral lubricants are beneficial for temporary relief of xerostomia (diminished salivation or loss of salivation) caused by head and neck radiation therapy or certain types of medications (e.g., pain medications). In addition, liquids and foods with sauces and gravies are usually well tolerated. Late effects of radiation therapy may include dental caries, permanent xerostomia, trismus (an inability to fully open the mouth), and osteoradionecrosis of the jaw (necrosis of the bone caused by exposure to radiation therapy).

Before beginning therapy, individuals should undergo a dental evaluation and thorough teeth cleaning and receive instruction in good oral hygiene and care, including daily brushing and rinsing (National Institute of Dental and Craniofacial Research [NIDCR], 2014). After therapy has been completed, individuals should continue to have close dental monitoring and follow-up. Individuals may also benefit from a referral to a speech therapist for assessment and evaluation of swallowing function.

Radiation to the Thorax

Nutrition-related symptoms of radiation therapy to the thorax (chest) can include heartburn and acute esophagitis, accompanied by dysphagia and odynophagia. Late effects include possible esophageal fibrosis and stenosis. When this occurs, individuals are generally able to swallow only liquids, and the use of medical food supplements and enteral nutrition support (EN) may be necessary to meet nutritional needs (see Chapter 13.) Often individuals undergo esophageal dilations or swallowing therapy and rehabilitation to improve swallowing function.

Radiation to the Abdomen or Pelvis

Radiation therapy to the abdomen or pelvis may cause gastritis or enteritis that can be accompanied by nausea, vomiting, diarrhea, and anorexia. Late effects can include lasting GI damage such as malabsorption of disaccharides (e.g., lactose), fats, vitamins, minerals, and electrolytes. Proactive management includes encouraging affected individuals to consume soluble fiber, to increase intake of hydrating liquids, and to avoid eating high nonsoluble fiber or lactose-containing foods. To alleviate symptoms, medications such as antidiarrheals like loperamide may be given to reduce intestinal motility.

TABLE 36-9　Nutrition-Related Effects of Radiation Therapy

Site of Radiation Therapy	Common Nutrition-Related Symptom
Central nervous system (brain and spinal cord)	**Acute Effects**
	Nausea, vomiting
	Fatigue
	Loss of appetite
	Hyperglycemia associated with corticosteroids
	Late Effects (>90 days after treatment)
	Headache, lethargy
Head and neck (tongue, larynx, pharynx, oropharynx, nasopharynx, tonsils, salivary glands)	**Acute Effects**
	Xerostomia
	Mucositis
	Sore mouth and throat
	Thick saliva/oral secretions
	Dysphagia, odynophagia
	Alterations in taste and smell
	Fatigue
	Loss of appetite
	Late Effects (>90 days after treatment)
	Mucosal atrophy and dryness
	Salivary glands—xerostomia, fibrosis
	Trismus
	Osteoradionecrosis
	Alterations in taste and smell
Thorax (esophagus, lung, breast)	**Acute Effects**
	Esophagitis
	Dysphagia, odynophagia
	Heartburn
	Fatigue
	Loss of appetite
	Late Effects (>90 days after treatment)
	Esophageal—fibrosis, stenosis, stricture, ulceration
	Cardiac—angina on effort, pericarditis, cardiac enlargement
	Pulmonary—dry cough, fibrosis, pneumonitis
Abdomen and pelvis (stomach, ovaries, uterus, colon, rectum)	**Acute Effects**
	Nausea, vomiting
	Changes in bowel function—diarrhea, cramping, bloating, gas
	Changes in urinary function—increased frequency, burning sensation with urination
	Acute colitis or enteritis
	Lactose intolerance
	Fatigue
	Loss of appetite
	Late Effects (>90 days after treatment)
	Diarrhea, malabsorption, maldigestion
	Chronic colitis or enteritis
	Intestinal—stricture, ulceration, obstruction, perforation, fistula
	Urinary—hematuria, cystitis

Data from Iwamoto RR et al: *Manual for radiation oncology and nursing practice and education*, ed 4, Pittsburgh, 2012, Oncology Nursing Society; Grant B: Nutritional effects of cancer treatment: chemotherapy, biotherapy, hormone therapy and radiation therapy. In Leser M et al, editors: *Oncology nutrition for clinical practice*, Chicago, 2013, Oncology Nutrition Dietetic Practice Group of the Academy of Nutrition and Dietetics.

Chronic radiation enteritis can develop with diarrhea, ulceration, or obstruction, intensifying the risk of malnutrition. Chronic radiation enteritis combined with or without significant bowel resection can result in bowel dysfunction and short bowel syndrome (SBS). The severity of this condition depends on the length and location of the nonfunctional or resected bowel and generally is diagnosed when the individual has less than 150 cm of small intestine remaining. The sequelae of SBS include malabsorption, malnutrition, dehydration, weight loss, fatigue, and lactose intolerance (Havrila et al, 2010) (see Chapter 28).

Initially parenteral nutrition (PN) may be required, and frequent monitoring of fluids and electrolytes may be necessary for weeks or months. Individuals with SBS may require an oral diet restricted to defined formula tube feedings or to frequent small meals high in protein, low in fat and fiber, and lactose free. Dietary supplements that contain vitamin B_{12}, folic acid, thiamin, calcium, and vitamins A, E, and K often are indicated to prevent deficiencies. Serum concentrations of various minerals also should be monitored and adjusted as needed.

Total-Body Irradiation

Total-body irradiation (TBI) is a technique of radiation therapy that is used in hematopoietic cell transplantation (HCT) to eliminate malignant cells, to ablate the bone marrow and make room for the engraftment of the infused hematopoietic cells, and to suppress the immune system to decrease the risk of rejection. Commonly encountered side effects are fever, nausea, vomiting, headache, mucositis, parotitis (inflammation of the parotid glands), xerostomia, diarrhea, anorexia, fatigue, and associated weight loss.

Surgery

The surgical resection or removal of any part of the alimentary tract (mouth to anus), as well as the malignant disease process, can potentially impair normal digestion and absorption. Surgery may be used as a single mode of cancer treatment, or it may be combined with preoperative or postoperative adjuvant chemotherapy or radiation therapy. After surgery, individuals commonly experience fatigue, and temporary changes in appetite and bowel function caused by anesthesia, and pain. They often require additional energy and protein for wound healing and recovery. Most side effects are temporary and dissipate after a few days after surgery. However, some surgical interventions have long-lasting nutritional implications (Table 36-10). When performing a nutrition assessment, it is very important to understand which part of the alimentary tract has been affected or surgically removed so that the appropriate nutrition intervention can be recommended. (Refer to Chapter 1 for a review gastrointestinal physiology).

Head and Neck Cancer

Individuals with head and neck cancer often have difficulty with chewing and swallowing caused by the cancer itself or the specific surgical intervention required to remove cancerous tissues. There can be additional problems because of history of smoking and alcohol abuse, illicit drug use, and subsequent poor nutrition intake, which place these individuals at high risk for malnutrition and postoperative complications. Surgery often necessitates temporary or long-term reliance on EN support (e.g., PEG tube feedings) (see Chapter 13). Individuals who resume oral intake often have prolonged dysphagia and require modifications of food consistency and extensive training in chewing and swallowing. Referrals to a speech therapist can yield dramatic positive results through evaluation and

TABLE 36-10	Nutrition-Related Effects of Surgery in Cancer Treatment
Anatomic Site	**Nutrition Impact Symptoms**
Oral cavity	Difficulty with chewing and swallowing
	Aspiration potential
	Sore mouth and throat
	Xerostomia
	Alteration in taste and smell
Larynx	Alterations in normal swallowing, dysphagia
	Aspiration potential
Esophagus	Gastroparesis
	Indigestion, acid reflux
	Alterations in normal swallowing, dysphagia
	Decreased motility
	Anastomotic leak
Lung	Shortness of breath
	Early satiety
Stomach	Dumping syndrome
	Dehydration
	Early satiety
	Gastroparesis
	Fat malabsorption
	Vitamin and mineral malabsorption (vitamin B_{12} and D; calcium, iron)
Gallbladder and bile duct	Gastroparesis
	Hyperglycemia
	Fluid and electrolyte imbalance
	Vitamin and mineral malabsorption (vitamin A, D, E, and K; magnesium, calcium, zinc, iron)
Liver	Hyperglycemia
	Hypertriglyceridemia
	Fluid and electrolyte malabsorption
	Vitamin and mineral malabsorption (vitamin A, D, E, K, B_{12} and folic acid, magnesium, zinc)
Pancreas	Gastroparesis
	Fluid and electrolyte imbalance
	Hyperglycemia
	Fat malabsorption (vitamin A, D, E, K, B_{12}; calcium, zinc, iron)
Small bowel	Chyle leak
	Lactose intolerance
	Bile acid depletion
	Diarrhea
	Fluid and electrolyte imbalance
	Vitamin and mineral malabsorption (vitamin A, D, E, K, B_{12}; calcium, zinc, iron)
Colon and rectum	Increased transit time
	Diarrhea
	Dehydration
	Bloating, cramping, gas
	Fluid and electrolyte imbalance
	Vitamin and mineral malabsorption (vitamin B_{12}, sodium, potassium, magnesium, calcium)
Ovaries and uterus	Early satiety
	Bloating, cramping, and gas
Brain	Nausea, vomiting
	Hyperglycemia associated with corticosteroids

Data from Leser M et al, editors: *Oncology nutrition for clinical practice*, Chicago, 2013, Oncology Nutrition Dietetic Practice Group of Nutrition of the Academy of Nutrition and Dietetics; Huhmann MB, August D: Surgical oncology. In Marian M, Roberts S, editors: *Clinical nutrition for oncology patients*, Sudbury, Mass, 2010, Jones and Bartlett.

individualized instruction in swallowing and positioning techniques, as well as evaluation for aspiration risk (see Chapter 40).

Esophageal Cancer

Surgical intervention for treatment of esophageal cancer often requires partial or total removal of the esophagus. The stomach is commonly used for esophageal reconstruction. A feeding jejunostomy tube, which allows for early postoperative tube feedings, can be placed before an individual undergoes surgery or at the time of surgery. Usually the individual is able to progress to oral intake with specific dietary recommendations to minimize nutrition-related symptoms, which include reflux, dumping syndrome (discussed later in this chapter), dysmotility, gastroparesis, early satiety, vomiting, and fluid and electrolyte imbalances (Huhmann and August, 2010). Postsurgical recommendations include a low-fat diet with small, frequent feedings of energy-dense foods and avoidance of large amounts of fluids at any one time (see Chapter 27).

Gastric Cancer

Surgery is the most common treatment for cancer of the stomach, although chemotherapy and radiation therapy can be used before or after surgery to improve survival. Surgical interventions include partial, subtotal, or total gastrectomy. Placement of a jejunostomy feeding tube at surgery is advisable, and enteral nutrition (EN) support using a jejunal feeding tube is generally feasible within a few days after surgery.

Postgastrectomy syndrome encompasses a myriad of symptoms, including dumping syndrome, fat malabsorption, gastric stasis, lactose intolerance, anemias, and metabolic bone disease (osteoporosis, osteopenia, osteomalacia). Dumping syndrome is a common complication of gastric surgery, manifested by the rapid transit of foods or liquids, and the dilutional response of the small remaining stomach to highly osmotic bolus feedings. Individuals may experience GI and vasomotor symptoms such as abdominal cramps, diarrhea, nausea, vomiting, flushing, faintness, diaphoresis, and tachycardia (Huhmann and August, 2010). Individuals experiencing dumping syndrome should limit simple carbohydrates and liquids at meal times (see Chapter 27).

Malabsorption is another complication of gastric surgery; deficiency of iron, folic acid, and less commonly vitamin B_{12} can lead to anemia. Micronutrient deficiencies of calcium and fat-soluble vitamins are also common (Huhmann and August, 2010). Individuals benefit from consumption of six to eight small meals per day, with fluids taken between meals. There may be fat intolerance, especially if the vagal nerve is severed. Administration of pancreatic enzymes with meals may help when the duodenal mixing of food and pancreatic juices is inadequate (see Chapter 27).

Pancreatic Cancer

Cancer of the pancreas, with or without surgical resection, can have significant nutritional consequences. The Whipple procedure and the pylorus-sparing pancreatic duodenectomy are the most common pancreatic cancer surgeries. Postsurgical complications include delayed gastric emptying, early satiety, glucose intolerance, bile acid insufficiency, diarrhea, and fat malabsorption. Pancreatic enzyme replacement, the use of small, more frequent low-fat meals and snacks, and avoidance of simple carbohydrates aid digestion and absorption (see Chapter 29).

Cancers of the Intestinal Tract

Partial or total resections of the intestinal tract because of colorectal cancer or carcinoid syndrome may induce profound losses of fluid and electrolytes secondary to decreased transit time and diarrhea, the severity of which are related to the length and site of the resection. Resections of as little as 15 cm of the terminal ileum can result in bile salt losses that exceed the liver's capacity for resynthesis, and vitamin B_{12} absorption is affected. With depletion of the bile salt pool, steatorrhea develops. Nutrition intervention strategies consist of a diet low in fat, osmolality, lactose, and oxalates (see Chapters 28 and 38).

Hematopoietic Cell Transplantation (HCT)

Hematopoietic cell transplantation (HCT) is performed for the treatment of certain hematologic cancers such as leukemia, lymphoma, and multiple myeloma. The stem cells used for HCT arise from bone marrow, peripheral blood, or umbilical cord blood. The preparative regimen includes cytotoxic chemotherapy, with or without total-body irradiation (TBI). This treatment regimen is followed by intravenous (IV) infusion of hematopoietic cells from the individual (autologous), or from a histocompatible related or unrelated donor (allogeneic), or from an identical twin (syngeneic) (National Marrow Donor Program, 2015).

Because HCT procedures can significantly affect nutrition status, the individual undergoing HCT should have a thorough nutrition assessment before the initiation of therapy and reassessments and monitoring throughout the entire transplant course. The acute toxicities of immunosuppression that can last for 2 to 4 weeks after the transplant include nausea, vomiting, anorexia, dysgeusia, stomatitis, oral and esophageal mucositis, fatigue, and diarrhea. In addition, immunosuppressive medications can also adversely affect nutrition status.

Depending upon the transplant regimen, individuals may have little or no oral intake, and the GI tract can be significantly compromised in the early post-transplant period. For many patients, parenteral nutrition (PN) is a standard component of care and is indicated for those who are unable to tolerate oral or enteral feeding (AND EAL, 2013; Macris Charuhas, 2013). In addition, administration of optimal levels of PN often is complicated by the frequent need to interrupt it for the infusion of antibiotics, blood products, and IV medications. Careful monitoring and the use of more concentrated nutrient solutions, increased flow rates and volumes, and double- or triple-lumen catheters often are needed to achieve optimal nutrition intakes.

Autologous HCT involves the use of the individual's own stem cells to reestablish hematopoietic stem cell function after the administration of high-dose chemotherapy. In some cases the use of mobilized stem cell progenitors has replaced autologous bone marrow as the source of hematopoietic progenitors for transplantation. Their use has shortened the period of pancytopenia (reduction in the cellular components of the blood), when individuals are at risk for bleeding, serious infections, or sepsis. These advances, along with improved prophylactic antibiotic regimens that are relatively easy to administer, have allowed individuals to receive autologous marrow transplantation in the outpatient setting. The reduced cost of transplantation has made it available to an increased number of people.

Because a majority of people receive much of their care outside the hospital, regular nutrition assessment and monitoring are important. The HCT procedure is associated with severe nutritional consequences that require prompt, proactive intervention. Nausea, vomiting, and diarrhea are caused by the cytotoxic conditioning regimen and may later accompany antibiotic administration. Complications of delayed-onset nutrition-related symptoms include varying degrees of mucositis, xerostomia, and dysgeusia. Mucositis, which is often severe and extremely painful, develops in more than 75% of transplant patients (see Figure 36-2).

Nutritional Precautions with Neutropenia

Individuals receiving HCT become immunocompromised and require supportive therapy, including medications and dietary changes to prevent infection. Some cancer centers continue to prescribe a low-microbial or low-bacteria diet for people with low white blood cell counts (neutropenia). However, there is no clear evidence that a strict "neutropenic" diet (only cooked foods) reduces overall rates of infection or death (AND, EAL, 2013). Current recommendations are for nutrition education to include dietary counseling on safe food handling and avoidance of foods that pose a risk of infection while patients are neutropenic and until immunosuppressive therapy has been completed (AND, EAL, 2013; SCCA, 2014) (see Box 36-3).

Graft-versus-Host Disease (GVHD)

Graft-versus-host disease (GVHD) is a major complication seen primarily after allogeneic transplants, in which the donated "donor" stem cells react against the tissues of the transplant recipient "host". The functions of several target organs (skin, liver, gut, lymphoid cells) are disrupted and are susceptible to infection. Acute GVHD can occur within the first 100 days after the transplant and may be seen as early as 7 to 10 days posttransplant. It may resolve, or it may develop into a chronic form that requires long-term treatment and dietary management. Skin GVHD is characterized by a maculopapular rash. GVHD of the liver, evidenced by jaundice and abnormal liver function tests, often accompanies gastrointestinal GVHD and further complicates nutrition management.

The symptoms of acute GI GVHD can be severe; individuals may experience gastroenteritis, abdominal pain, nausea, vomiting, and large volumes of secretory diarrhea. Immunosuppressive medications and a phased dietary regimen should be instituted (Macris Charuhas, 2013; SCCA, 2014). The first phase consists of total bowel rest and the use of PN until diarrhea subsides. Nitrogen losses associated with diarrhea can be severe and are compounded by the high-dose corticosteroids used to treat GVHD. The second phase reintroduces oral feedings of beverages that are isosmotic, low residue, and lactose free so as to compensate for the loss of intestinal enzymes secondary to alterations in the intestinal villi and mucosa. If these beverages are tolerated, phase three includes the reintroduction of solids that contain low levels of lactose, fiber, fat, and total acidity, and no gastric irritants. In phase four dietary restrictions are progressively reduced as foods are gradually introduced and tolerance is established. *Phase five* is the resumption of the individual's regular diet.

Chronic GVHD can develop up to 3 months after transplant and is observed with increased frequency in nonidentical related donors and unrelated donors. Chronic GVHD can affect the skin, oral mucosa (ulcerations, stomatitis, xerostomia), and the GI tract (anorexia, reflux symptoms, diarrhea) and can cause changes in body weight.

Another transplant-related complication is sinusoidal obstructive syndrome (SOS) (also known as venoocclusive disease), characterized by chemotherapy- or radiation therapy–induced damage to the hepatic venules. It can develop within 1 to 3 weeks after transplant, and symptoms of right upper quadrant discomfort, hepatomegaly, fluid retention, and jaundice can occur. In severe cases individuals may experience progressive hepatic failure leading to encephalopathy and multiple-organ system failure. Nutrition support requires PN, careful fluid and electrolyte management, close monitoring, and adjustment of macronutrients and micronutrients based on the tolerance and response of each individual.

Other acute or chronic complications of HCT include osteoporosis, pulmonary disease, impaired renal function, rejection of the graft, growth abnormalities in children, sepsis, and infection. Nutrition-related symptoms associated with HCT may persist; individuals receiving outpatient marrow transplantation require frequent monitoring and intervention.

NUTRITION MONITORING AND EVALUATION

Dietetic professionals must determine and quantify their patients' nutrition care goals by monitoring progress, measuring and evaluating outcomes and changes, and documenting this information throughout the process (Box 36-4). Monitoring and evaluation of these factors is needed to effectively diagnose nutrition problems that should be the focus of future nutrition interventions (AND, EAL, 2013) (see Chapter 10).

Physical Activity

Physical activity is an important part of cancer care. The effect of cancer and cancer treatment on the individual's quality of life should be addressed throughout cancer treatment and continue until the individual is able to successfully resume activities of daily living. Recovery from cancer treatment also requires physical activity to rebuild muscle; regain strength, energy, and flexibility; and help relieve symptoms of stress, anxiety, and even depression. Physical activity and exercise may be helpful in strengthening the immune system. However, before participating in any type of physical activity and exercise program, individuals should be advised to undergo evaluation by qualified professionals, who can then design an individualized physical assessment and activity plan. The STAR (Survivorship Training and Rehab) certified specialists are available around the country in large and small cancer centers; the program's goal is thealth care professionals seeking certification how rehab can help cancer patients and about the unique needs of cancer survivors after cancer treatment (ORP, 2015). In addition, the American College of Sports Medicine (ACSM) offers a certification program for trainers working with people diagnosed with cancer (a certified cancer exercise trainer) (ACSM, 2014). Finally, community-based programs such as the YMCA's LiveStrong (www.livestrong.org/LIVESTRONG-at-theYMCA) are available across the United States and offer physical activity and exercise opportunities to support cancer survivors.

PEDIATRIC CANCER

Like adults, children with cancer can experience malnutrition and nutrition-related symptoms as a result of their cancer and its treatment. Malnutrition can have long-term side effects with childhood cancer treatment such as slow or stunted growth and development, compromised bone health, eating disorders, and decreased quality of life (Fatemi et al, 2013).

Psychogenic food refusal in children requires interventions that address underlying psychological issues. Families and caregivers often express their fears of dying through an extreme preoccupation with eating and maintaining weight. Creative efforts are required to minimize the psychologic effects of fear, unpleasant hospital routines, unfamiliar foods, learned food aversions, and pain. Nutrition intervention strategies that use oral intake should stress the maximum use of favorite, nutrient-dense foods during times when intake is likely to be best, and food aversions are least likely to occur. Oral medical foods can be useful, but their acceptance is often a problem; thus children should be offered a selection from which to choose.

EN support by nasogastric tube (up to 3 months) or gastrostomy tube (more than 3 months) may be indicated for some children who are able to cooperate and who have functional GI tracts.

PN is indicated for children who are receiving intense treatment associated with severe GI toxicity (intractable vomiting and severe diarrhea) and for children with favorable prognoses who are malnourished or have a high risk of developing malnutrition. PN is seldom indicated for children with advanced cancer associated with significant deterioration or with diseases that are unresponsive to therapy.

Universally accepted, evidence-based guidelines for children diagnosed with cancer do not exist. However, the American Society for Parenteral and Enteral Nutrition (ASPEN) has established standards for the nutrition screening and specialized nutrition support for all hospitalized pediatric patients. The nutritional requirements of pediatric patients with cancer are similar, with an adjustment for activity, to those of normal growing children. Often pediatric patients with cancer are not bedridden but are as active as their healthy peers. Factors that may alter nutrient requirements in cancer include the effect of the disease on host metabolism, the catabolic effects of cancer therapy, and physiologic stress from surgery, fever, malabsorption, and infection. Fluid requirements are increased during anticancer therapy or in the presence of fever, diarrhea, or renal failure. Micronutrients may require supplementation during periods of poor intake, stress, or malabsorption.

The best long-term indicator of adequate nutrient intake is growth. Children have increased nutritional requirements for growth and development that must be met despite extended periods of cancer treatment (see Chapters 16 through 18). A special vulnerability exists during the adolescent growth spurt. Ewing sarcoma, common in adolescents and young adults, frequently is associated with malnutrition.

Another reason why children with advanced cancer are at greater risk of severe nutritional depletion than adults is the frequent use of more aggressive, multimodality treatment. Deficiencies in energy and protein can be expected to affect growth adversely, although the effects may be temporary, and catch-up growth depends on how much energy children are able to consistently consume (Fatemi et al, 2013). However, some cancer treatment regimens may have an effect on growth and development that is independent of nutritional deprivation. HCT is now an accepted and increasingly successful intensive therapy for a wide range of disorders in children. Many supportive therapies may be safely managed in the outpatient arena, thus reducing the period of hospitalization.

NUTRITION RECOMMENDATIONS FOR CANCER SURVIVORS

From the time of diagnosis through the balance of life, the ACS defines anyone living with a cancer diagnosis as a cancer survivor (Rock et al, 2012). The ACS guidelines as well as the WCRF and AICR recommendations provide sound diet, nutrition, and physical activity advice for primary cancer prevention and health for all individuals, including cancer survivors. In addition, the ACS published for the first time evidence-based nutrition and physical guidelines for cancer survivors in 2012 (Rock et al, 2012). Up until this point, the ACS specifically declined to call these a set of "guidelines" or "recommendations" because the evidence in this area of study is not as plentiful as in the primary prevention realm.

Cancer survivorship encompasses three phases: active treatment and recovery, living after recovery (including living disease free or with stable disease), and advance cancer and end of life (Rock et al, 2012). Cancer survivors represent one of the largest groups of people living with a chronic disease. It is estimated that there will be 13.7 million survivors in the United States in 2014; approximately 1 in every 25 Americans is a survivor (ACS, 2014a). The majority of individuals with cancer are able to return to full function and regain quality of life. This trend is expected to continue because of recent awareness in cancer prevention, advances in cancer detection, development of more effective cancer treatments, and advancements in determining the genetic causes of cancer. Long-term cancer survivors should now focus on healthy weight management, healthy diets, and physical activity geared toward secondary cancer and chronic disease prevention.

INTEGRATIVE ONCOLOGY

Complementary therapies are typically noninvasive and useful in controlling symptoms and improving quality of life during and after cancer treatment; they are used in addition to conventional medicine. **Integrative medicine** works to combine evidence-based complementary therapies into conventional cancer treatment (see Chapter 12). Integrative medicine uses strategies to promote self-empowerment, individual responsibility, and lifestyle changes that can potentially reduce risk for cancer recurrence and second primary tumors. Experts agree that a growing proportion of cancer survivors participate in these modalities with 40% to 50% participating in some form of complementary or integrative therapy during and after treatment (ASCO University, 2014).

The health care team working in oncology must be informed on the different therapies and knowledgeable regarding resources used to evaluate and educate the individuals in their care. Some cancer centers are fortunate; increasing consumer demand has encouraged health care institutions to create "Integrative Medicine" departments with onsite complementary services. Cancer survivors look for open, honest discussions or recommendations from their health care team. Medical, nursing, and nutrition assessments should include open-ended questions on dietary supplement use, such as, "What vitamins, minerals, herbs, or other dietary supplements are you currently taking?" and questions regarding the additional integrative or complementary therapies they are following at the time. The core components to discuss integrative or alternative therapies involve understanding and respecting the need people have to do something for themselves; having a willingness to listen to, explore, and respond frankly to questions; taking the time to discuss the options and offer advice; summarizing the discussion; documenting the dialog; and monitoring the progress of the therapy.

The NIH established a National Center for Complementary and Alternative Medicine (NCCAM) in 1999, renamed the National Center for Complementary and Integrative Health (NCCIH), which works to create a framework in which to evaluate and research these therapies (Box 36-5 and Figure 36-3).

Dietary Supplements

The most common form of integrative medicine practiced in the United States is the use of dietary supplements (see Chapter 12). Based on the last survey done by the National Center for Complementary and Integrative Health (NCCIH) in 2007, consumers spend in excess of $33.9 billion every year on complementary integrative medicine (CIM), of which $14.8 billion is spent on natural products marketed to maintain or enhance health

---

BOX 36-5 The National Center for Complementary and Integrative Health (NCCIH)

Natural Products: products such as herbs/botanicals, vitamins and minerals, glandulars, medicinal mushrooms, and probiotics
Mind and Body Practice: procedures or techniques delivered or instructed by a trained practitioner or teacher such as acupuncture, massage therapy, meditation, movement therapies, guided imagery, spinal manipulation, tai chi and qi gong, yoga, healing touch, and hypnotherapy
Other Complementary Health Approaches: practices of traditional healers, Ayurvedic medicine from India, traditional Chinese medicine, homeopathy, and naturopathy

Data from National Center for Complementary and Integrative Health (NCCIH): Main page (website): https://nccih.nih.gov/. Accessed February 20, 2015.

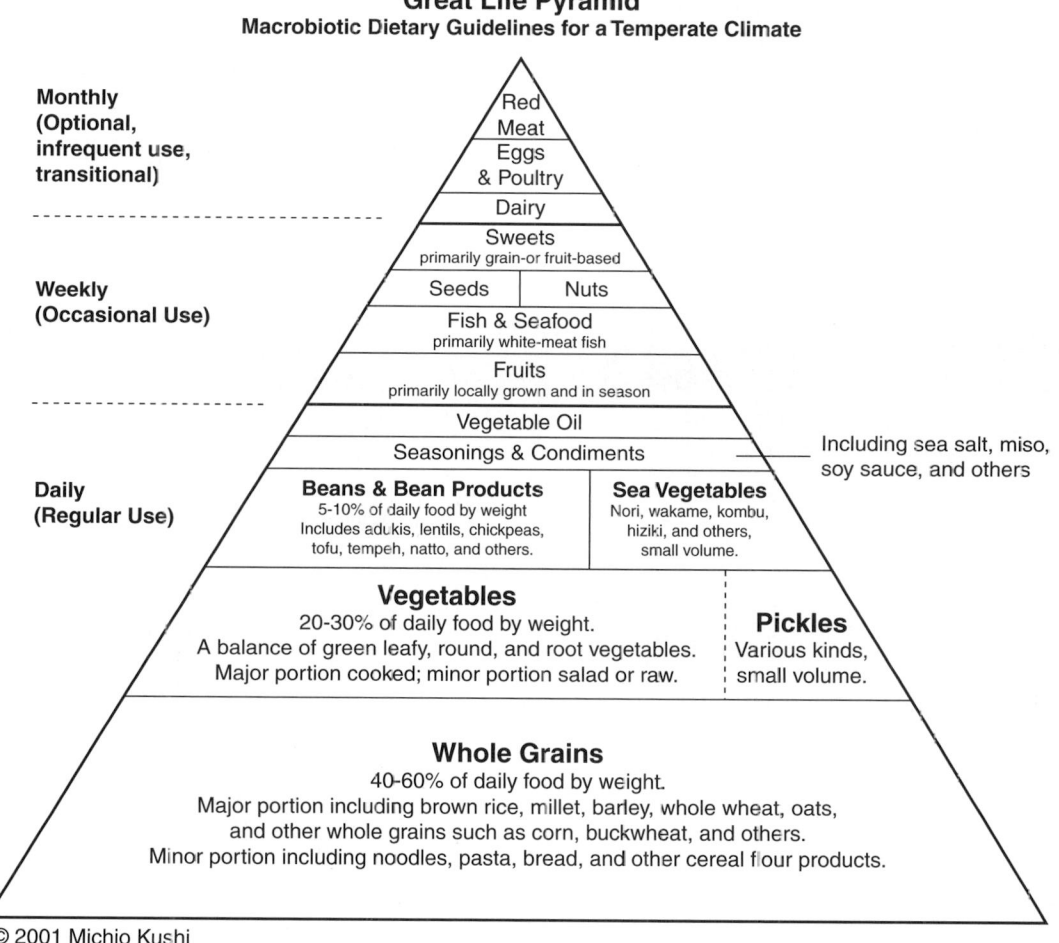

FIGURE 36-3 The Great Pyramid of Life.

(NCCIH, 2009). The largest percentage of use (18%) is nonvitamin, nonmineral natural products such as fish oil supplements and ginseng. That number jumps significantly when surveying cancer survivors, in whom significant use occurs. A primary motivation is symptom management but most also hope for tumor suppression.

Nondisclosure of use is a common occurrence, with a reported 53% of individuals receiving chemotherapy not discussing use of dietary supplements with their health care team (Davis et al, 2012; Hardy, 2008). People may view dietary supplements as a more natural alternative to prescription medications or a quick, easy remedy to an underlying medical problem. Distrust of the medical system, fear of being "fired" or dismissed by their doctor, or anticipated ignorance from the health care team may prevent cancer survivors from discussing use of dietary supplements. When discussing CIM use, the practitioner can take five steps: (1) inquire about use, (2) evaluate the supplement, (3) discuss any relevant regulatory issues, (4) discuss available safety and efficacy data, and (5) compare risks and benefits of use to available conventional therapies. Although time consuming, conversations that include most or all of these steps help open lines of communication between health care provider and survivor and prevent an adverse event or poor treatment decisions. Table 36-11 lists potential adverse effects of some of the commonly used supplements.

Orthomolecular Medicine

Orthomolecular medicine (OM) is the practice of restoring an optimal environment in the body by correcting nutritional imbalances and deficiencies, another alternative medicine practice in cancer care. The treatment is based on the theory that by correcting imbalances and deficiencies, the body will regain health. This has not been proven in clinical trials and instead is extrapolated from basic science. Infusions or supplementation may involve large doses of vitamins, minerals, essential fatty acids, fiber, amino acids, or enzymes. Orthomolecular practitioners (often medical doctors) consider a number of integrative medicine practices to be consistent with OM philosophy and may incorporate parts of naturopathic medicine, nutrition, acupuncture, mind-body therapies, and manipulative and body-based practices such as massage into their treatments.

Advanced Cancer and Palliative Care

Palliative care is the active total care of an individual when curative measures are no longer considered an option by either the medical team or the individual. Hospice care focuses on relieving symptoms and supporting individuals with a life expectancy of months, not years (NHPCO, 2014). The objectives are to provide for optimal quality of life; relieve physical symptoms; alleviate isolation, anxiety, and fear associated with advanced disease; and to help patients maintain independence as long as possible. The goals of nutrition intervention should focus on managing nutrition-related symptoms such as pain, weakness, loss of appetite, early satiety, constipation, weakness, dry mouth, and dyspnea (Trentham and Grant, 2013). Another important goal is maintaining strength and energy to enhance quality of life, independence, and the ability to perform activities of daily living. Nutrition should be provided "as tolerated or as desired" along with emotional support and awareness of and respect for individual needs and wishes. Thus the pleasurable aspects of eating should be emphasized, without concern for quantity or nutrient and energy content.

The use of nutrition support and hydration in individuals with advanced, incurable cancer is a difficult and often controversial issue and should be determined on a case-by-case basis. Advance directives are legal documents that guide health care providers regarding the specific wishes of individuals, outlining the extent of their desired medical care, including the provision of artificial nutrition and hydration. Whenever providing nutrition care, give consideration to advanced directives that may be in place.

TABLE 36-11   Potential Adverse Events with Dietary Supplements Commonly Used by Cancer Survivors

Dietary Supplement	Claim and Common Uses	Potential Adverse Event
Echinacea	Boosts the immune system	May cause gastrointestinal adverse effects; nausea, abdominal pain, diarrhea, and vomiting are the most common side effects reported
Garlic	Helps lower cholesterol	May increase risk for excessive bleeding, especially when used with certain anticlotting agents
Ginger	Helps with nausea	May increase risk for excessive bleeding, especially when used with certain anticlotting agents
Ginkgo	Helps increase blood circulation and oxygenation Enhances memory and mental concentration	May increase risk for excessive bleeding, especially when used with certain anticlotting agents
Licorice	Helps soothe the stomach	Certain licorice mixtures may cause high blood pressure, increase swelling, and cause electrolyte imbalances
Saw palmetto	Helps with enlarged prostate and urinary inflammation	May interact with other hormone therapies and may increase risk for excessive bleeding, especially when used with certain anticlotting agents
St. John's wort	Helps with mild to moderate depression, anxiety, or sleep disorders	May decrease effectiveness of all currently marketed medication using cytochrome P450 pathway in the liver: HIV and AIDS medications (NNRTIs and PIs), carbamazepine, cyclosporine, irinotecan (Camptosar) for chemotherapy, midazolam (Versed), nifedipine (Procardia), simvastatin (Zocor), theophylline, warfarin (Coumadin)
Valerian	Helps as mild sedative or sleep aid, or muscle relaxant	May increase effects of certain antiseizure medications or prolong effects of anesthetic agents

Natural Medicines Comprehensive Database: (website): http://naturaldatabase.therapeuticresearch.com/home.aspx?cs=&s=ND, 2015. Accessed February 20, 2015.

CLINICAL CASE STUDY 1

Rosa is a 62-year-old woman who has three adult daughters and eight grandchildren. Recently she was diagnosed with breast cancer (estrogen-receptor and progesterone-receptor negative and HER/2 neu positive). Surgery, followed by concurrent chemotherapy and biotherapy and then radiation therapy to her breast are planned for treatment of her disease. Anticipated side effects of her cancer therapy include treatment-related fatigue, mouth sores, nausea, vomiting, diarrhea, and peripheral neuropathy. She is 5'6" tall, weighs 168 lb, and has a history of hypercholesterolemia and hypertension that has been managed with dietary measures. She currently does not engage in regular physical activity other than helping to care for her grandchildren but is motivated to make changes in her lifestyle to improve her fitness and overall health. She also is attracted to the use of multiple vitamins/minerals and dietary supplements and complementary and alternative therapies for managing treatment-related side effects, reducing her cancer recurrence risk and managing her hypercholesterolemia and hypertension.

Nutrition Diagnostic Statement 1

Altered GI function related to prescribed cancer treatment as evidenced by anticipated nausea, vomiting, diarrhea, and mouth sores.

Nutrition Diagnostic Statement 2

Physical inactivity related to lack of a regular exercise plan as evidenced by patient reports of no exercise.

Nutrition Diagnostic Statement 3

Food- and nutrition-related knowledge deficit related to medical nutrition therapy related to cancer treatment and secondary prevention as evidenced by patient requesting more information.

Nutrition Care Questions

- What diet and nutrition recommendations would you give Rosa to prepare her for upcoming cancer treatment?
- List some dietary strategies Rosa may try if she experiences the following: fatigue, intermittent queasiness, mouth sores, and diarrhea.
- Is Rosa at her ideal body weight? If not, what suggestions would you recommend? Consider her lifestyle, hypertension, hypercholesterolemia, and planned cancer treatment.
- What guidance should be provided with regard to the appropriate use of vitamin and mineral supplements and ways to evaluate alternative therapies?

CLINICAL CASE STUDY 2

Daniel is a 54-year-old man with a recent diagnosis of cancer of the gastroesophageal junction. He has experienced gastroesophageal reflux (GERD) for the past 10 years and had been advised to undergo an endoscopic examination to rule out Barrett's esophagus, but he never followed up on his doctor's referral. He lost 30 pounds in the 3 months prior to his diagnosis because of lack of appetite and progressive dysphagia with solid foods. Pre-diagnosis, his diet consisted of drinking "muscle drinks" his son purchased at the local gym. He has been very pleased with his weight loss but knew something was wrong. His medical history also includes hypertension and sleep apnea.

Daniel underwent neo-adjuvant chemotherapy and radiation therapy, followed by an esophagogastrectomy 1½ months ago and recalls that he received some nutrition information from the inpatient registered dietitian nutritionist right before he was discharged. Daniel reports that he was anxious to go home and did not pay attention to the diet instruction and could not find the paperwork once he got home. While hospitalized, Daniel received enteral nutrition via a feeding tube, but the feedings were discontinued and the tube was removed just prior to discharge. He has lost an additional 25 pounds in the past month and has been admitted once for dehydration caused by lack of fluid intake and because of symptoms related to ongoing episodes of diarrhea after eating. He has also stopped using his C-Pap because he feels that it is no longer helpful; however, he states he is not sleeping well and never feels rested.

His current food and nutrition history includes small meals with a usual intake of approximately 1500 calories daily. He eats three times a day. He reports he does not have the energy to prepare food, so, while his wife is at work, he has started drinking the "muscle drinks" again and is warming canned soup in the microwave. He is also drinking sports drinks because he has been encouraged to increase his fluid intake. He has a sweet tooth, and because eating is difficult, he rewards himself with ice cream or sherbet. His beverages include whole milk, apple juice, and an occasional "finger" of scotch each night. He has been referred to see the outpatient registered dietitian nutritionist.

Biochemical Data

Pre-albumin: 14.0 mg/dl
Blood urea nitrogen: 18 mg/dl
Creatinine: 0.6 mg/dl
Blood pressure: 100/55
Pulse rate of 90

Anthropometric Data

Height: 70"
Weight history: Usual body weight: 220 lb, preoperative weight: 190 lb, 1 month postoperative weight: 165 lb
Current body mass index: 23

Medications

Metoclopramide (Reglan) 30 minutes before each meal
Metoprolol (Toprol)
Hydrochlorothiazide
Sildenafil (Viagra)

Dietary Supplements

One-A-Day for Men
Saw Palmetto
Lycopene

Nutrition Diagnostic Statement 1

Food- and nutrition-related knowledge deficit related to lack of education and counseling for appropriate medical nutrition therapy as evidenced by food history with inappropriate food choices.

Nutrition Diagnostic Statement 2

Altered gastrointestinal function related to esophagogastrectomy as evidenced by weight loss, dehydration, and dumping syndrome.

Nutrition Diagnostic Statement 3

Inadequate protein and energy intake related to postsurgery recovery as evidenced by decreased food and beverage intake, weight loss, and muscle wasting causing decreased creatinine.

Nutrition Care Questions

1. What kind of a daily eating plan would you design with Daniel so that he can take in enough food and fluid to meet his nutritional requirements?
2. After reviewing Daniel's medical, social and physical activity history, what other factors could be contributing to his difficulty with eating and his inability to regain weight?
3. Would you include Daniel's wife in your counseling sessions? If so, why? If not, why?
4. As Daniel continues to be seen for Survivorship Care at your clinic, what lingering or late-occurring side effects of cancer treatment should you anticipate and continue to monitor? Could any of these side effects affect his ongoing nutritional status? If so, should any laboratory tests be ordered or evaluated? What other factors should be monitored as a part of your nutritional care?

Nutrition Interventions

Nutrition prescription: Small, frequent meals consisting of energy-dense, lower-fat foods and limited simple carbohydrates; majority of fluid consumption between meals (sips during meals okay to aid in chewing and swallowing).

Continued

CLINICAL CASE STUDY 2—cont'd

Nutrition education: Update Daniel's knowledge of appropriate nutrition therapy after an esophagogastrectomy. Discuss tolerance of different food groups; sources of protein; energy-dense, easy-to-prepare menu options; and healthy beverage selections, including advising him to discontinue consumption of daily alcoholic beverage; and goal caloric intake needed for slow, steady weight gain. Suggest he consider eating every 2 hours, on the even hour, to create an external reminder to eat. Recommend he review his hypertension medication types and doses with his physicians because his need for medication may have changed with his significant weight loss.

At follow-up visits address weight stabilization and weight-gain progress, bowel function, food and beverage intake and tolerance; encourage physical activity (physician approved) starting with short walks to regain muscle strength. Daniel should be accompanied by a friend or family member on these walks. Encourage Daniel to follow-up with his primary care physician to discuss his problems sleeping and that he has stopped using his C-Pap.

Nutrition counseling: Coordinate with patient and wife to ensure appropriate foods and beverages are available for consumption. Discuss expected acute and long-term side effects from surgery. Establish slow, steady weight gain and physical activity goals for next 3 months.

Nutrition Monitoring and Evaluation

1. Body weight trends
2. Hydration status
3. Serum pre-albumin levels and creatinine levels (over 3 months)
4. Physical activity
5. Schedule follow-up session in 2 weeks, with optional phone call between visits

---

USEFUL WEBSITES AND RESOURCES

Academy of Nutrition and Dietetics Oncology Tool Kit
http://www.oncologynutrition.org/store/product/ebp-oncology-toolkit-electronic-format-115?returnBack=%2Fstore
Academy of Nutrition and Dietetics (AND) Standards of Practice and Standards of Professional Performance for Oncology Nutrition Practice
http://www.andjrnl.org/article/S0002-8223(09)01820-3/pdf
American Cancer Society (ACS)
www.cancer.org
American Institute for Cancer Research (AICR)
www.aicr.org
National Cancer Institute (NCI)
www.cancer.gov
National Center for Complementary and Integrative Health (NCCIH)
https://nccih.nih.gov
Oncology Nutrition Dietetic Practice Group (ONDPG)
www.oncologynutrition.org
World Cancer Research Fund (WCRF)
www.wcrf.org

REFERENCES

Academy of Nutrition and Dietetics (AND), Evidence Analysis Library (EAL): *Oncology nutrition evidence-based nutrition practice guidelines*, Chicago, 2013, Academy of Nutrition and Dietetics.

Academy of Nutrition and Dietetics (AND): *International dietetics and nutrition terminology (IDNT) reference manual: standard language for the nutrition care process*, ed 4, Chicago, 2012a, Academy of Nutrition and Dietetics.

Academy of Nutrition and Dietetics (AND): *Oncology Tool Kit*, Chicago, 2010, Academy of Nutrition and Dietetics.

Academy of Nutrition and Dietetics (AND): Position of the Academy of Nutrition and Dietetics: use of nutritive and nonnutritive sweeteners, *J Acad Nutr Diet* 112:739, 2012b.

American Cancer Society (ACS), McCullough M: *The Bottom Line on Soy and Breast Cancer Risk* (website): http://www.cancer.org/cancer/news/expert-voices/post/2012/08/02/the-bottom-line-on-soy-and-breast-cancer-risk.aspx, 2012a. Accessed January 29, 2015.

American Cancer Society (ACS): *Cancer Facts and Figures 2014*, Atlanta, 2014a, American Cancer Society, Available at: http://www.cancer.org/research/cancerfactsstatistics/cancerfactsfigures2014. Accessed February 20, 2015.

American Cancer Society (ACS): *Family Cancer Syndromes* (website): <http://www.cancer.org/cancer/cancercauses/geneticsandcancer/heredity-and-cancer>, 2014b. Accessed March 2, 2015.

American Cancer Society (ACS): *Folic Acid* (website): http://www.cancer.org/treatment/treatmentsandsideeffects/complementaryandalternativemedicine/herbsvitaminsandminerals/folic-acid, 2011. Accessed January 29, 2015.

American Cancer Society (ACS): *Food Additives, Safety and Organic Foods* (website): http://www.cancer.org/healthy/eathealthygetactive/acsguidelinesonnutritionphysicalactivityforcancerprevention/acs-guidelines-on-nutrition-and-physical-activity-for-cancer-prevention-food-additives, 2012b. Accessed January 29, 2015.

American Cancer Society (ACS): *Organizational Outcomes 2013* (website): http://www.cancer.org/acs/groups/content/

American Cancer Society (ACS): *Vitamin D* (website): http://www.cancer.org/treatment/treatmentsandsideeffects/complementaryandalternativemedicine/herbsvitaminsandminerals/vitamin-d, 2013b. Accessed March 2, 2015.

American College of Sports Medicine (ACSM): ACSM/ACS Certified Cancer Exercise Trainer. www.acsm.org; Accessed September 18, 2015.

American Institute for Cancer Research: *Continuous Update Projects 2015* (website): http://www.aicr.org/continuous-update-project/. Accessed January 29, 2015.

ASCO University: *Integrative Oncology: an Overview* (website): http://meetinglibrary.asco.org/content/114000233-144. Accessed January 26, 2015.

Ashar BH et al: Advising patients who use dietary supplements, *Am J Med* 121:91, 2008.

Ashrafian H et al: Metabolic surgery and cancer: protective effects of bariatric procedures, *Cancer* 117:1788, 2011.

Bailey RL et al: Total folate and folic acid intake from foods and dietary supplements in the United States: 2003-2006, *Am J Clin Nutr* 91:231, 2010.

Bender A et al: Nutrition and cancer prevention. In Leser M et al, editors: *Oncology nutrition for clinical practice*, Chicago, 2013, Oncology Dietetic Practice Group 2013.

Brown CG: *A guide to oncology symptom management*, Pittsburgh, 2009, Oncology Nursing Society.

Centers for Disease Control and Prevention (CDC): *Health, United States, 2012: with special feature on emergency care report*, Hyattsville, Md, 2013, US Department of Health and Human Services.

Choi SW, Friso S: Epigenetics: a new bridge between nutrition and health, *Adv Nutr* 1:8, 2010.

Davis EL et al: Cancer patient disclosure and patient-doctor communication of complementary and alternative medicine use: a systematic review, *Oncologist* 17:1475, 2012.

Edwards BK et al: Annual report to the nation on the status of cancer, 1975-2010, featuring prevalence of comorbidity and impact on survival among persons with lung, colorectal, breast, or prostate cancer, *Cancer* 120:1290, 2014.

Elliott L: Symptom management of cancer therapies. In Leser M et al, editors: *Oncology nutrition for clinical practice*, Chicago, 2013, Oncology Nutrition Dietetic Practice 2013.

Farhadian A et al: Determination of polycyclic aromatic hydrocarbons in grilled meat, *Food Control* 21:606, 2010.

Fatemi D et al: Nutritional management of the pediatric oncology patient. In Leser M et al, editors: *Oncology nutrition in clinical practice*, Chicago, 2013, Oncology Nutrition Dietetic Practice Group 2013.

Fearon KC: Cancer cachexia: developing multimodal therapy for a multidimensional problem, *Eur J Cancer* 44:1124, 2008.

Ferguson LR: Meat and cancer, *Meat Sci* 84:308, 2010.

Food and Drug Administration (FDA): *Bisphenol A (BPA): for Use in Food Content Application* (website): http://www.fda.gov/NewsEvents/PublicHealthFocus/ucm064437.htm, 2014. Accessed January 29, 2015.

Grant B: Nutritional effects of cancer treatment: chemotherapy, biotherapy, hormone therapy and radiation therapy. In Leser M et al, editors: *Oncology nutrition for clinical practice*, Chicago, 2013, Oncology Nutrition Dietetic Practice 2013.

Grant BL: *Academy of Nutrition and Dietetics pocket guide to the nutrition care process and cancer*, Chicago, 2015, Academy of Nutrition and Dietetics.

Guppy A et al: Anticancer effects of metformin and its potential as a therapeutic agent for breast cancer, *Future Oncol* 7:727, 2011.

Hamilton KK: Nutritional needs of the adult oncology patient. In Leser M et al, editors: *Oncology nutrition for clinical practice*, Chicago, 2013, Oncology Nutrition Dietetic Practice Group 2013.

Hardy ML: Dietary supplement use in cancer care: help or harm, *Hematol Oncol Clin North Am* 22:581, 2008.

Havrila C et al: Medical and radiation oncology. In Marian M, Roberts S, editors: *Clinical nutrition for oncology patients*, Sudbury, Mass, 2010, Jones and Bartlett.

Huhmann MB, August D: Surgical oncology. In Marian M, Roberts S, editors: *Clinical nutrition for oncology patients*, Sudbury, Mass, 2010, Jones and Bartlett.

Israel B: *How many cancers are caused by the environment?* (website): http://www.scientificamerican.com/article/how-many-cancers-are-caused-by-the-environment/, 2010. Accessed February 20, 2015.

Iwamoto RR et al: *Manual for radiation oncology and nursing practice and education*, ed 4, Pittsburgh, 2012, Oncology Nursing Society.

Kelsey MM et al: Age-related consequences of childhood obesity, *Gerontology* 60:222, 2014.

Kushi LH et al: American Cancer Society guidelines on nutrition and physical activity for cancer prevention: reducing the risk of cancer with healthy food choices and physical activity, *CA Cancer J Clin* 62:30, 2012.

Kwan ML et al: Alcohol consumption and breast cancer recurrence and survival among women with early–state breast cancer: the life after cancer epidemiology study, *J Clin Oncol* 28:4410, 2010.

Levine AJ et al: A candidate gene study of folate-associated one carbon metabolism genes and colorectal cancer risk, *Cancer Epidemiol Biomarkers Prev* 19:1812, 2010.

Ligibel JA et al: American Society of Clinical Oncology position statement on obesity and cancer, *J Clin Oncol* 32:3568, 2014.

Link A et al: Cancer chemoprevention by dietary polyphenols: promising role for epigenetics, *Biochem Pharmacol* 80:1771, 2010.

Longo V, Fontana L: Calorie restriction and cancer prevention: metabolic and molecular mechanisms, *Trends Pharmacol Sci* 31:89, 2010.

Macris Charuhas PM: Medical nutrition therapy for hematopoietic cell transplantation. In Leser M et al, editors: *Oncology nutrition for clinical practice*, Chicago, 2013, Oncology Nutrition Dietetic Group 2013.

Martinez et al: Dietary supplements and cancer prevention: balancing potential benefits against proven harm, *J Natl Cancer Inst* 104:732, 2012.

Medical News Today (MNT): *Folic Acid Linked to Breast Cancer Cell Growth in Animal Study* (website): http://www.medicalnewstoday.com/articles/271601.php, 2014. Accessed January 29, 2015.

Michalowicz J: Bisphenol A—sources, toxicity and biotransformation, *Environ Toxicol Pharmacol* 37:738, 2014.

Moyer VA: Vitamin, mineral and multivitamin supplements for the primary prevention of cardiovascular disease and cancer: US Preventive Services Task Force recommendation statement, *Ann Intern Med* 160:558, 2014.

National Center for Complementary and Integrative Health (NCCIH): *The use of complementary and alternative medicine in the United States: cost data* (website): https://nccih.nih.gov/news/camstats/costs/costdatafs.htm, 2009. Accessed February 20, 2015.

National Comprehensive Cancer Network (NCCN): *NCCN clinical practice guidelines for treatment of head and neck cancers (NCCN guidelines)* (website): http://oralcancerfoundation.org/treatment/pdf/head-and-neck.pdf, 2013. Accessed January 29, 2015.

National Comprehensive Cancer Network (NCCN): *NCCN Clinical Practice Guidelines in Oncology (NCCN Guidelines)* (website): http://www.nccn.org/clinical.asp. Accessed March 2, 2015.

National Hospice and Palliative Care Organization (NHPCO): *How can palliative care help?* (website): http://www.nhpco.org, 2014. Accessed March 2, 2015.

National Institute of Dental and Craniofacial Research (NIDCR): *Cancer Treatment and Oral Health* (website): http://www.nidcr.nih.gov/OralHealth/Topics/CancerTreatment/, 2014. Accessed March 2, 2015.

National Institutes of Health (NIH), National Cancer Institute (NCI): *Cancer Genetics Overview PDQ* (website): http://www.cancer.gov/cancertopics/pdq/genetics/overview/healthprofessional, 2014a. Accessed March 2, 2015.

National Institutes of Health (NIH), National Cancer Institute (NCI): *Cannabis and Cannabanoids PDQ* (website): http://www.cancer.gov/cancertopics/pdq/cam/cannabis/patient, 2014b. Accessed March 2, 2015.

National Institutes of Health (NIH), National Cancer Institute (NCI): *Chemotherapy and You* (website): http://www.cancer.gov/publications/patient-education/chemotherapy-and-you.pdf, 2011a (Accessed 01.29.15).

National Institutes of Health (NIH), National Cancer Institute (NCI): *Eating Hints Before, During, and After Treatment* (website): http://www.cancer.gov/publications/patient-education/eatinghints.pdf, 2011b. Accessed January 29, 2015.

National Institutes of Health (NIH), National Cancer Institute (NCI): *NCI Dictionary of Cancer Terms* (website): http://www.cancer.gov/dictionary/. Accessed January 29, 2015.

National Institutes of Health (NIH), National Cancer Institute (NCI): *Radiation Therapy and You* (website): http://www.cancer.gov/publications/patient-education/radiationtherapy.pdf, 2012. Accessed January 29, 2015.

National Institutes of Health (NIH), National Cancer Institute (NCI): *SEER Stat Fact Sheet: All Cancer Sites* (website): http://seer.cancer.gov/statfacts/html/all.html, 2014c. Accessed January 29, 2015.

National Institutes of Health (NIH), National Cancer Institute (NCI): *Tea and Cancer Prevention* (website): www.cancer.gov/cancertopics/factsheet/prevention/tea, 2010. Accessed March 2, 2015.

National Institutes of Health (NIH), National Institute of Environmental Health Services (NIEHS): Cancer and the Environment: What You Need to Know, What You Need to Do (website): http://www.niehs.nih.gov/health/materials/cancer_and_the_environment_508.pdf, 2003. Accessed 03.02.15.

National Marrow Donor Program (NMDP): *Transplant Basics* (website): http://bethematch.org/Transplant-Basics/. Accessed February 20, 2015.

Norat T et al:Fruits and vegetables: updating the epidemiologic evidence from the WCRF/AICR lifestyle recommendations for cancer prevention. *Cancer Treat Res* 159:35, 2014

Oaks BM et al: Folate intake, post folic acid grain fortification and pancreatic cancer risk in prostate, lung, colorectal and ovarian cancer screening trial, *Am J Clin Nutr* 91:449, 2010.

Oncology Rehab Partners (ORP): *STAR Program Information* (website): http://www.oncologyrehabpartners.com/star-certifications/. Accessed January 17, 2015.

Parekh N et al: Lifestyle, anthropometric, and obesity-related physiologic determinants of insulin-like growth factor-1 in the third National Health and Nutrition Examination Survey (1988-1994), *Ann Epidemiol* 20(3):182, 2010.

Pierce JP et al: Influence of a diet very high in vegetables, fruit and fiber and low in fat following treatment for breast cancer: the Women's Healthy Eating and Living (WHEL) randomized trial, *JAMA* 298:289, 2007.

Pollack M: Insulin, insulin-like growth factors and neoplasia, *Best Pract Res Clin Endocrinol Metab* 22:625, 2008.

Polovich M et al: Chemotherapy and biotherapy guidelines and recommendations for practice, ed 4, Pittsburgh, 2014, Oncology Nursing Society.

Quinn BJ et al: Repositioning metformin for cancer prevention and treatment, *Trends Endocrinol Metab* 24:469, 2013.

Rock CL et al: Nutrition and physical activity guidelines for cancer survivors, *CA Cancer J Clin* 62:243, 2012.

Santarpia L et al: Nutritional screening and early treatment of malnutrition in cancer patients, *J Cachexia Sarcopenia Muscle* 2:27, 2011.

Seattle Cancer Care Alliance (SCCA): *General Oncology Diet Guidelines* (website): http://www.seattlecca.org/general-oncology-diet-guidelines.cfm. Accessed March 2, 2015.

Thomson CA et al: Nutrition and physical activity cancer prevention guidelines, cancer risk and mortality in the women's health initiative, *Cancer Prev Res* 7:42, 2014.

Trentham K, Grant B: Nutritional management of oncology patients in palliative and hospice settings. In Leser M et al, editors: *Oncology nutrition for clinical practice*, Chicago, 2013, Oncology Nutrition Dietetic Practice Group 2013.

U.S. Department of Agriculture (USDA): *USDA Database for the Isoflavone Content of Selected Foods, release 2.0* (website): http://www.ars.usda.gov/Services/docs.htm?docid=6382, 2014. Accessed March 2, 2015.

Valavanidis A et al: 8-hydroxy-2'-deoxyguanosine (8-OHdG): a critical biomarker of oxidative stress and carcinogenesis, *J Environ Sci Health C Environ Carcinog Ecotoxical Rev* 27:120, 2009.

Voelker R: Even low, regular alcohol use increases the risk of dying from cancer, *JAMA* 309:970, 2013.

Wilkes GM, Barton-Burke M: *2013 Oncology nursing drug handbook*, Burlington, 2013, Jones and Bartlett.

World Cancer Research Fund (WCRF), American Institute for Cancer Research (AICR): *Food, nutrition, physical activity, and the prevention of cancer: a global perspective*, Washington, DC, 2007, AICR.

Zhou JR et al: Symposium introduction: metabolic syndrome and the onset of cancer, *Am J Clin Nutr* 86:817, 2007.

37

Medical Nutrition Therapy for HIV and AIDS

Kimberly R. Dong, MS, RDN
Cindy Mari Imai, PhD, RDN

KEY TERMS

acquired immune deficiency
  syndrome (AIDS)
acute HIV infection
antiretroviral therapy (ART)
asymptomatic HIV infection
CD4 + cells
CD4 count

clinical latency
drug resistance
HIV-associated lipodystrophy
  syndrome (HALS)
HIV ribonucleic acid (RNA)
human immunodeficiency virus
  (HIV)

lipoatrophy syndrome
long-term nonprogression
opportunistic infections (OIs)
seroconversion
symptomatic HIV infection
T-helper lymphocyte cells
viral load

Acquired immune deficiency syndrome (AIDS) is caused by the **human immunodeficiency virus (HIV)**. HIV affects the body's ability to fight off infection and disease, which ultimately can lead to death. Medications used to treat HIV have enhanced the quality of life and increased life expectancy of HIV-infected individuals. These **antiretroviral therapy (ART)** medications slow the replication of the virus but do not eliminate HIV infection. With increased access to ART, people are living longer with HIV (see *New Directions:* A New Era in HIV Prevention). Unfortunately, health issues such as cardiovascular disease and insulin resistance are increasingly prevalent, and people living with HIV are at risk of the same chronic diseases as the general population.

✳ NEW DIRECTIONS

A New Era in HIV Prevention

Michael J. Hahn, BA

Even before its identification as a retrovirus in 1983, the battle against HIV had been fought on two fronts: keeping people living with HIV healthy, and preventing new infections. By the time AZT (azidothymidine), the first antiretroviral drug approved by the FDA, was available in 1987, more than 29,000 cases of AIDS had been reported and the epidemic already had claimed more than 25,000 lives (AMFAR, 2014). Although antiretroviral treatment (ART) has been a revolutionary advance in keeping HIV+ individuals from progressing to AIDS, it is estimated that globally an average of 6300 new HIV infections occur daily (UNAIDS, 2014).

The primary route of HIV transmission remains sexual contact. Although prevention efforts have reduced sexual transmission significantly, the rate of new infection demonstrates the need for better tools. Much of the latest prevention efforts have focused on two areas: HIV vaccines and microbicides. Development of a prophylactic HIV vaccine has been difficult; numerous trials have been suspended because of lack of efficacy (National Institute of Allergy and Infectious Diseases, 2013). HIV's ability to elude the immune system makes traditional vaccines like those used for smallpox and measles ineffective. However, each trial has contributed to the body of knowledge to support development of a successful vaccine. Microbicide sponges and gels have shown some promise but to date trials have not led to an approved product because results have been inconsistent.

Three decades after the epidemic began, a new prevention strategy has emerged.

In 2012 the Food and Drug Administration approved an antiretroviral drug combination for preexposure prophylaxis, or PrEP. In a study of heterosexual partners in which one partner was HIV+ and one partner HIV−, consistent use of the drug Truvada (emtricitabine/tenofovir) reduced infections by at least 90% (Baeten et al, 2012). Similarly, in a study of 2500 HIV-negative men and transgender women who have sex with men, participants were randomly assigned to receive either Truvada or placebo once daily. Participants with detectable levels of the antiretrovirals in their blood showed a 92% to 99% greater protection against HIV (Grant et al, 2010).

Detractors of Truvada use contend that problems with adherence and high cost make preexposure prophylaxis an unrealistic solution to decreasing HIV transmission rates (Crary, 2014). A yearly supply of Truvada can cost up to $13,000 in the United States. However, recent estimates of the annual cost of HIV treatment averages $23,000, making the financial cost-benefit analysis still favorable for prophylaxis (Gebo et al, 2010).

The long-term health risks of PrEP are unknown. Short-term side effects have been reported to be gastric distress and diarrhea. Monitoring for lactic acidosis, liver damage, and renal issues is important. Common adverse effects of this class of ART also include low body levels of vitamin B_{12}, copper, zinc, and carnitine.

Nutritional status plays an important role in maintaining a healthy immune system and preventing the progression of HIV to AIDS. To develop appropriate nutrition recommendations, the nutrition professional should be familiar with the pathophysiology of HIV infection, the medication and nutrient interactions, and the barriers to adequate nutrition.

EPIDEMIOLOGY AND TRENDS

Global Status of HIV and AIDS

The first cases of AIDS related to HIV were described in 1981. In 1983 HIV was isolated and identified as the core agent leading to AIDS. Since then, the number of people with HIV has increased gradually, leading to a global pandemic affecting socioeconomic development worldwide. The continuing rise in the population of people living with HIV is reflective of new HIV infections and the widespread use of ART, which has delayed the progression of HIV infection to death. Globally, an estimated 35.3 million people were living with HIV or AIDS in 2012. The number of new HIV infections and related deaths has fallen in the last decade. In 2014, there were 2.0 million new HIV infections and 1.2 million AIDS-related deaths reported (Joint United Nations Programme on HIV/AIDS [UNAIDS] and the World Health Organization [WHO], 2013, 2015).

Despite increased prevention efforts and availability of ART, geographic variation in HIV infection is evident. The majority of infections continue to occur in the developing world (see Figure 37-1). Sub-Saharan Africa remains the region most heavily affected by HIV, accounting for 70% of new HIV infections and two-thirds of AIDS-related deaths (UNAIDS and WHO, 2014). However, increases in new infections are being seen in higher-income countries in Eastern Europe such as Ukraine and the Russian Federation. Within sub-Saharan Africa, heterosexual transmission is the most prevalent mode of HIV transmission. Other populations particularly at risk of HIV infection include injection drug users, men who have sex with men, sex workers, and clients of sex workers.

The United States

Within the United States, more than 1.2 million people are living with HIV infection and 13% may be unaware of their HIV status (Centers for Disease Control and Prevention [CDC], 2015). Although more people are living with a diagnosis of HIV or AIDS, incidence has remained relatively stable since the 1990s. In 2013, men accounted for 80% of all diagnoses of HIV infection, and the most common route of transmission was male-to-male sexual contact. The rate of new infections among women, primarily through heterosexual contact, has decreased since 2008 (CDC, 2015b). The largest percentage of persons living with HIV infection is among those aged 45 to 49; this same group accounts for the highest rate of new HIV infections. Ethnic populations disproportionately affected by HIV include African Americans and Latinos, who accounted for 44% and 21% of new HIV diagnoses, respectively, in 2010 (CDC, 2015a). The most common route of transmission among men is male-to-male sexual contact and among women is heterosexual contact (see Figure 37-2).

PATHOPHYSIOLOGY AND CLASSIFICATION

Primary infection with HIV is the underlying cause of AIDS. HIV invades the genetic core of the CD4 + cells, which are T-helper lymphocyte cells, and which are the principal agents involved in protection against infection. HIV infection causes a progressive depletion of CD4+ cells, which eventually leads to immunodeficiency.

HIV infection progresses through four clinical stages: acute HIV infection, clinical latency, symptomatic HIV infection, and progression of HIV to AIDS. The two main biomarkers used to assess disease progression are HIV ribonucleic acid (RNA) (viral load) and CD4+ T-cell count (CD4 count).

Acute HIV infection is the time from transmission of HIV to the host until the production of detectable antibodies against the virus (seroconversion) occurs. Half of individuals experience physical symptoms such as fever, malaise, myalgia, pharyngitis, or

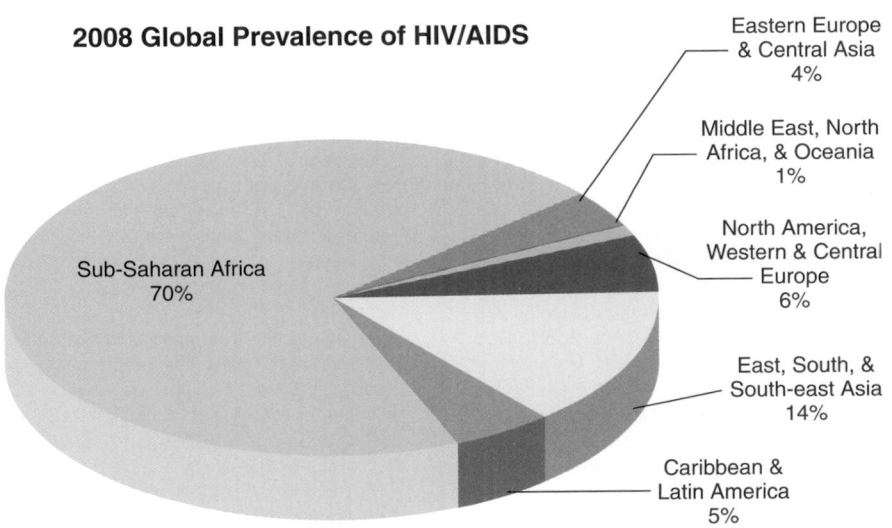

2008 Global Prevalence of HIV/AIDS

- Sub-Saharan Africa 70%
- Eastern Europe & Central Asia 4%
- Middle East, North Africa, & Oceania 1%
- North America, Western & Central Europe 6%
- East, South, & South-east Asia 14%
- Caribbean & Latin America 5%

FIGURE 37-1 Global prevalence of HIV/AIDS. (Joint United Nations Programme on HIV/AIDS [UNAIDS] and World Health Organization [WHO]: *UNAIDS 2014 Global Fact Sheet* [website]: http://www.unaids.org/sites/default/files/media_asset/20150714_FS_MDG6_Report_en.pdf, 2014. Accessed August 6, 2015.)

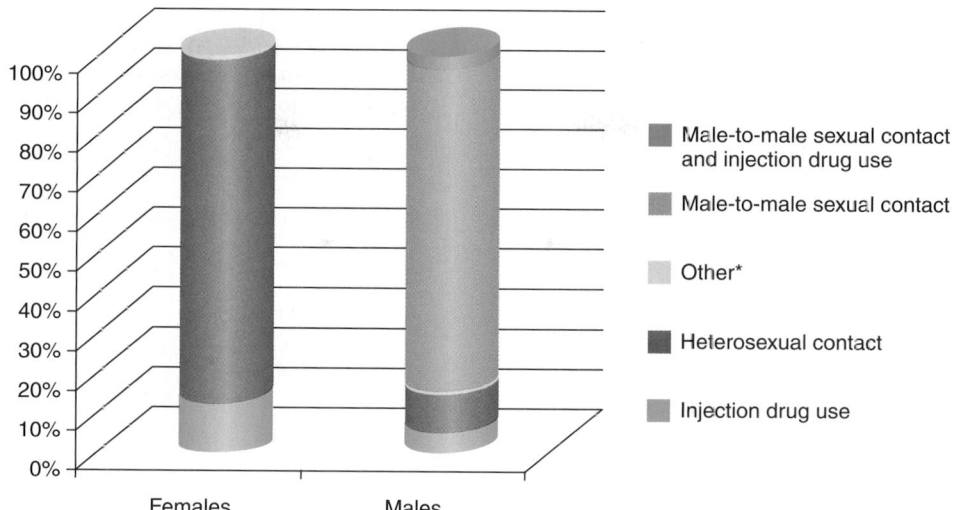

FIGURE 37-2 Estimated percentage of HIV diagnoses by route of transmission in the United States, 2013. (Centers for Disease Control and Prevention [CDC]: *HIV Surveillance Report* [website]: http://www.cdc.gov/hiv/library/reports/surveillance, 2015. Accessed August 6, 2015.)

swollen lymph glands at 2 to 4 weeks after infection, but these generally subside after 1 to 2 weeks. Because of the nonspecific clinical features and short diagnostic window, acute HIV infection is rarely diagnosed. HIV seroconversion occurs within 3 weeks to 3 months after exposure. If HIV testing is done before seroconversion occurs, a "false negative" may result despite HIV being present. During the acute stage, the virus replicates rapidly and causes a significant decline in CD4+ cell counts. Eventually, the immune response reaches a viral setpoint, when the viral load stabilizes and CD4+ cell counts return closer to normal.

A period of **clinical latency**, or **asymptomatic HIV infection**, then follows. Further evidence of illness may not be exhibited for as long as 10 years postinfection. The virus is still active and replicating, although at a decreased rate compared with the acute stage, and CD4+ cell counts continue to steadily decline. In 3% to 5% of HIV-infected individuals, **long-term nonprogression** occurs, in which CD4+ cell counts remain normal and viral loads can be undetectable for years without medical intervention (Department of Health and Human Services [DHHS], 2013). It has been suggested that this unique population has different and fewer receptor sites for the virus to penetrate cell membranes (Wanke et al, 2009).

In the majority of cases, HIV slowly breaks down the immune system, making it incapable of fighting the virus. When CD4+ cell counts fall below 500 cells/mm3 individuals are more susceptible to developing signs and symptoms such as persistent fevers, chronic diarrhea, unexplained weight loss, and recurrent fungal or bacterial infections, all of which are indicative of **symptomatic HIV infection**.

As immunodeficiency worsens and CD4 counts fall to even lower levels, the infection becomes symptomatic and progresses to AIDS. The progression of HIV to AIDS increases the risk of **opportunistic infections (OIs)**, which generally do not occur in individuals with healthy immune systems. The CDC classifies AIDS cases as positive laboratory confirmation of HIV infection in persons with a CD4+ cell count less than 200 cells/mm3 (or less than 14%) or documentation of an AIDS-defining condition (see Box 37-1).

BOX 37-1 2008 CDC Case Definition AIDS-Defining Clinical Conditions

Bacterial infections, multiple or recurrent (among children <13 years)
Candidiasis (bronchi, trachea, or lungs)
Candidiasis (esophagus)
Cervical cancer (invasive)
Coccidioidomycosis (disseminated or extrapulmonary)
Cryptococcosis (extrapulmonary)
Cryptosporidiosis (intestinal, >1 month duration)
Cytomegalovirus disease (other than liver, spleen, or nodes)
Cytomegalovirus retinitis (with loss of vision)
Encephalopathy (HIV related)
Herpes simplex: chronic ulcers (>1 month duration)
Herpes simplex: bronchitis, pneumonitis, or esophagitis
Histoplasmosis (disseminated or extrapulmonary)
Isosporiasis (intestinal, >1 month duration)
Kaposi sarcoma
Lymphoid interstitial pneumonia or pulmonary lymphoid hyperplasia complex
Lymphoma, Burkitt (or equivalent term)
Lymphoma, immunoblastic (or equivalent term)
Lymphoma, primary (brain)
Mycobacterium avium complex (disseminated or extrapulmonary)
Mycobacterium kansasii (disseminated or extrapulmonary)
Mycobacterium tuberculosis (any site, pulmonary, disseminated, or extrapulmonary)
Pneumocystis jiroveci pneumonia
Pneumonia (recurrent)
Progressive multifocal leukoencephalopathy
Salmonella septicemia (recurrent)
Toxoplasmosis (brain)
  Wasting syndrome attributed to HIV: >10% involuntary weight loss of baseline body weight plus (1) diarrhea (two loose stools per day for ≥30 days) or (2) chronic weakness and documented fever (≥30 days, intermittent or constant) in the absence of concurrent illness or condition other than HIV infection that could explain the findings (e.g., cancer, tuberculosis).

Schneider E et al: Revised surveillance case definitions for HIV infection among adults, adolescents, and children aged <18 months and for HIV infection and AIDS among children aged 18 months to <13 years—United States, 2008, *MMWR Recomm Rep* 57(RR-10):1, 2008. *AIDS,* Acquired immune deficiency syndrome; *CDC,* Centers for Disease Control and Prevention; *HIV,* human immunodeficiency virus.

HIV is transmitted via direct contact with infected body fluids such as blood, semen, preseminal fluid, vaginal fluid, and breast milk. Cerebrospinal fluid surrounding the brain and spinal cord, synovial fluid surrounding joints, and amniotic fluid surrounding a fetus are other fluids that can transmit HIV. Saliva, tears, and urine do not contain enough HIV for transmission. Sexual transmission is the most common way HIV is transmitted, and injection drug use is the second most prevalent method of transmission (see Figure 37-2).

Most people have HIV-1 infection, which, unless specified, is the type discussed in this chapter. HIV-1 mutates readily and has become distributed unevenly throughout the world in different strains, subtypes, and groups. HIV-2, first isolated in Western Africa, is less easily transmitted, and the time between infection and illness takes longer.

MEDICAL MANAGEMENT

HIV-related morbidity and mortality stem from the HIV virus weakening the immune system as well as the virus's effects on organs (such as the brain and kidney). If untreated, the HIV virion (virus particle) can replicate at millions of particles per day and rapidly progress through the stages of HIV disease. The introduction of three-drug combination ART in 1996 transformed the treatment of patients infected with HIV and has significantly decreased AIDS-defining conditions and mortality (see Box 37-1 for a list of these conditions). Most drugs are formulated as individual medications, but increasingly many are available as fixed-dose combinations to simplify treatment regimens, decrease pill burden, and potentially improve patient medication adherence.

CD4 count is used as the major indicator of immune function in people with HIV infection. It is used to determine when to initiate ART and is the strongest predictor of disease progression. CD4 counts generally are monitored every 3 to 4 months. In addition, HIV RNA (viral load) is monitored on a regular basis because it is the primary indicator to gauge the efficacy of ART. Table 37-1 provides the current guidelines on when to initiate ART.

The fundamental goals of ART are to achieve and maintain viral suppression, reduce HIV-related morbidity and mortality, improve the quality of life, and restore and preserve immune function. This generally can be achieved within 12 to 24 weeks if there are no complications with adherence or resistance to medications (DHHS, 2013). Because the guidelines for HIV management evolve rapidly, it is beneficial to frequently check for updated recommendations.

Classes of Antiretroviral Therapy Drugs

Currently ART includes more than 25 antiretroviral agents from six mechanistic classes of drugs:
- Nucleoside and nucleotide reverse transcriptase inhibitors (NRTIs)
- Nonnucleoside reverse transcriptase inhibitors (NNRTIs)
- Protease inhibitors (PIs)
- Integrase inhibitors (INSTIs)
- Fusion inhibitors
- CCR5 (chemokine receptor 5) antagonists.

TABLE 37-1   Indications for the Initiation of ART in HIV-infected Individuals

Clinical Category	CD4 Count	Recommendation
Asymptomatic, AIDS	<350 cells/mm^3	Treat
Asymptomatic	350-500 cells/mm^3	Treatment recommended
Asymptomatic	>500 cells/mm^3	Some clinicians recommend initiating therapy and some view treatment as optional
Symptomatic (AIDS, severe symptoms)	Any value	Treat
Pregnancy, HIV-associated nephropathy, HBV coinfection when treatment of HBV is indicated	Any value	Treat

From National Institutes of Health: *Guidelines for the Use of Antiretroviral Agents in HIV-1-Infected Adults and* Adolescents (website): http://www.aidsinfo.nih.gov/contentfiles/AdultandAdolescentGL.pdf>, 2009 (Accessed 14.10.23..
AIDS, Acquired immune deficiency syndrome; *ART,* antiretroviral therapy; *HBV,* hepatitis B virus; *HIV,* human immunodeficiency virus.

The most widely studied combination regimen for treatment of naïve patients (a general term to refer to individuals that have never started HIV drug therapy) consists of two NRTIs plus either one NNRTI or a PI (with or without ritonavir, used to increase drug levels and half-life in combination therapy, known as boosting). Recently a regimen consisting of raltegravir was approved for treatment-naïve patients, making the combination of an INSTI with two NRTIs another option (DHHS, 2013).

Although a reasonable number of different antiretroviral medications are currently available for the treatment of HIV infections, there is a growing need for new drugs that have fewer long-term toxicities and greater potency. Because eradication of HIV is not yet possible, and the need for treatment is lifelong, adverse effects of medications, including metabolic complications and other toxicities, become increasingly important as they may lead to nonadherence to the prescribed regimen. Nonadherence to ART can lead to drug resistance.

Predictors of Adherence

When initiating ART, patients must be willing and able to commit to lifelong treatment, and should understand the benefits and risks of therapy and the importance of adherence. The patient's understanding about HIV disease and the specific regimen prescribed is critical. A number of factors have been associated with poor adherence, including low levels of literacy, certain age-related challenges (e.g., vision loss, cognitive impairment), psychosocial issues (e.g., depression, homelessness, low social support, stressful life events, dementia, or psychosis), active substance use, stigma, difficulty with taking medication (e.g., trouble swallowing pills, daily schedule issues), complex regimens (e.g., pill burden, dosing frequency, food requirements), adverse drug effects, and treatment fatigue (DHHS, 2013). Food insecurity has been associated with increased behaviors that can transmit

HIV and decreased access to HIV treatment and care; it also can be a predictor of poor adherence (Anema, 2009; Musumari, 2014; Weiser, 2009) because medications are costly and they often compete with food for available resources.

With the use of boosted PIs and efavirenz, their longer half-lives may permit more lapses in adherence because drug levels stay high in the body for many days (Bangsberg, 2006; Raffa, 2008). However, these drugs are more likely to contribute to drug resistance if discontinued because of rapid viral mutation. Continued encouragement is needed to help patients adhere as closely as possible to the prescribed doses for all ART regimens.

Illicit Drug Use

In the United States, injection drug use is the second most common mode of HIV transmission after sexual contact. The most commonly used illicit drugs associated with HIV infection are heroin, cocaine, and methamphetamine. The chaotic lifestyle associated with drug use is associated with poor or inadequate nutrition, food insecurity, and depression. This complicates treatment of HIV if the individual is using drugs and potentially can lead to poor adherence with ART medications.

Injection drug use is linked strongly to transmission of bloodborne infections such as HIV, hepatitis B virus, and hepatitis C virus (HCV), especially if needles are reused or shared (see *Focus On:* HIV and Hepatitis C Virus Coinfection). Coinfection of HIV and HCV increases the risk of cirrhosis. Chronic HCV infection also complicates HIV treatment because of ART-associated hepatotoxicity. Special medical and nutrition treatment considerations should be taken into account if the liver is damaged from drug use, if there is coinfection with hepatitis, or increased nutrient excretion from diuresis and diarrhea (Hendricks, 2009; Tang, 2010).

◎ FOCUS ON

HIV and Hepatitis C Virus Coinfection

About one quarter of people in the United States who have human immunodeficiency virus (HIV) also are coinfected with hepatitis C virus (HCV). According to the CDC, 50% to 90% of HIV-infected injection drug users also have HCV (CDC, 2013). Although it is unknown if HCV accelerates HIV disease progression, it has been shown to damage the liver more quickly in HIV-infected persons. In the presence of hepatic impairment, the metabolism and excretion of antiretroviral medications may be impaired, affecting the efficacy of HIV treatment. In addition, three classes of anti-HIV medications (nucleoside and nucleotide reverse transcriptase inhibitors, nonnucleoside reverse transcriptase inhibitors, and protease inhibitors) are associated with hepatotoxicity. Therefore it is important for HIV-infected patients to be tested for HCV, preferably before starting ART, to appropriately manage treatment and prolong healthy liver function.

HCV is viewed as an OI (not an acquired immune deficiency syndrome–defining illness) in HIV-infected persons because there are higher titers of HCV, more rapid progression to liver disease, and increased risk of cirrhosis (DHHS, 2013). Nutrition recommendations and dosing and choice of HIV medications must be adjusted for those with liver failure (see Chapter 29).

Food-Drug Interactions

Some ART medications require attention to dietary intake. It is important to ask individuals with HIV to report all medications, including vitamins, minerals, other supplements, and recreational substances that they consume in order to assess their needs fully and prevent drug interactions and nutrient deficiencies. Some nutrients can affect how drugs are absorbed or metabolized (see Chapter 8). Interactions between food and drugs can influence the efficacy of the drug or may cause additional or worsening adverse effects. For example, grapefruit juice and PIs compete for the cytochrome P450 enzymes; thus individuals taking PIs who also drink grapefruit juice may have either increased or decreased blood levels of the drug. Table 37-2 provides potential nutrient interactions with ART medications (see Appendix 23).

Some ART medications can cause diarrhea, fatigue, gastroesophageal reflux, nausea, vomiting, dyslipidemia, and insulin resistance. Timing is also important for ART efficacy, so patients with HIV must take medications on a schedule. Some medications indicate that they must be taken with food or on an empty stomach. Sometimes food must be taken within a specific time frame of administering a medication. Refer to Table 37-2 for timing considerations with ART.

Medical Management

HIV infection should be confirmed by laboratory testing and not based on patient report (CDC, 2008). The presence of comorbidities such as heart disease, diabetes, hepatitis, and OIs may complicate the patient's treatment profile. The assessment should include the patient's past medical history and pertinent immediate family history for heart disease, diabetes, cancers, or other disorders. Metabolic issues such as dyslipidemia and insulin resistance are common in people with HIV and should be monitored. Biochemical measurements should be documented to determine the course of HIV treatment, need for ART, efficacy of ART, and underlying malnutrition and nutrient deficiencies. Some common biochemical measurements include CD4 count, viral load, albumin, hemoglobin, iron status, lipid profile, liver function tests, renal function tests, glucose, insulin, and vitamin levels. Table 37-3 discusses conditions associated with HIV and their nutritional implications.

MEDICAL NUTRITION THERAPY

For people living with HIV, adequate and balanced nutrition intake is essential to maintain a healthy immune system and prolong life. It has been documented that children and adults who are living with HIV have lower fat-free and total fat mass (American Dietetic Association, 2010). Proper nutrition may help maintain lean body mass, reduce the severity of HIV-related symptoms, improve quality of life, and enhance adherence to and effectiveness of ART. Therefore medical nutrition therapy (MNT) is integral to successfully manage HIV (see *Pathophysiology and Care Management Algorithm:* Human Immunodeficiency Virus Disease).

A registered dietitian nutritionist (RDN) can help the patient manage many of the necessary requirements for medications,

TABLE 37-2 Medication Interactions and Common Adverse Effects

Medication Name	Take with Meal or Snack	Take on Empty Stomach	Take without Regard to Food
NRTI			
emtricitabine (Emtriva, FTC)*			X
lamivudine (Epivir, 3TC)†			X
zidovudine (Retrovir, ZDV, AZT)†			X
abacavir, lamivudine, and zidovudine (Trizivir)†			X
didanosine (Videx, Videx EC, DDL)‡	Do not mix with acidic foods or antacids with magnesium or aluminum	X	
tenofovir (Viread, TDF)*			X
stavudine (Zerit, Zerit XR, d4T)‡			X
abacavir (Ziagen, ABC)†			X
NNRTI			
etravirine (Intelence, ETV)¶		X	
delavirdine (Rescriptor, DLV)¶			X
efavirenz (Sustiva)‡		X	
nevirapine (Viramune, NVP)§			X
rilpivirine (Edurant)¶			
Protease Inhibitors			
amprenavir (Agenerase)†		X	
tipranavir (Aptivus, TPV)§	Take with fatty meal		
indinavir (Crixivan)**		Unboosted	RTV-bocsted
lopinavir, ritonavir (Kaletra)††			X
fosamprenavir (Lexiva, fAPV)†			X
Ritonavir(Norvir, RTV)‖	X		
darunavir (Prezista)¶	X		
atazanavir (Reyataz, ATV)‡	Do not mix with antacids, H2 blockers, and proton pump inhibitors		
fortovase (FTV) soft gel, invirase (INV) (Saquinavir)‡‡	Avoid garlic supplements FTV: take with full meals INV: take within 2 hours after full meal		
nelfinavir (Viracept)‡‡	X		
Fusion inhibitors			
enfuvirtide (Fuzeon, T20)‡‡			X
CCR5 antagonists			
selzentry (Maraviroc, MVC)¶			X
Integrase inhibitors			
isentress (Raltegravir, RAL)**			X
Dolutegravir (Tivicay)†			Do not mix with antacid or laxatives, oral iron or calcium supplements
Combinations			
efavirenz, tenofovir, and emtrivitabine (Atripla)* ‡		X	
emtricitabine, rilpivirine, and tenofovir disoproxil fumarate (Complera)*	X		
elvitegravir, cobicistat, emtricitabine, tenofovir disoproxil fumarate (Stribild)*	X		

Abbreviations: NRTI, nucleoside and nucleotide reverse transcriptase inhibitor, NNRTI, non-nucleoside reverse transcriptase inhibitors

Notes: NRTI medications in general can potentially lead to anemia, loss of appetite, low vitamin B12, low copper, low zinc, and low carnitine. Taking NRTIs with snacks may help limit gastrointestinal upset.

Additional side effects may also be associated with these HIV medications. It is important to be aware of potential interactions with other medications and to be up-to-date with HIV medications by regularly checking the following sources:

Thomson MA et al: Antiretroviral Treatment of Adult HIV Infection2012 Recommendations of the International Antiviral Society–USA Panel, JAMA 308:387, 2012

National Institutes of Health: Guidelines for the Use of Antiretroviral Agents in HIV-1-Infected Adults and Adolescents, 2013. Accessed 31 March 2014 from http://aidsinfo.nih.gov/contentfiles/lvguidelines/adultandadolescentgl.pdf

United States Food and Drug Administration: Antiretroviral drugs used in the treatment of HIV infection, 2013. Accessed 31 March 2014 from http://www.fda.gov/ForConsumers/by Audience/ForPatientAdvocates/HIVandAIDSActivities/ucm118915.htm

*Made by Gilead (www.gilead.com).

†Made by Glaxosmithkl ne (www.gsk.com).

‡Made by Bristol-Myers Squibb Company (www.bms.com).

§Boehringer Ingelheim Pharmaceuticals, Inc (www.Boehringer-ingelheim.com).

¶Tibotec Therapeutics (www.tibotectherapeutics.com).

¶Pfizer (www.pfizer.com).

**Merck (www.merck.com).

††Abbott Laboratories (www.abbott.com).

‡Roche Laboratories, Inc (www.roche.com).

ADVERSE NUTRITION IMPLICATIONS

Nausea	Vomiting	Diarrhea	Hyperlipidemia	Hyperglycemia	Fat Maldistribution	Pancreatitis	Taste Alterations	Loss of Appetite	Anemia	Vitamins and/or Mineral Deficiencies	Liver Toxicity
								X	X	X	
								X	X	X	
							X	X	X	X	
X	X	X			X			X	X	X	
X					X	X		X	X	X	
X	X	X						X	X	X	
X	X	X	X			X		X	X	X	
X	X	X						X	X	X	
X											
		X	X	X	X			X			
			X				X	X			
								X			X
X	X	X			X				X		
			X	X	X						
X			X	X	X		X	X			X
X	X	X	X	X	X						
X	X	X	X	X	X						
X		X	X	X	X						
			X		X						
X		X	X	X	X						
		X	X	X	X						
X	X										
											X
X		X									
X	X										
X		X									
X		X									

PATHOPHYSIOLOGY AND CARE MANAGEMENT ALGORITHM

Human Immunodeficiency Virus Disease

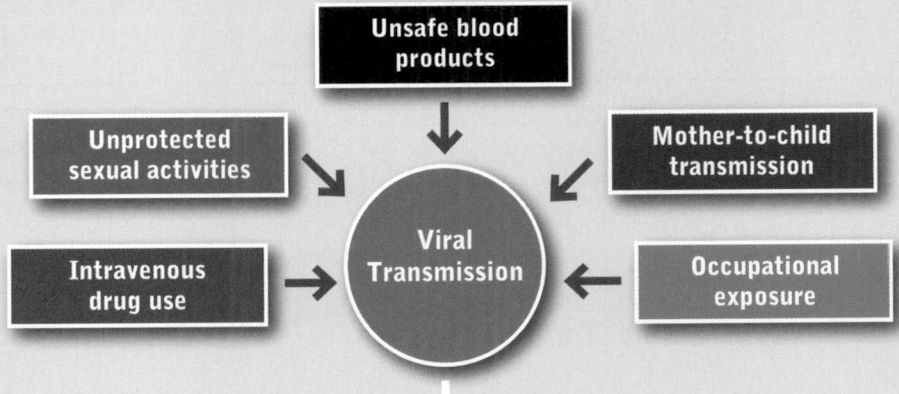

Unsafe blood products

Unprotected sexual activities

Mother-to-child transmission

Intravenous drug use

Viral Transmission

Occupational exposure

Clinical Findings

Acute HIV infection (Acute retroviral syndrome) Fever, fatigue, rash, headache, generalized lymphadenopathy, pharyngitis, myalgia, nausea/vomiting, diarrhea, night sweats, adenopathy, oral ulcers, genital ulcers, neurological symptoms, malaise, anorexia, weight loss, wasting syndrome

Seroconversion

HIV Positive Test HIV rapid tests; ELISA test, Western blot; PCR test

Asymptomatic HIV infection Abnormal metabolism, change of body composition (body cell mass loss with/without weight loss, lipoatrophy, lipohypertrophy), vitamin B_{12} deficiency, susceptibility to pathogens

Symptomatic HIV infection Weight loss, thrush, fever, loss of LBM with/without weight loss, diarrhea, oral hairy leukoplakia, herpes zoster, peripheral neuropathy, idiopathic thrombocytopenic purpura, pelvic inflammatory disease

Asymptomatic AIDS

Symptomatic AIDS (AIDS defined conditions) CD4 cell count $<200/mm^3$, opportunistic infectious diseases (pneumocystitis jirovecii, pneumonia, others), Kaposi's sarcoma, lymphoma, HIV-associated dementia, HIV-associated wasting, vitamins/minerals deficiencies

Medical Management

Treat possible co-morbidities
Hyperglycemia, hyperlipidemia, hypertension, body composition changes, pancreatitis, kidney and liver diseases, hypothyroidism, hypogonadism, osteopenia, hepatitis-C

Monitoring
Fasting blood lipid, fasting glucose/insulin level, protein status, blood pressure, TSH/testosterone level, CD4 cell count, and viral load

Medication
Antiretroviral therapy, lipid lowering agents, antidiabetic agents, antihypertensive agents, appetite stimulants, hormone replacement therapy, treatment for coinfectious diseases (i.e. hepatitis), prophylaxis and treatment for opportunistic infectious diseases

Nutrition Management

- Complete nutrition assessment 2-6 times/year. See Fig. 37-3
- Emphasize importance of early/ongoing nutritional intervention
- Promote adequate intake of nutrients and fluids
- Emphasize importance of food and water safety and sanitation
- Emphasize regular exercise and physical activity
- If psycho-social economic barriers to food, give resources
- Dietary multiple vitamin and mineral supplements
- Inform patient of possible side effects, symptoms, and/or complications
- Monitor/manage metabolic abnormalities
- Small, frequent, nutrient-dense meals
- If mouth ulcers present, foods made need to be mashed or ground
- Appetite stimulants if necessary
- Parenteral nutrition if necessary
- Anabolic therapies

TABLE 37-3   HIV-Related Conditions with Specific Nutrition Implications

Condition	Brief Description	Nutrition Implications
PCP	Potentially fatal fungal infection	Difficulty chewing and swallowing caused by shortness of breath
TB	Bacterial infection that attacks the lungs	Prolonged fatigue, anorexia, nutrient malabsorption, altered metabolism, weight loss
Cryptosporidiosis	Infection of small intestine caused by parasite	Watery diarrhea, abdominal cramping, malnutrition and weight loss, electrolyte imbalance
Kaposi sarcoma	Type of cancer causing abnormal tissue growth under the skin	Difficulty chewing and swallowing caused by lesions in oral cavity or esophagus
		Diarrhea or intestinal obstruction caused by lesions in intestine
Lymphomas	Abnormal, malignant growth of lymph tissue	
Brain	Changes in motor and cognitive abilities	Inability to prepare food and coordinate movement
Small bowel	Malabsorption	Weight loss, diarrhea, loss of appetite
Cytomegalovirus (disseminated)	Infection caused by herpes virus	Loss of appetite, weight loss, fatigue, enteritis, colitis
Candidiasis	Infection caused by fungi or yeast	Oral sores in mouth, difficulty chewing and swallowing, change in taste
HIV-induced enteropathy	Idiopathic, direct or indirect effect of HIV on enteric mucosa	Chronic diarrhea, weight loss, malabsorption, changes in cognition and behavior
HIV encephalopathy (AIDS dementia)	Degenerative disease of brain caused by HIV infection	Loss of coordination and cognitive function, inability to prepare food
Pneumocystis jiroveci pneumonia	Infection caused by fungi	Fever, chills, shortness of breath, weight loss, fatigue
Mycobacterium avium complex (disseminated)	Bacterial infection in lungs or intestine, spreads quickly through bloodstream	Fever, cachexia, abdominal pain, diarrhea, malabsorption

Coyne-Meyers K, Trombley LE: A review of nutrition in human immunodeficiency virus infection in the era of highly active antiretroviral therapy, *Nutr Clin Prac* 19:340, 2004; Falcone EL et al: Micronutrient concentrations and subclinical atherosclerosis in adults with HIV, *Am J Clin Nutr* 91:1213, 2010; McDermid JM et al: Mortality in HIV infection is independently predicted by host iron status and SLC11A1 and HP genotypes, with new evidence of a gene-nutrient interaction, *Am J Clin Nutr* 90:225, 2009; Pitney CL et al: Selenium supplementation in HIV-infected patients: is there any potential clinical benefit? *J Assoc Nurses AIDS Care* 20:326, 2009; Rodriguez M et al: High frequency of vitamin D deficiency in ambulatory HIV-positive patients, *AIDS Res Hum Retroviruses* 25:9, 2009.
AIDS, Acquired immune deficiency syndrome; *HIV*, human immunodeficiency virus; *PCP*, *Pneumocystis* pneumonia; *TB*, tuberculosis.

minimize adverse effects, and address nutritional concerns. Some common nutrition diagnoses in this population include the following:

- Inadequate oral food and beverage intake NI-2.1
- Increased nutrient needs NI-5.1
- Swallowing difficulty NC-1.1
- Altered gastrointestinal (GI) function NC-1.4
- Food-medication interaction NC-2.3
- Involuntary weight loss NC-3.2
- Overweight and obesity NC-3.3
- Food- and nutrition-related knowledge deficit NB-1.1
- Oversupplementation of nutrients
- Impaired ability to prepare foods or meals NB-2.4
- Inadequate access to food NB-3.2
- Intake of unsafe or undercooked foods NB-3.1.

All individuals with HIV infection should have access to an RDN or other qualified nutrition professional. Patients should undergo a baseline nutrition assessment once they are diagnosed with HIV (see Chapters 4 and 7). Follow-up should be ongoing and take into consideration the multifactorial complications that can affect patient care. The Academy of Nutrition and Dietetics (AND) recommends that an RDN should provide at least one to two MNT encounters per year for individuals with asymptomatic HIV infection and at least two to six MNT encounters per year for those with symptomatic, but stable HIV infection. Individuals diagnosed with AIDS usually need to be seen more often because they may require nutrition support (see Chapter 13).

Ultimately, MNT should be individualized, and frequency of nutrition counseling should be determined by the patient's needs. The major goals of MNT for persons living with HIV infection are to optimize nutritional status, immunity, and well-being; to maintain a healthy weight and lean body mass; to prevent nutrient deficiencies and reduce the risk of comorbidities; and to maximize the effectiveness of medical and pharmacologic treatments. Thus screening should be performed on all patients medically diagnosed with HIV to identify those at risk for nutritional deficiencies or in need of MNT.

Patients who exhibit the various HIV-related symptoms or conditions listed in Figure 37-3 should be referred to a RDN with expertise in managing this disease. A comprehensive nutrition assessment should be performed at the initial visit. In addition, regular monitoring and evaluation are essential to detect and manage any undesirable nutritional consequences of medical treatments or the disease process. Strategies for managing the adverse effects are given in Table 37-4. Key factors to assess are listed in Table 37-5.

Physical Changes

The physical presentation of the patient should be considered during initial and follow-up assessments. Patients with HIV are aware of changes in their body shape and are instrumental in identifying these changes. Health care professionals should remember to ask patients about body shape changes every 3 to 6 months. Changes in body shape and fat redistribution can be monitored by anthropometric measurements. Commonly these are taken as circumferences around the waist, hip, mid-upper arm, and thigh, and as skinfold measurements of the triceps, subscapular, suprailiac, thigh, and abdomen. If a dorsocervical fat pad (fat behind the neck) is present, measurement of the neck diameter can help track changes in this area. These physical changes are referred to as HIV-associated

I. Nutrition Screen and Referral Criteria for Adults with HIV/AIDS

Today's Date_____

Name _____ Phone _____ Messages: ☐ Yes ☐ No ☐ Discreet

Gender _____ Language _____ DOB ___/___/___ Age _____ File # _____

Medicaid Waiver Client? ☐ Yes ☐ No   Insurance _____ Case Managed By _____

Referred By _____ Date _____ Phone _____

Screen every six months and/or per status change. Automatically refer to a registered dietitian for any of the following:
(Check and circle all that apply)

A. Medical Diagnosis and Nutrition Assessment
1. ☐ Newly diagnosed HIV infection
2. ☐ Newly diagnosed with AIDS
3. ☐ Any change in disease, diet or nutritional status
4. ☐ No nutrition assessment by a registered dietitian or not seen by a registered dietitian in six months

B. Physical Changes and Weight Concerns
1. ☐ ≥3% unintentional weight loss from usual body weight in the last 6 months or since last visit
   (% wt. loss formula: usual body weight − current body wt/usual body wt × 100)
2. ☐ Visible wasting, <90% ideal body weight, BMI <20 kg/m², or decrease in body cell mass (BCM)
3. ☐ Uses anabolic steroids or growth hormone for weight, muscle gain or metabolic complications
4. ☐ Lipodystrophy: lipoatrophy, central fat adiposity and/or fat accumulation on the neck, upper back, breasts or other areas
5. ☐ Abdominal obesity: Waist circumference >102 cm or 40 inches (men) and >88 cm or 35 inches (women)
6. ☐ Client or MD initiated weight management, or obesity: BMI >30 kg/m²

C. Oral/GI Symptoms
1. ☐ Uses an appetite stimulant or suppressant
2. ☐ Loss of appetite, desire to eat or poor oral intake of food or fluid for >3 days
3. ☐ Missing teeth, severe dental caries, difficulty chewing and/or swallowing
4. ☐ Mouth sores, thrush, or mouth, tooth or gum pain
5. ☐ Persistant diarrhea, constipation or change in stools (color, consistency, frequency, smell)
6. ☐ Persistant nausea or vomiting
7. ☐ Persistant gas, bloating or heartburn
8. ☐ Changes in perception of taste or smell
9. ☐ Food allergies or food intolerances (fat, lactose, wheat, etc.)
10. ☐ Medication involving food or meal modification
11. ☐ Receives or needs evaluation for oral supplement or enteral or parental nutrition

D. Metabolic Complications and Other Medical Conditions
1. ☐ Diabetes mellitus, impaired glucose tolerance, impaired fasting glucose, insulin resistance, or history of hypoglycemia or hyperglycemia
2. ☐ Hyperlipidemia: cholesterol >200 mg/dL, triglycerides ≥150 mg/dL, LDL >100 g/dL, and/or HDL <40 mg/dL (men), <50 mg/dL (women)
3. ☐ Hypertension: two BP readings 120-139/80-90 mm Hg or diagnosed with HTN
4. ☐ Hepatic disease: Hepatitis C, Hepatitis B, cirrhosis, steatotosis, or other:_____
5. ☐ Osteopenia/osteoporosis risk, e.g., elevated alkaline phosphatase, DEXA of the hip and spine low T-scores
6. ☐ Other conditions: renal disease, anemia, heart disease, pregnancy, cancer or other:_____
7. ☐ Albumin <3.5 mg/dL, prealbumin <19 mg/dL, or cholesterol <120 mg/dL
8. ☐ Scheduled chemotherapy or radiation therapy

E. Barriers to Nutrition, Living Environment, Functional Status
Usually or always needs assistance with: Patient is:
1. ☐ Eating   4. ☐ Homebound   7. ☐ Has limited or no cooking skills
2. ☐ Preparing food   5. ☐ Homeless   8. ☐ Income at or below Federal Poverty Guidelines
3. ☐ Shopping for food and necessities   6. ☐ Unable to secure food 9. ☐ Has no stove or refrigerator

F. Behavioral Concerns or Unusual Eating Behaviors
1. ☐ Disordered eating, e.g., binges, purges, purposely skips meals, avoids eating when hungry, pica
2. ☐ Alcoholic consumption: >2/day (men), >1/day (women), or with contraindicated condition
3. ☐ Substance abuse, e.g., alcohol, tobacco, drugs
4. ☐ Vegetarianism
5. ☐ Client initiated vitamin and/or mineral supplementation, or complimentary or alternative diet or related therapies

FIGURE 37-3 Nutrition screen and referral criteria for adults with HIV and AIDS. (From ADA MNT Evidence Based Guides for Practice. Copyright 2005, American Dietetic Association, now Academy of Nutrition and Dietetics, March 2005. For interim revisions see http://andevidencelibrary. com/topic.cfm?cat=4458.

TABLE 37-4 Nutrition Recommendations for Typical Adverse Effects

Adverse Effect	Nutrition Recommendations
Nausea, vomiting	Eat small, frequent meals.
	Avoid drinking liquids with meals.
	Drink cool, clear liquids.
	Try dry crackers or toast.
	Try bland foods such as potatoes, rice, or canned fruits.
	Limit high-fat, greasy foods or foods that have strong odors such as ripe cheese or fish.
	Eat foods at room temperature or cooler.
	Wear loose-fitting clothes.
	Rest sitting up after meals.
	Keep a log of when nausea and vomiting occur and which foods seem to trigger it.
Diarrhea	Try plain carbohydrates such as white rice, rice congee, noodles, crackers, or white toast.
	Try low-fiber fruits like bananas and applesauce.
	Drink fluids that will replace electrolytes such as broths and oral hydration drinks.
	Try small, frequent meals.
	Avoid fatty, greasy foods.
	Avoid highly spiced foods.
	Avoid sugary items such as soda and fruit juice.
	Avoid milk and milk products.
	Limit caffeine.
Loss of appetite	Eat small, frequent meals.
	Focus on nutrient-dense foods such as milkshakes, lean protein, eggs, nut butters, vegetables, fruits, and whole grains.
	Try to eat in a pleasant environment.
Taste alterations	Add spices and herbs to foods.
	Avoid canned foods or canned oral supplements.
Hyperlipidemia	NCEP diet (see Chapter 33)
Hyperglycemia	Diet for patients with diabetes (see Chapter 30)
Mouth and esophageal ulcers and sore throat	Try soft foods such as oatmeal, rice, applesauce, scrambled eggs, milkshakes, or yogurt.
	Avoid acidic foods such as citrus, vinegar, spicy, salty, or hot foods.
	Moisten foods with gravy or sauces.
	Drink liquids with meals.
	Avoid acidic beverages.
	Try foods and beverages at room temperature.
Pancreatitis	Focus on low-fat foods and limit fat at each meal (see Chapter 29).
	May need pancreatic enzymes to aid in digestion.
Weight loss	Eat small, frequent meals (see Chapter 21).
	Focus on nutrient-dense foods such as milkshakes, lean protein, eggs, nut butters, vegetables, fruits, whole grains, trail mixes, and tofu.
	Add rice, barley, and legumes to soups.
	Add dry milk powder or protein powder to casseroles, hot cereals, and milkshakes.
	Try oral supplements.

NCEP, National Cholesterol Education Program.

TABLE 37-5 Factors to Consider in Nutrition Assessment

Medical	Stage of HIV disease
	Comorbidities
	Opportunistic infections
	Metabolic complications
	Biochemical measurements
Physical	Changes in body shape
	Weight or growth concerns
	Oral or gastrointestinal symptoms
	Functional status (i.e., cognitive function, mobility)
	Anthropometrics
Social	Living environment (support from family and friends)
	Behavioral concerns or unusual eating behaviors
	Mental health (i.e., depression)
Economical	Barriers to nutrition (i.e., access to food, financial resources)
Nutritional	Typical intake
	Food shopping and preparation
	Food allergies and intolerances
	Vitamin, mineral, and other supplements
	Alcohol and drug use

HIV, Human immunodeficiency virus.

experiencing neuropathy may be unable to work or be physically active.

Social and Economic Factors

Depending on a patient's mental status, psychosocial issues may take precedence over nutrition counseling. Depression is common, so the need to treat and provide services for mental health issues should be monitored. When individuals are unable to care for themselves, discussion with caretakers may be necessary to understand the patient's nutrition history. Particular habits, food aversions, timing of meals with medications, and related concerns should be documented.

Access to safe, affordable, and nutritious food should be evaluated. Common barriers include cost, location of supermarkets, lack of transportation, and lack of knowledge of healthier choices. Furthermore, stigma not only is a predictor of ART adherence, but also may prevent individuals with HIV from using nutrition programs and seeking support systems.

Nutrient Recommendations

When collecting the diet history, the clinician should include a review of current intake, changes in intake, limitations with food access or preparation, food intolerances or allergies, supplement use, current medications, and alcohol and recreational drug use to help determine the potential for any nutrient deficiencies and assist in making individualized recommendations (see Chapter 4).

Adequate nutrition intake can help patients with HIV with symptom management and improve the efficacy of medications, disease complications, and overall quality of life (see Figure 37-3 for a sample nutrition screening form). Note that a one-size-fits-all approach does not address the complexity of HIV. Recommendations in Box 37-2 to improve nutritional status, immunity, and quality of life, address drug-nutrient interactions or side effects, and identify barriers to desirable food intake should be personalized for the patient.

In the early years of nutrition therapy for HIV, the focus was on treatment and prevention of unintentional weight loss and wasting. Now with access to ART, new nutrition issues have

lipodystrophy syndrome (HALS). Unintentional weight changes should be monitored closely because they can indicate progression of HIV disease. Peripheral neuropathy is a potential side effect, most frequently associated with the use of NRTIs. The resulting nerve damage causes stiffness, numbness, or tingling, generally in the lower extremities. Patients

arisen caused by HALS. HIV-related death from OIs has shifted to other chronic disease conditions such as heart disease and diabetes in healthier individuals who are living with HIV (Leyes, 2008).

Energy and Fluid

When determining energy needs, the clinician must establish if the individual needs to gain, lose, or maintain weight. Other factors such as altered metabolism, nutrient deficiencies, severity of disease, comorbidities, and OIs should be taken into account when evaluating energy needs. Calculating energy and protein needs for this population is difficult because of other issues with wasting, obesity, HALS, and lack of accurate prediction equations. Some research suggests that resting energy expenditure is increased by approximately 10% in adults with asymptomatic HIV (Polo, 2007). After an OI, nutritional requirements increase by 20% to 50% in adults and children (WHO, 2005a). Continuous medical and nutrition assessment is necessary to make adjustments as needed. Individuals with well-controlled HIV are encouraged to follow the same principles of healthy eating and fluid intake recommended for the general population (see Chapter 11).

Protein

The current recommended dietary reference intake (DRI) is 0.8 g of protein per kilogram of body weight per day for healthy individuals. Deficiency of protein stores and abnormal protein metabolism occur in HIV and AIDS, but no evidence exists for increased protein intake over and above that necessary to accompany the required increase in energy (WHO, 2005b). For people with HIV who have adequate weight and are not malnourished, protein supplementation may not be sufficient to improve lean body mass (Sattler, 2008). However, with an OI, an additional 10% increase in protein intake is recommended because of increased protein turnover (WHO, 2005b). If other comorbidities such as renal insufficiency, cirrhosis, or pancreatitis are present, protein recommendations should be adjusted accordingly (see Chapter 29).

Fat

Evidence indicates that fat oxidation increases with HIV infection and thus, dietary fat requirements may be different (WHO, 2005b). However, the mechanism is multifaceted and at present, general heart-healthy guidelines should be the focus for dietary fat intake. Recent research has focused on immune function and omega-3 fatty acids. There is some research to suggest increasing the intake of omega-3 fatty acids in individuals with HIV who have elevated serum triglycerides may be beneficial.

Micronutrients

Vitamins and minerals are important for optimal immune function. Nutrient deficiencies can affect immune function and lead to disease progression. Micronutrient deficiencies are common in people with HIV infection as a result of malabsorption, drug-nutrient interactions, altered metabolism, gut infection, and altered gut barrier function. Vitamin A, zinc, and selenium serum levels are often low during a response to infection, so it is important to assess dietary intake to determine whether correction of serum micronutrients is warranted.

There are benefits to correcting some depleted serum levels of micronutrients. Low levels of vitamins A, B_{12}, and zinc are associated with faster disease progression. Higher intakes of vitamins C and B have been associated with increased CD4 counts and slower disease progression to AIDS (Coyne-Meyers and Trombley, 2004). The Nutrition for Healthy Living study found that minorities and women tend to have lower micronutrient intakes and may benefit from nutrition counseling and dietary assessment (Jones, 2006).

Studies on micronutrients are difficult to interpret because there are a variety of study designs and outcomes. Serum micronutrient levels reflect conditions such as acute infection, liver disease, technical parameters, and recent intake. Adequate micronutrient intake through consumption of a balanced, healthy diet should be encouraged. However, diet alone may not be sufficient in people with HIV. A multivitamin and mineral supplement that provides 100% of the DRI also may be recommended. Megadosing on some micronutrients such as vitamins A, B_6, D, E, and copper, iron, niacin, selenium, and zinc may be detrimental to health outcomes and may not protect against prevention of chronic diseases.

Research has been increasing in the area of micronutrient supplementation in people with HIV. It is important to consider the populations in which these studies have been conducted, and the findings should be individualized to the client's needs. Factors that should be considered are underlying nutritional status, the stage of HIV infection or AIDS, use of ART medications, the presence of coinfections, and indication of an actual micronutrient deficiency (preferably from laboratory documentation), as well as intended length of supplement use. Caution should be used when recommending micronutrient supplementation for all people with HIV, because megadosing on some micronutrients such as vitamin A and zinc can have adverse outcomes, such as disease progression.

Recent studies have suggested that selenium supplementation may slow HIV progression (Baum, 2013). Conversely, low serum 25-hydroxy vitamin D levels may hasten HIV disease progression, alluding to a possible benefit of vitamin D supplementation in people with HIV with a vitamin D deficiency (Shepherd, 2014). The challenging question is whether a low serum micronutrient laboratory value is indicative of a true deficiency or an acute phase response to the virus (Forrester, 2011). Because of these uncertainties, micronutrient supplementation should be thoroughly evaluated before being prescribed and if indicated, be monitored to determine the optimal length of time for supplementation.

The most beneficial levels of micronutrient supplementation have yet to be determined. There is evidence which supports micronutrient supplementation at the RDA amounts is as efficacious as supplementation at two to four times the RDA (Forrester, 2011). At this time, no evidence supports micronutrient supplementation in adults with HIV infection above the recommended levels of the DRI (Kawai, 2010, WHO, 2005c) (see Table 37-6).

SPECIAL CONSIDERATIONS

Wasting

Wasting implies unintentional weight loss and loss of lean body mass, and is strongly associated with an increased risk of disease progression and mortality. Despite the efficacy of ART, wasting continues to be a common problem in those with HIV. Wasting may be caused by a combination of factors, including inadequate dietary intake, malabsorption, and increased metabolic rates from viral replication or complications from the disease. Inadequate dietary intake can be caused by several issues related to conditions that affect the ability to chew or swallow food, gastrointestinal motility, neurologic diseases that affect perceptions of hunger or ability to eat, food insecurity related to psychosocial or economic factors, and anorexia from medications, malabsorption, systemic infections, or tumors (Mankal, 2014). Until the underlying cause of weight loss is discovered, it will remain difficult to target effective nutrition therapy.

Obesity

Obesity in people with HIV also has been noted. Unintentional weight loss in HIV infection has been associated with mortality, but more careful review in overweight or obese HIV-infected

TABLE 37-6 Common Micronutrient Deficiencies and Indications for Supplementation

Vitamin or Mineral	Potential Cause for Deficiency	Results of Vitamin Deficiency	Supplementation Indications
B$_{12}$	Malabsorption Inadequate intake	Increased risk of progression to AIDS Dementia Peripheral neuropathy Myelopathy Diminished performance (information processing and problem-solving skills)	Little evidence for benefits of supplementation beyond correcting low serum levels
A	Inadequate intake	Increased risk of progression to AIDS	Necessary to correct low levels Should not exceed DRI when serum levels are normal High intakes beyond correcting low levels can be detrimental to health and potentially increase risk of mortality from AIDS (Coyne-Meyers and Trombley, 2004) Needs more research
Beta-carotene	Inadequate intake Fat malabsorption	Potential relationship with oxidative stress Potentially weakens immune function	Recommend only amounts found in multivitamin supplement Needs more research
E	Inadequate intake	Potential increased progression to AIDS Oxidative stress Impaired immune response	High intake: may be associated with increased surrogate markers of atherosclerosis Needs more research
D	Inadequate intake Inadequate exposure to sunshine	Immune suppression	Correct low levels Needs more research
Selenium	Inadequate intake	Potential increased progression to AIDS Weakened immune function Oxidative stress	Multivitamin/mineral providing DRI Higher doses not recommended at this time until further research
Zinc	Inadequate intake	Increased risk for HIV-related mortality Weakened immune system Impaired healing processes Lower CD4 counts	Recommend supplementing to intakes of DRI High levels above DRI may lead to faster disease progression Needs more research
Iron	Low levels during initial asymptomatic HIV infection caused by inadequate absorption Inadequate intake	Anemia Progression and mortality in HIV infection Increased susceptibility to and severity from other infections such as TB	Correct low levels as needed Recommend intakes at DRI High levels potentially lead to increased viral load Needs more research

Coyne-Meyers K, Trombley LE: A review of nutrition in human immunodeficiency virus infection in the era of highly active antiretroviral therapy, *Nutr Clin Prac* 19:340, 2004; Falcone EL et al: Micronutrient concentrations and subclinical atherosclerosis in adults with HIV, *Am J Clin Nutr* 91:1213, 2010; McDermid JM et al: Mortality in HIV infection is independently predicted by host iron status and SLC11A1 and HP genotypes, with new evidence of a gene-nutrient interaction, *Am J Clin Nutr* 90:225, 2009; Pitney CL et al: Selenium supplementation in HIV-infected patients: is there any potential clinical benefit? *J Assoc Nurses AIDS Care* 20:326, 2009; Rodriguez M et al: High frequency of vitamin D deficiency in ambulatory HIV-positive patients, *AIDS Res Hum Retroviruses* 25:9, 2009.

AIDS, Acquired immune deficiency syndrome: *DRI*, dietary reference intake; *TB*, tuberculosis.

individuals is needed. Recently a lower risk of developing a noncommunicable disease was observed among overweight HIV-infected adults initiating ART compared with normal weight adults with HIV infection on ART (Koethe, 2014). However, excess adiposity is associated with cardiovascular risk factors and inflammation so weight changes in either direction should be monitored closely. In the era of ART, it is no longer believed that continuously gaining body weight is a protective cushion against HIV-related wasting and progression to AIDS.

Some of the ART medications increase the risk of hyperlipidemia, insulin resistance, and diabetes. It is important to monitor these risk factors and provide nutrition recommendations to maintain a healthy weight. Physical activity, aerobic exercise, and resistance training are recommended to work synergistically with optimal nutrition intake to achieve a healthy weight and maintain lean body mass.

HIV-Associated Lipodystrophy Syndrome (HALS)

HIV-associated lipodystrophy syndrome (HALS) refers to the metabolic abnormalities and body shape changes seen in patients with HIV, similar to the metabolic syndrome found in the general population. The typical body shape changes include fat deposition (generally visceral adipose tissue (VAT) in the abdominal region or as breast hypertrophy and a dorsocervical fat pad, see Figure 37-4, *A*) or fat atrophy (**lipoatrophy**) seen as loss of subcutaneous fat in the extremities, face, and buttocks (see Figure 37-5 which shows a facial lipoatrophy scale). The metabolic abnormalities include hyperlipidemia (particularly high triglycerides and low-density lipoprotein [LDL] cholesterol and low high-density lipoprotein [HDL] cholesterol) and insulin resistance. There is no consensus on the clinical definition of HALS and the manifestations vary greatly from patient to patient. Each part of the syndrome may occur independently or simultaneously.

The cause of HALS is multifactorial and includes duration of HIV infection, duration and type of ART medications, age, gender, race and ethnicity, increased viral load, and increased body mass index. Physical changes should be discussed with the health care team. It is important to monitor these changes by taking anthropometric measurements. Monitoring trends with body weight is important; however, doing so will not likely identify body shape changes. Generally, there is a shift in body composition even though weight remains stable. Taking waist, hip, arm,

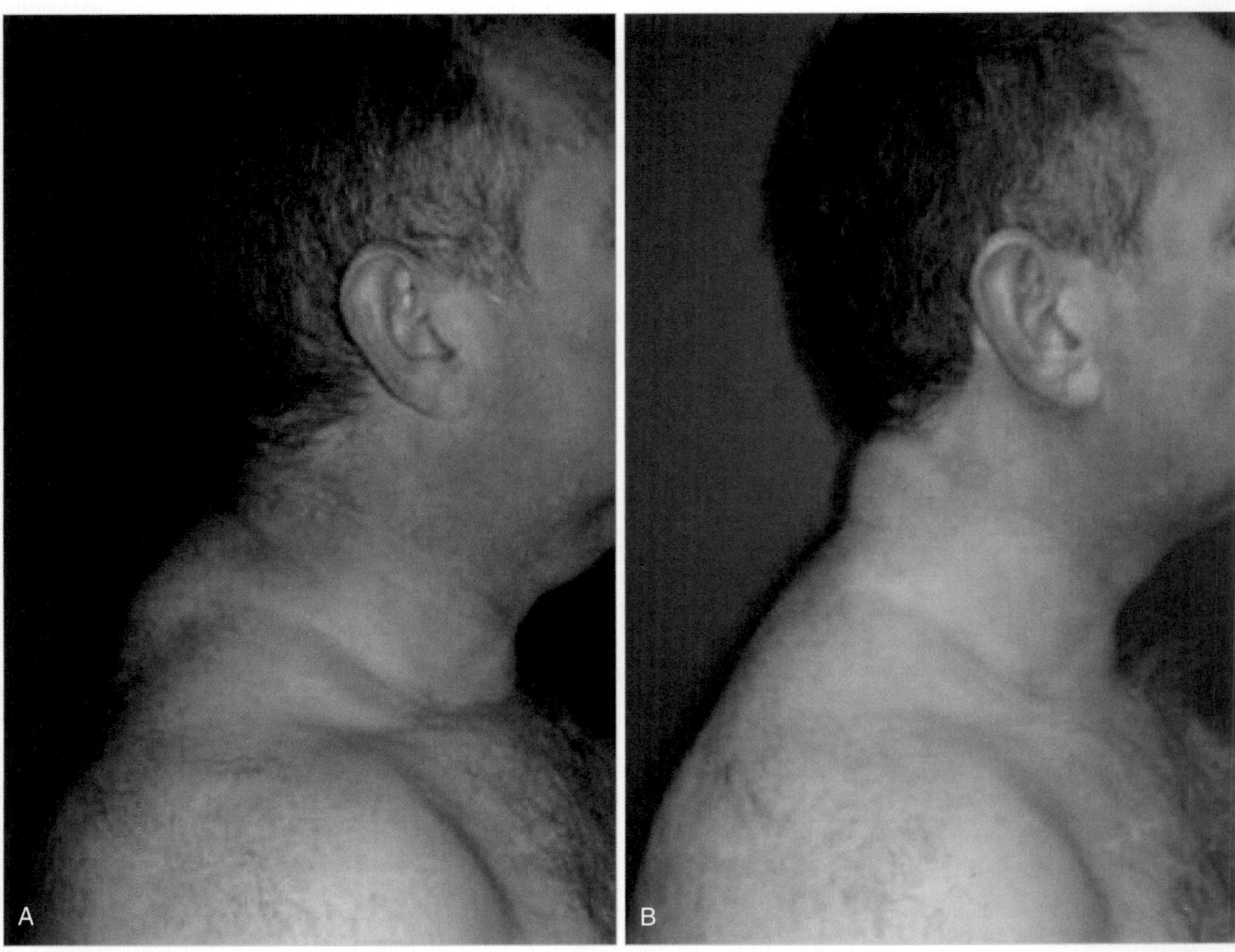

FIGURE 37-4 A, Preoperative view of a 48-year-old man with cervicodorsal lipodystrophy that developed 7 years before his initial consultation. He also complained of anterior neck lipodystrophy and facial lipoatrophy. **B,** Postoperative view 21 months after excisional lipectomy, SAL of the cervicodorsal fat pad, rhytidectomy, anterior neck lift with submental fat excision, and autologous fat transfer from the abdomen to the nasolabial folds bilaterally.

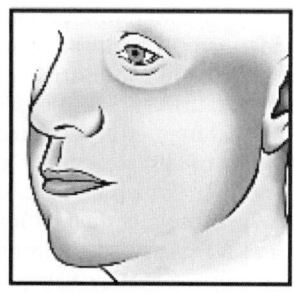
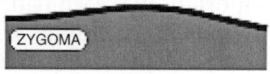
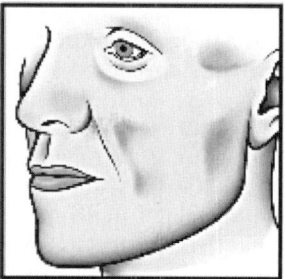
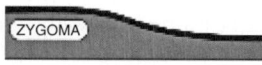
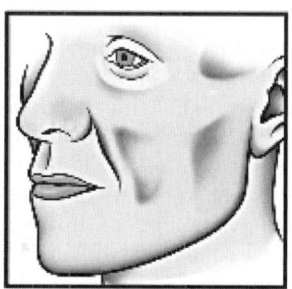
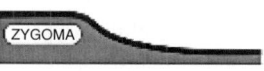
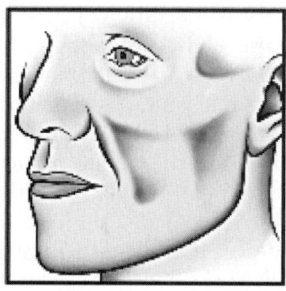
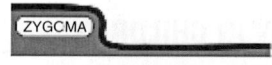

NORMAL
'Chubby' cheek
at or above the level of
the zygoma

MILD LIPOATROPHY
'Lean' cheek
just below the level of
the zygoma

MODERATE LIPOATROPHY
'Sunken' cheek
noticeably below the level of
the zygoma

SEVERE LIPOATROPHY
'Skeleton like' cheek
severely below the level of
the zygoma

FIGURE 37-5 Note: Zygoma = cheekbone. Source: St Stephens AIDS Trust, Chelsea and Westminster Hospital

mid-upper arm, and thigh circumference measurements and triceps, subscapular, suprailiac, abdominal, and thigh skinfold measurements are useful in monitoring exact locations of either fat hypertrophy or atrophy. Currently, some treatments address HALS-associated body shape changes, such as facial injections for lipoatrophy and surgical excisions for removal of dorsocervical fat pads (see Figure 37-4, *B*). The long-term efficacy of these procedures has yet to be determined, and most health care insurance companies do not provide coverage for these surgeries.

Nutrition interventions associated with HALS are limited (Loonam, 2012). For nutrition recommendations, the guidelines set by the National Cholesterol Education Program and American Diabetes Association are followed (see Chapters 30 and 33). Recommendations for physical activity, including aerobic exercise and resistance training, should complement dietary intake. In addition, special focus should be on achieving adequate dietary fiber intake. This can potentially decrease the risk of fat deposition (Dong et al, 2006; Moyle, 2010) and improve glycemic control.

For patients who have high triglycerides, omega-3 fatty acids may be useful. Omega-3 fatty acids decrease serum triglycerides and may reduce inflammation and improve depression. Studies focusing on the impact of omega-3 fatty acids in individuals with HIV are limited. Some studies have shown 2 to 4 g of fish oil supplements per day lower serum triglyceride levels in patients with HIV (Wohl, 2005; Woods, 2009). In a recent meta-analysis, which included four studies, omega-3 fatty acids intake lowered serum triglyceride concentrations in people with HIV on ART (Oliveira, 2011). However, because the studies were not homogenous with regards to dose, population, and length of intervention, it is challenging to determine the amount of omega-3 needed to see positive benefits, including the threshold of triglycerides with the most beneficial impact. In addition, optimal effects are seen with highly concentrated marine omega-3 fatty acids with high EPA and DHA levels. Potential side effects from supplementation include GI distress, hyperglycemia, and increased LDL cholesterol levels. Use of supplements should be monitored and discussed with the health care team.

HIV IN WOMEN

Around the world, women represent about half the people who are living with HIV or AIDS. In the United States women accounted for 9500 (20%) of the estimated number of new HIV infections in 2010 (CDC, 2013a). The highest rate of new HIV infection was seen in African American women, which was 20 times as high as that of Caucasian women, although the rate has decreased by 21% since 2008 (CDC, 2013a).

Women contract HIV less than men in the United States, but several factors put them at higher risk. Biologically, women are more likely to get HIV during unprotected vaginal sex because the lining of the vagina provides a larger area that can be exposed to HIV-infected semen. Barriers to receiving appropriate medical care also exist. Social and cultural stigma, lack of financial resources, responsibility of caring for others, and fear of disclosure may prevent women from seeking proper care.

Preconception and Prenatal Considerations

HIV-infected women of childbearing age should receive counseling before conception to learn how to decrease the risk of mother-to-child transmission. Current recommendations include prenatal screening for HIV, hepatitis C virus, and tuberculosis infection, initiation of ART during pregnancy, and ART for the child once he or she is born. In the United States these interventions have reduced the risk of mother-to-child transmission to less than 2% (DHHS, 2012). Similar to HIV-negative women, nutritional status and potential nutrient deficiencies should be monitored during pregnancy. Supplementation of vitamins B, C, and E have been shown to reduce the incidence of adverse pregnancy outcomes (e.g., low birth weight, fetal death) and decrease rates of mother-to-child transmission in women with compromised immune and nutrition status (Kawai, 2010). It is important to note if women have deficient serum vitamin A levels before supplementation, because different serum levels may affect risk of HIV transmission. Benefits may be noted only in those needing repletion to reach normal levels.

Postpartum and Other Considerations

In the United States breastfeeding is not recommended for HIV-infected women, including those on ART, or where safe, affordable, and feasible alternatives are available and culturally appropriate (DHHS, 2013). Banked milk from human milk banks is an option (see *Focus On:* What Is a Human Milk Bank? in Chapter 42). In developing countries, recommendations may differ depending on safety and availability of formula and access to clean drinking water and availability of human milk banks.

HIV IN CHILDREN

An estimated 260,000 new HIV infections occurred globally among children younger than the age of 15 in 2012 (UNAIDS and WHO, 2013). In the United States an estimated 200 HIV-infected children are born each year. The majority of these infections stem from mother-to-child transmission in utero, during delivery, or through consumption of HIV-infected breastmilk. Premastication (chewing foods or medicine before administering to a child) also has been reported as a route of transmission through blood in saliva (CDC, 2011).

Growth is the most valuable indicator of nutritional status in childhood. Poor growth may be an early indicator for progression of HIV disease. Growth failure can result from HIV infection itself and HIV-associated OIs (Guillen, 2007). Weight and height of HIV-infected children generally lags behind uninfected children of the same age. Loss of lean body mass with no changes in total body weight also can occur. To appropriately measure body changes, serial anthropometric measurements should be recorded, along with tracking of height and weight on growth charts (Sabery, 2009) (see Appendices 4 through 11).

HIV treatment has improved the clinical outcomes for children, with ART initiation resulting in significant catch-up in weight and height, but not to the level of uninfected children. The presence of HALS seen in adults is also common in children. With the increasing number of years on ART, more morphologic and metabolic abnormalities, as described in the section on HALS, are being documented in children (Dimock, 2011; Miller, 2012; Sabery and Duggan, 2009). Multivitamin and micronutrient supplementation may be beneficial at the DRI levels for children who are malnourished. Research does not currently support any supplementation at higher doses.

COMPLEMENTARY AND INTEGRATIVE THERAPIES

In general, any treatment method that is not practiced in conventional medicine is considered complementary and integrative medicine (CIM) or sometimes integrative medicine. Dietary supplements, herbal treatments, megavitamins, acupuncture, yoga, and meditation are just a few of the therapies that are categorized as CIM (see Chapter 12).

The use of CIM is prevalent in patients with HIV infection. National studies suggest CIM use in people living with HIV and AIDs is about 55%. Vitamins, herbs and supplements are the most common followed by prayer and other spiritual approaches (Lorenc, 2013). People experiencing greater HIV symptom severity and longer disease duration are more likely to use CIM (Lorenc, 2013).

Despite the high percentage of CIM use, only one third of patients disclose CIM use to their health care providers (Liu, 2009). Some patients with HIV have noted benefits with taking dietary supplements; however, potential interactions with ART medications should be addressed. In addition, caution with anecdote-based remedies should be monitored regarding credibility for a vulnerable population such as people living with HIV (Kalichman, 2012). Kalichman et al recruited more than 300 individuals from infectious disease clinics in Atlanta, Georgia, and discovered that one in four used at least one dietary supplement. Kalichman's cross-sectional study found that antioxidant supplements and teas were the common products used, and individuals spent approximately $50 per month on products. Therefore it is important that each patient be questioned carefully about use of integrative therapies, particularly those taken orally or subcutaneously. Information should be collected on the brands, dosage, frequency, timing, duration, and cost of the supplements. This should be compared with additional clinical information such as current medications, biochemical parameters, and nutrition intake. Each item should be researched for potential drug-drug and drug-nutrient interactions because there may interference with ART use. For example, garlic and St. John's wort (*Hypericum perforatum*) decrease blood levels of ART medications, decreasing the efficacy of ART and potentially leading to drug resistance.

A key point in counseling patients who are using integrative therapies is to understand why they choose to use them. Most studies have found that there may not be any additional benefit to supplementing beyond correcting deficiencies. Food should be recommended first.

CLINICAL CASE STUDY

Edwin is a 42-year-old male who has been HIV+ for 20 years. His viral load is undetectable and his CD4+ count is 643. His current HIV antiretroviral regimen is raltegravir (Isentress), atazanavir (Reyataz), ritonavir (Norvir), and emtricitabine (Emtriva); he also takes atorvastatin (Lipitor) and ranitidine (Zantac). His height is 5'9" and his weight is 188 lb. His fasting lipid profile shows a total cholesterol 184 mg/dl, triglycerides 304 mg/dl, high-density lipoprotein 25 mg/dl, and low-density lipoprotein 96 mg/dl. Since his last visit 6 months ago, he has noticed changes in his body composition including loss of buccal fat and increasing abdominal girth. Edwin lives by himself and doesn't like to cook; he also receives one meal per day from a community program. He walks for 30 minutes daily. Upon taking a 24-hour recall, you find his caloric intake to be 2700 kcal/day.

Nutrition Care Statements

Excessive dietary intake caused by frequent intake of prepackaged meals as evidenced by diet history. NB-1.7.

Altered nutrition laboratory values as evidenced by results of lipid profile assessment. NC-2.2

Unintended body composition change of increased adiposity as evidenced by increased abdominal girth. NC-3.4

Nutrition Care Questions

1. What factors may be contributing to the body shape changes that Edwin is experiencing?
2. What nutrition and lifestyle interventions would you recommend to address his nutrition diagnoses?
3. What are some biochemical and nutritional parameters you would monitor to determine whether the nutrition interventions are effective?
4. How would you evaluate the desired nutrition outcomes to determine whether they have been met?
5. Edwin has also been complaining of nausea and diarrhea. What recommendations do you suggest for these symptoms? Are there any drug-nutrient interactions of which you need to be aware?

USEFUL WEBSITES

Academy of Nutrition and Dietetics Infectious Diseases Nutrition Dietetic Practice Group
http://idndpg.org/

Centers for Disease Control and Prevention HIV Research, Prevention, and Surveillance
http://www.cdc.gov/hiv

Clinical Guidelines on HIV/AIDS Treatment, Prevention, and Research
http://www.aidsinfo.nih.gov

Joint United Nations Programme on HIV/AIDS
http://www.unaids.org/

National Center for Complementary and Alternative Medicine
http://www.nccam.nih.gov

Preexposure Prophylaxis and ART in Uninfected Individuals
http://www.cdc.gov/hiv/prevention/research/prep/

REFERENCES

American Dietetic Association: Position paper on nutrition intervention and human immunodeficiency virus infection, *J Am Diet Assoc* 110:1105, 2010.

AMFAR: *Thirty Years of HIV/AIDS: Snapshots of an Epidemic*, 2014. http://www.amfar.org/thirty-years-of-hiv/aids-snapshots-of-an-epidemic/. Accessed November 24, 2014.

Anema A, et al: Food insecurity and HIV/AIDS: current knowledge, gaps, and research priorities, *Curr HIV/AIDS Rep* 6(4):224, 2009.

Baeten JM, et al: Antiretroviral Prophylaxis for HIV Prevention in Heterosexual Men and Women, *New Engl J Med* 367:399, 2012.

Bangsberg DR: Less than 95% adherence to nonnucleoside reverse-transcriptase inhibitor therapy can lead to viral suppression, *Clin Infect Dis* 43:939, 2006.

Baum MK, et al: Effect of micronutrient supplementation on disease progression in asymptomatic antiretroviral-naïve, HIV-infected adults in Botswana: a randomized clinical trial, *JAMA* 310:2154, 2013.

Centers for Disease Control and Prevention (CDC): *HIV and Viral Hepatitis*, 2014. http://www.cdc.gov/hiv/pdf/library_factsheets_HIV_and_viral_Hepatitis.pdf. Accessed August 6, 2015.

Centers for Disease Control and Prevention (CDC): *HIV Surveillance Report*, 2015. http://www.cdc.gov/hiv/library/reports/surveillance. Accessed August 6, 2015.

Centers for Disease Control and Prevention (CDC): *HIV in the United States: At a Glance*, 2015a. http://www.cdc.gov/hiv/statistics/basics/ataglance.html. Accessed August 8, 2015.

Centers for Disease Control and Prevention (CDC): *HIV Among Women*, 2015b. http://www.cdc.gov/hiv/pdf/risk_women.pdf. Accessed August 6, 2015.

Centers for Disease Control and Prevention (CDC): *HIV surveillance – Epidemiology of HIV infection (through 2011)*. http://www.cdc.gov/hiv/pdf/statistics_surveillance_Epi-HIV-infection.pdf. Accessed March 14, 2014.

Centers for Disease Control and Prevention (CDC): Revised surveillance case definitions for HIV infection among adults, adolescents, and children aged <18 months and for HIV infection and AIDS among children aged 18 months to <13 years—United States, *MMWR* 57(No.RR-10):1, 2008.

Centers for Disease Control and Prevention (CDC): Premastication of food by caregivers of HIV-exposed children—nine U.S. sites, 2009–2010, *MMWR Morb Mortal Wkly Rep* 60(9):273, 2011.

Coyne-Meyers K, Trombley LE: A review of nutrition in human immunodeficiency virus infection in the era of highly active antiretroviral therapy, *Nutr Clin Prac* 19:340, 2004.

Crary D: *Gay Men Divided Over Use of HIV Prevention Drug, Associated Press*, 2014. http://bigstory.ap.org/article/gay-men-divided-over-use-hiv-prevention-drug. Accessed November 4, 2014.

Department of Health and Human Services (DHHS): *Panel on Antiretroviral Guidelines for Adults and Adolescents: Guidelines for the Use of Antiretroviral Agents in HIV-1-Infected Adults And Adolescents*, 2013.

http://aidsinfo.nih.gov/contentfiles/lvguidelines/AdultandAdolescentGL.pdf. Accessed March 2, 2014.

Department of Health and Human Services (DHHS): *Panel on Treatment of HIV-Infected Pregnant Women and Prevention of Perinatal Transmission. Recommendations for Use of Antiretroviral Drugs in Pregnant HIV-1-Infected Women for Maternal Health and Interventions to Reduce Perinatal HIV Transmission in U.S*, 2012. http://aidsinfo.nih.gov/contentfiles/lvguidelines/perinatalgl.pdf. Accessed March 2, 2014.

Dimock D, et al: Longitudinal assessment of metabolic abnormalities in adolescents and young adults with HIV-infection acquired perinatally or in early childhood, *Metabolism* 60(6):873, 2011.

Dong KR, et al: Dietary glycemic index of human immunodeficiency virus-positive men with and without fat deposition, *J Am Diet Assoc* 106:728, 2006.

Gebo KA, et al: Contemporary costs of HIV healthcare in the HAART era, *AIDS* 24(17):2705, 2010.

Grant RM, et al: Preexposure chemoprophylaxis for HIV prevention in men who have sex with men, *New Engl J Med* 363:2587, 2010.

Guillen S, et al: Impact on weight and height with the use of HAART in HIV-infected children, *Pediatr Infectious Dis J* 26:334, 2007.

Hendricks K, Gorbach S: Nutrition issues in chronic drug users living with HIV infection, *Addiction Sci Clin Prac* 5(1):16, 2009.

Hendricks KM, et al: Obesity in HIV-infection: dietary correlates, *J Am Coll Nutr* 25:321, 2006.

Jones CY, et al: Micronutrient levels and HIV disease status in HIV-infected patients on highly active antiretroviral therapy in the Nutrition for Healthy Living cohort, *J Acquir Immune Defic Syndr* 43:475, 2006.

Kalichman SC, et al: Use of dietary supplements among people living with HIV/AIDS is associated with vulnerability to medical misinformation on the internet, *AIDS Res Ther* 9:1, 2012.

Kawai K, et al: A randomized trial to determine the optimal dosage of multivitamin supplements to reduce adverse pregnancy outcomes among HIV-infected women in Tanzania, *Am J Clin Nutri* 91:391, 2010.

Koethe JR, et al: Body mass index and the risk of incident noncommunicable diseases after starting antiretroviral therapy, *HIV Medicine* 16:67, 2015.

Leyes P, et al: Use of diet, nutritional supplements and exercise in HIV-infected patients receiving combination antiretroviral therapies: a systematic review, *Antiretroviral Ther* 13:149, 2008.

Liu C, et al: Disclosure of complementary and alternative medicine use to health care providers among HIV-infected women, *Care STDS* 23:965, 2009.

Loonam CR, Mullen A: Nutrition and the HIV-associated lipodystrophy syndrome, *Nutr Res Rev* 25:267, 2012.

Lorenc A, Robinson N: A review of the use of complementary and alternative medicine and HIV: issues for patient care, *AIDS Patient Care STDS* 27:503, 2013.

Mankal PK, Kotler DP: From wasting to obesity, changes in nutritional concerns in HIV/AIDS, *Endocrinol Metab Clin N Am* 43:647, 2014.

Miller TL, et al: Metabolic abnormalities and viral replication are associated with biomarkers of vascular dysfunction in HIV-infected children, *HIV Med* 13(5):264, 2012.

Moyle G, et al: Epidemiology, assessment, and management of abdominal fat in persons with HIV infections, *AIDS Rev* 12:3, 2010.

Musumari PM, et al: Food insecurity is associated with increased risk of non-adherence to antiretroviral therapy among HIV-infected adults in the democractic republic of Congo: a cross-sectional study, *PLoS ONE* 9(1):e85327, 2014.

National Institute of Allergy and Infectious Diseases: *History of HIV Vaccine Research*, 2013. http://www.niaid.nih.gov/topics/HIVAIDS/Research/vaccines/Pages/history.aspx. Accessed November 24, 2014.

Oliveira JM, Rondó PHC: Omega-3 fatty acids and hypertriglyceridemia in HIV-infected subjects on antiretroviral therapy: systematic review and meta-analysis, *HIV Clin Trials* 12:268, 2011.

Polo R, et al: Recommendations from SPNS/GEAM/SENBA/SENPE/AEDN/SEDCA/GESIDA on nutrition in the HIV-infected patient, *Nutr Hosp* 22:229, 2007.

Raffa JD, et al: Intermediate highly active antiretroviral therapy adherence thresholds and empirical models for the development of drug resistance mutations, *J Acquir Immune Defic Syndr* 47:397, 2008.

Sabery N, Duggan C: A.S.P.E.N. clinical guidelines: nutrition support of children with human immunodeficiency virus infection, *J Parenteral Enteral Nutrition* 33:588, 2009.

Sabery N, et al: Pediatric HIV. In Hendricks K, et al, editors: *Nutrition management of HIV and AIDS*, Chicago, 2009, American Dietetic Association.

Sattler FR, et al: Evaluation of high-protein supplementation in weight-stable HIV-positive subjects with a history of weight loss: a randomized, double-blind, multicenter trial, *Am J Clin Nutr* 88:1313, 2008.

Shepherd L, et al: Prognostic value of vitamin D level for all-cause mortality, and association with inflammatory markers, in HIV-infected persons, *J Infect Dis* 210(2):234, 2014.

Tang AM, et al: Heavy injection drug use is associated with lower percent body fat in a multi-ethnic cohort of HIV-positive and HIV-negative drug users from three US cities, *Am J Drug Alcohol Abuse* 36:78, 2010.

Thomson MA, et al: Antiretroviral Treatment of Adult HIV Infection 2012. Recommendations of the International Antiviral Society-USA Panel, *JAMA* 308:387, 2012.

Joint United Nations Programme on HIV/AIDS (UNAIDS): *Global Report. UNAIDS Report on the Global AIDS Epidemic 2013*, 2013. http://www.unaids.org/en/media/unaids/contentassets/documents/epidemiology/2013/gr2013/UNAIDS_Global_Report_2013_en.pdf. Accessed March 2, 2014.

Joint United Nations Programme on HIV/AIDS (UNAIDS) and World Health Organization (WHO): *UNAIDS 2014 Global Fact Sheet*, 2014. http://www.unaids.org/sites/default/files/media_asset/20150714_FS_MDG6_Report_en.pdf. Accessed August 6, 2015.

United States Food and Drug Administration: *Antiretroviral Drugs Used in the Treatment of HIV Infection, 2013* http://www.fda.gov/ForConsumers/byAudience/ForPatientAdvocates/HIVandAIDSActivities/ucm118915.htm. Accessed March 31, 2014.

Wanke C, et al: Overview of HIV/AIDS today. In Hendricks K, et al, editors: *Nutrition management of HIV and AIDS*, Chicago, 2009, American Dietetic Association.

Weiser SD, et al: Food insecurity is associated with incomplete HIV RNA suppression among homeless and marginally housed HIV-infected individuals in San Francisco, *J Gen Intern Med* 24:14, 2009.

Wohl DA: Fish oils curb hypertriglyceridemia in HIV patients, *Clin Infect Dis* 41:1498, 2005.

Woods MN, et al: Effect of a dietary intervention and n-3 fatty acid supplementation on measures of serum lipid and insulin sensitivity in persons with HIV, *Am J Clin Nutr* 90:1566, 2009.

World Health Organization (WHO): *Executive Summary of a Scientific Review: Consultation on Nutrition and HIV/AIDS in Africa: Evidence, Lessons and Recommendations for Action*, 2005a. http://www.who.int/nutrition/topics/Executive_Summary_Durban.pdf. Accessed November 14, 2001.

World Health Organization (WHO): *Macronutrients and HIV/AIDS: a Review of Current Evidence: Consultation on Nutrition and HIV/AIDS in Africa: Evidence, Lessons, and Recommendations for Action*, 2005b. http://www.who.int/nutrition/topics/PN1_Macronutrients_Durban.pdf. Accessed November 1, 2014.

World Health Organization (WHO): *Micronutrients and HIV/AIDS: a Review of Current Evidence: Consultation on Nutrition and HIV/AIDS in Africa: Evidence, Lessons, and Recommendations for action*, 2005c. http://www.who.int/nutrition/topics/PN2_Micronutrients_Durban.pdf. Accessed November 1, 2014.

38

Medical Nutrition Therapy in Critical Care

Marion F. Winkler, PhD, RD, LDN, CNSC, FASPEN
Ainsley M. Malone, MS, RD, CNSC, FAND, FASPEN

KEY TERMS

abdominal compartment syndrome
acute-phase proteins
adrenocorticotropic hormone
catecholamines
cortisol
counterregulatory hormones
Curling ulcers
cytokines
ebb phase

epithelial barrier function (EBF)
flow phase
hemodynamic
ileus
interleukin-1 (IL-1)
interleukin-6 (IL-6)
multiple organ dysfunction syndrome
 (MODS)
nutrition support therapy

sepsis
shock
systemic inflammatory response
 syndrome (SIRS)
tight junctions
total body surface area (TBSA) burned
tumor necrosis factor (TNF)

Critical care is the complex medical management of a seriously ill or injured person. This level of illness or injury involves acute impairment of one or more vital organ systems with a high probability of life-threatening deterioration of the patient's condition. Critical care requires complex decision making and support of vital organ systems to prevent failure involving one or more of the following: the central nervous system, the circulatory system, the renal and hepatic systems, the metabolic and respiratory systems, and shock. Critical care patients are treated in an intensive care unit (ICU) that contains specialized equipment and highly trained staff. The presence of multiple monitors, tubes, catheters, and infusions makes these patients difficult to assess nutritionally (see Figure 38-1). Critical illness and injury results in profound metabolic alterations, beginning at the time of injury and persisting until wound healing and recovery are complete. Whether the event involves sepsis (infection), trauma, burns, or surgery, the systemic response is activated. The physiologic and metabolic changes that follow may lead to shock and other negative outcomes (see Figure 38-2). Disorders that frequently are treated in an ICU include, but are not limited to, acute respiratory distress syndrome (ARDS), asthma, burn, chronic obstructive pulmonary disease (COPD), pneumonia, respiratory distress syndrome, sepsis, and trauma.

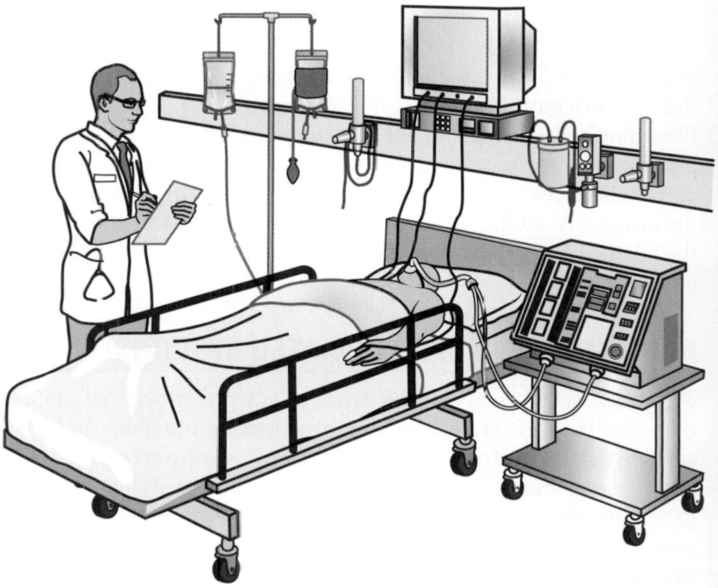

FIGURE 38-1 Common equipment used in the critically ill patient. (Courtesy of Afford Medical Technologies Pvt Ltd.)

METABOLIC RESPONSE TO STRESS

The metabolic response to critical illness, traumatic injury, sepsis, burns, or major surgery is complex and involves most metabolic pathways. Accelerated catabolism of lean body or skeletal mass occurs, which clinically results in net negative nitrogen balance and muscle wasting. The response to critical illness, injury, and sepsis characteristically involves ebb and flow phases. The ebb phase, occurring immediately after injury, is associated with hypovolemia, shock, and tissue hypoxia. Typically decreased cardiac output, oxygen consumption, and body temperature occur in this phase. Insulin levels fall in direct response to the increase in glucagon, most likely as a signal to increase hepatic glucose production. Increased cardiac output, oxygen consumption, body temperature, energy expenditure, and total body

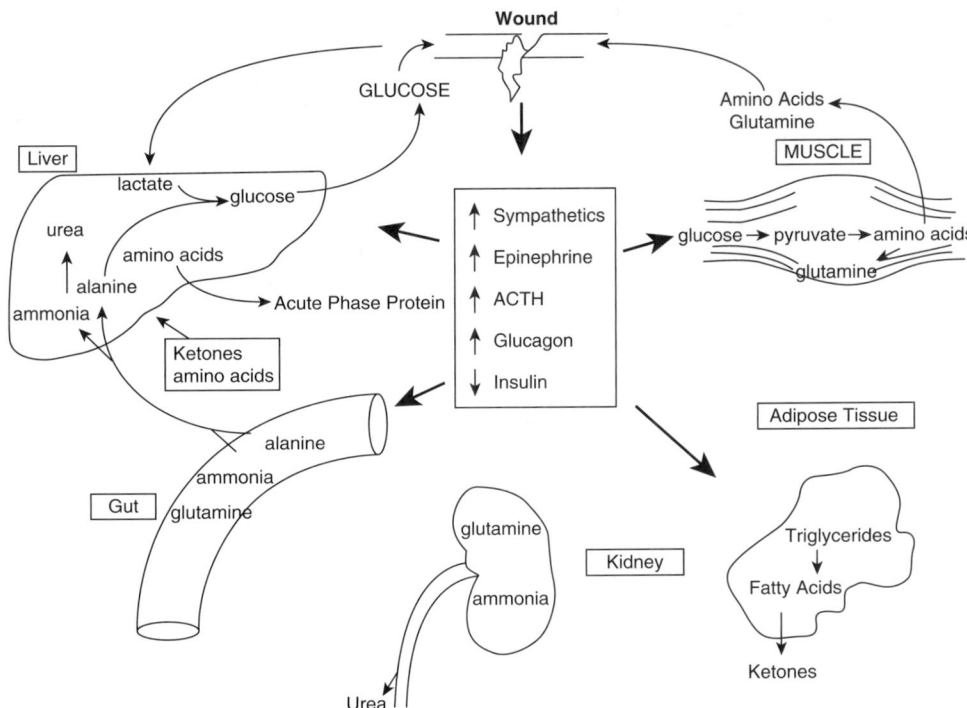

FIGURE 38-2 Neuroendocrine and metabolic consequences of injury. *ACTH,* adrenocorticotropic hormone. (Reprinted from Lowry SF, Perez JM: *Modern nutrition in health and disease,* Philadelphia, 2006, Lippincott Williams & Wilkins, pp 1381-1400.)

protein catabolism characterize the flow phase that follows fluid resuscitation and restoration of oxygen transport. Physiologically, in this phase is a marked increase in glucose production, free fatty acid release, circulating levels of insulin, catecholamines (epinephrine and norepinephrine released by the adrenal medulla), glucagon, and cortisol. The magnitude of the hormonal response appears to be associated with the severity of injury.

HORMONAL AND CELL-MEDIATED RESPONSE

Metabolic stress is associated with an altered hormonal state that results in an increased flow of substrate but poor use of carbohydrate, protein, fat, and oxygen. Counterregulatory hormones, which are elevated after injury and sepsis, play a role in the accelerated proteolysis. Glucagon promotes gluconeogenesis, amino acid uptake by the liver, ureagenesis, and protein catabolism. Cortisol, which is released from the adrenal cortex in response to stimulation by adrenocorticotropic hormone secreted by the anterior pituitary gland, enhances skeletal muscle catabolism and promotes hepatic use of amino acids for gluconeogenesis, glycogenolysis, and acute-phase protein synthesis (see Table 38-1).

After injury or sepsis, energy production increasingly depends on protein. Branched-chain amino acids (BCAAs leucine, isoleucine, and valine) are oxidized from skeletal muscle as a source of energy for the muscle; carbon skeletons are made available for the glucose-alanine cycle and muscle glutamine synthesis. The mobilization of acute-phase proteins, those secretory proteins in the liver that are altered in response to injury or infection, results in rapid loss of lean body mass and an increased net negative nitrogen balance, which

TABLE 38-1	The Metabolic Response to Injury
Physiologic Changes in Catabolism	
Carbohydrate metabolism	↑ Glycogenolysis
	↑ Gluconeogenesis
	Insulin resistance of tissues
	Hyperglycemia
Fat metabolism	↑ Lipolysis
	Free fatty acids used as energy substrate by tissues (except brain)
	Some conversion of free fatty acids to ketones in liver (used by brain)
	Glycerol converted to glucose in the liver
Protein metabolism	↑ Skeletal muscle breakdown
	Amino acids converted to glucose in liver and used as substrate for acute-phase proteins
	Negative nitrogen balance
Total energy expenditure is increased in proportion to injury severity and other modifying factors	
Progressive reduction in fat and muscle mass until stimulus for catabolism ends	

From Forsythe JLR, Parks RW: *The metabolic response to injury; principles and practice of surgery,* ed 6, 2012, Elsevier, Churchill Livingstone.

continues until the inflammatory response resolves. Breakdown of protein tissue also causes increased urinary losses of potassium, phosphorus, and magnesium. Lipid metabolism also is altered in stress and sepsis. Increased circulation of free fatty acids is thought to result from increased lipolysis caused by elevated catecholamines and cortisol, as well as a marked elevation in the ratio of glucagon to insulin.

Most notable is the hyperglycemia observed during stress. This initially results from a marked increase in glucose production and uptake secondary to gluconeogenesis and elevated levels of hormones, including epinephrine, that diminish insulin release. Stress also initiates the release of aldosterone, a corticosteroid that causes renal sodium retention, and vasopressin (antidiuretic hormone), which stimulates renal tubular water resorption. The action of these hormones results in conservation of water and salt to support the circulating blood volume.

The response to injury also is regulated by metabolically active **cytokines** (proinflammatory proteins) such as **interleukin (IL)-1, IL-6,** and **tumor necrosis factor (TNF)**, which are released by phagocytic cells in response to tissue damage, infection, inflammation, and some medications. IL-6 is secreted by T cells and macrophages to stimulate the immune response to trauma or other tissue damage leading to inflammation; it has proinflammatory and antiinflammatory actions (see Chapter 3). Cytokines are thought to stimulate hepatic amino acid uptake and protein synthesis, accelerate muscle breakdown, and induce gluconeogenesis. IL-1 appears to have a major role in stimulating the acute-phase response. The vagus nerve helps to regulate cytokine production through a cholinergic antiinflammatory pathway, releasing nicotinic acetylcholine receptor alpha-7 to reduce excessive cytokine activity.

As part of the acute-phase response, serum iron and zinc levels decrease, and levels of ceruloplasmin increase, primarily because of sequestration and, in the case of zinc, increased urinary zinc excretion. The net effect of the hormonally and cell-mediated response is an increase in oxygen supply and a greater availability of substrates for metabolically active tissues.

STARVATION VERSUS STRESS

The metabolic response to critical illness is very different from simple or uncomplicated starvation, in which loss of muscle is much slower in an adaptive response to preserve lean body mass. Stored glycogen, the primary fuel source in early starvation, is depleted in approximately 24 hours. After the depletion of glycogen, glucose is available from the breakdown of protein to amino acids, depicted in Figure 38-3. The depressed glucose levels lead to decreased insulin secretion and increased glucagon secretion. During the adaptive state of starvation, protein catabolism is reduced, and hepatic gluconeogenesis decreases.

Lipolytic activity is also different in starvation and in stress. After approximately a week of fasting or food deprivation, a state of ketosis develops, in which ketone bodies supply the bulk of energy needs, thus reducing the need for gluconeogenesis and conserving body protein to the greatest possible extent. In late starvation, as in stress, ketone body production is increased, and fatty acids serve as a major energy source for all tissues. Starvation is characterized by decreased energy expenditure, diminished gluconeogenesis, increased ketone body production, and decreased ureagenesis. Conversely, energy expenditure in stress is increased markedly, as are gluconeogenesis, proteolysis, and ureagenesis. As discussed, the stress response is activated by hormonal and cell mediators—counterregulatory hormones such as catecholamines, cortisol, and growth hormone. This mediator activation does not occur in starvation.

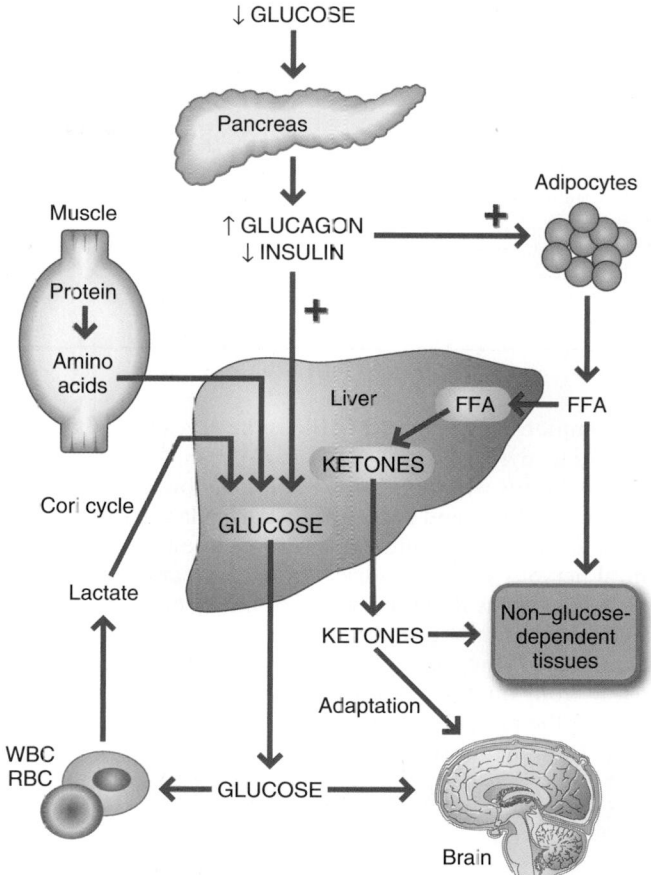

FIGURE 38-3 Metabolic changes in starvation. *FFAs,* Free fatty acids; *RBCs,* red blood cells; *WBCs,* white blood cells. (From Simmons RL, Steed DL: *Basic science review for surgeons,* Philadelphia, 1992, Saunders.)

SYSTEMIC INFLAMMATORY RESPONSE SYNDROME (SIRS) AND MULTIPLE ORGAN DYSFUNCTION SYNDROME (MODS)

Pathophysiology

Sepsis and the systemic inflammatory response syndrome (SIRS) often complicate the course of a critically ill patient. The term **sepsis** is used when a patient has a documented infection and an identifiable organism. Bacteria and their toxins lead to a stronger inflammatory response. Other microorganisms that lead to an inflammatory response include viruses, fungi, and parasites.

Systemic inflammatory response syndrome (SIRS) describes the widespread inflammation that can occur in infection, pancreatitis, ischemia, burns, multiple trauma, hemorrhagic shock, or immunologically mediated organ injury. The inflammation is usually present in areas remote from the primary site of injury, affecting otherwise healthy tissue. Each condition leads to release of cytokines, proteolytic enzymes, or toxic oxygen species (free radicals) and activation of the complement cascade. The American College of Chest Physicians (ACCP)–Society of Critical Care Medicine (SCCM) consensus conference definitions of sepsis are shown in Box 38-1.

A common complication of SIRS is the development of multiple organ dysfunction syndrome (MODS). The syndrome generally begins with lung failure and is followed by failure of the liver, intestines, and kidney in no particular order. Hematologic and myocardial failures usually manifest later; however, central nervous system changes can occur at any time. MODS can be primary as the direct result of injury to an organ from trauma. Examples of primary MODS include pulmonary contusion, acute kidney injury caused by hypoperfusion, or coagulopathy from multiple blood transfusions. Secondary MODS occurs in the presence of inflammation or infection in organs remote from the initial injury.

Patients with SIRS and MODS are clinically hypermetabolic and exhibit high cardiac output, low oxygen consumption, high venous oxygen saturation, and lactic acidemia. Patients generally have a strong positive fluid balance associated with massive edema and a decrease in plasma protein concentrations.

Multiple hypotheses have been proposed to explain the development of SIRS or MODS. In some studies, SIRS leading to MODS appears to be mediated by excessive production of proinflammatory cytokines and other mediators of inflammation. The gut hypothesis suggests that the trigger is injury or disruption of the gut barrier function, with corresponding translocation of enteric bacteria into the mesentery lymph nodes, liver, and other organs. Unique gut-derived factors carried in the intestinal lymph but not the portal vein usually lead to acute injury- and shock-induced SIRS and MODS. Shock results in gut hypoperfusion; the hypoperfused gut is a source of proinflammatory mediators. Early gut hypoperfusion causes an ileus or lack of peristalsis in the stomach and small bowel, and late infections cause further worsening of this gut dysfunction. Early enteral feeding is thought to restore gut function and influence the clinical course. The mechanism for this effect is due to the enhanced functional and structural integrity of the gut.

Enteral nutrition (EN) may have a role in maintaining tight junctions between the intraepithelial cells, stimulating blood flow and inducing the release of trophic factors (see Figure 38-4). Maintenance of villous height supports the secretory immunocytes that

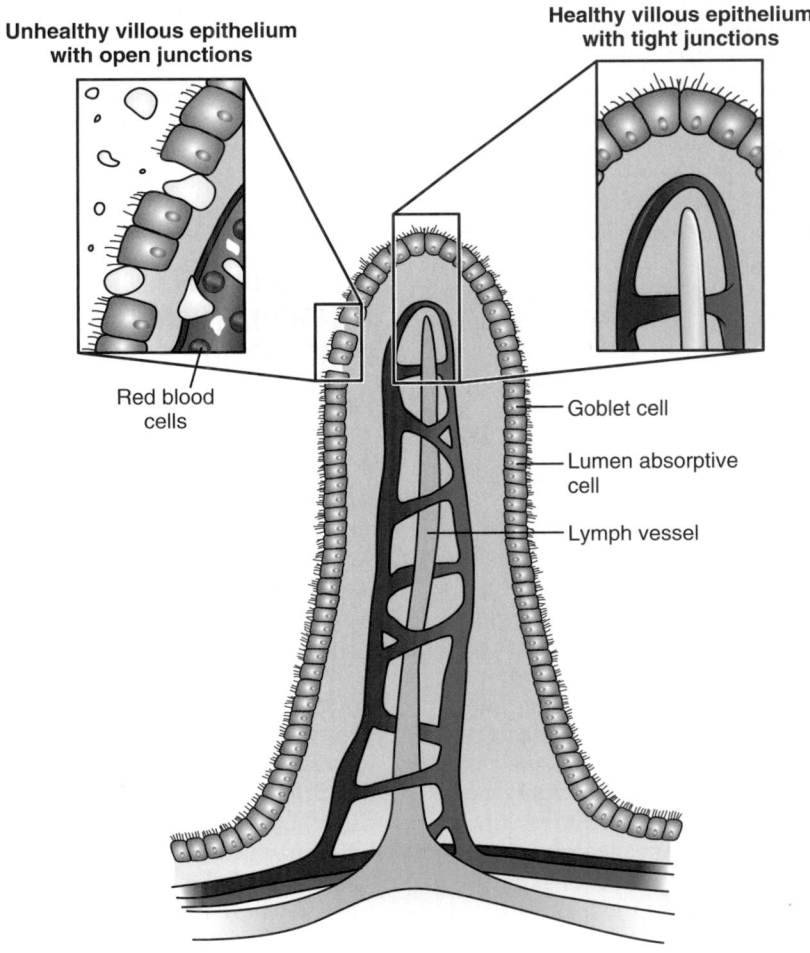

FIGURE 38-4 Tight junction in the intestinal villus, supporting gut membrane integrity.

make up the gut-associated lymphoid tissue. With central parenteral nutrition (PN), mucosal atrophy and a loss of epithelial barrier function (EBF) may occur. A rise in interferon gamma and decline in IL-10 contribute to the loss of EBF in animal models along with a dramatic decline in the expression of tight junction and adherens junction proteins (Yang et al, 2009). Studies in animals suggest that glutamine added to the parenteral solution may protect the EBF (Nose et al, 2010). However, clinicians should use caution when considering the addition of glutamine in EN and PN formulations for patients who have shock or multiple organ failure as research suggests the possibility of harm (Heyland et al, 2013). Although evidence is inconclusive to support the routine use of glutamine in critically ill patients, it could be considered in selected burn and trauma patients (Dhaliwal et al, 2014).

MALNUTRITION: THE ETIOLOGY-BASED DEFINITION

The historical approach to defining malnutrition in the patient undergoing the stress response has recently been reevaluated. In an effort to provide consistency in its definition, in 2009 an international group of nutrition support leaders developed an etiology basis for the definition of malnutrition for hospitalized adult patients (see Appendix 20). This approach focuses on the following three causes: starvation-related malnutrition, chronic disease–related malnutrition, or acute disease–related malnutrition (see Figure 38-5). Using this redefinition, a collaborative workgroup of the American Society for Parenteral and Enteral Nutrition (A.S.P.E.N.) and the Academy of Nutrition and Dietetics published a consensus document outlining specific criteria for diagnosing severe and nonsevere malnutrition. Each malnutrition cause is defined by specific criteria and thresholds (see Box 38-2 for criteria specific to the acute illness and injury malnutrition cause). This specific category includes those patients experiencing SIRS and MODS and is characterized by a heightened

---

BOX 38-2 Consensus Malnutrition Criteria for Acute Illness and Injury Cause

Severe Malnutrition
- Energy intake
  - ≤50% of estimated energy requirement for ≥5 days
- Weight loss (percentage of usual body weight over time period)
  - >2% over 1 week
  - >5% over 1 month
  - >7.5% over 3 months
- Loss of body fat
  - Moderate
- Loss of muscle mass
  - Moderate
- Fluid accumulation
  - Moderate to severe
- Hand grip strength
  - Measurably reduced

Non-Severe Malnutrition
- Energy intake
  - <75% of estimated energy requirement for >7 days
- Weight loss (percentage of usual body weight over time period)
  - 1% to 2% over 1 week
  - 5% over 1 month
  - 7.5% over 3 months
- Loss of body fat
  - Mild
- Loss of muscle mass
  - Mild
- Fluid accumulation
  - Mild
- Hand grip strength
  - Not applicable

From White JA et al: *J Parent Enteral Nutr* 36:275, 2012.

---

cytokine response, which in turn leads to profound losses in fat-free mass. Of note, in this setting, despite adequate provision of nutrition support therapy, repletion of lean body mass cannot occur (Jensen et al, 2009, 2010).

Medical Nutrition Therapy

The critically ill patient typically enters an intensive care unit (ICU) because of a cardiopulmonary diagnosis, intraoperative or postoperative complication, multiple trauma, burn injury, or sepsis. Traditional methods of assessing nutritional status are often of limited value in the ICU setting. The severely injured patient is usually unable to provide a dietary history. Values for weight may be erroneous after fluid resuscitation, and anthropometric measurements are not easily attainable,

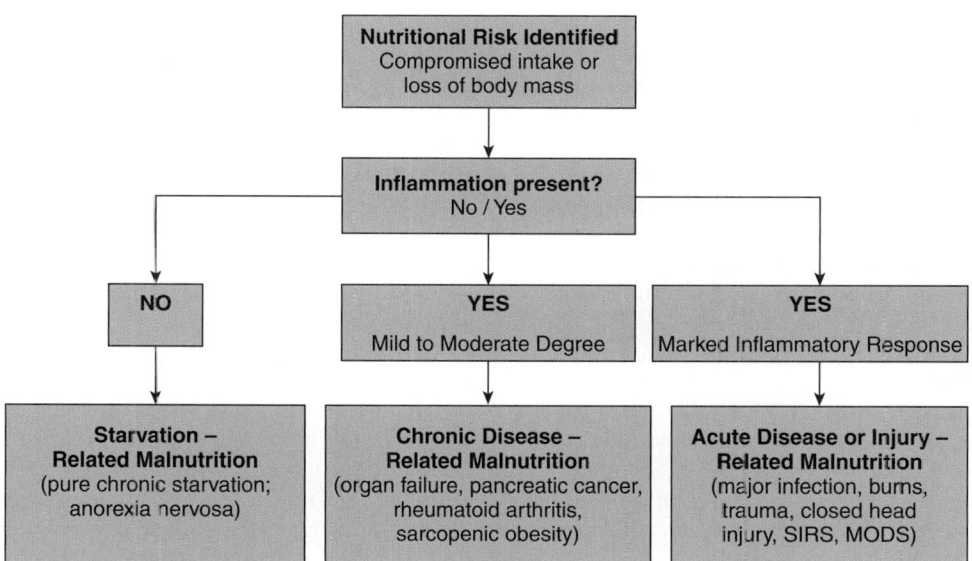

FIGURE 38-5 Diagram of malnutrition definitions. (Adapted from Jensen GL et al: Malnutrition syndromes: a conundrum versus continuum, *J Parenter Enteral Nutr* 33:710, 2009; Jensen G et al: Adult starvation and disease-related malnutrition: a proposal for etiology-based diagnosis in the clinical practice setting from the International Consensus Guideline Committee, *J Parenter Enteral Nutr* 34:156, 2010.)

nor are they sensitive to acute changes. Hypoalbuminemia reflects severe illness, injury, and inflammation; thus serum albumin should not be used as a marker of nutritional status. Other plasma proteins such as prealbumin and transferrin often drop precipitously, related not to nutrition status but to an inflammation-induced decrease in hepatic synthesis and changes caused by compartmental shifts in body fluid. This is part of the acute-phase response in which secretory and circulating proteins are altered in response to inflammation or injury (see Chapter 7).

The critical role of physical assessment cannot be overlooked. Loss of lean body mass and accumulation of fluid are common to the ICU patient, and the ability to recognize these, as well as other important physical parameters, is essential. In general, assessment and care planning focus on the preadmission, preoperative, or preinjury nutrition status; presence of any organ system dysfunction; the need for early nutrition support therapy; and options that exist for enteral or parenteral access. When designing and monitoring the nutrition prescription (see Chapter 13) for critically ill patients, focus should be on laboratory data, not on defining or determining nutrition status.

Because the patient is so ill, oral intake of food or fluid may be severely limited. Therefore some common nutrition diagnoses include the following:

- Inadequate oral food and beverage intake (requiring another mode of nutrient or fluid administration)
- Inadequate or excessive intake from EN or PN infusion
- Inappropriate infusion of EN or PN (e.g., using PN when EN is possible)
- Inadequate or excessive fluid intake (from intravenous [IV] infusions, nutrient solutions, tube flushes)
- Increased nutrient needs (such as protein for wound healing)
- Excessive carbohydrate intake (as when giving a parenteral solution to a chronically malnourished patient, with potential for refeeding syndrome)
- Abnormal nutrition-related laboratory values
- Altered gastrointestinal (GI) function (such as vomiting, diarrhea, constipation)

If malnutrition or an inflammatory response is present, the nutrition diagnosis should be framed around those conditions. The rationale for focusing on malnutrition and the inflammatory response is that these conditions increase the risk of complications related to nutritional status. An example of such a PES statement would be: Increased nutrient needs (energy and protein) *related to* an inflammatory response to injury *as evidenced by* elevated body temperature and minute ventilation.

Nutrition Support Therapy

Nutrition support therapy incorporates early EN when feasible, appropriate macro- and micronutrient delivery, and glycemic control. Favorable expected outcomes from these practices include reduced disease severity, decreased length of time in the ICU, and decreased infectious disease morbidity and overall mortality.

The traditional goals of nutrition support therapy during sepsis and after injury include minimization of starvation, prevention or correction of specific nutrient deficiencies, provision of adequate calories to meet energy needs while minimizing associated metabolic complications, and fluid and electrolyte management to maintain adequate urine output and normal homeostasis (see *Pathophysiology and Care Management Algorithm:* Hypermetabolic Response). We currently focus more on attenuating the metabolic response to stress, preventing oxidative cellular injury, and modulating the immune response. The first emphasis of care in the ICU is establishing hemodynamic stability (maintenance of airway and breathing, adequate circulating fluid volume and tissue oxygenation, and acid-base neutrality). It is important to follow the patient's heart rate, blood pressure, cardiac output, mean arterial pressure, and oxygen saturation to assess hemodynamic stability because this determines when nutrition support therapy can commence.

Glycemic control and its relationship to improved outcomes has been the focus of extensive study. It is now recognized that more moderate (blood glucose 150 to 180 mg/dL), rather than tight (blood glucose 80 to 110 mg/dL), control is associated with positive outcomes in critically ill patients (Academy Evidence Analysis Library – (EAL)). Dietitians must recognize the significant contribution of dextrose in PN formulas and its influence on glycemic control.

Nutritional Requirements

Energy. Ideally, indirect calorimetry (IC) should be used to determine energy requirements for critically ill patients (see Chapter 2). Oxygen consumption is an essential component in the determination of energy expenditure. Septic and trauma patients have substantial increases in energy expenditure associated with the magnitude of injury. IC can be performed serially as a patient's clinical status changes (EAL); this allows a more accurate assessment of energy requirements during a patient's stay in the ICU. IC is not appropriate for all patients, however, and should be performed and interpreted by experienced clinicians (EAL). High oxygen requirements, the presence of a chest tube, acidosis, and the use of supplemental oxygen, are factors that may lead to invalid results. In these situations measurement of energy expenditure by IC is not recommended (EAL).

In the absence of a metabolic cart for IC, energy requirements may be calculated as 25 to 30 kcal/kg/day (SCCM and A.S.P.E.N., 2009) or by using one of the many published predictive equations (see Chapter 2). Avoidance of overfeeding in the critically ill patient is important. Although adequate energy is essential for metabolically stressed patients, excess calories can result in complications such as hyperglycemia, hepatic steatosis, and excess carbon dioxide production, which can exacerbate respiratory insufficiency or prolong weaning from mechanical ventilation.

Some debate exists in practice regarding what value should be used for body weight in predictive equations. Actual body weight is a better predictor of energy expenditure than ideal body weight in obese individuals (Breen and Ireton-Jones, 2004). The 2012 Critical Illness Update recommends that when IC is unavailable, the Penn State University [PSU(2003b)] equation, using actual body weight, should be used in obese and nonobese patients who are younger than 60 years of age. For obese patients 60 years or older, the PSU (2010) equation should be used. Research indicates that these equations have the best prediction accuracy (EAL).

PATHOPHYSIOLOGY AND CARE MANAGEMENT ALGORITHM

Hypermetabolic Response

ETIOLOGY

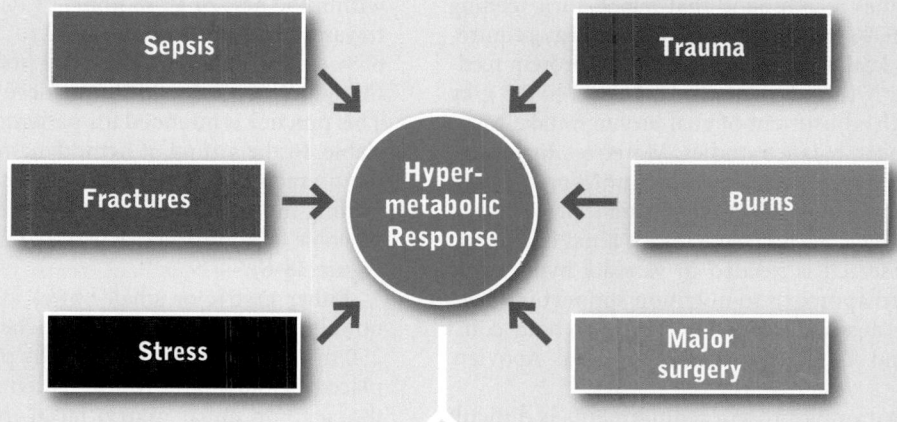

PATHOPHYSIOLOGY

EBB Phase

Hypovolemia
Shock
Tissue hypoxia
Decreased:
- Cardiac output
- O_2 consumption
- Body temperature

Flow Phase

Acute-phase proteins
Hormonal responses
Immune responses (cell-mediated and antibody)
Increased:
- Cardiac output
- O_2 consumption
- Body temperature
- Energy expenditure
- Protein catabolism

MANAGEMENT

Medical Management

- Treat cause of hypermetabolism
- Hemodynamic stability

Nutrition Management

- Minimize catabolism
- Meet energy requirements, but do not overfeed
  - Use indirect calorimetry if possible
  - Non-obese: 25-30 kcal/kg/day
  - Obese: 14-18 kcal/kg/day of actual body weight
- Meet protein, vitamin, and mineral needs
- Establish and maintain fluid and electrolyte balance
- Plan nutrition therapy (oral, enteral, and/or parenteral nutrition)
- Need for pharmaconutrients
- Physical therapy
- Exercise

Available research suggests that hypocaloric, high-protein nutrition support therapy or "permissive underfeeding" in critically ill obese patients results in achievement of net protein anabolism and minimizes complications resulting from overfeeding. A.S.P.E.N., in its 2013 Guidelines for Hospitalized Adult Patients with Obesity, suggests that clinical outcomes in patients supported with high-protein hypocaloric feeding are at least equivalent to those supported with high-protein eucaloric feeding. A trial of hypocaloric high-protein feeding is suggested in those patients who do not have severe renal or hepatic dysfunction. The Guidelines recommend that hypocaloric feeding may be started with 50% to 70% of estimated energy requirements or less than 14 kcal/kg actual weight. High-protein feeding may be started with 1.2 g/kg actual weight or 2 to 2.5 g/kg ideal body weight, with adjustment of goal protein intake based on the results of nitrogen balance studies. Moreover, hypocaloric low protein feedings are associated with unfavorable outcomes. Clinical vigilance for adequate protein provision is suggested in patients who do not have severe renal or hepatic dysfunction. More research is needed to validate hypocaloric feeding as the standard approach to nutrition support in obese patients, especially because of the wide variability in body composition (Choban and Dickerson, 2005; Port and Apovian, 2010).

Protein. Determination of protein requirements is difficult for critically ill patients. Patients typically require 1.2 to 2 g/kg/day depending on their baseline nutritional status, degree of injury and metabolic demand, and abnormal losses (e.g., through open abdominal wounds or burned skin) (Hoffer and Bistrian, 2012). Patients with acute kidney injury undergoing continuous renal replacement therapy (CRRT) may have a higher protein requirement because of the increased loss via the filtration process (see Chapter 35). A recent systematic review of protein requirements in critical illness concluded that protein delivery of 2.0 to 2.5 g/kg/day is safe and may be optimal for most critically ill patients except for those with refractory hypotension, overwhelming sepsis, or severe liver disease (Hoffer and Bistrian, 2012). Administration of excessive amounts of protein does not decrease the characteristic net negative nitrogen balance seen among hypermetabolic patients.

Vitamins, Minerals, and Trace Elements. No specific guidelines exist for the provision of vitamins, minerals, and trace elements in metabolically stressed individuals. Micronutrient needs are elevated during acute illness because of increased urinary and cutaneous losses and diminished GI absorption, altered distribution, and altered serum carrier protein concentrations. With increased caloric intake there may be an increased need for B vitamins, particularly thiamin and niacin. Catabolism and loss of lean body tissue increase the loss of potassium, magnesium, phosphorus, and zinc. GI and urinary losses, organ dysfunction, and acid-base imbalance necessitate that mineral and electrolyte requirements be determined and adjusted individually. Fluid and electrolytes should be provided to maintain adequate urine output and normal serum electrolytes.

Feeding Strategies. The preferred route for nutrient delivery is an orally consumed diet of whole foods. However, critically ill patients are often unable to eat because of endotracheal intubation and ventilator dependence. Furthermore, oral feeding may be delayed by impairment of chewing, swallowing, by anorexia induced by pain-relieving medications, or by posttraumatic shock and depression. Patients who are able to eat may not be able to meet the increased energy and nutrient requirements associated with metabolic stress and recovery. They often require combinations of oral nutritional supplements, enteral tube nutrition, and PN. When EN fails to meet nutritional requirements or when GI feeding is contraindicated, PN support should be initiated (see Figure 38-6).

Timing and Route of Feeding. EN is the preferred route of feeding for the critically ill patient who cannot eat food and yet has good intestinal function. Feedings should be initiated early within the first 24 to 48 hours of ICU admission and advanced toward goal during the next 48 to 72 hours. Intake of 50% to 65% of goal calories during the first week of hospitalization is thought to be sufficient to achieve the clinical benefit of EN. This practice is intended for patients who are hemodynamically stable. In the setting of hemodynamic instability (large volume requirements or use of high-dose catecholamine agents), tube feeding should be withheld until the patient is resuscitated fully or stable to minimize risk of ischemic or reperfusion injury (see Figure 38-6).

Either gastric or small-bowel feedings can be used. Small-bowel feedings are indicated when gastric residuals exceed 250 mL. Nasoenteric or surgically placed feedings tubes can be placed intraoperatively for patients with severe head, major thoracic, or spinal injury; facial injury requiring jaw wiring; proximal gastric or esophageal injuries, major pancreatic or duodenal injury; and severe trauma with plans for repeated surgeries.

Enteral tolerance should be monitored by assessing the level of pain, presence of abdominal distention, passage of flatus and stool, physical examination and, if appropriate, abdominal x-ray examination. Elevating the head of the bed and using promotility medication can reduce aspiration risk. The cause of diarrhea, when present, should be determined, including assessment for infectious diarrhea. Patients should be evaluated for intake of hyperosmolar medications and broad-spectrum antibiotics. PN is indicated for patients in whom EN is unsuccessful or contraindicated.

Formula selection, fluid, energy, and nutrient requirements, as well as GI function determine the choice of an enteral product. Most standard polymeric enteral formulas can be used to feed the critically ill patient. However, some are intolerant of these standard formulas because of the fat content and temporarily require a lower-fat formula or a product containing a higher ratio of medium-chain triglycerides. Several commercially available products are marketed specifically for patients with trauma and metabolic stress. These products typically have higher protein content and a higher ratio of BCAAs or additional glutamine or arginine.

Immune modulating enteral formulations that contain arginine, glutamine, nucleic acids, antioxidants, and omega-3 fatty acids potentially have beneficial effects and favorable outcomes for critically ill patients who have undergone GI surgery, as well as for trauma and burn patients. However, these formulations should not be used routinely for ICU patients with sepsis because they may worsen the inflammatory response (SCCM and A.S.P.E.N., 2009). Insoluble fiber should be avoided in critically ill patients; however, soluble fiber may be beneficial for the hemodynamically stable, critically ill patient who develops diarrhea (SCCM and A.S.P.E.N., 2009). Patients at high risk for bowel ischemia initially should not receive fiber-containing formulas or diets.

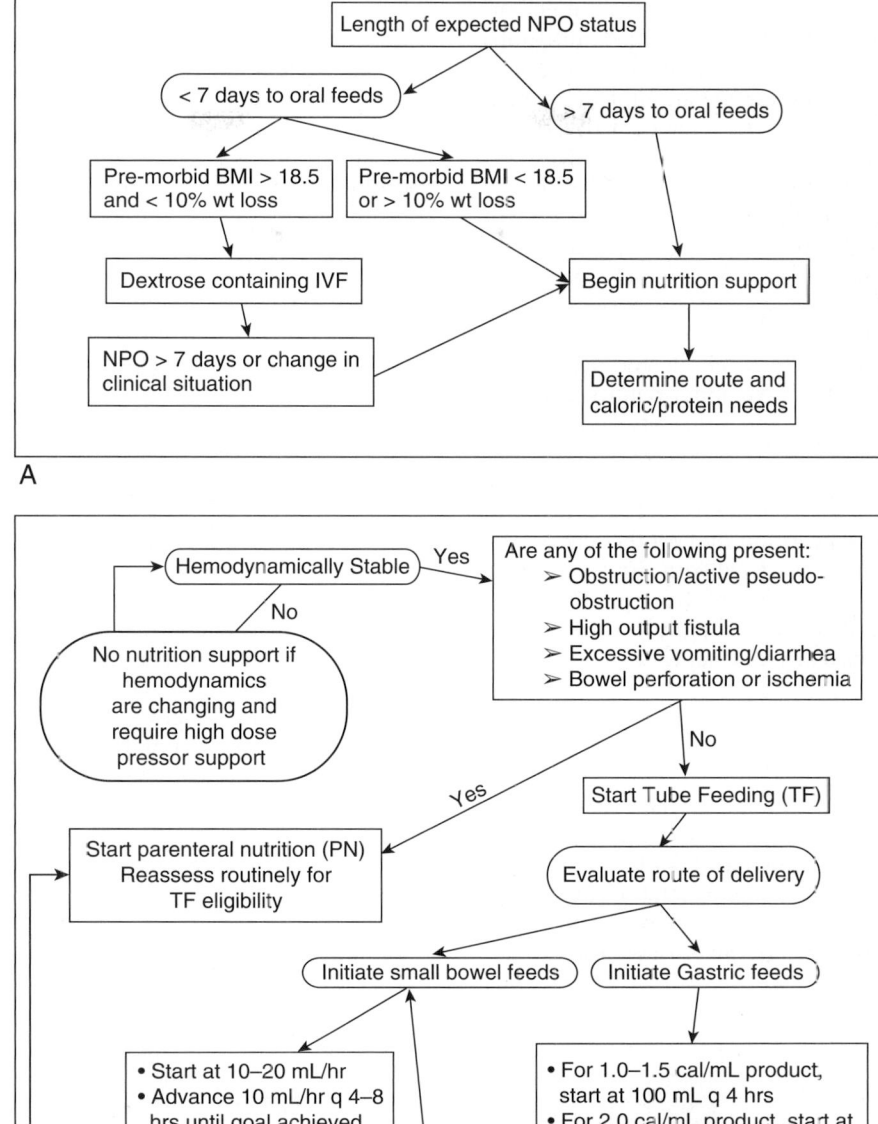

FIGURE 38-6 Timing and determining the route of nutrition support in the critically ill patient. **A,** Timing of nutrition support initiation. **B,** Determining optimal route of nutrition support. (Reprinted with permission from Beth Taylor.)

TRAUMA AND THE OPEN ABDOMEN

After major abdominal trauma, bowel distention, and states of shock, some patients experience increased intraabdominal pressure leading to hypoperfusion and ischemia of the intestines and other peritoneal and retroperitoneal structures. **Abdominal compartment syndrome** occurs with increased intraabdominal pressure, often after major abdominal trauma or sepsis. This condition has profound consequences, including hemodynamic instability and respiratory, renal, and neurologic abnormalities. Because the abdominal cavity has become too small, management consists of emergent decompressive laparotomy to relieve the intraabdominal pressure. Closure of the abdomen is not performed and instead a temporary sterile dressing may be applied.

Patients with an open abdomen have severe metabolic alterations, increased loss of fluids, and elevated nutritional requirements. The open abdomen also may be a significant source of protein loss depending on the amount of drainage (Hourigan et al, 2010). There has been some controversy as to whether patients with an open abdomen can be fed enterally. As long as the patient is hemodynamically stable and does not require large-volume fluid resuscitation or increasing doses of pressor agents, enteral feeding should be possible (Burlew et al, 2012). Ideally, a nasojejunal feeding tube should be positioned at the time of surgery to facilitate early EN support therapy.

Management of patients with intestinal fistulas and large draining wounds is also challenging surgically and nutritionally because these patients have metabolic abnormalities associated with losses of fluid, electrolytes, and nutrients (Friese, 2012; Majercik et al, 2012). The priorities for management of intestinal fistulas are to restore blood volume, replace fluid and electrolyte losses, treat sepsis, control fistula drainage, protect the surrounding skin, and provide optimal nutrition support therapy. The use of PN has decreased mortality associated with fistulas and is associated with spontaneous fistula closure; however, these same outcomes are possible with EN if a feeding tube can be placed through or distal to the fistula site (see Chapter 13).

MAJOR BURNS

Pathophysiology

Major burns result in severe trauma. Energy requirements can increase as much as 100% above resting energy expenditure (REE), depending on the extent and depth of the injury (see Figure 38-7). Exaggerated protein catabolism and increased urinary nitrogen excretion accompany this hypermetabolism. Protein also is lost through the burn wound exudate.

Burn patients are particularly susceptible to infection, and this markedly increases requirements for energy and protein. Because patients with major burns may develop an ileus and are anorexic, nutrition support therapy can be a real challenge. Inhalation injury may be present in those patients who sustained burns and have been in a smoke environment for prolonged periods of time. Patients who have airway compromise may require intubation and mechanical ventilation. These patients are at increased risk of dysphagia as a result of the inhalation injury or prolonged intubation and may require enteral nutrition. In children, healing after burn and trauma requires not only restoration of oxygen delivery and adequate calories to support metabolism and repair but also awareness of how children differ from adults in metabolic rate, growth requirements, and physiologic response (Cook and Blinman, 2010).

Medical Management
Fluid and Electrolyte Repletion

The first 24 to 48 hours of treatment for thermally injured patients are devoted to fluid resuscitation. The volume of resuscitation fluid is approximately 2 to 4 mL/kg body weight per percentage of burn depending on the patient's physiologic demands or response. Generally half of the calculated volume for the first 24 hours is given during the first 8 hours after burn injury and the remaining half in the next 16 hours. Urine output is used to titrate the rate of IV fluid replacement.

The volume of fluid needed is based on the age and weight of the patient and the extent of the injury designated by percentage of total body surface area (TBSA) burned. Once resuscitation is complete, ample fluids must be given to cover maintenance requirements and evaporative losses that continue through open wounds. Evaporative water loss can be estimated at 2 to 3.1 mL/kg

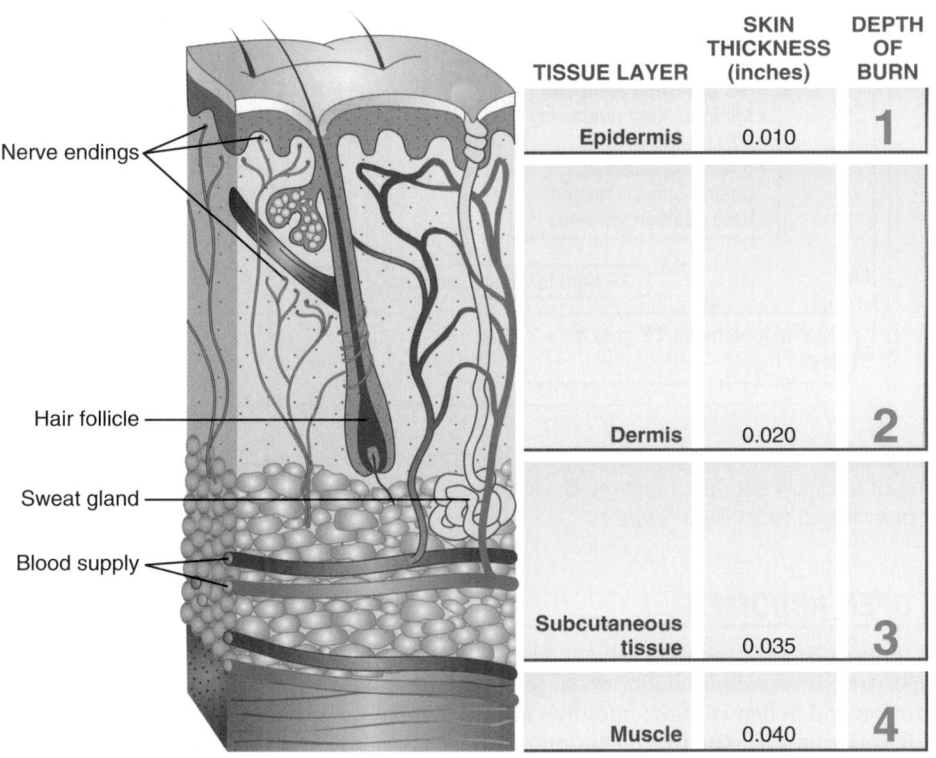

TISSUE LAYER	SKIN THICKNESS (inches)	DEPTH OF BURN
Epidermis	0.010	1
Dermis	0.020	2
Subcutaneous tissue	0.035	3
Muscle	0.040	4

FIGURE 38-7 Interpretation of burn classification based on damage to the integument.

of body weight per 24 hours per percent of TBSA burn. Serum sodium, osmolar concentrations, and body weight are used to monitor fluid status. Providing adequate fluids and electrolytes as soon as possible after injury is paramount for maintaining circulatory volume and preventing ischemia.

Wound Management

Wound management depends on the depth and extent of the burn. Current surgical management promotes use of topical antimicrobial agents and biologic and synthetic dressings, early debridement, excision, and grafting. Energy expenditure may be reduced slightly by the practice of covering wounds as early as possible to reduce evaporative heat and nitrogen losses and prevent infection.

Ancillary Measures

Passive and active range of motion exercises should be started early in the hospital to prevent contracture formation. Physical and occupational therapy helps maintain function and prevents muscle wasting and atrophy. A warm environment minimizes heat loss and the expenditure of energy to maintain body temperature. Thermal blankets, heat lamps, and individual heat shields often are used to maintain environmental temperature near 86° F. Minimizing fear and pain with reassurance from the staff and adequate pain medication also can reduce catecholamine stimulation and help avoid increases in energy expenditure. Treatments such as biofeedback, guided imagery, and good sleep hygiene are helpful. Finally, antacids are given to patients with major burns to prevent formation of stress-related **Curling ulcers,** which may occur because of reduced plasma volume and lead to ischemia and sloughing of gastric or duodenal mucosa. A number of pharmacologic strategies have been used to attenuate the hypermetabolic state and net protein loss sustained by burn patients (Abdullahi and Jeschke, 2014). These anabolic agents including insulin, oxandrolone, and propranolol improve lean body mass through metabolic effects on skeletal muscle or fat tissue. Insulin decreases protein breakdown and fat oxidation, oxandrolone decreases protein breakdown and fat oxidation, and propranolol decreases fat oxidation and promotes glucose homeostasis. These pharmacologic agents are used now in conjunction with nutrition support in the care of burn patients.

Medical Nutrition Therapy

A burn patient has greatly accelerated metabolism and needs increased energy, carbohydrates, proteins, fats, vitamins, minerals, and antioxidants to heal and prevent detrimental sequelae. A healthy liver is also essential. Hepatic acute phase proteins are strong predictors for postburn survival through their roles in gluconeogenesis, glycogenolysis, lipolysis, and proteolysis.

The goals of nutrition support therapy after major burn injury include provision of adequate calories to meet energy needs while minimizing associated metabolic complications, prevention or correction of specific nutrient deficiencies, and fluid and electrolyte management for adequate urine output and normal homeostasis. Adequate surgical care, infection control, and nutrition should be implemented as soon as possible after burn resuscitation. Delays in admission to an organized burn unit can be detrimental, especially for children, because malnutrition is a common concern. Nutritional assessment of the adult burn patient should include evaluation of any preexisting substance abuse, psychiatric illness, or chronic disease that may be associated with malnutrition and could influence energy and nutrient requirements.

Many burn patients will be able to eat food and nutrition counseling should focus on selection of high protein and calorically dense food and fluids. Enteral nutrition should be considered for those patients who are unable to eat or cannot achieve adequate intake by food alone. Achievement of enteral access and provision of a sufficient volume of enteral nutrients early in the hospital course of a critically ill burn patient affords an opportunity to improve the outcome of that patient (Mosier et al, 2011). Enteral feeding provides a conduit for the delivery of immune stimulants and serves as effective prophylaxis against stress-induced gastropathy and GI hemorrhage. Tube placement beyond the stomach into the small bowel in hypermetabolic, severely ill patients prone to ileus and disordered gut motility may aid delivery of enteral nutrients while reducing risk of aspiration. Placement of enteral tubes during surgery has been practiced at some burn centers in an effort to minimize the length of time a burn patient is without nutrition support therapy (see Box 38-3 for the nutritional care goals for the burned person).

Energy

Increased energy needs of the burn patient vary according to the size of the burn, with severely burned patients often approaching twice their predicted energy expenditure. Burn size makes the largest contribution to measured energy expenditure, followed by age (Shields et al, 2013). Most predictive equations used to calculate energy expenditure in severely burned adults do not correlate strongly with measured energy expenditure (Shields et al, 2013). Therefore measuring energy expenditure via indirect calorimetry is the most reliable method for assessing energy expenditure in burn patients. Increasing energy requirements by 20% to 30% is necessary to account for energy expenditure associated with wound care and physical therapy.

Additional calories may be required to meet the needs because of fever, sepsis, multiple traumas, or the stress of surgery. Although weight gain may be desirable for the severely underweight patient, this is generally not feasible until acute illness has resolved. Generally, caloric goals should not exceed more than two times the REE. Adjustments in caloric goals may be required when patients receive a large amount of intravenous dextrose solutions and propofol (an anesthetic in a lipid-delivery system).

BOX 38-3 Medical Nutrition Therapy Goals for Burn Patients

1. Minimize metabolic stress response by
   - Controlling environmental temperature
   - Maintaining fluid and electrolyte balance
   - Controlling pain and anxiety
   - Covering wounds early
2. Meet nutritional needs by
   - Providing adequate calories to prevent weight loss of greater than 10% of usual body weight
   - Providing adequate protein for positive nitrogen balance and maintenance or repletion of circulating proteins
   - Providing vitamin and mineral supplementation as indicated
3. Prevent Curling stress ulcer by
   - Providing antacids or continuous enteral feedings

Weight maintenance should be the goal for overweight patients until the healing process is complete. Obese individuals may be at higher risk of wound infection and graft disruption. The energy requirement for the obese burned person is probably more than that calculated when ideal body weight is used but less than that calculated when actual body weight is used. IC is the most accurate method of determining the energy needs of the obese person who is burned.

Protein

The protein needs of burn patients are elevated because of losses through urine and wounds, increased use in gluconeogenesis, and wound healing. Recent evidence promotes the feeding of high amounts of protein. Providing 20% to 25% of total calories as protein of high biologic value also is recommended.

The adequacy of energy and protein intake is best evaluated by monitoring wound healing, graft take, and basic nutrition assessment parameters. Wound healing or graft take may be delayed if weight loss exceeds 10% of the usual weight. An exact evaluation of weight loss may be difficult to obtain because of fluid shifts or edema, or because of differences in the weights of dressings or splints. The coordination of weight measurement with dressing changes or hydrotherapy may allow recording of a weight without dressings and splints. Generally the fluid gained during the resuscitation period is lost within 2 weeks. Trends in weight change then can be identified.

Nitrogen balance often is used to evaluate the efficacy of a nutritional regimen, but it cannot be considered accurate without accounting for wound losses, which is difficult to accomplish in a clinical setting. Nitrogen excretion should begin to decrease as wounds heal, are grafted, or are covered. However, serum albumin levels usually remain depressed until major burns are healed. Measurements of C-reactive protein in conjunction with shorter half-life proteins such as prealbumin and retinol binding protein (RBP) may help to assess the resolution of the inflammatory response and therefore allow interpretation of the adequacy of nutrition support therapy of burn patients.

Micronutrients and Antioxidants

Vitamin needs generally increase for burn patients, but exact requirements have not been established. Supplements may be needed for patients who are eating food; however, most patients who receive tube feeding or PN with vitamins and minerals receive amounts of vitamins and minerals in excess of the dietary reference intakes because of the high calorie intake. Vitamin C is involved in collagen synthesis, fibroblast and capillary formation, and immune system maintenance; it also acts as a powerful antioxidant (Nordlund et al, 2014). Furthermore, vitamin C levels decrease after burn injury and may be a result of cutaneous losses (Vinha et al, 2013). Vitamin C frequently is supplemented to promote wound healing, although not in high-doses, as results from studies are conflicting (Nordlund et al, 2014). A recent survey of 65 burn centers showed that 100% provided a multivitamin after burn injury and more than half of the centers also provided supplemental vitamin C and zinc (Graves et al, 2009).

Vitamin A is also an important nutrient for immune function and epithelialization. Vitamin A deficiency impairs collagen synthesis and may affect wound healing negatively. Few clinical data suggest routine supplementation of vitamin A in

burns. Some immune-modulating enteral formulas contain additional beta-carotene, therefore it is important to check the contents before recommending additional supplementation.

Vitamin D deficiency has been reported in pediatric burn patients; however, limited data are available for adult patients. Burn survivors have an increased risk of vitamin D deficiency because the major source of vitamin D synthesis is in the skin (Schumann et al, 2012).

Electrolyte imbalances that involve serum sodium or potassium usually are corrected by adjusting fluid therapy. Hyponatremia may be seen in patients whose evaporative losses are reduced drastically by the application of dressings or grafts; who have had changes in maintenance fluids; or who have been treated with silver nitrate soaks, which tend to draw sodium from the wound. Restricting the oral consumption of free water and sodium-free fluids may help correct hyponatremia. Hypokalemia often occurs after the initial fluid resuscitation and during protein synthesis. Slightly elevated serum potassium may indicate inadequate hydration.

Depression of serum calcium levels may be seen in patients with burns that involve more than 30% TBSA. Hypocalcemia often accompanies hypoalbuminemia. Calcium losses may be exaggerated if the patient is immobile or being treated with silver nitrate soaks. Early ambulation and exercise should help minimize these losses. Administration of calcium supplements may be necessary to treat symptomatic hypocalcemia.

Hypophosphatemia also has been identified in patients with major burns. This occurs most commonly in patients who receive large volumes of resuscitation fluid along with parenteral infusion of glucose solutions and large amounts of antacids for stress ulcer prophylaxis. Serum levels must be monitored and appropriate phosphate supplementation provided. Magnesium levels also may require attention because a significant amount of magnesium can be lost from the burn wound. Supplemental phosphorus and magnesium often are given parenterally to prevent GI irritation.

A depressed serum zinc level has been reported in burn patients, but whether this represents total body zinc nutriture or is an artifact of hypoalbuminemia is unclear, because zinc is bound to serum albumin. Zinc is a cofactor in energy metabolism and protein synthesis. Supplementation with 220 mg of zinc sulfate (50 mg elemental zinc) is common (Nordlund et al, 2014). The anemia initially seen after a burn usually is unrelated to iron deficiency and is treated with packed red blood cells.

Methods of Nutrition Support Therapy

Methods of nutrition support therapy must be implemented on an individual basis. Most patients with burns of less than 20% TBSA are able to meet their needs with a regular high-calorie, high-protein oral diet. Often the use of concealed nutrients such as protein added to puddings, milks, and gelatins is helpful because consuming large volumes of foods can be overwhelming to the patient. Patients should have immediate access to food and fluids at the bedside. They should be encouraged to consume calorically dense, high-protein drinks. Involving family and caregivers during mealtimes helps to promote good oral intake.

Patients with major burns, elevated energy expenditure, or poor appetites may require tube feeding or PN. Enteral feeding is the preferred method of nutrition support therapy for burn patients, but PN may be necessary with early excision and grafting to avoid the frequent interruptions of tube feeding required for anesthesia. Because ileus is often present only in the stomach, severely burned patients can be fed successfully by tube into the small bowel. PN may be needed for patients with persistent ileus who do not tolerate tube feedings or who have a high risk of aspiration. With careful monitoring, central lines for PN can be maintained through burn wounds (see Chapter 13).

SURGERY

The delivery of correctly formulated and safely administered nutritional and metabolic support is a matter of life or death in surgical and critical care units; obese patients have a higher surgical risk (Blackburn et al, 2010). Although surgical morbidity correlates best with the extent of the primary disease and the nature of the operation performed, malnutrition also may compound the severity of complications. A well-nourished patient usually tolerates major surgery better than a severely malnourished patient. Malnutrition is associated with a high incidence of operative complications, morbidity, and death. If a malnourished patient is expected to undergo major upper GI surgery and EN is not feasible, PN should be initiated 5 to 7 days preoperatively and continued into the postoperative period if the duration of therapy is anticipated to be longer than 7 days (SCCM and A.S.P.E.N., 2009; see Chapter 13).

Medical Nutrition Therapy
Preoperative Nutrition Care

The routine practice of requiring a patient take nothing by mouth (NPO) at midnight before surgery has been discontinued in many settings. The American Society of Anesthesiologists historically recommended withholding solids for 6 hours preoperatively and clear liquids for 2 hours before induction of anesthesia. This practice was intended to minimize aspiration and regurgitation. The use of a carbohydrate-rich beverage in the preoperative period has been shown to enhance glycemic control and decrease losses of nitrogen, lean body mass, and muscle strength after abdominal and colorectal surgery (Bilku et al, 2014).

Postoperative Nutrition Care

Postoperative patients who are critically ill and in the ICU should receive early EN unless there is an absolute contraindication (SCCM and A.S.P.E.N., 2009). This practice after major GI surgery is associated with reduced infection and decreased hospitalization. If the patient is malnourished (severe or nonsevere), however, the use of PN is indicated to provide perioperative support until patients are able to tolerate goal enteral feeding regimens (SCCM and A.S.P.E.N., 2009). The use of arginine-containing immune-enhanced enteral formulas is associated with a decrease in wound complications and a reduced hospital length of stay in patients who have undergone GI surgery (Drover, 2011; Marik and Zaloga, 2010).

If oral feeding is not possible or an extended NPO period is anticipated, an access device for enteral feeding should be inserted at the time of surgery. Combined gastrostomy-jejunostomy tubes offer significant advantages over standard gastrostomies because they allow for simultaneous gastric drainage from the gastrostomy tube and enteral feeding via the jejunal tube.

The timing of introduction of solid food after surgery depends on the patient's degree of alertness and condition of the GI tract. A general practice has been to progress over a period of several meals from clear liquids to full liquids and finally to solid foods. However, no physiologic reason exists for solid foods not to be introduced as soon as the GI tract is functioning and a few liquids are tolerated. Surgical patients can be fed a regular solid-food diet rather than a clear liquid diet.

CLINICAL CASE STUDY

Chronologic Clinical Case Study with Suggested Answers

First Assessment

A 44-year-old man was admitted to a hospital with an incarcerated ventral hernia and probable bowel compromise. He underwent a small bowel resection and hernia repair and required re-exploration 2 days later because of wound evisceration. His abdominal wound was left open. His postoperative course was complicated by acute respiratory distress syndrome and sepsis related to aspiration pneumonia. He was mechanically ventilated and sedated. On hospital day six, he underwent a third surgical procedure in which his recurrent hernia was repaired, his abdomen incision was closed, and a wound vacuum system was placed. He was (NPO) since admission with a nasogastric tube in place draining more than 1 L of green fluid.

Screening and Assessment Data

Height = 72″ (183 cm)
Weight = 364 lb (165 kg)
Body mass index = 49 kg/m²
Ideal body weight = 178 lb (81 kg)
Weight change in the 1 months before admission: no
Decreased intake in the previous month: no
Physical examination: bilateral severe pitting edema of ankles and upper extremities.
Abdominal examination: distended with absent bowel sounds
Radiologic examination: moderately dilated small bowel loops consistent with adynamic ileus
Currently receiving 0.45% normal saline @ 120 mL/hr
Intake/Output = 3305/3725 mL

Laboratory Values

Sodium: 138 mmol/dL
Potassium: 3 mmol/dL
Chloride: 105 mmol/dL
Carbon dioxide: 27 mmol/dL
Blood urea nitrogen: 13 mg/dL
Creatinine: 1.28 mg/dL

Glucose: 185 mg/dL

Ionized calcium: 1.12 mm/L
Magnesium: 1.6 mg/dL
Phosphorus: 2.1 mg/dL
Albumin: 1.9 gm/dL

1. Write pertinent nutrition diagnosis statements (problem, cause, and signs and symptoms [PES] format) in order of priority for this patient.
   Malnutrition in the context of acute illness as evidenced by energy intake <50% of requirements (≥ 5 days) and severe fluid accumulation.
   Altered nutrition-related laboratory values related to the metabolic response to stress and a lack of electrolyte intake in diet and intravenous fluids as evidenced by low serum sodium, potassium, and phosphorus.
2. Should he be started on parenteral nutrition (PN)? Explain.
   By the information presented in the case, he should be started on PN because he is malnourished, has been NPO for 6 days, and does not appear to be ready to begin enteral feeding (secondary to ileus). It will be important to discuss enteral feeding via jejunal access with the physicians once ileus has resolved.

Continued

CLINICAL CASE STUDY—cont'd

Chronologic Clinical Case Study with Suggested Answers

3. Calculate his nutritional needs.

His caloric requirement should be estimated using the hypocaloric, high-protein approach because he is morbidly obese (Grade III) and renal function is normal. Ideal body weight should be used.

Hypocaloric regimen for this patient is 14 kcal/kg actual body weight: 2310 kcal/day.

Protein requirement may be set at 2 to 2.5 g/kg ideal body weight or 162 to 203 g/day.

First Change of Status with Reassessment

On hospital day 10 the patient's body temperature spikes to 39° C, and he is found to have multiple infected abdominal abscesses. He goes to the operating room for abscess drainage. During this time his blood pressures (BP) and urine output drop considerably requiring initiation of fluid resuscitation and vasopressive agents for BP stabilization. His kidney function is noted to worsen. There is no plan for renal replacement therapy at the present.

Current status is noted:

T_{max} 39.3° C

VE = 15.6 L/min (minute ventilation)

PN continues

Intravenous fluids: 0.45% normal saline solution 150 mL/hr + additional fluid boluses

Sodium: 131 mmol/dL

Potassium: 5.1 mmol/dL

Chloride: 96 mmol/dL

Carbon dioxide: 15 mmol/dL

Blood glucose: 225 mg/dl

Ionized calcium: 1.01 mm/L

Magnesium: 2.8 mg/dL

Phosphorus: 4.8 mg/dL

Albumin: 1.2 gm/dL

Arterial blood gas: 7.31/24/115/11

4. Upon monitoring, what is his metabolic state?

He has become hypermetabolic, hypercatabolic and with worsening kidney function.

Hyperglycemia has worsened.

Electrolyte excess (potassium, phosphorus, magnesium).

5. What is his acid-base status?

He has a metabolic acidosis resulting from an impaired renal excretion of acid, and reabsorption and regeneration of bicarbonate.

6. Write updated PES statements:

Increased nutrient needs (energy and protein) related to a systemic inflammatory response as evidenced by fever and elevated minute ventilation.

Altered nutrition-related laboratory values (hyperglycemia) related to stress metabolism and glucose intake as evidenced by blood glucose of 225 mg/dL.

Altered nutrition-related laboratory values related to acute kidney injury as evidenced by elevated potassium, phosphorus, and magnesium.

7. Is the patient's blood glucose control adequate? If not, why and what should be done?

His blood glucose is not adequately controlled. There is evidence that when glucose levels are controlled between 180 to 215 mg/dL, survival is better.

The dextrose load in his PN should be reduced or a standardized insulin protocol should be instituted, or both. In addition, energy intake should be assessed to confirm absence of overfeeding because this could result in hyperglycemia.

8. Why is his serum albumin level falling?

Decreased acute-phase proteins are a response to the inflammatory process his body has mounted to try to reestablish homeostasis.

9. Recalculate his nutritional needs.

Energy assessment methodology will change due to the patient's acute kidney injury and the need to provide normal protein requirements.

Calorie requirement via Penn State Equation 2003b = 3035 kcal/day

Penn State Equation 2003b:

Mifflin-St. Jeor equation $\times$ (0.96) + Ve (31) + T_{max} (167) − 6212

Mifflin-St Jeor equation using actual weight, *Ve* is minute ventilation in L/min, T_{max} is maximum body temperature in the past 24 hours in degrees centigrade.

Protein requirement has decreased (1.2 to 1.3 g/kg ideal body weight or 97 to 105 g/day).

Second Change of Status with Reassessment

On hospital day 13, an abdominal film showed improvement in the patient's ileus picture. The patient has not yet stooled, but his abdomen is soft and he has hypoactive bowel sounds. His acute kidney injury continues, although hemodialysis has been initiated and electrolyte levels have normalized. On rounds, the dietitian asks whether the patient is stable enough to start tube feeding through the nasojejunal tube. The surgical and critical care teams believe that the patient's gastrointestinal status has improved sufficiently to initiate an enteral feeding.

10. What feeding formula should be used? Is an immune-enhancing tube feeding formula indicated?

Commercial immune-enhancing formulas that combine several nutrients thought to enhance immune function are not indicated for routine use, and may be contraindicated in the severely critically ill, such as this patient.

A polymeric nonfiber formula can be chosen. If a 1 kcal/mL formula is utilized, the infusion volume will be 3 L/day, if 1.5 kcal formula is used, the infusion volume will be approximately 2 L/day; and if a 2 kcal/mL formula is chosen, the volume will be approximately 1.5 L/day.

A polymeric enteral feeding was initiated via nasojejunal access and gradually advanced to goal rate during the next 3 to 4 days. Tolerance was demonstrated via no change in abdominal distention, pain, or nausea and vomiting. As the feeding advanced, the PN was gradually weaned, then discontinued when goal enteral feeding was achieved.

CLINICAL INSIGHT

Factors to consider when interpreting the literature with respect to conflicting data among nutrition support outcomes studies

- Study designs may differ
- Sample size may be too small
- Patient sample may be heterogeneous; subjects may differ by underlying illness or injury, acuity level, mortality risk
- Inclusion of well-nourished patients who would likely not show an effect of nutrition intervention
- Preexisting malnutrition may or may not be present and may or may not be diagnosed with similar criteria
- Length of ICU stay may vary
- Short interval time of nutrition therapy in the ICU

- Differences may be present with respect to timing of initiation of EN or PN
- Contribution of non-nutritional calorie sources such as D5W (5% dextrose in water) and medications in lipid delivery systems
- Differences in techniques to establish target energy goals (e.g., indirect calorimetry, predictive equations, kcal/kg)

Additional reading:

Jeejeebhoy KN: Parenteral nutrition in the intensive care unit, *Nutr Reviews* 70:623, 2012.

Singer P, Pichard C: Reconciling divergent results of the latest parenteral nutrition studies in the ICU. *Curr Opin Clin Nutr Metab Care* 16:187, 2013.

Wischmeyer P: Parenteral nutrition and calorie delivery in the ICU: Controversy, clarity, or call to action? *Curr Opin Crit Care* 18:164, 2012.

CLINICAL INSIGHT

Enhanced Recovery After Surgery (ERAS)

First presented in the late 1990s, this multimodal pathway for care of the surgical patient has become a standard of care for colon resections, complicated pancreatic procedures, and for bladder cancer procedures in many countries. This management approach involves aspects of the patient's care preoperatively, during the surgical procedure and postoperatively (see Figure 38-8). The central elements of the ERAS pathway address key factors including pain control, gut dysfunction and the need for intravenous fluids, and lastly, ambulation. The ERAS components help to clarify how these areas interact to affect patient recovery, and mounting evidence demonstrates that use of the ERAS pathway results in positive outcomes compared with standard surgical care.

In a recent meta-analysis, Varadhan and colleagues reported the ERAS pathway was shown to reduce surgical care time by more than 30% and reduce postoperative complications by up to 50% (Varadhan et al, 2010). An international ERAS society was formed in 2010 with its mission to "develop perioperative care and to improve recovery through research, audit education and implementation of evidence-based practice" (Gustafsson et al, 2012).

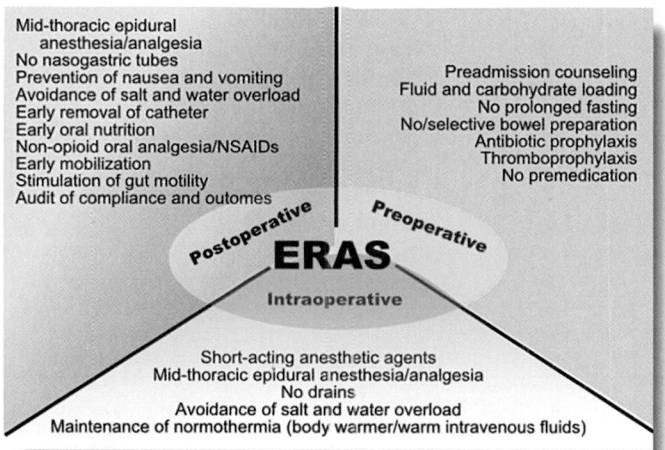

FIGURE 38-8 The ERAS Protocol. (http://www.erassociety.org/index.php/eras-care-system/eras-protocol. Accessed April 8, 2014.)

USEFUL WEBSITES

American Burn Association
http://www.ameriburn.org
American Society for Parenteral and Enteral Nutrition A.S.P.E.N.
http://www.nutritioncare.org
Critical Care Nutrition
http://www.criticalcarenutrition.com
Society of Critical Care Medicine
www.sccm.org
Surgical Nutrition: Tutorial
http://www.surgical-tutor.org.uk/default-home.htm?core/ITU/nutrition.htm~right

REFERENCES

Abdullahi A, Jeschke MG: Nutrition and anabolic pharmacotherapies in the care of burn patients, *Nutr Clin Pract*, October 2014; vol. 29, 5: pp. 621–630, May 14, 2014. doi: 10.1177/088453364533129.

Academy of Nutrition and Dietetics: *Critical Illness: Glucose Control. Evidence-Analysis Library*. http://www.adaevidencelibrary.com/topic.cfm?cat=4083&auth=1. Accessed March 14, 2015.

Academy of Nutrition and Dietetics: *Critical Illness: Determination of Resting Metabolic Rate*. http://andevidencelibrary.com/template.cfm?template=guide_summary&key=3200. Accessed April 13, 2014.

A.S.P.E.N. Society of Critical Care Medicine (SCCM) and American Society for Parenteral and Enteral Nutrition (A.S.P.E.N.): Guidelines for the provision and assessment of nutrition support therapy in the adult critically ill patient, *J Parenter Enteral Nutr* 33(3):277, May/June, 2009.

Bilku DK, et al: Role of preoperative carbohydrate loading: a systematic review, *Ann R Coll Surg Engl* 96:15, 2014.

Blackburn GL, et al: Nutrition support in the intensive care unit: an evolving science, *Arch Surg* 145:533, 2010.

Breen H, Ireton-Jones C: Predicting energy needs in obese patients, *Nutr Clin Pract* 19:284, 2004.

Burlew CC, et al: Who should we feed? A Western Trauma Association multi-institutional study of enteral nutrition in the open abdomen after injury, *J Trauma Acute Care Surg* 73:1380, 2012.

Choban PS, Dickerson RN: Morbid obesity and nutrition support: is bigger different? *Nutr Clin Pract* 20:480, 2005.

Cook RC, Blinman TA: Nutritional support of the pediatric trauma patient, *Semin Pediatr Surg* 19:242, 2010.

Dhaliwal R, et al: The Canadian Critical Care Nutrition Guidelines in 2013: An update on current recommendations and implementation strategies, *Nutr Clin Pract* 29:29, 2014.

Drover JW, et al: Perioperative use of arginine-supplemented diets: a systematic review of the evidence, *J Am Coll Surg* 212:385, 2011.

Friese RS: The open abdomen: definitions, management principles, and nutrition support considerations, *Nutr Clin Pract* 27:492, 2012.

Graves C, Saffle J, Cochran A: Actual burn nutrition care practices: an update, *J Burn Care Res* 2009;30:77–82.

Gustafsson UO, et al: Guidelines for perioperative care in elective colonic surgery: Enhanced Recovery After Surgery (ERAS) Society recommendations, *Clin Nutr* 31:783, 2012.

Heyland D, et al: A randomized trial of glutamine and antioxidants in critically ill patients, *N Engl J Med* 368:1489, 2013.

Hoffer LJ, Bistrian BR: Appropriate protein provision in critical illness: a systematic and narrative review, *Am J Clin Nutr* 96:591, 2012.

Hourigan LA, et al: Loss of protein, immunoglobulins, and electrolytes in exudates from negative pressure wound therapy, *Nutr Clin Pract* 25:510, 2010.

Jensen GL, et al: Malnutrition syndromes: a conundrum versus continuum, *JPEN J Parenter Enteral Nutr* 33:710, 2009.

Jensen GL, et al: Adult starvation and disease-related malnutrition: a proposal for etiology-based diagnosis in the clinical practice setting from the International Consensus Guideline Committee, *J Parenter Enteral Nutr* 34:156, 2010.

Majercik S, et al: Enteroatmospheric fistula: from soup to nuts, *Nutr Clin Pract* 27:507, 2012.

Marik PE, Zaloga GP: Immunonutrition in high-risk surgical patients: a systematic review and analysis of the literature, *J Parenter Ent Nutr* 34:378, 2010.

Mosier MJ, et al: Early enteral nutrition in burns: compliance with guidelines and associated outcomes in a multicenter study, *J Burn Care Res* 32:104, 2011.

Nordlund MJ, et al: Micronutrients after burn injury: a review, *J Burn Care Res* 35:121, 2014.

Nose K, et al: Glutamine prevents total parenteral nutrition-associated changes to intraepithelial lymphocyte phenotype and function: a potential mechanism for the preservation of epithelial barrier function, *J Interferon Cytokine Res* 30:67, 2010.

Port AM, Apovian C: Metabolic support of the obese intensive care unit patient: a current perspective, *Curr Opin Clin Nutr Metab Care* 13:184, 2010.

Schumann AD, et al: Vitamin D deficiency in burn patients, *J Burn Care Res* 33:731, 2012.

Shields BA, et al: Determination of resting energy expenditure after severe burn, *J Burn Care Res* 34:e22, 2013.

Varadhan KK, et al: The enhanced recover after surgery (ERAS) pathway for patients undergoing major elective open colorectal surgery: a meta-analysis of randomized trials, *Clin Nutr* 29:434, 2010.

Vinha PP, et al: Effect of acute thermal injury in status of serum vitamins, inflammatory markers, and oxidative stress markers: preliminary data, *J Burn Care Res* 34:e87, 2013.

Yang H, et al: Enteral versus parenteral nutrition: effect on intestinal barrier function, *Ann NY Acad Sci* 1165:338, 2009.

39

Medical Nutrition Therapy for Rheumatic Disease

F. Enrique Gómez, PhD
Martha Kaufer-Horwitz, DSc, NC
Gabriela E. Mancera-Chávez, MSc, NC

KEY TERMS

ankylosing spondylitis (AS)
antiinflammatory diet
antinuclear antibodies (ANA)
arachidonic acid (ARA)
arthritis
autoimmune arthritis
biologic response modifiers (BRM)
cyclooxygenase (COX)
C-reactive protein (CRP)
cytokines
dihomo-gamma-linolenic acid
    (DGLA)
disease-modifying antirheumatic
    drugs (DMARD)
docosahexaenoic acid (DHA)
eicosanoids

eicosapentaenoic acid (EPA)
gamma-linolenic acid (GLA)
gout
hyperuricemia
leukotrienes (LT)
lipoxygenase (LOX)
maresins
monosodium urate (MSU) crystals
osteoarthritis (OA)
polymyalgia rheumatic
polymyositis (PM)
polyunsaturated fatty acids (PUFAs)
prostaglandins (PG)
prostanoids
protectins
purines

Raynaud syndrome
resolvins
rheumatic fever
rheumatoid arthritis (RA)
rheumatic disease
rheumatoid factor (RF)
scleroderma
Sjögren syndrome (SS)
systemic lupus erythematosus (SLE)
temporomandibular disorders
    (TMDs)
thromboxanes (Tx)
uric acid
uricostatic
unicosuric

Rheumatic disease and related conditions include more than 100 different manifestations of inflammation and loss of function of connective tissue and supporting body structures, including joints, tendons, ligaments, bones, muscles, and sometimes internal organs. Some of these rheumatic diseases clearly have an autoimmune component, whereas the origin of others remains unknown. Therefore medical nutrition therapy (MNT), pharmacotherapy, and physical and occupational therapies must be tailored and designed to treat each disease and its symptoms. A diet with adequate protein and energy content, rich in vitamins, minerals, and omega-3 polyunsaturated fatty acids (PUFAs) can promote a beneficial protective effect against tissue damage and suppression of inflammatory activity. Table 39-1 provides an overview of these disorders and their nutritional management.

Arthritis and the related disorders are among the most prevalent chronic disease conditions in the United States. The annual cost for medical care to treat all forms of arthritis and joint pain is estimated to be $281.5 billion (American Academy of Orthopaedic Surgeons [AAOS], 2009).

Rheumatic disease affects all population groups. The Centers for Disease Control and Prevention (CDC) analyzed data from the 2010 to 2012 National Health Interview Survey (NHIS), and estimated that 52.5 million U.S. adults suffer from arthritis, equal to about 23%. Among persons with heart disease, diabetes, and obesity, the prevalence of doctor-diagnosed arthritis was 49.0%, 47.3%, and 31.2%, respectively (CDC, 2013).

The National Arthritis Data Workgroup reviewed data to estimate national prevalence rates of various rheumatic diseases based on 2005 U.S. census data, finding that in the United States rheumatoid arthritis (RA) affects 1.3 million adults; juvenile arthritis 294,000 people, spondylarthritides (the contemporary name of spondyloarthropathies) 0.6 to 2.4 million adults over 15, systemic lupus erythematosus (SLE) 161,000 to 322,000 adults, systemic sclerosis 49,000 adults, Sjögren syndrome (SS) 0.4 to 3.1 million adults, clinical osteoarthritis 27 million people aged 25 and older, polymyalgia rheumatic 711,000 people, gout 8 million adults, and fibromyalgia 5 million people (Helmick et al, 2008; Lawrence et al, 2008).

Arthritis is a generic term that comes from the Greek word *arthro*, which means "joint," and the suffix *-itis*, which means "inflammation." There are two distinct categories of disease: systemic, autoimmune **arthritis** and nonsystemic osteoarthritis (OA). The more debilitating autoimmune arthritis group includes RA, juvenile rheumatoid arthritis, gout, SS, fibromyalgia, SLE, and scleroderma. The OA group includes OA, bursitis, and tendonitis. Other rheumatic diseases include spondylarthritides, polymyalgia rheumatica, and polymyositis.

ETIOLOGY

Body changes associated with aging—including decreased somatic protein, body fluids, and bone density—and obesity may contribute to the onset and progression of arthritis. The

TABLE 39-1	Summary of Medical Nutrition Therapy for Rheumatic Diseases			
Disease	Medical Nutrition Therapy	Complementary and Alternative Medicine (CAM)	Supplements or Herbs that can be Safely Considered	Therapies Without Adequate Evidence
Rheumatoid arthritis	Vegan, Mediterranean diet; antiinflammatory diet; appropriate calories for maintenance of normal body weight; RDA for protein unless malnutrition present; moderate-fat diet with emphasis on omega-3 PUFAs and fish 1-2 times per week; modifications as needed for jaw pain, anorexia	Exercise, meditation, tai chi, spiritual practice, relaxation techniques; topical rubbing gels based on capsaicin.	Supplement diet as needed to meet DRI for antioxidant nutrients and, calcium, folate, vitamins B_6, B_{12}, D; GLA from evening primrose oil, black currant oil, and borage oil; fish oils; bromelain, rosemary, curcumin, curry, ginger, and other culinary herbs	China root, willow bark, valerian, feverfew, boswellia, copper or copper salts, devil's claw
Osteoarthritis	Weight management; diet adequate in calcium, folate, vitamins B_6, D, K; magnesium; antiinflammatory diet (see Box 39-2)	Exercise, acupuncture; SAM-e; topical rubbing gels based on capsaicin	Supplement diet as needed to meet DRI for antioxidant nutrients and, calcium, folate, vitamins B_6, B_{12}, and D; glucosamine, chondroitin; fish oils; diacerein; avocado soybean unsaponifiables, bromelain, hyaluronic acid	Shark cartilage
Gout	Weight management; purine-controlled diet; adequate fluid consumption; alcohol, particularly beer, restricted or eliminated; fructose from sweetened beverages and juices restricted.	Exercise; alkaline-ash foods; see *Clinical Insight* on Urinary pH in Chapter 35.	Cherry, cherry juice (see *New Directions: Can Cherries Prevent a Gout Attack?*)	
Lupus	Tailor diet to individual needs; calories to maintain IBW; restriction of protein, fluid, and sodium if renal involvement; check for gluten intolerance		Supplement diet as needed to meet DRI for antioxidant nutrients	
Scleroderma	Adequate fluid; high-energy, high-protein supplements as needed to prevent or correct weight loss; moist foods; modifications for GERD if needed			
Sjögren syndrome	Balanced diet with adequate B_6 or vitamin supplementation; restrict sugary foods and beverages; modify food portions to smaller size and soft consistency to improve chewing and swallowing processes		GLA improves eye discomfort and tear production	
TMD	Balanced diet with soft foods in small pieces to improve chewing and reduce pain			

DRI, Dietary reference intake; *GERD*, gastroesophageal reflux disease; *GLA*, Gamma-linolenic acid; *IBW*, ideal body weight; *RDA*, recommended dietary allowance; *SAM-e*, S-adenosyl-L-methionine; *TMD*, temporomandibular disorder.

aging body mass causes changes in neuroendocrine regulators, immune regulators, and metabolism, which affect the inflammatory process. Therefore recent increases in the frequency of these conditions may be the result of aging of the U.S. population. It is estimated that by 2030 approximately 67 million Americans will be at risk for rheumatic disease (CDC, 2013).

Rheumatic conditions are usually chronic and have no known cure but may present as acute episodes with short or intermittent duration. Chronic arthritic conditions are associated with alternating periods of remission without symptoms and flares with worsening symptoms that occur without any identifiable cause. Risk factors include repetitive joint injury, genetic susceptibility, and environmental factors, particularly smoking. Gender is a risk factor because women are more susceptible than men for most rheumatic diseases; the female/male ratio varies from 3:1 for RA, to 9:1 for SLE and SS. Only in gout, is there a clear dominance of male over female patients. Recently a transcriptome analysis of RNA levels showed that healthy women carry a "proinflammatory profile," particularly to develop RA (Jansen et al, 2014).

PATHOPHYSIOLOGY AND INFLAMMATION

Inflammation plays an important role in health and disease. The inflammatory process normally occurs to protect and repair tissue damaged by infections, injuries, toxicity, or wounds via accumulation of fluid and cells. Once the cause is resolved, the inflammation usually subsides. Whether inflammation is due to stress on the joints as in OA, or to an autoimmune response as in RA, an uncontrolled and long-lasting inflammatory reaction causes more damage than repair (see Chapter 3 for discussion of the Inflammation and the Pathophysiology of Chronic Disease) (see *Focus On: The Biochemistry of Inflammation*).

◎ FOCUS ON

The Biochemistry of Inflammation

COX, officially known as *prostaglandin-endoperoxide synthase (PTGS)*, has three isoforms: COX-1, COX-2, and COX-3 (the latter is a splice variant of COX-1, so it is sometimes called COX-1b or COX-1var). COX-1 is widely distributed and constitutively expressed in most tissues, whereas COX-2 is induced by inflammatory and proliferative stimuli. The difference in tissue distribution of COX expression may explain the existence of the two COX isoforms: COX-1 providing PG that are required for homeostatic functions (including gastric cytoprotection), and COX-2 playing the predominant role in PG formation during pathophysiologic states, such as in inflammation (Ricciotti and FitzGerald, 2011).

In the synthesis of prostanoids, COX consumes two double bonds from the original PUFA, whereas LOX consumes none; therefore, depending on the PUFA used as substrate, different eicosanoids are produced. For instance, **arachidonic acid (ARA)** (20:4, omega-6) has four double bonds and is the precursor of the series 2 of PG and Tx, and of the series 4 of LT, which are the most potent inflammatory eicosanoids (Patterson et al, 2012). The series 2 of prostanoids (PG_2 and Tx_2) are abundant because ARA is the most abundant in plasma membranes of cells involved in inflammation (macrophages, neutrophils, fibroblasts). If the substrate is **eicosapentaenoic acid (EPA)** (20:5, omega-3) that has five double bonds, series 3 of PG and Tx, and series 5 of LT are produced. **Dihomo-gamma-linolenic acid (DGLA)** (20:3, omega-6) has three double bonds and is the precursor of series 1 of PG and Tx, and of series 3 of LT that have antiinflammatory activities (Food and Agricultural Organization [FAO] of the United Nations [UN], 2010). Finally, **docosahexaenoic acid (DHA)** (22:6, omega-3) and EPA are converted to novel bioactive lipid mediators termed **resolvins (Rv), protectins**, and **maresins**, which promote the resolution of inflammation. Resolvins of the E series (RvE1 to 2) derived from EPA, and Rv of the D series (RvD1 to 6) derived from DHA, are produced by the sequential actions of the enzymes 15-lipoxygenase (15-LO) and 5-lipoxygenase (5-LO) (Norling and Perreti, 2013). Recent studies have shown that PUFAs also may regulate the expression of genes associated with the inflammatory response (Calder, 2013).

Based on this information, it is desirable to increase the omega-3/omega-6 ratio by increasing the consumption of antiinflammatory EPA, DGLA, and DHA (oily fish), while reducing the intake of ARA (vegetable oils and meat). Similarly, the increase in vegetables and fruits consumption also results in reduced risk of rheumatic diseases by contributing phytonutrients that have antiinflammatory effects (Boeing et al, 2012).

PUFAs play an important role in inflammation as precursors of a potent group of modulators of inflammation termed **eicosanoids** (*eicos* means "20" in Greek), which include the **prostanoids** and the **leukotrienes (LT)**. The prostanoids are the products of the enzyme **cyclooxygenase (COX)** and include the **prostaglandins (PG)** and **thromboxanes (Tx)**, whereas LTs are produced by the enzyme **lipoxygenase (LOX)** (see Box 39-1).

MEDICAL DIAGNOSIS AND TREATMENT

A thorough history of symptoms and a detailed physical examination are the cornerstones for an accurate diagnosis. However, laboratory testing can help to further refine the diagnosis and identify appropriate treatment.

BOX 39-1 Production of Bioactive Lipid Mediators from Omega-3 and Omega-6 PUFAs

Eicosapentaenoic acid EPA (20:5, omega-3)
Thromboxane A_3: Weak vasoconstrictor and weak platelet aggregator
Prostacyclin PGI_3: Vasodilator and platelet antiaggregator
Leukotriene B_5: Weak inflammation inducer and weak chemotactic agent
E-series resolvins (RvE1 and 2): promote resolution of inflammation

Arachidonic Acid (20:4, omega-6)
Thromboxane A_2: Vasoconstrictor and potent platelet aggregator
Prostaglandin E_2: Vasodilator and platelet antiaggregator
Leukotriene B_4: Inflammation inducer and potent leukocyte chemotaxis and adherence inducer

Dihomo-gamma-linolenic acid DGLA (20:3, omega-6)
Thromboxane A_1: Antiinflammatory and pain reducer
Prostaglandin E_1: Vasodilator, inhibits monocyte and neutrophil function, platelet antiaggregator
Leukotriene B_3: Very weak proinflammatory effects

Docosahexaenoic acid DHA (22:6, omega-3)
D-series resolvins (RvD 1 to 6): promote resolution of inflammation, analgesics, reduce leukocyte recruitment and activation, reduce IL-1 and TNF production
Protectin 1 (PD1) and Maresin 1 (MaR1): promote resolution of inflammation

Calder PC: Long chain fatty acids and gene expression in inflammation and immunity, *Curr Opin Clin Nutr Metab Care* 16:425, 2013.
Food and Agricultural Organization (FAO) of the United Nations: Fat and fatty acid intake and inflammatory and immune response. In *Fats and fatty acids in human nutrition. Report of an expert consulation,* Rome, 2010, Food and Agricultural Organization of the United Nations.
Norling LV, Perreti M: The role of omega-3 derived resolvins in arthritis, *Curr Opin Pharm* 13:476, 2013.

Biochemical Assessment

Acute-phase proteins are plasma proteins whose concentrations increase more than 25% during inflammatory states. Two acute-phase proteins traditionally used to screen for and monitor rheumatic disease are **rheumatoid factor (RF)** and **C-reactive protein (CRP)**, although they are nonspecific and, in the case of C-reactive protein, also may indicate an infection or even a recent cardiac event. The term **RF** is used to refer to a group of self-reacting antibodies (an abnormal IgM against normal IgG) found in the sera of rheumatic patients. The American College of Rheumatology (ACR) recommends periodic measurements of RF and CRP in addition to a detailed assessment of symptoms and functional status and radiographic examination to determine the current level of disease activity.

The detection of autoantibodies to a variety of antigens is important in the diagnosis of several rheumatic diseases (Watts, 2014). These antibodies can be directed against the nucleus (**antinuclear antibodies, ANA**) either to double-stranded DNA (dsDNA), ribonucleoproteins (RNPs), or other nuclear structures. Some autoantibodies recognize intracellular structures, or proteins that constitute extracellular matrices. Very often, the presence of a particular set of autoantibodies is a distinct characteristic of a rheumatic disease such as anti-dsDNA and anti-Sm for SLE, anticitrullinated protein antigens (ACPAs) for RA, and anti-Ro/SSA, and anti-La/SSB for SS (Demoruelle and Deane, 2011; Tincani et al, 2013). Routine blood testing also should include complement levels, a complete blood count, serum creatinine and hematocrit; urine or synovial fluid may be tested as well.

PHARMACOTHERAPY

Many of the drugs used in treating rheumatic disease provide relief from pain and inflammation, with hopes of controlling symptoms and slowing disease progress rather than providing a cure. Table 39-2 describes the commonly used drugs and their nutritional side effects (also see Appendix 31).

Analgesics

Analgesics are drugs designed specifically to relieve pain. There are several types of analgesics: acetaminophen (Tylenol) and a variety of opioid analgesics (also called narcotics). Some products combine acetaminophen with an opioid analgesic for added relief. Opioid analgesics work by binding to receptors on cells mainly in the brain, spinal cord, and gastrointestinal system.

TABLE 39-2 Medications Used in the Treatment of Rheumatic Diseases and their Nutritional Side Effects

Group/Name	Brand	Nutritional Side Effects*
Analgesics		
Acetaminophen	Excedrin, Tylenol Arthritis	
Acetaminophen with codeine	Tylenol with Codeine	Constipation, nausea, vomiting, urinary retention
Hydrocodone with acetaminophen	Hydrocet, Lorcet, Vicodin, Lortab	Constipation, nausea, vomiting, urinary retention
Hydrocodone with ibuprofen	Vicoprofen, Ibucoden	Abdominal pain, diarrhea, dry mouth, flatulence, infection, insomnia, urinary retention, vomiting
Methadone hydrochloride	Dolophine	Constipation, nausea, vomiting, urinary retention
Morphine sulfate	Avinza, Oramorph SR	Constipation, nausea, vomiting, urinary retention
Morphine sulfate with naltrexone	Embeda	Constipation, nausea, vomiting
Oxycodone	OxyContin, Roxycodone, OxyFAST, OxyIR	Constipation, nausea, vomiting, dry mouth
Oxycodone hydrochloride with acetaminophen	Percocet	Constipation, nausea, vomiting, dry mouth
Oxycodone with aspirin	Percodan	Abdominal or stomach cramps, constipation, diarrhea, heartburn or indigestion
Tapentadol	Nucynta ER	
Tramadol	Ultram, ConZyp, Rybix	Constipation, nausea, vomiting, urinary retention
Biologic Response Modifiers		
TNF Inhibitors		
Adalimumab	Humira	—
Certolizumab pegol	Cimzia	—
Etanercept	Enbrel	—
Golimumab	Simponi, Simponi Aria	—
Infliximab	Remicade	—
Selective B-Cell Inhibitors		
Belimumab	Benlysta	Nausea, vomiting
Rituximab	Rituxan	Abdominal pain
Selective Costimulation Modulator		
Abatacept	Orencia	—
IL-1 Inhibitors		
Anakinra	Kineret	—
Canakinumab	Ilaris	Diarrhea, stomach ache
IL-6 Inhibitors		
Tocilizumab	Actemra	—
IL-12 Inhibitors		
Ustekinumab	Stelara	Diarrhea
NSAIDs		
Traditional NSAID		
Diclofenac potassium	Cambia, cataflam, zipsor	Abdominal cramps, pain or discomfort, peptic ulcer, constipation, diarrhea, gastrointestinal bleeding, heartburn or indigestion, nausea or vomiting
Diclofenac sodium	Voltaren, Voltaren XR	Abdominal cramps, pain or discomfort, peptic ulcer, constipation, diarrhea, gastrointestinal bleeding, heartburn or indigestion, nausea or vomiting
Diclofenac sodium with misoprostol	Arthrotec	Abdominal cramps, pain or discomfort, diarrhea, (both with increased risk), constipation, gastrointestinal bleeding, heartburn or indigestion, nausea or vomiting, peptic ulcer (decreased risk)
Diflunisal	Generic only	Abdominal cramps, pain or discomfort, peptic ulcer, constipation, diarrhea, gastrointestinal bleeding, heartburn or indigestion, nausea or vomiting

TABLE 39-2 Medications Used in the Treatment of Rheumatic Diseases and their Nutritional Side Effects—cont'd

Group/Name	Brand	Nutritional Side Effects*
Etodolac	Generic only	Abdominal cramps, pain or discomfort, peptic ulcer, constipation, diarrhea, gastrointestinal bleeding, heartburn or indigestion, nausea or vomiting
Fenoprofen calcium	Nalfon	Abdominal cramps, pain or discomfort, peptic ulcer, constipation, diarrhea, gastrointestinal bleeding, heartburn or indigestion, nausea or vomiting
Ibuprofen	Motrin, Advil, Dyspel, Genpril	Abdominal cramps, pain or discomfort, peptic ulcer, constipation, diarrhea, gastrointestinal bleeding, heartburn or indigestion, nausea or vomiting
Indomethacin	Indocin	Abdominal cramps, pain or discomfort, peptic ulcer, constipation, diarrhea, gastrointestinal bleeding, heartburn or indigestion, nausea or vomiting
Ketoprofen	Generic only	Abdominal cramps, pain or discomfort, peptic ulcer, constipation, diarrhea, gastrointestinal bleeding, heartburn or indigestion, nausea or vomiting
Meloxicam	Mobic	Abdominal cramps, pain or discomfort, peptic ulcer, constipation, diarrhea, gastrointestinal bleeding, heartburn or indigestion, nausea or vomiting
Naproxen	Naprosyn	Abdominal cramps, pain or discomfort, peptic ulcer, constipation, diarrhea, gastrointestinal bleeding, heartburn or indigestion, nausea or vomiting
Naproxen sodium	Aleve, Naprelan	Abdominal cramps, pain or discomfort, peptic ulcer, constipation, diarrhea, gastrointestinal bleeding, heartburn or indigestion, nausea or vomiting
Piroxicam	Feldene	Abdominal cramps, pain or discomfort, peptic ulcer, constipation, diarrhea, gastrointestinal bleeding, heartburn or indigestion, nausea or vomiting.
Sulindac	Clinoril	Abdominal cramps, pain or discomfort, peptic ulcer, constipation, diarrhea, gastrointestinal bleeding, heartburn or indigestion, nausea or vomiting
COX-2 Inhibitors		
Celecoxib	Celebrex	Abdominal pain, acid reflux, diarrhea, nausea, vomiting, upset stomach
Salicylates		
Acetylsalicylic acid	Anacin, Ascriptin, Bayer, Bufferin, Ecotrin, Aspir-81, Aspirtab	Abdominal cramps, pain or discomfort, diarrhea, heartburn or indigestion, nausea or vomiting, stomach ulcers or bleeding
Choline and magnesium trisalicylates	Tricosal, Trilisate, CMT	Abdominal cramps, pain or discomfort, constipation, diarrhea, heartburn or indigestion; nausea or vomiting
Magnesium salicylate	MST 600	Abdominal cramps, pain or discomfort, constipation, diarrhea, heartburn or indigestion; nausea or vomiting
DMARD		
Azathioprine	Azasan, Imuran	Liver problems, loss of appetite, nausea or vomiting
Cyclophosphamide	Cytoxan	Loss of appetite, nausea or vomiting
Cyclosporine	Neoral, Gengraf	Abdominal pain, gingivitis, high blood pressure, kidney problems, loss of appetite, nausea
Gold sodium thiomalate	Myochrysine	Irritation and soreness of tongue, irritated or bleeding gums, metallic taste, ulcers or white spots on lips or in mouth or throat
Hydroxychloroquine	Plaquenil	Abdominal cramps, diarrhea, loss of appetite, nausea or vomiting
Leflunomide	Arava	Gastrointestinal problems, heartburn, high blood pressure, liver problems, stomach pain
Methotrexate	Otrexup, Rheumatrex, Trexall	Folic acid antagonist, abdominal pain, liver problems, mouth sores, nausea
Minocycline	Minocin	Diarrhea, gastrointestinal ulcers or bleeding, nausea, vomiting
Mycophenolate mofetil	CellCept	Diarrhea, stomach ulcers or bleeding
Sulfasalazine	Azulfidine	Abdominal discomfort, diarrhea, headache, loss of appetite, nausea and vomiting
Tofacitinib	Xeljanz	Diarrhea, hypertension, increased lipid level
Corticosteroids		
Betamethasone	Celestone	Elevated blood fats (cholesterol, triglycerides), elevated blood sugar, hardening of arteries (atherosclerosis), hypertension, increased appetite, indigestion, weight gain, ulcers
Cortisone acetate	Generic only	Elevated blood fats (cholesterol, triglycerides), elevated blood sugar, hardening of arteries (atherosclerosis), hypertension, increased appetite, indigestion, weight gain, ulcers
Dexamethasone	DexPak, ZemaPak, Baycadron	Elevated blood fats (cholesterol, triglycerides), elevated blood sugar, hardening of arteries (atherosclerosis), hypertension, increased appetite, indigestion, weight gain, ulcers
Hydrocortisone	Cortef	Elevated blood fats (cholesterol, triglycerides), elevated blood sugar, hardening of arteries (atherosclerosis), hypertension, increased appetite, indigestion, weight gain, ulcers
Methylprednisolone	Medrol	Elevated blood fats (cholesterol, triglycerides), elevated blood sugar, hardening of arteries (atherosclerosis), hypertension, increased appetite, indigestion, weight gain, ulcers
Prednisolone	AsmalPred, Flo-Pred, Millipred, Orapred, Pediapred, Prelone	Elevated blood fats (cholesterol, triglycerides), elevated blood sugar, hardening of arteries (atherosclerosis), hypertension, increased appetite, indigestion, weight gain, ulcers
Prednisone	Prednisone Intensol, Rayos	Elevated blood fats (cholesterol, triglycerides), elevated blood sugar, hardening of arteries (atherosclerosis), hypertension, increased appetite, indigestion, weight gain, ulcers

Arthritis Foundation: Arthritis today, Drug Guide. http://www.arthritistoday.org/arthritis-treatment/medications/drug-guide/, 2014. Accessed January 10, 2015.
*These side effects are usually short term and go away gradually after treatment stops.

Nonsteroidal Antiinflammatory Drugs (NSAIDs)

Nonsteroidal antiinflammatory drugs (NSAIDs) are used to relieve pain and inflammation associated with arthritis and related conditions. All NSAIDs work by blocking the synthesis of PG, which are involved in pain and inflammation, as well as many other bodily functions including protecting the stomach lining.

Traditional NSAIDs include more than twenty different drugs. They work by blocking PG synthesis by inhibiting COX-1 and COX-2, making the lining of the stomach vulnerable to ulcers and bleeding. Aspirin (acetylsalicylic acid) is the only NSAID that inhibits all COX proteins by covalent modification; all other NSAIDs act noncovalently.

Ibuprofen and naproxen slow down the body's production of PG by inhibiting COX-1. They are considered useful tools in the management of most rheumatic disorders; however, long-term use of NSAIDs may cause gastrointestinal problems such as gastritis, ulcers, abdominal burning, pain, cramping, nausea, gastrointestinal bleeding, or even renal failure.

Because of the damage to the gastric mucosa caused by COX-1 inhibitors, a new type of drug was developed to block only COX-2; among these drugs are the "coxibs," which include celecoxib (Celebrex), rofecoxib (Vioxx), and valdecoxib (Bextra). Because they only inhibit COX-2 without affecting COX-1, these drugs do not harm the stomach and are well tolerated by patients requiring long-term antiinflammatory therapy. However, the coxibs are not exempt from side effects, such as increased thrombotic events, skin reactions, and cardiotoxicity, so continuous medical monitoring is advised.

Calcitriol (1,25-dihydroxy-D_3, the active form of vitamin D), flavonoids, and BDMC33 (a curcumin derivative) are also specific blockers of COX-2, but they act by interfering with *COX-2* gene expression (Lee et al, 2013). In addition, calcitriol also blocks PG receptor expression in their target cells (Krishnan and Feldman, 2012).

Disease-Modifying Antirheumatic Drugs

Disease-modifying antirheumatic drugs (DMARD) is a category of otherwise unrelated drugs defined by their use in RA and other diseases such as SLE and SS, to slow down disease progression. Each DMARD works in different ways to slow or stop the inflammatory process that damages the joints and internal organs.

Of particular interest is the drug methotrexate (MTX), originally used to treat certain types of cancer, which is widely used to treat RA alone, or in combination with other DMARD. MTX works by competitively inhibiting dihydrofolate reductase (DHFR), an enzyme that converts folic acid to its active metabolite tetrahydrofolate (THF), which is required for nucleic acid (DNA and RNA) synthesis. Therefore patients taking MTX must consume supplemental folate to reduce the adverse effects caused by MTX such as abdominal pain, nausea, and mouth sores. Supplemental folate can be in the form of folic acid, folinic acid, or 5-methyltetrahydrofolate (5-MTHF) (see Appendix 46). Folinic acid (Leucovorin) is a folate derivative that is easily converted to THF and is unaffected by the inhibition of DHFR by MTX, while relieving some of the side effects of MTX (Shea et al, 2013). 5-MTHF (Metafolin) is the active form of folic acid used at the cellular level for DNA synthesis and also is not affected by MTX (Scaglione and Panzavolta, 2014). MTX should not be taken by pregnant and lactating women (Sammaritano and Bermas, 2014).

Biologic Response Modifiers (BRM) or Biologics

Biologic response modifiers (BRM), or biologics, are medications genetically engineered from a living organism, such as a virus, gene, or protein, to simulate the body's natural response to infection and disease. BRM target proteins, cells, and pathways responsible for the symptoms and damage of RA and other types of inflammatory arthritis.

The biologics used in arthritis treatment work in one of several ways: 1) by blocking proteins that are produced in response to injury such as interleukin-1 (IL-1), IL-6, tumor necrosis factor alpha (TNF-α); 2) by blocking B-cells, which produce antibodies that are produced excessively in some forms of arthritis; and 3) by inhibiting the activation of T-cells, thereby preventing the chain reactions that result in inflammation. These molecules are administered by injection (intravenously or subcutaneously) because they are proteins and oral administration would destroy their biologic activities. Patients taking these drugs should be monitored for chronic infections or malignancies (Ramiro et al, 2014). The main drawback is their high cost, on average $18,000 dollars per patient per year (see Arthritis Foundation [AF]).

Corticosteroids

Corticosteroids, sometimes called glucocorticoids, are medications that mimic the effects of the hormone cortisol, which is produced naturally by the adrenal glands. Cortisol affects many parts of the body, including the immune system. Corticosteroids are prescribed for patients who need quick relief from severe inflammation by lowering the levels of PG. In some cases of RA, corticosteroids pills are taken while waiting for other DMARD to start to take effect. Low-dose corticosteroids also may be prescribed long term for some patients with RA. However, the use of corticosteroids in RA is debated, because some doctors believe the long-term benefits do not outweigh the risk of side effects. If used alone, the immediate relief corticosteroids provide may defer the start of treatment, which could make a difference in the course of the disease.

As the most potent of the antiinflammatory drugs used to treat RA, steroids have extensive catabolic effects that can result in negative nitrogen balance. Hypercalciuria and reduced calcium absorption can increase the risk of osteoporosis (see Chapters 8 and 24). Concomitant calcium and vitamin D supplementation and monitoring of bone status should be considered to minimize osteopenia.

Vitamin D

Vitamin D deficiency has been linked to several autoimmune diseases, including type 1 diabetes, multiple sclerosis, Crohn's disease, dementia, cardiovascular diseases, and rheumatic disorders such as SLE and RA. Vitamin D acts by suppressing Th17 and Th1 cells that are proinflammatory, giving way to Th2 and T regulatory (T_{reg}) cells, which are antiinflammatory. As most studies indicate that vitamin D insufficiency is associated with high disease activity of RA, it would be logical to supplement these patients with vitamin D. In murine models of experimental arthritis, supplementation with 1,25-dihydroxyvitamin D_3 (calcitriol) prevents the onset and progression of the disease. Supplementation of 500 IU calcitriol daily given to previously DMARD-naïve patients with early RA along with triple DMARD therapy resulted in significant higher pain relief (50% vs. 30%) at the end of 3 months, compared with patients treated with triple DMARD and calcium (Haga, 2013). Most clinicians agree that with the increasing adverse health outcomes associated with hypovitaminosis D, screening and supplementation should be performed routinely in RA patients.

BOX 39-2　The Antiinflammatory Diet

General principles: Aims for variety, with plenty of fresh food, the least amount of processed foods and "fast foods," and abundant fruits and vegetables

Includes plenty of fruits and vegetables, except onions and potatoes, which contain the a kaloid solanine

Low in saturated fat and devoid of trans fats

Low in omega-6 fats, such as vegetable oils and animal fat

High in omega-3 PUFAs such as those found in olive oil, flax, walnuts, pumpkin seeds, and fatty cold-water oily fish such as salmon, sardines, mackerel, and herring. Other healthy oils include grapeseed, walnut, and canola.

Low in refined carbohydrates such as pasta, white bread, white rice, and other refined grains, and sucrose (table sugar) and sucrose-containing products such as pastries, cookies, cakes, energy bars, and candy

Favors intake of whole grains such as brown rice, bulgur wheat, and other unrefined grains such as amaranth, quinoa, and spelt

Includes lean protein sources such as chicken and fish

Low in eggs, red meat, butter, and other full-fat dairy products

Low in refined and processed foods

Includes spices such as ginger, curry, turmeric, and rosemary, which have antiinflammatory effects

Includes good sources of phytonutrients: fruits and vegetables of all bright and dark colors, especially berries, tomatoes, orange and yellow fruits, and dark leafy greens; cruciferous vegetables (cabbage, broccoli, brussels sprouts, cauliflower); soy foods, tea (especially white, green or oolong), dark plain chocolate in moderation

Additionally, weight should be maintained within healthy parameters, and exercise should be included.

Reference: Arthritis Foundation: Anti-inflammatory diet, 2014. Accessed August 2015 from: http://www.arthritis.org/living-with-arthritis/arthritis-diet/anti-inflammatory/anti-inflammatory-diet.php

Boeing H et al: Critical review: vegetables and fruits in the prevention of chronic diseases, *Eur J Nutr* 51:637, 2012.

ANTIINFLAMMATORY DIET

The antiinflammatory diet, a diet resembling the Mediterranean diet, has been useful for the treatment of inflammatory diseases, including RA. The diet aims for the inclusion of as much fresh food as possible, the least amount of processed foods and fast food, minimal amounts of sugar, particularly fructose and sucrose, and an abundance of fruits (especially berries) and vegetables, lean proteins, from animal sources such as chicken and fish, and vegetarian sources such as legumes and nuts, essential fatty acids, and dietary fiber. Although this diet is not intended for weight loss, people often lose weight on it (AF, 2014a) (see Box 39-2 and Appendix 31). Changing the dietary habits to a Mediterranean diet reduces the inflammatory status in healthy persons, as well as in patients with obesity, cardiovascular disease, and Crohn's disease (Castañer et al, 2013; Marlow et al, 2013; van Dijk et al, 2012). The antiinflammatory diet works by reducing the expression of genes involved in the inflammatory process such as IL-1, IL-6, and TNF-α.

COMPLEMENTARY OR INTEGRATIVE THERAPIES

Because of the chronic nature of arthritic diseases, their effects on quality of life, and the fact that most treatments result only in modest improvement in symptoms and function, patients commonly try alternative methods of treatment. Favorable effects of self-help treatments are often reported anecdotally, but usually no cause-and-effect relationships are documented. In addition, with unlimited access to the Internet, patients have greater exposure to remedies and controversial treatments. In a recent survey, rheumatologists in the United States showed a widespread favorable opinion toward complementary and alternative medicine (CAM) for patients with rheumatic diseases (Manek et al, 2010).

The World Health Organization (WHO) has defined CAM as "a broad set of health care practices that are not part of the country's own tradition and are not integrated into the dominant healthcare system" (WHO, 2014). The terms complementary and alternative refer to health-related products and practices that are not generally considered part of conventional medicine. Complementary medicine is used together with conventional medicine, and alternative medicine is used in place of conventional medicine. The term complementary integrative medicine (CIM) is being used more frequently to describe the new practice developing from conventional medicine (see Chapter 12).

There is not a lot scientific proof that CIM helps with some of the symptoms of arthritis, although this does not mean some CIM may work for all patients. Therapies vary from aromatherapy to reflexology, herbal, natural products and supplements, physical activities, body work, and many more. Some of the main categories in which CIM can be grouped are presented below. (National Institute of Health [NIH], National Center for Complementary and Integrative Health [NCCIH], 2014).

Mind and body practices include a large and diverse group of procedures or techniques administered or taught by a trained practitioner or teacher. These include acupuncture, massage therapies, meditation, movement therapies (Feldenkrais method, Alexander technique, Pilates), relaxation techniques (breathing exercises, guided imagery, progressive muscle relaxation), spinal manipulation, tai chi, qi gong, and yoga.

Natural products encompass herbs (botanicals), vitamins and minerals, and probiotics. They are widely marketed, available to consumers, and often sold as "dietary supplements," including glucosamine, chondroitin, S-adenosyl methionine (SAM-e), fish oil, extra virgin olive oil, curcumin, turmeric, boswellia, comfrey, alfalfa, cat's claw, thunder god vine, coenzyme Q10 (CoQ-10), Frankincense, and methylsulfonylmethane (MSM). Capsaicin, the compound responsible for the burning sensation produced by chili peppers, is used as a rubbing topical gel to relieve pain, particularly in joints of OA and RA patients (see Chapter 12 for further discussion of botanicals).

Other CIM includes the use of bracelets (usually made of copper), magnets, aromatherapy, and hypnotherapy.

A patient's decision to try any CIM should be discussed with his or her physician. If a type of CIM (or any combination of two or more) works, reduction of medication use can be considered. The main drawback for some patients is the additional costs of CIM.

Elimination Diets

Many people have the belief that certain foods may contain harmful substances that can worsen their arthritis symptoms. One theory is that they are having an allergic reaction to the food (see Chapter 26 for strategies for testing for food allergies or sensitivities and implementing an elimination diet). According to the NIH, the nightshade elimination diet for arthritis management is considered CIM and falls into this category of elimination diets. It is believed that nightshade plants aggravate the inflammation that causes pain, swelling, and stiffness in the joints of some patients with arthritis.

Nightshades are a diverse group of foods, herbs, shrubs, and trees that include more than 2800 species of plants of the *Solanaceae* family, such as potatoes, tomatoes, sweet and hot peppers, and eggplants. They contain a group of chemicals termed alkaloids, like solanine and chaconine, which are believed to cause damage to the joints and increase the loss of calcium from the bones. The night-shade elimination diet is believed to be safe, but there is always the risk that when eliminating certain foods from their diet, arthritis patients may not get enough of the necessary nutrients (vitamins, minerals, antioxidants; see Chapter 26). Although there are anecdotal claims of its effectiveness, the nightshade elimination diet has not been studied in depth, and no formal research has ever confirmed its beneficial effects (AF, 2014b).

MICROBIOTA AND ARTHRITIS

Increased levels of antibodies directed against antigens of certain species of gut bacteria point to the relationship between bacteria and arthritis. The idea that intestinal microorganisms are associated with the development of RA is not new: germ-free experiments have provided insight into host–microbial interactions and have shown that gut bacteria can induce autoimmunity in genetically predisposed animal models (Scher and Abramson, 2011). Mechanisms through which the microbiota may be involved in the pathogenesis of rheumatic diseases include altered epithelial and mucosal permeability, loss of immune tolerance to components of the indigenous microbiota, and trafficking of activated immune cells and antigenic material to the joints.

In 2007, based on phenotypic and phylogenetic analysis, a previously unrecognized bacterium termed *Prevotella copri* was recovered from human feces. *P. copri* is an obligate anaerobic, nonmotile, gram-negative rod. The importance of this discovery lies in that *P. copri* has been recovered in 75% of patients with new-onset untreated RA (NORA) and only in 21.4% of healthy individuals. Furthermore, there is an inverse correlation between HLA susceptibility alleles in patients with NORA and the abundance of *P. copri* detected in their fecal samples, which suggests a pathogenic role for *P. copri* in the development of RA, although its mechanism of damage remains unclear (Bernard, 2014).

Studies on the effect of diet on the microbiota, particularly with regard to the proinflammatory effects of the Western diet, are needed to gain insight into the treatment of rheumatic diseases. Potential future therapeutic approaches may include modification of the microbiota through the use of probiotics or prebiotics (Yeoh et al, 2013).

Some bacterial infections have been related to the development of reactive arthritis, the most widely documented from infection with *Streptococcus pyogenes,* a Group A beta-hemolytic bacteria that is the cause of streptococcal pharyngeal infection. Rheumatic fever is a systemic disease affecting the peri-arteriolar connective tissue and can occur after an untreated *S. pyogenes* infection. Acute rheumatic fever commonly appears in children between the ages of 6 and 15, with only 20% of first-time attacks occurring in adults. The illness is so named because of its similarity in presentation to RA.

Diagnosis of acute rheumatic fever is based on the presence of documented Group A streptococcal infection. The most common symptoms include arthritis (most of the time unilateral, instead of the common bilateral presentation in RA), carditis (inflammation of the heart tissue), and Sydenham chorea (involuntary movements of the face, hands, and feet, also known as "Saint Vitus' dance") (Burke and Chang, 2014). Heart complications may be long term and severe, particularly if valves are involved.

Molecular mimicry accounts for the tissue injury that occurs in rheumatic fever. In this process, the patient's immune responses are unable to distinguish between *S. pyogenes* structures and certain host tissues, attacking both. The resultant inflammation may persist well beyond the acute infection and produces the manifestations of rheumatic fever. The recurrence of rheumatic fever is relatively common in the absence of maintenance of low-dose antibiotics, especially during the first 3 to 5 years after the first episode. Survivors of rheumatic fever often have to take penicillin to prevent streptococcal infection, which could possibly lead to another case of rheumatic fever that could prove fatal.

OSTEOARTHRITIS

Osteoarthritis (OA), formally known as degenerative arthritis or degenerative joint disease, is the most prevalent form of arthritis. Obesity, aging, female gender, white ethnicity, greater bone density, and repetitive-use injury associated with athletics have been identified as risk factors. OA is not systemic or autoimmune in origin, but involves cartilage destruction with asymmetric inflammation. It is caused by joint overuse, whereas RA is a systemic autoimmune disorder that results in symmetric joint inflammation.

Pathophysiology

OA is a chronic joint disease that involves the loss of habitually weight-bearing articular (joint) cartilage. This cartilage normally allows bones to glide smoothly over one another. The loss can result in stiffness, pain, swelling, loss of motion, and changes in joint shape, in addition to abnormal bone growth, which can result in osteophytes (bone spurs) (see Figure 39-1 and *Pathophysiology and Care Management Algorithm:* Osteoarthritis).

A Healthy Joint

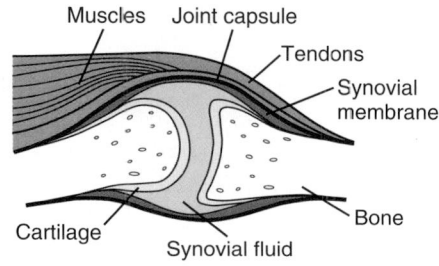

A Joint with Osteoarthritis

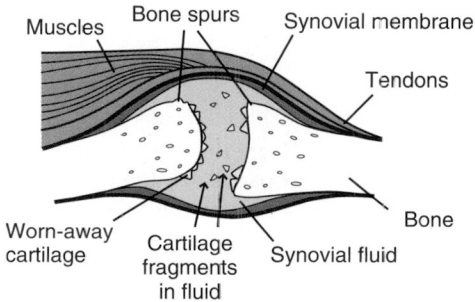

FIGURE 39-1 A healthy joint and a joint with severe osteoarthritis. (From National Institutes of Health, National Institute of Arthritis and Musculoskeletal and Skin Diseases: *Handout on health: osteoarthritis,* NIH Publication No. 13-4617, National Institutes of Health, August 2013, revised March 2014.)

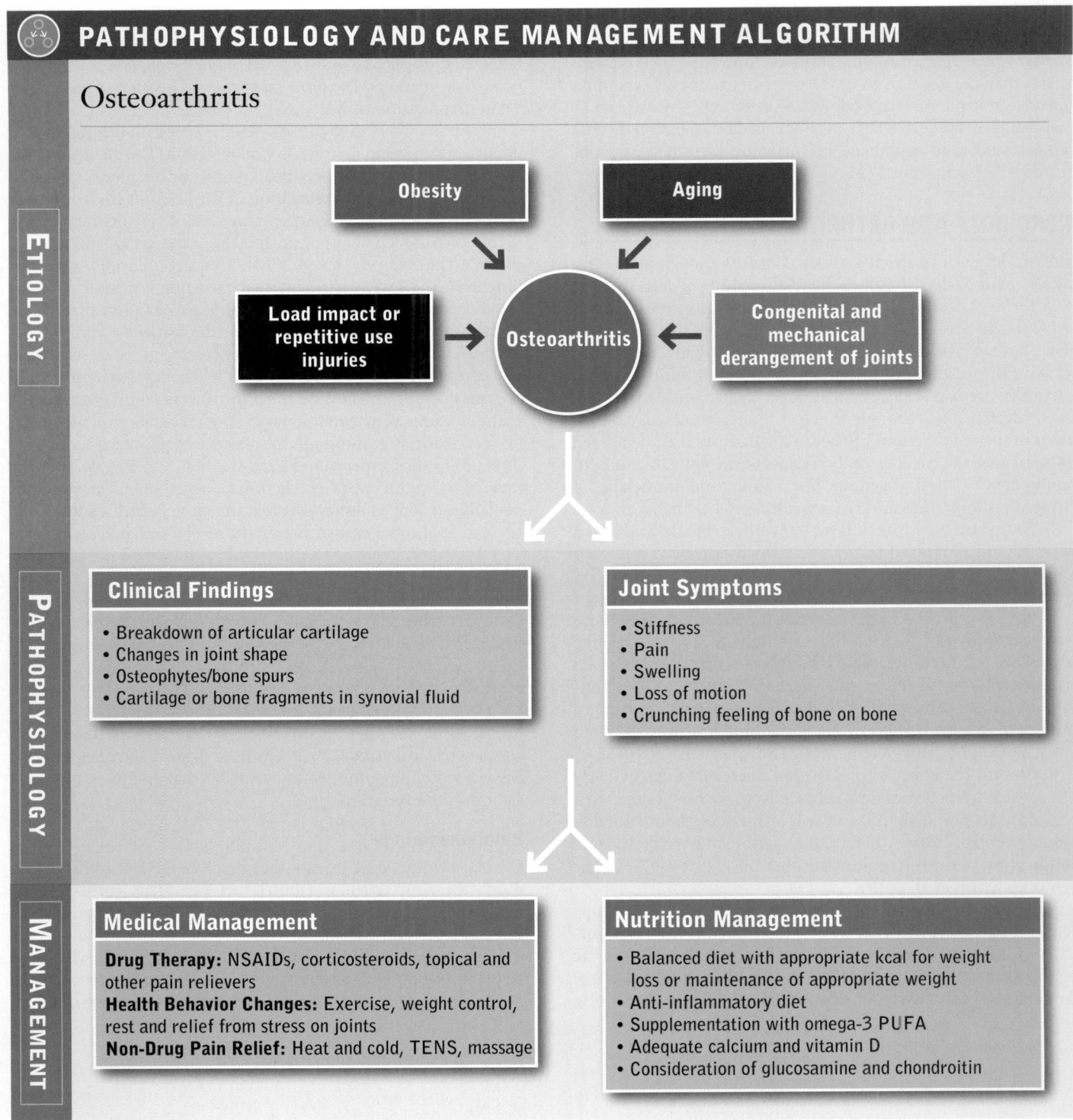

PATHOPHYSIOLOGY AND CARE MANAGEMENT ALGORITHM

Osteoarthritis

ETIOLOGY

Obesity

Aging

Load impact or repetitive use injuries

Osteoarthritis

Congenital and mechanical derangement of joints

PATHOPHYSIOLOGY

Clinical Findings

- Breakdown of articular cartilage
- Changes in joint shape
- Osteophytes/bone spurs
- Cartilage or bone fragments in synovial fluid

Joint Symptoms

- Stiffness
- Pain
- Swelling
- Loss of motion
- Crunching feeling of bone on bone

MANAGEMENT

Medical Management

Drug Therapy: NSAIDs, corticosteroids, topical and other pain relievers
Health Behavior Changes: Exercise, weight control, rest and relief from stress on joints
Non-Drug Pain Relief: Heat and cold, TENS, massage

Nutrition Management

- Balanced diet with appropriate kcal for weight loss or maintenance of appropriate weight
- Anti-inflammatory diet
- Supplementation with omega-3 PUFA
- Adequate calcium and vitamin D
- Consideration of glucosamine and chondroitin

The joints most often affected in OA are the distal interphalangeal joints, the thumb joint, and, in particular, the joints of the knees, hips, ankles, and spine, which bear the bulk of the body's weight (see Figure 39-2). The elbows, wrists, and ankles are less often affected. OA generally presents as pain that worsens with weight bearing and activity and improves with rest, and patients often report morning stiffness or "gelling" of the affected joint after periods of inactivity. Diseases of the joints influenced by congenital and mechanical derangements may contribute to OA as well. Inflammation occurs at times but is generally mild and localized.

Medical and Surgical Management

The patient's medical history and level of pain should determine the most appropriate treatment. This should include nonpharmacologic modalities (patient education, physical and occupational therapy), pharmacologic agents, and surgical procedures with the goals of pain control, improved function and

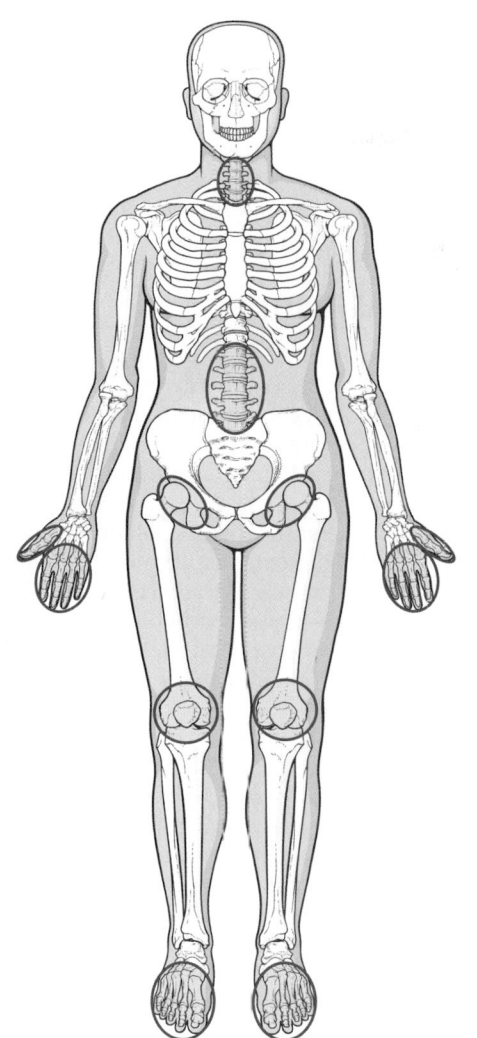

FIGURE 39-2 Joints commonly affected by osteoarthritis.

health-related quality of life, and avoidance of toxic effects from treatment. Weight loss and/or achievement of ideal body weight (body mass index [BMI] of 18.5 to 24.9 kg/m²) should be part of the medical treatment because it improves OA dramatically (see Chapter 21).

Patients with severe symptomatic OA pain who have not responded adequately to medical treatment and who have been progressively limited in their activities of daily living (ADLs), such as walking, bathing, dressing, and toileting, should be evaluated by an orthopedic surgeon. Surgical options include arthroscopic debridement (with or without arthroplasty), total joint arthroplasty, and osteotomy. Surgical reconstruction has been successful but should not be viewed as a replacement for overall good nutrition, maintenance of healthy body weight, and exercise.

Exercise

OA limits the ability to increase energy expenditure through exercise. It is critical that the exercise be done with correct form so as not to cause damage or exacerbate an existing problem. Physical and occupational therapists can provide unique expertise for OA patients by making individualized assessments and recommending appropriate exercise programs and assistive devices, in addition to offering guidance regarding

joint protection and energy conservation. Nonloading aerobic (swimming), range-of-motion, and weight-bearing exercises have been shown to reduce symptoms, increase mobility, and lessen continuing damage from OA. Non–weight-bearing exercise also may serve as an adjunct to NSAID use.

Sports or strenuous activities that subject joints to repetitive high impact and loading increase the risk of joint cartilage degeneration. Therefore increased muscle tone and strength, correct form, general flexibility, and conditioning help protect these joints in the habitual exerciser. A walking program and lower-extremity strength training are beneficial for individuals with knee OA.

Medical Nutrition Therapy
Weight and Adiposity Management

Excess weight puts an added burden on the weight-bearing joints. Epidemiologic studies have shown that obesity and injury are the two greatest risk factors for OA. The risk for knee OA increases as the BMI increases. Controlling obesity can reduce the burden of inflammation on OA and thus delay disease progression and improve symptoms. A well-balanced diet that is consistent with established dietary guidelines and promotes attainment and maintenance of a desirable body weight is an important part of MNT for OA.

The antiinflammatory diet combined with moderate exercise and diet-induced weight loss has been shown to be an effective intervention for knee OA. There is also an antiinflammatory effect from weight loss in OA management because the reduced fat mass results in the presence of less inflammatory mediators from adipose tissue (see Chapters 3 and 21).

Vitamins and Minerals

Cumulative damage to tissues mediated by reactive oxygen species has been implicated as a pathway that leads to many of the degenerative changes seen with aging. However, large doses of dietary antioxidants, including vitamins A, C, or D, alone or in combination, showed no benefit for the management of OA (Rosenbaum et al, 2010).

Many patients with OA consume deficient levels of calcium and vitamin D. Low serum levels of 25-OH-vitamin D are frequent and there is an inverse association between serum 25-OH-vitamin D and clinical findings (cartilage loss in the joint space) and joint pain (Cao et al, 2013). Calcitriol (1,25-dihydroxyvitamin D_3) functions as a transcription factor regulating the expression of several genes. Calcitriol binds to the vitamin D receptor (VDR) followed by their interaction with specific sequences in the DNA. However, the VDR gene also presents polymorphisms, and some of these have been associated with OA and another condition called intervertebral disc degeneration. Given the role of vitamin D in the cartilaginous tissue, the very common low levels of serum vitamin D, and the genetic polymorphism of the VDR, more studies are necessary to determine the role of vitamin D in the pathogenesis of OA (Colombini, et al, 2013).

Complementary Integrative Therapies

A meta-analysis have found that capsaicin gel and SAMe are useful in treating OA; articulin F (an ayurvedic mixture of withania, boswellia, curcuma, and zinc) improved pain and function; Indian Frankincense, MSM, and rose hip were somewhat effective; collagen, devil's claw, vitamin K, hyaluronic acid, and many more, proved to be ineffective for OA (De Silva et al, 2011).

Glucosamine and Chondroitin

Glucosamine and chondroitin are involved in cartilage production, but their mechanism for eliminating pain has not been identified. Limited data suggest that glucosamine sulfate administered orally, intravenously, intramuscularly, or intraarticularly may produce a gradual and progressive reduction in joint pain and tenderness, as well as improved range of motion and walking speed. Glucosamine has produced consistent benefits, including greater than 50% improvement in symptom scores in patients with OA, in some cases equal to or superior to ibuprofen. Together glucosamine and chondroitin rank third among all top-selling nutritional products in the United States.

The NIH undertook the Glucosamine/Chondroitin Arthritis Intervention Trial (GAIT), the first, large-scale, multicenter clinical trial in the United States to test the effects of these supplements on knee OA (NIH, NCCIH, 2008). A dose of 1500 mg of glucosamine (500 mg, three times daily) with 1200 mg of chondroitin (400 mg, three times daily) resulted in statistically significant pain relief for a small subset of participants who had moderate to severe pain, but not for those in the mild pain subset. Compared with 54% of those taking placebo, 79% of those taking glucosamine and chondroitin reported a 20% or greater reduction in pain. A more recent study over a 6-year period found that glucosamine/chondroitin prevented some cartilage loss when compared to placebo in patients with knee OA (Raynauld, 2016).

Although it is not effective for all afflicted individuals, a safe dose of glucosamine and chondroitin sulfate is 1500 mg/day and 1200 mg/day in divided doses, respectively. GAIT and other studies have found no change in glucose tolerance: a meta-analysis report that looked at more than 3000 human subjects found no adverse effects of oral glucosamine administration on blood, urine, or fecal parameters and no serious or fatal side effects (Anderson et al, 2005). In contrast, chondroitin is chemically similar to commonly used blood thinners and could cause excessive bleeding if used in combination with blood thinners; chondroitin also may elicit a reaction in those with shellfish allergies.

Another meta-analysis of the efficacy of glucosamine, chondroitin, and MSM for the treatment of spinal degenerative joint disease and degenerative disc disease (disc desiccation and retrolisthesis), reported that data are insufficient to support the use of any of these nutritional supplements for spinal degeneration (Stuber et al, 2011).

RHEUMATOID ARTHRITIS

Rheumatoid arthritis (RA) is a debilitating and frequently crippling autoimmune disease with overwhelming personal, social, and economic effects. Although less common than OA, RA is usually more severe, occurs more frequently in women than in men, with a peak onset commonly between 20 and 45 years.

RA affects the interstitial tissues, blood vessels, cartilage, bone, tendons, and ligaments, as well as the synovial membranes that line joint surfaces. Measurements of RF, and **antinuclear antibodies (ANA)** and antibodies to citrullinated protein antigens (ACPAs), are useful in the diagnosis as well as the prediction of the course and outcomes of RA (Demoruelle and Deane, 2011).

Numerous remissions and exacerbations generally follow its onset, although for some people it lasts just a few months or years and then goes away completely. Although any joint may be affected by RA, involvement of the small joints of the extremities—typically the proximal interphalangeal joints of the hands and feet—is most common (see Figure 39-3). Although the exact cause of RA is still unknown, certain genes have been discovered that play a role (Chatzikyriakidou et al, 2013).

Pathophysiology

RA is a chronic, autoimmune, systemic disorder in which **cytokines** and the inflammatory process play a role. RA has

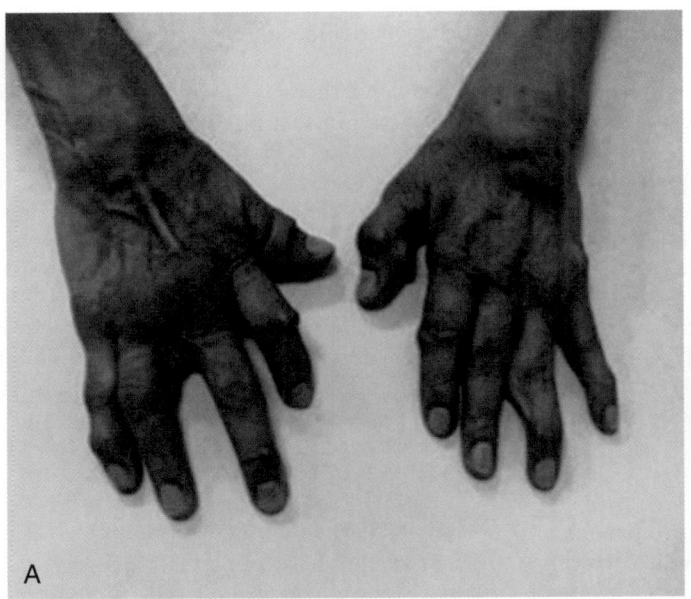
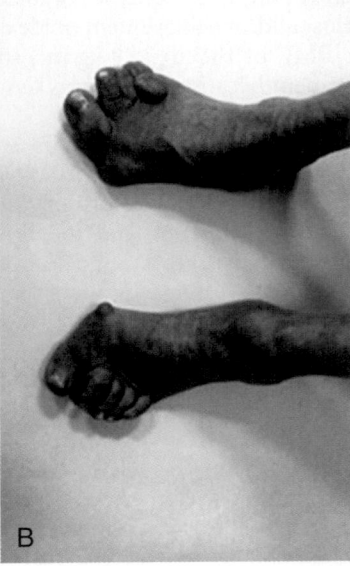

FIGURE 39-3 A female patient with advanced rheumatoid arthritis. The twisted hands (A) and feet (B), and the puffiness of the metacarpal joints are typical of the disease. (Photos courtesy Dr. F. Enrique Gómez. Instituto Nacional de Ciencias Médicas y Nutrición Salvador Zubirán. Mexico City, México, 2015.)

articular manifestations that involve chronic inflammation that begins in the synovial membrane and progresses to subsequent damage in the joint cartilage (see *Pathophysiology and Care Management Algorithm:* Rheumatoid Arthritis). Citrullination, also termed deimination, is a modification of arginine side chains catalyzed by peptidylarginine deiminase (PAD) enzymes. This posttranslational modification has the potential to alter the structure, antigenicity, and function of proteins. Four citrullinated antigens, fibrinogen, vimentin, collagen type II, and alpha-enolase, are expressed in the joints. In RA, antibodies to cyclic citrullinated peptides are now well established for clinical diagnosis (Demoruelle and Deane, 2011).

The appearance of rheumatoid factor (RF) may precede symptoms of RA. Pain, stiffness, swelling, loss of function, and anemia are common. The swelling or puffiness is caused by the accumulation of synovial fluid in the membrane lining the joints and inflammation of the surrounding tissues (see Figure 39-4).

Some controversy exists regarding green tea: it has been suggested that drinking large amounts of tea may increase the risk of developing RA, whereas other studies suggest a protective role (Walitt et al, 2010; Wu et al, 2012). Smoking is the environmental risk factor that is most associated with RA followed by coffee consumption, whereas dietary antioxidants and breastfeeding may be protective (Lahiri et al, 2012).

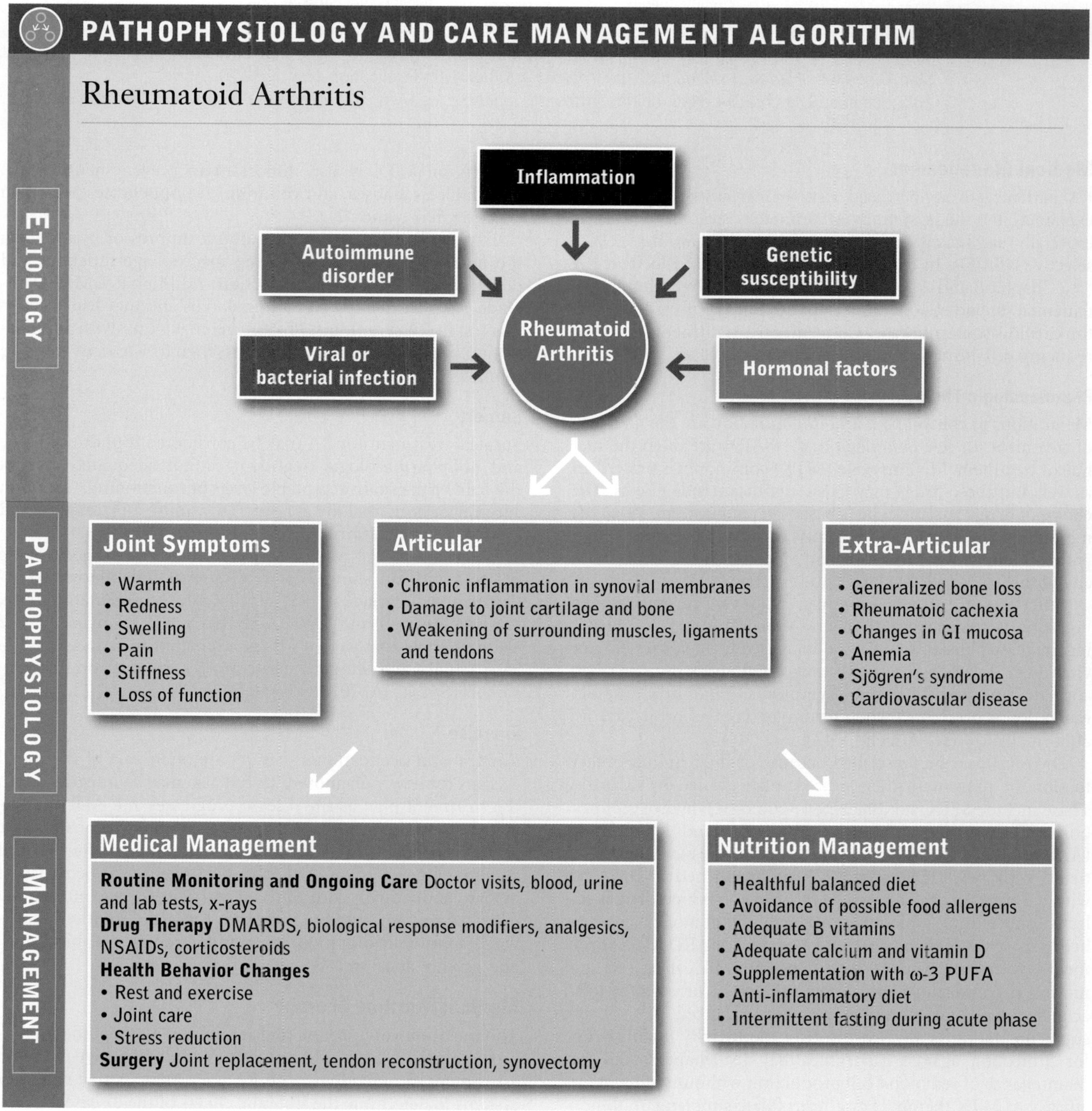

PATHOPHYSIOLOGY AND CARE MANAGEMENT ALGORITHM

Rheumatoid Arthritis

ETIOLOGY

Inflammation

Autoimmune disorder

Genetic susceptibility

Viral or bacterial infection

Rheumatoid Arthritis

Hormonal factors

PATHOPHYSIOLOGY

Joint Symptoms
- Warmth
- Redness
- Swelling
- Pain
- Stiffness
- Loss of function

Articular
- Chronic inflammation in synovial membranes
- Damage to joint cartilage and bone
- Weakening of surrounding muscles, ligaments and tendons

Extra-Articular
- Generalized bone loss
- Rheumatoid cachexia
- Changes in GI mucosa
- Anemia
- Sjögren's syndrome
- Cardiovascular disease

MANAGEMENT

Medical Management

Routine Monitoring and Ongoing Care Doctor visits, blood, urine and lab tests, x-rays
Drug Therapy DMARDS, biological response modifiers, analgesics, NSAIDs, corticosteroids
Health Behavior Changes
- Rest and exercise
- Joint care
- Stress reduction
Surgery Joint replacement, tendon reconstruction, synovectomy

Nutrition Management
- Healthful balanced diet
- Avoidance of possible food allergens
- Adequate B vitamins
- Adequate calcium and vitamin D
- Supplementation with ω-3 PUFA
- Anti-inflammatory diet
- Intermittent fasting during acute phase

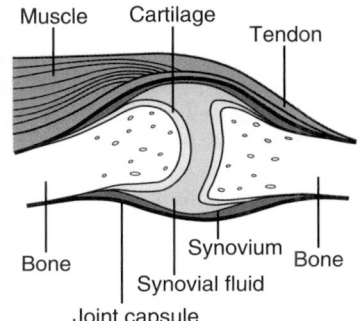

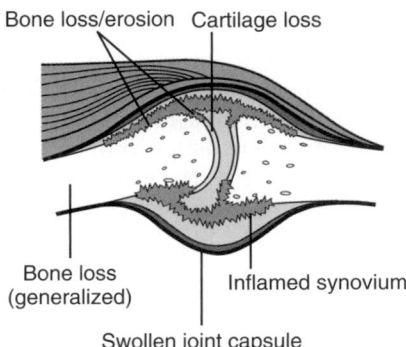

FIGURE 39-4 Comparison of a normal joint and one affected by rheumatoid arthritis, which has swelling of the synovium. (From National Institute of Arthritis and Musculoskeletal and Skin Diseases: *Handout on health: rheumatoid arthritis,* NIH Publication No. 12-4179, April 2013, Revised March 2014. National Institutes of Health.)

Medical Management

RA patients are at increased risk for cardiovascular disease, explained by the systemic inflammatory response. This is especially significant considering findings regarding COX-2 selective NSAIDs. In fact, many of the drugs used to treat RA (see Chapter 8 and Appendix 23) can result in hyperhomocysteinemia, hypertension, and hyperglycemia, all risk factors for cardiovascular disease. Conveniently, treatment aimed at reducing inflammation may benefit both diseases.

Pharmacologic Therapy

Medications to control pain and inflammation are the mainstay of treatment for RA. Salicylates and NSAIDs are often the first line of treatment. Methotrexate (MTX) commonly is prescribed as well, but these drugs may cause significant side effects. The choice of drug class and type is based on patient response to the medication, incidence and severity of adverse reactions, and patient compliance. Drug-nutrient side effects can occur with any of the drugs (see Chapter 8 and Appendix 23).

Salicylates are used commonly. However, chronic aspirin ingestion is associated with gastric mucosal injury and bleeding, increased bleeding time, and increased urinary excretion of vitamin C. Taking aspirin with milk, food, or an antacid often alleviates the gastrointestinal symptoms. Vitamin C supplementation is prescribed when serum levels of ascorbic acid are abnormally low (see Appendix 42).

DMARD may be prescribed because of their unique ability to slow or prevent further joint damage caused by arthritis. These include MTX, sulfasalazine (Azulfidine), hydroxychloroquine (Plaquenil), azathioprine (Imuran), and leflunomide (Arava). In fact, the ACR recommends that the majority of patients with newly diagnosed RA be prescribed a DMARD within 3 months of diagnosis. Depending on which drug is selected, side effects can include myelosuppression or macular or liver damage. A main adverse effect of the DMARD MTX treatment is folate antagonism. Treatment with MTX induces a significant rise in serum homocysteine, which is corrected by folic acid supplementation and a properly balanced diet. Folate supplementation is advised to offset the toxicity of this drug, for protection against gastrointestinal disturbances, and for maintenance of red blood cell production without reducing the efficacy of MTX therapy. Long-term folate supplementation in patients on MTX is also important to prevent neutropenia, mouth ulcers, nausea, and vomiting (see Appendices 31 and 46 and Chapters 8 and 32).

D-penicillamine acts as an immunosuppressor by reducing the number of T cells, inhibiting macrophage function, and decreasing IL-1 and RF production. Additional DMARD include gold salt therapy and antimalarials and may lead to a remission in RA symptoms. Proteinuria may occur with administration of gold and D-penicillamine; therefore toxicity must be monitored continually.

Surgery

Surgical treatment for RA may be considered if pharmacologic and nonpharmacologic treatment cannot adequately control the pain or maintain acceptable levels of functioning. Common surgical options include synovectomy, joint replacement, and tendon reconstruction.

After substantial weight loss from bariatric surgery, obese patients with RA showed lower disease activity, decreased inflammatory markers (CRP, erythrocyte sedimentation rate, total leukocytes) and less RA-related medication use. These findings show that weight loss is important to reduce RA disease activity and should be encouraged by nutrition professionals (Sparks JA, 2015).

Exercise

Physical and occupational therapy are often part of the initial therapy for newly diagnosed RA but also may be integrated into the treatment plan as the disease progresses and ADLs are affected. To maintain joint function, recommendations may be given for energy conservation, along with range-of-motion and strengthening exercises. Although the patient may be reluctant at first, individuals with RA can participate in conditioning exercise programs without increasing fatigue or joint symptoms while improving joint mobility, muscle strength, aerobic fitness, and psychological well-being.

Medical Nutrition Therapy

The nutrition care process and model serve as a guide for implementing MNT with RA patients. A comprehensive nutrition assessment of individuals with RA is essential, with a review of systems to determine the systemic effects of the disease process.

A physical examination provides diagnostic signs and symptoms of nutrient deficiencies (see Appendix 29). Current weight and history of weight change over time are the least expensive, least invasive, and most reliable assessment tools to use. Weight change is an important measure of RA severity. The characteristic progression of malnutrition in RA is attributed to excessive protein catabolism evoked by inflammatory cytokines and by disuse atrophy resulting from functional impairment.

The diet history should review the usual diet; the effect of the handicap; types of food consumed; and changes in food tolerance secondary to oral, esophageal, and intestinal disorders. The effect of the disease on food shopping and preparation, self-feeding ability, appetite, and intake also must be assessed. The use of elimination or other diets purported to treat or cure arthritis should be identified.

Articular and extraarticular manifestations of RA affect the nutrition status of individuals in several ways. Articular involvement of the small and large joints may limit the ability to perform nutrition-related ADLs, including shopping for, preparing, and eating food. Involvement of the temporomandibular joint can affect the ability to chew and swallow and may necessitate changes in diet consistency. Extraarticular manifestations include increased metabolic rate secondary to the inflammatory process, SS, and changes in the gastrointestinal mucosa.

Increased metabolic rate secondary to the inflammatory process leads to increased nutrient needs, often in the face of a diminishing nutrient intake. Taste alterations secondary to xerostomia and dryness of the nasal mucosa; dysphagia secondary to pharyngeal and esophageal dryness; and anorexia secondary to medications, fatigue, and pain may reduce dietary intake. Changes in the gastrointestinal mucosa affect intake, digestion, and absorption. The effect of RA and the medications used may be evident throughout the gastrointestinal tract. Based on the patient's unique profile, a registered dietitian nutritionist can determine the most appropriate nutrition intervention, followed by monitoring and evaluation.

The association of foods with disease flares should be discussed. Whether food intake can modify the course of RA is an issue of continued scientific debate and interest. Dietary manipulation by either modifying food composition or reducing body weight may give some clinical benefit in improving RA symptoms. A vegan, gluten-free diet causes improvement in some patients, possibly because of the reduction of immunoreactivity to food antigens (see Chapter 28). Identification of possible food allergies and use of an elimination diet may be useful (see Chapter 26).

Fasting has been practiced for millennia, but, only recently, studies have shed light on its role in adaptive cellular responses that reduce oxidative damage and inflammation. In humans it helps reduce hypertension, asthma, and symptoms of RA. Thus fasting has the potential to delay aging and help prevent and treat diseases while minimizing the side effects caused by medications (Longo and Mattson, 2014). Intermittent fasting during the acute phase of RA may provide some pain relief, but it has never been shown as an effective treatment for RA symptoms.

The antiinflammatory diet described in Box 39-2 should be considered. The similar Mediterranean-style eating plan includes foods that almost everyone should aim to consume on a daily basis, such as moderate amounts of lean meat, unsaturated fats instead of saturated fats, plenty of fruits and vegetables, and fish (AF, 2014a ; Boeing et al, 2012). These diets are also nutritionally adequate and cover all of the food groups (see Appendix 31 for additional description of the antiinflammatory diet).

Energy

There are three unique aspects of energy metabolism in RA. One is elevated resting energy expenditure. RA causes cachexia, a metabolic response characterized by loss of muscle mass and elevated resting energy expenditure. Another is elevated whole-body protein catabolism, a destructive form of muscle metabolism that translates to muscle wasting. And yet another is low body cell mass, which leads to increased fat mass. People with RA tend to be less active than people without it; the stiffness and swelling caused by inflammation naturally prompt them to pursue less physical, more sedentary lifestyles. Such habits lead in turn to overall gains in fat mass. Being overweight puts an extra burden on weight-bearing joints when they are already damaged or under strain.

Total energy expenditure is significantly lower in RA patients, mainly because of less moderate-intensity physical activity performance. Disease activity and fatigue are important contributing factors. Energy requirements should be adjusted according to the weight and activity level of the individual (Henchoz et al, 2012) (see Chapter 21).

People with RA should consume nutrient-rich diets and incorporate physical activity throughout the day to boost their total energy expenditure. This helps them improve their physical function and quality of life and maintain a healthy weight.

Protein

Protein requirements for individuals who are poorly nourished or who are in the inflammatory phase of the disease are 1.5 to 2.0 g protein/kg body weight. Well-nourished individuals do not have increased requirements.

Fat

Fat should contribute less than 30% of the total energy intake for the purposes of healthy eating and weight management. The type of fat included in the diet is important: an increase in the amount of omega-3 fatty acids primarily from fish oils and alpha-linolenic acid (found in flaxseed, soybean oils, and green leaves) have been shown to reduce inflammation in RA. The antiinflammatory diet (see Box 39-2) with higher omega-3 fatty acids can reduce inflammatory activity and allow for increased physical function, and improved vitality for RA patients.

There is evidence of a fairly consistent, but modest, benefit of marine omega-3 PUFAs on joint swelling and pain and duration of morning stiffness (Miles and Calder, 2012; Norling and Perreti, 2013). Fish oil at a high dose (3.5 g/day) has been shown to have additional benefits to those achieved by combination DMARD with similar MTX use, including reduced triple DMARD failure and a higher rate of remission (Proudman et al, 2015). Omega-3 fatty acids have increased in popularity in the management of RA because of their role in inflammatory pathways.

Some other oils of marine origin and a range of vegetable oils (olive and evening primrose oil) have indirect antiinflammatory actions probably mediated via PGE_1 (see *Clinical Insight: Fatty Acids and the Inflammatory Process*). The beneficial effects are generally delayed for up to 12 weeks after they are started, but last up to 6 weeks after discontinuing therapy (Bhangle and Kolasinski, 2011) (see Appendix 40 for omega-3 and omega-6 fatty acid content of foods). Although these benefits along with improved dietary habits are known, they usually cannot replace conventional drug therapies.

CLINICAL INSIGHT

Fatty Acids and the Inflammatory Process

Inflammation is the body's attempt at self-protection to remove harmful stimuli, including damaged cells, irritants, or pathogens, and begin the healing process. When the offending stimuli are removed, inflammation subsides. The resolving phase of inflammation is not a passive process, but actively "switches off" via the biosynthesis of endogenous antiinflammatory mediators. It could therefore be considered that chronic, nonresolving inflammation not only is associated with excessive production of proinflammatory mediators but also is attributed to a defect in the synthesis of antiinflammatory compounds.

Two classes of polyunsaturated omega-6 and omega-3 fatty acids are metabolized competitively, including conversion to their corresponding prostanoids (prostaglandins [PG] and thromboxanes [Tx]) and leukotrienes (LT). Eicosapentaenoic acid (EPA, 20:5) and docosahexaenoic acid (DHA, 22:6) are omega-3 polyunsaturated fatty acids (PUFA) that are abundant in cold-water fish such as salmon, sardines, mackerel, herring, tuna, fish oils, and some algae. Alpha-linolenic acid (ALA, 18:3) is also an omega-3 PUFA found in abundance in flaxseed, walnuts, and soy and canola (rapeseed) oils. EPA, DHA, and ALA have all been shown to replace the synthesis of inflammatory eicosanoids by competing with the conversion of arachidonic acid (ARA, 20:4 omega-6) to the series 2 of PG and Tx. Also, EPA and DHA are enzymatically converted to novel bioactive lipid mediators, termed resolvins, protectins, and maresins, which promote the resolution of inflammation. ARA comes exclusively from animal foods. Linoleic acid (LA, 18:2), an omega-6 PUFA found in safflower and other vegetable oils, is a precursor of ARA; therefore its consumption should be limited in rheumatic patients.

The type of mediator that is produced is determined by the type of PUFAs present in the phospholipids of the cell membrane, which in turn is influenced by the type of PUFAs in the diet. Theoretically, a person can replace omega-6 PUFAs with omega-3 PUFAs by increasing omega-3 PUFA consumption. This, in turn, will result in the synthesis of prostanoids (PG and Tx) with antiinflammatory effects. Similarly, reducing the amount of ARA minimizes inflammation and can enhance the benefits of fish oil supplementation.

Studies during the last 20 years clearly show beneficial changes in eicosanoid metabolism with fish oil supplementation in patients with RA, even when administered parenterally (Bahadori et al, 2010; Miles and Calder, 2012). Although fish oil seems to exert an antiinflammatory effect in short-term studies, these effects may vanish during long-term treatment because of decreased numbers of autoreactive T-cells via apoptosis.

These oils should be used in conjunction with improved eating that includes more omega-3 PUFA. This means a diet that includes baked or broiled fish one to two times per week. However, the Food and Drug Administration (FDA) has identified shark, swordfish, king mackerel, and tilefish as high-mercury fish that should be avoided (see *Focus On:* Childhood Methylmercury Exposure and Toxicity: Media Messaging in Chapter 17).

An average of 3.5 g/day of omega-3 PUFA (mainly EPA and DHA) can be recommended for RA patients (Lee et al, 2012; Norling and Perretti, 2013). Although the quality of fish oil supplements is steadily improving, these supplements are not without their own side effects, such as their fishy taste or odor, causing increased bleeding time or gastrointestinal distress; although these manifestations are usually dose dependent (Bhangle and Kolasinski, 2011).

The combination of fish oils with olive oil results in greater clinical improvements in RA patients than those consuming fish oils alone. These results are attributed to oleocanthal, a naturally occurring phenolic compound found in extra-virgin olive oil. Oleocanthal exerts its antiinflammatory activity by inhibiting COX-1 and COX-2, in a similar way as ibuprofen does, and by suppressing of MIP-1alpha and IL-6 (mRNA and protein synthesis) in macrophages and chondrocytes (Fezai et al, 2013; Scotece et al, 2012). Although these are promising results, further studies are required before oleocanthal can be recommended safely for human trials because its absorption, metabolism, and distribution are not known.

Minerals, Vitamins, and Antioxidants

Several vitamins and minerals function as antioxidants and therefore affect inflammation. Vitamin E is just such a vitamin, and along with omega-3 fatty acids and omega-6 fatty acids, may affect cytokine and eicosanoid production by decreasing proinflammatory cytokines and lipid mediators. Synovial fluid and plasma trace element concentrations, excluding Zn, change in inflammatory RA. Altered trace element concentrations in inflammatory RA may result from changes of the immunoregulatory cytokines. Degradation of collagen and eicosanoid stimulation are associated with oxidative damage.

RA patients often have nutritional intakes below the Dietary Reference Intakes (DRIs) for folic acid, calcium, vitamin D, vitamin E, zinc, vitamin B, and selenium. In addition, the commonly used drug MTX is known to decrease serum folate levels with the result of elevated homocysteine levels. Low serum level of pyridoxal-5-phosphate correlates with increased markers of inflammation (Sakakeeny et al, 2012) and continuous use of NSAID (Naproxen) also impairs pyridoxine metabolism by a mechanism related to COX inhibition (Chang et al, 2013).

Thus, in these patients, adequate intakes of folate and vitamins B_6 and B_{12} should be encouraged.

Calcium and vitamin D malabsorption and bone demineralization are characteristic of advanced stages of the disease, leading to osteoporosis or fractures. Prolonged use of glucocorticoids also can lead to osteoporosis. Therefore supplementation with calcium and vitamin D should be considered. Vitamin D status should be assessed and supplementation started if below normal. Indeed, vitamin D is a selective immunosuppressant and greater intakes of vitamin D may be beneficial. Because of drug-induced alterations in specific vitamin or mineral levels, mounting evidence supports supplementation beyond the minimum levels for vitamins D, E, folic acid, and vitamins B_6 and B_{12} (Haga, 2013).

Elevated levels of copper and ceruloplasmin in serum and joint fluid are seen in RA. Plasma copper levels correlate with the degree of joint inflammation, decreasing as the inflammation is diminished. Elevated plasma levels of ceruloplasmin, the carrier protein for copper, may have a protective role because of its antioxidant activity.

Complementary and Integrative Therapies

The increasing popularity of the use of complementary treatments appears to be particularly evident with people afflicted with RA. Herbal therapy is popular; however, concerns of toxicity must also be addressed because the Food and Drug Administration (FDA) provides relatively little regulation of herbal therapies.

Gamma-linolenic acid (GLA) is an omega-6 fatty acid found in the oils of black currant, borage, and evening primrose that can be converted into the antiinflammatory PGE_1 or into ARA, a precursor of the inflammatory PGE_2. Because of competition between omega-3 and omega-6 fatty acids for the same enzymes, the relative dietary contribution of these fats appears to affect which pathways are favored. The enzyme delta-5 desaturase converts GLA into ARA, but a diet high in omega-3 fats pulls more of this enzyme to the omega-3 pathway, allowing the body to use GLA to produce PGE_1 (see *Clinical Insight:* Fatty Acids and the Inflammatory Process). This antiinflammatory

PGE₁ may relieve pain, morning stiffness, and joint tenderness with no serious side effects. Further studies are required to establish optimum dosage and duration.

Thunder god vine (*Tripterygium wilfordii*) has been used for centuries in traditional Chinese medicine. Extracts are prepared from the skinned root of the herb, as other parts of the plant are highly poisonous. A systematic review of the research on thunder god vine for RA concluded that serious side effects occurred frequently enough that the risk of using it outweighs its benefits. Depending on the dose and type of extract, it affects the reproductive system, possibly causing menstrual changes in women and infertility in men and long-term use may decrease bone mineral density in women, potentially increasing the risk of osteoporosis. Other side effects can include diarrhea, upset stomach, hair loss, headache, and skin rash (NIH, NCCIH, 2013).

SJÖGREN SYNDROME (SS)

Sjögren syndrome (SS) is a chronic autoimmune inflammatory disease that affects the exocrine glands, particularly the salivary and the lacrimal glands, leading to dryness of the mouth (xerostomia) and of the eyes (xerophthalmia). SS can present alone (primary SS) or secondary as a result of a previous rheumatic disorder (commonly RA or SLE). It mainly affects middle-age women, with a female/male ratio of 9:1.

Common oral signs include thirst, burning sensation in the oral mucosa, inflammation of the tongue (glossitis), and lips (cheilitis), cracking of the corners of the lips (cheilosis), difficulties in chewing and swallowing (dysphagia), severe dental caries, oral infections (candidiasis), progressive dental decay, and nocturnal oral discomfort. Patients may also suffer from extraglandular disorders affecting the skin, lung, kidney, nerve, connective tissue, and digestive system (Ebert, 2012; Tincani et al, 2013). SS patients also may develop disturbances in smell perception (dysosmia) and in taste acuity (dysgeusia) (Ebert EC, 2012; Gomez et al, 2004).

Pathophysiology

Although the pathogenesis of SS remains elusive, environmental, genetic and hormonal contributors seem to be involved (Tincani et al, 2013). The majority of lymphocytes infiltrating the salivary glands are mostly CD4 T-cells. Increased levels of IL-1 and IL-6 in the saliva of SS patients suggest that a Th1 response participates in the pathogenesis of the disease. Although T-cells were originally considered to play the initiating role in SS, whereas B-cells were restricted to autoantibody production, it has been shown that B-cells play a central role in the development of the disease. A distinctive hallmark of SS is the presence of anti-Ro/SSA and anti-La/SSB autoantibodies. Interestingly, anti-Ro/SSA may be found either solely or concomitantly with anti-La/SSB antibodies, whereas exclusive anti-La/SSB positivity is rare (Huang et al, 2013).

Medical Management

The therapeutic management of SS is based on symptomatic treatment of glandular manifestations and on the use of DMARD for systemic involvement. Symptomatic treatment has beneficial effects on oral and ocular dryness and prevents further complications such as oral candidiasis, periodontal disease, and corneal ulceration and perforation.

Topical treatment of xerostomia begins by avoiding irritants such as caffeine, alcohol, and tobacco, followed by appropriate hydration (small sips of water) and the use of saliva substitutes, lubricating gels, mouth rinses, chewing gum, lozenges, or oils.

Any of these treatments is effective in the short term, but none improves saliva production. After consumption of sugary foods or beverages, the teeth should be brushed and rinsed with water immediately to prevent dental caries. Topical treatment for xerophthalmia starts by avoiding dry, smoky, or windy environments and prolonged reading or computer use. Artificial tears can be used. The muscarinic receptor agonists pilocarpine (Salagen) and cevimeline (Evoxac) may be used for the treatment of dry mouth and dry eyes only in patients with residual gland function (Tincani et al, 2013).

B-cell depletion therapy with rituximab (anti-CD20) improves the stimulated whole saliva flow rate and lacrimal gland function, as well as other variables including RF levels, extraglandular manifestations (arthritis, skin vasculitis), fatigue, and quality of life, indicating a major role of B-cells in the pathogenesis of SS (Tincani et al, 2013).

IL-1 and tumor necrosis factor-alpha (TNF-alpha) play a major role in the development of SS. Blocking IL-1 (anakinra) is beneficial in the treatment of SS, whereas blocking TNF-alpha (etanercept) is ineffective in controlling SS symptoms (Yamada et al, 2013; Yao et al, 2013). Etanercept exacerbated IFN-alpha and BAFF expression, providing a possible explanation for the lack of efficacy in blocking TNF-alpha in SS.

The management of extraglandular features must be tailored to the specific organs involved. Antimalarials (hydroxychloroquine), besides improving salivary flow, can help SS patients with arthromyalgia. The use of corticosteroids may be used in patients with extraglandular manifestations, although they have no effect in salivary or lacrimal flow rates.

Medical Nutrition Therapy

The first goal of dietary management for patients with SS is to help them relieve their oral symptoms and reduce the eating discomfort derived from the difficulty with chewing and swallowing. Very often SS patients modify their dietary habits on a "trial and error" basis to cope with their oral symptoms, particularly to improve biting (cutting fruits, vegetables, and meats in small pieces), chewing (making foods softer by preparing them as soups, broths, casseroles, or as tender cooked vegetables and meats), and swallowing (moistening foods with sauces, gravies, yogurts, or salad dressings). Foods that worsen oral symptoms should be limited, such as citrus fruits, as well as irritating, hot, or spicy foods (Sjögren's Syndrome Foundation, 2013).

Malnutrition or weight loss are not common in SS patients, although deficiencies of several nutrients are common. These include vitamin D, vitamin B₆, vitamin B₁₂, folate, and iron, which can be corrected easily by proper nutritional counseling or supplementation (Erten et al, 2014). More importantly single nutrient deficiencies in SS have been associated with other diseases, such as low levels of vitamin D with neuropathy and lymphoma, suggesting a possible role of vitamin D deficiency in the development of other symptoms, and the plausible beneficial effect for vitamin D supplementation (Tincani et al, 2013).

TEMPOROMANDIBULAR DISORDERS

Temporomandibular disorders (TMDs) affect the temporomandibular joint, which connects the lower jaw (mandible) to the temporal bone. TMDs can be classified as myofascial pain, internal derangement of the joint, or degenerative joint disease. One or more of these conditions may be present at the same time, causing pain or discomfort in the muscles or joint that control jaw function.

Pathophysiology

Besides experiencing a severe jaw injury, little scientific evidence suggests a cause for TMD. It is generally agreed that physical or mental stress may aggravate this condition.

Medical Nutrition Therapy

The goal of dietary management is to alter food consistency to reduce pain while chewing. According to the National Institute of Dental and Craniofacial Research (NIDCR), diet should be mechanically soft in consistency; all foods should be cut into bite-size pieces to minimize the need to chew or open the jaw widely; and chewing gum, sticky foods, and biting hard foods such as raw vegetables, candy, and nuts should be avoided (NIH, NIDCR, 2013). Nutrient intake of TMD patients appears to be the same as for the general population with regard to total calories, protein, fat, carbohydrates, vitamins, and minerals. However, during times of acute pain, intake of fiber is often reduced.

GOUT

Gout is one of the oldest diseases in recorded medical history. It is a disorder of purine metabolism in which abnormally high levels of uric acid accumulate in the blood (**hyperuricemia**). Contrary to what is observed in most rheumatic diseases, gout affects predominantly men. All studies have consistently shown that gout affects older men (older than 45 years) with a male to female ratio of 4:1. This ratio changes to 3:1 above 65 years, which reflects that gout rarely affects young women but the frequency increases in postmenopausal women. The incidence and prevalence of gout have increased markedly in the last few decades; in the United States gout is more prevalent than RA (Lawrence et al, 2008). The presence of metabolic syndrome that includes central obesity, hypertension, insulin resistance, and hyperlipidemia, occurs in approximately 60% of patients with gout. Gout is associated with significant morbidity, mortality (mainly because of coronary heart disease), functional impairment, and reduced quality of life (Suresh and Das, 2012).

Pathophysiology

Gout is a crystal deposition disease in which the clinical symptoms are caused by the formation of **monosodium urate (MSU) crystals** in the joints and soft tissues, and the elimination of these crystals "cures" the disease. **Uric acid** is the end-product of purine metabolism in humans, but it is an intermediary product in most other mammals. It is produced primarily in the liver by the action of the enzyme xanthine-oxidase, a molybdenum-dependent enzyme. In most mammals, uric acid is further degraded by the enzyme urate oxidase (uricase), to allantoin, which is more soluble than uric acid, and hence more readily excreted by kidneys. In humans and higher primates, the gene encoding for uricase is nonfunctional and due to this evolutionary event, uric acid levels are higher in humans than in many other mammals. Uric acid homeostasis is determined by the balance between production and renal excretion (Bobulescu and Moe, 2012). Endogenous production of uric acid from degradation of **purines** accounts for two thirds of the body urate pool, the remainder being of dietary origin. Because most uric acid is excreted via the kidney (approximately 70%), hyperuricemia results from reduced efficiency of renal urate clearance.

Two proteins have been well characterized in urate clearance: the urate transporter 1 (URAT1) and the glucose and fructose transporter (GLUT9). URAT1 localizes in the brush border membrane of the proximal tubule kidney and is responsible mainly for renal reabsorption of uric acid, whereas GLUT9 is located in the apical and basolateral membrane of the distal tubule where it functions as the main exit of urate from the body (Bobulescu and Moe, 2012).

In the vast majority of people with gout, hyperuricemia results from reduced renal urate clearance. MSU crystals preferentially form within cartilage and fibrous tissues; however if "shed" from these sites, they are highly immunogenic particles that are quickly phagocytosed by monocytes and macrophages, activating the NALP3 inflammasome and triggering the release of IL-1 and other cytokines, thus initiating an inflammatory response that affects the joint. MSU crystals act as a "danger signal" that can be recognized by pattern recognition receptors at the cell surface and in the cytoplasm, indicating the importance of innate immunity in gout (Rock et al, 2013). Persistent accumulation of MSU crystals causes joint damage through mechanical effects (pressure erosion) leading to chronic symptoms of arthritis (see Figure 39-5). MSU crystals can deposit in the small joints and surrounding tissues, producing recurrent episodes of extremely painful and debilitating joint and soft tissue inflammation (acute gout). In chronic gout, classic sites are the big toe, wrists and finger joints, elbow (see Figure 39-6), ankle, knee, and the helix of the ear.

Medical Management. Colchicine is used to treat the pain associated with acute flares of gout (within 12 to 24 hours) by reducing the inflammation caused by MSU crystals; it has no effect on serum urate levels. Colchicine may be used with other NSAIDs and only for a limited time because of its toxicity.

Because monocytes and macrophages produce IL-1 in response to MSU crystals, treatment with IL-1 antagonists (Anakinra) or with soluble IL-1 receptor (Rinolacept) results in rapid and complete pain relief (Suresh and Das, 2012).

Two classes of drugs have been used to lower serum urate: **uricostatic** drugs, which reduce the synthesis of uric acid by inhibiting xanthine oxidase, and **uricosuric** drugs, which increase the excretion of uric acid by blocking its renal tubular reabsorption. Allopurinol (Zyloprim) and febuxostat are uricostatic drugs; they are the drugs of choice for long-term treatment of hyperuricemia. On the other hand, sulfinpyrazone, probenecid, and benzbromarone are uricosuric drugs that act by inhibiting URAT1, therefore increasing the urinary excretion of uric acid (Bobulescu and Moe, 2012).

Pegloticase, a recombinant uricase, reduces serum urate levels by converting uric acid to allantoin, which is excreted rapidly in the urine. Pegloticase is used for rapid debulking of tophi and together with colchicine, in patients with severe and acute gout flares (Suresh and Das, 2012).

Medical Nutrition Therapy

Historically, gout has long been linked with a rich lifestyle involving excesses of meat and alcohol. There is an increased risk of gout associated with higher consumption of red meat (beef, pork, and lamb) and seafood, but not with consumption of vegetable protein. Diets high in purine-rich vegetables (beans, peas, lentils) do not increase the risk of gout.

On the other hand, diets high in low-fat dairy products and supplemental vitamin C have been associated with reduced risk of gout (Bobulescu and Moe, 2012). Consumption of coffee, but not green tea, is associated with low levels of serum urate, therefore, protective for gout.

Alcohol consumption, particularly beer (which is rich in purines), increases the risk of gout. Consumption of fructose, mainly as soft drinks sweetened with high fructose corn syrup, is associated with higher risk for gout. It is unclear whether this is a particular effect of fructose derived from corn, or whether

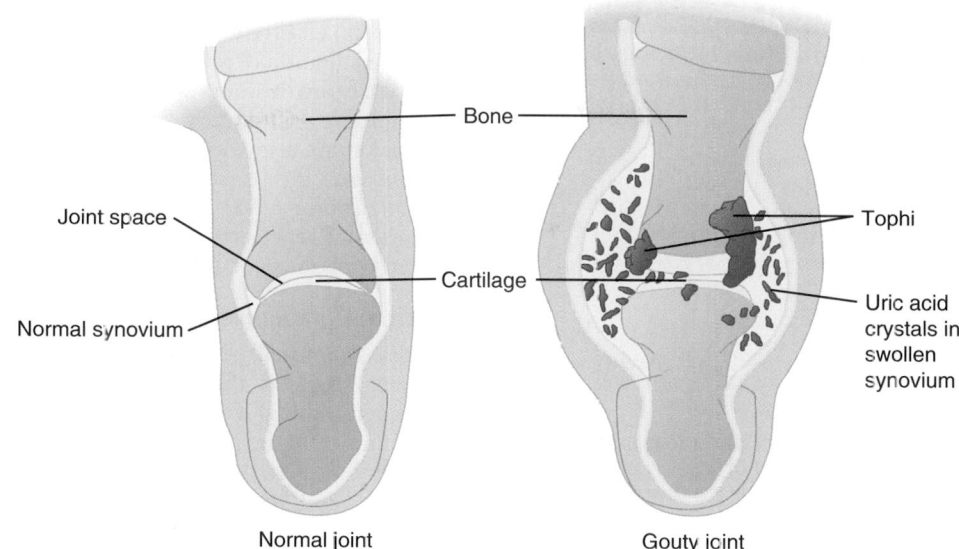

FIGURE 39-5 Comparison of a gouty joint and a normal joint in the toe. (From Black JM, et al: *Medical surgical nursing,* ed 7, Philadelphia, 2005, Saunders.)

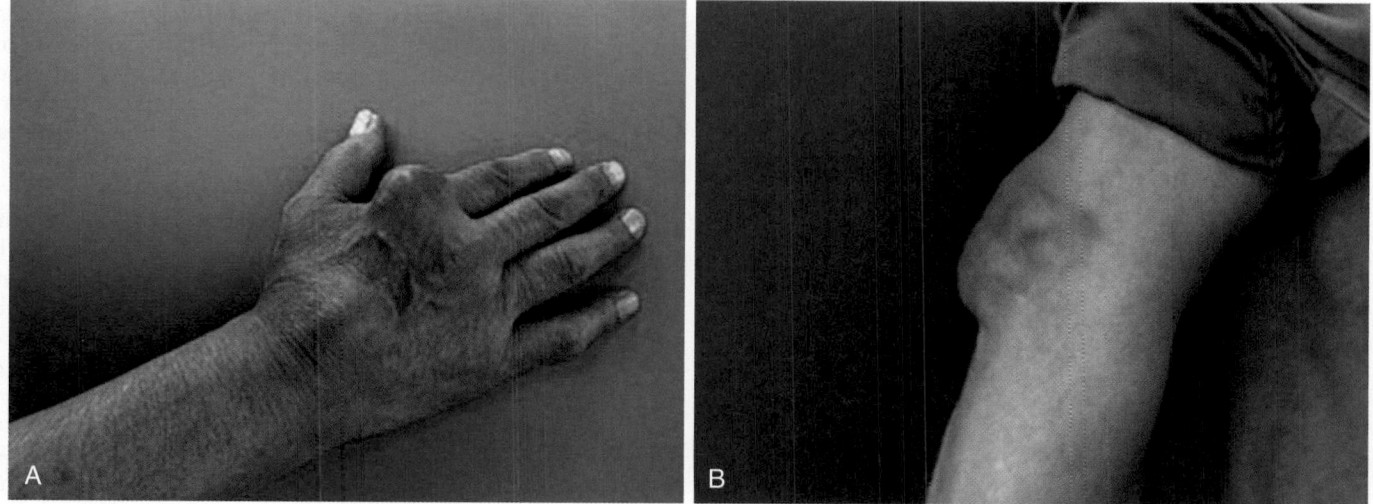

FIGURE 39-6 A male patient with advanced gout. Severe deposits of monosodium urate (MSU) crystals in the hand (A, wrist and fingers) and in the elbow (B). (Photos courtesy Dr. F. Enrique Gómez. Instituto Nacional de Ciencias Médicas y Nutrición Salvador Zubirán. Mexico City, México, 2015.)

it extends to sucrose. Fructose is known to raise the serum urate level by a mechanism recently linked to polymorphisms in GLUT9 (Dalbeth et al, 2013). Consumption of naturally occurring fructose such as in fruit or juices also may increase risk of gout, for example, eating an apple or orange a day, increase the risk by approximately 64% (Suresh and Das, 2012).

It is prudent to advise patients to consume a balanced meal plan with limited intake of animal foods and beer, avoidance of high-purine foods (see Box 39-3), limited consumption of sources of fructose (sweetened soft drinks and juices, candies, and sweet pastries), and controlled food portion sizes, and reduced noncomplex carbohydrate intake to achieve weight loss and improve insulin sensitivity (Li and Micheletti, 2011). Dairy products (milk or cheese), eggs, vegetable protein, cherries, (see *New Directions:* Can Cherries Prevent a Gout Attack?), and coffee appear to be protective, possibly because of the alkaline ash effect of these foods (Li and Micheletti, 2011). (see *Clinical Insight:* Urine pH—How Does Diet Affect It? in Chapter 35).

✳ **NEW DIRECTIONS**

Can Cherries Prevent a Gout Attack?

Over the past few decades, cherries have gained considerable public attention as a potentially effective option in the prevention and management of gout. The first study on the effect of cherries in gout attacks was conducted in 1950. Lately there have been a few studies using fresh and canned cherries, as well as cherry juice and cherry extract, to assess whether consumption of cherries lowers the risk of gout attacks. Small experimental studies have demonstrated that cherry intake lowers uric acid levels in healthy individuals. A recent study with gout patients showed that cherry intake was associated with a 35% lower risk of gout attacks compared with no intake; when cherry intake was combined with allopurinol, the risk of gout attacks was 75% lower (Zhang et al, 2012). The mechanism by which cherries and cherry juice concentrate prevent gout attack is still unclear, but is related to its potentially antiinflammatory properties. These findings suggest that cherry intake is associated with a lower risk of gout attacks but large, prospective randomized controlled trials are needed to further evaluate the efficacy of cherries and cherry juice concentrate for the prevention of attacks in patients with gout.

BOX 39-3   Purine Content of Foods

High Purine Content (100-1000 mg of Purine Nitrogen per 100 g of Food): Foods in this List Should be Omitted from the Diet of Patients Who have Gout (Acute and Remission Stages).

Anchovies	Meat extracts
Bouillon	Mincemeat
Brains	Mussels
Broth	Partridge
Consommé	Roe
Goose	Sardines
Gravy	Scallops
Heart	Sweetbreads
Herring	Yeast (baker's and brewer's), taken
Kidney	as supplement
Mackerel	

Moderate Purine Content (9-100 mg of Purine Nitrogen per 100 g of Food): One Serving (2-3 oz) of Meat, Fish, or Poultry or 1 Serving (½ C) of Vegetables from this Group is Allowed Daily.

Meat and fish	Vegetables
Fish	Asparagus
Poultry	Beans, dried
Meat	Lentils
Shellfish	Mushrooms
	Peas, dried
	Spinach

Negligible Purine Content: Foods Included in this Group may be Used Daily.

Bread (white) and crackers	Fruit
Butter or margarine (in moderation)*	Gelatin desserts
Cake and cookies	Herbs
Carbonated beverages†	Ice cream
Cereal beverage (e.g., Postum)	Milk
Cereals and cereal products	Macaroni products
Cheese	Noodles
Chocolate	Nuts
Coffee	Oil
Condiments	Olives
Cornbread	Pickles
Cream (in moderation)*	Popcorn
Custard	Puddings
Eggs	Relishes
Fats (in moderation)*	Rennet desserts
Vegetables (except those in group 2)	Rice
	Salt
	Sugar and sweets (in moderation)†
	Tea
	Vinegar
	White sauce

*Recommended in moderation because of fat content.
†Recommended in moderation because of fructose content.

SCLERODERMA

Scleroderma is a chronic, systemic sclerosis or hardening of the skin and visceral organs characterized by deposition of fibrous connective tissue. Women tend to be afflicted four times more often than men. **Raynaud syndrome** occurs, with ischemia or coldness in the small extremities, causing difficulty in preparation and consumption of meals. Sjögren syndrome is often also present, but there is variability among patients.

Pathophysiology

Scleroderma is considered an autoimmune rheumatic disease with a genetic component. Free-radical, oxidative damage from cytokines, in which fibroblast proteins are modified, is involved

(Pohl and Benseler, 2013). Gastrointestinal symptoms include gastroesophageal reflux, nausea and vomiting, dysphagia, diarrhea, constipation, fecal incontinence, and small intestine bacterial overgrowth. Joint stiffness and pain, renal dysfunction, hypertension, pulmonary fibrosis, and pulmonary arterial hypertension are also common (AF, 2014d). Renal crisis is a rare complication of scleroderma characterized by hypertension and oliguric or anuric acute renal failure. The occurrence of scleroderma renal crisis (SRC) is more common in patients treated with glucocorticoids (Guillevin et al, 2012).

Medical Management

The disease is usually, but not always, progressive, and no current treatment corrects the overproduction of collagen; therefore treatment is aimed at relieving symptoms and limiting damage. Some studies on the use of anti-TNF therapies have some promising results (Fett, 2013). SRC remains associated with severe morbidity and mortality despite treatment with angiotensin-converting enzyme inhibitors and dialysis (Guillevin et al, 2012).

Medical Nutrition Therapy

The dysphagia with this disease requires nutrition intervention (see Chapter 40 and Appendix 35). Dry mouth with resultant tooth decay, loose teeth, and tightening facial skin can also make eating difficult. Consuming adequate fluids, choosing moist foods, chewing sugarless gum, and using saliva substitutes help moisten the mouth and offer temporary relief. If gastroesophageal reflux is a concern, small, frequent meals are recommended along with avoidance of late-night eating, alcohol, caffeine, and spicy or fatty foods (see Chapter 27).

Malabsorption of lactose, vitamins, fatty acids, and minerals can cause further nutrition problems; supplementation may be required. A high-energy, high-protein supplement or enteral feeding may prevent or correct weight loss. Home enteral or parenteral nutrition often is required when problems such as chronic diarrhea persist (see Chapter 13).

SYSTEMIC LUPUS ERYTHEMATOSUS

Systemic lupus erythematosus (SLE) is known commonly as *lupus*. SLE is a chronic autoimmune disease characterized by production of autoantibodies directed against nuclear (anti-dsDNA, anti-SM, anti-nRNP) and cytoplasmic antigens affecting several organs (Fortuna and Brennan, 2013; Watts, 2014). SLE is most prevalent in women of childbearing age with a female to male ratio of 9:1, suggesting that sex-related factors are important in its development; and it has been shown that SLE is more common in African Americans and women of Hispanic, Asian, and Native American descent than in Caucasians.

Pathophysiology

The cause of SLE is multifactorial and involves multiple genes and environmental factors such as infections, hormones, and drugs. In SLE, circulating autoantibodies (ANA) can deposit in several tissues, causing inflammation and production of cytokines such as type 1 interferon (IFN) (Shrivastav and Niewold, 2013). This type 1-IFN, produced by cells of the innate immunity, activates B- and T-cells and propagates the signal to produce more IFN by dendritic cells. This up-regulation of the "type 1-IFN pathway" is critical in the severity and progression of SLE.

Common symptoms include extreme fatigue, painful or swollen joints, muscle pain, sensitivity to the sun, unexplained fever, skin rashes most commonly on the face, mouth ulcers, pale or purple fingers or toes from cold or stress (Raynaud phenomenon), and kidney problems (NIH, NIAMSD, 2013). SLE is characterized by periods of remission and relapse and may present with various constitutional and organ-specific symptoms.

Medical Management

General treatment of SLE includes sun protection, diet and nutrition, smoking cessation and exercise, whereas organ-specific treatments include use of steroids, NSAID, DMARD, and biologics (Fortuna and Brennan, 2013). Pharmacologic treatment includes the cytotoxic agents cyclophosphamide and azathioprine; their combination with corticosteroids must be employed early if there is major organ involvement in order to prevent or minimize irreversible damage.

The hallmark of SLE is B-cell activation and the production of harmful autoantibodies. Therefore B-cell depletion therapies, alone or combined with cytotoxic drugs, have been used to treat SLE. Treatment with rituximab and belimumab improved clinical and serologic parameters such as reduction in ANA (especially anti-dsDNA) and activated B-cells, as well as a reduction in SLE-related flares (Jordan et al, 2013).

Hydroxychloroquine (Plaquenil), an antimalarial drug, appears to be effective in clearing up skin lesions for some individuals with lupus, but has side effects that include nausea, abdominal cramping, and diarrhea. Immunosuppressives such as cyclophosphamide may be useful when there is renal involvement, but gastrointestinal and fertility problems may occur (Jordan et al, 2013).

Medical Nutrition Therapy

Because kidney problems are common in SLE, total protein intake must be adjusted accordingly (see Chapter 35). Although the total diet energy intake is normal, SLE patients tend to have higher consumption of carbohydrates, together with low intake of dietary fiber and omega-3 (EPA and DHA) and omega-6 fatty acids. The latter has been negatively associated with increased disease activity, altered serum profile, and increased carotid plaque presence (Elkan et al, 2012). In addition, SLE patients often have inadequate intakes of calcium, fruits, vegetables, and dairy products and high consumption of oils and fats (Borges et al, 2012).

Photosensitivity, sunlight avoidance, the use of sun protection and low dietary intake, in combination with medications prescribed to treat the symptoms of the disease, may be responsible for the observed low levels of vitamin D (Mok, 2013). Decreased conversion of 25-hydroxyvitamin D to its active form, 1,25-dihydroxyvitamin D (calcitriol), is possible because of renal impairment common in SLE, putting additional stress on vitamin D metabolism. Vitamin D supplementation (2000 IU/day) in patients with SLE is recommended because increased vitamin D levels seem to ameliorate inflammatory and hemostatic markers and show a tendency toward subsequent clinical improvement (Abou-Raya et al, 2013).

Diet therapy is a promising approach and nutritional counseling to improve the intake of vitamin D and calcium, omega-3 PUFA and fiber, may offer a better quality of life to patients with SLE.

Complementary Integrative Therapies

More than an estimated 50% of patients with SLE have used CIM to reduce symptoms and manage their health. Supplements of N-acetyl cysteine and turmeric reduce SLE activity and, together with mind-body methods (cognitive-behavioral therapy and other counseling interventions), improve mood and

quality of life of SLE patients (Greco et al, 2013). A mouse model of lupus nephritis treated with curcumin, showed promising clinical (reduced proteinuria) and serologic (reduced anti-ds-DNA antibodies) improvements. The depletion of regulatory T-cells (T-reg) eliminated the therapeutic effects of curcumin, suggesting a potential role of T-reg in the pathogenesis of SLE (Lee et al, 2013).

SPONDYLARTHRITIDES

The most important clinical features of this group of diseases are inflammatory back pain, asymmetric peripheral oligoarthritis, predominantly of the lower limbs, and enthesitis (inflammation at the site where the tendon attaches to the bone). Conventional medical treatment is based mainly on the use of NSAIDs (ibuprofen, COX-2 inhibitors), DMARD (sulfasalazine); patients with persistently active disease are also treated with blocking agents (TNF, IL-6). Physiotherapy is of major importance in the general approach to patients with any of these spondylarthritides. Nutritional therapy must emphasize keeping a healthy body weight, as well as increasing the consumption of foods rich in antioxidants and with antiinflammatory activities (see Box 39-2. and Appendix 31).

Ankylosing spondylitis (AS) is the major subtype of the spondylarthritides. AS (from Greek *ankylos,* fused; *spondylos,* vertebra; *-itis,* inflammation) affects joints in the spine and the sacroiliac joint in the pelvis and can cause eventual fusion of the spine. Ankylosing spondylitis most often develops in young adult men and it lasts a lifetime. Enthesitis accounts for much of the pain and stiffness of AS. This inflammation eventually can lead to bony fusion of the joints, where the fibrous ligaments transform to bone, and the joint permanently grows together. Other joints also can develop synovitis, with lower limb joints more commonly involved than upper-limb joints. Pain in the low back and buttocks are usually the first symptoms of AS. In contrast to mechanical low back pain, low back pain and stiffness in AS patients are worse after a period of rest or on waking up in the morning and improve after exercise, a hot bath, or a shower. Progressive stiffening of the spine is usual, with ankylosis occurring after some years of disease in many, but not all, patients. A majority of patients have mild or moderate disease with intermittent exacerbations and remissions and maintain some mobility and independence throughout life. Complete fusion results in a complete rigidity of the spine, a condition known as "bamboo spine."

Polymyalgia rheumatica (PMR) means "pain in many muscles", and is a syndrome with pain or stiffness, usually in the neck, shoulders, and hips. It may be caused by an inflammatory condition of blood vessels such as temporal arteritis (inflammation of blood vessels in the face, which can cause blindness if not treated quickly). Most PMR sufferers wake up in the morning with pain in their muscles; however, there have been cases in which the patient has developed the pain during the evenings. Treatment for PMR includes the use of corticosteroids (prednisone) alone or with a NSAID (ibuprofen) to relieve pain, exercises to strengthen the weak muscles, and a healthy diet (antiinflammatory diet) (see Box 39-2 and Appendix 31).

Polymyositis (PM) which means "inflammation of many muscles" is a type of chronic inflammation of the muscles (inflammatory myopathy) and is more common in adult women. Symptoms include pain, with marked weakness or loss of muscle mass in the muscles of the head, neck, torso, and upper arms and legs. The hip extensors are often severely affected, leading to particular difficulty in ascending stairs and rising from a seated position. Early fatigue while walking is caused by weakness in the upper leg muscles. Sometimes the weakness presents itself as an inability to raise from a seated position without help or an inability to raise one's arms above one's head. Dysphagia (difficulty swallowing) or other problems with esophageal motility occur in as many as one third of patients; foot drop in one or both feet can be a symptom of advanced PM.

Treatment for PM includes corticosteroids, specialized exercise therapy, and a healthy diet. Patients with dysphagia may benefit by changing the consistency of foods (softened, increased moisture) as in patients with Sjögren syndrome or with TMD (see Chapter 40).

CLINICAL CASE STUDY 1

Edith is a 33-year-old college teacher and mother of two. She is an active smoker with periodontal disease. Six months ago, she presented with chronic additive symmetrical polyarthritis, involving the wrists, hands, knees, and toes. Edith has morning stiffness for about an hour; symptoms improve with movement and worsen with rest. She has taken several NSAIDs with no major changes. At examination, the doctor noted inflammation in the joints.

Laboratory tests showed mild normocytic normochromic anemia, elevated erythrocyte sedimentation rate, and high C-reactive protein. She was positive for rheumatoid factor and antibodies to cyclic citrullinated peptide (ACPAs). Marginal erosions in the metacarpophalangeal joints were found by X-ray imaging.

Edith was diagnosed with rheumatoid arthritis. Based on polyarthritis, positivity of antibodies and erosions, it was determined to be a severe case, and she was started on DMARDs and corticosteroids.

Nutrition Assessment

Patient is 33-year-old woman with a recent diagnosis of rheumatoid arthritis.

Anthropometric Data

Ht 5′8″ (1.73m); Wt 152 lb (69 kg) (lost 6 lb over past 2 months)

BMI = 23

Biochemical data: Hgb 10.5 g/dL

Food and Nutrition History:

Changes in food preparation due to difficulty in shopping and cooking.

Caloric intake: 1600 kcal/day (less than energy requirements)

EER 2070 kcal (30 kcal/kg) and 104 g protein (1.5 g/kg BW for acute phase).

Nutrition Diagnostic Statements

1. Presence of iron deficiency anemia as evidenced by a serum hemoglobin of 10.5 g/dL. (NI-5.10.2)
2. Inadequate energy intake as evidenced by involuntary weight loss. (NI-2.1) (NC-3.2)

Nutrition Interventions

1. 2000 kcal diet, 104 g protein; emphasis on vegetables and whole grains, oily fish and fat free dairy.
2. Regular intake of green leaves and legumes as source of iron and folic acid; lean meats two or three times a week, increase consumption of extra-virgin olive oil to 1-2 oz daily as salad dressing.
3. Omega-3 fatty acid supplementation (3000 mg daily).
4. Advice to cease smoking and perform moderate intensity physical activity
5. Education to improve Edith′s cooking skills with a variety of easy recipes.

Nutritional Monitoring and Evaluation

Monthly weight measurements; although Edith′s BMI is currently adequate in spite of her weight loss, it is important to stop weight loss.

Repeat Hgb exam 3 months from date.

Evaluate energy, protein, iron and vitamin intake. If arthritis is not active, adjust protein to 1 g/kg BW.

CLINICAL CASE STUDY 2

Robert is a 55-year-old truck driver with a long-standing history of tophaceous gout and several recurrent episodes of severe pain during the past 10 years. He has been taking allopurinol. His episodes worsen with beer and red meat consumption. Sometimes he tries taking NSAIDs without improvement. Medical examination revealed multiple tophi overlying the first and second metacarpophalangeal joints of his left hand and the interphalangeal joints of his right hand, wrist, elbow, both ankles and interphalangeal and metatarsophalangeal joints of the feet and heels. The affected joints are swollen, erythematous and exquisitely painful, with a limited range of motion related to pain. Robert has a history of hypertension and hyperlipidemia. He continues to gain weight.

Nutrition assessment

Patient is a 55 year-old man with diagnosis of gout, hypertension and hyperlipidemia.

Anthropometric Data

Ht 6′3″ (1.90m) Wt 242 lb (110 kg) BMI 30 IBW 194 lb (88 kg)

BP: 155/90 mm Hg

Biochemical data:

Serum uric acid level is 10.2 mg/dL

Lipid profile
- TC: 228 mg/dL
- TG: 160 mg/dL
- HDL-C: 39 mg/dL
- LDL-C: 136 mg/dL
- Non-HDL-C: 189 mg/dL

Food and Nutrition History

Due to his job, Robert is often away from home for extended periods of time, when he eats at truck stop diners, where he selects hamburgers, fried eggs with bacon and deep fried foods; he eats large quantities of chips and beef jerky as snacks. He drinks almost no water. On weekends, when Robert is at home, he enjoys drinking beer (8 to 10 12-oz cans) and making barbecues. Diet is high in red meat, processed foods and refined carbohydrates, and low in fiber and vitamins.

EER: 2420 kcal (22 kcal/kg) and 110 g protein (1 g/kg BW)

Nutrition diagnostic statements

1. Obesity related to caloric intake higher to caloric expenditure as evidenced by elevated BMI. (NI-1.3)(NC-3.3)
2. Excessive alcohol and fat intake as evidenced from a diet history and flaring of gout symptoms. (NI- 4.3) (NI – 5.6.2)

Nutrition Interventions

Patient will include fruit and vegetables as frequently as possible in his diet, especially in substitution of high fat, high sugar snacks.

Patient will reduce alcohol consumption and increase non-sweetened drinks.

Education: Patient will be provided with guidelines for choosing meals and snacks with a low content of salt, processed sugars and saturated and *trans* fat.

Goals: Patient will be able to identify sources of purines from list of foods and make food choices for a low purine daily intake.

Patient will be physically active, taking 20-minute walks after dinner.

A weight loss of 6 lbs is desired the first month.

Monitoring and Evaluation:

Follow up a month from date to evaluate goal achievement.

Evaluate energy, water, alcohol, sugar, salt, fat and purine intake.

USEFUL WEBSITES

American Autoimmune Related Diseases Association
www.aarda.org
American College of Rheumatology
www.rheumatology.org
Arthritis Foundation
www.arthritis.org
Arthritis Research UK
www.arthritisresearchuk.org
Lupus Foundation of America
www.lupus.org
National Center for Complementary and Integrative Health
http://nccam.nih.gov/
National Institute of Arthritis and Musculoskeletal and Skin Diseases
www.niams.nih.gov
The Arthritis Society
www.arthritis.ca
Scleroderma Foundation
www.scleroderma.org
Sjögren's Syndrome Foundation
www.sjogrens.org

REFERENCES

Abou-Raya A, et al: The effect of vitamin D supplementation on inflammatory and hemostatic markers and disease activity in patients with systemic lupus erythematosus: a randomized placebo-controlled trial, *J Rheumatol* 40:265, 2013.

American Academy of Orthopaedic Surgeons (AAOS): *Arthritis and Related Conditions*, 2009. http://www.aaos.org/news/aaosnow/mar09/research6.asp. Accessed June 2014.

Anderson JW, et al: Glucosamine effects in humans: a review of effects on glucose metabolism, side effects, safety considerations and efficacy, *Food Chem Toxicol* 43:187, 2005.

Arthritis Foundation (AF): *Arthritis Food Myths*, 2014b. http://www.arthritis-today.org/what-you-can-do/eating-well/arthritis-diet/food-myths-arthritis-3.php. Accessed June 2014.

Arthritis Foundation (AF): *Can antibiotics really help in the treatment of RA?* 2014c. http://www.arthritistoday.org/about-arthritis/types-of-arthritis/rheumatoid-arthritis/treatment-plan/treatment-choices/ra-antibiotics.php. Accessed June 2014.

Arthritis Foundation (AF): *What Is Scleroderma?* 2014c. http://www.arthritis-today.org/about-arthritis/types-of-arthritis/more-types/about-scleroderma.php. Accessed June 2014.

Bahadori B, et al: Omega-3 fatty acids infusions as adjuvant therapy in rheumatoid arthritis, *J Parent Enter Nutr* 34:151, 2010.

Bernard NJ: Rheumatoid arthritis: Prevotella copri associated with new-onset untreated RA, *Nat Rev Rheumatol* 10:2, 2014.

Bhangle S, Kolasinski S: Fish oil in rheumatic diseases, *Rheum Dis Clin N Am* 37:77, 2011.

Bobulescu IA, Moe OW: Renal transport of uric acid: evolving concepts and uncertainties, *Adv Chronic Kidney Dis* 19:358, 2012.

Boeing H, et al: Critical review: vegetables and fruits in the prevention of chronic diseases, *Eur J Nutr* 51:637, 2012.

Borges MC, et al: Nutritional status and food intake in patients with systemic lupus erythematosus, *Nutrition* 28:1098, 2012.

Burke RJ, Chang C: Diagnostic criteria of acute rheumatic fever, *Autoimmun Rev* 13:503, 2014.

Calder PC: Long chain fatty acids and gene expression in inflammation and immunity, *Curr Opin Clin Nutr Metab Care* 16:425, 2013.

Cao Y, et al: Association between serum levels of 25-hydroxyvitamin D and osteoarthritis: a systematic review, *Rheumatology* 52:1323, 2013.

Castañer O, et al: In vivo transcriptomic profile after a Mediterranean diet in high-cardiovascular risk patients: a randomized controlled trial, *Am J Clin Nutr* 98:845, 2013.

Centers for Disease Control and Prevention (CDC): Prevalence of doctor-diagnosed arthritis and arthritis-attributable activity limitation – United States, 2010-2012. *MMWR* 62:44, 2013.

Chang HY, et al: Clinical use of cyclooxygenase inhibitors impairs vitamin B-6 metabolism, *Am J Clin Nutr* 98:1440, 2013.

Chatzikyriakidou A, et al: Genetics in rheumatoid arthritis beyond HLA genes: what meta-analysis have shown? *Semin Arthritis Rheum* 43:29, 2013.

Colombini A, et al: Relationship between vitamin D receptor gene (VDR) polymorphisms, vitamin D status, osteoarthritis and intervertebral disc degeneration, *J Steroid Biochem Mol Biol* 138:24, 2013.

Dalbeth N, et al: Population-specific influence of SLC2A9 genotype on the acute hyperuricaemic response to a fructose load, *Ann Rheum Dis* 72:1868, 2013.

Demoruelle MK, Deane K: Antibodies to citrullinated protein antigens (ACPAs): clinical and pathophysiologic significance, *Curr Rheumatol Rep* 13:421, 2011.

De Silva V, et al: Evidence for the efficacy of complementary and alternative medicines in the management of osteoarthritis: a systematic review, *Rheumatology* 50:911, 2011.

Ebert EC: Gastrointestinal and hepatic manifestations of Sjögren syndrome, *J Clin Gastroenterol* 46:25, 2012.

Elkan AC, et al: Diet and fatty acid pattern among patients with SLE: associations with disease activity, blood lipids and atherosclerosis, *Lupus* 21:1405, 2012.

Erten S, et al: Comparison of plasma vitamin D levels in patients with Sjögren's syndrome and healthy subjects, *Int J Rheum Dis* 18:70–75, 2015, Jan 28, [Epub ahead of print].

Fett N: Scleroderma: nomenclature, etiology, pathogenesis, prognosis, and treatment: facts and controversies, *Clin Dermatol* 31:432, 2013.

Fezai M, et al: Analgesic, anti-inflammatory and anticancer activities of extra virgin olive oil, *J Lipids* 2013, 129736, 2013, Epub, doi:10.1155/2013/129736.

Food and Agricultural Organization (FAO) of the United Nations: *Fat and fatty acid intake and inflammatory and immune response. In Fats and fatty acids in human nutrition. Report of an expert consultation*, Rome, 2010, Food and Agricultural Organization of the United Nations.

Fortuna G, Brennan MT: Systemic lupus erythematosus: epidemiology, pathophysiology, manifestations, and management, *Dent Clin North Am* 57:631, 2013.

Gomez FE, et al: Detection and recognition thresholds to the 4 basic tastes in Mexican patients with primary Sjögren's syndrome, *Eur J Clin Nutr* 58:629, 2004.

Greco CM, et al: Updated review of complementary and alternative medicine treatments for systemic lupus erythematosus, *Curr Rheumatol Rep* 15:378, 2013.

Guillevin L, et al: Scleroderma renal crisis: a retrospective multicentre study on 91 patients and 427 controls, *Rheumatology* 51:460, 2012.

Haga HJ: Vitamin D in rheumatoid arthritis, *Expert Rev Clin Immunol* 9:591, 2013.

Helmick CG, et al: Estimates of the prevalence of arthritis and other rheumatic conditions in the United States. Part I, *Arthritis Rheum* 58:15, 2008.

Henchoz Y, et al: Physical activity and energy expenditure in rheumatoid arthritis patients and matched controls, *Rheumatology* 51:1500, 2012.

Huang YF, et al: The immune factors involved in the pathogenesis, diagnosis, and treatment of Sjögren's syndrome, *Clin Dev Immunol* 2013:160491, 2013 Epub, doi: 10.1155/2013/160491.

Jansen R, et al: Sex differences in the human peripheral blood transcriptome, *BMC Genomics* 15:33, 2014.

Jordan N, et al: Novel therapeutic agents in clinical development for systemic lupus erythematosus, *BMC Medicine* 11:120, 2013.

Krishnan AV, Feldman D: Molecular pathways mediating the anti-inflammatory effects of calcitriol: implications for prostate cancer chemoprevention and treatment, *Endocr Relat Cancer* 17:R19, 2012.

Lahiri M, et al: Modifiable risk factors for RA: prevention, better than cure? *Rheumatology* 51:499, 2012.

Lawrence RC, et al: National Arthritis Data Workgroup. Estimates of the prevalence of arthritis and other rheumatic conditions in the United States: Part II, *Arthritis Rheum* 58:26, 2008.

Lee KH, et al: A curcumin derivative, 2,6-bis(2,5-dimethoxybenzylidene)-cyclohexanone (BDMC33) attenuates prostaglandin E2 synthesis via selective suppression of cyclooxygenase-2 in IFN-γ/LPS-stimulated macrophages, *Molecules* 16:9728, 2013.

Lee YH, et al: Omega-3 polyunsaturated fatty acids and the treatment of rheumatoid arthritis: a meta-analysis, *Arch Med Res* 43:356, 2012.

Li S, Michelleti R: Role of diet in rheumatic diseases, *Rheum Dis Clin N Am* 37:119, 2011.

Longo VD, Mattson MP: Fasting: molecular mechanisms and clinical applications, *Cell Metab* 19:181, 2014.

Manek NJ, et al: What rheumatologists in the United States think of complementary and alternative medicine: results of a national survey, *BMC Complement Altern Med* 10:5, 2010.

Marlow G, et al: Transcriptomics to study the effect of a Mediterranean-inspired diet on inflammation in Crohn's disease patients, *Hum Genomics* 7:24, 2013.

Miles EA, Calder PC: Influence of marine n-3 polyunsaturated fatty acids on immune function and a systematic review of their effects on clinical outcomes in rheumatoid arthritis, *Br J Nutr* 107(Suppl 2):S171, 2012.

Mok CC: Vitamin D and systemic lupus erythematosus: an update, *Expert Rev Clin Immunol* 9:453, 2013.

National Institutes of Health (NIH), National Center for Complementary and Alternative Medicine (NCCAM): *Complementary, alternative, or integrative health: What's in a Name?* 2014. http://nccam.nih.gov/health/whatiscam. Accessed March 2014.

National Institutes of Health (NIH), National Center for Complementary and Alternative Medicine (NCCAM): *Rheumatoid Arthritis and Complementary Health Approaches*, 2013. http://nccam.nih.gov/health/RA/getthefacts.htm. Accessed June 2, 2014.

National Institutes of Health (NIH), National Center for Complementary and Alternative Medicine (NCCAM): *Questions and Answers: NIH Glucosamine/Chondroitin Arthritis Intervention Trial Primary Study*, 2008. http://nccam.nih.gov/research/results/gait/qa.htm. Accessed March 20, 2011.

National Institutes of Health (NIH), National Institute of Arthritis and Musculoskeletal and Skin Diseases: Handout on health: *Systemic lupus erythematosus*, 2013. http://www.niams.nih.gov/Health_Info/Lupus/. Accessed March 2014.

National Institutes of Health (NIH), National Institute of Dental and Craniofacial Research: *TMJ disorders*, 2013. http://nidcr.nih.gov/OralHealth/Topics/TMJ/TMJDisorders.htm. Accessed June 2014.

Norling LV, Perreti M: The role of omega-3 derived resolvins in arthritis, *Curr Opin Pharm* 13:476, 2013.

Patterson E, et al: Health implications of high dietary omega-6 polyunsaturated fatty acids, *J Nutr Metab* 2012:539426, 2012.

Pohl D, Benseler S: Systemic inflammatory and autoimmune disorders, *Handb Clin Neurol* 112:1243, 2013.

Proudman SM, et al: Fish oil in recent onset rheumatoid arthritis: a randomized, double-blind controlled trial within algorithm-based drug use, *Ann Rheum Dis* 74:89, 2015.

Ramiro S, et al: Safety of synthetic and biological DMARDs: a systematic literature review informing the 2013 update of the EULAR recommendations for the management of rheumatoid arthritis, *Ann Rheum Dis* 73:529, 2014.

Raynauld JP, et al: Long-term effects of glucosamine/chondroitin sulfate on progression of structural changes in knee osteoarthritis: 6: year follow-up data from osteoarthritis initiative, *Arthritis Care Res* epub ahead of print, doi: 10.1002/acr.22866, Feb 16, 2016.

Ricciotti E, FitzGerald GA: Prostaglandins and inflammation, *Arterioscler Thromb Vasc Biol* 31:986, 2011.

Rock KL, et al: Uric acid as a danger signal in gout and its comorbidities, *Nat Rev Rheumatol* 9:13, 2013.

Rosenbaum CC, et al: Antioxidants and antiinflammatory dietary supplements for osteoarthritis and rheumatoid arthritis, *Altern Ther Health Med* 16:32, 2010.

Sakakeeny L, et al: Plasma pyridoxal-5-phosphate is inversely associated with systemic markers of inflammation in a population of U.S. adults, *J Nutr* 142:j1280, 2012.

Sammaritano LR, Bermas BL: Rheumatoid arthritis medications and lactation, *Curr Opin Rheumatol* 26:354, 2014.

Scaglione F, Panzavolta G: Folate, folic acid and 5-methyltetrahydrofolate are not the same thing, *Xenobiotica* 44:480, 2014.

Scher JU, Abramson SB: The microbiome and rheumatoid arthritis, *Nat Rev Rheumatol* 10:569, 2011.

Scotece M, et al: Further evidence for the anti-inflammatory activity of oleocanthal: inhibition of MIP-1α and IL-6 in J774 macrophages and in ATDC5 chondrocytes, *Life Sci* 91:1229, 2012.

Shea B, et al: Folic acid and folinic acid for reducing side effects in patients receiving methotrexate for rheumatoid arthritis, *Cochrane Database Syst Rev* 5:CD000951, 2013.

Shrivastav M, Niewold TB: Nucleic acid sensors and type 1 interferon production in systemic lupus erythematosus, *Front Immunol* 4:319, 2013.

Sjögren's Syndrome Foundation: *Diet & Food Tips*, 2013. http://www.sjogrens.org/home/about-sjogrens-syndrome/living-with-sjogrens/diet-a-food-tips. Accessed June 2014.

Sparks JA, et al: Impact of bariatric surgery on patients with Rheumatoid Arthritis, *Arthritis Care Res* 67:1619, 2015.

Stuber K, et al: Efficacy of glucosamine, chondroitin, and methylsulfonylmethane for spinal degenerative joint disease and degenerative disc disease: a systematic review, *J Can Chiropr Assoc* 55:47, 2011.

Suresh E, Das P: Recent advances in management of gout, *QJ Med* 105:407, 2012.

Tincani A, et al: Novel aspects of Sjögren's syndrome in 2012, *BMC Medicine* 11:93, 2013.

van Dijk SJ, et al: Consumption of a high monounsaturated fat diet reduces oxidative phosphorilation gene expression in peripheral blood mononuclear cells of abdominally overweight men and women, *J Nutr* 142:1219, 2012.

Walitt B, et al: Coffee and tea consumption and method of coffee preparation in relation to risk of rheumatoid arthritis and systemic lupus erythematosus in postmenopausal women, *Ann Rheum Dis* 69(Suppl 3):350, 2010.

Watts RA: Autoantibodies in the autoimmune rheumatic diseases, *Medicine* 42:121, 2014.

World Health Organization (WHO): *Traditional Medicine: Definitions*, 2014. http://www.who.int/medicines/areas/traditional/definitions/en/. Accessed March 2014.

Wu D, et al: Green tea EGCG, T cells and T cell-mediated autoimmune diseases, *Mol Aspects Med* 33:107, 2012.

Yamada A, et al: Targeting IL-1 in Sjögren's syndrome, *Expert Opin Ther Targets* 17:393, 2013.

Yao Y, et al: Type I interferons in Sjögren's syndrome, *Autoimmunity Rev* 12:558, 2013.

Yeoh N, et al: The role of the microbiome in rheumatic diseases, *Curr Rheumatol Rep* 15:314, 2013.

Zhang Y, et al: Cherry consumption and decreased risk of recurrent gout attacks, *Arthritis Rheum* 64:4004, 2012.

40

Medical Nutrition Therapy for Neurologic Disorders

Beth Zupec-Kania, RDN,
Therese O'Flaherty, MS, RDN

KEY TERMS

absence seizure (petit mal)
adrenomyeloleukodystrophy (ALD)
amyotrophic lateral sclerosis (ALS)
anosmia
aphasia
apraxia
areflexia
aspiration
aspiration pneumonia
chronic inflammatory demyelinating
   polyneuropathy (CIDP)
concussion
cortical blindness
deglutitory dysfunction
diffuse axonal injury
dysarthria
dysosmia
dysphagia

embolic stroke
epidural hematoma
epilepsy
Frazier Water Protocol
Glasgow Coma Score
Guillain-Barré syndrome (GBS)
hemiparesis
hemianopsia
hydrocephalus
hyperosmia
intracranial pressure (ICP)
intraparenchymal hemorrhage
ketogenic diet
medium-chain triglyceride (MCT) oil
multiple sclerosis (MS)
myasthenia gravis (MG)
myelin
neglect

otorrhea
paraplegia
paresthesia
Parkinson's disease (PD)
peripheral neuropathy
rhinorrhea
seizure
spinal cord injury (SCI)
stroke (cerebrovascular accident)
subarachnoid hemorrhage (SAH)
subdural hematoma
tetraplegia
thromboembolic event
thrombotic stroke
tonic-clonic (grand mal) seizure
transient ischemic attack (TIA)
traumatic brain injury (TBI)
Wernicke-Korsakoff syndrome (WKS)

Neurologic conditions arise from causes that vary in complexity. Some neurologic disorders result from a simple deficiency or excess of a nutrient, such as the neuropathy associated with thiamin deficiency, whereas others have more complex causes such as diabetic neuropathy, stroke, or trauma. Some conditions arise with the interaction of genetics and metabolic or environmental factors, as is the case with multiple sclerosis (MS), Parkinson's disease (PD), and alcoholism. Epilepsy, the most common neurologic condition, affecting 1% of the population, occurs as a symptom o f many neurologic disorders. The medical and health history is often the most important part of a neurologic evaluation.

Numerous symptoms and malnutrition may accompany neurologic diseases. Complaints of even minor symptoms such as headaches, dizziness, insomnia, fatigue, weakness, pain, or discomfort must be skillfully evaluated for the presence of a nutrition component in their cause and treatment. Although not all neurologic diseases have a nutritional cause, nutritional considerations are integral to effective medical and clinical management (see Table 40-1). Some neurologic dysfunctions such as peripheral neuropathy occur secondary to disease or a chronic deficiency of a single or several vitamins, whereas other diseases of the nervous system may be attributed to dietary deficiency or excess (see Table 40-2). This chapter emphasizes conditions with nutritionally significant dysfunction.

In those neurologic diseases with a nonnutritional cause, nutrition therapies are important adjuncts to effective medical management and are beginning to show promise in early studies. Therapeutic use of macro- and micronutrients will someday play a role in recovery from traumatic head, brain, and spinal cord injuries and are of increasing interest to some researchers secondary to athletic or sports trauma as well as injuries to military personnel. Many elements of nutrition care for neurologic diseases and conditions are similar regardless of the origin of the disease process.

THE CENTRAL NERVOUS SYSTEM

The central nervous system (CNS) in mammals is differentiated functionally into three segments, so lesions in the nervous system leave a unique "calling card" for localized dysfunction. Localizing the defect (lesion) to muscle, nerve, spinal cord, or brain is part of the medical diagnosis. Nerve tracts coming to and from the brain cross to opposite sides in the CNS (see Figure 40-1). Therefore a lesion in the brain that affects the right arm is found on the left side of the brain. Figure 40-2 shows the segments of the brain.

Signs of weakness are the most quantifiable clinical signs of nervous system disease. The neurons in the motor strip (upper motor neurons) receive input from all parts of the brain and project their axons all the way to their destinations in the spinal cord. Axons

TABLE 40-1 Nutritional Considerations for Neurologic Conditions

Medical Condition	Relevant Nutrition Therapy
Adrenoleukodystrophy	Dietary avoidance of VLCFAs has not been proven. Lorenzo's oil may lower VLCFA levels.
Alzheimer's disease (see Table 40-7)	Recommend antioxidants and antiinflammatory diet. Minimize distractions at mealtime. Initiate smell or touch of food. Guide hand to initiate eating. Provide nutrient-dense foods, omega-3 fatty acids.
Amyotrophic lateral sclerosis (see Table 40-9)	Intervene to prevent malnutrition and dehydration. Possibly ketogenic diet. Monitor dysphagia. Antioxidant use (vitamins C, E, selenium, methionine) is well tolerated, but not proven.
Epilepsy	Provide ketogenic diet (see Table 40-10).
Guillain-Barré	Attain positive energy balance with high-energy, high-protein tube feedings. Possibly gluten-free diet. Assess dysphagia.
Migraine headache	Follow general recommendations for food avoidance. Maintain adequate dietary and fluid intake. Keep extensive records of symptoms and foods.
Myasthenia gravis	Provide nutritionally dense foods at beginning of meal. Small, frequent meals are recommended. Limit physical activity before meals. Place temporary feeding tube.
Multiple sclerosis	Recommend antioxidants and antiinflammatory diet. Possibly recommend linoleic acid supplement. Evaluate health and especially vitamin D status of patient. Nutrition support may be needed in advanced stages. Distribute fluids throughout waking hours; limit before bed.
Neurotrauma	Enteral or parenteral nutrition support when needed.
Parkinson's disease (see Table 40-11)	Focus on drug-nutrient interactions. Minimize dietary protein at breakfast and lunch. Recommend antioxidants and antiinflammatory diet.
Pernicious anemia	Administer vitamin B$_{12}$ injections. Provide diet liberal in HBV protein. Provide diet supplemented with Fe$^+$, vitamin C, and B complex vitamins.
Spinal trauma	Provide enteral or parenteral nutrition support. Provide high-fiber diet, adequate hydration to minimize constipation. Provide dietary intake to maintain nutrition health and adequate weight.
Stroke	Dietary alterations for primary prevention. Maintain good nutrition status. Assess possible dysphagia. Nutrition support may be needed.
Wernicke-Korsakoff syndrome	Provide thiamin supplementation. Provide adequate hydration. Provide diet liberal in high-thiamin foods. Eliminate alcohol. Dietary protein may have to be restricted.

Fe$^+$, Iron; *HBV,* high biologic value; *MCT,* medium chain triglycerides fat; *VLCFA,* very-long-chain fatty acid.

TABLE 40-2 Neurologic Syndromes Attributed to Nutritional Deficiency or Excess

NUTRITIONAL DEFICIENCY

Site of Major Syndrome	Name
Encephalon	Hypocalcemia and tetany seizures from lack of vitamin D
	Impaired intellectual and cognitive function (protein-calorie deprivation)
	Cretinism (iodine deficiency)
	Wernicke-Korsakoff syncrome (thiamin deficiency)
Optic nerve	Nutritional deficiency optic neuropathy ("tobacco-alcohol amblyopia")
Brainstem	Central pontine myelinolysis (sodium)
Cerebellum	Alcoholic cerebellar degeneration
	Vitamin E deficiency caused by bowel disease
Spinal cord	Combined system disease (B$_{12}$ deficiency)
	Tropical spastic paraparesis
Peripheral nerves	Beriberi (thiamin deficiency), pellagra (nicotinic acid deficiency)
	Hypophosphatemia
	Tetany (vitamin D deficiency)
Muscle	Myopathy of osteomalacia

NUTRITIONAL EXCESS

Syndrome	Condition	Agent
Increased intracranial pressure	Self-medication	Vitamin A
Encephalopathy	Phenylketonuria	Phenylalanine
	Water intoxication	Water
	Hepatic encephalopathy	Protein (and NH$_3$)
	Ketotic or nonketotic coma in diabetes	Glucose, insulin
Stroke	Hyperlipidemia	Lipid
Peripheral neuropathy	Hypochondriasis	Pyridoxine
Myopathy	Insomnia, anxiety	Tryptophan
	Anorexia nervosa, bulimia	Emetine, ipecac
Myoglobinuria	Constipation	Licorice

connect to the spinal cord motor neurons (lower motor neurons). These neurons extend from the spinal cord to muscles without interruption. The location of a lesion in the nervous system often can be deduced clinically by observing stereotypical abnormalities and function of either upper or lower motor neurons (see Table 40-3).

Pathophysiology and Signs of Mass Lesions

The frontal lobes in the brain are the source of the most complex activities and commonly offer the most complex presentations. Psychiatric manifestations such as depression, mania, or personality change may herald a tumor or other frontal lobe mass, either right or left. With a lesion or tumor near the skull base, one may lose the sense of smell or have visual changes because olfactory and optic nerves track along the bottom of these frontal lobes. Chemosensory losses of smell have been described as **anosmia** (absence of smell), **hyperosmia** (increased sensitivity of smell), or **dysosmia** (distortion of normal smell).

Frontal lobes are larger and the posterior portions of the frontal lobes contain the motor strips, which control muscle movement. Lesions that develop in the central frontal lobe may present as motor apraxia. A person with **apraxia** cannot perform a complex activity such as independent eating despite a willingness to do so.

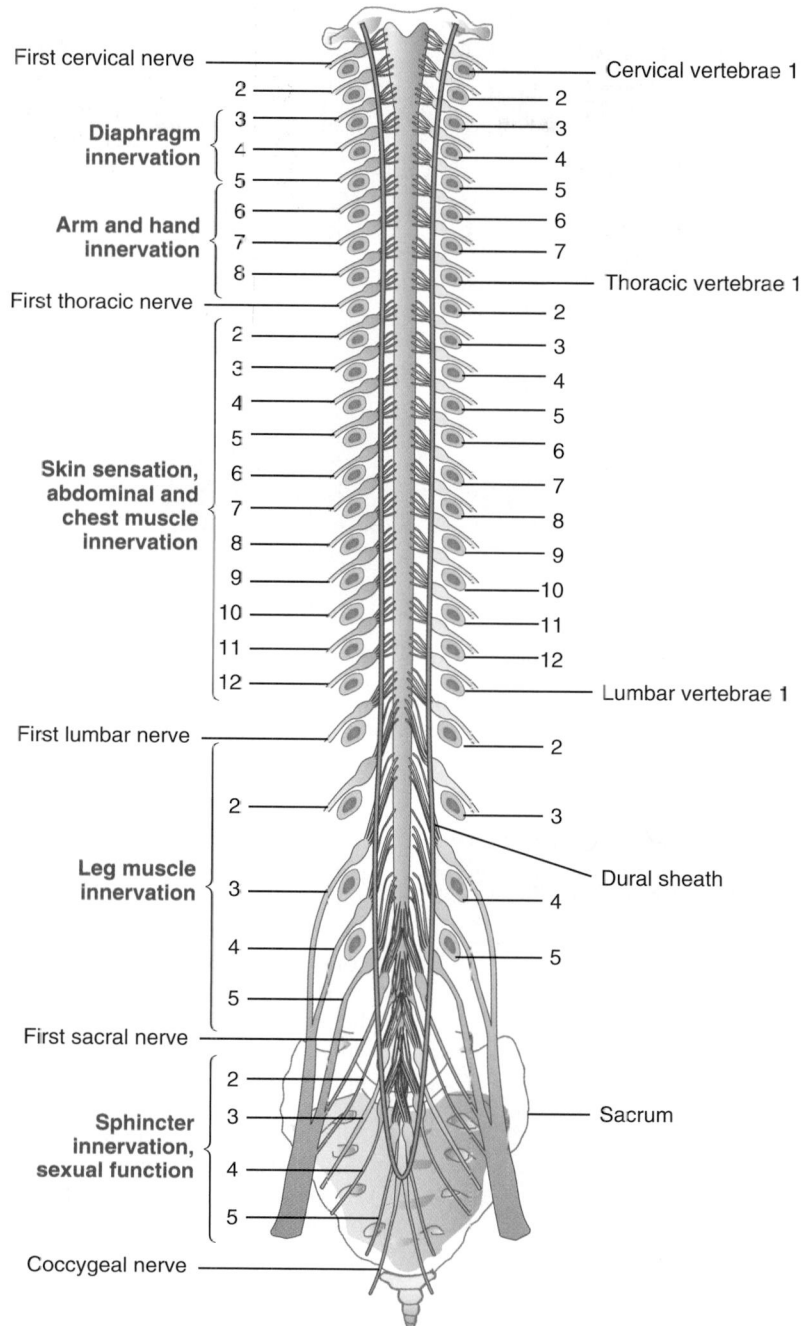

First cervical nerve

Diaphragm innervation

Arm and hand innervation

First thoracic nerve

Skin sensation, abdominal and chest muscle innervation

First lumbar nerve

Leg muscle innervation

First sacral nerve

Sphincter innervation, sexual function

Coccygeal nerve

Cervical vertebrae 1

Thoracic vertebrae 1

Lumbar vertebrae 1

Dural sheath

Sacrum

FIGURE 40-1 Spinal cord lying within the vertebral canal. Spinal nerves are numbered on the left side; vertebrae are numbered on the right side; body areas supplied by various levels are in blue.

Temporal lobes control memory and speech; lesions there may affect these abilities, as seen with the dementia of Alzheimer's and with stroke. Although any lesion of cerebral gray matter may produce seizures, the temporal lobes are particularly prone to seizures. A right parietal lobe mass or insult may result in chronic inability to focus attention, thus completely ignoring the body's left side. Because speech centers are located near the junction of the left temporal, parietal, and frontal lobes, pathologic conditions in this region may cause speech problems.

The occipital lobes are reserved for vision, and dysfunction here may bring about cortical blindness of varying degrees. In this condition the person is unaware that he or she cannot see.

Lesions of the cerebellum and brainstem may obstruct the ventricular system where it is the narrowest. This obstruction may precipitate life-threatening hydrocephalus, a condition of increased intracranial pressure (ICP) that may quickly result in death. Other signs of hydrocephalus include trouble with balance, walking and coordination, marked sleepiness, and complaints of a headache that is worse on awakening. Lesions in the brainstem may infiltrate any of the cranial nerves that innervate structures of the face and head, including the eyes, ears, jaw, tongue, pharynx, and facial muscles (see Table 40-3). These lesions have consequences for nutrition because the patient is often unable to eat without risking aspiration of food or liquids into the lung. Tumors or other lesions in the medulla

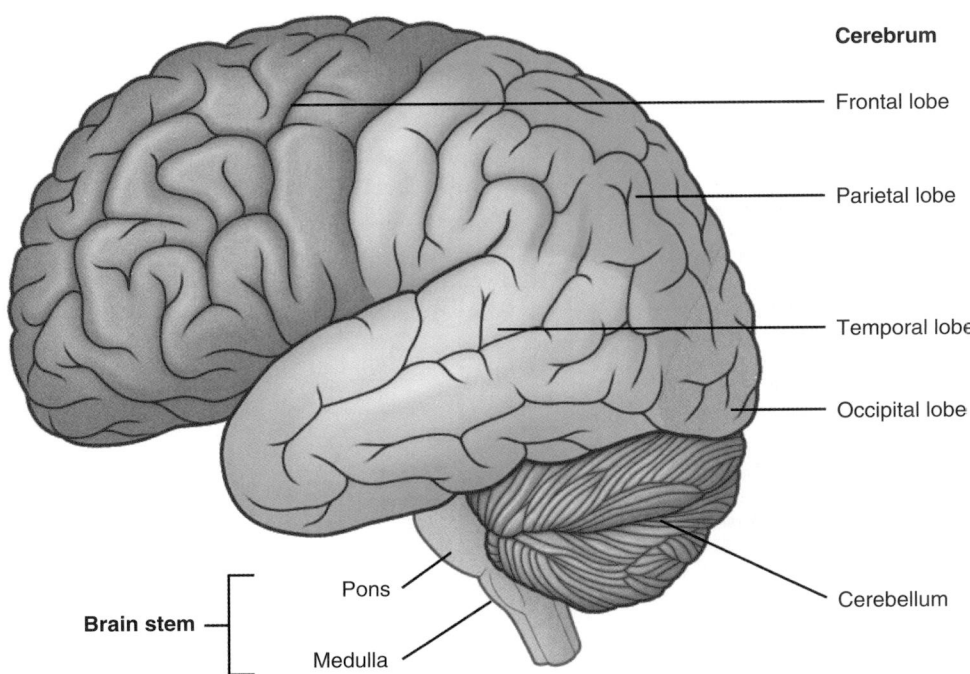

FIGURE 40-2 Parts of the brain. Trauma or disease in one area may affect speech, vision, movement or eating ability. (From http://projectflexner.sites.medinfo.ufl.edu/files/2009/04/brain-regions.jpg. From Scully C: Medical problems in dentistry, ed 6, 2010, Churchill Livingstone.)

TABLE 40-3 Basic Functions of Cranial Nerves

Number	Nerve Function
Olfactory (I)	Smell
Optic (II)	Vision
Oculomotor (III)	1. Eye movement 2. Pupil constriction
Trochlear (IV)	Eye movement
Trigeminal (V)	1. Mastication 2. Facial heat, cold, touch 3. Noxious odors 4. Input for corneal reflex
Abducens (VI)	Eye movement
Facial (VII)	1. All muscles of facial expression 2. Corneal reflex 3. Facial pain 4. Taste on anterior two thirds of tongue
Vestibulocochlear (VIII)	Hearing and head acceleration and input for oculocephalic reflex
Glossopharyngeal (IX)	1. Swallowing 2. Gag reflex 3. Palatal, glossal, and oral sensation
Vagus (X)	1. Heart rate, gastrointestinal activity, sexual function 2. Cough reflex 3. Taste on posterior third of tongue
Spinal accessory (XI)	1. Trapezius 2. Sternocleidomastoid muscle
Hypoglossal (XII)	Tongue movement

may infiltrate respiratory and cardiac centers, and dysregulation of these centers has grim consequences.

Lesions in the spinal cord are much less common than brain tumors and ordinarily cause lower motor neuron signs at the level of the lesion and upper motor signs in segments below the level of the lesion. Spinal cord injury (SCI) is the most common pathologic condition in this region. Other examples of spinal cord abnormalities are MS, amyotrophic lateral sclerosis (ALS), tumor, syrinx (fluid-filled neurologic cavity), chronic meningitis, vascular insufficiency, and mass lesions of the epidural space.

Lesions of the pituitary gland and hypothalamus are often heralded by systemic manifestations that may include electrolyte and metabolic abnormalities secondary to adrenocortical, thyroid, and antidiuretic hormone dysregulation. Because of the proximity to the visual pathways, changes may occur in visual field or acuity. The syndrome of inappropriate antidiuretic hormone secretion (SIADH) is often a complication; volume status and hyponatremia are part of the medical diagnosis (see Chapter 6). Because the hypothalamus is the regulatory center for hunger and satiety, lesions here may present as anorexia or overeating.

Finally, disorders of peripheral nerves and the neuromuscular junction affect one's ability to maintain proper nutrition. Disorders such as Guillain-Barré syndrome (GBS) or myasthenia gravis (MG) may counteract the efforts to maintain nutritional balance. To eat and drink effectively, many parts of the nervous system are required. A problem at any location of the nervous system can affect ability to meet nutritional requirements.

ISSUES COMPLICATING NUTRITION THERAPY

The nutritional management of patients with neurologic disease is complex. Severe neurologic impairments often compromise the mechanisms and cognitive abilities needed for adequate nourishment. A common result is dysphagia (difficulty swallowing), and the ability to obtain, prepare, and present food to the mouth can be compromised. Modified food textures are often required for the individual with swallowing problems. For an example of how diets are modified for dysphagia see Box 40-1. Early recognition of signs and symptoms, implementation of an appropriate care plan to

---

BOX 40-1   Development of Dysphagia Diets

Texture Modifications

Level 3: Dysphagia Advanced (Previously: Mechanical Soft):

- Soft-solid foods. Includes easy-to-cut whole meats, soft fruits and vegetables (i.e. bananas, peaches, melon without seeds, tender meat cut into small pieces and well moistened with extra gravy or sauce).
- Crusts should be cut off of bread.
- Most is chopped or cut into small pieces.

EXCLUDES hard, crunchy fruits and vegetables, sticky foods, and very dry foods. NO nuts, seeds, popcorn, potato chips, coconut, hard rolls, raw vegetables, pot Pudding-thick Liquids: also called pudding-thick; should hold their shape, and a spoon should stand up in them; they are not pourable and are eaten with a spoon. ato skins, corn, etc. Most food is chopped/cut into small pieces.

Level 2: Dysphagia Mechanically-Altered (Previously: Ground):

- Cohesive, moist, semisolid foods that require some chewing ability.
- Includes fork-mashable fruits and vegetables (i.e. soft canned, or cooked fruits with vegetables in pieces smaller than ½ inch).
- Meat should be ground and moist. Extra sauce and gravy should be served.

EXCLUDES most bread products, crackers, and other dry foods. No whole grain cereal with nuts, seeds and coconut. No food with large chunks. Most food should be ground texture.

Level 1: Dysphagia Puree:

- Smooth, pureed, homogenous, very cohesive, pudding-like foods that require little or no chewing ability.
- No whole foods.
- Includes mashed potatoes with gravy, yogurt with no fruit added, pudding, soups pureed smooth, pureed fruits and vegetables, pureed meat/poultry/fish, sauces/gravies, and pureed desserts without nuts, seeds, or coconut.

AVOID scrambled, fried, or hard boiled eggs.

Fluid Modifications

Thin Liquids: includes water, soda, juice broth, coffee, tea. This also includes foods like jello, ice cream and sherbet that melt and become thin when swallowed.

Nectar-thick Liquids: are pourable and the consistency of apricot nectar

Honey-thick Liquids: slightly thicker than nectar and can be drizzled; consistency of honey.

Pudding-thick Liquids: also called pudding-thick; should hold their shape, and a spoon should stand up in them; they are not pourable and are eaten with a spoon.

Courtesy : Clinical Nutrition Department, Providence Mt. St. Vincent , Seattle, WA.

meet the nutritional requirements of the individual, and counseling for the patient and family members on dietary choices are essential. Regular evaluation of the patient's nutrition status and disease management are priorities, with the ultimate goal of improving outcomes and the patient's nutritional quality of life.

Nutrition assessment requires detailed histories. The diet history and mealtime observations are used to assess patterns of normal chewing, swallowing, and rate of ingestion. Weight loss history establishes a baseline weight; a weight loss of 10% or more is indicative of nutritional risk. Assessment for nutrients involved in neurotransmitter synthesis is particularly important in these patients. Nutrition diagnoses common in the neurologic patient population include the following:

- Chewing difficulty
- Increased energy expenditure
- Inadequate energy intake
- Inadequate fluid intake
- Physical inactivity
- Poor nutritional quality
- Difficulty with independent eating
- Swallowing difficulty
- Underweight
- Elimination problems
- Inadequate access to food or fluid

Meal Preparation

Confusion, dementia, impaired vision, or poor ambulation may contribute to difficulty with meal preparation, thus hindering oral food and beverage intake. Assistance with shopping and meal planning are frequently necessary.

Eating Difficulties and Inadequate Access to Food or Fluid

With chronic neurologic diseases, a decline in function may hinder the ability for self-care and nourishment. Access to food and satisfying basic needs may depend on the involvement of family, friends, or professionals. With acute neurologic situations such as seizures, trauma, stroke, or GBS, the entire process of eating can be interrupted abruptly. The patient may require enteral nutrition for a time until overall function improves and adequate oral intake is resumed (see Chapter 13).

Eating Issues: Presentation of Food to the Mouth

The patient with neurologic disease may be unable to eat independently because of limb weakness, poor body positioning, hemianopsia, apraxia, confusion, or neglect. Tremors in PD, spastic movements, or involuntary movements that occur with cerebral palsy, Huntington disease, or tardive dyskinesia may further restrict dietary intake. The affected region of the CNS determines the resulting disability (see Table 40-4).

If limb weakness or paralysis occurs on the dominant side of the body, poor coordination resulting from a new reliance on the nondominant side may make eating difficult and unpleasant. The patient may have to adjust to eating with one hand and also to using the nondominant hand. Hemiparesis is weakness on one side of the body that causes the body to slump toward the affected side; it may increase a patient's risk of aspiration.

Hemianopsia is blindness for one half of the field of vision. The patient must learn to recognize that he or she no longer has a normal field of vision and must compensate by turning the head. Neglect is inattention to a weakened or paralyzed side of the body; this occurs when the nondominant (right) parietal side of the brain is affected. The patient ignores the affected body part, and his or her perception of the body's midline is shifted. Hemianopsia and neglect can occur together and severely impair the patient's function. A patient may eat only half of the contents of a meal because he or she recognizes only half of it (see Figure 40-3).

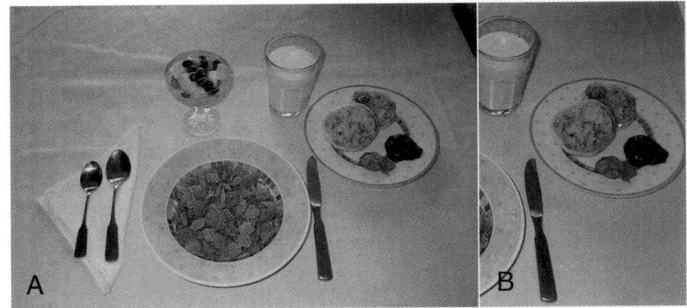

FIGURE 40-3 A, Normal vision. **B,** Vision with hemianopsia.

TABLE 40-4	Common Impairments with Neurologic Diseases	
Site in the Brain	**Impairment**	**Results**
Cortical lesions of the parietal lobe (perception of sensory stimuli)	Sensory deficits	Fine regulation of muscle activities impossible if the patient is unable to perceive joint position and motion and tension of contracting muscles
Lesions of the nondominant hemisphere	Hemi inattention syndrome (neglect)	Patient neglects that side of the body
Optic tract lesions (usually of the middle cerebral artery or the artery near the internal capsule)	Visual field cuts	Patient reads one half of a page, eats from only half of the plate, etc. (see Figure 40-3)
Loss of subcortically stored pattern of motor skills	Apraxia	Inability to perform a previously learned task (e.g., walking, rising from a chair), but paralysis, sensory loss, spasticity, and incoordination are not present
No identification with a particular brain disorder or a specifically located lesion	Language apraxia	Inability to produce meaningful speech, even though oral muscle function is intact and language production has not been affected
Lesion of Broca area	Nonfluent aphasia	Thought and language formulation are intact, but the patient is unable to connect them into fluent speech production
Lesion of Wernicke area	Fluent aphasia	Flow of speech and articulation seem normal, but language output makes little or no sense
Extensive brain damage	Global aphasia	Expression and speech perception are severely impaired
Brainstem lesions, bilateral hemispheric lesions, cerebellar disorders	Dysarthria	Inability to produce intelligible words with proper articulation

From Steinberg FU: Rehabilitating the older stroke patient: what's possible? *Geriatrics* 41:85, 1986.

Another potential deterrent to independent eating is apraxia because the person is unable to carry out an action and follow directions. Demonstration may make it possible for the action to occur; however, judgment may be affected as well and can result in the performance of dangerous tasks. This makes it unsafe to leave the patient alone.

DYSPHAGIA

Dysphagia often leads to malnutrition because of inadequate intake. Symptoms of dysphagia include drooling, choking, or coughing during or following meals; inability to suck from a straw; a gurgly voice quality; holding pockets of food in the buccal recesses (of which the patient may be unaware); absent gag reflex; and chronic upper respiratory infections. Patients with intermediate or late-stage PD, MS, ALS, dementia, or stroke are likely to have dysphagia.

A swallowing evaluation by a speech-language pathologist (SLP) is important in assessing and treating swallowing disorders. The SLP is often consulted for individual patients following traumatic brain injury (TBI), stroke, or cancers of the head and neck, and for those at risk of aspiration (inhaling foreign material into the lungs) or with other conditions that result in a lack of coordination in swallowing. Many registered dietitian nutritionists (RDNs) have acquired additional training in swallowing therapies to help coordinate this evaluative process.

Phases of Swallowing

Proper positioning for effective swallowing should be encouraged (i.e., sitting bolt upright with the head in a chin-down position). Concentrating on the swallowing process can also help reduce choking. Initiation of the swallow begins voluntarily but is completed reflexively. Normal swallowing allows for safe and easy passage of food from the oral cavity through the pharynx and esophagus into the stomach by propulsive muscular force, with some benefit from gravity. The process of swallowing can be organized into three phases, as shown in Figure 40-4.

Oral Phase

During the preparatory and oral phases of swallowing, food is placed in the mouth, where it is combined with saliva, chewed if necessary, and formed into a bolus by the tongue. The tongue pushes the food to the rear of the oral cavity by gradually squeezing it backward against the hard and soft palate. Increased ICP or intracranial nerve damage may result in weakened or poorly coordinated tongue movements and lead to problems in completing the oral phase of swallowing. Weakened lip muscles

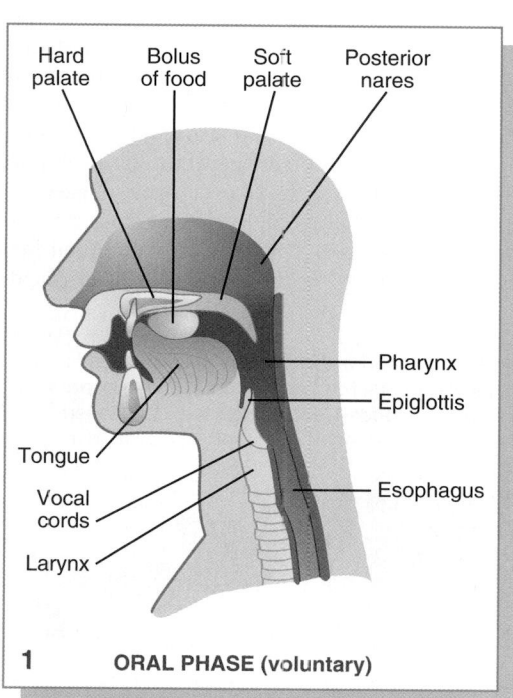
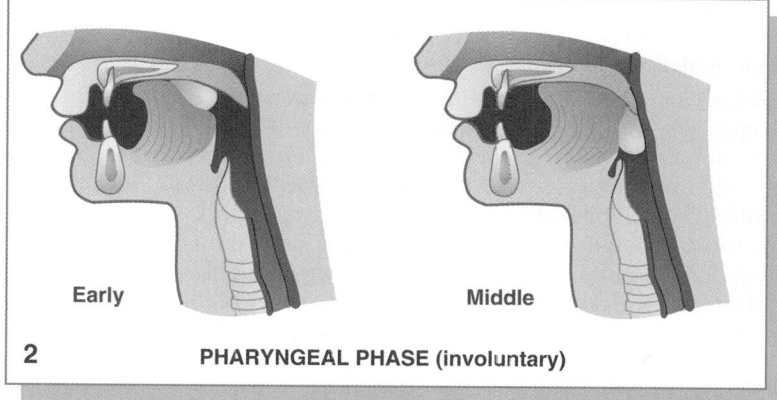
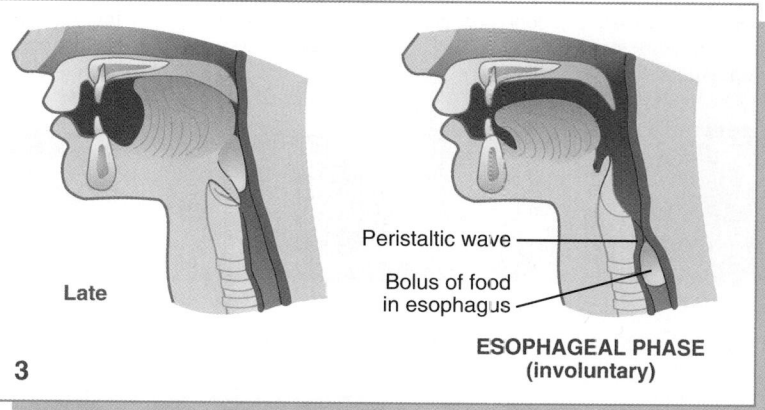

FIGURE 40-4 Swallowing occurs in three phases: Voluntary or oral phase: Tongue presses food against the hard palate, forcing it toward the pharynx. Involuntary, pharyngeal phase: Early: wave of peristalsis forces a bolus between the tonsillar pillars. Middle: soft palate draws upward to close posterior nares, and respirations cease momentarily. Late: vocal cords approximate, and the larynx pulls upward, covering the airway and stretching the esophagus open. Involuntary, esophageal phase: Relaxation of the upper esophageal (hypopharyngeal) sphincter allows the peristaltic wave to move the bolus down the esophagus.

result in the inability to completely seal the lips, form a seal around a cup, or suck through a straw. Patients are often embarrassed by drooling and may not want to eat in front of others. The patient may have difficulty forming a cohesive bolus and moving it through the oral cavity. Food can become pocketed in the buccal recesses, especially if sensation in the cheek is lost or facial weakness exists

Pharyngeal Phase

The pharyngeal phase is initiated when the bolus is propelled past the faucial arches. Four events must occur in rapid succession during this phase. The soft palate elevates to close off the nasopharynx and prevent oropharyngeal regurgitation. The hyoid bone and larynx elevate, and the vocal cords adduct to protect the airway. The pharynx sequentially contracts while the cricopharyngeal sphincter relaxes, allowing the food to pass into the esophagus. Breathing resumes at the end of the pharyngeal phase. Symptoms of poor coordination during this phase include gagging, choking, and nasopharyngeal regurgitation.

Esophageal Phase

The final or esophageal phase, during which the bolus continues through the esophagus into the stomach, is completely involuntary. Difficulties that occur during this phase are generally the result of a mechanical obstruction, but neurologic disease cannot be ruled out. For example, impaired peristalsis can arise from a brainstem infarct.

Medical Nutrition Therapy

Weight loss, anorexia, and dehydration are key concerns with dysphagia. Observation during meals allows the nurse or RDN to screen informally for signs of dysphagia and bring them to the attention of the health care team. Environmental distractions and conversations during mealtime increase the risk for aspiration and should be curtailed. Reports of coughing and unusually long mealtimes are associated with tongue, facial, and masticator muscle weakness. Changing the consistency of foods served may be beneficial while keeping the diet palatable and

nutritionally adequate also are important. A soft, blended, or pureed consistency can reduce the need for oral manipulation and conserve energy while eating.

In 2002, The Academy of Nutrition and Dietetics (formerly the American Dietetic Association) published the National Dysphagia Diet (NDD) developed through consensus from a panel of dietitians, speech pathologists and scientists. The NDD is prescribed by a speech pathologist that evaluates the individual's ability to safely swallow both food textures and liquids. Standard levels of dysphagia from severe to mild were designated with assigned diet texture modifications for each level to promote the safety of swallow (see Figure 40-5).

The levels of dysphagia (see Box 40-1) severity range from:
Severe Dysphagia: inability to clear the pharynx, nonfunctional volitional cough and silent aspiration
Moderate Dysphagia: moderate retention in the oral cavity requiring cues and or supervision to clear
Mild Dysphagia: retention in the pharynx that is able to be cleared through spontaneous cough

Liquids

Swallowing liquids of thin consistency such as juice or water is the most difficult swallowing task because of the coordination and control required. Liquids are easily aspirated into the lungs and may pose a life-threatening event because aspiration pneumonia may ensue, even from sterile water in the lungs. Sterile water is no longer sterile once it is introduced to the bacterial load of the oral cavity.

If a patient has difficulty consuming thin liquids, meeting fluid needs can become a challenge. Dry milk powder as a thickener alters the taste and might raise protein content too high for children, especially with limited free water. Commercial thickeners now have xanthan gum or modified food starches as ingredients. Benefits of xanthan gum include: it is tasteless, holds its thickening level over time, is easy to mix, and can be used on the ketogenic diet as it does not contain any carbohydrate or calories. It is not recommended for children less than 1 year of age because it has been implicated in

Level 2: Dysphagia Mechanically Altered Diet- This is a semisolid consistency, cohesive, moist food requiring some chewing. Fork mashed, well-cooked, drained cooked vegetables and fruit.

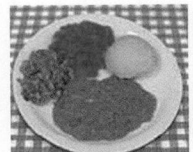 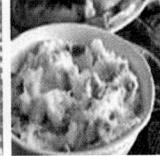 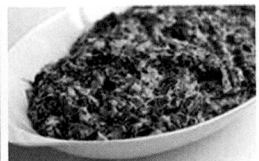

Level 3: Dysphagia–Advanced or Soft Diet- This is soft foods that require more chewing: thin-sliced, tender chunks or ground meats, eggs, casseroles, shredded lettuce, rice. Well-moistened breads. All canned or soft, ripe peeled fresh fruit, and all tender cooked vegetables.

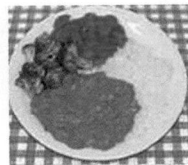 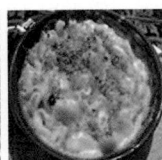 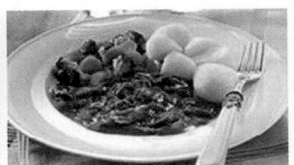

Regular Diet: All foods allowed.

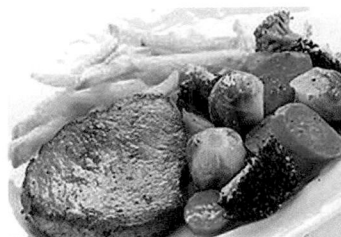 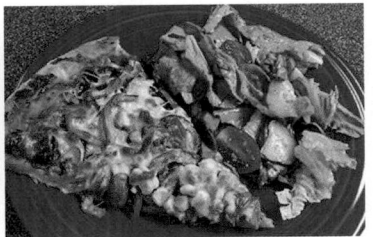

FIGURE 40-5 Levels of National Dysphagia Diet (NDD)

BOX 40-2   Levels of Thickening Liquids

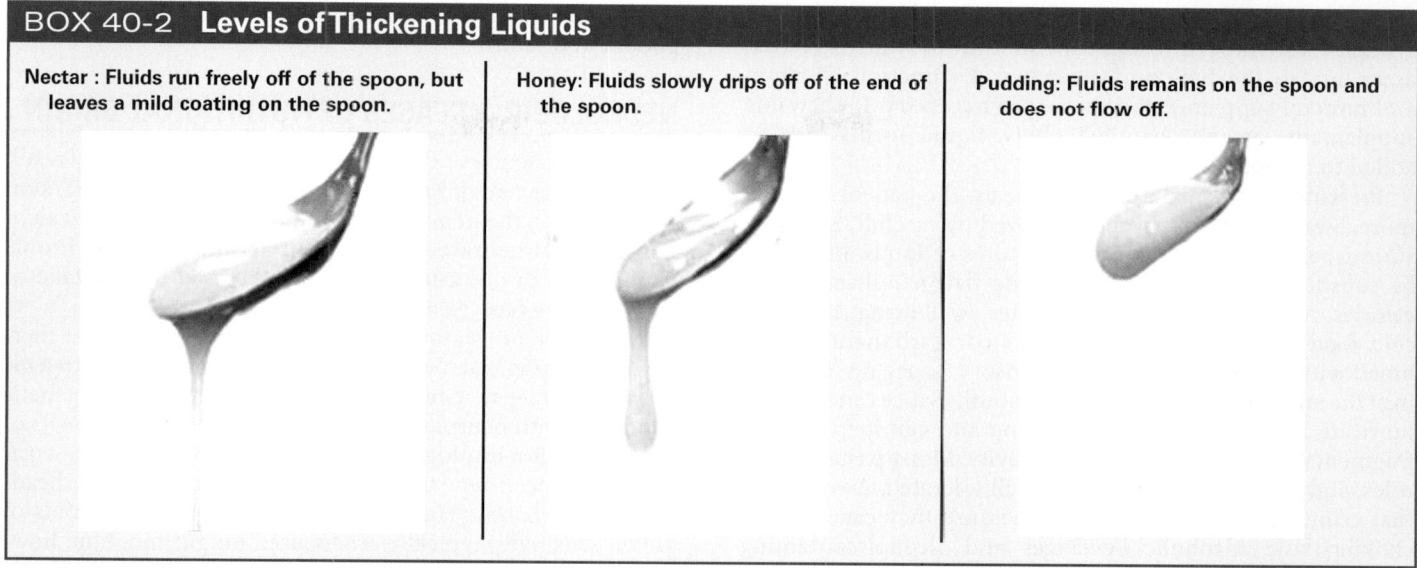

Nectar : Fluids run freely off of the spoon, but leaves a mild coating on the spoon.

Honey: Fluids slowly drips off of the end of the spoon.

Pudding: Fluids remains on the spoon and does not flow off.

(Chart created by Therese O'Flaherty MS, RD) adapted from the Dietitians Association and the Speech Pathology Association of Australia, 2007.

the development of necrotizing enterocolitis (NEC) (Beal et al., 2012). Modified food starches add calories and continue to thicken over time so it is more difficult to be accurate in the level of thickening. Modifications in fluids were also addressed in the NDD report and the four terms used to identify the viscosity level of fluids are thin, nectar-like, honey-like, and spoon-thick (McCullough, et.al., 2003):

Infant cereals, pudding or yogurt blend well into fluids, provide calories and protein, and are less expensive than commercial thickeners. Stage 2 baby fruits or applesauce can be added to juice to create a nectar or honey consistency, maintain a good flavor, and add calories, and they are less expensive than commercial supplements (see Box 40-2 and Table 40-5).

It is difficult to maintain adequate fluid intake with thickened liquids, especially if drinking skills are poor. Mild chronic dehydration resulting from limited water intake can cause fatigue and malaise. Encouraging soft or blended fruits and vegetables provide a good source of free water.

The Frazier Water Protocol, which allows for drinking water in those who otherwise require thickened liquids is being increasingly used in long term care. This protocol is based on the following assumptions:

1. Aspiration of water poses little risk to the patient if oral bacteria associated with the development of aspiration pneumonia can be minimized.
2. Allowing free water decreases the risk of dehydration.
3. Allowing free water increases patient compliance with swallowing precautions and improves quality of life.
4. Good oral hygiene is a key ingredient of the water protocol and offers other benefits to swallowing.

Liquid intake is a concern in those with neurogenic bladder and urinary retention, a common management issue in patients with a myelopathy (a pathologic condition of the spinal cord) or an SCI. This predisposes the individual to urinary tract infections (UTIs). Alternately, myelopathy and SCI may result in urinary urgency, frequency, or incontinence. To minimize these problems, distributing fluids evenly throughout the waking hours and limiting them before bedtime may help. Some patients limit fluid intake severely to decrease urgency or frequent urination. This practice increases the risk of UTI and is not recommended.

One nontraumatic cause of myelopathy and neurogenic bladder is MS, an unpredictable and severe, progressive disease of the CNS. Individuals with MS have a higher incidence of UTIs.

Milk is considered a liquid with unique properties. Some people associate consumption of milk with symptoms of excess mucus production; however, research evidence does not support this belief. When the dysphasic patient reports increased phlegm after milk consumption, it may actually be a consequence of poor swallowing ability rather than mucus production.

Textures

As chronic neurologic disease progresses, cranial nerves become damaged, leading to neurologic deficits often

TABLE 40-5

Thickening Infant or Pediatric Formulas with Rice Cereal

Formula	Nectar Consistency	Honey Consistency
4 ounces infant or 4 ounces pediatric	2 T rice cereal	3 T rice cereal

Thickening Juice with Pureed Stage 2 Fruit

Pureed Fruit	Nectar Consistency	Honey Consistency
2 ounces	6 T juice	2 T juice
3 ½ ounces	10 T juice	4 T juice
4 ounces	12 T juice`	5 T juice

Thickening Pediatric Formula with Pudding or Yogurt

Pureed fruit	Nectar Consistency	Honey Consistency
4 ounces pediatric formula	3 T pudding or yogurt	5 T pudding or yogurt

(Chart created by dietitians and speech therapists at Cincinnati Children's Hospital, 2011) Disclaimer: A viscometer, an instrument used to measure viscosity of a fluid, was not used.

manifested by dysphagia or elimination of entire food groups. Nutrition intervention should be individualized according to the type and extent of dysfunction. Vitamin and mineral supplementation may be necessary. If chewable supplements are not handled safely, liquid forms may be added to acceptable foods.

Presented with small, frequent meals, the patient may eat more. Swallowing can also be improved by carefully selecting various tastes, textures, and temperatures of foods. Juices can be substituted for water and provide flavor, nutrients, and calories. A cool temperature facilitates swallowing; therefore cold food items may be better tolerated. Carbonation combined with citrus, helps with the sensory issues by "awakening" the awareness sensation in the mouth. Sauces and gravies lubricate foods for ease in swallowing and can help prevent fragmentation of foods in the oral cavity. Moist pastas, casseroles, and egg dishes are generally well tolerated. Avoid foods that crumble easily in the mouth, because they can increase choking risk. Alcoholic beverages and alcohol-containing mouth washes should be avoided because they dry out the oral membranes.

Enteral Tube Nutrition

Patients with acute and chronic neurologic diseases may benefit from nutrition support. Well-managed nutrition support helps to prevent pneumonia and sepsis, which can complicate these diseases. Enteral tube feedings may be necessary if the risk of aspiration from oral intake is high, or if the patient cannot eat or drink enough to meet his or her nutritional needs. In the latter case nocturnal tube feedings can bridge the gap between oral intake and actual nutritional or fluid requirements. This should allow the normal sensation of hunger to be generated and provide freedom from tube feeding during the day. Depending on the lifestyle of the patient, caregivers, and family, it may be preferred to offer thickened liquids at meals, then bolus additional free water through the tube at the end of the meal. Assuring good fluid intake during the daytime might avoid nighttime continuous feedings and the need for a feeding pump and supplies.

In most instances the gastrointestinal tract function remains intact, and enteral nutrition is the preferred method of administering nutrition support. One noted exception occurs after SCI, in which ileus is common for 7 to 10 days after the insult, and parenteral nutrition may be necessary. Although a nasogastric (NG) tube can be a short-term option, a percutaneous endoscopic gastrostomy (PEG) tube, commonly known as a G-tube, or gastrostomy-jejunostomy (PEG/J) commonly known as a GJ-tube, is preferred for long-term management. These should be considered for patients whose swallowing is inadequate (see Chapter 13).

Malnutrition itself can produce neuromuscular weakness that negatively affects quality of life; it is a prognostic factor for poor survival. In the acutely ill but previously well-nourished individual who is unable to resume oral nourishment within 7 days, nutrition support is used to prevent decline in nutritional health and aid in recovery until oral intake can be resumed. Conversely, in the chronically ill, nutrition support is an issue that each patient must eventually address because it may result in prolonged therapy. However, adequate nutrition can promote health and may be a welcome relief to an overburdened patient. Tube feedings can relieve stress at mealtimes, encourage oral intake, and

should be scheduled based on the lifestyle needs of the patient and family.

NEUROLOGIC DISEASES OF NUTRITIONAL ORIGIN

Dietary deficiencies of thiamin and niacin can directly result in neurologic symptoms. With Wernicke-Korsakoff syndrome (WKS), the neurologic effect occurs secondary to alcoholism. Most neurologic symptoms arising from nutritional deficiencies can be corrected with increased food intake or supplements (see Tables 40-2 and Table 40-6).

A new era of treating neurologic disorders with diet therapy is emerging, stemming from the effective use of ketogenic diets for epilepsy. Gluten sensitivity is yet another genetic condition with neurologic implications. Numerous reports of patients with neurologic dysfunction related to gluten sensitivity have been reported since 1966 including ataxia, headache, and seizures (Hadijvassiliou et al, 2010). Symptoms of gluten sensitivity typically are focused on gut function; however, most patients who present with neurologic manifestations of gluten sensitivity have no gastrointestinal symptoms. Celiac disease is common in people with autism with and without gastrointestinal symptoms. A case study of a child with autism who had been maintained on a gluten and casein-free diet experienced significant gains in behavior and seizure control when her diet was additionally made ketogenic (Herbert and Buckley, 2013).

NEUROLOGIC DISORDERS FROM TRAUMA

Cerebrovascular Accident (Stroke)

Stroke (cerebrovascular accident) is defined as an acute onset of focal or global neurologic deficit lasting more than 24 hours; it is attributable to diseases of the intracranial or extracranial neurovasculature. Severe strokes are often

TABLE 40-6 Neurologic Diseases Arising from Nutritional Deficiencies

Disease	Nutrient	Physiologic Effect	Treatment
Wet beriberi	Thiamin	Peripheral or central neurologic dysfunction	Thiamin supplementation
Pellagra	Niacin	Memory loss, hallucinations, dementia	Niacin supplementation
Pernicious anemia	Vitamin B$_{12}$	Lesions occur in myelin sheaths of optic nerves, cerebral white matter, peripheral nerves	Monthly vitamin B$_{12}$ injections Oral vitamin B$_{12}$ supplements
Wernicke-Korsakoff syndrome	Thiamin	Encephalopathy, involuntary eye movements, impaired movement, amnesia	Eliminate alcohol, thiamin supplementation, adequate hydration

preceded by transient ischemic attacks (TIAs), brief attacks of cerebral dysfunction of vascular origin with no persistent neurologic defect. Stroke is a leading cause of death and the most common cause of disability in the United States (CDC, 2014b). Advanced age is the most significant risk factor for stroke. Among modifiable risk factors, hypertension and smoking are the major contributors (see Chapter 33). Other factors include obesity, coronary heart disease, diabetes, physical inactivity, and genetics. The high costs of stroke are attributed to the degree of disability imparted by these events.

Pathophysiology

Embolic stroke occurs when a cholesterol plaque is dislodged from a proximal vessel, travels to the brain, and blocks an artery, most commonly the middle cerebral artery (MCA). In patients with dysfunctional cardiac atria, clots may be dislodged from there and embolize. In thrombotic stroke a cholesterol plaque within an artery ruptures, and platelets subsequently aggregate to clog an already narrowed artery. Most strokes are incited by a thromboembolic event, which may be aggravated by atherosclerosis, hypertension, diabetes, and gout (see *Pathophysiology and Care Management Algorithm: Stroke*).

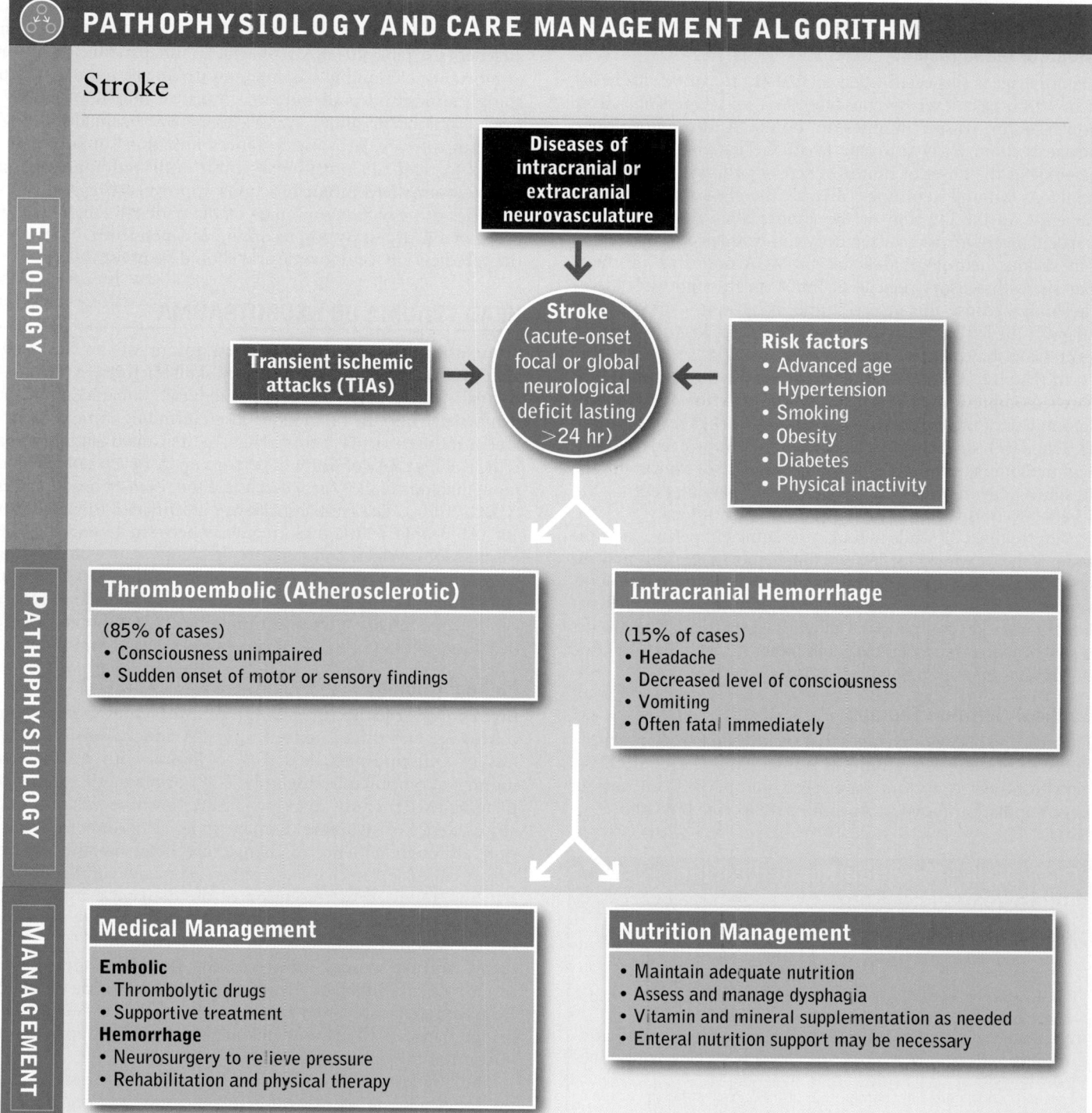

PATHOPHYSIOLOGY AND CARE MANAGEMENT ALGORITHM

Stroke

ETIOLOGY

Diseases of intracranial or extracranial neurovasculature

Transient ischemic attacks (TIAs) → Stroke (acute-onset focal or global neurological deficit lasting >24 hr) ←

Risk factors
- Advanced age
- Hypertension
- Smoking
- Obesity
- Diabetes
- Physical inactivity

PATHOPHYSIOLOGY

Thromboembolic (Atherosclerotic)
(85% of cases)
- Consciousness unimpaired
- Sudden onset of motor or sensory findings

Intracranial Hemorrhage
(15% of cases)
- Headache
- Decreased level of consciousness
- Vomiting
- Often fatal immediately

MANAGEMENT

Medical Management

Embolic
- Thrombolytic drugs
- Supportive treatment

Hemorrhage
- Neurosurgery to relieve pressure
- Rehabilitation and physical therapy

Nutrition Management
- Maintain adequate nutrition
- Assess and manage dysphagia
- Vitamin and mineral supplementation as needed
- Enteral nutrition support may be necessary

Intracranial hemorrhage occurs in only 15% of strokes but is often fatal immediately. Intracranial hemorrhage occurs more commonly in individuals with hypertension. In intraparenchymal hemorrhage, a vessel inside the brain ruptures. A variation of intraparenchymal hemorrhage is a lacunar (deep pool) infarct. These smaller infarcts occur in the deep structures of the brain such as the internal capsule, basal ganglia, pons, thalamus, and cerebellum. Even a small lacunar infarct can produce significant disability because the brain tissue in the deep structures is so densely functional. A second type of intracranial hemorrhage is subarachnoid hemorrhage (SAH). SAH occurs commonly as a result of head trauma but more often as a result of a ruptured aneurysm of a vessel in the subarachnoid space.

Medical Management

Hemorrhage is suspected when the patient presents with headache, decreased level of consciousness, and vomiting, all of which occur within minutes to hours. A thromboembolic stroke is more likely to occur when the patient is fully conscious, but the onset of motor or sensory changes occurs suddenly. As with all neurologic disease, the clinical presentation depends on the location of the abnormality. An infarct of a particular cerebrovascular territory can be suspected by seeking out various neurologic deficits. An MCA occlusion produces paresis, with sensory deficits of limbs on the opposite side of the body because this artery supplies the motor and sensory strips. If the left MCA is occluded, aphasia, or loss of speech or expression may be present.

In the past, treatment for embolic stroke was supportive; it focused on prevention of further brain infarction and rehabilitation. Use of thrombolytic, "clot-busting" drugs reverses brain ischemia by lysing the clots. Initiation of therapy needs to occur within 6 hours of the onset of symptoms. Use of aspirin may be of some value in preventing further cerebrovascular events, but its effectiveness varies from one patient to another.

Controlling ICP while maintaining sufficient perfusion of the brain is the treatment for intracranial hemorrhage. This may include surgical evacuation of large volumes of intracranial blood, ventricular drainage, or other neurosurgical interventions. Rehabilitation is a key component. Hemorrhage, particularly SAH, has severe functional consequences and therefore has a longer period of convalescence than ischemic stroke.

Medical Nutrition Therapy

Lifestyle and behavior changes that include diet are key components to primary prevention of stroke (Meschia et al, 2014). Nutrition-related factors have been compiled from various large population-based prospective studies (see Box 40-3).

Given the prevalence of stroke and its associated burden of disease, treatment for those afflicted with this disease cannot be ignored. In the United States in 2010 stroke-related medical costs and disability were estimated at $73.7 billion (American Heart Association, American Stroke Association, 2015).

Efforts should be directed toward maintaining the overall health of the patient. A diet high in omega-3 fatty acids has been shown in some studies to provide a protective benefit against stroke, however, omega-3 fat supplements have not shown the same benefit. Omega-3 fat supplements should be avoided by anyone taking a blood thinner such as warfarin or aspirin (NIH, NCCIH, 2013).

Eating difficulties and resulting behavioral problems are determined by the extent of the stroke and the area of the brain affected (see Table 40-7). Dysphagia, an independent predictor of mortality, commonly accompanies stroke and contributes to complications and poor outcome from malnutrition, pulmonary infections, disability, increased length of hospital stay, and institutional care. In some instances nutrition support is required to maintain nutritional health until oral alimentation can be resumed. As motor functions improve, eating and other activities of daily living are part of the patient's rehabilitation process and necessary for resuming independence. Malnutrition predicts a poor outcome and should be prevented.

HEAD TRAUMA OR NEUROTRAUMA

Traumatic brain injury (TBI) refers to any of the following, alone or in combination: brain injury, skull fractures, extraparenchymal hemorrhage—epidural, subdural, subarachnoid—or hemorrhage into the brain tissue itself, including intraparenchymal or intraventricular hemorrhage. In the United States trauma is the leading cause of death in persons up to 44 years of age, and more than one half of these deaths are the result of head injuries (CDC, 2014a). The annual incidence is estimated to be 200 per 100,000 people, with a peak frequency between 15 and 24 years of age. Motor vehicle collisions are the major source of injury.

Morbidity is high and headache is one of the most common complaints. It is difficult to accurately predict neurologic recovery. Despite intensive intervention, long-term disability occurs in a large portion of the survivors of severe head injury.

Pathophysiology

Brain injury can be categorized as three types: concussion, contusion, and diffuse axonal injury. A concussion is a brief loss of consciousness, less than 6 hours, with no damage found on computed tomography (CT) or magnetic resonance imaging (MRI) scans. Microscopic studies have failed to find any evidence of structural damage in areas of known concussion, although evidence of change in cellular metabolism exists. A contusion is characterized by damaged capillaries and swelling, followed by resolution of the damage. Large contusions may dramatically increase ICP and may lead to ischemia or herniation. Contusions can be detected by CT or MRI scans. Diffuse axonal injury results from the shearing of axons by a rotational acceleration of the brain inside the skull. Damaged areas are often found in the corpus callosum (the bridge between the two hemispheres) and the upper, outer portion of the brainstem.

Skull fractures of the calvarium and the base are described in the same manner as other fractures. Comminution refers to splintering of bone into many fragments. Displacement refers

---

BOX 40-3	Nutrition-Related Factors and Stroke Risk
Risk Factors for Stroke	**Protective Factors Against Stroke**
Body mass index >25 kg/m² in women	Daily consumption of fresh fruit
Weight gain >11 kg in 16 years in women	Flavonoid consumption >4.7 cups green tea/daily
Waist-to-hip ratio >0.92 in men	Fish consumption and fish oil use by white and black women and by black men
Diabetes	
Hypertension	
Elevated cholesterol in hemorrhagic stroke	High HDL cholesterol in ischemic stroke

TABLE 40-7   Practical Interventions for Eating-Related Behavioral Problems

Behavioral Problem	Intervention
Attention or concentration deficit	Verbally direct client through each step of eating process; place utensils in hand. Make food and fluids available and visible.
Combative, throws food	Identify provocative agent, remove. Dining assistant stands or sits on nondominant side. Provide nonbreakable dishes with suction holder. Give one food at a time. Reward appropriate mealtime behavior.
Chews constantly	Tell client to stop chewing after each bite. Serve soft foods to reduce the need to chew. Offer small bites.
Eats nonedible things	Remove nonedibles from reach; provide finger foods. Use edible centerpiece or table decorations.
Eats too quickly	Set utensils down between bites. Offer food items separately. Offer bulky foods that require chewing. Use a smaller spoon or cup.
Eats too slowly	Monitor eating pace and provide verbal cues: "chew," "take a bite." Serve first to allow more time. Use insulated dishes to maintain proper temperatures.
Forgetful or disoriented	Follow simple routines. Provide constant environment. Provide assigned seating. Minimize distractions and limit choices.
Forgets to swallow	Tell client to swallow. Feel for swallow before offering next bite. Stroke upward on larynx.
Inappropriate emotional expression	Engage in conversation; ignore emotional display. Provide a quiet environment.
Paces	Sit beside client at table. Change dining location. Provide aerobic exercise before meals. Offer finger foods. Use cups with covers or spouts.
Plays in food	Serve one food at a time. Fill glass or plate half full at refill. Offer finger foods. Use cups with covers or spouts.
Shows paranoia	Provide structured routine. Present food in consistent manner. Serve foods in closed containers. Do not put medicine in food.
Spits	Evaluate chewing and swallowing ability. Tell client not to spit. Place client away from others who would be offended. Provide mealtime supervision.
Will not go into dining room	Ask why; change dining location. Provide a single dining partner versus a group. Serve meals in room if needed.

Modified from National Institute on Aging (NIA) at http://www.nia.nih.gov/nia.nih.gov/templates/ADEAR. Accessed March 22, 2011.

to a condition in which bones are displaced from their original positions. *Open* or *closed* describes whether a fracture is exposed to air. Open fractures dramatically increase the risk of infection (osteomyelitis), and open skull fractures in particular carry an increased risk for meningitis because the dura mater is often violated.

Epidural and subdural hematomas are often corrected by surgical intervention. The volume of these lesions often displaces the brain tissue and may cause diffuse axonal injury and swelling. When the lesion becomes large enough, it may cause herniation of brain contents through various openings of the skull base. Consequent compression and ischemia of vital brain structures often rapidly lead to death.

Medical Management

The body's response to stress from TBI results in production of cytokines (interleukin-1, interleukin-6, interleukin-8, and tumor necrosis factor) and inflammation (see Chapter 3). These are elevated in the body after head injury and are associated with the hormonal milieu that negatively affects metabolism and organ function (see Chapter 38). Some of the metabolic events include fever, neutrophilia, muscle breakdown, altered amino acid metabolism, production of hepatic acute-phase reactants, increased endothelial permeability, and expression of endothelial adhesion molecules. Specific cytokines tend to cause organ demise; tissue damage has been observed in the gut, liver, lung, and brain. Overall, the molecular basis of functional recovery is poorly understood.

Clinical findings of brain injury often include a transient decrease in level of consciousness. Headache and dizziness are relatively common and not worrisome unless they become more intense or are accompanied by vomiting. Focal neurologic deficits, progressively decreasing level of consciousness, and penetrating brain injury demand prompt neurosurgical evaluation.

Skull fractures underneath lacerations often can be felt as a "drop off" or discontinuity on the surface of the skull and are readily identifiable by CT scan. Basilar skull fractures are manifested by otorrhea (fluid leaking from the ear) or rhinorrhea (salty fluid dripping from the nose or down the pharynx). Other signs include raccoon eyes and Battle's sign—blood behind the mastoid process. Basilar skull fractures may precipitate injuries to cranial nerves, which are essential for chewing, swallowing, taste, and smell.

Hematomas are neurosurgical emergencies because they may rapidly progress to herniation of brain contents through the skull base and to subsequent death. These lesions may present similarly, with decreased level of consciousness, contralateral hemiparesis, and pupillary dilation. These lesions damage brain tissue by gross displacement and traction. Classically the epidural hematoma presents with progressively decreasing consciousness after an interval of several hours during which the patient had only a brief loss of consciousness. Subdural hematoma usually features progressively decreasing consciousness from the time of injury.

Sequelae most often include epilepsy and the postconcussive syndrome, a constellation of headache, vertigo, fatigue, and memory difficulties. Treatment for these patients can be highly complex, but the two goals of any therapeutic intervention are to maintain cerebral perfusion and to regulate ICP. Perfusion and pressure control have implications for nutrition therapy.

Medical Nutrition Therapy

The goal of nutrition therapy is to oppose the hypercatabolism and hypermetabolism associated with inflammation (see Chapters 3 and 38). Hypercatabolism is manifested by protein degradation, evidenced by profound urinary urea nitrogen excretion. Nitrogen catabolism in a fasting normal human is only 3 to 5 g of nitrogen per day, whereas nitrogen excretion is 14 to 25 g of nitrogen per day in the fasting patient with severe head injury. In the absence of nutritional intake, this degree of nitrogen loss can result in a 10% decrease in lean mass within 7 days. A 30% weight loss increases mortality rate (Brain Trauma Foundation, 2007).

Hypermetabolism contributes to increased energy expenditure. Correlations between the severity of brain injury as measured by the Glasgow Coma Scale and energy requirements have been shown. The Glasgow Coma Scale is based on a 15-point scale for estimating and categorizing the outcomes of brain injury on the basis of overall social capability or dependence on others.

Replacement of 100% to 140% resting metabolism expenditure with 15% to 20% nitrogen calories reduces nitrogen loss (Brain Trauma Foundation, 2007). In patients medicated with barbiturates, metabolic expenditure may be decreased to 100% to 120% of basal metabolic rate. This decreased metabolic rate in pharmacologically paralyzed patients suggests that maintaining muscle tone is an important part of metabolic expenditure. See Chapter 38 for guidelines on care of the critically ill patient with head trauma.

An experimental dietary intervention based on a pyrazole curcumin derivative reestablishes membrane integrity and homeostasis after TBI (Sharma et al, 2010). The omega-3 fatty acids docosahexaenoic acid (DHA) and eicosapentaenoic acid (EPA) have antioxidative, antiinflammatory, and antiapoptosis effects, leading to neuron protection in the damaged brain (Su, 2010). Studies have shown that implementation of a ketogenic diet postinjury improves structural and functional outcome in TBI (Prins, 2014).

Immune enhancing nutrition formulas are available for critically ill head-injured patients that are enhanced with glutamine, arginine and omega-3 fatty acids. Data to support their use has not been consistent. One recent study did show increased prealbumin levels and some benefit of decreased infection in those patients using the immune-enhanced formula (Painter et al, 2015).

SPINE TRAUMA AND SPINAL CORD INJURY

Spine trauma encompasses many types of injuries, ranging from stable fractures of the spinal column to catastrophic transection of the spinal cord. A complete spinal cord injury (SCI) is defined as a lesion in which there is no preservation of motor or sensory function more than three segments below the level of the injury. With an incomplete injury there is some degree of residual motor or sensory function more than three segments below the lesion.

Pathophysiology

The spinal cord responds to insult in a manner similar to the brain. Bleeding, contusion, and shorn axons appear first, followed by a several-year remodeling process consisting of gliosis and fibrosis.

The location of the SCI and the disruption of the descending axons determines the extent of paralysis. Tetraplegia (formerly known as quadriplegia) exists when the injury to the spinal cord affects all four extremities. When the SCI location results in only lower extremity involvement, it is called paraplegia.

Medical Management

Spinal cord injuries have numerous clinical manifestations, depending on the level of the injury. Complete transection results in complete loss of function below the level of the lesion, including the bladder and sphincters. After the patient is stabilized hemodynamically, the doctor evaluates the degree of neurologic deficit. Patients with suspected SCI are usually immobilized promptly in the field. Complete radiographic evaluation of the spinal column is obligatory in multitrauma and unconscious patients.

In the awake patient, clinical evidence of spine compromise is usually sufficient to determine the need for further workup. CT and MRI are used to more accurately delineate bony damage and spinal cord compromise. A dismal 3% of patients with complete spinal cord insults recover some function after 24 hours. Failure to regain function after 24 hours predicts a poor prognosis for reestablishment of function in the future. Incomplete spinal cord syndromes may have somewhat better outcomes.

Morbidity and mortality rates associated with SCI have improved dramatically, particularly in the last two decades. Advances in acute-phase care have reduced early mortality and prevented complications frequently associated with early death, such as respiratory failure and pulmonary emboli. Today, fewer than 10% of patients with SCI die of the acute injury.

Medical Nutrition Therapy

Technologic advances in enteral and parenteral feeding techniques and formulas have played a role in maintaining nutrition status of these patients (see Chapter 13). Although the metabolic response to neurotrauma has been studied extensively, the acute metabolic response to SCI has not; but it is similar to other forms of neurotrauma during the acute phase. Initially paralytic ileus may occur but often resolves within 72 hours after injury. Because DHA and EPA have antioxidative, antiinflammatory, antiapoptosis effects, patients may benefit from fish oil supplementation (Su, 2010).

For those who survive the injury but are disabled for life, there are significant alterations in lifestyle as well as the possibility of secondary complications. In general the number and frequency of complications and the presence of constipation, pressure ulcers, obesity, and pain vary but will involve nutrition. Box 40-4 describes the rehabilitation potential based on the level of injury. Evidence-based practice guidelines for SCI were released in 2010 by the Academy of Nutrition and Dietetics.

Individuals with SCI have significantly higher fat mass and lower lean mass. Loss of muscle tone caused by skeletal muscle paralysis below the level of injury contributes to decreased metabolic activity, initial weight loss, and predisposition to osteoporosis. Guidelines for accepted weights adjusted for paraplegia and tetraplegia are as follows: the paraplegic should weigh 10 to 15 lb less than the ideal body mass index (BMI) would indicate; the tetraplegic should weigh 15 to 20 lb less than ideal weight dictated by the BMI. The higher the injury, the lower the metabolic rate; a lower energy requirement occurs.

Tetraplegic patients have lower metabolic rates than paraplegic patients, proportional to the amount of denervated muscle in their arms and legs, caused in part by the loss of residual motor function. In the rehabilitation phase, tetraplegics may

---

BOX 40-4 Key Guidelines for Managing Spinal Cord Injury

If the patient with spinal cord injury (SCI) is in the acute phase, the registered dietitian nutritionist (RDN) should assess energy needs by indirect calorimetry (IC).

Initial weight loss during the acute phase of injury may lead to weight gain in the chronic phase because of body mass redistribution.

Patients with SCI have reduced metabolic activity because of denervated muscle. Actual energy needs are at least 10% below predicted needs.

Because of decreased energy expenditure and caloric needs, secondary to lower levels of spontaneous physical activity and a lower thermic effect of food, adults in the chronic phase of SCI are often overweight or obese and therefore at risk for diabetes and cardiovascular disease.

Persons of all ages with SCI appear to be at high risk for cardiovascular disease, atherogenesis, and undesirable blood lipid values. Modifiable risk factors such as obesity, inactivity, dietary factors, and smoking must be addressed. Physical activity, including sports, swimming, electrically stimulated exercise, and body-weight supported treadmill training, may result in improvements in blood lipid parameters. Dietary intervention using the current evidence-based guide for lipid disorders should be provided by an RDN.

Nutrition care provided by the RDN as part of a multidisciplinary team results in improved nutrition-related outcomes in the acute care, rehabilitation, and community settings. SCI patients experience improvements in nutrient deficiencies, nutrition problems associated with social isolation and mobility issues, overweight and obesity, bowel management, swallowing, and nutrition-related chronic diseases.

Cranberry juice may be beneficial for prevention of urinary tract infections. One cup (250 ml) three times daily can be recommended, unless the patient has diabetes.

A minimum of 1.5 L of fluid is recommended per day. Therapeutic diets of high fiber and adequate water intake alone often do not suffice for treatment of constipation; a routine bowel preparation program may be required. For chronic bowel dysfunction, 15 g of fiber seems more beneficial than higher levels (20 to 30 g).

Maintenance of nutritional health is important because poor nutrition is a risk factor for infection and pressure ulcer development. Regular assessment of nutritional status, the provision of adequate nutritional intake, and the implementation of aggressive nutritional support measures are indicated. Reduced pressure ulcer development occurs in patients who maintain a normal weight, higher activity levels, and better serum levels of total protein, albumin, prealbumin, zinc, vitamin D, and vitamin A. Thus sufficient intake of calories, protein, zinc, and vitamins C, A, and B-complex is warranted.

When pressure ulcers are present, use 30 to 40 kcal/kg of body weight/day and 1.2 g to 1.5 g of protein/kg body weight/day (see Chapter 20). Fluid requirements should be at least 1 ml fluid per kcal provided; increase if air-fluidized beds are used and when losses are increased for any reason.

Data from American Dietetic Association: *Evidence Analysis Library: Spinal Cord Injury Guidelines* (website): http://www.adaevidencelibrary.com/topic.cfm?cat=3486&auth=1. Accessed October 31, 2010.

---

require approximately 25% to 50% fewer calories than conventional equations predict. Thus, these patients have the potential to become overweight. It has been proposed that obesity may slow the eventual rehabilitation process by limiting functional outcome.

As a consequence of bone loss resulting from the loss of mineralization caused by immobilization, SCI is associated with osteopenia and osteoporosis, and the prevalence of long-bone fractures increases. Adequate intake of vitamin D and calcium should be planned without excessive daily intakes.

NEUROLOGIC DISEASES

Adrenomyeloleukodystrophy
Pathophysiology

Adrenomyeloleukodystrophy (ALD) is a rare congenital enzyme deficiency that affects the metabolism of very-long-chain fatty acids (VLCFAs) in young men. This leads to accumulation of VLCFAs, particularly hexacosanoic acid (C26:0) and tetracosanoic acid (C24:0) in the brain and adrenal glands. The incidence is 1 in 21,000 male births and 1 in 14,000 female (Hung et al, 2013). It is an X-linked recessive disorder characterized by myelopathy, peripheral neuropathy, and cerebral demyelination. The adult variant, adrenomyeloneuropathy, has chronic distal axonopathy of spinal cord and peripheral nerves marked by cerebral inflammatory demyelination; head trauma is an environmental factor that is detrimental in those people genetically at risk. The mental and physical deterioration progresses to dementia, aphasia, apraxia, dysarthria, and blindness.

Medical Management

Clinical manifestations usually occur before age 7 and may manifest as adrenal insufficiency or cerebral decompensation.

Dysarthria (impairment of the tongue or other muscles needed for speech) and dysphagia may interfere with oral alimentation. Bronzing of the skin is a late clinical sign. With adrenal insufficiency, replacement of steroids is indicated (see Table 40-8), which may improve neurologic symptoms and prolong life. Numerous therapies have been directed at the root of the disorder but have been disappointing. The selective use of bone marrow transplant is one current therapy; gene therapy holds promise for the future.

Medical Nutrition Therapy

Nutritional therapy by dietary avoidance of VLCFAs does not lead to biochemical change because of endogenous synthesis. A specialty altered fatty acid product, Lorenzo's oil (C18:1 oleic acid and C22:1 erucic acid), lowers the VLCFA level. Although the clinical course is not significantly improved, a slower decline in function may result (Sassa et al, 2014).

Amyotrophic Lateral Sclerosis
Etiology

Amyotrophic lateral sclerosis (ALS), also known as Lou Gehrig disease, is a neurodegenerative disorder affecting the motor neurons in the central nervous system. There are 5000 people diagnosed annually in the United States (International Alliance of ALS/MND Associations, 2014). ALS involves a progressive denervation, atrophy, and weakness of muscles; hence the name amyotrophy. Men are affected more than women, and the average age of onset is the mid-50s with 90% having no family history of the disease.

The cause of ALS is not clear. Thus there is no cure, and survival is typically 3 to 5 years after disease onset. Risk factors related to occupation, trauma, diet, or socioeconomic status are not consistent, although environmental toxins have been suspected to play a role. One of the first clues that ALS may involve an environmental factor was obtained on the island of Guam in the Pacific, where an unusually high proportion of people over the past century have developed symptoms similar to ALS as they age. Studies are ongoing but thus far without proof of cause.

TABLE 40-8   Drugs Commonly Used in the Treatment of Neurologic Diseases

Disease or Condition	Drug	Basic Function	Nutrition-Related Side Effects
Adrenomyeloleukodystrophy	Adrenal hormones		Weight gain
Alzheimer's disease	Donepezil	Supports nerve cell communication	Anorexia, weight loss
	Galantamine		
	Axona	MCT energy source for mitochondria function	
	Rivastigmine	Delays worsening of symptoms	
	Tacrine		
	Memantine	May help improve attention, reasoning, language	
Amyotrophic lateral sclerosis	Riluzole	Decreases motor neuron damage	Suggests decreased use of caffeine
Epilepsy	Valproate	Anticonvulsant	Increased appetite and requirements of vitamin D
	Phenytoin	Anticonvulsant	Increased requirements of vitamin D and K
	Keppra	Anticonvulsant	Poor coordination
	Carbamazepine	Anticonvulsant	Nausea, increased vitamin D requirements
	Phenobarbital	Sedative, hypnotic	Increased requirements of vitamins D, K, and possibly folic acid
	Topamax	Anticonvulsant	Nausea
Guillain-Barré syndrome	Immunoglobulins or plasma-pheresis	Decreases immune attacks	Consider celiac disease
Migraine headache	NSAIDs	Antiinflammatory	
	Sympathomimetics		
	Serotonin agonists		
	Sumatriptan	Serotonin 5-HT1 receptor agonist	Dehydration, anorexia
Myasthenia gravis	Anticholinesterase inhibitors	Improve muscle contraction and strength	GI upset, increased urination
Multiple sclerosis	Corticosteroids: oral prednisone, IV methylprednisolone	Reduce inflammation	Increased appetite, weight gain
	Interferon: beta 1a –(Avonex, Rebif) beta 1b –(Betaseron)	Slow rate of symptom development	Anorexia, increased or decreased weight
	Novantrone (mitoxantrone) Anthracenedione	Immunosuppressants, anticancer antibiotics	Anorexia, harmful to heart, leukemia
	Natalizumab (formerly Antegran)	Monotherapy	Risk of progressive multifocal leukoencephalopathy
	Glatiramer acetate	Immunomodulator drug for relapsing-remitting MS	Flushing, sweating
	Symptomatic therapies: amantadine	Reduces fatigue, Reduces spasticity	Anorexia, weight loss Increased appetite, weight
	Diazepam	Decreases paroxysmal dystonia, sensory symptoms	Anorexia, N/V, diarrhea
	Carbamazepine		
	Amitryptyline	Reduces pain	
Parkinson's disease	Levodopa	Dopamine precursor	Anorexia
	COMT inhibitors: Entacapone Tolcapone	Prolongs effectiveness of levodopa	
	Exelon	Acetylcholinesterase inhibitor	Anorexia, weight loss
	MAO-B inhibitors	Reduces breakdown of dopamine	
	Trihexyphenidyl	Anticholinergics	
	Benztropine		
	Ethopropazine		
Stroke	Anticoagulants	Preventive	Bleeding, decreased platelets
	Antiplatelet agents		
	Thrombolytic therapy when acute: heparin	Dissolves clots	

Data from National Institute of Neurologic Disorders and Stroke: *Disorders Index* (website): http://www.ninds.nih.gov/disorders/disorder_index.htm. Accessed January 12, 2015; Mayo Clinic: *Patient Care and Health Information* (website): http://www.mayoclinic.com/health-information. Accessed January 11, 2015.

COMT (catechol-O-methyltransferase); *GI*, gastrointestinal; *IV*, intravenous; *MAO-B* (monoamine oxidase B); *MCT*, medium chain triglyceride; *MS*, multiple sclerosis; *NSAID*, nonsteroidal antiinflammatory drug; *N/V*, nausea and vomiting.

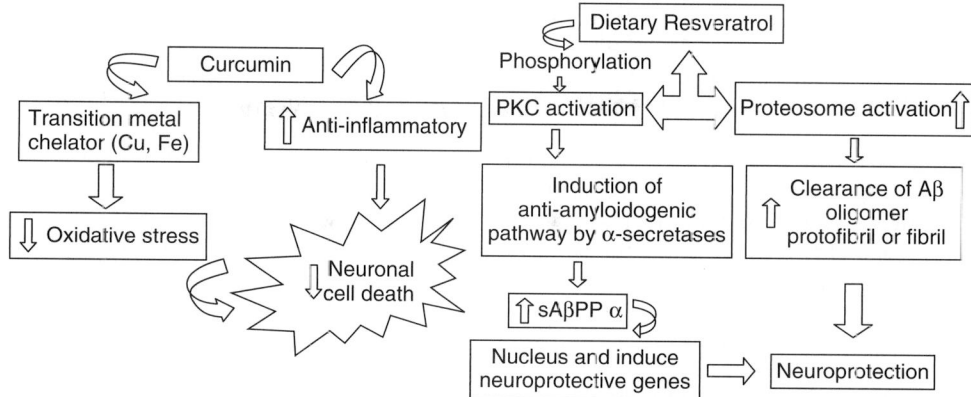

FIGURE 40-6 The role of curcumin and resveratrol in neuroprotection. Left: Curcumin has multiple biologic effects: it chelates transition metals (iron and copper) and acts as an antioxidant and antiinflammatory molecule, protecting from oxidative stress. Right: Resveratrol favors phosphorylation in protein kinase C, activating the nonamyloidogenic pathway of AβPP cleavage, and this leads to reduction in Aβ formation. sAβPPβ, a product of AβPP cleavage, gets translocated to the nucleus and modulates the genes. All these events favor neuronal cell survival. Aβ, Amyloid beta; PKC, protein kinase C; sAPPβ, secreted fragment of amyloid protein precursor beta. (From Ramesh BN et al: Neuronutrition and Alzheimer's disease, *J Alzheimers Dis* 19:1123, 2010. With permission from IOS Press.)

In 2014 the U.S. Department of Agriculture approved a randomized clinical trial of stem cell transplant in people with ALS, the most aggressive treatment attempted to date.

Pathophysiology

The pathologic basis of weakness in ALS is the selective death of motor neurons in the ventral gray matter of the spinal cord, brainstem, and in the motor cortex. Clinical manifestations are characterized by generalized skeletal muscular weakness, atrophy, and hyperreflexia (NIH, 2015).

The typical presentation is lower motor neuron (weakness, wasting, fasciculation) and upper motor neuron deficits (hyperactive tendon reflexes, Hoffman signs, Babinski signs, or clonus). Muscle weakness begins in the legs and hands and progresses to the proximal arms and oropharynx. As these motor nerves deteriorate, almost all of the voluntary skeletal muscles are at risk for atrophy and complete loss of function. The loss of spinal motor neurons causes the denervation of voluntary skeletal muscles of the neck, trunk, and limbs, resulting in muscle wasting, flaccid weakness, involuntary twitching (fasciculations), and loss of mobility.

Progressive loss of function in cortical motor neurons can lead to spasticity of jaw muscles, resulting in slurred speech and dysphagia. The onset of dysphagia is usually insidious. Swallowing difficulties usually follow speech difficulties. Although some weight loss is inevitable given the muscle atrophy, consistent or dramatic loss may be an indicator of chewing difficulties or dysphagia. Eye movement and eye blink are spared, as are the sphincter muscles of the bowel and bladder; thus incontinence is rare. Sensation remains intact and mental acuity is maintained.

Medical Management

No currently known therapy cures the disease. Treatment with a high dose of methylcobalamin (B₁₂) is being studied to preserve muscle integrity (NIH, 2014). The ketogenic diet has shown positive results in disease amelioration in mouse models (Paganoni, 2013). Although mechanical ventilation can extend the life of patients, most decline this option. Quality of life is poor in advanced ALS and supportive comfort measures are primarily used.

Medical Nutrition Therapy

There are decreases in body fat, lean body mass, muscle power, and nitrogen balance and an increase in resting energy expenditure as death approaches. Some of the nutritional changes during the different stages of ALS are noted in Table 40-9.

Hypermetabolic status and increased resting energy expenditure measurements have been noted. The relationship between dysphagia and respiratory status is important. As ALS progresses, a progressive loss of function in bulbar and respiratory muscles contributes to oral and pharyngeal dysphagia. This results in the need for nutrition support, generally via a gastrostomy tube. In late stages, when the respiratory status is

TABLE 40-9 Nutritional and Metabolic Changes During the Progression of Amyotrophic Lateral Sclerosis

	Early Phase	Late Phase
Pathophysiology	Cycles of muscle denervation, muscle catabolism and atrophy, reinnervation, and protein synthesis	Net muscle catabolism and atrophy
Functional status	Mild functional restriction of physical activity	Progressive limitation of physical activity
	Mild impairment of respiration	Increased work of ventilation
Nutritional and metabolic changes	Positive nitrogen balance	Negative nitrogen balance
	Normal resting energy expenditure	Increased resting energy expenditure
	Probable neutral energy balance	Decrease in body fat

From Kasarskis EJ et al: Nutritional status of patients with amyotrophic lateral sclerosis: relation to the proximity of death, *Am J Clin Nutr* 63:130, 1996.

impaired, feeding tube placement is associated with more risk. For that reason early feeding tube placement is recommended.

The clinician should become familiar with common clinical findings in ALS to prevent secondary complications of malnutrition and dehydration. The functional status of each patient should be monitored closely so that timely intervention with the appropriate management techniques can be started. In particular, dysphagia should be monitored closely. Oropharyngeal weakness affects survival in ALS by placing the patient at continuous risk of aspiration, pneumonia, and sepsis and by curtailing the adequate intake of energy and protein. These problems can compound the deteriorating effects of the disease. The Amyotrophic Lateral Sclerosis Severity Scale often is used to assess the functional level of swallowing, speech, and upper and lower extremities. Once the severity of deficits has been identified, appropriate interventions can be implemented (see *Focus On:* Dysphagia Intervention for Amyotrophic Lateral Sclerosis).

Epilepsy

Epilepsy is a chronic condition characterized by unprovoked, recurring seizures. Seizures are caused by abnormal electrical activity of a group of neurons. It is estimated that 3 million Americans have epilepsy (Epilepsy Foundation, 2014).

Pathophysiology

Most seizures begin in early life, but a resurgence occurs after age 60. The first occurrence of a seizure should prompt investigation into a cause. A clinical workup usually reveals no anatomic abnormalities, and the cause of the seizure may remain unknown (idiopathic). Seizures before age 2 are usually caused by fever, developmental defects, birth injuries, or a metabolic disease (see Chapters 43 and 44). The medical history is the key component for suggesting further avenues of diagnostic investigation and potential treatments, especially in children. An electroencephalogram can help to delineate seizure activity. It is most helpful in localizing partial complex seizures.

Medical Management

The dramatic tonic-clonic (grand mal) seizure is the most common image of a convulsive seizure, yet numerous classifications of seizures, each with a different and often less dramatic clinical presentation, exist. A generalized tonic-clonic seizure typically involves the entire brain cortex from its beginning phases. After such a seizure the patient wakes up slowly and will be groggy and disoriented for minutes to hours. This is termed the postictal phase and is characterized by deep sleep, headache, confusion, and muscle soreness.

◎ FOCUS ON

Dysphagia Intervention for Amyotrophic Lateral Sclerosis (ALS)

Strand and colleagues (1996) outlined dysphagia intervention on a continuum of five stages that correlate to the amyotrophic lateral sclerosis (ALS) severity scale. They include the following:

Normal Eating Habits (ALS Severity Scale Rating 10-9)

Early assessment and intervention are critical for maintaining nutritional health in ALS. This is the appropriate time to begin educating the patient, before the development of speech or swallowing symptoms. Hydration and maintenance of nutritional health are critical at this stage. Fluid intake of at least 2 qts/day is important. Dehydration contributes to fatigue and thickens saliva. For patients with spinal ALS, emphasis on fluids is important because they may intentionally limit fluid intake because of difficulties with toileting. The diet history is helpful to assess patterns of normal chewing, swallowing, and the rate of ingestion. Weight loss history establishes a baseline weight. A weight loss of 10% or more is indicative of nutritional risk.

Early Eating Problems (Severity Scale Rating 8-7)

At this point patients begin to report difficulties eating; reports of coughing and unusually long mealtimes are associated with tongue, facial, and masticator muscle weakness. Dietary intervention begins to focus on modification of consistency, avoidance of thin liquids, and use of foods that are easier to chew and swallow.

Dietary Consistency Changes (Severity Scale Rating 6-5)

As symptoms progress, the oral transport of food becomes difficult as dry, crumbly foods tend to break apart and cause choking. Foods that require more chewing (e.g., raw vegetables or steak) are typically avoided. As dysphagia progresses, ingestion of thin liquids, especially water, may become more problematic. Often the patient has fatigue and malaise, which may be associated with a mild chronic dehydration resulting from a decreased fluid intake. Dietary intervention should change food consistency to mechanically soft or pureed (see Appendix 28) to reduce the need for oral manipulation and to conserve energy. Small, frequent meals also may increase intake. Thick liquids that contain a high percentage of water, as well as attempts to increase fluid intake, must be emphasized to maintain fluid balance. Popsicles, gelatin, ice, and fresh fruit are additional sources of free water. Liquids can be thickened with a modified cornstarch thickener. Swallowing can be improved by emphasizing taste, texture, and temperature. Juices can be substituted for water

to provide taste, nutrients, and calories. A cool temperature facilitates the swallowing mechanism; therefore cold food items may be better tolerated; heat does not provide the same advantage. Carbonation also may be better tolerated because of the beneficial effect of texture. Instructions for preventing aspiration should be addressed: safe swallowing includes sitting bolt upright with the head in a chin-down position. Concentrating on the swallowing process can also help reduce choking. Avoid environmental distractions and conversation during mealtime; however, families should be encouraged to maintain a normal mealtime routine. As dysphagia progresses, the limitation of food consistencies may result in the exclusion of entire food groups. Vitamin and mineral supplementation may be necessary. If chewable supplements are not handled safely, liquid forms may be added to acceptable foods. Fiber also may have to be added along with fluids for constipation problems.

Tube Feeding (Severity Scale Rating 4-3)

Dehydration will occur acutely before malnutrition, a more chronic state, is exhibited. This may be an early indication of the need for nutrition support. Weight loss from muscle wasting and dysphagia eventually leads to placement of a percutaneous endoscopic gastrostomy (PEG) tube for nutrition and protection against aspiration caused by dysphagia. Enteral nutrition support is preferred because the gastrointestinal tract should be functioning properly. Given the progressive nature of ALS, placing feeding tubes when there are signs of dysphagia and dehydration is better than initiating this therapy later, after the patient has become overtly malnourished or when respiratory status is marginal. The decision of whether to place a feeding tube for nutrition support is part of the decision-making process each patient must face. Adequate nutriture can maintain health of the individual longer and may be a welcome relief for the patient. The purpose of nutrition support should be to enhance the quality of life. Long-term access should be considered via a PEG or percutaneous endoscope jejunostomy tube (see Chapter 13).

Nothing by Mouth (Severity Scale Rating 2-1)

The final level of dysphagia is reached when the patient can neither eat orally nor manage his or her own oral secretions. Although saliva production is not increased, it tends to pool in the front of the mouth as a result of a declining swallow response. Once the swallowing mechanism is absent, mechanical ventilation is required to manage saliva flow. Tube feeding is permanent at this stage.

The **absence seizure (petit mal)** is also generalized in nature. A patient with absence seizures may appear to be daydreaming during an episode, but he or she recovers consciousness within a few seconds and has no postictal fatigue or disorientation. Partial seizures occur when there is a discrete focus of epileptogenic brain tissue. A simple partial seizure involves no loss of consciousness, whereas a complex partial seizure is characterized by a change in consciousness. Failure of partial seizure control may prompt consideration of seizure surgery. A localized focus resected from nonessential brain renders a patient seizure free in 75% of cases.

Determining the seizure type is key to implementing effective therapy. Antiepileptic drugs control seizures in 70% of people; however, these drugs can have undesirable effects. Use of just one antiseizure medication is recommended initially, resorting to combination therapies only when needed. If seizures are not well controlled after a trial of two antiseizure drugs, the likelihood of control from an additional medication or combination of medications is minimal.

Medications used in anticonvulsant therapy may alter the nutrition status of the patient (see Table 40-8) (see Chapter 8 and Appendix 31). Phenobarbital has been associated with decreased intelligence quotient when used in children (Eddy et al, 2011). It occasionally is considered for use after failure of other antiepileptic drugs. Phenobarbital, phenytoin, and valproates interfere with intestinal absorption of calcium by interfering with vitamin D metabolism in the kidneys. Long-term therapy with these drugs may lead to osteomalacia in adults or rickets in children, and vitamin D supplementation is recommended. Folic acid supplementation

interferes with phenytoin metabolism; thus it contributes to difficulties in achieving therapeutic levels.

Phenytoin, valproates, and phenobarbital are bound primarily to albumin in the bloodstream. Decreased serum albumin levels limit the amount of drug that can be bound. This results in an increased free drug concentration and possible drug toxicity even with a standard dose.

Absorption of phenobarbital is delayed by the consumption of food; therefore administration of the drug must be staggered around mealtimes if it is used. Continuous enteral feeding slows the absorption of phenytoin, thus necessitating an increase in the dose to achieve a therapeutic level. Stopping the tube feeding 1 hour before and 1 hour after the phenytoin dose was common practice in the past but is no longer recommended. The phenytoin dose should be adjusted based on the tube feeding.

Medical Nutrition Therapy

The classic **ketogenic diet**, which has been in existence since the 1920s, can be used for treatment of all types of seizures (Zupec-Kania et al, 2013). Originally designed using ratios of 4:1 or 3:1 (grams of fat to nonfat) to achieve strong and consistent ketosis, less restrictive versions are now available that can also be effective. The modified ketogenic uses lower ratios (e.g., 1:1 and 2:1), modified Atkins, and the Low Glycemic Index Treatment (LGIT) are also available for those who may benefit from a less restricted approach (Kumada et al, 2013). Table 40-10 presents the classic ketogenic diet.

TABLE 40-10 Comparison of Ketogenic Diet Therapies

Questions	Ketogenic	MCT Oil	Low Glycemic Index Treatment	Modified Atkins
Is medical supervision required	Yes	Yes	Yes	Yes
Is diet high in fat?	Yes	Yes	Yes	Yes
Is diet low in carbohydrate?	Yes	Yes	Yes	Yes
What is the ratio of fat to carbohydrate & protein?	4:1 3:1, 2:1, 1:1	Approximately 1:1	Approximately 1:1	Approximately 1:1
How much carbohydrate is allowed on a 1000 Calorie diet?	8gm carb on a 4:1 16gm carb on a 3:1 30gm carb on a 2:1 40-60gm carb on a 1:1	40-50gm	40-60gm	10gm for 1 month 15-20gm afterwards
How are foods measured?	Weighed	Weighed or measured	Measured or estimated	Estimated
Are meal plans used?	Yes	Yes	Yes	Optional
Where is the diet started?	Hospital	Hospital	Home	Home
Are calories controlled?	Yes	Yes	Yes	No
Are vitamin and mineral supplements required?	Yes	Yes	Yes	Yes
Are liquids (fluids) restricted?	No	No	No	No
Is a pre-diet laboratory evaluation required?	Yes	Yes	Yes	Yes
Can there be side-effects?	Yes	Yes	Yes	Yes
What is the overall difference in design of these diets?	This is an individualized and structured diet that provides specific meal plans. Foods are weighed and meals should be consumed in their entirety for best results. The ratio of this diet can be adjusted to effect better seizure-control and also liberalized for better tolerance. This diet is also considered a low glycemic therapy and results in steady glucose levels.	An individualized and structured diet containing Medium Chain Triglycerides (MCT) which are highly ketogenic. This allows more carbohydrate and protein than the classic ketogenic diet. A source of essential fatty acids must be included with this diet.	This is individualized but less structured diet than the ketogenic diet. It uses exchange lists for meal planning and emphasizes complex carbohydrates. The balance of low glycemic carbohydrates in combination with fat result in steady glucose levels. It is not intended to promote ketosis.	This diet focuses on limiting the amount of carbohydrate while encouraging fat. Carbohydrate may be consumed at any time during the day as long as it is within limits and should be consumed with fat. Suggested meal plans are used as a guide. Protein is not limited but too much is discouraged.

Glucose Transporter Type I Deficiency Syndrome (Glut-1 DS) and pyruvate dehydrogenase deficiency (PDHD) are two genetically inherited disorders that typically include seizures and are treatable with ketogenic diet therapy. The diet also has been effective for other inherited disorders in which seizures are also typical: glycogen storage diseases, nonketotic hyperglycinemia, and respiratory chain defects. The common feature of each of these conditions is in the failure of the brain to derive adequate fuel from glucose. Ketones provided by ketogenic diet therapy offer an alternative fuel source which improves symptoms, preserves neurons, and can prevent further decline.

The ketogenic diet has minimal side effects, and risks of the diet are low blood sugar, upset stomach at first caused by the high amounts of fat, and constipation. The long-term risk of kidney stones is rare; elevated serum cholesterol is usually temporary and disappears with discontinuation of the diet; and growth, which is sometimes slowed while on the diet, resumes at the child's normal rate (Patel et al, 2010). Although the diet is restrictive and requires continued effort, it completely controls epilepsy in 10-15% of the children whose seizures are otherwise uncontrollable (Zupec-Kania et al, 2013). Practical guidelines for implementing the diet have been published in *Epilepsia* and are also available through The Charlie Foundation (Kossoff et al, 2009).

The diet is designed to create and maintain a state of ketosis. The beneficial effect in epilepsy may be caused by a change in neuronal metabolism; ketones may inhibit neurotransmitters, thus producing an anticonvulsant and neuroprotective effect in the brain. Initiation of the classic ketogenic diet in children typically begins under close medical supervision, while administration of the more liberal versions described earlier may begin at home with prior instructions. Fasting before starting diet therapies is sometimes used to stimulate ketosis especially in catastrophic epilepsies and in the overweight individual; however, it should not be prescribed in those with metabolic defects (which may result in a metabolic crisis). Improvement in seizure control can take up to 3 months after diet has been implemented. Antiepileptic drugs are not stopped but may be reduced before initiation, if medication toxicity occurs, or after it has been established that the diet therapy is effective.

The classic ketogenic diet is determined in a ratio of 3:1 or 4:1, meaning that there are 3 or 4 g of fat for every 1 g of protein and carbohydrate combined in the diet. With a 4:1 ratio, the diet is calculated so that at least 90% of the kilocalories are from fat. Protein is calculated to provide appropriate intake for growth (approximately 1 g/kg/day). Carbohydrates are added to make up the remaining small portion of calories that is typically less than 20 g in children (see Table 40-11).

The majority of the diet is composed of fresh meats, eggs, cheese, fish, heavy whipping cream, butter, oils, nuts, and seeds. Vegetables and fruits are added in small amounts, within the current diet prescription (see Table 40-11). Ketosis is monitored by regular measurements of urine ketones or serum beta-hydroxybutyrate.

Goal level of ketones are patient specific; some individuals need to be in the range of 35 to 60 mg/L (4 to 7 mmol/L) for seizure control while others may achieve control with little or no ketosis, which is typical with the liberal diets (modified ketogenic of 1:1 and 2:1 ratios, and LGIT). A carbohydrate-free multiple vitamin and mineral supplement is necessary to ensure that the diet is nutritionally complete. However, additional vitamins and minerals are often necessary, including calcium, vitamin D, and selenium.

TABLE 40-11   Typical Ketogenic Diet for a Child

Menu for 1 day	Amount (g)	Fat (g)	Protein (g)	Carbohydrate (g)	Energy Kcal & Ratio
Breakfast					
Keto pancakes (made with macadamia nuts and eggs)	54	25.19	5.41	1.72	255
Blueberries	10	0.06	0.04	0.95	5
Butter	10	8.11	0.09	0.01	73
Total		33.36	5.54	2.68	333 4:1
Lunch					
Cream–36%	45	16.2	0.9	1.35	155
Celery	10	0.02	0.07	0.14	1
Chicken breast, cooked—skin removed	17	0.61	5.27	0	27
Avocado	17	2.62	0.33	0.31	26
Olive oil	14	14	0	0	126
Total		33.45	6.57	1.8	335 4:1
Snack					
Cream—36% whipped	56	20.16	1.12	1.68	193
Strawberries	35	0.11	0.23	1.99	10
Total		20.27	1.35	3.67	203 4:1
Dinner					
Cream 36%	40	14.4	0.8	1.2	138
Tomato sauce	21	0.42	0.34	1.18	10
Ground beef 85% lean cooked	17	2.38	4.19	0	38
Spaghetti squash cooked	10	0.03	0.06	0.51	3
Olive oil	16	16	0	0	144
Total		33.23	5.39	2.89	333 4:1
Totals for the day		122.99	18.85	11.04	1204 4:1

Calculations from Ketodietalculator.org by Beth Zupec-Kania

All prescription and over-the-counter medications (e.g., pain relievers, cold remedies, mouthwash, toothpaste, and lotions) must be scrutinized for sugar content to minimize carbohydrate. It is important that the diet be strictly followed; the smallest amount of extra carbohydrate can cause a breakthrough seizure. Weight and height should be monitored, because a rapid rate of weight gain can decrease ketosis and reduce effectiveness. The nutritionists should work closely with the patient throughout the course of therapy to ensure nutritional adequacy and optimal seizure control benefit.

A variation of the ketogenic diet is the modified Atkins diet in which calories are not restricted, but carbohydrates are drastically limited to 10 to 20 g/day. The ratio of fat to protein and carbohydrate is usually 1:1. It appears that the best results are achieved when the diet begins with 10 g/day of carbohydrate and is then adjusted upward, always maintaining ketosis (Porta et al, 2009; Weber et al, 2009). Another variation of the ketogenic diet is the low glycemic index treatment, which aims for 60% of calories from fat and limits carbohydrate to 28% of calories; the remaining 12% of calories are allocated to protein. Foods are estimated in household measure and meal plans are used as a guide (Zupec-Kania et al, 2013).

The medium-chain triglyceride (MCT) oil–based ketogenic diet is yet another therapy, used frequently in the United Kingdom and Canada, in which 60% of the fat is provided by MCTs and 12% is provided by long-chain-fats. MCT oil is an odorless, colorless, tasteless oil and was originally used as a means of improving the palatability of the diet. A greater amount of nonketogenic foods such as fruits and vegetables and small amounts of bread and other starches can be allowed because ketosis from MCT can be more readily achieved with a lower percentage of fat in the diet. MCT can be added in to the classic ketogenic diet and modified Atkins diet to increase ketosis. Coconut oil also can be used as a source of MCT to increase palatability, but it contains only 45% to 50% MCT, so more may be needed. MCT oil or coconut oils also are added if the serum triglycerides are too high with the use of the traditional ketogenic diet.

Attention to the patient's health status, growth, and development is required during the course of therapy. For the child whose epilepsy is controlled by the diet, complying with the diet is much easier than dealing with devastating seizures and injuries.

As clinical and scientific research evolves, improvements in which diet to use, how long to use it, and specific guidelines for certain epilepsies will emerge. Some patients may benefit from a simple diet initially then graduate to the more restrictive ketogenic therapy based on their seizure outcome results. Others may start off with the most restrictive ketogenic therapy and transition to a less restrictive one for long term maintenance.

Discontinuation of the diet is individual and may vary from 1 to 3 years from the initiation period. The person is "weaned" off the ketogenic diet over a period of several months to a year as small amounts of carbohydrates are added with observation for seizure reoccurrence. Some patients choose to stay long term on the liberal versions of the ketogenic diet such as the LGIT for improved seizure control if they have not achieved seizure freedom on the more restrictive ketogenic diets.

Guillain-Barré Syndrome and Chronic Inflammatory Demyelinating Polyneuropathy

Guillain-Barré Syndrome (GBS) and chronic inflammatory demyelinating polyneuropathy (CIDP) are acquired immune-mediated inflammatory disorders of the peripheral nervous system. The incidence of GBS is approximately 2 in 100,000; the incidence of CIDP is far less prevalent (CDC, 2014).

Etiology

In 60% of GBS cases the disorder follows an infection, surgery, or an immunization. Some of the more common organisms are *Campylobacter jejuni* and *Mycoplasma* spp. Several pathologic varieties exist, and the nature of the distinction is related to the segment of the immune system that is inflicting nerve damage. The clinical course of GBS is similar regardless of subtype, although GBS after a *Campylobacter* infection tends to be more severe. Gluten sensitivity has been reported in some cases as a cause of GBS. The cause of CIDP is similar to GBS; however, the illness follows a longer course and was previously referred to as a chronic form of GBS (Eldar and Chapman, 2014).

Pathophysiology

Relatively symmetric weakness with paresthesia usually begins in the legs and progresses to the arms. The loss of function in affected nerves occurs because of demyelination. Myelin is the specialized fatty insulation that envelops the conducting part of the nerve, the axon. In GBS the immune system recognizes myelin and mounts an attack against it. Presumably myelin shares a common characteristic with the pathogen from the antecedent infection; thus the immune system cannot differentiate what is foreign (the pathogen) from what is native (myelin). When the nerve is demyelinated, its ability to conduct signals is severely impaired, resulting in neuropathy.

Medical Management

GBS reveals itself in a matter of days. The most common sequence of symptoms is areflexia (absence of reflexes), followed by proximal limb weakness, cranial nerve weakness, and respiratory insufficiency. These symptoms normally peak by 2 weeks but may progress up to 1 month. Medical diagnosis is ordinarily made on clinical grounds, but nerve conduction studies are also beneficial. Before the clinical course is apparent, myelopathic disorders must be considered.

Because of the precipitous progression of vital capacity and swallowing function may rapidly deteriorate such that intensive care is sometimes necessary. Intubation and respiratory support should be instituted early in respiratory decline to avoid the need for resuscitation. Plasmapheresis, the exchange of the patient's plasma for albumin, is often helpful to reduce the load of circulating antibodies. Intravenous immunoglobulin or steroids have been shown to be of benefit.

Medical Nutrition Therapy

Guillain-Barré syndrome evolves quickly; during the acute stage, the metabolic response of GBS is similar to the stress response that occurs in neurotrauma. Energy needs assessed by indirect calorimetry may be as high as 40 to 45 kcal/kg and protein needs twice the usual amount. Supportive nutritional care should be offered to attenuate muscle wasting.

For a small percentage of patients, oropharyngeal muscles may be affected, leading to dysphagia and dysarthria. In this situation, a visit by the RDN at mealtime can be a valuable way to observe difficulties the patient may have with chewing or swallowing. Specific difficulties warrant evaluation by a swallowing specialist. The speech therapist can evaluate the degree of dysphagia and make appropriate dietary recommendations pertaining to texture. As the patient recovers, it is important to discuss safe food handling and future prevention of *C. jejuni* infection.

Myasthenia Gravis

Myasthenia Gravis (MG) is the most well-known disorder of the neuromuscular junction. The neuromuscular junction is the site on the striated muscle membrane where a spinal motor neuron connects. Here the signal from the nerve is carried to the muscle via a submicron-size gap, a synapse. The molecule that carries the signal from the nerve ending to the muscle membrane is acetylcholine (Ach), and acetylcholine receptors (AchRs) populate the muscle membrane. These receptors translate the chemical signal of Ach into an electrical signal that is required for contraction of muscle fibers. MG is one of the most well-characterized autoimmune diseases, a class of disorders in which the body's immune system raises a response to AchRs. The incidence of MG is low, approximately 20 in 100,000 people (Myasthenia Gravis Foundation, 2014).

Pathophysiology

In MG the body unwittingly makes antibodies to AchR. These antibodies are the same that fight off colds and give immunity. The AchR antibodies bind to AchR and make them unresponsive to Ach. There is no disorder of nerve conduction and no intrinsic disorder of muscle. The characteristic weakness in MG occurs because the signal of the nervous system to the muscle is garbled at the neuromuscular junction. Patients with MG commonly have an overactive thymus gland. This gland resides in the anterior thorax and plays a role in the maturation of B-lymphocytes, the cells that are charged with synthesizing antibodies.

Relapsing and remitting weakness and fatigue, varying from minutes to days, characterize MG. The most common presentation is diplopia (double vision) caused by extraocular muscle weakness, followed by dysarthria, facial muscle weakness, and dysphagia. Dysphagia or swallowing disorders (resulting from fatigue after mastication) may cause malnutrition. Less commonly, proximal limb weakness in the hips and shoulders may be present. Severe diaphragmatic weakness can result in respiratory difficulty. No involvement of sensory nerves occurs.

Medical Management

Anticholinesterases are medicines that inhibit acetylcholinesterase, thus serving to increase the amount of Ach in the neuromuscular junction. Corticosteroids are immunosuppressive. Removal of the thymus results in symptomatic improvement in most patients.

Medical Nutrition Therapy

Chewing and swallowing often are compromised in MG. Because this compromise occurs with fatigue, it is important to provide nutritionally dense foods at the beginning of meals before the patient tires. Small, frequent meals that are easy to chew and swallow are helpful. Difficulties holding a bolus on the tongue also have been observed, suggesting that foods that do not fall apart easily may be better tolerated. For patients treated with anticholinesterase drugs, it is crucial to time medication with feeding to facilitate optimal swallowing.

Physical activity should be limited before mealtime to ensure maximum strength to eat a meal. It is also important not to encourage food consumption once the patient begins to fatigue because this may contribute to aspiration. If and when respiratory crisis occurs, it is usually temporary. Nutrition support via a tube may be implemented in the interim to assist in maintaining vital functions of the patient until the crisis subsides. Once extubated, a swallow evaluation using cinefluoroscopy is appropriate to assess the degree of deglutitory dysfunction (swallowing irregularity) or risk of aspiration associated with an oral diet.

Multiple Sclerosis

Multiple sclerosis (MS) is a chronic inflammatory disorder of the central nervous system (CNS) and is one of the most common causes of nontraumatic disability among young and middle-aged adults. MS-related health care costs are estimated to be more than $10 billion annually in the United States (US). MS affects the CNS and is characterized by destruction of the myelin sheath, the function of which is transmission of electrical nerve impulses. Multiple areas of optic nerves, spinal cord, and brain undergo "sclerosis," whereby myelin is replaced with sclera or scar tissue. No single test can ascertain whether a patient has MS; however, diagnostic criteria (McDonald criteria) were developed for use by practicing clinicians (Polman et al, 2011).

The signs and symptoms of MS are easily distinguished, and they recur over the natural history of this disease. In the worst scenario MS can render a person unable to write, speak, or walk. Fortunately, the majority of patients are only mildly affected. MS affects approximately 400,000 people in the United States and 2.5 million worldwide. In the United States, prevalence estimates are approximately 90 per 100,000 population. MS symptoms can start anywhere between 10 and 80 years of age, but onset is usually between 20 and 40 years, with a mean of 32 years. Although MS is more frequently seen in Caucasians than African Americans, the latter group appears to accumulate disability more quickly, suggesting more destructive tissue injury in this population. The prevalence of MS varies by geographic location and generally increases the further one travels from the equator in either hemisphere. It remains unclear whether this altered incidence represents an environmental influence, genetic difference, or variable surveillance (Hersh and Fox, 2015).

Pathophysiology

The precise cause of MS remains undetermined. A familial predisposition to MS has been noted in a minority of cases. It is more common in women and in people of Northern European ancestry (National MS Society, 2015). Geographic latitude and diet are therefore implicated. Epidemiologic studies have linked the incidence of MS to geographic location and sunshine exposure. Studies have shown that people born in an area with a high risk of MS who then move —or migrate—to an area with a lower risk before the age of 15 assume the risk of their new area. Such data suggest that exposure to some environmental agent before puberty may predispose a person to develop MS later on.

There is growing evidence that vitamin D may play a role. The degree of sunlight exposure catalyzes the production of vitamin D in the skin. Vitamin D produced by the skin is eventually metabolized to vitamin D_3 which is a selective immune system regulator and may inhibit MS progression (Lee et al, 2009). Further, in cross-sectional evaluations of MS and vitamin D, an increased prevalence of clinical vitamin D deficiency was associated with decreased bone density (Mark and Carson, 2006). Given the current evidence of the potential benefits of vitamin D, it appears to be reasonable and safe to consider vitamin D supplementation adequate to achieve normal levels in patients with MS (Solomon and Whitham, 2010).

The evidence is also growing that smoking plays an important role in MS. Studies have shown that smoking increases a person's risk of developing MS and is associated with more severe disease and more rapid disease progression. Fortunately, the evidence also suggests that stopping smoking—whether before or after the onset of MS—is associated with a slower progression of disability (National Multiple Sclerosis Society, 2015).

Medical Management

Fluctuating symptoms and spontaneous remissions make treatments difficult to evaluate. Currently no proven treatment for changing the course of MS, preventing future attacks, or preventing deterioration exists. Initially recovery from relapses is nearly complete, but over time, neurologic deficits remain. Therefore measures to maximize recovery from initial attacks or exacerbations, prevent fatigue and infection, and use all of the available rehabilitative measures to postpone the bedridden stage of disease are imperative. Physical and occupational therapies are standard for weakness, spasticity, tremor, uncoordination, and other symptoms.

Drugs for spasticity can be initiated at a low dose and cautiously increased until the patient responds. Physical therapy for gait training and range-of-motion exercises helps. Steroid therapy is used in treating exacerbations; adrenocorticotropic hormone (ACTH) and prednisolone are the drugs of choice. However, treatment is not consistently effective and tends to be more useful in cases of less than 5 years' duration. Side effects of short-term steroid treatment include increased appetite, weight gain, fluid retention, nervousness, and insomnia. Reduced cerebrospinal fluid and serum levels of vitamin B_{12} and folate have been noted in MS patients who receive high-dose steroids. Methotrexate also may be used with ACTH, causing anorexia and nausea.

Medical Nutrition Therapy

Several dietary regimens for managing MS have been studied, all of which have yielded equivocal results. Various diets such as allergen-free, gluten-free, pectin-free, fructose-restricted, raw food diet, megadoses of micronutrients, zinc phosphates with calcium, and other combinations have not been proven effective. Restriction of saturated fat has been evaluated by several researchers but with inconclusive results. The National Multiple Sclerosis Society has published a guide to vitamin, minerals, and herbs in 2011 that can be useful when working with an MS patient (Bowling and Stewart, 2011). The RDN's evaluation of the patient to maximize nutritional intake is imperative. Vitamin D status should be assessed by measuring 25-hydroxy vitamin D, and supplementation may be warranted (see Appendix 45). There is now some evidence that an anti-inflammatory diet (see Chapter 3 and Appendix 31) can be of use in treating MS. This is an active area of research.

As the disease progresses, neurologic deficits and dysphasia may occur as the result of damaged cranial nerves. Thus diet consistency may have to be modified from solids to mechanically soft or pureed items, even progressing to thick liquids to prevent aspiration. Impaired vision, dysarthria, and poor ambulation make meal preparation into a difficult task. In this situation reliance on comfort foods or prepackaged, single-serving, or convenience foods often permits independent preparation of meals. Given the chronic nature of this debilitating disease, patients may require enteral nutrition support.

Neurogenic bladder is common, causing urinary incontinence, urgency, and frequency. To minimize these problems, distributing fluids evenly throughout the waking hours and limiting them before bed is helpful. Some patients limit fluid intake severely to decrease frequency of urination but thereby increase the risk of urinary tract infections (UTIs). UTIs are common in patients with MS and are associated with MS relapse (Mahadeva et al, 2014).

Neurogenic bowel can cause either constipation or diarrhea, and incidence of fecal impaction is increased in MS. A diet that is high in fiber with additional prunes and adequate fluid can moderate both problems.

Parkinson's Disease

Parkinson's disease (PD) is a progressive, disabling, neurodegenerative disease, first described by James Parkinson in 1817. PD is characterized by slow and decreased movement, muscular rigidity, resting tremor, postural instability, and decreased dopamine transmission to the basal ganglia. Although the natural history of this disease can be remarkably benign in some cases, approximately 66% of patients are disabled within 5 years, and 80% are disabled after 10 years (Yao et al, 2013).

PD is one of the most common neurologic diseases in North America; it affects approximately 1% of the population older than 65 years of age. The incidence is similar across socioeconomic groups, although PD is less common in blacks and Asians in comparison with whites. It most commonly occurs between the ages of 40 and 70.

Pathophysiology

PD is caused by the progressive impairment or deterioration of neurons (nerve cells) in an area of the brain known as the substantia nigra. When functioning normally, these neurons produce the vital brain chemical known as dopamine. The cause of PD is unknown, but several factors appear to play a role. The presence of Lewy bodies, which are clumps of specific substances within brain cells, are microscopic markers of PD. Researchers believe these Lewy bodies hold an important clue to the cause of PD. Lewy bodies are proteins found in abundance in the brainstem area that deplete the neurotransmitter dopamine.

The role of endogenous toxins from cellular oxidative reactions has emerged because aging has been associated with a loss of neurons containing dopamine and an increase in monoamine oxidase. When metabolized (enzymatic oxidation and autoxidation), dopamine produces endogenous toxins (hydrogen peroxide and free radicals), causing peroxidation of membrane lipids and cell death. In the presence of an inherited or acquired predisposition, severe oxidative injury can lead to substantial loss of dopaminergic neurons similar to that observed in PD.

Several other environmental factors also have been implicated as causal factors of PD. The connection between smoking and a lowered risk for PD has been evaluated, but results are inconsistent (Ma et al, 2006). In older patients, drug-induced PD may occur as a side effect of neuroleptics or metoclopramide (see Chapter 8 and Appendix 23).

Dairy products have been linked to PD (Jiang et al, 2014). A meta-analysis of dairy intake and PD risk found a 17% increase in PD for every 200 g/day increment in milk intake. Environmental toxins in the dairy products consumed was not ruled out. Recent epidemiologic studies have shown a link between PD and environmental factors including drinking well water, rural living, farming, diet, and exposure to agricultural chemicals (Pan-Montojo and Reichmann, 2014). PD has also been linked to the exposure to different metals and industrial compounds. Many studies performed in the 1990s identified manganese, lead, copper, iron, zinc, aluminium, or amalgam. Higher incidence of PD has been reported in manganese miners. It was shown that manganese, a component of various pesticides, also reproduces PD symptoms after long and chronic exposure (between 6 months and 16 years). Remarkably, some populations have witnessed a decreasing prevalence of certain types of neurodegenerative diseases that coincide with the disappearance of an environmental factor unique to these populations (Pan-Montojo and Reichmann, 2014).

Nutrient-related findings are biologically plausible and support the hypothesis that oxidative stress may contribute to the pathogenesis of PD (Czlonkowska et al, 2011). The relationships of folate, elevated plasma homocysteine levels, and caloric deficits are being evaluated.

Medical Management

The "classic triad" signs—tremor at rest, rigidity, and bradykinesia—remain the criterion for medical diagnosis. However, it was well over a century before L-dopa (a precursor to dopamine) was introduced for controlling symptoms. Exelon, a cholinesterase inhibitor, was approved by the FDA in 2006 for use in mild to moderate PD dementia. Pharmacotherapy agents, surgical interventions, and physical therapy are the best adjunctive therapies.

Medical Nutrition Therapy

The primary focus of nutrition intervention is to optimize dietary intake particularly to maintain muscle mass for strength and mobility. Nutrition intervention should also focus on drug-nutrient interactions, especially between dietary protein and L-dopa. Side effects of medications for PD include anorexia, nausea, reduced sense of smell, constipation, and dry mouth. To diminish the gastrointestinal side effects of L-dopa, it should be taken with meals. Foods that contain natural L-dopa such as broad beans (fava beans) should be avoided. For some patients dyskinesia may be reduced by limiting dietary protein at breakfast and lunch and including it in the evening meal. Table 40-12 presents a sample menu for this diet.

Fiber and fluid adequacy lessen constipation, a common concern for persons with PD. Pyridoxine (vitamin B_6) has a possible interaction with L-dopa. Decarboxylase, the enzyme required to convert L-dopa to dopamine, depends on pyridoxine. If excessive amounts of the vitamin are present, L-dopa may be metabolized in the periphery and not in the CNS, where its therapeutic activity occurs. Therefore vitamin preparations containing pyridoxine should not be taken with doses of L-dopa. Interactions between pyridoxine and aspartame should be considered as well. In addition, manganese should be carefully monitored to avoid excesses above DRI levels.

The high demand for molecular oxygen, the enrichment of polyunsaturated fatty acids in membrane phospholipids, and the relatively low abundance of antioxidant defense enzymes are all relevant factors (Sun et al, 2008). Antiinflammatory and neuroprotective effects come from phenolic compounds, such as resveratrol from grapes and red wine, curcumin from turmeric, apocynin from *Picrorhiza kurroa*, and epigallocatechin from

TABLE 40-12 Dietary Protein Redistribution with L-Dopa Therapy	
	Amount of Protein (g)
BREAKFAST	
½ C oatmeal	2
1 orange	0.5
1 C Rice Dream beverage	0.5
Egg replacer (unlimited)	0
Low-protein bread toast	0
Margarine or butter (unlimited)	0
Jelly or jam (unlimited)	0
Sugar or sugar substitute (unlimited)	0
Coffee or tea (unlimited)	0
LUNCH	
½ C vegetable soup	2
1 C tossed salad	1
Salad dressing (unlimited)	0
1 banana	1
Low-protein pasta (unlimited)	0
Margarine or butter (unlimited)	0
Low-protein cookies (unlimited)	0
Juice, coffee, tea, or water	0
AFTERNOON SNACK	
Gum drops or hard candy (unlimited)	0
Apple or cranberry juice (unlimited)	0
TOTAL	7
DINNER	
4 oz (at least) beef, pork, veal, chicken	28 or more
1 C stuffing	4
Gravy	0
½ C peas	2
¾ C yogurt	8
1 C milk	8
EVENING SNACK	
1 oz cheese or deli meat	7
4 crackers	2
Juice, herbal tea, or water	0
DAILY TOTAL	66 or more

green tea (Sun et al, 2008). Sufficient intake of vitamin D_3 and omega-3 fatty acids should be recommended.

In a small clinical study seven volunteers with PD agreed to maintain a ketogenic diet for 1 month. Five had improvement in their postdiet test scores. Although this study did not include a control group, it has brought attention to the potential role of ketogenic diet therapy in this disease (Hashim and VanItallie, 2014).

As the disease progresses, rigidity of the extremities can interfere with the patient's ability to eat independently. Rigidity interferes with the ability to control the position of the head and trunk, necessary for eating. Eating is slowed; mealtimes can take up to an hour. Simultaneous movements such as those required to handle a knife and fork become difficult. Tremors in the arms and hands may make consuming liquids independently impossible without spilling. Perception and spatial organization can become impaired. Dysphagia is often a late complication. A large number of patients may be silent aspirators, which affects nutrition status.

Experimental treatment procedures are being tested and reported with increasing frequency. Deep brain penetration, other surgical interventions, and efforts with stem cell research continue in hopes that a "cure" is possible.

CLINICAL CASE STUDY

Clarence is a 74-year-old white man hospitalized for evaluation of dementia progression and recent hearing difficulty. He was diagnosed with Parkinson's disease 5 years ago. He has been taking L-dopa and furosemide (Lasix). He lives wife, who is his primary caregiver. Clarence is 5'10" and currently weighs 155 lb. His medical chart indicates that his weight was 170 lb at his last hospital visit 6 months ago, after a fall. Clarence's wife notes that his appetite and hearing seem to have changed and he shows little interest in food at meal times. They don't talk much during meals and staff have observed his wife helping him eat and suspect some problems with nutrition. His wife describes his eating is very slow, sometimes taking 2 hours for a meal. He coughs a lot after he eats. When asked about whether Clarence is losing weight his wife wasn't sure, but said his pants do seem to be getting looser.

Inadequate energy intake r/t decreased food intake as evidenced by weight loss and clothes getting looser.

Difficulty swallowing related to PD as evidenced by slow eating pace and coughing during meals.

Nutrition Care Questions

1. What dietary advice do you have for Clarence and his caregiver?
2. What changes in Clarence's diet would you recommend?
3. What other evaluations does Clarence need?
4. What possible food-drug interaction could be occurring?

USEFUL WEBSITES

Alzheimer's Association
http://alz.org/
American Stroke Association
http://www.strokeassociation.org
Center for Disease Control
http://www.cdc.gov
The Charlie Foundation for Ketogenic Therapies
http://www.charliefoundation.org/
Epilepsy Foundation
http://www.epilepsyfoundation.org
Migraine Awareness Group
http://www.migraines.org
Myasthenia Gravis Foundation of America, Inc
http://www.myasthenia.org
National Headache Foundation
http://www.headaches.org
National Human Genome Research Institute
http://www.genome.gov
National Institute of Neurological Disorders and Stroke
http://www.ninds.nih.gov/
National Institutes of Health: Swallowing Disorders
http://www.ninds.nih.gov/disorders/swallowing_disorders/
swallowing_disorders.htm
National Institute of Neurologic Disorders and Stroke: Stroke Page
http://www.ninds.nih.gov/disorders/stroke/stroke.htm
National Multiple Sclerosis Society
http://www.nationalmssociety.org/
The Michael J Fox Foundation for Parkinson's Research
https://www.michaeljfox.org/
Parkinson's Disease Foundation
http://www.pdf.org/en/symptoms

REFERENCES

American Dietetic Association (ADA): *Spinal Cord Injury and Nutrition Guideline.* http://www.adaevidencelibrary.com/category. cfm?cid=14&cat=0. Accessed October 30, 2010.

American Heart Association, American Stroke Association: *Impact of Stroke (Stroke Statistics).* http://www.strokeassociation.org/STROKEORG/About-Stroke/Impact-of-Stroke-Stroke-statistics_UCM_310728_Article.jsp. Accessed January 16, 2015.

Bowling A, Stewart T: *Vitamins, Minerals and Herbs in MS: an Introduction.* http://www.nationalmssociety.org/NationalMSSociety/media/MSNational-Files/Brochures/Brochure-Vitamins,-Minerals,-and-Herbs-in-MS_-An-Introduction.pdf. Accessed January 16, 2015.

Brain Trauma Foundation: *Guidelines for the management of severe traumatic brain injury,* ed 3, New York, NY, 2007, Brain Trauma Foundation. http://www.braintrauma.org/pdf/protected/Guidelines_Management_2007w_bookmarks.pdf. Accessed January 30, 2015.

Center for Disease Control and Prevention (CDC): *Rates of TBI-related Emergency Department Visits, Hospitalizations and Deaths-US 2001-2010,* 2014a. http://www.cdc.gov/traumaticbraininjury/data/rates.html. Accessed January 30, 2015.

Centers for Disease Control and Prevention (CDC): *Stroke Statistics and Maps,* 2014b. http://www.cdc.gov/stroke/statistics_maps.htm. Accessed May 16, 2015.

Czlonkowska A, Kurkowska-Jastrzebska I: Inflammation and gliosis in neurological diseases—clinical implications, *J Neuroimmunol* 231:78, 2011.

Eddy CM, et al: The cognitive impact of antiepileptic drugs, *Ther Adv Neuro Disord* 4:385, 2011.

Eldar AH, Chapman J: Guillain Barre syndrome and other immune mediated neuropathies: diagnosis and classification, *Autoimmun Rev* 13:525, 2014.

Epilepsy Foundation: *About Epilepsy, the Basics,* 2014. http://www.epilepsy.com/start-here/about-epilepsy-basics. Accessed January 30, 2015.

Hadijvassiliou M, et al: Gluten sensitivity: from gut to brain, *Lancet Neurol* 9:318, 2010.

Hashim SA, VanItallie TB: Ketone body therapy: from the ketogenic diet to the oral administration of ketone ester, *J Lipid Res* 55:1818, 2014.

Herbert MR, Buckley JA: Autism and dietary therapy: case report and review of the literature, *J Child Neurol* 28:975, 2013.

Hersh CM, Fox RJ: *Multiple Sclerosis.* http://www.clevelandclinicmeded.com/medicalpubs/diseasemanagement/neurology/multiple_sclerosis/Default.htm#top. Accessed January 16, 2015.

Hung KL, et al: Mutational analyses on X-linked adrenoleukodystrophy reveal a novel cryptic splicing and three missense mutations in the ABCD1 gene, *Pediatr Neurol* 49:185, 2013.

International Alliance of ALS/MND Associations: *What Is ALS/MND?* www.alsmndalliance.org/whatis.html. Accessed January 30, 2015.

Jiang W, et al: Dairy foods intake and risk of Parkinson's disease: a dose response meta-analysis of prospective cohort studies, *Eur J Epidemiol* 29:613, 2014.

Kossoff EH, et al: Optimal clinical management of children receiving the ketogenic diet: recommendations of the International Ketogenic Diet Study Group, *Epilepsia* 50:304, 2009.

Kumada T, et al: Modified Atkins Diet and low glycemic index treatment for medication-resistant epilepsy: current trends in ketogenic diet, *J Neurol Neurophysiol* S2:007, 2013. doi: 10.4172/2155-9562.S2-007.

Lee P, et al: Adequacy of vitamin D replacement in severe deficiency is dependent on body mass index, *Am J Med* 122:1056, 2009.

Ma L, et al: Dietary factors and smoking as risk factors for PD in a rural population in China: a nested case-control study, *Acta Neurol Scand* 113:278, 2006.

Mahadeva A, et al: Urinary tract infections in multiple sclerosis: underdiagnosed and under-treated? *Am J Clin Exp Immunol* 3:57, 2014.

Mark BL, Carson JA: Vitamin D and autoimmune disease—implications for practice from the multiple sclerosis literature, *J Am Diet Assoc* 106:418, 2006.

McCullough G, et al: National Dysphagia Diet: What to swallow? *The AHA Leader,* November 2003.

Meschia JF, et al: Guidelines for the Primary Prevention of Stroke; A Statement for Healthcare Professionals from the American Heart Association/American Stroke Association, *Stroke* 45:3754, 2014.

National Dysphagia Diet Task Force: *National Dysphagia Diet: Standardization for Optimal Care*, Chicago, IL, 2002, American Dietetic Association.

National Institutes of Health (NIH): *National Center for Complimentary and Integrative Health (NCCIH): Omega-3 supplements: an introduction*, 2013. https://nccih.nih.gov/health/omega3/introduction.htm. Accessed January 11, 2015.

National Multiple Sclerosis Society: *Smoking*. http://www.nationalmssociety.org/smoking. Accessed January 16, 2015.

Pan-Montojo F, Reichmann H: Considerations on the role of environmental toxins in idiopathic Parkinson's disease pathophysiology, *Transl Neurodegener* 3:10, 2014. http://www.ncbi.nlm.nih.gov/pmc/articles/PMC4019355. Accessed January 30, 2015.

Paganoni S, Wills AM: High-fat and ketogenic diets in amyotrophic lateral sclerosis, *J Child Neuro* 28:989, 2013.

Painter TJ, et al: Immune enhancing nutrition in traumatic brain injury – A preliminary study, *Int J Surg* 21:70, 2015.

Patel A, et al: Long-term outcomes of children treated with the ketogenic diet in the past, *Epilepsia* 51:1277, 2010.

Polman CH, et al: Diagnostic criteria for multiple sclerosis: 2010 revisions to the McDonald criteria, *Ann Neurol* 69:292, 2011.

Porta N, et al: The ketogenic diet and its variants: state of the art, *Rev Neurol* 165:430, 2009.

Prins M, Matsumoto JH: The collective therapeutic potential of cerebral ketone metabolism in traumatic brain injury, *J Lipid Res* 55:2450, 2014.

Sassa T, et al: Lorenzo's oil inhibits ELOVL1 and lowers the level of sphingomyelin with a saturated very long-chain fatty acid, *J Lipid Res* 55:524, 2014.

Sharma S, et al: A pyrazole curcumin derivative restores membrane homeostasis disrupted after brain trauma, *Exp Neurol* 226:191, 2010.

Solomon AJ, Whitham RH: Multiple sclerosis and vitamin D: a review and recommendations, *Curr Neurol Neurosci Rep* 10:389, 2010.

Strand EA, et al: Management of oral-pharyngeal dysphagia symptoms in amyotrophic lateral sclerosis, *Dysphagia* 11:129, 1996.

Su HM: Mechanisms of n-3 fatty acid-mediated development and maintenance of learning memory performance, *J Nutr Biochem* 21:364, 2010.

Sun AY, et al: Botanical phenolics and brain health, *Neuromolecular Med* 10:259, 2008.

Weber S, et al: Modified Atkins diet to children and adolescents with medical intractable epilepsy, *Seizure* 18:237, 2009.

Yao SC, et al: An evidence-based osteopathic approach to Parkinson disease, *Osteopath Fam Phys* 5:96, 2013.

Zupec-Kania BA, et al: An update on diets in clinical practice, *J Child Neuro* 28:1015, 2013.

41

MNT in Psychiatric and Cognitive Disorders

Jacob Teitelbaum, MD; Alan Weiss, MD;
Geri Brewster, RDN, MPH, CDN;
Ruth Leyse-Wallace, PhD

KEY TERMS

addiction
advanced glycation end products
  (AGEs)
alpha-linolenic acid
alpha-lipoic acid
alcoholism
Alzheimer's disease (AD)
anxiety
arachidonic acid
bipolar disorders
chronic fatigue syndrome (CFS)

dementia
depression
dopamine
Diagnostic and Statistical Manual of
  Mental Disorders (DSM-5)
docosahexaenoic acid (DHA)
dysthymia
eicosapentaenoic acid (EPA)
enteric nervous system (ENS)
epinephrine

fibromyalgia syndrome (FMS)
glutamate
leaky gut (intestinal hyperpermeability)
major depressive disorder (MDD)
mild cognitive impairment (MCI)
neurotransmission
norepinephrine
serotonin
serotonin syndrome
vascular dementia

Most illnesses reflect widespread disorders in many parts of the body and are a mix of physical and psychologic factors. For example, heart attacks are more common in those with higher levels of hostility (Izawa et al, 2011), and schizophrenia and autism have been associated with many factors, including food sensitivities (Jackson et al, 2012; Teitelbaum et al, 2011). Unfortunately, conditions may be labeled as psychologic from a mindset that views the condition as "less real" than other illnesses. This is especially common until a biologic marker or laboratory test is available for an illness. For example, multiple sclerosis was previously called "hysterical paralysis," thought to be caused by an oedipal complex; and lupus was once considered to be a neurosis, until tests for these conditions were developed. Chronic fatigue syndrome (CFS) and fibromyalgia (FMS) are now just moving beyond this same approach.

As this shift occurs, the artificial and unhealthy boundary between mental and physical illnesses is fading, being replaced with a more accurate reality that treatment in general is most effective when it treats the whole person, recognizing that physiologic underpinnings are causative in many mental health disorders. The psychologic consequences of suboptimal nutritional intake may occur before the physical signs. Suspicions may begin with a diet history indicating irregular eating habits and unhealthy food choices and progress through a nutrition-focused physical examination, to biochemical assessment and resolution of symptoms with supplementation.

The brain weighs approximately 3 lb (1.4 kg). Nerve cells (neurons) gather and transmit electrochemical signals via axons and dendrites. Neurons are the "gray matter" of the brain; dendrites and axons are the "white matter." The cerebrum is the largest part of the brain divided into two halves, which are divided into four lobes, in each hemisphere: (1) the frontal lobes involved with speech, thought, learning, emotion, and movement; (2) the parietal lobes, which process sensory information such as touch, temperature, and pain; (3) the occipital lobes, dealing with vision; and (4) the temporal lobes, which are involved with hearing and memory. The central nervous system consists of the brain and the spinal cord, which connect to the peripheral nervous system, which extends throughout the body (see Figure 41-1).

The brain is approximately 80% fat. The fatty acid composition of neuronal cell membrane phospholipids reflects their intake in the diet. The degree of a fatty acid's unsaturation determines its three-dimensional structure and thus membrane fluidity and function. The ratio between omega-3 and omega-6 polyunsaturated fatty acids (PUFAs) influences various aspects of serotoninergic and catecholaminergic neurotransmission. Beyond their role in brain structure, essential fatty acids (EFAs) are involved in the synthesis and functions of neurotransmitters and in the molecules of the immune system. Nutrition can impact multiple functions in most parts of the brain (see Box 41-1).

Nerve cells communicate through the release of molecules of neurotransmitters from the transmitting (releasing) end of one nerve cell, through the synapse between them, to the receiving end (receptors) of a nearby neuron. There are numerous neurotransmitters, including serotonin, acetylcholine, dopamine, norepinephrine, epinephrine, and glutamate. Amino acids such as tryptophan, tyrosine, and glycine are examples of nutrients necessary to the formation of neurotransmitters (see Table 41-1).

One of the most important contributions of nutrition to mental health is maintaining the structure and function of the

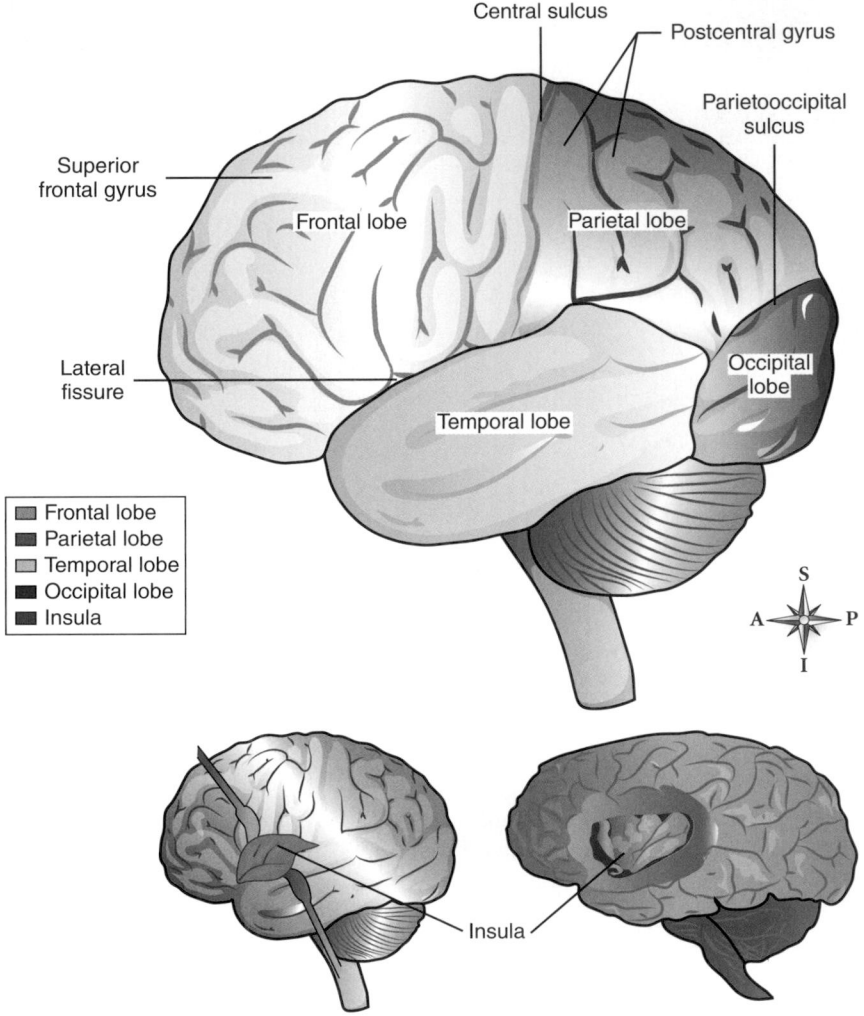

FIGURE 41-1 The human brain

neurons and neurotransmitters in the nervous system. The production of neurotransmitters requires adequate amounts of nutrients. Among these nutrients are amino acids (tryptophan, tyrosine, and glutamine), minerals (zinc, copper, iron, selenium, magnesium), and B vitamins (B_1, B_2, B_3, B_6, B_{12}, folic acid). These neurotransmitters and nutrients coordinate communication within the body and between the body and the environment. People often ask the question "Which nutrients are important for proper nervous system functioning, including mood?" The proper response is simply, "All of them".

Because the conditions discussed here largely reflect metabolic, biochemical and genetic derangements (e.g., nutritional deficiencies, food sensitivities, and alterations in neurotransmitter levels) rather than structural issues (e.g., cancers or heart attacks), they

✷ NEW DIRECTIONS

Brain-Derived Neurotrophic Factor (BDNF)

Brain-derived neurotrophic factor, also known as *BDNF*, is a protein found in the brain and the peripheral nerves. It plays a role in the growth, differentiation, and maintenance of nerve cells. In the brain, BDNF binds to receptors in the synapses between neurons, increasing voltage, and improving signal strength. The synapses can change and adapt over time in response to experience, a characteristic called *synaptic plasticity*. The BDNF protein helps regulate synaptic plasticity, which is important for learning and memory.

Inside the cells, BDNF activates genes that increase production of more BDNF and other important proteins, as well as serotonin, the neurotransmitter vital for learning and self-esteem. Low levels of BDNF have been associated with depression and even suicide.

The BDNF protein is found in regions of the brain that control eating, drinking, and body weight; and likely contributes to the management of these functions.

Certain common genetic variations (polymorphisms; see Chapter 5) in the BDNF gene have been associated with an increased risk of developing psychiatric disorders such as bipolar disorder, schizophrenia, anxiety, and eating disorders.

A particular polymorphism in the *BDNF* gene alters the amino acid sequence in the protein, replacing valine with methionine at position 66 (written at Val66Met or V66M), which impairs the protein's ability to function. Many studies report an association between the Val66Met polymorphism and psychiatric disorders; however, some studies have not supported these findings. It is still unclear how changes in the *BDNF* gene are related to these disorders. See http://ghr.nlm.nih.gov/gene/BDNF.

TABLE 41-1 Neurotransmitters: Precursors and Urinary Metabolites

Neurotransmitter	Precursors	Required Co-Factors	Urinary Metabolite
Norepinephrine	Phenylalanine and tyrosine	Copper, SAMe, vitamin C	Vanilmandelate (VMA)
Norepinephrine to epinephrine	Phenylalanine and tyrosine	Copper, SAMe, vitamin C	Vanilmandelate (VMA)
Dopamine	Phenylalanine and tyrosine	Tetrahydrobiopterin (BH4), vitamin B_6	Homovanillate (HVA)
Serotonin	Tryptophan	Tetrahydrobiopterin (BH4), vitamin B_6	5-Hydroxyindole-acetate (5-HIAA)

can often be dramatically improved through optimization of the diet. An example is hypothyroidism-induced depression or **dysthymia** that can be corrected by identification and treatment of iodine deficiency. This makes medical nutrition therapy (MNT) a very valuable component of treatment for these conditions.

THE ENTERIC NERVOUS SYSTEM (ENS)

The gut has a huge number of neurons, with the gut often being called the **enteric nervous system (ENS)** or "the second brain," which functions autonomously (Gershon, 1999). The ENS contains about 100 million neurons—fewer than the brain, but more than the spinal cord. Acetylcholine and norepinephrine are major neurotransmitters in the ENS. Neural activity in the gut is triggered by receptors that respond to mechanical, thermal, osmotic, and chemical stimuli. Bidirectional information continually passes between the gut and CNS. Factors such as psychologic stress, gender, and reproductive status influence transit time through the gut. Neurologic and gastrointestinal conditions may have gut and brain components (Sharkey and Savidge, 2014).

The gastrointestinal tract is colonized by more than 10 trillion bacteria, more than there are cells in the body. These bacteria and their by-products influence brain function and behavior. Gastrointestinal infections with unhealthy microbiota can influence brain function by causing increased gut membrane permeability, also called "**leaky gut**," which is discussed further in Chapters 26 and 28. Leaky gut can result from a host of bowel infections and medications and is associated with many illnesses such as Crohn's disease, celiac disease, multiple sclerosis, and irritable bowel syndrome. Because of this, both probiotics (which must be enteric coated to survive transit through the stomach acid), and prebiotics (e.g., chicory) which support the growth of heathy gut bacteria, should be included as a routine part of treatment.

BLOOD GLUCOSE REGULATION

Excessive sugar intake can cause wide fluctuations in blood glucose that can amplify aberrant moods and behavior (Young and Benton, 2014). Both high and low blood glucose have been found to have a strong association with a myriad of psychiatric conditions, including anxiety, depression, and schizophrenia (Balhara, 2011). Rapid and abrupt increases in blood sugar (glucose) can trigger rapid and excessive release of insulin. This is followed by a rapid drop in blood sugar as insulin drives glucose into the cells. The body compensates by raising levels of the compounds epinephrine and cortisol, both of which can trigger marked emotional changes and erratic behavior. The effects of insulin persist well beyond the

presence of sugar in the gastrointestinal tract (GIT). The natural response is to consume more sugar as it provides immediate relief of the symptoms of low blood sugar; this is the beginning of an emotional "sugar roller coaster" (Gaby, 2011).

The habit of eating sweets during stress may be physiologically rewarding, as it results in an increased movement of tryptophan into the brain. This occurs as insulin selectively drives other competing amino acids into muscles, leaving more tryptophan to enter the brain. This raises the level of serotonin, causing a soothing effect, the result being people learn to reach for sugar during stress (Page et al, 2011). Over time the increased sugar consumption combined with low fiber intake will cause increasing insulin resistance, paradoxically worsening the symptoms (see Chapter 30). With the average American consuming over 130 lb of sugar yearly (Walton, 2012), this is becoming a major health problem. On the other hand adequate *complex* carbohydrate intake is important because low-carbohydrate diets may have a negative effect on mood (Brinkworth et al, 2009).

To summarize, fluctuations in blood glucose can cause marked mood shifts, which can markedly accentuate psychiatric conditions and associated behavioral disorders. Reducing sugar intake can decrease these blood glucose fluctuations considerably. Higher protein as well as healthy fat intakes can contribute to stabilization of blood sugar levels, often with dramatic clinical and emotional improvement from balancing these three macronutrients (see *Clinical Insight*: Helping Your Client Consume Less Sugar).

CLINICAL INSIGHT

Helping Your Client Consume Less Sugar

- Instruct your client to reduce sugar intake by eliminating sodas and fruit juices, both of which have about ¾ tsp of sugar per ounce; a 64-ounce soda has 48 spoons of sugar: this message may effectively hit home.
- Recommend substituting healthy beverages such as vegetable juices, coconut water, and home-brewed herbal teas, which can be sweetened with sweeteners such as stevia (a processed plant-based sweetener) or erythritol (a sugar alcohol).
- Teach your client how to divide grams of sugar listed on the label by four to figure out how many teaspoons of sugar there are per serving of a food. So, if a serving contains 20 g of sugar as stated on the label – 20/4 = 5 tsp of sugar per serving. The American Heart Association (AHA) recommends adults consume no more than 6 to 9 teaspoons of sugar per day (AHA, 2014). This quick reality check is usually enough to change behavior.

Adapted from: Teitelbaum, J: Beat Sugar Addiction, Fair Winds Press, 2015.

FOOD ALLERGIES AND SENSITIVITIES

Adverse reactions to food (ARF), allergies, and intolerances may contribute to psychologic symptoms, as well as other neurologic issues (see Chapter 26 for a detailed discussion of ARF). Conditions associated with food intolerances include peripheral neuropathy, inflammatory myopathies (muscle dysfunction or inflammation), myelopathies (spinal cord dysfunction or inflammation), and headache, as well as anxiety, schizophrenia, epilepsy, ataxia, Attention-deficit/hyperactivity disorder (ADHD), depression, and autism spectrum disorders (Jackson et al, 2012a). Clinically, complex health conditions without known cause are often found to improve by treating food sensitivities.

THE ROLE OF NUTRIENTS IN MENTAL FUNCTION

Omega-3 Fatty Acids

Omega-3 polyunsaturated fatty acids are the preferred fatty acids in the brain and nervous system. From conception through maturity, the essential omega-3 fatty acids eicosapentaenoic acid (EPA) and docosahexaenoic acid (DHA) make unique and irreplaceable contributions to overall brain and nervous system functioning. Clinical research has shown effective and promising roles for EPA and DHA in various psychiatric conditions (see Box 41-2) (see _Focus On:_ Abbreviations for Fatty Acids).

FOCUS ON

Abbreviations for Fatty Acids

AA	Arachidonic acid
ALA	Alpha (α) linolenic acid
CLA	Conjugated linoleic acid
DGLA	Dihomo-_gamma_ (γ)-linolenic acid
DHA	Docosopentaneoic acid
EFA	Essential fatty acid
EPA	Eicosapentaenoic acid
GLA	Gamma-linolenic acid
HUFA	Highly unsaturated fatty acid
LA	Linoleic acid
LCFA	Long-chain fatty acids
MUFA	Monounsaturated fatty acids
PUFA	Polyunsaturated fatty acids

Alpha-linolenic acid (ALA), an omega-3 fat with 8 carbons and 3 double bonds (18:3), is found in the oil of some seeds and nuts (e.g., flax, chia, sunflower, soybean, and walnuts). **Eicosapentaenoic acid (EPA)** is a 20-carbon omega-3 fatty acid with 5 double bonds (20:5), and **docosahexaenoic acid (DHA)** is a 22-carbon fatty acid with 6 double bonds (22:6). EPA and DHA occur naturally in fatty fish and seafood.

ALA serves as a precursor for EPA and DHA, but the conversion of ALA to EPA is approximately 5% to 10%, and conversion of ALA to DHA is even lower (<3%). Health status, other nutritional factors, and genetic variations in the production of the delta-6 desaturase enzyme may influence the conversion rate. Studies have suggested possible differences in conversion rates between vegetarians and carnivores (Welch et al, 2010). Most nutrition and mental health experts do not recommend reliance on ALA as a source of EPA or DHA.

Arachidonic acid (ARA), a 20-carbon omega-6 fatty acid with 4 double bonds (20:4) serves as a precursor to the eicosanoids prostaglandins, thromboxanes, and leukotrienes, which are involved with inflammation, vasoconstriction, and a multitude of metabolic regulations, and also influence mood (see Chapter 3).

Although specific mechanisms remain unclear, clinical research has shown the importance of sufficient EPA intake for general mental health, and particularly as an adjunctive treatment for depression (Freeman et al, 2006). In general, EPA works better when ingested with DHA. They occur together naturally in foods. DHA is preferred and selectively stored in brain and nerve cells, and makes up much of the mass of brain tissue. It is required for normal brain growth, development, and

maturation and is involved with **neurotransmission** (brain cells communicating with each other), lipid messaging, genetic expression, and cell membrane synthesis. DHA also provides vital structural contributions; DHA is concentrated in the phospholipids of brain cell membranes.

Oily fish such as salmon, sardines, and tuna are high in EPA and DHA, with the freshest fish having the highest levels. Some canned tuna also has significant amounts and may be more practical for those who cannot get fresh fish. Omega-3 levels of canned albacore tuna are higher than "chunk light" canned tuna, and the tuna should be water and not oil packed, because otherwise the omega-3 oils, which are fat soluble, will be lost when the oil is poured off (see Appendix 34).

During Pregnancy and Lactation

Experts recommend that pregnant women consume at least 200 to 300 mg DHA during pregnancy for proper infant development. The role of DHA and EPA in pregnancy and lactation is discussed in Chapter 15. Up to 10% of pregnant women may experience depression, and there is considerable interest in finding effective alternatives to prescription medication. Several pilot trials using EPA and DHA from fish oil have been conducted in depressed pregnant women and women with postpartum depression. One dose-ranging study reported measurable improvements in women who consumed as little as 500 mg of combined EPA and DHA. Experts have also recently suggested that a daily intake of 900 mg DHA during pregnancy may be necessary to support infant and maternal needs.

A landmark study that followed more than 9000 pregnant women and their children for 8 years reported lower intelligence quotient and social development in the children of those women who consumed less than 12 ounces of fish a week while pregnant. In other words, the children of the women who ate fish two or more times a week during their pregnancy fared better emotionally and mentally (Hibbeln and Davis, 2009). Some concern has been raised about high mercury levels in fish during pregnancy (see Chapters 15 and 17); mercury-free omega-3 fatty acid supplements which also dramatically simplify supplementation are now available (see _New Directions:_ Fatty Acid Vectorization).

During Childhood

Depression among children is increasing. At the same time, the few studies measuring consumption of EPA and DHA in children report very low average intakes. The few clinical trials conducted in depressed children have shown significant benefit from EPA and DHA fish oil supplementation.

Some clinical trials using EPA and DHA supplements from fish oil in children with attention-deficit disorder (ADD) or attention-deficit hyperactivity disorder (ADHD) have reported benefit, but not all. The difference in findings may be due to many variables, including study design, dose, age of supplementation, the background diet, genetics, and teacher or family dynamics (Gillies, 2012). However, it has been shown that children with ADD, ADHD, behavior problems, or who are overweight, tend to have lower levels of EPA and DHA in their blood (Antalis et al, 2006). In one study, a total of 132 Australian children aged 7 to 12 years with ADHD participated in a randomized, placebo-controlled, double-blind intervention over 15 weeks, taking omega-3 fatty acids alone, omega-3 fatty acids + micronutrients, or placebo. Significant medium to strong positive treatment effects were found on parent ratings of core ADHD symptoms, inattention, hyperactivity/impulsivity, on the Conners Parent

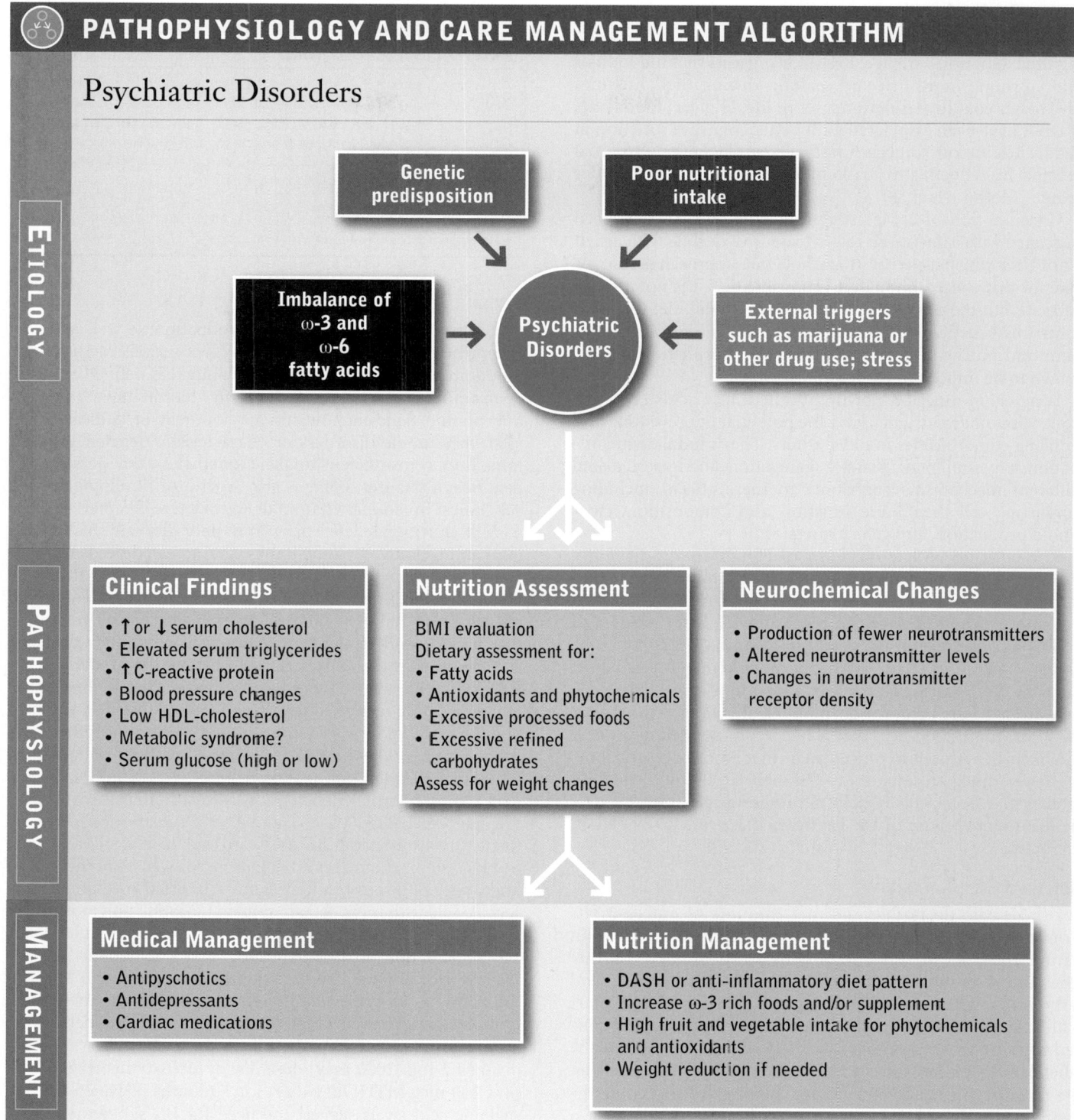

PATHOPHYSIOLOGY AND CARE MANAGEMENT ALGORITHM

Psychiatric Disorders

ETIOLOGY

- Genetic predisposition
- Poor nutritional intake
- Imbalance of ω-3 and ω-6 fatty acids
- Psychiatric Disorders
- External triggers such as marijuana or other drug use; stress

PATHOPHYSIOLOGY

Clinical Findings

- ↑ or ↓ serum cholesterol
- Elevated serum triglycerides
- ↑ C-reactive protein
- Blood pressure changes
- Low HDL-cholesterol
- Metabolic syndrome?
- Serum glucose (high or low)

Nutrition Assessment

BMI evaluation
Dietary assessment for:
- Fatty acids
- Antioxidants and phytochemicals
- Excessive processed foods
- Excessive refined carbohydrates
Assess for weight changes

Neurochemical Changes

- Production of fewer neurotransmitters
- Altered neurotransmitter levels
- Changes in neurotransmitter receptor density

MANAGEMENT

Medical Management

- Antipyschotics
- Antidepressants
- Cardiac medications

Nutrition Management

- DASH or anti-inflammatory diet pattern
- Increase ω-3 rich foods and/or supplement
- High fruit and vegetable intake for phytochemicals and antioxidants
- Weight reduction if needed

Rating Scale (CPRS) in both omega-3 fatty acid treatment groups compared with the placebo group (Sinn and Bryan, 2007) (see Chapter 44 for further discussion of ADD and ADHD).

During Adulthood

According to the World Health Organization (WHO) major depression is a leading cause of disability around the world (WHO, 2012). The intake of seafood has been shown to be inversely related to the incidence of depression in populations around the world. Increases in homicide occurrence have been associated with less seafood consumption. When EPA, DHA,

and multivitamins were given to prison inmates, antisocial behavior, including violence, fell significantly, compared with those on placebo. In another study, teens who had previously attempted suicide made fewer suicide attempts when given EPA and DHA (Hallahan et al, 2007).

With much of the brain composed of the fatty acids found in fish oil (DHA), it is not surprising that fish oil has been shown to be helpful in many conditions. These include depression and schizophrenia unresponsive to drug treatment alone. EPA was also found to be beneficial in treating the depression associated with bipolar illness (manic depressive illness) (Gaby, 2011).

During Senior Adulthood and Aging

Not surprisingly, omega-3 fatty acids assist in maintaining cognitive function with age. Research suggests that individuals who consume more fish and seafood during their lifetimes have better cognitive function later in life. Higher blood levels of DHA have been associated with better cognitive function in middle adulthood. Omega-3 fatty acids may have substantial benefits in reducing the risk of cognitive decline in older people (Molfino et al, 2014).

Consumption of a Mediterranean-type diet has also been associated with a decreased rate of cognitive decline with age. It is not clear which aspect of this whole diet approach is responsible for this effect, although it is possible that it is not a single nutrient, but the combined effects of the overall diet that produces this benefit. The Mediterranean diet is high in antioxidants and nutrients such as choline and phosphatidylcholine, known to be important for brain function.

Long-chain omega-3 polyunsaturated fatty acids (PUFAs), along with other nutrients, have the potential of preventing and reducing comorbidities in older adults. They modulate inflammation, hyperlipidemia, platelet aggregation, and hypertension. Different mechanisms contribute to these effects, including supporting cell membrane function and composition, eicosanoid production, and gene expression.

The position of The Academy of Nutrition and Dietetics (AND) includes a recommendation for children and adults to eat fish at least twice a week. The 2004 recommendation of the International Society for the Study of Fatty Acids and Lipids is consumption of a daily minimum of 500 mg combined of EPA and DHA. With caveats inherent for ecologic, nutrient disappearance analyses, a healthy dietary allowance for omega-3 fatty acids for current U.S. diets was estimated at 3.5 g/day for a 2000-kcal diet. This recommended allowance can likely be reduced to one tenth of that amount by consuming fewer omega-6 fatty acids (Hibbeln et al, 2006). Higher intakes may be especially helpful in neurologic and psychiatric disorders because of the key roles these omega-3s play in the brain.

Omega-3 Supplements

For those who do not get optimal amounts of omega-3 fats from their diet, supplements can be useful and effective. In nature 1000 mg of fish oil contains approximately 180 mg EPA and 120 mg DHA; the remainder is other oils and fatty acids. Therapeutic amounts of EPA and DHA start with around 400 mg of each. Supplement companies sell concentrates of varying dosages, so it is important to read the label. It is also important to make sure the label indicates that the fat is free of heavy metals such as mercury and contaminants such as organophosphates. Tasting the contents of a fish oil capsule can reveal rancid oil, which should not be consumed.

Omega-3 supplements containing krill oil have the added advantage of containing phosphatidylcholine and the phytonutrient astaxanthin, a natural antioxidant that gives krill oil its red color. An algal (vegetarian) source of DHA is also available for vegetarians and vegans. For most people, using a vectorized pure omega-3 with phospholipids is best, and allows optimal supplementation with one to two tablets a day instead of 8 to 16 capsules, while also avoiding problems of contamination with chemicals or heavy metals (see New Directions: Fatty Acid Vectorization).

✳ NEW DIRECTIONS

Fatty Acid Vectorization

A new process called "vectorization" yields a source of omega-3 fatty acids, in which the fatty acid is positioned in the center position of a glycerol (sn2) instead of position three (sn3). The COOH end of the fatty acid is phosphorylated, creating a phospholipid. Phospholipids have been shown to be a superior carrier of DHA and EPA, enhancing the absorption of the omega-3 fatty acids up to 50-fold over fish oil. One such product, "Vectomega" is available in Europe (Bourre, 2004; Parmentier et al, 2007). These products allow high levels of omega-3 fatty acid support with fewer pills or capsules.

Vitamins

Vitamins are critical for energy production as well as many other reactions, and deficiencies can cause serious cognitive and mood problems. Insufficient vitamin intake is defined as intake of an amount below the reference daily vitamin intake amounts, but vitamin deficiency means development of clinically relevant, measurable disorders or characteristic deficiency symptoms due to insufficient intake. Nonetheless, any person with insufficient vitamin intake is also at risk for development of a subclinical functional vitamin deficiency (see Chapter 7).

Mild nutritional deficiencies from poor diet can cause behavioral and cognitive dysfunction as can increased needs from altered metabolism resulting from gene mutations (see Chapter 5). Obtaining the levels of micronutrients shown in studies to change brain function often requires a pharmacologic, rather than an DRI level of supplementation, and cannot be reasonably achieved by diet alone. Described below are the function of selected vitamins and minerals involved in psychiatric conditions.

Studies have identified genetic mutations that alter the production and function of serotonin, dopamine, and other neurotransmitters. These alterations may sometimes be identified by various biochemical or deoxyribonucleic acid (DNA) tests. For example, the methylenetetrahydrofolate reductase (MTHFR) test can reveal alleles (C > T and A > C substitutions) that influence folate metabolism and can lead to a decrease in the production of serotonin and dopamine, as well as an increase in homocysteine levels resulting from a blocked metabolic pathway. People with these genetic single nucleotide polymorphisms (SNPs) (see Chapter 5) with active illness may require folate supplementation in a methylated (5-methyltetrahydrofolate -MTHF) form. Over half the adult population has an MTHFR mutation, so its presence is often not significant. An elevated homocysteine, or even a high folic acid level, should increase the index of suspicion and suggests there should be a clinical trial of giving a 2-mg (2000 mcg) dose/day of hydroxymethylcobalmin plus 200 mcg MTHF/day daily for 3 months. Elevated methylmalonic acid levels suggest the need for B_{12} supplementation, especially in the presence of elevated serum homocysteine levels (see Chapters 7 and 32) (see Appendix 40 for food sources of folic acid and vitamin B_{12}).

Thiamin (Vitamin B_1)

Thiamin diphosphate (TDP), the most bioactive form of thiamine, is an essential coenzyme in glucose metabolism and the biosynthesis of neurotransmitters, including acetylcholine, γ-aminobutyrate, glutamate, aspartate, and serotonin. Norepinephrine, serotonin, and glutamate, as well as their receptors, are potential targets for antidepressive therapies. The degradation rate of TDP, bound to its dependent enzymes, is directly proportional to the available amount of its main substrate, carbohydrate. Body stores of B_1 fall rapidly during fasting. Low TDP concentrations and impaired thiamin-dependent enzymatic activities have been detected in the brains of patients with Alzheimer's disease (AD), Parkinson's dementia (PD), and other neurodegenerative diseases (Zhang et al, 2013).

Wernicke encephalopathy (WE) is a potentially reversible, yet serious neurologic manifestation caused by vitamin B_1 (thiamin) deficiency. It is commonly associated with heavy alcohol consumption but is also reported with the excessive vomiting of hyperemesis gravidum, and vomiting after bariatric surgery. Most patients present with the triad of ocular signs (nystagmus), ataxia, and confusion (see Chapter 29).

Guidelines by the European Federation of Neurological Societies (EFNS) recommend that patients with alcoholism or the conditions mentioned above receive thiamin, 200 mg tid, administered IV, before starting any carbohydrate or glucose intake, and that it be continued until there is no further improvement in signs and symptoms (see Chapter 29). For nonalcoholic patients, an intravenous dose of thiamin, 100 to 200 mg once daily, may be sufficient (Galvin et al, 2010).

In a double-blind study 50 mg/day of thiamin (vs. placebo) was associated with reports of being more clearheaded, composed, and energetic. These influences took place in subjects whose thiamin status was adequate according to traditional criteria (Benton et al, 1997). Learning disorders as well as behavioral problems in young children (sometimes to the point of hospitalization) were shown to improve with a high-dose thiamin supplement (Fattal et al, 2011). People with AD were shown to have lower serum thiamin levels than those with other types of dementia (Lu'o'ng and Nguyen, 2011). Some medications may interact with thiamin (see Box 41-3).

Riboflavin (Vitamin B₂)

Biochemical signs of riboflavin depletion appear within a few days of dietary deprivation. Poor riboflavin status interferes with iron handling and contributes to the etiology of anemia when iron intakes are low. Riboflavin is involved in determining circulating concentrations of homocysteine and may exert some of its effects by reducing the metabolism of other B vitamins, notably folate and vitamin B_6, of particular interest in psychiatric disorders. In those with frequent migraines, supplementing with 400 mg of riboflavin a day decreased migraine frequency by 50% to 69% after 6 weeks of use (Markley, 2012).

BOX 41-3 Medications that May Cause Vitamin B1 Deficiency

- Digoxin—Laboratory studies suggest that digoxin (a medication used to treat heart conditions) may reduce the ability of heart cells to absorb and use vitamin B1; this may be particularly true when digoxin is combined with furosemide (Lasix, a loop diuretic).
- Diuretics—Diuretics (particularly furosemide, a loop diuretic) may reduce levels of vitamin B1 in the body.
- Phenytoin (Dilantin)—Some evidence suggests people taking phenytoin have lower levels of thiamin in their blood, and that may contribute to the side effects of the drug. However, that is not true of all people who take phenytoin.

Reference: University of Maryland Medical Center: *Possible interactions with vitamin B1* (thiamine) (website): http://umm.edu/health/medical/altmed/supplement-interact on/possible-interactions-with-vitamin-b1-thiamine, 2013. Accessec January 26, 2015.

Niacin (Vitamin B₃)

Niacin is a key component of the molecule NADH, which is important for production of the neurotransmitter dopamine. One of the signs of pellagra, the niacin-deficiency disease, is dementia. Pellagra can be a cause of delirium during alcohol withdrawal (Oldham and Ivkovic, 2012). Acute pellagra resembles sunburn in its first stages. Psychiatric manifestations are fairly common, but are easily overlooked due to their nonspecific nature. Examples include irritability, poor concentration, anxiety, fatigue, restlessness, apathy, and depression (Prakash et al, 2008).

A 5½-year, prospective, population study of more than 3700 people showed that those who had the lowest niacin intake (14 mg/day) were 70% more likely to develop AD than individuals who had the highest intake (45 mg/day). A benefit was shown with an increased intake up to 17 mg/day (Morris et al, 2004; Morris et al, 2005).

Vitamin B₁₂

The symptoms of vitamin B_{12} deficiency may include agitation, irritability, confusion, disorientation, amnesia, impaired concentration and attention, and insomnia. Mental symptoms may also include stupor, apathy, negativism, memory and judgment disorders or even psychoses, depression, and dementia (Grober et al, 2013). Catatonia is also described as a psychiatric form of vitamin B_{12} deficiency. Psychiatric disorders that may be diagnosed in patients having B_{12} deficiency include depression, bipolar disorder, panic disorder, psychosis, phobias, and dementia.

A vitamin B_{12} deficiency may express itself in a wide variety of neurologic manifestations such as paresthesias, coordination disorders, and reduced nerve conduction velocity and in the elderly, with progressive brain atrophy. Cobalamin contributes to hematopoiesis, myelin synthesis, and synthesis of epithelial tissue.

Seventy-five to ninety percent of persons with a clinically relevant B_{12} deficiency have neurologic disorders, and in about 25% of cases these are the only clinical manifestations of the B_{12} deficiency. Levels less than 200 ng/L are sure signs of a B_{12} deficiency, but a functional B_{12} deficiency may also be present at levels under 450 ng/L.

Moderately elevated concentrations of homocysteine (>10 μmol/L) have been associated with an increased risk of dementia, notably AD, in many cross-sectional and prospective studies. Raised plasma concentrations of homocysteine are associated with regional and whole-brain atrophy, not only in AD but also in healthy elderly people. Determination of methylmalonic acid and homocysteine are particularly recommended in cases of diagnostically unclarified B_{12} deficiency.

Possible nutrient-drug interactions occur with antibiotics, anticonvulsants, colchicine, metformin, and N_2O. Proton pump inhibitors reduce gastric acid secretion and thus the intestinal release of vitamin B_{12} from foods (see Chapter 8).

Hydroxycobalamin, methylcobalamin, and cyanocobalamin are suitable for treatment. The lowest dose of oral cyanocobalamin required to normalize mild vitamin B_{12} deficiency is more than 200 times the recommended dietary allowance of approximately 3 μg daily (i.e., >500 μg per day). For deficiency resulting from absorption disorders, doses of 500 to 2000 μg/day are required. A *Cochrane Group* review concluded that 1000 to 2000 μg/day, administered orally, was as effective as intramuscular B_{12} in achieving hematologic and neurologic responses (Vidal-Alaball et al, 2005), though IM B_{12} will achieve normalization more quickly and ensure compliance at the start of treatment.

In a recent randomized and double-blind interventional study (VITACOG study) involving 168 elderly persons with mild cognitive impairment (age >70 years), oral supplementation of vitamin B_{12}, folic acid, and vitamin B_6 over a period of 24 months slowed the progression of brain atrophy and the reduction of cognitive performance by 53.3% (Grober et al, 2013).

In a study of people being treated for depression, participants with higher levels of vitamin B_{12} tended to get a greater benefit from antidepressants (Moore et al, 2012).

Folic Acid

Folate deficiency is associated with depression, cognitive decline, and dementia. The NHANES 2010 data examined relations between folate and vitamin B_{12} status biomarkers for mental as well as physical conditions. These conditions included lead and neurobehavioral test performance, anemia and cognitive function, hypothyroidism, and gene-nutrient interactions.

Folate deficiency has been identified as a risk factor for schizophrenia through epidemiologic, biochemical, and gene association studies. Folate plus vitamin B_{12} supplementation can improve negative symptoms of schizophrenia. Negative symptoms imply the lack of something, such as social contacts, initiative, energy, motivation or display of emotion, but treatment response is influenced by genetic variation in folate absorption. These findings support a personalized medicine approach for the treatment of negative symptoms (Roffman et al, 2013).

Folate deficiency may be the result of decreased intake, or increased needs caused by common genetic defects (see MTHFR discussion above). Causes of decreased intake include poor diet, old age, poverty, and alcoholism. Less commonly, inadequate intake can arise through inappropriate and prolonged hyperalimentation or other use of synthetic diets that may be low in folate. Consequences of inadequate intake are compounded when there is an increased folate requirement, such as during pregnancy, lactation, premature birth, and chronic hemolytic anemias, for example, sickle cell anemia and thalassemias (see Chapter 32). Conditions associated with increased cell turnover such as leukemias, aggressive lymphomas, and tumors associated with a high proliferative rate can also cause increased folate demand.

Supplementing with folic acid may help memory. In one study, 818 cognitively healthy people ages 50 to 75 years took either folic acid, 800 mcg, or placebo for 3 years. On memory tests, those who took supplements had scores comparable to people $5\frac{1}{2}$ years younger (Durga et al, 2007).

In addition, low folate is associated with AD, with higher folate levels being associated with a 50% reduction in the risk of developing AD (Luchsinger et al, 2007). Not all studies have shown a protective effect, however, and one study showed a U-shaped curve, with very high folate levels being associated with higher homocysteine levels and a greater risk for developing AD (Faux et al, 2011).

Total homocysteine (tHcy), a nonspecific indicator of inadequate folate status, accumulates with folate inadequacy but is relatively stable across normal folate ranges (Yetley and Johnson, 2011). Folate biomarkers (serum, plasma, and red blood cell folate) increase in response to folic acid in a dose-response manner (Duffy et al, 2014).

Vitamin D

Vitamin D affects hundreds of genes in the human body and is recognized as an important nutrient for brain health as well as for bone and skeletal health. Clinical research has associated vitamin D deficiency with the presence of mood disorders, with aspects of cognitive disorders, as well as increased risk for major and minor depression in older adults (Stewart and Hirani, 2010). Supplementing with vitamin D, however, has shown mixed results (Bertone-Johnson et al, 2012; Kjærgaard et al, 2012).

Vitamin D has a crucial role in proliferation, differentiation, neurotrophism, neuroprotection, neurotransmission, and neuroplasticity of cells. Vitamin D exerts its biologic function not only by influencing cellular processes directly, but also by influencing gene expression. The brain has vitamin D receptors, which help to provide protection against, and even aid in reversal of, neurocognitive decline. In a study that combined vitamin D with the AD medication memantine, the combination therapy was associated with improvement when compared to memantine or vitamin D alone (Annweiler et al, 2012).

Serum levels of vitamin D are most often tested by assessing circulating levels of 25(OH)D, which is the combined product of skin synthesis from sun exposure and dietary sources (see Chapter 7 and Appendix 45). Currently, no "official" agreement has been reached regarding blood levels of 25(OH)D that indicate deficiency, insufficiency, and sufficiency of vitamin D, especially related to brain health. For example, serum levels of 25(OH)D may be low despite a person having an adequate diet or sufficient sun exposure, because of conversion to other forms such as 1,25(OH)D. Many practitioners favor 25(OH)D serum levels of at least 30 ng/ml or 75 nmol/L, although for treatment of cancer, diabetes, autoimmune illness or depression levels of 60 to 80 ng/ml may be beneficial.

The best sources of vitamin D are (1) exposure of a large amount of skin to sunlight for at least 15 to 20 min/day without sunscreen, (2) foods such as oily fish and egg yolks, and (3) vitamin D–fortified foods, such as cow, soy, or other fortified milks, and fortified cereals. The recommended advice regarding sun exposure is to "avoid sunburn—not sunshine" (see Appendix 45).

Minerals

Iron

Iron deficiency results in poor brain myelination and impaired monoamine metabolism. Glutamate and γ-aminobutyric acid homeostasis is modified by changes in brain iron status. Such changes not only produce deficits in memory, learning capacity, and motor skills but also result in emotional and psychologic problems (Kim and Wessling-Resnick, 2014).

Iron deficiency is associated with apathy, depression, and fatigue. Iron deficiency anemia in children is associated with a significantly increased risk of psychiatric disorders, including mood disorders, autism spectrum disorder, attention-deficit hyperactivity disorder, and developmental disorders (Chen et al, 2013) (see Chapters 32 and 44). At 10 years of age, children given iron supplements from 6 months to 12 months of age smiled and laughed more and needed less prompting to complete a social stress task. However, there were no differences in behaviors such as anxiety, depression, or social problems. Benefits in affect and response to reward may improve performance at school and work, mental health, and personal relationships (Lozoff et al, 2014). Anemia is a late sign of iron deficiency, and therefore a normal blood count in no way precludes its presence. In addition, a ferritin under 60 mcg/l (ng/ml), and when anemia is present a < 100 mcg/l (ng/ml), can reflect iron deficiency, even though this level is well within the normal range. (Vaucher 2012; Wang 2009; Kis 1998)

Iron plays a critical role in dopaminergic signaling. Atypical antipsychotic medications, increasingly used in children and adolescents, modulate brain dopamine. In a study of 115 children who had taken risperidone for 2.5 ± 1.7 years, 45% had iron depletion and 14% had iron deficiency. Iron status was inversely associated with weight gain during risperidone treatment. It was also inversely associated with the antipsychotic prolactin concentration, which was nearly 50% higher in the iron-deficient group (Calarge and Ziegler, 2013). Nutrition assessment should include evaluation of iron status. Prolactinemia is a challenging side effect of risperidone therapy, especially in males, that may be improved when iron status is normalized.

Selenium

The essential trace mineral selenium is a constituent of selenoproteins, which have important structural and functional roles. Known as antioxidants, they act as a catalyst for the production of active thyroid hormone and are needed for the proper functioning of the immune system. Deficiency has been linked to adverse mood states (Rayman, 2000). One study found that low dietary selenium intake was associated with an approximate tripling of the likelihood for developing de novo Major Depression Disorder (MDD) (Pasco et al, 2012).

Selenium is available in multivitamin/multimineral supplements and as a stand-alone supplement, often in the forms of selenomethionine or selenium-enriched yeast (grown in a high-selenium medium). An optimal dose for supplementation is ~ 55 mcg per day (Akbaraly T, 2010). Selenium poisoning from very large intakes is a concern (Nutall, 2006).

Selenium may have a moderate interaction with some medications. These include anticoagulants, aspirin, clopidogrel (Plavix), warfarin (Coumadin), and cholesterol-lowering drugs atorvastatin (Lipitor), fluvastatin (Lescol), lovastatin (Mevacor), and pravastatin (Pravachol). Selenium may decrease the clearance and excretion time of barbiturates. It may also interact with niacin, vitamins C and E, and beta-carotene (Web MD, 2009). See Chapter 8 and Appendix 23.

Zinc

Zinc imbalance can result not only from insufficient dietary intake but also from impaired activity of zinc transport proteins and zinc-dependent regulation of metabolic pathways. It is known that some neurodegenerative processes are connected with altered zinc homeostasis, and it may influence the state of AD, depression, and aging-related loss of cognitive function (Tyszka-Czochara et al, 2014). Zinc may play a role in regulating the production of dopamine in the brain. Mechanisms of action by which zinc reduces depressive symptoms include (1) decreasing dopamine reuptake (by binding to the dopamine receptor), (2) increasing the conversion of the thyroid hormone T4 to T3, and (3) the promotion of excitatory neurotransmitter function.

A study of older adults in Australia using a food-frequency questionnaire found those with the highest zinc intake had a 30% to 50% reduction of odds of developing depression. They also reported no association between the zinc-to-iron ratio and developing depression (Vashum et al, 2014).

A study of seventh graders showed that 20 mg a day of supplemental zinc improved school performance with improved memory and attention span (Teitelbaum, 2015). Children with attention-deficit hyperactivity disorder had lower blood levels of zinc, ferritin, and magnesium than children without ADHD, but had normal copper levels (Mahmoud et al, 2011).

Amino Acids

In addition to being the building blocks for the key neurotransmitters serotonin (from tryptophan), dopamine, and norepinephrine (both from tyrosine), amino acids are also critical precursors for the antioxidants glutathione (made from glutamine, glycine and N-acetyl cysteine [NAC]). Amino acid sufficiency can be measured either through plasma or urinary amino acids or by urinary organic acid testing, which measures by-products of the particular neurotransmitter pathways (see Table 41-1). As more of the neurotransmitters are found in the gut than in the brain, these tests may only be helpful but certainly are not absolute indicators of brain neurotransmitter levels or adequacy. Amino acid levels can be low due to inadequate protein intake.

The role of serotonin and dopamine in depression is widely known and it is targeted by many medications, but the role of antioxidants gets less attention, despite being important. For example, NAC has been shown to be helpful in a wide array of psychiatric conditions, including addiction, compulsive and grooming disorders, schizophrenia, and bipolar disorder (Dean et al, 2011). Doses of 500 to 2000 mg are commonly used safely and at low cost.

Phytochemicals

New research suggests that plant-based foods rich in bioactive phytochemicals make important nutritional and biochemical contributions to normal brain function and mental health. Promising phytochemicals include three subclasses of flavonoids: flavanols, anthocyanins, and flavanones (see *Focus On: Eating to Detoxify* in Chapter 19). These phytochemicals have antioxidant activity, but their more important contributions may be in protecting and preserving brain cell structure and metabolism through a complex cascade of cellular mechanisms, including signaling, transcription, phosphorylation, and gene expression (Spencer, 2010). Foods such as berries, citrus fruits, green tea, and some spices contain phytochemicals, as well as essential vitamins and minerals. Curcumin may be especially neuroprotective, being associated with lower risks of Alzheimer's and Parkinson's Disease (see Alzheimer's discussion below).

There is evidence that numerous other plant-based molecules have nutritional and possibly pharmacologic effects in the brain, and the mechanisms are sometimes unknown. These molecules appear to affect brain health through antioxidant, antiinflammatory, and nutragenomic influences. Other mechanisms are also plausible. Examples of these foods include onion, ginger, turmeric, oregano, sage, rosemary, and garlic. This is an exciting area of research to watch in the twenty-first century. In a study on sulforaphane treatment of autism spectrum disorder (ASD) by Singh et al (2014), participants receiving sulforaphane, a broccoli seed extract, had improvement in social interaction, abnormal behavior, and verbal communication. Sulforaphane, which showed negligible toxicity, was selected because it upregulates genes that protect aerobic cells against oxidative stress, inflammation, and DNA damage, all of which are prominent and possibly mechanistic characteristics of ASD (see Chapter 44).

Nutritional Supplements

People experiencing cognitive and mood dysfunction, or psychosis, often have difficulty maintaining a healthy diet despite guidance. Levels of some nutrients may require intakes in excess of the RDA, which often cannot be obtained through diet. A multivitamin is a reasonable solution (Davison and Kaplan, 2011).

There are hundreds of psychiatric disorders, which fall into general categories as shown in Table 41-2.

TABLE 41-2   Medical Nutrition Therapy (MNT) for Psychiatric Disorders

A psychiatric diagnosis is based on symptoms observed or reported. A psychoanalytic diagnosis involves the etiology and meaning of symptoms. *The Diagnostic and Statistical Manual of Mental Disorders*, Fifth Edition (DSM-5), is used by both groups of mental health professionals.
There are hundreds of psychiatric disorders, which fall into the thirteen categories below.
MNT therapy for psychiatric disorders requires a nutritional assessment, which takes into account the following:

1. Increase or decrease in appetite
2. Increase or decrease in activity level and therefore calorie requirements
3. Use of medications which cause dry mouth, thirst, and constipation
4. Decrease in ability to concentrate, understand, and follow directions
5. Altered nutritional needs due to use of alcohol, drugs, or tobacco
6. Possible decrease in ability for self-care such as adequate income, shopping, meal preparation
7. History of food choices or comorbid conditions that result in suboptimal or deficient nutritional intake, or supplement use while restoring healthy eating habits
8. Use of food or nutrition supplements as the "Magic Answer" in therapy

Psychiatric Disorder	Description	Examples	Nutrition Strategies
Adjustment disorders	A group of symptoms, such as stress, feeling sad or hopeless, and physical symptoms that can occur after a stressful life event. Difficulty coping can result in a stronger reaction than expected for the type of event that occurred.		Small, concrete steps and goals. Assess physical symptoms and changes (fatigue, diarrhea, activity level, etc.)
Anxiety disorders	Worry and fear are constant and overwhelming and can be crippling. Anxiety can cause such distress that it interferes with a person's ability to lead a normal life.	Includes panic disorder, social anxiety disorder, and specific phobias	Reassurance and verbal reward for successes. Gradual changes. Use healthy comfort foods. Support blood sugar stability.
Associative disorders	Escape from reality in ways that are involuntary and unhealthy, experience of disconnection and lack of continuity between thoughts, memories, surroundings, actions, and identity.	Symptoms include amnesia and not remembering previous alternate identities.	Support healthy food choices and eating habits. Omit foods with negative associations.
Eating disorders	A group of serious conditions in which preoccupation with food and weight results in focus on little else. Eating disorders can cause serious physical problems and can even be life-threatening. (see Chapter 22)	Includes anorexia nervosa, bulimia, and binge-eating disorders.	Support good food choices already in place. Enlist individual in goal-setting; Encourage use of multivitamin/mineral supplement. Include moderate activity level and social eating.
Impulse control disorders (ICD)	Repetitive or compulsive engagement in a specific behavior (e.g., gambling, hair-pulling) despite adverse consequences, diminished control over the problematic behavior, and tension, or urge state prior to engagement in the behavior.	Includes pathologic gambling, kleptomania, pyromania, and intermittent explosive disorder. Criteria for other ICDs (compulsive shopping, problematic Internet use, compulsive sexual behavior, and compulsive skin picking) are currently under consideration.	Steer away from over-focus on a single goal. Encourage variety in food choices. Moderate a regular schedule of meals and snacks.
Mood disorders	A general emotional state or mood that is distorted or inconsistent with the circumstances.	Includes: **Major depressive disorder**—prolonged and persistent periods of extreme sadness **Bipolar I and II disorders**—also called manic depression or bipolar affective disorders **Seasonal affective disorder (SAD)**—a form of depression associated with fewer hours of daylight **Cyclothymic disorder**— emotional ups and downs; less extreme than bipolar disorder **Premenstrual dysphoric disorder**—mood changes and irritability that occur during a woman's premenstrual phase and go away with the onset of menses **Persistent depressive disorder (dysthymia)**—a long-term (chronic) form of depression **Disruptive mood dysregulation disorder**—chronic, severe and persistent irritability in children, often includes frequent temper outbursts that are inconsistent with the child's developmental age	Inquire about history of weight changes. Ensure adequate folic acid (methyl folate), B_{12}, and omega-3 fatty acid intake. Encourage regular, simple meals and snacks Detailed planning Social eating if possible. Bipolar: Assess for consistent fluid and sodium intake. Plan designated income for food if necessary. Include plan for social exercise and activity.
Personality disorders	A class of mental disorders characterized by long-term rigid patterns of thought and behavior that deviate markedly from the expectations of the culture. They can cause serious problems and impairment of function.	Includes: behavioral pattern which causes significant distress or impairment in personal, social, or occupational situations. Similar situations do not affect most people's daily functioning to the same degree.	Flexible food choices. Variety of foods and beverages. Flexible eating times.

TABLE 41-2 Medical Nutrition Therapy (MNT) for Psychiatric Disorders—cont'd

Psychiatric Disorder	Description	Examples	Nutrition Strategies
Psychotic disorders	Serious illnesses that affect the mind and alter a person's ability to think clearly, make good judgments, respond emotionally, communicate effectively, understand reality, and behave appropriately.	Includes: **Schizophrenia**—symptoms such as hallucinations and difficulty staying in touch with reality. Often unable to meet the ordinary demands of dailylife. **Schizoaffective disorder**—have symptoms of schizophrenia and a mood disorder.	Social eating. Simple meals. Give shopping guidelines and healthy snack ideas. Assess for potential metabolic syndrome. Assess for excess supplement use or water intake. Support adequate nutrition for healthy physical function.
Sexual dysfunction	Inability to fully enjoy sexual intercourse; disorders that interfere with a full sexual response cycle rarely threaten physical health, but can take a heavy psychological toll, bringing on depression, anxiety, and debilitating feelings of inadequacy.		
Sexual disorders	Disorders involving sexual functioning, desire, or performance, must cause marked distress or interpersonal difficulty to rate as disorder.	Diagnosis made only when the situation persists, caused at least in part by psychological factors; could occur occasionally or be caused by a temporary factor such as fatigue, sickness, alcohol, or drugs.	
Sleep disorders	Disorders involving changes in sleeping patterns or habits. Signs and symptoms include excessive daytime sleepiness, irregular breathing or increased movement during sleep, difficulty sleeping, and abnormal sleep behaviors.	Includes insomnia, sleep apnea, restless leg syndrome and narcolepsy.	Food record with times of eating to increase awareness and presence of night eating syndrome.
Somatoform disorders	A group of disorders characterized by thoughts, feelings, or behaviors related to somatic (physical) symptoms, and are excessive for any medical disorder that may be present.	May accompany anxiety disorders and mood disorders, which commonly produce physical symptoms. Somatic symptoms improve with successful treatment of the anxiety or mood disorder.	Review physical symptoms and changes in frequency and severity (abdominal pain, diarrhea, constipation). Eating for comfort.
Substance disorders	Distinct, independent, co-occurring mental disorders, in that all or most of the psychiatric symptoms are the direct result of substance use.	Symptoms of **substance-induced disorders** go from mild anxiety and depression (the most common across all substances) to full-blown manic and other psychotic reactions (much less common). **Psychotic symptoms** can be caused by heavy and long-term amphetamine abuse. **Dementia** (problems with memory, concentration, and problem solving) may result from using substances directly toxic to the brain, which commonly include alcohol, inhalants like gasoline, and amphetamines.	Calculate calories from alcohol, mg of caffeine intake; % of calories from sugar and sweets to increase client awareness and track progress. Moderate goals. Gradual changes. Encourage use of vitamin/mineral supplements. Assess history of irregular food intake and weight changes. Challenge "magic answer" thinking re: supplements, etc.

ADDICTION AND SUBSTANCE ABUSE

Addiction is defined as the persistent compulsive use of a substance known by the user to be physically, psychologically, or socially harmful. Addiction to alcohol, or alcoholism, and other substances results in compulsive and relapsing behavior. Addiction may be accompanied by depression or anxiety.

Successful treatment requires attention to the contribution of nutrition in the perpetuation of and recovery from addiction. Addictions may result in poor appetite, craving for sugar and sweets, constipation, and lack of motivation to prepare meals. Poor nutritional status may result from primary malnutrition from insufficient food or nutrient intake, or secondary malnutrition due to alteration in absorption, digestion, metabolism, or excretion of nutrients.

Addiction involves numerous neurotransmitters. The master "pleasure" molecule, which links and involves most forms of addiction, is dopamine. Its production is triggered by use of heroin, amphetamines, marijuana, alcohol, nicotine, cocaine, and caffeine or the activities of gambling or sex. Some evidence links compulsive eating behavior to the same reward system. Other neurotransmitters demonstrated to be involved in addiction include serotonin and glutamate. Nutritional derangements associated with addiction may be severe and can perpetuate addiction, or intensify addiction-related health problems, and make recovery a more difficult process.

Screening for Alcoholism

A moderate intake is defined as no more than two drinks a day for men or one drink a day for women (CDC, 2014). Individuals with intakes larger than this should be assessed using a validated screening tool for **alcoholism.**

The CAGE questionnaire has been commonly been as a screening and evaluation tool for alcoholism (see Box 41-4).

However, the CAGE questionnaire has been largely replaced by the Alcohol Use Disorders Identification Test (AUDIT) screening instrument because of its improved sensitivity and specificity. The AUDIT tool, developed in 1982 by the World Health Organization, is a simple way to screen and identify people at risk of alcohol problems (see Box 41-5).

Pathophysiology

Alcohol can be both a tonic and a poison. Moderate drinking seems to be good for the heart and circulatory system and may protect against type 2 diabetes and gallstones. Heavy drinking is a major cause of preventable death in most countries; it is implicated in about half of fatal traffic accidents in the United States. Heavy drinking can damage the liver and heart, harm an unborn child, increase the chances of developing breast and some other cancers, contribute to depression and violence, and interfere with relationships (http://www.mayoclinic.org/healthy-living/nutrition-and-healthy-eating/in-depth/alcohol/art-20044551). When alcohol begins to create problems, and especially when one denies these issues or cannot change the course of them, alcohol addiction must be considered.

Nutrient deficiencies can exacerbate these negative consequences of chronic alcohol consumption:

1. Deficiency of vitamin B_1 can trigger confusion and psychosis (called Wernicke encephalopathy; see Chapter 29)
2. Magnesium deficiency may aggravate withdrawal symptoms such as delirium tremens (DTs) and cardiac arrhythmias. Red blood cell (RBC) magnesium levels are more useful in assessment than serum magnesium levels, which may remain "normal" even with severe magnesium deficiency. Because magnesium deficiency is so common in alcoholics, deficiency should be presumed to be present.
3. Osteoporosis can be a direct influence of alcohol use or due to the commonly associated poor diet of alcoholics. Key nutrients and recommended doses to improve bone density are shown below. Vitamin D inhibits strontium absorption, so it must be taken at a different time of day (Reginster et al, 2012).
Strontium: 340 to 680 mg/day
Vitamin D: 1000 to 2000 IU
Magnesium: 200 mg
Vitamin K: 150 mcg
Boron: 3 mg

Calcium is best obtained from food sources, such as dairy foods, sardines, dark green vegetables, and seeds.
4. Malnutrition, malabsorption, gastritis, and chronic diarrhea (see Chapter 28)
5. Hepatitis and cirrhosis (see Chapter 29)
6. Cardiomyopathy (see Chapter 33)
7. Bone marrow disorders
8. Neuropathy, which is also associated with B_{12} deficiency, and dementias

Medical Management

The science of treating addictions has evolved considerably. Treatment has progressed from viewing it as a character flaw or sign of weakness to thinking of addiction as a chronic brain disorder that results from genetic and environmental inputs.

Any patient or client with active substance abuse issues may be presumed to have nutritional deficiencies. It may be useful to do nutritional testing, especially to document the more dangerous conditions such as thiamin deficiency (see Chapter 7). However, in an acute setting it is critical and may even be lifesaving to presume that B vitamin and magnesium deficiencies are present, and treat them rather than wait for laboratory results.

Acute alcohol withdrawal is a unique case of an addiction-related medical emergency that requires prompt nutritional treatment. Other addictions and deficiencies may be addressed over a few weeks or months.

Medical Nutrition Therapy

Medical nutritional therapy for addictions should be individualized, taking into account the current nutritional status of the patient. Some addicts may be homeless and clearly malnourished, whereas others may have less visible deficiencies. Special attention must be given to B vitamins, magnesium, and amino acid deficiencies (see Chapter 29). When possible, the best approach is to evaluate each patient for deficiencies through blood work and then replete as needed or assume poor nutritional status and provide a broad multivitamin/mineral supplement and a diet containing high-quality protein and fats. When gastritis or other intestinal problems are evident, these must be treated to allow for adequate digestion and absorption of nutrients.

Providing adequate levels of amino acids, B vitamins, minerals and omega-3 fatty acids generally stabilizes function in a patient dealing with addiction of any kind. As seen with many psychiatric disorders, magnesium and NAC are also very helpful in addiction recovery (Bondi et al, 2014; McClure et al, 2014).

BOX 41-6 Summary of Medical Nutrition Therapy for Substance Abuse

If warranted by history, assess for high risk alcohol consumption.
Assess appetite, nausea, and potential changes in food consumption.
Assess oral health and missing teeth, and chewing ability.
Start multivitamin-mineral supplement: recommend use for 6 months.
Recommend supplement of omega-3 fatty acids: 800 to 1000 mg/day.
Recommend biochemical assessment of thiamin, iron, folic acid, Mg, Se.
Recommend 25% to 30% of calories in diet from high quality protein.
Liberal nutritionally adequate diet (300-450 mg caffeine, moderate use of desserts to mediate withdrawal, moderate fiber and adequate fluid intake, inclusion of dairy foods)
Recommend attendance at nutrition education group as early as possible during withdrawal

Reference: Weiss, D: *Nutrition interventions in addiction recovery: the role of the dietitian in substance abuse treatment.* Webinar, September 25, 2013.

Addressing specific neurotransmitter issues can be very useful. Whether a patient is self-medicating to overcome neurotransmitter imbalances or has imbalances brought on as a result of the addiction, bringing balance back to neurotransmitter levels is part of management and recovery. Providing amino acid supplementation can support neurotransmitter production. Specifically, tyrosine is essential for production of dopamine, whereas tryptophan is required for serotonin production. Using tyrosine at 500 mg twice a day, or adding tyrosine-rich foods may help boost dopamine levels and reduce the risk of relapse. Tyrosine-rich foods include duck, chicken, ricotta cheese, dark chocolate, and seaweed (see Box 8-4 for more foods rich in tyrosine and its decarboxylated product tyramine).

Protein malabsorption is common among alcoholics and addicts in general. Supporting digestive function using plant-based digestive enzymes, which work across a much wider pH range than animal-sourced enzymes, may also be helpful in promoting nutritional sufficiency.

Finally, educating addicts about brain function and nutrition enhances their ability to participate successfully in a recovery program, and empowers them to make healthy choices while also understanding the mechanism of addiction (see Box 41-6).

ANXIETY

According to the Centers for Disease Control (CDC), the prevalence rates for anxiety disorder in developed countries range from 13.6% to 28.8% of the population, and is higher in developed nations than in developing nations. The underlying etiology of anxiety is not well understood. Different forms of anxiety include generalized anxiety disorder (GAD), panic disorder, obsessive compulsive disorder (OCD), posttraumatic stress disorder (PTSD), and social anxiety disorder (see Table 41-2). Common to all these disorders are heightened and poorly controlled emotional, somatic, and neurologic symptoms triggered by a specific type of circumstance or situation, or in the case of GAD, not related to any specific trigger.

Etiology

At one level, **anxiety** expressed as a heightened awareness of one's surroundings and of potential danger can be seen as an evolutionary advantage in terms of dealing with threats. However, when this mechanism becomes pervasive and debilitating, it moves into the realm of pathology.

There is a clear genetic component to anxiety. Early life stress may constitute a significant etiologic factor for anxiety. It is felt that the anxiety and panic response becomes "hard-wired" responses at an early age that create hormonal and brain patterns that become entrenched.

Pathophysiology

The structure in the brain thought to generate anxiety is the amygdala (the threat center), which processes fear-related stimuli and then signals others parts of the brain (especially the locus ceruleus) to fire and release norepinephrine; corticotropin-releasing factor (CRF), which ultimately stimulates elevated cortisol levels; and other excitatory components of the sympathetic nervous system. Glutamate is being recognized as playing an increasing role in anxiety disorders (as well as in depression) and is a target for pharmacologic and nonpharmacologic treatment (European College of Neuropsychopharmacology, 2013).

BOX 41-7   MNT for Management of Anxiety

- Assess for vitamin D, magnesium, and B vitamin status (see Chapter 7).
- Reduce caffeine intake.
  Eliminating caffeine for 3 to 4 weeks is recommended to see if anxiety decreases. Warn the person about withdrawal for 7 to 10 days, including headaches. Cutting intake in half every 4 to 7 days may avoid this. Switching from coffee to green tea can also be helpful as it has less caffeine and contains theanine, a calming amino acid. Anxiety may be triggered by even low doses of caffeine (the amounts in decaffeinated coffee); a switch to caffeine-free teas may be necessary.
- Reduce intake of sucrose and other forms sugar.
- Add a multivitamin containing high doses of B vitamins and minerals including copper, chromium, zinc, and selenium plus 200 mg per day of magnesium.
- Increase high-quality protein intake throughout the day.

Complementary Therapies for Anxiety

- **Theanine:** Derived from green tea—doses of 200 mg 1 to 4× per day are helpful (Unno et al, 2013). L-theanine is involved in the formation of the calming neurotransmitter, gamma amino butyric acid (GABA), and also stimulates the release of serotonin and dopamine.
- **Passion flower extract:** Doses of 100 to 500 mg 1 to 4× per day can be helpful (Movafegh et al, 2008).
- **Magnolia:** Magnolia bark has a long history of use in traditional Chinese formulas that relieve both anxiety and depression without the feeling sedation (Talbott et al, 2013).

- **Lavender:** The smell of lavender is calming, so keeping a vase full of lavender flowers (even dried) around or using a lavender oil spray can be helpful. In addition, taking a lavender capsule can be calming and reduce the need for tranquilizers (Woelk and Schlafke, 2010).
- **Inositol:** Can be helpful in treating anxiety and panic disorders, and is very safe. In high doses may be valuable in controlling several other mental health disorders, including panic disorder, obsessive compulsive disorder, agoraphobia, and depression.
- **GABA:** Deficiency of the neurotransmitter GABA is associated with anxiety, with GABA being a primary counterbalance for the excitatory neurotransmitter glutamate (Lydiard, 2003).

Sources:

- Lydiard RB: The role of GABA in anxiety disorders, *J Clin Psychiatry* 64(Suppl 3):21, 2003.
- Movafegh A et al: Preoperative oral Passiflora incarnata reduces anxiety in ambulatory surgery patients: a double-blind, placebo-controlled study, *Anesth Analg* 106:1728, 2008.
- Talbott SM et al: Effect of Magnolia officinalis and Phellodendron amurense (Relora) on cortisol and psychological mood state in moderately stressed subjects, *J Int Soc Sports Nutr* 10:37, 2013.
- Unno K et al: Anti-stress effect of theanine on students during pharmacy practice: positive correlation among salivary α-amylase activity, trait anxiety and subjective stress, *Pharmacol Biochem Behav* 111:128, 2013.
- Woelk H, Schläfke S: A multi-center, double-blind, randomised study of the Lavender oil preparation Silexan in comparison to Lorazepam for generalized anxiety disorder, *Phytomedicine* 17:94, 2010.

Difficult life circumstances that provoke stress can exacerbate underlying anxiety disorders and may be helpful to address with counseling. These can include marital and relationship stress and job stress, as well as physiologic stressors such as sleep disorders, menopause, thyroid disease, and food allergies. Hormonal imbalances, including high or low thyroid, low progesterone, and high or low testosterone levels, can also trigger anxiety. Anxiety can be a presenting complaint of perimenopause and of high or low cortisol levels, reflecting adrenal gland dysfunction.

Anxiety provokes physical and emotional symptoms, including rapid heart rate, shallow breathing, diaphoresis, hypervigilance, and sleep disorders. It can be difficult at first to diagnose anxiety, because patients present with multiple somatic complaints, and only after somatic pathology is ruled out can a diagnosis of anxiety disorder be established.

Medical Management

The primary pharmacologic therapy for anxiety disorders includes benzodiazepines, selective serotonin reuptake inhibitors (SSRIs), and norepinephrine reuptake inhibitors. Medications used primarily for other conditions can be useful in the treatment of anxiety, such as gabapentin, buspirone, and antipsychotic medications. Each of these can be effective but not for everyone. Each of these treatments carries the potential for side effects.

Medical Nutritional Therapy

Nutritional therapies that target the underlying metabolic causes of anxiety can be effective. Reactive hypoglycemia can trigger anxiety and should be suspected if attacks are worse in the late morning or afternoon (i.e., after several hours without food) or 30 to 60 minutes after a sugary meal or drink. Caffeine aggravates this, causing even more severe hypoglycemic symptoms (Gaby, 2011).

Nutritional deficiencies are common, especially of vitamin D (Armstrong et al, 2007), B vitamins, and magnesium. Magnesium deficiency can cause anxiety and anxiety also can cause increased

magnesium losses. In hospitalized patients, two studies have shown that parenteral magnesium (e.g., 2 g IV over 1 hour, then 1 gm per hour for 1 to 3 days) significantly decreased severe anxiety and agitation in agitated psychiatric inpatients. A multivitamin with 100 mg magnesium and high-dose B vitamins was shown to decrease anxiety in a placebo-controlled study. Treatment with doses of B vitamins above RDA recommendations has also been shown to help a number of different types of anxiety, whether or not deficiency was present (Gaby, 2011). Box 41-7 presents MNT and herbal support for anxiety management.

Complementary therapies may also be helpful and usually carry much lower risks than medications (Alramadhan 2012).

BIPOLAR DISORDER

This is also called bipolar affective disorder, or manic depressive disorder. "Mood Disorders" in the *DSM-IV* has been replaced with separate sections for depressive disorders and bipolar disorders. Bipolar disorder is placed between the psychotic disorders and the depressive disorders in the *Diagnostic and Statistical Manual of Mental Disorders* (DSM5), "in recognition of its place as a bridge between the two diagnostic classes in terms of symptomatology, family history and genetics" (Parker, 2014). The criteria for the major psychotic disorders and mood disorders are largely unchanged in the *Diagnostic and Statistical Manual of Mental Disorders*, fifth edition.

Bipolar disorder is a disorder in which people experience episodes of an elevated or agitated mood known as mania alternating with episodes of depression. The National Institute of Mental Health (NIMH) reports the 12-month prevalence of bipolar disorder in the U.S. adult population is approximately 2.6% and the lifetime prevalence is about 4%. The average age of onset is 25 years (National Institute of Mental Health, 2015). There is a genetic component, but other factors, including hormones, neurotransmitter abnormalities, and stress, are likely to be factors in triggering this illness.

Pathophysiology

Symptoms occur with different levels of severity. At milder levels of mania, known as hypomania, individuals appear energetic, excitable, and may be highly productive. As mania becomes more severe, individuals begin to behave erratically and impulsively, and may have great difficulty with sleep. Behavior may include alcohol abuse, sexual indiscretion, and excessive spending. Eating disorders are a potential comorbidity. The manic phase may result in difficulty in planning and preparing food.

During the depressed phase, 25% to 50% of patients attempt suicide. At the most severe level, individuals can experience psychosis. Bipolar disorder has recently been subdivided into Bipolar I (involving cycles of severe mood episodes from mania to depression) and Bipolar II (in which milder episodes of mania are mixed with bouts of severe depression) (see Table 41-2). Some individuals experience a mixed state in which features of mania and depression are present at the same time. Manic and depressive episodes last from a few days to several months.

Medical Management

A number of medications are used with varying degrees of success. Medical treatment of bipolar disease is complex and requires frequent monitoring by skilled clinicians. Lithium, a classic treatment, is considered benign when used as lithium orotate at low doses (e.g., 5 mg a day), but when used at high doses as lithium carbonate, can cause marked toxicity, including hypothyroidism, renal toxicity, and tremor. Lithium carbonate has a narrow therapeutic index; there is not a large difference between a toxic and therapeutic dose, and blood levels must be closely observed. Other medications used to treat bipolar disorder are mood stabilizers, benzodiazepines, and antipsychotic medications.

The presence of MTHFR reductase genetic mutations should be determined. Some genetic mutations associated with a higher risk of bipolar disorder respond to nutritional treatments of methyl folate (5-MTHF) and methylated B_{12}.

Medical Nutritional Therapy

Lithium and sodium are similar in chemical binding; therefore a stable, moderate, intake of salt and sodium is necessary to help stabilize lithium levels. A diet low in sugar and caffeine may also be helpful and is worth exploring with individual patients.

Many people starting a course of lithium experience significant dose-dependent weight gain, often resulting in noncompliance with medication. Other side effects that may affect nutritional status include increased thirst, nausea, vomiting, and diarrhea.

Studies have shown that areas with lower levels of lithium in the tap water have higher suicide rates. The usual daily intake of lithium from the diet is 0.65 to 3.1 mg/day. (Kapusta et al, 2011).

New information relates bipolar disorder to mitochondrial dysfunction, which opens the door to treating bipolar disease with mitochondrial modulators such as coenzyme Q10, n-acetyl-cysteine (NAC), acetyl-l-carnitine (ALCAR), S-adenosylmethionine (SAMe), alpha lipoic acid, creatine monohydrate, and melatonin (Nierenberg et al, 2013). This suggests disruption of brain energy metabolism and its relationship to mood disorders and psychiatric disease.

Potentially useful supplements include the following:

Fish oil: high doses of 9.3 g a day of omega-3 oils have been helpful (Gaby, 2011).

NAC (N-acetylcysteine): 1000 mg twice per day. This significantly improved symptoms relative to placebo in 24 weeks (Berk et al, 2008).

Magnesium: 300 to 600 mg a day. Magnesium has effects that are similar to lithium, but without the toxicity (Gaby, 2011). Iron excess is also associated with an increased risk of bipolar disorder, so a screening serum ferritin level is warranted to ensure that it is within normal range (Serata et al, 2012).

Evaluation for mineral and trace element deficiencies is warranted and empiric therapy with a multimineral is likely to have limited risk and may indeed be helpful (Kaplan et al, 2001).

As with other mood and psychiatric disorders, evaluating for the presence of celiac disease or gluten sensitivity is warranted (Dickerson et al, 2011). In nonceliac gluten sensitivity (NCGS), serum and intestinal signs may be absent, but clinical symptoms are reported, and clear within a few days of starting a gluten-free diet. Emerging scientific literature contains several reports linking gluten sensitivity states with neuropsychiatric manifestations including autism, schizophrenia, and ataxia (Genuis and Lobo, 2014).

DEMENTIA AND ALZHEIMER'S DISEASE (AD)

Mild cognitive impairment (MCI) is an intermediate stage between the expected cognitive decline of normal aging and the more serious decline of dementia. It can involve problems with memory, language, thinking and judgment that are greater than normal age-related changes.

Dementia represents a serious loss of cognitive ability. It may be stable and nonprogressive, as may occur after brain injuries, or it may be progressive, resulting in long-term decline due to damage or disease in the body. Two of the most common causes are Alzheimer's disease (AD) and vascular disease (called multi-infarct dementia). Other less frequent causes are Parkinson's dementia and Lewy body dementia.

Three and a half million Americans have vascular dementia caused by poor circulation to the brain and multiple mini-strokes. This syndrome can result from (1) atherosclerotic vascular disease, (2) an embolism usually from the heart due to vascular or arrhythmic disease, (3) poorly controlled hypertension, or (4) an increased tendency to clotting for reasons either inherited or acquired. Recognition of vascular dementia with AD is often delayed until the syndrome is far into its course. Vascular dementia should be considered if the progression of the cognitive dysfunction has progressed in discrete steps, each representing another ministroke.

AD affects almost 5.3 million Americans (Alzheimer's Association, 2015). The most proven risk factor for AD is advanced age. Other factors that have been shown to be associated with higher risk of AD include a positive family history of AD, suboptimal folate intake or metabolism, the presence of APOE-4 alleles, female gender, cardiovascular disease, head injury, Down's syndrome, and low educational level. Recent research also links the oxidative stress of air pollution to AD risk (Zhao and Zhao, 2013). Diabetes mellitus is also a risk factor for the development of AD.

Pathophysiology

Alzheimer's disease is associated with loss of neurons, characterized by microscopic changes in the brain, which include deposition of amyloid plaques, tau proteins, and neurofibrillary tangles. The only definitive test for diagnosing AD is a brain biopsy, which, appropriately, is not done. For evaluating dementia the American Academy of Neurology recommends structural neuro-imaging, which may include CT or MRI, and screening for depression, vitamin B_{12} deficiency, and hypothyroidism. A recent study demonstrated potential use of a blood test for 10 lipids (eight phosphatidylcholines and two acetyl-carnitines) as the best combination lipid blood test panel. A sample of peripheral blood predicted with more than 90% accuracy the development of either amnestic mild cognitive impairment or AD within a 2- or 3-year time frame (Mapstone et al, 2014).

Medical Management

Only half of people with dementia seen by physicians in general practice receive even the basic workup discussed earlier. In only 35% is the correct cause of the dementia determined, and these workups are generally conducted in higher level (secondary care) hospital settings.

A study of autopsies showed that in half the people who had been diagnosed with AD, AD was not seen on their brain biopsy. Rather, they had other causes of dementia that were missed (White, 2011). Although problematic, this also suggests that by looking for and treating nutritional and other issues, function may be improved—sometimes markedly.

Even small changes in brain function can make the difference between being able to care for oneself versus not recognizing one's children. People with dementia can have marked day-to-day fluctuations in cognition. Several types of treatment, including nutritional support and attention to adequate hydration, may significantly improve cognitive function.

It is critical that the practitioner always consider the possible presence of a treatable condition when evaluating a patient for dementia. Examples of treatable and even reversible causes of cognitive decline and memory loss include hormonal imbalances, brain tumors, infections, nutritional deficiencies (e.g., folate and vitamin B_{12}), and the side effects of numerous medications (see *Focus On:* Polypharmacy in Older Adults in Chapter 8).

It is also important to distinguish between normal fluctuations in mental function and dementia. AD is not when one keeps forgetting where one left the keys. It's when one forgets how to USE the keys. In addition, the stress of hospitalization, with poor sleep, loss of routine and familiar surroundings, being restrained and given strong psychoactive medications to treat agitation, and poor diet (e.g., being kept repeatedly NPO for tests, or dietary restrictions from acute illness) may trigger disorientation that may be confused with dementia, and which, if addressed, may be reversible. Sometimes it is the hospitalization itself that triggers a self-perpetuating (and potentially entirely reversible) chain of events that leaves the patient delirious or cognitively impaired, which then comes to be labeled as dementia. Getting the person into familiar surroundings as early as possible, off potent psychoactive medications, out of restraints, and eating a nutritious diet are important keys to treatment, management, and potentially improvement. Other factors may also optimize cognitive function (see Box 41-8).

The medical management of vascular dementia involves decreasing or eliminating further vascular insults to the brain. Treatment may include using aspirin, cholesterol, and blood pressure–lowering agents, and medically managing heart disease when present.

The medical therapies available for AD are currently limited to (1) acetylcholinesterase inhibitors such as donepezil (Aricept), aimed at maintaining levels of acetylcholine in the brain, and (2) memantine (Nemanda), an N-methyl-D-aspartate (NMDA) receptor antagonist aimed at reducing glutamate activity, which is excitatory and destructive of brain tissue. Some benefit can be gained from combining these two classes of drugs. Although these medications are generally well tolerated and can modestly slow progression, they often do little to improve symptoms day to day.

BOX 41-8 Optimizing Cognition in DEMENTIA

Drugs: Wean the person off drugs that are not essential. Being on 10-15 drugs (polypharmacy) is not uncommon in the elderly and can result in abnormal behavior. Anticholinergic medications are especially problematic.

Emotional: Rule out depression and make sure the person gets adequate sleep. Nutritional support with theanine, herbals, and even the smell of lavender can help sleep without increasing the risk of falling and injury.

Metabolic: Hormonal deficiencies, especially thyroid and testosterone, dramatically increase the risk of Alzheimer's disease. Levels of these hormones must be optimized. Making sure that the person is getting at least the 150 µg RDA of iodine a day is important for maintaining optimal thyroid function (Carcaillon, 2013; Tan et al, 2008) (see Chapter 31).

Ears and eyes: Hearing and vision loss can mimic dementia.

Nutrition: Optimize nutritional intake.

Tumors and other brain lesions: An MRI or CT scan is appropriate if one is diagnosed with dementia.

Infections: Silent urine and sinus infections can impair mental function.

Anemia, diabetes, and other overt medical problems should be assessed for and treated.

Carcaillon L et al: Low testosterone and the risk of dementia in elderly men: impact of age and education, *Alzheimers Dement* 10(Suppl 5): S306, 2014.

Tan ZS et al: Thyroid function and the risk of Alzheimer disease: the Framingham study, *Arch Intern Med* 168:1514, 2008.

Medically managing diabetes and insulin resistance is critical to delaying progression of dementia of any type. Hyper- and hypoglycemia as well as unchecked insulin resistance can cause damage to brain structures (Northam and Cameron, 2013) (see *New Directions:* Insulin Resistance and AD and the SNIFF Study [Schiöth et al, 2012]).

✸ NEW DIRECTIONS

Insulin Resistance in AD and The SNIFF Study

Severe insulin resistance in some areas of the brain is present in AD. Brain tissue is one of the few tissues outside of the pancreas that produces insulin, and glucose is the fuel brain cells commonly use. If insulin resistance is present, glucose cannot enter brain cells and the cells essentially starve and cannot function, unless they switch to using ketones for fuel. This suggests that treatment of insulin resistance and metabolic syndrome may be useful in the prevention of or slowing the progression of AD (Willette et al, 2014).

This makes exercise, avoiding excess sugar and saturated fats, and increasing fiber intake especially important. Even just 4 weeks of cutting back on sugar and saturated fats was associated with increased insulin sensitivity and decreased amyloid (Hanson, 2013). Intranasal insulin at 10 or 20 IU 2×/day is currently being tested in an Alzheimer's Randomized Controlled Trial (the SNIFF (Study of Nasal Insulin to Fight Forgetfulness) study) (Claxton et al, 2015; Morris JK et al, 2014; Reger et al, 2008). See *http://www.alz.org/research/video/alzheimers_videos_and_media_insulin.asp*.

Another dietary goal may be to increase the level of ketones in the blood and brain. The brain can use ketones as fuel, and their metabolism does not require insulin (Paoli et al, 2014). Ketones can be increased by adding approximately 7 tsp a day of coconut oil to the diet, or even more effectively by using medium-chain triglyceride (MCT) oils. The role of ketones and ketogenic agents in prevention and management of AD continues to be researched (Sharma et al, 2014).

The "4 As" of AD point to the sequential changes in brain function, behavior, and performance that impair the individual

---

BOX 41-9   The 4 As of Alzheimer's Dementia

Amnesia: The inability to use or retain memory, including short-term and long-term memory.

The person may constantly repeat questions such as "Where am I?" and "Who are you?" and "When are we going to eat?" or accuse the caregiver of stealing or being an imposter. This type of behavior can continue for hours at a time. This occurs due to damage to the frontal lobes and the hippocampus. This is usually the first area of change noticed by others. At this level of amnesia, the person with dementia does not look ill, so the confusion and inability to remember can appear to be purposeful and is often interpreted as just "annoying" behavior.
NUTRITIONAL IMPACT: May forget to eat, or not trust the caretaker involved in meal preparation or service.

Aphasia: The inability to use or understand language.

The loss of the ability to speak and write is called *expressive aphasia*. An individual may forget words he has learned and will provide a lengthy description of an item because he or she cannot find the right word. He may call family members by the wrong names. With *receptive aphasia,* an individual may be unable to understand spoken or written words or may read and not understand a word of what is read. Sometimes an individual pretends to understand and even nods in agreement; this is to cover up aphasia. Although individuals may not understand words and grammar, they may still understand nonverbal behavior (i.e., smiling).
NUTRITIONAL IMPACT: May not articulate wants, needs, or requests when it comes to eating.

Apraxia: The inability to use or coordinate purposeful muscle movement or coordination.

In the early stages the person may reach for an item and miss it. He or she may have difficulty catching a ball or clapping his or her hands. The floor may appear to be moving to this person and balance becomes affected, increasing the risk for falls and injury. In time, this loss of ability to move affects the Activities of Daily Living (sleeping, ambulating, toileting, grooming, hygiene, dressing, and eating). In the end stage, the person is not able to properly chew or swallow food, increasing the risk of choking or aspiration. This is linked to damage to parietal lobes (pain, touch, temperature and pressure, sensory perception) and the cortex (skilled movement) and the Occipital lobes.
NUTRITIONAL IMPACT: Physically unable to eat, chew, or swallow.

Agnosia: The inability to recognize people, or use common objects.

The person may become lost in a familiar place because he or she doesn't recognize the items that alert us to our surroundings. He or she may confuse a fork with a spoon, a toothbrush with a hairbrush, or toothpaste with denture cream. Eventually the ability to recognize objects is lost completely. The person may also confuse a son with a husband or a father or an uncle, or a daughter may be confused with a mother or an aunt or a grandmother. This process is associated with increased damage to the frontal lobes, the occipital lobes (visual association, distance and depth perception), and the temporal lobes.
NUTRITIONAL IMPACT: May not be able to use normal eating utensils or may even forget how to feed him or herself.

Reference: *Alzheimer's Foundation of America:* About Alzheimer's. http://www.alzfdn.org/AboutAlzheimers/symptoms.html, 2014. Accessed January 30, 2015.

---

and ultimately can make adequate nutritional intake difficult to maintain (see Box 41-9). Specific techniques that take into account the brain deficits must be implemented to improve the ability to eat and enjoy food. An occupational therapist can offer assistance in a dining needs assessment.

Medical Nutritional Therapy

Recent evidence has emerged supporting the connection between dietary intake and cognitive health, particularly in regard to the ageing population. A healthier diet during middle-age years (adequate amounts of B vitamins, antioxidants, polyunsaturated fatty acids, phytonutrients [Valls-Pedret et al, 2012],

and nitrites and nitric oxide (Justice et al, 2015) has been associated with better cognitive function later in life. The MIND (Mediterranean-Dietary Approach to Systolic Hypertension (Dash) diet intervention for neurodegenerative delay) diet has been found to substantially slow cognitive decline with aging. (Morris et al, 2015) See Appendices 26 and 31.

Three parameters of cognition (delayed recall, learning ability, and memory) were significantly associated with Hb A_{1c} levels in the range of 4.3% to 6.5%, illustrating the effect of even moderate blood glucose levels (American Academy of Neurology, 2015; Kerti et al, 2013).

The metabolic consequences of a high fructose intake and a deficiency of omega-3 fatty acids on cognitive abilities was associated with insulin action, signaling mediators, and lower cognitive scores. Insulin is a vasodilator. This vasodilator function is blunted in insulin-resistant individuals, and decreases cerebral circulation (Agrawal and Gomez-Pinilla, 2012; Barrett et al, 2009). Insulin resistance and impairment of the insulin receptor signaling cascade in the hippocampus may be accompanied by decreasing regional blood flow and reduced memory. Vasoprotective effects that include improved cerebral bloodflow have been shown to be associated with a whole-food–based diet (Presley et al, 2011).

One of the most important nutrients for the prevention of AD is folic acid. A long-term study using data from the Baltimore Longitudinal Study of Aging, which was begun in 1958 and included more than 1400 participants, found that the participants who had intakes at or above the 400 mcg RDA for folate had a 55% reduction in the risk of developing AD (Corrada et al, 2005). Most people who reached that level did so by taking folic acid supplements, which suggests that many people do not get the recommended amounts of folate in their diets. In another study adding folate at 1 mg a day to the anticholinesterase medications used in AD resulted in improved functional status (Connelly et al, 2008). Overall, multivitamins were shown to result in improvement in immediate free recall memory (Grima et al, 2012). A multivitamin, preferably with higher than RDA doses of vitamin B_1 and 400 to 1000 mcg/day of folate, is recommended.

Inadequate levels of vitamin B_{12} can affect the risk for developing AD and dementia. Low vitamin D levels and function have also been implicated as playing a major role in AD (Gezen-Ak et al, 2014). Vitamin E may help slow progression, but only if a mixed natural tocopherol containing gamma tocopherol is used. Most vitamin E supplements are synthetic alpha tocopherols, which not only increase risk of vitamin E deficiency, but do not help AD. The high levels of alpha tocopherol (more than 100 IUs/day) can induce a relative deficiency of the other tocopherols. Because of this, supplementation with vitamin E at doses more than 100 IU is not recommended, unless a natural mixed tocopherol is used (Usoro and Mousa, 2010).

Proper probiotic and prebiotic support is also important. There is growing evidence in the literature that the microbiome composition, species, identity and combinations, density, and distribution of these bacteria may influence how well we age. As innate immunity predominates over time certain bacteria proliferate, triggering an inflammatory response such as from tumor necrosis factor-alpha (TNF-alpha).

The integrity of the blood-brain barrier (BBB) becomes more difficult to maintain as the bacterial load and sustained TNF-alpha response occurs. In conditions such as AD, genetic polymorphisms that favor jawbone resorption during inflammation result in increased periodontal pocket depth. This provides the perfect environment for oral anaerobes most closely associated with AD. These conditions in combination with predisposing genetic polymorphisms may increase the propensity for bacteria or endotoxins to gain access to the brain, triggering neuropathology and altering brain function (Shoemark and Allen, 2014).

Advanced glycation end products (AGEs) are implicated in the initiation and progression of Alzheimer-type dementia (Cai et al, 2014). Advanced glycation end products, also known as glycotoxins, are a diverse group of highly oxidant compounds created through a nonenzymatic reaction between reducing sugars and free amino groups of proteins, lipids, or nucleic acids. The formation of AGEs is a part of normal metabolism, but excessively high levels of AGEs in tissues and the circulation can become pathogenic. AGEs promote oxidative stress and inflammation by binding with cell surface receptors or cross-linking with body proteins, altering their structure and function. In addition to AGEs that form within the body, AGEs also exist in foods. AGEs in foods are formed during dry cooking of food, particularly baking, roasting, and frying. AGEs are absorbed and contribute significantly to the body's AGE pool (Uribarri et al, 2010).

Low levels of the omega-3 essential fatty acids DHA are present in those with dementia. Increasing omega-3 fat or fish oil intake is more likely to be helpful in those with mild cognitive defects than in those with severe AD (Freund et al, 2014). Krill oil is another substitute for fish oil in treating cognitive decline.

AD is 70% less common in India than in the United States, and this is thought to be due to a diet high in turmeric (curcumin—the spice that makes Indian curries yellow) (Rigacci and Stefani, 2015). A double-blind study, supplementing curcumin in the diets of people with AD is currently underway. Curcumin is poorly absorbed, however, so it is important to use a highly absorbed form such as BCM-95, whose absorption is 693% higher than 95% pure curcumin (Antony et al, 2008; Benny and Antony, 2006), and more than 35,000% higher than an equivalent weight of turmeric (Cuomo et al, 2011). Supplementing AD patients with BCM 95 curcumin resulted in blood amyloid changes suggestive of amyloid breakdown (Baum et al, 2008). Combining curcumin and vitamin D was also associated with increased amyloid clearance by macrophages (Masoumi et al, 2009; see Box 41-10). Curcumin may be generally neuroprotective, also showing benefit in Parkinson's disease(Pan 2012).

Other natural therapies that support brain and cognitive function include huperzine, acetylcholine, and alpha-lipoic acid, all of which are natural agonists of acetylcholine receptors (see *New Directions:* Something New in AD Management?)

 NEW DIRECTIONS

Something New in AD Management?

Phosphatidylserine may offer neuroprotection by inhibiting the formation of beta amyloid fragments. Early studies using bovine phosphatidylserine showed positive results in those with cognitive decline, but the compound was replaced with a soy-based phosphatidylserine because of fears of mad cow disease. However, the evidence supporting the improvement in age-related memory impairment associated with the soy-based compound is weaker; overall results are inconclusive and more research is needed (Wollen, 2010).

Phosphatidylcholine is a component in nerve cell membranes and may offer protection from degeneration. Cytidinediphosphocholine (CDP-choline), a precursor, has shown the most promise (Fioravanti and Yanagi, 2010). Research studies investigating the benefits of CDP-choline have been short but indicate possible positive effects on memory and behavior in patients with various forms of dementia, including AD. Longer-term studies are needed to investigate full benefits.

DEPRESSION

Major depressive disorder (MDD) is a common and costly disorder that is usually associated with severe and persistent symptoms, leading to social role impairment and increased mortality. Major depressive disorder is one of the most important causes of disability worldwide (WHO, 2012). There are multiple factors contributing to the development of depression, including genetics, nutrition, environmental stressors, hormonal disruption especially in the hypothalamic pituitary adrenal (HPA) axis, and alterations in neurotransmitter biology and function (the monoamine deficiency theory).

This range of factors and the relative contribution of each to the development of depression in an individual is likely an important reason for the variability of individual response to specific therapies. Thus viewing depression as a heterogeneous condition is useful and demands that the health care provider consider each patient's individuality (see Table 41-2 and Box 41-11).

BOX 41-10   MNT for Alzheimer's Disease

A multivitamin supplement containing at least 400 mcg of folate, 1000 IU of vitamin D, and 500 µg of B_{12}. If the serum vitamin B_{12} level is under 300 pg/ml or serum homocysteine or methylmalonic acid are elevated, a trial of vitamin B_{12} injections is reasonable.

Iron deficiency may be present despite technically normal ferritin (a key laboratory measure for iron) levels. Especially if anemia, cognitive dysfunction, or restless leg syndrome are present, it is reasonable to keep the ferritin level at least 60 mcg/l (ng/ml) or higher. Using the standard ferritin cutoffs of 12 and 20 mcg/l (ng/ml) (in females and males respectively) to diagnose iron deficiency is ill advised, as ferritin levels can be higher than this in as many as 92% of people with severe iron deficiency based on bone marrow biopsy.

Add 750 to 3000 mg a day of a highly absorbed BCM-95 curcumin product (Baum, 2008).

Manage blood glucose, lipid, and insulin levels to achieve normal levels.

Baum L et al: Six-month randomized placebo-controlled, double-bind, pilot clinical trial of curcumin in patients with Alzheimer's disease, *J Clin Psychopharmacol* 28:110, 2008.

BOX 41-11   Diagnostic Criteria for Major Depression

- Depressed mood or a loss of interest or pleasure in daily activities for more than 2 weeks.
- Mood representing a change from the person's baseline.
- Impaired function: social, occupational, educational.
- Specific symptoms, at least 5 of these 9, present nearly every day:
  1. Depressed mood or irritable most of the day, nearly every day, as indicated by subjective report (e.g., feels sad or empty) or observation made by others (e.g., appears tearful)
  2. Decreased interest or pleasure in most activities, most of each day
  3. Significant weight change (5%), or change in appetite
  4. Change in sleep: insomnia or hypersomnia
  5. Change in activity: psychomotor agitation or retardation
  6. Fatigue or loss of energy
  7. Guilt/worthlessness: feelings of worthlessness or excessive or inappropriate guilt
  8. Concentration: diminished ability to think or concentrate, or more indecisiveness
  9. Suicidality: Thoughts of death or suicide, or has suicide plan

American Psychiatric Association (APA): *Diagnostic and Statistical Manual of Mental Disorders*, ed 5, Arlington, Va, 2013, American Psychiatric Association.

Pathophysiology

The monoamine deficiency theory of depression suggests that a deficiency of the monoamines serotonin, dopamine, and norepinephrine, or altered monoamine receptor function in the central nervous system is the main pathophysiologic factor in depression. This theory has provided a target for the most common pharmacologic methods of treating depression.

In addition to the dietary decrease in fish oils and omega-3 fatty acids already discussed, other factors contribute to depression, including nutritional and hormonal deficiencies. In depression not responsive to antidepressants, a good response is seen using the T3 thyroid hormone despite normal thyroid tests. No significant improvement was seen with T4, the thyroid hormone most often used (Posternak et al, 2008). T3 has also been shown to be helpful in resistant bipolar depression (Kelly and Lieberman, 2009). Testosterone deficiency in men causes depression. Symptoms suggestive of depression can arise in the perimenopausal state and appropriate therapy including bioidentical hormone therapy can be a useful in addressing this (Joffe, 2011).

As discussed earlier, epidemiologic research has identified associations between lower seafood consumption and increased rates of depression around the world. Dozens of clinical studies using EPA and DHA omega-3 supplements for depression have been conducted, and results are mixed but generally positive (Martins, 2009).

Medical Management

Standard treatment of major depression includes pharmacotherapy as outlined in Box 41-12. Current pharmacologic therapy of depression is inconsistently effective (Garland, 2004).

Although a variable moderate percentage of depressed patients receive some benefit from pharmacologic therapy, a majority will not achieve full remission (see *New Directions*: Can Genes Help Determine Psychopharmacologic Therapy?)

There are pros and cons regarding whether antidepressant therapy surpasses the effect of placebo for mild to moderate depression (Insel, 2011; Kirsch et al, 2008). A thorough and instructive comparison of methods, assumptions, and the effect of media coverage written by Adrien Preda, MD, can be found at http://blogs.plos.org/mindthebrain/2012/12/26/the-antidepressant-wars-a-sequel-how-the-media-distort-findings-and-do-harm-to-patients/ (Coyne, 2012). Other therapies include cognitive behavioral therapy (CBT), light therapy, and transcranial magnetic stimulation.

❋ NEW DIRECTIONS

Can Genes Help Determine Psychopharmacologic Therapy?

Saliva-based genetic tests for genetic and biological markers can indicate the potential response to different psychiatric drugs. Analysis by a psychopharmacologist can help clinicians more quickly find effective treatment for patients with a range of psychiatric conditions, including depression, bipolar disorder, schizophrenia, anxiety disorders, obsessive compulsive disorders (OCD), and attention-deficit hyperactivity disorders (ADHD).

BOX 41-12   Common Medications Used to Treat Depression

- Selective serotonin reuptake inhibitors (SSRIs), such as fluoxetine, paroxetine, and sertraline among others
- Serotonin norepinephrine reuptake inhibitors, such as duloxetine and venlafaxine
- Norepinephrine-dopamine reuptake inhibitor-bupropion
- Older therapies including monoamine oxidase inhibitors and tricyclic antidepressants can be useful but are generally second-line therapies

---

Medical Nutritional Therapy

Fish oil supplements for treating depression are most effective with a composition of 60% EPA and 40% DHA. Supplements of fish oil with 60% EPA, using a dose of 200 to 2200 mg/day of EPA were effective against primary depression (Sublette and Ellis, 2011).

Curcumin appears to be a promising treatment for depression. A recent study showed a special highly absorbed form of curcumin (BCM 95 or CuraMed 500 mg 2×/day) to be effective for treating major depression after 8 weeks of use (Lopresti et al, 2014). Research has also shown this special, highly absorbed BCM 95 form of curcumin to be as effective as Prozac (Sanmukhani et al, 2014). Effectiveness of common curcumin is decreased because of poor absorption; the BCM 95 form used in these studies is needed for curcumin to be effective (Antony et al, 2008; Benny and Antony, 2006).

Vitamin B and magnesium deficiencies have also been linked to depression. Patients treated with 0.8 mg of folic acid/day or 0.4 mg of vitamin B$_{12}$/day show significant improvement (Young, 2007).

Several case reports also found that depressed patients treated with 125 to 300 mg of magnesium (as glycinate or taurinate) with each meal and at bedtime often had rapid improvement in cases of major depression in under a week (Eby and Eby, 2006).

For those with atypical depression, supplementation with chromium picolinate at 600 mcg/day was found helpful in decreasing cravings, but those treated with chromium and those receiving placebo demonstrated no difference in depression scores (Docherty et al, 2005). Key effects of chromium were on carbohydrate craving and appetite regulation.

Low serum zinc levels predispose people to treatment-resistance in depression. Repletion of zinc levels may augment otherwise ineffective therapies (Ranjbar and Shams, 2014). Mechanisms of action by zinc in reducing depressive symptoms include (1) decreasing dopamine reuptake (by binding to the dopamine receptor), (2) increasing the conversion of T4 to T3, and (3) the promotion of excitatory neurotransmitter function.

Nutritional approaches to augmenting serotonin and serotonin receptor response include the use of St John's Wort (see Chapter 12), 5-hydroxy-tryptophan (5-HTP), tryptophan, and vitamin D. S-adenosylmethionine (SAMe) can be an effective additive therapy to treat major depressive disorders. Caution must be used in treating depression with St. John's Wort, tryptophan, and 5-HTP in patients being treated with serotonergic drugs, such as SSRIs, SNRIs, or tramadol to avoid triggering the **serotonin syndrome** (see *Focus On*: Serotonin Syndrome).

Serotonin Syndrome

If brain serotonin levels go too high, the result is **serotonin syndrome**. Serotonin syndrome encompasses a wide range of clinical findings.

- Mild symptoms may consist of increased heart rate, anxiety, and sweating, along with dilated pupils, tremor or twitching, and hyper-responsive reflexes.
- Symptoms of moderate elevation include hyperactive bowel sounds, high blood pressure, and fever.
- Severe symptoms include increases in heart rate and blood pressure that may lead to shock.
- Most often, excess serotonin occurs from combining serotonin raising medications (typically selective serotonin reuptake inhibitors, SSRIs). It may also come from adding 5 HTP, tryptophan, or herbs (e.g., St. John's Wort, Panax, Ginseng, nutmeg, or yohimbe) to high doses of medications which raise serotonin. Treatment is to cut back or stop these adjunctive treatments. Abruptly stopping antidepressants can cause severe withdrawal, so, except in severe situations, dosing is usually lowered rather than stopped completely (Undurraga and Baldessarini, 2012).

BOX 41-13 **Effects of Insufficient, High-Quality Sleep**

Alteration in moods: irritability, anger, greater risk for depression
Lessened ability to cope with stress
Decreased ability to learn
Decreased memory
Poor insight
Impaired judgment
Increased pain
Immune dysfunction

Source: http://www.webmd.com/sleep-disorders/excessive-sleepiness-10/emotions-cognitive

---

Although many clinicians are trained to think that the only presentation of serotonin syndrome is a febrile rigid state requiring emergency medical care, in milder forms patients are simply agitated and have muscle spasms. There is no way to diagnose this other than by clinical suspicion and altering the therapy to reduce serotonin levels and note if symptoms resolve.

In those with vitamin B_{12} or folic acid deficiency and especially coexisting with a MTHFR (5-methyltetrahydrofolate reductase) methylation mutation or elevated homocysteine levels, optimizing B_{12} and folic acid levels can significantly improve depression by using 5-methyltetrahydrofolate (5-MTHF) to bypass the inefficient folate metabolism and activation. 5-MTHF crosses the blood-brain barrier more readily than does standard folic acid. It is important to evaluate all patients with longstanding mood disorders, especially those with a family history of mood disorders, for a genetic methylation mutation of either COMT (catechol-O-methyl transferase) or MTHFR (methylenetetrahydrofolate reductase) (see Chapter 5). These mutations are involved in inactivation of catecholamine neurotransmitters and are implicated in schizophrenia, OCD, ADHD, and depression as well as vascular disease, thrombotic stroke, homocysteinuria, and homocysteinemia.

FATIGUE, CHRONIC FATIGUE SYNDROME (CFS), AND FIBROMYALGIA SYNDROME (FMS)

Although research has shown that fatigue, chronic fatigue syndrome (CFS), and fibromyalgia syndrome (FMS) are physical conditions, discussion of them here is included because cognitive dysfunction (often called "brain fog") is a frequent symptom, and CFS and FMS are often poorly understood. Disorders such as CFS and FMS have a confusing array of diverse symptoms. Some experts believe that CFS and fibromyalgia are variations of the same process; they are discussed here as a single condition (CFS/FMS). Overt fibromyalgia affects approximately 2% of the population (Wolfe et al, 2013), and another approximately 2% have a milder intermediate form.

Women are affected twice as often as men. CFS and FMS can be caused by, and have overlapping symptoms with, autoimmune disorders such as systemic lupus erythematosus (SLE) or hypothyroidism. Viral pathogens, immune dysregulation, central nervous system dysfunction, musculoskeletal disorders, mitochondrial dysfunction, nutrient deficiencies, and other systemic abnormalities and allergies have been proposed as contributing factors in CSF/FMS.

Pathophysiology

Research suggests mitochondrial and hypothalamic dysfunction are common denominators in the syndromes of CFS/FMS (Cordero et al, 2010). Dysfunction of hormonal, sleep, and autonomic control (all centered in the hypothalamus), and energy production can explain the large number of symptoms and why most patients have a similar set of complaints.

Because the hypothalamus controls sleep, the hormonal and autonomic systems, and temperature regulation, it has very high energy needs for its size, so it malfunctions early in a shortage of energy. Similar to the circuit breaker in a house: if energy demands are too high, the body "blows a fuse." It is protective but must be reset. In addition, inadequate energy stores in a muscle results in muscle shortening (think of writer's cramp) and pain, which is further accentuated by the loss of deep sleep (see Box 41-13). The paradox of severe fatigue combined with insomnia, lasting more than 6 months, indicates the likelihood of a CFS-related process. If he or she also has widespread pain, fibromyalgia is probably present as well (see *Focus On:* Fibromyalgia Diagnostic Criteria).

Fibromyalgia Diagnostic Criteria

- Widespread pain index (WPI) ≥7 and symptom severity (SS) scale score ≥5, or WPI 3 to 6 and SS scale score ≥9.
- Symptoms have been present at a similar level for at least 3 months.
- The patient does not have a disorder that would otherwise explain the pain.

WPI (Widespread Pain Index)

Check each area below that you've had pain in over the last week. Score 1 point for each you check and enter the total score in the blank space provided.

- Shoulder girdle, left
- Shoulder girdle, right
- Upper arm, left
- Upper arm, right
- Lower arm, left
- Lower arm, right

- Hip (buttock, trochanter), left
- Hip (buttock, trochanter), right
- Upper leg, left
- Upper leg, right
- Lower leg, left
- Lower leg, right

- Jaw, left
- Jaw, right
- Chest
- Abdomen
- Upper back
- Lower back
- Neck

_____ **Total WPI** (score 1 point for each item checked above)

◎ FOCUS ON—cont'd

Fibromyalgia Diagnostic Criteria

SS (Symptom Severity)

a. Rate each of the three symptoms below according to their severity you've experienced over the past week using the scale shown.

0 = No problem

1 = Slight or mild problems, generally intermittent

2 = Moderate, considerable problems, often present and/or at a moderate level

3 = Severe: pervasive, continuous, life-disturbing problems

_____ Fatigue

_____ Waking unrefreshed

_____ Cognitive symptoms ("brain fog")

b. Rate each symptom below that you've experienced during the previous 6 months. Score 1 point for each you check.

0 = No problem

1 = Slight or mild problems, generally intermittent

2 = Moderate, considerable problems, often present and/or at a moderate level

3 = Severe: pervasive, continuous, life-disturbing problems

_____ Fatigue

_____ Waking unrefreshed

_____ Cognitive symptoms ("brain fog")

b. Check each symptom below that you've experienced during the previous 6 months. Score 1 point for each you check.

• Headaches

• Pain or cramps in lower abdomen

• Depression

_____ **Total SS** (add the scores you entered in step "a" plus 1 point for each symptom you checked in step "b")

American College of Rheumatology (ACR), 2010; Wolfe et al, 2011.

Diagnosis is based on the combination of chronic widespread pain and a symptom severity score based on the amount of fatigue, sleep disturbances, cognitive dysfunction, and other somatic symptoms. The diagnosis of fibromyalgia often overlaps with other chronic pain syndromes, including irritable bowel syndrome, temporomandibular disorders, and idiopathic low back pain. In CFS, chronic fatigue is the major symptom. It lasts 6 months or longer and is accompanied by hypotension, sore throat, multiple joint pains, headaches, postexertional fatigue, muscle pain, and impaired concentration (Avellaneda Fernández et al, 2009).

Medical Management

Standard medical therapy is aimed at addressing symptomatology but does not address the underlying metabolic, nutritional, and hormonal derangements. Medications such as low-dose Neurontin, Ambien, Flexeril, or Desyrel are used to initiate and deepen sleep. Neurontin can also be helpful in reducing pain and restless leg syndrome. Three medications are approved by the Food and Drug Administration (FDA) for treatment of fibromyalgia: duloxetine (Cymbalta), milnacipran (Savella), and the anticonvulsant pregabalin (Lyrica). These can be helpful in some patients suffering from FMS but can have significant side effects.

There are no FDA-approved medications for CFS, and clinicians generally attempt to improve sleep quality in these patients and may attempt a trial of stimulants such as modafinil or amphetamines to improve daytime function. Antiviral therapy targeted at addressing a possible viral etiology of CFS is sometimes attempted in a subset of patients, and this area is being actively researched (Johnson, 2014).

BOX 41-14   SHINE Protocol for Treating Chronic Fatigue and Fibromyalgia

Sleep support

Hormonal support

Infection treatment

Nutritional support

Exercise as able

Teitelbaum JE: Effective treatment of chronic fatigue syndrome, *Integr Med* 10:44, 2012.

Although there is still much to learn, effective treatment is now available for the majority of these patients. Restoring adequate energy production through nutritional, hormonal, and sleep support, and eliminating the stresses that overuse energy (e.g., infections, situational stresses) restores function in the hypothalamic "circuit breaker" and also allows muscles to release, thus allowing pain to resolve. A placebo-controlled study showed that with these measures, 91% of patients improve, with an average 90% improvement in quality of life, and the majority of patients no longer qualified as having FMS by the end of 3 months ($p < 0.0001$ vs. placebo) (Teitelbaum, 2012a).

The acronym *SHINE*, based on the integrated protocol used in the study, is a helpful way to structure treatment recommendations (see Box 41-14).

Disordered Sleep

A common element of CFS/FMS is a sleep disorder. Many patients sleep solidly for only 3 to 5 hours a night with multiple awakenings. Even more problematic is the loss of deep stage three and four "restorative" sleep. Besides the standard medications for sleep improvement, natural sleep remedies can also be very helpful (see Box 41-15).

Other sleep disturbances must be ruled out. Sleep apnea is suspected if the patient snores, is overweight, is hypertensive, and has a shirt collar size more than 17 inches. Restless leg syndrome (RLS), more accurately called periodic limb movement disorder of sleep (PLMD), is also fairly common in CFS/FMS. In addition to gabapentin, RLS is treated with supplemental iron, keeping ferritin levels more than 60 mcg/l (ng/ml) (Wang et al, 2009), and magnesium (Burke and Faulkner, 2012).

BOX 41-15   Natural Sleep Remedies and Recommended Dosages

1. Herbal: Use singly or in combination, once a day at HS (see Chapter 12 for possible interactions).

   Valerian (200-800 mg/day)

   Passion flower (90-360 mg)

   L-Theanine (50-200 mg)

   Hops (30-120 mg)

   Wild lettuce (18-64 mg)

   Lemon Balm Extract (20-80 mg)

   These are all combined in a product called the Revitalizing Sleep Formula (1-4 capsules at bedtime)

2. Melatonin: 0.5 - 5 mg at bedtime (0.5 mg is usually optimal for sleep, but higher doses may also decrease nighttime acid reflux).

3. Two to three spritzes or sprays of lavender on the pillow at bedtime helps sleep. Lavender is also available in capsule form.

Source: Teitelbaum JE: Effective treatment of chronic fatigue syndrome, *Integrative Medicine* 10:44, 2012.

Evaluation and Treatment of Associated Thyroid Hormonal Dysfunction

Hormonal dysfunctions are common in CFS/FMS. Sources of this dysfunction include hypothalamic and pituitary dysfunction and autoimmune conditions such as Hashimoto's thyroiditis (see Chapter 31).

If the thyroid is underactive because the hypothalamus is suppressed, as in CFS/FMS, the TSH test, which depends on normal hypothalamic function to be reliable, may appear to be normal or even suggest an overactive thyroid. Blood tests commonly use two standard deviations to define norms, making only the lowest or highest 2.5% of the population "abnormal" (i.e., viewed as requiring treatment). It is estimated that as many as 20% of women over 60 have positive antithyroperoxidase (TPO) antibodies and may be hypothyroid (see Chapter 31), showing the problem of relying on the normal range to determine the need for treatment.

In two studies by Dr. G.R. Skinner (Skinner, 1997) and his associates in the United Kingdom, patients thought to have hypothyroidism had technically normal thyroid blood tests. Yet, when treated with thyroid hormone, the large majority of patients with symptoms of low thyroid and yet normal testing, improved when given thyroid hormone (levothyroxine—T4) at an average dosage of 100 to 120 mcg/day. This is equivalent to the use of 1 to $1\frac{1}{4}$ grains of porcine or desiccated thyroid hormone (Teitelbaum, 2007).

The goal in CFS/FMS management is to restore optimal function while keeping laboratory values in the normal or reference range for safety. The optimal range may be different than the "normal range." Because the hypothalamus controls virtually the entire hormonal system, thyroid, adrenal, and ovarian and testicular support may be needed, with the decision to treat and adjust dosages is based on a mix of signs, symptoms, and laboratory results.

As noted earlier, treating with T_3 (but not T_4) hormone in major depression, even when thyroid tests are normal, also significantly improved depression (Teitelbaum, 2007).

Immune Dysfunction and Infections

Immune dysfunction is an integral part of CFS/FMS. Dozens of infections have been implicated in CFS/FMS, including viral, parasitic, *Candida albicans,* and antibiotic-sensitive infections. Most of these infections are known as "opportunistic infections," which means they will not survive in the presence of a healthy immune system. Many of them resolve on their own as the immune system recovers with the SHINE protocol (see Box 41-13).

Exercise

Because of decreased energy production, too much exercise may result in "postexertional fatigue," leaving the person bedridden for a day or two. After 2 to 3 months on the SHINE protocol, patients can usually begin conditioning. Water aerobics can be helpful for those too weak to walk.

General Pain Relief

Pain often resolves within 3 months of simply treating with the SHINE protocol (Teitelbaum, 2007). Nonsteroidal antiinflammatory drugs (NSAIDs) have been shown to be ineffective in fibromyalgia pain and can contribute to bleeding ulcers, and increased risk of heart attacks and strokes (Bhala et al, 2013; Trelle et al, 2010). Chronic use of acetaminophen depletes glutathione, a key antioxidant. The glutathione depletion from acetaminophen may be prevented by supplementing with N-acetylcysteine (NAC 500 to 1000 mg/d) (Woodhead et al, 2012).

Besides being effective in treatment of depression as already discussed, a unique form of curcumin (BCM 95) has been shown to be very helpful for pain (Antony et al, 2008; Benny and Antony, 2006).

Medical Nutritional Therapy

It is recommended that B_{12}, iron, total iron-binding capacity (TIBC), and ferritin levels be assessed, keeping in mind that elevated serum B_{12} may be a sign of an MTHFR mutation and inadequate utilization of B_{12}. Measurement of erythrocyte magnesium and zinc may be helpful, although the laboratory tests are not reliable indicators of nutritional status. Due to a probably low-nutrient-density diet and possible increased nutrient needs, other possible nutrient deficiencies are likely and must be treated with a healthy diet and nutritional supplements.

Healthy foods may not necessarily be the foods patients crave, but a routine of high protein, low-carbohydrate meals and snacks, along with avoidance of sugar, excessive caffeine, and alcohol are reasonable goals.

These patients often need to increase salt and water intake, especially in the presence of low blood pressure or orthostatic dizziness. Salt restriction is generally ill advised in these patients because of the adrenal dysfunction and orthostatic intolerance. Gluten avoidance may be helpful in a subset as well (Isasi et al, 2014; see Chapter 28).

Nutritional Supplements in Management of CFS and FMS

In addition to a healthy diet the following nutritional supplementation program may be helpful.

1. **A high-potency multivitamin.** A good broad-spectrum, high-potency, powdered multivitamin/multimineral is generally better tolerated, better absorbed, and less expensive than tablets. This supplement should include at least
   40 mg of each of the B vitamins
   400 mcg folate (with at least 200 mcg as the MTHF form)
   500 mcg of B_{12}
   1000 IU of vitamin D
   200 mg of magnesium glycinate
   15 mg of zinc (Teitelbaum, 2015).

2. **D-Ribose.** Because CFS/FMS represents an energy crisis, it is critical that patients have what is needed for optimal mitochondrial function. D-Ribose is natural sugar produced by the body in the pentose phosphate shunt to produce ATP, NADH, FADH, DNA, and RNA, and is a potentially critical rate-limiting nutrient in the production of energy. The key energy molecules ATP, FADH, and NADH are predominantly ribose plus B vitamins and phosphate. Two studies with a total of 298 CFS/FMS patients taking 5 g of D-ribose 3 x day for 3 weeks showed an average of 60% increase in energy at 3 weeks (Teitelbaum et al, 2006; Teitelbaum, 2012b). Improvement is usually seen within 1 month. Recommended dosing is 5 g three times per day for 3 weeks and then bid. It is well tolerated, although occasionally it can cause a mild drop in blood glucose.

3. **Iron.** If the iron percent saturation is under 22%, or serum ferritin is under 60 mcg/l (ng/ml), iron supplementation is recommended (Vaucher et al, 2012). It should not be taken within 6 hours of thyroid hormone, because iron blocks thyroid absorption. Treatment should be continued until the ferritin level is over 60 mcg/l (ng/ml).

4. **B_{12}.** If serum B_{12} is under 540 pg/ml, it is reasonable to consider a series of 10 weekly B_{12} injections, or prescribing

5 mg sublingual B_{12} daily. Studies on CFS show absent or near-absent spinal fluid B_{12} levels despite normal serum B_{12} levels.

5. **Coenzyme Q10.** Supplement with CoQ10 at 200 mg/day for 3 to 6 months, because blood levels of CoQ10 are often low in CFS/FMS (Maes et al, 2009). Side effects are rare.

6. **Acetyl L-carnitine (ALCAR).** Supplement with 1500 to 2000 mg daily for 4 months. Low carnitine levels are routinely seen in CFS/FMS. Supplementation to replace the deficits routinely present in CFS/FMS is limited to 4 months because of some concern about elevated carnitine levels being associated with increased risk of myocardial infarction (Teitelbaum, 2007).

SCHIZOPHRENIA

Schizophrenia is a severe mental disorder that presents as psychosis, often with paranoia and delusions. Diagnosis requires at least one of the symptoms to be delusions, hallucinations, or disorganized speech. A diagnosis of **schizoaffective disorder** requires that a person meet all of the criteria for schizophrenia and all of the criteria for an episode of bipolar disorder or depression, with the exception of impaired function (Parker, 2014).

Pathophysiology

The origins and causes of schizophrenia are not completely understood. Ultimately it may be understood as a heterogeneous disorder generated by a combination of biochemical, genetic, structural, nutritional, and environmental factors, including infections and toxins (Altamura et al, 2013). Schizophrenia is 83% inheritable (Cannon, 1998). Symptoms commonly begin to appear in males during their late teens and early twenties and appear in females in their twenties or early thirties.

In an ecological study higher sugar intake is associated with higher risk of developing schizophrenia (Peet, 2004).

A study of schizophrenic patients found that plasma copper was significantly higher than in the control group. Manganese and iron concentrations were significantly lower. These observations suggest that alterations in essential trace elements Mn, Cu, and Fe may play a role in the pathogenesis of schizophrenia. Variety in results of analysis are difficult to interpret (Yanik et al, 2004).

Medical Management

Pharmaceutical therapy revolves around the use of a combination of dopamine-blocking antipsychotic medications, antidepressants, and tranquilizers. Atypical antipsychotics, the newer, second-generation medications are generally preferred because they pose a lower risk of serious side effects than do conventional medications.

Conventional, or typical, first-generation antipsychotic medications have frequent and potentially significant neurologic side effects, including the possibility of developing a movement disorder (tardive dyskinesia) that may or may not be reversible. Other treatments include psychosocial interventions such as the following:

- Individual therapy
- Social skills training
- Family therapy
- Vocational rehabilitation and supported employment.

Side effects of antipsychotics may include dry mouth, constipation, and increased appetite. Some antipsychotics should not be used with grapefruit and some other citrus fruits (see Chapter 8). Use of alcohol is contraindicated.

Medical Nutritional Therapy

People with severe mental illnesses (SMI) are more likely than other groups to be overweight, to smoke, and to have hyperglycemia and diabetes, hypertension, and dyslipidemia. Metabolic syndrome and other cardiovascular risk factors, as well as a reduced life expectancy, are common in people with schizophrenia. (Vidovic et al, 2013.)

Schizophrenia appears to be associated with altered metabolism. A computed tomography study showed that with equal total body fat and equal subcutaneous fat, there was three times the amount of visceral fat stored by schizophrenic patients. Reduced energy needs have been found in this population. The energy needs of males taking clozapine, a potent anti-psychotic drug, was overestimated by 15% using the Harris-Benedict formula (Sharpe et al, 2005).

Weight gain after the start of antipsychotic medications is a common reason for patients to discontinue medication. Weight gains of 25 to 60 lb over the course of several years have been reported. Clinically meaningful weight gain was defined as a gain of 7% above baseline and may be the trigger for a nutrition consult (Alvarez-Jimenez et al, 2006). Many patients are willing, able, and successful with weight management programs when they are offered. The most frequently used interventions included regular visits with a dietitian, a self-directed diet, and a stated treatment goal of weight loss (O'Keefe et al, 2003). Behavioral group treatment has been shown successful in preventing weight gain and achieving weight loss.

Dietary factors that affect schizophrenia and depression are similar to those that predict illnesses such as coronary heart disease and diabetes. Low levels of membrane and erythrocyte essential fatty acids have been observed, but do not appear to be related to dietary intake, but rather related to phospholipid metabolism. Supplements have been shown effective in raising the levels of essential fatty acids in cell membranes and erythrocytes. A high intake of fish oil is also associated with a better prognosis, with the EPA fraction being more helpful than the DHA (Marano et al, 2013).

Evaluating for the presence of MTFHR mutations may also contribute to treatment (Zhang et al, 2013a). MTHFR and COMT polymorphisms may increase the predilection for schizophrenia, although the exact mechanism is currently unclear (Roffman et al, 2013). MTHFR defects and elevated plasma homocysteine concentration have been suggested as risk factors for schizophrenia, but the results of epidemiologic studies have been inconsistent (Nishi et al, 2014).

The role of gluten and casein in schizophrenia has been suspected for more than 40 years, with an early blinded, controlled study showing that patients with schizophrenia on a gluten- and casein-free diet were released from the hospital significantly earlier (Niebuhr et al, 2011). See *New Directions:* A1/A2 Milk Theory for a theory on how milk protein, casein, may be a problem. New research has also investigated the role of gluten. Studies of individuals in the Clinical Antipsychotic Trials of Intervention Effectiveness (CATIE) show that 5.5% of the those with schizophrenia have a high level of anti-tTG (transglutaminase) antibodies, a measure of gluten intolerance, compared with 1.1% of the healthy control sample (Jackson et al, 2012). Twenty-three percent of those with schizophrenia (age-adjusted) had antigliaden antibodies (AGA) compared with 3.1% in the comparison sample (Cascella et al, 2011). It is strongly recommended that those with schizophrenia have blood levels checked for IgA and IgG transglutaminase antibodies to screen for celiac disease or gluten sensitivity even in the absence of gastrointestinal symptoms (Jackson, 2012a). Antigliadin antibody levels, although not as specific, are also recommended for adequate assessment. A gluten-free trial is critical if these are positive, and reasonable even if the tests are negative (see Chapter 28).

✳ NEW DIRECTIONS

The A1/A2 Milk Theory

A1 and A2 variants are variants of beta casein that differ at amino acid position 67 with histidine (CAT) in A1 and proline (CCT) in A2 milk as a result of single nucleotide polymorphism which leads to a conformational change. Absorption by infants and adults may differ related to the maturity of the gastrointestinal system. The bioactive peptide, beta casomorphin 7, BCM-7, is estimated to be 4-fold higher in Type A1 milk (Cade, 2000; Sodhi et al, 2010), is suggested as a risk factor for human health as it can potentially affect numerous opioid receptors in the nervous, endocrine, and immune system. A1 milk has been suggested as a risk factor for Type 1 diabetes, coronary heart disease, arteriosclerosis, sudden infant death syndrome, autism, and schizophrenia. Some investigations have shown reduction in autistic and schizophrenic symptoms with decrease in A1 milk intake. A1 is the most frequent in Holstein-Friesian, Ayrshire, and Red cattle while A2 is more frequent in Jersey and Guernsey cows. Much more research is needed in this field (Kaminski et al, 2007).

Interactions between nutrition and medications may be unique in persons with schizophrenia. Plasma and red-cell selenium concentrations were measured in random venous blood samples from four groups: mood disorder ($n = 36$), schizophrenics treated with clozapine ($n = 54$), schizophrenics not treated with clozapine ($n = 41$), and a healthy control group ($n = 56$). Selenium concentrations in plasma and red cells were found to be significantly lower in schizophrenic patients treated with clozapine compared with all other groups (Vaddadi et al, 2003).

Schizophrenic patients who smoke have been found to have lower erythrocyte DHA and EPA compared with nonsmokers. Smoking status must be taken into account when studying essential fatty acids in this population (see Box 41-16).

BOX 41-16   MNT for Schizophrenia

Caution against use of grapefruit and/or grapefruit juice (can alter medication blood levels) and use of alcohol (see Chapter 8).

Assessment of blood levels for IgA and IgG transglutaminase antibodies to screen for celiac disease or gluten sensitivity even in the absence of gastrointestinal symptoms.

A gluten-free trial is critical if these are positive, and reasonable even if the tests are negative.

A milk-free trial period with assessment for symptom changes.

Monitor weight: a 7% weight gain should trigger assessment for metabolic syndrome.

Refer to a behavioral weight management program as needed. In addition to nutrition-related material, program should include education regarding smoking, exercise, and alcohol consumption.

Assess diet for quality of fat intake; recommend supplement of essential fatty acids EPA and DHA to replenish or maintain cell membrane and erythrocyte fatty acid status.

Relevant mineral status includes possible excess plasma copper and low plasma selenium.

Relevant vitamin status includes genetic polymorphism of MTFHR and adequacy of folic acid intake.

REFERENCES

Agrawal R, Gomez-Pinilla F: "Metabolic syndrome" in the brain: deficiency in omega-3 fatty acid exacerbates dysfunctions in insulin receptor signaling and cognition, *J Physiol* 590:2485, 2012.

Akbaraly T, Arnaud J, et al: Plasma Selenium and Risk of Dysglycemia in an Elderly French Population: Results from the Prospective Epidemiology of Vascular Ageing Study, *Nutr Metab* 7:21, 2010.

Alramadhan E, et al: Dietary and botanical anxiolytics, *Med Sci Monit* 18:RA40, 2012.

Altamura AC, et al: Neurodevelopment and inflammatory patterns in schizophrenia in relation to pathophysiology, *Prog Neuropsychopharmacol Biol Psychiatry* 42:63, 2013.

Alvarez-Jimenez M, et al: Attenuation of antipsychotic-induced weight gain with early behavioral intervention in drug-naïve first-episode psychosis patients: a randomized controlled trial, *J Clin Psychiatry* 67:1253, 2006.

Alzheimer's Association, www.alz.org, 2015. Accessed Feb, 2016.

American Academy of Neurology: *Press release: lower blood sugars may be good for the brain*, 2015. https://www.aan.com/PressRoom/home/PressRelease/1216. Accessed January 26, 2015.

American College of Rheumatology: *2010 fibromyalgia diagnostic criteria—exerpt*, 2014. https://www.rheumatology.org/practice/clinical/classification/fibromyalgia/fibro_2010.asp. Accessed January 26, 2015.

American Heart Association (AHA): *American Heart Association comments on the World Health Organization's "Guideline: Sugars intake for adults and children"*, 2014. www.heart.org/idc/groups/ahaeccpublic/@wcm/@adv/documents/downloadable/ucm_463487.pdf. Accessed January 29, 2015.

American Psychiatric Association (APA): *Diagnostic and Statistical Manual of Mental Disorders*, ed 5, Arlington, Va, 2013, American Psychiatric Association.

Annweiler C, et al: Effectiveness of the combination of memantine plus vitamin D on cognition in patients with Alzheimer disease: a pre-post pilot study, *Cogn Behav Neurol* 25:121, 2012.

Antalis CJ, et al: Omega-3 fatty acid status in attention-deficit/hyperactivity disorder, *Prostaglandins Leukot Essent Fatty Acids* 75:299, 2006.

Antony B, et al: A pilot cross-over study to evaluate human oral bioavailability of BCM-95CG (Biocurcumax), a novel bioenhanced preparation of curcumin, *Indian J Pharm Sci* 70:445, 2008.

Armstrong DJ, et al: Vitamin D deficiency is associated with anxiety and depression in fibromyalgia, *Clin Rheumatol* 26:551, 2007.

Avellaneda Fernández A, et al: Chronic fatigue syndrome: aetiology, diagnosis and treatment, *BMC Psychiatry* 9(Suppl 1):S1, 2009.

Balhara YP: Diabetes and psychiatric disorders, *Indian J Endocr Metab* 15:274, 2011.

Barrett EJ, et al: The vascular actions of insulin control its delivery to muscle and regulate the rate-limiting step in skeletal muscle insulin action, *Diabetologia* 52:752, 2009.

Baum L, et al: Six-month randomized placebo-controlled, double-blind, pilot clinical trial of curcumin in patients with Alzheimer's disease, *J Clin Psychopharmacol* 28:110, 2008.

Bell SJ, et al: Health implications of milk containing beta-casein with the A2 genetic variant, *Crit Rev Food Sci Nutr* 46:93, 2006.

Benny M, Antony B: Bioavailability of BioCurcumax™ (BCM-095™), *Spice India* 11:1, 2006.

Benton D: Diet, cerebral energy metabolism and psychological functioning. In Lieberman HR, et al, editors: *Nutritional neuroscience*, New York, 2005, CRC Taylor and Francis.

Benton D, et al: Thiamine supplementation mood and cognitive functioning, *Psychopharmacology (Berl)* 129:66, 1997.

Berk M, et al: N-acetyl cysteine for depressive symptoms in bipolar disorder- a double-blind randomized placebo-controlled trial, *Biol Psychiatry* 64:468, 2008.

Bertone-Johnson ER, et al: Vitamin D supplementation and depression in the women's health initiative calcium and vitamin D trial, *Am J Epidemiol* 176:1, 2012.

Bhala N, et al: Vascular and upper gastrointestinal effects of non-steroidal anti-inflammatory drugs: meta-analyses of individual participant data from randomised trials, *Lancet* 382:769, 2013.

Bondi CO, et al: Adolescent behavior and dopamine availability are uniquely sensitive to dietary omega-3 fatty acid deficiency, *Biol Psychiatry* 75:38, 2014.

Bourre JM: Roles of unsaturated fatty acids (especially omega-3 fatty acids) in the brain at various ages and during ageing, *J Nutr Health Aging* 8:163, 2004.

Brinkworth GD et al: Long-term effects of a very low-carbohydrate diet and a low-fat diet on mood and cognitive function, *Arch Intern Med* 169:1873, 2009.

Burke RA, Faulkner MA: Review of the treatment of restless legs syndrome: focus on gabapentin enacarbil, *J Cent Nerv Syst Dis* 4:147, 2012.

Cai W, et al: Oral glycotoxins are a modifiable cause of dementia and the metabolic syndrome in mice and humans, *Proc Natl Acad Sci U S A* 111:4940, 2014.

Calarge CA, Ziegler EE: Iron deficiency in pediatric patients in long-term risperidone treatment, *J Child Adolesc Psychopharmacol* 23:101, 2013.

Cannon TD, et al: The Genetic epidemiology of schizophrenia in a Finnish twin cohort, *Arch Gen Psychiatry* 55(1):67–74, Jan 1998.

Cascella NG, et al: Prevalence of celiac disease and gluten sensitivity in the United States clinical antipsychotic trials of intervention effectiveness study population, *Schizophr Bull* 37:94, 2011.

Centers for Disease Control and Prevention: *Alcohol & public health, frequently asked questions*, 2014. http://www.cdc.gov/alcohol/faqs.htm. Accessed January 30, 2015.

Chang CY, et al: Essential fatty acids and human brain, *Acta Neurol Taiwan* 18:231, 2009.

Chen MH, et al: Association between psychiatric disorders and iron deficiency anemia among children and adolescents: a nationwide population-based study, *BMC Psychiatry* 13:161, 2013.

Claxton A, et al: Long-acting intranasal insulin detemir improves cognition for adults with mild cognitive impairment or early-stage Alzheimer's disease dementia, *J Alzheimers Dis* 44:897, 2015.

Connelly PJ, et al: A randomized double-blind placebo-controlled trial of folic acid supplementation of cholinesterase inhibitors in Alzheimer's disease, *Int J Geriatr Psychiatry* 23:155, 2008.

Cordero MD, et al: Oxidative stress and mitochondrial dysfunction in fibromyalgia, *Neuro Endocrinol Lett* 31:169, 2010.

Corrada MM, et al: Reduced risk of Alzheimer's disease with high folate intake: the Baltimore Longitudinal Study of Aging, *Alzheimers Dement* 1:11, 2005.

Coyne J: *The antidepressant wars, a sequel: how the media distort findings and do harm to patients*, 2012. http://blogs.plos.org/mindthebrain/2012/12/26/the-antidepressant-wars-a-sequel-how-the-media-distort-findings-and-do-harm-to-patients/. Accessed January 26, 2015.

Cuomo J, et al: Comparative absorption of a standardized curcuminoid mixture and its lecithin formulation, *J Nat Prod* 74:664, 2011.

Davison KM, Kaplan BJ: Vitamin and mineral intakes in adults with mood disorders: comparisons to nutrition standards and associations with sociodemographic and clinical variables, *J Am Coll Nutr* 30:547, 2011.

Dean O, et al: N-acetylcysteine in psychiatry: current therapeutic evidence and potential mechanisms of action, *J Psychiatry Neurosci* 36:78, 2011.

Dickerson F, et al: Markers of gluten sensitivity and celiac disease in bipolar disorder, *Bipolar Disord* 13:52, 2011.

Docherty JP, et al: A double-blind, placebo-controlled, exploratory trial of chromium picolinate in atypical depression: effect on carbohydrate craving, *J Psychiatr Pract* 11:302, 2005.

Duffy ME, et al: Biomarker responses to folic acid intervention in healthy adults: a meta-analysis of randomized controlled trials, *Am J Clin Nutr* 99:96, 2014.

Durga J, et al: Effect of 3-year folic acid supplementation on cognitive function in older adults in the FACIT trial: a randomised, double blind, controlled trial, *Lancet* 369:208, 2007.

Eby GA, Eby KL: Rapid recovery from major depression using magnesium treatment, *Med Hypotheses* 67:362, 2006.

European College of Neuropsychopharmacology (ECNP): *Glutamatergic agents show promise for mood, anxiety disorders*, 2013. www.sciencedaily.com/releases/2013/10/131006142321.htm. Accessed January 26, 2015.

European Food Safety Authority: *Review of the potential health impact of β-casomorphins and related peptides*, 2009. http://www.efsa.europa.eu/en/efsajournal/pub/231r.htm. Accessed January 26, 2015.

Fattal I, et al: The crucial role of thiamine in the development of syntax and lexical retrieval: a study of infantile thiamine deficiency, *Brain* 134(Pt 6):1720, 2011.

Faux NG, et al: Homocysteine, vitamin B_{12}, and folic acid levels in Alzheimer's disease, mild cognitive impairment, and healthy elderly: baseline characteristics in subjects of the Australian Imaging Biomarker Lifestyle study, *J Alzheimers Dis* 27:909, 2011.

Fioravanti M, Yanagi M: *Cytidinediphosphocholine (CDP-choline) for cognitive and behavioral disturbances associated with chronic cerebral disorders in the elderly*, 2010. http://onlinelibrary.wiley.com/o/cochrane/clsysrev/articles/CD000269/pdf_fs.html. Accessed January 26, 2015.

Freeman MP, et al: Omega-3 fatty acids: evidence basis for treatment and future of research in psychiatry, *J Clin Psychiatry* 67:1954, 2006.

Freund LY, et al: Transfer of omega-3 fatty acids across the blood-brain barrier after dietary supplementation with a docosahexaenoic acid-rich omega-3 fatty acid preparation in patients with Alzheimer's disease: the OmegAD study, *J Intern Med* 275:428, 2014.

Gaby AR: *Nutritional medicine*, Concord, NH, 2011, Fritz Perlberg Publishing.

Galvin R, et al: EFNS guidelines for diagnosis, therapy and prevention of Wernicke encephalopathy, *Eur J Neurol* 17:1408, 2010.

Garland EJ: Facing the evidence: antidepressant treatment in children and adolescents, *CMAJ* 170:489, 2004.

Genuis SJ, Lobo RA: Gluten sensitivity presenting as a neuropsychiatric disorder, *Gastroenterol Res Pract* Feb. 12, 2014, doi.org/10.1155/2014/293206.

Gershon MD: The enteric nervous system: a second brain, *Hosp Pract (1995)* 34:31, 1999.

Gezen-Ak D, et al: Why vitamin D in Alzheimer's disease? The hypothesis, *J Alzheimers Dis* 40:257, 2014.

Gilbody S, et al: Methylenetetrahydrofolate reductase (MTHFR) genetic polymorphisms and psychiatric disorders: a HuGE review, *Am J Epidemiol* 165:1, 2007.

Gillies D, et al: Polyunsaturated fatty acids (PUFA) for attention deficit hyperactivity disorder (ADHD) in children and adolescents, *Cochrane Database Syst Rev* 7:CD007986, 2012.

Grima NA, et al: The effects of multivitamins on cognitive performance: a systematic review and meta-analysis, *J Alzheimers Dis* 29:561, 2012.

Grober U, et al: Neuroenhancement with vitamin B_{12}—underestimated neurological significance, *Nutrients* 5:5031, 2013.

Hallahan B, et al: Omega-3 fatty acid supplementation in patients with recurrent self-harm. Single-centre double-blind randomized controlled trial, *Br J Psychiatry* 190:188, 2007.

Haller J: Vitamins and brain function. In Lieberman HR et al, editors: *Nutritional neuroscience*, New York, 2005, CRC Taylor and Francis.

Hanson AJ, et al: Effect of apolipoprotein E genotype and diet on apolipoprotein E lipidation and amyloid peptides: randomized clinical trial, *JAMA Neurol* 70:972, 2013.

Haq MR, et al: Comparative evaluation of cow β-casein variants (A1/A2) consumption on Th2-mediated inflammatory response in mouse gut, *Eur J Nutr* 53:1039, 2014.

Henderson ST, et al: Study of the ketogenic agent AC-1202 in mild to moderate Alzheimer's disease: a randomized, double-blind, placebo-controlled, multicenter trial, *Nutr Metab (Lond)* 6:31, 2009.

Hibbeln JR, Davis JM: Considerations regarding neuropsychiatric nutritional requirements for intakes of omega-3 highly unsaturated fatty acids, *Prostaglandins Leukot Essent Fatty Acids* 81:179, 2009.

Hibbeln JR, et al: Healthy intakes of n-3 and n-6 fatty acids: estimations considering worldwide diversity, *Am J Clin Nutr* 83(Suppl 6):1483S, 2006.

Insel T: *Director's blog: antidepressants: a complicated picture*, 2011. http://www.nimh.nih.gov/about/director/2011/antidepressants-a-complicated-picture.shtml. Accessed January 26, 2015.

Isasi C, et al: Fibromyalgia and non-celiac gluten sensitivity: a description with remission of fibromyalgia, *Rheumatol Int* 34:1607, 2014.

Izawa S, et al: Cynical hostility, anger expression style, and acute myocardial infarction in middle-aged Japanese men, *Behav Med* 37:81, 2011.

Jackson JR, et al: A gluten-free diet in people with schizophrenia and anti-tissue transglutaminase or anti-gliadin antibodies, *Schizophr Res* 140:262, 2012.

Jackson JR, et al: Neurologic and psychiatric manifestations of celiac disease and gluten sensitivity, *Psychiatr Q* 83:91, 2012a.

Joffe RT: Hormone treatment of depression, *Dialogues Clin Neurosci* 13:127, 2011.

Johnson C: *Pridgen reports fibromyalgia antiviral trial results "very positive": predicts new approach will be "game-changer".* 2014. http://www.cortjohnson.org/blog/2014/03/24/pridgen-reports-fibromyalgia-antiviral-trial-results-positive/. Accessed January 26, 2015.

Justice JN et al: Improved motor and cognitive performance with sodium nitrite supplementation is related to small metabolite signatures: a pilot trial in middle-aged and older adults, *Aging (Albany NY)* 7:1004, 2015.

Kaminski S, et al: Polymorphism of bovine beta-cesein and its potential effect on human health, *J Appl Genet* 48:189, 2007.

Kaplan BJ, et al: Effective mood stabilization with a chelated mineral supplement: an open-label trial in bipolar disorder, *J Clin Psychiatry* 62:936, 2001.

Kapusta ND, et al: Lithium in drinking water and suicide mortality, *Br J Psychiatry* 198:346, 2011.

Kelly T, Lieberman DZ: The use of triiodothyronine as an augmentation agent in treatment-resistant bipolar II and bipolar disorder NOS, *J Affect Disord* 116:222, 2009.

Kerti L, et al: Higher glucose levels associated with lower memory and reduced hippocampal microstructure, *Neurology* 12:1746, 2013.

Kim JW, et al: The 5-item alcohol use disorders identification test (AUDIT-5): an effective brief screening test for problem drinking, alcohol use disorders and alcohol dependence, *Alcohol Alcohol* 48:68, 2013.

Kim J, Wessling-Resnick M: Iron and mechanisms of emotional behavior, *J Nutr Biochem* 25:1101, 2014.

Kirsch I, et al: Initial severity and antidepressant benefits: a meta-analysis of data submitted to the Food and Drug Administration, *PLoS Med* 5:e45, 2008.

Kis AM, Carnes M: Detecting iron deficiency in anemic patients with concomitant medical problems, *J Gen Intern Med* 13:455, 1998.

Kjærgaard M, et al: Effect of vitamin D supplement on depression scores in people with low levels of serum 25-hydroxyvitamin D: nested case-control study and randomised clinical trial, *Br J Psychiatry* 201:360, 2012.

Leyse-Wallace R: *Linking nutrition to mental health*, Lincoln, NE, 2008, iUniverse.

Li K, et al: Associations of dietary calcium intake and calcium supplementation with myocardial infarction and stroke risk and overall cardiovascular mortality in the Heidelberg cohort of the European Prospective Investigation into Cancer and Nutrition study (EPIC-Heidelberg), *Heart* 98:920, 2012.

Lopresti AL, et al: Curcumin for the treatment of major depression: a randomised, double-blind, placebo controlled study, *J Affect Disord* 167:368, 2014.

Lozoff B, et al: Iron supplementation in infancy contributes to more adaptive behavior at 10 years of age, *J Nutr* 144:838, 2014.

Luchsinger JA, et al: Relation of higher folate intake to lower risk of Alzheimer disease in the elderly, *Arch Neurol* 64:86, 2007.

Lu'o'ng Kv, Nguyen LT: Role of thiamine in Alzheimer's disease, *Am J Alzheimers Dis Other Demen* 26:588, 2011.

Maes M, et al: The gut-brain barrier in major depression: intestinal mucosal dysfunction with an increased translocation of LPS from gram negative enterobacteria (leaky gut) plays a role in the inflammatory pathophysiology of depression, *Neuro Endocrinol Lett* 29:117, 2008.

Maes M, et al: Coenzyme Q10 deficiency in myalgic encephalomyelitis/chronic fatigue syndrome (ME/CFS) is related to fatigue, autonomic and neuro-cognitive symptoms and is another risk factor explaining the early mortality in ME/CFS due to cardiovascular disorder, *Neuro Endocrinol Lett* 30:470, 2009.

Mahmoud MM, et al: Zinc, ferritin, magnesium and copper in a group of Egyptian children with attention deficit hyperactivity disorder, *Ital J Pediatr* 37:60, 2011.

Mapstone M, et al: Plasma phospholipids identify antecedent memory impairment in older adults, *Nat Med* 20:415, 2014.

Marano G, et al: Omega-3 fatty acids and schizophrenia: evidences and recommendations, *Clin Ter* 164:e529, 2013.

Markley HG: CoEnzyme Q10 and riboflavin: the mitochondrial connection, *Headache* 52(Suppl 2):81, 2012.

Martins JG: EPA but not DHA appears to be responsible for the efficacy of omega-3 long chain polyunsaturated fatty acid supplementation in depression: evidence from a meta-analysis of randomized controlled trials, *J Am Coll Nutr* 28:525, 2009.

Masoumi A, et al: 1 alpha,25-dihydroxyvitamin D3 interacts with curcuminoids to stimulate amyloid-beta clearance by macrophages of Alzheimer's disease patients, *J Alzheimers Dis* 17:703, 2009.

McClure EA, et al: Potential role of N-acetylcysteine in the management of substance use disorders, *CNS Drugs* 28:95, 2014.

Molfino A, et al: The role for dietary omega-3 fatty acids supplementation in older adults, *Nutrients* 6:4058, 2014.

Moore E, et al: Cognitive impairment and vitamin B_{12}: a review, *Int Psychogeriatr* 24:541, 2012.

Morris JK, et al: Impaired glycemia inceases disease progression in mild cognitive impairment, *Neurobiol Aging* 35:585, 2014.

Morris MC, et al: Dietary niacin and risk of incident Alzheimer's disease and of cognitive decline, *J Neurol Neurosurg Psychiatry* 75:1093, 2004.

Morris MC, et al: Fish consumption and cognitive decline with age in a large community study, *Arch Neurol* 62:1849, 2005.

Morris MC, et al: MIND diet slows cognitive decline with aging, *Alzheimers Dement,* 11:1015, 2015.

National Institute of Mental Health (NIMH): *Bipolar disorder.* http://www.nimh.nih.gov/health/statistics/prevalence/_148124.pdf. Accessed January 30, 2015.

Niebuhr DW, et al: Association between bovine casein antibody and new onset schizophrenia among US military personnel, *Schizophr Res* 128:51, 2011.

Nierenberg AA, et al: Mitochondrial modulators for bipolar disorder: a pathophysiologically informed paradigm for new drug development, *Aust N Z J Psychiatry* 47:26, 2013.

Nishi A, et al: Meta-analyses of blood homocysteine levels for gender and genetic association studies of the MTHFR C677T polymorphism in schizophrenia, *Schizophr Bull* 40:1154, 2014.

Northam EA, Cameron FJ: Understanding the diabetic brain: new technologies but old challenges, *Diabetes* 62:341, 2013.

Nuttall KL: Evaluating selenium poisoning, *Ann Clin Lab Sci* 36:409, 2006.

O'Keefe CD, et al: Reversal of antipsychotic-associated weight gain, *J Clin Psychiatry* 64:907, 2003.

Oldham MA, Ivkovic A: Pellagrous encephalopathy presenting as alcohol withdrawal delirium: a case series and literature review, *Addict Sci Clin Pract* 7:12, 2012.

Page KA, et al: Circulating glucose levels modulate neural control of desire for high-calorie foods in humans, *J Clin Invest* 121:4161, 2011.

Pan J: Curcumin inhibition of JNKs prevents dopaminergic neuronal loss in a mouse model of Parkinson's disease through suppressing mitochondria dysfunction, *Translational Neurodegeneration* 1:16, 2012.

Paoli A, et al: Ketogenic diet in neuromuscular and neurodegenerative diseases, *Biomed Res Int* July 3, 2014, doi: 10.1155/2014/474296.

Parker GF: DSM-5 and psychotic mood disorders, *J Am Acad Psychiatry Law* 42:182, 2014.

Parmentier M, et al: Polar lipids: n-3 PUFA carriers for membranes and the brain: nutritional interest and emerging processes, Oléagineux, Corps Gras, *Lipides* 14:224, 2007.

Pasco JA, et al: Dietary selenium and major depression: a nested case-control study, *Complement Ther Med* 20:119, 2012.

Peet M: International variations in the outcome of schizophrenia and the prevalence of depression in relation to national dietary practices: an ecological analysis, *Br J Psychiatry* 184:404, 2004.

Posternak M, et al: A pilot effectiveness study: placebo-controlled trial of adjunctive L-triiodothyronine (T3) used to accelerate and potentiate the antidepressant response, *Int J Neuropsychopharmacology* 11:15, 2008.

Prakash R, et al: Rapid resolution of delusional parasitosis in pellagra with niacin augmentation therapy, *Gen Hosp Psychiatry* 30:581, 2008.

Presley TD, et al: Acute effect of a high nitrate diet on brain perfusion in older adults, *Nitric Oxide* 24:34, 2011.

Ranjbar E, Shams J: Effects of zinc supplementation on efficacy of antidepressant therapy, inflammatory cytokines, and brain-derived neurotrophic factor in patients with major depression, *Nutr Neurosci* 17:65, 2014.

Rayman MP: The importance of selenium to human health, *Lancet* 356:233, 2000.

Reger MA, et al: Intranasal insulin administration dose-dependently modulates verbal memory and plasma amyloid-β in memory-impaired older adults, *J Alzheimers Dis* 13:323, 2008.

Reginster JY, et al: Maintenance of antifracture efficacy over 10 years with strontium ranelate in postmenopausal osteoporosis, *Osteoporos Int* 23:1115, 2012.

Rigacci S, Stefani M: Nutraceuticals and amyloid neurodegenerative diseases: a focus on natural phenols, *Expert Rev Neurother* 15:41, 2015.

Roffman JL, et al: Randomized multicenter investigation of folate plus vitamin B$_{12}$ supplementation in schizophrenia, *JAMA Psychiatry* 70:481, 2013.

Sanmukhani J, et al: Efficacy and safety of curcumin in major depressive disorder: a randomized controlled trial, *Phytother Res* 28:579, 2014.

Schiöth HB, et al: Brain insulin signaling and Alzheimer's disease: current evidence and future directions, *Mol Neurobiol* 46:4, 2012.

Serata D, et al: Hemochromatosis-induced bipolar disorder: a case report, *Gen Hosp Psychiatry* 34:101, 2012.

Sharkey KA, Savidge TC: Role of enteric neurotransmission in host defense and protection of the gastrointestinal tract, *Auton Neurosci* 181:94, 2014.

Sharma A, et al: Role of medium chain triglycerides (Axona (R)) in the treatment of mild to moderate Alzheimer's Disease, *Am J Alzheimers Dis and Other Dement*, 29:409, 2014.

Sharpe JK, et al: Resting energy expenditure is lower than predicted in people taking atypical antipsychotic medication, *J Am Diet Assoc* 105:612, 2005.

Shoemark DK, Allen SJ: The microbiome and disease: reviewing the links between the oral microbiome, aging and Alzheimer's disease, *J Alzheimers Dis* 43:725, 2015.

Sienkiewicz-Szłapkaa E, et al: Contents of agonistic and antagonistic opioid peptides in different cheese varieties, *International Dairy J* 19:258, 2009.

Singh K, et al: Sulforaphane treatment of autism spectrum disorder (ASD), *Proc Natl Acad Sci U S A* 111:15550, 2014.

Sinn N, Bryan J: Effects of supplementation with polyunsaturated fatty acids and micronutrients on learning and behavior problems associated with child ADHD, *J Dev Behav Pediatr* 28:82, 2007.

Skinner GR: Letter to the editor: thyroxine should be tried in clinically hypothyroid but biochemically euthyroid patients, *BMJ* 314:1760, 1997.

Spencer JP: The impact of fruit flavonoids on memory and cognition, *Br J Nutr* 104(Suppl 3): S40, 2010.

Stewart R, Hirani V: Relationship between vitamin D levels and depressive symptoms in older residents from a national survey population, *Psychosom Med* 72:608, 2010.

Sublette ME, Ellis SP: Meta-analysis of the effects of eicosapentaenoic acid (EPA) in clinical trials in depression, *J Clin Psychiatry* 72:1577, 2011.

Teitelbaum JE: Effective treatment of chronic fatigue syndrome, *Integr Med* 10:44, 2012a.

Teitelbaum JE: *From fatigued to fantastic!* ed 3, New York, 2007, Penguin/Avery.

Teitelbaum JE: Nutrition Primer. Cures A-Z (iPhone and Android App) and www.Vitality101.com, 2015.

Teitelbaum JE, et al: Improving communication skills in children with allergy-related Autism using Nambudripad's allergy elimination techniques: a pilot study, *Integr Medicine* 10:36, 2011.

Teitelbaum JE, et al: The use of D-ribose in chronic fatigue syndrome and fibromyalgia: a pilot study, *J Altern Complement Med* 12:857, 2006.

Teitelbaum JE, et al: Treatment of chronic fatigue syndrome and fibromyalgia with d-ribose, *Open Pain Jl* 5:32, 2012b.

Teitelbaum JE: *The Complete Guide to Beating Sugar Addiction,* 2015, Beverly, MA, Fairwinds Press.

Trelle S, et al: Cardiovascular safety of non-steroidal anti-inflammatory drugs: network meta-analysis, *BMJ* 342:c7086, 2011.

Tyszka-Czochara M, et al: The role of zinc in the pathogenesis and treatment of central nervous system (CNS) diseases. Implications of zinc homeostasis for proper CNS function, *Acta Pol Pharm* 71:369, 2014.

Undurraga J, Baldessarini RJ: Randomized, placebo-controlled trials of antidepressants for acute major depression: thirty-year meta-analytic review, *Neuropsychopharmacology* 37:851, 2012.

Uribarri J, et al: Advanced glycation end products in foods and a practical guide to their reduction in the diet, *J Am Diet Assoc* 110:911, 2010.

Usoro OB, Mousa SA: Vitamin E forms in Alzheimer's disease: a review of controversial and clinical experiences, *Crit Rev Food Sci Nutr* 50:414, 2010.

Vaddadi KS, et al: Low blood selenium concentrations in schizophrenic patients on clozapine, *Br J Clin Pharmacol* 55:307, 2003.

Vannice G, Rasmussen H: Position of the Academy of Nutrition and Dietetics: dietary fatty acids for healthy adults, *J Acad Nutr Diet* 114:136, 2014.

Valls-Pedret C, et al: Polyphenol-rich foods in the Mediterranean diet are associated with better cognitive function in elderly subjects at high cardiovascular risk, *J Alzheimers Dis* 29:773, 2012.

Vashum KP, et al: Dietary zinc is associated with a lower incidence of depression: findings from two Australian cohorts, *J Affect Disord* 166:249, 2014.

Vaucher P, et al: Effect of iron supplementation on fatigue in nonanemic menstruating women with low ferritin: a randomized controlled trial, *CMAJ* 184:1247, 2012.

Vermeulen RC, Scholte HR: Exploratory open label, randomized study of acetyl- and propionylcarnitine in chronic fatigue syndrome, *Psychosom Med* 66:276, 2004.

Vidal-Alaball J, et al: Oral vitamin B$_{12}$ versus intramuscular vitamin B$_{12}$ for vitamin B$_{12}$ deficiency, *Cochrane Database Syst Rev* 3:CD004655, 2005.

Vidovic B, et al: Selenium, zinc, and copper plasma levels in patients with schizophrenia: relationship with metabolic risk factors, *Biol Trace Elem Res* 156:22, 2013.

Walton AG: *How much sugar are Americans eating?* 2012. http://www.forbes.com/sites/alicegwalton/2012/08/30/how-much-sugar-are-americans-eating-infographic/. Accessed January 29, 2015.

Wang J, et al: Efficacy of oral iron in patients with restless legs syndrome and a low-normal ferritin: a randomized, double blind, placebo controlled study, *Sleep Med* 10:973, 2009.

WebMD: *Find a vitamin or supplement: selenium*, 2009. http://www.webmd.com/vitamins-supplements/ingredientmono-1003-SELENIUM.aspx?activeIngredientId=1003&activeIngredientName=SELENIUM&source=2&tabno=6. Accessed January 26, 2015.

Welch AA, et al: Dietary intake and status of n-3 polyunsaturated fatty acids in a population of fish-eating and non-fish-eating meat-eaters, vegetarians, and vegans and the precursor-product ratio of a-linolenic acid to long–chain n-3 polyunsaturated fatty acids: results from the EPIC-Norfolk cohort, *Am J Clin Nutr* 92:1040, 2010.

White L: *Alzheimer's Disease May Be Easily Misdiagnosed*, Honolulu, Hawaii, 2011, American Academy of Neurology- Contemporary and Clinical Issues and Case Studies Plenary Session Annual Meeting.

Willette AA, et al: Insulin resistance predicts brain amyloid deposition in late middle-aged adults, *Alzheimers Dement* 11:504, 2014.

Wolfe F, et al: Fibromyalgia criteria and severity scales for clinical and epidemiological studies: a modification of the ACR Preliminary Diagnostic Criteria for Fibromyalgia, *J Rheumatol* 38:1113, 2011.

Wolfe F, et al: Fibromyalgia prevalence, somatic symptom reporting, and the dimensionality of polysymptomatic distress: results from a survey of the general population, *Arthritis Care Res (Hoboken)* 65:777, 2013.

Wollen KA: Alzheimer's Disease: the pros and cons of pharmaceutical, nutritional, botanical, and stimulatory therapies, with a discussion of treatment strategies from the perspective of patients and practitioners, *Altern Med Rev* 15:223, 2010.

World Health Organization (WHO): *Depression*, 2012. http://www.who.int/mediacentre/factsheets/fs369/en/Fact sheet. Accessed January 29, 2015.

Woodhead JL, et al: An analysis of N-acetylcysteine treatment for acetaminophen overdose using a systems model of drug-induced liver injury, *J Pharmacol Exp Ther* 342:529, 2012.

World Health Organization (WHO): *Global Burden of Disease Study 2010*, 2012. http://www.thelancet.com/themed/global-burden-of-disease. Accessed January 29, 2015.

Yanik M, et al: Plasma manganese, selenium, zinc, copper, and iron concentrations in patients with schizophrenia, *Biol Trace Elem Res* 98:109, 2004.

Yetley EA, Johnson CL: Folate and vitamin B-12 biomarkers in NHANES: history of their measurement and use, *Am J Clin Nutr* 94: S322, 2011.

Young H, Benton D: The nature of the control of blood glucose in those with poorer glucose tolerance influences mood and cognition, *Metab Brain Dis* 29:721, 2014.

Young SN: Folate and depression–a neglected problem, *J Psychiatry Neurosci* 32:80, 2007.

Zhang G, et al: Thiamine nutritional status and depressive symptoms are inversely associated among older Chinese adults, *J Nutr* 143:53, 2013.

Zhang Y, et al: Association of MTHFR C677T polymorphism with schizophrenia and its effect on episodic memory and gray matter density in patients, *Behav Brain Res* 243:146, 2013a.

Zhao Y, Zhao B: Oxidative stress and the pathogenesis of Alzheimer's disease, *Oxid Med Cell Longev* 2013:316523, 2013.

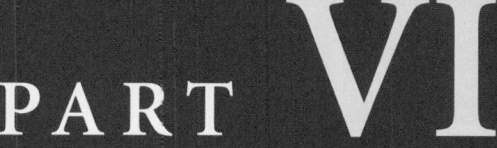

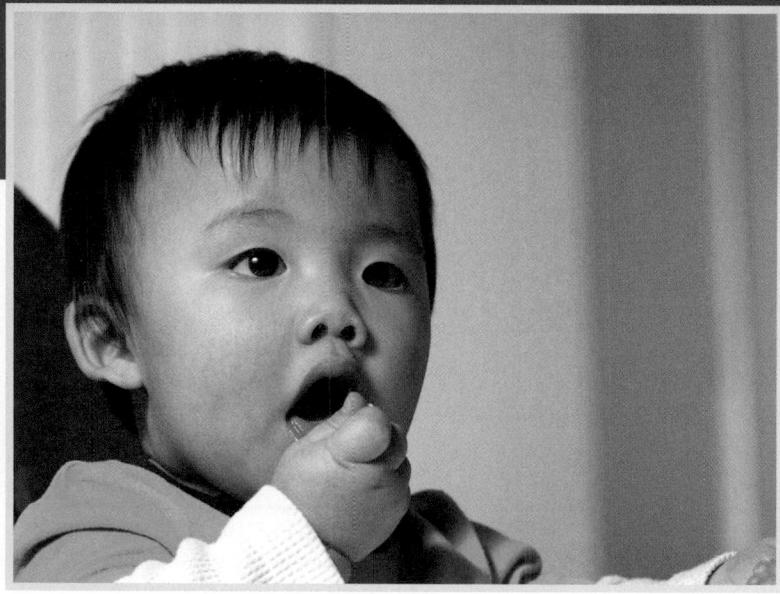

Pediatric Specialties

The unique, special roles of nutrition in the pediatric population cannot be underestimated. Pediatricians, nurses, and dietitian nutritionists all recognize that unusual feeding problems or disorders can negatively influence growth and health, especially in the very young. This section addresses the categories affecting the nutritional intake and growth velocity of infants and children. In some cases, adolescents are mentioned if relevant, but most of this section considers younger patients.

Whether in neonatal units, in hospital pediatric units, in out-patient clinics, in long-term care units, or in home care, children need to grow as well as cope with genetic or acquired disorders. More than ever, nutrition care in this specialty arena requires an understanding of the biochemical, physiological, social, and economic challenges that our youngest citizens face.

Medical Nutrition Therapy for Low-Birth-Weight Infants

Diane M. Anderson, PhD, RDN, FADA

KEY TERMS

apnea of prematurity
appropriate for gestational age (AGA)
bronchopulmonary dysplasia (BPD)
carnitine
extrauterine growth restriction (EUGR)
extremely low birthweight (ELBW)
gastric gavage
gestational age
glucose load

hemolytic anemia
human milk fortifiers
infancy
infant mortality rate
intrauterine growth restriction (IUGR)
kangaroo care
large for gestational age (LGA)
low birthweight (LBW)
necrotizing enterocolitis (NEC)

neonatal period
neutral thermal environment
osteopenia of prematurity
perinatal period
premature (preterm) infant
respiratory distress syndrome (RDS)
small for gestational age (SGA)
surfactant
term infant
very low birthweight (VLBW)

The management of low birthweight (LBW) infants requiring intensive care is continually improving. With new technologies, enhanced understanding of pathophysiologic conditions of the perinatal period (from 20 weeks of gestation to 28 days after birth), current nutrition management principles, and regionalization of perinatal care, the mortality rate during infancy—that period from birth to 1 year of age—has decreased in the United States. In particular, the development and use of surfactant—a mixture of lipoproteins secreted by alveolar cells into the alveoli and respiratory air passages that contributes to the elastic properties of pulmonary tissue—has increased the survival of preterm infants, as has the use of antepartum corticosteroids. Most premature infants have the potential for long and productive lives (Hack, 2013).

Nutrition can be provided to LBW infants in many ways, each of which has certain benefits and limitations. The infant's size, age, and clinical condition dictate the nutrition requirements and the way they can be met. Because of the complexities involved in the neonatal intensive care setting, a team that includes a registered dietitian nutritionist trained in neonatal nutrition should make the decisions necessary to facilitate optimal nutrition (Ehrenkranz, 2014). Neonatal nutritionists monitor compliance with standardized feeding guidelines; ensure that early, intense nutritional support is initiated; facilitate the smooth transition from parenteral to enteral nutrition; and monitor growth and individualized nutrition support to maintain steady infant growth. In regionalized perinatal care systems, the neonatal nutritionist also may consult with health care providers in community hospitals and public health settings.

INFANT MORTALITY AND STATISTICS

In 2011 the infant mortality rate in the United States decreased to 6.05 infant deaths per 1000 live births (MacDorman et al, 2013). More than 56% of these deaths occur in the neonatal period, with the leading causes being birth defects, prematurity, and LBW. The preterm birth rate was 11.7%, and the incidence of LBW was 8.1% (Hamilton et al, 2013). Both rates are decreased from the 2006 rate and mark a change from the previous 20-year increase in premature and LBW infants.

The US infant mortality rate still remains higher than that for many industrialized countries (Hamilton et al, 2013). This discrepancy may be attributable to the inconsistent collection of mortality data among nations, which may falsely lower mortality rates in other countries. However, the high incidence of premature and LBW infants born in the United States contributes to this high infant mortality rate (Hamilton et al, 2013; MacDorman et al, 2013).

PHYSIOLOGIC DEVELOPMENT

Gestational Age and Size

At birth an infant who weighs less than 2500 g (5½ lb) is classified as having a low birthweight (LBW); an infant weighing less than 1500 g (3⅓ lb) has a very low birthweight (VLBW); and an infant weighing less than 1000 g (2¼ lb) has an extremely low birthweight (ELBW). LBW may be attributable to a shortened period of gestation, prematurity, or a restricted intrauterine growth rate, which makes the infant small for gestational age (SGA).

The term infant is born between the 37th and 42nd weeks of gestation. A premature (preterm) infant is born before 37 weeks of gestation, whereas a postterm infant is born after 42 weeks of gestation.

Antenatally, an estimate of the infant's gestational age is based on the date of the mother's last menstrual period, clinical parameters of uterine fundal height, the presence of quickening (the first movements of the fetus that can be felt by the mother), fetal heart tones, or ultrasound evaluations. After birth, gestational age is determined by clinical assessment. Clinical parameters fall into two groups: (1) a series of neurologic signs, which depend primarily on postures and tone and (2) a series of external characteristics that reflect the physical maturity of the infant. The New Ballard Score examination is a frequently used clinical assessment tool (Ballard et al, 1991). An accurate assessment of gestational age is important for establishing nutritional goals for individual infants and differentiating the premature infant from the term SGA infant.

An infant who is **small for gestational age (SGA)** has a birth weight that is lower than the 10th percentile of the standard weight for that gestational age. An SGA infant whose intrauterine weight gain is poor, but whose linear and head growth are between the 10th and 90th percentiles on the intrauterine growth grid, has experienced asymmetric **intrauterine growth restriction (IUGR)**. An SGA infant whose length and occipital frontal circumference are also below the 10th percentile of the standards has symmetric IUGR. Symmetric IUGR, which usually reflects early and prolonged intrauterine deficit, is apparently more detrimental to later growth and development. Some infants can be SGA because they are genetically small, and these infants usually do well.

An infant whose size is **appropriate for gestational age (AGA)** has a birth weight between the 10th and 90th percentiles on the intrauterine growth chart. The obstetrician diagnoses IUGR when the fetal growth rate decreases. Serial ultrasound measurements document this reduction in fetal anthropometric measurements, which may be caused by maternal, placental, or fetal abnormalities. The future growth and development of infants who have had IUGR is diverse, depending on the specific cause of the IUGR and treatment. Some infants who suffered from IUGR are SGA, but many may plot as AGA infants at birth. Decreased fetal growth does not always result in an infant who is SGA.

An infant whose birth weight is above the 90th percentile on the intrauterine growth chart is **large for gestational age (LGA)**. Box 42-1 summarizes the weight classifications. Figure 42-1 shows the classification of neonates based on maturity and intrauterine growth.

Characteristics of Immaturity

The premature or LBW infant has not had the chance to develop fully in utero and is physiologically different from the term infant (see Figure 42-2). Because of this, LBW infants have various clinical problems in the early **neonatal period**, depending on their intrauterine environment, degree of prematurity, birth-related trauma, and function of immature or

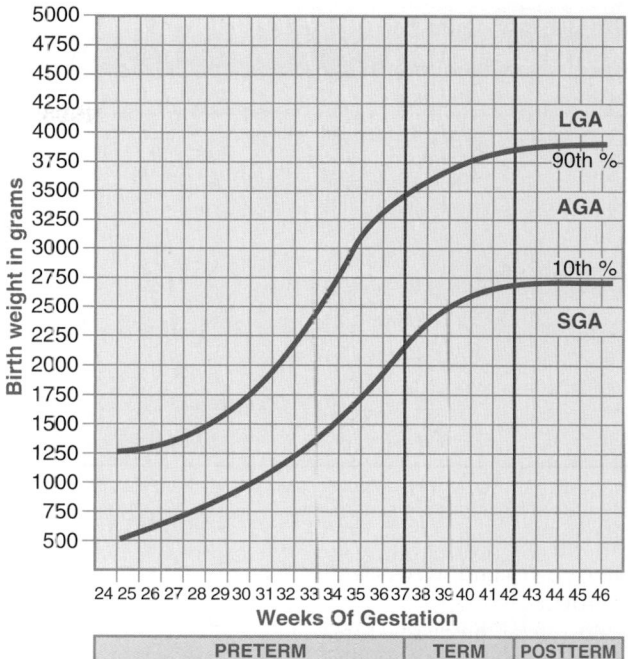

FIGURE 42-1 Classification of neonates based on maturity and intrauterine growth (small for gestational age [SGA], appropriate for gestational age [AGA], or large for gestational age [LGA]). (From Battaglia FC, Lubchenco LO: A practical classification of newborn infants by weight and gestational age, *J Pediatr* 71:159, 1967.)

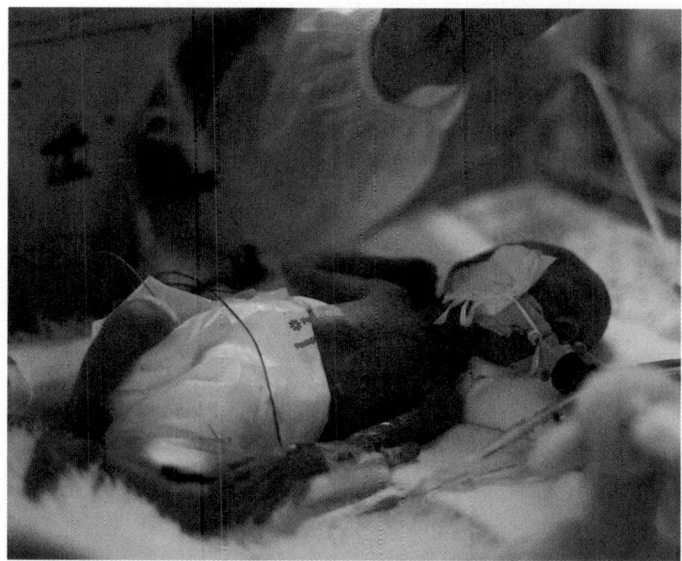

FIGURE 42-2 A.R., born at 27 weeks of gestation; birth weight of 870 g (1 lb, 14 oz).

BOX 42-1   Classification of Birth Weight and Intrauterine Growth

Low birth weight <2500 g
Very low birth weight <1500 g
Extremely low birth weight <1000 g
Small for gestational age = Birth weight <10th percentile of standard for gestational age
Appropriate for gestational age = Birth weight between the 10th and 90th percentile of standard for gestational age
Large for gestational age = Birth weight >90th percentile of standard for gestational age

stressed organ systems. Certain problems occur with such frequency that they are considered typical of prematurity (see Table 42-1). Premature infants are at high risk for poor nutrition status because of poor nutrient stores, physiologic immaturity, illness (which may interfere with nutritional

TABLE 42-1 Common Problems Among Premature Infants

System	Problem
Respiratory	Respiratory distress syndrome, chronic lung disease (bronchopulmonary dysplasia)
Cardiovascular	Patent ductus arteriosus
Renal	Fluid and electrolyte imbalance
Neurologic	Intraventricular hemorrhage, periventricular leukomalacia (cerebral necrosis)
Metabolic	Hypoglycemia, hyperglycemia, hypocalcemia, metabolic acidosis
Gastrointestinal	Hyperbilirubinemia, feeding intolerance, necrotizing enterocolitis
Hematologic	Anemia
Immunologic	Sepsis, pneumonia, meningitis
Other	Apnea, bradycardia, cyanosis, osteopenia

From Cloherty JP et al, editors: *Manual of neonatal care,* ed 7, Philadelphia, 2012, Wolters Kluwer/Lippincott Williams & Wilkins.

management and needs), and the nutrient demands required for growth.

Most fetal nutrient stores are deposited during the last 3 months of gestation; therefore, the premature infant begins life in a compromised nutritional state. Because metabolic (i.e., energy) stores are limited, nutrition support in the form of parenteral nutrition (PN), enteral nutrition (EN), or both should be initiated as soon as possible. In the preterm infant weighing 1000 g, fat constitutes only 1% of total body weight; by contrast the term infant (3500 g) has a fat percentage of approximately 16%. For example, a 1000-g AGA premature infant has a glycogen and fat reserve equivalent to approximately 110 kcal/kg of body weight. With basal metabolic needs of approximately 50 kcal/kg/day, it is obvious that this infant will rapidly run out of fat and carbohydrate fuel unless adequate nutrition support is established. The depletion time is even shorter for preterm infants weighing less than 1000 g at birth. Nutrient reserves also are depleted most quickly by tiny infants who have IUGR as a result of their decreased nutrient stores.

Theoretic estimates of survival time of starved and semi-starved infants are shown in Table 42-2. These estimates assume depletion of all glycogen and fat and approximately one third of body protein tissue at a rate of 50 kcal/kg/day. The effects of fluids such as intravenously provided water (which has no exogenous calories) and 10% dextrose solution ($D_{10}W$) are shown. Currently, PN fluids are started on the day of birth to provide energy and protein for the VLBW infant. Early protein intake promotes positive nitrogen balance, normal plasma amino acid levels, and glucose tolerance.

TABLE 42-2 Expected Survival Time of Starved (H_2O Only) and Semistarved ($D_{10}W$) Infants

| Birth Weight (g) | ESTIMATED SURVIVAL TIME (Days) | |
	H_2O	$D_{10}W$
1000	4	11
2000	12	30
3500	32	80

Data from Heird WC et al: Intravenous alimentation in pediatric patients, *J Pediatr* 80:351, 1972.
$D_{10}W$, Dextrose 10% in water; H_2O, water.

The small premature infant is particularly vulnerable to undernutrition. Malnutrition in premature infants may increase the risk of infection, prolong chronic illness, and adversely affect brain growth and function. Premature infants fed premature infant formula or human milk demonstrate better growth and development than premature infants fed standard infant formula. Milk from the infant's own mother fed the first month of life has been linked to improved growth and development. Premature infants fed their own mother's milk have improved neurodevelopment at 30 months of age and higher intelligence test scores at 8 years of age and have brains larger and more developed at 15 years of age (American Academy of Pediatrics [AAP], Section on Breastfeeding, 2012; Issacs et al, 2010).

NUTRITION REQUIREMENTS: PARENTERAL FEEDING

Many critically ill preterm infants have difficulty progressing to full enteral feedings in the first several days or even weeks of life. The infant's small stomach capacity, immature gastrointestinal tract, and illness make the progression to full enteral feedings difficult (see *Pathophysiology and Care Management Algorithm: Nutrition Support of Premature Infants*). PN becomes essential for nutrition support, either as a supplement to enteral feedings or as the total source of nutrition. Chapter 13 offers a complete discussion of PN; only aspects related to feeding of the preterm infant are presented here.

Fluid

Because fluid needs vary widely for preterm infants, fluid balance must be monitored. Inadequate intake can lead to dehydration, electrolyte imbalances, and hypotension; excessive intake can lead to edema, congestive heart failure, and possible opening of the ductus arteriosus. Additional neonatal clinical complications reported with high fluid intakes include necrotizing enterocolitis (NEC) and bronchopulmonary dysplasia (BPD) (see Chapter 34).

The premature infant has a greater percentage of body water (especially extracellular water) than the term infant (see Chapter 6). The amount of extracellular water should decrease in all infants during the first few days of life. This reduction is accompanied by a normal loss of 10% to 15% of body weight and improved renal function. Failure of this transition in fluid dynamics and lack of diuresis may complicate the course of preterm infants with respiratory disease.

Water requirements are estimated by the sum of the predicted losses from the lungs and skin, urine, and stool, and the water needed for growth. A major route of water loss in preterm infants is evaporation through the skin and respiratory tract. This insensible water loss is highest in the smallest and least mature infants because of their larger body surface area relative to body weight, increased permeability of the skin epidermis to water, and greater skin blood flow relative to metabolic rate. Insensible water loss is increased by radiant warmers and phototherapy lights and decreased by humidified incubators, heat shields and thermal blankets. Insensible water loss can vary from 50 to 100 ml/kg/day on the first day of life and increase up to 150 ml/kg/day, depending on the infant's size, gestational age, day of life, and environment. The use of humidified incubators can decrease insensible water losses and thereby reduce fluid requirements.

PATHOPHYSIOLOGY AND CARE MANAGEMENT ALGORITHM

Nutrition Support of Premature Infants

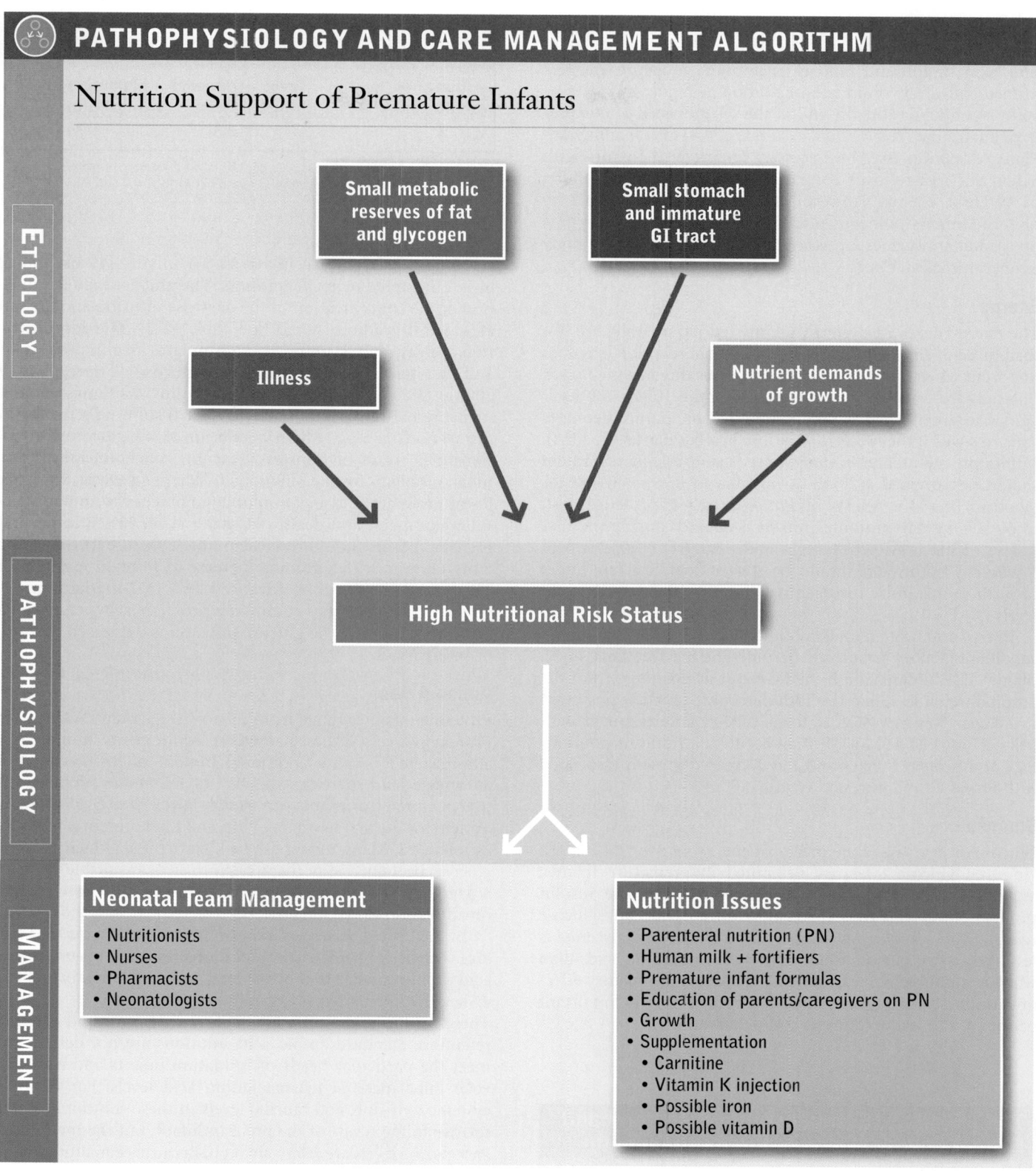

ETIOLOGY

Small metabolic reserves of fat and glycogen

Small stomach and immature GI tract

Illness

Nutrient demands of growth

PATHOPHYSIOLOGY

High Nutritional Risk Status

MANAGEMENT

Neonatal Team Management

- Nutritionists
- Nurses
- Pharmacists
- Neonatologists

Nutrition Issues

- Parenteral nutrition (PN)
- Human milk + fortifiers
- Premature infant formulas
- Education of parents/caregivers on PN
- Growth
- Supplementation
  - Carnitine
  - Vitamin K injection
  - Possible iron
  - Possible vitamin D

Excretion of urine, the other major route of water loss, varies from 1 to 3 ml/kg/hr (Doherty, 2012). This loss depends on the fluid volume and solute load presented to the kidneys. The infant's ability to concentrate urine increases with maturity. Stool water loss is generally 5 to 10 ml/kg/day, and 10 to 15 ml/kg/day is suggested as optimal for growth (Dell, 2011).

Because of the many variables affecting neonatal fluid losses, fluid needs must be determined on an individual basis. Usually fluid is administered at a rate of 60 to 100 ml/kg/day the first day of life to meet insensible losses and urine output. Fluid needs then are evaluated by assessing fluid intake and comparing it with the clinical parameters of urine output volume and serum electrolyte, creatinine, and urea nitrogen levels. Assessments of weight, blood pressure, peripheral perfusion, skin turgor, and mucous membrane moisture are performed daily. Daily fluid administration generally increases by 10 to 20 ml/kg/day. By the end of the second week of life, preterm infants may receive fluids at a rate of 140 to 160 ml/kg/day. Fluid restriction may be necessary in preterm infants with patent ductus arteriosus, congestive heart failure, renal failure, or cerebral edema. However, more fluids are needed by preterm infants who are placed under phototherapy lights or a radiant warmer or when the environmental or body temperature is elevated.

Energy

The energy needs of preterm infants fed parenterally are less than those of enterally fed infants because absorption loss does not occur when nutritional intake bypasses the intestinal tract. Enterally fed preterm infants usually require 105 to 130 kcal/kg/day to grow, whereas parenterally fed premature neonates can grow well if they receive 90 to 100 kcal/kg/day (AAP, 2014). Minimum maintenance energy needs and adequate protein should be provided as soon as possible to prevent tissue catabolism. Providing VLBW infants with 1.5 g of protein and 40 to 60 kcal/kg/day promotes nitrogen balance during the first 3 days of life (AAP, 2014; Rigo and Senterre, 2013). Two to 3 g/kg/day of protein should be started within a few hours of birth to maximize nitrogen balance and blood amino acid levels (AAP, 2014).

Energy and protein intake should be increased as the infant's condition stabilizes and growth becomes the goal (see Table 42-3). Many VLBW infants are born AGA but at discharge from the hospital weigh less than the 10th percentile for their postmenstrual age. This new SGA status is called extrauterine growth restriction (EUGR). EUGR may occur as a result of poor energy and protein intakes and the decreased growth associated with illness (Lapillonne and Griffin, 2013).

Glucose

Glucose or dextrose is the principal energy source (3.4 kcal/g). However, glucose tolerance is limited in premature infants, especially in VLBW infants, because of inadequate insulin production, insulin resistance, and continued hepatic glucose release while intravenous glucose is infusing. Hyperglycemia is less likely when glucose is administered with amino acids than when it is infused alone. Amino acids exert a stimulatory effect on insulin release. Prevention of hyperglycemia is important because it can lead to diuresis and dehydration.

TABLE 42-4 Guidelines for Glucose Load in Premature Infants

Initial Load (mg/kg/min)*	Daily Increments (mg/kg/min)	Maximum Load (mg/kg/min)
4-6	1-2	11-12

*Use the following formula to calculate glucose load: (% Glucose × ml/kg/day) × (1000 mg/g glucose) ÷ (1440 min/day). For example, (0.10 × 150 ml/kg/day) × (1000 mg/g glucose) ÷ (1440 min/day) = 10.4 mg/kg/min.

To prevent hyperglycemia in VLBW infants, glucose should be administered in small amounts. The glucose load is a function of the concentration of the dextrose infusion and the rate at which it is administered (see Table 42-4). The administration of intravenous amino acids stimulates insulin production and the tolerance of intravenous glucose (Thureen et al, 2003). The administration of exogenous insulin is avoided with premature infants (AAP, 2014). Insulin adheres to the intravenous tubing, which results in blood glucose fluctuations as a result of nonsteady insulin concentrations. Additional problems for the infant include hypoglycemia, decreased linear growth, the association of hypoglycemia with poor neurodevelopment, and death (Alsweiler et al, 2012). In general, preterm infants should receive an initial glucose load of 4.5 to 6 mg/kg/min, with a gradual increase to 11 to 12 mg/kg/min. The glucose load can be advanced by 1 to 2 mg/kg/min/day. Hypoglycemia is not as common a problem as hyperglycemia, but it may occur if the glucose infusion is decreased abruptly or interrupted.

Amino Acids

Protein guidelines range from 2.7 to 4.0 g/kg/day (AAP, 2014). Protein in excess of these parenteral requirements should not be administered because additional protein offers no apparent advantage, and increases the risk of metabolic problems. In practice preterm infants are usually given 2 to 3 g/kg/day of protein for the first few days of life, and then protein is provided as tolerated. Many nurseries stock starter PN, which is water, glucose, protein, and perhaps calcium and is available 24 hours a day. Infants then can be provided with protein immediately on admission to the nursery.

In the United States several pediatric PN solutions are available. The use of pediatric PN solutions results in plasma amino acid profiles similar to those of fetal and cord blood or to those of healthy infants fed breastmilk (van Goudoever et al, 2014). These solutions promote adequate weight gain and nitrogen retention. Standard amino acid solutions are not designed to meet the particular needs of immature infants and may provoke imbalances in plasma amino acid levels. For example, cysteine, tyrosine, and taurine levels in these solutions are low relative to the needs of the preterm infant, but the methionine and glycine levels are relatively high. Because premature infants do not effectively synthesize cysteine from methionine because of decreased concentrations of the hepatic enzyme cystathionase, a cysteine supplement has been suggested. Cysteine is insoluble and unstable in solution; thus it is added as cysteine hydrochloride when the PN solution is prepared.

In addition to plasma amino acid imbalances, other metabolic problems associated with amino acid infusions in preterm infants include metabolic acidosis, hyperammonemia, and azotemia. These problems can be minimized by using the crystalline

TABLE 42-3 Comparison of Parenteral and Enteral Energy Needs of Premature Infants

	Parenteral	Enteral
MAINTENANCE		
Gradually increase intake to meet energy needs by the end of the first week	30-50 kcal/kg/day	50 kcal/kg/day
GROWTH		
Meet energy needs as soon as the infant's condition is stable	90-100 kcal/kg/day	105-130 kcal/kg/day

TABLE 42-5 Guidelines for Administration of Parenteral Amino Acids for Premature Infants

Initial Rate (g/kg/day)*	Increments (g/kg/day)	Maximum Rate (g/kg/day)
2-3	Advance to meet needs	4

Data from American Academy of Pediatrics, Committee on Nutrition: Nutritional needs of preterm infants. In Kleinman RE, Greer FR, editors: *Pediatric nutrition handbook*, ed 7, Elk Grove, Ill, 2014, American Academy of Pediatrics.

*Use the following formula to calculate protein load: % Protein × ml/kg/day = Protein g/kg/day.

For example: 2% amino acid parenteral solution provided at 150 ml/kg/day *is* 0.02 × 150 ml/kg/day = 3 g/kg/day.

amino acid products that are available and by keeping the protein load within the recommended guidelines (see Table 42-5).

Lipids

Intravenous fat emulsions are used for two reasons: (1) to meet essential fatty acid (EFA) requirements and (2) to provide a concentrated source of energy. EFA needs can be met by providing 0.5 g/kg/day of lipids. Biochemical evidence of EFA deficiency has been noted during the first week of life in VLBW infants fed parenterally without fat. The clinical consequences of EFA deficiency may include coagulation abnormalities, abnormal pulmonary surfactant, and adverse effects on lung metabolism.

Lipids can be initiated at 1 to 2 g/kg/day and should be provided over 24 hours (AAP, 2014). Lipids can be advanced by 1 to 2 g/kg/day until a rate of 3 g/kg/day is reached (see Table 42-6). Plasma triglycerides should be monitored because elevated triglyceride levels may develop in infants with a decreased ability to hydrolyze triglycerides. These infants usually have lower gestational age, SGA status, infection, surgical stress, or liver disease. Monitoring of serum triglyceride levels is indicated, and a rate of less than 3 g/kg/day of fat may be required to keep serum triglyceride levels under 200 mg/dl (AAP, 2014). Once the infant is medically stable and additional energy is needed for growth, lipid loads can be increased slowly. Intralipids can be given to the infant with hyperbilirubinemia. At the present recommendation of 3 g/kg/day, given over 24 hours, the displacement of bilirubin from albumin-binding sites does not occur (AAP, 2014).

The total lipid load is usually 25% to 40% of nonprotein calories (AAP, 2014). (The lipid emulsions currently in use are described in Chapter 13.) In preterm infants 20% solutions providing 2 kcal/ml are recommended because plasma triglyceride, cholesterol, and phospholipid levels are generally lower

with these than with the 10% emulsions. The 10% emulsions contain more of the phospholipid emulsifier per gram of lipid and this emulsifier decreases the breakdown of triglycerides.

Intravenous fat emulsions are made from soybean oil and contain omega-6 fatty acids, linoleic acid, and arachidonic acid (ARA). These EFAs increase the production of inflammatory mediators and increase the infant's inflammatory state (Premkumar et al, 2014) (see Chapter 3 and *Focus On:* Biochemistry of Inflammation in Chapter 39). There is a fish-oil base intravenous fat and it contains omega-3 fatty acids: eicosapentaenoic acid (EPA) and docosahexaenoic acid (DHA). These omega-3 fatty acids are antiinflammatory and are helpful in the treatment of parenteral nutrition-associated liver disease (Premkumar et al, 2014). This fish-oil product is produced in Europe and requires approval for compassionate use by the Food and Drug Administration (FDA) for patients in the United States.

Clinical experience with the fish-oil base intravenous fat is positive with resolution of PN-associated liver disease in most premature infants (Premkumar et al, 2014). Investigations are needed to determine whether this product can be used to prevent PN-associated liver disease, which presents with an elevated conjugated bilirubin. Another European fat emulsion, SMOF (soy oil, medium-chain triglyceride, olive oil, and fish oil) has just become available in the United States and requires approval by the FDA for compassionate use. This blend of fat oils may also offer antiinflammatory properties (Vanek et al, 2012).

Carnitine is frequently added to PN solutions for premature infants. Carnitine facilitates the mechanism by which fatty acids are transported across the mitochondrial membrane, allowing their oxidation to provide energy. Because intravenous lipid does not contain carnitine and premature infants have limited ability to produce carnitine, carnitine supplementation may be helpful for preterm infants who are receiving only PN for 2 to 3 weeks (Hay et al, 2014).

Electrolytes

After the first few days of life, sodium, potassium, and chloride are added to parenteral solutions to compensate for the loss of extracellular fluid. To prevent hyperkalemia and cardiac arrhythmia, potassium should be withheld until renal flow is demonstrated. In general, the preterm infant has the same electrolyte requirements as the term infant, but actual requirements vary, depending on factors such as renal function, state of hydration, and the use of diuretics (see Table 42-7). Very immature infants may have a limited ability to conserve sodium and thus may require increased amounts of sodium to maintain a normal serum sodium concentration. Serum electrolyte levels should be monitored periodically.

TABLE 42-6 Guidelines for Administration of Parenteral Lipids for Premature Infants

Initial Rate (g/kg/day)*	Increments (g/kg/day)	Maximum Rate (g/kg/day)
1-2	1	3

Data from American Academy of Pediatrics, Committee on Nutrition: Nutritional needs of preterm infants. In Kleinman RE, Greer FR, editors: *Pediatric nutrition handbook*, ed 7, Elk Grove, Ill, 2014, American Academy of Pediatrics.

*Use the following formula to calculate lipid load: % Lipid × ml/kg/day = Lipid g/kg/day. For example, 0.20 × 15 ml/kg = 3 g/kg/day.

TABLE 42-7 Guidelines for Administration of Parenteral Electrolytes for Premature Infants

Electrolyte	Amount (mEq/kg/day)
Sodium	2-4
Chloride	2-4
Potassium	1.5-2

Data from American Academy of Pediatrics, Committee on Nutrition: Nutritional needs of preterm infants. In Kleinman RE, Greer FR, editors: *Pediatric nutrition handbook*, ed 7, Elk Grove, Ill, 2014, American Academy of Pediatrics.

Minerals

Calcium and phosphorus are important components of the PN solution. Premature infants who receive PN with low calcium and phosphorus concentrations are at risk for developing osteopenia of prematurity. This poor bone mineralization is most likely to develop in VLBW infants who receive PN for prolonged periods. Calcium and phosphorus status should be monitored using serum calcium, phosphorus, and alkaline phosphatase activity levels (see Appendix 22). Alkaline phosphatase activity levels in premature infants are greater than the levels seen with adults. It is common to see levels up to 600 IU/L, which may reflect rapid bone growth (Abrams, 2012). When alkaline phosphatase activity levels of 800 IU/L or more persist, knee or wrist radiographs should be examined for rickets (Abrams, 2012). Elevation in alkaline phosphatase activity also may be seen with liver disease.

Preterm infants have higher calcium and phosphorus needs than term infants. However, it is difficult to add enough calcium and phosphorus to parenteral solutions to meet these higher requirements without causing precipitation of the minerals. Calcium and phosphorus should be provided simultaneously in PN solutions. Alternate-day infusions are not recommended because abnormal serum mineral levels and decreased mineral retention develop.

Current recommendations for parenteral administration of additional calcium, phosphorus, and magnesium are presented in Table 42-8. The intakes are expressed at a volume intake of 120 to 150 ml/kg/day, with 2.5 g/100 ml of amino acids or protein. Lower fluid volumes or lower protein concentrations may cause the minerals to precipitate out of solution. The addition of cysteine hydrochloride increases the acidity of the fluid, which inhibits precipitation of calcium and phosphorus.

Trace Elements

Zinc should be given to all preterm infants receiving PN. If enteral feedings cannot be started by 2 weeks of age, additional trace elements should be added. However, the amount of manganese should be reduced for infants with obstructive jaundice; and the amounts of selenium, and chromium should be reduced in infants with renal dysfunction. Copper can be concentrated in the liver with cholestasis, and it is recommended to determine copper status by plasma copper levels or plasma ceruloplasmin levels (AAP, 2014). Parenteral iron is not routinely provided because infants often receive blood transfusions soon after birth, and enteral feedings, which provide a source of iron, often can be initiated. If necessary, the dosage for parenteral iron is approximately 10% of the enteral dosage; guidelines range from 0.2 to 0.25 mg/kg/day (Domellof, 2014). Table 42-9 provides guidelines for trace minerals.

TABLE 42-8 Guidelines for Administration of Parenteral Minerals for Premature Infants

Minerals	Amount (mg/kg/day)*
Calcium	60-80
Phosphorus	39-67
Magnesium	4.3-7.2

From American Academy of Pediatrics, Committee on Nutrition: Nutritional needs of preterm infants. In Kleinman RE, Greer FR, editors: *Pediatric nutrition handbook*, ed 7, Elk Grove, Ill, 2014, American Academy of Pediatrics.
*These recommendations assume an average fluid intake of 120 to 150 ml/kg/day with 2.5 g of amino acids per 100 ml. The amino acid concentration prevents the precipitation of these minerals.

TABLE 42-9 Guidelines for Administration of Parenteral Trace Elements for Premature Infants

Trace Elements	Amount (mcg/kg/day)
Zinc	400
Copper	20*
Manganese	1*
Selenium	1.5 – 4.5†
Chromium	0.05-0.3†
Molybdenum	0.25
Iodine	1

From American Academy of Pediatrics, Committee on Nutrition: Parenteral nutrition. In Kleinman RE, Greer FR, editors: *Pediatric nutrition handbook*, ed 7, Elk Grove, Ill, 2014, American Academy of Pediatrics.
*Reduced or not provided for infants with obstructive jaundice. Copper may have to be provided based on the infant's blood copper levels.
†Reduced or not provided for infants with renal dysfunction.

Vitamins

Shortly after birth all newborn infants receive an intramuscular (IM) injection of 0.3 to 1 mg of vitamin K to prevent hemorrhagic disease of the newborn from vitamin K deficiency. Stores of vitamin K are low in newborn infants, and there is little intestinal bacterial production of vitamin K until bacterial colonization takes place. Because initial dietary intake of vitamin K is limited, neonates are at nutritional risk if they do not receive this IM supplement.

Only intravenous multivitamin preparations currently approved and designed for use in infants should be given to provide the appropriate vitamin intake and prevent toxicity from additives used in adult multivitamin injections. The American Academy of Pediatrics recommends 40% of the infusion multivitamin (MVI)-pediatric 5-ml vial per kilogram of weight (AAP, 2014). The maximum dose of 5 ml is given to an infant with a weight of 2.5 kg (see Table 42-10).

Respiratory distress syndrome (RDS) is a disease that occurs in premature infants shortly after birth because these infants are deficient in the lung substance surfactant. Surfactant is responsible for keeping the lung elastic while breathing; thus surfactant supplements are given to the infant to prevent RDS or to lessen the illness. Lipids and proteins are components of surfactant, and phospholipids are the major lipid. Choline is required for phospholipid synthesis, but choline supplementation does not increase the production of phospholipids (van Aerde and Narvey, 2006). Choline is a conditionally essential nutrient because the

TABLE 42-10 Guidelines for Administration of Parenteral Vitamins for Premature Infants

	Preterm
Percentage of one 5-ml vial of MVI-Pediatric/INFUVITE*	40%/kg

MVI, multivitamin for infusion.
Maximum volume intake is 5 ml/day, which is achieved at 2.5 kg body weight.
Data from American Academy of Pediatrics, Committee on Nutrition: Nutritional needs of preterm infants. In Kleinman RE, Greer FR, editors: *Pediatric nutrition handbook*, ed 7, Elk Grove, Ill, 2014, American Academy of Pediatrics.
*MVI-Pediatric/INFUVITE (5 ml) contains the following vitamins: 80 mg of ascorbic acid, 2300 USP units of vitamin A, 400 USP units of vitamin D, 1.2 mg of thiamin, 1.4 mg of riboflavin, 1 mg of vitamin B_6, 17 mg of niacin, 5 mg of pantothenic acid, 7 USP units of vitamin E, 20 mcg of biotin, 140 mcg of folic acid, 1 mcg of vitamin B_{12}, and 200 mcg of vitamin K.

infant can synthesize choline (see Chapter 15 for a discussion of requirement for choline in pregnancy). Choline is added to premature infant formulas at the level contained in human milk. The upper level is extrapolated from the adult safe level of intake (Klein, 2002).

Bronchopulmonary dysplasia (BPD) is a chronic lung disease that commonly develops in the premature infant as a result of RDS and the mechanical ventilation and oxygen used to treat it. Because of the role of vitamin A in facilitating tissue repair, and because of reports of preterm infants having low vitamin A stores, large supplemental doses of vitamin A have been suggested for the prevention of BPD. One report suggests that providing ELBW premature infants with IM injections of vitamin A at 5000 units/day three times per week during the first month of life decreases the incidence of BPD (Tyson et al, 1999). Physicians may or may not use this supplementation. The decision will be based on the incidence of BPD in their nursery, the lack of proven additional benefits, the acceptability of using IM injections, and the availability of parenteral vitamin A (Darlow and Graham, 2011). See Chapter 34 for a discussion of BPD.

Apnea of prematurity is when the infant stops breathing for 20 seconds or longer. Apnea can be due to the infant's immature response to breathing. Bradycardia, slowness of the heart rate, and poor blood oxygenation may be associated with apnea. The medication, caffeine, can be given daily to prevent apnea of prematurity. Caffeine stimulates the infant to breathe by increasing the brain's sensitivity to carbon dioxide, stimulating the central respiratory drive, and improving skeletal muscle contraction of the diaphragm. Apnea also can be caused by a lack of oxygen, cold or hot environmental temperatures, medications, or illness. The cause of apnea must be determined to provide the correct treatment to the premature infant.

Oral sucrose is given to infants for pain management during procedures such as blood draws by heel stick or venipuncture. The taste of sucrose may release endorphins, but how sucrose aids in pain management is not clear.

TRANSITION FROM PARENTERAL TO ENTERAL FEEDING

It is beneficial to begin enteral feedings for preterm infants as early as possible because the feedings stimulate gastrointestinal enzymatic development and activity, promote bile flow, increase villous growth in the small intestine, and promote mature gastrointestinal motility. These initial enteral feedings also can decrease the incidence of cholestatic jaundice and the duration of physiologic jaundice and can improve subsequent feeding tolerance in preterm infants. At times small, initial feedings are used only to prime the gut and are not intended to optimize enteral nutrient intake until the infant demonstrates feeding tolerance or is clinically stable.

When making the transition from parenteral to enteral feeding, clinicians should maintain parenteral feeding until enteral feeding is well established to maintain adequate net intake of fluid and nutrients. In VLBW infants it may take 7 to 14 days to provide full enteral feeding, and it may take longer for infants with feeding intolerances or illness. The smallest, sickest infants usually receive increments of only 10 to 20 ml/kg/day. Larger, more stable preterm infants may tolerate increments of 20 to 30 ml/kg/day (see Chapter 13 for a more detailed discussion of transitional feeding).

NUTRITION REQUIREMENTS: ENTERAL FEEDING

Enteral alimentation is preferred for preterm infants because it is more physiologic than parenteral alimentation and is nutritionally superior. Initiating a tiny amount of an appropriate breastmilk feeding whenever possible is beneficial (Ahrabi and Schanler, 2013). However, determining when and how to provide enteral feedings is often difficult and involves consideration of the degree of prematurity, history of perinatal insults, current medical condition, function of the gastrointestinal tract, respiratory status, and several other individual concerns (see Table 42-11).

Preterm infants should be fed enough to promote growth similar to that of a fetus at the same gestational age, but not so much that nutrient toxicity develops. Although the exact nutrient requirements are unknown for preterm infants, several useful guidelines exist. In general the requirements of premature infants are higher than those of term infants because the preterm infant has smaller nutrient stores, decreased digestion and absorption capabilities, and a rapid growth rate. Stress, illness, and certain therapies for illness may further influence nutrient requirements. It is also important to remember that, in general, enteral nutrient requirements are different from parenteral requirements.

Energy

The energy requirements of premature infants vary with individual biologic and environmental factors. It is estimated that an intake of 50 kcal/kg/day is required to meet maintenance energy needs, compared with 105 to 130 kcal/kg/day for growth (see Table 42-12). However, energy needs may be increased by stress, illness, and rapid growth. Likewise, energy needs may be decreased if the infant is placed in a neutral thermal environment (the environmental temperature at which an infant expends the least amount of energy to maintain body temperature). It is important to consider the infant's rate of growth in relation to average energy intakes. Some premature infants may need greater than 130 kcal/kg/day to sustain an appropriate rate of growth. ELBW infants or those with BPD often require such increased amounts. To provide such a large number of calories to infants with a limited ability to tolerate large fluid volumes, it may be necessary to concentrate the feedings to a level of more than 24 kcal/oz (see Box 42-2).

TABLE 42-11 Factors to Consider Before Initiating or Increasing the Volume of Enteral Feedings

Category	Factors
Perinatal	Cardiorespiratory depression
Respiratory	Stability of ventilation, blood gases, apnea, bradycardia, cyanosis
Medical	Vital signs (heart rate, respiratory rate, blood pressure, temperature), lethargy
Gastrointestinal	Anomalies (gastroschisis, omphalocele), patency, gastrointestinal tract function (bowel sounds present, passage of stool), abdominal distension, risk of necrotizing enterocolitis
Infection	Sepsis or suspect sepsis

Data from Adamkin DH et al: Nutrition and selected disorders of the gastrointestinal tract. In Fanaroff AA, Fanaroff JM, editors: *Klaus and Fanaroff's Care of the high-risk newborn*, Philadelphia, 2013, Elsevier Saunders.

TABLE 42-12 Estimation of Energy Requirements of the Low Birthweight Infant

Activity	Average Estimation (kcal/kg/day)
Energy expended	40-60
Resting metabolic rate	40-50*
Activity	0-5*
Thermoregulation	0-5*
Synthesis	15†
Energy stored	20-30†
Energy excreted	15
Energy intake	90-120

Modified from American Academy of Pediatrics, Committee on Nutrition: Nutritional needs of preterm infants. In Kleinman RE, Greer FR, editors: *Pediatric nutrition handbook*, ed 7, Elk Grove, Ill, 2014, American Academy of Pediatrics; Committee on Nutrition of the Preterm Infant, European Society of Paediatric Gastroenterology and Nutrition (ESPGAN): *Nutrition and feeding of preterm infants*, Oxford, 1987, Blackwell Scientific.
*Energy for maintenance.
†Energy cost of growth.

BOX 42-2 Recipes for Preparing 90 ml (3 oz) of Concentrated Premature Infant Formula

Kcal/oz RTF* Formula	Ratio 24/30 kcal oz RTF Formula	Volume (ml) RTF* Premature 24	Volume RTF* (ml) Premature 30
24	1/0	90	0
26	2/1	60	30
27	1/1	45	45
28	1/2	30	60
30	0/1	0	90

RTF, Ready-to-feed formula.
*RTF (at 24 and 30 kcal/oz).
Example: Recipe for making a 26 kcal/oz formula:
Goal = 90 ml (3 oz) of formula
2 parts of 24 kcal/oz formula + 1 part of 30 kcal/oz formula = 3 parts of formula
90 ml ÷ 3 parts = 30 ml per part
30 ml × 2 parts = 60 ml of RTF Premature 24 kcal/oz formula + 30 ml × 1 part = 30 ml of Premature 30 kcal/oz = 90 ml (3 parts) of 26 kcal/oz formula

Protein

The amount and quality of protein must be considered when establishing protein requirements for the preterm infant. Amino acids should be provided at a level that meets demands without inducing amino acid or protein toxicity.

A reference fetus model has been used to determine the amount of protein that has to be ingested to match the quantity of protein deposited into newly formed fetal tissue (Ziegler, 2011). To achieve these fetal accretion rates, additional protein must be supplied to compensate for intestinal losses and obligatory losses in the urine and skin. Based on this method for determining protein needs, the advisable protein intake is 3.5 to 4 g/kg/day. This amount of protein is well tolerated. For the ELBW infant, up to 4.5 g/kg/day of protein has been recommended for milk feedings (Agostoni et al, 2010; Koletzko et al, 2014; Tudehope et al, 2013).

The quality or type of protein is an important consideration because premature infants have different amino acid needs than term infants because of immature hepatic enzyme pathways. The amino acid composition of whey protein, which differs from that of casein, is more appropriate for premature infants. The essential amino acid cysteine is more highly concentrated in whey protein, and premature infants do not synthesize cysteine well. In addition, the amino acids phenylalanine and tyrosine are lower, and the preterm infant has difficulty oxidizing them. Furthermore, metabolic acidosis decreases with consumption of whey-predominant formulas. Because of the advantages of whey protein for premature infants, breastmilk or formulas containing predominately whey proteins should be chosen whenever possible.

Taurine is a sulfonic amino acid that may be important for preterm infants. Human milk is a rich source of taurine, and taurine is added to most infant formulas. Term and preterm infants develop low plasma and urine concentrations of taurine without a dietary supply. The premature infant may have difficulty with synthesizing taurine from cysteine. Although no overt disease has been reported in infants fed low taurine formulas, low taurine may affect the development of vision and hearing (Klein, 2002).

Energy must be provided at sufficient levels to allow protein to be used for growth and not merely for energy expenditure. A range of 2.5 to 3.6 gms of protein per 100 kcal is recommended Inadequate protein intake is growth limiting, whereas excessive intake causes elevated plasma amino acid levels, azotemia, and acidosis.

Lipids

The growing preterm infant needs an adequate intake of well-absorbed dietary fat to help meet the high energy needs of growth, provide EFAs, and facilitate absorption of other important nutrients such as the fat-soluble vitamins and calcium. However, neonates in general, and premature and SGA infants in particular, digest and absorb lipids inefficiently.

Fat should constitute 40% to 50% of total calories. Furthermore, a diet that is high in fat and low in protein may yield more fat deposition than is desirable for the growing preterm infant. To meet EFA needs, linoleic acid should compose 3% of the total calories, and alpha-linolenic acid should be added in small amounts (AAP, 2014). Additional longer-chain fatty acids—ARA and DHA—are present in human milk and are added to infant formulas for term and premature infants to meet federal guidelines.

The premature infant has a greater need than the term infant for ARA and DHA supplementation. These fatty acids accumulate in fatty tissue and the brain during the last 3 months of gestation; thus the premature infant has decreased stores. Premature infants fed formulas supplemented with ARA and DHA frequently demonstrate greater gain in weight and length and higher psychomotor development scores than premature infants not receiving the fatty acid supplementation (Lapillonne et al, 2013). The DHA and ARA content of human milk is variable, and the premature infant may require supplements of ARA and DHA. However, research is needed to document supplementation use for the premature infants provided human milk (AAP, 2014).

Preterm infants have low levels of pancreatic lipase and bile salts, and this decreases their ability to digest and absorb fat. Lipases are needed for triglyceride breakdown, and bile salts solubilize fat for ease of digestion and absorption. Because medium-chain triglycerides (MCTs) do not require pancreatic lipase and bile acids for digestion and absorption, they have been added to the fat mixture in premature infant formulas.

Human milk and vegetable oils contain the EFA linoleic acid, but MCT oil does not. Premature infant formulas must contain vegetable oil and MCT oil to provide the essential long-chain fatty acids.

The composition of dietary fat also plays a role in the digestion and absorption of lipid. In general, infants absorb vegetable oils more efficiently than saturated animal fats, although one exception is the saturated fat in human milk. Infants digest and absorb human milk fat better than the saturated fat in cow's milk or the vegetable oil in standard infant formulas. Human milk contains two lipases that facilitate fat digestion and has a special fatty acid composition that aids absorption.

Carbohydrates

Carbohydrates are an important source of energy, and the enzymes for endogenous production of glucose from carbohydrate and protein are present in preterm infants. Approximately 40% of the total calories in human milk and standard infant formulas are derived from carbohydrates. Too little carbohydrate may lead to hypoglycemia, whereas too much may provoke osmotic diuresis or loose stools. The recommended range for carbohydrate intake is 40% to 50% of total calories.

Lactose, a disaccharide composed of glucose and galactose, is the predominant carbohydrate in almost all mammalian milks and may be important to the neonate for glucose homeostasis, perhaps because galactose can be used for either glucose production or glycogen storage. Generally galactose is used for glycogen formation first, and then it becomes available for glucose production as blood glucose levels decrease. Because infants born before 28 to 34 weeks of gestation have low lactase activity, the premature infant's ability to digest lactose may be marginal. In practice, malabsorption is not a clinical problem because lactose is hydrolyzed in the intestine or fermented in the colon and absorbed. Sucrose is another disaccharide that is found in commercial infant formula products. Because sucrase activity early in the third trimester is at 70% of newborn levels, sucrose is well tolerated by most premature infants. Sucrase and lactase are sensitive to changes in the intestinal milieu. Infants who have diarrhea, are undergoing antibiotic therapy, or are undernourished, may develop temporary intolerances to lactose and sucrose.

Glucose polymers are common carbohydrates in the preterm infant's diet. These polymers, consisting mainly of chains of five to nine glucose units linked together, are used to achieve the isoosmolality of certain specialized formulas. Glucosidase enzymes for digesting glucose polymers are active in small preterm infants.

Minerals and Vitamins

Premature infants require greater amounts of vitamins and minerals than term infants because they have poor body stores, are physiologically immature, are frequently ill, and will grow rapidly. Formulas and human milk fortifiers that are developed especially for preterm infants contain higher vitamin and mineral concentrations to meet the needs of the infant, obviating the need for additional supplementation in most cases (see Table 42-13). One major exception is infants receiving human milk with a fortifier that does not contain iron. An iron supplement of 2 mg/kg/day should be sufficient to meet their needs (AAP, 2014). The other exception is the use of donor human milk fortifier, which requires the addition of a multiple vitamin and an iron supplement.

TABLE 42-13 **Recommendations for Enteral Administration of Vitamins for the Premature Infant**	
Vitamin	**Amount (kg/day)**
Vitamin A	700-1500 IU
Vitamin D	150-400 IU*
Vitamin E	6-12 IU
Vitamin K	8-10 mcg
Ascorbic acid	18-24 mg
Thiamin	180-240 mcg
Riboflavin	250-360 mcg
Pyridoxine	150-210 mcg
Niacin	3.6-4.8 mg
Pantothenate	1.2-1.7 mg
Biotin	3.6-6 mcg
Folate	25-50 mcg
Vitamin B$_{12}$	0.3 mcg

Data from American Academy of Pediatrics, Committee on Nutrition: Nutritional needs of preterm infants. In Kleinman RE, Greer FR, editors: *Pediatric nutrition handbook,* ed 7, Elk Grove, Ill, 2014, American Academy of Pediatrics.
*Maximum of 400 IU/day.

Calcium and Phosphorus

Calcium and phosphorus are just two of many nutrients that growing premature infants require for optimal bone mineralization. Intake guidelines have been established at levels that promote the bone mineralization rate that occurs in the fetus. An intake of 150 to 220 mg/kg/day of calcium and 75 to 140 mg/kg/day of phosphorus is recommended (Abrams, AAP, 2013). Two thirds of the calcium and phosphorus body content of the term neonate is accumulated through active transport mechanisms during the last trimester of pregnancy. Infants who are born prematurely are deprived of this important intrauterine mineral deposition. With poor mineral stores and low dietary intake, preterm infants can develop osteopenia of prematurity, a disease characterized by demineralization of growing bones and documented by radiologic evidence of "washed-out" or thin bones. Very immature babies are particularly susceptible to osteopenia and may develop bone fractures or florid rickets with a prolonged dietary deficiency. Osteopenia of prematurity is most likely to develop in preterm infants who are (1) fed infant formula that is not specifically formulated for preterm infants, (2) fed human milk that is not supplemented with calcium and phosphorus, or (3) receiving long-term PN without enteral feedings.

Vitamin D

Human milk with human milk fortifier or infant formula for preterm infants provides adequate vitamin D when infants consume the entire calorie intake suggested. The current recommendations for intake range from 200 to 400 IU/day for preterm infants (Abrams, AAP, 2013).

Vitamin E

Preterm infants require more vitamin E than term infants because of their limited tissue stores, decreased absorption of fat-soluble vitamins, and rapid growth. Vitamin E protects biologic membranes against oxidative lipid breakdown. Because iron is a biologic oxidant, a diet high in either iron or polyunsaturated fatty acids (PUFAs) increases the risk of vitamin E deficiency. The PUFAs are incorporated into the red blood cell membranes and are more susceptible to oxidative damage than when saturated fatty acids compose the membranes.

A premature infant with vitamin E deficiency may experience hemolytic anemia (oxidative destruction of red blood cells). However, this anemia is now uncommon today because of improvements in human milk fortifiers and infant formula composition. The human milk fortifiers and premature infant formulas now contain appropriate vitamin E/PUFA ratios for preventing hemolytic anemia.

Because the dietary requirement for vitamin E depends on the PUFA content of the diet, the recommended intake of vitamin E is expressed commonly as a ratio of vitamin E to PUFA. The recommendation for vitamin E is 0.7 IU (0.5 mg of d-alpha-tocopherol) per 100 kcal, and at least 1 IU of vitamin E per gram of linoleic acid.

Pharmacologic dosing of vitamin E (50-100 mg/kg/day) has not proven to be helpful in preventing BPD or retinopathy of prematurity by reducing the toxic effects of oxygen. Furthermore, high doses of vitamin E have been associated with intraventricular hemorrhage, sepsis, NEC, liver and renal failure, and death.

Iron

Preterm infants are at risk for iron deficiency anemia because of the reduced iron stores associated with early birth. At birth most of the available iron is in the circulating hemoglobin. Thus frequent blood sampling further depletes the amount of iron available for erythropoiesis. Transfusions of red blood cells often are needed to treat the early physiologic anemia of prematurity. Recombinant erythropoietin (EPO) therapy has been used to prevent anemia. Iron supplementation is indicated to facilitate red blood cell production, and a dosage of 6 mg/kg/day of enteral iron has been used (AAP, 2014). This therapy has not consistently prevented anemia and the need for blood transfusions (AAP, 2014).

In general the recommendation for iron intake is 2 to 4 mg/kg/day (AAP, 2014). Infants fed human milk should be given ferrous sulfate drops beginning at 2 weeks of age (AAP, 2014). Formulas fortified with iron usually contain sufficient iron for preterm infants (AAP, 2014).

Folic Acid

Premature infants seem to have higher folic acid needs than infants born at term. Although serum folate levels are high at birth, they decrease dramatically, probably as a result of high folic acid use by the premature infant for deoxyribonucleic acid (DNA) and tissue synthesis needed for rapid growth.

A mild form of folic acid deficiency causing low serum folate concentrations and hypersegmentation of neutrophils is not unusual in premature infants. Megaloblastic anemia is much less common. A daily folic acid intake of 25 to 50 mcg/kg effectively maintains normal serum folate concentrations. Fortified human milk and formulas for premature infants meet these guidelines when full enteral feedings are established.

Sodium

Preterm infants, especially those with VLBW, are susceptible to hyponatremia during the neonatal period. These infants may have excessive urinary sodium losses because of renal immaturity and an inability to conserve adequate sodium. Furthermore, their sodium needs are high because of their rapid growth rate.

Daily sodium intakes of 2 to 3 mEq/kg meet the needs of most premature infants, but 4 to 5 mEq/kg or more may be required by some infants to prevent hyponatremia (Dell, 2011). Routine sodium supplementation of fortified human milk and infant formulas is not necessary. However, it is important to consider the possibility of hyponatremia and monitor infants by assessing serum sodium until the blood level is normal. Milk can be supplemented with sodium if repletion is necessary.

FEEDING METHODS

Decisions about breastfeeding, bottle feeding, or tube feeding depend on the gestational age and the clinical condition of the preterm infant. The goal is to feed the infant via the most physiologic method possible and supply nutrients for growth without creating clinical complications.

Gastric Gavage

Gastric gavage by the oral route often is chosen for infants who are unable to suck because of immaturity or problems with the central nervous system. Infants less than 32 to 34 weeks of gestational age, regardless of birthweight have poorly coordinated sucking, swallowing, and breathing abilities because of their developmental immaturity. Consequently they have difficulty with nipple feeding.

With the oral gastric gavage method, a soft feeding tube is inserted through the infant's mouth and into the stomach. The major risks of this technique include aspiration and gastric distention. Because of weak or absent cough reflexes and poorly developed respiratory muscles, the tiny infant may not be able to dislodge milk from the upper airway, which can cause reflex bradycardia or airway obstruction. However, electronic monitoring of vital functions and proper positioning of the infant during feeding minimize the risk of aspiration from regurgitation of stomach contents. Tiny, immature infants whose small gastric capacity and slow intestinal motility can impede the tolerance of large-volume bolus feeds may need bolus feedings provided with a pump for a 30 to 60 minute infusion to aid in feeding tolerance.

Occasionally, elimination of the distention and vagal bradycardia requires the use of an indwelling tube for continuous gastric gavage feedings rather than intermittent administration of boluses. Continuous feedings may lead to loss of milk fat, calcium, and phosphorus, which deposit in the feeding tubing so that the infant does not receive the total amount of nutrition provided. Bolus feedings provided with the use of the pump infusion can decrease nutrient loss and promote better weight gain (Rogers et al, 2010; Senterre, 2014).

Nasal gastric gavage is sometimes better tolerated than oral tube feeding. However, because neonates must breathe through the nose, this technique may compromise the nasal airway in preterm infants and cause an associated deterioration in respiratory function. This method is helpful for infants who are learning to nipple feed. An infant with a nasal gastric tube can still form a tight seal on the bottle nipple, but it can be difficult if an oral feeding tube is in place during feedings (see Chapter 13).

Transpyloric Feeding

Transpyloric tube feeding is indicated for infants who are at risk for aspirating milk into the lungs or who have slow gastric emptying. The goal of this method is to circumvent the often slow gastric emptying of the immature infant by passing the feeding tube through the stomach and pylorus and placing its tip within the duodenum or jejunum. Infants with severe gastrointestinal reflux do well with this method, which prevents aspiration of feedings into the lungs. This method also is used for infants whose respiratory function is compromised and who are at risk for milk aspiration. The possible disadvantages of transpyloric feedings include decreased fat absorption, diarrhea, dumping syndrome, alterations of the intestinal microflora, intestinal perforation, and bilious fluid in the stomach. In addition, the placement of transpyloric tubes also requires considerable expertise and radiographic confirmation of the catheter tip location. Although associated with many possible complications, transpyloric feedings are used when gastric feeding is not successful.

Nipple Feeding

Nipple feeding may be attempted with infants whose gestational age is greater than 32 weeks and whose ability to feed from a nipple is indicated by evidence of an established sucking reflex and sucking motion. Before this time they are unable to coordinate sucking, swallowing, and breathing. Because sucking requires effort by the infant, any stress from other causes such as hypothermia or hypoxemia diminishes the sucking ability. Therefore nipple feeding should be initiated only when the infant is under minimum stress and is sufficiently mature and strong to sustain the sucking effort. Initial oral feedings may be limited to one to three times per day to prevent undue fatigue or too much energy expenditure, either of which can slow the infant's rate of weight gain. Before oral feedings begin, a standardized oral stimulation program can help infants successfully nipple feed more quickly (Fucile et al, 2011).

Breastfeeding

When the mother of a premature infant chooses to breastfeed, nursing at the breast should begin as soon as the infant is ready. Before this time the mother must express her milk so that it can be tube-fed to her infant. These mothers need emotional and educational support for successful lactation. Studies report that premature breast-fed infants have better sucking, swallowing, and breathing coordination and fewer breathing disruptions than bottle-fed infants (Abrams and Hurst, 2014). Kangaroo care—allowing the mother to maintain skin-to-skin contact while holding her infant—facilitates her lactation. In addition, this type of contact promotes continuation of breastfeeding and enhances the mother's confidence in caring for her high-risk infant. The latter benefit also may apply to fathers who engage in kangaroo care with their infants (Kassity-Krich and Jones, 2014).

Feeding infants with cups instead of bottles to supplement breastfeeding has been suggested for preterm infants based on the rationale that it may prevent infant "nipple confusion" (i.e., confusion between nursing at the breast and from a bottle). Complications such as milk aspiration and low volume intakes have to be monitored. Cup feeding has been associated with successful breastfeeding at discharge, but increased length of stay in the hospital for the premature infant (AAP, American College of Obstetricians and Gynecologists [ACOG], 2014).

Tolerance of Feedings

All preterm babies receiving EN should be monitored for signs of feeding intolerance. Vomiting of feedings usually signals the infant's inability to retain the provided amount of milk. When not associated with other signs of a systemic illness, vomiting may indicate that feeding volumes were increased too quickly or are excessive for the infant's size and maturity. Simply reducing the feeding volume may resolve the problem. If not, or if the infant has signs of a systemic illness, feedings may have to be interrupted until the infant's condition has stabilized.

Abdominal distention may be caused by excessive feeding, organic obstruction, excessive swallowing of air, resuscitation, sepsis (i.e., systemic infection), or NEC. Observing infants for abdominal distention should be a routine practice for nurses. Abdominal distention often indicates the need to interrupt feeding until its cause is determined and resolved.

Gastric residuals, measured by aspiration of the stomach contents, may be determined routinely before each bolus gavage feeding and intermittently in all continuous drip feedings. Whether a residual amount is significant depends partly on its volume in relation to the total volume of the feeding. For example, a residual volume of more than 50% of a bolus feeding or equal to the continuous infusion rate may be a sign of feeding intolerance. However, when interpreting the significance of a gastric residual measurement, clinicians must consider other concurrent signs of feeding intolerance and the previous pattern of residual volumes established for a particular infant. Residuals are frequently present before feedings are initiated and as small volume feedings are started. As long as no signs of illness are present, feedings should not be withheld.

Bile-stained emesis or residuals frequently may be due to overdistention of the stomach with reflux of bile from the intestine, or to a feeding tube that has slipped into the intestine, or may indicate that the infant has an intestinal blockage and needs additional evaluation (Schanler, 2014). Bloody or bilious gastric residuals are more alarming than those that seem to be undigested milk.

The frequency and consistency of bowel movements should be monitored constantly when feeding preterm infants. Simple inspections can detect the presence of gross blood. All feeding methods for preterm infants have associated complications. Unless close attention is paid to symptoms that indicate poor feeding tolerance, serious complications may ensue. Certain diseases can be recognized by recognizing signs of feeding intolerance. For example, necrotizing enterocolitis (NEC) is a serious and potentially fatal disease associated with specific symptoms such as abdominal distention and tenderness, abnormal gastric residuals, and grossly bloody stools.

SELECTION OF ENTERAL FEEDING

During the initial feeding period, premature infants often require additional time to adjust to EN and may experience concurrent stress, weight loss, and diuresis. The primary goal of enteral feeding during this initial period is to establish tolerance to the milk. Infants seem to need a period of adjustment to be able to assimilate a large volume and concentration of nutrients. Thus parenteral fluids may be necessary until infants can tolerate adequate amounts of feedings by mouth.

After the initial period of adjustment, the goal of enteral feeding changes from establishing milk tolerance to providing complete nutrition support for growth and rapid organ development. All essential nutrients should be provided in quantities that support sustained growth. The following feeding choices are appropriate: (1) human milk supplemented with human milk fortifier and iron and vitamins as indicated by fortifier used, (2) iron-fortified premature infant formula for infants who weigh less than 2 kg, or (3) iron-fortified standard infant formula for infants who weigh more than 2 kg.

Premature infants who are discharged from the hospital can be given a transitional formula. Additional vitamin D may be indicated to provide 400 IU per day (Abrams, AAP, 2013). Breast-fed infants may be provided with two to three bottles of transitional formula daily to meet needs. The breast-fed premature infant also should receive 2 mg/kg/day of iron and a multiple vitamin for the first year of life (AAP, 2014). Premature infants discharged home on standard formula should receive a multivitamin until the infant reaches 3 kg in weight and then only vitamin D may be needed to provide 400 IU per day (AAP, 2014).

Human Milk

Human milk is the ideal food for healthy term infants and premature infants. Although human milk requires nutrient supplementation to meet the needs of premature infants, its benefits for the infant are numerous. During the first month of lactation, the composition of milk from mothers of premature infants differs from that of mothers who have given birth to term infants; the protein and sodium concentrations of breast-milk are higher in mothers with preterm infants (Klein, 2002). When premature infants are fed their own mother's milk, they grow more rapidly than infants fed banked, mature breastmilk (Ahrabi and Schanler, 2013).

In addition to its nutrient concentration, human milk offers nutritional benefits because of its unique mix of amino acids and long-chain fatty acids. The zinc and iron in human milk are more readily absorbed, and fat is more easily digested because of the presence of lipases. Moreover, human milk contains factors that are not present in formulas. These components include (1) macrophages and T and B lymphocytes; (2) antimicrobial factors such as secretory immunoglobulin A, lactoferrin, and others; (3) hormones; (4) enzymes; and (5) growth factors. It has been reported that human milk compared with premature infant formula fed to preterm infants reduces the incidence of NEC and sepsis, improves neurodevelopment, facilitates a more rapid advancement of enteral feedings, and leads to an earlier discharge (AAP, ACOG, 2014). The use of mother's own milk for her infant supplemented with liquid donor human milk fortifier and donor human milk is linked to decreased incidence of NEC (Sullivan et al, 2010). The use of donor milk and liquid donor human milk fortifier compared with premature infant formula decreases the incidence of NEC treated by surgery and decreases the days of parenteral nutrition (Cristofalo et al, 2013).

However, one well-documented problem is associated with feeding human milk to preterm infants. Whether it is preterm, term, or mature, human milk does not meet the calcium and phosphorus needs for normal bone mineralization in premature infants. Therefore calcium and phosphorus supplements are recommended for rapidly growing preterm infants who are fed predominantly human milk. Currently three human milk fortifiers are available: powder bovine milk base, liquid bovine milk base, and liquid donor human milk base. The bovine products contain calcium and phosphorus, as well as protein, carbohydrates, fat, vitamins, and minerals, and are designed to be added to expressed breastmilk fed to premature infants (see Table 42-14). Vitamin supplements are not

TABLE 42-14   Comparison of the Nutritional Content of Human Milk and Formulas

	Human Milk	Human Milk + Powder Bovine–Based Fortifier*	Human Milk + Liquid Bovine–Based Fortifier†	Human Milk + Liquid Donor Human Milk–Based Fortifier‡	Standard Formula§	Transitional Formula(ParaMarks)	Premature Formula¶
Caloric density (kcal/oz)	20	24	24	24	20	22	20, 24, 30
Protein whey/casein ratio	70:30	Whey predominates	Whey protein, or casein hydrolysate	Whey predominates	60:40, 48:52, 100:0	60:40, 50:50,	60:40;80:20:100:0
Protein(g/L)	9	19-20	24-26	19	14-15	21	20, 22, & 24,27, 29 & 30,33
Carbohydrate	Lactose	Lactose, glucose polymers	Lactose, glucose polymers	Lactose	Lactose or lactose and glucose polymers	Lactose, glucose polymers	Lactose, glucose polymers
Carbohydrate (g/L)	80	80-95	76-92	82	76-78	75-78	70-73, 79-88,78-109
Fat	Human fat	Human fat, MCT oil, vegetable oil	Human fat, MCT oil, vegetable oil, DHA, ARA	Human fat	Vegetable oil, DHA, ARA	Vegetable oil, MCT oil, DHA, ARA	Vegetable oil, MCT oil DHA, ARA
Fat (g/L)	35	38-45	36-48	46	34-37	39-41	34-37, 41-44, 51-67
Calcium (mg/L)	230	1130-1362	1158-1192	1214	450-530	780-890	1150, 1373, 1717
Phosphorus (mg/L)	130	630-778	633-675	642	260-290	460-490	620, 743, 927
Vitamin D (units/L)	10	1177-1510	1175-1575	268	405-507	520	1010-2000, 1210-2400, 1520-3000
Vitamin E (units/L)	6	37-52	38-52	9	10-14	27-30	37, 44, 51
Folic acid (mcg/L)	110	331-360	325-350	142	101-108	186-190	273, 329, 385
Sodium (mEq/L)	8	9-14	13-17	22	7-8	11	16, 20, 23

Data from American Academy of Pediatrics, Committee on Nutrition: Appendix R. Representative values for constituents of human milk. In Kleinman RE, Greer FR, editors: *Pediatric nutrition handbook*, ed 7, Elk Grove, Ill, 2014, American Academy of Pediatrics.

ARA, Arachidonic acid; *DHA*, docosahexaenoic acid; *MCT*, medium-chain triglyceride.

*Based on the composition of term human milk fortified with either powder Enfamil or Similac Human Milk Fortifiers at four packets per 100 ml.

†Based on the composition of term human milk fortified with liquid Enfamil or Similac Human Milk Fortifier at 1 vial/packet + 25 ml milk.

‡Based on the composition of term human milk fortified with Prolact +4.

§Based on the composition of Enfamil Premium, Similac Advance, and Gerber Good Start Gentle Plus formulas.

(ParaMarks)Based on the composition of Enfamil EnfaCare, and Similac Neosure formulas.

¶Based on the composition of Enfamil Premature , Gerber Good Start Premature, and Similac Special Care formulas.

needed. One bovine fortifier is iron fortified and the other requires the addition of iron. The human-milk base product is made from donor human milk that has been pasteurized, concentrated, and supplemented with calcium, phosphorous, zinc, and electrolytes. A multivitamin and an iron supplement is needed with the use of the human-milk base fortifier. The human-milk base fortifier comes as additives to make the milk 24, 26, 28 or 30 kcal/oz milk. The higher concentrations are used for infants who are volume restricted or not growing on lower caloric-dense milk (Hair et al, 2013). The calories and protein are higher with the increased concentrations, but the concentrations of calcium, phosphorous, and zinc remain the same with the donor human milk fortifier. Often the infant needs more energy and protein, but not increased mineral intake. A donor human milk cream supplement is available that is pasteurized human milk fat and can be added to human milk.

Providing human milk to a premature infant can be a very positive experience for the mother, one that promotes involvement and interaction. Because many preterm infants are neither strong enough nor mature enough to nurse at their mother's breast in the early neonatal period, their mothers usually express their milk for several days (and occasionally for several weeks) before nursing can be established. The proper technique of expression, storage, and transport of milk should be reviewed with the mother (see Table 15-19 in Chapter 15). Many summaries of the special considerations for nursing a preterm infant have been published (AAP, ACOG, 2014).

Donor Human Milk

Pasteurized donor human milk (DM) is recommended for the premature infant when the mother's own milk (MOM) is not available or is contraindicated (AAP, 2012; see *Focus On:* What Is a Human Milk Bank?). NICUs that use donor milk may have guidelines to ensure that the infants most at risk for NEC receive donor milk. For example, an infant with a birthweight less than 1500 g and a gestational age less than 34 weeks would qualify to receive donor milk. The risk for NEC is highest at 32 weeks' gestation (Yee et al, 2012). At 34 weeks, the infant can transfer to a discharge diet of mom's milk and supplementation with transitional formula if needed. Donor milk would not be used after discharge to home.

◎ FOCUS ON

What Is a Human Milk Bank?

By DeeAnna Wales VanReken, MS, RDN, CD

Human milk banks are nonprofit and for-profit establishments around the globe that work to pasteurize milk safely from healthy donor mothers and make it available to infants who need it most (PATH, 2013). Donors are screened carefully for medication and any supplement use, must be non-smokers, and will not be approved if they drink alcoholic beverages within defined exclusion periods.

For high-risk infants who are premature, immune compromised, or unable to breastfeed because of HIV-positive mothers, donor breastmilk is a life-saving resource when mother's own milk, the best choice, is not available (Arslanoglu et al, 2013). Because of its optimal nutrition profile and unique immunologic properties, no other source of nourishment compares when providing these vulnerable infants with the nutrition needed to get a healthy start in life. This precious commodity has saved lives and improved infant morbidity so greatly in Brazil, that the World Health Organization (WHO) has now asked that all nations advocate for the safe use of donor milk through human milk banking (WHO, 2000).

Hospitals with milk-banking systems are usually nonprofit and each have their own guidelines around distributing the milk so that it remains as a safe and altruistic option for all who need it. Recent research also has shown that unpasteurized sources of human milk can be purchased over the Internet and have a high probability for microbial contamination (Keim et al, 2013). Occasionally, mothers of healthy babies may seek out peer-to-peer sharing to avoid the cost, inconvenience, and depletion of resources for vulnerable babies who need pasteurized donor milk the most. If a mother expresses interest in these options, she should receive guidance to understand and mitigate the risks of sharing unpasteurized human milk (Gribble and Hausman, 2012).

Effective human milk banks protect, promote, and support breastfeeding at every level, and are cradled by governmental support (Arnold, 2006). The Human Milk Banking Association of North America (HMBANA) is the premier resource for information on the start up and management of this precious commodity in every community as a means to improve global health (HMBANA, 2014). Email info@hmbana.org for more information.

The use of donor milk has been linked with earlier initiation of feedings, less formula use and no change in the percentage of MOM use. DM frequently is used with the initiation of feedings before the mother's milk can be expressed. Neonatologists were concerned that the use of DM would lead to mothers not providing milk for their infant, but there was no change in mothers providing milk for their own infants (Marinelli et al, 2014).

Premature Infant Formulas

Formula preparations have been developed to meet the unique nutritional and physiologic needs of growing preterm infants. The quantity and quality of nutrients in these products promote growth at intrauterine rates. These formulas, which have caloric densities of 20, 24, and 30 kcal/oz, are available only in a ready-to-feed form. These premature formulas differ in many respects from standard cow's milk–based formulas (see Table 42-14). The types of carbohydrate, protein, and fat differ to facilitate digestion and absorption of nutrients. These formulas also have higher concentrations of protein, minerals, and vitamins.

Transitional Infant Formulas

Formulas containing 22 kcal/oz have been designed as transition formulas for the premature infant. Their nutrient content is less than that of the nutrient-dense premature infant formulas and more than that of the standard infant formula (see Table 42-14). These formulas can be introduced when the infant reaches a weight of 2000 g, and they can be used throughout the first year of life. Not all premature infants need these formulas to grow appropriately. It is not clear which premature infants need this specialized formula, because studies have not always demonstrated improved growth with the use of transitional formula (Young et al, 2012). Gain of weight, length, and head circumference for age and weight for length should be monitored on the World Health Organization growth curves (Lapillonne,

2014). Transitional formulas are available in powder form and in ready-to-feed form.

Formula Adjustments

Occasionally it may be necessary to increase the energy content of the formulas fed to small infants. This may be appropriate when the infant is not growing quickly enough and already is consuming as much as possible during feedings.

Concentration

One approach to providing hypercaloric formula is to prepare the formula with less water, thus concentrating all its nutrients, including energy. Concentrated infant formulas with energy contents of 24 kcal/oz are available to hospitals as ready-to-feed nursettes. However, when using these concentrated formulas, clinicians must consider the infant's fluid intake and losses in relation to the renal solute load of the concentrated feeding to ensure that a positive water balance is maintained. This method of increasing formula density often is preferred because the nutrient balance remains the same; infants who need more energy also need additional nutrients. As mentioned, the transitional formulas are available in ready-to-feed and powder form and can be concentrated from 24 to 30 kcal/oz. However, this formula is still inadequate for infants who need additional calcium (e.g., infants with osteopenia).

A ready-to-feed 30 kcal/oz premature infant formula is available. It meets the nutritional needs for premature infants who must be fluid restricted because of illness. This 30 kcal/oz formula can be diluted with premature infant formula (24 kcal/oz) to make 26, 27, or 28 kcal/oz milks (see Box 42-2). These milks are sterile and are the preferred source of providing concentrated milks to premature infants in the neonatal intensive care unit (NICU). Infant formula powder is not sterile and is not to be used with high-risk infants when a nutritionally adequate liquid, sterile product is available (Robbins and Meyers, 2011).

Caloric Supplements

Another approach to increasing the energy content of a formula involves the use of caloric supplements such as vegetable oil, MCT oil, or glucose polymers. These supplements increase the caloric density of the formula without markedly altering solute load or osmolality. However, they do alter the relative distribution of total calories derived from protein, carbohydrate, and fat. Because even small amounts of oil or carbohydrate dilute the percentage of calories derived from protein, adding these supplements to human milk or standard (20 kcal/oz) formulas is not advised. Caloric supplements should be used only when a formula already meets all nutrient requirements other than energy or when the renal solute load is a concern.

When a high-energy formula is needed, glucose polymers can be added to a base that has a concentration of 24 kcal/oz or greater (either full-strength premature formula or a concentrated standard formula), with a maximum of 50% of total calories from fat and a minimum of 10% of total calories from protein. Vegetable oil should be added to a feeding at the time or given as an oral medication. Vegetable oil added to a day's supply of formula that is chilled will separate out from the milk and cling to the milk storage container and will not be in the feeding to the infant.

NUTRITION ASSESSMENT AND GROWTH

Dietary Intake

Dietary intake must be evaluated to ensure that the nutrition provided meets the infant's needs. Parenteral fluids and milk feedings are advanced as tolerated, and the nutrient intakes must be reviewed to ensure that they are within the guidelines for premature infants and that the infant is thriving on the nutrition provided. Appropriate growth and growth charts are reviewed in the following paragraphs.

Laboratory Indices

Laboratory assessments usually involve measuring the following parameters: (1) fluid and electrolyte balance, (2) PN or EN tolerance, (3) bone mineralization status, and (4) hematologic status (see Table 42-15). Hemoglobin and hematocrit are monitored as medically indicated. The early decrease in hematocrit reflects the physiologic drop in hemoglobin after birth and blood drawings for laboratory assessments. Early low hemoglobins are treated with blood transfusions if needed. Dietary supplementation does not change this early physiologic drop in hemoglobin.

Growth Rates and Growth Charts

All neonates typically lose some weight after birth. Preterm infants are born with more extracellular water than term infants and thus tend to lose more weight than term infants. However, the postnatal weight loss should not be excessive. Preterm infants who lose more than 15% of their birth weight may become dehydrated from the inadequate fluid intake or experience tissue wasting from poor energy intake. An infant's birth weight should be regained by the second or third week of life. The smallest and sickest infants take the longest time to regain their birth weights.

TABLE 42-15 Monitoring of the Feeding of the Premature Infant

Monitor	Parenteral Nutrition	Enteral Nutrition
Fluid and electrolyte balance	Fluid intake	Fluid intake
	Urine output	Urine output
	Daily weights	Daily weights
	Serum sodium, potassium and chloride	
	Serum creatinine	
	BUN	
Glucose homeostasis	Serum glucose	Not routine
Fat tolerance	Serum triglycerides	Not indicated
Protein nutriture:		
BUN	Not helpful	Low levels with human milk–fed infants may indicate need for more protein
Osteopenia	Serum calcium	
	Serum phosphorous	Serum phosphorous
	Serum alkaline phosphatase activity	Serum alkaline phosphatase activity
Parenteral nutrition toxicity	Cholestasis: conjugated bilirubin	Not indicated
	Liver function: ALT	

ALT, Alanine aminotransferase; *BUN,* blood urea nitrogen.

Intrauterine growth curves have been developed using birth weight, birth length, and birth head circumference data of infants born at several successive weeks of gestation. The intrauterine growth curves are the standard of growth recommended for premature infants. During the first week of life premature infants fall away from their birth weight percentile, which reflects the normal postnatal weight loss of newborn infants. After an infant's condition stabilizes and the infant begins consuming all needed nutrients, the infant may be able to grow at a rate that parallels these curves. An intrauterine weight gain of 15 to 20 g/kg/day can be achieved.

Although weight is an important anthropometric parameter, measurements of length and head circumference also can be helpful. Premature infants should grow between 0.7 to 1 cm per week in body length and head circumference. A growth curve based on gender can be used to evaluate the adequacy of growth in all three areas (see Figures 42-3 and 42-4). This chart has a built-in correction factor for prematurity; the infant's growth can be followed from 22 to 50 weeks of gestation and it represents cross-sectional data from Canada, Australia, Germany, Italy, Scotland, and the United States (Fenton and Kim, 2013). The intrauterine curves are smooth into the World Health Organization Charts.

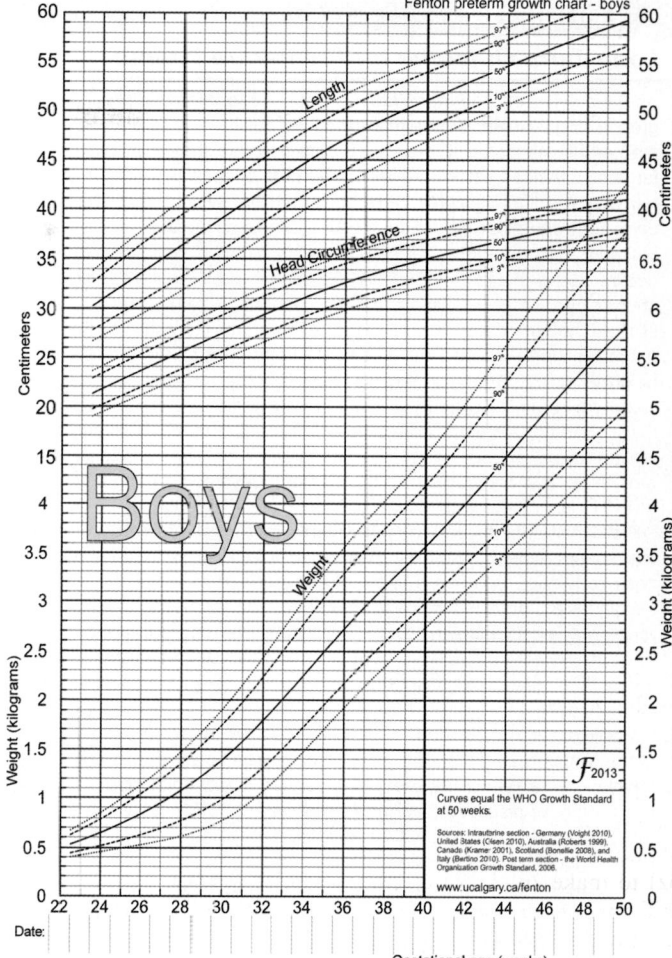

FIGURE 42-4 Example of a growth record of weight, length, and head circumference for male infants from 22 to 50 weeks of gestation. This chart has a built-in correction factor for prematurity. http://ucalgary.ca/fenton (From Fenton TR, Kim JH: A systematic review and meta-analysis to revise the Fenton growth chart for preterm infants, *BMC Pediatr* 13:59, 2013.

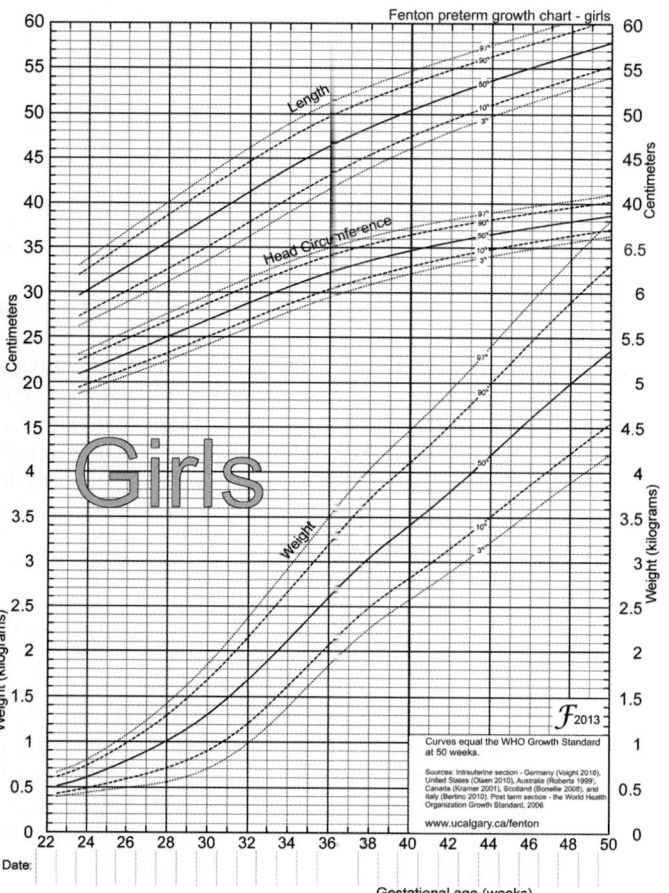

FIGURE 42-3 Example of a growth record of weight, length, and head circumference for female infants from 22 to 50 weeks of gestation. This chart has a built-in correction factor for prematurity. http://ucalgary.ca/fenton (From Fenton TR and Kim JH: A systematic review and meta-analysis to revise the Fenton growth chart for preterm infants, *BMC Pediatr* 13:59, 2013.)

Additional intrauterine growth charts based on the birthweight, birth length, and head circumferences of infants born in the United States have been developed (Olsen et al, 2010). Separate charts for male and female infants are available and infants can be plotted from 23 to 41 weeks' gestation.

The 2006 World Health Organization Growth Charts designed for children from birth to 2 years of age also should be used for preterm infants once they reach 40 weeks' gestation, as long as the age is adjusted (see *Focus On:* Long-Term Outcome for Premature Infants). For example, an infant born at 28 weeks of gestation is 12 weeks premature (40 weeks of term gestation minus 28 weeks of birth gestational age). Four months after birth, the growth parameters of a premature infant born at 28 weeks of gestation can be compared with those of a 1-month-old infant born at term (see Box 42-3). When using growth grids, age should be adjusted for prematurity until at least 2½ to 3 years of corrected age. In Figure 42-5 A.R.'s pattern of growth is shown through 18 years of age. These charts are based on term, healthy infants who were breast fed the first year of life (Grummer-Strawn et al, 2010). By using this chart, the infant's growth can be compared with the term infant to assess catch-up growth.

Long-Term Outcome for Premature Infants

As the survival of premature infants continues to improve, their physical growth, cognitive development, health, and quality of life are being evaluated and investigated. Previously it was believed that, if premature infants experienced catch-up growth, it would occur only during the first few years of life. However, catch-up growth for weight and length can continue throughout childhood. Head circumference catch up growth is limited to 6 to 12 months corrected age (Hack, 2013). Brain development occurs during the first year of life. As adults, ELBW infants tend to be shorter and weigh the same as infants born at term (Roberts et al, 2013a). The parents of the premature infants are often shorter than the parents of term infants, and this could contribute to the infant's adult height.

Growth in the NICU for ELBW infants is linked to growth and development at 18 to 22 months corrected age (Ehrenkranz, 2014). Infants with weight gains greater than 18 grams/kg/day or head circumference growth of 0.9 cm/week had better neurodevelopment and physical growth than infants with slower growth.

Premature infants and very low birthweight infants often develop adult-onset type 2 diabetes. Premature infants have decreased glucose regulation compared with infants born at term. Higher fasting insulin levels, impaired glucose tolerance, and increased insulin resistance may occur (Kajantie and Hovi, 2014). Premature infants or very low birthweight infants have been reported to have higher blood pressures than infants born at term and normal weight (Lapillonne and Griffin, 2013).

More research is needed. What is the optimal rate of growth for premature infants in the NICU and postdischarge to maximize cognitive/developmental outcomes and decrease their risk of adult cardiovascular and metabolic diseases (Lapillonne and Griffin, 2013)? How fast should the premature infant grow? What should the body composition be? When should catch-up growth occur?

Tools have been developed and validated that assess how adults report their health status and quality of life. The evaluations may be conducted by interviews or completion of written questionnaires (Saigal, 2014). As adults, premature and very low birthweight infants rate their quality of life to be similar to adults who were born at term. Roberts and colleagues (2013b) reported on 194 ELBW infants and 148 term infants who completed written evaluations at 18 years. Both groups were the same in their reported quality of life, health status, and self-esteem. Quality of life did not differ for the adults with the smallest birth weight or youngest gestational age. Premature infants not completing the evaluation at 18 years were more likely to have a neurosensory disability at 8 years of age, such as cystic periventricular leukomalacia, blindness, cerebral palsy, and a lower intelligent quotient.

Therefore not only are more premature infants surviving, but they also are growing into adults who are enjoying and living productive lives (Hack, 2013; Saigal, 2013). The medical and nutrition care in the hospital nursery continues to progress, which improves outcome in the nursery and sets the stage for later development.

BOX 42-3 Steps for Adjusting Age for Prematurity on Growth Charts

Calculate the number of weeks the infant was premature:
- 40 weeks (term) – Weeks of birth gestational age = Number of weeks premature
- The resulting number of weeks is the correction factor.
- Calculate the adjusted age for prematurity:
- Chronologic age – Correction factor = Adjusted age for prematurity

For example:
- 40 weeks – 28 weeks of gestation = 12 weeks premature
- Therefore 12 weeks (3 months) is the correction factor.
- 4 months (chronologic age) – 3 months (correction factor) = 1 month adjusted age

---

Commonly used PES (problem, etiology, signs and symptom) statements for infants are provided in Box 42-4. Assessment of nutrient intakes and infant growth are reviewed.

DISCHARGE CARE

Establishment of successful feeding is a pivotal factor determining whether a preterm infant can be discharged from the hospital nursery. Preterm infants must be able to (1) tolerate their feedings and usually obtain all of their feedings from the breast or bottle, (2) grow adequately on a modified-demand feeding schedule (usually every 3-4 hours during the day for bottle-fed infants or every 2-3 hours for breast-fed infants), and (3) maintain their body temperature without the help of an incubator. Medically stable premature infants who have delayed feeding development go home on gavage feedings for a short period. In addition, it is important that any ongoing chronic illnesses, including nutrition problems, be manageable at home.

Most important, the parents must be ready to care for their infant. In hospitals that allow parents to visit their infants in the nursery 24 hours a day, staff can help parents develop their caregiving skills and learn to care for their infant at home. Often, parents are permitted to "room in" with their infant (i.e., stay with the infant all day and night) before discharge, which helps build confidence in their ability to care for a high-risk infant (see Figure 42-6).

Many preterm infants who are discharged from the hospital weigh less than 5½ lb. Although these infants must meet certain discharge criteria before they can go home, the stress of a new environment may lead to setbacks. Small preterm infants should be followed very closely during the first month after discharge, and parents should be given as much information and support as possible. Within the first week of discharge, a home visit by a nurse, dietitian, or both and a visit to the pediatrician can be extremely helpful educationally; and they can provide opportunity for early intervention for developing problems.

Factors that affect the feeding skills and behavior of preterm infants are particularly important after the infants have been discharged. Physical factors such as a variable heart rate, a rapid respiratory rate, and tremulousness are examples of physiologic events that interfere with feeding. In addition, infants weighing less than 5½ lb have poor muscle tone. Although muscle tone gradually improves as an infant becomes larger and more mature, it can deteriorate quickly in infants who are tired or weak. Feeding is often difficult for infants who have limited muscle flexion and strength and poor head and neck control, which are needed to maintain a good feeding posture. Positioning these infants in a manner that supports normal body flexion and ensures proper alignment of the head and neck during feedings is helpful. Premature infants may also need their chin and cheeks supported while bottle feeding.

Small infants tend to sleep more than larger and term infants. It is much easier for preterm infants to feed effectively if they are fully awake. To awaken a preterm infant, the caregiver should provide one type of gentle stimulation for a few minutes and then change to a different type, repeating this pattern until the infant is fully awake. Lightly swaddling of the infant and then placing him or her in a semi upright position also may help.

The feeding environment should be as quiet as possible. Preterm infants are easily distracted and have difficulty focusing on feeding when noises or movements interrupt their attention. They also tire quickly and are easily overstimulated. When they are overstimulated, they may show only subtle signs of distress. It is important to teach parents of premature infants to

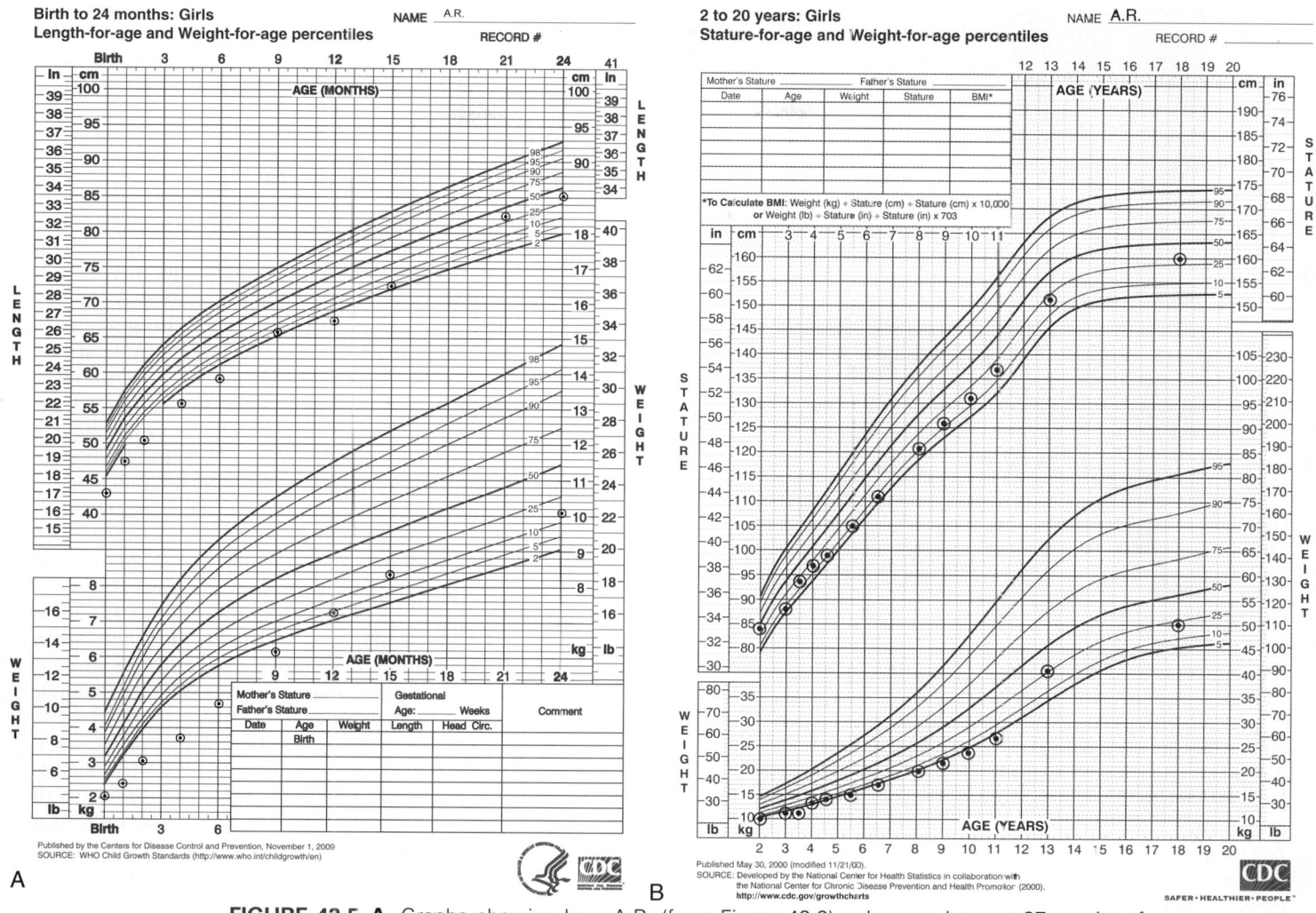

FIGURE 42-5 A, Graphs showing how A.R. (from Figure 42-2), who was born at 27 weeks of gestation, grew after leaving the neonatal unit 1 day before her due date at a weight of 4½ lb. Heights and weights until age of 24 months are plotted on the grid at "corrected age" points. A.R. experienced catch-up growth during the first 12 months. **B,** A.R.'s growth pattern from the age of 2 to 18 years. During the first 10 years she grew at the 5th percentile for weight and the 10th percentile for height. She followed her channel of growth but did not experience catch-up growth. However, between the ages of 10 and 13 she began to change growth channels and moved to the 25th percentile for weight and the 25th percentile for height (catch-up growth). At 18 years she crossed the 25th percentile for height and fell slightly below the 25th percentile for weight.

BOX 42-4 PES Statements Commonly Used for Infants

- Increased nutrient (multinutrient) needs related to increased metabolic demand as evidenced by weight gain <15 g/kg/day despite intake meeting estimated needs
- Suboptimal growth rate related to nutrient provision not meeting estimated needs as evidenced by weight gain <20 g/day
- Suboptimal mineral (iron) intake related to low iron-fortified human milk intake as evidenced by iron intake less than estimated needs for premature infants (guideline is 2-4 mg/kg/day)
- No nutrition diagnosis at this time as enteral nutrition meeting estimated needs and weight gain/growth appropriate overall

Data taken from commonly used PES Statements used by Neonatal Dietitians at Texas Children's Hospital, Houston, Texas, December, 2014.

recognize the subtle cues that indicate the need for rest or comfort and to respond to them appropriately.

The premature infant may be able to breastfeed all feedings to meet nutritional needs. Infants with a birthweight less than 1500 g may need formula supplementation of human milk to meet their nutritional needs for adequate growth. Two to three feedings of the transitional formula can be provided, and the mother can breastfeed the other feedings or provide expressed human milk in bottles. Transitional formula is available as a liquid ready-to-feed formula. The use of powder formula as a supplement can be avoided. Infant formula powders are not sterile and have been linked with *Cronobacter sakazakii* infections. The use of two or three bottles of ready-to-feed formula provides more protein and minerals than provided when human milk is fortified with infant formula powder (AAP, 2014). A multivitamin and iron

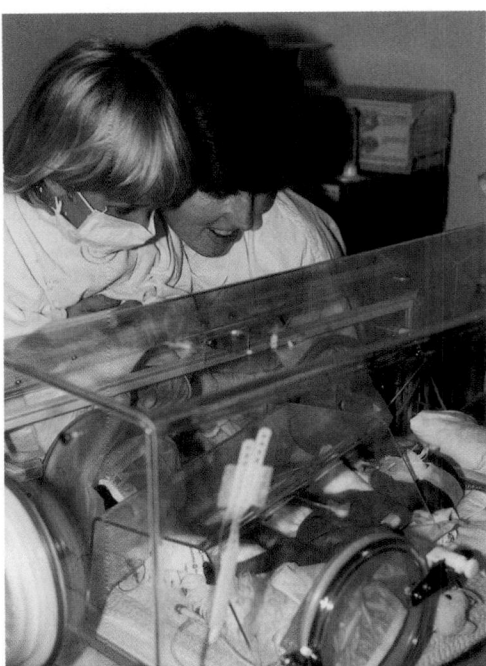

FIGURE 42-6 Family in the nursery with their premature infant.

supplementation should be provided to meet the infant's vitamin D and increased iron demands.

After discharge, most preterm infants need approximately 180 ml/kg/day (2¾ oz/lb/day) of breastmilk or standard infant formula containing 20 kcal/oz. This amount of milk provides 120 kcal/kg/day (55 kcal/lb/day). Alternatively, transitional formula with a concentration of 22 kcal/oz can be provided at a rate of 160 ml/kg/day (or 2.5 oz/lb/day). The best way to determine whether these amounts are adequate for individual infants is to compare their intake with their growth progress over time. Some infants may need a formula that provides 24 kcal/oz. As mentioned previously, powdered transitional formula can be readily altered to a concentration of 24 kcal/oz.

It is important to evaluate needs based on the three growth parameters: weight, length, and head circumference. Patterns of growth should be assessed to determine whether (1) individual growth rate curves at least parallel reference curves, (2) growth curves are shifting inappropriately across growth percentiles, (3) weight is appropriate for length, and (4) growth is proportionate in all three areas.

NEURODEVELOPMENTAL OUTCOME

It is possible to meet the metabolic and nutritional needs of premature infants sufficiently to sustain life and promote growth and development. In fact, more tiny premature infants are surviving than ever before because of adequate nutrition support and the recent advances in neonatal intensive care technology. There is concern that the ELBW infant is often smaller at discharge than the infant of the same postmenstrual age who was not born prematurely. One report suggests that providing appropriate protein intake during week 1 of life to ELBW infants leads to improved growth of weight, length, and head circumference at 36 weeks' gestation, and improved head circumference in male infants at 18 months' corrected age (Poindexter, 2014). Improved neurodevelopment and growth at 18 months has been reported with ELBW infants who gained more weight and had greater head circumference growth during their stay in the nursery (Ehrenkranz, 2014). The developmental outcome scores for ELBW infants have been higher as the intakes of mother's own milk increase (Ahrabi and Schanler, 2013). Research on the neurodevelopment of premature infants who receive fortified donor human milk is needed (Arslanoglu et al, 2013).

The increased survival rate of ELBW infants has increased concerns about their short- and long-term neurodevelopmental outcomes. Many questions have been raised about the quality of life awaiting infants who receive neonatal intensive care. As a rule, VLBW infants should be referred to a follow-up clinic to evaluate their development and growth and begin early interventions (Hack, 2013). The survival of ELBW infants has increased, with an increase in the number of children who are developmentally normal who attend school and live independent lives as adults (Hack, 2013). Many of these premature infants reach adulthood with no evidence of any disability (see Figure 42-7).

CLINICAL CASE STUDY 1

Heather, an infant born at 26 weeks of gestation, was admitted to the neonatal intensive care unit. Her birth weight was 850 g (appropriate for gestational age). Heather had respiratory distress syndrome and had to receive a tube for mechanical ventilation. During the first few hours of her life, she was given surfactant, and her ventilator settings were lowered. She was also placed in a humidified incubator and given 100 ml/kg/day of starter parenteral nutrition (dextrose 10% in water with amino acids) intravenously.

On the second day after her birth, she had gained 20 g, and her serum sodium concentration and urine volume output were low. She was diagnosed with excessive fluid intake. Her blood pressure was low and the drug dopamine was provided to increase her urine output.

On the fourth day after birth, her body weight had decreased 50 g—6% of her birth weight—and her serum electrolyte levels were normal. The protein concentration of her parenteral fluids was increased, as was the volume of intravenous fat being provided.

By the fifth day, Heather was clinically stable. She began receiving feedings of milk from her mother—1.0 ml every 3 hours (10 ml/kg of her birth weight)—via bolus oral gastric tube. The feedings were tolerated well. She then began receiving daily a larger volume of her mother's breastmilk and less parenteral fluids.

On day eleven, full enteral feedings were established, and after extubation Heather was successfully breathing on her own.

Nutrition Diagnostic Statement, Day 2

Excessive fluid intake related to intravenous fluids administered as evidenced by gain of 20 g and low serum sodium level.

Nutrition Diagnostic Statement, Day 11

Inadequate intake of protein and minerals related to increased needs due to prematurity as evidenced by unfortified human milk not meeting established nutritional needs of premature infants.

Nutrition Care Questions

1. On the second day after birth, should Heather's intravenous fluid volume have been (1) increased because she needed more calories, (2) decreased because she was overhydrated, or (3) changed to enteral feedings because she was clinically stable?

2. How should the intravenous fat that was given to Heather have been administered?

3. The breastmilk from Heather's mother may have inadequate amounts of which nutrients? What do you recommend to resolve this?

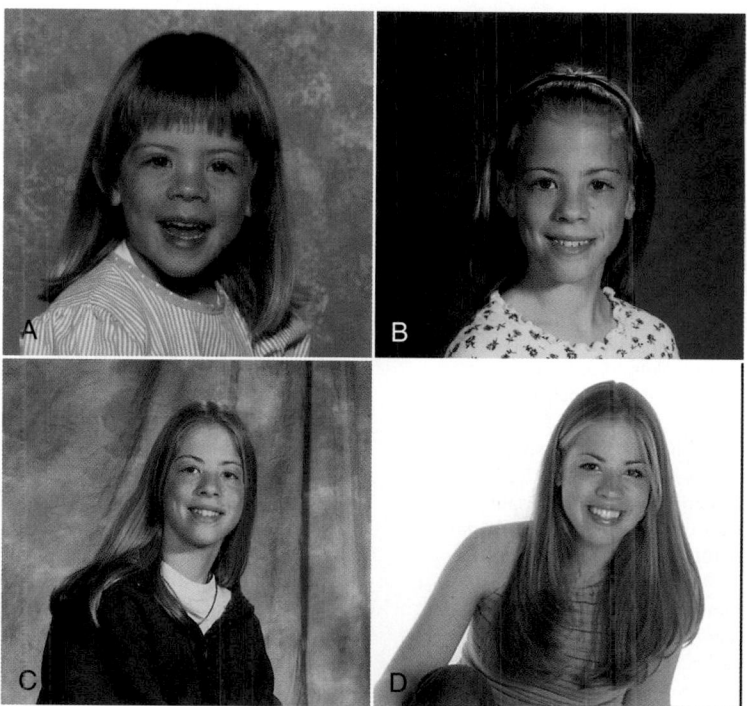

FIGURE 42-7 The premature infant A.R. (see Figures 42-2 and 42-6) as she grows up. **A,** 3½ years. **B,** 10 years. **C,** 14 years. **D,** 18 years. (*D,* Courtesy Yuen Lui Studio, Seattle, Wash.)

CLINICAL CASE STUDY 2

Baby Le was born at 29 weeks of gestation, and his birthweight was 1400 g. He is now 1 week old or 30 weeks' postmenstrual age and weighs 1375 g. He is receiving parenteral nutrition at 130 ml/kg/day that contains 12.5% dextrose and 3.5% amino acids and a 20% intravenous fat emulsion at 15 ml/kg per day. The registered dietitian nutritionist (RDN) assesses the nutrient intake, and calculations are given in the following table. The patient's intakes are compared with the parenteral guidelines of the American Academy of Pediatrics (AAP, 2014) for premature infants.

Nutrient	Nutrient (kg/day)	Guidelines (kg/day)
Kilocalories kcal/kg/day	103	90-100
Glucose mg/kg/min	11.3	11-12
Protein g/kg	4.6	2.7-4.0
Fat g/kg	3	1-3

Nutrition Diagnostic Statement

Excessive protein intake related to excessive provision in parenteral nutrition as evidenced by protein intake greater than recommendation of 4.0 g of protein per kilogram established by the AAP in 2014.

Nutrition Care Questions

1. The RDN chooses the nutrition diagnosis and writes the problem-etiology-signs and symptoms statement. Interventions include decreasing the amino acid concentration to 3%, which will provide 4.0 g of protein per kilogram per day.
2. In how many days would you monitor and evaluate Baby Le's nutrition status?
3. What guidance is needed for the staff to evaluate him for signs of dehydration?

USEFUL WEBSITES

American Academy of Pediatrics
www.aap.org
Fenton Growth Chart
http://ucalgary.ca/fenton
Human Milk Banking Association of North American
www.hmbana.org
March of Dimes
www.marchofdimes.org
National Center for Education in Maternal and Child Health
www.ncemch.org
Olsen Growth Chart
http://www.nursing.upenn.edu/media/infantgrowthcurves/
  Documents/Olsen-NewIUGrowthCurves_2010permission.pdf
World Health Organization Growth Curves
http://www.cdc.gov/growthcharts/who_charts.htm

REFERENCES

Abrams SA: Osteopenia (metabolic bone disease) of prematurity. In Cloherty JP et al, editors: *Manual of neonatal care,* Philadelphia, 2012, Wolters Kluwer/Lippincott Williams & Wilkins, p 555.

Abrams SA, American Academy of Pediatrics, Committee on Nutrition: Calcium and vitamin D requirements of enterally fed preterm infants, *Pediatrics* 131:e1676, 2013.

Abrams SA, Hurst NM: Breastfeeding the preterm infant. In Garcia-Prats JA, Kim MS, editors: *UpToDate* (website): www.uptodate.com. Accessed June 1, 2014.

Agostoni C et al: Enteral nutrient supply for preterm infants: Commentary from the European Society for Paediatric Gastroenterology, Heapatology, and Nutrition Committee on Nutrition, *J Pediatr Gastroenterol Nutr,* 50:85, 2010.

Ahrabi AF, Schanler RJ: Human milk is the only milk for premies in the NICU! *Early Hum Dev* 89(Suppl 2):S51, 2013.

Alsweiler JM et al: Tight glycemic control with insulin in hyperglycemic preterm babies: A randomized controlled trial, *Pediatrics* 129;639, 2012.

American Academy of Pediatrics (AAP), American College of Obstetricians and Gynecologists (ACOG): Lactation support technology. In Schanler RJ et al, editors: *Breastfeeding handbook for physicians*, ed 2, Evanston, Ill, 2014, American Academy of Pediatrics.

American Academy of Pediatrics (AAP), Committee on Nutrition: Nutritional needs of the preterm infant. In Kleinman RE, Greer FR, editors: *Pediatric nutrition handbook*, ed 7, Elk Grove, Ill, 2014, American Academy of Pediatrics.

American Academy of Pediatrics (AAP), Section on Breastfeeding: Breastfeeding and the use of human milk, *Pediatrics* 129:e827, 2012.

Arnold LDW: Global health policies that support the use of banked donor human milk: a human rights issue, *Int Breastfeed J* 1:26, 2006.

Arslanoglu S et al: Donor human milk for preterm infants: current evidence and research directions, *J Pediatr Gastroenterol Nutr*, 57:535, 2013.

Ballard JL et al: New Ballard score, expanded to include extremely premature infants, *J Pediatr* 119:417, 1991.

Cristofalo EA et al: Randomized trial of exclusive human milk versus preterm formula diets in extremely premature infants, *J Pediatr* 163:1592, 2013.

Darlow BA, Graham PJ: Vitamin A supplementation to prevent mortality and short- and long-term morbidity in very low birthweight infants, *Cochrane Datab Syst Rev* 10:CD000501, 2011, DOI:10.1002/14651858.CD000501.pub 3.

Dell KM: Fluid, electrolyte, and acid-base homeostasis. In Martin RJ et al, editors: *Fanaroff and Martin's Neonatal-perinatal medicine diseases of the fetus and infant*, ed 9, St Louis, 2011, Elsevier.

Doherty EG: Fluid and electrolyte management. In Cloherty JP et al, editors: *Manual of neonatal care*, ed 7, Philadelphia, 2012, Wolters Kluwer/Lippincott Williams & Wilkins.

Domellof M: Nutritional care of premature infants: microminerals. In Koletzko B et al, editors: *Nutritional care of preterm infants: scientific basis and practical guidelines (World Rev Nutr Diet, Vol. 110)*, Germany, 2014, S. Karger AG.

Ehrenkranz RA: Nutrition, growth and clinical outcomes. In Koletzko B et al, editors: *Nutritional care of preterm infants: scientific basis and practical guidelines (World Rev Nutr Diet, Vol. 110)*, Germany, 2014, S. Karger AG.

Fenton TR, Kim JH: A systematic review and meta-analysis to revise the Fenton growth chart for preterm infants, *BMC Pediatrics* 13:59, 2013.

Fucile S et al: Oral and non-oral sensorimotor interventions enhance oral feeding performance in preterm infants, *Dev Med Child Neurology* 53:829, 2011.

Gribble KD, Hausman BL: Milk sharing and formula feeding: Infant feeding risks in comparative perspective? *Australas Med J* 5:275, 2012.

Grummer-Strawn LM et al: Centers for Disease Control and Prevention, Use of World Health Organization and CDC growth charts for children aged 0-59 months in United States, *MMWR* 59(No. RR-9):1, 2010. Erratum in *MMWR Recomm Rep* 59(36):1184, 2010.

Hack M: The outcome of neonatal intensive care. In Fanaroff AA, Fanaroff JM, editors: *Klaus and Fanaroff's care of the high-risk newborn*, Philadelphia, 2013, Elsevier Saunders.

Hair AB et al: Human milk feeding supports adequate growth in infants ≤1250 grams birth weight, *BMC Research Notes* 6:459, 2013.

Hamilton BE et al: Annual summary of vital statistics: 2010-2011, *Pediatrics* 131:548, 2013.

Hay WW et al: Energy requirements, protein-energy metabolism and balance, and carbohydrates in preterm infants. In Koletzko B et al, editors: *Nutritional care of preterm infants: scientific basis and practical guidelines (World Rev Nutr Diet, Vol. 110)*, Germany, 2014, S. Karger AG.

Human Milk Banking Association of North America (HMBANA): https://www.hmbana.org/. Accessed March 2, 2014.

Isaacs EB et al: Impact of breast milk on intelligence quotient, brain size, and white matter development, *Pediatr Res* 67:357, 2010.

Kajantie E, Hovi P: Is very preterm birth a risk factor for adult cardiometabolic disease? *Semin Fetal Neonatal Med* 19:112, 2014.

Kassity-Krich NA, Jones JJ: Complementary and integrative therapies. In Kenner C, Lott JW, editors: *Comprehensive neonatal nursing care*, New York, 2014, Springer Publishing Co.

Keim SA et al: Microbial contamination of human milk purchased via the internet, *Pediatrics* 132:e1227, 2013.

Klein CJ: Nutrient requirements for preterm infant formula, *J Nutr* 132(6 Suppl 1):1395S, 2002.

Koletzko B et al: Recommended nutrient intake levels for stable, fully enterally fed very low birth weight infants. In Koletzko B et al, editors: *Nutritional care of preterm infants: scientific basis and practical guidelines* (World Rev Nutr Diet, 110:297, Germany, 2014, S. Karger AG.

Lapillonne A: Feeding the preterm infant after discharge. In Koletzko B et al, editors: *Nutritional care of preterm infants: Scientific basis and practical guidelines, World Rev Nutr Diet, Vol. 110*, Germany, 2014, S. Karger AG.

Lapillonne A et al: Lipid needs of preterm infants: Updated recommendations, *J Pediatr* 162(Suppl 3):S37, 2013.

Lapillonne A, Griffin IJ: Feeding preterm infants today for later metabolic and cardiovascular outcomes, *J Pediatr* 162(Suppl 3):S7, 2013.

MacDorman MF et al: Recent declines in infant mortality in the United States, 2005-2011. *NCHS Data Brief* 120, Hyattsville, Md, 2013, National Center for Health Statistics.

Marinelli KA et al: The effect of a donor milk policy on the diet of very low birth weight infants, *J Hum Lact* 30:310, 2014.

Olsen IE et al: New intrauterine growth curves based on United States data, *Pediatrics* 125:e214, 2010.

PATH: *Strengthening human milk banking: a global implementation framework*, version 1, Seattle, Wa, 2013, Bill and Melinda Gates Foundation Grand Challenges Initiative, PATH.

Poindexter B: Approaches to growth faltering. In Koletzko B et al, editors: *Nutritional care of preterm infants: scientific basis and practical guidelines(World Rev Nutr Diet, Vol. 110)*, Germany, 2014, S. Karger AG.

Premkumar MH et al: Fish oil-based lipid emulsions in the treatment of parenteral nutrition-associated liver disease: An ongoing positive experience, *Adv Nutr* 5:65, 2014.

Rigo J, Senterre T: Intrauterine-like growth rates can be achieved with premixed parenteral nutrition solution in preterm infants, *J Nutr* 143(Suppl 12); 2966S, 2013.

Robbins ST, Meyers R, editors: *Infant feedings: guidelines for preparation of formula and human milk in health care facilities*, ed 2, Chicago, 2011, American Dietetic Association.

Roberts G et al: Growth of extremely preterm survivors from birth to 18 years of age compared with term controls, *Pediatrics* 131:e439, 2013a.

Roberts G et al: Quality of life at age 18 after extremely preterm birth in the post-surfactant era, *J Pediatr* 163:1008, 2013b.

Rogers SP et al: Continuous feedings of fortified human milk lead to nutrient losses of fat, calcium and phosphorous, *Nutrients* 2:230, 2010.

Saigal S: Quality of life of former premature infants during adolescence and beyond, *Early Hum Dev* 89:209, 2013.

Saigal S: Functional outcomes of very premature infants into adulthood, *Semin Fetal Neonatal Med*, 19:125, 2014.

Schanler RJ: Approach to enteral nutrition in the premature infant. In Abrams SA, Kim MS, editors: *UpToDate*, Wolters Kluwer Health. www.uptodate.com. Accessed June 1, 2014.

Senterre T: Practice of enteral nutrition in very low birth weight and extremely low birth weight infants. In Koletzko B et al, editors: *Nutritional care of preterm infants: scientific basis and practical guidelines (World Rev Nutr Diet, Vol. 110)*, Germany, 2014, S. Karger AG.

Sullivan S et al: An exclusively human milk-based diet is associated with a lower rate of necrotizing enterocolitis than a diet of human milk and bovine milk-based products, *J Pediatr* 156:562, 2010.

Thureen PJ et al: Effect of low versus high intravenous amino acid intake on very low birth weight infants in the early neonatal period, *Pediatr Res* 53:24, 2003.

Tudehope D et al: Nutritional needs of the micropreterm infant, *J Pediatr* 162(Suppl 3):S72, 2013.

Tyson JE et al: Vitamin A supplementation for extremely-low-birth-weight infants, *N Engl J Med* 340:1962, 1999.

van Aerde JE, Narvey M: Acute respiratory failure. In Thureen PJ, Hay WW, editors: *Neonatal nutrition and metabolism*, ed 2, Cambridge, 2006, Cambridge University Press.

van Goudoever JB et al: Amino acids and proteins. In Koletzko B et al, editors: *Nutritional Care of Preterm Infants: Scientific basis and practical guidelines*(*World Rev Nutr Diet, Vol. 110*), Germany, 2014, S. Karger AG.

Vanek VW et al: A.S.P.E.N. position paper: Clinical role for alternative intravenous fat emulsions, *Nutr Clin Pract* 27:150, 2012.

World Health Organization (WHO) Collaborative study team on the role of breastfeeding in the prevention of infant mortality: effect of breastfeeding on infant and child mortality due to infectious diseases in less developed countries: a pooled analysis, *Lancet 355:451, 2000.*

Yee WH et al: Incidence and timing of presentation of necrotizing enterocolitis in preterm infants, *Pediatrics* 129:e298, 2012.

Young L et al: Nutrient-enriched formula versus standard term formula for preterm infants following hospital discharge, *Cochrane Datab Syst Rev*3:CD004696, 2012, DOI: 10.1002/14651858.CD004696.pub4.

Ziegler EE: Meeting the nutritional needs of the low-birth-weight infant, *Ann Nutr Metab* 58(Suppl 1):8, 2011.

43

Medical Nutrition Therapy for Genetic Metabolic Disorders

Beth N. Ogata, MS, RDN, CD, CSP,
Cristine M. Trahms, MS, RDN, FADA

KEY TERMS

argininosuccinic aciduria (ASA)
autosomal-recessive
branched-chain ketoaciduria
carbamyl-phosphate synthetase (CPS) deficiency
citrullinemia
fatty acid oxidation disorders
galactokinase deficiency
galactosemia
galactose-1-phosphate uridyltransferase (GALT) deficiency

genetic metabolic disorders
gluconeogenesis
glycogen storage diseases (GSDs)
glycogenolysis
hereditary fructose intolerance
ketone utilization disorder
L-carnitine
long-chain 3-hydroxyacyl-CoA dehydrogenase (LCHAD) deficiency

maple syrup urine disease (MSUD)
medium-chain acyl-CoA dehydrogenase (MCAD) deficiency
methylmalonic acidemia
ornithine transcarbamylase (OTC) deficiency
phenylketonuria (PKU)
propionic acidemia
urea cycle disorders (UCds)

Genetic metabolic disorders are inherited traits that result in the absence or reduced activity of a specific enzyme or cofactor necessary for optimal metabolism. Most genetic metabolic disorders are inherited as autosomal-recessive traits; autosomal means that the gene is located on a chromosome other than the X or Y chromosomes (see Chapter 5). The treatment for many metabolic disorders is medical nutrition therapy (MNT), with intervention specific to the disorder. The goals of MNT are to maintain biochemical equilibrium for the affected pathway, provide adequate nutrients to support typical growth and development, and support social and emotional development. Nutrition interventions are designed to circumvent the missing or inactive enzyme by (1) restricting the amount of substrate available, (2) supplementing the amount of product, (3) supplementing the enzymatic cofactor, or (4) combining any or all of these approaches. The primary conditions commonly found in the United States are discussed here, and Table 43-1 outlines other disorders by the enzymatic defects, distinctive clinical and biochemical features, and current approaches to dietary therapy.

In some instances, when treatment is initiated early in the newborn period and meticulously continued for a lifetime, the affected individual can be cognitively and physically normal. For other conditions, cognitive and physical damage can occur despite early and meticulous treatment. Biochemical disorders range from variations in enzyme activity that are benign, to severe manifestations that are incompatible with life. For many, significant questions related to diagnosis and treatment remain.

NEWBORN SCREENING

Most inherited metabolic disorders are associated with severe clinical illness that often appears soon after birth. Intellectual disability and severe neurologic involvement may be immediately apparent. Diagnosis of a specific disorder may be difficult, and appropriate treatment measures may be uncertain. Prenatal diagnosis is available for many metabolic disorders, but it usually requires the identification of a family at risk, which can be done only after the birth of an affected child. Effective newborn screening programs, as well as advanced diagnostic techniques and treatment modalities have improved the outcome for many of these infants.

Infants suspected of having a metabolic disorder should be afforded access to care offered by centers with expertise in treating these disorders. Infants who are afebrile for no apparent reason, lethargic, vomiting, in respiratory distress, or having seizures should be evaluated for an undiagnosed metabolic disorder. The initial assessment should include blood gas measurements, electrolyte values, glucose and ammonia tests, and a urine test for ketones.

Advances in newborn screening technology offer opportunities for earlier diagnosis, prevention of neurologic crisis, and improved intellectual and physical outcomes. When tandem mass spectrometry techniques are used in newborn screening laboratories, infants with a broader range of metabolic disorders can be detected, and the disorder can be identified earlier (see *Focus On:* Newborn Screening and Figure 43-1).

TABLE 43-1 Selected Genetic Metabolic Disorders That Respond To Dietary Treatment

Disorder	Affected Enzyme	Prevalence	Clinical and Biochemical Features	Medical Nutrition Therapy	Adjunct Treatment
Urea Cycle Disorders (UCDs)					
Carbamyl-phosphate synthetase deficiency	Carbamy-phosphate synthetase	1:30,000 (all UCDs)	Vomiting, seizures, sometimes coma → death. Survivors usually have ID. ↑ plasma ammonia and glutamine	Food: low protein. Formula: without nonessential amino acids	L-carnitine, phenylbutyrate,* L-citrulline, L-arginine. Hemodialysis or peritoneal dialysis during acute episodes
Ornithine trans-carbamylase deficiency	Ornithine trans-carbamylase (x-linked)	1:30,000 (all UCDs)	Vomiting, seizures, coma → death as a newborn. ↑ plasma ammonia, glutamine, glutamic acid and alanine	Food: low protein. Formula: without nonessential amino acids	L-carnitine, phenylbutyrate,* L-citrulline, L-arginine
Citrullinemia	Argininosuccinate synthetase	1:30,000 (all UCDs)	*Neonatal:* vomiting, seizures, coma → death. *Infantile:* vomiting, seizures, progressive developmental delay. ↑ plasma citrulline and ammonia, alanine	Food: low protein. Formula: without nonessential amino acids	L-carnitine, phenylbutyrate,* L-arginine
Argininosuccinic aciduria	Argininosuccinate lyase	1:30,000 (all UCDs)	*Neonatal:* hypotonia, seizures. *Subacute:* vomiting, FTT, progressive developmental delay. ↑ plasma argininosuccinic acid, citrulline and ammonia	Food: low protein. Formula: lower protein SF (without nonessential amino acids)	L-carnitine, phenylbutyrate*
Argininemia	Arginase	1:30,000 (all UCDs)	Periodic vomiting, seizures, coma. Progressive spastic diplegia, developmental delay. ↑ arginine and ammonia related to protein intake	Food: low protein. Formula: lower protein SF (without nonessential amino acids)	L-carnitine, phenylbutyrate*
Organic Acidemias					
Methylmalonic acidemia	Methylmalonyl-CoA mutase or similar	1:80,000	Metabolic acidosis, vomiting, seizures, coma, often death. ↑ organic urine acid and plasma ammonia levels	Food: low protein. Formula: lower protein SF (without isoleucine, methionine, threonine, valine)	L-carnitine, vitamin B$_{12}$. IV fluids, bicarbonate during acute episodes
Propionic acidemia	Propionyl-CoA carboxylase or similar	1:80,000	Metabolic acidosis, ↑ plasma ammonia and propionic acid, ↑ urine methylcitric acid	Food: low protein. Formula: lower protein SF (without isoleucine, methionine, threonine, valine)	L-carnitine, biotin. IV fluids, bicarbonate during acute episodes
Isovaleric acidemia	Isovaleryl-CoA dehydrogenase	1:80,000	Poor feeding, lethargy, seizures, metabolic ketoacidosis, hyperammonemia	Food: low protein. Formula: SF (without leucine)	L-carnitine, L-glycine
Ketone utilization disorder	2-methylacetoace-tyl-CoA-thiolase or similar	Unknown	Vomiting, dehydration, metabolic ketoacidosis	Food: low protein. Formula: SF (without isoleucine). Avoid fasting, high complex carbohydrates	L-carnitine, Bicitra

Continued

TABLE 43-1   Selected Genetic Metabolic Disorders That Respond To Dietary Treatment—cont'd

Disorder	Affected Enzyme	Prevalence	Clinical and Biochemical Features	Medical Nutrition Therapy	Adjunct Treatment
Biotinidase deficiency	Biotinidase or similar	1:60,000	In *infancy*, seizures, hypotonia, rash, stridor, apnea; in *older children*, also see alopecia, ataxia, developmental delay, hearing loss		Supplemental oral biotin
Carbohydrate Disorders					
Galactosemia	Galactose-1-phosphate uridyltransferase	1:50,000	Vomiting, hepatomegaly, FTT, cataracts, ID, often early sepsis ↑ urine and blood galactose	Eliminate lactose, low galactose, use soy protein isolate formula	
Hereditary fructose intolerance	Fructose-1-phosphate aldolase	1:20,000	Vomiting; hepatomegaly; hypoglycemia, FTT, renal tubular defects after fructose introduction ↑ blood and urine fructose after fructose feeding	No sucrose, fructose	
Fructose 1,6-diphosphatase deficiency	Fructose 1,6-diphosphatase	Unknown	Hypoglycemia, hepatomegaly, hypotonia, metabolic acidosis upon fructose introduction No ↑ blood/urine fructose	No sucrose, fructose	
Glycogen storage disease, type Ia	Glucose-6-phosphatase	1:60,000	Profound hypoglycemia, hepatomegaly	Low lactose, fructose, sucrose; low fat; high complex carbohydrate; avoid fasting	Raw cornstarch, iron supplements
Amino Acid Disorders					
Hyperphenylalaninemias					
Phenylketonuria	Phenylalanine hydroxylase	1:15,000		Food: low protein Formula: SF (without Phe, supplemented with tyrosine)	
Mild phenylketonuria	Phenylalanine hydroxylase	1:24,000	↑ blood Phe	Food: low protein Formula: SF (without Phe, supplemented with tyrosine)	
Dihydropteridine reductase deficiency	Dihydropteridine reductase	Rare	↑ blood Phe, Irritability, developmental delay, seizures	Food: low protein Formula: SF (without Phe, supplemented with tyrosine)	Biopterin, 5-hydroxytryptophan, L-dopa, folinic acid
Biopterin synthase defect	Biopterin synthase	Rare	Mild ↑ blood Phe, irritability, developmental delay, seizures	None	L-dopa, tetrahydrobiopterin, 5-hydroxytryptophan
Tyrosinemia, type I	Fumarylacetoacetate hydrolase	<1:120,000	Vomiting, acidosis, diarrhea, FTT, hepatomegaly, rickets ↑ blood and urine tyrosine, methionine; ↑ urine parahydroxy derivatives of tyrosine; liver cancer	Food: low protein Formula: SF (without tyrosine, Phe, methionine)	Nitisinone[†]
Maple Syrup Urine Disease					
MSUD	Branched-chain ketoacid decarboxylase complex (<2% activity)	1:200,000	Seizures, acidosis Plasma leucine, isoleucine, valine 10× normal	Food: low protein Formula: SF (without leucine, isoleucine, valine)	Thiamin[‡]

TABLE 43-1   Selected Genetic Metabolic Disorders That Respond To Dietary Treatment—cont'd

Disorder	Affected Enzyme	Prevalence	Clinical and Biochemical Features	Medical Nutrition Therapy	Adjunct Treatment
Intermittent MSUD	Branched-chain ketoacid decarboxylase complex (<20% activity between episodes)	Rare	Intermittent symptoms Plasma leucine, isoleucine, valine 10× normal during illness	Food: low protein Formula: SF (without leucine, isoleucine, valine)	
Homocystinuria	Cystathionine synthase or similar	1:200,000	Detached retinas; thromboembolic and cardiac disease; mild to moderate ID; bony abnormalities; fair hair and skin; ↑ methionine, homocysteine	Food: low protein Formula: SF (without methionine, supplemented with L-cystine)	Betaine, folate, vitamin B$_{12}$, vitamin B$_6$[‡] if folate levels are normal
Fatty Acid Oxidation Disorders					
Long chain acyl-CoA dehydrogenase deficiency	Long-chain acyl-CoA dehydrogenase	Rare	Vomiting, lethargy, hypoglycemia	Low fat, low long-chain fatty acids; avoid fasting	MCT oil, L-carnitine[§]
Long-chain 3-hydroxy-acyl-CoA dehydrogenase deficiency	Long-chain 3-hydroxy-acyl-CoA dehydrogenase	Rare	Vomiting, lethargy, hypoglycemia	Low fat, low long-chain fatty acids; avoid fasting	MCT oil, L-carnitine[§]
Medium chain acyl-CoA dehydrogenase deficiency	Medium-chain acyl-CoA dehydrogenase	1:20,000	Vomiting, lethargy, hypoglycemia	Low fat, low medium-chain fatty acids, avoid fasting	L-carnitine[§]
Short chain acyl-CoA dehydrogenase deficiency	Short-chain acyl-CoA dehydrogenase	Rare	Vomiting, lethargy, hypoglycemia	Low fat, low short-chain fatty acids, avoid fasting	L-carnitine[§]
Very long chain acyl-CoA dehydrogenase deficiency	Very-long-chain acyl-CoA dehydrogenase	Rare	Vomiting, lethargy, hypoglycemia	Low fat, low long-chain fatty acids, avoid fasting	L-carnitine,[§] MCT oil

CoA, Coenzyme A; *FTT,* failure to thrive; *ID,* intellectual disability; *IV,* intravenous; *MCT,* medium-chain triglyceride; *MSUD,* maple syrup urine disease; *Phe,* phenylalanine; *SF,* specialized formulas are available for medical nutrition therapy for this disorder; *UCD,* urea cycle disorder.

*Phenylbutyrate is a chemical administered to enhance waste ammonia excretion; other compounds producing the same effect are also used.

[†]*Nitisinone,* formerly *NTBC,* 2-(2-nitro-4-trifluoro-methyl-benzoyl-1,3-cyclohexanedione, commercially available as Orfadin.

[‡]Patient may or may not respond to the compound.

[§]Use depends on clinic.

⊚ FOCUS ON

Newborn Screening (NBS)

Since the 1960s, states across the United States have adopted mandatory newborn screening (NBS) as law (Waisbren, 2006). These programs were developed as a result of the efficacy of the Guthrie bacterial inhibition assay, in which dried blood spots were used to identify PKU. This simple, sensitive, and inexpensive screening test became the basis for population-based screening systems for newborns. Hemoglobinopathies, endocrine disorders, metabolic disorders, and some infectious diseases can be identified effectively with the use of dried blood spots.

Tandem mass spectrometry was first used in the 1990s and is now used across the United States. This technology makes it possible to identify multiple disorders from a single dried blood spot. The number of disorders screened for varies by state, and expanded screening also is offered by private, for-profit companies. Follow-up programs also vary; some states have single, organized programs, whereas follow-up in other states is less centralized. Conditions successfully screened for by early NBS programs include congenital hypothyroidism, phenylketonuria, congenital adrenal hyperplasia, galactosemia, sickle cell disease, and maple syrup urine disease (Brosco et al, 2006).

The Maternal and Child Health Bureau (MCHB) of the US Health Resources and Services Administration commissioned a report from the American College of Medical Genetics (ACMG). This expert panel identified 29 conditions for which newborn screening should be mandated and 25 secondary conditions that may be detected incidentally (MCHB, 2007). The ACMG developed a series of ACTion (ACT) sheets and confirmatory algorithms for disorders that are identified by NBS screening. The ACT sheets describe the steps health professionals should follow in communicating with the family and determining follow-up. They are available at http://www.ncbi.nlm.nih.gov/books/NBK55827/.

Other groups, including the World Health Organization, March of Dimes, and Massachusetts Newborn Screening Advisory Committee, also have issued recommendations.

Providers who may be involved in the care and follow-up of families identified by NBS should have a good understanding of their state's system, as well as the confounding factors that may affect results. Communication among families, primary health care providers, and tertiary clinics is critical to timely identification and treatment. Follow-up, including referral to the appropriate specialists, is important for any family who receives positive NBS results. NBS fact sheets from the Committee on Genetics of the American Academy of Pediatrics describe (1) newborn screening; (2) follow-up of abnormal screening results to facilitate timely diagnostic testing and management; (3) diagnostic testing; (4) disease management, which requires coordination with the medical home and genetic counseling; and (5) continuous evaluation and improvement of the NBS system (Kaye et al, 2006).

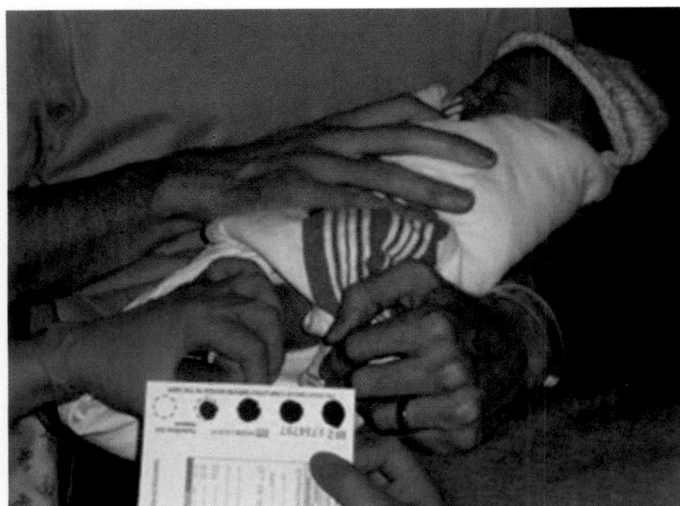

FIGURE 43-1 Blood spots are collected from a newborn for newborn screening. (Courtesy Kelly McKean.)

DISORDERS OF AMINO ACID METABOLISM

Nutrition therapy for amino acid disorders most commonly consists of substrate restriction, which involves limiting one or more essential amino acids to the minimum requirement while providing adequate energy and nutrients to promote typical growth and development (e.g., restricting phenylalanine [Phe] in phenylketonuria). An inadequate intake of an essential amino acid is often as detrimental as excess. Supplementation of the product of the specific enzymatic reaction usually is required in nutrition therapy for amino acid

disorders; for example, tyrosine (Tyr) is supplemented in formulas for treatment of PKU.

Requirements for individual amino acids are difficult to determine because typical growth and development can be achieved over a wide range of intake. The data of Holt and Snyderman (1967) often are used as the basis for prescribing amino acid intakes (see Table 43-2). Careful and frequent monitoring is required to ensure the adequacy of the nutritional prescription. Although nitrogen studies are the most precise, weight gain in infants is a sensitive and easily monitored index of well-being and nutritional adequacy.

PHENYLKETONURIA

Etiology

Phenylketonuria (PKU) is the most common of the hyperphenylalaninemias. In this disorder phenylalanine (Phe) is not metabolized to tyrosine (Tyr) because of a deficiency or inactivity of phenylalanine hydroxylase (PAH) as shown in Figure 43-2. Of the amino acid disorders, PKU provides a reasonable model for detailed discussion because it (1) occurs relatively frequently and most neonates are screened for it; (2) has a successful MNT treatment; and (3) has a predictable course, with available documentation of "natural" and "intervention" history (see *Focus On:* Time Line of Events in the Diagnosis and Treatment of Phenylketonuria).

Nutritional treatment involves restricting the substrate (Phe) and supplementing the product (Tyr) (see *Pathophysiology and Care Management Algorithm:* Phenylketonuria). Most affected infants exhibit PAH deficiency; the remainder (less than 3%) have defects in associated pathways. Low-Phe nutrition therapy does not prevent the neurologic deterioration present in the disorders of these other associated pathways.

TABLE 43-2 Approximate Daily Requirements for Selected Dietary Components and Amino Acids in Infancy and Childhood

Dietary Component or Amino Acid	AGE AND REQUIREMENT Birth to 12 mo (mg/kg)	1-10 yr (mg/day)	Dietary Component or Amino Acid	AGE AND REQUIREMENT Birth to 12 mo (mg/kg)	1-10 yr (mg/day)
Phenylalanine	1-5 mo: 47-90 6-12 mo: 25-47	200-500*	Lysine	90-120	1200-1600
			Threonine	45-87	800-1000
Histidine	16-34		Tryptophan	13-22	60-120
Tyrosine†	1-5 mo: 60-80 6-12 mo: 40-60	25-85 (mg/kg)	Energy	1-5 mo: 108 kcal/kg 6-12 mo: 98 kcal/kg	70-102 kcal/kg
Leucine	76-150	1000	Water	100 mL/kg	1000 mL
Isoleucine	1-5 mo: 79-110 6-12 mo: 50-75	1000	Carbohydrate	kcal × 0.5 ÷ 4 = g/day	kcal × 0.5 ÷ 4 = g/day
Valine	1-5 mo: 65-105 6-12 mo: 50-80	400-600	Total protein	1-5 mo: 2.2 g/kg 6-12 mo: 1.6 g/kg	16-18
Methionine‡	20-45	400-800	Fat	kcal × 0.35 ÷ 9 = g/day	kcal × 0.35 ÷ 9 = g/day
Cyst(e)ine§	15-50	400-800			

Modified from American Academy of Pediatrics, Committee on Nutrition: Special diets for infants with inborn errors of metabolism, *Pediatrics* 57:783, 1976.

Compiled from amino acid data of Holt and Snyderman. Information on amino acid requirements of infants and children at different ages is limited; the figures given here are in excess of minimum requirements. Consequently, this table should be used only as a guide and should not be regarded as an authoritative statement to which individual patients must conform.

*More phenylalanine (>800 mg) is required in the absence of tyrosine.

†Total phenylalanine plus tyrosine should be considered in the prescription because most phenylalanine is converted to tyrosine.

‡More methionine is required in the absence of cyst(e)ine.

§More cyst(e)ine is required in presence of a blocked *trans*-sulfuration outflow pathway for methionine metabolism.

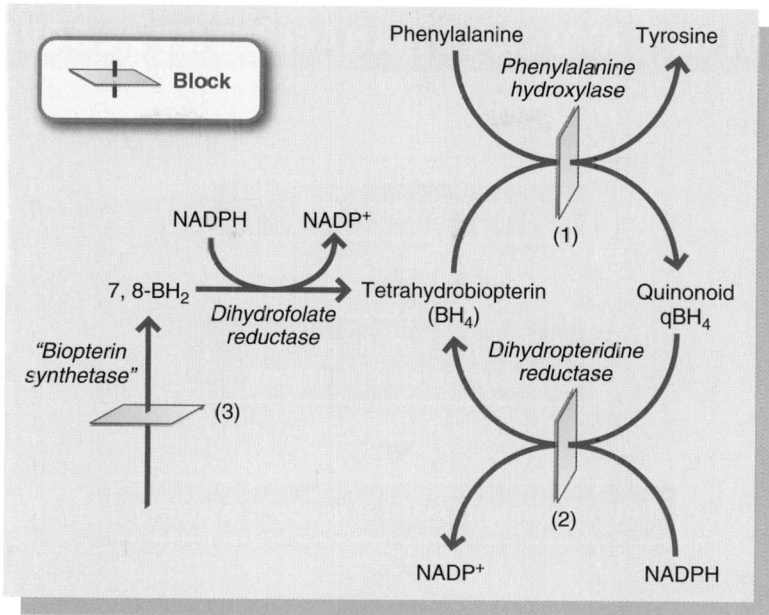

FIGURE 43-2 Hyperphenylalaninemias. **1,** Phenylalanine hydroxylase deficiency; **2,** Dihydropteridine reductase deficiency; **3,** Biopterin synthetase deficiency. *NADPH,* Nicotinamide-adenine dinucleotide phosphate (reduced form); *NADP+,* nicotinamide-adenine dinucleotide phosphate (oxidized form).

◎ FOCUS ON

Time Line of Events in the Diagnosis and Treatment of Phenylketonuria

1934: A. Folling identifies phenylpyruvic acid in the urine of mentally retarded siblings.

1950s: G. Jervis demonstrates a deficiency of phenylalanine oxidation in the liver tissue of an affected patient. H. Bickel demonstrates that dietary phenylalanine restrictions lower the blood concentration of phenylalanine.

1960s: R. Guthrie develops a bacterial inhibition assay for measuring blood phenylalanine levels.

Mid-1960s: Semisynthetic formulas restricted in phenylalanine content become commercially available.

1965-1970: States adopt newborn screening programs to detect phenylketonuria (PKU).

1967-1980: Collaborative Study of Children Treated for Phenylketonuria is conducted. Data from this study form the basis for treatment protocols for PKU clinics in the United States.

Late-1970s: Detrimental effects of maternal PKU are recognized as a significant public health problem.

1980s: Lifelong restriction of phenylalanine intake becomes the standard of care in PKU clinics in the United States.

1983: The Maternal PKU Collaborative Study begins to study the effects of treatment on the pregnancy outcome of women with phenylketonuria.

1987: Techniques for carrier detection and prenatal diagnosis of PKU are developed.

Late-1980s: The gene for phenylalanine hydroxylase deficiency (MIM No. 261600) is located on chromosome 12q22-q24.1. DNA mutation analysis is accomplished with peripheral leukocytes.

1990s: Phenylalanine level of 2-6 mg/dl (120-360 μmol/L), lower than the previous level of less than 10 mg/dL (600 μmol/L), becomes the new standard of care for treatment of PKU.

2000s: Tetrahydrobiopterin-responsive forms of PKU are recognized, especially those with mild mutations.

2010: Research into alternative and adjunct therapies such as the use of large neutral amino acids, BH4 supplementation, enzyme substitution, and somatic gene therapy.

2014: Clinical trials for enzyme replacement therapy using pegylated phenylalanine ammonia lyase (PEG-PAL) injections are underway.

Data from Maternal Child Health Bureau: Newborn screening: toward a uniform screening panel and system, *Genet Med* 8(Suppl 1):1S, 2006; Saugstad LF: From genetics to epigenetics, *Nutr Health* 18:285, 2006; Mitchell JJ, Scriver CR: Phenylalanine hydroxylase deficiency. In Pagon RA et al, editors: GeneReviews [Internet]. Seattle, 1993-2000, University of Washington, Seattle [updated January 31, 2013].

Medical Treatment

All states have newborn screening programs for PKU and other metabolic disorders. Diagnostic criteria for PKU include an elevated blood concentration of Phe and an elevated (i.e., greater than 3) Phe:Tyr ratio. The diagnostic process also should include evaluation for hyperphenylalaninemia that results from the deficiency of enzymes other than PAH, including defects in tetrahydrobiopterin (BH_4) synthesis or regeneration

(Vockley et al, 2014). An effective newborn screening program and access to an organized follow-up program are critical to early identification and treatment of infants with PKU.

The advantage of rigorous nutrition therapy has been demonstrated by measurements of intellectual function. Individuals who do not receive diet therapy have severe intellectual disability, whereas individuals who are on therapy from the early neonatal period have normal intellectual function (McPheeters et al,

PATHOPHYSIOLOGY AND CARE MANAGEMENT ALGORITHM

Phenylketonuria

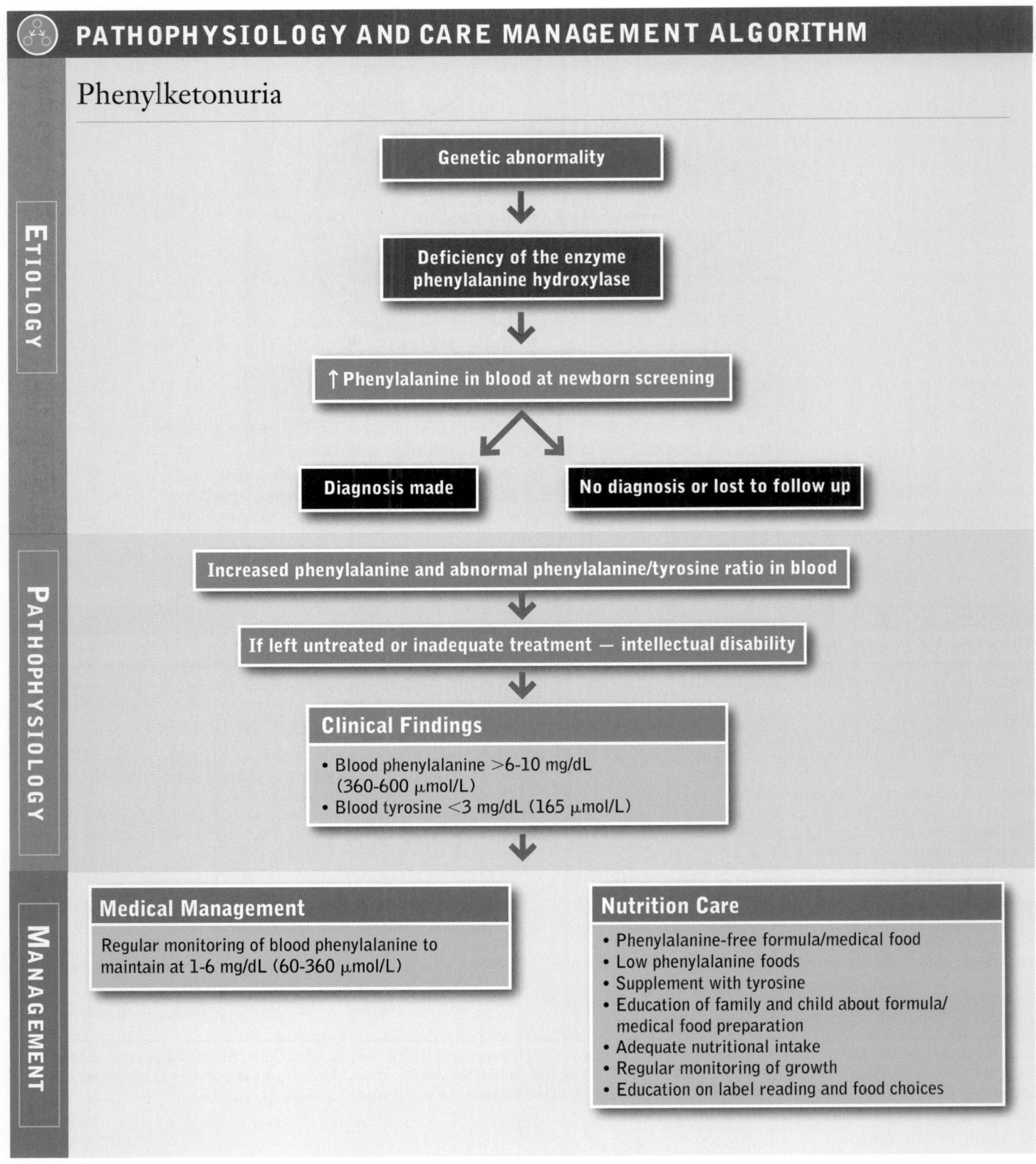

ETIOLOGY

Genetic abnormality

↓

Deficiency of the enzyme phenylalanine hydroxylase

↓

↑ Phenylalanine in blood at newborn screening

Diagnosis made   No diagnosis or lost to follow up

PATHOPHYSIOLOGY

Increased phenylalanine and abnormal phenylalanine/tyrosine ratio in blood

↓

If left untreated or inadequate treatment — intellectual disability

↓

Clinical Findings

- Blood phenylalanine >6-10 mg/dL (360-600 μmol/L)
- Blood tyrosine <3 mg/dL (165 μmol/L)

MANAGEMENT

Medical Management

Regular monitoring of blood phenylalanine to maintain at 1-6 mg/dL (60-360 μmol/L)

Nutrition Care

- Phenylalanine-free formula/medical food
- Low phenylalanine foods
- Supplement with tyrosine
- Education of family and child about formula/ medical food preparation
- Adequate nutritional intake
- Regular monitoring of growth
- Education on label reading and food choices

2012). Outcome, measured as intellectual function, depends on the age of the infant at diagnosis and start of nutrition therapy, as well as the individual's biochemical control over time.

BH$_4$ has been studied to evaluate its effectiveness as an alternative treatment to severe dietary Phe restriction, since BH$_4$ is a cofactor needed for proper activity of the enzyme. Treatment with sapropterin (a synthetic form of BH$_4$) is used as an adjunct therapy for some milder mutations; observations on long-term outcome are needed (Lindgren et al, 2013). Those individuals who respond have what is called

BH4-responsive PKU. However, even for BH$_4$-responsive individuals, ongoing intervention and nutrition monitoring is needed (Singh et al, 2010).

Other studies have examined the possibility of enzyme substitution with phenylalanine ammonia lyase (PAL) to degrade Phe, or gene therapy to restore PAH activity (Blau et al, 2010).

Blood Phenylalanine Control. Blood Phe concentration must be checked regularly, depending on the age and health status of the child, to be sure it remains within the range of 2 to 6 mg/dl or 120 to 360 μmol/L (McPheeters et al, 2012). Phe-containing foods are offered as tolerated as long as the blood concentration of Phe remains in the range of good biochemical control. The child's rate of growth and mental development must be monitored carefully.

Effective management requires a team approach in which the child, parents, registered dietitian nutritionist, pediatrician, psychologist, social worker, and nurse work together to achieve and maintain biochemical control in an atmosphere promoting normal mental and emotional development. An essential management tool for parents, children, and clinicians is the food diary used to monitor Phe intake. Daily record keeping supports compliance with treatment and builds self-management skills. An accurate record of food and formula intake (see Figure 4-6) for at least the 3 days before a laboratory specimen is obtained is critical for accurate interpretation of the results and subsequent adjustment of the Phe prescription.

Elevations in blood Phe concentration generally are caused by either excessive Phe intake or tissue catabolism. Intake of Phe in excess of the amount required for growth accumulates in the blood. Deficient energy intake or the stress of illness or infection can result in protein breakdown and the release of amino acids, including Phe, into the blood. In general, the anorexia of illness limits energy intake. Preventing tissue catabolism by maintaining intake of the formula/medical food as much as possible is essential. Although it occasionally may be necessary to offer only clear liquids during an illness, the Phe-free formula/medical food should be reintroduced as soon as it is feasible. Tube-feeding is an option if oral intake is not possible.

Continuing the restricted-Phe dietary therapy throughout childhood, adolescence, and beyond is recommended (McPheeters et al, 2012; Vockley et al, 2014). Progressively decreasing IQs, learning difficulties, poor attention span, and behavioral difficulties have been reported in children who have discontinued the dietary regimen. Children who maintain well-controlled blood Phe levels demonstrate comparatively higher intellectual achievement than those who do not. Good dietary control of blood Phe concentrations is the best predictor of IQ, whereas "off-diet" blood Phe concentrations of greater than 20 mg/dl (1200 μmol/L) are the best predictors of IQ loss. Subtle deficits in higher-level cognitive function may persist even at blood Phe levels of 6 to 10 mg/dl (360 to 600 μmol/L). Thus most clinics recommend treatment blood levels of 2 to 6 mg/dl (120 to 360 μmol/L). *Restricted-Phe therapy should be continued for life to maintain normal cognitive function.*

Medical Nutrition Therapy

Nutrition management guidelines for PKU have been published (Singh et al, 2014).

Formula. For PKU, dietary therapy is planned around the use of a formula/medical food with Phe removed from the protein. Formulas or medical foods provide a major portion of the daily protein and energy needs for affected infants, children, and adults. In general, the protein source in the formula/medical food is L-amino acids, with the critical amino acid (i.e., Phe) omitted. Glycomacropeptide (GMP), a whey protein with very little Phe, is used in a few medical foods as an alternative to L-amino acids (van Calcar and Ney, 2012). Carbohydrate sources are corn syrup solids, modified tapioca starch, sucrose, and hydrolyzed cornstarch. Fat is provided by a variety of oils.

Some formula/medical foods contain no fat or carbohydrate, so these components must be provided from other sources. If using formulas without fat, clinicians must provide sources of essential fatty acids. Essential fatty acid deficiencies have been noted among individuals consuming fat-free formulas (Camp et al, 2014; Singh et al, 2014). Most formulas and medical foods contain calcium, iron, and all other necessary vitamins and minerals and are a reliable source of these nutrients. When others are devoid of these nutrients, supplementation is needed to ensure nutritional adequacy.

Phe-free formula is supplemented with regular infant formula or breastmilk during infancy and cow's milk in early childhood to provide high-biologic value protein, nonessential amino acids, and sufficient Phe to meet the individualized requirements of the growing child. The optimal amount of protein substitute depends on the individual's age (and thus requirements for growth) and enzyme activity; thus it must be prescribed individually. Because the protein in specialized formulas is synthetic, it is provided in amounts greater than the Dietary Reference Intake (DRI) (Singh et al, 2014).

The Phe-free formula and milk mixture often provides approximately 90% of the protein and 80% of the energy needed by infants and toddlers. A method for calculating the appropriate quantities of a low-Phe food pattern is shown in Table 43-3. Calculations should provide adequate but not excessive energy for the infant, as well as appropriate fluid to maintain hydration. To support metabolic control effectively, formula/medical foods must be consumed in three or four nearly equal portions throughout the day.

Low-Phenylalanine Foods. Foods of moderate- or low-Phe content are used as a supplement to the formula or medical food mixture. These foods are offered at the appropriate ages to support developmental readiness and to meet energy needs. Puréed foods from a spoon may be introduced at 5 to 6 months of age, finger foods at 7 to 8 months, and the cup at 8 to 9 months, using the same timing and progression of texture recommended for typical children (see Chapters 16 and 17). Table 43-4 lists typical low-Phe food patterns for young children.

Low-protein pastas, breads, and baked goods made from wheat starch add variety to the food pattern and allow children to eat some foods "to appetite." A variety of low-protein pastas, rice, baked goods, egg replacers, and other foods are available. Wheat starch and a variety of low-protein baking mixes for breads, cakes, and cookies are also available. Table 43-5 compares low-protein and regular food items.

In many cases parents create recipes or adapt family favorites to meet the needs of their children. These recipes offer the children a variety of textures and food choices, allowing them to participate in family meals. Families are also able to meet the energy and Phe needs of their children without resorting to excessive intakes of sugars and concentrated sweets.

TABLE 43-3   Guidelines for Low-Phenylalanine Food Pattern Calculations

Step 1: Calculate the child's needs for phenylalanine, protein, and energy (kcal).

Phenylalanine

7.7 kg × 40* mg phenylalanine = 308 mg phe/kg/d

Protein

7.7 kg × 2.5-3† g pro = 19-25 g pro/kg/d

Energy

7.7 kg × 100‡ kcal = 770 kcal/kg/d

Step 2: Estimate the amount of phenylalanine, protein, and energy to be obtained from foods other than the formula mixture.

	APPROXIMATE NEEDS		
	Phenylalanine (mg/d)	Protein (g/d)	Energy (kcal/d)
Foods	30	1-2	100
Formula	~288	18-24	670
Total	*318*	*19-25*	*770*

Step 3: Confirm that a reasonable food pattern is provided with the estimated phenylalanine from food guideline. A sample food pattern:

	Phenylalanine (mg)	Protein (g)	Energy (kcal)
Green beans, strained, 2 Tbsp	15	0.4	8
Banana, mashed, 2 Tbsp	10	0.3	28
Carrots, strained, 2 Tbsp	6	0.2	7
Total	*30*	*0.9*	*33*

Step 4: Determine the amount of standard infant formula to be included in the formula. This information is determined from the infant's estimated phenylalanine needs.

Step 5: Determine the amount of phenylalanine-free formula required per day. This information is determined from the infant's estimated protein and energy needs.

Step 6: Determine the amount of water to mix with the formula. The consistency of the formula will vary according to the infant's age and fluid requirements. For example, for the infant described in the case study, add water to make a total volume of 32 oz.

Step 7: Determine the amounts of phenylalanine, protein, and energy provided by formulas and foods.

	Phenylalanine (mg/d)	Protein (g/d)	Energy (kcal/d)
Phenex-1 powder (70 g)	0	10.5	325
Enfamil powder (70 g)	294	7.4	350
Food	30	1-2	100
Total	*324*	*18.9-19.9*	*775*

Step 8: Determine the actual amounts of phenylalanine, protein, and energy per kilogram body weight.

Phenylalanine

324 ÷ 7.7 kg = 42 mg phe/kg/d

Protein

19.4 ÷ 7.7 kg = 2.5 g pro/kg/d

Energy

774 ÷ 7.7 kg = 101 kcal/kg/d

*A phenylalanine intake of 40 mg/kg/day is chosen as a moderate intake level. The prescription for phenylalanine must be adapted to individual needs as judged by growth and blood levels.

†Although these intakes are higher than the recommended dietary allowance, they are the intakes found by the Collaborative Study to promote normal growth with consumption of protein hydrolysate-based formula.

‡Total energy intake must be adjusted to meet individual needs, and an excess must be avoided.

Acosta PB: Recommendations for protein and energy intakes by patients with phenylketonuria, *Eur J Pediatr* 155(Suppl 1):S121, 1996 and Singh RH et al: Recommendations for the nutrition management of phenylalanine hydroxylase deficiency, *Genet Med* 16:121, 2014.

TABLE 43-4   Typical Menus for a 3-Year-Old with Phenylketonuria

Tolerance: 300 mg phenylalanine/day

Formula/medical food for 24 hours: 120 g Phenyl-Free-2, 100 g 2% milk, water to 24 oz

This formula mixture provides 30 g protein, 460 kcal, 170 mg phenylalanine.

Tolerance: 400 mg phenylalanine/day

Formula/medical food for 24 hours: 120 g Phenyl-Free-2, 100 g 2% milk, water to 24 oz

This formula mixture provides 30 g protein, 460 kcal, 170 mg phenylalanine.

Menu for 100 mg Phenylalanine from Food	Phenylalanine (mg)	Menu for 200 mg Phenylalanine from Food	Phenylalanine (mg)
Breakfast		Breakfast	
Formula mixture, 6 oz		Formula mixture, 6 oz	
Kix cereal, ¼ cup	22	Rice Krispies, 20 g (¼ cup)	25
Peaches, canned, 60 g (¼ cup)	9	Nondairy creamer, 2 Tbsp	9
Lunch		Lunch	
Formula mixture, 6 oz		Formula mixture, 6 oz	
Low protein bread, ½ slice	6	Vegetable soup, ½ cup	82
Jelly, 1 tsp	0	Grapes, 50 g (10)	9
Carrots, cooked, 40 g (¼ cup)	14	Low-protein crackers, 5	3
Apricots, canned, 25 g (½ cup)	32	Low-protein cookie, 2	8
Snack		Snack	
Apple slice, peeled, ½ cup	3	Rice cakes, 6 g (2 min)	25
Goldfish crackers, 10	18 mg	Jelly, 1 tsp	0
Formula mixture, 6 oz		Formula mixture, 6 oz	
Dinner		Dinner	
Formula mixture, 6 oz		Formula mixture, 6 oz	
Low-protein pasta, ½ C, cooked	5	Potato, diced, 50 g (5 Tbsp)	39
Tomato sauce, 2 Tbsp	12	Dairy-free margarine, 1 tsp	0 mg
Green beans, cooked, 17 g (2 Tbsp)	9	Zucchini, sauteed, ¼ cup (45 g)	10
Total phenylalanine from food	*130 mg*	*Total phenylalanine from food*	*180*

A formula or medical food that is free of Phe and has a more appropriate amino acid, vitamin, and mineral composition for an older child is generally introduced in the toddler or preschool period. The criteria for introduction of these "next-step" formulas are that the child accept the food pattern and formula well and reliably consume a wide variety of foods from the low-Phe food list. Successful management with consistently low blood Phe levels is based on habit (i.e., the formula/medical food is offered and consumed without negotiation or threat). Children respond favorably to the regularity

TABLE 43-5 Comparison of Protein and Energy Content of Foods Used in Low-Protein Diets

Food Item	Energy (kcal)	Protein (g)
Pasta, ½ cup, cooked		
Low-protein	107	0.15
Regular	72	2.4
Bread, 1 slice		
Low-protein	135	0.2
Regular	74	2.4
Cereal, ½ cup, cooked		
Low-protein	45	0.0
Regular	80	1.0
Egg, 1		
Low-protein egg replacer	30	0.0
Regular	67	5.6

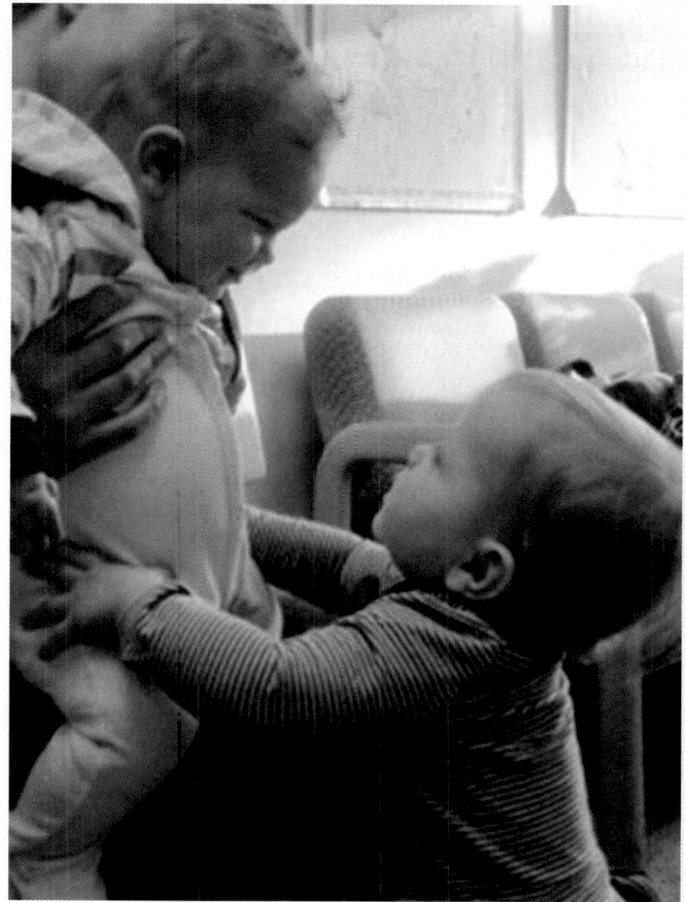

FIGURE 43-3 Two young children, both with phenylketonuria, who were identified by a newborn screening program and started on treatment by 7 days of age, demonstrate typical growth and development. (Courtesy Beth Ogata, Seattle.)

of the time of ingestion of the formula/medical food and the familiarity of its taste and presentation. Table 43-6 compares a restricted Phe food pattern with a typical food pattern for a child of the same age.

Education About Therapy Management. The energy needs and amino acid requirements of children with PKU do not differ appreciably from those of children in general. With proper management, typical growth can be expected (see Figure 43-3). However, parents may tend to offer excessive energy as sweets because they feel their child is being deprived of food experiences. Health care providers should support families in recognizing that children with PKU are healthy children who must make careful food choices for themselves, not chronically ill children who require food indulgences.

Appropriate clinical interaction with family members provides them with the information and skills to differentiate between food behaviors that are typical for the age and developmental level of the child and those related specifically to PKU. To avoid power struggles and conflicts over food, it is advisable to involve the child in choosing appropriate foods at an early age. Children who are 2 to 3 years old can master the concept of appropriate choices when foods are categorized as "yes foods"

and "no foods." The concept of an appropriate quantity of a food can be introduced to a 3- or 4-year-old child in terms of "how many" by counting crackers or raisins and then in terms of "how much" by weighing or measuring foods such as cereal or fruit. The child then moves to more complex tasks

TABLE 43-6 Comparison of Menus Appropriate for Children with and without Phenylketonuria

Meal	Menu for PKU	Phenylalanine (mg)	Regular menu	Phenylalanine (mg)
Breakfast	Phenylalanine-free formula	0	Milk	450
	Puffed rice cereal	19	Puffed rice cereal	19
	Orange juice	11	Orange juice	11
Lunch	Jelly sandwich with low-protein bread	18	Peanut butter and jelly sandwich with regular bread	625
	Banana	49	Banana	49
	Carrot and celery sticks	12	Carrot and celery sticks	12
	Low-protein chocolate chip cookies	4	Chocolate chip cookies	60
	Juice	0	Juice	0
Snack	Phenylalanine-free formula	0	Milk	450
	Orange	16	Orange	16
	Potato chips (small bag)	44	Potato chips	44
Dinner	Phenylalanine-free formula	0	Milk	450
	Salad	10	Salad	10
	Low-protein spaghetti with tomato sauce	8	Spaghetti with tomato sauce and meatballs	240 600
	Sorbet	10	Ice cream	120
	Estimated intake	201		3156

PKU, Phenylketonuria.

TABLE 43-7   Tasks Expected of Children with Phenylketonuria by Age Level

Age (yr)	School Level	Task
2-3	Preschool	Distinguishing between "yes" and "no" foods
3-4	Preschool	Counting: how many?
4-5	Preschool	Measuring: how much?
5-6	Kindergarten	Preparing own formula; using scale
6-7	Grade 1-2	Writing basic notes in food diary
7-8	Grade 2	Making some decisions on after-school snack
8-9	Grade 3	Preparing breakfast
9-10	Grade 4	Packing lunches
10-14	Middle school	Managing food choices with increasing independence
14-18	High school	Independently managing phenylketonuria

TABLE 43-8   Frequency of Abnormalities in Children Born to Mothers with Phenylketonuria

Complication (% of Offspring)	MATERNAL PHENYLALANINE LEVELS (mg/dl)				
	20	16-19	11-15	3-10	Non-PKU Mother
Mental retardation	92	73	22	21	5.0
Microcephaly	73	68	35	24	4.8
Congenital heart disease	12	15	6	0	0.8
Low birth weight	40	52	56	13	9.6

Modified from Lenke RR, Levy HL: Maternal phenylketonuria and hyper-phenylalaninemia: an international survey of the outcome of untreated and treated pregnancies, *N Engl J Med* 303:1202, 1980.
PKU, Phenylketonuria.

(e.g., formula and food preparation) and planning of meals (e.g., breakfast or a packed lunch). Responsibility for planning a full day's menu by calculating the quantity of Phe in portions of food and compiling the daily total is the ultimate goal. These age-related tasks are shown in Table 43-7.

Psychosocial Development. The necessity of carefully controlling food intake may prompt parents to overprotect their children and perhaps to restrict their social activities. The children, in turn, may react negatively to their parents and to their nutrition therapy. The ability of the family to respond to the stresses of PKU, as reflected by adaptability and cohesion scores, is demonstrated by improved blood Phe concentrations and the positive coping behaviors of older children with PKU. Thus continuing nutrition therapy beyond early childhood requires that children become knowledgeable about and responsible for managing their own food choices. The health care team becomes responsible for working with families and children to provide strategies that enable children and adolescents to participate in social and school activities, interact with peers, and progress through the typical developmental stages with self-confidence and self-esteem.

Children require parental and professional support as they assume responsibility for their food management. Self-management of food choices is a strategy to prevent the child using dietary noncompliance as a wedge against parental restrictions. Normal intellectual development is a laudable goal of management of PKU, but to be entirely successful children with PKU concomitantly need to develop self-assurance and a strong self-image. This can be achieved in part by fostering self-management, problem-solving skills, independence, and a typical lifestyle.

Maternal PKU

A pregnant woman with elevated blood Phe concentrations endangers her fetus because of the active transport of amino acids across the placenta. The fetus is exposed to approximately twice the Phe level contained in normal maternal blood. Babies whose mothers have elevated blood Phe concentrations have an increased occurrence of cardiac defects, retarded growth, microcephaly, and intellectual disability, as presented in Table 43-8. The fetus appears to be at risk of damage even with minor elevations in maternal

blood Phe levels, and the higher the level, the more severe the effect. Strict control of maternal Phe levels before conception and throughout pregnancy offers the best opportunity for normal fetal development (Koch et al, 2010; Martino et al, 2013).

Nutrition management for pregnant women with hyper-phenylalaninemia is complex. The changing physiology of pregnancy and fluctuating nutritional needs are difficult to monitor with the precision required to maintain appropriately low blood-Phe concentrations. Even with meticulous attention to Phe intake, blood concentrations, and the nutrient requirements of pregnancy, a woman cannot be ensured a normal infant (Lee et al, 2005). The risks of abnormal development of the fetus, even with therapeutic dietary management and maintenance of blood Phe concentrations at 1 to 5 mg/dl (60-300 μmol/L), are an important consideration for young women with PKU considering pregnancy (Waisbren and Azen, 2003).

Nutritional management during pregnancy is challenging, even for women who have consistently followed a low-Phe dietary regimen since infancy. Women who have discontinued Phe dietary treatment find that reinstituting medical food consumption and limiting food choices can be difficult and overwhelming. Inadequate maternal nourishment (i.e., inadequate intakes of total protein, fat, and energy) may contribute to poor fetal development and should be prevented. Adherence to nutrition therapy during pregnancy for even the well-motivated woman requires family and professional support, as well as frequent monitoring of biochemical and nutritional aspects of pregnancy and PKU.

Adults Living with Phenylketonuria

Many adults with PKU have had the benefits of early diagnosis and treatment and are less likely to be affected by neurologic damage. However, among those who have had some degree of intellectual disability, hyperactivity and self-abuse are often major concerns. Not all patients respond to late initiation of treatment with improved behavioral or intellectual function. For the difficult-to-manage older patient, a trial of a low-Phe food pattern is recommended. If successful, continued Phe restriction therapy may facilitate behavioral management.

Reinstituting a Phe-restricted food pattern is difficult after the eating pattern has been liberalized. However, the current recommendation of most clinics is effective management of blood Phe concentration throughout a lifetime. This recommendation is based on reports of declining intellectual capabilities and changes in the brain after prolonged, significant elevation of Phe concentrations (Camp et al, 2014). The efficacy of continued treatment throughout adulthood has been documented by reports of improved intellectual performance and problem-solving abilities when blood Phe levels are kept low. Dietary management of PKU throughout the life span is similar to that of other chronic disorders, and prudent MNT results in a normal quality of life.

Maple Syrup Urine Disease

Maple syrup urine disease (MSUD), or branched-chain ketoaciduria, results from a defect in enzymatic activity, specifically the branched-chain alpha-ketoacid dehydrogenase complex. It is an autosomal-recessive disorder. Infants appear normal at birth, but by 4 or 5 days of age they demonstrate poor feeding, vomiting, lethargy, and periodic hypertonia. A characteristic sweet, malty odor from the urine and perspiration can be noted toward the end of the first week of life.

Pathophysiology

The decarboxylation defect of MSUD prevents metabolism of the branched-chain amino acids (BCAAs) leucine, isoleucine, and valine (see Figure 43-4). Leucine tends to be more problematic than the others. The precise mechanism for the com-

plete decarboxylase reaction and the resultant neurologic damage is not known. Neither is the reason why leucine metabolism is significantly more abnormal than that of the other two BCAAs (Strauss et al, 2013).

Medical Treatment

Failure to treat this condition leads to acidosis, neurologic deterioration, seizures, and coma, proceeding eventually to death. Management of acute disease often requires peritoneal dialysis and hydration (see Chapter 35).

Depending on the severity of the enzyme defect, early intervention and meticulous biochemical control can provide a more hopeful prognosis for infants and children with MSUD. Reasonable growth and intellectual development in the normal-to-low-normal range have been described. Diagnosis before 7 days of age and long-term metabolic control are critical factors in long-term normalization of intellectual development. Maintenance of plasma leucine concentrations in infants and preschool children should be as close to physiologically normal as possible. Concentrations greater than 10 mg/dl (760 μmol/L) often are associated with alpha-ketoacidemia and neurologic symptoms.

Because the liver is the central site of metabolic control for amino acids and other compounds that cause acute degeneration of the brain during illness, therapeutic liver transplantation has been proposed as an option in MSUD. Studies are underway to assess the long-term effects of this procedure on stabilization of biochemical and neurologic status (Mazariegos et al, 2012).

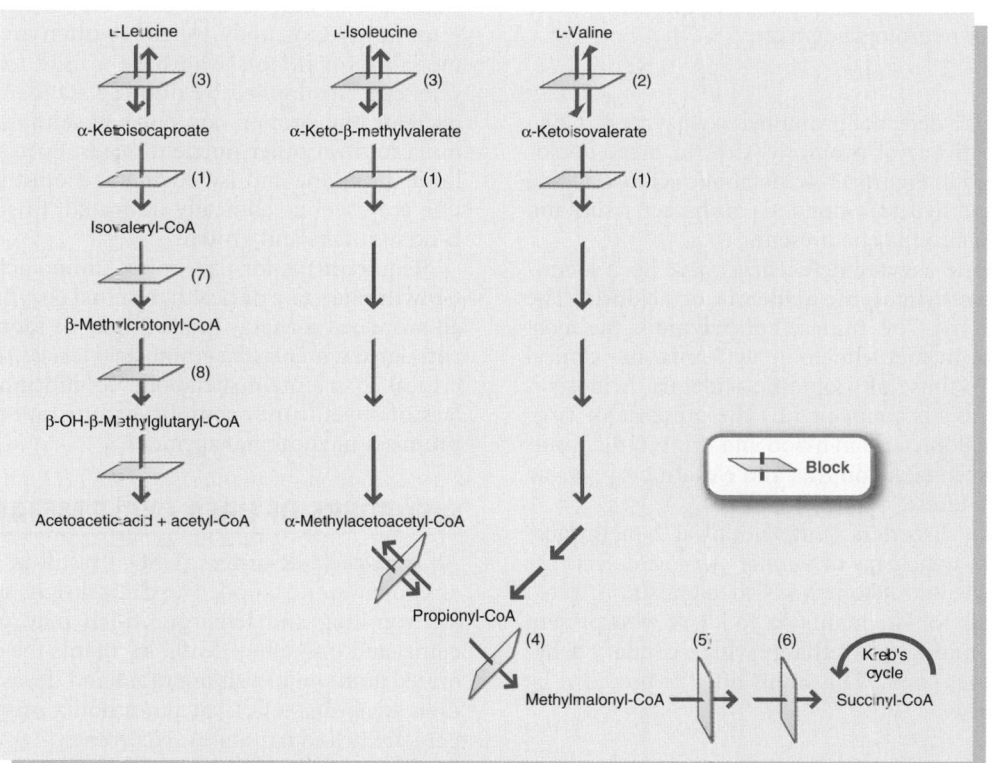

FIGURE 43-4 Organic acidemias and maple syrup urine disease (MSUD). **1,** Branched-chain ketoacid decarboxylase (MSUD); **2,** Valine aminotransferase; **3,** Leucine-isoleucine aminotransferase; **4,** Propionyl-CoA carboxylase (propionic acidemia); **5,** Methylmalonyl-CoA racemase (methylmalonic aciduria); **6,** Methylmalonyl-CoA mutase (methylmalonic aciduria); **7,** Isovaleryl-CoA dehydrogenase (isovaleric acidemia); **8,** Beta-methylcrotonyl-CoA carboxylase (biotin-responsive multiple carboxylase deficiency). **CoA,** Coenzyme A.

Medical Nutrition Therapy

Nutrition therapy requires very careful monitoring of blood concentrations of leucine, isoleucine, and valine as well as growth and general nutritional adequacy. Several formulas specifically designed for the treatment of this disorder are available to provide a reasonable amino acid and vitamin mixture. These generally are supplemented with a small quantity of standard infant formula or cow's milk to provide the BCAAs needed to support growth and development. Some infants and children may require additional supplementation with L-valine or L-isoleucine to maintain biochemical balance.

BCAAs may be introduced gradually into the diet when plasma leucine concentrations are decreased sufficiently (Chuang and Shih, 2010; Frazier et al, 2014). Clinical relapse is related most often to the degree of elevation of leucine concentrations, and these relapses often are related to infection. Acute infections represent life-threatening medical emergencies in this group of children. If the plasma leucine concentration increases rapidly during illness, BCAAs should be removed from the diet immediately and intravenous therapy can be started.

DISORDERS OF ORGANIC ACID METABOLISM

The organic acid disorders are a group of disorders characterized by the accumulation in the blood of non-amino acid organic acids. Usually most of the organic acids are excreted efficiently in the urine. Diagnosis is based on excretion of compounds not normally present or the presence of abnormally high amounts of other compounds in the urine. The clinical course can vary but is generally marked by vomiting, lethargy, hypotonia, dehydration, seizures, and coma. Survivors often have permanent neurologic damage.

Pathophysiology

Propionic acidemia is a defect of propionyl–coenzyme A (CoA) carboxylase in the pathway of propionyl-CoA to methylmalonyl-CoA, as illustrated in Figure 43-4. Metabolic acidosis with a marked anion gap and hyperammonemia is characteristic, and long-chain ketonuria also may be present.

At least five separate enzyme deficiencies have been identified that result in methylmalonic acidemia or aciduria. The defect of methylmalonyl-CoA mutase apoenzyme is the most frequently identified. In methylmalonic acidemia, the clinical features are similar to those of propionic acidemia. Acidosis is common, and diagnosis is confirmed by the presence of large amounts of methylmalonic acid in blood and urine. Other findings include hypoglycemia, ketonuria, and elevation of plasma ammonia and lactate levels.

Ketone utilization disorders (mitochondrial 2-methylacetoacetyl-CoA thiolase deficiency or similar enzyme defect) are disorders of isoleucine and ketone body metabolism. Affected individuals are usually older infants or toddlers who present with ketoacidosis, vomiting, and lethargy with secondary dehydration and sometimes coma. This event often is preceded by febrile illness or fasting.

Medical Treatment

Some patients with propionic acidemia may respond to pharmacologic doses of biotin. Long-term outcome in propionic acidemia is variable; hypotonia and cognitive delay may result even in children who are diagnosed early and who receive rigorous treatment. Liver damage and cardiomyopathy are possible sequelae. Liver transplantation may limit intellectual disability and cardiac changes (Sutton et al, 2012).

Individuals with methylmalonic acidemia may respond to pharmacologic doses of vitamin B_{12}. Responsiveness should be determined as part of the diagnostic process (Manoli and Venditti, 2010). Progressive renal insufficiency is often a long-term outcome. Developmental delay is often caused by early and/or prolonged hyperammonemia.

For ketone use disorders, the treatment is dietary protein restriction (usually 1.5 g/kg of body weight per day); supplementation with L-carnitine, a carrier of fatty acids across the mitochondrial membranes; avoidance of fasting by providing small, frequent meals that consist primarily of complex carbohydrates; and the use of Bicitra (sodium citrate-citric acid) to treat ketoacidosis.

Medical Nutrition Therapy

The goals of managing acute episodes of propionic acidemia and methylmalonic acidemia are to achieve and maintain normal nutrient intake and biochemical balance. Maintenance of energy and fluid intake is important to prevent tissue catabolism and dehydration. Intravenous fluids correct electrolyte imbalances, and abnormal metabolites are removed through urinary excretion, promoted by a high fluid intake. Relapses of metabolic acidosis may result from excessive protein intake, infection, constipation, or unidentified factors. Treatment for these episodes must be rapid because coma and death can occur quickly. Parents become skilled at identifying early signs of illness.

Restricted protein intake is an essential component of the treatment of organic acid disorders. A daily protein intake of 1 to 1.5 g/kg of body weight is often an effective treatment modality for infants who have a mild form of the disorder. This can be supplied by diluting standard infant formula to decrease the protein content and adding a protein-free formula to meet other nutrient needs. Specialized formulas that limit threonine and isoleucine and omit methionine and valine are used, as clinically indicated, to support an adequate protein intake and growth.

Requirements for the limited amino acids may vary widely. Growth rate, state of health, residual enzyme activity, and overall protein and energy intakes must be monitored carefully and correlated with plasma amino acid levels. Adequate hydration is critical to maintain metabolic equilibrium. Food refusal and lack of appetite may complicate nutrition therapy, which compromises medical management.

DISORDERS OF UREA CYCLE METABOLISM

All urea cycle disorders (USDs) result in an accumulation of ammonia in the blood. The clinical signs of elevated ammonia are vomiting and lethargy, which may progress to seizures, coma, and ultimately death. In infants the adverse effects of elevated ammonia levels are rapid and devastating. In older children symptoms of elevated ammonia may be preceded by hyperactivity and irritability. Neurologic damage may result from frequent and severe episodes of hyperammonemia. The severity and variation of the clinical courses of some urea cycle defects may be related to the degree of residual enzyme activity. The common urea cycle defects are discussed in a progression that proceeds around the urea cycle, as shown in Figure 43-5.

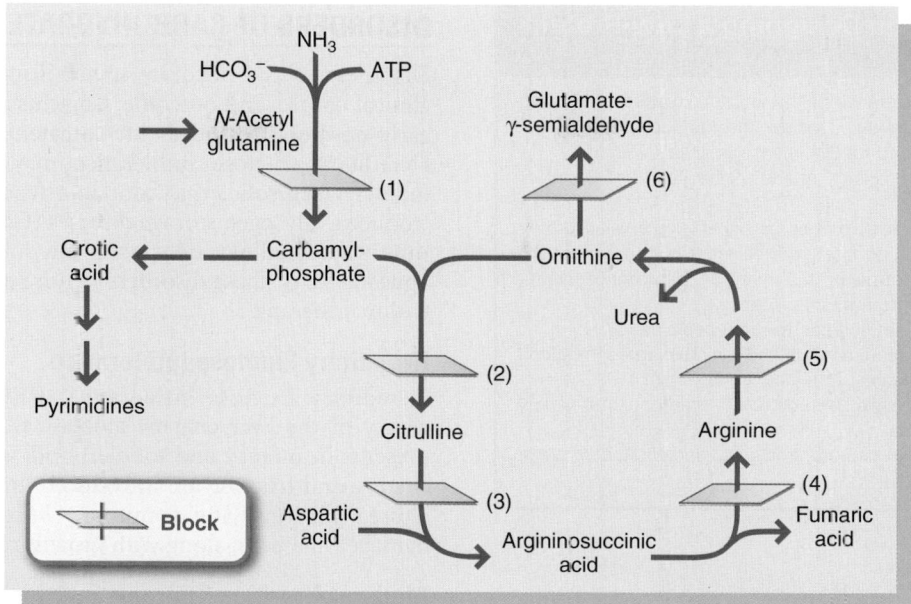

FIGURE 43-5 Urea cycle disorders. **1,** Carbamyl-phosphate synthetase deficiency; **2,** Ornithine carbamyl transferase deficiency; **3,** Argininosuccinic acid synthetase (citrullinemia); **4,** Argininosuccinic acid lyase (argininosuccinic aciduria); **5,** Arginase deficiency (arginemia); **6,** Adenosine triphosphate.

Pathophysiology

Ornithine transcarbamylase (OTC) deficiency is an X-linked disorder marked by blockage in the conversion of ornithine and carbamyl phosphate to citrulline. OTC deficiency is identified by hyperammonemia and increased urinary orotic acid, with normal levels of citrulline, argininosuccinic acid, and arginine. Severe OTC deficiency is usually lethal in males. Heterozygous females with various degrees of enzyme activity may not demonstrate symptoms until they are induced by stress, as from an infection, or a significant increase in protein intake.

Citrullinemia is the result of a deficiency of argininosuccinic acid synthetase in the metabolism of citrulline to argininosuccinic acid. Citrullinemia is identified by markedly elevated citrulline levels in the urine and blood. Symptoms may be present in the neonatal period, or they may develop gradually in early infancy. Poor feeding and recurrent vomiting occur which, without immediate treatment, progress to seizures, neurologic abnormalities, and coma.

Argininosuccinic aciduria (ASA) results from deficiency of argininosuccinate lyase, which is involved in the metabolism of argininosuccinic acid to arginine. ASA is identified by the presence of argininosuccinic acid in urine and blood. L-arginine must be supplemented to provide an alternative pathway for waste nitrogen excretion.

Carbamyl-phosphate synthetase (CPS) deficiency is the result of deficient activity of CPS. The onset is usually in the early neonatal period, with vomiting, irritability, marked hyperammonemia, respiratory distress, altered muscle tone, lethargy, and often coma. Specific laboratory findings usually include low plasma levels of citrulline and arginine and normal orotic acid levels in urine.

Medical Treatment

Acute episodes of illness are managed by discontinuing protein intake and administering intravenous fluids and glucose to correct dehydration and provide energy. If hyperammonemia is severe, peritoneal dialysis, hemodialysis, or exchange transfusion may be required. Intravenous sodium benzoate or other alternative pathway compounds have been beneficial in reducing the hyperammonemia.

Neurologic outcome and intellectual development in individuals with urea cycle disorders vary, with a range from normal IQ and motor function to severe intellectual disability and cerebral palsy. Although information on long-term follow-up is limited, the use of alternative pathways for waste nitrogen excretion and a protein-restricted food pattern may improve the outcome.

Medical Nutrition Therapy

Nutritional management of patients who have urea cycle disorders is a challenging task. The aim of therapy for the urea cycle disorders is to prevent or decrease hyperammonemia and the detrimental neurologic consequences associated with it. Treatment is similar for all of the disorders. For mildly affected infants a standard infant formula can be diluted to provide protein at 1 to 1.5 g/kg body weight per day. The energy, vitamin, and mineral concentrations can be brought up to recommended intake levels with the addition of a protein-free formula that contains these nutrients. However, for most individuals, specialized formulas are needed to adjust protein composition in an effort to limit ammonia production.

The amount of protein tolerated is affected by variables such as the specific enzyme defect, age-related growth rate,

BOX 43-1   Steps in Designing a Low-Protein Eating Plan

1. Determine the protein tolerance of the individual based on (1) diagnosis, (2) age, and (3) growth. Consider the metabolic stability and total protein intake required for the infant's or child's weight.
2. Calculate the protein and energy needs of the individual based on age, activity, and weight.
3. Provide at least 70% of total protein as high-biologic value protein from formula for infants, and from milk or dairy foods for older children. Use a specialized formula if the infant or child cannot tolerate the entire protein intake from intact protein.
4. Provide energy and nutrient sources to meet basic needs.
5. Add water to meet fluid requirements and maintain appropriate concentration of formula mixture.
6. For the older infant and child, provide foods to meet food variety, texture, and energy needs.
7. Provide adequate intake of calcium, iron, zinc, and all other vitamins and minerals for age.

health status, level of physical activity, amount of free amino acids administered, energy needs, residual enzyme function, and the use of nitrogen-scavenging medications. Recommendations must take family lifestyle and the individual's eating behaviors into consideration. Long-term therapy consists of restricting dietary protein to 1 to 2 g/kg/day, depending on individual tolerance. For most infants and children with these disorders, L-arginine supplements are required to prevent arginine deficiency and assist in waste nitrogen excretion. L-arginine is supplemented based on individual needs, except in the case of arginase deficiency (Brusilow and Horwich, 2010). Phenylbutyrate or other compounds that enhance alternative metabolic pathways usually are required to normalize ammonia levels.

Protein-Restricted Diets

Infants and children with urea cycle defects or organic acidemias generally require restricted-protein intakes and specialized formulas. The amount of protein prescribed is based on the individual's tolerance or residual enzyme activity, age, and projected growth rate. The highest protein level tolerated should be given to ensure adequate growth and a margin of nutritional safety. The steps for effective planning of a low-protein food pattern are shown in Box 43-1.

In general, low-protein or restricted-protein food patterns can be formulated from readily available, lower-protein infant, toddler, and table foods. Special low-protein foods (see Table 43-5) can be used to provide energy, texture, and variety in the food pattern without appreciably increasing the protein load. The prescribed protein level can be met by adding a protein-free or specialized formula product to standard infant formula. Supplementing carbohydrate and fat makes up the resultant energy deficit.

Specialty formulas are available when needed. The appropriate choice depends on the level of protein restriction, age, and condition of the child. The usual recommendations for energy density and vitamin and mineral composition are generally appropriate to support growth for the infant or child. Osmolarity of the formula and the individual's ability to tolerate hyperosmolar solutions must be considered.

DISORDERS OF CARBOHYDRATE METABOLISM

Disorders of carbohydrate metabolism vary in presentation, clinical course, and outcome. Galactosemia may present in the early newborn period as life-threatening seizures and sepsis. Hereditary fructose intolerance may present during mid-infancy when solids that contain offending ingredients are introduced. Glycogen storage diseases (GSDs) may present at the time when feedings are spaced and subsequent hypoglycemia appears. All of these disorders require early and aggressive nutritional therapy.

Hereditary Fructose Intolerance

Hereditary fructose intolerance (HFI) results from a deficiency of the liver enzyme aldolase B. The disorder typically presents in infancy and toddlerhood, when dietary sources of sucrose and fructose are introduced. Initial symptoms include nausea, bloating, and vomiting. Untreated, liver and kidney damage can occur, along with growth restriction.

Medical Nutrition Therapy

Current management for HFI is restriction of dietary sources of fructose (including disaccharides composed of fructose) and some sugar alcohols, such as sorbitol. HFI (incidence of about 1 in 20,000 to 30,000 in Europe) is different than the more common fructose malabsorption, in which individuals experience gastrointestinal symptoms after ingesting large amounts of fructose (Ali et al, 1998; Bouteldja and Timson, 2010; see Chapter 28).

Galactosemia

Galactosemia, an elevated level of plasma galactose-1-phosphate combined with galactosuria, is found in two autosomal-recessive metabolic disorders: galactokinase deficiency and galactose-1-phosphate uridyltransferase (GALT) deficiency, which is also called "classic galactosemia." Illness generally occurs within the first 2 weeks of life. Symptoms are vomiting, diarrhea, lethargy, failure to thrive, jaundice, hepatomegaly, and cataracts. Infants with galactosemia may be hypoglycemic and susceptible to infection from gram-negative organisms. If the condition is not treated, death frequently ensues secondarily to septicemia.

Pathophysiology

Galactosemia results from a disturbance in the conversion of galactose to glucose because of the absence or inactivity of one of the enzymes shown in Figure 43-6. The enzyme deficiency causes an accumulation of galactose, or galactose and galactose-1-phosphate, in body tissues. In addition, expanded newborn screening programs have identified many newborns with Duarte galactosemia. These infants have one allele for galactosemia and one for Duarte galactosemia and are often said to have "D/G galactosemia." The Duarte allele produces approximately 5% to 20% of the GALT enzyme. Little is known about the natural history of D/G galactosemia; apparently infants and children develop normally without medical complications.

Medical Treatment

When diagnosis and therapy are delayed, intellectual disability can result (Waisbren, 2006). With early diagnosis and treatment,

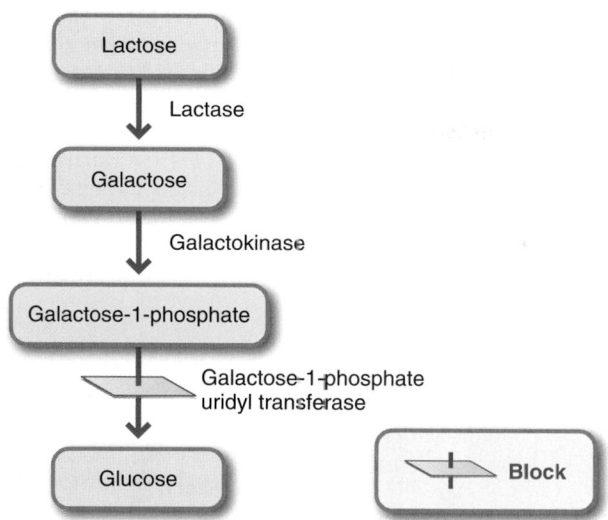

FIGURE 43-6 Schematic diagram of the metabolism of galactose in galactosemia.

physical and motor development should proceed normally. However, intellectual achievement may be depressed. Patients often have IQs of 85 to 100, visual-perceptual and speech difficulties, and problems with executive function (Doyle et al, 2010; Kaufman et al, 1995). Ovarian failure affects approximately 75% to 95% of women with galactosemia (Forges et al, 2006).

Medical Nutrition Therapy

Galactosemia is treated with lifelong galactose restriction. Although galactose is required for the production of galactolipids and cerebrosides, it can be produced by an alternative pathway if galactose is omitted from the diet. Galactose restriction mandates strict avoidance of all milk and milk products and lactose-containing foods because lactose is hydrolyzed into galactose and glucose. Effective galactose restriction requires careful reading of food product labels (see Box 26-9). Milk is added to many products, and lactose often appears in the coating of the tablet form of medications. Infants with galactosemia are fed soy-based formula (see Box 26-9). Some fruits and vegetables contain significant amounts of galactose. Whether these sources of galactose contribute to the pathophysiology characteristics of the disorder is unclear. Table 43-9 presents a low-galactose food pattern.

Medical opinions differ about the intensity and duration of treatment for Duarte galactosemia (Berry, 2012). Many centers eliminate galactose from the diets of these children for the first year of life; other centers do not.

Glycogen Storage Diseases

Glycogen storage diseases (GSDs) reflect an inability to metabolize glycogen to glucose. There are a number of possible enzyme defects along the pathway. The most common of the GSDs are types I and III. Their symptoms are poor physical growth, hypoglycemia, hepatomegaly, and abnormal biochemical parameters, especially for cholesterol and triglycerides. Advances in the treatment of GSDs may improve the quality of life for affected children (Bali et al, 2013).

TABLE 43-9 Food Lists for Low-Galactose Food Pattern	
Allowable Foods	**Galactose-Containing Foods to be Avoided***
Milk and Milk Substitutes Similac Sensitive Isomil Soy Enfamil Prosobee Gerber Good Start Soy Plus	All forms of animal milk Imitation or filled milk Cream, butter, some margarines Cottage cheese, cream cheese Hard cheeses Yogurt Ice cream, ice milk, sherbet Breastmilk
Fruits All fresh, frozen, canned, or dried fruits except those processed with unsafe ingredients[†]	
Vegetables All fresh, frozen, canned, or dried vegetables except those processed with unsafe ingredients,[†] seasoned with butter or margarine, breaded, or creamed	
Meat, Poultry, Fish, Eggs, Nuts Plain beef, lamb, veal, pork, ham, fish, turkey, chicken, game, fowl, Kosher frankfurters, eggs, nut butters, nuts	
Breads and Cereals Cooked and dry cereals, bread or crackers without milk or unsafe ingredients,[†] macaroni, spaghetti, noodles, rice, tortillas	
Fats All vegetable oils; all shortening, lard, margarines, and salad dressings except those made with unsafe ingredients[†]; mayonnaise; olives	

*Lactose is often used as a pharmaceutical bulking agent, filler, or excipient; thus tablets, tinctures, and vitamin and mineral mixtures should be evaluated carefully for galactose content. The *Physician's Desk Reference* now lists active and inactive ingredients in medications, as well as manufacturers' telephone numbers.
[†]Unsafe ingredients include milk, buttermilk, cream, lactose, galactose, casein, caseinate, whey, dry milk solids, or curds. Labels should be checked regularly and carefully because formulations of products change often (see Box 26-9).

Pathophysiology

GSD type Ia (25% of GSDs) is a defect in the enzyme glucose-1-6-phosphatase, which impairs the formation of new glucose (gluconeogenesis) and the breakdown of glycogen from storage (glycogenolysis). The affected person is unable to metabolize glycogen stored in the liver. Severe hypoglycemia can result and cause irreparable damage.

Amylo-1, 6-glucosidase deficiency (GSD III or debrancher enzyme deficiency) prevents glycogen breakdown beyond branch points. This disorder is similar to GSD Ia in that glyco-genolysis is inefficient but gluconeogenesis is amplified to help maintain glucose production. The symptoms of GSD III are usually less severe and range from hepatomegaly to severe hy-poglycemia (Dagli et al, 2012).

Medical Treatment

The outcome of treatment has been good. The hazard of severe hypoglycemic episodes is diminished, physical growth is im-proved, and liver size is decreased. The risk of progressive renal dysfunction is not entirely eliminated by current treatment, but liver transplantation for some types of GSD (e.g., type Ib) is sometimes an option. Treatment protocols for the GSDs are still evolving. The protocols include various kinds of carbohydrates at various doses during the day and night. Individual tolerance, body weight, state of health, ambient temperature, and physical activity are important considerations when designing the spe-cific pattern of carbohydrate administration. The goal for all of the protocols remains the same: normalization of blood glucose levels.

Medical Nutrition Therapy

The rationale for intervention is to maintain plasma glucose in a normal range and prevent hypoglycemia by providing a constant supply of exogenous glucose. Administration of raw cornstarch (e.g., a slurry of cornstarch mixed with cold water) at regular intervals and a high–complex carbohy-drate, low-fat dietary pattern are advocated to prevent hypo-glycemia. Some infants and children do very well with oral cornstarch administration, whereas others require glucose polymers administered via continuous-drip gastric feedings to prevent hypoglycemic episodes during the night (Bali et al, 2013; Dagli et al, 2012). The dose of cornstarch should be individualized; doses of 1.6 to 2.5 g/kg at 4- to 6-hour intervals are generally effective for young children with GSD I (Bali et al, 2013). Iron supplementation is required to maintain adequate hematologic status because cornstarch interferes with iron absorption.

DISORDERS OF FATTY ACID OXIDATION

Recent laboratory advancements have enabled identification of fatty acid oxidation disorders such as medium-chain acyl-CoA dehydrogenase (MCAD) deficiency and long-chain 3-hydroxyacyl-CoA dehydrogenase (LCHAD) deficiency (see Figure 43-7). Children who are not identified by newborn screening usually present during periods of fasting or illness with symptoms of variable severity, including failure to thrive, episodic vomiting, and hypotonia.

Pathophysiology

Children with MCAD deficiency who present clinically typi-cally have hypoglycemia without urine ketones, lethargy, sei-zures, and coma. Children with LCHAD deficiency become hypoglycemic and demonstrate abnormal liver function, re-duced or absent ketones in the urine, and often secondary carnitine deficiency. They also may have hepatomegaly and acute liver disease. Hypoglycemia can progress quickly and be fatal (Matern and Rinaldo, 2012; Roe and Ding, 2010). Both disorders are included in the newborn screening panels in all U.S. states.

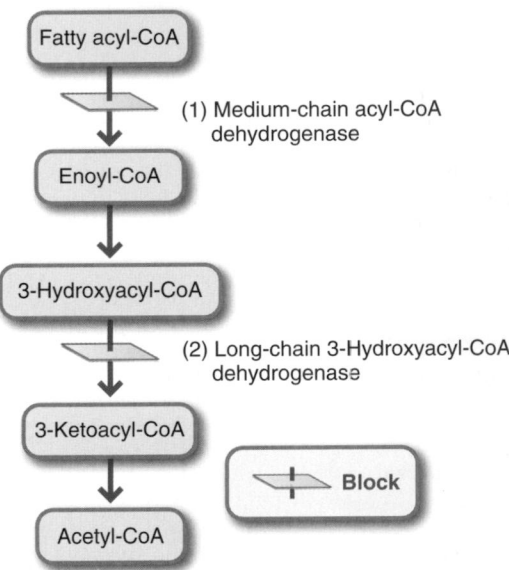

FIGURE 43-7 Mitochondrial fatty acid oxidation disorders: **1,** Medium-chain acyl-Coenzyme A dehydrogenase deficiency, the most common fatty acid oxidation disorder. **2,** Long-chain 3-hydroxyacyl-CoA dehydrogenase deficiency.

Medical Nutrition Therapy

The concept underlying effective treatment for fatty acid oxida-tion disorders is straightforward: avoidance of fasting. This is accomplished by the regularly spaced intake of foods that pro-vide an adequate energy intake and are high in carbohydrates. A low-fat diet is advocated because fats are not effectively me-tabolized. Consumption of not more than 30% of energy as fat has been recommended; some individuals require more restric-tion. Supplementation with L-**carnitine**, a substance that func-tions as a carrier of fatty acids across the mitochondrial membranes, is recommended by some clinics.

Children often do very well with three meals and three snacks offered at regular intervals. Most children may require additional carbohydrate before bed, based on individual ability to maintain blood glucose levels throughout the night (Matern and Rinaldo, 2012). Depending on the disorder, supplementation with specific fatty acids (e.g., medium-chain fats for disorders that involve blocks of long-chain metabolism) may be indicated.

ROLE OF THE NUTRITIONIST IN GENETIC METABOLIC DISORDERS

The role of the pediatric nutrition specialist in the treatment of metabolic disorders is a complex one that requires expertise in MNT for the specific disorder. Preparation and competency requires access to detailed information about the disorders and treatment modalities. A family-centered approach, knowledge of feeding-skill development, and understanding of behavior modification techniques, as well as the support and counsel of a team of health care providers involved in the care of the pa-tient, are also required. Nutrition intervention is often a lifelong consideration. Specific objectives of nutrition care are shown in Box 43-2.

BOX 43-2 Intervention Objectives for the Nutritionist Involved in the Treatment of Genetic Metabolic Disorders

In the clinic the registered dietitian nutritionist (RDN) has a major role in ongoing therapy and planning for each child. These responsibilities include gathering of objective food intake data from the family, assessing the adequacy of the child's intake, and working with the family to incorporate appropriate ways to monitor the restricted food intake pattern. The child with a metabolic disorder often presents with a wide range of concerns, which may include unstable biochemical markers, failure to gain weight, excessive weight gain, difficulty adhering to the diet, and behaviors that cause an adverse feeding situation. Thus managing a child with a metabolic disorder requires input from the entire health care team. The nutritionist uses skills and knowledge of foods as sources of nutrients, parent-child relationships, growth, development, and interviewing to obtain the necessary information for assessing and planning for the child with a genetic metabolic disorder.

I. The RDN functions as an effective interdisciplinary team member by doing the following:
   A. Becoming familiar with the background and current status of the child by reviewing the medical record
   B. Recognizing and accepting the responsibility as the nutritionist by doing the following:
      1. Identifying appropriate intake of nutrients for growth, activity, and biochemical balance
      2. Identifying developmental stages of feeding behavior
      3. Understanding the concept of food as a support of developmental progress
      4. Identifying behavior as it affects nutrient intake
   C. Understanding, respecting, and using the expertise of the team disciplines in providing care for the child
II. The RDN provides adequate and supportive patient services by doing the following:
   A. Establishing a positive, cooperative working relationship with the parent, child, and other family members

   B. Interviewing the family about dietary intake and the feeding situation in a nonjudgmental manner
   C. Assessing the parent-child relationship as it relates to dietary management and control of the disorder
   D. Developing a plan for appropriate dietary management based on growth, biochemical levels, nutrient needs, developmental progress and nutrition diagnosis, such as:
      Excessive protein intake
      Altered nutrition-related laboratory values
      Intake of inappropriate amino acids
      Inadequate vitamin intake
      Inadequate mineral intake
      Food medication interaction
      Food- and nutrition-related knowledge deficit
      Limited adherence to nutrition-related recommendations
   E. Developing a plan that includes appropriate foods and recognizes the family's skills in food preparation, as well as family routines
   F. Working with the family to establish a method to deal effectively with negative feeding behaviors, if necessary
   G. Contacting the family after receiving laboratory results and calculating food records to make necessary and appropriate changes in diet prescription
III. Supporting families in their efforts at effective dietary and behavior management
IV. The RDN develops a professional knowledge base by doing the following:
   A. Being familiar with the current literature on the treatment of metabolic disorders
   B. Understanding the genetic basis of metabolic disorders
V. The RDN works with team members to understand the long-term patient care and create a written care plan for the patient.

CLINICAL CASE STUDY

Adelaide was born weighing 6-lb, 7 oz and her 1-day newborn screening test result for phenylalanine was 3.7 mg/dl (222 μmol/L). She was breast-fed with no supplemental formula. A repeat sample was requested to further document the phenylalanine concentration in her blood. The result from this sample, collected on day 4 of life, was 6.2 mg/dl (372 μmol/L). To confirm the diagnosis for this child, which was considered to be "presumptive positive," a quantitative sample was obtained, and phenylalanine and tyrosine levels were both measured. On day of life 9 the serum phenylalanine concentration was 16.6 mg/dl (1328 μmol/L), and the tyrosine level was 1.1 mg/dl (60.5 μmol/L); the phenylalanine to tyrosine ratio was 22.0:1. Blood and urine were collected for biopterin screening; results were later found to be normal.

To provide adequate protein and energy intake and at the same time decrease the serum phenylalanine concentration, a phenylalanine-free formula was introduced at standard dilution without a phenylalanine supplement. Within 24 hours Adelaide's serum phenylalanine concentration had decreased to 8.3 mg/dl (498 μmol/L) while she was being provided an intake of 12 to 14 oz of the Phe-free formula. Breastfeedings were reintroduced; she was offered 3 breastfeedings and Phe-free formula ad lib. Within 48 hours the level was 6.6 mg/dl (396 μmol/L), with an intake of 4 oz of the formula.

Adelaide's phenylalanine concentrations were measured every 4 days, and the levels were 3.6 mg/dl (216 μmol/L) and 2.2 mg/dl (132 μmol/L). In subsequent weeks growth and serum phenylalanine concentrations continued to be monitored carefully, and energy and phenylalanine intakes

were adjusted as necessary to maintain blood phenylalanine concentrations between 2 and 6 mg/dl (120 to 360 μmol/L) and to maintain growth in appropriate channels.

By age 2 months, Adelaide's intake had increased to approximately 12 oz formula along with three breastfeedings daily (alternating breastmilk and formula feedings), and her feeding pattern was fairly consistent. Blood phenylalanine was measured at 8.7 mg/dl (522 μmol/L), which is outside the desired range. Her Phe-free formula was increased to 14 oz/d to effectively decrease the amount of phenylalanine provided by breastmilk.

Nutrition Diagnostic Statement

Altered nutrition-related laboratory values (phenylalanine) related to phenylketonuria and dietary phe intake, as evidenced by blood phenylalanine outside desired range.

Nutrition Care Questions

1. What is the expected energy requirement for Adelaide?
2. What are the baseline expectations for intake for a 6-lb, 7-oz neonate? If breastmilk is expected to provide about half of this amount, how much phenylalanine-free formula would you use to provide protein and energy intakes at recommended levels?
3. What are the growth expectations for Adelaide?
4. What steps would you take if Adelaide's plasma phenylalanine concentration exceeded 6 mg/dl (360 μmol/L) on subsequent measurements?

USEFUL WEBSITES

American College of Medical Genetics (ACMG)
http://www.acmg.net
Gene Reviews
http://www.genetests.org/by-genereview/
Genetics Home Reference
http://ghr.nlm.nih.gov
Genetic Metabolic Dietitians International (GMDI)
http://www.gmdi.org
MedlinePlus: Metabolic Disorders
http://www.nlm.nih.gov/medlineplus/metabolicdisorders.html
National Newborn Screening and Genetics Resource Center
http://genes-r-us.uthscsa.edu/
National PKU Alliance
http://npkua.org/
National PKU News
http://www.pkunews.org

REFERENCES

Ali M, et al: Hereditary fructose intolerance, *J Med Genet* 35:353, 1998.

Bali S, et al: Glycogen storage disease type 1. In Pagon RA et al, editors: *GeneReviews*. 2013. http://www.geneclinics.org. Accessed January 29, 2014.

Berry GT: Galactosemia: when is it a newborn screening emergency? *Mol Genet Metab* 106:7, 2012.

Blau N, et al: Optimizing the use of sapropterin (BH4) in the management of phenylketonuria, *Molec Genet Metab* 96:158, 2010.

Bouteldja N, Timson DJ: The biochemical basis of hereditary fructose intolerance, *J Inherit Metab Dis* 33:105, 2010.

Brosco JP, et al: Universal newborn screening and adverse medical outcomes: a historical note, *Ment Retard Dev Disabil Res Rev* 12:262, 2006.

Brusilow SW, Horwich AL: Urea cycle enzymes. In Valle D et al, editors: *The online metabolic and molecular bases of inherited disease*, New York, 2010, McGraw Hill.

Camp KM, et al: Phenylketonuria Scientific Review Conference: State of the science and future research needs, *Mol Genet Metab* 112:87, 2014.

Chuang DT, Shih VE: Maple syrup urine disease (branched-chain ketoaciduria). In Valle D, et al, editors: *The online metabolic and molecular bases of inherited disease*, New York, 2010, McGraw Hill.

Dagli A, et al: Glycogen storage disease type III. In Pagon RA et al, editors: *GeneReviews*, Seattle, Wash, 2012, University of Washington, Seattle. http://www.geneclinics.org. Accessed January 29, 2014.

Doyle CM, et al: The neuropsychological profile of galactosemia, *J Inherit Metab Dis* 33:603, 2010.

Forges T, et al: Pathophysiology of impaired ovarian function in galactosaemia, *Human Reprod Update* 12:573, 2006.

Frazier DM, et al: Nutrition management guideline for maple syrup urine disease: an evidence- and consensus-based approach, *Mol Genet Metab* 112:210, 2014.

Holt LE, Snyderman SE: The amino acid requirements of children. In Nyhan WL, editor: *Amino acid metabolism and genetic variation*, New York, 1967, McGraw-Hill.

Kaufman FR, et al: Cognitive functioning, neurologic status and brain imaging in classical galacotsemia, *Eur J Pediatr* 154(7 Suppl 2):S2, 1995.

Kaye CI, et al: Newborn screening fact sheets, *Pediatrics* 118:e934, 2006.

Koch R, et al: Psychosocial issues and outcomes in maternal PKU, *Mol Genet Metab* 99 (Suppl 1):S68, 2010.

Lee PJ, et al: Maternal phenylketonuria: report from the United Kingdom Registry 1978-1997, *Arch Dis Child* 90:143, 2005.

Lindgren ML, et al: A systematic review of BH4 (sapropterin) for the adjuvant treatment of phenylketonuria, *JIMD Rep* 8:109, 2013.

Manoli I, Venditti CP: Methylmalonic acidemia. In Pagon RA et al, editors: *GeneReviews*, Seattle, Wash, 2010, University of Washington Seattle. http://www.geneclinics.org. Accessed January 26, 2014.

Martino, et al: Maternal hyperphenylalaninemia: rapid achievement of metabolic control predicts overall control throughout pregnancy, *Mol Genet Metab* 109:3, 2013.

Matern D, Rinaldo P: Medium-chain acyl-coenzyme A dehydrogenase deficiency. In Pagon RA et al, editors: *GeneReviews*. Seattle, Wash, 2012, University of Washington, Seattle. http://www.geneclinics.org. Accessed January 29, 2014.

Maternal Child Health Bureau (MCHB): *Advisory Committee on Heritable Disorders and Genetic Diseases in Newborns and Children*, 2013. http://www.hrsa.gov/heritabledisorderscommittee/default.htm. Accessed January 5, 2015.

Maternal Child Health Bureau (MCHB): Newborn screening: toward a uniform screening panel and system, *Genet Med* 8(Suppl 1):1S, 2006.

Mazariegos GV, et al: Liver transplantation for classical maple syrup urine disease: long-term follow-up in 37 patients and comparative United Network for Organ Sharing experience, *J Pediatr* 160:116, 2012.

McPheeters ML, et al: *Adjuvant Treatment for Phenylketonuria: Future Research Needs: Identification of Future Research Needs From Comparative Effectiveness Review No. 56 [Internet]*, Rockville, Md, 2012, Agency for Healthcare Research and Quality (US).

Mitchell JJ, Scriver CR: Phenylalanine hydroxylase deficiency. In Pagon RA et al, editors: *GeneReviews*, Seattle, Wash, 2013, University of Washington, Seattle, http://www.geneclinics.org. Accessed December 30, 2014.

Roe CR, Ding J: Mitochondrial fatty acid oxidation disorders. In Valle D et al, editors: *The online metabolic and molecular bases of inherited disease*, New York, 2010, McGraw Hill.

Saugstad LF: From genetics to epigenetics, *Nutr Health* 18:285, 2006.

Singh RH, et al: BH4 therapy impacts the nutrition status and intake in children with phenylketonuria: 2-year follow-up, *J Inherit Metab Dis* 33:689, 2010.

Singh RH, et al: Recommendations for the nutrition management of phenylalanine hydroxylase deficiency, *Genet Med* 16(20):121, 2014.

Strauss, et al: Maple syrup urine disease. In Pagon RA, et al, editors: *GeneReviews*, Seattle, Wash, 2013, University of Washington, Seattle, http://geneclinics.org. Accessed December 30, 2014.

Sutton VR, et al: Chronic management and health supervision of individuals with propionic academia, *Mol Genet Metab* 105:26, 2012.

van Calcar SC, Ney DM: Food products made with glycomacropeptide, a low phenylalanine whey protein, provide a new alternative to amino acid-based medical foods for nutrition management of phenylketonuria, *J Acad Nutr Diet* 112:1201, 2012.

Vockley J, et al: Phenylalalnine hydroxylase deficiency: diagnosis and management guideline, *Genet Med* 16:188, 2014.

Waisbren SE: Newborn screening for metabolic disorders, *J Am Med Assoc* 296:993, 2006.

Waisbren SE, Azen C: Cognitive and behavioral development in maternal phenylketonuria offspring, *Pediatrics* 112:1544, 2003.

44

Medical Nutrition Therapy for Intellectual and Developmental Disabilities

Harriet Cloud, MS, RDN, FAND

KEY TERMS

alcohol-related birth defects (ARBD)
alcohol-related neurodevelopmental disorders (ARND)
Arnold Chiari malformation of the brain
Asperger syndrome
attention-deficit/hyperactivity disorder (ADHD)
autism spectrum disorders (ASD)
cerebral palsy (CP)

cleft lip and cleft palate (CL/CP)
developmental disability
Down's syndrome (DS)
fetal alcohol spectrum disorders (FASD)
hypotonia
individualized education plan (IEP)
individualized family plan
intellectual disability
midfacial hypoplasia

mosaicism
myelomeningocele (MM)
nondysjunction
oral-motor problems
pervasive developmental disorder (PDD)
Prader-Willi syndrome (PWS)
spina bifida
translocation

Individuals with developmental disabilities were generally housed in institutions for the first half of the 20th century. Little attention was paid to their education, or medical or nutritional care. In 1963 the Developmental Disabilities Assistance and Bill of Rights Act was passed. Through this Act federal funds supported the development and operation of state councils, protection and advocacy systems, university centers, and projects of national significance. This Act provided the structure to assist people with developmental disabilities to pursue meaningful and productive lives. The institutions that housed these individuals gradually were closed or reduced in size. By 1975 these individuals were cared for at home, in schools, or in small residential facilities. In 1975 Public Law (P.L.) 94-142 was passed, opening public schools to children with developmental disabilities. In 1985 P.L. 99-487 (102-119 in 1992), the Early Intervention Act, was passed, bringing services to children from birth to school age.

A developmental disability is defined as a severe chronic disability that is attributable to a mental or physical impairment or combination of mental and physical impairments. It is manifested before the person attains age 22; is likely to continue indefinitely; results in substantial functional limitations in three or more areas of major life activity (self-care, receptive and expressive language, learning, mobility, self-direction, capacity for independent living, and economic self-sufficiency); and reflects the person's need for a combination of generic or specialized interdisciplinary care, treatments, or other services that are lifelong or of extended duration and individually planned and coordinated. Developmental disabilities affect individuals of all ages and are not a disease state. They are conditions that are caused by fetal abnormalities, birth defects, and metabolic and chromosomal disorders.

Intellectual disability replaced the term *mental retardation* in the 11th edition of the *Definition Manual of the American Association on Intellectual and Developmental Disabilities* (AAIDD, 2013). Intellectual disability is the most common developmental disability, characterized by significantly below-average intellectual functioning along with related limitations in areas such as communication, self-care, functional academics, home living, self-direction, health and safety, leisure, or work and social skills. An estimated 1% to 3% of the population have this diagnosis.

Developmental disabilities have been traced to many causes: chromosomal aberrations, congenital anomalies, specific syndromes, neuromuscular dysfunction, neurologic disorders, prematurity, cerebral palsy (CP), untreated inborn errors of metabolism, toxins in the environment, and nutrient deficiencies. The Centers for Disease Control and Prevention (CDC) reports that 3% of all live births have a birth defect (CDC, 2014), and there are 4.5 million Americans living with developmental disabilities (Van Riper et al, 2010).

MEDICAL NUTRITION THERAPY

Medical nutrition therapy (MNT) services vary depending on the individual's physical or mental problem, and much has been learned about the role of nutrition in the prevention of disabilities and intervention. The role of the registered dietitian nutritionist (RDN) is essential. Because there is an abundance of information that parents and caretakers use from support groups and websites that are untested scientifically, RDNs often are providing evidence-based counseling to counteract misinformation.

Numerous nutrition problems have been identified in the individual with developmental disabilities. Growth retardation, obesity, failure to thrive, feeding problems, metabolic disorders, gastrointestinal disorders, medication-nutrient interactions, constipation, and cardiac and renal problems may be present. Other health problems exist, depending on the disorder. Table 44-1 lists the most common developmental disabilities and their associated nutrition problems.

The Academy of Nutrition and Dietetics confirms that nutrition services provided by RDNs are essential components of comprehensive care for infants, children, and adults with intellectual and developmental disabilities. Nutrition services should be provided throughout the life cycle. Educational and vocational programs should provide MNT in a manner that is interdisciplinary, family centered, community based, and culturally competent (Van Riper et al, 2010).

TABLE 44-1	Selected Syndromes and Developmental Disabilities: Frequent Nutrition Diagnoses				
Syndrome or Disability	**Underweight or Overweight/Obesity**	**Altered Energy Requirements**	**Altered GI function**	**Feeding Problems**	**Other Issues**
Cerebral Palsy A disorder of muscle control or coordination resulting from injury to the brain during its early (fetal, perinatal, and early childhood) development; there may be associated problems with intellectual, visual, or other functions.	Growth problems	Failure to thrive	Constipation	Oral/motor problems	Central nervous system involvement; orthopedic problems; medication-nutrient interactions related to seizure disorder treatment
Down's Syndrome (Genetic Disorder) Results from an extra chromosome 21, causing developmental problems such as congenital heart disease, intellectual disability, small stature, and decreased muscle tone	Risk for obesity	Related to short stature and limited activity	Constipation	Poor suck in infancy	Gum disease; increased risk of heart disease; osteoporosis; Alzheimer's disease risk
Prader-Willi Syndrome (Genetic Disorder) A disorder characterized by uncontrollable eating habits, inability to distinguish hunger from appetite; severe obesity; poorly developed genitalia; and moderate to severe intellectual disability	Risk for obesity	Failure to thrive in infancy	N/A	Weak suck in infancy; abnormal food-related activities	Risk of diabetes mellitus
Autism Classified as a type of pervasive developmental disorder; diagnostic criteria include communication problems, ritualistic behaviors, and inappropriate social interactions	N/A	N/A	Possible dysfunction	Limited food selections; strong food dislikes	Pica; medication-nutrient interactions
Spina Bifida (Myelomeningocele) Results from a midline defect of the skin, spinal column, and spinal cord; characterized by hydrocephalus, intellectual disability, and lack of muscular control	Risk for obesity	Altered energy needs based on short stature and limited mobility	Constipation	Swallowing problems caused by Arnold Chiari malformation of the brain	Urinary tract infections

Data from American Dietetic Association: Position of the American Dietetic Association: providing nutrition services for people with developmental disabilities and special health care needs, *J Am Diet Assoc* 110:297, 2010.

GI, Gastrointestinal; *N/A,* not applicable.

Nutrition Assessment
Anthropometric Measures

Anthropometric measures are altered when an individual is unable to stand, suffers from contractions, or has other gross motor problems. Measuring body weight may require special equipment such as chair scales or bucket scales. Wheelchair scales are used in some clinics but require that the wheelchair weight be known. Obtaining height for the nonambulatory individual requires a recumbent board that can be purchased or constructed. Other measures of height include arm span, knee-to-ankle height, or sitting height (see Figure 44-1 and Appendix 15).

Although growth charts for children with various syndromes do exist, most clinicians recommend using the general CDC charts (see Appendices 4 through 11) because the information in the specialized charts is often based on small numbers, mixed populations, and old data (CDC, 2014). For the infant with a developmental disability, the WHO growth charts are recommended from birth to 24 months.

Other measures that can be used to explore weight issues include arm circumference, triceps skinfold measures, and body mass index (BMI). BMI is a part of the CDC growth charts and can also be found in Appendices 7, 11, and 18. Using the BMI for age can be controversial. For example, BMI is limited for identifying overweight in children with developmental disabilities who are overly fat because of decreased muscle mass and short stature.

Biochemical Measures

Laboratory assessment for the child and adult with developmental disabilities is generally the same as that discussed in Chapter 7 and Appendix 22. Additional tests may be indicated for the individual with epilepsy or seizures who is receiving an anticonvulsant medication such as phenytoin, divalproex sodium, topiramate, or carbamazepine. Use of these medications can lead to low blood levels of folic acid, carnitine, ascorbic acid, calcium, vitamin D, alkaline phosphatase, phosphorus, and pyridoxine (see Chapter 8 and Appendix 23).

Assessment of thyroid status is part of the protocol for children with Down's syndrome (DS), and a glucose tolerance test is recommended for evaluation of the child with Prader-Willi syndrome (PWS). As appropriate, genetic testing may be encouraged for affected individuals and their biological family members.

Dietary Intake and Feeding Problems

Dietary information should be obtained for the child with a developmental disability through a diet history or a food frequency

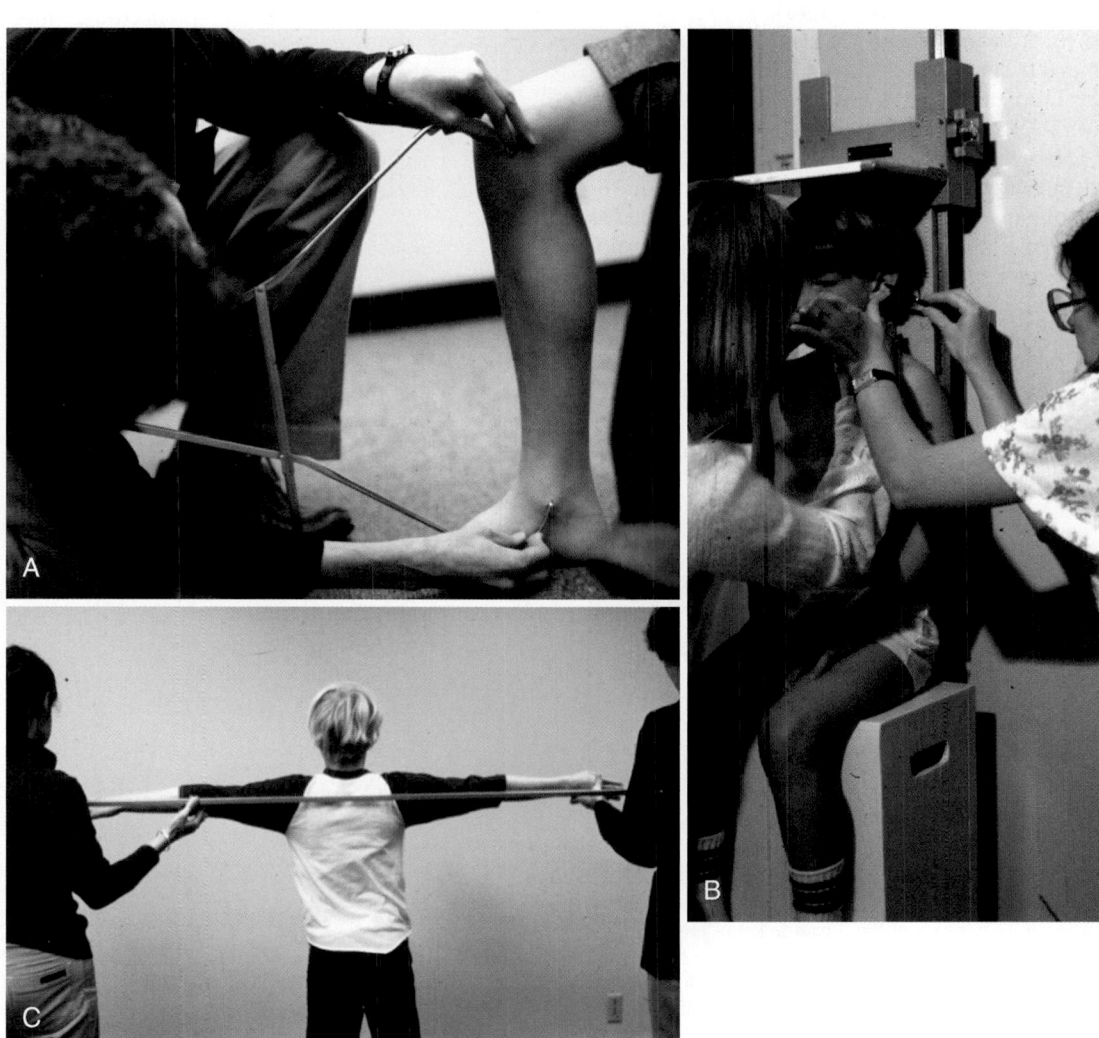

FIGURE 44-1 A, Knee height measure. **B,** Sitting height measure. **C,** Arm span measure. (Courtesy Cristine M. Trahms, 2002.)

questionnaire (see Chapter 4). However, obtaining an accurate recall is difficult when the child is in a day care center. Written diaries are also difficult to obtain when the child has multiple caretakers or when he or she is in school. When working with an adult with developmental disabilities, it is often difficult to obtain accurate information unless the individual has supervision, such as in special residential housing. Use of pictures and food models often can help in obtaining an estimate of the individual's intake (see *Focus On: Does Your App Know What You Are Eating?* in Chapter 4).

Many children and adults with developmental disabilities display feeding problems that seriously decrease their ability to eat an adequate diet. Feeding problems are defined as the inability or refusal to eat certain foods because of neuromotor dysfunction, obstructive lesions such as strictures, and psychosocial factors. Other causes of feeding problems in this population include oral-motor difficulties, dysphagia, positioning problems, conflict in parent-child relationships, sensory issues, and tactile resistance from previous intubation (Heiss et al, 2010). The nutritional consequences of feeding problems include inadequate weight gain, poor growth in length, lowered immunity, anemia, vitamin and mineral deficiencies, dental caries, and psychosocial problems. Feeding problems should be assessed with an understanding of the normal development of feeding and the physical makeup of the mouth and pharynx (see Chapters 16 through 18 and Chapter 40).

Estimates are that feeding problems are found in 40% to 70% of children with special health care needs and 80% of children with developmental delays. Feeding problems are classified as oral motor, positioning, behavioral, and self-feeding. **Oral-motor problems** include difficulty with suckling, sucking, swallowing, and chewing. They also include sensory motor integration and problems with self-feeding and are described as exaggerations of normal neuromotor mechanisms that disrupt the rhythm and organization of oral-motor function and interfere with the feeding process (see Box 44-1).

Children with developmental disabilities such as Down's syndrome (DS), cerebral palsy (CP), or cleft lip and palate (CL/CP) often have oral-motor feeding problems that may be related to the cleft, muscle tone, and inability to accept texture changes. The oral-motor problem also can be related to the developmental level, which may be delayed.

Positioning a child for feeding relates to his or her motor development, head control, trunk stability, and ability to have hips and legs at a right angle (see Figures 44-2 and 44-3). This is frequently a problem for individuals with CP, spina bifida, and DS. Without proper positioning, oral-motor problems are difficult to correct.

The ability to self-feed may be delayed in the child with developmental disabilities and requires training by a feeding specialist. A feeding evaluation is best completed with actual

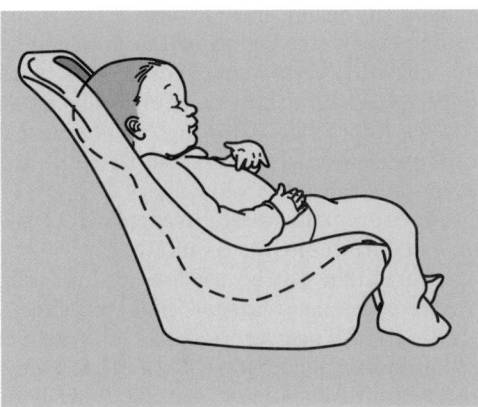

FIGURE 44-2 Proper feeding position for the infant. (From Cloud H: *Team approach to pediatric feeding problems,* Chicago, 1987, American Dietetic Association. © American Dietetic Association. Reprinted with permission.)

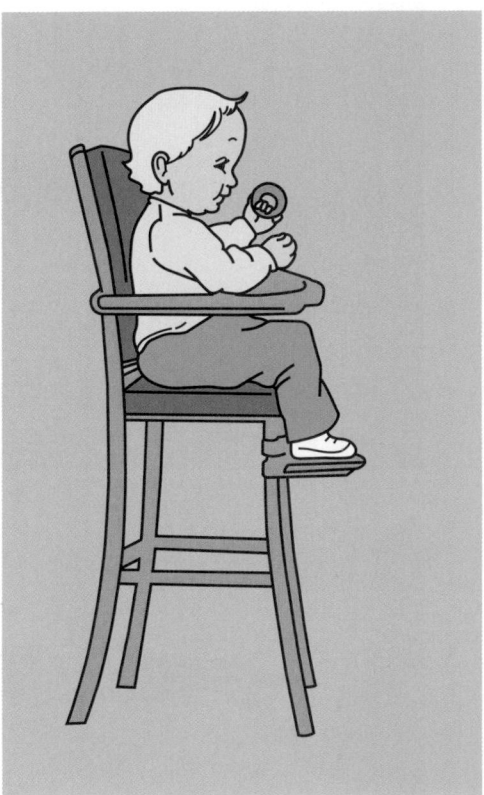

FIGURE 44-3 Good feeding position for a child ages 6 to 24 months, showing hip flexion, trunk in midline, and head in midline. Good foot support with a stool should continue throughout childhood. (From Cloud H: *Team approach to pediatric feeding problems,* Chicago, 1987, American Dietetic Association. © American Dietetic Association. Reprinted with permission.)

BOX 44-1	Oral-Motor Problems
Problem	**Description**
Tonic bite reflex	Strong jaw closure when teeth and gums are stimulated
Tongue thrust	Forceful and often repetitive protrusion of an often bunched or thick tongue in response to oral stimulation
Jaw thrust	Forceful opening of the jaw to the maximum extent during eating, drinking, attempting to speak, or general excitement
Tongue retraction	Pulling back the tongue within the oral cavity at the presentation of food, spoon, or cup
Lip retraction	Pulling back the lips in a very tight smile-like pattern at the approach of the spoon or cup toward the face
Sensory defensiveness	A strong adverse reaction to sensory input (touch, sound, light)

observation by a team composed of a speech therapist, a dentist, a physical therapist, an occupational therapist, and an RDN. An excellent interdisciplinary feeding evaluation form is the Developmental Feeding Tool shown in Figure 44-4. Frequently, adaptive feeding equipment is needed.

Behavioral issues may result from oral-motor or sensory problems, medical problems, certain medications, and the amount of emphasis placed on feeding. Issues such as control of the feeding process along with lack of autonomy in the child may create negative behavior. Environmental factors also

---

Developmental Feeding Tool (DFT)

Parent/Guardian_____   Date_____
Address_____   Staff member_____
City_____ State_____ Zip _____   Child's name_____
County_____ Telephone_____   Birth date_____ Age_____ Sex_____ Race_____
Referrer_____   Head circumference (cm)____ (%ile NCHS)____ Hand dominance _____
                                                             Height (cm)_____ (%ile NCHS)_____ Weight (kg)_____ (%ile NCHS)____
                                                             Weight for height (%ile NCHS)_____ Hematocrit_____ Urine screen_____

		PHYSICAL			NEUROMOTOR/MUSCULAR			ORAL/MOTOR
Yes	No	Size	Yes	No	Tonicity	Yes	No	Facial Expression
		1. Weight (avg. %ile NCHS)			34. Body tone (normal)*			62. Symmetrical structure/function*
		2. Underweight			Head and Trunk Control			63. Muscle tone lips/cheeks (normal)
		3. Overweight			35. Head control (normal)*			
		4. Stature (avg. %ile NCHS)			36. Lifts head in prone			64. Hypertonic muscle tone of lips
		5. Short (below 5th %ile for ht. NCHS)			37. Head lags when pulled to sitting			65. Hypotonic muscle tone of lips
		6. Tall (above 95th %ile for ht. NCHS)			38. Head drops forward			Oral Reflexes
					39. Head drops backward			66. Gag (normal)*
		7. Abnormal body proportions*			40. Trunk control (normal)*			67. Bite (normal)*
					Upper Extremity Control			68. Rooting (normal)*
		8. Head circumference (avg. %ile NCHS)			41. Range of motion (normal)*			69. Suck/swallow (normal)*
		9. Microcephalic			42. Approach to object (normal)*			Respiration
		10. Macrocephalic			43. Grasp of object (normal)*			70. Mouth
		Laboratory			44. Release of object (normal)*			71. Nose
		11. Hematocrit (normal)			45. Brings hand to mouth			72. Thoracic
		12. Urine screen (normal)*			46. Dominance established			73. Abdominal
		Health Status			Reflexes			74. Regular rhythm*
		13. Bowel problems*			47. Grossly normal			Oral Sensitivity
		14. Diabetes			48. Asymmetrical tonic neck reflex*			75. Inside mouth (normal)*
		15. Vomiting			49. Symmetical tonic neck reflex*			76. Outside mouth (normal)*
		16. Dental caries						77. Hypersensitivity*
		17. Anemia			50. Moro reflex*			78. Hyposensitivity*
		18. Food allergies/intolerance*			51. Grasp reflex*			79. Intolerance to brushing teeth
		19. Medications*			Body Alignment			
		20. Vitamin/mineral supplements*			52. Scoliosis			FEEDING PATTERNS
		21. Ingests non-food items			53. Kyphosis	Yes	No	Bottle-feeding
		22. Therapeutic diet*			54. Lordosis			80. Suckling tongue movements
		23. General appearance (normal)*			55. Hip subluxation or dislocation, suspected			81. Sucking tongue movements
		24. Head (normal)*			Position in Feeding			82. Firm lip seal*
		25. Eyes (normal)*			56. Mother's lap			83. Coordinated suck-swallow-breathing
		26. Ears (normal)*			57. Infant seat			84. Difficulty swallowing*
		27. Nose (normal)*			58. High chair			Cup-drinking
		28. Teeth/gums (normal)*			59. Table and chair			85. Adequate lip closure*
		29. Palate (normal)*			60. Wheelchair			86. Loses less than 1/2 total amount*
		30. Skin (normal)*			61. Other adaptive chair*			
		31. Muscles (normal)*						
		32. Arms/hands (normal)*						
		33. Legs/feet (normal)*						

Yes	No		Yes	No		Yes	No	
		87. Wide up-and-down jaw movements			91. Suckles as food approaches			96. When food placed in center of tongue
		88. Stabilizes jaw by biting edge of cup			92. Cleans food off lower lip			97. To move food from side to side
		89. Stabilizes jaw through muscle control			93. Cleans food off spoon with upper lip			98. Vertical jaw movements
		90. Drinks through a straw			94. Munching pattern			99. Rotary jaw movements
		Feeding Patterns—Spoon-feeding			Lateralizes Tongue:			Feeding Patterns—Chewing
					95. When food placed between molars			100. Lip closure during chewing*

Continued

Developmental Feeding Tool (Cont'd)

Yes	No	Isolated, Voluntary Tongue Movements
		101. Protrudes/retracts tongue
		102. Elevates tongue outside mouth
		103. Elevates tongue inside mouth
		104. Depresses tongue outside mouth
		105. Depresses tongue inside mouth
		106. Lateralizes tongue outside mouth
		107. Lateralizes tongue inside mouth

Special Oral Problems

Yes	No	
		108. Drools*
		109. Thrusts tongue when utensil placed in mouth*
		110. Thrusts tongue during chewing/swallowing*
		111. Other oral-motor problem*

NUTRITION HISTORY

Yes	No	Past Status
		112. Feeding problems birth—1 year*
		113. Breast fed
		114. Bottle fed
		115. Weaned

Current Status

		116. Eats blended food
		117. Eats limited texture
		118. Eats chopped table foods
		119. Eats table foods
		120. Feeds unassisted
		121. Feeds with partial guidance
		122. Feeds with complete guidance
		123. Drinks from a cup unassisted
		124. Drinks from a cup assisted
		125. Finger-feeds
		126. Uses a spoon
		127. Uses a fork
		128. Uses a knife

Yes	No	
		129. Average rate of eating
		130. Fast rate of eating
		131. Slow rate of eating

Diet Review

		132. Appetite normal
		133. Eats 3 meals/day
		134. Snacks daily

Dietary Intake, Current

		135. Milk/dairy products, 3-4/day
		136. Vegetables, 2-3/day
		137. Fruit, 2-3/day
		138. Meat/meat substitute, 2-3/day
		139. Bread/cereal, 3-4/day
		140. Sweets/snacks, 1-2/day
		141. Liquids, 2 cups/day

SOCIAL/BEHAVIORAL

Yes	No	Child-Caregiver Relationship
		142. Child responds to caregiver
		143. Caregiver affectionate to child

Social Skills

		144. Eye contact
		145. Smiles
		146. Gestures, i.e. waves byebye
		147. Clings to caregiver
		148. Interacts with examiner
		149. Responds to simple directions
		150. Seeks approval
		151. Toilet trained
		152. Knows own sex

Behavior Problems

		153. Self abusive
		154. Hyperactive
		155. Aggressive
		156. Withdrawn
		157. Other*

Play

		158. Plays infant games, i.e., pat-a-cake
		159. Solitary play
		160. Parallel play
		161. Cooperative play
		162. Additional comments*

Number COMMENTS

FIGURE 44-4 Developmental feeding tool. (Smith MAH et al: *Feeding management for a child with a handicap: a guide for professionals,* Memphis, 1982, University of Tennessee: The Boling Child Development Center, University of Tennessee Center for Health Sciences). *-list or specify on comments section

influence the eating behavior of the child (see Chapter 17). Examples include where the child is fed, distractibility, serving sizes, delayed weaning, and frequency of feeding.

Nutrition Diagnosis

Once the nutrition assessment has been completed, problems should be identified related to growth. Excessive or inadequate weights; inadequate dietary intake; excessive or inadequate fluid intake; altered gastrointestinal problems such as constipation, vomiting, and diarrhea; intake of foods that are unsafe because of contamination or food allergies; food-medication interactions; chewing and swallowing difficulties; and problems with self-feeding may be issues. The nutrition diagnoses should be listed and priorities established. When possible, this information is shared with the parent, caregiver, or the adult client before the intervention process begins.

Interventions

Once the nutrition diagnoses are identified and prioritized, short- and long-term goals should be set. Consideration must be given to the motivational level of the parent or client, his or her cultural background, and how the therapy can be community based and family centered. This means that consideration must be given to where the client will be served so that it becomes a part of the individualized education plan (IEP) or the individualized family plan.

Intervention plans should include all aspects of an individual's treatment program to avoid issuing an isolated set of instructions relevant to only one treatment goal. In some cases MNT may not be the family's first priority in the care of the child or adult, making it important for the RDN to recognize the family's cues (see Chapter 14). Even when the family is ready for an intervention, such as weight management for a child with spina bifida, many factors require consideration. The parent or caregiver's educational level and income, language barriers, access to safe and appropriate food, and family coping strategies always should be identified (see Chapter 14).

Monitoring and Evaluation

Once MNT has been initiated, the need for follow-up evaluation and monitoring by either the RDN or another health care professional is important. Giving information in writing, followed by a phone call, gives the chance to repeat some of the discussion and to answer any questions not asked during the initial session. Clarification of suggestions often is needed when monitoring nutrition changes that affect growth and development; a follow-up visit also may be needed.

A case manager may be involved who communicates with the adult with the disability. The RDN may need to find appropriate resources to pay for supplemental nutrition products, tube feedings, and special food products as a part of the follow-up process. Community and agency resources are discussed.

CHROMOSOMAL ABERRATIONS

Down's Syndrome

Down's syndrome (DS) is a chromosomal aberration of chromosome 21 (trisomy 21). It has an incidence of 1 in 600 to 800 live births and results from the presence of an extra chromosome in each cell of the body. This anomaly causes the physical and developmental features of short stature; congenital heart disease; mental retardation; decreased muscle tone; hyperflexibility of joints; speckling of the iris (Brushfield spots); upward slant of the eyes; epicanthal folds; small oral cavity; short, broad hands with the single palmar crease; and a wide gap between the first and second toes (Bull and Committee on Genetics, 2011; see Figure 44-5).

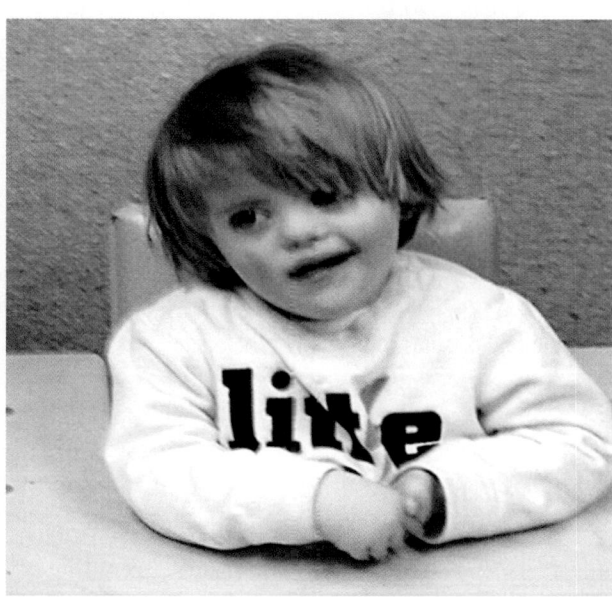

FIGURE 44-5 Child with Down's syndrome.

Pathophysiology

Normally every cell of the human body except for the gametes (sperm or ova) contains 46 chromosomes, which are arranged in pairs (see Chapter 5). With DS there is one extra chromosome for a total of 47. This anomaly can occur by one of these three processes: nondysjunction, translocation, and mosaicism. In nondysjunction, chromosome 21 fails to separate before conception and the abnormal gamete joins with a normal gamete at conception to form a fertilized egg with three of chromosome 21. This also may occur during the first cell division after conception. This type of DS is usually sporadic and has a recurrence rate of 0.5% to 1%. In translocation, the extra chromosome is attached to another chromosome (usually 14, 15, or 22). Approximately half the time, this type of DS is inherited from a parent who is a carrier; it has a much higher risk of recurrence in another pregnancy. In mosaicism the abnormal separation of chromosome 21 occurs sometime after conception. All future divisions of the affected cell result in cells with an extra chromosome. Therefore the child has some cells with the normal number of chromosomes and other cells with an extra chromosome. Frequently the child with this type of DS lacks some of the more distinctive features of the syndrome (Bull and Committee on Genetics, 2011) (see *Pathophysiology and Care Management Algorithm:* Down's Syndrome).

Medical Treatment

The National Down Syndrome Congress has published a listing of the health concerns for individuals with DS; many have nutrition implications (see Table 44-2).

TABLE 44-2	Health Concerns of Children with Down's Syndrome	
Health Concern	**Implications**	**Treatment**
Congenital heart disease	40%-50% of population	Medication or surgical repair
Hypotonia	Reduced muscle tone, increased range of joints	
Motor function problem	Poor physical function	Early intervention for physical therapy, occupational therapy
Delayed growth	Short stature	In some cases growth hormone
Developmental delays	Poor physical, emotional function	Early intervention
Hearing concerns	Small ear canals, otitis media, conductive impairment	Early intervention
Dental problems	Decreased saliva, reflux, and vomiting	Low sucrose intake
Ocular problems	Refractive errors, strabismus, cataracts	Corrective glasses
Cervical spine abnormality		None
Thyroid disease	Hypothyroidism	Thyroid supplement, tests repeated annually
Overweight	Excessive weight gain, inactivity	Decrease energy intake, increase activity
Seizure disorders	Variable nutrient intake	Medications
Emotional disorders	May occur late in childhood	Medication, counseling

Updated from Saenz RB: Primary care of infants and young children with Down syndrome, *Am Fam Phys* 59:381, 1999.

PATHOPHYSIOLOGY AND CARE MANAGEMENT ALGORITHM

Down's Syndrome

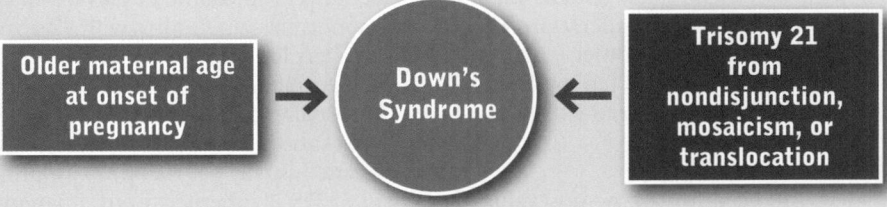

Older maternal age at onset of pregnancy → **Down's Syndrome** ← Trisomy 21 from nondisjunction, mosaicism, or translocation

Clinical Findings

- Hypotonia
- Hyperflexibility/mobility of the joints
- Hip subluxation or dislocation
- Scoliosis
- Foot deformity
- Microbrachycephaly
- Short neck
- Depressed nasal bridge and small nose
- Upward slanting eyes
- Abnormally shaped ear

- Enlarged, protruding tongue
- Single simian crease in center of the palm
- Excessive space between large and second toe
- Mental retardation
- Speech and motor delay
- Cardiac anomalies
- GI atresia or stenosis
- Hearing loss
- Hypothyroidism
- Dental problems
- Cataracts

Nutrition Assessment

- Feeding problems
- Nutritional intake
- Fluid intake
- BMI compared with Down's syndrome standards
- Weight changes
- Dysphagia
- Hemoglobin concentration

Medical Management

- Monitor for leukemia
- Management of infections
- Management of respiratory problems
- Signs of Alzheimer's disease later
- Annual monitoring of hypothyroidism

Nutrition Care

- Feeding management
- Feeding environment
- Use of adaptive feeding utensils
- Monitor weight changes
- Monitor for signs of nutrient deficiencies

Medical Nutrition Therapy

Anthropometric Measures. Height, weight, head circumference, triceps skinfold, and arm circumference are obtained for the child with DS with the usual measurements (see Chapter 7). BMI can be taken but may be higher than normal because of short stature. Growth measures are an important part of the assessment and ongoing nutrition therapy because these individuals tend to be short. Muscle tone is low and gross motor ability is often delayed, leading to the possibility of the individual becoming overweight. Monitoring should be frequent, and growth is plotted on the CDC charts or the WHO charts for the younger child (see Appendices 4 through 11).

Biochemical Measures. Numerous studies have shown biochemical and metabolic abnormalities in individuals with DS; however, many have involve small samples and were difficult to interpret (Bull and Committee on Genetics, 2011). Although serum concentrations of albumin have been found to be low, the guidelines from the Down Syndrome Medical Congress do not list serum albumin assessment as routine. Increased glucose levels have been reported, with an increased incidence of diabetes mellitus.

Current guidelines for the treatment of infants and children with DS include evaluation of thyroid function at birth and thereafter annually. A number of studies have looked at zinc, copper, and selenium as possible deficiencies but concluded that they do not usually exist in children with Down's syndrome (Lima et al, 2010).

Dietary Intake. During infancy the food intake of the infant with DS may differ from that of the normal infant. Although human breastmilk is recommended, many infants with DS are formula fed. Infant illnesses, admission to the neonatal unit, frustration, depression, perceived milk insufficiency, and difficulty in suckling by the infant are reasons why formula feeding is used.

Progression to solid food has been found to be delayed in children with DS, mostly as a result of delays in feeding and motor development. Introduction of solid food may not be offered at 6 months if the infant has poor head control or is not yet sitting. Low tone and sucking problems also delay weaning from the breast or bottle to the cup. IEPs include feeding and feeding progression instruction and practice.

An important part of evaluating the dietary intake is determining energy and fluid needs, because children with DS have a high prevalence of obesity. Studies have indicated that the resting energy expenditure (REE) of the child with DS is lower than for children without DS—and may be as much as 10% lower than the dietary reference intake (DRI) for energy. For the child older than the age of 5, calculations for energy requirements may have to be based on height rather than weight (see Table 44-3 and Chapter 2).

Feeding Skills. Feeding skills are delayed in the infant and child with DS. Some parents find difficulty in initiating oral motor skills such as suckling and sucking. The infant with DS often has difficulty in coordinating sucking, swallowing, and breathing, which are the foundations for early feeding. When the infant has a congenital heart defect, which occurs in 40% to 60% of DS infants, sucking is weakened, and fatigue interferes with the feeding process. Gastrointestinal anomalies are found in 8% to 12% of infants with DS, and these infants often require nasogastric or gastrostomy feedings.

Other physical factors that make feeding difficult in the first years of life include a midfacial hypoplasia (a craniofacial deformity common in cleft palate), a small oral cavity, a small mandible, delayed or abnormal dentition, malocclusion, nasal congestion,

TABLE 44-3 Estimated Caloric Needs for Special Conditions

Condition	kcal/cmhgt	Comments
Normal child	Average 16	
Prader-Willi	Maintain growth: 10-11	For all children and adolescents
	Promote weight loss: 8.5	
Cerebral palsy		
Mild	14	For children ages 5-11 yr
Severe, limited mobility	11	For children ages 5-11 yr
Down's syndrome	Girls: 14.3	For children ages 5-11 yr
	Boys: 16.1	
Motor dysfunction		
Nonambulatory	7-11	For children ages 5-12 yr
Ambulatory	14	For children ages 5-12 yr
Spina bifida	Maintain weight: 9-11	For all children older than 8 years of age and minimally active
	Promote weight loss: 7	

Modified from Weston S, Murray P: Alternative methods of estimating daily energy requirements based on health condition. In Devore J, Shotton A, editors: *Pocket guide to children with special health care and nutritional needs,* Chicago, 2012, Academy of Nutrition and Dietetics.

facial hypotonia, small hands and short fingers. Weaning and self-feeding are usually late compared with the normal infant and frequently do not emerge until 15 to 18 months of age. The DS infant strives for independence and autonomy approximately 6 months later than the child without DS.

Intervention Strategies

Overweight. The most effective intervention for the overweight child with DS is to design a calorie-controlled eating plan based on kilocalories per centimeter of height as shown in Table 44-3 (Murray and Ryan-Krause, 2010). Dietary management includes assessing the feeding developmental level of the child, working with a physical therapist related to gross motor skills and physical activity levels, and making environmental changes. Environmental changes should include following a regular eating schedule that includes three meals at regular times with the child sitting either in a high chair or at the table. Planned snacks should be low in fat and sugar. Soft drinks should be eliminated, and milk should be low fat (after age 2). Physical activity should be encouraged.

Counseling in which the parent helps determine a realistic plan should focus on serving sizes and food preparation and decreasing the number of times meals are purchased in fast-food restaurants. If the child or adolescent is school age, a prescription for a special meal at school can be obtained by using the school food service prescription (to be discussed later in the chapter). Recent studies involving adolescents and young adults have addressed the success of exercise and healthy lifestyles for obese participants with Down's syndrome. Successful programs include parent training in behavioral intervention, and nutrition and activity education over multiple sessions (Curtin et al, 2013).

Eating Skills. Often parents wrongly expect different eating development for the child with DS. Behavioral problems related to feeding may develop based on what happens between the parent and child at mealtime. An example of this is the unnecessary delay of weaning to a cup or progression of food textures because of inadequate effort or education. During intervention programs the feeding team can guide the parent in positioning the child and working toward attainable feeding skills related to the developmental level of the child.

Constipation. This is a frequent problem for the child with DS because of overall low tone followed by lack of fiber and fluid in the diet. Treatment should involve increasing fiber and fluid, with water consumption emphasized. Fiber content of the diet for children after age 3, is 5 to 6 g per year of age per day. For adults the recommendation is for 25 to 30 g of dietary fiber daily (see Chapter 28).

Prader-Willi Syndrome

Prader-Willi syndrome (PWS) was first described in 1956 by Prader, Willi, and Lambert. It is a genetic condition caused by the absence of chromosomal material. PWS occurs with a frequency of 1 in 10,000 to 1 in 25,000 live births. Characteristics of the syndrome include developmental delays, poor muscle tone, short stature, small hands and feet, incomplete sexual development, and unique facial features. Insatiable appetite leading to obesity is the classic feature of PWS; however, in infancy the problem of hypotonia (low muscle tone) interferes with feeding and leads to failure to thrive (Miller et al, 2011; see Figure 44-6). Developmental delays (affecting 50% of the population), learning disabilities, and mental retardation (affecting 10%) are associated with PWS.

The genetic basis of PWS is complex. Individuals with PWS have a portion of genetic material deleted from chromosome 15 received from the father. Of the cases of PWS, 70% are caused from the paternal deletion, occurring in a specific region on the q arm of the chromosome. PWS also can develop if a child receives both chromosome 15s from the mother. This is seen in approximately 25% of the cases of PWS and is called maternal uniparental disomy. Early detection of PWS is now possible because of the use of DNA methylation analysis, which correctly diagnoses 99% of the cases (Miller et al, 2011). This is an important development in the early identification and subsequent treatment of these children to prevent obesity and growth retardation, and is used to identify the infant born with features and characteristics described previously.

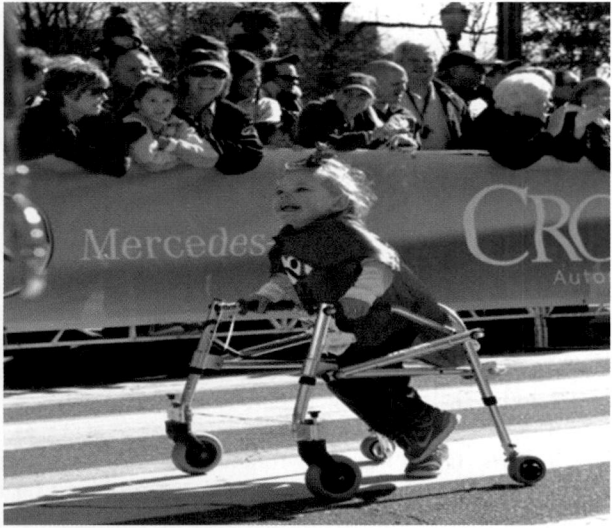

FIGURE 44-6 Child with Prader Willi syndrome.

Pathophysiology

Metabolic Abnormalities. Short stature in the individual with PWS has been attributed to growth hormone deficiency. In addition to decreased growth hormone release, children have low serum insulin-like growth factor (IGF)-1, low IGF-binding protein-1, and low insulin compared with normal obese children. Growth hormone (GH) therapy was approved by the Food and Drug Administration in 2000, and in one 5-year study in Japan 37 patients from age 3 to 21 years experienced significant increase in height gain velocity when given growth hormone (Obata et al, 2003). A more recent study found that GH therapy of infants and toddlers for 12 months significantly improved body composition and mobility skill acquisition (Carrel et al, 2010).

In addition to the growth hormone deficiency, individuals have a deficiency in the hypothalamic-pituitary-gonadal axis, causing delayed and incomplete sexual development. Finally there is a decreased insulin response to a glucose load in children with PWS compared with age-matched non-PWS obese children (Haqq et al, 2011).

Appetite and Obesity. Appetite control and obesity are common problems for individuals with PWS. After the initial period of failure to thrive, children begin to gain excessively between the ages of 1 and 4, and appetite slowly becomes excessive. Based on longitudinal study, Miller et al describe this gradual and complex progression in terms of seven nutritional phases based on levels of appetite, metabolic changes, and growth. In fact, some adults with PWS may progress to the last phase, with no insatiable appetite, and the person is able to feel full (Miller et al, 2011).

This uncontrollable appetite, a classic feature of PWS, when combined with overeating, a low basal metabolic rate, and decreased activity, leads to the characteristic obesity. The cause of the uncontrollable appetite is suspected to involve the hypothalamus and altered levels of satiety hormones and peptides such as ghrelin (Scerif et al, 2011).

Body composition is an important consideration in the evaluation of individuals with PWS. They have decreased lean body mass and increased body fat, even in infancy (Reus et al, 2011). Body fat generally is deposited in the thighs, buttocks, and abdominal area. The lowered energy expenditure is found in young children, adolescents, and adults with PWS, with one study showing adolescents with PWS having a total energy expenditure (TEE) 53% of that of normal obese adolescents (McCune and Driscoll, 2005). The low muscle tone contributes greatly to the lack of interest in physical activity.

Nutrition Assessment

Anthropometric Measures. Height measurements tend to be lower in PWS infants and young children, with the rate of height gain tapering off between the ages of 1 and 4. The usual measurements of length or height, weight, and head circumference should be taken and plotted on the CDC growth curves. Other measures of interest include arm circumference and triceps skinfold measures. BMI may be distorted for the individual with PWS because of the short stature; however, plotting the BMI over time is useful in determining unusual changes (see Appendices 7 and 11). It is important that anthropometric measures be taken frequently and reported to the parents or caregiver.

Biochemical Measures. Biochemical studies are generally the same for the PWS individual, with the exception of either fasting blood glucose tests or glucose tolerance tests. These are added because of the risk for diabetes mellitus, possibly related to the decreased insulin response and obesity that usually company PWS.

Dietary Intake. Dietary information varies for individuals with PWS, depending on their age. In infancy the dietary information should be obtained with a careful dietary history and analyzed for energy and nutrient intake. Infants are commonly difficult to feed because of their hypotonia, poor suck, and delayed motor skills. Generally their feeding development is slower than in the normal infant, and transitioning to food at 4 to 6 months of age may be difficult. Many of these infants have gastroesophageal reflux, requiring medication or thickening of their formula.

During the toddler years, weight gain may increase rapidly as dietary intake increases. This requires careful assessment of portion sizes, frequency of feeding, and types of foods served. Although some parents may report that the child with PWS does not eat more than other children in the family, they have to be educated that the energy needs of the child are lower because of the reduced lean muscle mass and slow development of motor skills and activity. As the child gets older, interest in food increases; and, starting around ages 5 through 12, the child may be hungry all the time and display difficult behaviors such as tantrums, stubbornness, and food stealing. Information gathered during the dietary interview should include asking about environmental control techniques.

Determination of energy needs for the infant with PWS is the same as for a normal infant. However, as the child enters the toddler years, he or she will need fewer calories to maintain weight gain along the growth curve. This will apply in adulthood when fewer calories are needed to maintain weight. Energy needs have been calculated according to centimeters of height from 2 years on. It has been recommended that the macronutrient intake of the diet be 25% protein, 50% carbohydrate, and 25% fat (see Table 44-3).

Feeding Skills. The infant with PWS often presents with weak oral skills and poor sucking skills in the first year of life. As the child matures, feeding skills are not a problem, but they may be delayed. Chewing and swallowing problems usually are not seen, although they may be associated with the low muscle tone. Behavioral feeding issues are associated with an insatiable appetite and not being provided with food. This can bring about tantrums.

Intervention Strategies

Intervention for PWS should occur at each developmental stage: infancy, toddler, preschool age, school age, and adult.

Infancy. Providing adequate nutrition as established by the American Academy of Pediatrics (AAP) related to breastfeeding or formula feeding is recommended. Because feeding may be difficult related to sucking, concentrating the formula or breastmilk may be necessary to promote adequate weight gain. Feeding intervention will assist in improving the sucking problems caused by hypotonia. As the infant matures, a concentrated formula is not necessary, and foods can be added when head control and trunk stability are achieved, usually at approximately ages 4 to 6 months.

Toddler and Preschool Age. Most children begin to gain excessive weight between 1 and 4 years of age. Beginning a structured dietary protocol for the child and the family is important so that the toddler learns that meals are provided at specified times so that a pattern of grazing doesn't develop. Parents should be taught to provide small servings of meats, vegetables, grains, and fruits and limited amounts of sweets. Early intervention for these children in the preschool years is very important in working with feeding issues and intake control as they grow older. Weight, height, and nutrient intake should be monitored monthly and energy needs adjusted if weight gain becomes excessive. Concurrently physical activity must be encouraged as a part of the IEP, and physical therapy services made available if necessary.

School Age. For the school-age child, collaboration with the school food service program becomes important. Energy needs should be calculated per centimeter of height (see Table 44-3) and are generally 50% to 75% of the energy needs of unaffected children. This may require using the prescription for special meals through the school food service program.

At home environmental controls may be required, with cupboards and even kitchens being locked, because the child and adolescent have limited satiety, and will search for food away from mealtime. Some parents report that growth hormone therapy for their child helps, but it doesn't seem to change the child's lack of satiety. Appetite-suppressing medications have been used but are largely unsuccessful.

Adulthood. Prevention of obesity is truly the key for successful treatment of PWS; however, many adults who are not identified early become very obese. Weight management programs providing a very low 6 to 8 kcal per centimeter of height may be required. Nutrient values should be calculated, and vitamin-mineral supplements added, as well as essential fatty acids (EFAs) if indicated. Many dietary treatments have been tried such as the ketogenic diet (see Chapter 40) and the protein-sparing modified-fast diets. However, with any approach strict supervision is usually required, and great emphasis must be placed on physical activity. A behavior management approach also has been recommended to implement the dietary management and physical activity plans. In many states there are group homes for adults with PWS, in which supervised independent living is possible and meals can be very structured and exercise programs implemented.

MNT of children and adults with PWS requires follow-up with many health care providers and schools. Fortunately parents of the individual with PWS now have access to a number of support groups and organizations dedicated to education, research, and establishing treatment programs.

NEUROLOGIC DISORDERS

Spina Bifida

Spina bifida is a neurologic tube defect that presents in a number of ways: meningocele, myelomeningocele (MM), and spina bifida occulta. MM is the most common derangement in the formation of the spinal cord and generally occurs between 26 to 30 days of gestation, with the date of occurrence affecting the location of the lesion. The lesion may occur in the thoracic, lumbar, or sacral area and influences the amount of paralysis. The higher the lesion, the greater is the paralysis. Manifestations range from weakness in the lower extremities to complete paralysis and loss of sensation. Other manifestations include incontinence and hydrocephalus. The incidence of spina bifida is about 2.7 to 3.8 per 10,000 live births in the US per year, with Hispanics having the highest incidence (Canfield et al, 2014).

Prevention of spina bifida is now possible. In the 1980s, studies reported a positive effect from supplementation of mothers with folic acid plus multivitamins (Smithells et al, 1983). This reduced the risk of a second pregnancy with spina bifida as an outcome. As a result of numerous studies showing folic acid supplementation before conception to be effective, the national recommendation is 400 mcg/day for all women of childbearing age. Through their Public Health Program, the World Health Organization advocates globally for folic acid supplementation. Folic acid has been added to many flours and other cereal and grain products in the food supply since 1996 (CDC, 2010). These public health measures have resulted in increased folic acid blood levels in U.S. women of childbearing age and a decrease of 20% in the national rate of spina bifida (Das et al, 2013; see Chapter 15).

Pathophysiology

The spinal lesion may be open and can be repaired surgically shortly after birth, usually within 24 hours, to prevent infection. Although the spinal opening can be repaired surgically, the nerve damage is permanent, resulting in the varying degrees of paralysis of the lower limbs. In addition to physical and mobility issues, most individuals have some form of learning disability.

The spinal lesion affects many systems of the body and can result in weakness in the lower extremities, paralysis, and nonambulation; poor skin condition caused by pressure sores; loss of sensation and bladder incontinence; hydrocephalus; urinary tract infections; constipation; and obesity. Seizures also occur in approximately 20% of children with MM and may require medication. If medication fails, a ketogenic diet can be tried (see Chapter 40). Chronic medication is required for prevention and treatment of urinary tract infections and for bladder control. The resultant nutrition problems include obesity, feeding problems, constipation, and drug-nutrient interaction problems. Children with spina bifida may be allergic to latex. It has been recommended that they avoid certain foods such as bananas, kiwi, and avocados. Mild reactions can occur from apples, carrots, celery, tomatoes, papaya, and melons (Blumchen et al, 2010; see Box 26-5).

Nutrition Assessment

Anthropometric Measures. Infants and children with neural tube defects are usually shorter because of reduced length and atrophy of the lower extremities, although other problems such as hydrocephalus, scoliosis, renal disease, and malnutrition may contribute. The level of the lesions also can affect the length and height of the individual.

Obtaining accurate length and height measures can be difficult, especially as the child grows older. An alternate measure for determining height, the arm span/height ratio, is used and modified, depending on leg muscle mass. Arm span can be used directly as a height measure (arm span $\times$ 1) if there is no leg muscle mass loss, as in a sacral lesion. Arm span $\times$ 0.95 can be used to determine height if there is partial leg muscle loss, and arm span $\times$ 0.90 is used for a height measurement when there is complete leg muscle loss, such as with a thoracic spinal lesion (Kreutzer et al, 2013; see Figure 44-1 and Appendix 15).

Weight measures can be obtained for the child unable to stand by using chair scales, bucket scales, and wheelchair scales. To monitor the weight accurately, it should be obtained in a consistent manner, with the person in light clothing or undressed. Triceps skinfold measures can also be used, along with subscapular measures and abdominal and thorax measures, to determine the amount of body fat. They may be used as adjuncts to stature and weight measurements (Krick et al 2012).

Head circumference should be measured in infants and toddlers up to age 3. A high percentage of children with spina bifida have head shunts as a result of their hydrocephalus. Unusual changes in the size of the head may indicate a problem with the shunt.

Biochemical Measures. Most protocols in the treatment of spina bifida include iron status tests, measurements of vitamin C and zinc levels, and other tests related to the nutritional consequences of medications needed for seizures and urinary tract infection control (see Chapters 7 and 8 and Appendices 30 and 31).

Dietary Intake. Many children with spina bifida eat a limited variety of foods, and they are frequently described as "picky eaters" by the parents. When doing a dietary history, it is important to ask about the variety of foods, particularly of high-fiber foods. The school-age child may be prone to skipping breakfast because early morning preparations for school require more time than for the nonaffected child.

Energy needs are lower for the child with spina bifida (see Table 44-3), and calorie requirements must be determined carefully to prevent the obesity to which many are prone. Ekvall and Cerniglia (2005) found that for MM children 8 years or older, the caloric need is 7 cal/cm of height for weight loss and 9 to 11 cal/cm of height to maintain weight. It is important to evaluate how the mother or caretaker perceives food for the child because it represents sympathy and love for many parents.

It is important to evaluate fluid intake because so many children have urinary tract infections and may be drinking inadequate amounts of water and excessive amounts of soft drinks or tea. Cranberry juice can be offered. Physical activity also must be evaluated and may be found to be very limited, particularly when the child is nonambulatory. Ambulatory individuals with a shunt may be restricted from contact sports but can be involved in walking and running.

Feeding skills need to be evaluated, along with oral motor function in particular. Many children with spina bifida are born with Arnold Chiari malformation of the brain, which affects the brainstem and swallowing (see Chapter 40 and Appendix 28 for dietary recommendations for dysphagia). Difficulty in swallowing may contribute to the child avoiding certain foods later in life. Because of this there may be delays in weaning from the breast or bottle to the cup, but there should be no delays in gaining self-feeding skills.

Clinical Evaluation. Evaluation should include looking for pressure sores and signs of dehydration, along with asking about the amount and type of fluids consumed. Constipation may be caused by the neurogenic bowel combined with a diet low in fiber and fluids. The evaluation should include a review of food intake, fiber content, and fluids.

Intervention Strategies

Many children with spina bifida are overweight. It usually occurs when ambulation is a problem leading to decreased energy needs. Refusal to accept a wide variety of foods is common. Frequent feeding is an oral-motor and a behavioral problem. Counseling should include introducing foods around age 6 months, limiting the intake of high-sucrose infant jar foods, and training the child to accept a wide variety of flavors and textures.

Obesity prevention should include addressing the problems of limited physical activity, increasing fluids and fiber, and calculating the appropriate amount of calories. Once the child is in school, the food service manager should be provided with a prescription for a low-calorie breakfast and lunch, and weight management program should be listed as a part of the IEP. Enrollment in a group weight management program has been used successfully with modification of the accompanying physical exercise. The ideal program uses a team approach with involvement of the RD, nurse, occupational therapist, physical therapist, educator, and psychologist (see Chapter 21).

In many clinics the child or adult with spina bifida is seen on a semiannual or annual basis. This frequent follow-up is necessary and should include monitoring of growth, particularly weight; food and fluid intake; and medication use. School programs and IEPs are excellent follow-up tools; however, the school often lacks appropriate scales for weighing a nonambulatory student. In this situation the parent should be encouraged to bring the child to the clinic for weight checks or, if distance is a problem, find a long-term care facility that will permit use of its scales. Follow-up by phone contact or e-mail can be done for evaluating dietary intake and fluid management.

Cerebral Palsy

Cerebral palsy (CP) is a group of disorders of motor control or coordination resulting from injury to the brain during its early development. Among the causative agents of CP are prematurity; blood-type incompatibility; placental insufficiency; maternal infection that includes German measles; other viral diseases; neonatal jaundice; anoxia at birth; and other bacterial infections of the mother, fetus, or infant that affect the central nervous system.

The problem in CP lies in the inability of the brain to control the muscles, even though the muscles themselves and the nerves connecting them to the spinal cord are normal. The extent and location of the brain injury determine the type and distribution of CP. The incidence of CP varies with different studies, but the most commonly used rate is 1.5 to 4 in 1000 live births. The prevalence of premature births has contributed to maintenance of this figure despite electronic fetal monitoring (see Figure 44-7).

Pathophysiology

There are various types of CP, which are classified according to the neurologic signs involving muscle tone and abnormal motor patterns and postures. The diagnosis of CP is generally made between 9 to 12 months of age and as late as 2 years with some types (see Box 44-2).

Poor nutrition status and growth failure, often related to feeding problems, are common in children with CP. Meeting energy and nutrient needs is particularly difficult in children and adults with more severe forms of CP such as spastic quadriplegia and athetoid CP. For example, bone mineral density of children and adolescents with moderate to severe CP is reduced in those with gross motor function and feeding difficulties (Andrew and Sullivan, 2010).

Other health problems include constipation, usually caused by inactivity and lack of fiber and fluids, often connected to feeding problems. Dental problems occur and often are related to malocclusion, dental irregularities, and fractured teeth. Lengthy and prolonged bottle-feedings of milk and juice promote the decay of the primary upper front teeth and molars (see Chapter 25). Hearing problems and especially visual impairments, mental retardation, respiratory problems, and seizures affect nutrition status. Seizures are controlled with anticonvulsants, and a number of drug-nutrient interaction problems occur (see Chapter 8).

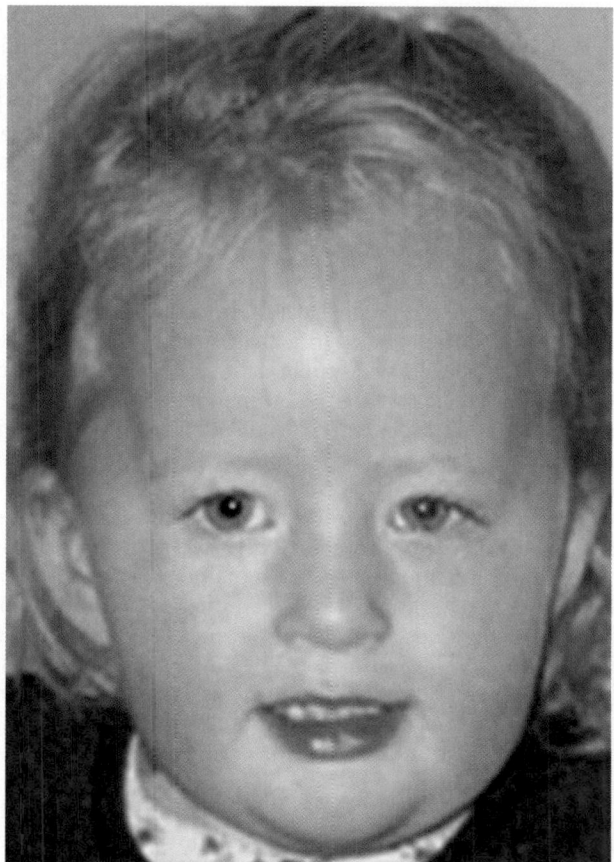

FIGURE 44-7 Child with cerebral palsy.

BOX 44-2 Different Types of Cerebral Palsy

Spastic CP: Increased muscle tone, persistent infant reflexes, increased deep tendon reflexes in one of three patterns: hemiplegia (arm and leg on one side of the body), diplegia (involving the lower extremities), and quadriplegia (all four extremities and may include the trunk, head, and neck)

Dyskinetic CP: Abnormalities in muscle tone that affect the entire body; includes athetoid CP, which includes uncontrolled and continuous involuntary movements

Mixed CP: A condition in which both athetosis and spasticity are present

Ataxic CP: Abnormalities of voluntary movement and balance such as unsteady gait

Athetoid dyskinetic CP: Normal intelligence but difficulty walking, sitting, speaking clearly

---

CP, Cerebral palsy.
Data from MYCHILD: Types of Cerebral Palsy (website): http://www.cerebralpalsy.org/types-of-cerebral-palsy/, 2015. Accessed January 7, 2015.

Nutrition Assessment

Anthropometric Measures. This is an important area of assessment because of the growth failure of the more severely involved child or adult with CP. Children with CP are often shorter, and, depending on the level of severity, some children with CP may have to be measured for length using recumbent length boards or standing boards even as they grow older (see Appendix 15). However, some of the measuring devices are inappropriate for the child with contractures and inability to be stretched out full length. Arm span can be used when the individual's arms are stretchable, as well as upper arm and lower leg length. Stevenson (2005) has recommended lower leg length or knee height as a possible measure for determining height for children and adults with lower-leg CP (see Figure 44-1). The CDC recommends using the CDC/WHO curves designed for nonaffected children, plotting sequentially for indications of malnutrition rather than using the disease-specific curves.

Weight measures should be collected over time. Scales may require modifications, with positioning devices for the individual with CP who has developed scoliosis, contractures, and spasticity. Working with a physical therapist to find a positioning device that can be placed in a chair scale or using a bucket scale often works well. Mid–upper arm circumference and triceps skinfold measures are recommended reliable ways to screen for fat stores in children with CP. Head circumference should be measured regularly from birth to 36 months and plotted on the CDC growth curves.

Biochemical Measures. Although no specific laboratory tests are indicated for the child with CP, a complete blood count, including hemoglobin and hematocrit, should be done when food intake is limited and malnutrition is a possibility. Because bone fractures are a significant problem for many children and adults with spastic quadriplegia, bone mineral density may require evaluating. Medications for seizures may be given; many have nutrition interaction problems (see Appendix 23). Evaluation of vitamin D, calcium, carnitine, and vitamin K levels is recommended.

Dietary Intake. Feeding methods can result in limiting the intake of food and fluid; caretakers may not provide sufficient food to meet nutritional needs. The energy needs of the individual with CP vary according to the type of CP. Studies show that the REE and TEE are lower in those with spastic quadriplegic CP than in normal controls (see Table 44-3).

Intervention Strategies

A high percentage of children with CP have feeding problems that are largely the result of oral-motor, positioning, and behavioral factors. As infants they have difficulty swallowing and co-ordinating swallowing and chewing, so the normal progression to solid foods is later than usual. All this may lead to inadequate intake and growth limitations. For those infants and children with IEPs, the team of dietitian nutritionist, speech therapist, occupational therapist, and physical therapist should evaluate the problem and work together in planning therapy.

Gastroesophageal reflux frequently is seen in these infants and toddlers. A tube feeding may be required if a modified barium swallow reveals aspiration. Alternative techniques in feeding should be considered, which could include thickening all beverages or placing a gastrostomy tube (Mahant et al, 2011). RDNs should evaluate gastrostomy feedings for caloric and nutritional value, volume required, and osmolality and offer directions for inclusion of solid foods in addition to the formula if possible.

Usual problems identified in the evaluation will be altered growth, inadequate energy or fluid intakes, drug-nutrient interaction problems, constipation, and feeding problems. Working out an intervention plan is most successful when it involves the parent as part of the team, addresses cultural issues, and recognizes the importance of the feeding problem. Children with CP have complex problems that require continuing follow-up with the family in the community and will take time to correct. State agencies provide tube-feeding formulas and special wheelchairs

TABLE 44-4	Pervasive Developmental Disorders (PDD)
Disorder	**Characteristics**
Autistic disorder	Impairment in social interaction Poor communication skills Repetitive and stereotypical behavior
Rett syndrome	Normal until 6-18 months Loss of motor skill abilities Loss of social interaction Deceleration of head growth between 5 and 48 months
Childhood disintegrative disorder	Before age 10 years Loss of expressive language, social skills, bowel or bladder control, play motor skills
Asperger syndrome	Impairment in social interaction Restricted repetitive or stereotypical behavior Normal language development Normal cognitive development
Pervasive developmental disorder not otherwise specified	Deficits in social behavior Impairment in understanding speech and in speech development Does not meet the criteria for the other four disorders

and equipment to assist with feeding problems. These agencies vary from state to state.

Autism

Autism is one of five disorders under the category **pervasive developmental disorder (PDD)**. PDD was first used in the 1980s to describe a class of disorders as shown in Table 44-4. All types of PDD are neurologic disorders that are usually evident by age 3. In general, children who have a type of PDD have difficulty in talking, playing with other children, and relating to others, including their families. In a recent report CDC estimated that 1 in 68 children has been identified with autism spectrum disorder. This estimate is roughly 30% higher than a previous estimate in 2012 (www.cdc.gov/mmwr, CDC, 2015).

Pathophysiology

Autism spectrum disorders (ASD) are diagnosed by the presence of qualitatively impaired reciprocal social interaction; impaired communication skills; and restricted, repetitive, stereotypical interests and behaviors. Many children with autism also have intellectual compromise. ASD is four times more common in boys than in girls.

Asperger syndrome describes children with the problems of ASD but who have normal to high cognitive levels. These children have a difficult time socializing but may otherwise be able to attend school successfully.

ASD may occur with other developmental or physical disabilities. They have been associated with tuberous sclerosis and maternal rubella. Macrocephaly has been a common finding in large surveys of individuals with autism and also among their relatives. Overall growth is usually normal, and medical problems nonexistent. However, with the limited variety of foods usually eaten by these children, phytonutrient, vitamin and mineral intake could be inadequate.

Efforts to find the cause of ASD have led to many studies looking at a possible toxic environment or food, a nutritionally deficient diet, immune system problems, oxidative stress, and pesticide exposure as important factors. Other studies have studied neurotransmitters such as elevated serotonin levels and disturbances in gamma-amino butyric acid (GABA) receptors, glutamate transmitters, and cholinergic activity. A number of prenatal causes have been evaluated, including pesticides. In one California study women in the first 8 weeks of pregnancy who lived near farm fields sprayed with dicofol and endosulfan were several times more likely to give birth to children with autism (Roberts et al, 2007). More research is needed with greater numbers of mothers included.

Some treatment and research programs are using genomic panels to identify specific intervention protocols. The genomic panel identifies single-nucleotide polymorphisms (SNPs), which are identified from blood samples or cell cultures (see Chapter 5). This work has revealed that the child with autism may need additional omega-3 or EFAs; nutrients with antioxidant qualities such as vitamins A, C, E, and selenium; mineral supplementation with zinc, calcium, and magnesium; a mercury-free diet; or an allergy-elimination diet (see Chapter 26).

Interest in a neurochemical cause of ASD has noted gluten and casein as the suspected sources. Intestinal inflammation has been reported in children with ASD and has improved with dietary restriction of gluten and casein (Elder, 2008; Whiteley et al, 2013). Antibodies to casein, gluten, and soy have been noted in some children with ASD.

Nutrition Assessment

Anthropometric Measures. Height and weight are determined for the child and adult with ASD using the equipment and growth charts for nonaffected individuals. Head circumference has been found to be larger than that of the non-ASD individual.

Biochemical Measures. There is no standard pattern of tests that should be given other than the regular blood work for health monitoring. However, amino acid screening shortly after birth, thyroid testing, and allergy testing may be indicated (see Chapter 26).

Dietary Intake. Dietary evaluations are sometimes difficult to complete for the child with a very limited intake. An effective measure may be provided by having the parents and caregivers keep a food diary for several days to determine the macronutrient intake in addition to the vitamin and mineral intake (see Chapter 4). Obtaining information related to when food is presented and the amount eaten is important, along with fluid consumption. Often excessive fluids are provided to compensate for limited food consumption.

Evaluations should include an observation of the child during mealtime. Some children are slow in arriving at developmental milestones for self-feeding, and require feeding. Others finger feed or insist on self-feeding. The texture of the food presented should be recorded because sensory integration is difficult for children with ASD, and they may be very resistant to texture progression or variety. This is reflected in their fixation on one food (e.g., crackers, dry cereal, or chips). Food jags and picky eating are common. Evaluation should include a description of the feeding environment, whether there is a high chair or age-appropriate toddler chair, the timing of meals, and the location for meals.

Medical Nutrition Therapy

No one therapy or method works for all individuals with ASD. Many professionals and families use a range of treatments simultaneously, including behavior modification, structured educational approaches, medication, speech therapy, occupational therapy, and counseling. Popular nutrition interventions include mineral and vitamin therapy and elimination diets such as a gluten-free (see Chapter 28), casein-free diet (see Chapter 26); allergy diets (see Chapter 26); supplementation with essential fatty acids (EFAs) and megavitamins. A recent double-blind, placebo-controlled, randomized study involved the use of sulforaphane, a phytochemical found in broccoli seed extract, to treat 29 males with ASD, aged 13 to 27 yrs. The results showed its use improved social interaction and verbal communication, and reduced abnormal behavior based on three widely accepted behavioral measures. Dietary sulforaphane was selected because it upregulates genes that protect cells against oxidative stress, inflammation and DNA-damage, all of which are prominent and possibly mechanistic characteristics of ASD (Singh et al, 2014).

There are anecdotal reports of success. The exclusion diets are now used in some treatment centers and are publicized on various websites (http://www.autismndi.com). Table 44-5 describes some exclusion diets. It is important for the RDN to understand these various forms of therapy in order to counsel the parent effectively. Because of the increasing prevalence of ASD, research on potential MNT should be promoted. One of the problems with the gluten-, casein-free diet is cost, because special foods needed to provide sufficient food choices are expensive and sometimes difficult to find (see Chapters 26 and 28).

When MNT is used, taking a team approach and working with the occupational therapist, speech therapist, and others is important for success. Parents also should be members of the team and counseled that changes will take time. Unfortunately, there have been no double-blind, randomized, controlled studies.

Follow-up is an important component of all therapy. From a nutritional standpoint, routine measures of height and weight should be scheduled, and there should be regular evaluation of eating and feeding behavior related to increasing the ability to self-feed and accept new and different foods.

Attention-Deficit/Hyperactivity Disorder

Attention-deficit/hyperactivity disorder (ADHD) is a neurobehavioral problem seen in children with increasing frequency. It has been associated with learning disorders, inappropriate degrees of impulsiveness, hyperactivity, and attention deficit. Diagnostic criteria, developed by the American Psychiatric Association, designate three types: (1) combined type of hyperactivity and attention deficit, (2) predominately inattentive type, and (3) predominately hyperactive-impulse type. ADHD affects the child at home, in school, and in social situations. The causes of ADHD are not well understood, but environmental and genetic factors may be indicated. A long-term study of 64,322 children and their mothers found that use of acetaminophen during pregnancy was a contributing factor to ADHD in the children at the age of 7 (Liew Z et al, 2014).

Nutrition Assessment

Many factors should be considered, along with the usual anthropometric measures, particularly when the individual is on medication.

Anthropometric Measures. Measurements of height and weight should be taken and recorded on a regular basis because the medications used in treatment may cause anorexia if given at inappropriate times, resulting in inadequate

TABLE 44-5   Comparison of Foods Allowed in the Gluten-Free and Casein-Free Diet, Specific Carbohydrate Diet, and Body Ecology Diet

Food	Gluten- and Casein-Free	Specific Carbohydrate Diet	Body Ecology Diet
Gluten-containing grains (wheat, rye, barley, spelt, kamut, possibly oats) and any products from those grains	Not allowed	Not allowed	Not recommended
Rice	Unlimited	Not allowed	Not recommended
Corn	Unlimited	Not allowed	Some OK if tolerated
Millet, quinoa, amaranth, buckwheat	Unlimited	Not allowed	Unlimited (80/20 rule)*, presoaked
Eggs and meat (beef, fish, lamb, chicken, turkey)	Unlimited	Allowed, processed not permitted	Recommended, organic free range or wild caught preferred, use 80/20 rule*
Vegetables	Unlimited	Fresh or frozen allowed, no canned, no potatoes and yams	Unlimited, fermented vegetables highly recommended
Fruits	Unlimited	Allowed, cooked in initial phase, no canned	Not recommended except lemon, lime, cranberry or black currants; no tomatoes
Milk products	Not allowed	Not initially; then 24-hr goat yogurt, dry curd cottage cheese, specific cheeses and butter	Raw butter and cream initially, kefir in 1 month
Sweeteners	Unlimited	Honey and saccharin	Stevia only
Vinegar	Unlimited	White or apple cider	Raw apple cider only
Juice	Unlimited	Those with no added sugar	Only those from fruits listed previously
Oils	Unlimited	Unlimited	Olive, coconut, pumpkin seed
Condiments	Unlimited	No added sugars, spices	Wheat-free tamari, herbs and spices, Celtic sea salt
Nuts and seeds	Unlimited	Most nuts, no seeds for 3 months	Unlimited raw and soaked
Seaweed	Unlimited	Not allowed	Highly recommended
Beans	Unlimited	Allowed after 3 months and then soaked 12 hr	Not recommended
Coffee and tea	Unlimited	Allowed weak	Only herb tea or green tea
Coconut products	Unlimited	Fresh only	All recommended
Gelatin	Unlimited	Allowed	Not recommended. Use agar-agar instead

Developed by Houston-Ludlam GA: Reprinted with permission from The ANDI News, Autism Network for Dietary Intervention, 2005.

*80/20 = meal contains: (1) 80% land and ocean vegetables and 20% either protein or a grain and (2) 80% alkaline-forming foods and 20% acid forming foods.

energy intake and potential slowing of growth. However, a 10-year prospective study of more than 250 children with and without ADHD, treated or not treated with medication, found no evidence of limited growth in height over time (Biederman et al, 2010).

Biochemical Measures. These measurements should include a complete blood count and blood and tissue levels of vitamin and minerals if megavitamin therapy is used.

Dietary Intake. A detailed dietary history would include infant feeding history, food likes and dislikes, behavior at mealtimes, snacking behavior, presence of food allergies or food intolerances, or use of special diets. If the individual is on medications, the time of administration in relation to mealtime is important. Information should be obtained regarding any specific diet for the child or individual and how closely it is being followed.

Feeding evaluations should include observing the individual at mealtime. Generally the problems around feeding will be behavioral and will not include oral-motor or positioning peculiarities. Evaluating the environment around mealtime is important because distractions can be problematic.

Medical Nutrition Therapy

Current treatment may include psychotropic medications and the use of consistent behavioral management techniques. The timing and type of medication must be adjusted so that there is minimum influence on the child's dietary intake.

Specific diets have been used for many years, but they are not based on scientific research. For example, parents have been advised to use the Feingold diet, which states that foods containing synthetic food colors and naturally occurring salicylates be removed from the diet because of their neurologic effect.

Recently there has been renewed interest in the role of artificial food colorings (previously identified by Feingold) as exacerbating hyperactivity in some children. Eight dyes are included: FD&C Blue 1 and 2, FD&C green 3, Orange B, FD&C Red 3, Red 40, FD&C Yellow 5 and 6 (see Table 44-6). The outcome of current interest involves the Food and Drug Administration and committee discussion related to removing food coloring from the food supply (Pelsser et al 2011). A study by Purdue University reported that many children could be consuming far more dyes than previously thought (Stevens et al, 2014). A major source of the artificial food dyes are beverages such as sports drinks, powdered beverages, and fruit drinks, not juice. The recommended amount of artificial food dyes for children has been set at 12 mg per day; however high usage of beverages, colored cereals, and candies can result in 100 mg per day (Stevens et al, 2014). Some manufacturers are now reducing the amount of artificial food colorings in their food products for children.

TABLE 44-6	**Food Dyes and Where They are Found**
FD&C Blue No. 1 – Brilliant Blue (dye and lake)	Ice cream, canned processed peas, packet soups, bottled food colorings, icings, ice pops, blue raspberry flavored products, dairy products, sweets and drinks
FD&C Blue No. 2 – Indigotine (dye and lake)	Gelatin desserts, ice cream, biscuits, soda pop, candies, cereals, sports drinks, soft drinks, and pet foods
FD&C Green No. 3 – Fast Green (dye and lake)	Jellies, sauces, fish, desserts, and dry bakery mixes
FD&C Red No. 3 – Erythrosine (dye)	Candies and popsicles, and even more widely used in cake-decorating gels. It is also used to color pistachio shells
FD&C Red No. 40 – Allura Red (dye and lake)	Soft drinks, children's medications, and cotton candy. It is by far the most commonly used red dye in the united states
FD&C Yellow No. 5 – Tartrazine (dye and lake)	Desserts and sweets: ice cream, ice pops and popsicles, confectionery and hard candy (such as gummy bears, Peeps marshmallow treats, etc.), cotton candy, instant puddings and gelatin (such as Jell-O), cake mixes, pastries (such as Pillsbury pastries), custard powder, marzipan, biscuits, and cookies
	Beverages: soft drinks (such as Mountain Dew), energy and sports drinks, powdered drink mixes (such as Kool-aid), fruit cordials, and flavored/mixed alcoholic beverages
	Snacks: flavored corn chips (such as Doritos, nachos), chewing gum, popcorn (microwave and cinema-popped), and potato chips
	Condiments and spreads: jam, jelly (including mint jelly), marmalade, mustard, horseradish, pickles (and other products containing pickles such as tartar sauce and dill pickle dip), and processed sauces
	Other processed foods: cereal (such as corn flakes, muesli), instant or "cube" soups), rice (e.g., paella, risotto), noodles (such as some varieties of Kraft dinner) and pureed fruit
FD&C Yellow No. 6 – Sunset Yellow (dye and lake)	Orange sodas, marzipan, Swiss rolls, apricot jam, citrus marmalade, lemon curd, sweets, beverage mix and packet soups, margarine, custard powders, packaged lemon gelatin desserts, energy drinks such as Lucozade, breadcrumbs, snack chips such as Doritos, packaged instant noodles, cheese sauce mixes and powdered marinades, bottled yellow and green food coloring, ice creams, pharmaceutical pills and prescription medicines, over-the-counter medicines (especially children's medicines) cake decorations and icings. squashes, and other products with artificial yellow, orange, or red colors

Stevens LJ et al: Amounts of artificial food dyes and added sugars in foods and sweets commonly consumed by children, *Clin Pediatr (Phila),* 2014 (Epub ahead of print).
MCT, Medium-chain triglyceride.

Other recommendations have included the elimination of sugar, the elimination of caffeine, or the addition of large doses of vitamins (megavitamin therapy). A series of well-designed studies to evaluate the effectiveness of these recommendations have generally had negative results, and successful outcomes are largely anecdotal (American Academy of Pediatrics [AAP], 2013).

For the child or adult who is up and down throughout the meal, behavior modification may be indicated, and it should be a part of the overall behavioral management program. Distractions should be eliminated.

The most effective treatment for the individual with ADHD is a diet based on wholesome foods as outlined in the Dietary Guidelines or MyPlate and in Chapter 11. The food should be served at regular times, with small servings followed by refills. This is an important concept because of the tendency of the child or individual to eat very small amounts and leave the table, planning to return or graze throughout the day. Some programs recommend removing the food and returning it only once after explaining why this is being done. The intervention requires that the child or individual sit at the table or in the high chair away from television or other distractions. These suggestions are most applicable to children in preschool settings and in the school cafeteria or classroom.

One suggestion is that a lack of EFAs is a possible cause of hyperactivity in children. It is more likely the result of varying biochemical influences. These children have a deficiency of EFAs because they cannot metabolize linoleic acid normally, they cannot absorb EFAs effectively from the intestine, or their EFA requirements are higher than normal. A recent study in Germany of 810 children ages 5 to 12 provided a food supplement containing omega-3 and omega-6 fatty acids plus zinc

and magnesium, and it resulted in considerable reduction in attention deficit and hyperactivity in the children after 12 weeks of supplementation (Huss et al, 2010). This type of supplementation can be considered. Other clinical trials using EPA and DHA from fish oil supplements in children with ADD or ADHD have reported benefit, but this is not true for all the studies. The difference in findings may be due to many variables including study design, dose, age of supplementation, the present nutritional status, genetics, and teacher or family dynamics (Gillies et al, 2012).

Cleft Lip and Palate

Cleft lip and cleft palate (CL/CP) are the most commonly occurring craniofacial birth defects (Shkoukani et al, 2013). Cleft lip is a condition that creates an opening of the upper lip. It can range from a slight notch to complete separation in one or both sides of the lips, and extending upward. If it occurs on one side of the lip, it is called a unilateral cleft lip; if it occurs on both sides, it is called a bilateral cleft lip. The cleft palate occurs when the roof of the mouth has not joined completely; it can be either unilateral or bilateral. Cleft palate can range from just an opening at the back of the soft palate or separation of the roof of the mouth with both soft and hard palate involved. CL/CP result from incomplete merging and fusion of embryonic processes during formation of the face. There is also a condition called submucous cleft palate in which there is incomplete fusion of the muscular layers of the soft palate with fusion of the overlying mucosa (see Figures 44-8 and 44-9).

Lip and palate development occur between 5 and 12 weeks of gestation. Lip development begins first, usually at

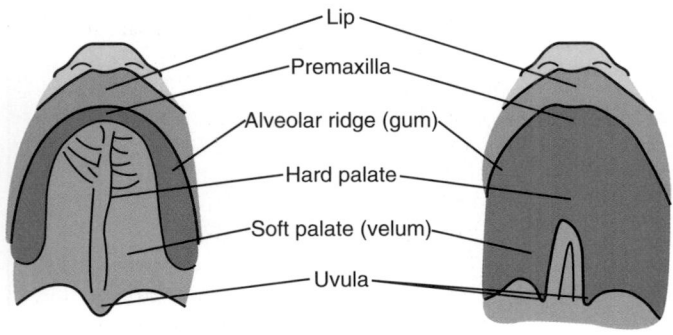

FIGURE 44-8 Cleft palate. (From the Cleft Palate Foundation: www.cleftline.org, 2014. Accessed January 7, 2015.)

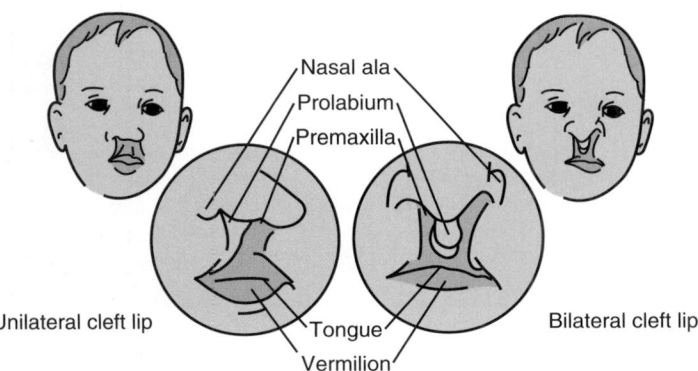

FIGURE 44-9 Cleft lip. (From the Cleft Palate Foundation: www.cleftline.org, 2014. Accessed January 7, 2015.)

5 weeks of gestation, followed by the development of the maxilla prominences and the primary palate. Fusion of the hard palate is completed by 10 weeks of gestation and the soft palate by 12 weeks.

The incidence of CL/CP varies, but is generally 1 in 1000 live births. CL/CP have multiple causes and often are associated with underlying syndromes such as Pierre Robin sequence. The Pierre Robin syndrome or complex is a birth condition that involves the lower jaw being either small in size (micrognathia) or set back from the upper jaw (retrognathia) (Cleft Palate Foundation, 2007). As a result, the tongue tends to be displaced back toward the throat, where it can fall back and obstruct the airway. Most infants with Pierre Robin will have a cleft palate, but none will have a cleft lip. The incidence of Pierre Robin ranges from 1 in 2000 to 30,000 births, based on how strictly the diagnosis is made. The basic cause appears to be the failure of the lower jaw to develop normally before birth.

Approximately 50% of children with cleft palate have an underlying syndrome or multiple anomalies. Wide ranges of studies in developmental biology have shown that genetics and environmental factors are involved in causing oral clefts. Some of the risk factors from the environment include maternal folic acid deficiency, smoking, alcohol use, anticonvulsant use, and some maternal illnesses. Genetic counseling can now identify high-risk families.

Nutrition Assessment

Nutrition assessment for CL/CP includes the usual anthropometric measures for all infants and children. Biochemical measures are also those used with nonaffected children, and dietary intake information depends on the feeding problems that exist. Other problems include dental abnormalities and missing teeth, speech difficulties, and increased incidence of middle ear infections. The feeding evaluation is a major part of the assessment and is best accomplished with a team approach, including the parents. Because the major problem in CL/CP is feeding and providing adequate intake, growth can be jeopardized and must be assessed regularly.

Medical Nutrition Therapy

Surgical repair of the cleft lip generally is performed at 2 to 3 months of age, and cleft palate repair at 9 months. Other operations may involve minor improvements to the lip or nose and usually are completed before the child starts school.

Breastfeeding is difficult for these infants because of problems with sucking, although those infants with just the cleft lip may be successful. It is generally recommended that the mother who wishes to breastfeed express her milk and give it to her baby from a specialized bottle and nipple. Parents and caregivers must be educated in the positioning of the child for feeding, nipple selection, bottle selection, and monitoring of intake (Goyal et al, 2014).

Energy needs are generally the same as for a nonaffected infant or child, but, if the feeding process is too difficult, the energy needs may not be met. Strategies for solving that problem vary, with some professionals advising tube feeding, whereas others recommend continuing with appropriate bottles and nipples but using more concentrated formula or breastmilk (see Chapter 42 and Table 44-7).

Effective feeding requires that the infant be able to form a vacuum inside the mouth and form a seal around the nipple

TABLE 44-7	Increasing Calories Through Concentration of Formulas and Addition of Oils and Carbohydrates	
Using 20 cal/oz		
Formula Caloric Density Required Per Ounce	**Measures of Powder**	**Water Added**
20 calories	1 scoop	2 fl oz
22 calories	2 scoops	3.5 fl oz
24 calories	3 scoops	5 fl oz
27 calories	3 scoops	4.25 fl oz
Using 22 cal/oz Formula		
22 cal	1 scoop	2 fl oz
24 cal	3 scoops	5.5 fl oz
27 cal	5 scoops	8 fl oz
Adding Oil or Carbohydrates		
Product	**kcal**	**Source**
Corn oil or safflower oil	9/g or 8.3/ml	Corn or safflower oil
Microlipid	4.5/mL	Safflower oil
MCT oil	8.3/g or 7.6/ml	Fractionated coconut oil
Karo syrup	1 Tbsp = 58 kcal	Polysaccharides
Polycose liquid	2/mL or 60/fl oz	Glucose polymers
Polycose powder	3.8/g; 8/tsp; 23/Tbsp	Glucose polymers
Moducal powder	30/Tbsp	Glucose polymers

with the lips. This is achieved through the proper bottle, nipple, and position for feeding. Some of the acceptable nipples and bottles include a regular newborn nipple with enlarged holes, a Ross cleft palate assembly, an obturator nipple, and the orthodontic vented nipple. Bottles can vary from a very soft bottle with a cross-cut nipple to a Haberman feeder, squeeze bottle, or an Asepto feeder.

Individuals with CL/CP are different; thus it is extremely important that the feeding team evaluate various types of equipment and carefully educate the parent in their use. Palate obturators have been used to cover the cleft palate until the child can have surgery to close it; their use results in improved intake, better feeding skills, increased weight gain, and growth of the dental arches. Disadvantages include cost and the inconvenience of refabricating the devices as the infant grows to maintain effectiveness. One review article (Goyal et al, 2014) measured growth and the length of feeding, looking at all the various nipples and bottles and the obturator, and found no significant differences in growth, leading the researchers to conclude that the obturator along with special bottles and nipples were all effective. Positioning in an upright position, choosing the appropriate nipple, and directing the liquid flow to the side or back of the mouth seem to be just as effective in promoting optimal feeding and are recommended. The baby should be given ample opportunities for frequent burping in an upright position.

Introduction of solid foods for the CL/CP infant can follow the usual protocol at 4 to 6 months of age. By this time the cleft lip should have been repaired, and the child has achieved good head control and trunk stability. Care that the food is presented slowly is important, allowing the infant to control each bite while gradually learning how to direct the food around the cleft if it hasn't been repaired yet. After the repair and healing of the cleft palate, feeding along the developmental pathway should progress slowly but normally (see Chapter 16 and Table 44-6).

FETAL ALCOHOL SYNDROME

Fetal alcohol spectrum disorders (FASD) are a group of conditions that can develop in the fetus of a woman who drinks alcohol during pregnancy. The effects of the alcohol consumption include growth retardation and usually characteristic facial stigmata, damaged neurons, and brain structures, which can result in psychologic or behavioral problems and other physical problems. The prevalence rate in the US and Europe is estimated to be between 0.2 and 1.5 in every 1000 live births. Fetal alcohol syndrome (FAS) was named in 1973 by Drs. Kenneth Jones and David Smith at the University of Washington School of Medicine after identifying a pattern of craniofacial, limb, and cardiovascular defects in eight unrelated children of three ethnic groups all born to women who were alcoholics (Jones et al, 1973).

Diagnosis of fetal alcohol syndrome requires that the following criteria are fully met: (1) growth deficiency, (2) FAS facial features, (3) central nervous system damage, and (4) prenatal alcohol exposure. The three facial features include smooth filtrum (the groove between the upper lip and the nose); thin upper lip; and small palpebral (between the upper and lower eyelid) fissures (see Figure 15-4). There are two other terms used to describe FASD: **alcohol-related neurodevelopmental disorders (ARND)** and **alcohol-related birth defects (ARBD)**.

Children with ARND may have intellectual disabilities and problems with behavior and learning, particularly with math, memory, attention, judgment, and poor impulse control. Children with ARBD may have problems with the heart, kidney, bones, or with hearing.

Nutrition Assessment

Anthropometric measures are very important in the assessment of the FASD child because growth deficiency is part of the diagnosis. In severe growth deficiency the height and weight are below the 3rd percentile, whereas in moderate cases of growth deficiency, either the height or weight is below the 3rd percentile, but not both. Growth should be evaluated frequently and plotted on the CDC and WHO growth curves. Studies have shown that the prenatal growth retardation of the infant may persist postnatally, and some infants have failure to thrive (Huber and Ekvall, 2005). Feeding problems have also been associated with FAS, including having a week suck and oral motor problems, making these babies difficult to feed. This would contribute to failure to thrive.

Medical Nutrition Therapy

Nutritional intervention for the child with FASD is focused on the specific nutrition problem that exists for that child. Working with growth deficiency, failure to thrive, and feeding problems requires the usual evaluation and intervention used in other infants and children with developmental disabilities. Energy and nutrient needs are the same as for nonaffected children, although strategies for increasing calories would be required for those who have failure to thrive. For some children ADHD has been reported, and the treatment should be the same as already described.

CONTROVERSIAL NUTRITION THERAPY

An important factor in providing MNT for children and adults with developmental disabilities is realizing that counseling may have been inadequate in helping the parent accept the limitations of the disorder - limitations such as growth, feeding problems, and cognitive ability. As a result, many parents look for unusual medical or nutrition therapies. Major sources of information are often the Internet and parent support groups. Recent media coverage has promoted the use of antioxidant vitamins (A, C, and E) and minerals (zinc, copper, manganese, and selenium) along with the amino acids glutamine, tyrosine, and tryptophan. The expected outcomes are improved growth; increased cognition, alertness, and attention span; and changed facial features.

Little scientific information validates these therapies. Research studies have addressed the vitamin needs of children with DS, spina bifida, fragile X syndrome, and autism, and findings do not indicate that the vitamin and mineral needs of these children with developmental disabilities are higher than normal. Numerous historical studies have searched for nutritional deficiencies as causative factors in DS (Tenenbaum et al, 2011). Traditionally, the studies have included numerous vitamins, minerals, fatty acids, digestive enzymes, lipotropic nutrients, and numerous drugs, with no definitive results (Solar Marin and Xandri Graupera, 2011).

The key concept in the proposed nutrition interventions for DS is metabolic correction of genetic overexpression. It is postulated that presence of the third chromosome 21 causes overproduction of superoxide dismutase and cystathionine-β[SPC1]-synthase, which disrupts active methylation pathways. Vitamin supplements of folic acid and antioxidants counteract this and are considered key to the treatment. However, these are just theories, and at this point nutrition supplements are considered an expensive, questionable approach.

Parents of children with ADHD report that omitting sugar from the children's diets decreases hyperactivity, but no scientific evidence supports this. However, it is a good idea to eliminate or at least reduce the sugar intake in any child's diet to promote better nutritional intake. Blue-green algae has been promoted for children with DS and other developmental disabilities, purportedly to increase attention span and concentration. High-dose supplementation of vitamin B_6 and magnesium has been proposed for autism to diminish tantrums and self-stimulation activities and improve attention and speech. Another proposed treatment is dimethyl glycine. Limited research is available.

COMMUNITY RESOURCES

For many types of nutrition problems and MNT, the school system is an excellent resource through the school lunch and school breakfast programs. Children and adolescents may receive modified meals at school. Child and adult care food programs must provide meals at no extra cost for children and adolescents with special needs and developmental disabilities. School food service is required to offer special meals at no additional cost to children whose disabilities restrict their diets as defined in the U.S. Department of Agriculture's nondiscrimination regulations.

The term "child with a disability" under Part B of the Individuals with Disabilities Education Act (IDEA) refers to a child evaluated in accordance with IDEA as having one of the 13 recognized disability categories: (1) autism; (2) deaf-blindness; (3) deafness; (4) mental retardation; (5) orthopedic impairments; (6) other health impairments caused by chronic or acute health problems such as asthma, nephritis, diabetes, sickle cell anemia, a heart condition, epilepsy, rheumatic fever, hemophilia, leukemia, lead poisoning, or tuberculosis; (7) emotional disturbances; (8) specific learning disabilities; (9) speech or language impairment; (10) traumatic brain injury; (11) visual impairment; (12) multiple disabilities; and (13) developmental delays. Attention deficit disorder may fall under 1 of the 13 categories.

When a referral is made to the school system for a special meal related to a developmental disability, it must be accompanied by a medical statement for a child with special dietary needs. The request requires an identification of the medical or other special dietary condition, the food or foods to be omitted, and the food or choice of foods to be substituted. The statement requires the signature of the physician or recognized medical authority. The school food service may make food substitutions for individual children who do not have a disability but who are medically certified as having a special medical or dietary need. An example is the child with severe allergies or an inborn error of metabolism. The availability of school food service for children with developmental disabilities is an important resource in the long-term implementation of MNT.

CLINICAL CASE STUDY - CHILD WITH DOWN SYNDROME

Nutrition Assessment

Client History

Colin is a 21-month-old boy with Down's syndrome. He was born prematurely (30 weeks of gestation) and was started on gastrostomy tube feeding at 10 days of age because of his poor weight gain and severe gastroesophageal reflux. The poor weight gain was caused by a poor suck, although swallowing was not a problem. He was first seen by a nutritionist in an early intervention program at 4 months of age when he was 22.5 in long and weighed 10 lb 7 oz.

Food/Nutrition-Related History

At 16 months Colin was tube fed Pediasure and started eating table foods. His usual intake is 1 jar of baby food a day along with the tube-feeding formula.

Anthropometric Measurements

At 4 months of age he was 22.5 in long and weighed 10 lb. 7 oz.
At 21 months, height was 28," weight was 18.5 lb and he was in the 5% for length and weight.

Physical Findings

He is crawling but not yet walking, and he has very limited self-feeding skills. Now at age 21 months his mother's highest priority is to stop the tube feeding and have Colin continue to grow well. She is concerned about his rate of weight gain. She also is concerned that constipation has become a problem requiring use of the medication lactulose. He also has respiratory problems and extreme hypotonia.

Feeding problems identified:
   Weak suck, and swallow

Hyperactive gag reflex
Refusal to drink formula from a bottle or cup due to g-tube
Poor appetite
Not self-feeding

Nutrition Diagnostic Statements

Tube-fed toddler with caloric intake estimated at 100 kcal per kg. NI-1.4
Self-feeding difficulty related to developmental delays as evidenced by inability to feed himself most foods offered. NB-2.6
Inadequate intake of baby food and table food. NI-2.1
Refusal to drink his formula or other beverages from a cup. NC-1.1

Nutrition Intervention

1. Introduction of drinking from a cup with a straw using formula and water.
2. Introduction of soft table foods before gastrostomy feedings.
3. Reduction of size of servings of food offered.
4. Work with occupational therapy in promoting eating of finger foods.

Nutrition Care Questions

1. What would be your approach in working with this mother and the other team members?
2. What do you think would be his nutritional needs, starting with energy?
3. How many ounces of a 30 cal/oz tube-feeding formula would you recommend for Colin to promote weight gain?
4. What steps should be taken to increase his oral intake and decrease the tube feeding?
5. What would you recommend for management of his constipation?

CLINICAL CASE STUDY - ADOLESCENT WITH DOWN SYNDROME AND OBESITY

Nutrition Assessment

History

Alicia, a 14-year-old girl with Down's syndrome, is admitted to a mental health services facility for treatment of sleep apnea, prediabetes, and severe behavioral activities. The contributing factor to the medical problems is her severe obesity. Before her admission to the facility she had been in public school in a special education program, but her behavior was so difficult to control that the school transferred her to this mental health facility. She is the only individual in her family with Down's syndrome, and was born when her mother was 40. There is a history of diabetes in the family and food has always been used as a reward for Alicia.

Food/Nutrition-Related History

Alicia's birthweight was 7 lb 8 oz, her birth length was 19," and she was full term. She was breast fed until age 3 months when she was transferred to Similac formula and reportedly had no feeding problems other than consuming more than 36 oz of milk daily, and eating baby food in unusually large amounts. Her weaning to a cup was late, at 18 months, and her motor-skill development was late; she did not walk until 28 months of age. She also had low muscle tone.

By the time she was 12 months of age her weight was 28 lb, placing her above the 95th percentile. Each subsequent year she remained between the 75th and 95th percentile for her weight but at the 10th percentile for her height.

During her preschool and school years Alicia's intake was reported as very limited in variety with a heavy concentration of foods from fast food restaurants, and little intake of fruits and vegetables. She drank milk, but preferred soft drinks and sweetened tea. She also consumed many sweetened desserts, cookies, and bakery products. Although her mother reported trying to control Alicia's overeating behavior, a grandparent was very indulgent. Alicia also developed behavioral problems with a great deal of acting out at home and at school. It was this behavior that led to her referral to the mental health facility.

Anthropometric measurements:

Weight 247 # > 97th%
Height: 56"- 50% to 75%
H/W relationship: > 97th%
BM index: > 97%
Estimated energy needs: 1716 kcal
Estimated energy intake at home: 3000 kcal (based on maternal report)
Estimated protein need: 52 g

Biochemical Data

Hgb: 14 gm/dL —(12-14.9)
Hct: 36% (39.) low
Cholesterol: 210 mg/dL (high) <170 acceptable

Glucose: 120 mg/dL (high) 70-100 acceptable
Medications: Topomax and Clonidine, for seizures and behavioral problems.
Diet order after physical examination: 1500 calories per day and exercise.

Nutrition-Focused Physical Findings

Excessive appetite
Dry skin
Inactivity with behavioral outbursts related to walking
Feeding problems—very rapid eating with possibility of choking
Low muscle tone
Constipation

Nutrition Diagnostic Statements

Obesity: NC 3.3
Excessive intake of carbohydrates: N1-53.2
Excessive oral food/beverage intake: NI-2.2

Intervention Goals

1. Weight loss and acceptance of difference in food provided.
2. Increase consumption of high fiber foods.
3. Limit between meal to fruit and vegetables. ND-1
4. Counsel parents related to meal management and poor behavior related to food. FH 3.1
5. Increase physical activity at school and home. FH 6.3

Nutrition Intervention

1. Modify the menus to provide 1500 calories including snacks. ND-1
2. Provide copies of menu to group home staff and parents. ND 1.2
3. Increase availability of fresh fruit and raw vegetables for snacks. ND 1.2
4. Increase water intake. ND 1.3

Monitoring and Evaluation

1. Weigh monthly and plot on growth grid with report to parents.
2. Counsel parents monthly or as necessary related to food intake and exercise at home.
3. Record amount of walking at school with teachers and other students.

Nutrition Care Questions

1. Teachers report that student eats only part of the meal provided and refuses the snacks offered. What would be your response?
2. The parents report in their monthly conference that Alicia is very rebellious and refuses to participate in the family activities unless provided with a trip to a fast food restaurant for hamburgers and French fries. What could you suggest?
3. Monthly weights show a loss of 2 to 3 pounds each month. Should there be a reward system? Could you use motivational interviewing with the family? How would you modify this approach with Alicia?

USEFUL WEBSITES

Centers for Disease Control and Prevention Birth Defects Research
http://www.cdc.gov/ncbddd/birthdefects/research.html
March of Dimes
http://www.modimes.org
National Center for Education in Maternal and Child Health
http://www.ncemch.org/
National Dissemination Center for Children with Disabilities
http://www.nichcy.org
National Folic Acid Campaign
http://www.cdc.gov/folicacid/promote.htm

REFERENCES

American Academy of Pediatrics (AAP): *Your child's diet: a cause and a cure of ADHD?*, 2013. http://www.healthychildren.org/English/health-issues/conditions/adhd/Pages/Your-Childs-Diet-A-Cause-and-a-Cure-of-ADHD.aspx. Accessed January 5, 2015.

American Association on Intellectual and Developmental Disabilities (AAIDD): *Definitions*, 2013. http://www.aaidd.org/content_100.cfm?navID=21. Accessed January 5, 2015.

Andrew MJ, Sullivan PB: Growth in cerebral palsy, *Nutr Clin Pract* 25:357, 2010.

Biederman J, et al: A naturalistic 10-year prospective study of height and weight in children with attention-deficit hyperactivity disorder grown up: sex and treatment effects, *J Pediatr* 157:635, 2010.

Blumchen K, et al: Effects of latex avoidance on latex sensitization, atopy and allergic disease in patients with spina bifida, *Allergy* 65:1585, 2010.

Bull MJ, Committee on Genetics: Health supervision for children with Down syndrome, Pediatrics 128:393, 2011.

Canfield MA, et al: The association between race/ ethnicity and major birth defects in the United States, 1999-2007), *Am J Pub Hlth* 104:e-14, 2014. www.cdc.gov/ncbddd/spinabifida/data.html

Carrel AL, et al: Long-term growth hormone therapy changes the natural history of body composition and motor function in children with Prader-Willi syndrome, *J Clin Endocrinol Metab* 95:1131, 2010.

Centers for Disease Control and Prevention (CDC): CDC Grand Rounds: additional opportunities to prevent neural tube defects with folic acid fortification, *MMWR Morb Mortal Wkly Rep* 59:980, 2010. Accessed Jan. 26, 2016.

Centers for Disease Control and Prevention (CDC): *Key Findings: Updated National Birth Prevalence Estimates for Selected Birth Defects in the United States, 2004-2006,* 2014. http://www.cdc.gov/ncbddd/birthdefects/features/birthdefects-keyfindings.html. Accessed Jan. 26, 2016.

Centers for Disease Control and Prevention (CDC): *Autism and Developmental Disabilities Monitoring Network, 2015,* 2015. http://www.cdc.gov/ncdd/autism/addm.html.

Cleft Palate Foundation: *Pierre Robin Sequence,* 2007. http://www.cleftline.org/publications/pierre_robin. Accessed January 5, 2015.

Curtin C, et al: Parent support improves weight loss in adolescents and young adults with Down syndrome, *J Pediatr* 163:1402, 2013.

Das JK, et al: Micronutrient fortification of food and its impact on woman and child health: a systematic review, *Syst Rev* 2:67, 2013.

Ekvall SW, Cerniglia F: Myelomeningocele. In Ekvall SW, Ekvall VK, editors: *Pediatric nutrition in developmental disabilities and chronic disorders,* ed 2, New York, 2005, Oxford University Press.

Gillies D, et al: Polyunsaturated fatty acids (PUFA) for attention deficit hyperactivity disorder (ADHD) in children and adolescents, *Cochrane Database Syst Rev* 7:CD007986, 2012.

Goyal M, et al: Role of obturators and other feeding inventions in patients with cleft lip and palate: a review, *Eur Arch Paediatr Dent* 15:1, 2014.

Haqq AM, et al: The metabolic syndrome of Prader Willi syndrome in childhood: heightened insulin sensitivity relative to body mass index, *J Clin Endocrinol Metab* 96:E225, 2011.

Heiss CJ, et al: Registered dietitians and speech-language pathologists: an important partnership in dysphagia management, *J Am Diet Assoc* 110:1290, 2010.

Huber A, Ekvall SW: Fetal alcohol sSyndrome. In Ekvall SV, Ekvall VK, editors: *Pediatric nutrition in chronic disease and developmental disorders,* ed 2, New York, 2005, Oxford University Press.

Huss M, et al: Supplementation of polyunsaturated fatty acids, magnesium and zinc in children seeking medical advice for attention-deficit/hyperactivity problems—an observational cohort study, *Lipids Health Dis* 9:105, 2010.

Jones KL, et al: Pattern of malformation in offspring of chronic alcoholic mothers, *Lancet* 1:1267, 1973.

Kreutzer C, et al: *Nutrition issues in children with myelomeningocele (Spina Bifida), in Nutrition Focus for Children with Special Health Care Needs* 28:5, Seattle, Wash, 2013, University of Washington Center on Human Developmental Disability.

Liew Z, et al: Acetominophen use during pregnancy, behavioral problems and hyperkinetic disorders, *JAMA Pediatr* 168:313, 2014.

Lima AS, et al: Nutritional status of zinc in children with Down Syndrome, *Biol Trace Elem Res* 133:20, 2010.

Mahant S, et al: Decision-making around gastrostomy-feeding in children with neurologic disabilities. Pediatrics 127:e1471, 2011.

McCune H and Driscoll D: Prader-Willi syndrome. In Ekvall SW, Ekvall VK, editors: *Pediatric nutrition in chronic disease and developmental disorders,* ed 2, New York, 2005, Oxford University Press.

Miller JL, et al: Nutritional phases in Prader-Willi syndrome, *Am J Med Genet A* 155:1040, 2011.

Murray J, Ryan-Krause P: Obesity in children with Down syndrome: background and recommendations for management, *Pediatr Nurs* 36:314, 2010.

Obata K, et al: Effects of 5 years growth hormone treatment in patients with Prader-Willi syndrome, *J Pediatr Endocrinol Metab* 16:155, 2003.

Pelsser LM, et al: Effects of a restricted elimination diet on the behavior of children with attention-deficit hyperactivity disorder (INCA study): a randomised controlled trial, *Lancet* 377:494, 2011.

Reus L, et al: Motor problems in Prader-Willi syndrome: a systematic review on body composition and neuromuscular functioning, *Neurosci Biobehav Rev* 35:956, 2011.

Roberts EM, et al: Maternal residence near agricultural pesticide applications and autism spectrum disorders among children in the California Central Valley, *Environ Health Perspect* 115:1482, 2007.

Scerif M, et al: Ghrelin in obesity and endocrine diseases, *Mol Cell Endocrinol* 340:15, 2011.

Shkoukani MA, et al: Cleft lip—a comprehensive review, *Front Pediatr* 1:53, 2013.

Singh K, et al: Sulforaphane treatment of autism spectrum disorder (ASD), *Proc Natl Acad Sci USA* 111:15550, 2014.

Solar Marin A, Xandri Graupera JM: Nutrtional status of intellectual disabled persons with Down Syndrome, *Nutr Hosp* 26:1059, 2011.

Smithells RW, et al: Further experience of vitamin supplementation for prevention of neural tube defect recurrences, *Lancet* 1:1027, 1983.

Stevens LJ, et al: Amounts of artificial food dyes and added sugars in foods and sweets commonly consumed by children, *Clin Pediatr (Phila)* 54:309, 2015.

Stevenson RD: Use of segmental measures to estimate stature in children with cerebral palsy, *Arch Paediatr Adolesc Med* 149:658, 1995.

Tenenbaum A, et al: Anemia in children with Down syndrome, *Int J Pediatr* 2011:813541, 2011.

Van Riper CL, et al: Position of the American Dietetic Association: providing nutrition services for people with developmental disabilities and special health care needs, *J Am Diet Assoc* 110:297, 2010.

Whiteley P, et al: Gluten and casein-free dietary intervention for autism spectrum conditions, *Front Hum Neurosci* 6:344, 2013.

Unit Abbreviations

Along with the specialized vocabulary that is used in the medical, dietetic, and nursing fields, there are acceptable forms of abbreviations.

The following is a list of abbreviations commonly used.

aa:	Gr. *ana*; of each	mEq:	milliequivalent
ac:	L. *ante cibum*, before meals	mg:	milligram
ad, add:	L. *adde, addatus,* or *addantur;* add or added	mil or mL:	milliliter
ad lib:	L. *ad libitum;* at pleasure, as desired	mM:	millimole
aq:	L. *aqua;* water	μmol:	micromol
aq dest:	L. *aqua destillata;* distilled water	mOsm:	milliosmole
bid, bis in d:	L. *bis in die* twice a day	oz:	ounce
c̄:	L. *cum;* with	prn:	L. *pro re nata;* as needed
c:	cup	pt:	pint
Cent; cent; C:	centigrade, Celsius	pulv:	L. *pulvis;* powder
cm:	centimeter	qd:	L. *quaque die;* every day
dilut:	L. *dilutus;* dilute	QID, qid:	L. *quater in die;* four times daily
div:	L. *divide;* divide	q3h:	every 3 hours
fac:	make	qs:	L. *quantum satis;* a sufficient quantity
g:	gram	qt:	quart
gr:	L. *granum;* grain	RE:	retinal equivalent
gtt:	L. *guttae;* drops	s̄:	L. *sine;* without
hs:	L. *hora somni;* at hour of sleep	sol:	solution
IU:	international unit	ss:	L. *semis;* half
kcal:	kilocalorie	stat:	L. *statim;* immediately
kg:	kilogram	t, tsp:	teaspoon
kJ:	kilojoule	T, Tbsp:	tablespoon
lb:	pound	tid:	L. *ter in die:* three times a day
mcg:	microgram		

Milliequivalents and Milligrams of Electrolytes

To Convert Milligrams to Milliequivalents: Divide milligrams by atomic weight and then multiply by the valence.

$$\text{Example}: \frac{\text{Milligrams}}{\text{Atomic weight}} \; \text{Valence} = \text{Milliequivalents}$$

Mineral Element	Chemical Symbol	Atomic Weight (mg)	Valence
Calcium	Ca	40	2
Chlorine	Cl	35	1
Magnesium	Mg	24	2
Phosphorus	P	31	2
Potassium	K	39	1
Sodium	Na	23	1
Sulfate	SO_4	96	2
Sulfur	S	32	

To Convert Specific Weight of Sodium to Sodium Chloride: Multiply by 2.54.

Example 1000 mg Sodium 1000 2.54 = 2540 mg Sodium chloride (2.5g)

To Convert Specific Weight of Sodium Chloride to Sodium: Multiply by 0.393.

Example 2.5 g Sodium chloride 2.5 0.393 = 1000 mg sodium

Milligrams	Sodium in Milliequivalents (mEq)	Grams of Sodium Chloride
500	21.8	1.3
1000	43.5	2.5
1500	75.3	3.8
2000	87.0	5.0

Modified from Merck Manual, Ready Reference Guide. Accessed 22 March 2011 from http://www.merckmanuals.com/professional/print/appendixes/ap1/ap1a.html; Nelson JK et al: Mayo Clinic diet manual, ed 7, St Louis 1994, Mosby.

Equivalents, Conversions,* and Portion (Scoop) Sizes

LIQUID MEASURE—VOLUME EQUIVALENTS

1 tsp = ⅓ Tbsp = 5 mL or cc
1 Tbsp = 3 tsp = 15 mL or cc
2 Tbsp = 1 fluid oz = ⅛ cup = 30 mL or cc
2 Tbsp + 2 tsp = ⅙ cup = 40 mL or cc
4 Tbsp = ¼ cup = 2 fluid oz = 60 mL or cc
5 Tbsp + 1 tsp = ⅓ cup = 80 mL or cc
6 Tbsp = 3 fluid oz = ⅜ cup = 90 mL or cc
8 Tbsp = ½ cup = 120 mL or cc
10 Tbsp + 2 tsp = ⅔ cup = 160 mL or cc
12 Tbsp = ¾ cup = 180 mL or cc
48 tsp = 16 Tbsp = 1 cup (8 fluid ounces) = ½ pint = 240 mL or cc
2 cups = 1 pint (16 fluid oz) = 0.4732 L
4 cups = 2 pints = 1 quart (32 fluid oz) = 0.9462 L
1.06 quarts = 34 fluid oz = 1000 mL or cc
4 quarts = 1 gallon = 3785 mL or cc

DRY MEASURE

1 quart = 2 pints = 1.101 L
Dry measure and quarts are approximately ⅙ larger than liquid measure pints and quarts.

WEIGHTS	
English (Avoirdupois)	Metric
1 oz	Approx 30 g
1 lb (16 oz)	454 g
2.2 lb	1 kg

SCOOP SIZES

It is important to use the proper scoop size when portioning out foods to serve to patients.

Number	Approximate Liquid Volume
6	⅔ cup (5 fluid oz)
8	½ cup (4 fluid oz)
10	⅜ cup (3¼ fluid oz)
12	⅓ cup (2⅔ fluid oz)
16	¼ cup (2 fluid oz)
20	3⅕ Tbsp (1⅗ fluid oz)
24	2⅔ Tbsp (1⅓ fluid oz)
30	2⅕ Tbsp (1 fluid oz)
40	1⅗ Tbsp (0.3 fluid oz)
60	1 Tbsp (0.5 fluid oz)

Metric Conversion Factors		
Multiply	By	To Get
Fluid ounces	29.57	Grams
Ounces (dry)	28.35	Grams
Grams	0.0353	Ounces
Grams	0.0022	Pounds
Kilograms	2.21	Pounds
Pounds	453.6	Grams
Pounds	0.4536	Kilograms
Quarts	0.946	Liters
Quarts (dry)	67.2	Cubic inches
Quarts (liquid)	57.7	Cubic inches
Liters	1.0567	Quarts
Gallons	3.785	Cubic centimeters
Gallons	3.785	Liters

From North Carolina Dietetic Association: *Nutrition care manual*, 2011, Raleigh, NC, The Association.
*Note: In the U.S. measuring systems the same word may have two meanings. For example, an ounce may mean 1/16 of a pound and 1/16 of a pint; but the former is strictly a weight measure, and the latter is a volume measure. Except in the case of water, milk, or other liquids of the same density, a fluid ounce and an ounce of weight are two completely different quantities. These measures are not to be used interchangeably.

Birth to 24 Months: Boys Length-for-Age and Weight-for-Age Percentiles

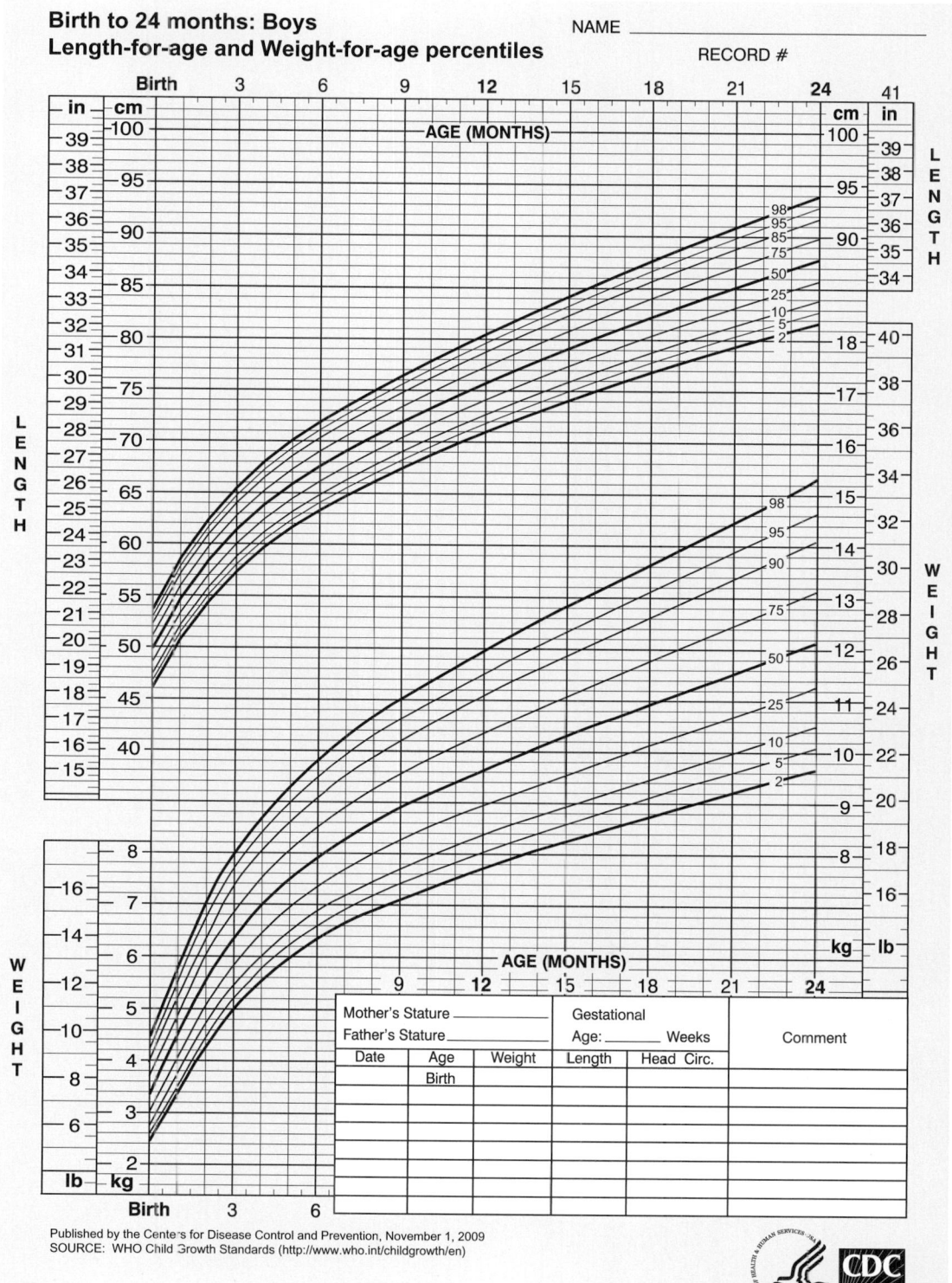

Birth to 24 months: Boys
Length-for-age and Weight-for-age percentiles

NAME _____

RECORD # _____

Published by the Centers for Disease Control and Prevention, November 1, 2009
SOURCE: WHO Child Growth Standards (http://www.who.int/childgrowth/en)

Birth to 24 Months: Boys Head Circumference-for-Age and Weight-for-Length Percentiles

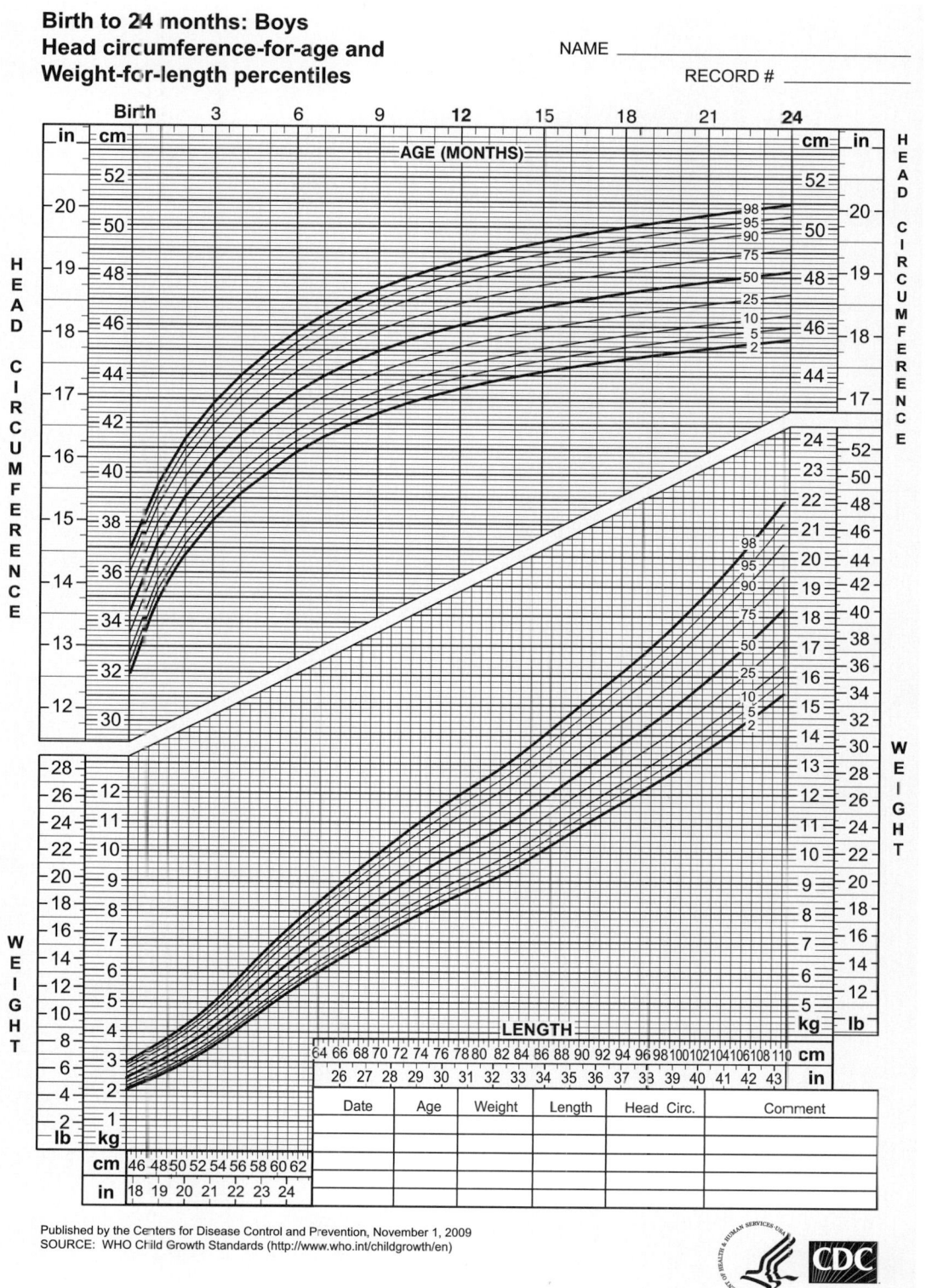

Birth to 24 months: Boys
Head circumference-for-age and
Weight-for-length percentiles

NAME _____

RECORD # _____

Published by the Centers for Disease Control and Prevention, November 1, 2009
SOURCE: WHO Child Growth Standards (http://www.who.int/childgrowth/en)

2 to 20 Years: Boys Stature-for-Age and Weight-for-Age Percentiles

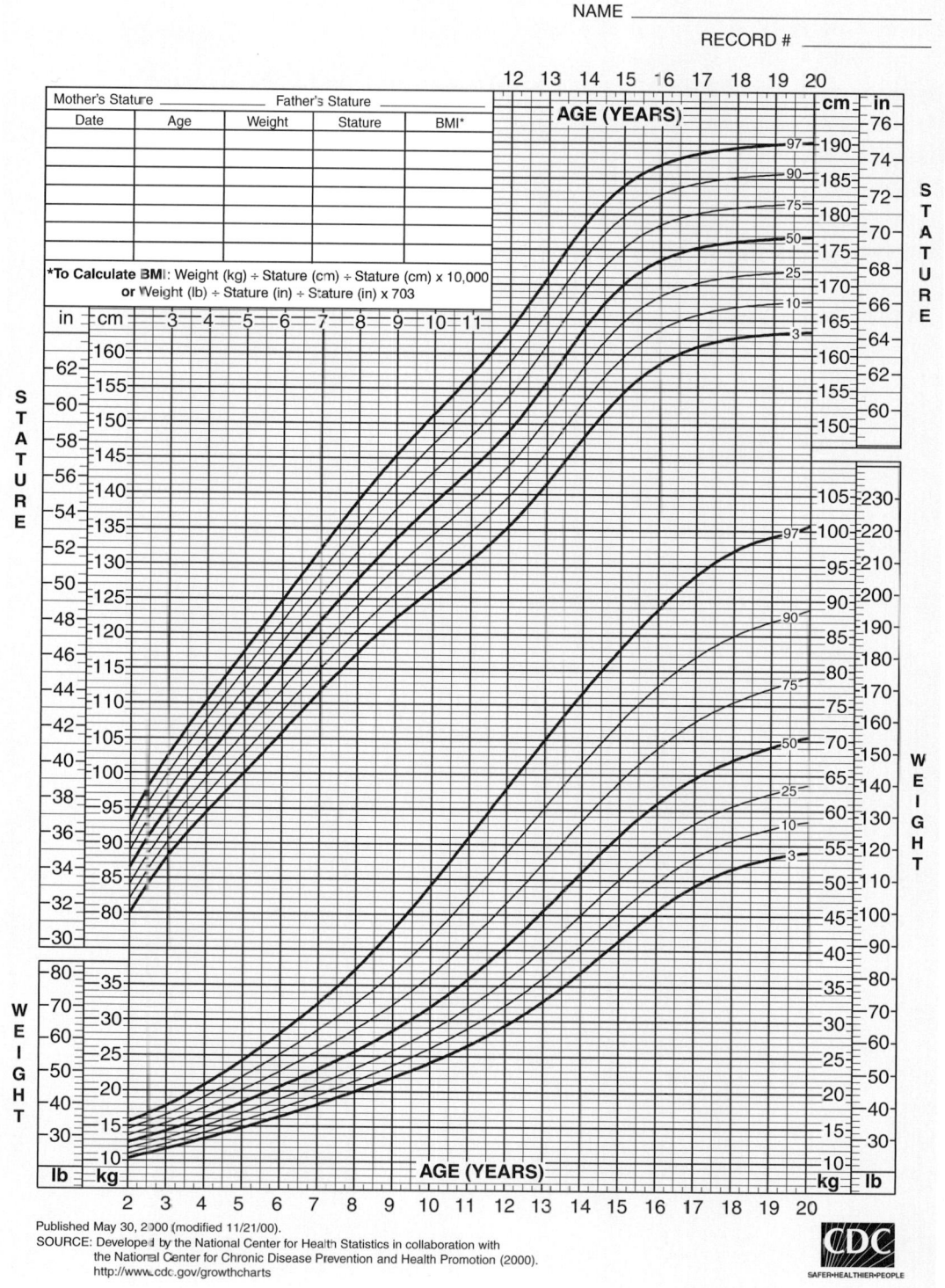

NAME _____

RECORD # _____

Mother's Stature _____ Father's Stature _____

Date	Age	Weight	Stature	BMI*

*To Calculate BMI: Weight (kg) ÷ Stature (cm) ÷ Stature (cm) x 10,000
or Weight (lb) ÷ Stature (in) ÷ Stature (in) x 703

AGE (YEARS)

STATURE

WEIGHT

Published May 30, 2000 (modified 11/21/00).
SOURCE: Developed by the National Center for Health Statistics in collaboration with
the National Center for Chronic Disease Prevention and Health Promotion (2000).
http://www.cdc.gov/growthcharts

CDC
SAFER·HEALTHIER·PEOPLE

Body Mass Index-for-Age Percentiles: Boys, 2 to 20 Years

NAME _____

RECORD # _____

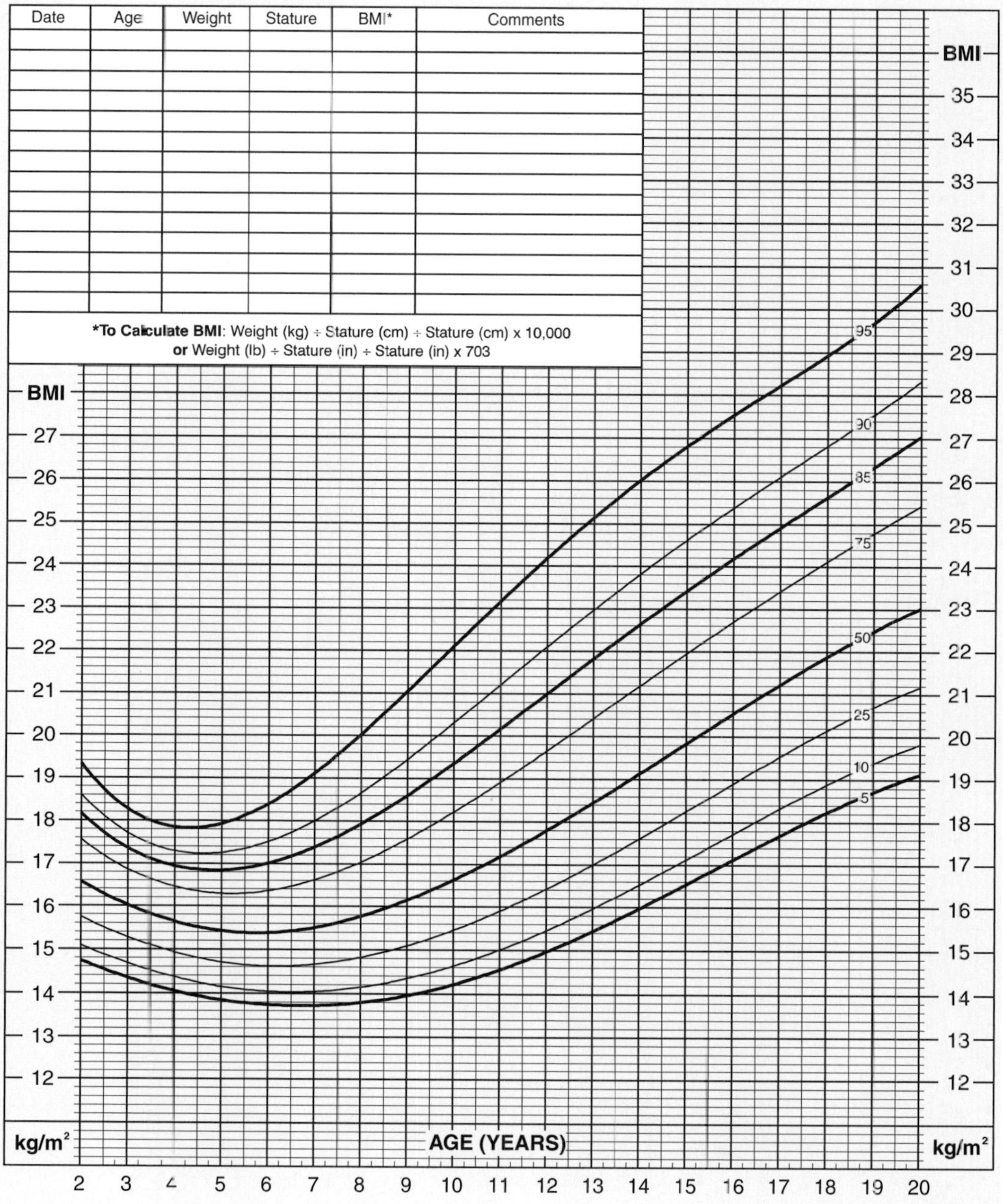

Date	Age	Weight	Stature	BMI*	Comments

*To Calculate BMI: Weight (kg) ÷ Stature (cm) ÷ Stature (cm) x 10,000
or Weight (lb) ÷ Stature (in) ÷ Stature (in) x 703

BMI

35
34
33
32
31
30 — 95
29
28
27 — 90
26 — 85
25
24 — 75
23
22 — 50
21
20 — 25
19 — 10
18 — 5

BMI — 27, 26, 25, 24, 23, 22, 21, 20, 19, 18, 17, 16, 15, 14, 13, 12

kg/m² — AGE (YEARS) — kg/m²

2 3 4 5 6 7 8 9 10 11 12 13 14 15 16 17 18 19 20

Published May 30, 2000 (modified 10/16/00).
SOURCE: Developed by the National Center for Health Statistics in collaboration with
the National Center for Chronic Disease Prevention and Health Promotion (2000).
http://www.cdc.gov/growthcharts

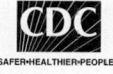
SAFER·HEALTHIER·PEOPLE

Birth to 24 Months: Girls Length-for-Age and Weight-for-Age Percentiles

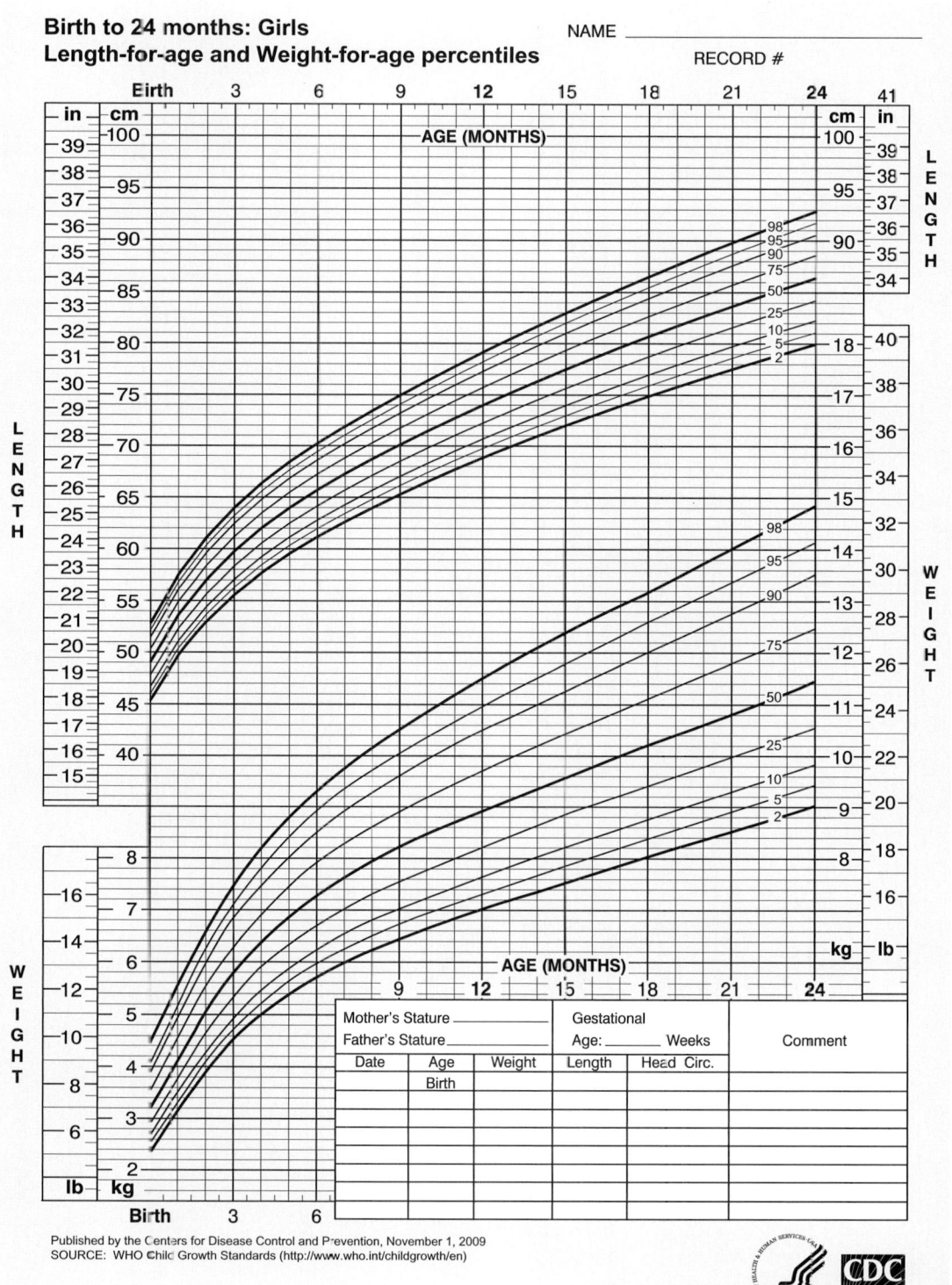

Birth to 24 months: Girls
Length-for-age and Weight-for-age percentiles

NAME _____

RECORD # _____

Published by the Centers for Disease Control and Prevention, November 1, 2009
SOURCE: WHO Child Growth Standards (http://www.who.int/childgrowth/en)

Birth to 24 Months: Girls Head Circumference-for-Age and Weight-for-Length Percentiles

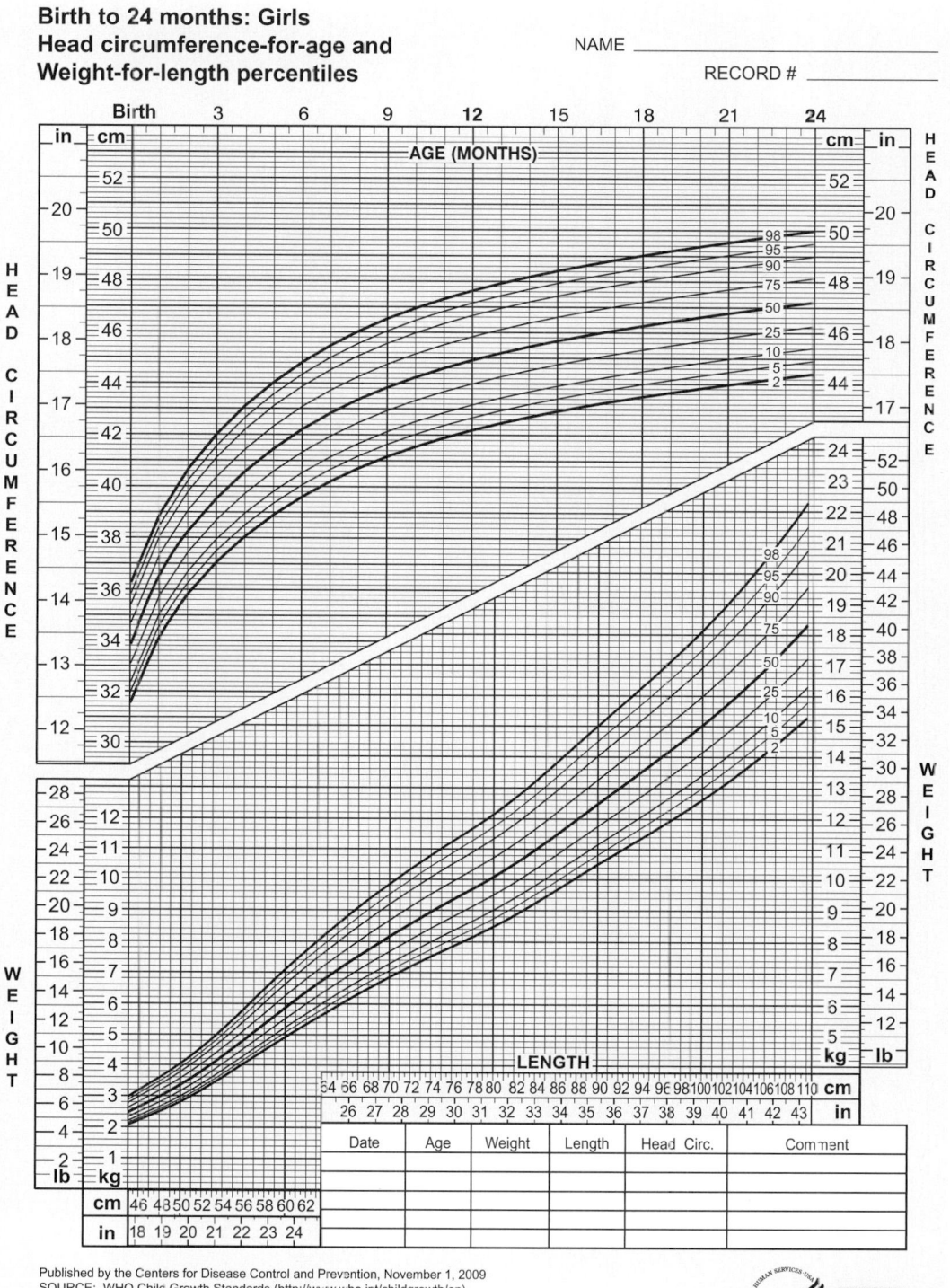

Birth to 24 months: Girls
Head circumference-for-age and
Weight-for-length percentiles

NAME _____

RECORD # _____

Date	Age	Weight	Length	Head Circ.	Comment

Published by the Centers for Disease Control and Prevention, November 1, 2009
SOURCE: WHO Child Growth Standards (http://www.who.int/childgrowth/en)

947

2 to 20 Years: Girls Stature-for-Age and Weight-for-Age Percentiles

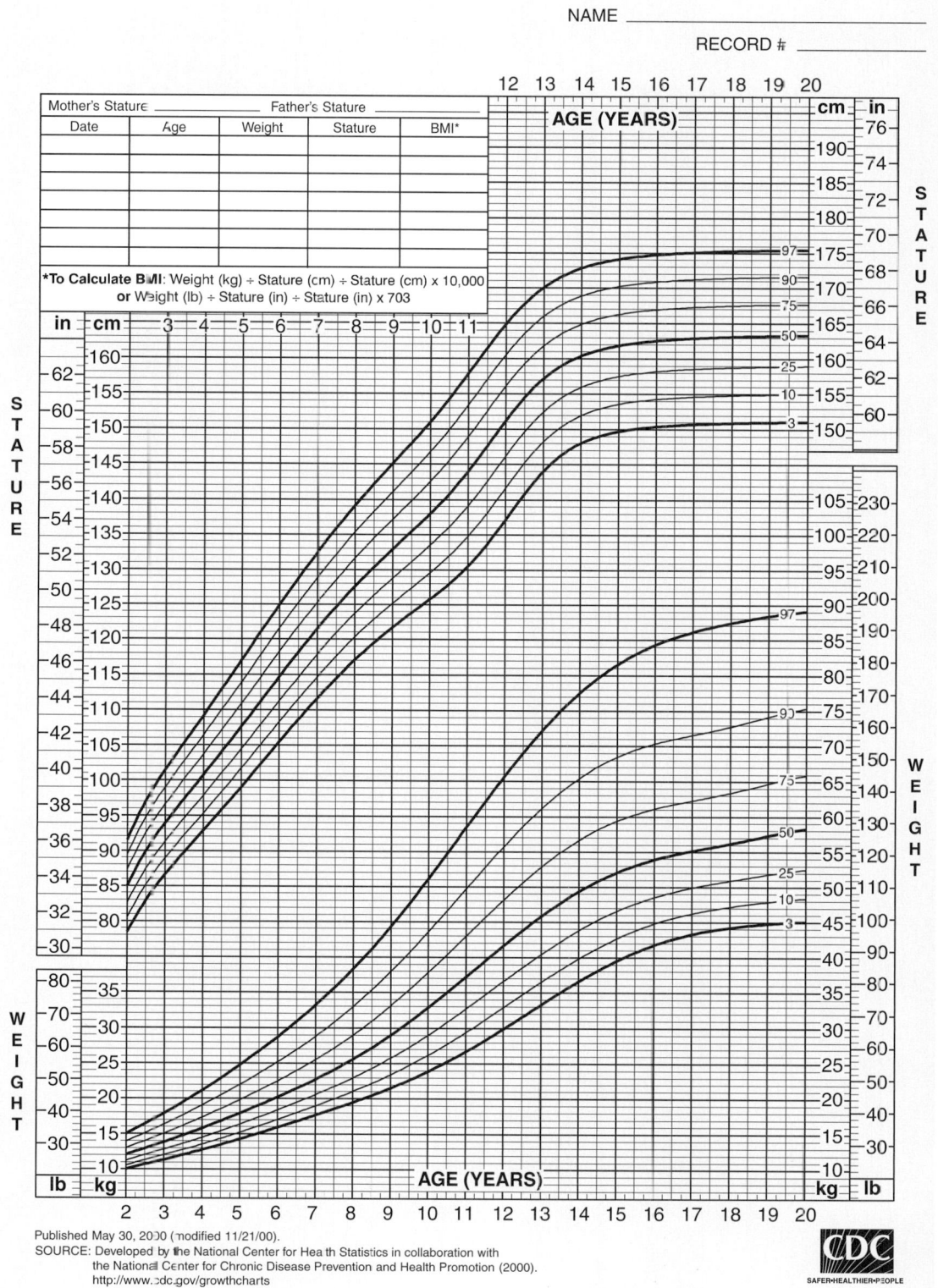

NAME _____

RECORD # _____

Mother's Stature _____ Father's Stature _____

Date	Age	Weight	Stature	BMI*

*To Calculate BMI: Weight (kg) ÷ Stature (cm) ÷ Stature (cm) x 10,000
or Weight (lb) ÷ Stature (in) ÷ Stature (in) x 703

AGE (YEARS)

STATURE

WEIGHT

Published May 30, 2000 (modified 11/21/00).
SOURCE: Developed by the National Center for Health Statistics in collaboration with
the National Center for Chronic Disease Prevention and Health Promotion (2000).
http://www.cdc.gov/growthcharts

CDC
SAFER•HEALTHIER•PEOPLE

949

Body Mass Index-for-Age Percentiles: Girls, 2 to 20 Years

NAME _____

RECORD # _____

Date	Age	Weight	Stature	BMI*	Comments

*To Calculate BMI: Weight (kg) ÷ Stature (cm) ÷ Stature (cm) x 10,000
or Weight (lb) ÷ Stature (in) ÷ Stature (in) x 703

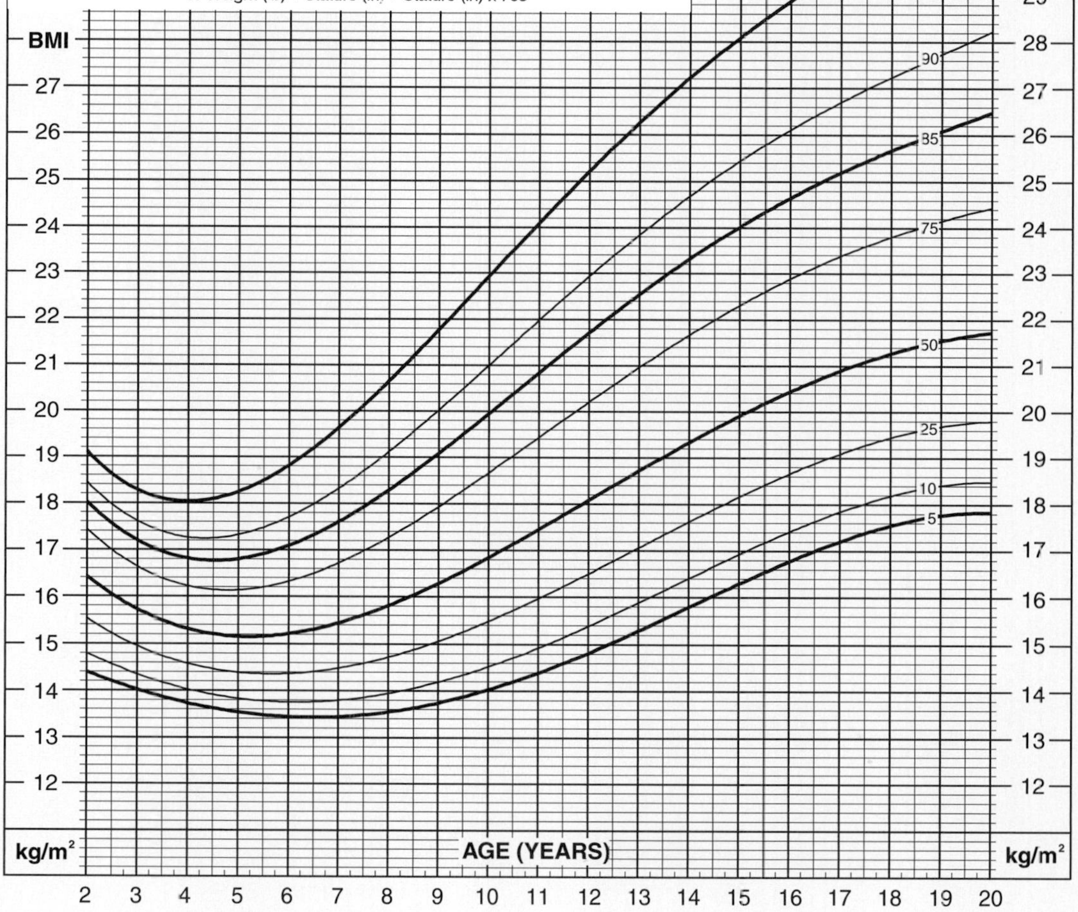

BMI

95
90
85
75
50
25
10
5

BMI

kg/m²

AGE (YEARS)

kg/m²

2 3 4 5 6 7 8 9 10 11 12 13 14 15 16 17 18 19 20

Published May 30, 2000 (modified 10/16/00).
SOURCE: Developed by the National Center for Health Statistics in collaboration with
the National Center for Chronic Disease Prevention and Health Promotion (2000).
http://www.cdc.gov/growthcharts

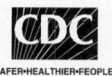

Tanner Stages of Adolescent Development for Girls

Chronologic age is not always the best way to assess adolescent growth because of individual variations in beginning and completing the growth sequence. A more useful way of describing pubertal development, and thus the varying needs for nutrients throughout adolescence, is to divide growth into stages of breast and pubic hair development in girls. These are termed the *Tanner Stages of Adolescent Development.* Nutritional requirements vary, depending on the stage of development.

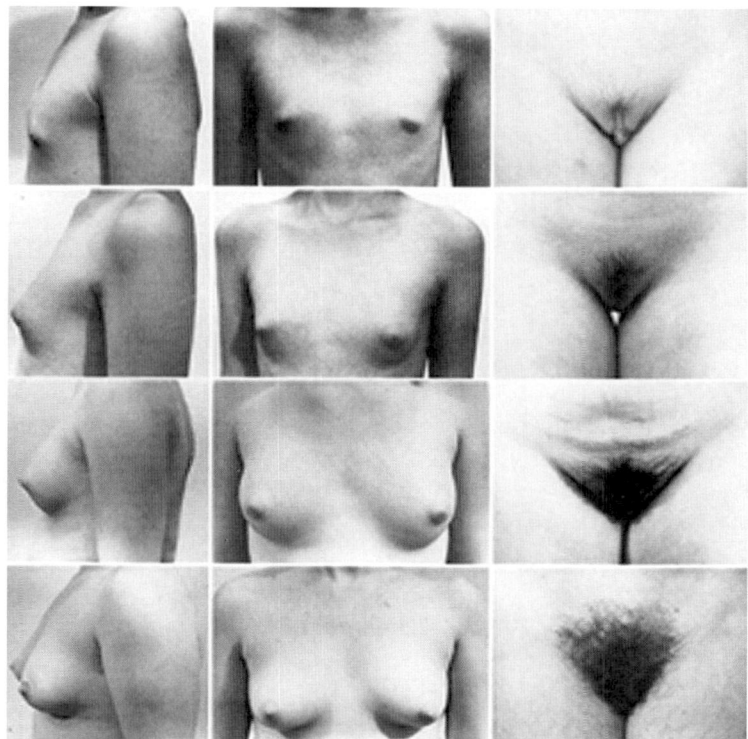

From Mahan LK, Rees JM: Nutrition in adolescence, St Louis, 1984, Mosby.

Tanner Stages of Adolescent Development for Boys

Chronologic age is not always the best way to assess adolescent growth because of individual variations in beginning and completing the growth sequence. A more useful way of describing pubertal development, and thus the varying needs for nutrients throughout adolescence, is to divide growth into stages pubic hair and penis and testicle development in boys. These are termed the *Tanner Stages of Adolescent Development*. Nutritional requirements vary, depending on the stage of development.

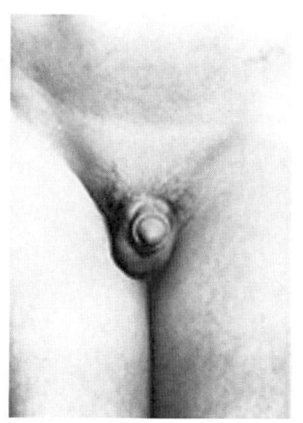 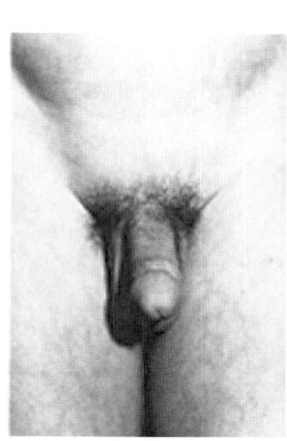 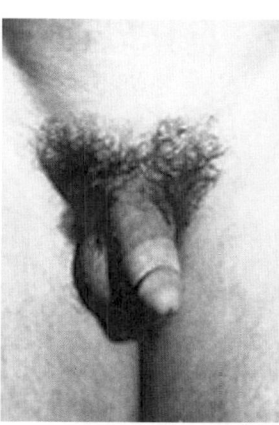 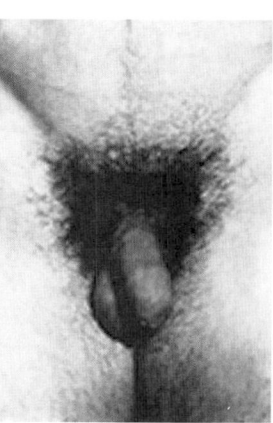

From Mahan LK, Rees JM: *Nutrition in adolescence*, St. Louis, 1984, Mosby.

Direct Methods for Measuring Height and Weight

HEIGHT

1. Height should be measured without shoes.
2. The individual's feet should be together, with the heels against the wall or measuring board.
3. The individual should stand erect, neither slumped nor stretching, looking straight ahead, without tipping the head up or down. The top of the ear and outer corner of the eye should be in a line parallel to the floor (the "Frankfort plane").
4. A horizontal bar, a rectangular block of wood, or the top of the statiometer should be lowered to rest flat on the top of the head.
5. Height should be read to the nearest ¼ inch or 0.5 cm.

WEIGHT

1. Scale accuracy must be determined. Frequent calibration is required.
2. Use a beam balance scale, not a spring scale, whenever possible.
3. Weigh the subject in light clothing without shoes.
4. Record weight to the nearest ½ lb or 0.2 kg for adults and ¼ lb or 0.1 kg for infants. Measurements above the 90th percentile or below the 10th percentile warrant further evaluation.

*When weighing patients on bed scales, see manufacturer guidelines for directions.

Indirect Methods for Measuring Height

MEASURING ARM SPAN

Steps:

1. The arms are extended straight out to the sides at a 90-degree angle from the body.
2. The distance from the longest fingertip of one hand to the longest finger of the other hand is measured.

ADULT RECUMBENT

Steps:

1. Stand on right side of the body.
2. Align body so that the lower extremities, trunk, shoulders, and head are straight.
3. Place a mark at the top of the sheet in line with the crown of the head and one at the bottom of the sheet in line with the base of the heels.
4. Measure length between marks with measuring tape.

KNEE HEIGHT

Knee height measurement is highly correlated with upright height. It is useful in those who cannot stand and in those who may have curvatures of the spine.

Steps:

1. Use the left leg for measurements.
2. Bend the left knee and the left ankle to 90-degree angles. A triangle may be used if available.
3. Using knee height calipers, open the caliper and place the fixed part under the heel. Place the sliding blade down against the thigh (approximately 2 inches behind the patella).
4. Measure from the heel to the anterior surface of the thigh, using a cloth measuring tape.

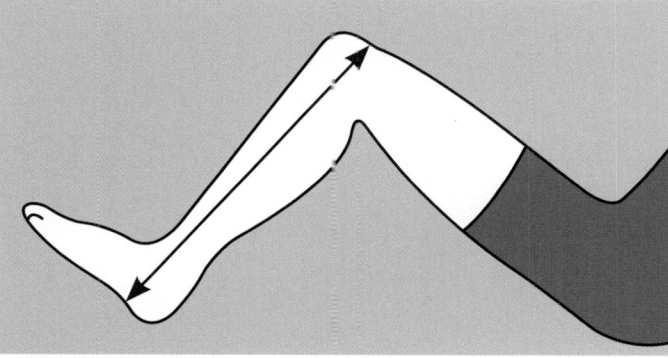

5. Obtain the measurement and convert it to centimeters by multiplying by 2.54.
6. Formulas to use to calculate estimated height from knee height:

Men (height in centimeters) 64.19 (0.04 Age) + (2.02 × Knee height in centimeters)

Women (height in centimeters) 84.8 (0.24 Age) + (1.83 × Knee height in centimeters)

Using Population-Specific Formula, Calculate Height from Standard Formula:

Population and Gender Group	Equation: Stature (cm) =
Non-Hispanic white men (U.S.)[11] [SEE = 3.74 cm]	78.31 + (1.94 × knee height) − (0.14 × age)
Non-Hispanic black men (U.S.)[11] [SEE = 3.80 cm]	79.69 + (1.35 × knee height) − (0.14 × age)
Mexican-American men (U.S.)[11] [SEE = 3.68 cm]	82.77 + (1.83 × knee height) − (0.16 × age)
Non-Hispanic white women (U.S.)[11] [SEE = 3.98 cm]	82.21 + (1.85 × knee height) − (0.21 × age)
Non-Hispanic black women (U.S.)[11] [SEE = 3.82 cm]	89.58 + (1.61 × knee height) − (0.17 × age)
Mexican-American women (U.S.)[11] [SEE = 3.77 cm]	84.25 + (1.82 × knee height) − (0.26 × age)
Taiwanese men[12] [SEE = 3.86 cm]	85.10 + (1.73 × knee height) − (0.11 × age)
Taiwanese women[12] [SEE = 3.79 cm]	91.45 + (1.53 × knee height) − (0.16 × age)
Elderly Italian men[13] [SEE = 4.3 cm]	94.87 + (1.58 × knee height) − (0.23 × age) + 4.8
Elderly Italian women[13] [SEE = 4.3 cm]	94.87 + (1.58 × knee height) − (0.23 × age)
French men[14] [SEE = 3.8 cm]	74.7 + (2.07 × knee height) − (−0.21 × age)
French women[14] [SEE = 3.5 cm]	67.00 + (2.2 × knee height) − (0.25 × age)
Mexican Men[15] [SEE = 3.31 cm]	52.6 + (2.17 × knee height)
Mexican Women[15] [SEE = 2.99 cm]	73.70 + (1.99 × knee height) − (0.23 × age)
Filipino Men[16]	96.50 + (1.38 × knee height) − (0.08 × age)
Filipino Women[16]	89.63 + (1.53 × knee height) − (0.17 × age)
Malaysian men[17] [SEE = 3.51 cm]	(1.924 × knee height) + 69.38
Malaysian women[17] [SEE = 3.40]	(2.225 × knee height) + 50.25

SEE = Standard Error of Estimate[11]

REFERENCES

Guigoz Y, Vellas B, Garry PJ: Assessing the nutritional status of the elderly: The Mini Nutritional Assessment as part of the geriatric evaluation, *Nutr Rev* 54:S59–S65, 1996.

Fallon C, Bruce I, Eustace A, et al: Nutritional status of community dwelling subjects attending a memory clinic, *J Nutr Health Aging* 6(Suppl):21, 2002.

Kagansky N, Berner Y, Koren-Morag N, Perelman L, Knobler H, Levy S: Poor nutritional habits are predictors of poor outcomes in very old hospitalized patients, *Am J Clin Nutr* 82:784–791, 2005.

Vellas B, Villars H, Abellan G, et al: Overview of the MNA® – It's history and challenges, *J Nutr Health Aging* 10:456–463, 2006.

Guigoz Y, Vellas J, Garry P: Mini Nutritional Assessment: A practical assessment tool for grading the nutritional state of elderly patients, *Facts Res Gerontol* 4(Suppl 2):15–59, 1994.

Guigoz Y: The Mini-Nutritional Assessment (MNA®) review of the literature – what does it tell us? *J Nutr Health Aging* 10:466–485, 2006.

Murphy MC, Brooks CN, New SA, Lumbers ML: The use of the Mini Nutritional Assessment (MNA) tool in elderly orthopaedic patients, *Eur J Clin Nutr* 54:555–562, 2000.

Kaiser MJ, Bauer JM, Ramsch C, et al: Validation of the Mini Nutritional Assessment Short-Form(MNA®-SF): A practical tool for identification of nutritional status, *J Nutr Health Aging* 13:782–788, 2009.

HIckson M, Frost G: A comparison of three methods for estimating height in the acutely ill elderly population, *J Hum Nutr Diet* 6:1–3, 2003.

Kwok T, Whjitelaw MN: The use of armspan in nutritional assessment of the elderly, *J Am Geriatric Soc* 39:492–496, 1991.

Chumlea WC, Guo SS, Wholihan K, Cockram D, Kuczmarski RJ, Johnson CL: Stature prediction equations for elderly non-Hispanic white, non-Hispanic black, and Mexican-American persons developed from NHANES III data, *J Am Diet Assoc* 98:137–142, 1998.

Cheng HS, See LC, Sheih YH: Estimating stature from knee height for adults in Taiwan, *Chang Gung Med J* 24:547–556, 2001.

Donini LM, de Felice MR, De Bernardini L, et al: Prediction of stature in the Italian elderly, *J Nutr Health Aging* 4:72–76, 2000.

Guo SS, Wu X, Vellas B, Guigoz Y, Chumlea WC: Prediction of stature in the French elderly, *Age & Nutr* 5:169–173, 1994.

Mendoza-Nunez VM, Sanchez-Rodrigez MA, Cervantes-Sandoval A, et al: Equations for predicting height for elderly Mexican-Americans are not applicable for elderly Mexicans, *Am J Hum Biol* 14:351–355, 2002.

Tanchoco CC, Duante CA, Lopez ES: Arm span and knee height as proxy indicators for height, *J Nutritionist-Dietitians' Assoc Philippines* 15:84–90, 2001.

Shahar S, Pooy NS: Predictive equations for estimation of statue in Malaysian elderly people, *Asia Pac J Clin Nutr* 12(1):80–84, 2003.

Lefton J, Malone A: Anthropometric Assessment. In Charney P, Malone A, editors: *ADA Pocket Guide to Nutrition Assessment*, ed 2, Chicago, IL, 2009, American Dietetic Association, pp 160–161.

Osterkamp LK: Current perspective on assessment of human body proportions of relevance to amputees, *J Am Diet Assoc* 95:215–218, 1995.

Determination of Frame Size

Method 1: Height is recorded without shoes. Wrist circumference is measured just distal to the styloid process at the wrist crease on the right arm, using a tape measure. The following formula is used (From Grant JP: Handbook of total parenteral nutrition, Philadelphia, 1980, Saunders):

$$r = \frac{\text{Height (cm)}}{\text{Wrist circumstance (cm)}}$$

Frame size can be determined as follows:

Males	Females
r >10.4 small	r >11.0 small
r = 9.6-10.4 medium	r = 10.1-11.0 medium
r < 9.6 large	r <10.1 large

Method 2: The patient's right arm is extended forward perpendicular to the body, with the arm bent so the angle at the elbow forms 90 degrees with the fingers pointing up and the palm turned away from the body. The greatest breadth across the elbow joint is measured with a sliding caliper along the axis of the upper arm on the two prominent bones on either side of the elbow. This is recorded as the elbow breadth. The following tables give the elbow breadth measurements for medium-framed men and women of various heights (from Metropolitan Life Insurance Co., 1983). Measurements lower than those listed indicate a small frame size; higher measurements indicate a large frame size.

MEN		WOMEN	
Height in 1" Heels	**Elbow Breadth (inches)**	**Height in 1" Heels**	**Elbow Breadth (inches)**
5'2"-5'3"	2½-2⅞	4'10"-4'11"	2¼-2½
5'4"-5'7"	2⅝-2⅞	5'0"-5'3"	2¼-2½
5'8"-5'11"	2¾-3	5'4"-5'7"	2⅜-2⅝
6'0"-6'3"	2¾-3⅛	5'8"-5'11"	2⅜-2⅝
6'4"	2⅞-3¼	6'0"	

Adjustment of Desirable Body Weight for Amputees

The percentages listed here are estimates because body proportions vary in individuals. Use of these percentages provides an approximation of desirable body weight, which is more accurate than a comparison with the standards for adults without amputations. Ideal body weight (IBW) must be adjusted downward to compensate for missing limbs or paralysis. It is estimated that 5% to 10% should be subtracted from IBW for a paraplegic and from 10% to 15% subtracted for a tetraplegic (quadriplegic.)

Adjustment of Ideal Body Weight for Amputees

Body Segment	Average % of Total Weight
Lower arm and hand	2.3
Trunk without extremities	50.0
Entire arm	5.0
Hand	0.7
Entire lower leg	16.0
Below knee including foot	5.9
Lower leg without foot	4.4
Foot	1.5

Lefton J., Malone A. Anthropometric Assessment. In Charney P, Malone A, eds. ADA Pocket Guide to Nutrition Assessment, 2nd edition. Chicago, IL: American Dietetic Association; 2009:160.

$$\text{Estimated IBW} = \frac{100 - \% \text{ amputation}}{100} \times \text{IBW for original height}$$

To use this information, determine the patient's approximate height before the amputation. Span measurement is a rough estimate of height at maturity and is calculated as follows: with the upper extremities, including the hands, fully extended and parallel to the ground, measure the distance between the tip of one middle finger and the tip of the other middle finger. Use this height or actual measurement to calculate the desirable body weight for the normal body size; then adjust the figures according to the type of amputation performed.

Example: To determine the desirable body weight for a 5'10" male with a below-the-knee amputation:

1. Calculate desirable body weight for a 5'10" male:	166 lb
2. Subtract weight of amputated limb (6%) = 166 × 0.06:	$\dfrac{-9.96}{156\,\text{lb}}$ (approx. 10 lb)
3. Desirable weight of a 5'10" male with a below-knee amputation:	

From North Carolina Dietetic Association: Nutrition care manual, 2011, Raleigh, NC, The Association.

Body Mass Index Table

BMI	NORMAL WEIGHT						OVERWEIGHT					OBESE					
	19	20	21	22	23	24	25	26	27	28	29	30	31	32	33	34	35
Height									Weight (in pounds)								
4'10" (58")	91	96	100	105	110	115	119	124	129	134	138	143	148	153	158	162	167
4'11" (59")	94	99	104	109	114	119	124	128	133	138	143	148	153	158	163	168	173
5' (60")	97	102	107	112	118	123	128	133	138	143	148	153	158	163	168	174	179
5'1" (61")	100	106	111	116	122	127	132	137	143	148	153	158	164	169	174	180	185
5'2" (62")	104	109	115	120	126	131	136	142	147	153	158	164	169	175	180	186	191
5'3" (63")	107	113	118	124	130	135	141	146	152	158	163	169	175	180	186	191	197
5'4" (64")	110	116	122	128	134	140	145	151	157	163	169	174	180	186	192	197	204
5'5" (65")	114	120	126	132	138	144	150	156	162	168	174	180	186	192	198	204	210
5'6" (66")	118	124	130	136	142	148	155	161	167	173	179	186	192	198	204	210	216
5'7" (67")	121	127	134	140	146	153	159	166	172	178	185	191	198	204	211	217	223
5'8" (68")	125	131	138	144	151	158	164	171	177	184	190	197	203	210	216	223	230
5'9" (69")	128	135	142	149	155	162	169	176	182	189	196	203	209	216	223	230	236
5'10" (70")	132	139	146	153	160	167	174	181	188	195	202	209	216	222	229	236	243
5'11" (71")	136	143	150	157	165	172	179	186	193	200	208	215	222	229	236	243	250
6' (72")	140	147	154	162	169	177	184	191	199	206	213	221	228	235	242	250	258
6'1" (73")	144	151	159	166	174	182	189	197	204	212	219	227	235	242	250	257	265
6'2" (74")	148	155	163	171	179	186	194	202	210	218	225	233	241	249	256	264	272
6'3" (75")	152	160	168	176	184	192	200	208	216	224	232	240	248	256	264	272	279

Data from National Institutes of Health and National Heart, Lung, and Blood Institute: Evidence report of clinical guidelines on the identification, evaluation, and treatment of overweight and obesity in adults, Bethesda, MD, 1998, NIH/NHLBI. For a BMI of greater than 35, please go to http://www.nhlbi.nih.gov/health/educational/lose_wt/BMI/bmi_tbl2.htm.

Percentage of Body Fat Based on Four Skinfold Measurements*

Sum of Skinfolds (mm)	MALES (AGE IN YEARS)				FEMALES (AGE IN YEARS)			
	17-29	30-39	40-49	50+	16-29	30-39	40-49	50+
15	4.8	—	—	—	10.5	—	—	—
20	8.1	12.2	12.2	12.6	14.1	17.0	19.8	21.4
25	10.5	14.2	15.0	15.6	16.8	19.4	22.2	24.0
30	12.9	16.2	17.7	18.6	19.5	21.8	24.5	26.6
35	14.7	17.7	19.6	20.8	21.5	23.7	26.4	28.5
40	16.4	19.2	21.4	22.9	23.4	25.5	28.2	30.3
45	17.7	20.4	23.0	24.7	25.0	26.9	29.6	31.9
50	19.0	21.5	24.6	26.5	26.5	28.2	31.0	33.4
55	20.1	22.5	25.9	27.9	27.8	29.4	32.1	34.6
60	21.2	23.5	27.1	29.2	29.1	30.6	33.2	35.7
65	22.2	24.3	28.2	30.4	30.2	31.6	34.1	36.7
70	23.1	25.1	29.3	31.6	31.2	32.5	35.0	37.7
75	24.0	25.9	30.3	32.7	32.2	33.4	35.9	38.7
80	24.8	26.6	31.2	33.8	33.1	34.3	36.7	39.6
85	25.5	27.2	32.1	34.8	34.0	35.1	37.5	40.4
90	26.2	27.8	33.0	35.8	34.8	35.8	38.3	41.2
95	26.9	28.4	33.7	36.6	35.6	36.5	39.0	41.9
100	27.6	29.0	34.4	37.4	36.4	37.2	39.7	42.6
105	28.2	29.6	35.1	38.2	37.1	37.9	40.4	43.3
110	28.8	30.1	35.8	39.0	37.8	38.6	41.0	43.9
115	29.4	30.6	36.4	39.7	38.4	39.1	41.5	44.5
120	30.0	31.1	37.0	40.4	39.0	39.6	42.0	45.1
125	30.5	31.5	37.6	41.1	39.6	40.1	42.5	45.7
130	31.0	31.9	38.2	41.8	40.2	40.6	43.0	46.2
135	31.5	32.3	38.7	42.4	40.8	41.1	43.5	46.7
140	32.0	32.7	39.2	43.0	41.3	41.6	44.0	47.2
145	32.5	33.1	39.7	43.6	41.8	42.1	44.5	47.7
150	32.9	33.5	40.2	44.1	42.3	42.6	45.0	48.2
155	33.3	33.9	40.7	44.6	42.8	43.1	45.4	48.7
160	33.7	34.3	41.2	45.1	43.3	43.6	45.8	49.2
165	34.1	34.6	41.6	45.6	43.7	44.0	46.2	49.6
170	34.5	34.8	42.0	46.1	44.1	44.4	46.6	50.0
175	34.9	—	—	—	—	44.8	47.0	50.4
180	35.3	—	—	—	—	45.2	47.4	50.8
185	35.6	—	—	—	—	45.6	47.8	51.2
190	35.9	—	—	—	—	45.9	48.2	51.6
195	—	—	—	—	—	46.2	48.5	52.0
200	—	—	—	—	—	46.5	48.8	52.4
205	—	—	—	—	—	—	49.1	52.7
210	—	—	—	—	—	—	49.4	53.0

From Durnin JVGA, Wormersley J: Body fat assessed from total body density and its estimation from skinfold thickness: measurements on 481 men and women ages 16-72 years, Br J Nutr 32:77, 1974.

Measurements made on the right side of the body, using biceps, triceps, subscapular, and suprailiac skinfolds.

Physical Activity and Calories Expended per Hour

Activity	Type	BODY WEIGHT (110 lb)	(130 lb)	(150 lb)	(170 lb)	(190 lb)	(210 lb)	(230 lb)	(250 lb)
Aerobics class	Water	210	248	286	325	364	401	439	477
Aerobics class	Low impact	263	310	358	406	455	501	549	596
Aerobics class	High impact	368	434	501	568	637	702	768	835
Aerobics class	Step with 6- to 8-inch step	446	527	609	690	774	852	933	1014
Aerobics class	Step with 10- to 12-inch step	525	621	716	812	910	1003	1097	1193
Backpack	General	368	434	501	568	637	702	768	835
Badminton	Singles and doubles	236	279	322	365	410	451	494	537
Badminton	Competitive	368	434	501	568	637	702	768	835
Baseball	Throw, catch	131	155	179	203	228	251	274	298
Baseball	Fast or slow pitch	263	310	358	406	455	501	549	596
Basketball	Shooting baskets	236	279	322	365	410	451	494	537
Basketball	Wheelchair	341	403	465	528	592	652	713	775
Basketball	Game	420	496	573	649	728	802	878	954
Bike	10-11.9 mph, slow	315	372	430	487	546	602	658	716
Bike	12-13.9 mph, moderate	420	496	573	649	728	802	878	954
Bike	14-15.9 mph, fast	525	621	716	812	910	1003	1097	1193
Bike	16-19.9 mph, very fast	630	745	859	974	1092	1203	1317	1431
Bike	>20 mph, racing	840	993	1146	1299	1457	1604	1756	1908
Bike	50 watts, stationary, very light	158	133	215	243	273	301	329	358
Bike	100 watts, stationary, light	289	341	394	446	501	552	603	656
Bike	150 watts, stationary, moderate	368	434	501	568	637	702	768	835
Bike	200 watts, stationary, vigorous	551	652	752	852	956	1053	1152	1252
Bike	250 watts, stationary, very vigorous	656	776	895	1015	1138	1253	1372	1491
Bike	BMX or mountain	446	527	609	690	774	852	933	1014
Boxing	Punching bag	315	372	430	487	546	602	658	716
Boxing	Sparring	473	558	644	730	819	902	988	1074
Calisthenics	Back exercises	184	217	251	284	319	351	384	417
Calisthenics	Pull-ups, jumping jacks	420	496	573	649	728	802	878	954
Calisthenics	Push-ups or sit-ups	420	496	573	649	728	802	878	954
Circuit training	General	420	496	573	649	728	802	878	954
Football	Flag or touch	420	496	573	649	728	802	878	954
Football	Competitive	473	558	644	730	819	902	988	1074
Frisbee	General	158	133	215	243	273	301	329	358
Frisbee	Ultimate	420	496	573	649	728	802	878	954
Golf	Power cart	184	217	251	284	319	351	384	417
Golf	Pull clubs	226	267	308	349	391	431	472	513
Golf	Carry clubs	236	279	322	365	410	451	494	537
Handball	General	630	745	859	974	1092	1203	1317	1431
Hike	General	315	372	460	487	546	602	658	716
Hockey	Ice, field hockey	420	496	573	649	728	802	878	954
Jog	General	368	434	501	568	637	702	768	835
Jog	Jog-walk combination	315	372	430	487	546	602	658	716
Jump rope	Slow	420	496	573	649	728	802	878	954
Jump rope	Moderate	525	621	716	812	910	1003	1097	1193
Jump rope	Fast	630	745	859	974	1092	1203	1317	1431
Kayak	General	263	310	358	406	455	501	549	596

Continued

Activity	Type	BODY WEIGHT							
		(110 lb)	(130 lb)	(150 lb)	(170 lb)	(190 lb)	(210 lb)	(230 lb)	(250 lb)
Martial arts	General	525	621	716	812	910	1003	1097	1193
Racquetball	Casual	368	434	501	568	637	702	768	835
Racquetball	Competition	525	621	716	812	910	1003	1097	1193
Rafting	Whitewater	263	310	358	406	455	501	549	596
Rock climb	General	420	496	573	649	728	802	878	954
Rugby	General	525	621	716	812	910	1003	1097	1193
Run	5 mph, 12 min/mile	420	496	573	649	728	802	878	954
Run	5.2 mph, 11.5 min/mile	473	558	644	730	819	902	988	1074
Run	6 mph, 10 min/mile	525	621	716	812	910	1003	1097	1193
Run	6.7 mph, 9 min/mile	578	683	788	893	1001	1103	1207	1312
Run	7 mph, 8.5 min/mile	604	714	824	933	1047	1153	1262	1372
Run	7.5 mph, 8 min/mile	656	776	895	1015	1138	1253	1372	1491
Run	8 mph, 7.5 min/mile	709	838	967	1096	1229	1354	1481	1610
Run	8.6 mph, 7 min/mile	735	869	1003	1136	1274	1404	1536	1670
Run	9 mph, 6.5 min/mile	788	931	1074	1217	1366	1504	1646	1789
Run	10 mph, 6 min/mile	840	993	1146	1299	1457	1604	1756	1908
Run	10.9 mph, 5.5 min/mile	945	1117	1289	1461	1639	1805	1975	2147
Run	Cross country	473	558	644	730	819	902	988	1074
Skate, ice	General	368	434	501	568	637	702	768	835
Skate, inline	Inline, general	656	776	895	1015	1138	1253	1372	1491
Skateboard	General	263	310	358	406	455	501	549	596
Ski, downhill	Light	263	310	358	406	455	501	549	596
Ski, downhill	Moderate	315	372	430	487	546	602	658	716
Ski, downhill	Vigorous, race	420	496	573	649	728	802	878	954
Ski machine	General	368	434	501	568	637	702	768	835
Ski, cross-country	2.5 mph, slow	368	434	501	568	637	702	768	835
Ski, cross-country	4-4.9 mph, moderate	420	496	573	649	728	802	878	954
Ski, cross-country	5-7.9 mph, brisk	473	558	644	730	819	902	988	1074
Snowboard	General	394	465	537	609	683	752	823	895
Snowshoe	General	420	496	573	649	728	802	878	954
Soccer	Casual	368	434	501	568	637	702	768	835
Soccer	Competitive	525	621	716	812	910	1003	1097	1193
Softball	General	263	310	358	406	455	501	549	596
Stair stepper	General	473	558	644	730	819	902	988	1074
Stationary rower	50 watts, light	184	217	251	284	319	351	384	417
Stationary rower	100 watts, moderate	368	434	501	568	637	702	768	835
Stationary rower	150 watts, vigorous	446	527	609	690	774	852	933	1014
Stationary rower	200 watts, very vigorous	630	745	859	974	1092	1203	1317	1431
Stretch, yoga	General, Hatha	131	155	179	203	228	251	274	298
Swim	Lake, ocean, or river	315	372	430	487	546	602	658	716
Swim	Laps freestyle, slow or moderate	368	434	501	568	637	702	768	835
Swim	Laps freestyle, fast	525	621	716	812	910	1003	1097	1193
Swim	Backstroke	368	434	501	568	637	702	768	835
Swim	Sidestroke	420	496	573	649	728	802	878	954
Swim	Breaststroke	525	621	716	812	910	1003	1097	1193
Swim	Butterfly	578	683	788	893	1001	1103	1207	1312
Tennis	Doubles	315	372	430	487	546	602	658	716
Tennis	Singles	420	496	573	649	728	802	878	954
Treadmill, run	6 mph, 10 min/mile, 0% incline	525	621	716	812	910	1003	1097	1193
Treadmill, run	6 mph, 10 min/mile, 2% incline	578	683	788	893	1001	1103	1207	1312
Treadmill, run	6 mph, 10 min/mile, 4% incline	620	732	845	958	1074	1183	1295	1408
Treadmill, run	6 mph, 10 min/mile, 6% incline	667	788	909	1031	1156	1273	1394	1515
Treadmill, run	7 mph, 8.5 min/mile, 0% incline	604	714	824	933	1047	1153	1262	1372
Treadmill, run	7 mph, 8.5 min/mile, 2% incline	667	788	909	1031	1156	1273	1394	1515
Treadmill, run	7 mph, 8.5 min/mile, 4% incline	719	850	981	1112	1247	1374	1503	1634
Treadmill, run	7 mph, 8.5 min/mile, 6% incline	767	906	1046	1185	1329	1464	1602	1741
Treadmill, run	8 mph, 7.5 min/mile, 0% incline	709	838	967	1096	1229	1354	1481	1610

Activity	Type	BODY WEIGHT							
		(110 lb)	(130 lb)	(150 lb)	(170 lb)	(190 lb)	(210 lb)	(230 lb)	(250 lb)
Treadmill, run	8 mph, 7.5 min/mile, 2% incline	756	894	1031	1169	1311	1444	1580	1718
Treadmill, run	8 mph, 7.5 min/mile, 4% incline	814	962	1110	1258	1411	1554	1701	1849
Treadmill, run	8 mph, 7.5 min/mile, 6% incline	872	1030	1189	1347	1511	1665	1821	1980
Treadmill, run	3 mph, 20 min/mile, 0% incline	173	205	236	268	300	331	362	394
Treadmill, run	3 mph, 20 min/mile, 2% incline	194	230	265	300	337	371	406	441
Treadmill, run	3 mph, 20 min/mile, 4% incline	215	254	293	333	373	411	450	489
Treadmill, run	3 mph, 20 min/mile, 6% incline	236	279	322	365	410	451	494	537
Treadmill, run	4 mph, 15 min/mile, 0% incline	263	310	358	406	455	501	549	596
Treadmill, run	4 mph, 15 min/mile, 2% incline	294	348	401	455	510	562	614	668
Treadmill, run	4 mph, 15 min/mile, 4% incline	326	385	444	503	564	622	680	740
Treadmill, run	4 mph, 15 min/mile, 6% incline	352	416	480	544	610	672	735	799
Tread water	Moderate	210	248	286	325	364	401	439	477
Tread water	Vigorous	525	621	716	812	910	1003	1097	1193
Volleyball	Noncompetitive	158	133	215	243	273	301	329	358
Volleyball	Competitive	420	496	573	649	728	802	878	954
Walk	<2 mph	105	124	143	162	182	201	219	239
Walk	2 mph, 30 min/mile	131	155	179	203	228	251	274	298
Walk	2.5 mph, 24 min/mile	158	133	215	243	273	301	329	358
Walk	3 mph, 20 min/mile	173	205	236	268	300	331	362	394
Walk	3.5 mph, 17 min/mile	200	236	272	308	346	381	417	453
Walk	4 mph, 15 min/mile	263	310	358	406	455	501	549	596
Walk	4.5 mph, 13 min/mile	331	391	451	511	574	632	691	751
Walk	Race walking	341	403	465	528	592	652	713	775
Water polo	General	525	621	716	812	910	1003	1097	1193
Weight training	Free, nautilus, light/ moderate	158	133	215	243	273	301	329	358
Weight training	Free, nautilus, vigorous	315	372	430	487	546	602	658	716
Wind surf	Casual	158	133	215	243	273	301	329	358

NOTE: This chart is not intended to be a comprehensive list for all nutritional or metabolic deficiencies or nonnutrition examples.
From Hammond K: Physical assessment: a nutritional perspective, Nurs Clin North Am 32(4):779, 1997.

Nutrition-Focused Physical Assessment

PART 1: Parameters Useful in the Assessment of General Nutritional Status and the Presence of Malnutrition

Exam Areas	Tips	Severe Malnutrition	Mild-Moderate Malnutrition	Well Nourished
Subcutaneous Fat Loss				
Orbital Region – Surrounding the Eye	View patient when standing directly in front of them, touch above cheekbone	Hollow look, depressions, dark circles, loose skin	Slightly dark circles, somewhat hollow look	Slightly bulged fat pads. Fluid retention may mask loss
Upper Arm Region – Triceps/biceps	Arm bent, roll skin between fingers, do not include muscle in pinch	Very little space between folds, fingers touch	Some depth pinch, but not ample	Ample fat tissue obvious between folds of skin
Thoracic and Lumbar Region – Ribs, Lower Back, Midaxillary line	Have patient press hands hard against a solid object	Depression between the ribs very apparent. Iliac Crest very prominent	Ribs apparent, depressions between them less pronounced. Iliac Crest somewhat prominent	Chest is full, ribs do not show. Slight to no protrusion of the iliac crest.
Muscle Loss				
Temple Region – Temporalis Muscle	View patient when standing directly in front of them, ask patient to turn head side to side	Hollowing, scooping, depression	Slight depression	Can see/feel well-defined muscle
Clavicle Bone Region – Pectoralis Major, Deltoid, Trapezius Muscles	Look for prominent bone. Make sure patient is not hunched forward	Protruding, prominent bone	Visible in male, some protrusion in female	Not visible in male, visible but not prominent in female
Clavicle and Acromion Bone Region – Deltoid Muscle	Patient arms at side; observe shape	Shoulder to arm joint looks square. Bones prominent. Acromion protrusion very prominent	Acromion process may slightly protrude	Rounded, curves at arm/shoulder/neck
Scapular Bone Region – Trapezius, Supraspinus, Infraspinus Muscles	Ask patient to extend hands straight out, push against solid object	Prominent, visible bones, depressions between ribs/scapula or shoulder/spine	Mild depression or bone may show slightly	Bones not prominent, no significant depressions
Dorsal Hand – Interosseous Muscle	Look at thumb side of hand; look at pads of thumb when tip of forefinger touching tip of thumb	Depressed area between thumb-forefinger	Slightly depressed	Muscle bulges, could be flat in some well nourished people
Lower Body Less Sensitive to Change				
Patellar Region – Quadricep Muscle	Ask patient to sit with leg propped up, bent at knee	Bones prominent, little sign of muscle around knee	Kneecap less prominent, more rounded	Muscles protrude, bones not prominent
Anterior Thigh Region – Quadriceps Muscles	Ask patient to sit, prop leg up on low furniture. Grasp quads to differentiate amount of muscle tissue from fat tissue	Depression/line on thigh, obviously thin	Mild depression on inner thigh	Well rounded, well developed
Posterior Calf Region- Gastrocnemius Muscle	Grasp the calf muscle to determine amount of tissue	Thin, minimal to no muscle definition	Not well developed	Well-developed bulb of muscle

Continued

PART 1: Parameters Useful in the Assessment of General Nutritional Status and the Presence of Malnutrition—cont'd

Exam Areas	Tips	Severe Malnutrition	Mild-Moderate Malnutrition	Well Nourished
Edema Rule out other causes of edema, patient at dry weight	View scrotum/vulva in activity restricted patient; ankles in mobile patient	Deep to very deep pitting, depression lasts a short to moderate time (31-60 sec) extremity looks swollen (3-4+)	Mild to moderate pitting, slight swelling of the extremity, indentation subsides quickly (0-30 sec)	No sign of fluid accumulation

Notes:
1. Introduce yourself to the patient/family
2. Provide rationale for examination request
3. Ask the patient for permission to examine them
4. Wash/dry hands thoroughly; wear gloves
5. Use standard precautions to prevent disease transmission

References:
1. McCann L. Subjective global assessment as it pertains to the nutritional status of dialysis patients. *Dialysis & Transplantation.* 1996; 25(4):190-202.
2. Council on Renal Nutrition of the National Kidney Foundation. *Pocket Guide to Nutrition Assessment of the Patient with Chronic Kidney Disease,* 3rd ed. (McCann, L, ed.) 2005 Last accessed 5/30/12 at http://www.scribd.com/doc/6991983/Pocket-Guide-to-Nut-Crd
3. Secker DJ, JeeJeebhoy KN. How to perform subjective global nutritional assessment in children. *J Acad Nutr Diet* 2012;(112):424-431.
This table was developed by Jane White, PhD, RD, FADA, LDN, Louise Merriman, MS, RD, CDN, Terese Scollard, MBA, RD and the Cleveland Clinic Center for Human Nutrition, Content was approved by the Adult Malnutrition Education and Outreach Committee, a joint effort of the Academy of Nutrition and Dietetics and the American Society of Parenteral and Enteral Nutrition.
©2013 Academy of Nutrition and Dietetics. Malnutrition Coding in Biesemeier, C.. Ed. Nutrition Care Manual, October, 2013 release.

Part 2: Clinical Characteristics That the Clinician Can Obtain and Document to Support a Diagnosis of Malnutrition (Academy/A.S.P.E.N.)

Clinical Characteristic	MALNUTRITION IN THE CONTEXT OF SOCIAL OR ENVIRONMENTAL CIRCUMSTANCES		MALNUTRITION IN THE CONTEXT OF CHRONIC ILLNESS		MALNUTRITION IN THE CONTEXT OF ACUTE ILLNESS OR INJURY	
	Nonsevere (Moderate) Malnutrition	Severe Malnutrition	Nonsevere (Moderate) Malnutrition	Severe Malnutrition	Nonsevere (Moderate) Malnutrition	Severe Malnutrition
(1) Energy intake[1] Malnutrition is the result of inadequate food and nutrient intake or assimilation; thus, recent intake compared with estimated requirements is a primary criterion defining malnutrition. The clinician may obtain or review the food and nutrition history, estimate optimum energy needs, compare them with estimates of energy consumed, and report inadequate intake as a percentage of estimated energy requirements over time.	<75% of estimated energy requirement for >7 days	≤50% of estimated energy requirement for ≥5 days	<75% of estimated energy requirement for ≥1 month	≤75% of estimated energy requirement for ≥1 month	<75% of estimated energy requirement for ≥3 months	≤50% of estimated energy requirement for ≥1 month

(2) Interpretation of weight loss [2-5]	%	Time	%	Time	%	Time	%	Time	%	Time	%	Time
The clinician may evaluate weight in light of other clinical findings, including the presence of under- or over-hydration. The clinician may assess weight change over time reported as a percentage of weight lost from baseline.	1–2	1 wk	>2	1 wk	5	1 mo	>5	1 mo	5	1 mo	>5	1 mo
	5	1 mo	>5	1 mo	7.5	3 mo	>7.5	3 mo	7.5	3 mo	>7.5	3 mo
	7.5	3 mo	>7.5	3 mo	10	6 mo	>10	6 mo	10	6 mo	>10	6 mo
					20	1 y	>20	1 y	20	1 y	>20	1 y

Physical Findings[5,6]
Malnutrition typically results in changes to the physical exam. The clinician may perform a physical exam and document any one of the physical exam findings below as an indicator of malnutrition

Part 2: Clinical Characteristics That the Clinician Can Obtain and Document to Support a Diagnosis of Malnutrition (Academy/A.S.P.E.N.)—cont'd

Clinical Characteristic	MALNUTRITION IN THE CONTEXT OF SOCIAL OR ENVIRONMENTAL CIRCUMSTANCES		MALNUTRITION IN THE CONTEXT OF CHRONIC ILLNESS		MALNUTRITION IN THE CONTEXT OF ACUTE ILLNESS OR INJURY	
	Nonsevere (Moderate) Malnutrition	Severe Malnutrition	Nonsevere (Moderate) Malnutrition	Severe Malnutrition	Nonsevere (Moderate) Malnutrition	Severe Malnutrition
(3) **Body fat** Loss of subcutaneous fat (eg, orbital, triceps, fat overlying the ribs)	Mild	Moderate	Mild	Severe	Mild	Severe
(4) **Muscle mass** Muscle loss (eg, wasting of the temples [temporalis muscle], clavicles [pectoralis and deltoids], shoulders [deltoids], interosseous muscles, scapula [latissimus dorsi, trapezious, deltoids], thigh [quadriceps], and calf [gastrocnemius])	Mild	Moderate	Mild	Severe	Mild	Severe
(5) **Fluid accumulation** The clinician may evaluate generalized or localized fluid accumulation evident on exam (extremities, vulvar/scrotal edema, or ascites). Weight loss is often masked by generalized fluid retention (edema), and weight gain may be observed.	Mild	Moderate to severe	Mild	Severe	Mild	Severe
(6) **Reduced grip strength**[7] Consult normative standards supplied by the manufacturer of the measurement device	NA	Measurably reduced	NA	Measurably reduced	NA	Measurably reduced

A minimum of 2 of the 6 characteristics above is recommended for diagnosis of either severe or nonsevere malnutrition. *NA*, not applicable.

Notes:
Height and weight should be measured rather than estimated to determine body mass index (BMI).
Usual weight should be obtained to determine the percentage and to interpret the significance of weight loss.
Basic indicators of nutrition status such as body weight, weight change, and appetite may substantively improve with refeeding in the absence of inflammation. Refeeding and/or nutrition support may stabilize but not significantly improve nutrition parameters in the presence of inflammation.
The National Center for Health Statistics defines *chronic* as a disease/condition lasting 3 months or longer.[8]
Serum proteins such as serum albumin and prealbumin are not included as defining characteristics of malnutrition because recent evidence analysis shows that serum levels of these proteins do not change in response to changes in nutrient intake.[9-12]

References
1. Kondrup J. Can food intake in hospitals be improved? *Clin Nutr.* 2001;20:153-160.
2. Blackburn GL, Bistrian BR, Maini BS, Schlamm HT, Smith MF. Nutritional and metabolic assessment of the hospitalized patient. *JPEN J Parenter Enteral Nutr.* 1977;1:11-22.
3. Klein S, Kinney J, Jeejeebhoy K, et al. Nutrition support in clinical practice: review of published data and recommendations for future research directions. National Institutes of Health, American Society for Parenteral and Enteral Nutrition, and American Society for Clinical Nutrition. *JPEN J Parenter Enteral Nutr.* 1977;21:133-156.
4. Rosenbaum K, Wang J, Pierson RN, Kotler DP. Time-dependent variation in weight and body composition in healthy adults. *JPEN J Parenter Enteral Nutr.* 2000;24:52-55.
5. Keys A. Chronic undernutrition and starvation with notes on protein deficiency. *JAMA.* 1948;138:500-511.
6. Sacks GS, Dearman K, Replogle WH, Cora VL, Meeks M, Canada T. Use of subjective global assessment to identify nutrition-associated complications and death in long-term care facility residents. *J Am Coll Nutr.* 2000;19:570-577.
7. Norman K, Stobaus N, Gonzalez MC, Schulzke J-D, Pirlich M. Hand grip strength: outcome predictor and marker of nutritional status. *Clin Nutr.* 2011;30:135-142.
8. Hagan JC. Acute and chronic diseases. In: Mulner RM, ed. *Encyclopedia of Health Services Research.* Vol 1. Thousand Oaks, CA: Sage; 2009:25.
9. American Dietetic Association Evidence Analysis Library. Does serum prealbumin correlate with weight loss in four models of prolonged protein-energy restriction: anorexia nervosa, non-malabsorptive gastric partitioning bariatric surgery, calorie-restricted diets or starvation. http://www.adaevidencelibrary.com/conclusion.cfm?conclusion_statement_id=251313&highlight=prealbumin&home=. Accessed August 1, 2011.
10. American Dietetic Association Evidence Analysis Library. Does serum prealbumin correlate with nitrogen balance? http://www.adaevidencelibrary.com/conclusion.cfm?conclusion_statement_id=251315&highlight=prealbumin&home=1. Accessed August 1, 2011.
11. American Dietetic Association Evidence Analysis Library. Does serum albumin correlate with weight loss in four models of prolonged protein-energy restriction: anorexia nervosa, non-malabsorptive gastric partitioning bariatric surgery, calorie-restricted diets or starvation. http://www.adaevidencelibrary.com/conclusion.cfm?conclusion_statement_id=251263&highlight=albumin&home=. Accessed August 1, 2011.
12. American Dietetic Association Evidence Analysis Library. Does serum albumin correlate with nitrogen balance? http://www.adaevidencelibrary.com/conclusion.cfm?conclusion_statement_id=251265&highlight=albumin&home=1. Accessed August 1, 2011.

This table was developed by Annalynn Skipper PhD, RD, FADA. The content was developed by an Academy workgroup composed of Jane White, PhD, RD, FADA, LDN, Chair; Maree Ferguson, MBA, PhD, RD; Sherri Jones, MS, MBA, RD, LDN; Ainsley Malone, MS, RD, LD, CNSD; Louise Merriman, MS, RD, CDN; Terese Scollard, MBA, RD; Annalynn Skipper, PhD, RD, FADA; and Academy staff member Pam Michael, MBA, RD. Content was approved by an A.S.P.E.N. committee consisting of Gordon L. Jensen, MD, PhD, Co-Chair; Ainsley Malone, MS, RD, CNSD, Co-Chair; Rose Ann Dimaria, PhD, RN, CNSN; Christine M. Framson, RD, PHD, CSND; Nilesh Mehta, MD, DCH; Steve Plogsted, PharmD, RPh, BCNSP; Annalynn Skipper, PhD, RD, FADA; Jennifer Wooley, MS, RD, CNSD; Jay Mirtallo, RPh, BCNSP, Board Liaison; and A.S.P.E.N. staff member Peggi Guenter, PhD, RN. Subsequently, it was approved by the A.S.P.E.N. Board of Directors. The information in the table is current as of February 1, 2012. Changes are anticipated as new research becomes available.
Adapted from Skipper A. Malnutrition coding. In: Skipper A, ed. *Nutrition Care Manual.* Chicago, IL: Academy of Nutrition and Dietetics; 2012. **FROM: White, JV et al: Consensus Statement: Academy of Nutrition and Dietetics and American Society for Parenteral and Enteral Nutrition: Characteristics Recommended for the Identification and Documentation of Adult Malnutrition (Undernutrition), JPEN, 36:275, 2012.**

PART 3: Nutrition-Focused Physical Examination

Mary D. Litchford, PHD, RDN, LDN
Kathleen A. Hammond, MS, RN, BSN, BSHE, RD, LD

System	Normal Findings	Abnormal Findings	Possible Nutrition and Metabolic Etiologies	Nonnutritional Etiologies
Body Habitus – See Part 1. General survey	Weight for height appropriate, well-nourished, alert, and cooperative with good stamina	Loss of weight, muscle mass and fat stores, skeletal muscle wasting (hands, face, quadriceps, and deltoids), subcutaneous fat loss (face, triceps, thighs, waist) or overall weight loss, sarcopenia (loss of lean body mass in older adults). See Part 1 Growth retardation in children Inappropriate rates of height and weight gain in children and adolescents	Sub-optimal energy and protein intakes Non-severe malnutrition Severe malnutrition	Endocrine disorders, osteogenic disorders, menopausal disorders secondary to estrogen depletion Sarcopenia related to decreased physical activity, increased cytokine (interleukin-6) and decreased levels of growth hormone and insulin-like growth factor
Skin	Healthy color, soft, moist turgor with instant recoil, smooth appearance	Excess fat stores	Excess energy intake	Diabetes, steroids
		Poor or delayed wound healing, pressure ulcers	Protein deficiency Vitamin C deficiency Zinc deficiency	Poor vascular perfusion
		Dry with fine lines and shedding, scaly (xerosis)	Essential fat deficiency Vitamin A deficiency	Environmental or hygiene factors
		Spinelike plaques around hair follicles on buttocks, thighs, or knees (follicular hyperkeratosis)	Vitamin A deficiency Essential fat deficiency	
		Pellagrous dermatitis (hyperpigmentation of skin exposed to sunlight)	Niacin deficiency Tryptophan deficiency	Thermal, sun, or chemical burns; Addison's disease
		Pallor	Iron deficiency Folic acid deficiency Vitamin B_{12} deficiency	Skin pigmentation disorders, hemorrhage, low volume, low perfusion state
		Generalized dermatitis	Zinc deficiency Essential fatty acid deficiency	Atopic dermatitis, contact dermatitis, allergic or medication rash, psoriasis, connective tissue disease
		Yellow pigmentation	Carotene excess Vitamin B_{12} deficiency	Jaundice
		Poor skin turgor	Fluid loss	Aging process
		Petechiae, ecchymoses	Vitamin K deficiency Vitamin C deficiency	Aspirin overdose, liver disease, or trauma
Nails	Smooth, translucent, slightly curved nail surface and firmly attached to nail bed; nail beds with brisk capillary refill	Spoon-shaped (koilonychia)	Iron deficiency Non-severe malnutrition Severe malnutrition	COPD, heart disease, aortic stenosis, diabetes, lupus, chemotherapy
		Dull, lackluster	Protein deficiency Iron deficiency	Chemical effects
		Pale, mottled, poor blanching	Vitamin A deficiency Vitamin C deficiency	Infection, chemical effects
		Ridging, transverse-more than one extremity	Protein deficiency	Beau's lines, grooves caused by trauma, coronary occlusion, skin disease, transient illness
Scalp	Pink, no lesions, tenderness; fontanels without softening, bulging	Softening or craniotabes	Vitamin D deficiency	
		Open anterior fontanel (usually closes by $\approx$ 18 months of age)	Vitamin D deficiency	Hydrocephalus
Hair	Natural shine, consistency in color and quantity, fine to coarse texture	Lack of shine and luster, thin, sparse	Protein deficiency Zinc deficiency Biotin deficiency, Linoleic acid deficiency	Hypothyroidism, chemotherapy, psoriasis, color treatment

PART 3: Nutrition-Focused Physical Examination—cont'd

System	Normal Findings	Abnormal Findings	Possible Nutrition and Metabolic Etiologies	Nonnutritional Etiologies
		Easily pluckable	Protein deficiency Biotin deficiency	Hypothyroidism, chemotherapy, psoriasis, color treatment
		Alternating bands of light and dark hair in young children (flag sign)	Protein deficiency	Chemically processed or bleached hair
		"Corkscrew" hair	Copper deficiency Vitamin C deficiency	Menkes disease Chemical alteration
		Premature whitening	Selenium deficiency Vitamin B_{12} deficiency	Graves disease, medications
Face	Skin warm, smooth, dry, soft, moist with instant recoil	Diffuse depigmentation, swollen	Protein deficiency	Steroids and other medications
		Pallor	Iron deficiency Folic acid deficiency Vitamin B_{12} deficiency	Low-perfusion, low-volume states
		Moon face	Protein deficiency	Cushing's disease, steroids
		Bilateral temporal wasting. See Part 1	Protein deficiency Energy deficit	Neuromuscular disorders
		Undifferentiated mucocutaneous border	Riboflavin deficiency	
Eyes	Evenly distributed brows, lids, lashes; conjunctiva pink without discharge; sclerae without spots; cornea clear; skin without cracks or lesions	Pale conjunctiva	Iron deficiency Folate deficiency Vitamin B_{12} deficiency	Low output states
		Night blindness	Vitamin A deficiency	
		Dry, grayish, yellow or white foamy spots on whites of eyes (Bitot's spots)	Vitamin A deficiency	Pterygium, Gaucher's disease
		Dull, milky, or opaque cornea (corneal xerosis)	Vitamin A deficiency	
		Dull, dry, rough appearance to whites of eyes and inner lids (conjunctival xerosis)	Vitamin A deficiency	Chemical, environmental
		Softening of cornea (keratomalacia)	Vitamin A deficiency	
		Cracked and reddened corners of eyes (angular palpebritis)	Riboflavin deficiency Niacin deficiency	Infection, foreign objects
Nose	Uniform shape, septum slightly to left of midline, nares patent bilaterally, mucosa pink and moist, able to identify aromas	Scaly, greasy, with gray or yellowish material around nares (nasolabial seborrhea)	Riboflavin deficiency Niacin deficiency Pyridoxine deficiency	
		Inflammation, redness of sinus tract, discharge, obstruction or polyps	Irritation of skin membranes	Need to reconsider if placing nasoenteric feeding tube; evaluate for nonfood allergies
Oral Cavity				
Lips, mouth	Pink, symmetric, smooth intact	Angular Stomatitis (Bilateral cracks, redness of lips)	Riboflavin deficiency Niacin deficiency Pyridoxine deficiency Dehydration	Poor-fitting dentures, herpes, syphilis. HIV, environmental exposure,
		Cheilosis (Vertical cracks of lips or fissuring)	Riboflavin deficiency Niacin deficiency Dehydration	HIV (Kaposi's sarcoma), environmental exposure,
		Chapped or peeling	Dehydration	Environmental exposure
		General inflammation	Protein, energy, folic acid	Xerostomia

Continued

PART 3: Nutrition-Focused Physical Examination—cont'd

System	Normal Findings	Abnormal Findings	Possible Nutrition and Metabolic Etiologies	Nonnutritional Etiologies
Tongue	Pink, moist, midline, symmetric with rough texture	Magenta (purplish-red color), inflammation of the tongue (glossitis)	Riboflavin deficiency, B_6 deficiency Niacin deficiency Folate deficiency Vitamin B_{12} deficiency Riboflavin deficiency, Iron deficiency	Crohn's Disease, uremia, Infectious disease state, antibiotics, malignancy, Irritants (excess tobacco, alcohol, spices), generalized skin disorder
		Smooth, slick, loss of papillae (atrophic filiform papillae)	Folate deficiency Niacin deficiency Riboflavin deficiency Iron deficiency Vitamin B_{12} deficiency Non-Severe Malnutrition Severe Malnutrition	
		Distorted taste (dysgeusia)	Zinc deficiency	Cancer therapy, medications, advanced age, trauma, syphilis, xerostomia, poor-fitting dentures, poor hygiene
		Decreased taste (hypogeusia)	Zinc deficiency, Vitamin A deficiency	Cancer therapy, advanced age, medications, xerotomia
Gums	Pink, moist without sponginess	Spongy, bleeding, receding	Vitamin C deficiency Riboflavin deficiency	Dilantin and other medication, poor hygiene, lymphoma, polycythemia, thrombocytopenia
		Red, swollen interdental gingival hypertrophy	Vitamin C deficiency Folic acid deficiency, vitamin B_{12} deficiency	Dilantin, poor oral hygiene, lymphoma, vitamin A toxicity
Teeth	Repaired, no loose teeth; color may be various shades of white	Missing, poor repair, caries, loose teeth	Excess sugar intake	Trauma, syphilis, aging, poor dental hygiene
		White or brownish patches (mottled)	Excess fluoride	Enamel hypoplasia, erosion
Cranial nerves	Intact	Abnormal	Feeding route	
Gag reflex	Intact	Absent	Route of feeding	
Jaw	Proper alignment, movement from side to side	Improper alignment and movement	Ability to chew properly	
Parotid gland	Located anterior to earlobe, no enlargement	Bilateral enlargement	Non-Severe Malnutrition Severe Malnutrition	Bulimia, cysts, tumors, hyperparathyroidism
Neck nodules	Trachea midline, freely movable without enlargement or nodules	Enlarged thyroid	Iodine deficiency	Cancer, allergy, cold infection
Cardiopulmonary				
Chest, lungs	Anterior and posterior thorax; adequate muscle and fat stores, respirations even and unlabored, symmetric rise and fall of chest during inspiration and expiration, lung sounds clear	Somatic muscle- and fat-wasting; labored respirations; breath sounds such as crackles, ronchi, and wheezing: evaluate for fluid status vs. tenacious secretions that may labor breathing and increase energy expenditure; also consider increased rate and depth, decreased rate and depth	Non-Severe Malnutrition Severe Malnutrition Metabolic acidosis Metabolic alkalosis	Respiratory disease (e.g., COPD)
Heart	Rhythm regular and rate within normal range; S_1 and S_2 heart sounds	Irregular rhythm	Potassium deficiency or excess Calcium deficiency Magnesium deficiency or excess Phosphorus deficiency	Cardiopulmonary disease states, stress
		Enlarged heart	Thiamin deficiency associated with anemia and beriberi	

PART 3: Nutrition-Focused Physical Examination—cont'd

System	Normal Findings	Abnormal Findings	Possible Nutrition and Metabolic Etiologies	Nonnutritional Etiologies
		Pitting edema	Retention of sodium chloride, which causes the body to retain water Edema-associated disease of heart, liver, kidneys Fluid leaking into the interstitial tissue spaces	
Vascular access devices intact	No swelling, redness, drainage	Purulent drainage, swelling, excessive redness	Nutrition effects if device has to be removed	
Abdomen	Soft, nondistended, symmetric, bilateral without masses, umbilicus in midline, no ascites, bowel sounds present and normoactive; tympanic on percussion; feeding device intact without redness, swelling	Generalized symmetric distention	Obesity	Enlarged organs, fluid, or gas, ileus from other disease
		Protruding, everted umbilicus; tight glistening appearance (ascites)	Effects on protein, fluid, sodium concerns of feeding	
		Scaphoid appearance	Non-Severe Malnutrition Severe Malnutrition	
		Increased bowel sounds	Nutrition effects in gastroenteritis (normal if hunger pains)	
		High-pitched tinkling	Nutrition effects if intestinal fluid and air present, indicating early obstruction	
		Decreased bowel sounds	Nutrition effects if peritonitis or paralytic ileus present	
Kidney, ureter, bladder	Urine golden yellow (ranges from pale yellow to deep gold), clear without cloudiness, adequate output	Decreased output, extremely dark, concentrated	Dehydration	
Musculoskeletal	Full range of motion without joint swelling or pain, adequate muscle strength	Inability to flex, extend, and rotate neck adequately	Interference with ability to feed or make hand-to-mouth contact	
		Decreased range of motion, swelling, impaired joint mobility of upper extremities; muscle wasting on arms, legs; skin folding on buttocks	Non-Severe Malnutrition Severe Malnutrition	
		Swollen, painful joints	Vitamin C deficiency Vitamin D deficiency	Connective tissue disease
		Bone tenderness	Vitamin A deficiency	
		Enlargement of epiphyses at wrist, ankle, or knees	Vitamins D deficiency Vitamin C deficiency	Trauma, deformity, or congenital cause
		Bowed legs	Vitamin D deficiency Calcium deficiency	
		Beading of ribs	Vitamin D deficiency Calcium deficiency	Renal rickets, malabsorption
		Pain in calves, thighs	Thiamin deficiency	Deep vein thrombosis, other neuropathy or other
Neurologic	Alert, oriented, hand-to-mouth coordination; no weakness or tremors	Decreased or absent mental alertness; inadequate or absent hand-to-mouth coordination	Interference with the ability to feed or make hand-to-mouth contact	

Continued

PART 3: Nutrition-Focused Physical Examination—cont'd

System	Normal Findings	Abnormal Findings	Possible Nutrition and Metabolic Etiologies	Nonnutritional Etiologies
		Psychomotor changes, cognitive and sensory deficits, memory loss, confusion, peripheral neuropathy	Non-Severe Malnutrition Severe Malnutrition; Thiamin deficiency, Pyridoxine deficiency, Vitamin B_{12} deficiency	Trauma, neurologic disease, brain injury, brain tumor, chemotherapy
		Dementia	Thiamin deficiency Niacin deficiency Vitamin B_{12} deficiency	Trauma, neurologic disease, vascular disease, brain injury, brain tumor, chemotherapy
		Tetany	Calcium deficiency Magnesium deficiency	
		Paresthesias or numbness in stocking-glove distribution	Vitamin B_{12} deficiency Thiamin deficiency	Diabetic neuropathy
	Cranial nerves intact: primary nutritionally focused ones include trigeminal, facial, glossopharyngeal, vagus, and hypoglossal			
	Reflexes (biceps, brachioradialis patella, and Achilles common in examination), functioning within normal range of 2^{++}	Hyperactive reflexes	Hypocalcemia	Tetany, upper motor neuron disease
	Hypoactive reflexes	Hypokalemia		Associated with metabolic diseases such as diabetes mellitus and hypothyroidism
		Hypoactive Achilles, patellar reflex	Thiamin deficiency, Vitamin B_{12} deficiency	Neurologic disorder

From
Litchford, MD. *Nutrition-Focused Physical assessment: Making Clinical Connections.* Greensboro, NC: CASE Software & Books, 2012.
Hammond K: Physical assessment: a nutritional perspective, *Nurs Clin North Am* 32(4):779, 1997. Modified, 2010; Hammond K: History and physical examination. In Matarese LE and Gottschlich M., editors: *Contemporary Nutrition Support Practice*, Philadelphia, 2003, Saunders Company; Porter RS, Kaplan JL (eds.): *Nutrition disorders, Merck Manual Online.* Accessed May 2015 from http://www.merckmanuals.com/professional/nutritional-disorders/undernutrition/overview-of-undernutrition *This chart is not intended to be a comprehensive list for all nutritional or metabolic deficiencies or non-nutrition examples.*

Laboratory Values for Nutritional Assessment and Monitoring

Diana Noland, MPH, RD, CCN,
Mary Litchford, PhD, RDN, LDN

I. PRINCIPLES OF NUTRITIONAL LABORATORY TESTING

A. Purpose

Laboratory-based testing is used to estimate nutrient availability in biologic fluids and tissues. It is critical for assessment of both nutrient insufficiencies and frank deficiencies. Laboratory data are the only objective data used in nutrition assessment that are "controlled"—that is, the validity of the method of the measurement is checked each time a specimen is assayed by also assaying a sample with a known value. The known sample is called a *control,* and if the value obtained for the sample is outside the range of normal analytic variability, both the specimen and control are measured again.

The nutrition professional can use laboratory test results to support subjective data and clinical findings to determine a personalized nutritional assessment leading to more targeted interventions and successful outcomes. The lab values provide objective data useful in regular monitoring and can be used to assess progress and manage side effects such as inflammation, aberrant lipid and glucose metabolism, and poor immune health. Furthermore, because numeric values do not themselves connote personal judgment, this kind of data can often be passed on to a patient or client without implicit or perceived blame.

B. Specimen Types

Ideally the specimen to be tested reflects a high percentage of total body content of the nutrient to be assessed. However, often the best specimen is not readily available. The most common specimens for analysis are the following:

Whole blood—Must be collected with an anticoagulant if entire content of the blood is to be evaluated. The two common anticoagulants for whole blood analyses are ethylenediaminetetraacetic acid, a calcium chelator used in hematologic analyses, and heparin (maintains the blood in its most natural state).

Blood cells—Separated from uncoagulated whole blood for measurement of cellular analyte content: Red blood cells (indicate a 120-day window into intracellular and membrane composition), various blood components like white blood cells, protein-bound molecules, and others.

Plasma—The uncoagulated fluid that bathes the formed elements (blood cells).

Serum—The fluid that remains after whole blood or plasma has coagulated. Coagulation proteins and related substances are missing or significantly reduced.

Urine—Contains a concentrate of excreted metabolites and potential toxins.

Feces—Important in identifying various gastrointestinal functional parameters including inflammatory markers, microbiology, mycology, parasitology, digestive markers and nutritional analyses when nutrients are not absorbed and therefore are present in fecal material.

Saliva—laboratory analysis to identify endocrine, inflammatory, infectious, immunologic, some nutrients and other parameters with buccal cell or whole saliva samples.

Genomic—expanding beyond the historical metabolic macro- and micronutrient testing, genomic polymerase chain reaction (PCR) assays are emerging genomic clinical indicators for nutrigenetic and nutrigenomic influences on the metabolism of an individual (see Chapter 5).

Expired Air— Concentration of expired gases is a noninvasive and useful estimate of bacterial metabolism. Emerging measurements of expired nitric oxide and ketosis may be useful in estimating inflammatory or ketotic status in selected medical conditions.

Hair—An easy-to-collect tissue; most commonly measuring minerals; usually a poor indicator of actual body levels.

Other tissues—Fat biopsies have been used to estimate vitamin D stores in research studies.

C. Interpretation of Laboratory Data

As with all data, nutrition data may be quantitative (e.g., how much, how often, how fast), semiquantitative (e.g., many, most, few, a lot, usually, majority, several), or qualitative (e.g., color, shape, species). The advantage of quantitative data is that they are less ambiguous or more objective than other types of observations. Although objective laboratory data are extremely important resources in nutrition assessment, one should be extremely cautious about using a single isolated laboratory test value to make an assessment. An isolated value

---

*Samples obtained for blood coagulation tests are diluted with solutions containing sodium citrate (a calcium chelator). Because of the dilutional effect of the anticoagulant solutions, citrated samples are not suitable for measurement of the concentrations of analytes.

†Clark GH, Fraser CG: Biological variation of acute phase proteins, *Ann Clin Biochem* 30:373, 1993.

is often misleading, especially when used without the context of an individual's lifestyle habits, clinical status, dietary, medical and genomic histories. Besides the importance of identifying frank deficiencies or excesses of nutrients, the best data are obtained from analysis of changes in laboratory values. It is especially important to monitor laboratory values when contemplating nutritional interventions that involve potentially unsafe levels beyond upper limits (UL), such as fat-soluble vitamins or a mineral like selenium.

When monitoring patients for changes in nutrition test values, one must consider how much change is necessary to give confidence that a difference is significant. The change required for statistical significance has been called the *critical difference.* It is calculated from measurement of the variances calculated from repeated measurements of an analyte: (1) specimens that have been obtained, at several different times, from each of several healthy persons (intrasubject variation); and (2) separate samples from a large specimen pool (analytic variation).

In practice, assessments are not based on the measurement of a single analyte at one point in time except in the case of severe deficiencies or dangerous excesses. Changes in laboratory tests may have biologic significance (e.g., patient's condition is improving) long before statistical significance is achieved. The changes in laboratory data may precede changes in other nutritional indices, but generally, although not always, the data available should point to the same conclusion.

D. Reference Ranges

To determine whether a particular laboratory value is abnormal, particularly when serial data are not available, the value is generally compared to a diagnostic reference range. The reference range is constructed from a large number of test values (20 to >1000). The average value and the standard deviation for these data are determined, and the reference range is calculated from the mean ±2 standard deviations. If the sample group is representative of the reference population, the reference range will include values that reflect those found in approximately 95% of the reference population. Approximately 2.5% of this normal population will have values greater than the upper end of the reference range, and 2.5% will have values less than the lower end. This means that one normal individual in 20 would have a value below or above the reference range.

Reference ranges can be made for different populations. For example, reference ranges based on gender, age, race, and so forth, can be developed. In practice, the differences between populations are often ignored because the importance of small differences in a nutrient analyte is not usually significant. However, in the event of borderline values, the possible influence of differences between the patient's population and the reference population may need to be considered. Reference ranges are often determined by obtaining blood from personnel working in or near the clinical laboratory. This population is often skewed toward younger persons, has few minorities, and is overrepresented by women.

As the science of nutrition continues to rapidly evolve due to technological and scientific advances, changes in laboratory values can be interpreted as indicating metabolic trends, even within the reference range of a test. The nutritionist's skill in perceiving nutrient insufficiencies or imbalances related to nutritional influences can provide a more targeted assessment resulting in improved outcomes from therapy.

E. Units

Many types of units are used in reporting nutrient-dependent laboratory values. Two basic systems of units are in common use: the conventional system and the Système Internationale d'Unités (SI) system. The conventional system sometimes lacks convention; thus different laboratories adopt different units to report the same analyte. For example, the conventional report of an ionized calcium value could be 2.3 mEq/L, 46 mg/L or 4.6 mg/dL. However, in the SI system only 1.15 mmol/L is allowed.

F. Nature of Nutritional Testing and Types of Tests

Typically laboratory tests are static assays (i.e., the concentration of an analyte is measured in a biologic fluid [e.g., a fasting blood specimen] at a point in time). Assessment of nutrient status made by this approach is often inaccurate or distorted. Some nutrients can be assessed by tests that are based on measurements that reflect the endogenous availability of a nutrient to a measurable biologic function (e.g., biochemical, tissue, or organ). Most often, functional assessment of nutrient status may be done by measurement of a biochemical marker (i.e., a normal or abnormal metabolite) of function. The results of this type of testing can be reliably considered to reflect the adequacy of a nutrient pool or possible individual genomic nutrient requirements.

✳ NEW DIRECTIONS

Bioelectrical Impedance Analysis (BIA) and Bioimpedance Spectroscopy (BIS)— A New Functional Test

Nutrition assessment is taking on a new level of specificity with the explosion of technology and discoveries of the pathophysiology of disease and functions of the human body. These breakthroughs assist in molecular level identification of nutrition status. Bioelectrical Impedance Analysis (BIA) and Bioimpedance Spectroscopy (BIS) have a credible history of use in research, but recently have found an increasing use as a clinical tool in nutrition assessment.

BIA estimates body composition and cellular activity by measuring the bulk electrical impedance of the body. The testing procedure involves application of conductors (electrodes) to a person's hand and foot, and sending a small alternating electric current through the body (see figure on next page). The different electrical conductive properties of various body tissues (adipose, muscular and skeletal) and hydration affect the impedance measurement. An algorithm derived from statistical analysis of BIA measurements is used to calculate the various parameters that can be measured by this technique.

Normal hydration is critical for results to be valid, with these guidelines prior to testing:

1) Drink water (16-24 oz during 4 hours prior to test)
2) No alcohol for 12 hours prior to test
3) No food or caffeine drinks for 4 hours before test
4) No moderate to intense exercise for 12 hours prior to test.

Contraindications to BIA testing are pregnancy, or the presence of implants like pacemakers or defibrillators. Follow-up monitoring of BIA testing should attempt to be near the same time of day.

There are commercially available BIA devices that measure only body fat % and weight. But professional BIA or BIS instruments are available

✳ NEW DIRECTIONS—cont'd

Bioelectrical Impedance Analysis (BIA) and Bioimpedance Spectroscopy (BIS)— A New Functional Test

that provide reliable, more comprehensive full body data, and automatically calculate total body water, intracellular and extracellular water, fat-free mass, percent body fat, phase angle, capacitance and body cell mass. They are very useful in tracking changes in an individual's progress over time. Research in the past decade has shown promise for the BIA Phase Angle as a prognostic indicator of some cancers (Norman 2010,) and other chronic conditions (Maddocks et al, 2014).

The multiple parameters measured in a BIA or BIS test provide three categories of data:

1. *Anthropometry:* BMI (body mass index), BMR (basal metabolic rate), body fat percentage, and lean body mass percentage. These measurements are used with weight management, monitoring of wasting syndromes, and acute care formulation of dietary prescriptions. Weight/height/age/gender date must be entered to obtain these results.

2. *Cellular metabolism:* Phase angle, which measures cell membrane fluidity and is a prognostic marker of mortality, capacitance (electrical resistance of the cell membrane) and body cell mass (the number or amount of metabolically active cells). Using these three measurements provides an easy-to-use, non-invasive, and reproducible technique to evaluate changes in body composition and nutritional status. Phase angle (BIA) detects changes in tissue electrical properties, and is hypothesized as a marker of malnutrition for investigating various diseases in the clinical setting. Lower phase angles suggest cell death or decreased cell integrity, while higher phase angles suggest large quantities of intact cell membranes (Selberg and Selberg, 2002).

3. *Hydration:* Total body water (in pounds and as a percentage), intracellular water (in pounds and as a percentage), and extracellular water (in pounds and as a percentage).

Every professional practicing nutrition therapy can now consider adding a reasonably priced BIA or BIS instrument to their nutritional assessment tool box to assist in the management of a client or patient. The four companies from which professional BIA or BIS instruments can currently be obtained are:

www.impedimed.com
www.inbody.com
www.biodynamics.com
www.rjlsystems.com

These companies also provide informative education on the technology and operation of their bioimpedance or bioimpedance spectroscopy instruments.

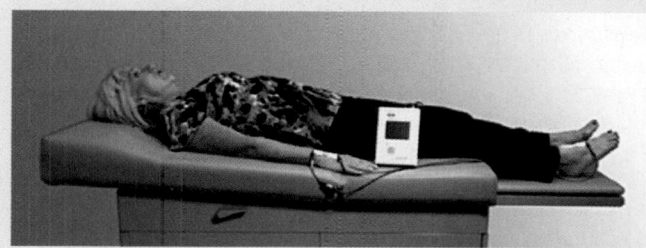

Image reproduced with permission of ImpediMed Limited.

Bauer JM, et al: The Mini Nutritional Assessment (R)—its history, today's practice, and future perspectives, *Nutr Clin Pract* 23:388, 2008.

Davis MP, et al: Bioelectrical impedance phase angle changes during hydration and prognosis in advanced cancer, *Am J Hosp Palliat Care* 26(3):180, 2009.

Ellis, KJ, et al: Bioelectrical impedance methods in clinical research: a follow-up to the NIH Technology Assessment Conference. Nutrition, 12(11-12): 874, 1999.

Gupta D, et al: The relationship between bioelectrical impedance phase angle and subjective global assessment in advanced colorectal cancer, *Nutrition Journal* 7:19, 2008.

Gupta D, et al: Bioelectrical impedance phase angle as a prognostic indicator in breast cancer, *BMC Cancer* 8:249, 2008.

Hengstermann S, et al: Nutrition status and pressure ulcer: what we need for nutrition screening, *JPEN J Parenter Enteral Nut* 31:288, 2007.

Jaffrin MY, Morel H. Body fluid volumes measurements by impedance: A review of bioimpedance spectroscopy (BIS) and bioimpedance analysis (BIA) methods. Med Eng Phys. 30:1257, 2008.

Khalil SF, et al: The theory and fundamentals of bioimpedance analysis in clinical status monitoring and diagnosis of diseases. Sensors 14:10895, 2014.

Kyle UG: Bioelectrical impedance analysis-part II: utilization in clinical practice, *Am J Clin Nutr* 23:1226, 2004.

Methods of Body Composition Tutorials (Interactive). Dept. of Nutrition and Food Sciences, University of Vermont. http://nutrition.uvm.edu/bodycomp/ Accessed May 19, 2011.

Maddocks M et al: Bioelectrical impedance phase angle relates to function, disease severity and prognosis in stable chronic obstructive pulmonary disease. Clin Nutr. 34:1245, 2015, doi: 10.1016/j.clnu.2014.12.020.

Norman K, et al: Cutoff percentiles of bioelectrical phase angle predict functionality, quality of life, and mortality in patients with cancer, *Am J Clin Nutr* 92:612, 2010.

Selberg O, Selberg D: Norms and correlates of bioimpedance phase angle in healthy human subjects, hospitalized patients, and patients with liver cirrhosis, *Eur J Appl Physiol* 86:509, 2002.

Van Loan MD, et al: Use of bioimpedance spectroscopy (BIS) to determine extracellular fluid (ECF), intracellular fluid (ICF), total body water (TBW), and fat free mass (FFM). In Ellis K, editor: *Human Body Composition: In Vivo Measurement and Studies*, New York, 1993, Plenum Publishing Co., pp 6770.

Varan HD, et al: Phase angle assessment by bioelectrical impedance analysis and its predictive value for malnutrition risk in hospitalized geriatric patients. Aging Clin Exp Res, Jan 19, 2016, pp 1-6, Epub ahead of print.

II. Clinical Chemistry
A. Protein Markers

Test	Principles	Interpretation	Reference Range	Limitations and Implications
Normalized Protein Catabolic Rate (nPCR)	nPCR is determined by measuring the intradialytic appearance of urea in body fluids plus any urea lost in the urine in patients with residual renal function. nPCR = 0.22 + (0.036 x *intradialytic rise in BUN x × 24)/ (intradialytic interval). (also called: Protein Nitrogen Appearance rate (PNA) (g/day) = 13 + 7.31 UNA (mmol/day) [UNA (mmol/day) = Vd(ml) x Cd (mmol/L) + Vu (ml) + Cu (mmol/L)]	Useful in assessing Dietary Protein Intake (DPI) in patients who are in a steady state on hemodialysis, as a means toward determining adequate nutrition status.	0.81-1.02 g UN/kg per day	nPCR considered superior to sAlb for monitoring nutrition protein status due to sAlb influence by processes other than nutrition status.[2] During hemodialysis the PCR can also reflect inadequate dialysis. For CAPD patients the nPCR value has not been consistently predictive of outcome.[3]

Test	Principles	Interpretation	Risk	Ratio
Urine creatinine (U : Cr)	U : Cr concentration in fasting, first-void urine used to compare amino acid catabolism (BUN) with muscle mass (creatinine).	Urine concentration (mg/dL) U : Cr = Urine area (mg/dL) ÷ Urine creatinine (mg/dL). The U : Cr is used in comparing other markers like microablbumin, albumin, GFR ratios.	Low Medium High	>12.0 6.0-12.0 <6.0

Test	Principles	Interpretation	Reference Range	Limitations and Implications
Urea Urinary Nitrogen (UUN)	The protein pool (visceral and somatic) N is catabolized to urea; urine urea represents ~80% of N catabolized; requires accurate estimate of protein intake; thus usually used only for PN or tube-feeding patients.	UUN is compared with the actual N intake. Nitrogen Balance = Nitrogen intake (Protein g/day÷6.25) – Nitrogen Losses (UUN (g)+ 4)[a]	– = Catabolism 0 = Catabolism + = Anabolism (3-6 g/24 hr = optimal use range)	24 hour urine collection must be quantitative (complete); UUN not appropriate in renal insufficiency; does not account for wound leakage, cell losses, or diarrhea; inaccurate in metabolically stressed patients.
Total Urinary Nitrogen (TUN)	Some N is excreted as non-urea N (e.g., ammonia and creatinine); 24-hour TUN reflects total protein catabolism, accounting for all sources of urinary N; as for UUN, requires accurate protein intake. Used primarily to accurately follow the protein catabolic response during disease and response to nutritional support.	TUN is compared with the actual N intake; Nitrogen Balance = Nitrogen intake (Protein g/day÷6.25) – Nitrogen Losses (TUN (g)+ 2)[b]	– = Catabolism 0 = Catabolism + = Anabolism (3-6 g/24 hr = optimal use range)	Urine 24 hour collection must be quantitative (complete); TUN not appropriate in renal insufficiency; not done in many institutions; does not account for wound leakage, cell losses, or diarrhea.
Urea Kinetic Modeling (UKM)	Formulas used to estimate nPCR (normalized protein catabolic rate) from changes in BUN concentration in patients with impaired renal function.	Urinary urea (KrU) and BUN levels (urea generation rate—UG) are used to determine nPCR; 1- to 3-day diet intake compared with nPCR. Urea kinetic Modeling (Kt/V_{urea} and nPCR)	In protein balance, nPRC = protein intake (g/kg/day)	Urea lost in dialysis must be accounted for in calculating urea nitrogen appearance. Dietary protein intake hard to estimate.

B. Inflammatory Markers

Test	Principles	Interpretation	Reference Range	Limitations and Implications
Albumin (ALB)	Easily and quickly measured colorimetrically; large body pool (3-5 g/kg body weight), ~60% is outside the plasma in the extravascular pool; long half-life of 3 weeks.	Decreased levels can occur following acute and chronic inflammatory states; often associated with other deficiencies (i.e., zinc, iron, and vitamin A) reflecting that ALB transports (many small molecules.	3.5-5 g/dL) (35-50 g/L)	Stable half life ~3 weeks. A negative phase reactant, impacted by inflammatory stress, (protein losing conditions and hemodilution. Hepatic proteins are indicators of morbidity and mortality:
Globulin (GLOB)	Large body pool (3-5 g/kg body weight), ~35% is outside the plasma in the extravascular pool; long half-life averages 23 days, but varies with particular globulins.	Globulin proteins include enzymes and carriers that transport proteins including antibodies that primarily assist in immune function and fight infection.	2.3-3.4 g/dL (23-34 g/L)	Significance confounded by acute stress reaction, infection, inflammatory conditions.
A/G Ratio	Calculated from ALB and GLOB values by direct measurement of TP and ALB.	It represents the relative amounts of ALB and GLOB	A/G Ratio 1 : 1 - normal <1 : 1 - disease state	Albumin levels fall and globulin levels rise with inflammatory stress.

Transferrin (Tf or TFN)	The iron bound globulin protein that responds to the need for iron. Can be calculated from TIBC and serum iron; half-life ~9 days. See Chapter 7.	Tf increased with low iron stores, and prevents build up of highly toxic excess unbound iron in circulation. In iron overload states Tf levels decrease. Because B_6 is required for iron to bind to Hgb, B_6 deficiency promotes ↑Tf from the ↑ circulating iron that binds to Tf; smaller extravascular pool than albumin.	Adult male: 215-365 mg/dL (2.15-3.65 g/L) Adult female: 250-380 mg/dL (2.50-3.80 g/L) Newborn: 130-275 mg/dL (1.3-2.75 g/L) Child: 203-360 mg/dL (2.03-3.6 g/L) Pregnancy and estrogen HRT associated with ↑Tf.	Lead can biologically mimic and displace iron thus releasing Fe into circulation and ↑Tf. Tf is a negative acute phase reactant diminished in chronic illness and hypoproteinemia.
Transferrin Saturation (Tf-sat or TSAT)	Tf-sat (%) = Serum iron level ÷ TIBC × 100%	Tf-sat decreases to <15% in Fe deficiency; useful in diagnosis of iron toxicity or Fe overload (hemochromatosis). See Chapter 32.	M: 20%-50% F: 15%-50% Chronic illness: normal Tf-sat%. Late pregnancy: low Tf-sat%.	Increased Tf-sat when low vitamin B_6 as in aplastic anemia.
PreAlbumin (PAB)/ Transthyretin (TTR)	Transports T_4 and acts as a carrier for retinol-binding protein; PAB also called thyroxin-binding protein; half-life 2 days.	Measure of inflammatory status. Zinc deficiency reduces PAB levels.	15-36 mg/dL or 150-360 mg/L (15-36 mg/dL female 21-43 mg/dL male) Malnutrition: <8 mg/dL (<0.8 g/L or <80 mg/L)	Sensitive to acute zinc deficiency and acute stress reaction. PAB values do not reflect protein status, but is a prognostic index for mortality and morbidity.[4]
Retinol-binding protein (RBP)	Transport retinol; because of low molecular weight, RBP is filtered by glomerulus and catabolized by the kidney tubule; half-life = 12 hours	Measure of inflammatory status.	2.6-7.6 mg/dL (1.43-2.86 mmol/L)	Sensitive to stress response; vitamin A and zinc deficiencies, and hemodilution; increased in chronic renal disease.
C-Reactive Protein high sensitivity (hs-CRP)	A nonspecific acute phase reactant; short half life 5-7 hr; CRP responds to inflammation in 6-10 hours. (also called CRP-ultra sensitivity and CRP-card o)	A sensitive marker of bacterial disease and systemic inflammation; associated with periodontitis, trauma, cardiovascular disease, neoplastic proliferation and bacterial infections.	Low Risk for CVD = Less than 1.0 mg/L Intermediate Risk for CVD = 2.9 mg/L High Risk for CVD = Greater than 3.0 mg/L Seek inflammatory cause if >10 mg/L	Useful metabolic indicator for adults.[9] Acute-phase reactant; relates mostly to bacterial infection, central adiposity, trauma and neoplastic activity.
Fibrinogen	Acute-phase reactant protein essential to blood-clotting mechanism/coagulation system.	Decreased fibrinogen related to prolonged Pro Time (PT) and Partial Thromboplastin Time (PTT); produced in liver; rises sharply during tissue inflammation or necrosis; association with CHD, stroke, myocardial infarction and peripheral arterial disease.	200-400 mg/dL If <100 mg/dL, increased risk of bleeding. Should be monitored in conjunction with blood platelet levels involved with coagulation status.	Good test and retest reliability and covariance is stable over time; diets rich in Omega 3/6 fatty acids reduce fibrinogen blood levels.

C. Metabolic Indicators

Insulin-like growth factor-1 (IGF-1) or Somatomedin C	The peptide mediator of growth hormone activity produced by the liver; half-life of a few hours; much less sensitive to stress response than other proteins.	Low in chronic undernutrition; increases rapidly during nutrition repletion; TSAT, PAB, and RBP are not affected. Elevated levels associated with elevated GH in acromegaly and neoplastic activity.	Adult: 42-110 ng/mL Children age 0-19: can vary with age, gender and Tanner Stages (Appendices 17 & 18) used for references per age	Reduced levels seen in hypopituitarism, hypothyroidism, liver disease, and with estrogen use. Growing evidence of elevated IGF-1 as a prognostic biomarker of neoplastic activity.[5,6]
Hemoglobin A1C (HgbA1C)	Glycosylated hemoglobin; dependent on blood glucose level over life span of RBC (120 days); the more glucose the Hgb is exposed to, the greater the % HgbA1C.	Assessment of the mean glycemic blood level and of chronic diabetic control detecting for the previous 2-3 months.[7]	Non-diabetic adult/child: 4%-5.9% Controlled diabetes (DM): 4-7% Fair DM control: 7-8% Poor DM control: >8%	HbgA1 measurement is a simple, rapid, and objective procedure. Home testing available.

Continued

Insulin, fasting	Pancreatic hormone signaling cell membrane insulin receptors to initiate glucose transport into cell; test fasting 7 hours, or 1 or 2 hours post prandial; usually ordered with blood glucose test.	Elevated levels associated with hyperinsulinemia related to metabolic syndrome; diagnosis of insulin-producing neoplasms; excess insulin associated with inflammatory conditions.	Adult values: Fasting 6-27 μ IU/mL 1 or 2 hour PP: see lab reference	Good to test and retest reliability, and covariance is stable over time.[8] Insulin antibodies may invalidate the test.

D. Immune Dysregulation Tests
Allergies/Sensitivity

Immunoglobulins (IgA, IgG, IgE, IgM,)	Serologic antibody screening tests; testing of Immunoglobulins; Total IgE ELISA; RAST (radioallergosorbent-blood IgE); Bloodspot: IgG Provocative specific antigen skin prick: (IgE related skin response) used to diagnose allergy and identify the allergen.	Used to determine immunodeficiency states; measurement of +IgE = allergic disorders; (see Table 27-3) +IgG = delayed immunologic sensitivity or intolerance response (see Table 27-3). IgA = largest % Ig primarily made in GI lymphoid tissue and marker of immune strength and response.	Total IgA: Adults = 85-463 mg/dL Children = 1-350 mg/dL Total IgG: < 2.0 mcg/mL Total IgE = <10 IU/mL RAST IgE = <1 IU/mL low allergic risk Total IgM: Adults 48-271 mg/dL Children 17-200 mg/dL Total IgD = < 15.3 mg/dL	NSAIDS, glucocorticosteroids, vitamin C, bioflavonoids can suppress the immunologic response and promote a false negative. IgA used as a biomarker reference of adequate immune response to enable measurement of IgG, IgE, IgM, IgD

Innate Immune Factors

Total Leukocyte Count (TLC)	Calculated from the percentage of lymphocytes reported in the hemogram and the WBC count. Units = cells/μl or cells/mm³	Decreased in protein-energy malnutrition and immunocompromised state.	Normal: >2700 Moderate depletion: 900-1800 Severe depletion: <900	
Delayed cutaneous hypersensitivity	Anergy for antigens, such as mumps and Candida; occurs in malnutrition; antigens intradermal injection; redness (erythema) and hardness (induration) read 1, 2, or 3 days later.	Response affected by protein-energy status and vitamin A, iron, zinc, and vitamin B₆ deficiencies.	Induration 1+: <5 mm 2+: 6-10 mm 3+: 11-20 mm 4+: >20 mm Erythema present or absent	Usefulness in acute care limited by drugs, effect of aging and disease (metabolic, malignant, and infectious diseases); difficult to administer and interpret results; semiquantitative.
Cytokines	Serum or joint fluid proteins tested from venous blood. They include lymphocytes, (T & B cells), monocytes, leukocytes (interleukins), eosinophils, interferon and growth factors. (See Chapter 3)	A group of immune reactant proteins that have many functions even from one cell to another. They respond to the environmental influences to communicate and orchestrate the immune response to protect from cancer, infection and inflammation.	Cytokine examples: Interleukins: IL-1, IL-6, IL-8, IL-10, TNF-α, TH-1, TH-2 (per lab references)	

Adaptive Immune Factors

Eosinophils (Eosinophil leukocyte)	Blood: **Bronchoalveolar lavage** (BAL) fluid CSF specimen to rule out eosinophilic meningitis.	Blood: Wide range of clinical conditions reflect nonspecific eosinophilia; elevated related to possible allergies, asthma, sensitivities, or cancers; particularly elevated eosinophils are found with intestinal parasites; noninfectious conditions.	Blood: 1% to 3% 50-500/mm³ BAL negative for infection CSF < 10 mm³	Because of the nonspecific nature of blood eosinophilia, it can require further clinical investigation to determine the causal agent.

Food Intolerance/Sensitivity Panels

Antigen Leucocyte Cellular Antibody Test (ALCAT)	Measurement of leukocyte cellular reactivity in whole blood, measures levels of mediators by blood cells presented with food or chemical antigens; measures relative changes in cell size (see Table 26-4)	Food and chemical non-IgE sensitivity (intolerance) testing for up to 350 foods plus gliadin/gluten, casein/whey, and candida albicans; food additives, molds, environmental chemicals, pharmacoactive agents, and other suspected items upon request.	350 Foods: Acceptable Foods Normal = no response Mild Intolerance Moderate Intolerance Severe Intolerance Candida/gluten-gliadin/ casein-whey, chemicals/molds: No Reaction Mild, Moderate or Severe Reaction	NSAIDS, glucocorticosteroids, vitamin C, bioflavonoids can suppress the immunologic response and promote a false negative. IgA used as a biomarker reference of adequate immune response.

Mediator Release Test (MRT) (immunologic food reaction test)	Untreated whole blood assay; sample is divided into 150 aliquots plus control samples and incubated with a precise dilution of pure extract of a specific food or food additive[c] (see Chapter 26)	Non IgE-mediated reactions; measurement of blood components; blood specimen checked against the specific signs of cell-mediated reactivity to the antigen challenged (imminent or actual mediator release). See Table 26-4.	Normal = no response Mild, moderate or severe reactions are delineated.	NSAIDS, glucocorticosteroids, vitamin C, bioflavonoids can suppress the immunologic response and promote a false negative. IgA used as a biomarker of adequate immune response.
Celiac Panel/ Gluten Sensitivity Panel	1. Immunologic and genomic for celiac or gluten sensitivity–related genes	Measurements to identify a possible genetic or immunologic disease of the small bowel in response to exposure to gluten or gliadin molecules in diet. Continued long-term exposure to gluten or gliadin molecules leads to nutrient deficiencies and insufficiencies.	See celiac tests 2.- 10.	Any of the celiac tests 2-10 tests should be compared with baseline IgA serum levels and presence of immune suppressive medications to rule out IgA deficiency, which can skew test results to false negative because of compromised or suppressed immune response. Undiagnosed celiac is associated with increased incidence of all chronic diseases and shortened lifespan[10,11,12]
	2. Endomysial antibodies (EMA)	High specificity for celiac disease; may obviate need for small bowel biopsy for diagnosis; become negative on gluten-free diet;	EMA negative	Sensitivity/Specificity 90+%/95%
	3. TissueTransglutaminase (tTG-IgA, tTG-IgG)	Autoantigen of celiac disease, tTG is indicative of villous atrophy secondary to gluten exposure causing damage to GI small intestine villi. tTG negative test results indicate gluten-free diet compliance; marker of restoration of GI villi tight junctions and small bowel villi integrity.	tTG IgA negative tTG IgG negative	Sensitivity/specificity 98%/95% in adults; 96%/99% in children. Best age to begin measuring tTG is age 2-3 years.[13]
	4. Antigliadin antibodies (AGA IgA, AGA IgG)	Positive results are evidence of immune response to the gliadin proteins in gluten-containing foods.	AGA IgA negative AGA IgG negative	Lowest sensitivity among celiac panel (70%-85%) and specificity (70%-90%) for celiac. Also useful for non-celiac gluten sensitivity.
	5. Deamidated gliadin peptide (DGP)	DGP antibodies improves[14] diagnostic accuracy for diagnosis of CD when tested with tTG; proteins present in the submucosa of affected person's bond to deamidated peptides to form molecular complexes that stimulate the immune system.	DGP negative	Specificity varied between 97.3% and 99.3%. Sensitivity of IgG anti-DGP significantly better than that of IgG anti-tTG (p < 0.05). Specificity was significantly better than IgA and IgG AGA[15]
	6. Celiac genetic HLA haplotype HLA-DQ2 HLA-DQ8 Cellular assay/MLC to test HLA class II types	HLA-DQ2 and HLA-DQ8 positive indicates a low positive predictive value but a very high negative predictive value for celiac disease. Higher prevalence of CD in patients with Type 1 DM or autoimmune thyroid disease (2%-4%) than in general population	Genotype: HLA DQ2 negative HLA DQ8 negative	More than 97% of individuals with celiac disease share the two HLA markers DQ2 and DQ8, which have high sensitivity and poor specificity. One of the markers can increase possible non-celiac gluten sensitivity (e.g., Type 1 DM DQA1*0501:DQB1*0201 haplotype).[14,15,16]

Continued

7. Wheat/Gluten Proteome Reactivity & Autoimmunity	Functional medicine serum lab tests to broaden the view of celiac and gluten sensitivity by assessing antibody production against an array of protein, enzyme and peptide antigens; includes *glutens, lectins, opioids* and the enzyme *glutamic decarboxylase* (GAD65) IgG, IgA. Available from www.cyrexlabs.com.	ELISA Index
		Wheat
		  IgG 0.30-1.30 mcg/mL
		  IgA 0.40-2.40 mg/dL
		Agglutinin
		  IgG 0.30-1.50 mcg/mL
		  IgA 0.90-1.90 mg/dL
		Alpha Gliadin 17 MER
		  IgG 0.30-1.50 mcg/mL
		  IgA 0.60-2.00 mg/dL
		Alpha Gliadin 33 MER
		  IgG 0.30-1.40 mcg/mL
		  IgA 0.60-1.80 mg/dL
		Gamma Gliadin 15 MER
		Omega Gliadin
		  IgG 0.50-1.60 mcg/mL
		  IgA 0.60-1.80 mg/dL
		Glutenin
		  IgG 0.20-1.50 mcg/mL
		  IgA 0.50-1.70 mg/dL
		Gluteomorphin
		  IgG 0.30-1.50 mcg/mL
		  IgA 0.60-1.80 mg/dL
		Prodynorphin
		  IgG 0.40-1.70 mcg/mL
		  IgA 0.60-1.80 mg/dL
		GAD65
		  IgG 0.40-1.30 mcg/mL
		  IgA 0.80-1.50 mg/dL
			Enhances clinical sensitivity and specificity in detection of celiac and gluten sensitivity reactions

8. Gluten-Associated Cross-Reactive Foods and Foods Sensitivity IgG + IgA Combined Cow's Milk Alpha-Casein & Beta-Casein Casomorphin Milk Butyrophilin American Cheese Chocolate (Others available)	Functional medicine serum lab tests to assess IgG and IgA immune antibody reactions to known cross-reactive food antigens, with the most common being casein. Other foods included are: sesame, hemp, rye, barley, wheat, buckwheat, sorghum, millet, spelt, amaranth, quinoa, yeast, tapioca, oats, coffee, corn, rice, potato.	ELISA Index: IgG & IgA combined 0.20 mcg/mL /0.40 mg/dL -1.80 mcg/mL /2.00 mg/dL	Assists further dietary evaluation for celiac or gluten sensitive individuals that are non-responsive to a gluten-free diet; can relate to gut dysbiosis and continued GI inflammation. Available from cyrexlabs.com.

III. Tests of Carbohydrate Absorption
Lactose Intolerance

Hydrogen Breath Test for Lactose (HBT-lactose)	Lactose loading (2 g/kg) in lactase deficiency allows bacterial metabolism of lactose with production of H_2 gas. Breath analyzed for H_2 by gas chromatography.	Breath H_2 measured fasting and 0.5 and 2 hours after dosing with lactose; a significant increase is associated with malabsorption.	Normal increase: <50 parts/million (i.e., <50 ppm) Lactose intolerance: 50 ppm or greater	Bacterial overgrowth can cause false-positive results; consumption of soluble fiber or legumes, and smoking are associated with H_2 production; false-negative results caused by antibiotics.
Lactose tolerance test	Lactose loading (50 g) followed by blood sampling at 5, 10, 30, 60, 90, and 120 min after dose; glucose produced from lactose is assayed.	Lactase deficiency associated with <20 mg/dL increase in serum glucose.	Normal serum glucose Lactose increase >20 mg/dL	Test is not specific (many false positives) or sensitive (many false negatives).

Fructose Intolerance

Hydrogen Breath Test-Fructose (HBT-fructose)	An assessment for the change in the level of hydrogen and/or methane gas is diagnostic for fructose malabsorption.	HBT-fructose can be used to diagnose a mutation in the aldolase B gene. If hereditary fructose intolerance, may result in gastrointestinal symptoms and hypoglycemia.	Normal increase <20 parts/million (<20 ppm) Positive BHT-fructose >20 parts per million (>20 ppm)	Positive test results indicate probable benefit of a fructose-restricted diet; research supports use in abdominal pain, IBS, gout.
Fructose Sensitivity	Blood lymphocyte specimen grown with a mitogen to measure growth by incorporating tritiated radioactive thymidine into the DNA of the cells A functional test of fructose metabolism.	Functional intracellualar metabolic test of possible genetic errors compromising fructose metabolism like fructose-6-phospate	>34% patient's growth response test media measured by DNA synthesis compared to optimal growth observed in 100% media. (valid for male and female of 12 years or older)	Rule out fructose sensitivity in hypoglycemia of unknown etiology, overweight, obesity.

IV. Tests of Lipid Status

Lipids

Cholesterol, Total serum or plasma (CHOL)	CHOL is enzymatically released from cholesterol esters; fasting test	Total CHOL correlated with risk for cardiovascular diseases.	AHA/ACC/NHLBI 2014 Guidelines do not have target levels for cholesterol. Generally < than 200 mg/dL is desirable (see Chapter 33).	Cholesterol measurements have considerable within-subject variability. May partly result from variability in specimen collection or handling.
High Density Lipoproteins (HDL-c)	LDL-c (and VLDL-c) are precipitated from the serum before measurement of residual HDL-c particle size; direct measurement of HDL-c is now done in some laboratories.	HDL-c is called "good cholesterol" to indicate that it is protective against atherosclerotic vascular development	Generally, levels should be above 40 mg/dL. The higher the better.	Some precipitation methods cause underestimation of HDL;HDL can be divided into classes: HDL_1, HDL_2, and HDL_3; Elevated HDL_3 correlates with risk of CVD.
Low Density Lipoproteins (LDL-c)	LDL-c is estimated by the Friedewald formula, LDL-c = total cholesterol – HDL-c – TG/5, or by new direct assays. Available lipid particle size testing examples: www.privateMDLab.com(VAP Lipid Profile) www.BerkeleyHeartLab.com	LDL-c is called "bad cholesterol" to indicate that it is a positive risk factor for CVD. See NCEP guidelines in Chapter 33. Lipoprotein particle (LPP) size: Pattern B (small, dense LDL-C) is associated with increased risk of CHD and is responsive to diet. Pattern A (larger, buoyant LDL) is not associated with risk. LPP are not recommended in new ATP4.	Generally, below 130 mg/dL is considered desirable.	Calculation only valid when TG concentration is <400 mg/dL, cannot be determined in non-fasting serum or plasma. Direct assay methods preferred.
Triglycerides (TGs)	Lipases release glycerol and fatty acids from TGs.	The association of TGs and CHD has been shown. Elevated TG increases blood viscosity.	<150 mg/dL normal >500 mg/dL high	Fasting specimen is essential: sugar concentrated foods and alcohol ingestion can increase TG level; some anticoagulants may affect TG level; carnitine-dependent fatty acids synthesis.

Fat Malabsorption

Fecal fat screening	Microscopic inspection of fat-stained (Sudan stain) specimens for the presence of lipid droplets.	Trained observers are able to identify excessive fat in ~80% of persons with fat malabsorption.	Qualitative results	Patient must be consuming sufficient fat for analysis to reveal malabsorption. Semiquantitative.
Prothrombin time (PT)	Fat malabsorption decreases absorption of fat-soluble vitamins A,E,D,K,Beta-Carotene; low vitamin K levels impair coagulation, causing a prolonged PT. (also can be called INR (international normalized ratio))	A prolonged PT is a relatively sensitive but nonspecific indicator of the fat-soluble vitamin K from fat malabsorption.	10-15 sec INR: 0.8-1.1 Possible critical value: > 20 sec. INR: > 5.5	Tests affected by oral anticoagulants and other drugs, reduced platelet count, acquired and hereditary bleeding diseases, and liver disease PT.

Continued

Quantitative fecal fat determination	Patient must consume 100 g fat/day (4-8 oz whole milk/day, and 2 Tbsp vegetable oil/meal/day) for 2 days before collection	Quantitative 72-hour stool collection required for accurate assessment; average daily discharge used for interpretation.	Normal: <5 g fat/24 hr Malabsorption: >10 g/24 hr	Failure to adhere to the diet invalidates the results.
Vitamin A, D, E, K	See V. Tests of Micronutrient Status.			
Fatty acid analysis	Whole blood or RBC levels of ALA (C18 : 3n3) and LA (C18 : 2n6) reflect essential fatty acid status; Also, complex relationships regarding fatty acid analysis are related to neurological and inflammatory diseases, cell membrane dysfunction and genetic disorders [17,18]	RBC fatty acid shown to be associated with fatty acid tissue composition. Plasma fatty acid levels are associated with dietary fat or supplement intake or fat digestion and absorption.	Arachidonic Acid (AA)/Eicosapentanoic acid (EPA) = 1.5-3.0 = Normal AA/EPA = High Risk >15 Omega-3 (EP+DHA) Index Risk: Index <2.2 High Index 2.2-3.2 Moderate Index >3.2 Low Omega 6/Omega-3 Ratio 5.7-21 EPA/AA Ratio </= 0.2 Arachidonic Acid 520-1490 nmol/mL 5.2-12.9% EPA 14-100 nmol/mL 0.2-1.5% DHA 30-250 nmol/mL 0.2-3.9% GLA 16-150 nmol/mL Omega-6 : omega-3 optimal between 1 : 1 and 4 : 1.	Is not specific for risk of atherosclerotic disease; inflammation influences this fatty acid test. Likely causes are minor injuries, trauma, and bacterial infections, periodontal/cavitations, orodental disease,[19] chlamydia pneumoniae,[20] dietary fats and central adiposity[21]

V. Tests of Micronutrient Status
A. Vitamins

Thiamin (B₁)[c]	Thiamin status is usually assessed by measuring the amount of TPP needed to fully activate the RBC enzyme transketolase.	The TPP needed to fully activate transketolase is inversely related to B₁ status; percent stimulation by TTP.	Normal: 70-200 nmol/L (for individuals not taking thiamine (B1)) Stimulation >20% (index >1.2) indicates deficiency	Amount (and activity) of enzyme affected by drugs, iron, folate, or vitamin B₁₂ status, malignant or GI diseases, and diabetes.
Riboflavin (B₂)	Riboflavin status is assessed by measuring the amount of FAD needed to fully activate RBC enzyme GR	The FAD needed to fully activate GR is inversely related to B₂ status; percent stimulation.	% Stimulation >40% (index >1.4) indicates deficiency	Amount or activity of enzyme may change with age, iron status, liver disease, and glucose-6-phosphate dehydrogenase deficiency.
Niacin (B3)	Urinary excretion of N¹-methylnicotinamide (NMN) is decreased; <0.8 mg/day (<5.8 μmol/day) suggests a niacin deficiency.	Blood: Liquid Chromatography/Tandem Mass Spectrometry (LC/MS/MS) Niacin (nicotinic acid) is a water-soluble vitamin that is also referred to as vitamin B₃.	Nicotinic acid: 0.0–5.0 ng/mL Nicotinamide: 5.2–72.1 ng/mL	Niacin (nicotinic acid) is a water-soluble vitamin that is also referred to as vitamin B₃. Nicotinamide (nicotinic acid amide) is the derivative of niacin
Pyridoxine (B₆)[e] PLP (pyridoxal-5-phosphate) compounds	1. RBC enzymes, ALT (SGPT) or AST (SGOT),[e] are assayed for the presence of PLP as the enzymes' cofactor. 2. Plasma PLP can be directly measured by High-pressure liquid chromatography (HPLC) with fluorescence detection	1. Difference between enzyme activities before and after addition of PLP is inversely related to B₆ status. 2. PLP is major transport form of B₆; therefore serum levels reflect body stores.	1. % ALT stimulation of >25% or AST activity of >50% in deficiency 2. Normal: 0.50-3.0 mcg/dL (20-120 nmol/L) Male: 5.3–46.7 μg/L Female: 2.0–32.8 μg/L	1. Disease and drugs that affect the liver and heart, and pregnancy confound interpretation. 2. Deficiency may be seen clinically before plasma PLP levels decrease.

	3. Trp load test, measures excretion of the PLP-dependent metabolite xanthurenate acid (XA). 24 hour urine collection required.	3. Functional test indicating marginal vitamin B_6 status when the levels of urinary XA decrease significantly following the ingestion of 3-5 g of L-Trp	3. Marginal status: Level of urinary XA decreases <50 mg/24 hr	3. Steroid drugs and estrogen enzyme activity and some drugs cause analytic errors. Trp load test most sensitive and responsive to functional adequacy of B_6.
Folate[g]	1. Because of ↓ DNA synthesis, large RBCs are produced. See Chapter 32.	1. Deficiency leads to increase in MCV (mean corpuscular volume) and macrocytic RBCs	1. Normal: MCV 80-100 fL	1. Not sensitive or specific for folate. Possible involvement with B_6, B_{12}, SAMe and other cofactors in the methionine pathway.
	2. Shape of neutrophil nucleus affected by folate deficiency.	2. Increased neutrophil lobe count seen in folate deficiency.	2. Normal: < or equal 4 lobes per neutrophil	2. Lobe count sensitive but not specific.
	3. Blood folate levels can be directly measured by radioimmunoassay.	3. Both RBC and serum folate are indicators of body stores.	3. 2-10 mcg/L serum; 140-960 ng/L RBC (3.2-22 nmol/L)	3. Plasma from non-fasting subjects may reflect recent intake; RBC folate is not measured accurately.
	4. Functional folate status assayed by FIGLU in 24-hour urine or after oral histicine loading.	4. After 2-15 g loading dose, 10-50 mg of FIGLU should be excreted in 8 hours.	4. Normal: <7.4 mg/24 hours (<42.6 mmol/24 hr) without loading	4. FIGLU affected by vitamin B_{12}, drugs, liver disease, cancer, tuberculosis, and pregnancy.
	5. Single Nucleotide Polymorphisms (SNPs) MTHFR 677C MTHFR1298C	5. SNPs of compromised methylation (transfer of methyl groups in metabolism) potential in use and conversion of folate or folic acid intracellularly. See Chapter 5.	MTHF 677C/1298C Normal = Wild type −/−	Other SNPs are known that affect methylation metabolism: COMT, CYP1B1, and other cytochrome enzymes. See Chapter 5.
Cobalamin (B_{12})	1. Because of low B_{12} resulting in decreased DNA synthesis, large RBCs are produced.	1. Deficiency leads to increase in MCV	1. Normal: MCV 80-100 fL	1. Not sensitive or specific for B_{12}.
	2. Shape of neutrophil nucleus is affected by B_{12} deficiency.	2. Increased neutrophil lobe count in B_{12} deficiency.	2. Normal: < or equal 4 lobes per neutrophil	2. Lobe count sensitive but not specific.
	3. B_{12} can be directly measured by radioimmunoassay.	3. Levels <150 ng/L indicate deficiency (age affects level).	3. 130-950 pg/mL (118-701 pmol/L)	3. Marginal deficiency not correlated with level.
	4. Methylmalonic acid excretion (MMA) reflects a functional test of B_{12} availability for BCAA (branched chain amino acid) metabolism.	4. MMA excretion >300 mg/24 hr in B_{12} deficiency. Sensitive test without being overly specific.	4. Normal excretion: 5 mg/24 hr (<2 mmol/24 hr) Serum MMA - 0 08-0.56 mmol/L (Normal < 105 ng/mL)	4. Specific for B_{12} but requires normal BCAA levels; available at most laboratories.
	5. Schilling test for intrinsic factor and B_{12} absorption assesses radiolabeled B_{12} absorption as reflected by urinary excretion.	5. Abnormal B_{12} absorption indicated by excretion <3% of B_{12} radioactivity per 24 hours.	5. Normal excretion: ~3% of radioactivity per 24 hours	5. Test must be repeated with oral administration of intrinsic factor (IF) to differentiate IF deficiency and malabsorption. Rarely used because of necessity of radioactive B_{12}.
	6. Homocysteine (Hcy)	Hcy level is an independent risk factor for CVD, venous thrombotic disease, and other diseases; folic acid and vitamins B_{12} and B_6 reduce plasma Hcy levels. Total Hcy (oxidized + reduced forms) is an intermediate amino acid in methionine metabolism.	Normal: 4-14 mmol/L Suggested optimal levels: 4-7 mmol/L	Cardiovascular event risk is increased even at slightly elevated levels. Hcy has a strong association with degenerative neurologic conditions like Parkinson's disease and dementias. Hcy suggests poor methylating capacity of client with need for increased intake of folic acid, B_6, B_{12}, and SAMe.

Continued

Ascorbic acid (vitamin C)	Plasma or leukocyte vitamin C measured by (1) chromatography; (2) by ascorbate oxidase; (3) spectrophotometrically by reaction with 2,4-dinitrophenylhydrazine.	Leukocyte C is less affected by recent intake, but plasma levels in fasting person parallel leukocyte levels; plasma preferred for acutely ill patients because leukocyte level is affected by infection,[22] some drugs, and hyperglycemia;	Normal: 0 to 11 months: Not established 1 to 12 years: 0.2–2.3 mg/dL 13+ years: 0.2–2.0 mg/dL (30-80 mmol/L) Adult: 0.2-1.5 mg/dL (12–90 mmol/L) Leukocyte vitamin C: 20-50 mcg/10^8	Blood samples must be carefully prepared for assay to prevent vitamin C breakdown. Oxalate, glucose, and proteins interfere with some assays; recent intake can mask deficiency.
Retinols (vitamin A)	Serum retinol and retinol esters; functional tests (e.g., dark adaptation) only detect severe deficiency; Age and sex important determining factors for normal retinol levels.	Retinol levels <20 mcg/dL (<0.7 mmol/L) indicate severe deficiency; specific levels are being determined for placental/newborn deficiency serum levels.	Normal: 20 to 100 mcg/dL (0.7-3.5 mmol/L) Suboptimum (NHANES II/ Gibson): Age 3-11 y: < 0.35 mmol/L Age 12-17 y <0.70 mmol/L Age 18-74 y 0.70-1.05 mmol/L Pregnancy 0.79-1.91 mmol/L Upper Limit: 3.5 mmol\L	Exposure of serum to bright light or oxygen destroys vitamin A; low RBP (retinol binding protein) level is associated with low vitamin A, zinc and iron (see protein-energy section). Vitamin A's gene transcription is on the nuclear RXR;[22] the vitamin D receptor forms a heterodimer, requiring balance between vitamins A and D for optimum function.
Carotene, Serum Total (CARO)	Carotenoids, fat-soluble pigments in plant foods, poorly absorbed in fat malabsorption; light sensitive; transport specimen in amber transport tube; Quantitative Spectrophotometry testing. See Raman Spectroscopy, Chapter 7.	A CARO level of less than 50 mg/dL is seen in ~85% of patients with fat malabsorption.	50-200 mcg/dL (0.74-3.72 mmol/L)	Decreased CARO levels or low spectrophotometry score are also seen in those with low vegetable and fruit diets (e.g., in PN or tube feeding), liver failure, celiac disease, cystic fibrosis, human immunodeficiency virus, and some lipoprotein disorders.
Tocopherols (vitamin E)	Serum alpha- and beta-gamma-tocopherols serve different antioxidant functions. Growing evidence that beta and gamma tocopherols may be more important than alpha-tocopherol for human vitamin E nutrition.	Lower values found in infants. Interpretation requires monitoring lipid levels; if hyperlipidemia calculate plasma alpha-tocopherol: cholesterol mmol/L ratio <2.2 or alpha-tocopherol <5 mg/L indicates risk of vitamin E deficiency[23]	Normal: alpha-tocopherol 5.7-20 mg/L beta-gamma-tocopherol 4.3 or less mg/L	Plasma level depends on recent intake and level of lipids, especially TGs, in blood. Smoking and BMI also negatively affect tocopherol levels.
Cholecalciferol (D$_3$) and (D$_2$) ergocalciferol	1. Alkaline phosphatase activity reflects level of bone activity and indirectly vitamin D status. (see further discussion of ALP in Liver Enzymes section).		Adult: 25-100 U/L Child 1-12 yr: <350 U/L	1. Not specific, but a sensitive indicator; serum Ca and PO$_4$ should also be evaluated. Zinc and B$_{12}$ are rate-limiting cofactors for production of alkaline phosphatase;, therefore low levels of < 40 U/L suggest possible zinc or B$_{12}$ or intrinsic factor insufficiencies.
	2. Cholecalcidiol (D3 25-OH-D) and ergocalciferol (D2 25-OH-D).	2. <20 ng/mL (<50 nmol/L) indicates deficiency; >200 ng/mL (500 nmol/L) indicates hypervitaminosis D.	2. 30 – 100 ng/mL (75 – 250 nmol/L)	2. Best indicator of status (liver stores), but marginal levels hard to interpret.[24] Increased BMI and body fat % may reduce serum D3 25-OH vit D.
	3. Calcitriol (1,25-[OH]2-D$_3$)	3. Used to show that vitamin D metabolism is occurring normally; Active vitamin D to signal nuclear RXR receptor.	3. 2.5-4.5 ng/dL (60-108 pmol/L) (little seasonal change)	3. Poor indicator of status because of tight control of synthesis independent of body stores.

25-hydroxyvitamin D (25-OH-D) / Calcifediol/ Calcidiol	Prohormone Vitamin D malabsorption can lead to secondary malabsorption of calcium. Vitamin D supplementation can lead to increased absorption of calcium and phosphorus; supplementation contraindicated for individuals with kidney or gall stones, sarcoidosis, tuberculosis, lymphoma, or when become hypercalcemic with vitamin D supplementation.	Vitamin D insufficiency is defined as the lowest threshold value for plasma 25-OH-D that prevents secondary hyperparathyroidism, bone turnover, bone mineral loss, or seasonal variations in plasma PTH.	25-OH-D: 30-100 ng/mL (85-160 nmol/L) Deficiency: <20 ng/mL (<50 nmol/L (lab references vary per individual laboratory)	Available at all laboratories. If elevated serum calcium, further evaluation recommended by testing vitamin 1,25 DOH, PTH, ionized or free calcium, vitamin A retinol and osteocalcin (as a vitamin K2 marker) before supplementation.
Phylloquinone (K$_1$) and Menaquinone (K$_2$) Menadione (K$_3$)	Normal coagulation factor synthesis requires K1. PT assesses coagulation status. K2 primarily involved with calcium metabolism, including bone health.	In K1 deficiency, PT increases with increasing production of abnormal coagulation factors.[h] K1 vegetable plant source; drug-nutrient interaction with blood thinners. K2 animal and bacterial fermented sources. K3 synthetic form of Vitamin K; vitamin precursor to Vitamin K2 known as a provitamin.	K1: 0.13-1.19 ng/mL (0.29-2.64 nmol/L K2: (not commercially available—see K2 marker, Osteocalcin, below)	The level of vitamin K available for vitamin K–dependent bone proteins may not be reflected by the PT; test references vary significantly with method.
Osteocalcin (OC) / undercarboxylated osteocalcin (ucOC) (K2 marker)	Serum noncollagenous protein specific for bone and dentin formation and turnover. Functional marker of vitamin K2, a rate-limiting cofactor of formation of osteocalcin. One of the osteocalcin fragments, undercarboxylated osteocalcin, is most sensitive K2 marker and associated with risk of fracture.	Can be used as a marker of metabolic trend, suggesting low or high vitamin K2; useful in assessing need for a vitamin K2 rich diet or K2 supplementation to optimize formation of intracellular bone osteocalcin. K2 inhibits soft tissue calcification. OC and ucOC are considered more sensitive markers of bone activity than alkaline phosphatase during corticosteroid therapy.	OC: 11-50 ng/mL ucOC: Normal < 1.65 ng/mL High > 1.65 ng/mL NOTE: Elevated levels associated with low 25-OH-vit D levels	Vitamin K2 is not as involved with coagulation as K1. Vitamin K2 is important in calcium metabolism and therefore calcium and vitamin D status. There is a synthetic vitamin K3, usually administered IV that has similar actions as K2, and is being used as adjunctive to integrative cancer therapy.

B. Minerals
Electrolytes

Sodium (Na$^+$) Potassium (K$^+$) Chloride (Cl$^-$) Bicarbonate or total CO$_2$	Serum electrolytes, including bicarbonate, are usually measured together by ion-specific electrodes in autoanalyzers; sometimes Na and K are measured by flame emission spectrophotometry.[i]	Elevated serum Na seen in water loss; decreased serum Na and K occurs in diarrhea and with poor dietary intake or cellular uptake. Decreased chloride levels are seen with cation and osmotic changes in the body. Bicarbonate levels reflect acid-base balance.	Na: 135-145 mEq/L (135-145 mmol/L) K: 3.5-5 mEq/L (3.5-5 mmol/L) Cl: 100-110 mEq/L (100-110 mmol/L) Bicarb or total CO2: 21-30 mEq/L (21-30 mmol/L)	Electrolytes change rapidly in response to changes in physiology (e.g., hormonal stimulus, renal and other organ dysfunction, acid-base balance changes, and drug action. Serum electrolytes are minimally affected by diet.

Major Minerals

Calcium (Ca^{2+})	1. Total serum Ca^{2+} (bound and unbound)	Usually slightly more than half of the serum Ca^{2+} is bound to albumin or complexed with other molecules; the remaining Ca^{2+} is called *ionized Ca (ICA)*; ICA is available physiologically. Elevated IgE and mast cell release increases intracellular calcium ion levels and negatively distributes ICA.	1. 8.6 - 10 mg/dL (2.15-2.5 mmol/L)	Calcium status is related to many factors, including vitamin D, vitamin K2, phosphate, parathyroid function, renal function: medications (thiazide diuretics, lithium), vitamin A toxicity, presence of malignancy
	2. Ionized (free) Ca^{2+}	Interpretation of ionized calcium levels requires consideration of other related markers: osteocalcin, vitamin D25-OH vit D and D1,25-OH vit D, and serum retinol (vit A.)	2. 4.64-5.28 mg/dL (1.16-1.32 mmol/L)	Ionized calcium depends on vitamin K2 to enter the bone matrix and to prevent calcification of soft tissue. If phosphate <3.0 mg/dL, check intake of phosphate-binding medications.

Continued

Phosphate (H_2PO_4, (Phosphorus)	Phosphorus in body as phosphate form; test measures inorganic phosphate. Most phosphate is part of organic compounds; small part is inorganic.	Abnormal P level is most closely associated with disturbed intake, distribution, or renal function.	2. 7-4.5 mg/dL (0.87-1.45 mmol/L) (higher in children)	Reported as phosphorus (P), not phosphate; hemolyzed blood cannot be used because of high RBC phosphate levels.
Magnesium (Mg^{2+})	1. Total serum Mg^{2+} measured after reaction to form chromogenic or fluorescent complexes. 2. Ionized (free) Mg^{2+}	Neuromuscular function. Hyperirritability, tetany, convulsion, and electrocardiographic changes occur when levels of total serum Mg^{2+} fall to <1 mEq/L.	1. 1.3-2.5 mEq/L (0.65-1.25 mmol/L) 2. 0.7-1.2 mEq/L (0.35-0.60 mmol/L)	Usually 45% of the serum Mg^{2+} is complexed with other molecules; the remaining Mg^{2+} is called ionized magnesium. Serum levels remain constant until body stores are nearly depleted.
Trace Minerals Iron CBC[k] and RBC indices	1. HCT = % RBC in whole blood 2. Hgb = blood hemoglobin concentration 3. MCV = mean RBC volume = mean corpuscular volume	A CBC with RBC indices is one of the first set of tests that a patient receives; although CBC data are not specific for nutrition status, their universal and repeated presence in the patient's record makes them very important.	1. Females: 35%-47% (0.35-0.47)[l] Males: 42%-52% (0.42-0.52) 2. Females: 12-15 g/dL (7.45-9.31 mmol/L) Males: 14-17 g/dL (8.44-10.6 mmol/L) 3. 82-99 mm³ (82-99 fL)	These tests are affected only when iron stores are essentially depleted. HCT and Hgb are sensitive to hydration status; low MCV also occurs in thalassemias and lead poisoning as well as with iron and copper deficiencies; high MCV suggests macrocytic RBCs and possible inadequate folate, vitamins B_6, or B_{12}.
Serum iron (Fe)	Serum Fe^{3+} reduced to Fe^{2+} and then complexed with chromogen.	Slightly higher in males than in premenopausal females; reflects recent Fe intake.	F: 40-150 mcg/dL (7.2-26.9 mmol/L) M: 50-160 mg/dL (8.9-28.7 mmol/L)	Very insensitive index of total Fe stores; extremely variable (day-to-day and diurnal).
Total Iron Binding Capacity (TIBC)	TIBC determined by saturating serum transferrin with Fe and then remeasuring serum Fe.	Reflects transferrin concentration.	250-400 mcg/dL (45-71 mmol/L)	TIBC does not increase until Fe stores are essentially completely depleted. TIBC decreases with increased Fe stores; used to rule out excess iron intake or hemochromatosis. See Chapter 32
Transferrin (Tf or TFN)	The iron bound globulin protein that responds to the need for iron; half-life ~9 days. (see Chapter 7)	(see Section I:A. Protein Status : Tf)	Females: 250-380 mg/dL (2.15-3.80 g/L) Males: 215-365 mg/dL (2.15-3.65 g/L) Newborn: 130-275 mg/dL Child: 203-360 mg/dL	Transferrin is low when Fe stores essentially depleted. Transferrin is low with low vitamin B_6 and low Tf-sat in aplastic anemia.
Transferrin Saturation (Tf-sat or TSAT)	Tf-sat (%) = Serum iron level ÷ TIBC x 100%	(see Section I:A. Protein Status : Tf-sat)	Females: 15%-50% Males: 20%-50% Chronic illness - normal Tf-sat%. Late pregnancy low Tf-sat%.	
RBC Distribution Width (RDW)	Measurement of variation in RBC diameter (anisocytosis); reported to be helpful in distinguishing Fe deficiency from anemia associated with chronic inflammation.	Very sensitive indicator of Fe status; normal RDW reportedly rules out anemia caused by chronic inflammatory diseases.[m] Thalassemia (low MCV, normal RDW) differentiated from iron-deficiency (low MCV, high RDW)	Normal value: 11.0-14.5% Microscopic electronic interpretation required.	Specificity of RDW for Fe deficiency is relatively low; interpretation confounded by RBC transfusion; measurement usually not reported.

Ferritin	The primary intracellular Fe-storage protein stored mostly in liver; serum levels parallel iron stores;	Best biochemical index of uncomplicated iron deficiency or overload (iron toxicity) and excess storage. Rule out hemochromatosis or pancreatitis if Ferritin >1000 ng/dL (>1000 mcg/L).	Iron overload: >400 ng/mL (mcg/L) With anemia of chronic disease: <100 ng/mL (<100 mcg/L) F: 10-150 ng/mL (10-150 mcg/L) M: 12-300 ng/mL (12-300 mcg/L) Females with anemia of chronic disease: <20 ng/mL (<20 mcg/L) 6 mos.-15 yr: 7-142 ng/mL (7-142 mcg/L) <1 mo. - 5 mos.: 50-200 ng/mL (50-200 mcg/L) Newborn: 25-200 ng/mL (25-200 mcg/L)	A positive acute phase reactant that increases during metabolic response to injury, even when Fe stores are adequate; not useful in anemia of chronic and inflammation diseases.
Zinc (Zn)[n]	Serum levels measured by atomic absorption spectrophotometry.	Serum levels affected by diet and the inflammatory response. Zinc deficiency associated with many diseases and trauma.	0.7-1.2 mg/L (11-18 mmol/L)	Serum levels detect frank—but not marginal—deficiency; blood must be collected in zinc-free tubes.
Copper (Cu)	1. Serum levels measured by flame emission atomic absorption spectrophotometry (AS) or Inductively-Coupled Plasma/Mass Spectrometry (ICP/MS). 2. Ceruloplasmin is the major Cu-containing plasma protein; measured by immunoassay (e.g., nephelometry).	1. Cu deficiency is associated with neutropenia, anemia, and scurvy-like bone disease and megadoses of zinc. 2. Ceruloplasmin is required for conversion of Fe^{3+} to Fe^{2+} during cellular Fe uptake. Anemia can result from low ceruloplasmin. Ceruloplasmin is useful biomarker to follow Tetrathiomolybdate ™ (T.M.) copper chelation for Wilson's Disease and cancer anti-angiogenesis copper chelation therapy.[25]	Adult: 70-175 mcg/dL (11-28 mmol/L) 20 to 35 mg/dL (1-4 mmol/L)	1. Serum levels detect frank but not marginal deficiency; use of oral contraceptives lowers serum Cu. 2. Ceruloplasmin not a useful marker of Cu status, but can be used to assess changes in status after supplementation; useful to calculate free copper index with serum zinc and serum copper as a cancer biomarker.[26,28,29]
Selenium (Se)	1. Serum selenium test 2. Whole blood levels better reflect long-term status.	Margin between deficiency and toxicity is narrower for Se than any other trace component of the antioxidant enzyme element; important in glutathione peroxidase.	(1) 80-320 mcg/L (1-4 mmol/L) (2) 60-340 mcg/L (0.75-4.3 mmol/L)	Cutoff points for deficiency or toxicity are not well established.
Iodine (I)	Urinary excretion is best indicator of I status, either mcg/24 hr or mcg/g creatinine; thyroid hormone level related to I status. Urine test can use 50 mg I/KI challenge.	Excretion should be 24-hour urine >70 mcg/g creatinine. It can be beneficial to test thyroid hormone and antibodies (TSH, T_3-free, T_4-free, thyroid peroxidase and thyroglobulin antibodies) for improved interpretation. Iodine important for other metabolic functions.	No urinary I reference range; T_4 reference range: F: 5-12 mcg/dL (64-154 mmol/L) M: 4-12 mcg/dL (51-154 mmol/L)	Thyroid hormone levels are affected by many factors besides iodine status. Other halogen elements (Br+, Fl+, Cl+) are known antagonists to iodine metabolism; when completing the iodine urine testing, some laboratories will also test for bromine, fluorine, and chlorine.
Creatinine (Cr)	Urinary excretion usually tested by atomic absorption spectrophotometry.	Excretion should be 0.63-2.50 g/24 hr; deficiency reported in patients on long-term PN; decreased levels in diabetes mellitus.	10-200 ng/dL (1.9-38 nmol/L)	Test not available in most clinical laboratories; special handling required to prevent specimen contamination during collection.

Continued

VI. Blood Gases and Hydration Status

pH	$pH = -\log[H^+]$; H^+ depends mainly on the CO_2 from respiration: $CO_2 + H_2O \Leftrightarrow H_2CO_3 \Leftrightarrow HCO_3 + H^+$ Measured by ion-selective electrodes (like those found in common pH meters)	Acidosis: pH <7.35 Alkalosis: pH >7.45 pH compatible with life: 6.80-7.80.	Whole blood: Arterial pH: 7.35-7.45 Venous pH: 7.32-7.42	Blood must not be exposed to air before or during measurement.
Po_2 and O_2 saturation (SaO_2)	Whole blood O_2 measured by oxygen electrode. $Po_2 =$ "pressure" contributed by O_2 to the total "pressure" of all the gases dissolved in blood. O_2 Content (CaO2) = O_2/gm SaO_2 x Hgb (gm/dl) x 1.34 ml + PaO_2 x (.003 ml O_2/mm Hg/dl) $PaO_2 = FIO_2$(PB-47) − 1.2($PaCO_2$)	Affected by alveolar gas exchange, ventilation-perfusion inequalities, and generalized alveolar hypoventilation.	Arterial blood: PaO_2: 83-108 mm Hg <40 mm Hg = critical value (gravely dangerous) O_2 saturation: 0.95-0.98 (95%-98%) Elderly = 95% Newborn = 40-90%	Blood must not be exposed to air before or during measurement.
PCO_2	Measured by ion-selective electrode; "pressure" contributed by CO_2 to the total "pressure" of all the gases dissolved in blood.	Increased in respiratory acidosis (increased CO_2 in inspired air or decreased in alveolar ventilation) and decreased in respiratory alkalosis (e.g., in hyperventilation from anxiety, mechanical ventilator, or closed head injury [damaged respiratory center]).	Whole blood: Arterial F: 32-45 mm Hg M: 35-48 mm Hg Venous 6-7 mm Hg higher	Blood must not be exposed to air before or during measurement.
Bicarbonate (HCO_3^-) and total CO_2 (tCO_2)	For whole blood (HCO_3^-) is calculated from the equation given in pH section.	Increased in compensated respiratory acidosis and in metabolic acidosis; decreased in metabolic acidosis and in compensated respiratory alkalosis.	Whole blood, arterial: 21-28 mEq/L (21-28 mmol/L)	Blood must not be exposed to air before or during measurement.
Osmolality (Osmol), serum	Osmol depends on amount of particles (solutes) dissolved in a solution; measurement based on relationship between solute concentration and freezing point; serum osmol assesses hydration status and solute load.	Serum Osmol increases in dehydration, diabetic coma, diabetic ketoacidosis; also estimated from the formula: mOsmol/L = 2 (Na^+) + (Glucose mg/dL)/18 + (BUN mg/dL)/2.8	282-300 mOsm/kg H_2O (1 Osmol = 1 mol of solute particles; 1 kg serum/L)	Freezing point depression gives a more accurate estimate of osmol than the calculated value (e.g., in ketoacidosis).
Urinalysis: Specific Gravity (Sp.Gr.)	Specimen midstream clean-catch if infection suspected, or regular collection. Dip Stick or laboratory testing for Specific Gravity.	One of a multiple of tests on a urine specimen. Sp.Gr. is a measure of concentration of particles and electrolytes in the urine.	Adult: 1.005-1.030 Sp.Gr. Newborn: 1.001-1.020 Sp.Gr.	Appearance can also give subjective indication of fluid concentration; darker color = higher concentration.

VII. Tests of Antioxidant Status and Oxidative Stress

Water-soluble compounds	See Vitamin C above.			
Lipid-soluble compounds: see Vitamin E, Carotenoids, and Coenzyme Q_{10}	The carotenoids: lutein, xanthine zeaxanthin, alpha- and beta-carotene, and lycopene; carotenoids and coenzyme Q_{10} (ubiquinone-10) are measured chromatographically	Reference ranges for these compounds vary greatly, depending on the method used for their assay.	See reference for carotenoid range under fat malabsorption	Tests for carotenoids and coenzyme Q are not yet available for routine clinical use.
Total antioxidant capacity (e.g., ORAC, TEAC, FRAP)	ORAC: Oxygen radical absorbance capacity TEAC: Trolox-equivalent antioxidant capacity FRAP: Ferric-reducing ability of plasma. See Raman Spectroscopy in Chapter 7 for carotenoid assessment.	These assays reflect the presence of all of plasma or serum antioxidants, including vitamins C and E, carotenoids, coenzyme Q_{10}, glutathione, uric acid, bilirubin, superoxide dismutase, catalase, glutathione peroxidase, and albumin.		These assays are now commercially available but are currently performed only in specialized laboratories. Testing botanicals also available.

Oxidative stress markers:	Free radical oxidation products of lipids	8-Isoprostane (also called 8-epiprostaglandin F$_{2a}$) increases in plasma or urine of patients with lung disease, hypercholesterolemia, or diabetes mellitus. 8HDG represents whole-body cytosolic and nuclear free radical activity, including status of DNA. Lipid peroxides is a marker of membrane oxidative damage by reactive oxygen species (ROS) to PUFAs of cell membranes.	Examples: o-tyrosine nitro-tyrosine 8-isoprostane 4-hydroxynonenal maondialdehyde Lipid Peroxides 8-hydroxy-2-deoxyguanosine (8-CHDG) (refer to Laboratory references)	8-Isoprostane assays are now commercially available. Markers of oxidative stress are currently assayed only in specialized laboratories.

VIII. Tests for Monitoring Nutrition Support

CRP (see section V. hs-CRP)	CRP is an acute-phase protein used to assess inflammatory status.	Large increases in CRP are associated with development of a catabolic state during the stress response; CRP levels begin to fall when the anabolic phase is entered.	CRP <10 mg/L	Serial values rather than a single value must be used to specify the stage of the stress response.
Chemistry panel with phosphate and Mg^{2+}	Panel includes electrolytes, glucose, creatinine, BUN, and total CO$_2$ (bicarbonate); see earlier discussion for additional test information.	Used to monitor carbohydrate tolerance, hydration status, and major organ system function.	See earlier discussion on phosphate and magnesium.	Very frequently ordered test panel.
Osmolality	(see discussion in VII. Blood Gases and Hydration Status)			
Protein-Energy Balance	(see earlier discussion on PAB, RBP, Tf, ALB, nPCR, Nitrogen Balance, UUN and TUN)			
Minerals: Zn, Cu, Se, Cr	(see earlier discussion of serum zinc, serum copper, ceruloplasmin, and lymphocyte micronutrient testing)			
Vitamins C, D and A	(see earlier discussion of vitamins C, D and A) Because vitamins C, 25-OH-D, and A are important in immune function and wound healing, they should be assessed regularly.	Note regarding TPN nutritional monitoring: Vitamin C levels can ↓ sharply in response to stress. Vitamin D and A nuclear receptors share the same connection with the RXR receptor which have synergistic function and should be monitored congruently.[27,28]		Note regarding TPN nutritional monitoring. Systematic, regular monitoring protocol should be followed. 25-OH-vit D is produced in the liver and can be suppressed with hepatic stress conditions.[29]
Vitamin K1 & K2 status	(TPN only) (see earlier discussion) Contribution of the gut flora to vitamin K status is absent during TPN, and basic TPN formulas are devoid of it.			Important to differentiate between vitamin K1 and K2.

IX. Liver Function Tests

Bilirubin (BILI T/D) (Direct and Indirect)	Total serum bilirubin represents both conjugated or direct bilirubin, and unconjugated or indirect bilirubin. Elevated levels suggest medical problem.	Conjugated bilirubin levels are elevated with cancer of pancreas or liver and bile duct obstruction; unconjugated bilirubin level elevated with hepatitis and jaundice anemias	Total bilirubin: 0.3-1 mg/dL (5.1-17 mmol/L) Direct bilirubin: 0.1-0.3 mg/dL; (1.7-5.1 mmol/L) Indirect bilirubin: 0.2-0.8 mg/dL (3.4-12 mmol/L)	Many medications are associated with elevated bilirubin levels.
Alanine Amino Transferase (ALT)	Enzyme found primarily in the liver (also called serum glutamic pyruvic transaminase (SGPT).	Injury to the liver results in elevated levels of ALT. Depressed in malnutrition.	4-36 U/L Infant: 2 x adult levels	Many medications and alcohol intake are associated with elevated ALT levels. ALT levels are often compared with AST for differential diagnosis.
Gamma-glutamyl transferase (GGT)	Biliary excretory enzyme involved in transfer of amino acids across cell membranes.	Used to evaluate progression of liver disease and screening for alcoholism	F: 4-25 U/L M: 12-38 U/L	Many medications are associated with elevated GGT levels.

Continued

Test	Description	Clinical significance	Reference values	Notes
Alkaline phosphatase (ALP)	Enzyme found primarily in the bone, liver, and biliary tract; increased in an alkaline environment.	Elevated levels noted in liver and bone disorders.	30-120 U/L	Nonspecific test; other tests need to confirm diagnosis. Many medications are associated with elevated ALP levels.
Aspartate Amino Transferase (AST)	Enzyme primarily found in the heart, liver, and skeletal muscle cells. (Also called serum glutamic oxaloacetic transaminase (SGOT))	Diagnostic tool when coronary occlusive heart disease or hepatocellular disease is suspected.	0-35 U/L	Many medications are associated with elevated AST levels. AST levels are often compared with ALT for differential diagnosis.
Alpha 1 Antitrypsin (A1AT)	A1AT is a serine protease inhibitor secreted primarily by hepatocytes. Most common genetic A1AT variants are ZZ, SS, MZ, SZ. Measured by serum electrophoresis.	Decreased or absent Alpha-1-band in serum electrophoresis; A1AT is an acute-phase reactant associated with emphysema, COPD and cirrhosis of the liver; A1AT elevated with states of inflammation, infection or malignancy.	85-213 mg/dL (0.85-2.13 g/L) Homozygous + + variants: severe disease early in life. 80 known variants of A1AT gene: heterozygous ZZ and SS gene variants: majority have hepatic or pulmonary symptoms MZ and SZ milder gene variants: rarely have symptoms.[o,p]	There are 100 known variants of the A1AT gene.[o,p] If a person is not diagnosed with a severe form as a child, an individual may not be identified until an adult with end-stage lung and liver disease..

X. Thyroid Function Tests

Test	Description	Clinical significance	Reference values	Notes
Thyroxine Total T_4, and free T_4	Measures the total amount of T_4 in the blood; free T_4 is the active form. See Chapter 31.	T_4 increased in hyperthyroidism; T_4 decreased in hypothyroidism and malnutrition	T_4, Total F: 5-12 mcg/dL; (64-154 nmol/L) M: 4-12 mcg/dL (51-154 nmol/L) Free T_4 = 0.7-1.9 ng/dl (10-23 pmol/L)	Tests are ordered to distinguish between euthyroidism, or hyperthyroidism and hypothyroidism. Can be related to iodine deficiencies.
Triiodothyronine T_3, Total and free T_3	Measures the total amount of T_3 in the blood; free T_3 active form. See Chapter 31.	Hyperthyroidism-usually elevated; hypothyroidism-usually decreased and can show low function of thyroid peroxidase enzyme when T_4 normal or high, and T_3 low (poor conversion).	Total T_3 20-50 yr: 70-205 ng/dL (1.2-3.4 nmol/L) >50 yr: 40-180 ng/dL (0.6-2.8 nmol/L) Free T_3: 230-619 pg/mL	Tests are ordered to distinguish between euthyroidism, or hyperthyroidism and hypothyroidism. If low T_3 levels, consider insufficient nutrient cofactors (selenium, vitamin E) for thyroid peroxidase enzyme conversion of T_4 to T_3.
Thyroid-stimulating hormone (TSH)	Used to monitor exogenous thyroid replacement or thyroid suppression; also used as a screening test for thyroid function. See Chapter 31.	Decreased TSH in hyperthyroidism; elevated TSH in hypothyroidism	0.5-5 mIU/L AACE Standards: Target TSH: 0.3-3.0 µIU/mL[o]	Tests are ordered to distinguish between euthyroidism, hyperthyroidism and hypothyroidism. If depressed, use caution with iodine intake. If elevated, consider assessing nutrient cofactors: iodine, selenium, vitamin E, A.
Antithyroglobulin antibody (anti-TG)	Anti-TG blood test used as a marker for autoimmune thyroiditis and related diseases.[30] High prevalence of thyroid autoantibodies in celiac and rheumatoid arthritis patients	Anti-TG autoantibodies bind to thyroglobulin and affect thyroid hormone synthesis, storage and release. Recommend investigation of gluten intolerance if elevated Anti-TG.	Titer <4 IU/mL Anti-TG often tested in conjunction with Anti-TPO test.	Resulting disordered thyroid function seen most with common related conditions: Hashimoto's thyroiditis and autoimmune hypothyroid.
Antithyroid peroxidase antibody (Anti-TPO or TPO-AB)	Anti-TPO blood test used in the diagnosis of thyroid diseases, such as Hashimoto's thyroiditis or chronic lympocytic thyroiditis (in children). High prevalence of thyroid autoantibodies in celiac and rheumatoid arthritis patients	Thyroid microsomal antibodies act on section of the microsome in the thyroid cell and initiate inflammatory and cytotoxic effects on the thyroid follicle. Recommend investigation of gluten intolerance if elevated Anti-TPO.	TPO AB <9 IU/mL Anti-TPO often tested in conjunction with Anti-TG test.	Most sensitive assay for antimicrosomal antibody. Nutritional considerations are vitamin E and selenium cofactors for production of TPO enzyme.

XI. Tests for Metabolic Disease

Amino acidurias	Dietary treatment is the major therapy for many of these genetic diseases: phenylketonuria, cystinuria, maple syrup urine disease, tyrosinemia, homocystinuria, Hartrup disease. See Chapter 42. Urine or plasma amino acid testing.	Monitoring amino acid level in urine or serum is necessary to assess adequacy of treatment.	Examples: Phe: 2-6 g/L (120-360 mmol/L) Phe (during pregnancy): 2-6 mg/dL (120-360 mmol/L) Cys: 2-22 g/L (10-90 mmol/L) Val: 17-37 g/L (145-315 mmol/L) Tyr: 4-16 g/L (20-90 mmol/L)	There are several methods used to measure (e.g., phenylalanine); these usually do not have exactly equivalent reference ranges.
Organic Acids Panel	Urine organic acids panel; home collection of 10 ml sample of nocturnal and first morning urine, frozen and then shipped to lab.[q]	Sensitive, broad range test that evaluates comprehensive functional markers for metabolic nutrient pathway functions that can suggest early markers for risk of disease or metabolic imbalances.	(see particular lab references)	Excellent for overview of metabolic function and non-invasive pediatric testing.

Diabetes Mellitus (See Chapter 31)

Prediabetes diagnosis	Fasting Blood Glucose (FBG)	Prediabetes, blood glucose levels are higher than normal but not high enough for a diagnosis of diabetes.	Non-diabetic FBG = < 99 mg/dL Impaired fasting glucose: 100-125 mg/dL	American Diabetes Association recommends testing for prediabetes in adults without symptoms who are overweight or obese, and who have one or more additional risk factors for diabetes.
Diabetes diagnosis	1. Serum or whole blood glucose: after fasting 8-16 hours or on a random blood sample.	1. Two or more FBG levels >126 mg/dL are diagnostic; random level >200 mg/dL followed by fasting level >126 mg/dL are diagnostic. Fasting levels of 110 to 126 mg/dL indicate impaired glucose tolerance (IGT.)		1. Elevated glucose levels normally appear with physiologic stress; whole blood gives slightly lower values.
	2. Glucose tolerance test (GGT); 75 g glucose (100 g during pregnancy) given after fasting; serum glucose measured by before and five times during the next 3 hours after oral dosing. Glucose measured by automated chemistry procedure.	2. Serum levels FBG >200 mg/dL at 2-hour point is diagnostic; 2-hour level <140 and all 0- to 2-hour levels <200 are normal; 140-199 at 2 hours indicates IGT. Gestational diabetes: fasting >105; 1-hour GGT >190; 2 hour GGT >165; and 3-hour GGT >145 mg/dL.	2. Serum: Fasting: <110 mg/dL (<6.1 mmol/L) 30 min: <200 mg/dL (<11.1 mmol/L) 1 hour: <200 mg/dL (<11.1 mmol/L) 2 hours: <140 mg/dL (<7.8 mmol/L) 3 hours: 70-115 mg/dL (<6.4 mmol/L) 4 hours: 70-115 mg/dL (<6.4 mmol/L) Urine: glucose negative	2. Often used for confirmation; ambulatory patient only; bed rest or stress impairs GGT; inadequate carbohydrate consumption before test invalidates results.

Continued

| Diabetes monitoring | 1. Blood glucose—monitoring requires that *the patient* monitor blood glucose level. 2. Serum fructosamine—assesses medium-term glucose control by measured glycated serum proteins; currently testing available in the laboratory and home tests. 3. Serum glycated hemoglobin or HgbA1C—assesses longer-term glucose control. 4. Porphyrin urine or whole blood testing for dioxin,[31] a toxin with significant association with promoting diabetes | 1. Tight diabetes control requires frequent monitoring of glucose levels. 2. Allows assessment of average glucose levels for previous 2-3 weeks. 3. Allows assessment of average glucose levels for previous 2-3 months and verification of patient's serum glucose log. | 1. 70-99 mg/dL (3.9-5.5 mmol/L) 2. Normal levels: 1%-2% of total protein Ranges vary according to method used. 3. Normal levels: Nondiabetic: 4-5.9% Good diabetic control: 4-7% Fair diabetic control: 6%-8% Poor diabetic control: >8%; Mean blood sugar 205 mg/dL or greater is associated with increased risk of side effects | A combination of glucose monitoring (by patient) and laboratory measurement of glycated proteins are needed to effectively monitor glucose control; fructosamine must be interpreted in light of plasma protein half-lives, and HgbA1C must be interpreted in light of RBC ha f-life. Department of Defense study (July 2005) 47% percent increase in diabetes among veterans with the highest levels of dioxin.[31] |

A1AT, alpha 1 antitypsin; *AACE*, American Association of Clinical Endocrinologists; *A/C ratio*, albumin/globulin ratio; *AGA*, antigliadian antibodies; *ALA*, alpha linolenic acid; *ALB*, albumin; *ALP*, alkaline phosphatase; *ALT*, alanine amino transferase; *Anti-TG*, antithyroglobulin antibody; *Anti-TPO*, antithyroid peroxidase antibody; *AST*, aspartate aminotransferase; *BAL*, bronchoalveolar lavage; *BCAA*, branched-chain amino acid; *BILI T/D*, Bilirubin Total/Direct: *BUN*, blood urea nitrogen; *CAPD*, continuous ambulatory peritoneal dialysis; *CBC*, complete blood count; *CD*, cardiac disease *CHD*, coronary heart disease; *Cr*, chromium; *CRP*, C-reactive protein; *CSF*, cerebrospinal fluid; *CVD*, cardiovascular disease; *DGLA*, dihomo-gammalinolenic acid; *DGP*, deamidated gliadin peptide antibody; *DHA*, docosahexaenoic acid; *DNA*, deoxyribonucleic acid; *DRI*, dietary reference intake; *DRT*, diet readiness test; *EDTA*, ethylenediaminetetraacetic acid; *EFA*, essential fatty acid; *EMA*, endomysium antibody; *EPA*, eicosapentaenoic acid; *FAD*, flavin adenine dinucleotide; *FIGLU*, formiminoglutamic acid; *FBG*, fasting blood glucose; *FBS*, fasting blood sugar; *FPG*, fasting plasma glucose; *FRAP*, ferric-reducing ability of plasma; *GGT*, gamma glutamyl transferase; *GH*, growth hormone; *GI*, gastrointestinal; *GLOB*, globulin; *GOT*, glutamic-oxalacetic transaminase; *GPT*, glutamic-pyruvate transaminase; *GR*, glutathione reductase; *GU*, urea generation rate; *HBT-lactose*, hydrogen breath test-lactose; *HBT-fructose*, hydrogen breath test-fructose; *HCT*, hematocrit; *Hcy*, homocysteine; *Hgb*, hemoglobin; *HLA*, human leukocyte antigen; *HPLC*, high performance liquid chromotography; *hs-CRP*, high-sensitivity C-reactive protein; *I*, iodine; *ICA*, ionized calcium; *Ig*, immunoglobulin; *IGF*, insulin-like growth factor; *IGT*, impaired glucose tolerance; *IV*, intravenously; *KrU*, residual renal urea clearance; *Kt/V*$_{urea}$, urea kinetics(kinetic dialyzer) x time(min)/volume urea(ml); *LA*, linoleic acid; *LDL*, low-density lipoprotein; *MCV*, mean cell volume; *MLC*, mixed lymphocyte culture; *N*, nitrogen; *NCEP*, National Cholesterol Education Program; *NSAID*, nonsteroidal antiinflammatory disease; *nPCR*, normalized protein catabolic rate; *ORAC*, oxygen radical absorbance capacity; *PAB*, prealbumin; *PCR*, protein catabolic rate; *PEM*, protein-energy malnutriton; *PLP*, pyridoxal phosphate; *PNA*, protein equivalent of nitrogen appearance; *PT*, prothrombin time; *PTH*, parathyroid hormone; *PTT*, partial thromboplastin time; *PUFA*, polyunsaturated fatty acid; *RBC*, red blood cell; *RBP*, retinol-binding protein; *RDW*, RBC distribution width; *ROS*, reaction oxygen species; *RXR*, retinoid X receptor; *SAMe*, s-adenosylmethionine; *SNP*, single nucleotide polymorphism; *T*$_3$, triiodothyronine; *T*$_4$, thyroxine; *T1DM*, type 1 diabetes mellitus; *TEAC*, trolox-equivalent antioxidant capacity; *Tf-sat*, transferrin saturation; *TG*, triglyceride; *TIBC*, total iron-binding capacity; *TLC*, total lymphocyte count; *TP*, total protein; *TPN*, total parenteral nutrition; *TPP*, thiamin pyrophosphate; *Trp*, tryptophan; *TSAT*, transferrin saturation; *tTG*, tissue transglutaminase; *TUN*, total urinary nitroger; *U*: Cr, urea/creatine ratio; *UUN*, urea urinary nitrogen; *VLDL*, very-low-density lipoprotein; *WBC*, white blood cell; *XA*, xanthuric acid.

[a]Factor = 5.95 for TPN; reflects severity of metabolic stress.

[b]Factor = 5.95 for TPN; reflects severity of metabolic stress; TUN gives the most accurate estimation of total protein catabolism.

[c]Red blood cells are separated from plasma by centrifugation and washed with saline; after hemolyzing the cells, the intracellular material is analyzed for vitamin availability.

[d]No biochemical tests have been developed to assess B$_3$ status; the fraction of whole blood niacin as NAD is a potentially useful test (see Powers HJ: Current knowledge concerning optimum nutritional status of riboflavin, niacin, and pyridoxine, *Proc Nutr Soc* 58:435, 1999).

[e]ALT and GPT are the same enzyme; AST and GOT are the same enzyme.

[f]PLP is a rate-limiting co-enzyme in the transamination of amino acids (ALT and AST). PLP found primarily in liver and muscles.

[g]Microbiologic growth assays, the deoxyuridine suppression test, and recently developed research tests for folate and vitamin B$_{12}$ are not generally offered in the contemporary clinical laboratory.

[h]More sensitive procedures for measurement of vitamin K include serum chromatography and determination of the serum level of vitamin K–dependent bone protein called osteocalcin. Deficiency significantly increases the amount of abnormal forms of this protein. These tests are not yet widely available.

[i]These substances are measured by similar techniques when the concentration in urine or other body fluids is determined.

[j]These tests are combined with serum glucose, creatinine, and BUN on a test battery or panel. This set of tests is among the first and most frequently administered laboratory tests.

[k]The CBC includes the red cell count, the red cell indices, Hb concentration, HCT, MCV, mean cell hemoglobin (MCH), mean cell hemoglobin concentration (MCHC), and white cell and platelet counts. Only HCT, Hb, and MCV are discussed here (see Savage RA: The red cell indices: yesterday, today, and tomorrow, *Clin Lab Med* 13:773-785, 1993).

[l]Ranges are for adult men and premenopausal women. Pregnant women, infants, and children have different reference ranges.

[m]See van Zeben D et al: Evaluation of microcytosis using serum ferritin and red cell distribution width, *Eur J Haematol* 44:106-109, 1990.

[n]Taste acuity tests can be used to supplement laboratory methods (see, e.g., Gibson RS et al: A growth limiting mild zinc deficiency syndrome in some Southern Ontario boys with low growth percentiles, *Am J Clin Nutr* 49:1266,1989)

[o]AACE supports target TSH level between 0.3- and 3.0 mIU/mL to reduce the incidence of risks associated with subclinical hypothyroidism. AACE Task Force Thyroid Guidelines, *Endocr Pract.* 8:466, 2002.

[p]More recent awareness of the highly undiagnosed common disease of A1AT is improving education of healthcare providers regarding this condition. Kohnlein, T, Welte T: alpha-1 antitrypsin deficiency: pathogenesis, clinical presentation, diagnosis, and treatment, *The Am J of Med* 121:3, 2008.

[q]Organic acid functional markers for metabolic effects of micronutrient inadequacies, toxic exposure, neuroendocrine activity and intestinal bacterial overgrowth. Lord R, Bralley J: Organics in urine: assessment of gut dysbiosis, nutrient deficiencies and toxemia. *Nutr Pers* 1997:20:25.

1. Parrish CR, Series Ed: Serum proteins as markers of nutrition: what are we treating? Nutr Issues in Gastroenterology, Series 43, *Prac Gastroenterol* October, 2006.
2. Juarez-Congelosi M et al: Normalized protein catabolic rate versus serum albumin as a nutrition status marker in pediatric patients receiving hemodialysis, *J Renal Nutr* 17 (4):269, 2007.
3. Harty JC et al: The normalized protein catabolic rate is a flawed marker of nutrition in CAPD patients, *Kidney Int* 45:103, 1994.
4. Beck FK, Rosenthal TC: Prealbumin: a marker for nutritional evaluation, *Am Fam Physician* 65:1575, 2002.
5. Wu X et al: Joint effect of insulin-like growth factors and mutagen sensitivity in lung cancer risk, *J Natl Cancer Inst* 92:737, 2000.
6. Rowlands MA: Circulating insulin-like growth factor peptides and prostate cancer risk: a systematic review and meta-analysis, *Int J Cancer* 124:2416, 2009.
7. Gonen B et al: Haemoglobin A1: An indicator of the metabolic control of diabetic patients, *Lancet* 2(8041):734, 1977.
8. Riese H et al: Covariance of metabolic and hemostatic risk indicators in men and women, *Fibrinolysis Proteolysis* 15(1):9, 2001.
9. Bo S et al: Dietary magnesium and fiber intakes and inflammatory and metabolic indicators in middle-aged subjects from a population-based cohort 1,2,3, *Am J Clin Nutr* 84:1062, 2006.

10. Douglas D: MedScape Today News. Improved Diagnosis Does Not Change Celiac Mortality, Reuters Health Information, Feb 1, 2011.
11. Grainge MJ et al: Causes of Death in People With Celiac Disease Spanning the Pre- and Post-Serology Era: A Population-Based Cohort Study From Derby, UK, *Am J of Gastroenterol* 106:933, 2011.
12. Lewis NR: Risk of Morbidity in Contemporary Celiac Disease, *Expert Rev Gastroenterol and Hepatol* 4:767, 2010.
13. Donaldson MR et al: Strongly positive tissue transglutaminase antibodies are associated with Marsh 3 histopathology in adult and pediatric celiac disease. *J Clin Gastroenterol* 42:256, 2008.
14. Vermeersch P et al: Use of likelihood ratios improves clinical interpretation of IgG and IgA anti-DGP antibody testing for celiac disease in adults and children, *Clin Biochem* 44:248, 2011.
15. Vermeersch P et al: Diagnostic performance of IgG anti-deamidated gliadin peptide antibody assays is comparable to IgA anti-tTG in celiac disease, *Clin ChimActa* 411:931, 2010.
16. Sharifi N et al: Celiac disease in patients with type-1 diabetes mellitus screened by tissue transglutaminase antibodies in northwest of Iran, *Int J Diab Dev Ctries* 28:95, 2008.
17. Lampasona V et al: Antibodies to tissue transglutaminase C in type I diabetes, *Diabetologia* 42:1195, 1999.
18. Holopainena P et al: Candidate gene regions and genetic heterogeneity in gluten sensitivity, *Gut* 48:696, 2001.
19. Feingold KR et al: Infection decreases fatty acid oxidation and nuclear hormone receptors in the diaphragm, *J Lipid Res* 50:2055, 2009.
20. Lord R, Bralley JA, editors: *Laboratory evaluations for integrative and functional medicine*, ed 2, Duluth, GA, 2008, MetaMetrix Institute.
21. Sypniewska G: *Pro-inflammatory and prothrombotic factors and metabolic syndrome*, Department of Laboratory Medicine, Collegium Medicum, Nicolae Copernicus University, Bydgoszcz, Poland, 2007.
22. Ng KY et al: Vitamin D and vitamin A receptor expression and the proliferative effects of ligand activation of these receptors on the development of pancreatic progenitor cells derived from human fetal pancreas, *Stem Cell Rev* 7:53, 2011.
23. Aslam A et al: Vitamin E deficiency induced neurological disease in common variable immunodeficiency: two cases and a review of the literature of vitamin E deficiency, *Clin Immunol* 112(1):24, 2004.
24. Kim K et al: Associations of visceral adiposity and exercise participation with C-reactive protein, insulin resistance, and endothelial dysfunction in Korean healthy adults, *Metabolism* 57:1181, 2008.
25. Finney L et al: Copper and angiogenesis: unravelling a relationship key to cancer progression, *Clin Exp Pharmacol Physiol* 36:88, 2009.
26. Charney P, Malone AM: *ADA pocket guide to nutrition assessment*, ed 2, Chicago, IL, 2009, American Dietetic Association.
27. Snellman G et al: Determining vitamin D status: a comparison between commercially available assays, *PLoS One* 5(7):e11555, 2010.
28. Katz K et al: Suspected Nonalcoholic Fatty Liver Disease Is Not Associated with Vitamin D Status in Adolescents after Adjustment for Obesity, *J Obes* 2010; 2010. Published online Feb. 2011.
29. Ahmed A: *The role of 11b-hydroxysteroid dehydrogenase type 1 and hepatic glucocorticoid metabolism in the metabolic syndrome*, Doctoral thesis to College of Medical and Dental Sciences, University of Birmingham, 2010.
30. Yu W et al: RXR: a coregulator that enhances binding of retinoic acid, thyroid hormone, and vitamin D receptors to their cognate response elements, *Cell* 67:1251, 1991.
31. Longnecker MP, Michalek JE: Serum dioxin level in relation to diabetes mellitus among Air Force veterans with background levels of exposure, *Epidemiol* 11:44, 2000.
32. Norman K, et al. Cutoff percentiles of bioelectrical phase angle predict functionality, quality of life, and mortality in patients with cancer[1,2] First published July 14, 2010, doi. 10.3945/ajcn.2010.29215 *Am J Clin Nutr September 2010 vol. 92 no. 3 612-619*.
33. Maddocks M, Kon SS, Jones SE, Canavan JL, Nolan CM, Higginson IJ, Gao W, Polkey MI, Man WD. Clin Nutr. 2015 Jan 7. pii: S0261-5614(15)00003-5. doi: 10.1016/j.clnu.2014.12.020. [Epub ahead of print]

Nutritional Implications of Selected Drugs

Doris Dudley Wales BA, BS, RPh,
DeeAnna Wales VanReken, MS, RDN, CD

Drug	Drug Effect	Nutritional Implications and Cautions
Selected Antiinfective Drugs		
Antibacterial Agents		
Penicillins • amoxicillin (Amoxil) • amoxicillin/clavulanic acid (Augmentin)	Long-term use may lead to oral candidiasis, diarrhea, epigastric distress. Some products contain high amounts of potassium or sodium. May cause *Clostridium difficile*.	Use caution with low-sodium diet or potassium supplements. **Augmentin:** take with food to ↓ GI distress. Replace fluids & electrolytes for diarrhea. Probiotic is advised.
Macrolides • azithromycin (Zithromax) • clarithromycin (Biaxin) • erythromycin (Ery-Tab)	May cause GI distress, anorexia, stomatitis, dysgeusia, or diarrhea. May increase sedative effect of alcohol. May cause *Clostridium difficile*.	Take with food to ↓ GI distress. Eat frequent, small, appealing meals to counteract anorexia. Use mouth rinses, fresh mint, or lemon water for dysgeusia. Replace fluids & electrolytes for diarrhea. Avoid alcohol. Probiotic is advised.
Sulfonamide Combination • sulfamethoxazole/ trimethoprim (Bactrim)	May interfere with folate metabolism, especially with long-term use. May cause stomatitis, anorexia, nausea and vomiting, severe allergic reactions. May cause *Clostridium difficile*.	Take with food and 8 oz fluid to ↓ nausea, vomiting, and anorexia. Replace fluids & electrolytes for diarrhea. Supplement folic acid as needed. Discontinue and consult physician at first sign of allergic reaction. Probiotic is advised.
Cephalosporins • cephalexin (Keflex) • cefprozil (Cefzil) • ceftriaxone (Rocephin) • cefuroxime (Ceftin) • cefdinir (Omnicef)	May cause stomatitis, sore mouth and tongue and interfere with eating. May cause diarrhea and *Clostridium difficile*. Food ↑ bioavailability of tablets and suspension. Antacids, Ca, and Mg supplements may ↓ bioavailability.	Replace fluids & electrolytes for diarrhea. Eat moist, soft, low-salt foods and cold foods such as ice chips, sherbet, and yogurt for stomatitis and sore mouth. Probiotic is advised. Take with a meal for optimal bioavailability. Take separately from antacids, Ca, or Mg supplements. Probiotic may be advised.
Fluoroquinolones • ciprofloxacin (Cipro) • levafloxacin (Levaquin) • moxifloxacin (Avelox)	Drug may rarely precipitate in renal tubules. Drug will bind to magnesium, calcium, zinc, and iron, forming an insoluble, unabsorbable complex. May cause *Clostridium difficile*. **Cipro:** Inhibits metabolism of caffeine, and can therefore ↑ CNS stimulation.	Take drug with 8 oz of fluid and maintain adequate hydration. Limit caffeine intake. Take at least 4 hours before or 8 hours after antacids, Mg, Ca, Fe, Zn supplements or multivitamin with minerals. Replace fluids & electrolytes for diarrhea. Hold tube feeds 1 hour before and 1 hour after drug. Probiotic is advised.
Antimicrobial Agents		
Oxazolidinone • linezolid (Zyvox)	Drug exhibits mild monoamine oxidase inhibition. May cause taste change, oral candidiasis, and *Clostridium difficile*.	Avoid significant amounts (>100 mg) of high tyramine/pressor foods. See chart in 18th ed. of *Food Medication Interactions*. Eat small, frequent, appealing meals f tastes change. Replace fluids & electrolytes for diarrhea. Probiotic is advised
Tetracyclines • tetracycline (Sumycin) • doxycycline (Vibramycin)	Often used to treat Lyme disease; may cause anorexia. Binds to Mg, Ca, Zn, and Fe, forming an insoluble unabsorbable complex. May ↓ bacterial production of vitamin K in GI tract. Long-term use may cause B vitamin deficiencies. Combining with vitamin A may ↑ risk of benign intracranial hypertension. May cause *Clostridium difficile*.	Take supplements separately by 3 hours. Eat frequent, small, appealing meals to ↓ anorexia. Avoid excessive vitamin A while taking drug. Long-term use may warrant Vitamins K and B supplementation. Probiotic is advised. Replace fluids & electrolytes for diarrhea. **Sumycin:** Take drug 1 hour before or 2 hours after food or milk.
Antiprotozoal/Antibacterial • metronidazole (Flagyl)	May cause anorexia, GI distress, stomatitis, and metallic taste in mouth. May cause disulfiram-like reaction when ingested with alcohol. Often used to treat *Clostridium difficile*.	Take with food to ↓ GI distress. Eat small, frequent, appealing meals to decrease anorexia. Avoid all alcohol during use and for 3 days after discontinuation. Probiotic is advised.
• clindamycin (Cleocin)	May cause weight loss, increased thirst, esophagitis, nausea, vomiting, cramps, flatulence, bloating, or diarrhea. May cause severe *Clostridium difficile*.	Take oral forms with food or 8oz water to decrease esophageal irritation. Replace fluids & electrolytes for diarrhea. Probiotic is advised.

Continued

Drug	Drug Effect	Nutritional Implications and Cautions
Nitrofuran • nitrofurantoin (Macrobid)	Peripheral neuropathy, muscle weakness and wasting may occur with preexisting anemia, vitamin B deficiency or electrolyte abnormalities. May cause *Clostridium difficile*.	Drug should be taken with adequate calories, protein, and vitamin B complex. Avoid in G-6-PD deficiency because of increased risk of hemolytic anemia. Replace fluids & electrolytes for diarrhea. Probiotic is advised.
Antituberculars • isoniazid (Nydrazid)	Drug may cause pyridoxine (vitamin B_6) and niacin (vitamin B_3) deficiency resulting in peripheral neuropathy and pellagra. Drug may affect vitamin D metabolism and ↓ calcium and phosphate absorption. Drug has MAO inhibitor–like activity.	Avoid in malnourished individuals and others at ↑ risk for peripheral neuropathy. Supplement with 25-50 mg of pyridoxine and possibly B-complex if skin changes occur. Avoid foods high in tyramine (e.g., aged cheeses). Maintain adequate calcium and vitamin D intake.
• rifampin (Rifadin)	Drug may increase metabolism of vitamin D. Rare cases of osteomalacia have been reported.	May need vitamin D supplement with long-term use.
• ethambutol (Myambutol) • pyrazinamide (Rifater)	Drug may ↓ the excretion of uric acid, leading to hyperuricemia and gout. **Myambutol:** may ↓ copper and zinc.	Maintain adequate hydration and purine-restricted diet. **Myambutol:** ↑ foods high in Cu and Zn; daily multivitamin with long term use.
Antifungal Agents • amphotericin B (Fungizone)	Drug may cause anorexia and weight loss. Drug causes loss of potassium, magnesium, and calcium.	Eat frequent, small, appealing meals high in magnesium, potassium, and calcium. Ensure adequate hydration.
• ketoconazole (Nizoral)	Drug does not dissolve at pH >5.	Take with food to ↑ absorption. Take with acidic liquid (e.g., cola), especially individuals with achlorhydria.
• terbinafine (Lamisil)	Drug may cause taste changes or loss, dyspepsia, abdominal pain, and diarrhea, weight loss, and headaches.	Avoid taking with acidic foods such as applesauce or fruit based foods. Limit alcohol and caffeine.
Selected Antithrombotic/Hematologic Drugs *Anticoagulant Agents* **Vitamin K Antagonist** • warfarin (Coumadin)	Prevents the conversion of oxidized vitamin K to the active form. Produces systemic anticoagulation. May inhibit mineralization of newly formed bone.	Consistent intake of vitamin K containing foods and supplements is needed to achieve desired state of anticoagulation. Monitor bone mineral density in individuals on long-term therapy.
Direct Thrombin Inhibitor • dabigatran (Pradaxa)	Drug may cause dyspepsia, abdominal pain, GERD, esophagitis, erosive gastritis, diarrhea, gastric hemorrhage, or GI ulcer. Alcohol may cause bleeding.	Avoid alcohol and supplements. SJW can ↓ drug effectiveness. Chewing can ↓ bioavailability by 75%. Take with food if GI distress occurs.
Factor Xa Inhibitors • rivaroxaban (Xarelto) • apixavan (Eliquis)	Drug may cause abdominal pain, oropharyngeal pain, toothaches, dyspepsia, and anemia. Excess alcohol can ↑ bleeding risk.	Avoid Vitamin E and herbal products with antiplatelet or anticoagulant effects. Avoid SJW and grapefruit/related citrus (limes, pomelo, Seville oranges). Minimize alcohol intake.
Antiplatelet Agents **Platelet Aggregation Inhibitors** • aspirin/salicylate (Bayer)	Drug may cause GI irritation and bleeding; ↓ systemic levels of iron, folic acid, sodium, and potassium with high dose long-term use. Drug may ↓ uptake of vitamin C and ↑ urinary loss.	Incorporate foods high in vitamin C and folate Monitor electrolytes and hemoglobin to determine need for potassium or iron supplements. Avoid alcohol consumption.
• clopidogrel (Plavix)	Drug may cause dyspepsia, nausea and vomiting, abdominal pain, GI bleeding/hemorrhage, diarrhea, and constipation.	Food ↑ bioavailability. Take with food if GI distress occurs. Avoid grapefruit/related citrus (limes, pomelo, Seville oranges). Replace fluids & electrolytes for diarrhea.
Selected Antihyperglycemic Drugs *Insulin Sensitizing Agents* **Biguanide** • metformin (Glucophage)	Drug may ↓ absorption of vitamin B_{12} and folic acid. May cause lactic acidosis. Drug does not cause hypoglycemia.	Follow American Diabetes Association dietary guidelines. ↑ foods high in vitamin B_{12} and folate; supplement if necessary. Avoid alcohol to ↓ risk of lactic acidosis.
Thiazolidinedione (TZD) • rosiglitizone (Avandia) • pioglitizone (Actos)	Drugs may lead to ↑ weight and insulin sensitivity, and ↓ gluconeogenesis. **Avandia** may ↑ total cholesterol, LDL, triglycerides and ↓ HDL. **Actos** may ↓ total cholesterol, LDL, triglycerides, and ↑ HDL. Rarely, drugs may cause hypoglycemia.	Follow American Diabetes Association dietary guidelines. Reduce calorie intake if weight loss is the goal. Avoid SJW. Monitor blood lipid levels closely and encourage anti-inflammatory diet to manage undesirable fluctuations.
Insulin Stimulating Agents **Sulfonylureas** • glipizide (Glucotrol) • glyburide (Diabeta) • glimepiride (Amaryl)	Drug may cause ↑ or ↓ in appetite, weight gain, dyspepsia, nausea, diarrhea, or constipation. Drugs may lead to hypoglycemia.	Follow American Diabetes Association dietary guidelines and encourage regular exercise. Time food intake according to pharmaceutical recommendations.

Drug	Drug Effect	Nutritional Implications and Cautions
Meglitinides • repaglinide (Prandin)	Drug stimulates the release of insulin and may lead to weight gain. May also cause nausea, vomiting, diarrhea, or constipation. Drug may cause hypoglycemia.	Follow American Diabetes Association dietary guidelines and encourage exercise. Reduce calories if weight loss is the goal. Time food intake according to drug recommendations. Limit alcohol intake.
Enzyme Inhibitor Agents **Alpha-glucosidase Inhibitors** • miglitol (Glycet) • acarbose (Precose)	Drugs may delay the absorption of dietary disaccharides and complex carbohydrates. May also cause abdominal pain, diarrhea, and gas. **Glycet:** may reduce Iron absorption. Drugs do not cause hypoglycemia.	Follow American Diabetes Association dietary guidelines. Avoid digestive enzymes and limit alcohol. **Precose:** Monitor liver enzymes (AST, ALT) quarterly during the first year. **Glycet:** Monitor Iron levels and supplement as needed.
Dipeptidyl Peptidase-4 (DPP-4) Inhibitors (Gliptins) • sitagliptin (Januvia) • saxagliptin (Onglyza) • linagliptin (Tradjenta)	Drugs may lead to weight gain, abdominal pain, constipation, diarrhea, gastroenteritis, nausea, vomiting, and rarely, pancreatitis. Drug may cause hypoglycemia.	Follow American Diabetes Association dietary guidelines. ↓ calories if weight loss is the goal. **Onglyza:** Avoid grapefruit/related citrus (limes, pomelo, Seville oranges). **Onglyza/Tradjenta:** Avoid SJW.
Glucose Reabsorption Inhibitor Agents **SGLT-2 Inhibitors (Gliflozins)** • canagliflozin (Invokana) • dapagliflozin (Farxiga)	Drugs ↓ reabsorption of glucose and ↑ urinary glucose excretion. Drugs may lead to weight loss, polydypsia, ↑ LDL, hypovolemia, and dehydration. Drugs may cause hypoglycemia.	Follow American Diabetes Association dietary guidelines. Reduce calorie intake if weight loss is the goal. Monitor LDL and encourage appropriate fat intake. **Invokana:** Avoid SJW.
Selected Steroidal/Hormonal Drugs **Corticosteroids** • prednisone (Deltasone) • methylprednisolone (Medrol)	Drug induces protein catabolism, resulting in muscle wasting, and atrophy of bone protein matrix, delayed wound healing. Drug ↓ intestinal absorption of calcium; ↑ urinary loss of calcium, potassium, zinc, vitamin C, and nitrogen; causes sodium retention.	Maintain diet high in Ca, vitamin D, protein, K+, Zn, and vitamin C, and low in sodium. Ca and vitamin D supplements recommended to prevent osteoporosis with long-term use of drug.
Bisphosphonates • alendronate (Fosamax) • ibandronate (Boniva)	Drug may induce mild ↓ in serum calcium. Long-term use may cause zinc deficiency.	Pair with diet high in Ca or use Ca/Vitamin D supplement. Monitor for signs of zinc deficiency. Drug must be taken 30 minutes to 1 hour before first intake of day with plain water only. Take zinc supplements 2 hours away from drug.
Sex Hormones • estrogen (Premarin) • Oral Contraceptives	Drug may ↓ absorption and tissue uptake of vitamin C but may ↑ absorption of vitamin A. May inhibit folate conjugate and decrease serum folic acid. Drug may ↓ serum vitamin B6, B12, riboflavin, magnesium, zinc.	Maintain diet with adequate Mg, folate, vitamin B6 and B12, riboflavin, and zinc. Calcium and vitamin D supplements may be advised with estrogen as hormone replacement for postmenopausal women.
Thyroid Hormones • levothyroxine (Synthroid)	Drug may cause appetite changes, weight loss, and nausea/diarrhea. Iron, Calcium or Magnesium may ↓ absorption of drug. Soy, walnuts, cottonseed oil, or high fiber foods may also ↓ absorption.	Take Fe, Ca, or Mg supplements away from drug by ≥ 4 hours; take drug 2-3 hours before soy. Eat walnuts, cottonseed oil, or high fiber foods away from medication. Use caution with grapefruit/related citrus (limes, pomelo, Seville oranges). Take drug 30 minutes before a meal.
Selected Cardiovascular Drugs **Cardiac Glycoside Agent** • digoxin (Lanoxin)	Drug may ↑ urinary loss of magnesium and ↓ serum levels of potassium.	Hypokalemia, hypomagnesemia, and hypercalcemia ↑ drug toxicity. Maintain diet high in potassium and magnesium. Monitor magnesium levels and use caution with calcium supplements and antacids.

Continued

Drug	Drug Effect	Nutritional Implications and Cautions
Beta Blocking Agents • metoprolol (Lopressor, Toprol XL) • atenolol (Tenormin) • carvedilol (Coreg)	Drugs may mask signs of or prolong hypoglycemia. Drug may ↓ insulin release in response to hyperglycemia. Drug may cause wt gain, nausea, vomiting, and diarrhea. May mask symptoms of diabetic hyperglycemia.	Monitoring of blood glucose levels for hypoglycemia or hyperglycemia may be recommended upon initiation of drugs. Avoid natural licorice and encourage low sodium diet. ↓ calories if weight loss is the goal. Patients with diabetes should monitor glucose regularly.
ACE Inhibitor Agents • enalapril (Vasotec) • lisinopril (Zestril) • benazepril (Lotensin) • ramipril (Altace)	Drugs may ↑ serum potassium. Drugs may cause abdominal pain, constipation, or diarrhea.	Caution with high potassium diet or supplements. Avoid salt substitutes. Ensure adequate fluid intake. Avoid natural licorice. Limit Alcohol.
Angiotensin II Receptor Antagonists • losartan (Cozaar) • valsartan (Diovan) • irbesartan (Avapro) • telmisartan (Micardis)	Drugs may ↑ serum potassium.	Caution with high-potassium diet or supplements. Ensure adequate hydration. Avoid natural licorice and salt substitutes. **Cozaar:** avoid grapefruit/related citrus (limes, pomelo, Seville oranges).
Calcium Channel Blocking Agents • amlodipine (Norvasc) • diltiazem (Cardizem)	Drug may cause dysphagia, nausea, cramps, and edema. Drug may cause anorexia, dry mouth, dyspepsia, nausea, vomiting, constipation, and diarrhea.	If GI distress occurs, take with food. Avoid natural licorice. Reduce sodium intake. Avoid natural licorice. Strict adherence to a low sodium diet may ↓ antihypertensive effect.
Alpha Adrenergic Agonist • clonidine (Catapres)	Drug commonly causes dizziness, drowsiness, and sedation.	Avoid alcohol and alcohol products. Drug ↑ sensitivity to alcohol, which may ↑ sedation caused by drug alone.
Peripheral Vasodilator • hydralazine (Apresoline)	Drug interferes with pyridoxine (vitamin B_6) metabolism and may result in pyridoxine deficiency.	Maintain a diet high in pyridoxine. Supplementation may be necessary.
Antiarrhythmic Agent • amiodarone (Pacerone)	Drug may cause anorexia, nausea, vomiting, taste changes, or increases in liver enzymes or thyroid hormones.	Avoid grapefruit/related citrus (limes, pomelo, Seville oranges) and SJW. Monitor hepatic and thyroid function. Encourage appealing foods.
Selected Antihyperlipidemic Drugs **HMG Co-A Reductase Inhibitors** • atorvastatin (Lipitor) • simvastatin (Zocor) • pravastatin (Pravachol) • rosuvastatin (Crestor)	Drug may cause significant reduction in Co Q_{10}. Drug lowers LDL cholesterol; raises HDL cholesterol.	Supplementation with Co Q_{10} has not been shown to ↓ statin myopathy but may still be advisable for repletion of the nutrient. Encourage anti-inflammatory diet for optimal drug effect. **Lipitor/Zocor:** Avoid grapefruit/related citrus (limes, pomelo, Seville oranges)
Fibric Acid Derivative • gemfibrozil (Lopid) • fenofibrate (Tricor)	Drug decreases serum triglycerides. **Lopid:** Taste changes may occur.	Encourage anti-inflammatory diet for optimal drug effect. Avoid alcohol. **Lopid:** encourage small appealing meals.
Bile Acid Sequestrant • cholestyramine (Questran)	Drug binds fat-soluble vitamins (A, E, D, K), β-carotene, calcium, magnesium, iron, zinc, and folic acid.	Take fat-soluble vitamins in water-miscible form or take vitamin supplement at least 1 hour before first dose of drug daily. Maintain diet high in folate, Mg, Ca, Fe, Zn or supplement as needed. Monitor serum nutrient levels for long-term use.
Nicotinic Acid • niacin (Niaspan)	High dose may elevate blood glucose and uric acid.	Low-purine diet as recommended. Monitor blood glucose with diabetes.

Drug	Drug Effect	Nutritional Implications and Cautions
Selected Diuretic Drugs *Loop Diuretics* • furosemide (Lasix) • bumetanide (Bumex)	Drug ↑ urinary excretion of sodium, potassium, magnesium, and calcium. Long-term use can lead to ↑ urinary zinc excretion.	Maintain diet high in zinc, potassium, magnesium, and calcium. Avoid natural licorice, which may counteract diuretic effect of drug. Monitor electrolytes; supplement as needed.
Thiazide Diuretic • hydrochlorothiazide (Hydrodiuril)	Drug ↑ urinary excretion of sodium, potassium, magnesium and ↑ renal resorption of calcium. Long-term use can lead to ↑ urinary zinc excretion.	Maintain diet high in zinc, potassium, and magnesium. Avoid natural licorice, which may counteract diuretic effect of drug. Monitor electrolytes and supplement as needed. Use caution with Ca supplements.
Potassium-Sparing Diuretics • triamterene (Dyrenium) • spironolactone (Aldactone)	Drug ↑ renal resorption of potassium. Long-term use can lead to ↑ urinary zinc excretion.	Avoid salt substitutes. Use caution with potassium supplements. Avoid excessive potassium intake in diet. Monitor for signs of zinc deficiency.
Selected Analgesic Drugs *Non-Narcotic Analgesics* • acetaminophen (Tylenol)	Drug may cause hepatotoxicity at high dose. Chronic alcohol ingestion ↑ risk of hepatotoxicity.	Maximum safe adult dose is ≤ 3 g/day Avoid alcohol or limit to ≤ 2 drinks/day.
Non-Steroidal Anti-Inflammatory Drugs (NSAIDs) • ibuprofen (Motrin) • naproxen (Naprosyn) • meloxicam (Mobic) • ketorolac (Toradol)	**Standard warning with NSAIDs:** **GI** ↑ risk of serious GI events (bleeding, ulceration, perforation of stomach & intestines) can occur at anytime during use without warning. The elderly are at greater risk. **Cardiovascular:** ↑ risk of serious cardiovascular thrombotic events, myocardial infarction & stroke.	Take drug with food or milk to decrease risk of GI toxicity. Avoid use in the elderly or in individuals with severe cardiovascular disease.
Cox-2 Inhibitor • celecoxib (Celebrex)	Drug may cause GI distress, weight gain, taste changes, dyspepsia, nausea, abdominal pain, diarrhea, and flatulence. Rare sudden, serious GI bleeding and colitis can occur.	If GI distress occurs, take with food and limit caffeine. High fat meals can delay concentration, but ↑ absorption.
Narcotic Analgesic Agents (Opioids) • morphine (MS Contin) • codeine/apap (Tylenol #3) • hydrocodone/apap (Norco) • oxycodone (OxyContin) • hydromorphone (Dilaudid) • fentanyl (Duragesic) • methadone (Dolophine)	Narcotics can be highly addictive and may cause severe dose-related sedation, respiratory depression, dry mouth, and constipation. Drugs cause slowing of digestion.	Monitor respiratory function and bowel function (not with paralytic ileus). Do not crush or chew sustained-release. **OxyContin/Fentanyl/Methadone:** Caution with grapefruit/related citrus (limes, pomelo, Seville oranges).
Synthetic Opioid Analgesic • tramadol (Ultram)	Drug may cause anorexia, dry mouth, dyspepsia, nausea/vomiting, abdominal pain, constipation, diarrhea, or gas.	Avoid alcohol. Use caution with SJW.
Selected Antidepressant Drugs *Selective Serotonin Reuptake Inhibitors (SSRIs)* • sertraline (Zoloft) • citalopram (Celexa) • escitalopram (Lexapro) • fluoxetine (Prozac) • paroxetine (Paxil)	Drugs may ↑ weight, appetite. Some herbs and supplements may ↑ toxicity. **Prozac:** may cause weight loss; may ↓ absorption of leucine.	Avoid tryptophan, SJW. Additive effects may produce adverse effects or serotonin syndrome. Monitor weight trends as appropriate. Avoid alcohol.
Serotonin Antagonist/Reuptake Inhibitor (SARI) & Serotonin-Norepinephrine Reuptake Inhibitors (SNRIs) • trazodone (Desyrel) - SARI • venlafaxine (Effexor XR) - SNRI • desvenlafaxine (Pristiq) - SNRI	Some herbal and natural products may ↑ toxicity.	Avoid tryptophan and SJW. Additive effects may produce adverse effects or serotonin syndrome.

Continued

Drug	Drug Effect	Nutritional Implications and Cautions
TriCyclic Antidepressants (TCAs)		
• amitriptyline (Elavil)	Drug may cause ↑ appetite (especially for carbo-hydrates/sweets) and weight gain. High fiber may ↓ drug absorption.	Monitor caloric intake. Maintain consistent amount of fiber in diet.
Noradrenergic/Specific Serotonic Antidepressants (NaSSA)		
• mirtazapine (Remeron)	Some herbal and natural products may ↑ toxicity. Drug can also be used as an appetite stimulant and may cause significant ↑ in appetite/weight gain.	Avoid tryptophan and SJW. Additive effects may produce adverse effects or serotonin syndrome.
Norepinephrine/Dopamine Reuptake Inhibitor (NDRI)		
• bupropion (Wellbutrin)	Drug may cause anorexia, weight loss or gain, ↑ appetite, dry mouth, stomatitis, taste changes, dysphagia, pharyngitis, nausea/vomiting, dyspepsia, or GI distress.	Minimize or avoid alcohol. Take with food to decrease GI irritation. Avoid mixing with SJW.
Monoamine Oxidase Inhibitors (MAOIs)		
• phenelzine (Nardil)	Drug may cause ↑ appetite (especially for carbo-hydrates and sweets) and weight gain. Risk for severe reaction with dietary tyramine.	Avoid foods high in tyramine during drug use and for 2 weeks after discontinuation to prevent hypertensive crisis. Monitor caloric intake to avoid weight gain.
Mood Stabilizers		
• lithium (Lithobid)	Sodium intake affects drug levels. May cause dry mouth, dehydration, and thirst, reflective of ↑ drug toxicity. Drug may cause GI irritation.	Drink 2 to 3 L of fluid daily to avoid dehydration. Maintain consistent dietary sodium intake. Take with food to ↓ GI irritation. Limit caffeine.
Selected Antipsychotic & Antianxiety/Hypnotic Drugs		
Typical Antipsychotic Agent		
• haloperidol (Haldol)	May cause ↑ appetite, weight gain or loss, constipation, or dry mouth. Risk for tardive dyskinesia.	Monitor weight and calorie count. Tardive dyskinesia may interfere with biting, chewing, swallowing.
Atypical Antipsychotic Agents		
• risperidone (Risperdal) • quetiapine (Seroquel) • olanzapine (Zyprexa)	Drugs may cause ↑ appetite and weight gain. May also cause ↑ blood sugar, HbA1c, or lipids/triglycerides.	Monitor weight, fasting blood sugar, HbA1c, and lipids/triglycerides. Do not use in elderly dementia patients; may ↑ risk of stroke.
Antianxiety/Hypnotic Agents		
• lorazepam (Ativan) • alprazolam (Xanax) • clonazepam (Klonopin) • diazepam (Valium) • temazepam (Restoril) • zolpidem (Ambien)	Drugs may cause significant sedation. Benzodiazepine drugs are highly addictive.	Avoid concurrent ingestion of alcohol, which will produce CNS depression. Limit or avoid caffeine, which may decrease the therapeutic effect of the drug. Use caution with herbal and natural products that cause CNS stimulation or sedation.
Selected Anticonvulsant Drugs		
Caboxamides		
• carbamazepine (Tegretol)	Drug may ↓ biotin, folic acid, and vitamin D levels. Long-term therapy (>6 months) may cause loss of bone mineral density.	Maintain diet high in folate and vitamin D. Calcium and vitamin D supplements may be necessary for long-term therapy. Use caution with grapefruit/related citrus (limes, pomelo, Seville oranges). Star fruit or pomegranate may ↑ drug levels and lead to toxicity. Avoid alcohol.
Hydantoin		
• phenytoin (Dilantin)	Drug may ↓ serum folic acid, calcium, vitamin D, biotin, and thiamine. Drug can cause altered taste, dysphagia, nausea, vomiting, and constipation. Alcohol intake disrupts drug function. Ca and Mg may ↓ absorption.	May be paired with daily folic acid supplement; monitor levels. Consider Ca, vitamin D and B vitamin supplements with long-term use. Ca, Mg, or antacids should be taken 2 hours away from drug. Holding tube feeds 1 hour before & 1 hour after drug is recommend. Avoid alcohol and SJW.

Drug	Drug Effect	Nutritional Implications and Cautions
Barbiturate • phenobarbital (Luminal)	Drug may induce rapid metabolism of vitamin D, leading to Vitamin D and Calcium deficiencies. May also ↑ the metabolism of vitamin K and ↓ serum folic acid and vitamin B_{12}.	Encourage ↑ dietary intake of Ca, vitamin D, and folate. Consider Ca, vitamin D, folic acid, and vitamin B_{12} supplementation with long-term use.
GABA Analogues • gabapentin (Neurontin) • pregabalin (Lyrica)	Drugs used for neuropathy, hot flashes, migraines, and as mood stabilizers. Mg can interfere with drug efficacy by ↓ absorption. Can cause ↑ weight and appetite, nausea, gingivitis, constipation, vomiting and diarrhea.	Take Mg supplements separately by 2 hours.
Fructose Derivative • topiramate (Topamax)	May cause weight loss, anorexia, dry mouth, gingivitis, taste changes, GERD, nausea, dyspepsia, constipation, or diarrhea.	Encourage adequate fluid intake to ↓ risk of kidney stones. Replace fluids & electrolytes for diarrhea. Avoid alcohol.
Selected Anti-Dementia Drugs **Cholinesterase Inhibitors** • donepezil (Aricept) • rivastigmine (Exelon)	Drug is highly cholinergic; may cause weight loss, diarrhea, nausea/vomiting, ↑ gastric acid, and GI bleeding.	Take with food to prevent GI irritation. Monitor food intake and weight trends.
NMDA Receptor Antagonist • memantine (Namenda)	Drug is cleared from the body almost exclusively by renal excretion. Urine pH >8 decreases renal excretion by 80%.	Avoid diet that alkalinizes the urine (predominantly milk products, citrus fruit) to avoid drug toxicity.
Selected Gastrointestinal Drugs **H_2 Receptor Antagonist** • ranitidine (Zantac) • famotidine (Pepcid)	Drug may reduce the absorption of vitamin B_{12} and iron.	Monitor iron studies, vitamin B_{12} level on long-term therapy. Supplement as needed.
Proton Pump Inhibitors • omeprazole (Prilosec) • lansoprazole (Prevacid) • esompeprazole (Nexium) • pantoprazole (Protonix) • dexlansoprazole (Dexilant)	Long-term ↓ acid secretion may inhibit the absorption of iron and vitamin B_{12}; ↓ calcium absorption may lead to osteoporosis. Low Mg may occur. Inhibition of acid secretion may also ↑ the risk of *Clostridium difficille*. Some studies have also shown correlation between PPI therapy, Small Intestine Bacterial Overgrowth (SIBO), and IBS	Monitor iron studies, vitamin B_{12}, magnesium levels, and bone density with long-term use; supplement as needed. Consider alternatives in those with a diagnosis of SIBO and/or IBS. **Prilosec:** Avoid SJW & Gingko. Hold tube feeds 1 hour before and 1 hour after drug.
Prokinetic Agent • metoclopramide (Reglan)	Drug ↑ gastric emptying; may change insulin requirements in persons with diabetes; may ↑ CNS depressant effects of alcohol. Drug may cause tardive dyskinesia with extended use.	Monitor blood glucose in persons with diabetes carefully when drug is initiated. Avoid alcohol. Tardive dyskinesia may interfere with biting, chewing, swallowing.
Selected Antineoplastic Drugs **Folate Antagonist** • methotrexate (Rheumatrex)	Drug inhibits dihydrofolate reductase; decreased formation of active folate. Drug may cause GI irritation or injury. All antineoplastic drugs are cytotoxic; potential to damage intestinal mucosa. Drug also used as an antirheumatic.	Maintain diet high in folate and vitamin B_{12}. Daily folic acid supplement may be recommended with antirheumatic doses but is not advised with antineoplastic. Leucovorin rescue may be necessary with antineoplastic doses.
Alkylating Agent • cyclophosphamide (Cytoxin)	Drug metabolite causes bladder irritation, acute hemorrhagic cystitis. All antineoplastic drugs are cytotoxic; potential to damage intestinal mucosa.	Maintain high fluid intake (2-3 L daily) to induce frequent voiding.

Continued

Drug	Drug Effect	Nutritional Implications and Cautions
Epidermal Growth Factor Inhibitor		
• erlotinib (Tarceva)	Drug may cause anorexia, weight loss, stomatitis, nausea, vomiting, diarrhea. Rarely, GI bleeding can occur.	Avoid SJW and grapefruit/related citrus (limes, pomelo, Seville oranges). Hold tube feeds 2 hour before and 1 hour after drug.
Selected Anti-Parkinson's Drugs		
Dopamine Precursor		
• carbidopa/levodopa (Sinemet)	Carbidopa protects levodopa against pyridoxine-enhanced peripheral decarboxylation to dopamine.	Pyridoxine supplements > 10-25 mg daily may ↑ carbidopa requirements and ↑ adverse effects of levodopa.
Dopamine Agonist		
• bromocriptine (Parlodel)	Drug may cause GI irritation, nausea, vomiting, and GI bleeding.	Take with food to prevent GI irritation. Take at bedtime to ↓ nausea.
MAO-B Inhibitor		
• selegiline (Eldepryl)	Drug selectively inhibits MAO-B at 10 mg or less per day. Drug loses selectivity at higher doses.	Avoid high-tyramine foods at doses > 10 mg/day. May precipitate hypertension.
COMT Inhibitor		
• entacopone (Comtan)	Drug chelates iron, which for some patients, may ↓ serum iron and make the drug less effective.	Monitor iron levels. Take iron supplement as needed 2-3 hours away from drug. Avoid alcohol.
Selected ADHD Treatment Drugs		
CNS Stimulants		
• methylphenidate (Ritalin, Concerta) • dextroamphetamine & amphetamine (Acderall)	Drugs may cause anorexia, weight loss, and ↓ growth in children. Dry mouth, metallic taste and GI upset can occur. May be habit forming.	Monitor children's weight/growth; ensure adequate calories. Limit caffeine & alcohol. **Ritalin/Concerta:** Avoid SJW. **Adderall:** High-dose vitamin C and acidifying foods may ↓ absorption and ↑ excretion.

ACE, Angiotensin-converting enzyme; *CNS,* central nervous system; *Co-A,* coenzyme A; *COMT,* catechol-o-methyl transferase; *G-6-PD,* glucose-6-phosphate dehydrogenase; *GI,* gastrointestinal; *HbA1c,* hemoglobin A1c; *HMG,* 3-hydroxy-3-methyl-glutaryl; *MAO,* monoamine oxidase; *NSAID,* nonsteroidal antiinflammatory drug; *PKU,* phenylketonuria; ↓↑, increase/decrease; *SJW,* St. John's Wort.

Copyright retained by Waza, Inc. T/A Food Medication Interactions, Birchrunville, PA.

*Some sections of this table were copied verbatim from the previous version of the table listed as Resource #1, how do I note this?

REFERENCES

Crowe, Sr. Jeanne P, PharmD, Rph: Krause's Food and the Nutrition Care Process, ed 13, Nutritional Implications of Selected Drugs, Appendix 31. 2012, pp 1100–1106

Pronsky, Zaneta M, Dean Elbe, Keith Ayoob: *Food Medication Interactions.* Birchrunville, Penn, 2015, Food-Medication Interactions. Print.

Nieminen TH, Hagelberg NM, Saari TI, et al: Grapefruit juice enhances the exposure to oral Oxycodone, *Basic Clin Pharmacol Toxicol* 107:782–788, 2010.

Bailey DG, Dresser G, Arnold JM: Grapefruit-medication interactions: forbidden fruit or avoidable consequences? *CMAJ* 2012; doi:10.1503/cmaj.120951

Drugs.com web site: Drug Interactions Checker. www.drugs.com_interactions.php. Accessed June, 2015.

Higdon J: *Linus Pauling Institute Micronutrient Information Center: Zinc.* http://lpi.oregonstate.edu/mic/minerals/zinc#drug-interactions. Updated 06/11/2015. Accessed June 19, 2015.

PL Detail-Document, Potential Drug Interactions with Grapefruit. Pharmacist's Letter/Prescriber's Letter. January 2013.

Banach M, Serban C, Sahebkar A, et al: Effects of coenzyme Q10 on statin-induced myopathy: a meta-analysis of randomized controlled trials, *Mayo Clin Proc* 90(1):24–34, Jan 2015.

Novartis Pharmaceuticals: Product information: Comtan (entacapone), East Hanover, NJ, July 2014, Novartis pharmaceuticals. https://www.pharma.us.novartis.com/product/pi/pdf/comtan.pdf. Accessed June 22, 2015.

Pattani R, Palda VA, Hwang SW, Shah PS: Probiotics for the prevention of antibiotic-associated diarrhea and Clostridium difficile infection among hospitalized patients: systematic review and meta-analysis, *Open Med* 7(2):e56–67, May 28, 2013.

Enteral (Tube Feeding) Formulas for Adults Marketed in the USA

This table does not reference products marketed only for oral use or not intended to provide complete nutrition support. Product composition and availability are subject to change.

Consult Abbott Nutrition, http://abbottnutrition.com/, and Nestlé Nutrition, www.nestle-nutrition.com for current, detailed information.

See **http://www.medicine.virginia.edu/clinical/departments/ medicine/divisions/digestive-health/nutrition-support-team/ clinician-resources/BLENDERIZED_TUBE_FEEDING.pdf** for safety tips, use suggestions, and recipes that may be used to create hoe blenderized feedings.

Enteral Formulas	kcal/ mL	Protein (g/L)	CHO (g/L)	Fat (g/L)	mOsm/kg water	Water (mL/L)	Notes
Whole food based (commercial)	1.06	48	132	40	340	854	Contains chicken, peas, carrots, tomatoes, cranberry juice with added vitamins/minerals
Polymeric, standard	1-1.5	44-68	144-216	35-65	300-650	760-1260	Suitable for most patients; higher caloric density products provide less volume; some contain fiber
Polymeric, high-protein	1-1.2	53-63	130-160	26-39	340-490	818-839	Higher protein content relative to energy; some contain fiber
Polymeric, low electrolyte	1.8-2	35-81	161-290	83-100	600-960	700-736	Volume restricted; lower concentrations of some vitamins/minerals
Polymeric, modified carbohydrate	1-1.5	40-83	96-100	48-75	280-875	859-854	Proprietary carbohydrate blends; some with pureed fruits and vegetables and without sugar alcohols; some with fiber
Polymeric; reduced carbohydrate	1.5	63-68	100-106	93-95	330-785	535-785	Lower carbohydrate with MCT oil; marketed as possible option to reduce diet-induced carbon dioxide production
Peptide-based	1-1.5	40-94	78-188	39-64	345-610	759-848	Di- and tri-peptides from whey or casein; MCT oil; some with MCT combined with fish oil; some with fructooligosaccharides; varying protein to energy ratios
Critical Care (polymeric or free amino acid options)	1-1.5	50-78	134-176	28-94	460-630	759-868	Various formulations marketed as support for the immune system and healing; some with omega-3 fatty acids, fiber, and/or free amino acids

Modular Additives	kcal	Protein (g)	CHO (g)	Fat (g)			
Liquid Protein & Carbohydrate/30 mL	100	10	14 (glycerin)	0			Hydrolyzed collagen fortified with tryptophan
Powdered Protein/7 g	25	6	0	0			Whey protein
Fat & Carbohydrate blend/10g	49	0	7.3	2.2			Cornstarch, vegetable oil, MCT oil

Sample Stepwise Method to Calculate a PN Formula

1. Determine total calories needed (see energy equations in Ch 3)
2. Determine total protein need: Recommendations - Range of 1-2 gm protein/kg or provide 20% of total calories as protein
3. Determine total fat needs: Recommendations -1 gm/kg/day or 20-30% of total calories
4. Balance kcals with carbohydrate (dextrose)

PN FORMULA

EX: Female, Ht: 65 in (165 cm), Wt: 145 pounds (65.9 kg), Age: 43

Recommended Energy Intake: 1800 calories (kcals)/day with 1.4 gm protein/kg (moderate stress)

Macronutrients:

1. <u>Protein (amino acids)</u> = 90 gm
   (Using a 10% amino acid solution - 100gm amino acids/liter)
   EX: 20% of 1800 kcal = 360 kcal from protein * 4 kcal/gm = 90 gm protein = 900 ml
2. <u>Fat -(lipid emulsion)</u> = ~50-55 gm
   (Using 20% lipid emulsion which provides 2 kcal/ml)
   EX: 25% of 1800 kcal = 450 kcal = 225 ml

3. <u>Balance of kcals as carbohydrate</u> = 990 kcal = 291 gm
   (Using 70% dextrose = 700 g/1000mL * 3.4 kcal/g = 2380 kcal/1000 mL)
   EX: 990 kcal needed * 2380 kcal/1000ml = 415 mL

Macronutrients:

10% amino acids	= 900 ml
20% lipid	= 225 ml
70% dextrose	= 415 ml
Total	=1540 ml

4. Micronutrients:
   add multivitamin infusion (MVI) + trace elements = 12-15 ml = 1555 ml
5. Electrolytes/additives: (~100 ml) = 100 ml = 1665 ml (to balance - based on current labs*)
6. Total nutritional fluids: 1665 ml
7. Fluids needs 2000 ml/day = add 335 ml sterile water to equal = 2000 ml/day

---

*labs that are significantly below normal due to disease fluctuations may need to be treated outside the PN solution.
**Infuvite® adult Baxter Healthcare Corporation.

DASH Diet

The DASH diet is an eating pattern that reduces high blood pressure. It is not the traditional low-salt diet. DASH uses foods high in the minerals calcium, potassium, and magnesium, which, when combined, help lower blood pressure. It is also low in fat and high in fiber, an eating style recommended for everyone.

The Healthy Eating Pattern is the template for the DASH eating pattern, with inclusion of ½ to 1 serving of nuts, seeds, and legumes daily, limited fats and oils, and use of nonfat or low-fat milk. The eating pattern is reduced in saturated fat, total fat, cholesterol, and sweet and sugar-containing beverages; and provides abundant servings of fruits and vegetables.

Although the DASH eating plan is naturally lower in salt because of the emphasis on fruits and vegetables, all adults should still make an effort to reduce packaged and processed foods and high-sodium snacks (such as salted chips, pretzels, and crackers) and use less or no salt at the table.

DASH can be an excellent way to lose weight. Because weight loss can help lower blood pressure, it is often suggested. In addition to following DASH, try adding in daily physical activity such as walking or other exercise. You may want to check with your doctor first.

Current recommendations include:

THE DASH DIET

Food Group	1600 kcal Servings/Day	2000 kcal Servings/Day	2600 kcal Servings/Day	3100 kcal Servings/Day
Grains (whole grains)	6	7-8	10-11	12-13
Vegetables	3-4	4-5	5-6	6
Fruits and juices	4	4-5	5-6	6
Milk, nonfat or low-fat	2-3	2-3	3	3-4
Meats, poultry, and fish	1-2	2 or less	6	2-3
Nuts, seeds, and legumes	3/week	½-1	1	1
Fats and oils	2	2-3	3	4
Sweets	0	5/week	Less than 2	2

DIETARY GUIDELINES

Food Group	Servings/Day	Serving Sizes	Examples	Significance of Each Food Group
Grains	6-13	1 slice bread ½ cup (1 oz) dry cereal* ½ cup cooked rice, pasta, or cereal and fiber	Whole-wheat bread, English muffin, pita bread, bagel, cereals, grits, oatmeal, crackers, unsalted pretzels, and popcorn	Major sources of energy
Vegetables	3-6	1 cup raw, leafy veg ½ cup cooked veg 6 oz veg juice	Tomatoes, potatoes, carrots, peas, kale, squash, broccoli, turnip greens, collards, spinach, artichokes, beans, sweet potatoes	Rich sources of potassium, magnesium, antioxidants, and fiber
Fruits	4-6	6 oz fruit juice 1 medium fruit ¼ cup dried fruit ½ cup fresh, frozen, or canned fruit	Apricots, bananas, dates, grapes, oranges and juice, tangerines, strawberries, mangoes, melons, peaches, pineapples, prunes, raisins, grapefruit and juice	Important sources of energy, potassium, magnesium, and fiber
Low-fat dairy	2-4	8 oz milk, 1 cup yogurt, or 1.5 oz cheese	Fat-free or 1% milk, fat-free or low-fat buttermilk, yogurt, or cheese	Major sources of calcium, vitamin D, and protein

Continued

1015

DIETARY GUIDELINES

Food Group	Servings/Day	Serving Sizes	Examples	Significance of Each Food Group
Meat, poultry, fish	1-3	3 oz cooked meats, poultry, or fish 1 egg white[†]	Select only lean meats; trim away visible fats, broil, roast, boil, instead of frying; remove skin from poultry	Rich sources of protein, zinc, and magnesium
Nuts, seeds, legumes	3/wk–1/day	1.5 oz (½ cup) nuts, ½ oz or 2 tbsp seeds, ½ cup cooked legumes	Almonds, filberts, mixed nuts, walnuts, sunflower seeds, kidney beans, lentils	Rich sources of energy, magnesium, protein, monounsaturated fats, and fiber
Fat	2-4	1 tsp soft margarine, veg oil, 1 Tbsp low-fat mayo or salad dressing, or 2 Tbsp light salad dressing[‡]	Soft margarine, low fat mayo, veg oil, light salad dressing	The DASH study had 27% of calories as fat, including fat in or added to foods Sweets should be low in fat

National Institutes of Health, National Heart, Lung, and Blood Institute: YOUR GUIDE TO Lowering Your Blood Pressure With DASH, U.S. Department of Health and Human Services, NIH Publication No. 06-4082, 2006.

*Serving sizes vary between ½ cup and 1¼ cup, depending on cereal type. Check the product's Nutrition Facts label.

[†]Because eggs are high in cholesterol, limit egg yolk intake to no more than four per week; two egg whites have the same protein content as 1 oz of meat.

[‡]Fat content changes serving amount for fats and oils. For example, 1 Tbsp of regular salad dressing equals one serving; 1 Tbsp of a low-fat dressing equals one-half serving; 1 Tbsp of a fat-free dressing equals zero servings.

SAMPLE MENU

Breakfast

1 cup calcium-fortified orange juice
¾ cup Raisin Bran
1 cup skim milk
Mini –whole-wheat bagel
1½ tsp soft margarine
1 cup coffee
2 tsp sugar

Lunch

3-oz boneless skinless chicken breast
2 slices reduced-fat cheese
2 large leaves lettuce
2 slices tomato
1 Tbsp light mayonnaise
2 slices whole wheat bread
1 medium apple
½ cup raw carrot sticks
1 cup iced tea

Dinner

1 cup spaghetti with vegetarian/low-sodium tomato sauce
3 Tbsp Parmesan cheese
½ cup green beans
1 cup spinach, raw
½ cup mushrooms, raw
2 Tbsp croutons
2 Tbsp low-fat Italian dressing
1 slice Italian bread
½ cup frozen yogurt

Midmorning Snack

1 cup apple juice
2 oz walnuts

Nutritional Analysis:

Midafternoon Snack

1 large banana

Kilocalories: 1980
Protein: 78 g
Fat: 56 g
Saturated fat: 13 g
Carbohydrates: 314 g

Sodium: 2377 mg
Potassium: 4129 mg
Fiber: 32 g
Magnesium: 517 g

Exchange Lists for Meal Planning

Menu Plan						
					Grams	Percent
				Carbohydrate	_____	_____
Meal Plan for: _____		Date: _____		Protein	_____	_____
				Fat	_____	_____
Dietitian: _____		Phone: _____		Calories	_____	_____

Time	Number of Exchanges and Choices	Menu Ideas	Menu Ideas
	_____ Carbohydrate group		
	_____ Starch		
	_____ Fruit		
	_____ Milk _____		
	_____ Meat group _____		
	_____ Fat group _____		
	_____ _____		
	_____ _____		
	_____ _____		
	_____ Carbohydrate group		
	_____ Starch		
	_____ Fruit		
	_____ Milk _____		
	_____ Vegetables		
	_____ Meat group		
	_____ Fat group		
	_____ _____		
	_____ _____		
	_____ _____		
	_____ Carbohydrate group		
	_____ Starch		
	_____ Fruit		
	_____ Milk _____		
	_____ Vegetables		
	_____ Meat group		
	_____ Fat group		

HOW THIS EXCHANGE LIST WORKS WITH MEAL PLANNING

There are three main groups of foods in this exchange list. They are based on the three major nutrients: carbohydrates, protein (meat and meat substitutes), and fat. Each food list contains foods grouped together because they have similar nutrient content and serving sizes. Each serving of a food has about the same amount of carbohydrate, protein, fat, and calories as the other foods on the same list.

- Foods on the **Starch** list, **Fruits** list, **Milk** list, and **Sweets, Desserts, and Other Carbohydrates** list are similar because they contain 12 to 15 grams of carbohydrate per serving.
- Foods on the **Fat** list and **Meat and Meat Substitutes** list usually do not have carbohydrate (except for the plant-based meat substitutes such as beans and lentils).

- Foods on the Starchy Vegetables list (part of the **Starch** list and including foods (such as potatoes, corn, and peas) contain 15 grams of carbohydrate per serving.
- Foods on the **Nonstarchy Vegetables** list (such as green beans, tomatoes, and carrots) contain 5 grams of carbohydrate per serving.
- Some foods have so little carbohydrate and calories that they are considered "free," if eaten in small amounts. You can find these foods on the **Free Foods** list.
- Foods that have different amounts of carbohydrates and calories are listed as **Combination Foods** (such as lasagna) or **Fast Foods.**

Foods are listed with their serving sizes, which are usually measured after cooking. When you begin, measuring the size of each serving will help you learn to "eyeball" correct serving sizes. The following chart shows the amount of nutrients in one serving from each list:

Food List	Carbohydrate (grams)	Protein (grams)	Fat (grams)	Calories
Carbohydrates				
Starch: breads, cereals and grains, starchy vegetables, crackers and snacks, and beans, peas, and lentils	15	0-3	0-1	80
Fruits	15	—	—	60
Milk				
Fat-free, low-fat, 1%	12	8	0-3	100
Reduced fat, 2%	12	8	5	120
Whole	12	8	8	160
Sweets, desserts, and other carbohydrates	15	Varies	Varies	Varies
Nonstarchy Vegetables	5	2	—	25
Meat and Meat Substitutes				
Lean	—	7	0-3	45
Medium-fat	—	7	4-7	75
High-fat	—	7	8+	100
Plant-based proteins	Varies	7	Varies	Varies
Fats	—	—	5	45
Alcohol	Varies	—	—	100

STARCH

Cereals, grains, pasta, breads, crackers, snacks, starchy vegetables, and cooked beans, peas, and lentils are starches. In general, 1 starch is:

- ½ cup of cooked cereal, grain, or starchy vegetable
- ½ cup of cooked rice or pasta
- 1 oz of a bread product, such as 1 slice of bread
- ¾ oz to 1 oz of most snack foods (some snack foods may also have extra fat)

Nutrition Tips

1. A choice on the **Starch** list has 15 grams of carbohydrate, 0-3 grams of protein, 0-1 grams of fat, and 80 calories.
2. For maximum health benefits, eat three or more servings of whole grains each day. A serving of whole grain is about ½ cup of cooked cereal or grain, 1 slice of whole-grain bread, or 1 cup of whole-grain cold breakfast cereal.

Selection Tips

1. Choose low-fat starches as often as you can.
2. Starchy vegetables, baked goods, and grains prepared with fat count as 1 starch and 1 fat.
3. For many starchy foods (bagels, muffins, dinner rolls, buns), a general rule of thumb is 1 oz equals 1 serving. Always check the size you eat. Because of their large size, some foods have a lot more carbohydrate (and calories) than you might think. For example, a large bagel may weigh 4 oz and equal 4 carbohydrate servings.
4. For specific information, read the Nutrition Facts panel on the food label.

Food	Serving Size	Food	Serving Size
Bread		**Cereals and Grains**	
Bagel, large (about 4 oz)	¼ (1 oz)	Barley, cooked	⅓ cup
Biscuit, 2½ inches across†	1	Bran, dry	
Bread		Oat*	¼ cup
Reduced-calorie*	2 slices (1½ oz)	Wheat*	½ cup
White, whole-grain, pumpernickel, rye, unfrosted raisin	1 slice (1 oz)	Bulgar (cooked)*	½ cup
Chapatti, small, 6 inches across	1	**Cereals**	
Cornbread, 1¾ inch cube†	1 (1½ oz)	Bran*	½ cup
English muffin	½	Cooked (oats, oatmeal)	½ cup
Hot dog bun or hamburger bun	½ (1 oz)	Puffed	1½ cup
Naan, 8 inches by 2 inches	¼	Shredded wheat, plain	½ cup
Pancake, 4 inches across, ¼ inch thick	1	Sugar-coated	½ cup
Pita, 6 inches across	½	Unsweetened, ready-to-eat	¾ cup
Roll, plain, small	1 (1 oz)	Couscous	⅓ cup
Stuffing, bread†	⅓ cup		
Taco shell, 5 inches across†	2	**Granola**	
Tortilla, corn, 6 inches across	1	Low-fat	¼ cup
Tortilla, flour, 6 inches across	1	Regular†	¼ cup
Tortilla, flour, 10 inches across	⅓ tortilla	Grits, cooked	½ cup
Waffle, 4-inch square or 4 inches across†	1	Kasha	½ cup
		Millet, cooked	⅓ cup
		Muesli	¼ cup
		Pasta, cooked	⅓ cup
		Polenta, cooked	⅓ cup

Food	Serving Size	Food	Serving Size
Quinoa, cooked	⅓ cup	Sandwich-style, cheese or peanut butter filling†	3
Rice, white or brown, cooked	⅓ cup	Whole-wheat regular†	2-5 (¾ oz)
Tabbouleh (tabouli), prepared	½ cup	Whole-wheat lower fat or	2-5 (¾ oz)
Wheat germ, dry	3 Tbsp	crispbreads*	
Wild rice, cooked	½ cup	Graham cracker, 2½-inch square	3
		Matzoh	¾ oz
Starchy Vegetables		Melba toast, about 2-inch by 4-inch piece	4 pieces
Cassava	⅓ cup	Oyster crackers	20
Corn	½ cup		
On cob, large	½ cob (5 oz)	***Popcorn (Microwave Popped)***	***3 cups***
Hominy, canned*	¾ cup	With butter†*	3 cups
Mixed vegetables with corn, peas or pasta*	1 cup	No fat added*	3 cups
Parsnips*	½ cup	Lower fat*	3 cups
Peas, green*	½ cup	Pretzels	¾ oz
Plantain, ripe	⅓ cup	Rice cakes, 4 inches across	2
Potato		***Snack Chips***	
Baked with skin	¼ large (3 oz)	Fat-free or baked (tortilla, potato), baked pita chips	15-20 (¾ oz)
Boiled, all kinds	½ cup or ½ medium (3 oz)	Regular (tortilla, potato)†	9-13 (¾ oz)
Mashed, with milk and fat†	½ cup		
French fried (oven-baked)	1 cup (2 oz)	**Beans, Peas, and Lentils**	
Pumpkin, canned, no sugar added*	1 cup	**The Choices on this List Count as 1 Starch + 1 lean meat.**	
Spaghetti/pasta sauce	½ cup	Baked beans*	⅓ cup
Squash, winter (acorn, butternut)*	1 cup	Beans, cooked (black, garbanzo,	½ cup
Succotash*	½ cup	kidney, lima, navy, pinto, white)*	
Yam, sweet potato, plain	½ cup	Lentils, cooked (brown, green, yellow)*	½ cup
		Peas, cooked (black-eyed, split)*	½ cup
Crackers and Snacks		Refried beans, canned‡*	½ cup
Animal crackers	8		
Crackers			
Round-butter type†	6		
Saltine-type	6		

*More than 3 grams of dietary fiber per serving.
†Extra fat, or prepared with added fat. (Count as 1 starch + 1 fat.)
‡480 milligrams or more of sodium per serving.

Fresh, frozen, canned, and dried fruits and fruit juices are on this list. In general, 1 fruit choice is:

- ½ cup of canned or fresh fruit or unsweetened fruit juice
- 1 small fresh fruit (4 oz)
- 2 tablespoons of dried fruit

Nutrition Tips

1. A choice on the **Fruits** list has 15 grants of carbohydrate, 0 grants of protein, 0 grants of fat, and 60 calories.
2. Fresh, frozen, and dried fruits are good sources of fiber. Fruit juices contain very little fiber. Choose fruits instead of juices whenever possible.
3. Citrus fruits, berries, and melons are good sources of vitamin C.

Selection Tips

1. Use a food scale to weigh fresh fruits. Practice builds portion skills.
2. The weight listed includes skin, core, seeds, and rind.
3. Read the Nutrition Facts on the food label. If 1 serving has more than 15 g of carbohydrate, you may need to adjust the size of the serving.
4. Portion sizes for canned fruits are for the fruit and a small amount of juice (1 to 2 tablespoons).
5. Food labels for fruits may contain the words *no sugar added* or *unsweetened*. This means that no sucrose (table sugar) has been added; it *does not* mean the food contains no sugar.
6. Fruit canned in *extra light syrup* has the same amount of carbohydrate per serving as the *no sugar added* or the *juice pack*. All canned fruits on the **Fruits** list are based on one of these three types of pack. Avoid fruit canned in heavy syrup.

The weight listed includes skin, core, seeds, and rind.

Food	Serving Size
Fruit	
Apple, unpeeled, small	1 (4 oz)
Apples, dried	4 rings
Applesauce, unsweetened	½ cup
Apricots	
Canned	½ cup
Dried	8 halves
Fresh*	4 whole (5½ oz)
Banana, extra small	1 (4 oz)
Blackberries*	¾ cup
Blueberries	¾ cup
Cantaloupe, small	⅓ melon or 1 cup cubed (11 oz)
Cherries	
Sweet, canned	½ cup
Sweet fresh	12 (3 oz)
Dates	3
Dried fruits (blueberries, cherries, cranberries, mixed fruit, raisins)	2 Tbsp
Figs	
Dried	1½
Fresh*	1½ large or 2 medium (3½ oz)
Fruit cocktail	½ cup
Grapefruit	
Large	½ (11 oz)
Sections, canned	¾ cup
Grapes, small	17 (3 oz)
Honeydew melon	1 slice or 1 cup cubed (10 oz)
Kiwi*	1 (3½ oz)
Mandarin oranges, canned	¾ cup
Mango, small	½ fruit (5½ oz) or ½ cup
Nectarine, small	1 (5 oz)
Orange, small*	1 (6½ oz)
Papaya	½ fruit or 1 cup cubed (8 oz)
Peaches	
Canned	½ cup
Fresh, medium	1 (6 oz)
Pears	
Canned	½ cup
Fresh, large	½ (4 oz)
Pineapple	
Canned	½ cup
Fresh	¾ cup
Plums	
Canned	½ cup
Dried (prunes)	3
Small	2 (5 oz)
Raspberries*	1 cup
Strawberries*	1¼ cup whole berries
Tangerines, small*	2 (8 oz)
Watermelon	1 slice or 1¼ cups cubes (13½ oz)
Fruit Juice	
Apple juice/cider	½ cup
Fruit juice blends, 100% juice	⅓ cup
Grape juice	⅓ cup
Grapefruit juice	½ cup
Orange juice	½ cup
Pineapple juice	½ cup
Prune juice	⅓ cup

*More than 3 grams of dietary fiber per serving.

MILK

Different types of milk and milk products are on this list. However, 2 types of milk products are found in other lists:

- Cheeses are on the **Meat and Meat Substitutes** list (because they are rich in protein).
- Cream and other dairy fats are on the **Fats** list.

Milks and yogurts are grouped in 3 categories (fat-free/low-fat, reduced-fat, or whole) based on the amount of fat they have. The following chart shows you what 1 milk choice contains:

	Carbohydrate (grams)	Protein (grams)	Fat (grams)	Calories
Fat-free (skim), low-fat (1%)	12	8	0-3	100
Reduced-fat (2%)	12	8	5	120
Whole	12	8	8	160

Nutrition Tips

1. Milk and yogurt are good sources of calcium and protein.
2. The higher the fat content of milk and yogurt, the more saturated fat and cholesterol it has.
3. Children over the age of 2 and adults should choose lower-fat varieties such as skim, 1%, or 2% milks or yogurts.

Selection Tips

1. 1 cup equals 8 fluid oz or ½ pint.
2. If you choose 2%, or whole-milk foods, be aware of the extra fat.

Food	Serving Size	Count As
Milk and Yogurts		
Fat-free or low-fat (1%)		
Milk, buttermilk, acidophilus milk, Lactaid	1 cup	1 fat-free milk
Evaporated milk	½ cup	1 fat-free milk
Yogurt, plain or flavored with an artificial sweetener	⅔ cup (6 oz)	1 fat-free milk
Reduced-fat (2%)		
Milk, acidophilus milk, kefir, Lactaid	1 cup	1 reduced-fat milk
Yogurt, plain	⅔ cup (6 oz)	1 reduced-fat milk
Whole		
Milk, buttermilk, goat's milk	1 cup	1 whole milk
Evaporated milk	½ cup	1 whole milk
Yogurt, plain	8 oz	1 whole milk
Dairy-Like Foods		
Chocolate milk		
Fat-free	1 cup	1 fat-free milk + 1 carbohydrate
Whole	1 cup	1 whole milk + 1 carbohydrate

Food	Serving Size	Count As
Eggnog, whole milk	½ cup	1 carbohydrate + 2 fats
Rice drink		
Flavored, low-fat	1 cup	2 carbohydrates
Plain, fat-free	1 cup	1 carbohydrate
Smoothies, flavored, regular	10 oz	1 fat-free milk + 2½ carbohydrates
Soy milk		
Light	1 cup	1 carbohydrate + ½ fat
Regular, plain	1 cup	1 carbohydrate + 1 fat
Yogurt		
And juice blends	1 cup	1 fat-free milk + 1 carbohydrate
Low carbohydrate (less than 6 grams carbohydrate per choice)	⅔ cup (6 oz)	½ fat-free milk
With fruit, low-fat	⅔ cup (6 oz)	1 fat-free milk + 1 carbohydrate

Common Measurements

Dry:

3 tsp = 1 Tbsp
4 oz = ½ cup
8 oz = 1 cup

Liquid:

4 Tbsp = ¼ cup
8 oz = ½ pint

Nutrition Tips

1. A carbohydrate choice has 15 grams of carbohydrate, variable grams of protein, variable grams of fat, and variable calories.
2. The foods on this list do not have as many vitamins, minerals, and fiber as the choices on the **Starch, Fruits,** or **Milk** lists. When choosing sweets, desserts, and other carbodrate foods, you should also eat foods from other food lists to balance out your meals.
3. Many of these foods don't equal a single choice. Some will also count as one or more fat choices.
4. If you are trying to lose weight, choose foods from this list less often.
5. The serving sizes for these foods are small because of their fat content.

SWEETS, DESSERTS, AND OTHER CARBOHYDRATES

You can substitute food choices from this list for other carbohydrate-containing foods (such as those found on the **Starch, Fruit,** or **Milk** lists) in your meal plan, even though these foods have added sugars or fat.

Selection Tips

1. Read the Nutrition facts on the food label to find the serving size and nutrient information.
2. Many sugar-free, fat-free, or reduced-fat products are made with ingredients that contain carbohydrate. These types of food usually have the same amount of carbohydrate as the regular foods they are replacing. Talk with your RD and find out how to fit these foods into your meal plan.

Food	Serving Size	Count As
Beverages, Soda, and Energy/Sports Drinks		
Cranberry juice cocktail	½ cup	1 carbohydrate
Energy drink	1 can (8.3 oz)	2 carbohydrates
Fruit drink or lemonade	1 cup (8 oz)	2 carbohydrates
Hot Chocolate		
Regular	1 envelope added to 8 oz water	1 carbohydrate + 1 fat
Sugar-free or light	1 envelope added to 8 oz water	1 carbohydrate
Soft drink (soda), regular	1 can (12 oz)	2½ carbohydrates
Sports drink	1 cup (8 oz)	1 carbohydrate
Brownies, Cake, Cookies, Gelatin, Pie, and Pudding		
Brownie, small, unfrosted	1¼-inch square, ⅞ inch high (about 1 oz)	1 carbohydrate + 1 fat
Cake		
Angel food, unfrosted	1/12 of cake (about 2 oz)	2 carbohydrates
Frosted	2-inch square (about 2 oz)	2 carbohydrates + 1 fat
Unfrosted	2-inch square (about 2 oz)	1 carbohydrate + 1 fat

Food	Serving Size	Count As
Cookies		
Chocolate chip	2 cookies (2¼ inches across)	1 carbohydrate + 2 fats
Gingersnap	3 cookies	1 carbohydrate
Sandwich, with creme filling	2 small (about ⅔ oz)	1 carbohydrate + 1 fat
Sugar-free	3 small or 1 large (¾-1 oz)	1 carbohydrate + 1-2 fats
Vanilla wafer	5 cookies	1 carbohydrate + 1 fat
Cupcake, frosted	1 small (about 1¾ oz)	2 carbohydrates + 1-1½ fats
Fruit cobbler	½ cup (3½ oz)	3 carbohydrates + 1 fat
Gelatin, regular	½ cup	1 carbohydrate
Pie		
Commercially prepared fruit, 2 crusts	⅙ of 8-inch pie	3 carbohydrates + 2 fats
Pumpkin or custard	⅛ of 8-inch pie	1½ carbohydrates + 1½ fats
Pudding		
Regular (made with reduced-fat milk)	½ cup	2 carbohydrates
Sugar-free or sugar- and fat-free (made with fat-free milk)	½ cup	1 carbohydrate

Continued

Food	Serving Size	Count As
Candy, Spreads, Sweets, Sweeteners, Syrups, and Toppings		
Candy bar, chocolate/peanut	2 "fun size" bars (1 oz)	1½ carbohydrates + 1½ fats
Candy, hard	3 pieces	1 carbohydrate
Chocolate "kisses"	5 pieces	1 carbohydrate + 1 fat
Coffee Creamer		
Dry, flavored	4 tsp	½ carbohydrate + ½ fat
Liquid, flavored	2 Tbsp	1 carbohydrate
Fruit snacks, chewy (pureed fruit concentrate)	1 roll (¾ oz)	1 carbohydrate
Fruit spreads, 100% fruit	1½ Tbsp	1 carbohydrate
Honey	1 Tbsp	1 carbohydrate
Jam or jelly, regular	1 Tbsp	1 carbohydrate
Sugar	1 Tbsp	1 carbohydrate
Syrup		
Chocolate	2 Tbsp	2 carbohydrates
Light (pancake type)	2 Tbsp	1 carbohydrate
Regular (pancake type)	1 Tbsp	1 carbohydrate
Condiments and Sauces		
Barbeque sauce	3 Tbsp	1 carbohydrate
Cranberry sauce, jellied	¼ cup	1½ carbohydrates
Gravy, mushroom, canned‡	½ cup	½ carbohydrate + ½ fat
Salad dressing, fat-free, low fat, cream-based	3 Tbsp	1 carbohydrate
Sweet and sour sauce	3 Tbsp	1 carbohydrate
Doughnuts, Muffins, Pastries, and Sweet Breads		
Banana nut bread	1-inch slice (1 oz)	2 carbohydrates + 1 fat
Doughnut		
Cake, plain	1 medium (1½ oz)	1½ carbohydrates + 2 fats
Glazed	3¾ inches across (2 oz)	2 carbohydrates + 2 fats

Food	Serving Size	Count As
Muffin (4 oz)	¼ muffin (1 oz)	1 carbohydrate + ½ fat
Sweet roll or Danish	1 (2½ oz)	2½ carbohydrates + 2 fats
Frozen Bars, Frozen Desserts, Frozen Yogurt, and Ice Cream		
Frozen pops	1	½ carbohydrate
Fruit juice bars, frozen, 100% juice	1 bar (3 oz)	1 carbohydrate
Ice Cream		
Fat-free	½ cup	1½ carbohydrates
Light	½ cup	1 carbohydrate + 1 fat
No sugar added	½ cup	1 carbohydrate + 1 fat
Regular	½ cup	1 carbohydrate + 2 fats
Sherbet, sorbet	½ cup	2 carbohydrates
Yogurt, Frozen		
Fat-free	⅓ cup	1 carbohydrate
Regular	½ cup	1 carbohydrate + 0-1 fat
Granola Bars, Meal Replacement Bars/Shakes, and Trail Mix		
Granola or snack bar, regular or low-fat	1 bar (1 oz)	1½ carbohydrates
Meal replacement bar	1 bar (1⅓ oz)	1½ carbohydrates + 0-1 fat
Meal replacement bar	1 bar (2 oz)	2 carbohydrates + 1 fat
Meal replacement shake, reduced calorie	1 can (10-11 oz)	1½ carbohydrates + 0-1 fat
Trail Mix		
Candy/nut-based	1 oz	1 carbohydrate + 2 fats
Dried fruit-based	1 oz	1 carbohydrate + 1 fat

‡480 mg or more of sodium per serving.

NONSTARCHY VEGETABLES

Vegetable choices include vegetables in this **Nonstarchy Vegetables** list and the Starchy Vegetables list found within the **Starch** list. Vegetables with small amounts of carbohydrate and calories are on the **Nonstarchy Vegetables** list. Vegetables contain important nutrients. Try to eat at least 2 to 3 nonstarchy vegetable choices each day (as well as choices from the Starchy Vegetables list). In general, 1 nonstarchy vegetable choice is:

- ½ cup of cooked vegetables or vegetable juice
- 1 cup of raw vegetables

If you eat 3 cups or more of raw vegetables or 1½ cups of cooked vegetables in a meal, count them as 1 carbohydrate choice.

Nutrition Tips

1. A choice on this list (½ cup cooked or 1 cup raw) equals 5 grams of carbohydrate, 2 grams of protein, 0 grams of fat, and 25 calories.
2. Fresh and frozen vegetables have less added salt than canned vegetables. Drain and rinse canned vegetables to remove some salt.

3. Choose dark green and dark yellow vegetables each day. Spinach, broccoli, romaine, carrots, chilies, squash, and peppers are great choices.
4. Brussels sprouts, broccoli, cauliflower, greens, peppers, spinach, and tomatoes are good sources of vitamin C.
5. Eat vegetables from the cruciferous family several times each week. Cruciferous vegetables include bok choy, broccoli, brussels sprouts, cabbage, cauliflower, collards, kale, kohlrabi, radishes, rutabaga, turnip, and watercress.

Selection Tips

1. Canned vegetables and juices are also available without added salt.
2. A 1-cup portion of broccoli is a portion about the size of a regular light bulb.
3. Starchy vegetables such as corn, peas, winter squash, and potatoes that have more calories and carbohydrates are on the Starchy Vegetables section in the **Starch** list.
4. The tomato sauce referred to in this list is different from spaghetti/pasta sauce, which is on the Starchy Vegetables list.

Nonstarchy Vegetables

Amaranth or Chinese spinach	Cucumber	Peppers (all varieties)*
Artichoke	Eggplant	Radishes
Artichoke hearts	Gourds (bitter, bottle, luffa, bitter melon)	Rutabaga
Asparagus	Green onions or scallions	Sauerkraut‡
Baby corn	Greens (collard, kale, mustard, turnip)	Soybean sprouts
Bamboo shoots	Hearts of palm	Spinach
Beans (green, wax, Italian)	Jicama	Squash (summer, crookneck, zucchini)
Bean sprouts	Kohlrabi	Sugar pea snaps
Beets	Leeks	Swiss chard*
Borscht‡	Mixed vegetables (without corn, peas, or pasta)	Tomato
Broccoli	Mung bean sprouts	Tomatoes, canned
Brussels sprouts*	Mushrooms, all kinds, fresh	Tomato sauce‡
Cabbage (green, bok choy, Chinese)	Okra	Tomato/vegetable juice‡
Carrots*	Onions	Turnips
Cauliflower	Oriental radish or daikon	Water chestnuts
Celery	Pea pods	Yard-long beans
Chayote*		
Coleslaw, packaged, no dressing		

*More than 3 grams of dietary fiber per serving.
‡480 milligrams or more of sodium per serving.

MEAT AND MEAT SUBSTITUTES

Meat and meat substitutes are rich in protein. Foods from this list are divided into 4 groups based on the amount of fat they contain. These groups are lean meat, medium-fat meat, high-fat meat, and plant-based proteins. The following chart shows you what one choice includes:

	Carbohydrate (grams)	Protein (grams)	Fat (grams)	Calories
Lean meat	—	7	0-3	45
Medium-fat meat	—	7	4-7	75
High-fat meat	—	7	8+	100
Plant-based protein	Varies	7	Varies	Varies

Nutrition Tips

1. Read labels to find foods low in fat and cholesterol. Try for 3 grams of fat or less per serving.
2. Read labels to find "hidden" carbohydrate. For example, hot dogs actually contain a lot of carbohydrate. Most hot dogs are also high in fat, but are often sold in lower-fat versions.

3. Whenever possible, choose lean meats.
   a. Select grades of meat that are the leanest.
   b. Choice grades have a moderate amount of fat.
   c. Prime cuts of meat have the highest amount of fat.
4. Fish such as herring, mackerel, salmon, sardines, halibut, trout, and tuna are rich in omega-3 fats, which may help reduce risk for heart disease. Choose fish (not commercially fried fish fillets) two or more times each week.
5. Bake, roast, broil, grill, poach, steam, or boil instead of frying.

Selection Tips

1. Trim off visible fat or skin.
2. Roast, broil, or grill meat on a rack so that the fat will drain off during cooking.
3. Use a nonstick spray and a nonstick pan to brown or fry foods.
4. Some processed meats, seafood, and soy products contain carbohydrate. Read the food label to see if the amount of carbohydrate in the serving size you plan to eat is close to 13 grams. If so, count it as 1 carbohydrate choice and 1 or more meat choice.
5. Meat or fish that is breaded with cornmeal, flour, or dried bread crumbs contain carbohydrate. Count 3 Tbsp of one of these dry grains as 15 grams of carbohydrate.

Food	Amount
Lean Meats and Meat Substitutes	
Beef: Select or Choice grades trimmed of fat: ground round, roast (chuck, rib, rump), round, sirloin, steak (cubed, flank, porterhouse, T-bone), tenderloin	1 oz
Beef jerky‡	1 oz
Cheeses with 3 grams of fat or less per oz	1 oz
Cottage cheese	¼ cup
Egg substitutes, plain	¼ cup
Egg whites	2
Fish, fresh or frozen, plain: catfish, cod, flounder, haddock, halibut, orange roughy, salmon, tilapia, trout, tuna	1 oz
Fish, smoked: herring or salmon (lox)‡	1 oz
Game: buffalo, ostrich, rabbit, venison	1 oz
Hot dog with 3 grams of fat or less per oz‡ (8 dogs per 14 oz package) *(Note: Maybe high in carbohydrate)*	1
Lamb: chop, leg, or roast	1 oz
Organ meats: heart, kidney, liver *(Note: Maybe high in cholesterol)*	1 oz
Oysters, fresh or frozen	6 medium
Pork, Lean	
Canadian bacon‡	1 oz
Rib or loin chop/roast, ham, tenderloin	1 oz
Poultry, without skin: Cornish hen, chicken, domestic duck or goose (well-drained of fat), turkey	1 oz
Processed sandwich meats with 3 grams of fat or less per oz: chipped beef, deli thin-sliced meats, turkey ham, turkey kielbasa, turkey pastrami	1 oz
Salmon, canned	1 oz
Sardines, canned	2 medium
Sausage with 3 grams of fat or less per oz‡	1 oz
Shellfish: clams, crab, imitation shellfish, lobster, scallops, shrimp	1 oz
Tuna, canned in water or oil, drained	1 oz
Veal, loin chop, roast	1 oz

Food	Amount
Medium-Fat Meat and Meat Substitutes	
Beef: corned beef, ground beef, meatloaf, Prime grades trimmed of fat (prime rib), short ribs, tongue	1 oz
Cheeses with 4-7 grams of fat per oz: feta, mozzarella, pasteurized processed cheese spread, reduced-fat cheeses, string	1 oz
Egg (Note: High in cholesterol, so limit to 3 per week)	1
Fish, any fried product	1 oz
Lamb: ground, rib roast	1 oz
Pork: cutlet, shoulder roast	1 oz
Poultry: chicken with skin; dove, pheasant, wild duck, or goose; fried chicken; ground turkey	1 oz
Ricotta cheese	2 oz or ¼ cup
Sausage with 4-7 grams of fat per oz‡	1 oz
Veal, cutlet (no breading)	1 oz

‡480 milligrams or more of sodium per serving.

The following foods are high in saturated fat, cholesterol, and calories and may raise blood cholesterol levels if eaten on a regular basis. Try to eat 3 or fewer servings from this group per week.

High-Fat Meat and Meat Substitutes

Food	Amount
Bacon	
Pork‡	2 slices (16 slices per lb or 1 oz each, before cooking)
Turkey‡	3 slices (½ oz each before cooking)
Cheese, regular: American, bleu, brie, cheddar, hard goat, Monterey jack, queso, and Swiss	1 oz
Hot dog: beef, pork, or combination (10 per lb-sized package)‡†	1
Hot dog: turkey or chicken (10 per lb-sized package)‡	1
Pork: ground, sausage, spareribs	1 oz
Processed sandwich meats with 8 grams of fat or more per oz: bologna, pastrami, hard salami	1 oz
Sausage with 8 grams fat or more per oz: bratwurst, chorizo, Italian, knockwurst, Polish, smoked, summer‡†	1 oz

†Extra fat, or prepared with added fat. (Add an additional fat choice to this food.)
‡480 milligrams or more of sodium per serving.

Because carbohydrate content varies among plant-based proteins, you should read the food label.

Food	Amount	Countas
Plant-Based Proteins		
"Bacon" strips, soy-based	3 strips	1 medium-fat meat
Baked beans*	⅓ cup	1 starch + 1 lean meat
Beans, cooked: black, garbanzo, kidney, lima, navy, pinto, white*	½ cup	1 starch + 1 lean meat

Food	Amount	Countas
"Beef" or "sausage" crumbles, soy-based*	2 oz	½ carbohydrate + 1 lean meat
"Chicken" nuggets, soy-based	2 nuggets (1½ oz)	½ carbohydrate + 1 medium-fat meat
Edamame*	½ cup	½ carbohydrate + 1 lean meat
Falafel (spiced chickpea and wheat patties)	3 patties (about 2 inches across)	1 carbohydrate + 1 high-fat meat
Hot dog, soy-based	1 (1½ oz)	½ carbohydrate + 1 lean meat
Hummus*	⅓ cup	1 carbohydrate + 1 high-fat meat
Lentils, brown, green, or yellow*	½ cup	1 carbohydrate + 1 lean meat
Meatless burger, soy-based*	3 oz	½ carbohydrate + 2 lean meats
Meatless burger, vegetable- and starch-based*	1 patty (about 2½ oz)	1 carbohydrate + 2 lean meats
Nut spreads: almond butter, cashew butter, peanut butter, soy nut butter	1 Tbsp	1 high-fat meat
Peas, cooked: black-eyed and split peas*	½ cup	1 starch + 1 lean meat
Refried beans, canned‡*	½ cup	1 starch + 1 lean meat
"Sausage" patties, soy-based	1 (1½ oz)	1 medium-fat meat
Soy nuts, unsalted	¾ oz	½ carbohydrate + 1 medium-fat meat
Tempeh	¼ cup	1 medium-fat meat
Tofu	4 oz (½ oz)	1 medium-fat meat
Tofu, light	4 oz (½ oz)	1 lean meat

*More than 3 grams of dietary fiber per serving.
‡480 milligrams or more of sodium per serving.

FATS

Fats are divided into 3 groups, based on the main type of fat they contain:

- **Unsaturated fats** (omega-3, monounsaturated, and polyunsaturated) are primarily vegetable and are liquid at room temperature. These fats have good health benefits.
  - **Omega-3 fats** are a type of polyunsaturated fat and can help lower triglyceride levels and the risk of heart disease.
  - **Monounsaturated fats** also help lower cholesterol levels and may help raise HDL (good) cholesterol levels.
  - **Polyunsaturated fats** can help lower cholesterol levels.
- **Saturated fats** have been linked with heart disease. They can raise LDL (bad) cholesterol levels and should be eaten in small amounts. Saturated fats are solid at room temperature.
- *Trans* fats are made in a process that changes vegetable oils into semi-solid fats. These fats can raise blood cholesterol levels and should be eaten in small amounts. Partially hydrogenated and hydrogenated fats are types of man-made *trans* fats and should be avoided. *Trans* fats are also found naturally occurring in some animal products such as meat, cheese, butter, and dairy products.

Nutrition Tips

1. A choice on the **Fats** list contains 5 grams of fat and 45 calories.
2. All fats are high in calories. Limit serving sizes for good nutrition and health.
3. Limit the amount of fried foods you eat.
4. Nuts and seeds are good sources of unsaturated fats if eaten in moderation. They have small amounts of fiber, protein, and magnesium.
5. Good sources of omega-3 fatty acids include:
   a. Fish such as albacore tuna, halibut, herring, mackerel, salmon, sardines, and trout
   b. Flaxseeds and English walnuts
   c. Oils such as canola, soybean, flaxseed, and walnut.

Selection Tips

1. Read the Nutrition Facts on food labels for serving sizes. One fat choice is based on a serving size that has 5 grams of fat.

2. The food label also lists total fat grams, saturated fat, and *trans* fat grams per serving. When most of the calories come from saturated fat, the food is part of the Saturated Fats list.
3. When selecting fats, consider replacing saturated fats with monounsaturated fats and omega-3 fats. Talk with your RD about the best choices for you.
4. When selecting regular margarine, choose those that list liquid vegetable oil as the first ingredient. Soft or tub margarines have less saturated fat than stick margarines and are a healthier choice. Look for *trans* fat-free soft margarines.
5. When selecting reduced-fat or lower-fat margarines, look for liquid vegetable oil (*trans* fat-free). Water is usually the first ingredient.

Fats and oils have mixtures of unsaturated (polyunsaturated and monounsaturated) and saturated fats. Foods on the Fats list are grouped together based on the major type of fat they contain. In general, 1 fat choice equals:
- 1 teaspoon of regular margarine, vegetable oil, or butter
- 1 tablespoon of regular salad dressing

Food	Serving Size
Unsaturated Fats—Monounsaturated Fats	
Avocado, medium	2 Tbsp (1 oz)
Nut butters (*trans* fat-free): almond butter, cashew butter, peanut butter (smooth or crunchy)	1½ tsp
Nuts	
Almonds	6 nuts
Brazil	2 nuts
Cashews	6 nuts
Filberts (hazelnuts)	5 nuts
Macadamia	3 nuts
Mixed (50% peanuts)	6 nuts
Peanuts	10 nuts
Pecans	4 halves
Pistachios	16 nuts
Oil: canola, olive, peanut	1 tsp
Olives	
Black (ripe)	8 large
Green, stuffed	10 large
Polyunsaturated Fats	
Margarine: lower-fat spread (30%-50% vegetable oil, *trans* fat-free)	1 Tbsp
Margarine: stick, tub (*trans* fat-free), or squeeze (*trans* fat-free)	1 tsp
Mayonnaise	
Reduced-fat	1 Tbsp
Regular	1 tsp
Mayonnaise-Style Salad Dressing	
Reduced-fat	1 Tbsp
Regular	2 tsp
Nuts	
Walnuts, English	4 halves
Pignolia (pine nuts)	1 Tbsp
Oil: corn, cottonseed, flaxseed, grape seed, safflower, soybean, sunflower	1 tsp
Oil: made from soybean and canola oil—Enova	1 tsp
Plant Stanol Esters	
Light	1 Tbsp
Regular	2 tsp
Salad Dressing	
Reduced-fat (Note: May be high in carbohydrate)‡	2 Tbsp
Regular‡	1 Tbsp

Food	Serving Size
Seeds	
Flaxseed, whole	1 Tbsp
Pumpkin, sunflower	1 Tbsp
Sesame seeds	1 Tbsp
Tahini or sesame paste	2 tsp
Saturated Fats	
Bacon, cooked, regular or turkey	1 slice
Butter	
Reduced-fat	1 Tbsp
Stick	1 tsp
Whipped	2 tsp
Butter Blends Made with Oil	
Reduced-fat or light	1 Tbsp
Regular	1½ tsp
Chitterlings, boiled	2 Tbsp (½ oz)
Coconut, sweetened, shredded	2 Tbsp
Coconut Milk	
Light	⅓ cup
Regular	1½ Tbsp
Cream	
Half and half	2 Tbsp
Heavy	1 Tbsp
Light	1½ Tbsp
Whipped	2 Tbsp
Whipped, pressurized	¼ cup
Cream Cheese	
Reduced-fat	1½ Tbsp (¾ oz)
Regular	1 Tbsp (½ oz)
Lard	1 tsp
Oil: coconut, palm, palm kernel	1 tsp
Salt pork	¼ oz
Shortening, solid	1 tsp
Sour Cream	
Reduced-fat or light	3 Tbsp
Regular	2 Tbsp

‡480 milligrams or more of sodium per serving.

FREE FOODS

A "free" food is any food or drink choice that has less than 20 calories and 5 grams or less of carbohydrate per serving.

Selection Tips

1. Most foods on this list should be limited to 3 servings (as listed here) per day. Spread out the servings throughout the day. If you eat all 3 servings at once, it could raise your blood glucose level.

2. Food and drink choices listed here without a serving size can be eaten whenever you like.

Food	Serving Size	Food	Serving Size
Low Carbohydrate Foods		***Mayonnaise-style Salad Dressing***	
Cabbage, raw	½ cup	Fat-free	1 Tbsp
Candy, hard (regular or sugar-free)	1 piece	Reduced-fat	1 tsp
Carrots, cauliflower, or green beans, cooked	¼ cup	***Salad Dressing***	
Cranberries, sweetened with sugar substitute	½ cup	Fat-free or low-fat	1 Tbsp
Cucumber, sliced	½ cup	Fat-free, Italian	2 Tbsp
		Sour cream, fat-free or reduced-fat	1 Tbsp
Gelatin			
Dessert, sugar-free		***Whipped Topping***	
Unflavored		Light or fat-free	2 Tbsp
Gum		Regular	1 Tbsp
Jam or jelly, light or no sugar added	2 tsp	**Condiments**	
Rhubarb, sweetened with sugar substitute	½ cup	Barbecue sauce	2 tsp
Salad greens		Catsup (ketchup)	1 Tbsp
Sugar substitutes (artificial sweeteners)		Honey mustard	1 Tbsp
Syrup, sugar-free	2 Tbsp	Horseradish	
		Lemon juice	
Modified Fat Foods with Carbohydrate		Miso	1½ tsp
Cream cheese, fat-free	1 Tbsp (½ oz)	Mustard	
		Parmesan cheese, freshly grated	1 Tbsp
Creamers		Pickle relish	1 Tbsp
Nondairy, liquid	1 Tbsp		
Nondairy, powdered	2 tsp	***Pickles***	
		Dill‡	1½ medium
Margarine Spread		Sweet, bread and butter	2 slices
Fat-free	1 Tbsp	Sweet, gherkin	¾ oz
Reduced-fat	1 tsp	Salsa	¼ cup
		Soy sauce, light or regular‡	1 Tbsp
Mayonnaise		Sweet and sour sauce	2 tsp
Fat-free	1 Tbsp	Sweet chili sauce	2 tsp
Reduced-fat	1 tsp	Taco sauce	1 Tbsp
		Vinegar	
		Yogurt, any type	2 Tbsp

‡480 milligrams or more of sodium per serving.

Free Snacks

These foods in these serving sizes are perfect free-food snacks:
- 5 baby carrots and celery sticks
- ¼ cup blueberries
- ½ oz sliced cheese, fat-free
- 10 goldfish-style crackers
- 2 saltine-type crackers
- 1 frozen cream pop, sugar-free
- ½ oz lean meat
- 1 cup light popcorn
- 1 vanilla wafer

Drinks/Mixes

Any food on this list—without a serving size listed—can be consumed in any moderate amount:
- Bouillon, broth, consommé‡
- Bouillon or broth, low-sodium
- Carbonated or mineral water
- Club soda
- Cocoa powder, unsweetened (1 Tbsp)
- Coffee, unsweetened or with sugar substitute
- Diet soft drinks, sugar-free
- Drink mixes, sugar-free
- Tea, unsweetened or with sugar substitute
- Tonic water, diet
- Water
- Water, flavored, carbohydrate free

Seasonings

Any food on this list can be consumed in any moderate amount:
- Flavoring extracts (for example, vanilla, almond, peppermint)
- Garlic
- Herbs, fresh or dried
- Nonstick cooking spray
- Pimento
- Spices
- Hot pepper sauce
- Wine, used in cooking
- Worcestershire sauce

COMBINATION FOODS

Many of the foods you eat are mixed together in various combinations, such as casseroles. These "combination" foods do not fit into any one choice list. This is a list of choices for some typical combination foods. This list will help you fit these foods into your meal plan. Ask your RD for nutrient information about other combination foods you would like to eat, including your own recipes.

Food	Serving Size	Count As
Entrees		
Casserole type (tuna noodle, lasagna, spaghetti with meatballs, chili with beans, macaroni and cheese)‡	1 cup (8 oz)	2 carbohydrates + 2 medium-fat meats
Stews (beef/other meats and vegetables)‡	1 cup (8 oz)	1 carbohydrate + 1 medium-fat meat + 0-3 fats
Tuna salad or chicken salad	½ cup (3½ oz)	½ carbohydrate + 2 lean meats + 1 fat
Frozen Meals/Entrees		
Burrito (beef and bean)‡*	1 (5 oz)	3 carbohydrates + 1 lean meat + 2 fats
Dinner-type meal‡	Generally 14-17 oz	3 carbohydrates + 3 medium-fat meats + 3 fats
Entree or meal with less than 340 calories‡	About 8-11 oz	2-3 carbohydrates + 1-2 lean meats
Pizza		
Cheese/vegetarian, thin crust‡	¼ of a 12 inch (4½-5 oz)	2 carbohydrates + 2 medium-fat meats
Meat topping, thin crust‡	¼ of a 12 inch (5 oz)	2 carbohydrates + 2 medium-fat meats + 1½ fats
Pocket sandwich‡	1 (4½ oz)	3 carbohydrates + 1 lean meat + 1-2 fats
Pot pie‡	1 (7 oz)	2½ carbohydrates + 1 medium-fat meat + 3 fats
Salads (Deli-Style)		
Coleslaw	½ cup	1 carbohydrate + 1½ fats
Macaroni/pasta salad	½ cup	2 carbohydrates + 3 fats
Potato salad‡	½ cup	1½-2 carbohydrates + 1-2 fats
Soups		
Bean, lentil, or split pea‡	1 cup	1 carbohydrate + 1 lean meat
Chowder (made with milk)‡	1 cup (8 oz)	1 carbohydrate + 1 lean meat + 1½ fats
Cream (made with water)‡	1 cup (8 oz)	1 carbohydrate + 1 fat
Instant‡	6 oz prepared	1 carbohydrate
With beans or lentils‡	8 oz prepared	2½ carbohydrates + 1 lean meat
Miso soup‡	1 cup	½ carbohydrate + 1 fat
Oriental noodle‡	1 cup	2 carbohydrates + 2 fats
Rice (congee)	1 cup	1 carbohydrate
Tomato (made with water)‡	1 cup (8 oz)	1 carbohydrate
Vegetable beef, chicken noodle, or other broth-type‡	1 cup (8 oz)	1 carbohydrate

FAST FOODS

The choices in the **Fast Foods** list are not specific fast food meals or items, but are estimates based on popular foods. You can get specific nutrition information for almost every fast food or restaurant chain. Ask the restaurant or check its website for nutrition information about your favorite fast foods.

Food	Serving Size	Count As
Breakfast Sandwiches		
Egg, cheese, meat, English muffin‡	1 sandwich	2 carbohydrates + 2 medium-fat meats
Sausage biscuit sandwich‡	1 sandwich	2 carbohydrates + 2 high-fat meats + 3½ fats
Main Dishes/Entrees		
Burrito (beef and beans)‡*	1 (about 8 oz)	3 carbohydrates + 3 medium-fat meats + 3 fats
Chicken breast, breaded and fried‡	1 (about 5 oz)	1 carbohydrate + 4 medium-fat meats
Chicken drumstick, breaded and fried	1 (about 2 oz)	2 medium-fat meats
Chicken nuggets‡	6 (about 3½ oz)	1 carbohydrate + 2 medium-fat meats + 1 fat
Chicken thigh, breaded and fried‡	1 (about 4 oz)	½ carbohydrate + 3 medium-fat meats + 1½ fats
Chicken wings, hot‡	6 (5 oz)	5 medium-fat meats + 1½ fats
Oriental		
Beef/chicken/shrimp with vegetables in sauce‡	1 cup (about 5 oz)	1 carbohydrate + 1 lean meat + 1 fat
Egg roll, meat‡	1 (about 3 oz)	1 carbohydrate + 1 lean meat + 1 fat
Fried rice, meatless	½ cup	1½ carbohydrates + 1½ fats
Meat and sweet sauce (orange chicken)‡	1 cup	3 carbohydrates + 3 medium-fat meats + 2 fats
Noodles and vegetables in sauce (chow mein, lo mein)‡*	1 cup	2 carbohydrates + 1 fat
Pizza		
Cheese, pepperoni, regular crust‡	⅛ of a 14 inch (about 4 oz)	2½ carbohydrates + 1 medium-fat meat + 1½ fats
Cheese/vegetarian, thin crust‡	¼ of a 12 inch (about 6 oz)	2½ carbohydrates + 2 medium-fat meats + 1½ fats
Sandwiches		
Chicken sandwich, grilled‡	1	3 carbohydrates + 4 lean meats
Chicken sandwich, crispy‡	1	3½ carbohydrates + 3 medium-fat meats + 1 fat
Fish sandwich with tartar sauce	1	2½ carbohydrates + 2 medium-fat meats + 2 fats

*More than 3 grams of dietary fiber per serving.
‡600 milligrams or more of sodium per serving (for combination food main dishes/meals).

Continued

Food	Serving Size	Count As
Hamburger		
Large with cheese‡	1	2½ carbohydrates + 4 medium-fat meats + 1 fat
Regular	1	2 carbohydrates + 1 medium-fat meat + 1 fat
Hot dog with bun‡	1	1 carbohydrate + 1 high-fat meat + 1 fat
Submarine sandwich		
Less than 6 grams fat‡	6-inch sub	3 carbohydrates + 2 lean meats
Regular‡	6-inch sub	3½ carbohydrates + 2 medium-fat meats + 1 fat
Taco, hard or soft shell (meat and cheese)	1 small	1 carbohydrate + 1 medium-fat meat + 1½ fats
Salads		
Salad, main dish (grilled chicken type, no dressing or croutons)‡*	Salad	1 carbohydrate + 4 lean meats
Salad, side, no dressing or cheese	Small (about 5 oz)	1 vegetable
Sides/Appetizers		
French fries, restaurant style†	Small	3 carbohydrates + 3 fats
	Medium	4 carbohydrates + 4 fats
	Large	5 carbohydrates + 6 fats
Nachos with cheese‡	Small (about 4½ oz)	2⅓ carbohydrates + 4 fats
Onion rings‡	1 serving (about 3 oz)	2½ carbohydrates + 3 fats
Desserts		
Milkshake, any flavor	12 oz	6 carbohydrates + 2 fats
Soft-serve ice cream cone	1 small	2½ carbohydrates + 1 fat

*More than 3 grams of dietary fiber per serving.
†Extra fat, or prepared with extra fat.
‡600 milligrams or more of sodium per serving (for fast food main dishes/meals).

ALCOHOL

Nutrition Tips

1. In general, 1 alcohol choice (½ oz absolute alcohol) has about 100 calories.

Selection Tips

1. If you choose to drink alcohol, you should limit it to 1 drink or less per day for women, and 2 drinks or less per day for men.
2. To reduce your risk of low blood glucose (hypoglycemia), especially if you take insulin or a diabetes pill that increases insulin, always drink alcohol with food.
3. While alcohol, by itself, does not directly affect blood glucose, be aware of the carbohydrate (for example, in mixed drinks, beer, and wine) that may raise your blood glucose.
4. Check with your RD if you would like to fit alcohol into your meal plan.

Alcoholic Beverage	Serving Size	Count As
Beer		
Light (4.2%)	12 fl oz	1 alcohol equivalent + ½ carbohydrate
Regular (4.9%)	12 fl oz	1 alcohol equivalent + 1 carbohydrate
Distilled spirits: vodka, rum, gin, whiskey 80 or 86 proof	1½ fl oz	1 alcohol equivalent
Liqueur, coffee (53 proof)	1 fl oz	1 alcohol equivalent + 1 carbohydrate
Sake	1 fl oz	½ alcohol equivalent
Wine		
Dessert (sherry)	3½ fl oz	1 alcohol equivalent + 1 carbohydrate
Dry, red or white (10%)	5 fl oz	1 alcohol equivalent

Development of Standardized Dysphagia Diets

TEXTURE MODIFICATIONS

Level 3: Dysphagia Advanced (Previously: Mechanical Soft):

- Soft-solid foods. Includes easy-to-cut whole meats, soft fruits and vegetables (i.e. bananas, peaches, melon without seeds, tender meat cut into small pieces and well moistened with extra gravy or sauce).
- Crusts should be cut off of bread.
- Most is chopped or cut into small pieces.
  EXCLUDES hard, crunchy fruits and vegetables, sticky foods, and very dry foods. NO nuts, seeds, popcorn, potato chips, coconut, hard rolls, raw vegetables, potato skins, corn, etc. Most food is chopped/cut into small pieces.

Level 2: *Dysphagia Mechanically-Altered (Previously: Ground):

- Cohesive, moist, semisolid foods that require some chewing ability.
- Includes fork-mashable fruits and vegetables (i.e. soft canned, or cooked fruits with vegetables in pieces smaller than ½ inch).
- Meat should be ground and moist. Extra sauce and gravy should be served.
  EXCLUDES most bread products, crackers, and other dry foods. No whole grain cereal with nuts, seeds and coconut.

No food with large chunks. Most food should be ground texture.

Level 1: *Dysphagia Puree:

- Smooth, pureed, homogenous, very cohesive, pudding-like foods that require little or no chewing ability.
- No whole foods.
- Includes mashed potatoes with gravy, yogurt with no fruit added, pudding, soups pureed smooth, pureed fruits and vegetables, pureed meat/poultry/fish, sauces/gravies, and pureed desserts without nuts, seeds, or coconut.
  AVOID scrambled, fried, or hard boiled eggs.

FLUID MODIFICATIONS

Thin Liquids: includes water, soda, juice broth, coffee, tea. This also includes foods like jello, ice cream and sherbet that melt and become thin when swallowed.

Nectar-thick Liquids: are pourable and the consistency of apricot nectar

Honey-thick Liquids: slightly thicker than nectar and can be drizzled; consistency of honey.

Pudding-thick Liquids: also called pudding-thick; should hold their shape, and a spoon should stand up in them; they are not pourable and are eaten with a spoon.

Courtesy: Clinical Nutrition Department, Providence Mt. St. Vincent, Seattle, WA.

Renal Diet for Dialysis

Your diet depends on your kidney function. Most of the information here relates to people on dialysis. What is right for others is not always right for you. As your kidney function changes, your diet may change as well. This guide will help you do two things: plan nutritious meals you enjoy and keep your body working at its best. Your renal dietitian will work with you to make any changes needed to your usual meal plan, but this appendix contains helpful guidelines.

1. Increase Protein

   You will need to eat a high-protein diet. Beef, pork, lamb, fish, shellfish, chicken, eggs, and other animal foods provide most of the protein in your diet. Your protein needs are based on your weight. Most people need at least 6 to 8 oz of protein per day. A deck of cards is about the size of a 3-oz serving of protein.

2. Limit Potassium

   Most foods contain some potassium, but fruits and vegetables are the easiest to control. Limit fruits, vegetables, and juices to 6 servings per day. A serving is usually ½ cup.

   Do not use salt substitute or "lite" salt because they are made with potassium.

3. Limit Salt

   Limit the salt you eat. Don't add salt during cooking or at the table. Avoid high-salt foods such as frozen meals; canned or dried foods; "fast foods"; and salted meats such as ham, sausage, and luncheon meats. Use salt-free spices or spice mixes such as Mrs. Dash instead of salt to add flavor to your food.

4. Limit Phosphorus

   Use only 1 serving of milk or dairy food per day. A serving is usually ½ to 1 cup. Take phosphate binders such as Tums, PhosLo, Renagel, or Fosrenol with your meals as prescribed by your doctor.

5. Fluid

   A safe amount of fluid to drink is different for everyone. It depends on how much urine you are making. Try not to drink more than 3 cups (24 oz) of fluid each day plus the amount equal to your urine output. If you are limiting your salt intake, you should not feel thirsty.

   Fluids include all beverages and foods that are liquid at room temperature such as Jell-O, ice cream, ice, and soup.

6. Poor Appetite and Weight Loss

   It is common to have a poor appetite if you are new to dialysis. If your appetite has been poor, try eating small frequent meals and extra snacks.

   Try adding high-calorie fats such as butter, margarine, and oils; sauces and gravies; and sour cream, cream cheese, or whipped cream for extra calories. Adding rice, pasta, bread, and rolls to meals also adds calories.

   Sugar and sweets such as cakes, candies, and pastries are also a good source of calories if you are not following a diabetic diet.

   Talk to your nutritionist about trying a nutritional supplement.

PROTEIN

When on dialysis, you need to eat a high-protein diet. This is because you lose protein during each dialysis treatment. To stay healthy, you need to eat enough protein for your daily needs and also make up for the amount lost during dialysis. Meat, fish, poultry, eggs, and other animal foods provide most of the protein in your diet. Your body uses protein to build and repair muscles, skin, blood, and other tissues.

ALBUMIN

Albumin is a protein found in blood. Each month a laboratory test measures your albumin. It is a good way to know how healthy you are. Your albumin level should be more than 3.4 mg/dL.

KEEPING A HEALTHY ALBUMIN LEVEL

Make sure that you eat enough protein every day. How much protein you need daily depends on how much you weigh.

Find your weight on the chart below to see how many protein servings you need each day.

PROTEIN SERVINGS FOR YOU

If you weigh:	You need:
40 kg	4-5 servings
50 kg	5-6 servings
60 kg	6-7 servings
70 kg	7-8 servings
80 kg	8-9 servings
90 kg	9-10 servings
Your weight: _____ kg	
You need: _____ protein servings each day	

ONE SERVING OF PROTEIN IS:

1 egg
1 oz cooked meat, fish, poultry
¼ cup cooked or canned fish, seafood

½ cup tofu
1 cup milk
1 oz cheese
¼ cup cottage cheese
¾ cup pudding or custard
2 Tbsp peanut butter
1 scoop protein powder
½ protein bar

COMMON SERVING SIZES

Most people eat protein foods in portions larger than 1 serving. Here are some examples:
Average hamburger patty (3 oz) = 3 protein servings
Small beefsteak (3 in × 4 in) = 4 protein servings
Half chicken breast (3 oz) = 3 protein servings
Chicken drumstick or thigh (2 oz) = 2 protein servings
Average pork chop (3 oz) = 3 protein servings
Fish fillet (3 in × 3 in) = 3 protein servings

ESTIMATING SERVING SIZES

Here are some other easy ways to estimate protein serving sizes:
- Your whole thumb is about the size of 1 oz.
- Three stacked dice are about the size of 1 oz.
- A deck of cards is about the size of 3 oz.
- The palm of your hand is about the size of 3 to 4 oz.
- Your clenched fist is about the size of 1 cup.

TIPS FOR EATING MORE PROTEIN

Some people on dialysis dislike the taste of protein. Some people find cooking smells unpleasant. Still others are not able to eat enough protein each day.
The following tips will be helpful:
- Use gravy, sauces, seasonings, or spices to improve or hide flavors.
- Prepare meals ahead of time, or stay away from kitchen smells if they spoil your appetite.
- Eat cooked protein foods cold. Try cold fried chicken, a roast beef sandwich, or shrimp salad.
- Add cut-up meats or beans to soups or salads.
- Use more eggs. Try hardboiled eggs, egg salad sandwiches, custards, or quiches. Stir beaten eggs into casseroles and soups.
- Try other protein foods such as angel food cake, peanut butter, or bean salads.
- Eat a protein bar. Your nutritionist can help you choose one.
- Use a protein powder. Your nutritionist can help you choose one and give you ideas for using it.

NUTRITIONAL SUPPLEMENTS

Nutritional supplements provide extra calories and protein. In general, use one can of supplement as a snack each day. Add one extra can for each meal you miss.
Not all nutritional supplements are safe for dialysis patients. Check with your nutritionist before using any supplement. Here are some of the supplements that are used by people on dialysis:

MALNUTRITION

If you are not eating enough meat, fish, poultry, eggs, and other high-protein foods, your albumin level will drop below the recommended level.
If your albumin level is low, the cells in your body cannot hold fluid well. This leads to swelling (edema) and low blood pressure during dialysis. Low albumin increases your risk of death. Patients with albumin levels above 4 have the lowest death rate.
It is also important to eat enough calories. Your nutritionist can help you make sure you are getting plenty of protein and calories.

EXERCISE

Try to be active in some way each day (e.g., walk, swim, garden, stretch). Using your muscles helps keep them strong. Protein that is stored in your muscles helps support your albumin level.

POTASSIUM FOR PEOPLE ON HEMODIALYSIS

- Most foods have some potassium, but fruits and vegetables are the easiest form to control in your diet. The following list groups vegetables and fruits by the amount of potassium in one serving.
- Remember, there are no foods that you cannot eat on your diet. What is important is the amount of foods you eat and how often you eat them. Keep this list handy for shopping or eating out.
- If there are fruits and vegetables you enjoy that are not on the list, ask your nutritionist about them.

MOST PEOPLE ON HEMODIALYSIS MAY HAVE

- 1 serving per day from the high-potassium group
- 2 servings per day from the medium-potassium group
- 2 to 3 servings per day from the low-potassium group

This is approximately 2000 to 3000 mg of potassium per day with the other foods you eat. Check the serving size for each food, listed in parentheses next to the item.

SOAKING VEGETABLES AND BEANS

Soaking works well for high-potassium foods such as potatoes, parsnips, sweet potatoes, winter squash, and beans. The procedure for soaking follows.
1. Peel vegetables and slice thinly (⅛ inch). Rinse well. Place them in a bowl of warm water, using four times more water than vegetable. For example, soak 1 cup of sliced vegetables in 4 cups of water. Soak at least 1 hour. Drain and rinse again.
2. Vegetables that have been soaked this way can then be fried, mashed, scalloped, put in soups or stews, or served fresh. If you are boiling the food, use four times more water than food and cook as usual.
3. Dried beans should be cooked and then chopped and soaked, using the preceding directions. Canned beans can simply be chopped, rinsed, and soaked.

	Low-Potassium Foods 5-150 mg	Medium-Potassium Foods 150-250 mg	High-Potassium Foods 250-500 mg
		Food Category	
Fruits	Applesauce (½ cup)	Apple (1 medium), cherries (8-10)	Apricots (3)
	Blackberries (½ cup)	Fruit cocktail (½ cup)	Avocados (¼)
	Blueberries (1 cup)	Grapes (10-15)	Banana (1 medium)
	Grapefruit (½ cup)	Mango (½ medium)	Dates (5)
	Pears, canned (½ cup)	Melons: cantaloupe, honeydew	Figs (3)
	Pineapple (½ cup	(½ cup), papaya (½ cup)	Kiwi (1)
	Plums, canned (½ cup)	Peaches, canned (½ cup)	Nectarine (1 medium)
	Raspberries (½ cup)	Pear, fresh (1 medium)	Orange (1 medium)
	Rhubarb, cooked (½ cup	Plums (2)	Peach, fresh (1 medium)
	Strawberries (½ cup	Watermelon (1 cup)	Prunes (5)
	Tangerine (1)		Raisins and dried fruit (¼ cup)
Vegetables	Asparagus (4 spears)	Broccoli (½ cup)	Artichoke (1 medium)
	Bean sprouts (½ cup)	Brussels sprouts (4-6)	Beans: lima, kidney, navy, pinto (½ cup)
	Cabbage (½ cup)	Beets (½ cup)	Greens: beet, collard, mustard, spinach, turnip (½ cup)
	Cauliflower (½ cup)	Carrots (½ cup)	Lentils, split peas, chickpeas, black-eyed peas (½ cup)
	Corn (½ cup)	Celery (½ cup)	Nuts: all kinds (½ cup)
	Cucumber (½)	Eggplant (½ cup)	Parsnips (½ cup)
	Green and wax beans (½ cup)	Mixed vegetables (½ cup)	Potatoes (½ cup or 1 small)
	Lettuce (1 cup)	Mushrooms (½ cup)	Pumpkin (½ cup)
	Okra (3 pods)	Peanut butter (2 Tbsp)	Spinach (½ cup)
	Onions (½ cup)	Pepper, green (1)	Tomato (1 medium)
	Peas (½ cup)	Potato chips (10)	Tomato sauce, tomato salsa (¼ cup)
	Radishes (5)	Soaked potatoes (½ cup)	Winter squash (½ cup)
	Rutabagas (½ cup		Yams, sweet potatoes (½ cup)
	Summer squash (½ cup)		
	Turnips (½ cup)		
	Water chestnuts (4)		
Juices	Apple juice (½ cup)	Apricot nectar (½ cup)	Pomegranate juice (½ cup)
	Cranberry juices (1 cup)	Grape juice, canned (½ cup)	Prune juice (½ cup)
	Grape juice, frozen (1 cup)	Grapefruit juice (½ cup)	Tomato juice (½ cup)
	Tang, Hi-C and other fruit drinks (1 cup), Kool-Aid (1 cup)	Pineapple juice (½ cup)	V-8 juice (½ cup)
	Lemonade and limeade (1 cup)		
	Peach or pear nectar (½ cup)		

OTHER HIGH-POTASSIUM FOODS

- Milk is high in potassium. Limit milk to 1 cup per day unless you are told to do otherwise.
- Supplements such as Ensure Plus and Enhancer Plus also contain a lot of potassium. Always speak to your nutritionist before using supplements.
- Most salt substitutes and "lite" salt products are made with potassium. Do not use these products. If you are unsure, ask your nutritionist.

SHAKING THE SALT HABIT

Salt, or "sodium chloride," is found in convenience and preserved foods. Foods that do not spoil easily are usually high in sodium. The more sodium you eat, the thirstier you will be. The following list of foods is grouped by sodium levels.

Following a low-sodium diet can be challenging. This list of sodium levels of foods is meant to help you learn what foods and how much of them you can enjoy.

Remember, there are no foods that you cannot eat on your diet. What is important is the amount of foods you eat and how often you eat them. Keep this list handy for shopping or dining.

MOST PEOPLE ON DIALYSIS MAY HAVE

- 1 serving per day from the high group
- 1 serving per day from the medium group
- As many servings as desired from the low group
- 3 servings per day from the medium group
- As many servings as you want from the low group
  This is 2000 to 3000 mg of sodium per day. Check the serving size for each food, listed in parentheses next to the item.

RINSING CANNED FOODS TO LOWER SODIUM (CANNED VEGETABLES, CHUNK OR FLAKED FISH OR SHELLFISH, POULTRY OR MEATS)

1. Empty can into colander or sieve.
2. Drain brine and discard.
3. Break up chunks into flakes or smaller pieces.
4. Rinse under running water for 1 min.
5. Drain food until most moisture is gone.

	Low-Sodium Foods 1-150 mg	Medium-Sodium Foods 150-250 mg	High-Sodium Foods 250-700 mg
		Food Category	
Breads and cereals	Breads, white, whole grain Cakes, cookies, crepes, doughnuts Cereals: cooked, granola, puffed rice, puffed wheat, Shredded Wheat, Sugar Pops, Sugar Smacks, Sugar Crisps Crackers: graham, low salt, melba toast Macaroni, noodles, spaghetti, rice	Biscuits, rolls, muffins: homemade (1) Pancakes (1) "Ready-to-eat" cereals (¾ cup) Saltine crackers (6) Sweet roll (1)	All Bran (¼ cup) Instant mixes: noodles, potatoes, rice (½ cup) Instant mixes: biscuits, breads, muffins, rolls (1 serving) Waffles (1)
Condiments	Butter, margarine, oil Horseradish, mustard, spices, herbs, sugar, syrup, Tabasco, vinegar, Worcestershire	Bacon (2 slices) Catsup, steak sauce (1 Tbsp) Commercial salad dressing (1 Tbsp) Gravy (2 Tbsp) Low-sodium soy sauce (2 tsp) Mayonnaise (2 Tbsp) Pickle relish (2 Tbsp) Sweet pickles (2 small)	Salt (¼ tsp)
Dairy products	Cheeses: cream, Monterey, Mozzarella, Ricotta, low-salt types Cream: half-and-half, sour, whipping Custard, ice cream, sherbet Milk: all kinds, yogurt Nondairy creamer	Cheeses (1-oz slice) Cottage cheese (½ cup) Pudding (¾ cup)	Buttermilk (1 cup) Processed cheeses and cheese spreads (1 slice or 2 Tbsp)
Main dishes	All unprocessed meats, fish, poultry Eggs Peanut butter Tuna: low-sodium or rinsed		Broth (½ cup) Canned fish, meat (¼ cup) Canned soups (½ cup) Hot dog (1) Luncheon meat (1 slice) Canned entrees (e.g., pork and beans, spaghetti, stew) (1 cup) Sausage (1 oz)
Fruits and vegetables	All fresh or frozen vegetables All fruits and juices Canned tomatoes, tomato paste Canned vegetables: low-sodium or rinsed	Vegetables (½ cup) Juices: tomato, vegetable (½ cup)	Canned tomato sauce or puree (¼ cup) Frozen vegetables with special sauce (½ cup) Sauerkraut (¼ cup)
Beverages and snacks	Beer, wine, coffee, tea Candy: all kinds Fruit drinks, Popsicles, soda pop, Kool-Aid, Tang Low-salt products: without potassium substitutes Unsalted nuts, unsalted popcorn	Potato and corn chips (1 cup) Snack crackers (5-10)	Commercial dips (¼ cup) Dill pickle chips (3 slices) Olives (5) Salted nuts (½ cup)

PHOSPHORUS

Low-Phosphorus Diet

When phosphorus is high for too long, bones become brittle and weak. You may have joint and bone pain. Extra phosphorus may go into your soft tissue, causing hard or soft lumps. Also, you may have severe itching.

The good news is that with diet, binders, and good dialysis, you can keep your phosphorus level under control.

Phosphorus is a mineral found in most foods. Dialysis does not remove it easily. Your phosphorus level depends on the foods you eat and your medications. Keeping your phosphorus at a safe level will help keep your bones healthy.

Each month your phosphorus level will be measured. High phosphorus is a common problem for people on dialysis. A good phosphorus level in your blood is between 3 and 6 g/dL.

High-Phosphorus Foods

Phosphorus is found in most foods you eat, especially protein foods. The foods that are highest in phosphorus are milk and things made from milk (dairy foods).

By limiting these foods you can cut down on the phosphorus you are eating. Most people on dialysis can have one serving daily from this list of dairy foods. The serving size is also noted.

You can also eat part of a serving of different foods to add up to 1 serving.

Milk (1 cup)
Cheese (2 oz)
Cottage cheese (⅔ cup)
Yogurt (1 cup)
Ice cream (1½ cup)
Frozen yogurt (1½ cup)
Milkshake (1 cup)
Hot chocolate (1 cup)
Pudding or custard (1 cup)

Other High-Phosphorus Foods

When your phosphorus level is high, you may need to limit these foods to once a week.
Bran cereals (1 oz)
Dried beans or peas (½ cup cooked)
Chili (½ cup)

Nuts (½ cup)
Frozen waffles (1)

Phosphorus and Potassium

High-phosphorus foods are often high in potassium as well. This is another reason to limit dairy foods and other high-phosphorus foods.

Phosphate Binders

Phosphate binders are pills you take when you eat. Binders help keep phosphorus in your food from going into your blood.

Your doctor will decide which binder is best for you and how many you should take each time you eat.

It is important to take all your binders planned for each day.

You can take your binders just before you start a meal, during the meal, or right after eating.

If you forget to take them or skip a meal, it may be difficult to get your full binder dose. Ask your doctor what to do if this happens.

It may take some hard work to remember to take binders each time you eat. Try these ideas:

- Each morning take out the number of binders you need that day. Put them in a small container to carry with you. It should be empty at the end of the day.
- Carry a spare container of binders for when you travel or eat out.
- Take your binders with high-protein snacks such as sandwiches or dairy foods.
- Binders may cause constipation. Talk with your nutritionist about ideas to help with bowel movements.
- There are many types of binders. If you don't like the kind you are taking, talk with your doctor, pharmacist, or nutritionist about other kinds.

Lower-Phosphorus Ideas

Following are some lower-phosphorus choices you can make in the place of milk and other creamy dairy products. Check those you will try.

- Use nondairy creamer such as Mocha Mix or Coffee Rich on cereal, for creamy sauces or soups, and in shakes.
- Try rice milk or soymilk. They are lower in potassium too.
- Try soy cheese or soy yogurt. They are available in a variety of flavors.
- Use cream cheese in the place of regular cheese or cottage cheese.
- Use sour cream or imitation sour cream on fruits or to replace yogurt in dips.
- Try a nondairy frozen ice cream made from soy, rice, or nondairy creamer such as Mocha Mix.
- Enjoy sorbet or sherbet instead of ice cream.

High Phosphorus Levels

Following are some reasons for a high phosphorus level. Check the ones that you think may apply to you:

- Eating too many high-phosphorus foods
- Forgetting to take your binders
- Not taking all the phosphate binders ordered for you
- Not taking your phosphate binders at the right times

Even if you follow your diet and take your binders, your phosphorus level may be high. When calcium and phosphorus are out of balance, your parathyroid gland becomes overactive. High levels of parathyroid hormone damage your bones. Your doctor can test for this problem and recommend treatment.

Appendix created by Katy G. Wilkens, MS, RD.
NOTE: Some foods are very high in sodium and should be used only once a week. These include Chinese, Oriental foods; corned beef, ham, pastrami; fast foods (e.g., commercial hamburgers, pizza, tacos); pickles; soy sauce; and TV dinners and frozen entrees.

Sodium in Food

The 2015 US Dietary Guidelines specify an upper limit of 2300 mg/day of sodium for adults. This is approximately a teaspoon of table salt. In the past this level of sodium was considered to be a restriction. Currently, the average American eats almost double the recommended daily amount of sodium, so sodium restrictions continue to be commonly prescribed for patients with heart disease, kidney disease and liver disease.

The sodium in food is added in processing. Virtually no food is naturally high in sodium (see selected food list below). Food manufacturers have been responding to the call from health professionals and consumers to lower the amount of sodium in processed foods, but processed foods remain the main source of sodium in the US diet.

SPECIAL CONSIDERATIONS

A therapeutic sodium-restricted meal plan should be prescribed in terms of milligrams of sodium desired on a daily basis. The following are the commonly used levels of sodium restrictions:

No Added Salt (NAS): This is the least restrictive of the sodium-restricted diets. Table salt should not be used, and salt should not be added in cooking. High-sodium foods such as smoked, cured, or dried meats and cheeses; condiments and seasonings, salted snacks, and canned and dried soups and bouillon are restricted. The NAS diet provides no more than 3000 mg of sodium daily. It is desirable to be closer to the 2300 mg of sodium when possible.

2000 mg sodium: This diet may be appropriate for people with some types of liver disease and renal disease. It is no longer recommended for patients with heart failure (see chapter 33). This diet *eliminates* processed and prepared foods and beverages that are high in sodium. In addition to limiting all the foods in the NAS diet, baked products must also be limited. Milk and milk products are limited to 16 oz daily. Only salt-free commercially prepared foods should be used.

GUIDELINES FOR SODIUM RESTRICTION

Salt substitutes containing potassium chloride should be recommended only if approved by a physician. Potassium is generally contraindicated for patients with renal disease. Salt-free, herb-based seasoning products are readily available in most grocery stores and should be suggested instead.

- Instruct patients/clients on reading the Nutrition Facts food label for sodium content of foods.
- Encourage patients to prepare food at home without adding salt and to limit eating in restaurants.
- Recommend baked products, using sodium-free baking powder, potassium bicarbonate (instead of sodium bicarbonate or baking soda), and salt-free shortening in place of those containing sodium.
- Avoid obviously salted foods such as bouillon, soup and gravy bases, canned soups and stews; bread and rolls with salt toppings, salted crackers; salted nuts or popcorn, potato chips, pretzels, and other salted snack foods. Avoid buying vegetables prepared in sauce.
- Avoid smoked or cured meats, such as bacon, bologna, cold cuts, other processed meats, chipped or corned beef, frankfurters, ham, koshered or kosher style meats, and canned meat poultry.
- Avoid salted and smoked fish such as cod, herring, and sardines.
- Avoid sauerkraut, olives, pickles, relishes, kimchi, and other vegetables prepared in brine, tomato, and vegetable cocktail juices.
- Avoid seasonings such as celery salt, garlic salt, Worcestershire sauce, fish sauce and soy sauce. Reduced sodium versions of items like soy sauce can still be very high in sodium.
- Serve cheeses in limited amounts. Swiss cheese and cream cheese are relatively low in sodium.
- Monitor the sodium content of various medications, including over-the-counter brands.

The front of the food package can be used to quickly identify foods that may contain less sodium, but it is important to understand the terminology. For example, look for foods with claims such as:

- **Salt/Sodium-Free** → Less than 5 mg of sodium per serving
- **Very Low Sodium** → 35 mg of sodium or less per serving
- **Low Sodium** → 140 mg of sodium or less per serving
- **Reduced Sodium** → At least 25% less sodium than in the original product
- **Light in Sodium or Lightly Salted** → At least 50% less sodium added than in the regular product
- **No-Salt-Added or Unsalted** → No salt is added during processing, but not necessarily sodium-free. Check the Nutrition Facts Label.

Seasoning without salt: Flavorings or seasonings will make food more appetizing. For example:

- Lemon or vinegar is excellent with fish or meat and with many vegetables such as broccoli, asparagus, green beans, or salads.
- Meat may be seasoned with onion, garlic, green pepper, nutmeg, ginger, dry mustard, sage, cumin and marjoram. It may be cooked with fresh mushrooms or unsalted tomato juice. Curries made without salt are a good way to season meats and lentils.

- Cranberry sauce, applesauce, or jellies make appetizing accompaniments to meats and poultry.
- Vegetables can be flavored by the addition of onion, mint, ginger, mace, dill seed, parsley, green pepper, or fresh mushrooms.
- Unsalted cottage cheese can be flavored with minced onion, chopped chives, raw green pepper, grated carrots, chopped parsley, or crushed pineapple.
- A number of salt-free seasonings for use in cooking are available in the spice section of most supermarkets.

Sodium Content of Selected Common Foods	
1 cup of whole or reduced fat milk	107 mg
1 slice whole wheat bread	110-170 mg
1 hamburger bun	300-375 mg
1 slice American cheese	270-280 mg
1 slice Swiss cheese (non-processed)	50-65 mg
2 oz. mozzarella cheese, part skim	350 mg
2 oz. cream cheese	178 mg
3 oz corned beef (brisket)	900-1100 mg
3 oz. lean ground beef	55-60 mg
3 oz. chicken, raw broiler without the skin	65 mg
1 slice bacon, pork	185 mgR
1 cup kidney beans, cooked without salt	2 mg
1 cup canned kidney beans, drained	230-250 mg
1 tbsp soy sauce (tamari)	1000 mg
1 tbsp reduced sodium soy sauce	450 mg
1 cup chopped celery, raw	80 mg
1 cup chopped onion, raw	6 mg
1 tbsp garlic	0 mg
1 med banana	1 mg
1 avocado	11 mg
1 small potato with skin, baked	12 mg
1 cup chopped broccoli, raw	30 mg
½ cup broccoli in cheese sauce (Green Giant)	420 mg
1 cup brown rice, cooked	8 mg
1 cup white rice, cooked	0 mg
1 cup prepared rice pilaf (Rice-a-Roni)	970 mg
1 cup pasta, enriched	3-8 mg
1 large egg, raw	71 mg
1 large olive, ripe	65 mg
1 tbsp olive oil	0 mg
2 tbsp ranch dressing	270 mg
2 tbsp balsamic vinegar	8 mg
2 tbsp sour cream, cultured	8 mg
12 oz cola, regular	11 mg
1 slice cheese pizza (Domino's)	565 mg
1 slice pepperoni pizza (Pizza Hut)	769 mg
1 Big Mac (McDonald's)	460 mg
1 6-in Subway Club on white bread	720 mg

References: USDA Agriculture Research Service National Nutrient Data Base http://www.ricearoni.com/Products/ http://www.greengiant.com/Products

The Anti-Inflammatory Diet

Kelly Morrow, MS, RDN,
Mary Purdy, MS, RDN

DIETARY APPROACHES TO REDUCE INFLAMMATION

Inflammation is thought to underlie most chronic health conditions including metabolic syndrome, type 2 diabetes, cancer, cardiovascular disease, arthritis, autoimmune diseases, atopic conditions, inflammatory bowel disease, and there is now evidence linking it to cognitive decline. Various nutrients, foods and dietary patterns have been shown to reduce inflammatory markers as well as subjective and objective measures of inflammation.

Multiple iterations of an anti-inflammatory diet exist: DASH (Dietary Approaches to Stop Hypertension), Mediterranean, MIND (Mediterranean-DASH Intervention for Neurodegenerative Delay), vegetarian, food allergy elimination, calorie restriction, and low histamine. In most cases, overall dietary and lifestyle habits are more important to consider rather than any single change. Which diet is right for any individual often depends on trial and error (Saneei, et al. 2014) (Rajaie et al, 2013).

The Dietary Inflammatory Index (DII) has been developed and validated as a tool to evaluate the overall inflammatory potential of the diet based on evaluation of over 6500 peer reviewed research articles. The DII consists of 45 foods, spices, nutrients and bioactive compounds in relation to six inflammatory biomarkers IL-1β, IL-4, IL-6, IL-10, TNF-α and C-reactive protein (Shivappa et al., 2014) (Garcia-Arellano et al. 2014).

Dietary components with the most anti-inflammatory effect are included as negative numbers in the Overall Inflammatory Effect Score as shown in the table below.

Food Parameters in the Dietary Inflammatory Index and Overall Inflammatory Effect Score

Food Parameter	Overall Inflammatory Effect Score	Food Parameter	Overall Inflammatory Effect Score
Alcohol (g)	−0-278	Riboflavin (mg)	−0-068
Vitamin B$_{12}$ (μg)	0-106	Saffron (g)	−0-140
Vitamin B$_6$ (mg)	−0-365	Saturated fat (g)	0-373
β-Carotene (μg)	−0-584	Se (μg)	−0-191
Caffeine (g)	−0-110	Thiamin (mg)	−0-098
Carbohydrate (g)	0-097	*Trans* fat (g)	0-229
Cholesterol (mg)	0-110	Turmeric (mg)	−0-785
Energy (kcal)	0-180	Vitamin A (RE)	−0-401
Eugenol (mg)	−0-140	Vitamin C (mg)	−0-424
Total fat (g)	0-298	Vitamin D (μg)	−0-446
Fibre (g)	−0-663	Vitamin E (mg)	−0-419
Folic acid (μg)	−0-190	Zn (mg)	−0-313
Garlic (g)	−0-412	Green/black tea (g)	−0-536
Ginger (g)	−0-453	Flavan-3-ol (mg)	−0-415
Fe (mg)	0-032	Flavones (mg)	−0-616
Mg (mg)	−0-484	Flavonols (mg)	−0-467
MUFA (g)	−0-009	Flavonones (mg)	−0-250
Niacin (mg)	−0-246	Anthocyanidins (mg)	−0-131
n-3 Fatty acids (g)	−0-436	Isoflavones (mg)	−0-593
n-6 Fatty acids (g)	−0-159	Pepper (g)	−0-131
Onion (g)	−0-301	Thyme/oregano (mg)	−0-102
Protein (g)	0-021	Rosemary (mg)	−0-013
PUFA (g)	−0-337		

RE, retnol equivalents.

Adapted from Shivappa N et al. Designing and developing a literature derived population based dietary inflammatory index. *Public Health Nutrition*, 17:1689, 2013.

The following recommendations reflect an effort to consolidate similarities among the various anti-inflammatory diets.

CONSUME AN ABUNDANCE OF FRUITS, VEGETABLES, HERBS AND SPICES

Colorful fruits and vegetables contain a myriad of anti-inflammatory phytochemicals and fiber and are thought to be the cornerstone of an anti-inflammatory diet due to their ability to down-regulate markers such as C-reactive protein (CRP), Nuclear Factor-kappa Beta (NFkB), histamine and other inflammatory cytokines in vivo and in vitro. (Jungberger and Medjakovic, 2012),(Habauzit, 2012), (Hagenlocher, 2014) (Jiang et al., 2014).

Although most plant based foods contain anti-inflammatory properties, the following fruits and vegetables appear to be the most anti-inflammatory based on their mention in research: cruciferous vegetables, onions, berries, purple grapes, cherries, citrus fruits, tomatoes, and pomegranates. Anti-inflammatory herbs and spices include: green and black tea, turmeric, garlic, ginger, rosemary, oregano, fenugreek, caraway, anise, cocoa, mint, clove, coriander, cinnamon, nutmeg, red chili powder, lemongrass, fennel, saffron, black pepper, parsley, sage, dill, Bay leaf, and basil. (Jiang et al.,2014), (Aggarwal, 2004), (Habauzit, 2012),(Galland, 2010), (Jungbauer and Medjakovic, 2011)

EAT A LOW GLYCEMIC DIET

Excessive amounts of refined carbohydrates and sugars may be pro-inflammatory. Regular consumption of these high glycemic foods can increase blood glucose and insulin levels which, when chronically elevated, can trigger an inflammatory response. Choosing low glycemic foods has been shown to reduce post prandial glucose and insulin levels and "modestly lower" concentrations of the insulin-like growth factor and improve the inflammatory and adipokine (inflammatory proteins secreted by adipose tissue) profiles (Runchey, 2012) (Neuhouser, 2012). It's important to look at the glycemic load of a food versus the glycemic index because the load is a better indicator of the actual portion of food. See Appendix 37. For example, beets have a high glycemic index: 64, but a low glycemic load: 5.

High Glycemic Foods	Low Glycemic Foods
Cookies, cakes, pastries*, chips, white flour breads, crackers, tortillas, pasta, white rice	Whole and unprocessed grains, (like oats, brown rice, quinoa, whole wheat) high fiber or whole grain pastas
Large amounts of fruit juice and dried fruits	Fresh fruit
White (russet potatoes) mashed or baked without the skin	Sweet potatoes, pumpkin, squashes, beans and lentils, nuts and seeds
Sugar-sweetened sodas and other beverages	Most vegetables**

*cookies, cakes etc, can be made using low glycemic ingredients like oats and nuts which can reduce their glycemic load
**Consuming large amounts of certain juiced vegetables like carrots or beets will produce a higher glycemic load.

HAVE NUTS AND SEEDS OR NUT AND SEED BUTTERS EVERY DAY

Nuts and seeds not only provide anti-inflammatory and valuable phenolic compounds, but they provide a beneficial ratio of polyunsaturated fats (omega-6 and omega-3) that helps to support a healthy inflammatory response in the body. (Sears et al., 2011) Consume a variety of nuts in order to gain the spectrum of nutrients that each has to offer. Especially beneficial are pumpkin seeds, sunflower seeds, almonds, cashews, Brazil nuts, flaxseed, sesame seeds, and walnuts.

ADJUST THE QUALITY AND QUANTITY OF DIETARY FAT AND OILS

Increase:
Unsaturated fats high in omega-3 fatty acids (alpha-linolenic acid) which are anti-inflammatory. Best sources include cold water fish, flax, chia and hemp seeds, and walnuts. Flaxseed and walnut oil are excellent plant sources of omega-3 fatty acids, and are great for salad dressings, but should not be heated. Canola is also a price-friendly option for obtaining more omega 3's in the diet, but is considered by some to be more processed.
Monounsaturated fats:
Use extra virgin olive oil as the main ingredient for sauces, salad dressings, and marinades. Unrefined coconut oil can be used for sautéing.
Avocados can replace cheese or mayonnaise on sandwiches, and can be added to dips, smoothies and salads.

Decrease:
Excessive amounts of animal protein contain arachidonic acid, which can increase inflammation in excess.
Processed foods and oils are high in omega-6 fatty acids (linoleic acid) such as soybean, corn, safflower, and sunflower oils. Omega-6 fatty acids can increase pro-inflammatory markers in the body if eaten in excess. Many of these oils are widely used in processed foods.
Avoid hydrogenated fats and trans fats that are found in many baked and prepackaged foods and are in hydrogenated vegetable shortening and many margarines. Trans fat consumption has been shown to increase markers of systemic inflammation and is particularly associated with coronary artery disease. (Bendsen et al, 2011). Trans fats were banned in processed foods in the US in July of 2015, but manufacturers have 3 years to completely remove it.

GET ADEQUATE SOURCES OF PROBIOTICS

Supporting the gut ecology helps to keep the digestive tract healthy and balance the immune system, which may reduce inflammation. Fermented and cultured foods are an excellent source of probiotic bacteria. Sources include miso, sauerkraut, yogurt, kefir, and kimchi, tempeh and kombucha (a fermented beverage). Getting sufficient pre-biotics to feed the good bacteria is also important. Inulin and fructooligosaccharides are examples of prebiotics and can be found in bananas, asparagus, maple syrup, onions, garlic, chicory, artichoke and many other plant foods.

CONSIDER FOOD ALLERGY OR SENSITIVITY ELIMINATION

A food allergy is a systemic immune mediated response that involves both the innate (macrophages, mast cells) and adaptive immune system (antibodies). A food intolerance or sensitivity happens within the gut and can be the result of an enzyme deficiency or a reaction to a food additive or to naturally occurring chemicals in foods. These adverse reactions to food can induce the production of a variety of inflammatory mediators including immunoglobulins, cytokines and histamine. Reactions can be either immediate or delayed, and their intensity may depend on dose and individual tolerance. Risk may depend on timing and composition of food exposure in early life, diet quality and gastrointestinal microflora balance. See Chapter 26.

The 8 common food allergens that must be listed on food labels are: milk, eggs, fish, wheat, tree nuts, peanuts, soybeans and shellfish.

Common food intolerances are non-celiac gluten, lactose, soy, histamine and salicylate intolerances

Common food additive intolerances are to sulfites, tartrazine (Yellow 5), benzoic acid, and monosodium glutamate (MSG) (Wilson, 2005)

Eliminating these foods and additives, or even *some* of these foods and additives for a period of two weeks and assessing any improvement in symptoms, may help determine whether there is an adverse food reaction. Additionally some individuals find themselves to be sensitive to a compound called "solanine" found in nightshade family of fruits and vegetables. One can try removing nightshade foods (eggplant, peppers, tomatoes, tomatillos, goji berries and potatoes) from the diet temporarily to assess the impact on inflammation, especially in the joints. See Chapter 39.

AVOID CHEMICALS

Many industrial chemicals and pesticides can irritate or disrupt the immune system and cause inflammation. Choose organic or low pesticide foods and "green" personal care and cleaning products to reduce exposure. Many canned foods contain bisphenol A in their linings. Bisphenol A (aka "BPA"), which is also found in many plastic bottles and food containers, is an endocrine disruptor, impairs the action of insulin in the body, and up-regulates inflammatory pathways. (Valentino, R, et al., 2013) Seek out "BPA-Free" cans, and use glass containers and bottles as often as possible. Refer to the Environmental Working Group www.ewg.org for more information.

DRINK ALCOHOL IN MODERATION

Alcohol can have the effect of both increasing and decreasing markers of inflammation, depending on the individual person and the amount consumed. High intake, especially for prolonged periods, can increase inflammatory cytokines (Miller et al. 2011). In the PREDIMED trial, moderate alcohol consumption was associated with improved lipid profiles, blood pressure, endothelial function and reduced reactive oxygen species (ROS) and was associated with about a 1 drink equivalent (10g) per day. Red wine is the most commonly featured alcoholic beverage with its high anti-inflammatory polyphenol content and can be found in discussions about the Mediterranean diet and MIND diet. (Widmer et al., 2015) (Garcia-Arellano et al., 2015)

STRESS AND SLEEP

High stress levels and lack of adequate sleep are both associated with inflammation. Elevated circulating cortisol levels found under conditions of psychological stress are associated with elevated inflammatory cytokines. Sustained sleep restriction has also been associated with an inflammatory state and an elevation of TNF- α, IL -1β, IL-2, IL-4 and monocyte chemo-attractant protein-1 (MCP-1). (Axelsson et al, 2013) Intentionally practicing stress reduction techniques such as meditation has been shown to reduce the inflammatory response in human experimental models (Kox et al, 2014).

EXAMPLE OF AN ANTI-INFLAMMATORY 1 DAY DIET BASED ON THE DASH*, MIND AND MEDITERRANEAN MEAL PATTERNS*

Breakfast: Vegetable frittata with onions, garlic, basil, spinach, artichoke hearts and tomato. Baked sweet potato wedges. Herbal tea.

Lunch: Lentil vegetable soup and a green salad with arugula, purple cabbage, red onion, cucumber, carrot, walnuts and a mustard vinaigrette. Whole grain bread or crackers. Iced black tea with lemon

Snack: Greek yogurt with berries and green tea

Dinner: Lemon dill baked fish over brown rice with garlic sautéed kale and a glass of red wine

Dessert: Dark chocolate and cherries

REFERENCES

Aggarwal B, Shishodia S: Suppression of Nuclear Factor Kappa-B Activation Pathway by Spice-Derived Phytochemicals, *Ann NY Acad Sci* 1030: 434–441, 2004.

Axelsson J, et al: Effects of Sustained Sleep Restriction on Mitogen-Stimulated Cytokines, Chemokines and T Helper 1/T Helper 2 Balance in Humans, *PLOS One* 8(12):e82291, 2013.

Bendsen NT, et al: Effect of industrially produced trans fat on markers of systemic inflammation: evidence from a randomized trial in women, *J Lipid Res* 52(10):1821-1828, 2011.

Galland L: Diet and Inflammation, *Nutr Clin Prac* 25:634–640, 2010.

Garcia-Arellano A, et al: Dietary Inflammatory Index and Incidence of Cardiovascular Disease in the PREDIMED Study, *Nutrients* 7(6): 4124–4138, 2015.

Habauzit V, Morand C: Evidence for a protective effect of polyphenolscontaining foods on cardiovascular health: an update for clinicians, *Ther Adv Chronic Dis* 3(2):87–106, 2012.

Hagenlocher Y, Lorentz A: Immunomodulation of mast cell nutrients, *Mollecular Immunol* 63:25–31, 2015.

Jiang Y, et al: Cruciferous vegetable intake is inversely correlated with circulating levels of proinflammatory markers in women, *J Acad Nutr Diet* 114(5):700-8.e2, 2014.

Jungbauer A, Medjakovic S: Anti-inflammatory properties of culinary herbs and spices that ameliorate the effects of metabolic syndrome, *Maturitas* 71:227–239, 2012.

Kox M, et al: Voluntary activation of the sympathetic nervous system and attenuation of the innate immune response in humans, *Proc Natl Acad Sci USA* 111(20):7379–7384, 2014.

Miller A, et al: Molecular Mechanisms of Alcoholic Liver Disease: Innate Immunity and Cytokines, *Alcoholism Clin and Exp Res* 35(5):787–793, 2011.

*Diet could be modified for multiple ethnicities based on incorporation of the basic principles outlined in this appendix

Morris, et al: MIND diet slows cognitive decline with aging, *Alzheimer's Dement* 9:1015, 2015.

Neuhouser ML, Schwarz Y, Wang C, et al: A low-glycemic load diet reduces serum C-reactive protein and modestly increases adiponectin in overweight and obese adults, *J Nutr* 142(2):369–374, Feb 2012.

Rajaie S, et al: Comparative Effects of Carbohydrate Versus fat Restriction on Serum Adipocytokines, Markers of Inflammation and Endothelial Function Among Women with Metabolic Syndrome: A Randomized Cross-Over Clinical trial, *Ann Nutr Metab* 63:159–167, 2013.

Runchey SS, Pollak MN, Valsta LM, et al: Glycemic load effect on fasting and post-prandial serum glucose, insulin, IGF-1 and IGFBP-3 in a randomized, controlled feeding study, *Eur J Clin Nutr* 66(10):1146–1152, 2012.

Saneei P, et al: The Dietary Approaches to Stop Hypertension (DASH) Affects Inflammation in Childhood Metabolic Syndrome: A Randomized Cross Over Clinical Trial, *Ann Nutr Metab* 64:20–27, 2014.

Sears B, et al: Anti-Inflammatory Nutrition as a Pharmacological Approach to Treat Obesity, *Journal of Obesity* 2011. pii: 431985. Doi:10.1155/2011/431985.

Shivappa N, et al: Designing and developing a literature derived population based dietary inflammatory index, Public Health Nutrition, 17(8): 1689–1696, 2013.

Valentino R, et al: Bisphenol-A Impairs Insulin Action and Up-Regulates Inflammatory Pathways in Human Subcutaneous Adipocytes and 3T3-L1 Cells, *PLoS ONE* 8(12):e82099, 2013. doi:10.1371/journal.pone.0082099.

Widmer J, et al: The Mediterranean Diet, its Components and Cardiovascular Disease, *Am Jour of Medicine* 128(3):229–238, 2015.

Wilson B, Bahna S: Adverse reactions to food additives, *Annals of Allergy, Asthma & Immunology* 95(6):499–507, 2005.

Nutritional Facts on Alcoholic Beverages

Alcohol may have beneficial effects when consumed in moderation. The lowest all-cause mortality occurs at an intake of one to two drinks per day. The lowest coronary heart disease mortality also occurs at an intake of one to two drinks per day. Morbidity and mortality are highest among those drinking large amounts of alcohol. Guidelines:

- Alcoholic beverages should not be consumed by some individuals, including those who cannot restrict their alcohol intake, women of childbearing age who may become pregnant, pregnant and lactating women, children and adolescents, individuals taking medications that can interact with alcohol, and those with specific medical conditions.
- Those who choose to drink alcoholic beverages should do so sensibly and in moderation—defined as the consumption of up to one drink per day for women and up to two drinks per day for men.
- Alcoholic beverages should be avoided by individuals engaging in activities that require attention, skill, or coordination, such as driving or operating machinery.

CALORIES IN SELECTED ALCOHOLIC BEVERAGES*

This table is a guide to estimate the caloric intake from various alcoholic beverages. A sample serving volume and the calories in that drink are shown for beer, wine, and distilled spirits. Higher alcohol content (higher percent alcohol or higher proof) and mixing alcohol with other beverages such as sweetened soft drinks, tonic water, fruit juice, or cream increase the amount of calories in the beverage. Alcoholic beverages supply calories but provide few essential nutrients.

Beverage	Serving (oz)	Alcohol (g)	Carbohydrate (g)	Calories	Exchanges for Calorie or Diabetes Control
Beer					
Regular	12	13	13	150	1 starch, 2 fat
Light	12	11	5	100	2 fat
Near beer	12	1.5	12	60	1 starch
Distilled Spirits					
80-Proof (gin, rum, vodka, whiskey, scotch)	1.5	14	Trace	100	2 fat
Dry brandy, cognac	1	11	Trace	75	1.5 fat
Table Wines					
Dry white	4	11	Trace	80	2 fat
Red or rose	4	12	2	85	2 fat
Sweet wine	4	12	5	105	⅓ starch, 2 fat
Light wine	4	6	1	50	1 fat
Wine cooler	12	13	30	215	2 fruit, 2 fat
Dealcoholized wines	4	Trace	6-7	25-35	0.5 fruit
Sparkling Wines					
Champagne	4	12	4	100	2 fat
Sweet kosher wine	4	12	12	132	1 starch, 2 fat
Appetizer and Dessert Wines					
Sherry	2	9	2	74	1.5 fat
Sweet sherry, port, muscatel	2	9	7	90	0.5 starch, 1.5 fat
Cordials, liqueurs	1	13	18	160	1 starch, 2 fat
Vermouth					
Dry	3	13	4	105	2 fat
Sweet	3	13	14	140	1 starch, 2 fat

Continued

Beverage	Serving (oz)	Alcohol (g)	Carbohydrate (g)	Calories	Exchanges for Calorie or Diabetes Control
Cocktails					
Bloody Mary	5	14	5	116	1 vegetable, 2 fat
Daiquiri	2	14	2	111	2 fat
Manhattan	2	17	2	178	2.5 fat
Martini	2.5	22	Trace	156	3.5 fat
Old-fashioned	4	26	Trace	180	4 fat
Tom Collins	7.5	16	3	120	2.5 fat
Mixes					
Mineral water	Any	0	0	0	Free
Sugar-free tonic	Any	0	0	0	Free
Club soda	Any	0	0	0	Free
Diet soda	Any	0	0	0	Free
Tomato juice	4	0	5	25	1 vegetable
Bloody Mary mix	4	0	5	25	1 vegetable
Orange juice	4	0	15	60	1 fruit
Grapefruit juice	4	0	15	60	1 fruit
Pineapple juice	4	0	15	60	1 fruit

From Franz MJ: Alcohol and diabetes: its metabolism and guidelines for its occasional use. Part TI, Diabetes Spectrum 3(4):210-216, 1990.

The caloric contribution from alcohol of an alcoholic beverage can be estimated by multiplying the number of ounces by the proof and then again by the factor 0.8. For beers and wines, kilocalories from alcohol can be estimated by multiplying ounces by percentage of alcohol (by volume) and then by the factor 1.6.

Nutritional Facts on Caffeine-Containing Products

Caffeine is similar in structure to adenosine, a chemical found in the brain that slows down its activity. Because the two compete, the more caffeine that is consumed, the less adenosine that is available up to a point. Caffeine temporarily heightens concentration and wards off fatigue. Within 30 to 60 minutes of drinking a cup of coffee, caffeine reaches peak concentrations in the bloodstream and takes 4 to 6 hours for its effects to wear off. The average American adult consumes about 200 mg of caffeine a day, and many may consume twice that level. It is generally safe to consume no more than the equivalent amount of caffeine in 1 to 2 cups of coffee daily during pregnancy or lactation. Individuals with heart disease and hypertension may benefit from a reduction in caffeine consumption. To reduce caffeine and its stimulant effects, monitor intake from foods and beverages listed below.

Selected Food and Beverage Sources of Caffeine

Caffeine-Containing Products	Serving (mg)
Coffee	
Starbucks coffee (in store), 16 oz.	330
Starbucks coffee (at home), 16 oz.	260
Brewed, drip method, 6 oz	103
Brewed, percolator method, 6 oz	75
Instant, 1 rounded tsp	57
Flavored, regular and sugar-free, 6 oz	26-75
Espresso, 1 oz	40
Café Latte, short (8 oz) or tall (12 oz) (Starbucks)	35
Decaffeinated, 6 oz	2
Tea	
Black or green tea, 16 oz	60-100
3-minute brew, 12-oz	72
Lipton, Arizona, or Snapple tea, 16 oz	30-60
Instant, 1 rounded tsp in 8 oz of water	25-35
Tea, green brewed, 8 oz	30
Tea, bottles (12 oz) or from instant mix, 8 oz	14
Decaffeinated, 5- minute brew, 6-oz cup	1
Carbonated Beverages	
7-Eleven Big Gulp cola, 64 oz	190
Mountain Dew MDX or Vault, 12 oz	120
Diet Pepsi Max, 20 oz	70
Mountain Dew, 12 oz, regular or diet	54
Mellow Yellow, 12 oz, regular or diet	52

Caffeine-Containing Products	Serving (mg)
Regular or diet cola, cherry colas, Dr. Pepper, Mr. Pibb, 12 oz	35-50
Decaffeinated drinks, 12 oz	Trace
Cocoa and Chocolate	
Chocolate, baking, unsweetened, 1 oz	58
Chocolate, sweet, semisweet, dark, milk, 1 oz	8-20
Milk chocolate bar, 1.5 oz	10
Chocolate milk, 8 oz	8
Cocoa beverage, 6-oz cup	4
Chocolate-flavored syrup, 1 oz	5
Chocolate pudding, ½ cup	4-8
Miscellaneous	
Powershot (8 oz)	800
Rock Star, 16 oz	240
NoDoz, Maximum Strength (1), or Vivarin (1)	200
Pit Bull Energy Bar, 2 oz	165
Excedrin (2)	130
NoDoz, Regular Strength (1)	100
Red Bull (8.3 oz)	80
Water, caffeinated (Edge 2 O), (8 oz)	70
Anacin (2)	65
Bud Extra Beer, 10 oz	55
Propel Invigorating water	50
Jolt (8 oz)	48

Nutritional Facts on Essential (Omega) Fatty Acids

Essential fatty acids (EFAs) are fatty acids that are required in the human diet. They must be obtained from food because human cells have no biochemical pathways capable of producing them internally. There are two closely related families of EFAs: **omega-3 (Ω-3 or ω-3)** and **omega-6 (Ω-6 or ω-6)**. Only one substance in each of these families is truly essential, because, for example, the body can convert one ω-3 to another ω-3 but cannot create an ω-3 from scratch.

In the body essential fatty acids serve multiple functions. In each of these the balance between dietary ω-3 and ω-6 strongly affects function. They are modified to make the eicosanoids (affecting inflammation and many other cellular functions); the endogenous cannabinoids (affecting mood, behavior, and inflammation); the lipoxins from ω-6 EFAs and resolvins from ω-3 (in the presence of aspirin, down-regulating inflammation); the isofurans, isoprostanes, hepoxilins, epoxyeicosatrienoic acids, and neuroprotectin D; and the lipid rafts (affecting cellular signaling). They also act on deoxyribonucleic acid (activating or inhibiting transcription factors for nuclear factor–κ-B [NFκB], a proinflammatory cytokine).

Between 1930 and 1950 arachidonic and linolenic acids were termed *essential* because each was more or less able to meet the growth requirements of rats given fat-free diets. Further research has shown that **human metabolism requires both fatty acids**. To some extent any ω-3 and any ω-6 can relieve the worst symptoms of fatty acid deficiency. However, in many people the ability to convert the ω-3 α-linolenic acid (ALA) to the ω-3 eicosapentaenoic (EPA) and docosahexaenoic acid (DHA) is only 5% efficient. Therefore it is important to incorporate the EPA and DHA directly into the diet usually as fish or a fish oil supplement. Particular fatty acids such as DHA are needed at critical life stages (e.g., infancy and lactation) and in some disease states.

The essential fatty acids are:
- ALA (18:3)-ω-3
- Linoleic acid (18:2)- ω-6

These two fatty acids cannot be synthesized by humans because humans lack the desaturase enzymes required for their production. They form the starting point for the creation of longer and more desaturated fatty acids, which are also referred to as long-chain polyunsaturates:

Ω-3 FATTY ACIDS:

- EPA (20:5) eicosapentanoic acid
- DHA (22:6) docosahexanoic acid
- ALA (18:) alpha-linolenic acid

Ω-6 FATTY ACIDS:

- γ-Linolenic acid (GLA) (18:3)
- Dihomo-γ-linolenic acid (DGLA) (20:3)
- Arachidonic acid (AA) (20:4)

Ω-9 Fatty acids are not essential in humans, because humans possess all the enzymes required for their synthesis.

ADEQUATE INTAKES FOR Ω-3 FATTY ACIDS FOR CHILDREN AND ADULTS				ADEQUATE INTAKES FOR Ω-6 FATTY ACIDS FOR CHILDREN AND ADULTS			
Age (years)	Males and Females (g/day)	Pregnancy (g/day)	Lactation (g/day)	Age (years)	Males and Females (g/day)	Pregnancy (g/day)	Lactation (g/day)
1-3	0.7	N/A	N/A	1-3	7	N/A	N/A
4-8	0.9	N/A	N/A	4-8	10	N/A	N/A
9-13	1.2 for boys; 1 for girls	N/A	N/A	9-13	12 for boys; 10 for girls	N/A	N/A
14-18	1.6 for boys;1.1 for girls	1.4	1.3	14-18	16 for boys; 11 for girls	13	13
19+	1.6 for men; 1.1 for women	1.4	1.3	19+	17 for men; 12 for women	13	13

N/A, Not applicable.

DIETARY SOURCES

Some of the food sources of ω-3 and ω-6 fatty acids are fish and shellfish, flaxseed (linseed), soya oil, canola (rapeseed) oil, hemp oil, chia seeds, pumpkin seeds, sunflower seeds, leafy vegetables, and walnuts.

EFAs play a part in many metabolic processes, and there is evidence to suggest that low levels of EFAs or the wrong balance of types among the EFAs may be a factor in a number of illnesses.

Plant sources of ω-3s do not contain EPA and DHA. This is thought to be the reason that absorption of EFAs is much greater from animal rather than plant sources.

EFA content of vegetable sources varies with cultivation conditions. Animal sources vary widely, both with the animal's feed and that the EFA makeup varies markedly with fats from different body parts.

OMEGA-3 FATTY ACIDS

There is some evidence that suggests that ω-3s may:
- Help lower elevated triglyceride levels. High triglyceride levels can contribute to coronary heart disease.
- Reduce the blood's tendency to clot, which may relate to the clogging that occurs with atherosclerosis.
- Reduce the inflammation involved in conditions such as rheumatoid arthritis.
- Improve symptoms of depression and other mental health disorders in some individuals.

Dietary sources of ω-3 fatty acids include fish oil and certain plant and nut oils. Fish oil contains both DHA and EPA, whereas some nuts (English walnuts) and vegetable oils (canola, soybean, flaxseed and linseed, olive) contain only the ω-3 ALA.

There is evidence from multiple large-scale population (epidemiologic) studies and randomized controlled trials that intake of recommended amounts of DHA and EPA in the form of fish or fish oil supplements lowers triglycerides; reduces the risk of death, heart attack, dangerous abnormal heart rhythms, and strokes in people with known cardiovascular disease; slows the buildup of atherosclerotic plaques ("hardening of the arteries"); and lowers blood pressure slightly. However, high doses may have harmful effects such as an increased risk of bleeding. Some species of fish carry a higher risk of environmental contamination such as with methyl mercury.

COMMON FOOD SOURCES OF OMEGA-3 FATS

Omega-3 Fat	Food Source
ALA	Ground flaxseed and walnuts and soybeans
	Flaxseed, walnut, soybean and canola oils, and nonhydrogenated canola and soy margarines
DHA and EPA	Mackerel, salmon, herring, trout and sardines, and other fish and shellfish
	Marine algae supplements

Fish or Other Food Source	Omega-3 Content in a 4-oz Serving
English walnuts	6.8 g
Chinook salmon	3.6 g
Sockeye salmon	2.3 g
Mackerel	1.8-2.6 g
Herring	1.2-2.7 g
Rainbow trout	1.0 g
Wheat germ and oat germ	0.7-1.4 g
Halibut	0.5-1.3 g
White tuna	0.97 g
Light tuna	0.35 g
Whiting	0.9 g
Spinach	0.9 g
Flounder	0.6 g
King crab	0.6 g
Shrimp	0.5 g
Tofu	0.4 g (probably much less in "lite" tofu)
Clam	0.32 g
Cod	0.3 g
Scallop	0.23 g

Supplements*	
Cod liver oil	800-100 mg/tsp
Fish body oil	1200-1800 mg/tsp
Omega-3 fatty acid concentrate	250 mg/capsule

Enhancing Intake of Omega-3 Fats
- Eat fish at least two times each week.
- Include canned fish in your diet (examples: salmon, sardines, light tuna). Try sardines on toast.
- Add ground flaxseed to foods such as hot or cold cereal or yogurt. NOTE: Pregnant women should limit their intake of ground flaxseed to occasional use (not daily). Ground flaxseeds contain lignans. There is not enough information about their safety in pregnancy.
- Eat walnuts. Add walnuts to salads, cereals, baking (examples, muffins, cookies, breads) and pancakes.
- Have fresh or frozen soybeans (edamame) as a vegetable at meals.
- Use soybean oil or canola oil in salad dressings and recipes.
- Use nonhydrogenated margarine made from canola or soybean as a spread or in baking.
- Cook with ω-3 liquid eggs or eggs in the shell. Enjoy scrambled eggs or try a homemade egg sandwich.
- Use other ω-3 fortified products such as milk, yogurt, bread, and pasta.
- Substitute ¼ cup ground flaxseed for ¼ cup flour in bread, pizza dough, muffin, cookie, or meatloaf recipes.
- Replace 1 egg with 1 Tbsp ground flaxseed and 3 Tbsp water in recipes.

*Exact omega-3 content varies per manufacturer. Check label.

Nutritional Facts on a High-Fiber Diet

This diet is a modification of the regular diet. The purpose of this diet is to decrease transit time through the intestine, promote more frequent bowel movements, and softer stools. This diet may be prescribed as a treatment for diverticulosis, irritable bowel syndrome, hemorrhoids, or constipation. A high fiber diet is prescribed for weight loss and prevention of heart disease. It includes all the foods on a regular diet, with emphasis on the proper planning and selection of foods to increase the daily intake of fiber. Fluid intake should be increased. The Academy of Nutrition and Dietetics recommends that the average adult have a daily fiber intake of 20 to 35 g from a variety of sources. For children the child's age plus 5 g of fiber is recommended daily. In cases of severe constipation more fiber is recommended.

Dietary Reference Intakes for Fiber for Children and Adults

Age (years)	Males and Females (g/day)	Pregnancy (g/day)	Lactation (g/day)
1-3	19	N/A	N/A
4-8	25	N/A	N/A
9-13	31 for boys; 26 for girls	N/A	N/A
14-18	38 for boys; 26 for girls	28	29
19+	38 for men; 25 for women	28	29

N/A, Not applicable.

Although numerous over-the-counter fiber supplements are available, food sources provide many nutrients and are the preferred method of increasing dietary fiber. Adequate liquid consumption (at least eight 8-oz glasses per day) is recommended. Fiber should be added to the diet slowly because of possible cramps, bloating, and diarrhea with a sudden fiber increase. Maximum therapeutic benefits of fiber are obtained after several months of compliance. There are two components of dietary fiber, each providing health benefits: insoluble and soluble.

TYPES OF DIETARY FIBER

Type of Fiber	Components of Cells	Food Sources	Health Benefits
Soluble fibers	Gums, mucilages, pectin, certain hemicelluloses	Vegetables, fruits, barley, legumes, oats, and oat-bran	Decrease total blood cholesterol. Guard against diabetes. Prevent constipation. May help manage irritable bowel syndrome. May protect against colon cancer and gallstones.

TYPES OF DIETARY FIBER

Type of Fiber	Components of Cells	Food Sources	Health Benefits
Insoluble fibers	Cellulose, lignin, some hemicelluloses	Whole-wheat products, wheat and corn bran, and many vegetables (including cauliflower, green beans, potatoes, and skins of root vegetables)	May prevent diverticular disease. Prevents constipation. May delay glucose absorption (probably insignificant). May increase satiety and therefore assist with weight loss. Lower cholesterol. May protect against colon cancer.

GUIDELINES FOR HIGH-FIBER DIET

1. Increase consumption of whole-grain breads, cereals, flours, and other whole-grain productions to 6 to 11 servings daily.
2. Increase consumption of vegetables, legumes and fruits, nuts, and edible seeds to 5 to 8 servings daily.
3. Consume high-fiber cereals, granolas, and legumes as needed to bring fiber intake to 25 g or more daily.
4. Increase consumption of fluids to at least 2 L (or approximately 2 qt) daily.
5. For a high-fiber diet of approximately 24 g of dietary fiber: use 12 or more servings of the foods from the groups below (each food contains approximately 2 g of dietary fiber). For example, ½ cup of baked beans (8 Tbsp) would count as 4 servings.

EACH OF THESE FOODS IN THIS AMOUNT CONTAINS 2 G OF DIETARY FIBER

Apple, 1 small	Strawberries, ½ cup
Orange, 1 small	Pear, ½ small
Banana, 1 small	Cherries, 10 large
Peach, 1 medium	Plums, 2 small
Whole-wheat bread, 1 slice	Oatmeal, dry, 3 Tbsp
All Bran, 1 Tbsp	Shredded wheat, ½ biscuit
Rye bread, 1 slice	Wheat bran, 1 tsp
Corn flakes, ⅔ cup	Grape-nuts, 3 Tbsp
Cracked wheat bread, 1 slice	Puffed wheat, 1½ cup
Broccoli, ½ stalk	Potato, 2-in diameter
Lettuce, raw, 2 cups	Celery, 1 cup
Brussels sprouts, 4	Tomato, raw, 1 medium
Green beans, ½ cup	Corn on the cob, 2 in
Carrots, ⅔ cup	Baked beans, canned, 2 Tbsp

SELECTED FOOD SOURCES OF FIBER

Food	Grams per Serving	% Daily Value*
Navy beans, cooked, ½ cup	9.5	38
Bran ready-to-eat cereal (100%), ½ cup	8.8	35
Kidney beans, canned, ½ cup	8.2	33
Split peas, cooked, ½ cup	8.1	32
Lentils, cooked, ½ cup	7.8	31
Black beans, cooked, ½ cup	7.5	30
Pinto beans, cooked, ½ cup	7.7	31
Lima beans, cooked, ½ cup	6.6	26
Artichoke, globe, cooked, 1 each	6.5	26
White beans, canned, ½ cup	6.3	25
Chickpeas, cooked, ½ cup	6.2	24
Great northern beans, cooked, ½ cup	6.2	24
Cowpeas, cooked, ½ cup	5.6	22
Soybeans, mature, cooked, ½ cup	5.2	21
Bran ready-to-eat cereals, various, 1 oz	2.6-5.0	10-20
Crackers, rye wafers, plain, 2 wafers	5.0	20
Sweet potato, baked, with peel, I medium (146 g)	4.8	19
Asian pear, raw, 1 small	4.4	18
Green peas, cooked, ½ cup	4.4	18
Whole-wheat English muffin, 1 each	4.4	18
Pear, raw, 1 small	4.3	17
Bulgur, cooked, ½ cup	4.1	16
Mixed vegetables, cooked, ½ cup	4.0	16
Raspberries, raw, ½ cup	4.0	16
Sweet potato, boiled, no peel, 1 medium (156 g)	3.9	15.5
Blackberries, raw, ½ cup	3.8	15
Potato, baked, with skin, 1 medium	3.8	15
Soybeans, green, cooked, ½ cup	3.8	15
Stewed prunes, ½ cup	3.8	15
Figs, dried, ¼ cup	3.7	14.5
Dates, ¼ cup	3.6	14
Oat bran, raw, ¼ cup	3.6	14
Pumpkin, canned, ½ cup	3.6	14
Spinach, frozen, cooked, ½ cup	3.5	14
Shredded wheat ready-to-eat cereals, various, ≈ 1 oz	2.8-3.4	11-13
Almonds, 1 oz	3.3	13
Apple with skin, raw, 1 medium	3.3	13
Brussels sprouts, frozen, cooked, ½ cup	3.2	13
Whole-wheat spaghetti, cooked, ½ cup	3.1	12
Banana, 1 medium	3.1	12
Orange, raw, 1 medium	3.1	12
Oat bran muffin, 1 small	3.0	12
Guava, 1 medium	3.0	12

SELECTED FOOD SOURCES OF FIBER

Food	Grams per Serving	% Daily Value*
Pearled barley, cooked, ½ cup	3.0	12
Sauerkraut, canned, solids, and liquids, ½ cup	3.0	12
Tomato paste, ¼ cup	2.9	11.5
Winter squash, cooked, ½ cup	2.9	11.5
Broccoli, cooked, ½ cup	2.8	11
Parsnips, cooked, chopped, ½ cup	2.8	11
Turnip greens, cooked, ½ cup	2.5	10
Collards, cooked, ½ cup	2.7	11
Okra, frozen, cooked, ½ cup	2.6	10
Peas, edible-podded, cooked, ½ cup	2.5	10

*Daily values (DVs) are reference numbers based on the recommended dietary allowance. They were developed to help consumers determine if a food contains a lot or a little of a specific nutrient. The DV for fiber is 25 g. The percent DV (%DV) listed on the Nutrition Facts panel of food labels states the percentage of the DV provided in 1 serving. %DVs are based on a 2000-calorie diet.

Food Sources of Dietary Fiber ranked by grams of dietary fiber per standard amount. (All are ≥10% of adequate intake for adult women, which is 25 g/day.)

HIGH-FIBER MEAL PLAN

Breakfast	Lunch	Dinner
1 orange ¾ cup raisin bran 2 slices whole wheat toast 2 tsp margarine 1 cup skim milk 1 cup coffee 2 tsp sugar	3-oz boneless, skinless chicken breast ½ cup broccoli ½ cup long grain and wild rice 1 whole wheat roll ½ cup chocolate pudding ½ Tbsp whipped topping 2 tsp margarine 1 cup iced tea ¼ tsp salt ¼ tsp pepper 2 tsp sugar	1 cup spaghetti with meat sauce 1 cup tossed salad with assorted vegetables and ¼ cup chickpeas* 1 slice Italian bread ½ cup apple crisp 2 tsp margarine 1 cup skim milk 1 cup coffee ¼ tsp salt ¼ tsp pepper 2 tsp sugar

Nutritional Analysis
Kilocalories: 2074
Protein: 84 g
Fat: 52 g
Carbohydrate: 313 g
Sodium: 4647 mg
Potassium: 3706 mg
Fiber: 28 g

*Fiber content may be higher, depending on vegetables selected for salad.

Nutritional Facts on Fluid and Hydration

Adequate **hydration** is essential for life. Body water is necessary to regulate body temperature, transport nutrients, moisten body tissues, compose body fluids, and make waste products soluble for excretion. **Principles:** As the most plentiful substance in the human body, water is also the most plentiful nutrient in the diet. The amount of water recommended for an individual varies with age, activity, medical condition, and physical condition. The water in juice, tea, milk, decaffeinated coffee, and carbonated beverages contributes the majority of water in the diet. Solid foods also contribute water to the diet but usually are not counted in the amount of water provided per day.

Water deficiency, or **dehydration,** is characterized by dark urine; decreased skin turgor; dry mouth, lips, and mucous membranes; headache; a coated, wrinkled tongue; dry or sunken eyes; weight loss; a lowered body temperature; and increased serum sodium, albumin, blood urea nitrogen (BUN), and creatinine values. Dehydration may be caused by inadequate intake in relation to fluid requirements or excessive fluid losses caused by fever, increased urine output, diarrhea, draining wounds, ostomy output, fistulas, environmental temperature, or vomiting. Concentrated or high-protein tube feeding formulas may increase the water requirement.

Thirst is often the first noticed sign of the need for more water. However, athletes or workers exercising or working hard in hot climates may be significantly dehydrated before they realize they are thirsty. In these situations they should be drinking at regular intervals; they may not be able to rely on thirst to determine their need to drink.

Water excess or **overhydration** is rare and may be the result of inadequate output or excessive intake. Overhydration is characterized by increased blood pressure; decreased pulse rate; edema; and decreased serum sodium, potassium, albumin, BUN, and creatinine values. Fluid restrictions may be necessary for certain medical conditions such as kidney or cardiac disease. For those on fluid restrictions, the fluid needs should be calculated on an individual basis. The usual diet provides approximately 1080 mL (36 oz), a little more than a quart of fluid per day.

Estimating Daily Fluid Requirements for Healthy Individuals

Children	Body Weight	Daily Fluid Requirement
Infants		140 to 150 mL/kg
Children		
Method 1		50 to 60 mL/kg
Method 2	3 to 10 kg of body weight	100 mL/kg
	11 to 20 kg of body weight	1000 mL + 50 mL/kg >10
	More than 20 kg	1500 mL + 20 mL/kg >20
Adults*		
Method 1	30 to 35 mL per weight in kilograms	
Method 2	1 mL fluid per calorie consumed	
Method 3	First 10 kg of body weight	100 mL/kg
	Second 10 kg of body weight	+50 mL/kg
	Remaining kg of body weight (age <50)	+20 mL/kg
	Remaining kg of body weight (age >50)	+15 mL/kg
Method 4	Age in years	
	16-30 (active)	40 mL/kg
	20-55	35 mL/kg
	55-75	30 mL/kg
	>75	25 mL/kg

*The 1 mL of fluid per calorie method should be used with caution because it will underestimate the fluid needs of those with low-calorie needs. Persons who are significantly obese may best be evaluated by Method 3 because it adjusts for high body weight.
From the California Diet Manual, ©2003, State of California Department of Developmental Services, revised 2004.
Note: 3 oz is approximately ⅓ cup; 6 oz is approximately ⅔ cup.

Approximate Fluid Content of Common Foods

Food	Fluid Ounces	Household Measure	Metric Measure
Juice	2	¼ cup	60 mL
	3	⅓ cup	90 mL
	4	½ cup	120 mL
	8	1 cup	240 mL
Coffee, tea, decaffeinated coffee	6	⅔ cup	180 mL
Gelatin	4	½ cup	120 mL
Ice cream, sherbet	3	⅓ cup	90 mL
Soup	6	⅔ cup	180 mL
Liquid coffee creamer	1	2 Tbsp	30 mL

©2003, State of California Department of Developmental Services, revised 2004.

Glycemic Index and Glycemic Load of Selected Foods*

	GI	GL
Breakfast Cereals		
Kellogg's All-Bran	30	4
Kellogg's Cocoa Puffs	77	20
Kellogg's Corn Flakes	92	24
Kellogg's MiniWheats	58	12
Kellogg's Nutrigrain	66	10
Old-fashioned oatmeal	42	9
Kellogg's Rice Krispies	82	22
Kellogg's Special K	69	14
Kellogg's Raisin Bran	61	12
Grains and Pastas		
Buckwheat	54	16
Bulgur	48	12
Rice		
Basmati	58	22
Brown	50	16
Instant	87	36
Uncle Ben's	39	14
Converted, white	4	
Noodles—instant	7	19
Pasta		
Egg fettuccine (avg)	40	18
Spaghetti (avg)	38	18
Vermicelli	35	16
Tortellini, Stouffer's	50	1
Bread		
Bagel	72	25
Croissant[†]	67	17
Crumpet	69	13
"Grainy" breads (avg)	49	6
Pita bread	57	10
Pumpernickel (avg)	50	6
Rye bread (avg)	58	8
White bread (avg)	70	10
Whole-wheat bread (avg)	77	9
Crackers and Crispbread		
Kavli	71	12
Puffed crisp bread	81	15
Ryvita	69	11
Water cracker	78	14
Cookies		
Oatmeal	55	12
Milk Arrowroot	69	12
Shortbread (commercial)[†]	64	10
Cake		
Chocolate, frosted, Betty Crocker	38	20
Oat bran muffin	69	24
Sponge cake	46	17
Waffles	76	10

	GI	GL
Vegetables		
Beets, canned	64	5
Carrots (avg)	47	3
Parsnip	97	12
Peas (green, avg)	48	3
Potato		
Baked (avg)	85	26
Boiled	88	16
French fries	75	22
Microwaved	82	27
Pumpkin	75	3
Sweet corn	60	11
Sweet potato (avg)	61	17
Rutabaga	72	7
Yam (avg)	37	13
Legumes		
Baked beans (avg)	48	7
Broad beans	79	9
Butter beans	31	6
Chickpeas (avg)	28	8
Cannellini beans (avg)	38	12
Kidney beans (avg)	28	7
Lentils (avg)	29	5
Soy beans (avg)	18	1
Fruit		
Apple (avg)	38	6
Apricot (dried)	31	9
Banana (avg)	51	13
Cherries	22	3
Grapefruit	25	3
Grapes (avg)	46	8
Kiwi fruit (avg)	53	6
Mango	51	8
Orange (avg)	48	5
Papaya	59	10
Peach (avg)		
Canned (natural juice)	38	4
Fresh (avg)	42	5
Pear (avg)	38	4
Pineapple	59	7
Plum	39	5
Raisins	64	28
Cantaloupe	65	4
Watermelon	72	4
Dairy Foods		
Milk		
Full-fat	27	3
Skim	32	4
Chocolate-flavored	42	13
Condensed	61	33
Custard	43	7

Continued

	GI	GL		GI	GL
Ice cream			Split-pea	60	16
Regular (avg)	61	8	Tomato	38	6
Low-fat	50	3	Sushi (avg)	52	19
Yogurt, low-fat	33	10	Pizza, cheese	60	16
Beverages			**Sweets**		
Apple juice	40	12	Chocolate[†]	44	13
Coca Cola	63	16	Jelly beans (avg)	78	22
Lemonade	66	13	Life Savers	70	21
Fanta	68	23	Mars Bar	68	27
Orange juice (avg)	52	12	Kudo whole-grain chocolate-chip bar	62	20
Snack Foods			**Sugars**		
Tortilla chips[†] (avg)	63	17	Honey (avg)	55	10
Fish sticks	38	7	Fructose (avg)	19	2
Peanuts[†] (avg)	14	1	Glucose*	100	10
Popcorn	72	8	Lactose (avg)	46	5
Potato chips[†]	57	10	Sucrose (avg)	68	7
Convenience Foods			**Sports Bars**		
Macaroni and cheese	64	32	Clif bar (cookies and cream)	101	3
Soup			PowerBar (chocolate)	83	35
Lentil	44	9	METRx bar (vanilla)	74	37

From Brand Miller J et al: The new glucose revolution, New York, 2003, Avalon/Marlowe & Company.
*Glucose = 100.
[†]These foods are high in saturated fat.

Nutritional Facts on a High-Protein Diet

A diet high in protein is recommended most often for increased needs for healing. A diet of 1.2gm/kg to 1.5 gm/kg is recommended for healing by the National Pressure Ulcer Advisory Panel. It is now recommended for people on dialysis and for those with some types of liver disease. High protein diets are recommended for athletes who are building muscle. Historically, a high protein diet has been defined as one with at least 100 g of protein per day. This has been replaced by recommendations based on weight. How to accurately determine protein needs in an obese person remains debatable. Some researchers and practitioners recommend a high protein diet provide 1.75 gm/kg of ideal body weight (IBW) for those with obesity.

BEST FOOD SOURCES OF PROTEIN

Meat: most types of meat provide 7 gm per ounce
Fish and shellfish: 7 gm per ounce
Eggs: 6-7 gm per egg, depends on the egg size
Cow's Milk: 8 gm per cup
Goat's Milk: 9 gm per cup
Soy Milk: 7-8 gm per cup
Non-fat milk powder:
Plain yogurt: 6-7 gm per ½ cup
Greek yogurt: 11-15 gm per ½ cup
Cheese: 7 gm per ¼ C. of cottage cheese OR 1 ounce hard cheese.

Peanut butter or nut butter: 8 gm per 2 Tbsp.
Tofu: 4.6 gm per ounce
Lentils: 10 gm per ½ cup, cooked
Chickpeas: 8 gm per ½ cup, cooked
Quinoa: 4 gm per ½ cup, cooked
Teff: 5 gm per ½ cup, cooked
Chia seeds: 5 gm per ounce

PROTEIN SUPPLEMENTS

Nonfat dry milk (NFDM) may be added to cooked foods to increase protein intake. However, when it is added, carbohydrate is also added as the sugar lactose. NFDM can be added to regular milk to create more concentrated milk. Protein powders are a popular way to increase the protein content of the diet, either by adding it to foods or by using it in smoothies or shakes. Whey-based supplements are the most common because they are water-soluble and provide complete protein. Soy-based supplements are also popular, especially for those avoiding animal products. For other vegetable protein sources, see Appendix 39. There are now hundreds of products available, most with other added nutrients.

It is important to note that almond milk, hemp milk and coconut milk in their fluid forms are relatively low in protein. If used for high nutrition impact drinks, an added source of powdered protein may be necessary to meet nutrition goals.

Nutritional Facts on Vegetarian Eating

A well-planned vegetarian diet can meet nutritional needs and can be a healthy way to meet the dietary guidelines. Vegetarian diets are chosen for nutritional, religious, ecologic, or personal reasons. It is the position of the Academy of Nutrition and Dietetics (AND) that "Appropriately planned vegetarian diets are healthful, nutritionally adequate and provide health benefits in the prevention and treatment of certain diseases."

AND's practice guideline contains recommendations, based on scientific evidence, designed to assist practitioners on the appropriate nutrition care for vegetarians. The guideline includes recommendations for children, adolescents, adults and women who are pregnant or lactating, providing more than 30 nutrition recommendations related to vegetarian nutrition, including:

- Macronutrients, including protein
- Micronutrients, including vitamin B_{12}
- Knowledge, beliefs and motivations
- Diet diversity
- Nutrition counseling
- Treatment of hyperlipidemia, obesity, Type 2 diabetes
- Adherence to a vegetarian diet

Vegetarian adaptations of the USDA food patterns are included in the 2010 *Dietary Guidelines for Americans*, with sample vegetarian food patterns that allow for additional flexibility in food group choices.

Vegetarian diets are usually classified into one of the following three types:

1. Lacto-ovo-vegetarian is a modification of the diet, which eliminates all dietary sources of animal protein except dairy products and eggs. This is the most common type of vegetarian diet and is the easiest of the vegetarian diets to prepare.
2. Lacto-vegetarian is a modification of the diet, which eliminates all dietary sources of animal protein except dairy products. This requires that baked products be made without eggs and the elimination of egg noodles.
3. Strict vegetarian (vegan diet) is a modification of the diet, which eliminates all dietary sources of animal protein.

Adequacy: The more restrictive the diet, the more challenging it is to ensure adequacy. Lacto-ovo and lacto-vegetarian diets require the same planning as any other diet. The vegan diet is a little more difficult, but can be adequate with some planning. The *Power Plate* is a tool developed by Physicians Committee for Responsible Medicine to assist in planning a nutritionally complete vegan diet and can be accessed at PCRM.org.

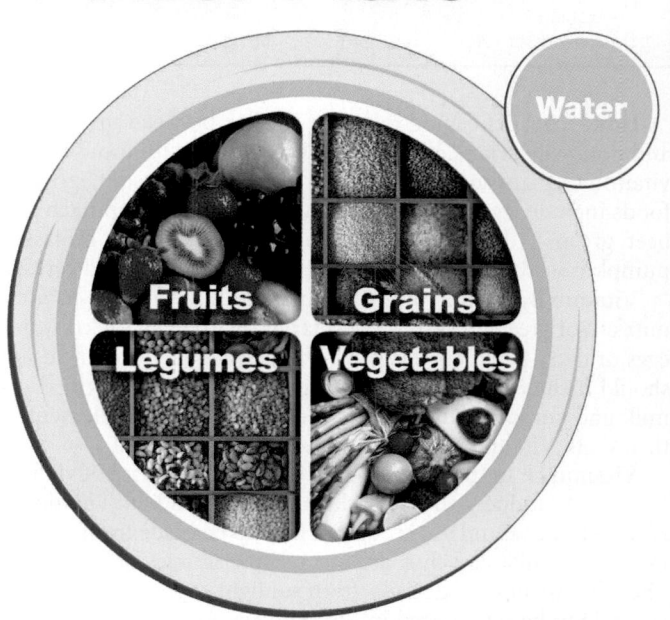

The Sustainable Power Plate

Water
Fruits
Grains
Legumes
Vegetables

SustainablePowerPlate.org

NUTRIENTS TO CONSIDER WHEN PLANNING A VEGETARIAN MENU

Protein

Foods that provide approximately 7 grams of protein per serving:

¼ cup cottage cheese	½ cup legumes, cooked
1 cup cow's milk, goat's milk or soy milk	¼ cup soy beans
	¾ cup of almonds
1 oz cheese	¼ cup tofu (soy cheese)
⅓ cup mixed nuts	¾ cup yogurt
1 egg	¼ cup plain, Greek style yogurt
2 Tbsp peanut butter	1 cup of quinoa

Foods that contain the essential amino acids are considered complete proteins. However, foods that are incomplete proteins can be combined to make a complete protein. These are known as complementary proteins. They do not have to be eaten together at the same meal. The most common combination of complementary proteins is beans (legumes) combined with rice or corn.

Calcium: All vegetarians, especially young women, should ensure adequate calcium intake for development and maintenance of strong bones. In place of dairy products, choose abundant amounts of dark, leafy greens (e.g., kale, mustard and turnip greens, collards); bok choy; broccoli; legumes; tofu processed with calcium; dried figs; sunflower seeds; and calcium-fortified cereals and juices can be incorporated into the diet. The following foods provide approximately the same amount of calcium as 1 cup of cow's milk (approximately 300 mg).

1 cup calcium-fortified soy milk, nut milk, grain, or hemp milk	3 cups cooked dried beans
1⅔ cups sunflower seeds	1 cup almonds
1 cup collards or kale, cooked	1.5 oz chia seeds

Iron: Iron deficiency rates are similar between vegetarians and non-vegetarians. When consumed along with foods rich in vitamin C, plant sources of iron are better absorbed. High-iron foods include legumes, dark green vegetables (i.e., spinach and beet greens), dried fruits; prune juice, blackstrap molasses, pumpkin seeds, soy nuts, and iron-fortified breads and cereals.

Vitamin B_{12}. Found only in animal foods, vitamin B_{12} is not a nutrient of great concern for vegetarians who regularly consume eggs or dairy products (lacto-ovo-vegetarians). However, vegans should include vitamin B_{12}–fortified foods such as fortified soy milk and commercial breakfast cereals, or a B_{12} supplement in their diets. Vitamin B_{12} is also found in Brewer's yeast.

Vitamin D: In the United States the primary source of vitamin D is dairy products, most of which are fortified with vitamin D. However, cheese and yogurt do not have to be made from vitamin D–fortified milk and thus are not reliable sources of vitamin D. The other main source results from sunlight exposure, causing vitamin D to be synthesized in the skin. See Appendix 45. If dairy products are not consumed and direct sunlight exposure is limited, supplementation is warranted. Foods containing vitamin D include fortified cow's milk, soy milk, rice milk, or nut milk. Supplementation (at least 1000 IU/day) is needed for individuals who do not consume milk products or who spend little time in the sun.

Zinc: Because zinc is found in animal foods, the vegetarian diet may be limited. The following foods can be included in the diet to increase zinc intake:

Wheat germ
Tofu
Nuts including cashews and almonds
Seeds including sunflower, flax, poppy and chia seeds
Dried beans,
Breakfast cereals, fortified

SPECIAL NOTES

Pregnancy and Lactation: Well-planned vegan and lacto-ovo-vegetarian eating patterns adequately provide for the nutritional needs of pregnant and lactating women (American Dietetic Association, 2009). Folate supplements are recommended for all pregnant women, including vegetarians. Vegans must ensure daily intake of 2 mcg of vitamin B_{12} daily during pregnancy and 2.6 mcg during lactation, whether through supplements or fortified foods. Women with limited sun exposure should include vitamin D–fortified foods and possibly a vitamin D supplement. Caution should be used with vitamin D supplementation because excess vitamin D can cause fetal abnormalities.

Infants, Children, and Adolescents: According to the AND, well-planned vegan and lacto-ovo-vegetarian eating patterns adequately provide for the nutritional needs of infants, children, and adolescents. Because of the high bulk of low-fat vegetarian eating patterns, it may be difficult for children and adolescents to consume enough food to provide for their energy needs. Frequent meals and snacks with nutrient-dense foods can help meet energy and nutrient needs. If sun exposure is limited, vitamin D fortified–foods or supplements should be used. For vegan children a reliable source of vitamin B_{12} should be included in their diets. To provide for growth, calcium, iron, and zinc intakes deserve special attention. It is recommended that parents of vegetarian infants and youth consult a registered dietitian nutritionist (RDN) with expertise in the vegetarian eating pattern.

Meal Pattern: Lacto-Vegetarian

Breakfast	Lunch	Dinner	Snack
½ cup orange juice	Vegetarian chili	Quinoa patties	½ peanut butter
Whole grain cereal and milk	Corn bread	Brown rice	sandwich and 8 oz
Berry Yogurt Parfait	Green Salad	Fresh spinach served with lemon and butter if desired	milk
	Fresh fruit	Banana pudding made with coconut milk	

Meal Pattern: Lacto-Ovo Vegetarian

Breakfast	Lunch	Dinner	Snack
Fresh fruit	Egg Salad sandwich on whole wheat bread with lettuce	Black bean burritos with cheese, avocado and salsa	Apple and cheese
½ cup oatmeal served with Greek yogurt	Cup of tomato soup	Lettuce salad	
1 cup (8 oz) milk	Carrot sticks	Peanut Butter cookie and 8oz milk	
	Fresh fruit		

Meal Pattern: Vegan

Breakfast	Lunch	Dinner	Snack
½ cup orange juice (calcium fortified)	Bean Burritos served with guacamole and salsa	Tofu-Vegetable Stir-fry (include bok choy and spinach for calcium) Top with cashews	½ peanut butter sandwich or ½ cup of edamame
3 whole grain pancakes topped with walnuts, applesauce and cinnamon	Green salad with oil and vinegar salad dressing	Brown rice	
1 cup fortified soy milk or soy yogurt	1 fresh apple	Cardamom-flavored chia pudding made with soy milk	
	1 cup fortified soy milk	Beverage of choice	

Reference: AND Evidence Analysis Library, Vegetarian Nutrition Guideline, 2011.

Nutritional Facts on Folic Acid, Vitamin B$_6$, and Vitamin B$_{12}$

FOLATE

Folate is a water-soluble B vitamin that occurs naturally in food. Folic acid is the synthetic form of folate that is found in supplements and is added to fortified foods. Folate, formerly known as folacin, is the generic term to refer to both folate and folic acid. Folate functions as an enzyme in single carbon transfers, and is involved in the production and maintenance of new cells, which is especially important during periods of rapid cell division and growth such as infancy, adolescence, and pregnancy. See Chapter 15. Folate is needed to make deoxyribonucleic acid (DNA) and ribonucleic acid, the building blocks of cells. Both adults and children need folate to make normal red blood cells and prevent anemia. See Chapter 32. Folate is also essential for the conversion of homocysteine to methionine in the synthesis of s-adenosyl-methionine, and important methyl donor.

A genetic mutation of a folate-metabolizing enzyme (5,10-methylenetetrahydrofolate) results in the inability to convert dietary folate or folic acid into the active form, 5-methyltetrahydrofolate (5-MTHFA). The result is folate deficiency unless folate is consumed in the methylated form as methyltetrahydrofolic acid (MTHFA). See Chapter 5.

Recommended Intakes

Intake recommendations for folate and other nutrients are provided in the Dietary Reference Intakes (DRIs) developed by the Food and Nutrition Board (FNB), Institute of Medicine (IOM) of the National Academies (formerly National Academy of Sciences). DRI is the general term for a set of reference values used for planning and assessing nutrient intakes of healthy people. These values, which vary by age and gender, include:

- Recommended Dietary Allowance (RDA): average daily level of intake sufficient to meet the nutrient requirements of nearly all (97%–98%) healthy individuals.
- Adequate Intake (AI): established when evidence is insufficient to develop an RDA and is set at a level assumed to ensure nutritional adequacy.
- Tolerable Upper Intake Level (UL): maximum daily intake unlikely to cause adverse health effects. ULs for folic acid are listed on the inside back cover of this text.

The table lists the current RDAs for folate as micrograms (mcg) of dietary folate equivalents (DFEs). The FNB developed DFEs to reflect the higher bioavailability of folic acid than that of food folate. At least 85% of supplemental folic acid is estimated to be bioavailable when taken with food, whereas only about 50% of folate naturally present in food is bioavailable. Based on these values, the FNB defined DFE as follows:

- 1 mcg DFE = 1 mcg food folate
- 1 mcg DFE = 0.6 mcg folic acid from fortified foods or dietary supplements consumed with foods
- 1 mcg DFE = 0.5 mcg folic acid from dietary supplements taken on an empty stomach

For infants from birth to 12 months of age, AIs were established that are equivalent to the mean intake of folate in healthy, breastfed infants in the United States.

Recommended Dietary Allowances (RDAs) for Folate

Age	Male	Female	Pregnant	Lactating
Birth to 6 months*	65 mcg DFE*	65 mcg DFE*	N/A	N/A
7–12 months*	80 mcg DFE*	80 mcg DFE*	N/A	N/A
1–3 years	150 mcg DFE	150 mcg DFE	N/A	N/A
4–8 years	200 mcg DFE	200 mcg DFE	N/A	N/A
9–13 years	300 mcg DFE	300 mcg DFE	N/A	N/A
14–18 years	400 mcg DFE	400 mcg DFE	600 mcg DFE	500 mcg DFE
19+ years	400 mcg DFE	400 mcg DFE	600 mcg DFE	500 mcg DFE

*Adequate Intake (AI)
N/A, Not applicable.

Selected Food Sources of Folate and Folic Acid

Food	mcg DFE per Serving	Percent DV*	Food	mcg DFE per Serving	Percent DV*
Beef liver, braised, 3 ounces	215	54	Rice, white, medium-grain, cooked, ½ cup†	90	23
Spinach, boiled, ½ cup	131	33	Asparagus, boiled, 4 spears	89	22
Black-eyed peas (cowpeas), boiled, ½ cup	105	26	Spaghetti, cooked, enriched, ½ cup†	83	21
Breakfast cereals, fortified with 25% of the DV†	100	25	Brussels sprouts, frozen, boiled, ½ cup	78	20
			Lettuce, romaine, shredded, 1 cup	64	16

Continued

Selected Food Sources of Folate and Folic Acid—cont'd

Food	mcg DFE per Serving	Percent DV*	Food	mcg DFE per Serving	Percent DV*
Avocado, raw, sliced, ½ cup	59	15	Turnip greens, frozen, boiled, ½ cup	32	8
Spinach, raw, 1 cup	58	15	Orange, fresh, 1 small	29	7
Broccoli, chopped, frozen, cooked, ½ cup	52	13	Papaya, raw, cubed, ½ cup	27	7
Mustard greens, chopped, frozen, boiled, ½ cup	52	13	Banana, 1 medium	24	6
			Yeast, baker's, ¼ teaspoon	23	6
Green peas, frozen, boiled, ½ cup	47	12	Egg, whole, hard-boiled, 1 large	22	6
Kidney beans, canned, ½ cup	46	12	Vegetarian baked beans, canned, ½ cup	15	4
Bread, white, 1 slice†	43	11	Cantaloupe, raw, 1 wedge	14	4
Peanuts, dry roasted, 1 ounce	41	10	Fish, halibut, cooked, 3 ounces	12	3
Wheat germ, 2 tablespoons	40	10	Milk, 1% fat, 1 cup	12	3
Tomato juice, canned, ¾ cup	36	9	Ground beef, 85% lean, cooked, 3 ounces	7	2
Crab, Dungeness, 3 ounces	36	9	Chicken breast, roasted, ½ breast	3	1
Orange juice, ¾ cup	35	9			

*DV = Daily Value. The FDA developed DVs to help consumers compare the nutrient contents of products within the context of a total diet. The DV for folate is 400 mcg for adults and children aged 4 and older. However, the FDA does not require food labels to list folate content unless a food has been fortified with this nutrient. Foods providing 20% or more of the DV are considered to be high sources of a nutrient.
†Fortified with folic acid as part of the folate fortification program.

VITAMIN B$_6$

Vitamin B$_6$ is a water-soluble vitamin that exists in three major chemical forms: pyridoxine, pyridoxal, and pyridoxamine and their respective esters. Pyridoxal 5' phosphate (PLP) and pyridoxamine 5' phosphate (PMP) are the active coenzyme forms of vitamin B$_6$. Vitamin B$_6$ is naturally present in many foods, is added to others, and also exists as a dietary supplement.

Vitamin B$_6$ performs a wide variety of functions in the body. It is needed for more than 100 enzymes involved in protein metabolism and is essential for red blood cell metabolism. The nervous and immune systems need vitamin B$_6$ to function efficiently, and it is also needed for the conversion of tryptophan (an amino acid) to niacin. A vitamin B$_6$ deficiency can result in a form of anemia that is similar to iron deficiency anemia. See Chapter 32.

Through its involvement in protein metabolism and cellular growth, vitamin B$_6$ is important to the immune system. It helps maintain the health of lymphoid organs (thymus, spleen, and lymph nodes) that make white blood cells. It is also important for maintaining normal blood glucose levels.

Recommended Intakes

Intake recommendations for vitamin B$_6$ and other nutrients are provided in the Dietary Reference Intakes (DRIs) developed by the Food and Nutrition Board (FNB) of the Institute of Medicine (IOM) of the National Academies. DRI is the general term for a set of reference values used for planning and assessing nutrient intakes of healthy people. These values, which vary by age and gender, include:

- Recommended Dietary Allowance (RDA): average daily level of intake sufficient to meet the nutrient requirements of nearly all (97%–98%) healthy individuals.
- Adequate Intake (AI): established when evidence is insufficient to develop an RDA and is set at a level assumed to ensure nutritional adequacy.
- Tolerable Upper Intake Level (UL): maximum daily intake unlikely to cause adverse health effects. The ULs for vitamin B$_6$ are listed on the inside back cover of this text.

Recommended Dietary Allowances for Vitamin B$_6$ for Children and Adults

Age (years)	Males (mg/day)	Females (mg/day)	Pregnancy (mg/day)	Lactation (mg/day)
0 – 6 mos	.1*	.1*	N/A	N/A
7 – 12 mos	.3*	.3*	N/A	N/A
1-3	0.5	.5	N/A	N/A
4-8	0.6	.6	N/A	N/A
9-13	1.0	1.0	N/A	N/A
14-18	1.3	1.2	1.9	2.0
19 - 50	1.3	1.3	1.9	2.0
51+	1.7	1.5	N/A	N/A

N/A, Not applicable.
*Adequate Intake (AI). AI for vitamin B$_6$ is equivalent to the mean intake of vitamin B$_6$ in healthy, breastfed infants.

Substantial proportions of the naturally occurring pyridoxine in fruits, vegetables, and grains exist in glycosylated forms that exhibit reduced bioavailability.

Selected Food Sources of Vitamin B$_6$

Food	Milligrams (mg) per Serving	Percent DV*
Chickpeas, canned, 1 cup	1.1	55
Beef liver, pan fried, 3 ounces	0.9	45
Tuna, yellowfin, fresh, cooked, 3 ounces	0.9	45
Salmon, sockeye, cooked, 3 ounces	0.6	30
Chicken breast, roasted, 3 ounces	0.5	25
Breakfast cereals, fortified with 25% of the DV for vitamin B$_6$	0.5	25
Potatoes, boiled, 1 cup	0.4	20
Turkey, meat only, roasted, 3 ounces	0.4	20
Banana, 1 medium	0.4	20
Marinara (spaghetti) sauce, ready to serve, 1 cup	0.4	20
Ground beef, patty, 85% lean, broiled, 3 ounces	0.3	15

Selected Food Sources of Vitamin B₆—cont'd

Food	Milligrams (mg) per Serving	Percent DV*
Waffles, plain, ready to heat, toasted, 1 waffle	0.3	15
Bulgur, cooked, 1 cup	0.2	10
Cottage cheese, 1% low-fat, 1 cup	0.2	10
Squash, winter, baked, ½ cup	0.2	10
Rice, white, long-grain, enriched, cooked, 1 cup	0.1	5
Nuts, mixed, dry-roasted, 1 ounce	0.1	5
Raisins, seedless, ½ cup	0.1	5
Onions, chopped, ½ cup	0.1	5
Spinach, frozen, chopped, boiled, ½ cup	0.1	5
Tofu, raw, firm, prepared with calcium sulfate, ½ cup	0.1	5
Watermelon, raw, 1 cup	0.1	5

*DV = Daily Value. DVs were developed by the U.S. Food and Drug Administration (FDA) to help consumers compare the nutrient contents of products within the context of a total diet. The DV for vitamin B₆ is 2 mg for adults and children age 4 and older. However, the FDA does not require food labels to list vitamin B₆ content unless a food has been fortified with this nutrient. Foods providing 20% or more of the DV are considered to be high sources of a nutrient.

VITAMIN B₁₂

Vitamin B₁₂ is a member of the vitamin B complex. It contains cobalt; thus it is also known as *cobalamin.* Methylcobalamin and 5-deoxyadenosylcobalamin are the active forms of vitamin B₁₂. Like folate, vitamin B₁₂ is involved in the conversion of homocysteine to methionine.

Vitamin B₁₂ is necessary for the synthesis of red blood cells, the maintenance of the nervous system, DNA synthesis and growth. Deficiency can cause anemia. See Chapter 32. Vitamin B₁₂ neuropathy, involving the degeneration of nerve fibers and irreversible neurologic damage, can also occur.

Proper vitamin B₁₂ absorption requires the presence of hydrochloric acid (HCL) and gastric protease, which cause its release from the protein it is bound to in food, allowing it to be absorbed. B₁₂ then combines with intrinsic factor (IF), secreted by the stomach's parietal cells, and travels down the GI tract where it is absorbed as the B₁₂-IF complex in the distal ileum. See Chapter 1. Because HCL production tends to diminish with age, B₁₂ supplementation where the B₁₂ is already separated from the protein molecule and is in its free form can be useful in treating or preventing a deficiency. Total body store of B₁₂ is 2 to 5 mg in adults. Approximately 80% of this is stored in the liver.

Along with folate and vitamin B₆, vitamin B₁₂ is helpful in lowering the level of the amino acid homocysteine in the blood. It has been hypothesized that at high levels homocysteine might damage coronary arteries or make it easier for blood-clotting cells to clump together and form a clot. This could increase risks for a heart attack or stroke.

Recommended Intakes

- Recommended Dietary Allowance (RDA): average daily level of intake sufficient to meet the nutrient requirements of nearly all (97%–98%) healthy individuals.
- Adequate Intake (AI): established when evidence is insufficient to develop an RDA and is set at a level assumed to ensure nutritional adequacy.

- Tolerable Upper Intake Level (UL): maximum daily intake unlikely to cause adverse health effects. The ULs for vitamin B₁₂ are listed on the inside back cover of this text.

The table below lists the current RDAs for vitamin B₁₂ in micrograms (mcg). For infants aged 0 to 12 months, there are AIs that are equivalent to the mean intake of vitamin B₁₂ in healthy, breastfed infants.

Recommended Dietary Allowances for Vitamin B₁₂ for Children and Adults

Age (years)	Males and Females (mcg/day)	Pregnancy (mcg/day)	Lactation (mcg/day)
0 – 6 mos	0.4*	N/A	N/A
7 – 12 mos	0.5*	N/A	N/A
1-3	0.9	N/A	N/A
4-8	1.2	N/A	N/A
9-13	1.8	N/A	N/A
14 +	2.4	2.6	2.8

N/A, Not applicable.
*Adequate Intake (AI)

Vitamin B₁₂ is found primarily in animal foods such as fish, meat, poultry, eggs, and dairy products. However, it is also synthesized by bacteria and there has been considerable research into proposed plant sources of vitamin B₁₂. Fermented soy products, seaweeds, and algae (spirulina) have all been suggested as containing significant B₁₂. However, the present consensus is that any B₁₂ present in plant foods is likely to be unavailable to humans; thus these foods should not be relied on as safe sources. Vegans need B₁₂ from fortified foods or as a supplement. Fortified breakfast cereals are a readily available source of vitamin B₁₂ with high bioavailability for vegans. Some nutritional yeast products also contain vitamin B₁₂. Fortified foods vary in formulation, so it is important to read product labels.

Many vegan foods are supplemented with B₁₂.

Selected Food Sources of Vitamin B₁₂

Food	Micrograms (mcg) per Serving	Percent DV*
Clams, cooked, 3 ounces	84.1	1,402
Liver, beef, cooked, 3 ounces	70.7	1,178
Breakfast cereals, fortified with 100% of the DV for vitamin B₁₂, 1 serving	6.0	100
Trout, rainbow, wild, cooked, 3 ounces	5.4	90
Salmon, sockeye, cooked, 3 ounces	4.8	80
Trout, rainbow, farmed, cooked, 3 ounces	3.5	58
Tuna fish, light, canned in water, 3 ounces	2.5	42
Cheeseburger, double patty and bun, 1 sandwich	2.1	35
Haddock, cooked, 3 ounces	1.8	30
Breakfast cereals, fortified with 25% of the DV for vitamin B₁₂, 1 serving	1.5	25

Continued

Selected Food Sources of Vitamin B$_{12}$—cont'd

Food	Micrograms (mcg) per Serving	Percent DV*
Beef, top sirloin, broiled, 3 ounces	1.4	23
Milk, low-fat, 1 cup	1.2	18
Yogurt, fruit, low-fat, 8 ounces	1.1	18
Cheese, Swiss, 1 ounce	0.9	15
Beef taco, 1 soft taco	0.9	15
Ham, cured, roasted, 3 ounces	0.6	10
Egg, whole, hard boiled, 1 large	0.6	10
Chicken, breast meat, roasted, 3 ounces	0.3	5

*DV = Daily Value. DVs were developed by the U.S. Food and Drug Administration (FDA) to help consumers determine the level of various nutrients in a standard serving of food in relation to their approximate requirement for it. The DV for adults and children aged 4 and older is 6.0 mcg. The %DV listed on the Nutrition Facts label states the percentage of the DV provided per serving. However, the FDA does not require food labels to list vitamin B$_{12}$ content unless a food has been fortified with this nutrient. Foods providing 20% or more of the DV are considered to be high sources of a nutrient, but foods providing lower percentages of the DV also contribute to a healthful diet.

REFERENCES

Institute of Medicine. Food and Nutrition Board: *Dietary Reference Intakes: Thiamin, Riboflavin, Niacin, Vitamin B$_6$, Folate, Vitamin B$_{12}$, Pantothenic Acid, Biotin, and Choline.* Washington, DC, 1998, National Academy Press.

Folate Dietary Supplement Fact Sheet: https://ods.od.nih.gov/factsheets/Folate-HealthProfessional/. Accessed January 30, 2016.

U.S. Department of Agriculture Agricultural Research Service: (2012) USDA National Nutrient Database for Standard Reference, Release 25, 2012.

Vitamin B$_6$ Dietary Supplement Fact Sheet. https://ods.od.nih.gov/factsheets/VitaminB$_6$-HealthProfessional/. Accessed January 30, 2016.

U.S. Department of Agriculture, Agricultural Research Service: USDA National Nutrient Database for Standard Reference, Release 24, 2011, Nutrient Data Laboratory Home Page. http://www.ars.usda.gov/ba/bhnrc/ndl. Accessed January 30, 2016.

Vitamin B$_{12}$ Dietary Supplement Fact Sheet. https://ods.od.nih.gov/factsheets/VitaminB$_{12}$-HealthProfessional/. Accessed January 31, 2016.

Nutritional Facts on Vitamin A and Carotenoids

Vitamin A includes a group of compounds that affect vision, bone growth, reproduction, cell division, immunity, and healthy surface linings of the respiratory tract and mucous membranes. There are two categories of vitamin A, depending on whether the food source is an animal or a plant. Vitamin A found in animal foods is called *preformed vitamin A* and is absorbed as retinol. Sources include liver, whole milk, and some fortified food products. In the body retinol can be made into retinal and retinoic acid (other active forms of vitamin A).

Plant sources of vitamin A provide the provitamin A, called *carotenoids.* They can be made into retinol in the body and then into the other active forms of vitamin A. In the United States approximately 26% to 34% of vitamin A consumed is in the form of provitamin A carotenoids. Common provitamin A carotenoids which give plants their color, and are β-carotene, α-carotene, and β-cryptoxanthin. Among these, β-carotene is most efficiently made into retinol. The darker the color of a fruit or vegetable, the greater is its carotenoid content.

Vitamin A deficiency rarely occurs in the United States. Vitamin A deficiency is more common in developing countries, where access to sufficient animal and beta-carotene containing plant sources is limited. Vitamin A deficiency is a leading cause of preventable blindness in children. Children with measles or diarrhea can significantly benefit from increased vitamin A. Fat malabsorption can result in diarrhea and prevent normal absorption of vitamin A; this may result in vitamin A deficiency in celiac disease, Crohn's disease, and pancreatic disorders. The best absorbed form of vitamin A is in the oil form such as in cod liver oil.

RECOMMENDED DIETARY ALLOWANCES (RDA)

The RDA is the average daily dietary intake level that is sufficient to meet the nutrient requirement of the vast majority (97 - 98%) of healthy individuals in a particular gender and age group, with special considerations for pregnancy or lactation, where applicable.

All dietary sources of vitamin A are converted to retinol. Intake recommendations for Vitamin A in foods are expressed as micrograms of retinol activity equivalents (RAEs) as a way to standardize the variation in bioactivities of retinol and provitamin A carotenoids, and account for the differences based on source. International Units (IU) are a helpful guideline, but conversion rates also vary based on source:

- 1 IU retinol = 0.3 mcg RAE
- 1 IU beta-carotene from dietary supplements = 0.15 mcg RAE
- 1 IU beta-carotene from food = 0.05 mcg RAE
- 1 IU alpha-carotene or beta-cryptoxanthin = 0.025 mcg RAE

Recommended Daily Allowances

Age (years)	Males and Females (mcg RAEs/day)	Pregnancy (mcg RAEs/day)	Lactation (mcg RAEs/day)
0 6 mos	400*	N/A	N/A
0 – 7 mos	500*	N/A	N/A
1-3	300	N/A	N/A
4-8	400	N/A	N/A
9-13	600	N/A	N/A
14-18	900 for boys; 700 for girls	750	1200
19+	900 for men; 700 for women	770	1300

N/A, Not applicable; *RAE*, Retinol activity equivalent.
*Adequate Intakes

FOOD SOURCES OF VITAMIN A

Selected Animal Sources of Vitamin A

Food	Vitamin A (IU)	% Daily Value
Liver, beef, cooked, 3 oz	27,185	545
*Liver, chicken, cooked, 3 oz	12,325	245
Milk, fortified skim, 1 cup	500	10
Cheese, cheddar, 1 oz	284	6
Milk, whole (3.25% fat), 1 cup	249	5
Egg substitute, ¼ cup	226	5

Selected Plant Sources of Vitamin A (from β-Carotene)

Food	Vitamin A (IU)	% Daily Value*	Food	Vitamin A (IU)	% Daily Value*
Carrot juice, canned, ½ cup	22,567	450	Papaya, 1 cup cubes	1532	30
Carrots, boiled, ½ cup slices	13,418	270	Mango, 1 cup sliced	1262	25
Spinach, frozen, boiled, ½ cup	11,458	230	Oatmeal, instant, fortified, plain, prepared with water, 1 cup	1252	25
Kale, frozen, boiled, ½ cup	9558	190			
Carrots, 1 raw (7½ in)	8666	175	Peas, frozen, boiled, ½ cup	1050	20
Vegetable soup, canned, chunky, ready-to-serve, 1 cup	5820	115	Tomato juice, canned, 6 oz	819	15
			Peaches, canned, juice pack, ½ cup halves or slices	473	10
Cantaloupe, 1 cup cubes	5411	110			
Spinach, raw, 1 cup	2813	55	Peach, 1 medium	319	6
Apricots with skin, juice pack, ½ cup	2063	40	Pepper, sweet, red, raw, 1 ring (3 inches diameter by ¼ inch thick)	313	6
Apricot nectar, canned, ½ cup	1651	35			

*Daily values (DVs) are reference numbers based on the RDA. They were developed to help consumers determine if a food contains a lot or a little of a nutrient. **The DV for vitamin A is 5000 IU.** Most food labels do not list vitamin A content. The %DV column in this table indicates the percentage of the DV provided in one serving. A food providing 5% or less of the DV is a low source, whereas a food that provides 10% to 19% of the DV is a good source. A food that provides 20% or more of the DV is high in that nutrient. It is important to remember that foods that provide lower percentages of the DV also contribute to a healthful diet.

Carotenoids in Fruits and Vegetables (mole %)

	Neoxanthins and Violaxanthins	Lutein and Zeaxanthin	Lutein	Zeaxanthin	Cryptoxanthins	Lycopenes	α-carotene	β-carotene
Egg yolk	8	89	54	35	4	0	0	0
Maize (corn)	9	86	60	26	5	0	0	0
Kiwi	38	54	54	0	0	0	0	8
Red seedless grapes	23	53	43	10	4	5	3	16
Zucchini squash	19	52	47	5	24	0	0	5
Pumpkin	30	49	49	0	0	0	0	21
Spinach	14	47	47	0	19	4	0	16
Orange pepper	4	45	8	37	22	0	8	21
Yellow squash	19	44	44	0	0	0	28	9
Cucumber	16	42	38	4	38	0	0	4
Pea	33	41	41	0	21	0	0	5
Green pepper	29	39	36	3	20	0	0	12
Red grape	27	37	33	4	29	0	1	6
Butternut squash	24	37	37	0	34	0	5	0
Orange juice	28	35	15	20	25	0	3	8
Honeydew	18	35	17	18	0	0	0	48
Celery (stalks, leaves)	12	34	32	2	40	1	13	0
Green grapes	10	31	25	6	52	0	0	7
Brussels sprouts	20	29	27	2	39	0	0	11
Scallions	32	29	27	2	35	4	0	0
Green beans	27	25	22	3	42	0	1	5
Orange	36	22	7	15	12	11	8	11
Broccoli	3	22	22	0	49	0	0	27
Apple (red delicious)	22	20	19	1	23	13	5	17
Mango	52	18	2	16	4	6	0	20
Green lettuce	33	15	15	0	36	0	16	0
Tomato juice	0	13	11	2	2	57	12	16
Peach	20	13	5	8	8	0	10	50
Yellow pepper	86	12	12	0	1	0	1	0
Nectarine	18	11	6	5	23	0	0	48
Red pepper	56	7	7	0	2	8	24	3
Tomato (fruit)	0	6	6	0	0	82	0	12
Carrots	0	2	2	0	0	0	43	55
Cantaloupe	9	1	1	0	0	3	0	87
Dried apricots	2	1	1	0	9	0	0	87
Green kidney beans	72	0	0	0	28	0	0	0

Table from Sommerburg O et al: Fruits and vegetables that are sources for lutein and zeaxanthin: the macular pigment in human eyes, Br J Ophthalmol 82:907, 1998.
The content of the major carotenoids are given in mole%. The amounts of the carotenoids were shown in seven major groups, as 1) neoxanthins and violaxanthins (neoxanthin, violaxanthin, and their related isomers, lutein 5, 6 epoxide), 2) lutein, 3) zeaxanthin, 4) cryptoxanthins (α-cryptoxanthin, β-cryptoxanthins, and related isomers), 5) lycopenes (lycopene and related isomers), 6) alpha- carotenes, and 7) β-carotene (all trans β-carotene and cis isomers. Lutein and zeaxanthin are given combined and as single amounts. The data are sorted by the combined amount of lutein and zeaxanthin.

Nutritional Facts on Vitamin C

Vitamin C is a nutrient naturally present in foods (mainly fruits and vegetables) and is also known by the chemical name of its principal form, L-ascorbic acid or simply ascorbic acid. Unlike most animals humans are unable to synthesize vitamin C. Vitamin C is principally known as a water-soluble antioxidant, preventing the damaging effects of free radicals, and it regenerates other antioxidants in the body including vitamin E or alpha-tocopherol. See Chapter 3.

Vitamin C is required for the biosynthesis of collagen, L-carnitine, and certain neurotransmitters; it is also involved in protein metabolism. Collagen is an essential component of connective tissue, which plays a vital role in wound healing, and it plays an important role in immune function. It also improves the absorption of nonheme iron, the form of iron present in plant-based foods. See Chapter 32. Vitamin C prevents scurvy, characterized by fatigue or lassitude, widespread connective tissue weakness, and capillary fragility.

RECOMMENDED INTAKES

Dietary Recommended Intakes for vitamin C were developed by the Food and Nutrition Board (FNB), Institute of Medicine (IOM) of the National Academies (formerly National Academy of Sciences). DRI is the general term for a set of reference values used for planning and assessing nutrient intakes of healthy people. These values include:
- Recommended Dietary Allowance (RDA): average daily level of intake sufficient to meet the nutrient requirements of nearly all (97%–98%) healthy individuals.
- Adequate Intake (AI): established when evidence is insufficient to develop an RDA and is set at a level assumed to ensure nutritional adequacy.
- Tolerable Upper Intake Level (UL): maximum daily intake unlikely to cause adverse health effects. ULs for vitamin C are listed on the inside back cover of this text.

The RDAs for vitamin C are based on its known physiological and antioxidant functions in white blood cells and are much higher than the amount required for protection from deficiency. For infants from birth to 12 months, the FNB established an AI for vitamin C that is equivalent to the mean intake of vitamin C in healthy, breastfed infants

Fruits and vegetables are the best sources of vitamin C especially citrus fruits, red and green peppers, kiwi fruit and tomatoes and tomato juice. Other good food sources include broccoli, strawberries Brussels sprouts, and cantaloupe. Some fortified breakfast cereals are also good sources of vitamin C.

Recommended Dietary Allowances (RDAs) for Vitamin C for Children and Adults

Age (years)	Males and Females (mg/day)	Pregnancy (mg/day)	Lactation (mg/day)
0 – 6 mos	40*	N/A	N/A
7 – 12 mos	50*	N/A	N/A
1-3	15	N/A	N/A
4-8	25	N/A	N/A
9-13	45	N/A	N/A
14-18	75 for boys; 65 for girls	80	115
19+	90 for men; 75 for women	85	120
Smokers	Individuals who smoke require 35 mg/day more vitamin C than nonsmokers.		

N/A, Not applicable.

The vitamin C content of food can be lessened by prolonged storage and by cooking because ascorbic acid is water soluble and is destroyed by heat. Steaming or microwaving vegetables rather than boiling them may reduce cooking losses. Fortunately, many of the best food sources of vitamin C, such as fruits and vegetables, are usually consumed raw.

Selected Food Sources of Vitamin C

Food	Milligrams (mg) per Serving	Percent (%) DV*
Red pepper, sweet, raw, ½ cup	95	158
Orange juice, ¾ cup	93	155
Orange, 1 medium	70	117
Grapefruit juice, ¾ cup	70	117
Kiwifruit, 1 medium	64	107
Green pepper, sweet. raw, ½ cup	60	100
Broccoli, cooked, ½ cup	51	85
Strawberries, fresh, sliced, ½ cup	49	82
Brussels sprouts, cooked, ½ cup	48	80
Grapefruit, ½ medium	39	65
Broccoli, raw, ½ cup	39	65
Tomato juice, ¾ cup	33	55
Cantaloupe, ½ cup	29	48
Cabbage, cooked, ½ cup	28	47
Cauliflower, raw, ½ cup	26	43
Potato, baked, 1 medium	17	28
Tomato, raw, 1 medium	17	28
Spinach, cooked, ½ cup	9	15
Green peas, frozen, cooked, ½ cup	8	13

*DV = Daily Value. DVs were developed by the U.S. Food and Drug Administration (FDA) to help consumers compare the nutrient contents of products within the context of a total diet. **The DV for vitamin C is 60 mg for adults and children aged 4 and older**. The FDA requires all food labels to list the percent DV for vitamin C. Foods providing 20% or more of the DV are considered to be high sources of a nutrient.

Dietary Supplements

Supplements typically contain vitamin C in the form of ascorbic acid, which has equivalent bioavailability to that of naturally occurring ascorbic acid in foods, such as orange juice and broccoli. Other forms of vitamin C supplements include sodium ascorbate; calcium ascorbate; other mineral ascorbates; ascorbic acid with bioflavonoids; and combination products, such as Ester-C®, which contains calcium ascorbate, dehydroascorbate, calcium threonate, xylonate and lyxonate. It is still controversial whether Ester-C® is more bioavailable or effective than ascorbic acid in improving vitamin C status.

REFERENCES

Vitamin C Fact Sheet for Health Professionals. https://ods.od.nih.gov/factsheets/VitaminC-HealthProfessional/. Accessed Feb 1, 2016.

Institute of Medicine, Food and Nutrition Board: *Dietary Reference Intakes for Vitamin C, Vitamin E, Selenium, and Carotenoids.* Washington, DC, 2000, National Academy Press.

U.S. Department of Agriculture, Agricultural Research Service: *USDA National Nutrient Database for Standard Reference,* Release 24, 2011 Nutrient Data Laboratory Home Page. http://www.ars.usda.gov/ba/bhnrc/ndl. Accessed Feb 1, 2016.

Nutritional Facts on Vitamin E

Vitamin E is a naturally occurring fat-soluble vitamin that exists in eight different forms: alpha-, beta-, gamma-, and delta-tocopherol, and alpha-, beta-, gamma-, and delta-tocotrienol that have varying levels of biological activity. Alpha- (or α-) tocopherol appears to be the most active form, and is the only form that is recognized to meet human requirements. Serum concentrations of alpha-tocopherol depend on the liver, which takes up the nutrient after absorption of all the forms from the small intestine. The liver then preferentially secretes only alpha-tocopherol, and metabolizes and excretes the other vitamin E forms. As a result, blood and cellular concentrations of other forms of vitamin E are lower than those of alpha-tocopherol and thus have been less studied.

Vitamin E has powerful antioxidant activities which protect cells from the damaging effects of free radicals. Free radicals combine with oxygen and form reactive oxygen species (ROS) that damage cells. Free radicals are produced endogenously when the body metabolizes food to energy. Exogenous sources come from exposure to cigarette smoke, air pollution, and ultraviolet radiation from the sun. ROS are part of signaling mechanisms among cells and antioxidant vitamin E protects the cells against free radical damage. See Chapter 3. Scientists are investigating whether, by limiting free-radical production and possibly through other mechanisms, vitamin E might help prevent or delay the chronic diseases associated with free radicals. Besides functioning as an antioxidant, vitamin E is also involved in immune function and, as shown primarily by *in vitro* studies of cells, cell signaling, regulation of gene expression, and other metabolic processes .

Vitamin E in supplements is usually sold as α-tocopheryl acetate, a form of α-tocopherol that protects its ability to function as an antioxidant. The synthetic form is labeled *dl*, whereas the natural form is labeled *d*. The synthetic form is only half as active as the natural form. It is important to include foods high in vitamin E on a daily basis to get enough vitamin E from foods alone. Vegetable oils, nuts, green leafy vegetables, and fortified cereals are common food sources of vitamin E.

RECOMMENDED INTAKES

Recommendations for vitamin E are provided in the Dietary Reference Intakes (DRIs) developed by the Food and Nutrition Board (FNB), Institute of Medicine (IOM), The National Academies (formerly National Academy of Sciences). DRI is the general term for a set of reference values used to plan and assess nutrient intakes of healthy people. These values, which vary by age and gender, include:

- Recommended Dietary Allowance (RDA): average daily level of intake sufficient to meet the nutrient requirements of nearly all (97%–98%) healthy people.

- Adequate Intake (AI): established when evidence is insufficient to develop an RDA and is set at a level assumed to ensure nutritional adequacy.
- Tolerable Upper Intake Level (UL): maximum daily intake unlikely to cause adverse health effects. ULs for vitamin E are listed inside the cover of this text.

The FNB's vitamin E recommendations are for alpha-tocopherol alone, the only form maintained in plasma. Acknowledging "great uncertainties" in these data, the FNB has called for research to identify other biomarkers for assessing vitamin E requirements.

RDAs in the table are for vitamin E are for alpha-tocopherol in both milligrams (mg) and IU of the natural form. For example, 15 mg x 1.49 IU/mg = 22.4 IU in the natural form. The corresponding value for synthetic alpha-tocopherol would be 33.3 IU (15 mg x 2.22 IU/mg).

Because insufficient data are available to develop RDAs for infants, AIs were developed based on the amount of vitamin E consumed by healthy breastfed babies.

Recommended Dietary Allowances (RDAs) for Vitamin E (in milligrams) of α-TE for Children and Adults

Age	Males and Females (mg/day)	Pregnancy (mg/day)	Lactation (mg/day)
0 – 6 mos	4 mg (6 IU)*	N/A	N/A
7 – 12 mos	6 mg (7.5 IU)*	N/A	N/A
1-3 years	6 (9 IU)	N/A	N/A
4-8 years	7 (10.4 IU)	N/A	N/A
9-13 years	11 (16.4 IU)	N/A	N/A
14-18 years	15 (22.4 IU)	15 (22.4 IU)	19 (28.4 IU)
19+ years	15 (22.4 IU)	15 (22.4 IU)	19 (28.4 IU)

N/A, Not applicable.
*Adequate Intake (AI)

Vitamin E content of food is stated as milligrams of α-tocopherol, milligrams of α-tocopherol equivalents (mg α-TE), or as international units (IUs) on supplement labels. 1 unit = 0.67 α-TE in the *d* form and approximately ½ of that in the *dl* or synthetic form. The vitamin E content of foods and dietary supplements is listed on labels in international units (IUs), a measure of biological activity rather than quantity. Naturally sourced vitamin E is called d-alpha-tocopherol; the synthetically produced form is dl-alpha-tocopherol. Conversion rules are as follows:

- To convert from mg to IU: 1 mg of alpha-tocopherol is equivalent to 1.49 IU of the natural form or 2.22 IU of the synthetic form.

- To convert from IU to mg: 1 IU of alpha-tocopherol is equivalent to 0.67 mg of the natural form or 0.45 mg of the synthetic form.

Numerous foods provide vitamin E. Nuts, seeds, and vegetable oils are among the best sources of alpha-tocopherol, and significant amounts are available in green leafy vegetables and fortified cereals. See Table. Most vitamin E in American diets is in the form of gamma-tocopherol from soybean, canola, corn, and other vegetable oils and food products.

Selected Food Sources of Vitamin E (Alpha-Tocopherol)

Food	Milligrams (mg) per Serving	Percent DV*
Wheat germ oil, 1 tablespoon	20.3	100
Sunflower seeds, dry roasted, 1 ounce	7.4	37
Almonds, dry roasted. 1 ounce	6.8	34
Sunflower oil, 1 tablespoon	5.6	28
Safflower oil, 1 tablespoon	4.6	25
Hazelnuts, dry roasted, 1 ounce	4.3	22
Peanut butter, 2 tablespoons	2.9	15
Peanuts, dry roasted, 1 ounce	2.2	11
Corn oil, 1 tablespoon	1.9	10
Spinach, boiled, ½ cup	1.9	10
Broccoli, chopped, boiled, ½ cup	1.2	6
Soybean oil, 1 tablespoon	1.1	6
Kiwifruit, 1 medium	1.1	6
Mango, sliced, ½ cup	0.7	4
Tomato, raw, 1 medium	0.7	4
Spinach, raw, 1 cup	0.6	3

*DV = Daily Value. DVs were developed by the U.S. Food and Drug Administration (FDA) to help consumers compare the nutrient content of different foods within the context of a total diet. The DV for vitamin E is 30 IU (approximately 20 mg of natural alpha-tocopherol) for adults and children age 4 and older. However, the FDA does not require food labels to list vitamin E content unless a food has been fortified with this nutrient. Foods providing 20% or more of the DV are considered to be high sources of a nutrient, but foods providing lower percentages of the DV also contribute to a healthful diet.

The U.S. Department of Agriculture's (USDA's) Nutrient Database Web site lists the nutrient content of many foods, including, in some cases, the amounts of alpha-, beta-, gamma-, and delta-tocopherol. The USDA also provides a comprehensive list of foods containing vitamin E arranged by nutrient content and by food name.

SAMPLE MEAL PLAN

Breakfast

¾ cup ready-to-eat cereal, fortified with vitamin E
   ½ cup low-fat or fat-free milk
   1 red delicious apple
   2 Tbsp peanut butter (2.5 mg vitamin E)

Lunch

1 cup mixed salad greens
   3 oz tuna steak
   2 slices multigrain bread
   ½ cup fruit salad

Dinner

3 oz grilled chicken breast
   ½ cup fresh steamed spinach (1.9 mg vitamin E)
   ½ cup whole grain rice
   Side salad

Snack

1 oz dry roasted almonds (6.8 mg vitamin E)
   1 Tbsp low-fat granola
   ½ cup low-fat or fat-free yogurt
   1 tsp wheat germ oil (6.7 mg vitamin E).

REFERENCES

Vitamin E Fact Sheet for Health Professionals: https://ods.od.nih.gov/factsheets/VitaminE-HealthProfessional/. Accessed January 31, 2016.

Institute of Medicine, Food and Nutrition Board: *Dietary Reference Intakes: Vitamin C, Vitamin E, Selenium, and Carotenoids.* Washington, DC, 2000, National Academy Press.

U.S. Department of Agriculture, Agricultural Research Service: *USDA National Nutrient Database for Standard Reference,* Release 24, 2011. Nutrient Data Laboratory Home Page. http://www.ars.usda.gov/ba/bhnrc/ndl.

Dietrich M, Traber MG, Jacques PF, Cross CE, Hu Y, Block G: Does γ-tocopherol play a role in the primary prevention of heart disease and cancer? A review, *Am J Coll Nutr* 25:292–299, 2006.

Nutritional Facts on Vitamin K

Vitamin K refers to a family of compounds with a common chemical structure. These compounds include phylloquinone (vitamin K1) and a series of menaquinones known as vitamin K2. They are further designated as MK-4 through MK-13 depending on the length of their individual side chains. Vitamin K is fat soluble and is naturally present in some foods, is produced by the bacteria naturally present in the gastrointestinal tract, and is available as a dietary supplement. Vitamin K1, the main dietary form of vitamin K, is present mainly in green leafy vegetables. Menaquinones, primarily of bacterial origin, are found in some animal based foods and in fermented foods. Natto, a Japanese fermented soy food is an excellent source of vitamin K2. Menaquinones are also produced by the naturally occurring bacteria in the gut. However, MK-4 is unique in that it is produced from phylloquinone by a conversion process that does not involve bacteria.

Vitamin K functions as a coenzyme for vitamin K-dependent carboxylase, an enzyme required for the synthesis of proteins involved in hemostasis (blood clotting) and bone metabolism, and other diverse physiological functions. Prothrombin (clotting factor II) is a vitamin K-dependent protein in plasma that is directly involved in blood clotting. https://ods.od.nih.gov/factsheets/VitaminK-HealthProfessional/.

Matrix Gla-protein, is another vitamin K-dependent protein present in vascular smooth muscle, bone, and cartilage, is the focus of considerable scientific research because it might help reduce abnormal calcification. Osteocalcin is another vitamin K-dependent protein, and is present in bone and may be involved in bone mineralization or turnover. See Chapter 24.

The Dietary Reference Intakes for vitamin K are adequate intakes and are listed in the table.
- Adequate Intake (AI): established when evidence is insufficient to develop a Recommended Dietary Allowance (RDA); intake at this level is assumed to ensure nutritional adequacy.
- Tolerable Upper Intake Level (UL): maximum daily intake unlikely to cause adverse health effects. ULs for vitamin K are listed on the inside cover of this text.

Antibiotics may interfere with this normal production. Circumstances that may lead to vitamin K deficiency include liver disease, serious burns, health problems that can prevent the absorption of vitamin K (such as gallbladder or biliary disease, which may alter the absorption of fat), cystic fibrosis, celiac disease, Crohn's disease, and chronic antibiotic therapy. Excess vitamin E can inhibit vitamin K activity and precipitate signs of deficiency. The classic sign of a vitamin K deficiency is a prolonged prothrombin time, which increases the risk of spontaneous hemorrhage. Because vitamin K is stored in the liver, clinical deficiencies are rare.

Vitamin K is needed to make clotting factors that help the blood to clot and prevent bleeding. The amount of vitamin K in food may affect drug therapy, such as that from warfarin or other anticoagulants. Warfarin (Coumadin®) and some anticoagulants used primarily in Europe antagonize the activity of vitamin K and, in turn, prothrombin. For this reason, individuals who are taking these anticoagulants need to maintain consistent vitamin K intakes. When taking these medications, it is necessary to eat a normal, balanced diet, maintaining a consistent amount of vitamin K, and avoiding large changes in vitamin K intake.

In general, leafy green vegetables and certain legumes and vegetable oils contain high amounts of vitamin K. Foods that contain a significant amount of vitamin K include beef liver, green tea, turnip greens, broccoli, kale, spinach, cabbage, asparagus, and dark green lettuce. Chlorophyll, which is water soluble, is the substance in plants that gives them their green color and provides vitamin K; thus chlorophyll supplements need to be considered when assessing vitamin K intake. Foods that appear to contain low amounts of vitamin K include roots, bulbs, tubers, the fleshy portion of fruits, fruit juices and other beverages, and cereal grains and their milled products.

Dietary Reference Intakes: Adequate Intakes (AIs) for Vitamin K for Children and Adults

Age (years)	Males and Females (mcg/day)	Pregnancy (mcg/day)	Lactation (mcg/day)
Birth to 6 mos	2	N/A	N/A
7 – 12 mos	2.5	N/A	N/A
1-3	30	N/A	N/A
4-8	55	N/A	N/A
9-13	60	N/A	N/A
14-18	75	75	75
19+	120 for men; 90 for women	90	90

N/A, Not applicable.

Selected Food Sources of Vitamin K (Phylloquinone, Except as Indicated)

Food	Micrograms (mcg) per Serving	Percent DV*	Food	Micrograms (mcg) per Serving	Percent DV*
Natto, 3 ounces (as MK-7)	850	1,062	Canola oil, 1 tablespoon	10	13
Collards, frozen, boiled, ½ cup	530	662	Cashews, dry roasted, 1 ounce	10	13
Turnip greens, frozen, boiled ½ cup	426	532	Carrots, raw, 1 medium	8	10
Spinach, raw, 1 cup	145	181	Olive oil, 1 tablespoon	8	10
Kale, raw, 1 cup	113	141	Ground beef, broiled, 3 ounces (as MK-4)	6	8
Broccoli, chopped, boiled, ½ cup	110	138	Figs, dried, ¾ cup	6	8
Soybeans, roasted, ½ cup	43	54	Chicken liver, braised, 3 ounces (as MK-4)	6	8
Carrot juice, ¾ cup	28	34	Ham, roasted or pan-broiled, 3 ounces (as MK-4)	4	5
Soybean oil, 1 tablespoon	25	31			
Edamame, frozen, prepared, ½ cup	21	26	Cheddar cheese, 1½ ounces (as MK-4)	4	5
Pumpkin, canned, ½ cup	20	25	Mixed nuts, dry roasted, 1 ounce	4	5
Pomegranate juice, ¾ cup	19	24			
Okra, raw, ½ cup	16	20	Egg, hard boiled, 1 large (as MK-4)	4	5
Salad dressing, Caesar, 1 tablespoon	15	19	Mozzarella cheese, 1½ ounces (as MK-4)	2	3
Pine nuts, dried, 1 ounce	15	19	Milk, 2%, 1 cup (as MK-4)	1	1
Blueberries, raw, ½ cup	14	18	Salmon, sockeye, cooked, 3 ounces (as MK-4)	0.3	0
Iceberg lettuce, raw, 1 cup	14	18			
Chicken, breast, rotisserie, 3 ounces (as MK-4)	13	17	Shrimp, cooked, 3 ounces (as MK-4)	0.3	0
Grapes, ½ cup	11	14			
Vegetable juice cocktail, ¾ cup	10	13			

*DV = Daily Value. DVs were developed by the U.S. Food and Drug Administration (FDA) to help consumers compare the nutrient contents of products within the context of a total diet. **The DV for vitamin K is 80 mcg for adults and children age 4 and older.** However, the FDA does not require food labels to list vitamin K content unless a food has been fortified with this nutrient. Foods providing 20% or more of the DV are considered to be high sources of a nutrient.

The U.S. Department of Agriculture's (USDA's) Nutrient Database website (https://ods.od.nih.gov/pubs/usdandb/MK-4_Nutrient_Content_SR27.pdf) lists the nutrient content of many foods and provides comprehensive lists of foods containing vitamin K (phylloquinone) arranged by nutrient content and by food name, and of foods containing vitamin K (MK-4) arranged by nutrient content and food name.

REFERENCES

Schurgers LJ: Vitamin K: key vitamin in controlling vascular calcification in chronic kidney disease, *Kidney Int* 83:782, 2013.

Health Professionals Fact Sheet for Vitamin K. ods.od.nih.gov/factsheets/VitaminK-HealthProfessional/. Accessed January 30, 2016.

Nutritional Facts on Vitamin D

Vitamin D is a fat-soluble vitamin that is naturally present in very few foods, is added to some foods, is available as a nutritional supplement, and is made when ultraviolet light, specifically UVB rays from the sun, strike the skin and stimulate its synthesis. Both the vitamin D that is absorbed from food and supplements, and that is made by the skin is biologically inert. It must be hydroxylated twice in the body – first into 25(OH) vitamin D (calcidiol) by the liver, and again into $1,25(OH)^2$ vitamin D (calcitriol.) by the kidney.

Vitamin D is needed for the absorption of calcium from the small intestine and for the functioning of calcium in the body. Vitamin D also acts like a hormone and has many functions unrelated to its co-functions with calcium absorption and bone growth and remodeling. (See Chapter 24) Besides being in bone, receptors for vitamin D have been identified in the gastrointestinal tract, brain, breast, nerve, and many other tissues. Vitamin D maintains adequate serum calcium and phosphate concentrations to prevent hypocalcemic tetany. It also modulates cell growth, neuromuscular and immune function, and reduction of inflammation. Many genes that encode for the regulation of cell proliferation, differentiation and apoptosis are modulated by vitamin D (see Chapter 5.) https://ods.od.nih.gov/factsheets/VitaminD-HealthProfessional/. RDAs were established for vitamin D in 2011, and are presented in Table 1.

VITAMIN D SYNTHESIZED FROM SUNLIGHT EXPOSURE

Vitamin D made in the skin lasts twice as long in the blood as vitamin D ingested from the diet. The skin not only makes vitamin D upon exposure to UVB rays, but also makes other photoproducts that cannot be obtained from food or supplements. It is unknown if any of these products have unique benefits to health, but research continues in this area.

UVB light cannot pass through glass; exposure of the skin to sunlight through glass will not result in vitamin D synthesis. Another deterrent to vitamin D synthesis by the skin is sunscreen. A sunscreen with an SPF 15 reduces skin synthesis of vitamin D by 95%, and an SPF30 reduces it by 99%.

How much sun exposure is the correct amount to maintain optimal vitamin D levels in the body? A person sunbathing in a bathing suit will have received a dose of between 10,000 and 25,000 IU of vitamin D when he or she has sunbathed long enough to be slightly pink 24 hours later (technically called a minimal erythemal dose or "1 MED.") Exposing 25% of the body (arms and legs) for ¼ to ½ the time it takes to get slightly pink will allow the body to make 2,000 to 4,000 IU of vitamin D with each exposure.

The amount of time necessary for sunlight exposure to produce adequate vitamin D depends on the person's skin type (pale skin requires less time than dark skin with a lot of the burn protecting pigment melanin), season of the year (the lower the sun on the horizon in the winter, the greater the time needed), the latitude (within + or – 35 degrees from the equator, the most vitamin D can be produced when skin is exposed to UVB rays), and the time of day (more vitamin D is synthesized by the skin when the sun is directly overhead between 11:00 am and 3:00 pm.) A person should be exposed to sunlight 2 to 3 times per week from March through October in northern climates to accumulate enough vitamin D to get through the winter with adequate vitamin D. See Holick for tables of time of sun exposure needed to make adequate amounts of vitamin D. Several apps are also available to determine this – Vitamin D Calculator, Vitamin D Pro, and D-Minder.

VITAMIN D IN FOODS

Vitamin D is measured in international units (IUs). 1 mcg = 40 IU of vitamin D or calciferol. IUs are used on food and supplement labels and both are used in the 2011 RDAs for vitamin D. The vitamin D in foods is measured as calciferol. There are only a few food sources of vitamin calciferol. Fish such as salmon, tuna and mackerel and fish oils are one of the few natural sources of vitamin D. Beef liver, cheese and egg yolks contain small amounts of vitamin D3, a metabolite of vitamin D which appears to be approximately five times more potent than the parent vitamin (calciferol) in raising serum 25(OH)D concentrations. At the present time, the USDA's Nutrient Database does not include this vitamin D metabolite when reporting the vitamin D content of foods. Actual vitamin D intakes in the U.S. population may be underestimated for this reason.

TABLE 1 Recommended Dietary Allowances (RDAs) for Vitamin D				
Age	Male	Female	Pregnancy	Lactation
0–12 months*	400 IU (10 mcg)	400 IU (10 mcg)	N/A	N/A
1–13 years	600 IU (15 mcg)	600 IU (15 mcg)	N/A	N/A
14–18 years	600 IU (15 mcg)	600 IU (15 mcg)	600 IU (15 mcg)	600 IU (15 mcg)
19–50 years	600 IU (15 mcg)	600 IU (15 mcg)	600 IU (15 mcg)	600 IU (15 mcg)
51–70 years	600 IU (15 mcg)	600 IU (15 mcg)	N/A	N/A
>70 years	800 IU (20 mcg)	800 IU (20 mcg)	N/A	N/A

Adequate Intake (AI)

Mushrooms are the only plant food known to contain vitamin D, and the amount varies widely depending on the type of mushroom and amount of sunlight exposure during growth. Commercially raised mushrooms are now being grown with controlled UVB exposure so that they synthesize and thus contain much more vitamin D than if grown in the wild. In fact, grown with lots of UVB exposure, 4-5 button or crimini mushrooms may contain as much as 400 IU of vitamin D.

Good sources of vitamin D are fortified foods and beverages such as milk, fortified soy, rice and nut beverages, some yogurts and margarine fortified breakfast cereals, fortified orange juice and other juices, and fortified products. (check the labels on these foods.) These fortified foods supply most of the calcium in the American diet. Cow's milk in the US is voluntarily fortified to 100 IU/cup and in Canada is fortified by law to 35-40 IU/100 ml (84 – 96 IU/cup). Yogurt, cheese, cottage cheese, quark and other milk products, unless made with vitamin D fortified milk (which is not required), or are fortified with vitamin D during production, are not good sources of vitamin D. See Table 2 for the vitamin D content of selected foods.

TABLE 2 Selected Food Sources of Vitamin D

Food	IUs per Serving*	Percent DV**
Cod liver oil, 1 tablespoon	1,360	340
Swordfish, cooked, 3 ounces	566	142
Salmon (sockeye), cooked, 3 ounces	447	112
Mushrooms, maitake, raw, 3 ounces	943	235
Mushrooms, portabella, exposed to UV light, raw, 3 ounces	375	94
Mushrooms, chanterelle, raw, 3 ounces	15	4
Mushrooms, shitake, raw, 3 ounces	178	45
Mushrooms, white, raw, 3 ounces	6	2
Tuna fish, canned in water, drained, 3 ounces	100	39
Orange juice fortified with vitamin D, 1 cup (check product labels, as amount of added vitamin D varies)	137	34
Milk, nonfat, reduced fat, and whole, vitamin D-fortified, 1 cup	115	29-31
Yogurt, fortified, with 20% of the daily value (DV) for vitamin D, 6 ounces (some yogurts are more heavily fortified – check label)	80	20
Margarine, fortified, 1 tablespoon	60	15
Sardines, canned in oil, drained, 2 sardines	46	12
Liver, beef, cooked, 3 ounces	42	11
Egg, 1 large (vitamin D is found in yolk)	41	10
Ready-to-eat cereal, fortified with 10% of the DV for vitamin D, 0.75-1 cup (more heavily fortified cereals might provide more of the DV)	40	10
Cheese, Swiss, 1 ounce	6	2

DV for vitamin D is 400 IU (10 mcg).
*IUs = International Units.
The U.S. Department of Agriculture's (USDA's) Nutrient Database Web site lists the nutrient content of many foods and provides a comprehensive list of foods containing vitamin D arranged by nutrient content and by food name.

VITAMIN D IN SUPPLEMENTS

In supplements, as well as in fortified foods, vitamin D is available in two forms, D_2 (ergocalciferol) and D_3 (cholecalciferol). Vitamin D_2 is manufactured by the UV irradiation of ergosterol in yeast, and vitamin D_3 is manufactured by the irradiation of 7-dehydrocholesterol from lanolin and the chemical conversion of cholesterol. Both forms effectively raise serum 25(OH)D levels. Firm conclusions about any different effects of these two forms of vitamin D cannot be drawn at this time. However, it appears that at nutritional doses vitamins D_2 and D_3 are equivalent, but at high doses vitamin D_2 appears to be less potent. https://ods.od.nih.gov/factsheets/VitaminD-HealthProfessional/ It also appears that frequent smaller dosing (daily) rather than much, much larger bolus dosing (weekly or monthly) of vitamin D may be more effective in improving 25(OH) vitamin D levels.

REFERENCES

Institute of Medicine, Food and Nutrition Board: *Dietary Reference Intakes for Calcium and Vitamin D*. Washington, DC, 2010, National Academy Press.

Holick MF: *The Vitamin D Solution*, 2010, Penguin Group, pp 180-188.

Taylor CL, et al: Including food 25-hydroxyvitamin D in intake estimates may reduce the discrepancy between dietary and serum measures of vitamin D status, *J Nutr* 144:654, 2014.

U.S. Department of Agriculture, Agricultural Research Service: *USDA National Nutrient Database for Standard Reference*, Release 24, 2011. Nutrient Data Laboratory Home Page. http://www.ars.usda.gov/ba/bhnrc/ndl.

Hollis BW, Wagner CL: Clinical review: The role of the parent compound vitamin D with respect to metabolism and function: Why clinical dose intervals can affect clinical outcomes, *J Clin Endocrinol Metab* 98:4619, 2013. doi: 10.1210/jc.2013-2653. Epub 2013 Oct 8.

Nutritional Facts on Calcium

Calcium, the most abundant mineral in the body, is found in some foods, is added to others, is available as a dietary supplement, and is present in some medications such as antacids. Less than 1% of total body calcium supports critical metabolic functions required for vascular contraction and vasodilation, muscle function, nerve transmission, intracellular signaling and hormonal secretion. The remaining 99% of the body's calcium supply is stored in the bones and teeth where it supports their structure and function. See Chapters 24 and 25.

Serum calcium is very tightly regulated and does not fluctuate with changes in dietary intakes; the body uses bone tissue as a reservoir for and source of calcium, in order to maintain constant concentrations of calcium in blood, muscle, and intercellular fluids. https://ods.od.nih.gov/factsheets/Calcium-Health Professional is an excellent resource for additional calcium nutrition information.

RECOMMENDED INTAKES

- Recommended Dietary Allowance (RDA): average daily level of intake sufficient to meet the nutrient requirements of nearly all (97%–98%) healthy individuals.
- Adequate Intake (AI): established when evidence is insufficient to develop an RDA; intake at this level is assumed to ensure nutritional adequacy.
- Estimated Average Requirement (EAR): average daily level of intake estimated to meet the requirements of 50% of healthy individuals. It is usually used to assess the adequacy of nutrient intakes in population groups but not individuals.
- Tolerable Upper Intake Level (UL): maximum daily intake unlikely to cause adverse health effects.

Recommended Dietary Allowances (RDAs) for Calcium

Age	Male	Female	Pregnancy	Lactating
0-6 months*	200 mg	200 mg		
7-12 months*	260 mg	260 mg		
1-3 years	700 mg	700 mg		
4-8 years	1,000 mg	1,000 mg		
9-13 years	1,300 mg	1,300 mg		
14-18 years	1,300 mg	1,300 mg	1,300 mg	1,300 mg
19-50 years	1,000 mg	1,000 mg	1,000 mg	1,000 mg
51–70 years	1,000 mg	1,200 mg		
71+ years	1,200 mg	1,200 mg		

*Adequate Intake (AI)

CALCIUM IN FOODS

There are many dietary sources of calcium, but low-fat milk or yogurt or fortified substitutes are the most efficient and readily available. The lactose in mammalian milks appears to improve the absorption of calcium from milk. Lactose-free milk and soy, nut, rice and other grain milks fortified with calcium and vitamin D are now available. They are usually fortified to 300 mg calcium per cup, equivalent to the amount of calcium in cow's or goat's milk, but the nutrition label should be checked.

In addition to milk, a variety of foods and calcium-fortified juices contain calcium and can help children, teens, and adults get sufficient levels of calcium in their diets. If it is difficult to get the recommended amounts of calcium from foods alone, a combination of food sources and supplements may be needed.

The absorption of calcium from the gut is increased when there is high body need such as during pregnancy and lactation, growth in infancy, childhood and adolescence, and when there is adequate vitamin D. Absorption is decreased by the presence of phytic acid and oxalic acid containing foods in the gut (see Chapter 35), alcohol and caffeine.

SELECTED FOOD SOURCES OF CALCIUM

See Table Selected Food Sources of Calcium. See http://ndb.nal.usda.gov/ndb/nutrients/index for a complete list of the calcium content of foods.

Selected Food Sources of Calcium

Food	Milligrams per Serving
Dairy Foods	
Milk, with added calcium, 1 cup	420
Milk, whole, 2%, 1% skim, 1 cup	300
Yogurt, low fat, plain, ¾ cup	300
Cheese, processed slices, 2 slices	265
Yogurt, fruit on the bottom, ¾ cup	250
Processed cheese spread, 3 Tbsp	250
Cheese, hard, 1 oz	240
Milk, evaporated, ¼ cup	165
Cottage cheese, ¾ cup	120
Frozen yogurt, soft serve, ½ cup	100
Ice cream, ½ cup	85
Macaroni and Cheese, prepared as per box instructions, ½ cup	80
Beans and Bean Products	
Soy cheese substitutes, 1 oz	0-200
Tofu, firm, made with calcium sulfate, 3½ oz	125
White beans, ½ cup	100

Continued

Selected Food Sources of Calcium—cont'd

Food	Milligrams per Serving
Navy beans, ½ cup	60
Black turtle beans, canned, ½ cup	42
Pinto beans, chickpeas, ½ cup	40
Nuts and Seeds	
Almonds, dry roasted, ¼ cup	95
Whole sesame seeds (black or white), 1 Tbsp	90
Tahini (sesame seed butter), 1 Tbsp	63
Brazil, hazelnuts, ¼ cup	55
Almond butter, 1 Tbsp	43
Meats, Fish, and Poultry	
Sardines, canned, 3½ oz (8 med)	370
Salmon, canned with bones, 3 oz	180
Oysters, canned, ½ cup	60
Shrimp, canned, ½ cup	40
Turnip greens, boiled, ½ cup	99
Okra, frozen, ½ cup	75
Chinese cabbage or bok choy, ½ cup	75
Kale, raw, chopped, ½ cup	50
Mustard greens, boiled, ½ cup	76
Chinese broccoli (gai lan), ½ cup	44
Broccoli, raw, ½ cup	21
Fruit	
Orange, 1 med	55
Dried figs, 2 med	54
Nondairy Drinks	
Calcium enriched orange juice, 1 cup	300
Fortified rice milk, 1 cup	300
Fortified almond milk, 1 cup	300
Fortified soy milk, 1 cup	300
Regular soy milk, 1 cup	20
Grains	
Amaranth, raw, ½ cup	150
Whole wheat flour, 1 cup	40
Pizza, cheese, 1 small slice (l oz)	120
Macaroni and cheese, boxed mix, prepared as per label, 1 cup	80
Other	
Blackstrap molasses, 1 Tbsp	80
Regular molasses, 1 Tbsp	41
Asian Foods	
Sea cucumber, fresh, 3 oz	285
Shrimp, small, dried, 1 oz	167
Dried fish, smelt, 2 Tbsp	140
Seaweed, dry (hijiki), 10 g	140
Seaweed, dry (agar), 10 g	76
	70
	69
	50
Boiled bone soup, ½ cup	Negligible
Laver, nori, and wakame seaweeds are low in calcium.	
Native Foods	
Oolichan, salted, cooked, 3 oz	210
Fish head soup, 1 cup	150
Native American ice cream (whipped soapberries), ½ cup	130

CALCIUM SUPPLEMENTS

Calcium carbonate is the most common and least expensive calcium supplement. It can be difficult to digest and causes gas and constipation in some people. Calcium carbonate is 40% elemental calcium; 1000 mg will provide 400 mg of calcium. This supplement should be taken with food to aid in absorption. Taking magnesium with it can help to prevent constipation.

Calcium citrate is more easily absorbed (bioavailability is 2.5 times higher than calcium carbonate), easier to digest, and less likely to cause constipation and gas than calcium carbonate. It also has a lower risk of contributing to the formation of kidney stones. However, it is less concentrated, providing approximately 21% elemental calcium; 1000 mg will provide 210 mg of calcium. It is more expensive than calcium carbonate, and more of it must be taken to get the same amount of calcium, but it is better absorbed. It can be taken with or without food.

Calcium phosphate costs more than calcium carbonate but less than calcium citrate. It is easily absorbed and is less likely to cause constipation and gas.

Calcium lactate and calcium aspartate are both more easily digested but more expensive than calcium carbonate.

As the dose of calcium supplement increases, the percentage absorbed decreases. Because it appears that absorption is highest with dosages of <500 mg at a time, it is best to take calcium supplements in at least two dosages per day.

CALCIUM IN MEDICATIONS

Many over the counter antacids such as Tums and Rolaids contain calcium carbonate because of calcium carbonate's ability to neutralize stomach acid. Depending on the product, each chewable pill or soft chew contains 200 – 300 mg of elemental calcium, which can be a significant source of calcium supplementation for the person with normal levels of stomach acid.

REFERENCES

Committee to Review Dietary Reference Intakes for Vitamin D and Calcium, Food and Nutrition Board, Institute of Medicine: *Dietary Reference Intakes for Calcium and Vitamin D*. Washington, DC, 2010, National Academy Press, 2010.

Nutritional Facts on Chromium

Chromium is known to enhance the action of insulin; chromium was identified as the active ingredient in the "glucose tolerance factor" many years ago. Chromium also appears to be directly involved in carbohydrate, fat, and protein metabolism; but more research is needed to determine the full range of its roles in the body.

Chromium is widely distributed in the food supply, but most foods provide only small amounts (less than 2 mcg per serving). Meat and whole-grain products, as well as some fruits, vegetables, and spices, are relatively good sources, but Brewer's yeast is by far the most concentrated food source. Foods high in simple sugars (such as sucrose and fructose) are low in chromium. Dietary intakes of chromium cannot be reliably determined because the content of the mineral in foods is substantially affected by agricultural and manufacturing processes and food-composition databases are inadequate. Chromium values in foods are approximate and should only serve as a guide. It appears that chromium picolinate and chromium nicotinate used in supplements are more bioavailable than chromic chloride.

Dietary Reference Intakes for Chromium are Adequate Intakes (AIs). See table.

Dietary Reference Intakes (AIs) for Chromium for Children and Adults

Age (years)	Males and Females (mcg/day)	Pregnancy (mcg/day)	Lactation (mcg/day)
0-6 months	.2		
7-12 months	5.5		
1-3	11	N/A	N/A
4-8	15	N/A	N/A
9-13	25 for boys, 21 for girls	N/A	N/A
14-18	35 for men, 24 for women	29	44
19+	35 for men, 25 for women	30	45
50+	30 for men, 29 for women	N/A	N/A

N/A, Not applicable.

Selected Food Sources of Chromium

Food	Micrograms per Serving
Broccoli, ½ cup	11
Grape juice, 1 cup	8
English muffin, whole wheat, 1	4
Potatoes, mashed, 1 cup	3
Garlic, dried, 1 tsp	3
Basil, dried, 1 Tbsp	2

Selected Food Sources of Chromium—cont'd

Food	Micrograms per Serving
Beef cubes, 3 oz	2
Orange juice, 1 cup	2
Turkey breast, 3 oz	2
Whole wheat bread, 2 slices	2
Red wine, 5 oz	1-13
Apple, unpeeled, 1 med	1
Banana, 1 med	1
Green beans, ½ cup	1

DV = Daily Value. DVs were developed by the FDA to help consumers compare the nutrient contents of products within the context of a total diet. **The DV for chromium is 120 mcg**. The percentage DV listed on the label indicates the percentage of the DV provided in one serving. A food providing 5% of the DV or less is a source, whereas a food that provides 10% to 19% of the DV is a good source. A food that provides 20% or more of the DV is high in that nutrient.

Interactions Between Chromium and Medications

Medications	Nature of Interaction
Antacids Corticosteroids H₂ blockers (e.g., cimetidine, famotidine, nizatidine, and ranitidine) Proton-pump inhibitors (e.g., omeprazole, lansoprazole, rabeprazole, pantoprazole, and esomeprazole)	These medications alter stomach acidity and may impair chromium absorption or enhance excretion.
β-blockers (such as atenolol or propranolol) Corticosteroids Insulin Nicotinic acid Nonsteroidal antiinflammatory drugs Prostaglandin inhibitors (e.g., ibuprofen, indomethacin, naproxen, piroxicam, and aspirin)	These medications may have their effects enhanced if taken together with chromium, or they may increase chromium absorption.

Citations:
National Institutes of Health: *Office of Dietary Supplements* (website). https://ods.od.nih.gov/factsheets/Chromium-HealthProfessional/ Accessed August 29, 2015.

Nutritional Facts on Iodine

Iodine is an important mineral that is naturally found in some foods and added to others (primarily iodized salt). It is most concentrated in foods from the ocean. More than 70 countries, including the US and Canada, have salt iodization programs.

Iodine is an essential component of thyroid hormones, thyroxine (T4) and triiodothyroxine (T3), which help to regulate metabolic rate, body temperature, growth, reproduction, blood cell production, muscle function, nerve function, and even gene expression. Iodine appears to have physiological functions including a role in the immune response and possibly a beneficial effect on mammary dysplasia and fibrocystic breast disease. See Chapter 31.

The most useful clinical tool for measuring thyroid function and thus iodine sufficiency is to measure thyroid-stimulating hormone (TSH), which is released from the pituitary gland and stimulates thyroid hormone production and release. If the TSH is high, thyroid function should be evaluated further. Selenium-dependent enzymes are also required for the conversion of thyroxine (T4) to the biologically active thyroid hormone, triiodothyronine (T3); thus deficiencies of selenium, vitamin A, or iron may also affect iodine status. Another method to assess iodine status is the urinary iodine excretion test.

DEFICIENCY

Iodine deficiency is an important health problem throughout much of the world. Most of the earth's iodine is found in its oceans and soils; thus parts of the world away from the oceans exposed for millions of years longer, have iodine-deficient soils, and the food grown in these soils have low iodine content. Thus, large percentages of people eating foods from those iodine deficient soils, and not able to consume fish, can become iodine deficient unless public health measures are taken. Iodine deficiency can cause mental retardation, hypothyroidism, goiter, and varying degrees of other growth and developmental abnormalities. Iodine is now recognized as the most common cause of preventable brain damage in the world, with millions living in iodine-deficient areas.

The major source of dietary iodine in the United States is "iodized" salt, which has been fortified with iodine. In the United States assume that any salt in processed foods is iodized unless the product label shows that it is not iodized. In the United States and Canada iodized salt contains 77 mcg of iodine per gram of salt. Iodine is also added in the diet because it is used in the feed of animals and in many processed or preserved foods as a stabilizer and as a component of red food dyes.

Vegetarian and nonvegetarian diets that exclude iodized salt, fish, and seaweed have been found to contain very little iodine. Urinary iodine excretion studies suggest that iodine intakes are declining in the United States, possibly as a result of increased adherence to dietary recommendations to reduce salt intake.

GOITROGENS

Substances that interfere with iodine use or thyroid hormone production are known as goitrogens and occur in some foods. Some species of millet and cruciferous vegetables (e.g., cabbage, broccoli, cauliflower, and Brussels sprouts) contain goitrogens; and the soybean isoflavones genistein and daidzein have also been found to inhibit thyroid hormone synthesis. Most of these goitrogens are not of clinical importance unless they are consumed in large amounts or there is a coexisting iodine or selenium deficiency.

RECOMMENDED INTAKES

- Recommended Dietary Allowance (RDA): average daily level of intake sufficient to meet the nutrient requirements of nearly all (97%–98%) healthy individuals.
- Adequate Intake (AI): established when evidence is insufficient to develop an RDA; intake at this level is assumed to ensure nutritional adequacy.
- Estimated Average Requirement (EAR): average daily level of intake estimated to meet the requirements of 50% of healthy individuals. It is usually used to assess the adequacy of nutrient intakes in population groups but not individuals.
- Tolerable Upper Intake Level (UL): maximum daily intake unlikely to cause adverse health effects. ULs are listed on the inside back cover of this text.

Recommended Dietary Allowances (RDAs) for Iodine

Age	Male mcg/day	Female mcg/day	Pregnancy mcg/day	Lactation mcg/day
0-6 months	110*	110*	N/A	N/A
7-12 months	130*	130*	N/A	N/A
1-3 years	90	90	N/A	N/A
4-8 years	90	90	N/A	N/A
9-13 years	120	120	N/A	N/A
14-18 years	150	150	220	290
19+	150	150	220	290

*Adequate intake.
N/A not applicable

The World Health Organization, United Nations Children's Fund and the International Council for the Control of Iodine Deficiency Disorders recommend a slightly higher iodine intake for pregnant women of 250 mcg per day. See Chapter 15.

The iodine contents of some common foods containing iodine are given in the table. As already mentioned, the iodine content of fruits and vegetables depends on the soil in which they were grown; the iodine content of animal foods, outside of those from the ocean, depends on where they were raised and which plants they consumed. Therefore these values are average approximations.

Selected Food Sources of Iodine

Food	Serving	Micrograms (mcg) per Serving	% Daily Value*
Salt (iodized)	1 g	47.5	31.3%
Cod	3 oz	99	66
Shrimp	3 oz	35	23
Fish sticks	2 fish sticks (2 oz)	54	36
Tuna, canned in oil	3 oz (½ can)	17	11
Milk (cow's), reduced fat	1 cup (8 fluid oz)	56	37
Egg, boiled	1 large	24	16
Navy beans, cooked	½ cup	35	23
Potato with peel, baked	1 medium	63	42
Seaweed	1 g, dried	Variable; 16 to 2,984; may be greater than 18,000 mcg (18 mg)	11 to 1,989

National Institutes of Health: *Office of Dietary Supplements* (website). https://ods.od.nih.gov/factsheets/Iodine-HealthProfessional/ Accessed January 27, 2016.
DV = Daily Value. DVs were developed by the Food and Drug Administration (FDA) to help consumers to compare the nutrient content of products. The DV for iodine is 150 mcg for adults and children 4 years and older. Foods containing 20% or more of the DV are considered to be excellent sources. However, the FDA does not require food labels to list iodine content unless the food has been fortified with iodine.

Nutritional Facts on Iron

Iron is a nutrient found in trace amounts in every cell of the body. Iron is part of hemoglobin in red blood cells and myoglobin in muscles. The role of both of these molecules is to carry oxygen. Iron also makes up part of many proteins and enzymes in the body. Iron deficiency anemia is common in children, adolescent girls, and women of childbearing age. It is usually treated with an iron-rich diet as well as iron supplements. Iron exists in foods in two forms: heme iron and nonheme iron. Vitamin C containing foods (See Appendix 42) enhance the absorption of nonheme iron and should be consumed at the same time as an iron-rich food or meal. The presence of heme iron in the meal also enhances the absorption of nonheme iron. Substances that decrease the absorption of nonheme iron are:

Oxalic acid, found in raw spinach and chocolate
Phytic acid, found in wheat bran and beans (legumes)
Tannins, found in commercial black or pekoe teas
Polyphenols, found in coffee
Calcium carbonate supplements

Heme iron found in animal foods is absorbed more efficiently than nonheme iron. The richest dietary sources of heme iron are: oysters, liver, lean red meat (especially beef), poultry (the dark red meat), tuna and salmon. Less rich sources are lamb, pork, shellfish and eggs (especially the yolks).

Non-heme iron is harder for the body to absorb. Sources of non-heme iron are: iron-fortified cereals, dried beans, whole grains (wheat, millet, oats, brown rice), legumes (lima beans, soybeans, dried beans and peas, kidney beans), nuts (almonds, brazil nuts), dried fruits (especially prunes, raisins, apricots), vegetables and greens (broccoli, spinach, kale, collards, asparagus, dandelion greens). See Table Selected Food Sources of Iron.

Breast milk contains a highly bioavailable form of iron that is well absorbed by infants, but the amount is not enough to meet the needs of the infant older than 4 to 6 months, so a food source of iron (usually as infant cereal) should be offered to the older infant.

RECOMMENDED INTAKES

- Recommended Dietary Allowance (RDA): average daily level of intake sufficient to meet the nutrient requirements of nearly all (97%–98%) healthy individuals.
- Adequate Intake (AI): established when evidence is insufficient to develop an RDA; intake at this level is assumed to ensure nutritional adequacy.
- Estimated Average Requirement (EAR): average daily level of intake estimated to meet the requirements of 50% of healthy individuals. It is usually used to assess the adequacy of nutrient intakes in population groups but not individuals.
- Tolerable Upper Intake Level (UL): maximum daily intake unlikely to cause adverse health effects. ULs are listed on the inside cover of this text.

See Table RDA for Iron.

Recommended Dietary Allowances for Iron for Children and Adults

Age	Male	Female	Pregnancy	Lactation
0-6 months	0.27 mg*	0.27 mg*		
7-12 months	11 mg	11 mg		
1-3 years	7 mg	7 mg		
4-8 years	10 mg	10 mg		
9-13 years	8 mg	8 mg		
14-18 years	11 mg	15 mg	27 mg	10 mg
19-50 years	8 mg	18 mg	27 mg	9 mg
51+ years	8 mg	8 mg		

*Adequate Intake (AI)

Selected Food Sources of Iron

Food	Milligrams Per Serving	% Daily Value*
Clams, canned, drained, 3 oz	2.28	12.67
Fortified ready-to-eat cereals (various), ≈1 oz	18-19.2	10-107
Oysters, eastern, wild, cooked, moist heat, 3 oz	8	44
Organ meats (liver, giblets), various, cooked, 3 oz†	5.2-9.9	29-55
	1.77-33.46	9.83-185.9
Fortified instant cooked cereals (various), 1 packet	3.40-10.55	18.9-58.6
Soybeans, mature, cooked, ½ cup	4.4	24
White beans, canned, ½ cup	3.9	22
Molasses, 1 Tbsp	3.5	19
Lentils, cooked, ½ cup	3.3	18
Spinach, cooked from fresh, ½ cup	3.2	18
Beef, chuck, blade roast, lean, cooked, 3 oz	3.1	17
Beef, bottom round, lean, 0 in fat, all grades, cooked, 3 oz	2.8	15.5
Kidney beans, cooked, ½ cup	2.6	14
Sardines, canned in oil, drained, 3 oz	2.5	14
Beef, rib, lean, ¼ in. fat, all grades, 3 oz	2.4	13
Chickpeas, cooked, ½ cup	2.4	13
Pumpkin and squash seed kernels, roasted, 1 oz	2.3	12.7
Duck, meat only, roasted, 3 oz	2.3	13
Lamb, shoulder, arm, lean, ¼ in fat, choice, cooked, 3 oz	2.3	13
Prune juice, ¾ cup	2.3	13
Shrimp, canned, 3 oz	1.3	10
Cowpeas, cooked, ½ cup	2.2	12
Ground beef, 15% fat, cooked, 3 oz	2.2	12
Tomato puree, ½ cup	2.2	12
Lima beans, cooked, ½ cup	2.2	12
Soybeans, green, cooked, ½ cup	2.3	13

Continued

Selected Food Sources of Iron—cont'd

Food	Milligrams Per Serving	% Daily Value*
Navy beans, cooked, ½ cup	2.2	12
Refried beans, ½ cup	2.1	11.5
Beef, top sirloin, lean, 0 in fat, all grades, cooked, 3 oz	2.0	11
Tomato paste, ¼ cup	2.0	11

†High in cholesterol.

DV = Daily Value. DVs were developed by the Food and Drug Administration to help consumers compare the nutrient content of products. The %DV listed on the Nutrition Facts panel of food labels states the percentage of the DV provided in one serving. **The DV for iron is 18 mg.** Foods containing 20% or more of the DV are considered to be excellent sources of the nutrient.

TIPS FOR INCREASING IRON INTAKE

The amount of iron the body absorbs varies, depending on several factors. For example, the body will absorb more iron from foods when iron stores are low and will absorb less when stores are sufficient. In addition, use these tips to enhance absorption:

- Include heme and non-heme iron at the same meal
- Include a vitamin C rich food in a meal
- Drink coffee or tea between meals rather than with a meal
- Cook acidic foods in cast iron pots; which can increase the iron content of food up to 30 times.

WHAT ABOUT TOO MUCH IRON?

It is unlikely that a person would take iron at toxic (too high) levels. However, children can sometimes develop iron toxicity by eating iron supplements, mistaking them for candy. Symptoms include the following: fatigue, anorexia, dizziness, nausea, vomiting, headache, weight loss, shortness of breath, and grayish color to the skin.

Hemochromatosis is a genetic disorder that affects the regulation of iron absorption. Treatment consists of a low-iron diet, no iron supplements, and phlebotomy (blood removal) on a regular basis. See Chapter 32.

Excess storage of iron in the body is known as hemosiderosis. The high iron stores come from eating excessive iron supplements or from receiving frequent blood transfusions, not from increased iron intake in the diet. See Chapter 32.

To reduce the iron from dietary sources, review the list of foods and exclude or severely limit their intake until the iron overload is alleviated. Pay particular attention to sports drinks, energy bars, fortified cereals, and multivitamin mineral supplements that have significant amounts of added iron.

SAMPLE MEAL PLAN

Breakfast
Spinach and red pepper omelet with at least 1 egg yolk (1.6 mg)
1 whole wheat English muffin with I T. molasses (3.5 mg)
1 Tbsp almond butter
Prune juice, ¾ c (2.3 mg)

Lunch

2 grilled steak fajitas (with mixed peppers) (2.8)
1 oz shredded low-fat pepper jack cheese
½ cup black refried beans (2.1 mg)
Side salad with low-fat dressing

Dinner

3 oz grilled turkey breast
½ cup mashed potatoes
½ cup fresh steamed green beans topped with almonds
1 small whole wheat dinner roll
½ cup fresh strawberries

Snack

1 med orange
1 oz roasted pumpkin seeds (2.3 mg)

Citations:
USDA Agricultural Research Service: *National Nutrient Database for Standard Reference Release 27* (website). http://ndb.nal.usda.gov/ndb/search Accessed August 29, 2015.
Same as:
USDA Agricultural Research Service: *National Nutrient Database for Standard Reference Release 27* (website). https://ods.od.nih.gov/pubs/usdandb/Iron-Food.pdf Accessed August 29, 2015.
National Institutes of Health: *Office of Dietary Supplements* (website). https://ods.od.nih.gov/factsheets/Iron-HealthProfessional/ Accessed January 27, 2016.

Nutritional Facts on Magnesium

The mineral magnesium is important for every organ in the body, particularly the heart, muscles, and kidneys. It also contributes to the composition of teeth and bones. Most important, it is a cofactor in hundreds of enzyme systems, contributing to energy production and DNA synthesis, and it helps regulate calcium levels, as well as copper, zinc, potassium, vitamin D, and other important nutrients in the body.

DIETARY SOURCES

Rich sources of magnesium include tofu, legumes, whole grains, green leafy vegetables, wheat bran, Brazil nuts, soybean flour, almonds, cashews, blackstrap molasses, pumpkin and squash seeds, pine nuts, and black walnuts. Other good dietary sources of this mineral include peanuts, whole-wheat flour, oat flour, beet greens, spinach, pistachio nuts, shredded wheat, bran cereals, oatmeal, bananas, baked potatoes (with skin), chocolate, and cocoa powder. Many herbs, spices, and seaweeds supply magnesium, such as agar seaweed, coriander, dill weed, celery seed, sage, dried mustard, basil, cocoa powder, fennel seed, savory, cumin seed, tarragon, marjoram, and poppy seed. See Table - Selected Food Sources of Magnesium.

DIETARY RECOMMENDED INTAKES

- Recommended Dietary Allowance (RDA): average daily level of intake sufficient to meet the nutrient requirements of nearly all (97%–98%) healthy individuals.
- Adequate Intake (AI): established when evidence is insufficient to develop an RDA and is set at a level assumed to ensure nutritional adequacy.
- Estimated Average Requirement (EAR): average daily level of intake estimated to meet the requirements of 50% of healthy individuals. It is usually used to assess the adequacy of nutrient intakes in population groups but not individuals.
- Tolerable Upper Intake Level (UL): maximum daily intake unlikely to cause adverse health effects. The ULs for magnesium are listed on the inside back cover of this text.

See Table for RDA for Magnesium.

Recommended Dietary Allowance (RDA) for Magnesium for Children and Adults

Age	Males and Females (mg/day)	Females (mg/day)	Pregnancy (mg/day)	Lactation (mg/day)
0-6 months	30	30	N/A	N/A
7-12 months	75	75	N/A	N/A
1-3	80	80	N/A	N/A
4-8	130	130	N/A	N/A

Recommended Dietary Allowance (RDA) for Magnesium for Children and Adults—con'd

Age	Males and Females (mg/day)	Females (mg/day)	Pregnancy (mg/day)	Lactation (mg/day)
9-13 years	240	240	N/A	N/A
14-18 years	410	360	400	360
19-30 years	400	310	350	310
31-50 years	420	320	360	320
51+ years	420	320	N/A	N/a

N/A, Not applicable.

Selected Food Sources of Magnesium

Food	Milligram per Serving	% Daily Value*
Pumpkin and squash seed kernels, roasted, 1 oz	156	39
Brazil nuts, 1 oz	107	27
Bran ready-to-eat cereal (100%), ≈1 oz	103	25.5
Quinoa, dry, ¼ cup	84	21
Mackerel, baked, 3 oz	82	20.5
Spinach, canned, ½ cup	81	20
Almonds, 1 oz	78	19.5
Spinach, cooked from fresh, ½ cup	78	19.5
Buckwheat flour, ¼ cup	75	19
Cashews, dry roasted, 1 oz	74	18.5
Soybeans, mature, cooked, ½ cup	74	18.5
Pine nuts, dried, 1 oz	71	17.5
Pollock, walleye, cooked, 3 oz	69	17
White beans, canned, ½ cup	67	17
Mixed nuts, oil roasted, with peanuts, 1 oz	65	16.5
Black beans, cooked, ½ cup	60	15
Bulgur, dry, ¼ cup	57	14
Oat bran, raw, ¼ cup	55	13.5
Soybeans, green, cooked, ½ cup	54	13.7
Lima beans, baby, cooked from frozen, ½ cup	50	12.5
Peanuts, dry roasted, 1 oz	50	12.5
Beet greens, cooked, ½ cup	49	12
Navy beans, cooked, ½ cup	48	12
Tofu, firm, prepared with nigari,† ½ cup	47	11.7
Soy Milk, not fortified 1 cup	61	15.2
Cowpeas, cooked, ½ cup	46	11.5
Hazelnuts, 1 oz	46	11.5
Oat bran muffin, 1 oz	45	11.3
Great northern beans, cooked, ½ cup	44	11
Oat bran, cooked, ½ cup	44	11
Buckwheat groats, roasted, cooked, ½ cup	43	10.7
Brown rice, cooked, ½ cup	42	10.5
Okra, cooked from frozen, ½ cup	37	9.2
Tuna, yellowfin, cooked, 3 oz	36	9

Continued

Selected Food Sources of Magnesium—cont'd

Food	Milligram per Serving	% Daily Value*
Cod, baked, 3 oz	36	9
Artichokes (hearts), cooked, ½ cup	35	9
Turkey, roasted, white meat, 3 oz	27	6.8
Halibut, cooked, 3 oz	24	6
Veal, cutlet, cooked, 3 oz	24	6
Haddock, cooked, 3 oz	22.1	5.5
Chicken, cooked, 3 oz	22	6
T-bone steak, broiled, lean only, 3 oz	22	5.7
Beef, ground, cooked, extra lean, 17% fat, 3 oz	17	4

†Calcium sulfate and magnesium chloride.

DV = Daily Value. DVs were developed by the Food and Drug Administration to help consumers compare the nutrient content of products. The %DV listed on the Nutrition Facts panel of food labels states the percentage of the DV provided in one serving. **The DV for magnesium is 400 mg.** Foods containing 20% or more of the DV are considered to be excellent sources of the nutrient.

Common and Important Magnesium-Drug Interactions

Drug	Potential Interaction
Loop and thiazide diuretics (e.g., Lasix, Bumex, edecrin, and hydrochlorothiazide) Antineoplastic drugs (e.g., cisplatin) Antibiotics (e.g., gentamicin and amphotericin)	These drugs may increase the loss of magnesium in urine; thus taking these medications for long periods may contribute to magnesium depletion.
Tetracycline antibiotics	Magnesium binds tetracycline in the gut and decreases the absorption of tetracycline.
Magnesium-containing antacids and laxatives	Many antacids and laxatives contain magnesium. When frequently taken in large doses, these drugs can inadvertently lead to excessive magnesium consumption and hypermagnesemia.

SAMPLE MEAL PLAN

Breakfast

1 med oat bran muffin (45 mg magnesium)
1 small banana
½ cup low-fat or fat-free milk

Lunch

½ cup penne pasta with the following:
3 oz grilled chicken breast
½ cup fresh cooked spinach (78 mg magnesium)
2 oz toasted pine nuts (142 mg magnesium)
1 cup mixed salad greens topped with spinach leaves, tomatoes, shredded lettuce
1 oz shredded low-fat mozzarella cheese

Dinner

2 Cajun shrimp skewers
½ cup fresh steamed green beans
½ cup brown rice (42 mg magnesium)
½ cup fresh pineapple

Snack

1 cup soy fruit smoothie (47 mg magnesium)
1 oz Brazil nuts (107 mg magnesium)
Note: Take one multivitamin or multimineral supplement daily.

Citation:
USDA Agricultural Research Service: *National Nutrient Database for Standard Reference Release 27* (website). http://ndb.nal.usda.gov/ndb/search Accessed August 29, 2015.
Same as:
USDA Agricultural Research Service: *National Nutrient Database for Standard Reference Release 27* (website). https://ods.od.nih.gov/pubs/usdandb/Magnesium-Food.pdf Accessed August 29, 2015.
National Institutes of Health: *Office of Dietary Supplements* (website). https://ods.od.nih.gov/factsheets/Magnesium-HealthProfessional/Accessed January 27, 2016.

Nutritional Facts on Potassium

A potassium-rich diet is useful for cardiac patients who are trying to lower their blood pressure using diet. If diuretics are also used, it is important to know if potassium is retained or depleted by the diuretic, and it should be monitored. Most patients with chronic kidney disease or on renal dialysis may need to restrict potassium in their diets. See Chapter 35. Because potassium is lost in sweat, athletes need to pay attention to the potassium in their diets. See Chapter 23.

There is no RDA for potassium. Dietary Reference Intake (DRI) is a general term for a set of reference values used to plan and assess nutrient intakes of healthy people. The DRIs for potassium are stated as Adequate Intakes (AIs). For breastfed infants the AI is the mean intake; for older individuals the AI is believed to cover the needs of all individuals in the group, but there is a lack data to be more specific. AIs are given in the table.

Dietary Reference Intakes: Adequate Intakes (AIs) for Potassium for Children and Adults

Age	Males and Females (g/day)	Pregnancy (g/day)	Lactation (g/day)
0-6 months	0.4	N/A	N/A
7-12 months	0.7	N/A	N/A
1-3m years	3	N/A	N/A
4-8 years	3.8	N/A	N/A
9-13 years	4.5	N/A	N/A
14-18 years	4.7	4700	5100
19+ years	4.7	4700	5100

N/A, Not applicable.

Selected Food Sources of Potassium

Food	Milligrams (mg) per Serving	% Daily Value*	Food	Milligrams (mg) per Serving	% Daily Value*
Sweet potato, baked, 1 potato (143 g)	694	19.8	Rockfish, Pacific, cooked, 3 oz	397	11.3
Tomato paste, ¼ cup	669	19	Tomato juice, ¾ cup	395	11.3
Beet greens, cooked, ½ cup	655	18.7	Milk, nonfat, 1 cup	382	10.9
Potato, baked, flesh, 1 potato (156 g)	610	17.4	Pork chop, center loin, cooked, 3 oz	382	10.9
White beans, canned, ½ cup	595	17	Rainbow trout, farmed, cooked, 3 oz	382	10.9
Yogurt, plain, non-fat, 8-oz container	579	16.5	Apricots, dried, uncooked, ¼ cup	378	10.8
Tomato puree, ½ cup	549	15.7	Orange juice, ¾ cup	372	10.6
Clams, canned, 3 oz	534	15.3	Buttermilk, cultured, low-fat, 1 cup	370	10.5
Yogurt, plain, low-fat, 8-oz container	531	15.2	Cantaloupe, ¼ med	368	10.5
Prune juice, ¾ cup	530	15.1	1%-2% milk, 1 cup	366	10.4
Carrot juice, ¾ cup	517	14.8	Honeydew melon, ⅛ med	365	10.4
Soybeans, green, cooked, ½ cup	485	13.9	Lentils, cooked, ½ cup	365	10.4
Lima beans, cooked, ½ cup	484	13.8	Tomato sauce, ½ cup	364	10.4
Halibut, cooked, 3 oz	449	12.8	Pork loin, center rib (roasts), lean, roasted, 3 oz	358	10.2
Tuna, yellow fin, cooked, 3 oz	448	12.8			
Winter squash, cooked, ½ cup	448	9.5	Plantains, cooked, ½ cup slices	358	10.2
Soybeans, mature, cooked, ½ cup	443	12.8	Kidney beans, cooked, ½ cup	358	10.2
Bananas, 1 med	422	12.1	Split peas, cooked, ½ cup	355	10.1
Spinach, cooked, ½ cup	419	12	Yogurt, plain, whole milk, 8-oz container	352	10.0
Peaches, dried, uncooked, ¼ cup	398	11.4	Cod, Pacific, cooked, 3 oz	246	7.0
Prunes, stewed, ½ cup	398	11.4			

*Daily values (DVs) are reference numbers based on the recommended dietary allowance. They were developed to help consumers determine if a food contains a lot or a little of a specific nutrient. **The DV for potassium is 3500 mg**. The %DV listed on the Nutrition Facts panel of food labels states the percentage of the DV provided in one serving. Percent DVs are based on a 2000-calorie diet.

Citations:
Oregon State University: *Linus Pauling Institute* (website). http://lpi.oregonstate.edu/mic/minerals/potassium Accessed August 29, 2015.
USDA Agricultural Research Service: *National Nutrient Database for Standard Reference Release 27* (website). http://ndb.nal.usda.gov/ndb/nutrients/index Accessed January 27, 2016.

Nutritional Facts on Selenium

Selenium is incorporated into proteins to make selenoproteins, which are important antioxidant enzymes. The antioxidant properties of selenoproteins prevent cellular damage from free radicals. Other selenoproteins help regulate thyroid function and play a role in the immune system. Selenium, as a nutrient that functions as an antioxidant, may be protective against some types of cancer. Its role in heart disease is not clear, but it may have a preventive role.

Plant foods are the major dietary sources of selenium. The content of selenium in food depends on the selenium content of the soil where plants are grown or animals are raised. Soil in Nebraska and the Dakotas has very high levels of selenium. The southeast coastal areas in the United States have very low levels; selenium deficiency is often reported in these regions. Selenium is also found in some meats and seafood. Animals that eat grains or plants that were grown in selenium-rich soil have higher levels of selenium in their muscle. In the United States meats, bread, and Brazil nuts are common sources of dietary selenium.

Most food labels do not list the selenium content of a food however, if they do, it is listed as a % Daily Value (DV). DVs were developed by the Food and Drug Administration to help consumers compare the nutrient content of products. The % Daily Value (DV) listed on the label indicates the percentage of the DV provided in one serving. A food providing 5% of the DV or less is a source, whereas a food that provides 10% to 19% of the DV is a good source. A food that provides 20% or more of the DV is high in that nutrient. It is important to remember that foods that provide lower percentages of the DV also contribute to a healthful diet.

Dietary Reference Intakes for Selenium for Children and Adults

Age (years)	Males and Females (mcg/day)	Pregnancy (mcg/day)	Lactation (mcg/day)
1-3	20	N/A	N/A
4-8	30	N/A	N/A
9-13	40	N/A	N/A
14-18	55	60	70
19+	55	60	70

N/A, Not applicable.

Selected Food Sources of Selenium

Food	Micrograms per Serving	% DV	Food	Micrograms per Serving	% DV
Brazil nuts, dried, unblanched, 1 oz	544	777	Macaroni, elbow, enriched, boiled, 1 cup	37	53
Tuna, yellowfin, cooked, dry heat, 3 oz	92	131	Egg, whole, 1 med	15	21
Ground Beef, 25% fat, cooked, oz	18	26	Cottage cheese, 1% fat , 1 cup	20	29
Spaghetti sauce, marinara, 1 cup	4	6	Oatmeal, instant, fortified, cooked, 1 cup	13	19
Corn Flakes, 1 cup	2	3	Milk, 1 %, 1 cup	8	11
Turkey, light meat, roasted, 3 oz	31	44	Lentils, boiled, 1 cup	6	9
Spinach, frozen, boiled, 1 cup	11	16	Bread, whole wheat, 1 slice	13	19
Chicken breast, meat only, roasted 3 oz	22	31	Rice, brown, long grain, cooked, 1 cup	19	27
Noodles, enriched, boiled, ½ cup	19	27	Cashew nuts, dry roasted, 1 oz	3	4

DV = Daily Value. DVs were developed by the Food and Drug Administration to help consumers compare the nutrient content of products. The %DV listed on the Nutrition Facts panel of food labels states the percentage of the DV provided in one serving. **The DV for selenium for adults and children aged 4 and over is 70 mcg**. Foods containing 20% or more of the DV are considered to be excellent sources of the nutrient.

Citations:
National Institutes of Health: *Office of Dietary Supplements* (website).https://ods.od.nih.gov/factsheets/Selenium-HealthProfessional/ Accessed August 29, 2015.
National Institutes of Health: *Office of Dietary Supplements* (website).https://ods.od.nih.gov/factsheets/Selenium-Consumer/ Accessed August 29, 2015.
USDA Agricultural Research Service: *National Nutrient Database for Standard Reference Release 27* (website). http://ndb.nal.usda.gov/ndb/search Accessed August 29, 2015.
Same as:
USDA Agricultural Research Service: *National Nutrient Database for Standard Reference Release 27* (website). https://ods.od.nih.gov/pcubs/usdandb/Selenium-Content.pdf Accessed January 27, 2016.

SAMPLE MEAL PLAN

Breakfast

½ cup oatmeal (6 mcg selenium)
1 medium scrambled egg (14 mcg selenium)
1 small banana
½ cup low-fat or fat-free milk

Lunch

1 turkey sandwich (36 mcg selenium)
½ cup carrot sticks
1 bag baked chips

Dinner

3 oz meatloaf
½ cup macaroni and cheese (20 mcg selenium)
½ cup fresh steamed green beans

Snack

½ cup cottage cheese (12 mcg selenium)
½ cup fresh sliced peaches

Nutritional Facts on Zinc

Zinc is an essential mineral that is found in almost every cell. It stimulates the activity of approximately 100 enzymes, which are substances that promote biochemical reactions in the body. Zinc supports immunity; is needed for wound healing; helps maintain the sense of taste and smell; is needed for deoxyribonucleic acid (DNA) synthesis; and supports normal growth and development during pregnancy, childhood, and adolescence.

Zinc is found in a wide variety of foods. Atlantic oysters contain more zinc per serving than any other food, but red meat and poultry provide the majority of zinc in the American diet. Other good food sources include beans, nuts, certain seafood, whole grains, fortified breakfast cereals, and dairy products.

Because zinc absorption is greater from a diet high in animal protein than a diet rich in plant proteins, vegetarians may become deficient if they are not monitored carefully. Phytates from whole-grain breads, cereals, legumes, and other products can decrease zinc absorption.

DIETARY RECOMMENDED INTAKES

- Recommended Dietary Allowance (RDA): average daily level of intake sufficient to meet the nutrient requirements of nearly all (97%–98%) healthy individuals.
- Adequate Intake (AI): established when evidence is insufficient to develop an RDA; intake at this level is assumed to ensure nutritional adequacy.
- Estimated Average Requirement (EAR): average daily level of intake estimated to meet the requirements of 50% of healthy individuals. It is usually used to assess the adequacy of nutrient intakes in population groups but not individuals.
- Tolerable Upper Intake Level (UL): maximum daily intake unlikely to cause adverse health effects. ULs are listed on the inside back cover of this text.

Recommended Dietary Allowance (RDA) for Zinc for Children and Adults

Age	Males and Females (mg/day)	Pregnancy (mg/day)	Lactation (mg/day)
0-6 months	2	N/A	N/A
7-12 months	2	N/A	N/A
1-3	3	N/A	N/A
4-8	5	N/A	N/A
9-13	8	N/A	N/A
14-18	11 for boys, 9 for girls	12	13
19+	11 for men, 8 for women	11	12

N/A, Not applicable.
DV = daily value. **The DV for zinc is 15 mg.**

Selected Food Sources of Zinc

Food	Milligrams (mg) per Serving	% Daily Value*
Oysters, battered and fried, 6 med	16.0	100
RTE breakfast cereal, fortified with 100% of the DV for zinc per serving, ¾ cup serving	15.0	100
Beef shank, lean only, cooked 3 oz	8.9	60
Beef chuck, arm pot roast, lean only, cooked, 3 oz	7.1	47
Beef tenderloin, lean only, cooked, 3 oz	4.8	30
Beef, eye of round, lean only, cooked, 3 oz	4.0	25
RTE breakfast cereal, fortified with 25% of the DV for zinc per serving, ¾ cup	3.8	25
RTE breakfast cereal, complete wheat bran flakes, ¾ cup serving	3.7	25
Pork shoulder, arm picnic, lean only, cooked, 3 oz	3.5	25
Baked beans, canned, plain or vegetarian, ½ cup	2.9	19
Chicken leg, meat only, roasted, 1 leg	2.7	20
Pork tenderloin, lean only, cooked, 3 oz	2.5	15
Pork loin, sirloin roast, lean only, cooked, 3 oz	2.2	15
Yogurt, plain, low fat, 1 cup	2.2	15
Baked beans, canned, with pork, ½ cup	1.8	10
Cashews, dry roasted without salt, 1 oz	1.6	10
Yogurt, fruit, low fat, 1 cup	1.6	10
Raisin bran, ¾ cup	1.5	9
Chickpeas, mature seeds, canned, ½ cup	1.5	9
Pecans, dry roasted without salt, 1 oz	1.4	10
Oatmeal, instant, low sodium, 1 packet	1.3	9
Cheese, Swiss, 1 oz	1.2	8
Mixed nuts, dry roasted with peanuts, without salt, 1 oz	1.1	8
Walnuts, black, dried, 1 oz	1.0	6
Almonds, dry roasted, without salt, 1 oz	1.0	6
Milk, fluid, any kind, 1 cup	0.9	6
Chicken breast, meat only, roasted, ½ breast with bone and skin removed	0.9	6
Cheese, cheddar, 1 oz	0.9	6

Continued

Selected Food Sources of Zinc—cont'd

Food	Milligrams (mg) per Serving	% Daily Value*
Cheese, mozzarella, part skim, low moisture, 1 oz	0.9	6
Beans, kidney, California red, cooked, ½ cup	0.9	6
Peas, green, frozen, boiled, ½ cup	0.5	4
Flounder or sole, cooked, 3 oz	0.3	2

RTE, Ready to eat.

DV = Daily Value: developed by the Food and Drug Administration to help consumers compare the nutrient content of products. Foods containing 20% or more of the DV are considered to be excellent sources.

SAMPLE MEAL PLAN

Breakfast

¼ cup scrambled eggs
¾ cup ready-to-eat breakfast cereal with 25% DV (3.8 mg zinc)
½ cup sliced peaches
½ cup low-fat or fat-free milk

Lunch

1 chicken salad sandwich
½ cup carrot sticks
2 Tbsp Ranch dressing
1 bag baked chips

Snack

Yogurt, plain (2.2 mg zinc)

Dinner

3 oz grilled beef shank (8.9 mg zinc)
½ cup fresh steamed peas (**0.95** mg zinc)

Side Salad

1 small sweet potato
½ cup fresh pineapple

Snack

½ cup Trail mix (raisins, pecans, cashews, dried cranberries)

Citations:
USDA Agricultural Research Service: *National Nutrient Database for Standard Reference Release 27* (website). http://ndb.nal.usda.gov/ndb/search Accessed August 29, 2015.
Same as:
USDA Agricultural Research Service: *National Nutrient Database for Standard Reference Release 27* (website). https://ods.od.nih.gov/pubs/usdandb/Zinc-Content.pdf Accessed August 29, 2015.
National Institutes of Health: *Office of Dietary Supplements* (website). https://ods.od.nih.gov/factsheets/Zinc-HealthProfessional/ Accessed January 26, 2016.